British National Formulary

BNF 55

March 2008

bnf.

Published jointly by
BMJ Group
Tavistock Square, London WC1H 9JP, UK
and
RPS Publishing
RPS Publishing is the wholly-owned publishing organisation of the Royal Pharmaceutical Society of Great Britain
1 Lambeth High Street, London, SE1 7JN, UK

ISBN: 978 085369 776 3

ISSN: 0260-535X

Printed by GGP Media GmbH, Poessneck, Germany

A catalogue record for this book is available from the British Library.

Copies may be obtained through any bookseller or direct from:

RPS Publishing
c/o Turpin Distribution
Stratton Business Park
Pegasus Drive
Biggleswade
Bedfordshire
SG18 8TQ
UK
Tel: +44 (0) 1767 604 971
Fax: +44 (0) 1767 601 640
E-mail: custserv@turpin-distribution.com
www.pharmpress.com

RPS Publishing also supplies the BNF in digital formats suitable for standalone use or for small networks, for use over an intranet and for use on a personal digital assistant (PDA).

Distribution of BNFs
The UK health departments distribute BNFs to NHS hospitals, doctors, dental surgeons, and community pharmacies. In England, BNFs are mailed individually to NHS general practitioners and community pharmacies; contact the DH Publication Orderline for extra copies or changes relating to mailed BNFs.
Tel: 08701 555 455
In Wales, telephone the Business Services Centre
Tel: 01495 332 000

For further information on the supply of copies of the BNF to NHS organisations, see http://tinyurl.com/2uebpp

The BNF is designed as a digest for rapid reference and it may not always include all the information necessary for prescribing and dispensing. Also, less detail is given on areas such as obstetrics, malignant disease, and anaesthesia since it is expected that those undertaking treatment will have specialist knowledge and access to specialist literature. *BNF for Children* should be consulted for detailed information on the use of medicines in children. The BNF should be interpreted in the light of professional knowledge and supplemented as necessary by specialised publications and by reference to the product literature. Information is also available from medicines information services (see inside front cover).

Preface

The BNF is a joint publication of the British Medical Association and the Royal Pharmaceutical Society of Great Britain. It is published biannually under the authority of a Joint Formulary Committee which comprises representatives of the two professional bodies and of the UK Health Departments. The Dental Advisory Group oversees the preparation of advice on the drug management of dental and oral conditions; the Group includes representatives of the British Dental Association. The Nurse Prescribers' Advisory Group advises on the content relevant to nurses.

The BNF aims to provide prescribers, pharmacists and other healthcare professionals with sound up-to-date information about the use of medicines.

The BNF includes key information on the selection, prescribing, dispensing and administration of medicines. Medicines generally prescribed in the UK are covered and those considered less suitable for prescribing are clearly identified. Little or no information is included on medicines promoted for purchase by the public.

Information on drugs is drawn from the manufacturers' product literature, medical and pharmaceutical literature, UK health departments, regulatory authorities, and professional bodies. Advice is constructed from clinical literature and reflects, as far as possible, an evaluation of the evidence from diverse sources. The BNF also takes account of authoritative national guidelines and emerging safety concerns. In addition, the editorial team receives advice on all therapeutic areas from expert clinicians; this ensures that the BNF's recommendations are relevant to practice.

The BNF is designed as a digest for rapid reference and it may not always include all the information necessary for prescribing and dispensing. Also, less detail is given on areas such as obstetrics, malignant disease, and anaesthesia since it is expected that those undertaking treatment will have specialist knowledge and access to specialist literature. *BNF for Children* should be consulted for detailed information on the use of medicines in children. The BNF should be interpreted in the light of professional knowledge and supplemented as necessary by specialised publications and by reference to the product literature. Information is also available from medicines information services (see inside front cover).

It is **vital** to use the most recent edition of the BNF for making clinical decisions. The more important changes for this edition are listed on p. xi.

The BNF on the internet (bnf.org) includes additional information of relevance to healthcare professionals dealing with medicines. Other digital versions of the BNF—including intranet and personal digital assistant (PDA) versions—are produced in parallel with the paper version.

The BNF welcomes comments from healthcare professionals. Comments and constructive criticism should be sent to:
Executive Editor, British National Formulary,
Royal Pharmaceutical Society of Great Britain,
1 Lambeth High Street, London SE1 7JN.
Email: editor@bnf.org

Contents

Preface iii
Acknowledgements iv
How the BNF is constructed vii
How to use the BNF ix
Changes for this edition xi
Significant changes xi
Dose changes xi
Classification changes xii
Discontinued preparations xii
New preparations included in this edition xii
Late additions xiii
Name changes xiv
Guidance on prescribing 1
General guidance 1
Prescription writing 4
Emergency supply of medicines 6
Controlled drugs and drug dependence 7
Adverse reactions to drugs 11
Prescribing for children 13

For detailed advice on medicines used for children consult *BNF for Children*

Prescribing in palliative care 15
Prescribing for the elderly 19
Prescribing in dental practice 21
Drugs and sport 26
Emergency treatment of poisoning 27
Notes on drugs and Preparations
1: Gastro-intestinal system 37
2: Cardiovascular system 70
3: Respiratory system 145
4: Central nervous system 179
5: Infections 277
6: Endocrine system 358
7: Obstetrics, gynaecology, and urinary-tract disorders 418
8: Malignant disease and immunosuppression 448
9: Nutrition and blood 490
10: Musculoskeletal and joint diseases 534
11: Eye 565
12: Ear, nose, and oropharynx 582
13: Skin 597
14: Immunological products and vaccines 641
15: Anaesthesia 665
Appendixes and indices
Appendix 1: **Interactions** 686
Appendix 2: **Liver disease** 762
Appendix 3: **Renal impairment** 772
Appendix 4: **Pregnancy** 787
Appendix 5: **Breast-feeding** 807
Appendix 6: **Intravenous additives** 821
Appendix 7: **Borderline substances** 833
Appendix 8: **Wound management products and elastic hosiery** 850
Appendix 9: **Cautionary and advisory labels for dispensed medicines** 867
Dental Practitioners' Formulary 882
Nurse Prescribers' Formulary 884
Index of manufacturers 888
Index 904

Acknowledgements

The Joint Formulary Committee is grateful to individuals and organisations that have provided advice and information to the BNF.

The principal contributors for this edition were:

I.H. Ahmed-Jushuf, K.W. Ah-See, S.P. Allison, S. Almond, J.C. Atherton, M.N. Badminton, T.P. Baglin, P.R.J. Barnes, D.N. Bateman, S.L. Bloom, D. Bowsher, R.J. Buckley, I.F. Burgess, D.J. Burn, J.J. Coleman, J. Cox, R. Dinwiddie, P.N. Durrington, T.S.J. Elliott, B.G. Gazzard, A.M. Geretti, A.H. Ghodse, N.J.L. Gittoes, P.J. Goadsby, E.C. Gordon-Smith, J. Guillebaud, B.G. Higgins, S.H.D. Jackson, A. Jones, J.R. Kirwan, P.G. Kopelman, A.J. Krentz, T.H. Lee, D.N.J. Lockwood, L. Luzzatto, A.G. Marson, P.D. Mason, K.E.L. McColl, G.M. Mead, E. Miller, N.S. Morton, J.P. Neilson, J.M. Neuberger, D.J. Nutt, L.P. Ormerod, W.J. Penny, P.A. Poole-Wilson, M.M. Ramsey, J. Reynolds, D.J. Rowbotham, P.C. Rubin, J.W. Sander, R.S. Sawers, G.J. Shortland, S. Thomas, J.P. Thompson, D.G. Waller, D.A. Worrell, A. Wilcock, C.E. Willoughby, M.M Yaqoob.

Expert advice on the management of oral and dental conditions was kindly provided by M. Addy, P. Coulthard, A. Crighton, M.A.O. Lewis, J.G. Meechan, N.D. Robb, R.A. Seymour, R. Welbury, and J.M. Zakrzewska. R.S. Gasser and S. Kaur provided valuable advice on dental prescribing policy.

Members of the British Association of Dermatologists Therapy Guidelines and Audit Subcommittee, H.K. Bell, R.H. Bull, D.J. Eedy, L.C. Fuller, D. Joseph, D. Mitchell, A.D. Ormerod, M.J. Tidman, P.D. Yesudian, and M. Donoghue (Secretariat) have provided valuable advice.

Members of the Advisory Committee on Malaria Prevention, B.A. Bannister, R.H. Behrens, P.L. Chiodini, F. Genasi, J. Gibson, A.D. Green, D. Hill, G. Kassianos, D.G. Lalloo, G. Lea, C. Lucas, G. Pasvol, M. Powell, D.V. Shingadia, D.A. Warrell, C.J.M. Whitty, and C.A. Swales (Secretariat) have also provided valuable advice.

The Joint British Societies' Coronary Risk Prediction Charts have been reproduced with the kind permission of P.N. Durrington who has also provided the BNF with access to the computer program for assessing coronary and stroke risk.

R Suvarna and colleagues at the MHRA have provided valuable assistance.

Correspondents in the pharmaceutical industry have provided information on new products and commented on products in the BNF. The Prescription Pricing Authority has supplied the prices of products in the BNF.

Numerous doctors, pharmacists, nurses and others have sent comments and suggestions.

The BNF has valuable access to the *Martindale* data banks by courtesy of S. Sweetman and staff.

J.E. Macintyre and staff provided valuable technical assistance.

C. Adetola, A. Breewood, M. Davis, R. Fisher, E.H. Glover, D.T.H. Griffiths, J.M. James, S. Kakar, E. Laughton, G. Meier, H.M.N. Neill, P. Patel, and R.G. Taljaard provided considerable assistance during the production of this edition of the BNF.

Xpage have provided technical assistance with the editorial database and typesetting software.

Dinesh K. Mehta *BPharm, MSc, FRPharmS*

The Joint Formulary Committee wish to record their deep appreciation to Dinesh K. Mehta, who left the *BNF* in November 2007, for his outstanding tenure as Executive Editor. Under his guidance BNF publications have grown from strength to strength. He spearheaded the development of the new digital versions and launched the *Nurse Prescribers' Formulary*, the *WHO Model Formulary*, and the *BNF for Children*. He ensured that the BNF remains a byword for authority and relevance among all those who seek guidance on the safe and effective use of medicines.

The editorial team join the Committee in paying tribute to an exceptional editor; it is a rare privilege to work with a person with such commitment and passion.

Editorial Staff

Managing Editor: Knowledge Creation
John Martin *BPharm, PhD, MRPharmS*

Assistant Editors
Bryony Jordan *BSc, DipPharmPract, MRPharmS*
Colin R. Macfarlane *BPharm, MSc, MRPharmS*
Rachel S. M. Ryan *BPharm, MRPharmS*
Shama M. S. Wagle *BPharm, DipPharmPract, MRPharmS*

Staff Editors
Onatefe Akporobaro-Iwudibia *MPharm, MRPharmS*
Shaistah J. Ali *MPharm, MRPharmS*
Sejal Amin *BPharm, MSc, MRPharmS*
Lisa M. Britton *BPharm, MRPharmS*
Irene Chiwele *BPharm, MRPharmS*
Leigh Anne Claase *BSc, PhD, MRPharmS*
Allison F. Corbett *BPharm, MRPharmS*
Julia A. Dickin *MPharm, MRPharmS*
Laura K. Glancy *MPharm, MSc, MRPharmS*
Manjula Halai *BScChem, MPharm, MRPharmS*
Amy E. Harvey *MPharm, PGDipCommPharm, MRPharmS*
Paul S. Maycock *MPharm, DipPharmPract, MRPharmS*
Elizabeth Nix *DipPharm(NZ), MRPharmS*
Claire L. Preston *BPharm, MRPharmS*
Vinaya K. Sharma *BPharm, MSc, PGDipPIM, MRPharmS*
Rajeshree Sooriakumaran *BPharm, DipPharmPract, MRPharmS*

Editorial Assistant
Gerard P. Gallagher *MSc, MRSH, MRIPH*

Senior BNF Administrator
Heidi Homar *BA*

Administrative Assistant
Eliana Carranza-Pitcher *BA*

Knowledge Systems
Robert C. Buckingham *BSc*
Digital Development Assistant
Philip D. Lee *BSc, PhD*
Digital Development Editor
Sarah Peck *BSc*
Terminologist
Anne Spence *BSc*
Digital Development Assistant

Head of Publishing Services
John Wilson

BNF Publishing Director
Dominic Vaughan *MBA, MIoD*

Director of Publications
Charles Fry

Joint Formulary Committee 2007–2008

Chairman
Martin J. Kendall
OBE, MB ChB, MD, FRCP, FFPM

Deputy Chairman
Alison Blenkinsopp
PhD, BPharm, FRPharmS

Committee Members
Jeffrey K. Aronson
MA, MB ChB, DPhil, FRCP, FBPharmacolS, FFPM
Anthony J. Avery
BMedSci, MB ChB, DM, FRCGP
Tawfique K. Daneshmend
MB ChB, MD, FRCP
Wendy Harris
BScPharm, MRPharmS
Beth Hird
BPharm, MSc, MRPharmS, SP, IP
W. Moira Kinnear
BSc, MSc, MRPharmS
Frank P. Marsh
MA, MB, BChir, FRCP
Gul Root
BPharm, MRPharmS, DMS
Rafe Survana
MBBS, BSc, MFPM, DAvMed, DipIMC
Carwen Wynne Howells
BPharm, FRPharmS

Executive Secretary
Heidi Homar
BA

Dental Advisory Group 2007–2008

Chairman
David Wray
MD, BDS, MB ChB, FDSRCPS, FDSRCS Ed, F MedSci

Committee Members
Shaistah J. Ali
MPharm, MRPharmS

Christine Arnold
BDS, DDPHRCS, MCDH

Simon J. Carruthers
LDSRCS, BDS, MFGDP(UK)

Barry Cockcroft
BDS, FFDS (Eng)

Martin J. Kendall
OBE, MB ChB, MD, FRCP, FFPM

Lesley P. Longman
BSc, BDS, FDSRCS Ed, PhD

John Martin
BPharm, PhD, MRPharmS

Michelle Moffat
BDS, MFDS RCS Ed, M Paed Dent RPCS, FDS (Paed Dent) RSC Ed
(from January 2008)

David B. Murphy
BDS, DGDP(UK)
(until January 2008)

Richard J. Oliver
BDS, BSc, PhD, FDSRCPS, FDS (OS) RCPS
(from January 2008)

Shama M.S. Wagle
BPharm, DipPharmPract, MRPharmS

Dominic Vaughan
MBA, MIoD

Joint Secretary
Sally E. Cartwright
BSc, MSc
(from January 2008)

J. Claire Lowe
BSc, DPhil

Executive Secretary
Heidi Homar
BA

> Advice on dental practice
> The **British Dental Association** has contributed to the advice on medicines for dental practice through its representatives on the Dental Advisory Group.

Nurses Prescribers' Advisory Group 2007–2008

Chairman
Nicky A. Cullen
PhD, RGN

Committee Members
Una J. Adderley
MSc, BA, RGN, DN

Michele L. Cossey
BPharm, MSc, MRPharmS

Molly Courtenay
PhD, MSc, Cert Ed, BSc, RGN

Margaret F. Helliwell
MB, BS, BSc, MFPHM

Bryony Jordan
BSc, DipPharmPract, MRPharmS

Martin J. Kendall
OBE, MB ChB, MD, FRCP, FFPM

John Martin
BPharm, PhD, MRPharmS

Paul S. Maycock
MPharm, DipPharmPract, MRPharmS

Maureen P. Morgan
RN, RHV, MBA

Elizabeth J. Plastow
RMN, RGN, RSCPHN(HV), MSc, PGDipEd

Paul G.H. Robinson

Gul Root
BSc, MRPharmS, DMS

Jill M. Shearer
BSc, RGN, RM

Rabina Tindale
RN, RSCN, BSc, DipAEN, PGCE

Dominic Vaughan
MBA, MIoD

Vicky Vidler
MA, RGN, RSCN

Executive Secretary
Heidi Homar
BA

How the BNF is constructed

The BNF is unique in bringing together authoritative, independent guidance on best practice with clinically validated drug information enabling healthcare professionals to select safe and effective medicines for individual patients.

Information in the BNF has been validated against emerging evidence, best-practice guidelines, and advice from a network of clinical experts.

While hundreds of changes are made between editions, the most clinically significant changes are listed at the front of each edition (pp. xi-xiii).

Joint Formulary Committee

The Joint Formulary Committee (JFC) is responsible for the content of the BNF. The JFC includes doctors appointed by the BMJ Publishing Group, pharmacists appointed by the Royal Pharmaceutical Society of Great Britain, and representatives from the Medicines and Healthcare products Regulatory Agency (MHRA) and the UK health departments. The JFC decides on matters of policy and reviews amendments to the BNF in the light of new evidence and expert advice. The Committee meets quarterly and each member also receives proofs of all BNF chapters for review before publication.

Editorial team

BNF staff editors are pharmacists with a sound understanding of how drugs are used in clinical practice. Each staff editor is responsible for editing, maintaining and updating specific chapters of the BNF. During the publication cycle the staff editors review information in the BNF against a variety of sources (see below).

Amendments to the text are drafted when the editors are satisfied that any new information is reliable and relevant. The draft amendments are passed to expert advisers for comment and then presented to the Joint Formulary Committee for consideration. Additionally, for each edition, sections are chosen from every chapter for thorough review. These planned reviews aim to verify all the information in the selected sections and to draft any amendments to reflect the current best practice.

Staff editors prepare the text for publication and undertake a number of checks on the knowledge at various stages of the production.

Expert advisers

The BNF uses about 60 expert clinical advisers (including doctors, pharmacists, nurses, and dentists) throughout the UK to help with the production of each edition. The role of these expert advisers is to review existing text and to comment on amendments drafted by the staff editors. These clinical experts help to ensure that the BNF remains reliable by:

- commenting on the relevance of the text in the context of best clinical practice in the UK;
- checking draft amendments for appropriate interpretation of any new evidence;
- providing expert opinion in areas of controversy or where reliable evidence is lacking;
- advising on areas where the BNF diverges from summaries of product characteristics;
- providing independent advice on drug interactions, prescribing in hepatic impairment, renal impairment, pregnancy, breast-feeding, children, the elderly, palliative care, and the emergency treatment of poisoning.

In addition to consulting with regular advisers, the BNF calls upon other clinical specialists for specific developments when particular expertise is required.

The BNF also works closely with a number of expert bodies that produce clinical guidelines. Drafts or prepublication copies of guidelines are routinely received for comment and for assimilation into the BNF.

Sources of BNF information

The BNF uses a variety of sources for its information; the main ones are shown below.

Summaries of product characteristics The BNF receives summaries of product characteristics (SPCs) of all new products as well as revised SPCs for existing products. The SPCs are the principal source of product information and are carefully processed, despite the ever-increasing volume of information being issued by the pharmaceutical industry. Such processing involves:

- verifying the approved names of all relevant ingredients including 'non-active' ingredients (the BNF is committed to using approved names and descriptions as laid down by the Medicines Act);
- comparing the indications, cautions, contra-indications and side-effects with similar existing drugs. Where these are different from the expected pattern, justification is sought for their inclusion or exclusion;
- seeking independent data on the use of drugs in pregnancy and breast-feeding;
- incorporating the information into the BNF using established criteria for the presentation and inclusion of the data;
- checking interpretation of the information by two staff editors before submitting to a senior editor; changes relating to doses receive an extra check;
- identifying potential clinical problems or omissions and seeking further information from manufacturers or from expert advisers;
- careful validation of any areas of divergence of the BNF from the SPC before discussion by the Committee (in the light of supporting evidence);
- constructing, with the help of expert advisers, a comment on the role of the drug in the context of similar drugs.

Much of this processing is applicable to the following sources as well.

Expert advisers The role of expert clinical advisers in providing the appropriate clinical context for all BNF information is discussed above.

Literature Staff editors monitor core medical and pharmaceutical journals. Research papers and reviews relating to drug therapy are carefully processed. Where a difference between the advice in the BNF and the paper is noted, the new information is assessed for reliability and relevance to UK clinical practice. If necessary, new text is drafted and discussed with expert advisers and the Joint Formulary Committee. The BNF enjoys a close working relationship with a number of national information providers.

Systematic reviews The BNF has access to various databases of systematic reviews (including the Cochrane Library and various web-based resources). These are used for answering specific queries, for reviewing existing text and for constructing new text. Staff editors receive training in critical appraisal, literature evaluation and search strategies. Reviews published in Clinical Evidence are used to validate BNF advice.

Consensus guidelines The advice in the BNF is checked against consensus guidelines produced by expert bodies. A number of bodies make drafts or pre-publication copies of the guidelines available to the BNF; it is therefore possible to ensure that a consistent message is disseminated. The BNF routinely processes guidelines from the National Institute for Health and Clinical Excellence (NICE), the Scottish Medicines Consortium (SMC) and the Scottish Intercollegiate Guidelines Network (SIGN).

Reference sources Textbooks and reference sources are used to provide background information for the review of existing text or for the construction of new text. The BNF team works closely with the editorial team that produces *Martindale: The Complete Drug Reference*. The BNF has access to Martindale information resources and each team keeps the other informed of significant developments and shifts in the trends of drug use.

Statutory information The BNF routinely processes relevant information from various Government bodies including Statutory Instruments and regulations affecting the Prescription only Medicines Order. Official compendia such as the British Pharmacopoeia and its addenda are processed routinely to ensure that the BNF complies with the relevant sections of the Medicines Act. The BNF itself is named as an official compendium in the Medicines Act.

The BNF maintains close links with the Home Office (in relation to controlled drug regulations) and the Medicines and Healthcare products Regulatory Agency (including the British Pharmacopoeia Commission). Safety warnings issued by the Commission on Human Medicines (CHM) and guidelines on drug use issued by the UK health departments are processed as a matter of routine.

Relevant professional statements issued by the Royal Pharmaceutical Society of Great Britain are included in the BNF as are guidelines from bodies such as the Royal College of General Practitioners.

The BNF reflects information from the Drug Tariff, the Scottish Drug Tariff and the Northern Ireland Drug Tariff.

Pricing information The Prescription Pricing Division provides information on prices of medicinal products and appliances in the BNF. The BNF also receives and processes price lists from product suppliers.

Comments from readers Readers of the BNF are invited to send in comments. Numerous letters and emails are received during each edition. Such feedback helps to ensure that the BNF provides practical and clinically relevant information. Many changes in the presentation and scope of the BNF have resulted from comments sent in by users.

Comments from industry Each manufacturer is provided with a complimentary copy of the BNF and invited to comment on it. Close scrutiny of the BNF by the manufacturers provides an additional check and allows them an opportunity to raise issues about the BNF's presentation of the role of various drugs; this is yet another check on the balance of the BNF's advice. All comments are looked at with care and, where necessary, additional information and expert advice are sought.

Virtual user groups The BNF is setting up virtual user groups across various healthcare professions (e.g. doctors, pharmacists, nurses, dentists). The aim of these groups will be to provide feedback to the editors and publishers to ensure that BNF publications continue to serve the needs of its users.

Market research Market research is conducted at regular intervals to gather feedback on specific areas of development, such as drug interactions or changes to the way information is presented in digital formats.

> The BNF is an independent professional publication that is kept up-to-date and which addresses the day-to-day prescribing information needs of healthcare professionals. Use of this resource throughout the health service helps to ensure that medicines are used safely, effectively and appropriately.

How to use the BNF

Notes on conditions, drugs and preparations

The main text consists of classified notes on clinical conditions, drugs and preparations. These notes are divided into 15 chapters, each of which is related to a particular system of the body or to an aspect of medical care. Each chapter is then divided into sections which begin with appropriate *notes for prescribers*. These notes are intended to provide information to doctors, dental surgeons, pharmacists, nurses, and other healthcare professionals to facilitate the selection of suitable treatment. Guidance on dental and oral conditions is identified by means of a relevant heading (e.g. Dental and Orofacial pain) in the appropriate sections of the BNF. The notes are followed by details of relevant drugs and preparations. Preparations which can be prescribed by dental surgeons using NHS form FP10D (GP14 in Scotland, WP10D in Wales) are identified within the BNF by means of a note headed Dental Prescribing on NHS.

For information available since publication of this edition see bnf.org

Guidance on prescribing

This part includes information on prescription writing, controlled drugs and dependence, prescribing for children and the elderly, and prescribing in palliative care. Advice is given on the reporting of adverse reactions. The BNF also includes advice on medical emergencies

DRUG NAME 

Indications details of uses and indications

Cautions details of precautions required (with cross-references to appropriate Appendixes) and also any monitoring required

Counselling Verbal explanation to the patient of specific details of the drug treatment (e.g. posture when taking a medicine)

Contra-indications details of any contra-indications to use of drug

Side-effects details of common and more serious side-effects

Dose

- Dose and frequency of administration (max. dose); CHILD and ELDERLY details of dose for specific age group
- By alternative route, dose and frequency

***Approved Name** (Non-proprietary) PoM
Pharmaceutical form colour, coating, active ingredient and amount in dosage form, net price, pack size = basic NHS price. Label: (as in Appendix 9)

Proprietary Name® (Manufacturer) PoM NHS
Pharmaceutical form sugar-free, active ingredient mg/mL, net price, pack size = basic NHS price. Label: (as in Appendix 9)
Excipients include clinically important excipients or electrolytes

*exceptions to the prescribing status are indicated by a note or footnote.

Note Specific notes about the product e.g. handling

Preparations

Preparations usually follow immediately after the drug which is their main ingredient.

Preparations are included under a non-proprietary title, if they are marketed under such a title, if they are not otherwise prescribable under the NHS, or if they may be prepared extemporaneously.

If proprietary preparations are of a distinctive colour this is stated.

In the case of compound preparations the indications, cautions, contra-indications, side-effects, and interactions of all constituents should be taken into account for prescribing.

Drugs

Drugs appear under pharmacopoeial or other non-proprietary titles. When there is an *appropriate current monograph* (Medicines Act 1968, Section 65) preference is given to a name at the head of that monograph; otherwise a British Approved Name (BAN), if available, is used (see also p. xiv).

The symbol ◢ is used to denote those preparations considered by the Joint Formulary Committee to be less suitable for prescribing. Although such preparations may not be considered as drugs of first choice, their use may be justifiable in certain circumstances.

Prescription-only medicines PoM

This symbol has been placed against those preparations that are available only on a prescription issued by an appropriate practitioner. For more detailed information see *Medicines, Ethics and Practice*, No. 31, London, Pharmaceutical Press, 2007 (and subsequent editions as available).

The symbol CD indicates that the preparation is subject to the prescription requirements of the Misuse of Drugs Act. For regulations governing prescriptions for such preparations see pages 7–10.

Preparations not available for NHS prescription NHS

This symbol has been placed against those preparations included in the BNF that are not prescribable under the NHS. Those prescribable only for specific disorders have a footnote specifying the condition(s) for which the preparation remains available. Some preparations which are not *prescribable* by brand name under the NHS may nevertheless be *dispensed* using the brand name providing that the prescription shows an appropriate non-proprietary name.

Prices

Prices have been calculated from the basic cost used in pricing NHS prescriptions dispensed in November 2007 see p. x for details.

and other medical problems in dental practice, together with a review of the oral side-effects of drugs.

An index of conditions relevant to dental surgeons is included.

Emergency treatment of poisoning

This chapter provides information on the management of acute poisoning when first seen in the home, although aspects of hospital-based treatment are mentioned.

Appendixes and indexes

The appendixes include information on interactions, liver disease, renal impairment, pregnancy, breast-feeding, intravenous additives, borderline substances, wound management products, and cautionary and advisory labels for dispensed medicines. They are designed for use in association with the main body of the text.

The Dental Practitioners' List and the Nurse Prescribers' List are also included in this section. The indexes consist of the Index of Manufacturers and the Main Index.

Patient packs

Directive 92/27/EEC specifies the requirements for the labelling of medicines and outlines the format and content of patient information leaflets to be supplied with every medicine; the directive also requires the use of Recommended International Non-proprietary Names for drugs (see p. xiv).

All medicines have approved labelling and patient information leaflets; anyone who supplies a medicine is responsible for providing the relevant information to the patient (see also Appendix 9).

Many medicines are available in manufacturers' original packs complete with patient information leaflets. Where patient packs are available, the BNF shows the number of dose units in the packs. In particular clinical circumstances, where patient packs need to be split or medicines are provided in bulk dispensing packs, manufacturers will provide additional supplies of patient information leaflets on request.

During the revision of each edition of the BNF careful note is taken of the information that appears on the patient information leaflets. Where it is considered appropriate to alert a prescriber to some specific limitation appearing on the patient information leaflet (for example, in relation to pregnancy) this advice now appears in the BNF.

The patient information leaflet also includes details of all inactive ingredients in the medicine. A list of common E numbers and the inactive ingredients to which they correspond is now therefore included in the BNF (see inside back cover).

PACT and SPA

PACT (Prescribing Analyses and Cost) and SPA (Scottish Prescribing Analysis) provide prescribers with information about their prescribing.

The *PACT Standard Report*, or in Scotland SPA *Level 1 Report*, is sent to all general practitioners on a quarterly basis. The PACT Standard Report contains an analysis of the practitioner's prescribing and the practice prescribing over the last 3 months, and gives comparisons with the local Primary Care Trust equivalent practice and with a national equivalent. The report also contains details of the practice prescribing for a specific topic; a different topic is chosen each quarter.

The *PACT Catalogue*, or in Scotland SPA *Level 2 Report*, provides a full inventory of the prescriptions issued by a prescriber. The PACT catalogue is available on request for periods between 1 and 24 months. To allow the prescriber to target specific areas of prescribing, a Catalogue may be requested to cover individual preparations, BNF sections, or combinations of BNF chapters.

PACT is also available electronically (ePACT.net). This system gives users on-line access through NHSnet to the 3 years' prescribing data held on the Prescription Pricing Authority's database; tools for analysing the data are also provided.

Prices in the BNF

Basic **net prices** are given in the BNF to provide an indication of relative cost. Where there is a choice of suitable preparations for a particular disease or condition the relative cost may be used in making a selection. Cost-effective prescribing must, however, take into account other factors (such as dose frequency and duration of treatment) that affect the total cost. The use of more expensive drugs is justified if it will result in better treatment of the patient or a reduction of the length of an illness or the time spent in hospital.

Prices have generally been calculated from the net cost used in pricing NHS prescriptions dispensed in November 2007. Unless an original pack is available these prices are based on the largest pack size of the preparation in use in community pharmacies. The price for an extemporaneously prepared preparation has been omitted where the net cost of the ingredients used to make it would give a misleadingly low impression of the final price. In Appendix 8 prices stated are per dressing or bandage.

The unit of 20 is still sometimes used as a basis for comparison, but where suitable original packs or patient packs are available these are priced instead.

Gross prices vary as follows:

1. Costs to the NHS are greater than the net prices quoted and include professional fees and overhead allowances;
2. Private prescription charges are calculated on a separate basis;
3. Over-the-counter sales are at retail price, as opposed to basic net price, and include VAT.

BNF prices are NOT, therefore, suitable for quoting to patients seeking private prescriptions or contemplating over-the-counter purchases.

A fuller explanation of costs to the NHS may be obtained from the Drug Tariff. Separate drug tariffs are applicable to England and Wales, Scotland, and Northern Ireland; prices in the different tariffs may vary.

Changes for this edition

Significant changes

The BNF is revised twice yearly and numerous changes are made between issues. All copies of BNF No. 54 (September 2007) should therefore be withdrawn and replaced by BNF No. 55 (March 2008). Significant changes have been made in the following sections for BNF No. 55:

Midazolam [classification change], Controlled drugs and drug dependence

Prevention of endocarditis [updated advice on the prevention of endocarditis in dental procedures], Prescribing in dental practice

Updated advice on management of dental patients taking anticoagulants, Prescribing in dental practice

Replacement of pralidoxime mesilate with pralidoxime chloride for the treatment of poisoning by organophosphorus insecticide or nerve agent, Emergency Treatment of Poisoning

Adalimumab [for the treatment of severe active Crohn's disease], section 1.5

Diltiazem for the management of anal fissures, section 1.7.4

Heart failure, section 2.5.5.1

Angina and non-ST-segment-elevation myocardial infarction, section 2.6

Management of myocardial infarction, section 2.10.1

Omalizumab for severe persistent allergic asthma [NICE guidance], section 3.4.2

Anaphylaxis [updated advice], section 3.4.3

Treatment of depression, section 4.3

Opioid analgesics [section updated and reorganised], section 4.7.2

Levodopa, section 4.9.1

Varenicline for smoking cessation [NICE guidance], section 4.10

Benzathine benzylpenicillin for the treatment of syphilis, section 5.1, Table 1

Prevention of endocarditis [NICE guidance], section 5.1, Table 2

Rosiglitazone and pioglitazone [updated MHRA/CHM advice], section 6.1.2.3

Glucocorticoid therapy [section updated and reorganised], section 6.3.2

HRT [updated MHRA/CHM advice], section 6.4.1.1

Strontium ranelate [updated advice on severe allergic reactions], section 6.6.2

Pemtrexed for the treatment of non-small cell lung cancer [NICE guidance], section 8.1.3

Carmustine implants and temozolomide for the treatment of newly diagnosed high-grade glioma [NICE guidance], section 8.1.5

Bortezomib monotherapy for relapsed multiple myeloma [NICE guidance], section 8.1.5

Natalizumab for the treatment of adults with highly active relapsing-remitting multiple sclerosis [NICE guidance], section 8.2.4

Folic acid and prevention of neural tube defects [updated advice], section 9.1.2

Erythropoietins [MHRA/CHM advice on target haemoglobin concentration], section 9.1.3

Erythropoietins [MHRA/CHM advice on tumour progression and survival in patients with cancer], section 9.1.3

Drugs unsafe for use in acute porphyrias [updated advice], section 9.8.2

Azapropazone [application of 'less suitable for prescribing' symbol], section 10.1.1

Piroxicam [application of 'less suitable for prescribing' symbol], section 10.1.1

Adalimumab for the treatment of psoriatic arthritis [NICE guidance], section 10.1.3

Adalimumab, etanercept and infliximab for the treatment of rheumatoid arthritis [NICE guidance], section 10.1.3

Rituximab for the treatment of rheumatoid arthritis [NICE guidance], section 10.1.3

Chlorhexidine mouthwash [updated advice on prevention of endocarditis], section 12.3.4

Photodamage [updated advice for treatment of actinic keratosis and basal cell carcinoma], section 13.8.1

Metformin for hirsutism in women with polycystic ovary syndrome, section 13.9

Table of arbitrary grading system for renal impairment (mild, moderate, severe) removed, Appendix 3

Dose changes

Changes in dose statements introduced into BNF No. 55:

Sodium calcium edetate [repeated courses], p. 34

Metronidazole [treatment of active Crohn's disease], p. 53

Infliximab [severe active Crohn's disease], p. 57

Magnesium Hydroxide Mixture, BP, p. 63

Mannitol [cerebral oedema and raised intraocular pressure], p. 78

Nadolol, p. 89

Iloprost, p. 94

Lisinopril [hypertension, diabetic nephropathy], p. 102

Valsartan [hypertension], p. 107

Alteplase [myocardial infarction], p. 134

Novolizer®, p. 162

Adrenaline [anaphylaxis], p. 171

Chlorpromazine hydrochloride [schizophrenia and autism in children], p. 190

Citalopram [depression and panic disorder], p. 209

Fluvoxamine maleate [obsessive compulsive disorder in children], p. 210

Durogesic® *DTrans*, p. 232

Lamotrigine, p. 248

NiQuitin®, p. 272

Benzylpenicillin, p. 285

Azithromycin, p. 302

Trimethoprim, p. 309

Fluconazole [intravenous dose for prevention of relapse of cryptococcal meningitis in AIDS patients], p. 323

Epivir® [paediatric dose], p. 330

Combivir® [paediatric dose], p. 331

Fosamprenavir, p. 332

Dasatinib, p. 468

Mitotane, p. 465

Bicalutamide, p. 487

Etoricoxib [osteoarthritis], p. 539

Ibuprofen, p. 540

Mefenamic acid, p. 542

Infliximab, p. 554

Alfentanil [assisted ventilation, by intravenous injection], p. 675

Ropivacaine [surgical anaesthesia, by lumbar epidural], p. 684

Classification changes

Classification changes have been made in the following sections for BNF No. 55:

Section 2.5.5.3 Renin inhibitors [new section]

Section 2.12 Bile acid sequestrants [sub-section title change]

Section 4.7.1 Non-opioid analgesics [*Midrid*® moved from section 4.7.4.1]

Section 6.7.4 Somatomedins [new section]

Section 10.1.5 Other drugs for rheumatic diseases [new section]

Section 13.8.1 Sunscreen preparations [*Efudix*® moved from section 8.1.3]

Section 15.1.5 Neuromuscular blocking drugs [title change]

New names

Name changes introduced into BNF 55 (see also p. xiv):

NiQuitin® [formerly *Niquitin CQ*®], p. 272

TicoVac® [formerly *FSME-IMMUN*®], p. 658

Discontinued preparations

Preparations discontinued during the compilation of BNF No. 55:

Amoxil® syrup

Betadine® alcoholic solution

Betadine® antiseptic paint

Betadine® antiseptic solution

Betadine® mouthwash

Betadine® pessaries

Betadine® shampoo

Betadine® skin cleanser solution

Betadine® surgical scrub

Betadine® vaginal cleansing kit

Calciparine®

Carylderm® lotion

Cicatrin®

Combivent® aerosol inhalation

Cromogen Easi-Breathe®

Deteclo®

Exubera®

Glurenorm®

Helicobacter Test Hp-Plus®

Hibicet Hospital Concentrate®

Intal® aerosol inhalation

Menogon®

Menoring®

Minims® Rose Bengal

Minulet®

Mixtard® 10

Mixtard® 20

Mixtard® 40

Mixtard® 50

Moditen®

Netillin®

Ortho-creme®

Pork Mixtard® 30

Prexige®

Rimactazid 300®

Salazopyrin® retention enema

Securon® tablets

Semi-Daonil®

Sustac®

Tertroxin®

Trasylol®

Tri-Minulet®

Zoton® suspension

New preparations included in this edition

Preparations included in the relevant sections of BNF No. 55:

Acea®, p. 630

Adcal D_3 Dissolve®, p. 526

Advagraf®, p. 477

Alateris®, p. 557

Atriance®, p. 460

ATryn®, p. 136

Canesten® Cream Combi, p. 426

Cardioxane®, p. 450

Celsentri®, p. 335

Cervarix®, p. 650

Cholestagel®, p. 138
ChloraPrep®, p. 638
CitraFleet®, p. 63
Clipper®, p. 56
Dynepo®, p. 498
Ecalta®, p. 323
Emollin®, p. 600
Etopan XL®, p. 539
Etrivex®, p. 608
Exelon® patches, p. 276
Fostair®, p. 162
Fostimon®, p. 399
Gygel®, p. 435
Halothane, p. 669
Increlex®, p. 417
Inovelon®, p. 251
Invega®, p. 196
Katya 30/75®, p. 432
Merional®, p. 399
Mezavant® XL, p. 54
Mircera®, p. 498
Mini TT 380® Slimline, p. 436
Pergoveris®, p. 399
Rasilez®, p. 107
Revlimid®, p. 482
Sebivo®, p. 341
Soliris®, p. 500
Spiriva Respimat®, p. 154
Sunya 20/75®, p. 431
Tostran®, p. 395
Utrogestan®, p. 394
Yondelis®, p. 472

Late additions

Ambrix® (GSK) ▼ PoM

Injection, suspension of inactivated hepatitis A virus (grown in human diploid cells) 720 ELISA units and recombinant (DNA) hepatitis B surface antigen [illegible] micrograms/mL adsorbed onto aluminium hydro- [illegible] aluminium phosphate, net price 1-mL pre-filled sy[illegible] £31.18

BNF section 1[illegible] [illegible] prevention of hepatitis A and hepatitis B in non-immune in[illegible]

Atripla® (Gilead) PoM

Tablets, pink, f/c, efavirenz [illegible] [illegible]tricitabine 200 mg, tenofovir disoproxil (as [illegible]mg, net price 30-tab pack = £626.90. Label: [illegible]

BNF section 5.3.1. For the treatment of HIV-1 inf[illegible] who have had HIV-1 RNA levels of less than 50 copies[illegible] more than 3 months on their current combination antiretro[illegible] drugs

IONSYS® (Janssen-Cilag) ▼ CD

Iontophoretic transdermal system, fentanyl 40 micrograms/dose, net price 1 unit (80 doses) = £62.00 (hosp. only)

BNF section 4.7.2. For the treatment of moderate to severe postoperative pain

ISENTRESS® (MSD) ▼ PoM

Tablets, pink, f/c, raltegravir (as potassium) 400 mg, net price 60-tab pack = £647.29. Label: 25

BNF section 5.3.1. For the treatment of HIV-1 infection in combination with other antiretroviral drugs in patients with evidence of ongoing HIV-1 replication despite treatment

Nicopass® (Fabre)

Lozenges, sugar-free, fresh mint (beige) and liquorice mint (brown) flavours, nicotine (as resinate complex) 1.5 mg, net price pack of 12 = £1.68, pack of 36 = £4.18, pack of 96 = £8.94

Excipients include aspartame (section 9.4.1)

BNF section 4.10. For use as an adjunct to smoking cessation therapy

Nicopatch® (Fabre)

Patches, self-adhesive, nicotine *'7 mg patch'* (releasing approx. 7 mg/24 hours), net price 7 = £8.95; *'14 mg patch'* (releasing approx. 14 mg/24 hours), 7 = £8.95; *'21 mg patch'* (releasing approx. 21 mg/24 hours), 7 = £8.95

BNF section 4.10. For use as an adjunct to smoking cessation therapy

Name changes

European Law requires use of the Recommended International Non-proprietary Name (rINN) for medicinal substances. In most cases the British Approved Name (BAN) and rINN were identical. Where the two diff... the BAN was modified to accord with the rIN... which the ...d with the rINN.

The following list shows those subst... as synonyms in the former BAN has been modifie... Former BANs have be... BNF. ... **noradrenaline** Adrenaline and ... are the terms used in the titles of mono-... **Adr...** the European Pharmacopoeia and are thus the ...cial names in the member states. For these substances, BP 2008 shows the European Pharmacopoeia names and the rINNs at the head of the monographs; the BNF has adopted a similar style.

Former BAN	New BAN
adrenaline	*see above*
amethocaine	tetracaine
aminacrine	aminoacridine
amoxycillin	amoxicillin
amphetamine	amfetamine
amylobarbitone sodium	amobarbital sodium
beclomethasone	beclometasone
bendrofluazide	bendroflumethiazide
benzhexol	trihexyphenidyl
benzphetamine	benzfetamine
benztropine	benzatropine
busulphan	busulfan
butobarbitone	butobarbital
carticaine	articaine
cephalexin	cefalexin
cephradine	cefradine
chloral betaine	cloral betaine
chlorbutol	chlorobutanol
chlormethiazole	clomethiazole
chlorpheniramine	chlorphenamine
chlorthalidone	chlortalidone
cholecalciferol	colecalciferol
cholestyramine	colestyramine
clomiphene	clomifene
colistin sulphomethate sodium	colistimethate sodium
corticotrophin	corticotropin
cyclosporin	ciclosporin
cysteamine	mercaptamine
danthron	dantron
dexamphetamine	dexamfetamine
dibromopropamidine	dibrompropamidine
dicyclomine	dicycloverine
dienoestrol	dienestrol
dimethicone(s)	dimeticone
dimethyl sulphoxide	dimethyl sulfoxide
dothiepin	dosulepin
doxycycline hydrochloride (hemihydrate hemiethanolate)	doxycycline hyclate
eformoterol	formoterol
etha...ylate	etamsylate
...inyloestradiol	ethinylestradiol
ethynodiol	etynodiol
flumethasone	flumetasone
flupenthixol	flupentixol
flurandrenolone	fludroxycortide
frusemide	furosemide
guaiphenesin	guaifenesin
hexachlorophane	hexachlorophene
hexamine hippurate	methenamine hippurate
hydroxyurea	hydroxycarbamide
indomethacin	indometacin
lignocaine	lidocaine
methotrimeprazine	levomepromazine
methyl cysteine	mecysteine
methylene blue	methylthioninium chloride
methicillin	meticillin
mitozantrone	mitoxantrone
nicoumalone	acenocoumarol
noradrenaline	*see above*
oestradiol	estradiol
oestriol	estriol
oestrone	estrone
oxpentifylline	pentoxifylline
phenobarbitone	phenobarbital
pipothiazine	pipotiazine
polyhexanide	polihexanide
pramoxine	pramocaine
procaine penicillin	procaine benzylpenicillin
prothionamide	protionamide
quinalbarbitone	secobarbital
riboflavine	riboflavin
salcatonin	calcitonin (salmon)
sodium calciumedetate	sodium calcium edetate
sodium cromoglycate	sodium cromoglicate
sodium ironedetate	sodium feredetate
sodium picosulphate	sodium picosulfate
sorbitan monostearate	sorbitan stearate
stibocaptate	sodium stibocaptate
stilboestrol	diethylstilbestrol
sulphacetamide	sulfacetamide
sulphadiazine	sulfadiazine
sulphamethoxazole	sulfamethoxazole
sulphapyridine	sulfapyridine
sulphasalazine	sulfasalazine
sulphathiazole	sulfathiazole
sulphinpyrazone	sulfinpyrazone
tetracosactrin	tetracosactide
thiabendazole	tiabendazole
thioguanine	tioguanine
thiopentone	thiopental
thymoxamine	moxisylyte
thyroxine sodium	levothyroxine sodium
tribavirin	ribavirin
trimeprazine	alimemazine
urofollitrophin	urofollitropin

Guidance on prescribing

General guidance

Medicines should be prescribed only when they are necessary, and in all cases the benefit of administering the medicine should be considered in relation to the risk involved. This is particularly important during pregnancy when the risk to both mother and fetus must be considered (for further details see Prescribing in Pregnancy, Appendix 4).

It is important to discuss treatment options carefully with the patient to ensure that the patient is content to take the medicine as prescribed (see also Taking Medicines to Best Effect, below). In particular, the patient should be helped to distinguish the side-effects of prescribed drugs from the effects of the medical disorder. When the beneficial effects of the medicine are likely to be delayed, the patient should be advised of this.

Taking medicines to best effect Difficulties in compliance with drug treatment occur regardless of age. Factors contributing to poor compliance with prescribed medicines include:

- prescription not collected or not dispensed;
- purpose of medicine not clear;
- perceived lack of efficacy;
- real or perceived side-effects;
- patients' perception of the risk and severity of side-effects may differ from that of the prescriber;
- instructions for administration not clear;
- physical difficulty in taking medicines (e.g. with swallowing the medicine, with handling small tablets, or with opening medicine containers);
- unattractive formulation (e.g. unpleasant taste);
- complicated regimen.

The prescriber and the patient should agree on the health outcomes that the patient desires and on the strategy for achieving them ('concordance'). The prescriber should be sensitive to religious, cultural, and personal beliefs that can affect patients' acceptance of medicines.

Taking the time to explain to the patient (and relatives) the rationale and the potential adverse effects of treatment may improve compliance. Reinforcement and elaboration of the physician's instructions by the pharmacist also helps. Advising the patient of the possibility of alternative treatments may encourage the patient to seek advice rather than merely abandon unacceptable treatment.

Simplifying the drug regimen may help; the need for frequent administration may reduce compliance although there appears to be little difference in compliance between once-daily and twice-daily administration. Combination products reduce the number of drugs taken but this may be at the expense of the ability to titrate individual doses.

Complementary and alternative medicine An increasing amount of information on complementary and alternative medicine is becoming available. The scope of the BNF is restricted to the discussion of conventional medicines but reference is made to complementary treatments if they affect conventional therapy (e.g. interactions with St John's wort—see Appendix 1). Further information on herbal medicines is available at www.mhra.gov.uk.

Abbreviation of titles In general, titles of drugs and preparations should be written *in full*. Unofficial abbreviations should not be used as they may be misinterpreted.

Non-proprietary titles Where non-proprietary ('generic') titles are given, they should be used in prescribing. This will enable any suitable product to be dispensed, thereby saving delay to the patient and sometimes expense to the health service. The only exception is where bioavailability problems are so important that the patient should always receive the same brand; in such cases, the brand name or the manufacturer should be stated. Non-proprietary titles should **not** be invented for the purposes of prescribing generically since this can lead to confusion, particularly in the case of compound and modified-release preparations.

Titles used as headings for monographs may be used freely in the United Kingdom but in other countries may be subject to restriction.

Many of the non-proprietary titles used in this book are titles of monographs in the European Pharmacopoeia, British Pharmacopoeia, or British Pharmaceutical Codex 1973. In such cases the preparations must comply with the standard (if any) in the appropriate publication, as required by the Medicines Act (Section 65).

Proprietary titles Names followed by the symbol® are or have been used as proprietary names in the United Kingdom. These names may in general be applied only to products supplied by the owners of the trade marks.

Marketing authorisation and BNF advice In general the *doses, indications, cautions, contra-indications,* and *side-effects* in the BNF reflect those in the manufacturers' data sheets or Summaries of Product Characteristics (SPCs) which, in turn, reflect those in the corresponding marketing authorisations (formerly known as Product Licences). The BNF does not generally include proprietary medicines that are not supported by a valid Summary of Product Characteristics or when the marketing authorisation holder has not been able to supply essential information.

Where an unlicensed drug is included in the BNF, this is indicated in square brackets after the entry. Where the BNF suggests a use (or route) that is outside the licensed indication of a product ('off-label' use), this too is indicated. Unlicensed use of medicines becomes necessary if the clinical need cannot be met by licensed medicines; such use should be supported by appropriate evidence and experience. When a preparation is available from more than one manufacturer, the BNF reflects advice that is the most clinically relevant regardless of any variation in the marketing authorisations.

The doses stated in the BNF are intended for general guidance and represent, unless otherwise stated, the usual range of doses that are generally regarded as being suitable for adults.

> Prescribing medicines outside the recommendations of their marketing authorisation alters (and probably increases) the doctor's professional responsibility and potential liability. The prescriber should be able to justify and feel competent in using such medicines.

Oral syringes An **oral syringe** is supplied when oral liquid medicines are prescribed in doses other than multiples of 5 mL. The oral syringe is marked in 0.5-mL divisions from 1 to 5 mL to measure doses of less than 5 mL. It is provided with an adaptor and an instruction leaflet. The *5-mL spoon* is used for doses of 5 mL (or multiples thereof).

Strengths and quantities The strength or quantity to be contained in capsules, lozenges, tablets, etc. should be stated by the prescriber.

If a pharmacist receives an incomplete prescription for a systemically administered preparation and considers it would not be appropriate for the patient to return to the doctor, the following procedures will apply[1]:

(a) an attempt must always be made to contact the prescriber to ascertain the intention;

(b) if the attempt is successful the pharmacist must, where practicable, subsequently arrange for details of quantity, strength where applicable, and dosage to be inserted by the prescriber on the incomplete form;

(c) where, although the prescriber has been contacted, it has not proved possible to obtain the written intention regarding an incomplete prescription, the pharmacist may endorse the form 'p.c.' (prescriber contacted) and add details of the quantity and strength where applicable of the preparation supplied, and of the dose indicated. The endorsement should be initialled and dated by the pharmacist;

(d) where the prescriber cannot be contacted and the pharmacist has sufficient information to make a professional judgement the preparation may be dispensed. If the quantity is missing the pharmacist may supply sufficient to complete up to 5 days' treatment; except that where a combination pack (i.e. a proprietary pack containing more than one medicinal product) or oral contraceptive is prescribed by name only, the smallest pack shall be dispensed. In all cases the prescription must be endorsed 'p.n.c.' (prescriber not contacted), the quantity, the dose, and the strength (where applicable) of the preparation supplied must be indicated, and the endorsement must be initialled and dated;

(e) if the pharmacist has any doubt about exercising discretion, an incomplete prescription must be referred back to the prescriber.

1. These recommendations are acceptable for **prescription-only medicines** (PoM). For items marked CD see also Controlled Drugs and Drug Dependence, p. 7.

Excipients Branded oral liquid preparations that do not contain *fructose, glucose,* or *sucrose* are described as 'sugar-free' in the BNF. Preparations containing hydrogenated glucose syrup, mannitol, maltitol, sorbitol, or xylitol are also marked 'sugar-free' since there is evidence that they do not cause dental caries. Patients receiving medicines containing cariogenic sugars should be advised of appropriate dental hygiene measures to prevent caries. Sugar-free preparations should be used whenever possible.

Where information on the presence of *aspartame, gluten, tartrazine, arachis (peanut) oil* or *sesame oil* is available, this is indicated in the BNF against the relevant preparation.

Information is provided on *selected excipients* in skin preparations (section 13.1.3), in vaccines (section 14.1), and on *selected preservatives* and *excipients* in eye drops and injections. Pressurised metered aerosols containing *chlorofluorocarbons* (CFCs) have also been identified throughout the BNF (see section 3.1.1.1).

The presence of *benzyl alcohol* and *polyoxyl castor oil* (polyethoxylated castor oil) in injections is indicated in the BNF. Benzyl alcohol has been associated with a fatal toxic syndrome in preterm neonates, and therefore, parenteral preparations containing the preservative should not be used in neonates. Polyoxyl castor oils, used as vehicles in intravenous injections, have been associated with severe anaphylactoid reactions.

The presence of *propylene glycol* in oral or parenteral medicines is indicated in the BNF; it can cause adverse effects if its elimination is impaired, e.g. in renal failure, in neonates and young children, and in slow metabolisers of the substance. It may interact with disulfiram and metronidazole.

> In the absence of information on excipients in the BNF and in the product literature, contact the manufacturer (see Index of Manufacturers) if it is essential to check details.

Extemporaneous preparation A product should be dispensed extemporaneously only when no product with a marketing authorisation is available.

The BP direction that a preparation must be *freshly prepared* indicates that it must be made not more than 24 hours before it is issued for use. The direction that a preparation should be *recently prepared* indicates that deterioration is likely if the preparation is stored for longer than about 4 weeks at 15–25° C.

The term **water** used without qualification means either potable water freshly drawn direct from the public supply and suitable for drinking or freshly boiled and cooled purified water. The latter should be used if the public supply is from a local storage tank or if the potable water is unsuitable for a particular preparation (Water for injections, section 9.2.2).

Drugs and driving Prescribers should advise patients if treatment is likely to affect their ability to drive motor vehicles. This applies especially to drugs with sedative effects; patients should be warned that these effects are increased by alcohol. General information about a patient's fitness to drive is available from the Driver and Vehicle Licensing Agency at www.dvla.gov.uk (see also Appendix 9).

Patents In the BNF, certain drugs have been included notwithstanding the existence of actual or potential patent rights. In so far as such substances are protected by Letters Patent, their inclusion in this Formulary neither conveys, nor implies, licence to manufacture.

Health and safety When handling chemical or biological materials particular attention should be given to the possibility of allergy, fire, explosion, radiation, or poisoning. Substances such as corticosteroids, some antimicrobials, phenothiazines, and many cytotoxics, are irritant or very potent and should be handled with caution. Contact with the skin and inhalation of dust should be avoided.

Safety in the home Patients must be warned to keep all medicines out of the reach of children. All solid dose and all oral and external liquid preparations must be dispensed in a reclosable *child-resistant container* unless:

- the medicine is in an original pack or patient pack such as to make this inadvisable;
- the patient will have difficulty in opening a child-resistant container;
- a specific request is made that the product shall not be dispensed in a child-resistant container;
- no suitable child-resistant container exists for a particular liquid preparation.

All patients should be advised to dispose of *unwanted medicines* by returning them to a supplier for destruction.

Name of medicine The name of the medicine should appear on the label unless the prescriber indicates otherwise.

(a) The strength is also stated on the label in the case of tablets, capsules, and similar preparations that are available in different strengths.

(b) If it is the wish of the prescriber that a description such as 'The Sedative Tablets' should appear on the label, the prescriber should write the desired description on the prescription form.

(c) The arrangement will extend to approved names, proprietary names or titles given in the BP, BPC, BNF, DPF, or NPF.

(d) The name written on the label is that used by the prescriber on the prescription.

(e) When a prescription is written other than on an NHS prescription form the name of the prescribed preparation will be stated on the label of the dispensed medicine unless the prescriber indicates otherwise.

(f) The Council of the Royal Pharmaceutical Society advises that the labels of dispensed medicines should indicate the total quantity of the product dispensed in the container to which the label refers. This requirement applies equally to solid, liquid, internal, and external preparations. If a product is dispensed in more than one container, the reference should be to the amount in each container.

> Non-proprietary names of **compound preparations** which appear in the BNF are those that have been compiled by the British Pharmacopoeia Commission or another recognised body; whenever possible they reflect the names of the active ingredients.
>
> Prescribers should avoid creating their own compound names for the purposes of generic prescribing; such names do not have an approved definition and can be misinterpreted.
>
> Special care should be taken to avoid errors when prescribing compound preparations; in particular the hyphen in the prefix 'co-' should be retained.
>
> Special care should also be taken to avoid creating generic names for **modified-release** preparations where the use of these names could lead to confusion between formulations with different lengths of action.

Security and validity of prescriptions The Councils of the British Medical Association and the Royal Pharmaceutical Society have issued a joint statement on the security and validity of prescriptions.

In particular, prescription forms should:

- not be left unattended at reception desks;
- not be left in a car where they may be visible; and
- when not in use, be kept in a locked drawer within the surgery and at home.

Where there is any doubt about the authenticity of a prescription, the pharmacist should contact the prescriber. If this is done by telephone, the number should be obtained from the directory rather than relying on the information on the prescription form, which may be false.

Patient group direction (PGD) In most cases, the most appropriate clinical care will be provided on an individual basis by a prescriber to a specific individual patient. However, a Patient Group Direction for supply and administration of medicines by other healthcare professionals can be used where it would benefit patient care without compromising safety.

A Patient Group Direction is a written direction relating to the supply and administration (or administration only) of a licensed prescription-only medicine by certain classes of healthcare professionals; the Direction is signed by a doctor (or dentist) and by a pharmacist. Further information on Patient Group Directions is available in Health Service Circular HSC 2000/026 (England), HDL (2001) 7 (Scotland), and WHC (2000) 116 (Wales).

NICE and Scottish Medicines Consortium Advice issued by the National Institute for Health and Clinical Excellence (NICE) and by the Scottish Medicines Consortium (SMC) is included in the BNF when relevant. If advice within a NICE Single Technology Appraisal differs from SMC advice, the Scottish Executive expects NHS Boards within NHS Scotland to comply with the SMC advice. Details of the advice together with updates can be obtained from www.nice.org.uk and from www.scottishmedicines.org.uk.

Prescription writing

Shared care

In its guidelines on responsibility for prescribing (circular EL (91) 127) between hospitals and general practitioners, the Department of Health has advised that legal responsibility for prescribing lies with the doctor who signs the prescription.

Prescriptions[1] should be written legibly in ink or otherwise so as to be indelible[2], should be dated, should state the full name and address of the patient, and should be signed in ink by the prescriber[3]. The age and the date of birth of the patient should preferably be stated, and it is a legal requirement in the case of prescription-only medicines to state the age for children under 12 years.

The following should be noted:

(a) The unnecessary use of decimal points should be avoided, e.g. 3 mg, not 3.0 mg.
Quantities of 1 gram or more should be written as 1 g etc.
Quantities less than 1 gram should be written in milligrams, e.g. 500 mg, not 0.5 g.
Quantities less than 1 mg should be written in micrograms, e.g. 100 micrograms, not 0.1 mg.
When decimals are unavoidable a zero should be written in front of the decimal point where there is no other figure, e.g. 0.5 mL, not .5 mL.
Use of the decimal point is acceptable to express a range, e.g. 0.5 to 1 g.

(b) 'Micrograms' and 'nanograms' should **not** be abbreviated. Similarly 'units' should **not** be abbreviated.

Pharmacy Stamp | Age: 1yr 11mths | Title, Forename, Surname & Address: Master Peter Patient
D.o.B: 2/4/2004 | Flat 1, 50 Stanhope Street, Newtown TE22 1ST
Please don't stamp over age box
Number of days' treatment N.B. Ensure dose is stated: 5
Endorsements:
Amoxicillin oral suspension
125mg/5ml sugar-free
125mg three times daily
Supply 100ml
[No more items on this prescription]

SAMPLE

Signature of Prescriber | Date: 02/03/06
For dispenser No. of Prescns. on form
Anyborough Health Authority
Dr D O Good 345543
7 High Street
Anytown KB1 CD2
Tel: 0111 222 333
NHS FP10NC0105

(c) The term 'millilitre' (ml or mL)[4] is used in medicine and pharmacy, and cubic centimetre, c.c., or cm^3 should not be used.

(d) Dose and dose frequency should be stated; in the case of preparations to be taken 'as required' a **minimum dose interval** should be specified.
When doses other than multiples of 5 mL are prescribed for *oral liquid preparations* the dose-volume will be provided by means of an **oral syringe**, see p. 2 (except for preparations intended to be measured with a pipette).
Suitable quantities:

Elixirs, Linctuses, and Paediatric Mixtures (5-mL dose), 50, 100, or 150 mL

Adult Mixtures (10-mL dose), 200 or 300 mL

Ear Drops, Eye drops, and Nasal Drops, 10 mL (or the manufacturer's pack)

Eye Lotions, Gargles, and Mouthwashes, 200 mL

(e) For suitable quantities of dermatological preparations, see section 13.1.2.

(f) The names of drugs and preparations should be written clearly and **not** abbreviated, using approved titles **only** (see also advice in box on p. 3 to **avoid** creating generic titles for modified-release preparations).

(g) The quantity to be supplied may be stated by indicating the number of days of treatment required in the box provided on NHS forms. In most cases the exact amount will be supplied. This does not apply to items directed to be used as required—if the dose and frequency are not given then the quantity to be supplied needs to be stated.
When several items are ordered on one form the box can be marked with the number of days of treatment provided the quantity is added for any item for which the amount cannot be calculated.

(h) Although directions should preferably be in **English without abbreviation**, it is recognised that some Latin abbreviations are used (for details see Inside Back Cover).

(i) Medical and dental practitioners may prescribe unlicensed medicines (i.e. those without marketing authorisation) or withdrawn medicines. The prescriber should inform the patient or the patient's carer that the product does not have a marketing authorisation.

Prescribing by dental surgeons Until new prescribing arrangements are in place for NHS prescriptions, dental surgeons should use form FP10D (GP14 in Scotland, WP10D in Wales) to prescribe only those items listed in the Dental Practitioners' Formulary.

1. These recommendations are acceptable for **prescription-only medicines** (PoM). For items marked CD see also Controlled Drugs and Drug Dependence, p. 7.
2. It is permissible to issue carbon copies of NHS prescriptions as long as they are signed in ink.
3. Computer-generated facsimile signatures do not meet the legal requirement.
4. The use of capital 'L' in mL is a printing convention throughout the BNF; both 'mL' and 'ml' are recognised SI abbreviations.

The Act and Regulations do not set any limitations upon the number and variety of substances which the dental surgeon may administer to patients in the surgery or may order by private prescription—provided the relevant legal requirements are observed the dental surgeon may use or order whatever is required for the clinical situation. There is no statutory requirement for the dental surgeon to communicate with a patient's medical practitioner when prescribing for dental use. There are, however, occasions when this would be in the patient's interest and such communication is to be encouraged. For legal requirements relating to prescriptions for Controlled Drugs, see p. 7.

Computer-issued prescriptions

For computer-issued prescriptions the following advice, based on the recommendations of the Joint GP Information Technology Committee, should also be noted:

1. The computer must print out the date, the patient's surname, one forename, other initials, and address, and may also print out the patient's title and date of birth. The age of children under 12 years and of adults over 60 years must be printed in the box available; the age of children under 5 years should be printed in years and months. A facility may also exist to print out the age of patients between 12 and 60 years.
2. The doctor's name must be printed at the bottom of the prescription form; this will be the name of the doctor responsible for the prescription (who will normally sign it). The doctor's surgery address, reference number, and Primary Care Trust (PCT[1]) are also necessary. In addition, the surgery telephone number should be printed.
3. When prescriptions are to be signed by general practitioner registrars, assistants, locums, or deputising doctors, the name of the doctor printed at the bottom of the form must still be that of the responsible principal.
4. Names of medicines must come from a dictionary held in the computer memory, to provide a check on the spelling and to ensure that the name is written in full. The computer can be programmed to recognise both the non-proprietary and the proprietary name of a particular drug and to print out the preferred choice, but must not print out both names. For medicines not in the dictionary, separate checks are required—the user must be warned that no check was possible and the entire prescription must be entered in the lexicon.
5. The dictionary may contain information on the usual doses, formulations, and pack sizes to produce standard predetermined prescriptions for common preparations, and to provide a check on the validity of an individual prescription on entry.
6. The prescription must be printed in English without abbreviation; information may be entered or stored in abbreviated form. The dose must be in numbers, the frequency in words, and the quantity in numbers in brackets, thus: 40 mg four times daily (112). It must also be possible to prescribe by indicating the length of treatment required, see (h) above.
7. The BNF recommendations should be followed as in (a), (b), (c), (d), and (e) above.
8. Checks may be incorporated to ensure that all the information required for dispensing a particular drug has been filled in. For instructions such as 'as directed' and 'when required', the maximum daily dose should normally be specified.
9. Numbers and codes used in the system for organising and retrieving data must never appear on the form.
10. Supplementary warnings or advice should be written in full, should not interfere with the clarity of the prescription itself, and should be in line with any warnings or advice in the BNF; numerical codes should not be used.
11. A mechanism (such as printing a series of non-specific characters) should be incorporated to cancel out unused space, or wording such as 'no more items on this prescription' may be added after the last item. Otherwise the doctor should delete the space manually.
12. To avoid forgery the computer may print on the form the number of items to be dispensed (somewhere separate from the box for the pharmacist). The number of items per form need be limited only by the ability of the printer to produce clear and well-demarcated instructions with sufficient space for each item and a spacer line before each fresh item.
13. Handwritten alterations should only be made in exceptional circumstances—it is preferable to print out a new prescription. Any alterations must be made in the doctor's own handwriting and countersigned; computer records should be updated to fully reflect any alteration. Prescriptions for drugs used for contraceptive purposes (but which are not promoted as contraceptives) may need to be marked in handwriting with the symbol ♀ (or endorsed in another way to indicate that the item is prescribed for contraceptive purposes).
14. Prescriptions for controlled drugs can be printed from the computer, but the prescriber's signature must be handwritten[2].
15. The strip of paper on the side of the FP10SS[3] may be used for various purposes but care should be taken to avoid including confidential information. It may be advisable for the patient's name to appear at the top, but this should be preceded by 'confidential'.
16. In rural dispensing practices prescription requests (or details of medicines dispensed) will normally be entered in one surgery. The prescriptions (or dispensed medicines) may then need to be delivered to another surgery or location; if possible the computer should hold up to 10 alternatives.
17. Prescription forms that are reprinted or issued as a duplicate should be labelled clearly as such.

1. Health Board in Scotland, Local Health Board in Wales.
2. See Controlled Drugs and Drug Dependence p. 7; the prescriber may use a date stamp.
3. GP10(COMP) and GP10SS in Scotland, WP10SS in Wales.

Emergency supply of medicines

Emergency supply requested by member of the public

Pharmacists are sometimes called upon by members of the public to make an emergency supply of medicines. The Prescription Only Medicines (Human Use) Order 1997 allows exemptions from the Prescription Only requirements for emergency supply to be made by a person lawfully conducting a retail pharmacy business provided:

(a) that the pharmacist has interviewed the person requesting the prescription-only medicine and is satisfied:
  - (i) that there is immediate need for the prescription-only medicine and that it is impracticable in the circumstances to obtain a prescription without undue delay;
  - (ii) that treatment with the prescription-only medicine has on a previous occasion been prescribed by a doctor, a supplementary prescriber, a community practitioner nurse prescriber (formerly a district nurse or health visitor prescriber), a nurse independent prescriber, or a pharmacist independent prescriber, for the person requesting it;
  - (iii) as to the dose that it would be appropriate for the person to take;

(b) that no greater quantity shall be supplied than will provide 5 days' treatment except when the prescription-only medicine is:
  - (i) insulin, an ointment or cream, or a preparation for the relief of asthma in an aerosol dispenser when the smallest pack can be supplied;
  - (ii) an oral contraceptive when a full cycle may be supplied;
  - (iii) an antibiotic in liquid form for oral administration when the smallest quantity that will provide a full course of treatment can be supplied;

(c) that an entry shall be made by the pharmacist in the prescription book stating:
  - (i) the date of supply;
  - (ii) the name, quantity and, where appropriate, the pharmaceutical form and strength;
  - (iii) the name and address of the patient;
  - (iv) the nature of the emergency;

(d) that the container or package must be labelled to show:
  - (i) the date of supply;
  - (ii) the name, quantity and, where appropriate, the pharmaceutical form and strength;
  - (iii) the name of the patient;
  - (iv) the name and address of the pharmacy;
  - (v) the words 'Emergency supply';
  - (vi) the words 'Keep out of the reach of children' (or similar warning);

(e) that the prescription-only medicine is not a substance specifically excluded from the emergency supply provision, and does not contain a Controlled Drug specified in Schedules 1, 2, or 3 to the Misuse of Drugs Regulations 2001 except for phenobarbital or phenobarbital sodium for the treatment of epilepsy: for details see *Medicines, Ethics and Practice*, No. 31, London, Pharmaceutical Press, 2007 (and subsequent editions as available).

Emergency supply requested by prescriber

Emergency supply of a prescription-only medicine may also be made at the request of a doctor, a supplementary prescriber, a community practitioner nurse prescriber (formerly a district nurse or health visitor prescriber), a nurse independent prescriber, or a pharmacist independent prescriber provided:

(a) that the pharmacist is satisfied that the prescriber by reason of some emergency is unable to furnish a prescription immediately;

(b) that the prescriber has undertaken to furnish a prescription within 72 hours;

(c) that the medicine is supplied in accordance with the directions of the prescriber requesting it;

(d) that the medicine is not a substance specifically excluded from the emergency supply provision, and does not contain a Controlled Drug specified in Schedules 1, 2, or 3 to the Misuse of Drugs Regulations 2001 except for phenobarbital or phenobarbital sodium for the treatment of epilepsy: for details see *Medicines, Ethics and Practice*, No. 31, London, Pharmaceutical Press, 2007 (and subsequent editions as available);

(e) that an entry shall be made in the prescription book stating:
  - (i) the date of supply;
  - (ii) the name, quantity and, where appropriate, the pharmaceutical form and strength;
  - (iii) the name and address of the practitioner requesting the emergency supply;
  - (iv) the name and address of the patient;
  - (v) the date on the prescription;
  - (vi) when the prescription is received the entry should be amended to include the date on which it is received.

Royal Pharmaceutical Society's Guidelines

1. The pharmacist should consider the medical consequences of *not* supplying a medicine in an emergency.
2. If the pharmacist is unable to make an emergency supply of a medicine the pharmacist should advise the patient how to obtain essential medical care.

For conditions that apply to supplies made at the request of a patient see *Medicines, Ethics and Practice*, No. 31, London Pharmaceutical Press, 2007 (and subsequent editions).

Controlled drugs and drug dependence

The Misuse of Drugs Act, 1971 prohibits certain activities in relation to 'Controlled Drugs', in particular their manufacture, supply, and possession. The penalties applicable to offences involving the different drugs are graded broadly according to the *harmfulness attributable to a drug when it is misused* and for this purpose the drugs are defined in the following three classes:

Class A includes: alfentanil, cocaine, diamorphine (heroin), dipipanone, lysergide (LSD), methadone methylenedioxymethamfetamine (MDMA, 'ecstasy'), morphine, opium, pethidine, phencyclidine, remifentanil, and class B substances when prepared for injection

Class B includes: oral amphetamines, barbiturates, codeine, ethylmorphine, glutethimide, pentazocine, phenmetrazine, and pholcodine

Class C includes: certain drugs related to the amphetamines such as benzfetamine and chlorphentermine, buprenorphine, cannabis, cannabis resin, diethylpropion, mazindol, meprobamate, pemoline, pipradrol, most benzodiazepines, zolpidem, androgenic and anabolic steroids, clenbuterol, chorionic gonadotrophin (HCG), non-human chorionic gonadotrophin, somatotropin, somatrem, and somatropin

The Misuse of Drugs Regulations 2001 define the classes of person who are authorised to supply and possess controlled drugs while acting in their professional capacities and lay down the conditions under which these activities may be carried out. In the regulations drugs are divided into five schedules each specifying the requirements governing such activities as import, export, production, supply, possession, prescribing, and record keeping which apply to them.

Schedule 1 includes drugs such as cannabis and lysergide which are not used medicinally. Possession and supply are prohibited except in accordance with Home Office authority.

Schedule 2 includes drugs such as diamorphine (heroin), morphine, remifentanil, pethidine, secobarbital, glutethimide, amfetamine, and cocaine and are subject to the full controlled drug requirements relating to prescriptions, safe custody (except for secobarbital), the need to keep registers, etc. (unless exempted in Schedule 5).

Schedule 3 includes the barbiturates (except secobarbital, now Schedule 2), buprenorphine, diethylpropion, mazindol, meprobamate, midazolam, pentazocine, phentermine, and temazepam. They are subject to the special prescription requirements (except for temazepam) but not to the safe custody requirements (except for buprenorphine, diethylpropion, and temazepam) nor to the need to keep registers (although there are requirements for the retention of invoices for 2 years).

Schedule 4 includes in Part I benzodiazepines (except temazepam and midazolam which are in Schedule 3) and zolpidem, which are subject to minimal control. Part II includes androgenic and anabolic steroids, clenbuterol, chorionic gonadotrophin (HCG), non-human chorionic gonadotrophin, somatotropin, somatrem, and somatropin. Controlled drug prescription requirements do not apply and Schedule 4 Controlled Drugs are not subject to safe custody requirements.

Schedule 5 includes those preparations which, because of their strength, are exempt from virtually all Controlled Drug requirements other than retention of invoices for two years.

Prescriptions Preparations in Schedules 2 and 3 of the Misuse of Drugs Regulations 2001 (and subsequent amendments) are identified throughout the BNF by the symbol CD (Controlled Drug). The principal legal requirements relating to medical prescriptions are listed below (see also Department of Health Guidance, p. 8).

Prescription requirements

Prescriptions for Controlled Drugs that are subject to prescription requirements[1] must be indelible,[2] and must be *signed* by the prescriber, *be dated,* and specify the prescriber's *address.* The prescription must always state:

- the name and address of the patient;
- in the case of a preparation, the form[3] and where appropriate the strength[4] of the preparation,
- either the total quantity (in both words and figures) of the preparation[5], or the number (in both words and figures) of dosage units, as appropriate, to be supplied; in any other case, the total quantity (in both words and figures) of the Controlled Drug to be supplied;
- the dose;[6]
- the words 'for dental treatment only' if issued by a dentist.

A pharmacist is **not** allowed to dispense a Controlled Drug unless all the information required by law is given on the prescription. In the case of a prescription for a Controlled Drug in Schedule 2 or 3, a pharmacist can amend the prescription if it specifies the total quantity only in words or in figures or if it contains minor typographical errors, provided that such amendments are indelible and clearly attributable to the pharmacist making them[7]. Failure to comply with the regulations concerning the writing of prescriptions will result in inconvenience to patients and delay in supplying the necessary medicine.

1. All preparations in Schedules 2 and 3, except temazepam.
2. A machine-written prescription is acceptable. The prescriber's signature must be handwritten.
3. The dosage form (e.g. tablets) must be included on a Controlled Drugs prescription irrespective of whether it is implicit in the proprietary name (e.g. *MST Continus*) or whether only one form is available.
4. When more than one strength of a preparation exists the strength required must be specified.
5. The Home Office has advised that quantities of liquid preparations such as methadone mixture should be written in millilitres.
6. The instruction 'one as directed' constitutes a dose but 'as directed' does not.
7. Implementation date for *N. Ireland* not confirmed.

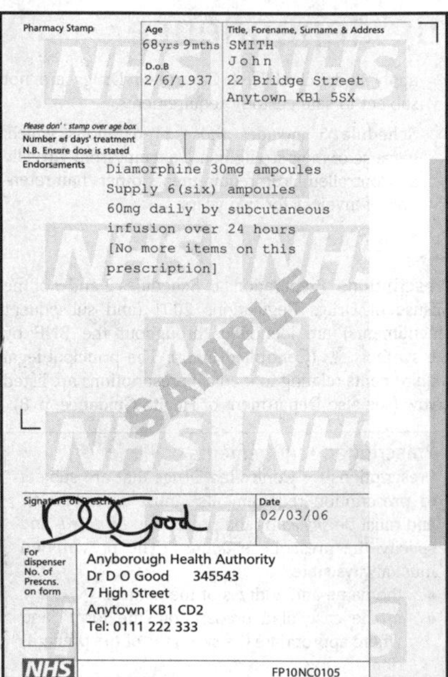

Pharmacy Stamp

Age: 68yrs 9mths

D.o.B: 2/6/1937

Title, Forename, Surname & Address: SMITH John 22 Bridge Street Anytown KB1 5SX

Please don't stamp over age box

Number of days' treatment N.B. Ensure dose is stated

Endorsements

Diamorphine 30mg ampoules
Supply 6(six) ampoules
60mg daily by subcutaneous
infusion over 24 hours
[No more items on this
prescription]

SAMPLE

Signature of Prescriber

Date: 02/03/06

For dispenser No. of Prescns. on form

Anyborough Health Authority
Dr D O Good 345543
7 High Street
Anytown KB1 CD2
Tel: 0111 222 333

NHS

FP10NC0105

A prescription may order a Controlled Drug to be dispensed by instalments; the amount of instalments and the intervals to be observed must be specified.[1] Prescriptions ordering 'repeats' on the same form are **not** permitted for Controlled Drugs in Schedules 2 or 3. A prescription for a Controlled Drug in Schedules 2, 3, or 4 is valid for 28 days from the date stated thereon[2].

Private prescriptions Private prescriptions for Controlled Drugs in Schedules 2 and 3 must be written on specially designated forms provided by Primary Care Trusts in England, Health Boards in Scotland, Local Health Boards in Wales or the Northern Ireland Central Services Agency; in addition, prescriptions must specify the *prescriber's identification number*. Prescriptions to be supplied by a pharmacist in hospital are exempt from the requirement for private prescriptions.

Department of Health guidance Guidance (June 2006) issued by the Department of Health in England on prescribing and dispensing of Controlled Drugs requires:

- in general, prescriptions for Controlled Drugs in Schedules 2, 3, and 4 to be limited to a supply of up to 30 days' treatment; exceptionally, to cover a justifiable clinical need and after consideration of any risk, a prescription can be issued for a longer period, but the reasons for the decision should be recorded on the patient's notes;
- the patient's identifier to be shown on NHS and private prescriptions for Controlled Drugs in Schedules 2 and 3.

Further information is available at www.dh.gov.uk/controlleddrugs.

Dependence and misuse The most serious drugs of addiction are **cocaine**, **diamorphine** (heroin), **morphine**, and the **synthetic opioids**. For arrangements for prescribing of diamorphine, dipipanone, or cocaine for addicts, see p. 10.

Despite marked reduction in the prescribing of **amphetamines** there is concern that abuse of illicit amfetamine and related compounds is widespread.

The benzodiazepine **temazepam** has commonly been associated with misuse. The misuse of **barbiturates** is now less common, in line with declining prescription numbers.

Cannabis (Indian hemp) has no approved medicinal use and cannot be prescribed by doctors. Its use is illegal but has become widespread. Cannabis is a mild hallucinogen seldom accompanied by a desire to increase the dose; withdrawal symptoms are unusual. **Lysergide** (lysergic acid diethylamide, LSD) is a much more potent hallucinogen; its use can lead to severe psychotic states which can be life-threatening.

Prescribing drugs likely to cause dependence or misuse The prescriber has three main responsibilities:

- To avoid creating dependence by introducing drugs to patients without sufficient reason. In this context, the proper use of the morphine-like drugs is well understood. The dangers of other controlled drugs are less clear because recognition of dependence is not easy and its effects, and those of withdrawal, are less obvious.
- To see that the patient does not gradually increase the dose of a drug, given for good medical reasons, to the point where dependence becomes more likely. This tendency is seen especially with hypnotics and anxiolytics (for CSM advice see section 4.1). The prescriber should keep a close eye on the amount prescribed to prevent patients from accumulating stocks. A minimal amount should be prescribed in the first instance, or when seeing a new patient for the first time.
- To avoid being used as an unwitting source of supply for addicts. Methods include visiting more than one doctor, fabricating stories, and forging prescriptions.

Patients under temporary care should be given only small supplies of drugs unless they present an unequivocal letter from their own doctors. Doctors should also remember that their own patients may be doing a collecting round with other prescribers, especially in hospitals. It is sensible to decrease dosages steadily or to issue weekly or even daily prescriptions for small amounts if it is apparent that dependence is occurring.

The stealing and misuse of prescription forms could be minimised by the following precautions:

---

1. A total of 14 days' treatment by instalment of any drug listed in Schedule 2 of the Misuse of Drugs Regulations, buprenorphine and diazepam may be prescribed in England. In *England*, forms FP10(MDA) (blue) and FP10H(MDA) (blue) should be used. In *Scotland*, forms GP10, HBP, or HBP(A) should be used. In *Wales* a total of 14 days' treatment by instalment of any drug listed in Schedules 2–5 of the Misuse of Drugs Regulations may be prescribed. In Wales, form WP10(MDA) or form WP10HP(AD) should be used.
2. The prescriber may forward-date the prescription; the start date may also be specified in the body of the prescription.

- do not leave unattended if called away from the consulting room or at reception desks; do not leave in a car where they may be visible; when not in use, keep in a locked drawer within the surgery and at home;
- draw a diagonal line across the blank part of the form under the prescription;
- write the quantity in words and figures when prescribing drugs prone to abuse; this is obligatory for controlled drugs (see Prescriptions, above);
- alterations are best avoided but if any are made they should be clear and unambiguous; add initials against altered items;
- if prescriptions are left for collection they should be left in a safe place in a sealed envelope.

Travelling abroad Prescribed drugs listed in Schedule 4 Part II (CD Anab) and Schedule 5 of the Misuse of Drugs Regulations 2001 are not subject to export or import licensing. However, patients intending to travel abroad for more than 3 months carrying any amount of drugs listed in Schedules 2, 3, or 4 Part I (CD Benz) will require a personal export/import licence. Further details may be obtained at www.drugs.homeoffice.gov.uk/drugs-laws/licensing/personal, or from the Home Office by contacting (020) 7035 0467 or licensing_enquiry.aadu@homeoffice.gsi.gov.uk.

Applications must be supported by a covering letter from the prescriber and should give details of:

- the patient's name and address;
- the quantities of drugs to be carried;
- the strength and form in which the drugs will be dispensed;
- the country of destination;
- the dates of travel to and from the United Kingdom.

Applications for licences should be sent to the Home Office, Drugs Licensing, Peel Building, 2 Marsham Street, London, SW1P 4DF. Alternatively, completed application forms can be emailed to licensing_enquiry.aadu@homeoffice.gsi.gov.uk with a scanned copy of the covering letter from the prescriber. A minimum of two weeks should be allowed for processing the application.

Patients travelling for less than 3 months do not require a personal export/import licence for carrying Controlled Drugs, but are advised to carry a letter from the prescribing doctor. Those travelling for more than 3 months are advised to make arrangements to have their medication prescribed by a practitioner in the country they are visiting.

Doctors who wish to take Controlled Drugs abroad while accompanying patients may similarly be issued with licences. Licences are not normally issued to doctors who wish to take Controlled Drugs abroad solely in case a family emergency should arise.

Personal export/import licences do not have any legal status outside the UK and are only issued to comply with the Misuse of Drugs Act and facilitate passage through UK Customs and Excise control. For clearance in the country to be visited it would be necessary to approach that country's consulate in the UK.

Notification of drug misusers

Doctors should report cases of drug misuse to their regional or national drug misuse database or centre—see below for contact telephone numbers. The National Drugs Treatment Monitoring System (NDTMS) was introduced in England in April 2001; regional (NDTMS) centres replace the Regional Drug Misuse Databases. A similar system has been introduced in Wales.

Notification to regional (NDTMS) or national centre should be made when a patient starts treatment for drug misuse. All types of problem drug misuse should be reported including opioid, benzodiazepine, and CNS stimulant.

The regional (NDTMS) or national centres are now the only national and local source of epidemiological data on people presenting with problem drug misuse; they provide valuable information to those working with drug misusers and those planning services for them. The databases cannot, however be used as a check on multiple prescribing for drug addicts because the data are anonymised.

Enquiries about the regional (NDTMS) or national centres (including information on how to submit data) can be made to one of the centres listed below:

ENGLAND

Eastern
Tel: (01223) 767 904
Fax: (01223) 597 601

South East
Tel: (01865) 334 725
Fax: (01865) 334 733

London
Tel: (020) 7261 8820
Fax: (020) 7261 8883

North West
Tel: (0151) 231 4533
Fax: (0151) 231 4515

North East
Tel: (0191) 334 0372
Fax: (0191) 334 0391

Yorkshire and the Humber
Tel: (0113) 295 3714
Fax: (0113) 295 3720

South Western
Tel: (0117) 970 6474 ext 311
Fax: (0117) 970 7021

East Midlands
Tel: (0115) 971 2738
Fax: (0115) 971 2740

West Midlands
Tel: (0121) 415 8556
Fax: (0121) 414 8197

SCOTLAND

Tel: (0131) 275 6655
Fax: (0131) 275 7511

WALES

Tel: (029) 2050 3343
Fax: (029) 2050 2330

In **Northern Ireland**, the Misuse of Drugs (Notification of and Supply to Addicts) (Northern Ireland) Regulations 1973 require doctors to send particulars of persons whom they consider to be addicted to certain controlled drugs to the Chief Medical Officer of the Department of Health and Social Services. The Northern Ireland contacts are:

Medical contact:

Dr Ian McMaster
C3 Castle Buildings
Belfast, BT4 3FQ
Tel: (028) 9052 2421
Fax: (028) 9052 0718

Administrative contact:

Drug & Alcohol Information & Research Unit
Annex 2
Castle Building
Belfast, BT4 3SQ
Tel: (028) 9052 2520

The Drug & Alcohol Information & Research Unit also maintains the Northern Ireland Drug Misuse Database (NIDMD) which collects detailed information on those presenting for treatment, on drugs misused and injecting behaviour; participation is not a statutory requirement.

Prescribing of diamorphine (heroin), dipipanone, and cocaine for addicts

The Misuse of Drugs (Supply to Addicts) Regulations 1997 require that only medical practitioners who hold a special licence issued by the Home Secretary may prescribe, administer or supply diamorphine, dipipanone (*Diconal*®) or cocaine in the treatment of drug addiction; other practitioners must refer any addict who requires these drugs to a treatment centre. Whenever possible the addict will be introduced by a member of staff from the treatment centre to a pharmacist whose agreement has been obtained and whose pharmacy is conveniently sited for the patient. Prescriptions for weekly supplies will be sent to the pharmacy by post and will be dispensed on a daily basis as indicated by the doctor. If any alterations of the arrangements are requested by the addict, the portion of the prescription affected must be represcribed and not merely altered.

General practitioners and other doctors do not require a special licence for prescribing diamorphine, dipipanone, and cocaine for patients (including addicts) for *relieving pain* from organic disease or injury.

For guidance on prescription writing, see p. 7.

Adverse reactions to drugs

Any drug may produce unwanted or unexpected adverse reactions. Rapid detection and recording of adverse reactions is of vital importance so that unrecognised hazards are identified promptly and appropriate regulatory action is taken to ensure that medicines are used safely. Doctors, dentists, coroners, pharmacists, and nurses (see also self-reporting below) are urged to report suspected adverse reactions directly to the Medicines and Healthcare products Regulatory Agency (MHRA) through the Yellow Card Scheme using the electronic form at www.yellowcard.gov.uk. Alternatively, prepaid Yellow Cards for reporting are available from the address below and are also bound in this book (inside back cover).

Medicines and Healthcare products Regulatory Agency
CHM
Freepost
London SW8 5BR
Tel: (0800 731 6789)

Suspected adverse reactions to *any* therapeutic agent should be reported, including drugs *(self-medication* as well as those *prescribed)*, blood products, vaccines, radiographic contrast media, complementary and herbal products.

A 24-hour Freefone service is available to all parts of the UK for advice and information on suspected adverse drug reactions; contact the National Yellow Card Information Service at the MHRA on 0800 731 6789. Outside office hours a telephone-answering machine will take messages.

The following Yellow Card Centres may *follow up* reports:

Yellow Card Centre Mersey
Freepost
Liverpool L3 3AB
Tel: (0151) 794 8206

Yellow Card Centre Wales
Freepost
Cardiff CF4 1ZZ
Tel: (029) 2074 4181
(direct line)

Yellow Card Centre Northern & Yorkshire
Freepost 1085
Newcastle upon Tyne NE1 1BR
Tel: (0191) 232 1525
(direct line)

Yellow Card Centre West Midlands
Freepost SW2991
Birmingham B18 7BR
Tel: (0121) 507 5672

Yellow Card Centre Scotland
CARDS
Freepost NAT3271
Edinburgh EH16 4BR
Tel: (0131) 242 2919

The MHRA's database facilitates the monitoring of adverse drug reactions.

More detailed information on reporting and a list of products currently under intensive monitoring can be found on the MHRA website: www.mhra.gov.uk.

> *Drug Safety Update* is a monthly newsletter from the MHRA and the Commission on Human Medicines (CHM); it is available at www.mhra.gov.uk/mhra/drugsafetyupdate.

Self-reporting Patients, parents, and carers can also report suspected adverse reactions to the MHRA. Reports can be submitted directly to the MHRA through the Yellow Card Scheme using the electronic form at www.yellowcard.gov.uk or by telephone on 0808 100 3352. Alternatively, patient Yellow Cards are available from pharmacies or can be downloaded from www.mhra.gov.uk, where more detailed information on patient reporting is available.

Prescription-event monitoring In addition to the MHRA's Yellow Card Scheme, an independent scheme monitors the safety of new medicines using a different approach. The Drug Safety Research Unit identifies patients who have been prescribed selected new medicines and collects data on clinical events in these patients. The data are submitted on a voluntary basis by general practitioners on green forms. More information about the scheme and the Unit's educational material is available from www.dsru.org.

Newer drugs and vaccines Only limited information is available from clinical trials on the safety of new medicines. Further understanding about the safety of medicines depends on the availability of information from routine clinical practice.

The black triangle symbol (▼) identifies newly licensed medicines that are monitored intensively by the MHRA. Such medicines include those that have been licensed for administration by a new route or drug delivery system, or for significant new indications which may alter the established risks and benefits of that drug. There is no standard time for which products retain a black triangle; safety data are usually reviewed after 2 years.

Spontaneous reporting is particularly valuable for recognising possible new hazards rapidly. For medicines showing the black triangle symbol, the MHRA asks that **all** suspected reactions (including those considered not to be serious) are reported through the Yellow Card Scheme. An adverse reaction should be reported even if it is not certain that the drug has caused it, or if the reaction is well recognised, or if other drugs have been given at the same time.

Established drugs and vaccines Doctors, dentists, coroners, pharmacists and nurses are asked to report *all* serious suspected reactions, including those that are fatal, life-threatening, disabling, incapacitating, or which result in or prolong hospitalisation; they should be reported even if the effect is well recognised. Examples include anaphylaxis, blood disorders, endocrine disturbances, effects on fertility, haemorrhage from any site, renal impairment, jaundice, ophthalmic disorders, severe CNS effects, severe skin reactions, reactions in pregnant women, and any drug interactions. Reports of serious adverse reactions are required to enable comparison with other drugs of a similar class. Reports of overdoses (deliberate or accidental) can complicate the assessment of adverse drug reactions, but provide important information on the potential toxicity of drugs.

For established drugs there is no need to report well-known, relatively minor side-effects, such as dry mouth with tricyclic antidepressants or constipation with opioids.

Adverse reactions to medical devices Suspected adverse reactions to medical devices including dental or surgical materials, intra-uterine devices and contact lens fluids should be reported. Information on reporting these can be found at: www.mhra.gov.uk.

Side-effects in the BNF The BNF includes clinically relevant side-effects for most drugs; an exhaustive list is not included for drugs that are used by specialists (e.g. cytotoxic drugs and drugs used in anaesthesia). Where causality has not been established, side-effects in the manufacturers' literature may be omitted from the BNF.

Recognising that hypersensitivity reactions can occur with virtually all medicines, this effect is not generally listed, unless the drug carries an increased risk of such reactions. The BNF also omits effects that are likely to have little clinical consequence (e.g. transient increase in liver enzymes).

Side-effects are generally listed in order of frequency and arranged broadly by body systems. Occasionally a rare side-effect might be listed first if it is considered to be particularly important because of its seriousness.

In the product literature the frequency of side-effects is generally described as follows:

Very common	greater than 1 in 10
Common	1 in 100 to 1 in 10
Uncommon ['less commonly' in BNF]	1 in 1000 to 1 in 100
Rare	1 in 10 000 to 1 in 1000
Very rare	less than 1 in 10 000

Special problems

Delayed drug effects. Some reactions (e.g. cancers, chloroquine retinopathy, and retroperitoneal fibrosis) may become manifest months or years after exposure. Any suspicion of such an association should be reported directly to the MHRA through the Yellow Card Scheme.

The elderly. Particular vigilance is required to identify adverse reactions in the elderly.

Congenital abnormalities. When an infant is born with a congenital abnormality or there is a malformed aborted fetus doctors are asked to consider whether this might be an adverse reaction to a drug and to report all drugs (including self-medication) taken during pregnancy.

Children. Particular vigilance is required to identify and report adverse reactions in children, including those resulting from the unlicensed use of medicines; **all** suspected reactions should be reported directly to the MHRA through the Yellow Card Scheme.

Prevention of adverse reactions

Adverse reactions may be prevented as follows:

- never use any drug unless there is a good indication. If the patient is pregnant do not use a drug unless the need for it is imperative;
- allergy and idiosyncrasy are important causes of adverse drug reactions. Ask if the patient had previous reactions;
- ask if the patient is already taking other drugs *including self-medication drugs, health supplements, complementary and alternative therapies*; interactions may occur;
- age and hepatic or renal disease may alter the metabolism or excretion of drugs, so that much smaller doses may be needed. Genetic factors may also be responsible for variations in metabolism, notably of isoniazid and the tricyclic antidepressants;
- prescribe as few drugs as possible and give very clear instructions to the elderly or any patient likely to misunderstand complicated instructions;
- whenever possible use a familiar drug; with a new drug, be particularly alert for adverse reactions or unexpected events;
- warn the patient if serious adverse reactions are liable to occur.

Oral side-effects of drugs

Drug-induced disorders of the mouth may be due to a local action on the mouth or to a systemic effect manifested by oral changes. In the latter case urgent referral to the patient's medical practitioner may be necessary.

Oral mucosa

Medicaments left in contact with or applied directly to the oral mucosa can lead to inflammation or ulceration; the possibility of allergy should also be borne in mind.

Aspirin tablets allowed to dissolve in the sulcus for the treatment of toothache can lead to a white patch followed by ulceration.

Flavouring agents, particularly **essential oils**, may sensitise the skin, but mucosal swelling is not usually prominent.

The oral mucosa is particularly vulnerable to ulceration in patients treated with cytotoxic drugs, e.g. **methotrexate**. Other drugs capable of causing oral ulceration include **captopril** (and other ACE inhibitors), **gold**, **nicorandil**, **NSAIDs**, **pancreatin**, **penicillamine**, **proguanil**, and **protease inhibitors**.

Erythema multiforme (including Stevens-Johnson syndrome) may follow the use of a wide range of drugs including **antibacterials**, **antiretrovirals**, **sulphonamide derivatives**, and **anticonvulsants**; the oral mucosa may be extensively ulcerated, with characteristic target lesions on the skin. Oral lesions of *toxic epidermal necrolysis* (Lyell's syndrome) have been reported with a similar range of drugs.

Lichenoid eruptions are associated with **ACE inhibitors**, **NSAIDs**, **methyldopa**, **chloroquine**, **oral antidiabetics**, **thiazide diuretics**, and **gold**.

Candidiasis can complicate treatment with **antibacterials** and **immunosuppressants** and is an occasional side-effect of **corticosteroid inhalers**, see also p. 160.

Teeth and Jaw

Brown staining of the teeth frequently follows the use of **chlorhexidine** mouthwash, spray or gel, but can readily be removed by polishing. **Iron** salts in liquid form can stain the enamel black. Superficial staining has been reported rarely with **co-amoxiclav** suspension.

Intrinsic staining of the teeth is most commonly caused by **tetracyclines**. They will affect the teeth if given at any time from about the fourth month *in utero* until the age of twelve years; they are contra-indicated in pregnancy, breast-feeding women, and in children under 12 years. All tetracyclines can cause permanent, unsightly staining in children, the colour varying from yellow to grey.

Excessive ingestion of **fluoride** leads to *dental fluorosis* with mottling of the enamel and areas of hypoplasia or pitting; fluoride supplements occasionally cause mild mottling (white patches) if the dose is too large for the child's age (taking into account the fluoride content of the local drinking water and of toothpaste).

Osteonecrosis of the jaw has been reported in patients receiving a bisphosphonate by the intravenous route and, rarely, in those taking a biphosphonate orally. If possible, dental surgical procedures should be avoided during and after bisphosphonate treatment, see also p. 406.

Periodontium

Gingival overgrowth (gingival hyperplasia) is a side-effect of **phenytoin** and sometimes of **ciclosporin** or of **nifedipine** (and some other calcium-channel blockers).

Thrombocytopenia may be drug related and may cause bleeding at the gingival margins, which may be spontaneous or may follow mild trauma (such as toothbrushing).

Salivary glands

The most common effect that drugs have on the salivary glands is to *reduce flow* (xerostomia). Patients with a persistently dry mouth may have poor oral hygiene; they are at an increased risk of dental caries and oral infections (particularly candidiasis). Many drugs have been implicated in xerostomia, particularly **antimuscarinics** (anticholinergics), **antidepressants** (including tricyclic antidepressants, and selective serotonin re-uptake inhibitors), **alpha-blockers**, **antihistamines**, **antipsychotics**, **baclofen**, **bupropion**, **clonidine**, **5HT$_1$ agonists**, **opioids**, **sibutramine**, and **tizanidine**. Excessive use of **diuretics** can also result in xerostomia.

Some drugs (e.g. clozapine, neostigmine) can *increase saliva production* but this is rarely a problem unless the patient has associated difficulty in swallowing.

Pain in the salivary glands has been reported with some **antihypertensives** (e.g. clonidine, methyldopa) and with **vinca alkaloids**.

Swelling of the salivary glands can occur with **iodides**, **antithyroid drugs**, **phenothiazines**, **ritodrine**, and **sulphonamides**.

Taste

There can be *decreased* taste acuity or *alteration* in taste sensation. Drugs implicated include **amiodarone**, **calcitonin**, **captopril** (and other ACE inhibitors), **carbimazole**, **clarithromycin**, **gold**, **griseofulvin**, **lithium salts**, **metformin**, **metronidazole**, **penicillamine**, **phenindione**, **propafenone**, **protease inhibitors**, **terbinafine**, and **zopiclone**.

Defective medicines

During the manufacture or distribution of a medicine an error or accident may occur whereby the finished product does not conform to its specification. While such a defect may impair the therapeutic effect of the product and could adversely affect the health of a patient, it should **not** be confused with an Adverse Drug Reaction where the product conforms to its specification.

The Defective Medicines Report Centre assists with the investigation of problems arising from licensed medicinal products thought to be defective and co-ordinates any necessary protective action. Reports on suspect defective medicinal products should include the brand or the non-proprietary name, the name of the manufacturer or supplier, the strength and dosage form of the product, the product licence number, the batch number or numbers of the product, the nature of the defect and an account of any action already taken in consequence.

The Centre can be contacted at:

The Defective Medicines Report Centre
Medicines and Healthcare products Regulatory Agency
Room 18–159
1 Nine Elms Lane
London SW8 5NQ
(020) 7084 2574 (weekdays 9.00 am–5.00 pm)
or (020) 7210 3000 (outside office hours)

Prescribing for children

For detailed advice on medicines used for children, consult *BNF for Children*

Children, and particularly neonates, differ from adults in their response to drugs. Special care is needed in the neonatal period (first 30 days of life) and doses should always be calculated with care. At this age, the risk of toxicity is increased by reduced drug clearance and differing target organ sensitivity.

Whenever possible, intramuscular injections should be **avoided** in children because they are painful.

Where possible, medicines for children should be prescribed within the terms of the marketing authorisation (product licence). However, many children may require medicines not specifically licensed for paediatric use.

Although medicines cannot be promoted outside the limits of the licence, the Medicines Act does not prohibit the use of unlicensed medicines. It is recognised that the informed use of unlicensed medicines or of licensed medicines for unlicensed applications ('off-label' use) is often necessary in paediatric practice.

Adverse drug reactions in children The reporting of all suspected adverse drug reactions in children is **strongly encouraged** through the Yellow Card Scheme (see p. 11) even if the intensive monitoring symbol (▼) has been removed, because experience in children may still be limited.

The identification and reporting of adverse reactions to drugs in children is particularly important because:

- the action of the drug and its pharmacokinetics in children (especially in the very young) may be different from that in adults;
- drugs are not extensively tested in children;
- many drugs are not specifically licensed for use in children and are used 'off-label';
- suitable formulations may not be available to allow precise dosing in children;
- the nature and course of illnesses and adverse drug reactions may differ between adults and children.

Prescription writing Prescriptions should be written according to the guidelines in Prescription Writing (p. 4) Inclusion of age is a legal requirement in the case of prescription-only medicines for children under 12 years of age, but it is preferable to state the age for **all** prescriptions for children.

It is particularly important to state the strengths of capsules or tablets. Although liquid preparations are particularly suitable for children, they may contain sugar which encourages dental decay. Sugar-free medicines are preferred for long-term treatment.

Many children are able to swallow tablets or capsules and may prefer a solid dose form; involving the child and parents in choosing the formulation is helpful.

When a prescription for a liquid oral preparation is written and the dose ordered is smaller than 5 mL an **oral syringe** will be supplied (for details, see p. 2). Parents should be advised not to add any medicines to the infant's feed, since the drug may interact with the milk or other liquid in it; moreover the ingested dosage may be reduced if the child does not drink all the contents.

Parents must be warned to keep **all** medicines out of reach of children, see Safety in the Home, p. 3.

Rare paediatric conditions

Information on substances such as *biotin* and *sodium benzoate* used in rare metabolic conditions is included in *BNF for Children*; further information can be obtained from:

Alder Hey Children's Hospital
Drug Information Centre
Liverpool L12 2AP
Tel: (0151) 252 5381

Great Ormond Street Hospital for Children
Pharmacy
Great Ormond St
London WC1N 3JH
Tel: (020) 7405 9200

Dosage in Children

Children's doses in the BNF are stated in the individual drug entries as far as possible, except where paediatric use is not recommended, information is not available, or there are special hazards.

Doses are generally based on body-weight (in kilograms) or the following age ranges:

first month (neonate)
up to 1 year (infant)
1–5 years
6–12 years

Unless the age is specified, the term 'child' in the BNF includes persons aged 12 years and younger.

Dose calculation Many children's doses are standardised by **weight** (and therefore require multiplying by the body-weight in kilograms to determine the child's dose); occasionally, the doses have been standardised by **body-surface area** (in m^2). These methods should be used rather than attempting to calculate a child's dose on the basis of doses used in adults.

For most drugs the adult maximum dose should not be exceeded. For example if the dose is stated as 8 mg/kg (max. 300 mg), a child weighing 10 kg should receive 80 mg but a child weighing 40 kg should receive 300 mg (rather than 320 mg).

Young children may require a higher dose per kilogram than adults because of their higher metabolic rates. Other problems need to be considered. For example, calculation by body-weight in the overweight child may result in much higher doses being administered than necessary; in such cases, dose should be calculated from an ideal weight, related to height and age (see inside back cover).

Body-surface area (BSA) estimates are more accurate for calculation of paediatric doses than body-weight since many physiological phenomena correlate better with body-surface area. Body-surface area can be estimated from weight by means of a table. For more information, refer to *BNF for Children*.

Where the dose for children is not stated, prescribers should consult *BNF for Children* or seek advice from a medicines information centre.

Dose frequency Antibacterials are generally given at regular intervals throughout the day. Some flexibility should be allowed in children to avoid waking them during the night. For example, the night-time dose may be given at the parent's bedtime.

Where new or potentially toxic drugs are used, the manufacturers' recommended doses should be carefully followed.

Prescribing in palliative care

Palliative care is the active total care of patients whose disease is not responsive to curative treatment. Control of pain, of other symptoms, and of psychological, social and spiritual problems, is paramount to provide the best quality of life for patients and their families. Careful assessment of symptoms and needs of the patient should be undertaken by a multidisciplinary team.

Specialist palliative care is available in most areas as day hospice care, home-care teams (often known as Macmillan teams), in-patient hospice care, and hospital teams. Many acute hospitals and teaching centres now have consultative, hospital-based teams.

Hospice care of terminally ill patients has shown the importance of symptom control and psychosocial support of the patient and family. Families should be included in the care of the patient if they wish.

Many patients wish to remain at home with their families. Although some families may at first be afraid of caring for the patient at home, support can be provided by community nursing services, social services, voluntary agencies and hospices together with the general practitioner. The family may be reassured by the knowledge that the patient will be admitted to a hospital or hospice if the family cannot cope.

Drug treatment The number of drugs should be as few as possible, for even the taking of medicine may be an effort. Oral medication is usually satisfactory unless there is severe nausea and vomiting, dysphagia, weakness, or coma, when parenteral medication may be necessary.

Pain

Analgesics are more effective in preventing pain than in the relief of established pain; it is important that they are given regularly.

The non-opioid analgesic **paracetamol** or an **NSAID** (section 10.1.1) given regularly will often make the use of opioids unnecessary. An NSAID may also control the pain of *bone secondaries*; if necessary, flurbiprofen or indometacin can be given rectally. Radiotherapy, bisphosphonates (section 6.6.2), and radioactive isotopes of **strontium** (*Metastron*® available from GE Healthcare) may also be useful for pain due to bone metastases.

An opioid such as **codeine**, alone or in combination with a non-opioid analgesic at adequate dosage, may be helpful in the control of moderate pain if non-opioids alone are not sufficient. Alternatively, **tramadol** can be considered for moderate pain. If these preparations do not control the pain, **morphine** is the most useful opioid analgesic. Alternatives to morphine include **hydromorphone**, **methadone**, **oxycodone**, and transdermal **fentanyl** (see below and section 4.7.2); these drugs are best initiated by those with experience in palliative care. Initiation of an opioid analgesic should not be delayed by concern over a theoretical likelihood of psychological dependence (addiction).

Equivalent single doses of opioid analgesics

These equivalences are intended **only** as an approximate guide; patients should be carefully monitored after **any** change in medication and dose titration may be required

Analgesic	Dose
Morphine salts (oral)	10 mg
Diamorphine hydrochloride (intramuscular)	3 mg
Hydromorphone hydrochloride	1.3 mg
Oxycodone (oral)	5 mg

Oral route Morphine is given *by mouth* as an oral solution or as standard ('immediate release') tablets regularly every 4 hours, the initial dose depending largely on the patient's previous treatment. A dose of 5–10 mg is enough to replace a weaker analgesic (such as paracetamol), but 10–20 mg or more is required to replace a strong one (comparable to morphine itself). If the first dose of morphine is no more effective than the previous analgesic, the next dose should be increased by 50%, the aim being to choose the lowest dose that prevents pain. The dose should be adjusted with careful assessment of the pain, and the use of adjuvant analgesics (such as NSAIDs) should also be considered. Although morphine in a dose of 5–20 mg is usually adequate there should be no hesitation in increasing it stepwise according to response to 100 mg or occasionally up to 500 mg or higher if necessary. It may be possible to omit the overnight dose if double the usual dose is given at bedtime.

If pain occurs between regular doses of morphine ('breakthrough pain'), an additional dose ('rescue dose') should be given. An additional dose should also be given 30 minutes before an activity that causes pain (e.g. wound dressing). Fentanyl lozenges are also licensed for breakthrough pain.

When the pain is controlled and the patient's 24-hour morphine requirement is established, the daily dose can be given as a *modified-release preparation* in a single dose or in two divided doses.

Preparations suitable for twice-daily administration include *Morphgesic SR*® tablets, *MST Continus*® tablets or suspension, and *Zomorph*® capsules. *MXL*® capsules allow administration of the total daily morphine requirement as a single dose.

The starting dose of modified-release morphine preparations designed for twice daily administration is usually 10–20 mg every 12 hours if no other analgesic (or only paracetamol) has been taken previously, but to replace a weaker opioid analgesic (such as co-codamol) the starting dose is usually 20–30 mg every 12 hours. Increments should be made to the dose, not to the frequency of administration, which should remain at every 12 hours.

The effective dose of modified-release preparations can alternatively be determined by giving the oral solution of morphine every 4 hours in increasing doses until the pain has been controlled, and then transferring the patient to the same total 24-hour dose of morphine given as the modified-release preparation (divided into two portions for 12-hourly administration). The first dose of the modified-release preparation is given 4 hours after the last dose of the oral solution.[1]

Morphine, as oral solution or standard formulation tablets, should be prescribed for breakthrough pain; the dose should be about one-sixth of the total daily dose of oral morphine repeated every 4 hours if necessary (review pain management if analgesic required more frequently).

Parenteral route If the patient becomes unable to swallow, the equivalent intramuscular dose of morphine is half the oral solution dose; in the case of the modified-release tablets it is half the total 24-hour dose (which is then divided into 6 portions to be given every 4 hours). **Diamorphine** is preferred for injection because, being more soluble, it can be given in a smaller volume. The equivalent intramuscular (or subcutaneous) is approximately a third of the oral dose of morphine. *Subcutaneous infusion* of diamorphine via syringe driver can be useful (for details, see p. 17).

If the patient can resume taking medicines by mouth, then oral morphine may be substituted for subcutaneous infusion of diamorphine. See table of approximate equivalent doses of morphine and diamorphine, p. 19.

Oxycodone (p. 235) is used in patients who require an opioid but cannot tolerate morphine. If the patient is already receiving an opioid, oxycodone should be started at a dose equivalent to the current analgesic (see p. 15).

Rectal route Morphine is also available for *rectal administration* as suppositories; alternatively **oxycodone** suppositories can be obtained on special order.

Transdermal route Transdermal preparations of fentanyl and buprenorphine are available (section 4.7.2); they are not suitable for acute pain or in those patients whose analgesic requirements are changing rapidly because the long time to steady state prevents rapid titration of the dose.

The following 24-hour doses of morphine are considered to be approximately equivalent to the fentanyl patches shown:

Morphine salt 45 mg daily ≡ fentanyl '12' patch
Morphine salt 90 mg daily ≡ fentanyl '25' patch
Morphine salt 180 mg daily ≡ fentanyl '50' patch
Morphine salt 270 mg daily ≡ fentanyl '75' patch
Morphine salt 360 mg daily ≡ fentanyl '100' patch

Morphine (as oral solution or standard formulation tablets) is given for breakthrough pain.

Gastro-intestinal pain The pain of *bowel colic* may be reduced by loperamide 2–4 mg 4 times daily. *Hyoscine hydrobromide* may also be helpful, given sublingually at a dose of 300 micrograms 3 times daily as *Kwells*® (Roche Consumer Health) tablets. For the dose by subcutaneous infusion using a syringe driver, see p. 18).

Gastric distension pain due to pressure on the stomach may be helped by a preparation incorporating an antacid with an antiflatulent (section 1.1.1) and by domperidone 10 mg 3 times daily before meals.

1. Studies have indicated that administration of the last dose of the *oral solution* with the first dose of the *modified-release tablets* is not necessary.

Muscle spasm The pain of muscle spasm can be helped by a muscle relaxant such as diazepam 5–10 mg daily or baclofen 5–10 mg 3 times daily.

Neuropathic pain Patients with neuropathic pain (section 4.7.3) may benefit from a trial of a tricyclic antidepressant for several weeks. An anticonvulsant may be added or substituted if pain persists; gabapentin and pregabalin (both section 4.8.1) are licensed for neuropathic pain.

Pain due to nerve compression may be reduced by a corticosteroid such as dexamethasone 8 mg daily, which reduces oedema around the tumour, thus reducing compression.

Nerve blocks can be considered when pain is localised to a specific area. **Transcutaneous electrical nerve stimulation** (TENS) may also help.

Miscellaneous conditions

Unlicensed indications or routes
Several recommendations in this section involve unlicensed indications or routes.

Raised intracranial pressure Headache due to raised intracranial pressure often responds to a high dose of a corticosteroid, such as dexamethasone 16 mg daily for 4 to 5 days, subsequently reduced to 4–6 mg daily if possible; dexamethasone should be given before 6 p.m. to reduce the risk of insomnia.

Intractable cough Intractable cough may be relieved by moist inhalations or by regular administration of oral morphine in an initial dose of 5 mg every 4 hours. Methadone linctus should be avoided because it has a long duration of action and tends to accumulate.

Dyspnoea Breathlessness at rest may be relieved by regular oral morphine in carefully titrated doses, starting at 5 mg every 4 hours. Diazepam 5–10 mg daily may be helpful for dyspnoea associated with anxiety. A corticosteroid, such as dexamethasone 4–8 mg daily, may also be helpful if there is bronchospasm or partial obstruction.

Excessive respiratory secretion Excessive respiratory secretion (death rattle) may be reduced by subcutaneous injection of hyoscine hydrobromide 400–600 micrograms every 4 to 8 hours; however, care must be taken to avoid the discomfort of dry mouth. Alternatively glycopyrronium can be given by subcutaneous or intramuscular injection in a dose of 200 micrograms every 4 hours. For the dose by subcutaneous infusion using a syringe driver, see p. 18.

Restlessness and confusion Restlessness and confusion may require treatment with haloperidol 1–3 mg by mouth every 8 hours. Levomepromazine (methotrimeprazine) is also used occasionally for restlessness. For the dose by subcutaneous infusion using a syringe driver, see p. 18.

Hiccup Hiccup due to gastric distension may be helped by a preparation incorporating an antacid with an antiflatulent (section 1.1). If this fails, metoclopramide 10 mg every 6 to 8 hours by mouth or by subcutaneous or intramuscular injection can be added; if this also fails, baclofen 5 mg twice daily, or nifedipine 10 mg three times daily, or chlorpromazine 10–25 mg every 6 to 8 hours can be tried.

Anorexia Anorexia may be helped by prednisolone 15–30 mg daily or dexamethasone 2–4 mg daily.

Constipation Constipation is a very common cause of distress and is almost invariable after administration of an opioid. It should be prevented if possible by the regular administration of laxatives; a faecal softener with a peristaltic stimulant (e.g. co-danthramer) or lactulose solution with a senna preparation should be used (section 1.6.2 and section 1.6.3).

Fungating growths Fungating growths can be treated by regular dressing and oral administration of metronidazole (section 5.1.11); topical application of metronidazole (section 13.10.1.2) is also used.

Capillary bleeding Capillary bleeding can be treated with tranexamic acid (section 2.11) by mouth; treatment is usually discontinued one week after the bleeding has stopped, or, if necessary, it can be continued at a reduced dose. Alternatively, gauze soaked in tranexamic acid 100 mg/mL or adrenaline (epinephrine) solution 1 mg/mL (1 in 1000) can be applied to the affected area.

Dry mouth Dry mouth may be relieved by good mouth care and measures such as the sucking of ice or pineapple chunks or the use of artificial saliva (section 12.3.5); dry mouth associated with candidiasis can be treated by oral preparations of nystatin or miconazole (section 12.3.2); alternatively, fluconazole can be given by mouth (section 5.2). Dry mouth may be caused by certain medications including opioids, antimuscarinic drugs (e.g. hyoscine), antidepressants and some anti-emetics; if possible, an alternative preparation should be considered.

Pruritus Pruritus, even when associated with obstructive jaundice, often responds to simple measures such as application of emollients (section 13.2.1). In the case of obstructive jaundice, further measures include administration of colestyramine (section 1.9.2).

Convulsions Patients with cerebral tumours or uraemia may be susceptible to convulsions. Prophylactic treatment with phenytoin or carbamazepine (section 4.8.1) should be considered. When oral medication is no longer possible, diazepam as suppositories 10–20 mg every 4 to 8 hours, or phenobarbital by injection 50–200 mg twice daily is continued as prophylaxis. For the use of midazolam by subcutaneous infusion using a syringe driver, see below.

Dysphagia A corticosteroid such as dexamethasone 8 mg daily may help, temporarily, if there is an obstruction due to tumour. See also under Dry Mouth.

Nausea and vomiting Nausea and vomiting are common in patients with advanced cancer. Ideally, the cause should be determined before treatment with an anti-emetic (section 4.6) is started.

Nausea and vomiting may occur with opioid therapy particularly in the initial stages but can be prevented by giving an anti-emetic such as haloperidol or metoclopramide. An anti-emetic is usually necessary only for the first 4 or 5 days and therefore combined preparations containing an opioid with an anti-emetic are not recommended because they lead to unnecessary anti-emetic therapy (and associated side-effects when used long-term).

Metoclopramide has a prokinetic action and is used in a dose of 10 mg 3 times daily by mouth for nausea and vomiting associated with gastritis, gastric stasis, and functional bowel obstruction. Drugs with antimuscarinic effects antagonise prokinetic drugs and, if possible, should not therefore be used concurrently.

Haloperidol is used by mouth in an initial dose of 1.5 mg once or twice daily (can be increased if necessary to 5–10 mg daily in divided doses) for most metabolic causes of vomiting (e.g. hypercalcaemia, renal failure).

Cyclizine is given in a dose of 50 mg up to 3 times daily by mouth. It is used for nausea and vomiting due to mechanical bowel obstruction, raised intracranial pressure, and motion sickness.

Anti-emetic therapy should be reviewed every 24 hours; it may be necessary to substitute the anti-emetic or to add another one.

Levomepromazine (methotrimeprazine) can be used if first-line anti-emetics are inadequate; it is given by mouth in a dose of 6–25 mg daily [6-mg tablets available on named-patient basis] in 1–2 divided doses. Dexamethasone 8–16 mg daily by mouth can be used as an adjunct.

For the administration of anti-emetics by subcutaneous infusion using a syringe driver, see below.

For the treatment of nausea and vomiting associated with cancer chemotherapy, see section 8.1.

Insomnia Patients with advanced cancer may not sleep because of discomfort, cramps, night sweats, joint stiffness, or fear. There should be appropriate treatment of these problems before hypnotics are used. Benzodiazepines, such as temazepam (section 4.1.1), may be useful.

Hypercalcaemia See section 9.5.1.2.

Syringe drivers

Although drugs can usually be administered *by mouth* to control the symptoms of advanced cancer, the parenteral route may sometimes be necessary. Repeated administration of *intramuscular injections* can be difficult in a cachectic patient. This has led to the use of a portable syringe driver to give a *continuous subcutaneous infusion*, which can provide good control of symptoms with little discomfort or inconvenience to the patient.

> **Syringe driver rate settings**
> Staff using syringe drivers should be **adequately trained** and different rate settings should be **clearly identified** and **differentiated**; incorrect use of syringe drivers is a common cause of drug errors.

Indications for the **parenteral route** are:

- the patient is unable to take medicines by mouth owing to *nausea and vomiting, dysphagia, severe weakness,* or *coma;*
- there is *malignant bowel obstruction* in patients for whom further surgery is inappropriate (avoiding the need for an intravenous infusion or for insertion of a nasogastric tube);
- occasionally when the patient *does not wish* to take regular medication by mouth.

Prescribing in palliative care

Nausea and vomiting Haloperidol is given in a *subcutaneous infusion dose* of 2.5–10 mg/24 hours.

Levomepromazine (methotrimeprazine) is given in a *subcutaneous infusion dose* of 5–25 mg/24 hours but sedation can limit the dose.

Cyclizine is particularly likely to precipitate if mixed with diamorphine or other drugs (see under Mixing and Compatibility, below); it is given in a *subcutaneous infusion dose* of 150 mg/24 hours.

Metoclopramide can cause skin reactions; it is given in a *subcutaneous infusion dose* of 30–100 mg/24 hours.

Octreotide (section 8.3.4.3), which stimulates water and electrolyte absorption and inhibits water secretion in the small bowel, can be used by subcutaneous infusion in a dose of 300–600 micrograms/24 hours to reduce intestinal secretions and vomiting.

Bowel colic and excessive respiratory secretions Hyoscine hydrobromide effectively reduces respiratory secretions and is sedative (but occasionally causes paradoxical agitation); it is given in a *subcutaneous infusion dose* of 0.6–2.4 mg/24 hours.

Hyoscine butylbromide is effective in bowel colic, is less sedative than hyoscine hydrobromide, but is not always adequate for the control of respiratory secretions; it is given in a *subcutaneous infusion dose* of 20–60 mg/24 hours (**important:** this dose of *hyoscine butylbromide* must not be confused with the much lower dose of *hyoscine hydrobromide*, above).

Glycopyrronium 0.6–1.2 mg/24 hours by subcutaneous infusion may also be used.

Restlessness and confusion Haloperidol has little sedative effect; it is given in a *subcutaneous infusion dose* of 5–15 mg/24 hours.

Levomepromazine (methotrimeprazine) has a sedative effect; it is given in a *subcutaneous infusion dose* of 12.5–200 mg/24 hours.

Midazolam is a sedative and an antiepileptic that may be suitable for a very restless patient; it is given in a *subcutaneous infusion dose* of 20–100 mg/24 hours.

Convulsions If a patient has previously been receiving an antiepileptic drug *or* has a primary or secondary cerebral tumour *or* is at risk of convulsion (e.g. owing to uraemia) antiepileptic medication should not be stopped. Midazolam is the benzodiazepine antiepileptic of choice for *continuous subcutaneous infusion*, and it is given initially in a dose of 20–40 mg/24 hours.

Pain control Diamorphine is the preferred opioid since its high solubility permits a large dose to be given in a small volume (see under Mixing and Compatibility, below). The table on p. 19 shows approximate equivalent doses of morphine and diamorphine.

Mixing and compatibility The general principle that injections should be given into separate sites (and should not be mixed) does not apply to the use of syringe drivers in palliative care. Provided that there is evidence of compatibility, selected injections can be mixed in syringe drivers. Not all types of medication can be used in a subcutaneous infusion. In particular, chlorpromazine, prochlorperazine, and diazepam are **contra-indicated** as they cause skin reactions at the injection site; to a lesser extent cyclizine and levomepromazine (methotrimeprazine) also sometimes cause local irritation.

In theory injections dissolved in water for injections are more likely to be associated with pain (possibly owing to their hypotonicity). The use of physiological saline (sodium chloride 0.9%) however increases the likelihood of precipitation when more than one drug is used; moreover subcutaneous infusion rates are so slow (0.1–0.3 mL/hour) that pain is not usually a problem when water is used as a diluent.

Diamorphine can be given by subcutaneous infusion in a strength of up to 250 mg/mL; up to a strength of 40 mg/mL either *water for injections* or *physiological saline* (sodium chloride 0.9%) is a suitable diluent—above that strength only *water for injections* is used (to avoid precipitation).

The following can be mixed with *diamorphine*:

Cyclizine[1]
Dexamethasone[2]
Haloperidol[3]
Hyoscine butylbromide
Hyoscine hydrobromide
Levomepromazine
Metoclopramide[4]
Midazolam

Subcutaneous infusion solution should be monitored regularly both to check for precipitation (and discoloration) and to ensure that the infusion is running at the correct rate.

Problems encountered with syringe drivers The following are problems that may be encountered with syringe drivers and the action that should be taken:

- if the subcutaneous infusion runs *too quickly* check the rate setting and the calculation;
- if the subcutaneous infusion runs *too slowly* check the start button, the battery, the syringe driver, the cannula, and make sure that the injection site is not inflamed;
- if there is an *injection site reaction* make sure that the site does not need to be changed—firmness or swelling at the site of injection is not in itself an indication for change, but pain or obvious inflammation is.

1. Cyclizine may precipitate at concentrations above 10 mg/mL *or* in the presence of sodium chloride 0.9% *or* as the concentration of diamorphine relative to cyclizine increases; mixtures of diamorphine and cyclizine are also likely to precipitate after 24 hours.
2. Special care is needed to avoid precipitation of dexamethasone when preparing it.
3. Mixtures of haloperidol and diamorphine are likely to precipitate after 24 hours if haloperidol concentration is above 2 mg/mL.
4. Under some conditions metoclopramide becomes discoloured; such solutions should be discarded.

Equivalent doses of morphine sulphate and diamorphine hydrochloride

These equivalences are *approximate only* and should be adjusted according to response

MORPHINE		PARENTERAL DIAMORPHINE	
Morphine sulphate oral solution or standard tablets	Morphine sulphate by subcutaneous infusion	Diamorphine hydrochloride by intramuscular injection	Diamorphine hydrochloride by subcutaneous infusion
every 4 hours	***every 24 hours***	***every 4 hours***	***every 24 hours***
5 mg	15 mg	1.25–2.5 mg	10 mg
10 mg	30 mg	2.5–5 mg	20 mg
15 mg	45 mg	5 mg	30 mg
20 mg	60 mg	7.5 mg	40 mg
30 mg	90 mg	10 mg	60 mg
40 mg	120 mg	12.5 mg	80 mg
60 mg	180 mg	20 mg	120 mg
80 mg	240 mg	27.5 mg	160 mg
100 mg	300 mg	35 mg	200 mg
130 mg	390 mg	42.5 mg	260 mg
160 mg	480 mg	55 mg	320 mg
200 mg	600 mg	65 mg	400 mg

If breakthrough pain occurs give a subcutaneous (preferable) or intramuscular injection equivalent to one-sixth of the total 24-hour subcutaneous infusion dose. It is kinder to give an intermittent bolus injection *subcutaneously*—absorption is smoother so that the risk of adverse effects at peak absorption is avoided (an even better method is to use a subcutaneous butterfly needle).

To minimise the risk of infection no individual subcutaneous infusion solution should be used for longer than 24 hours.

Prescribing for the elderly

Old people, especially the very old, require special care and consideration from prescribers. *Medicines for Older People*, a component document of the National Service Framework for Older People,[1] describes how to maximise the benefits of medicines and how to avoid excessive, inappropriate, or inadequate consumption of medicines by older people.

Appropriate prescribing Elderly patients often receive multiple drugs for their multiple diseases. This greatly increases the risk of drug interactions as well as adverse reactions, and may affect compliance (see Taking medicines to best effect under General guidance). The balance of benefit and harm of some medicines may be altered in the elderly. Therefore, elderly patients' medicines should be reviewed regularly and medicines which are not of benefit should be stopped.

Non-pharmacological measures may be more appropriate for symptoms such as headache, sleeplessness, and lightheadedness when associated with social stress as in widowhood, loneliness, and family dispersal.

In some cases prophylactic drugs are inappropriate if they are likely to complicate existing treatment or introduce unnecessary side-effects, especially in elderly patients with poor prognosis or with poor overall health. However, elderly patients should not be denied medicines which may help them, such as anticoagulants or antiplatelet drugs for atrial fibrillation, antihypertensives, statins, and drugs for osteoporosis.

1. Department of Health. National Service Framework for Older People. London: Department of Health, March 2001.

Form of medicine Frail elderly patients may have difficulty swallowing tablets; if left in the mouth, ulceration may develop. They should always be encouraged to take their tablets or capsules with enough fluid, and whilst in an upright position to avoid the possibility of oesophageal ulceration. It can be helpful to discuss with the patient the possibility of taking the drug as a liquid if available.

Manifestations of ageing In the very old, manifestations of normal ageing may be mistaken for disease and lead to inappropriate prescribing. In addition, age-related muscle weakness and difficulty in maintaining balance should not be confused with neurological disease. Disorders such as lightheadedness not associated with postural or postprandial hypotension are unlikely to be helped by drugs.

Sensitivity The nervous system of elderly patients is more sensitive to many commonly used drugs, such as opioid analgesics, benzodiazepines, antipsychotics, and antiparkinsonian drugs, all of which must be used with caution. Similarly, other organs may also be more susceptible to the effects of drugs such as antihypertensives and NSAIDs.

Pharmacokinetics

The most important effect of age is reduction in renal clearance. Many aged patients thus *excrete drugs slowly*, and are *highly susceptible to nephrotoxic drugs*. Acute illness can lead to rapid reduction in renal clearance, especially if accompanied by dehydration. Hence, a patient stabilised on a drug with a narrow margin between the therapeutic and the toxic dose (e.g. digoxin) can rapidly develop adverse effects in the aftermath of a myocardial infarction or a respiratory-tract infection. The metabolism of some drugs is reduced in the elderly.

Pharmacokinetic changes can markedly increase the tissue concentration of a drug in the elderly, especially in debilitated patients.

Adverse reactions

Adverse reactions often present in the elderly in a vague and non-specific fashion. *Confusion* is often the presenting symptom (caused by almost any of the commonly used drugs). Other common manifestations are *constipation* (with antimuscarinics and many tranquillisers) and postural *hypotension* and *falls* (with diuretics and many psychotropics).

Hypnotics Many hypnotics with long half-lives have serious hangover effects including drowsiness, unsteady gait, slurred speech, and confusion. Hypnotics with short half-lives should be used but they too can present problems (section 4.1.1). Short courses of hypnotics are occasionally useful for helping a patient through an acute illness or some other crisis but every effort must be made to avoid dependence. Benzodiazepines impair balance, which may result in falls.

Diuretics Diuretics are overprescribed in old age and should **not** be used on a long-term basis to treat simple gravitational oedema which will usually respond to increased movement, raising the legs, and support stockings. A few days of diuretic treatment may speed the clearing of the oedema but it should rarely need continued drug therapy.

NSAIDs Bleeding associated with aspirin and other NSAIDs is more common in the elderly who are more likely to have a fatal or serious outcome. NSAIDs are also a special hazard in patients with cardiac disease or renal impairment which may again place older patients at particular risk.

Owing to the *increased susceptibility of the elderly* to the *side-effects of NSAIDs* the following recommendations are made:

- for *osteoarthritis, soft-tissue lesions,* and *back pain*, first try measures such as weight reduction (if obese), warmth, exercise, and use of a walking stick;
- for *osteoarthritis, soft-tissue lesions, back pain,* and *pain in rheumatoid arthritis,* paracetamol should be used first and can often provide adequate pain relief;
- alternatively, a low-dose NSAID (e.g. ibuprofen up to 1.2 g daily) may be given;
- for pain relief when either drug is inadequate, paracetamol in a full dose plus a low-dose NSAID may be given;
- if necessary, the NSAID dose can be increased or an opioid analgesic given with paracetamol;
- do not give two NSAIDs at the same time.

For advice on prophylaxis of NSAID-induced peptic ulcers if continued NSAID treatment is necessary, see section 1.3.

Other drugs Other drugs which commonly cause adverse reactions are *antiparkinsonian drugs, antihypertensives, psychotropics*, and *digoxin*. The usual maintenance dose of digoxin in very old patients is 125 micrograms daily (62.5 micrograms in those with renal disease); lower doses are often inadequate but toxicity is common in those given 250 micrograms daily.

Drug-induced blood disorders are much more common in the elderly. Therefore drugs with a tendency to cause bone marrow depression (e.g. *co-trimoxazole, mianserin*) should be avoided unless there is no acceptable alternative.

The elderly generally require a lower maintenance dose of *warfarin* than younger adults; once again, the outcome of bleeding tends to be more serious.

Guidelines

Always consider whether a drug is indicated at all.

Limit range It is a sensible policy to prescribe from a limited range of drugs and to be thoroughly familiar with their effects in the elderly.

Reduce dose Dosage should generally be substantially lower than for younger patients and it is common to start with about 50% of the adult dose. Some drugs (e.g. long-acting antidiabetic drugs such as glibenclamide and chlorpropamide) should be avoided altogether.

Review regularly Review repeat prescriptions regularly. In many patients it may be possible to stop some drugs, provided that clinical progress is monitored. It may be necessary to reduce the dose of some drugs as renal function declines.

Simplify regimens Elderly patients benefit from simple treatment regimens. Only drugs with a clear indication should be prescribed and whenever possible given once or twice daily. In particular, regimens which call for a confusing array of dosage intervals should be avoided.

Explain clearly Write full instructions on every prescription (*including* repeat prescriptions) so that containers can be properly labelled with full directions. Avoid imprecisions like 'as directed'. Child-resistant containers may be unsuitable.

Repeats and disposal Instruct patients what to do when drugs run out, and also how to dispose of any that are no longer necessary. Try to prescribe matching quantities.

If these guidelines are followed most elderly people will cope adequately with their own medicines. If not then it is essential to enrol the help of a third party, usually a relative or a friend.

Prescribing in dental practice

The following is a list of topics of particular relevance to dental surgeons.

> Advice on the drug management of dental and oral conditions has been integrated into the BNF. For ease of access, guidance on such conditions is usually identified by means of a relevant heading (e.g. Dental and Orofacial Pain) in the appropriate sections of the BNF.

General guidance
- Prescribing by dental surgeons, p. 4
- Oral side-effects of drugs, p. 12
- Medical emergencies in dental practice, below
- Medical problems in dental practice, p. 23

Drug management of dental and oral conditions
- **Dental and orofacial pain,** p. 224
  - Neuropathic pain, p. 23[illegible]
  - Non-opioid analgesics, p. 225
  - Opioid analgesics, p. 230
  - Non-steroidal anti-inflammatory drugs, p. 536
- **Oral infections**
  - Bacterial infections, p. 278
    - Phenoxymethylpenicillin, p. 285
    - Broad-spectrum penicillins (amoxicillin and ampicillin), p. 287
    - Cephalosporins (cefalexin and cefradine), p. 291
    - Tetracyclines, p. 297
    - Macrolides (erythromycin and azithromycin) , p. 301
    - Clindamycin, p. 303
    - Metronidazole, p. 315
    - Fusidic acid p. 629
  - Fungal infections, p. 592
    - Local treatment, p. 592
    - Systemic treatment, p. 321
  - Viral infections
    - Herpetic gingivostomatitis, local treatment, p. 593
    - Herpetic gingivostomatitis, systemic treatment, p. 335 and p. 593
    - Herpes labialis, p. 633
- **Anaesthetics, anxiolytics and hypnotics**
  - Anaesthesia, sedation, and resuscitation in dental practice, p. 666
  - Hypnotics, p. 180
  - Peri-operative anxiolytics, p. 672
  - Local anaesthesia, p. 681
- **Oral ulceration and inflammation,** p. 590
- **Mouthwashes, gargles and dentifrices,** p. 594
- **Dry mouth,** p. 595
- **Vitamins and minerals**
  - Fluorides, p. 521
  - Oral vitamin B complex preparations, p. 522 and p. 524
  - Ascorbic acid (vitamin C), p. 524
- **Antihistamines,** p. 166
- **Aromatic inhalations,** p. 176
- **Nasal decongestants,** p. 568

Dental Practitioners' Formulary, p. 882

Changes to Dental Practitioners' Formulary, p. 883

Medical emergencies in dental practice

This section provides guidelines on the management of the more common medical emergencies which may arise in dental practice. Dental surgeons and their staff should be familiar with standard resuscitation procedures, but in all circumstances it is advisable to summon medical assistance as soon as possible. For an **algorithm** of the procedure for **cardiopulmonary resuscitation,** see inside back cover.

> **The drugs referred to in this section include:**
> Adrenaline Injection (Epinephrine Injection), adrenaline 1 in 1000, (adrenaline 1 mg/mL as acid tartrate), 1-mL amps
> Aspirin Dispersible Tablets 300 mg
> Glucagon Injection, glucagon (as hydrochloride), 1-unit vial (with solvent)
> Glucose (for administration by mouth)
> Glyceryl Trinitrate Spray
> Midazolam Buccal Liquid, midazolam 10 mg/mL *or* Midazolam Injection, midazolam (as hydrochloride) 2 mg/mL, 5-mL amps, or 5 mg/mL, 2-mL amps
> Oxygen
> Salbutamol Aerosol Inhalation, salbutamol 100 micrograms/metered inhalation

Adrenal insufficiency

Adrenal insufficiency may follow prolonged therapy with corticosteroids and can persist for years after stopping. A patient with adrenal insufficiency may become hypotensive under the stress of a dental visit (important: see also p. 380 for details of corticosteroid cover before dental surgical procedures under general anaesthesia).

Management

- Lay the patient flat
- Give oxygen
- Transfer patient urgently to hospital

Anaphylaxis

A severe allergic reaction may follow oral or parenteral administration of a drug. Anaphylactic reactions in dentistry may follow the administration of a drug or contact with substances such as latex in surgical gloves. In general, the more rapid the onset of the reaction the more profound it tends to be. Symptoms may develop within minutes and rapid treatment is essential.

Anaphylactic reactions may also be associated with *additives* and *excipients* in foods and medicines (see Excipients, p. 2). Refined arachis (peanut) oil, which may be present in some medicinal products, is unlikely to cause an allergic reaction—nevertheless it is wise to check the full formula of preparations which may contain allergenic fats or oils (including those for topical application, particularly if they are intended for use in the mouth or for application to the nasal mucosa).

Prescribing in dental practice

Symptoms and signs

- Paraesthesia, flushing, and swelling of face
- Generalised itching, especially of hands and feet
- Bronchospasm and laryngospasm (with wheezing and difficulty in breathing)
- Rapid weak pulse together with fall in blood pressure and pallor; finally cardiac arrest

Management

First-line treatment includes securing the airway, restoration of blood pressure (laying the patient flat and raising the feet, or in the recovery position if unconscious or nauseous and at risk of vomiting), and administration of **adrenaline** (epinephrine) injection. This is given **intramuscularly** in a dose of 500 micrograms (0.5 mL adrenaline injection 1 in 1000); a preparation delivering a dose of 300 micrograms (0.3 mL adrenaline injection 1 in 1000) is available for immediate *self-administration*. The dose is repeated if necessary at 5-minute intervals according to blood pressure, pulse, and respiratory function. **Oxygen** administration is also of primary importance. Arrangements should be made to transfer the patient to hospital urgently.

For further details on the management of anaphylaxis including details of paediatric doses of adrenaline, see p. 170

Asthma

Patients with asthma may have an attack while at the dental surgery. Most attacks will respond to 2 puffs of the patient's short-acting $beta_2$-adrenoceptor stimulant inhaler such as **salbutamol** 100 micrograms/puff (or **terbutaline** 250 micrograms/puff); further puffs are required if the patient does not respond rapidly. If the patient is unable to use the inhaler effectively, further puffs should be given through a large-volume spacer device (or, if not available, through a plastic or paper cup with a hole in the bottom for the inhaler mouthpiece). If the response remains unsatisfactory, or if further deterioration occurs, then the patient should be transferred urgently to hospital. Whilst awaiting transfer, **oxygen** should be given with salbutamol 2.5–5 mg by nebuliser. If a nebuliser is unavailable, then 4–6 puffs of salbutamol inhaler or terbutaline inhaler should be given (preferably by a large-volume spacer device), and repeated every 10 minutes if necessary. If asthma is part of a more generalised anaphylactic reaction, an intramuscular injection of **adrenaline** (as detailed under Anaphylaxis above) should be given.

For a table describing the management of Acute Severe Asthma, see p. 147

Patients with severe chronic asthma or whose asthma has deteriorated previously during a dental procedure may require an increase in their prophylactic medication before a dental procedure. This should be discussed with the patient's medical practitioner and may include increasing the dose of inhaled or oral corticosteroid.

Cardiac emergencies

If there is a history of *angina* the patient will probably carry **glyceryl trinitrate** spray or tablets (or isosorbide dinitrate tablets) and should be allowed to use them. Hospital admission is not necessary if symptoms are mild and resolve rapidly with the patient's own medication. See also Coronary Artery Disease on p. 24.

Arrhythmias may lead to a sudden reduction in cardiac output with loss of consciousness. Medical assistance should be summoned. For advice on pacemaker interference, see also Pacemakers, p. 24.

The pain of *myocardial infarction* is similar to that of angina but generally more severe and more prolonged. For general advice see also Coronary Artery Disease on p. 24

Symptoms and signs of myocardial infarction

- Progressive onset of severe, crushing pain across front of chest; pain may radiate towards the shoulder and down arm, or into neck and jaw
- Skin becomes pale and clammy
- Nausea and vomiting are common
- Pulse may be weak and blood pressure may fall
- Breathlessness

Initial management of myocardial infarction

Call immediately for medical assistance and an ambulance, as appropriate.

Allow the patient to rest in the position that feels most comfortable; in the presence of breathlessness this is likely to be sitting position, whereas the syncopal patient should be laid flat; often an intermediate position (dictated by the patient) will be most appropriate. Oxygen may be administered.

Sublingual glyceryl trinitrate may relieve pain. Intramuscular injection of drugs should be avoided because absorption may be too slow (particularly when cardiac output is reduced) and pain relief is inadequate. Intramuscular injection also increases the risk of local bleeding into the muscle if the patient is given a thrombolytic drug.

Reassure the patient as much as possible to relieve further anxiety. If available, aspirin in a single dose of 300 mg should be given. A note (to say that aspirin has been given) should be sent with the patient to the hospital. For further details on the initial management of myocardial infarction, see p. 132.

If the patient collapses and loses consciousness attempt standard resuscitation measures. For an **algorithm** of the procedure for **cardiopulmonary resuscitation**, see inside back cover.

Epileptic seizures

Patients with epilepsy must continue with their normal dosage of anticonvulsant drugs when attending for dental treatment. It is not uncommon for epileptic patients not to volunteer the information that they are epileptic but there should be little difficulty in recognising a tonic-clonic (grand mal) seizure.

Symptoms and signs

- There may be a brief warning (but variable)
- Sudden loss of consciousness, the patient becomes rigid, falls, may give a cry, and becomes cyanotic (tonic phase)
- After 30 seconds, there are jerking movements of the limbs; the tongue may be bitten (clonic phase)
- There may be frothing from mouth and urinary incontinence
- The seizure typically lasts a few minutes; the patient may then become flaccid but remain unconscious. After a variable time the patient regains consciousness but may remain confused for a while

Management

During a convulsion try to ensure that the patient is not at risk from injury but make no attempt to put anything in the mouth or between the teeth (in mistaken belief that this will protect the tongue). Give oxygen to support respiration if necessary.

Do not attempt to restrain convulsive movements.

After convulsive movements have subsided place the patient in the coma (recovery) position and check the airway.

After the convulsion the patient may be confused ('post-ictal confusion') and may need reassurance and sympathy. The patient should not be sent home until fully recovered. Seek medical attention or transfer the patient to hospital if it was the first episode of epilepsy, or if the convulsion was atypical, prolonged (or repeated), or if injury occurred.

Medication should only be given if convulsive seizures are prolonged (convulsive movements lasting 5 minutes or longer) or repeated rapidly.

Either **midazolam** buccal liquid or midazolam injection solution can be given by the buccal route [unlicensed use] in a single dose of 10 mg. For further details on the management of status epilepticus, including details of paediatric doses of midazolam, see p. 257.

Partial seizures similarly need very little active management (in an automatism only a minimum amount of restraint should be applied to prevent injury). Again, the patient should be observed until post-ictal confusion has completely resolved.

Hypoglycaemia

Insulin-treated diabetic patients attending for dental treatment under local anaesthesia should inject insulin and eat meals as normal. If food is omitted the blood glucose will fall to an abnormally low level (hypoglycaemia). Patients can often recognise the symptoms themselves and this state responds to sugar in water or a few lumps of sugar. Children may not have such prominent changes but may appear unduly lethargic.

Symptoms and signs

- Shaking and trembling
- Sweating
- 'Pins and needles' in lips and tongue
- Hunger
- Palpitation
- Headache (occasionally)
- Double vision
- Difficulty in concentration
- Slurring of speech
- Confusion
- Change of behaviour; truculence
- Convulsions
- Unconsciousness

Management

Initially glucose 10–20 g is given by mouth either in liquid form or as granulated sugar or sugar lumps. Glucose 10 g is available from 2 teaspoons sugar, 3 sugar lumps, *GlucoGel*® (formerly known as *Hypostop*® *Gel*; glucose 10 g/25 g tube, available from BBI Healthcare), and non-diet versions of *Lucozade*® *Energy Original* 55 mL, *Coca-Cola*® 90 mL, *Ribena*® *Original* 15 mL (to be diluted). If necessary this may be repeated in 10–15 minutes.

If glucose cannot be given by mouth, if it is ineffective, or if the hypoglycaemia causes unconsciousness, **glucagon** 1 mg (1 unit) should be given by intramuscular (or subcutaneous) injection; a child under 8 years or of body-weight under 25 kg should be given 500 micrograms. Once the patient regains consciousness oral glucose should be administered as above. If glucagon is ineffective or contra-indicated, the patient should be transferred urgently to hospital. The patient must also be admitted to hospital if hypoglycaemia is caused by an oral antidiabetic drug.

Syncope

Insufficient blood supply to the brain results in loss of consciousness. The commonest cause is a vasovagal attack or simple faint (syncope) due to emotional stress.

Symptoms and signs

- Patient feels faint
- Low blood pressure
- Pallor and sweating
- Yawning and slow pulse
- Nausea and vomiting
- Dilated pupils
- Muscular twitching

Management

- Lay the patient as flat as is reasonably comfortable and, in the absence of associated breathlessness, raise the legs to improve cerebral circulation
- Loosen any tight clothing around the neck
- Once consciousness is regained, give sugar in water or a cup of sweet tea

Other possible causes

Postural hypotension can be a consequence of rising abruptly or of standing upright for too long; antihypertensive drugs predispose to this. When rising, susceptible patients should take their time. Management is as for a vasovagal attack.

Under stressful circumstances, some patients hyperventilate. This gives rise to feelings of faintness but does not usually result in syncope. In most cases reassurance is all that is necessary; rebreathing from cupped hands or a bag may be helpful but calls for careful supervision.

Adrenal insufficiency or arrhythmias are other possible causes of syncope, see p. 21 and p. 24.

Medical problems in dental practice

Individuals presenting at the dental surgery may also suffer from an unrelated medical condition; this may require modification to the management of their dental condition. If the patient has systemic disease or is taking other medication, the matter may need to be discussed with the patient's general practitioner or hospital consultant.

For advice on adrenal insufficiency, anaphylaxis, asthma, cardiac emergencies, epileptic seizures, hypoglycaemia and syncope see under Medical Emergencies in Dental Practice.

Allergy

Patients should be asked about any history of allergy; those with a history of atopic allergy (asthma, eczema, hay fever, etc.) are at special risk. Those with a history of a severe allergy or of anaphylactic reactions are at high risk—it is essential to confirm that they are not allergic to any medication, or to any dental materials or equipment (including latex gloves). See also Anaphylaxis on p. 21.

Arrhythmias

Patients, especially those who suffer from heart failure or who have sustained a myocardial infarction, may have irregular cardiac rhythm. Atrial fibrillation is a common arrhythmia even in patients with normal hearts and is of little concern except that dental surgeons should be aware that such patients may be receiving anticoagulant therapy. The patient's medical practitioner should be asked whether any special precautions are necessary. Premedication (e.g. with temazepam) may be useful in some instances for very anxious patients.

See also Cardiac emergencies, p. 22 and Dental Anaesthesia, p. 681.

Cardiac prostheses

For an account of the risk of infective endocarditis in patients with prosthetic heart valves, see Infective Endocarditis, below. For advice on patients receiving anticoagulants, see Thromboembolic disease, below.

Coronary artery disease

Patients are vulnerable for at least 4 weeks following a myocardial infarction or following any sudden increase in the symptoms of angina. It would be advisable to check with the patient's medical practitioner before commencing treatment. See also Cardiac Emergencies on p. 22.

Treatment with low-dose aspirin (75 mg daily), clopidogrel, or dipyridamole should not be stopped routinely nor should the dose be altered before dental procedures.

A Working Party of the British Society for Antimicrobial Chemotherapy has not recommended antibiotic prophylaxis for patients following coronary artery bypass surgery.

Cyanotic heart disease

Patients with cyanotic heart disease are at risk in the dental chair, particularly if they have pulmonary hypertension. In such patients a syncopal reaction increases the shunt away from the lungs, causing more hypoxia which worsens the syncopal reaction—a vicious circle that may prove fatal. The advice of the cardiologist should be sought on any patient with congenital cyanotic heart disease. Treatment in hospital is more appropriate for some patients with this condition.

Hypertension

Patients with hypertension are likely to be receiving antihypertensive drugs such as those described in section 2.5. Their blood pressure may fall dangerously low under general anaesthesia, see also under Dental Anaesthesia on p. 681.

Immunosuppression and indwelling intraperitoneal catheters

See Table 2, section 5.1

Infective endocarditis

While almost any dental procedure can cause bacteraemia, there is no clear association with the development of infective endocarditis. Routine daily activities such as tooth brushing also produce a bacteraemia and may present a greater risk of infective endocarditis than a single dental procedure.

Antibacterial prophylaxis and chlorhexidine mouthwash are **not** recommended for the prevention of endocarditis in patients undergoing dental procedures. Such prophylaxis may expose patients to the adverse effects of antimicrobials when the evidence of benefit has not been proven.

Reduction of oral bacteraemia Patients at risk of endocarditis[1] should be advised to maintain the highest possible standards of oral hygiene in order to reduce the:

- need for dental extractions or other surgery;
- chances of severe bacteraemia if dental surgery is needed;
- possibility of 'spontaneous' bacteraemia.

Postoperative care Patients at risk of endocarditis[1] should be warned to report to the doctor or dental surgeon any unexplained illness that develops after dental treatment. Any infection in patients at risk of endocarditis[1] should be investigated promptly and treated appropriately to reduce the risk of endocarditis.

Patients on anticoagulant therapy For general advice on dental surgery in patients receiving oral anticoagulant therapy see Thromboembolic Disease, below.

Joint prostheses

See Table 2, section 5.1

Liver disease

Liver disease may alter the response to drugs and drug prescribing should be kept to a minimum in patients with severe liver disease. Problems are likely mainly in patients with *jaundice*, *ascites*, or evidence of *encephalopathy*.

For a table of drugs to be avoided or used with caution in liver disease see Appendix 2.

Pacemakers

Pacemakers prevent asystole or severe bradycardia. Some ultrasonic scalers, electronic apex locators, electro-analgesic devices, and electrocautery devices interfere with the normal function of pacemakers (including shielded pacemakers) and should not be used. The manufacturer's literature should be consulted whenever

1. Patients at risk of endocarditis include those with valve replacement, acquired valvular heart disease with stenosis or regurgitation, structural congenital heart disease (including surgically corrected or palliated structural conditions, but excluding isolated atrial septal defect, fully repaired ventricular septal defect, fully repaired patent ductus arteriosus, and closure devices considered to be endothelialised), hypertrophic cardiomyopathy, or a previous episode of infective endocarditis.

possible. If severe bradycardia occurs in a patient fitted with a pacemaker, electrical equipment should be switched off and the patient placed supine with the legs elevated. If the patient loses consciousness and the pulse remains slow or is absent, cardiopulmonary resuscitation (see inside back cover) may be needed. Call immediately for medical assistance and an ambulance, as appropriate.

A Working Party of the British Society for Antimicrobial Chemotherapy does not recommend antibacterial prophylaxis for patients with pacemakers.

Pregnancy

Drugs taken during pregnancy can be harmful to the fetus and should be prescribed only if the expected benefit to the mother is thought to be greater than the risk to the fetus; all drugs should be avoided if possible during the first trimester.

Appendix 4 includes information on drug treatment during pregnancy.

Breast-feeding

Some drugs taken by the mother whilst breast-feeding can be transferred to the breast milk, and may affect the infant.

Appendix 5 includes information on drug treatment during breast-feeding.

Renal impairment

The use of drugs in patients with reduced renal function can give rise to many problems. Many of these problems can be avoided by reducing the dose or by using alternative drugs.

Special care is required in renal transplantation and immunosuppressed patients; if necessary such patients should be referred to specialists.

For a table of drugs to be avoided or used with caution in renal impairment see Appendix 3.

Thromboembolic disease

Patients receiving **heparin** or oral anticoagulants such as **warfarin**, **acenocoumarol** (nicoumalone), or **phenindione** may be liable to excessive bleeding after extraction of teeth or other dental surgery. Often dental surgery can be delayed until the anticoagulant therapy has been completed.

For a patient requiring long-term oral anticoagulant therapy, the patient's medical practitioner should be consulted and the International Normalised Ratio (INR) should be assessed 72 hours before the dental procedure. This allows sufficient time for dose modification if necessary. In those with an unstable INR (including those who require weekly monitoring of their INR, or those who have had some INR measurements greater than 4.0 in the last 2 months), the INR should be assessed within 24 hours of the dental procedure. Patients requiring minor dental procedures (including extractions) who have an INR below 4.0 may continue warfarin without dose adjustment. There is no need to check the INR for a patient requiring a non-invasive dental procedure.

If possible, a single extraction should be done first; if this goes well further teeth may be extracted at subsequent visits (two or three at a time). Measures should be taken to minimise bleeding during and after the procedure. This includes the use of sutures and a haemostatic such as oxidised cellulose, collagen sponge or resorbable gelatin sponge. Scaling and root planing should initially be restricted to a limited area to assess the potential for bleeding.

For a patient on long-term anticoagulation treatment, the advice of the clinician responsible for the patient's anticoagulation should be sought if:

- the INR is unstable, or if the INR is greater than 4.0;
- the patient has thrombocytopenia, haemophilia, or other disorders of haemostasis, or suffers from liver impairment, alcoholism, or renal failure;
- the patient is receiving antiplatelet drugs, cytotoxic drugs or radiotherapy.

Intramuscular injections are *contra-indicated* in patients on anticoagulant therapy, and in those with any disorder of haemostasis.

A local anaesthetic containing a vasoconstrictor should be given by infiltration or by intraligamentary injection if possible. If regional nerve blocks cannot be avoided the local anaesthetic should be given cautiously using an aspirating syringe.

Drugs which have potentially serious interactions with anticoagulants include aspirin and other NSAIDs, carbamazepine, imidazole and triazole antifungals (including miconazole), erythromycin, clarithromycin, and metronidazole; for details of these and other interactions with anticoagulants, see Appendix 1 (heparin, phenindione, and coumarins). Although studies have failed to demonstrate an interaction, common experience in anticoagulant clinics is that the INR can be altered following a course of an oral broad-spectrum antibiotic, such as ampicillin or amoxicillin.

Drugs and sport

UK Sport advises that athletes are personally responsible should a prohibited substance be detected in their body. Information and advice, including the status of specific drugs in sport, can be obtained from UK Sport's Drug Information Database at www.didglobal.com. An advice card listing examples of permitted and prohibited substances is available from:

Drug-Free Sport
UK Sport
40 Bernard Street
London WC1N 1ST
Tel: 0800 528 0004
drug-free@uksport.gov.uk
www.uksport.gov.uk

A similar card detailing classes of drugs and doping methods prohibited in football is available from the Football Association.

General Medical Council's advice

Doctors who prescribe or collude in the provision of drugs or treatment with the intention of improperly enhancing an individual's performance in sport contravene the GMC's guidance, and such actions would usually raise a question of a doctor's continued registration. This does not preclude the provision of any care or treatment where the doctor's intention is to protect or improve the patient's health.

Emergency treatment of poisoning

These notes provide only an overview of the treatment of poisoning, and it is strongly recommended that either **TOXBASE** or the **UK National Poisons Information Service** (see below) be consulted when there is doubt about the degree of risk or about management.

Hospital admission Patients who have features of poisoning should generally be admitted to hospital. Patients who have taken poisons with delayed action should also be admitted, even if they appear well. Delayed-action poisons include aspirin, iron, paracetamol, tricyclic antidepressants, co-phenotrope (diphenoxylate with atropine, *Lomotil*®), and paraquat; the effects of modified-release preparations are also delayed. A note of all relevant information, including what treatment has been given, should accompany the patient to hospital.

Further information and advice

TOXBASE, the primary clinical toxicology database of the National Poisons Information Service, is available on the internet to registered users at www.toxbase.org. It provides information about routine diagnosis, treatment, and management of patients exposed to drugs, household products, and industrial and agricultural chemicals.

> Specialist information and advice on the treatment of poisoning is available day and night from the **UK National Poisons Information Service** on the following number:
> Tel: 0844 892 0111

Advice on laboratory analytical services can be obtained from TOXBASE or from the National Poisons Information Service.

Help with identifying capsules or tablets may be available from a regional medicines information centre (see inside front cover).

General care

It is often impossible to establish with certainty the identity of the poison and the size of the dose. Fortunately this is not usually important because only a few poisons (such as opioids, paracetamol, and iron) have specific antidotes; few patients require active removal of the poison. In most patients, treatment is directed at managing symptoms as they arise. Nevertheless, knowledge of the type and timing of poisoning can help in anticipating the course of events. All relevant information should be sought from the poisoned individual and from carers or parents. However, such information should be interpreted with care because it may not be complete or entirely reliable. Sometimes symptoms arise from other illnesses and patients should be assessed carefully. Accidents may involve domestic and industrial products (the contents of which are not generally known). The **National Poisons Information Service** should be consulted when there is doubt about any aspect of suspected poisoning.

Respiration

Respiration is often impaired in unconscious patients. An obstructed airway requires immediate attention. In the absence of trauma, the airway should be opened with simple measures such as chin lift or jaw thrust. An oropharyngeal or nasopharyngeal airway may be useful in patients with reduced consciousness to prevent obstruction, provided ventilation is adequate. Intubation and ventilation should be considered in patients whose airway cannot be protected or who have respiratory acidosis because of inadequate ventilation; such patients should be monitored in a critical care area.

Most poisons that impair consciousness also depress respiration. Assisted ventilation (either mouth-to-mouth or using a bag-valve-mask device) may be needed. Oxygen is not a substitute for adequate ventilation, although it should be given in the highest concentration possible in poisoning with carbon monoxide and irritant gases.

Respiratory stimulants do not help and should be **avoided**.

Blood pressure

Hypotension is common in severe poisoning with central nervous system depressants. A systolic blood pressure of less than 70 mmHg may lead to irreversible brain damage or renal tubular necrosis. Hypotension should be corrected initially by tilting down the head of the bed and administration of either sodium chloride intravenous infusion or a colloidal infusion. Vasoconstrictor sympathomimetics (section 2.7.2) are rarely required and their use may be discussed with the National Poisons Information Service.

Fluid depletion without hypotension is common after prolonged coma and after aspirin poisoning due to vomiting, sweating, and hyperpnoea.

Hypertension, often transient, occurs less frequently than hypotension in poisoning; it may be associated with sympathomimetic drugs such as amphetamines, phencyclidine, and cocaine.

Heart

Cardiac conduction defects and arrhythmias can occur in acute poisoning, notably with tricyclic antidepressants, some antipsychotics, and some antihistamines. Arrhythmias often respond to correction of underlying hypoxia, acidosis, or other biochemical abnormalities. Ventricular arrhythmias that cause serious hypotension require treatment. If the QT interval is prolonged, specialist advice should be sought because the use of some anti-arrhythmic drugs may be inappropriate. Supraventricular arrhythmias are seldom life-threatening and drug treatment is best withheld until the patient reaches hospital.

Body temperature

Hypothermia may develop in patients of any age who have been deeply unconscious for some hours, particularly following overdose with barbiturates or phenothiazines. It may be missed unless core temperature is measured using a low-reading rectal thermometer or by some other means. Hypothermia is best treated by wrapping the patient (e.g. in a 'space blanket') to conserve body heat.

Hyperthermia can develop in patients taking CNS stimulants; children and the elderly are also at risk when taking therapeutic doses of drugs with antimuscarinic properties. Hyperthermia is initially managed by removing all unnecessary clothing and using a fan. Sponging with tepid water will promote evaporation; iced water should **not** be used. Advice should be sought from the National Poisons Information Service on the management of severe hyperthermia resulting from conditions such as the serotonin syndrome.

Both hypothermia and hyperthermia require **urgent** hospitalisation for assessment and supportive treatment.

Convulsions

Single short-lived convulsions do not require treatment. If convulsions are protracted or recur frequently, lorazepam 4 mg or diazepam (preferably as emulsion) 10 mg should be given by slow intravenous injection into a large vein (section 4.8.2). Benzodiazepines should not be given by the intramuscular route for convulsions. If the intravenous route is not readily available, diazepam can be administered as a rectal solution or midazolam [unlicensed use] can be given by the buccal route (section 4.8.2).

Removal and elimination

Removal from the gastro-intestinal tract

Gastric lavage is rarely required; for substances that cannot be removed effectively by other means (e.g. iron), it should be considered only if a life-threatening amount has been ingested within the previous hour. It should be carried out only if the airway can be protected adequately. Gastric lavage is contra-indicated if a corrosive substance or a petroleum distillate has been ingested, but it may occasionally be considered in patients who have ingested drugs that are not adsorbed by charcoal, such as iron or lithium. Induction of *emesis* (e.g. with ipecacuanha) is **not** recommended because there is no evidence that it affects absorption and it may increase the risk of aspiration.

Whole bowel irrigation (by means of a bowel cleansing solution) has been used in poisoning with certain modified-release or enteric-coated formulations, in severe poisoning with iron and lithium salts, and if illicit drugs are carried in the gastro-intestinal tract ('body-packing'). However, it is not clear that the procedure improves outcome and advice should be sought from the National Poisons Information Service.

Prevention of absorption

Given by mouth, **activated charcoal** can bind many poisons in the gastro-intestinal system, thereby *reducing their absorption*. The **sooner** it is given the **more effective** it is, but it may still be effective up to 1 hour after ingestion of the poison—longer in the case of modified-release preparations or of drugs with antimuscarinic (anticholinergic) properties. It is relatively safe and is particularly useful for the prevention of absorption of poisons that are toxic in small amounts, e.g. antidepressants.

For the use of charcoal in active elimination techniques, see below.

CHARCOAL, ACTIVATED

Indications adsorption of poisons in the gastro-intestinal system; see also active elimination techniques, below

Cautions drowsy or comatose patient (risk of aspiration); reduced gastro-intestinal motility (risk of obstruction); **not** for poisoning with petroleum distillates, corrosive substances, alcohols, clofenotane (dicophane, DDT), malathion, and metal salts including iron and lithium salts

Side-effects black stools

Dose

- See under preparations below

Actidose-Aqua® Advance (Cambridge)

Oral suspension, activated charcoal, net price 50-g pack (240 mL) = £8.69

Note The brand name *Actidose-Aqua®* was formerly used

Dose reduction of absorption, 50–100 g; INFANT under 1 year 1 g/kg (approx. 5 mL/kg), CHILD 1–12 years 25–50 g

Active elimination (see below for ADULT dose); INFANT under 1 year, 1 g/kg (approx. 5 mL/kg) every 4–6 hours; CHILD 1–12 years, 25–50 g every 4–6 hours

Carbomix® (Beacon)

Powder, activated charcoal, net price 25-g pack = £8.50, 50-g pack = £11.90

Dose reduction of absorption, 50 g, repeated if necessary; CHILD under 12 years 25 g (50 g in severe poisoning)

Active elimination, see below

Charcodote® (PLIVA)

Oral suspension, activated charcoal, net price 50-g pack = £11.88

Dose reduction of absorption, 50 g; CHILD under 12 years 25 g (50 g in severe poisoning)

Active elimination, see below

Active elimination techniques

Repeated doses of **activated charcoal** by mouth *enhance the elimination* of some drugs after they have been absorbed; repeated doses are given after overdosage with:

Carbamazepine	Quinine
Dapsone	Theophylline
Phenobarbital	

The usual adult dose of activated charcoal is 50 g initially then 50 g every 4 hours. Vomiting should be treated (e.g. with an anti-emetic drug) since it may reduce the efficacy of charcoal treatment. In cases of intolerance, the dose may be reduced and the frequency increased (e.g. 25 g every 2 hours *or* 12.5 g every hour) but this may compromise efficacy.

Other techniques intended to enhance the elimination of poisons after absorption are only practicable in hospital and are only suitable for a small number of severely poisoned patients. Moreover, they only apply to a limited number of poisons. Examples include:

- haemodialysis for salicylates, phenobarbital, methyl alcohol (methanol), ethylene glycol, and lithium,
- alkalinisation of the urine for salicylates and phenoxyacetate herbicides (e.g. 2,4-dichloro-phenoxyacetic acid).

Forced diuresis is potentially harmful and no longer recommended.

Specific drugs

Alcohol

Acute intoxication with alcohol (ethanol) is common in adults but also occurs in children. The features include ataxia, dysarthria, nystagmus, and drowsiness, which may progress to coma, with hypotension and acidosis. Aspiration of vomit is a special hazard and hypoglycaemia may occur in children and some adults. Patients are managed supportively, with particular attention to maintaining a clear airway and measures to reduce the risk of aspiration of gastric contents. The blood glucose is measured and glucose given if indicated.

> The **National Poisons Information Service** (Tel: 0844 892 0111) will provide specialist advice on all aspects of poisoning day and night

Analgesics (non-opioid)

Aspirin The chief features of salicylate poisoning are hyperventilation, tinnitus, deafness, vasodilatation, and sweating. Coma is uncommon but indicates very severe poisoning. The associated acid-base disturbances are complex.

Treatment must be in hospital where plasma salicylate, pH, and electrolytes can be measured; absorption of aspirin may be slow and the plasma-salicylate concentration may continue to rise for several hours, requiring repeated measurement of plasma-salicylate concentration. Activated charcoal can be given within 1 hour of ingesting more than 125 mg/kg of aspirin. Fluid losses are replaced and intravenous sodium bicarbonate given to enhance urinary salicylate excretion when the plasma-salicylate concentration is greater than:

500 mg/litre (3.6 mmol/litre) in adults *or*

350 mg/litre (2.5 mmol/litre) in children.

Haemodialysis is the treatment of choice for severe salicylate poisoning and should be considered when the plasma-salicylate concentration exceeds 700 mg/litre (5.1 mmol/litre) or in the presence of severe metabolic acidosis.

NSAIDs Mefenamic acid has important consequences in overdosage because it can cause convulsions, which if prolonged or recurrent require treatment, see p. 28.

Overdosage with ibuprofen may cause nausea, vomiting, epigastric pain, and tinnitus, but more serious toxicity is very uncommon. Activated charcoal followed by symptomatic measures are indicated if more than 400 mg/kg has been ingested within the preceding hour.

Paracetamol As little as 10–15 g (20–30 tablets) or 150 mg/kg of paracetamol taken within 24 hours may cause severe hepatocellular necrosis and, much less frequently, renal tubular necrosis. Nausea and vomiting, the only early features of poisoning, usually settle within 24 hours. Persistence beyond this time, often associated with the onset of right subcostal pain and tenderness, usually indicates development of hepatic necrosis. Liver damage is maximal 3–4 days after ingestion and may lead to encephalopathy, haemorrhage, hypoglycaemia, cerebral oedema, and death.

Therefore, despite a lack of significant early symptoms, patients who have taken an overdose of paracetamol should be transferred to hospital urgently.

Administration of activated charcoal should be considered if paracetamol in excess of 150 mg/kg or 12 g, **whichever is the smaller**, is thought to have been ingested within the previous hour.

Acetylcysteine protects the liver if infused within 24 hours of ingesting paracetamol. It is most effective if given within 8 hours of ingestion, after which effectiveness declines sharply; if more than 24 hours have elapsed advice should be sought from the National Poisons Information Service or from a liver unit on the management of serious liver damage. In remote areas **methionine** by mouth is an alternative only if acetylcysteine cannot be given promptly. Once the patient reaches hospital the need to continue treatment with the antidote will be assessed from the plasma-paracetamol concentration (related to the time from ingestion).

Patients at risk of liver damage and therefore requiring treatment can be identified from a single measurement of the plasma-paracetamol concentration, related to the time from ingestion, provided this time interval is not less than 4 hours; earlier samples may be misleading. The concentration is plotted on a paracetamol treatment graph, with a reference line ('normal treatment line') joining plots of 200 mg/litre (1.32 mmol/litre) at 4 hours and 6.25 mg/litre (0.04 mmol/litre) at 24 hours (see p. 30). Those whose plasma-paracetamol concentration is above the *normal treatment line* are treated with acetylcysteine by intravenous infusion (or, if acetylcysteine is not available, with methionine by mouth, provided the overdose has been taken **within 10–12 hours** *and* the patient is not vomiting).

Patients taking enzyme-inducing drugs (e.g. carbamazepine, phenobarbital, phenytoin, primidone, rifampicin, alcohol, and St John's wort) or who are malnourished (e.g. in anorexia, in alcoholism, or those who are HIV-positive) may develop toxicity at **lower** plasma-paracetamol concentration and should be treated if the concentration is above the *high-risk treatment line* (which joins plots that are at 50% of the plasma-paracetamol concentrations of the normal treatment line).

The prognostic accuracy of plasma-paracetamol concentration taken after 15 hours is uncertain, but a concentration above the relevant treatment line should be regarded as carrying a serious risk of liver damage.

The plasma-paracetamol concentration may be difficult to interpret when paracetamol has been ingested over several hours. If there is doubt about timing or the need for treatment then the patient should be treated with an antidote.

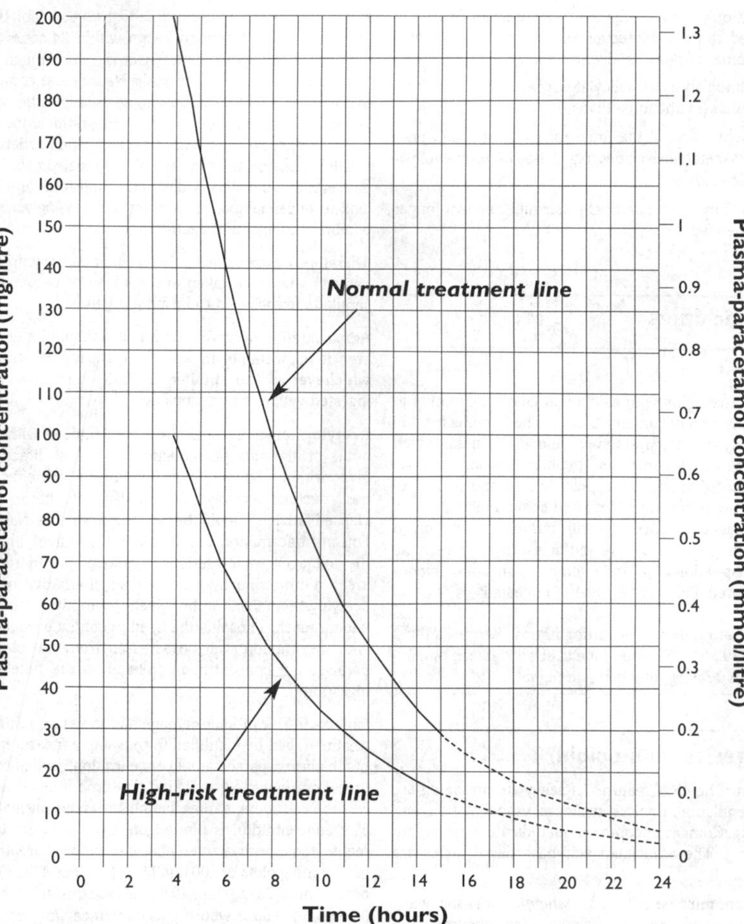

Patients whose plasma-paracetamol concentrations are above the **normal treatment line** should be treated with acetylcysteine by intravenous infusion (or, if acetylcysteine cannot be used, with methionine by mouth, provided the overdose has been taken **within 10–12 hours** and the patient is not vomiting).

Patients on enzyme-inducing drugs (e.g. carbamazepine, phenobarbital, phenytoin, primidone, rifampicin, alcohol, and St John's wort) or who are malnourished (e.g. in anorexia, in alcoholism, or those who are HIV-positive) should be treated if their plasma-paracetamol concentration is above the **high-risk treatment line**.

The prognostic accuracy after 15 hours is uncertain but a plasma-paracetamol concentration above the relevant treatment line should be regarded as carrying a serious risk of liver damage.

Graph reproduced courtesy of University of Wales College of Medicine Therapeutics and Toxicology Centre

ACETYLCYSTEINE

Indications paracetamol overdosage, see notes above

Cautions asthma (see side-effects below but do not delay acetylcysteine treatment)

Side-effects hypersensitivity-like reactions managed by reducing infusion rate or suspending until reaction settled—contact the National Poisons Information Service if reaction severe (rash also managed by giving antihistamine; acute asthma managed by giving nebulised short-acting beta$_2$ agonist)

Dose

- By intravenous infusion, ADULT and CHILD, initially 150 mg/kg (max. 16.5 g) over 15 minutes, then 50 mg/kg (max. 5.5 g) over 4 hours then 100 mg/kg (max. 11 g) over 16 hours

Administration Dilute requisite dose in glucose intravenous infusion 5% as follows: ADULT and CHILD over 12 years, initially 200 mL given over 15 minutes, then 500 mL over 4 hours, then 1 litre over 16 hours; CHILD under 12 years, body-weight over 20 kg, initially 100 mL given over 15 minutes, then 250 mL over 4 hours, then 500 mL over 16 hours; CHILD body-weight under 20 kg, initially 3 mL/kg given over 15 minutes, then 7 mL/kg over 4 hours, then 14 mL/kg over 16 hours

Note Manufacturer also recommends other infusion fluids, but glucose 5% is preferable

Acetylcysteine (Non-proprietary) PoM
Injection, acetylcysteine 200 mg/mL, net price 10-mL amp = £2.50

Parvolex® (UCB Pharma) PoM
Injection, acetylcysteine 200 mg/mL, net price 10-mL amp = £2.50

METHIONINE

Indications paracetamol overdosage, see notes above
Cautions hepatic impairment (Appendix 2)
Side-effects nausea, vomiting, drowsiness, irritability
Dose
- ADULT and CHILD over 6 years initially 2.5 g, followed by 3 further doses of 2.5 g every 4 hours, CHILD under 6 years initially 1 g, followed by 3 further doses of 1 g every 4 hours

Methionine (Pharma Nord) PoM
Tablets, f/c, methionine 500 mg, net price 20-tab pack = £9.95

Methionine (UCB Pharma)
Tablets, DL-methionine 250 mg, net price 200-tab pack = £87.76

With paracetamol (co-methiamol)
Section 4.7.1

Analgesics (opioid)

Opioids (narcotic analgesics) cause coma, respiratory depression, and pinpoint pupils. The specific antidote **naloxone** is indicated if there is coma or bradypnoea. Since naloxone has a shorter duration of action than many opioids, close monitoring and repeated injections are necessary according to the respiratory rate and depth of coma. When repeated administration of naloxone is required, it can be given by continuous intravenous infusion instead and the rate of infusion adjusted according to vital signs. The effects of some opioids, such as buprenorphine, are only partially reversed by naloxone. Dextropropoxyphene and methadone have very long durations of action; patients may need to be monitored for long periods following large overdoses.

Naloxone reverses the opioid effects of dextropropoxyphene; the long duration of action of dextropropoxyphene calls for prolonged monitoring and further doses of naloxone may be required. Norpropoxyphene, a metabolite of dextropropoxyphene, also has cardiotoxic effects which may require treatment with **sodium bicarbonate**, or **magnesium sulphate**, or both; arrhythmias may occur for up to 12 hours.

> The **National Poisons Information Service** (Tel: 0844 892 0111) will provide specialist advice on all aspects of poisoning day and night

NALOXONE HYDROCHLORIDE

Indications overdosage with opioids; postoperative respiratory depression (section 15.1.7)
Cautions physical dependence on opioids; cardiac irritability; naloxone is short-acting, see notes above
Dose
- By intravenous injection, 0.4–2 mg repeated at intervals of 2–3 minutes to a max. of 10 mg if respiratory function does not improve (then question diagnosis); CHILD 10 micrograms/kg; subsequent dose of 100 micrograms/kg if no response
- By subcutaneous *or* intramuscular injection, ADULT and CHILD dose as for intravenous injection but use only if intravenous route not feasible (onset of action slower)
- By continuous intravenous infusion using an infusion pump, 4 mg diluted in 20 mL intravenous infusion solution [unlicensed concentration] at a rate adjusted according to response (initial rate may be set at 60% of initial intravenous injection dose (see above) and infused over 1 hour)

Important Doses used in acute opioid overdosage may not be appropriate for the management of opioid-induced respiratory depression and sedation in those receiving palliative care and in chronic opioid use; see also section 15.1.7 for management of postoperative respiratory depression

[1] **Naloxone** (Non-proprietary) PoM
Injection, naloxone hydrochloride 400 micrograms/mL, net price 1-mL amp = £4.10; 1 mg/mL, 2-mL prefilled syringe = £6.61

[1] **Min-I-Jet® Naloxone** (Celltech) PoM
Injection, naloxone hydrochloride 400 micrograms/mL, net price 1-mL disposable syringe = £9.00, 2-mL disposable syringe = £11.78, 5-mL disposable syringe = £11.53

Antidepressants

Tricyclic and related antidepressants Tricyclic and related antidepressants cause dry mouth, coma of varying degree, hypotension, hypothermia, hyperreflexia, extensor plantar responses, convulsions, respiratory failure, cardiac conduction defects, and arrhythmias. Dilated pupils and urinary retention also occur. Metabolic acidosis may complicate severe poisoning; delirium with confusion, agitation, and visual and auditory hallucinations are common during recovery.

Transfer to hospital is strongly advised in case of poisoning by *tricyclic and related antidepressants* but symptomatic treatment and activated charcoal can be given before transfer. Supportive measures to ensure a clear airway and adequate ventilation during transfer are mandatory. Intravenous lorazepam or intravenous diazepam (preferably in emulsion form) may be required to control convulsions. Although arrhythmias are worrying, some will respond to correction of hypoxia and acidosis. The use of anti-arrhythmic drugs is best avoided, but intravenous infusion of sodium bicarbonate can arrest arrhythmias or prevent them in those with an extended QRS duration. Diazepam given by mouth is usually adequate to sedate delirious patients but large doses may be required.

Selective serotonin re-uptake inhibitors (SSRIs)
Symptoms of poisoning by selective serotonin re-uptake inhibitors include nausea, vomiting, agitation, tremor, nystagmus, drowsiness, and sinus tachycardia; convulsions may occur. Rarely, severe poisoning results in the serotonin syndrome, with marked neuropsychiatric effects, neuromuscular hyperactivity, and autonomic instability; hyperthermia, rhabdomyolysis, renal failure, and coagulopathies may develop.

Management of SSRI poisoning is supportive. Activated charcoal given within 1 hour of the overdose reduces absorption of the drug. Convulsions can be treated with

1. PoM restriction does not apply where administration is for saving life in emergency

lorazepam, diazepam, or buccal midazolam [unlicensed use] (see p. 28). Contact the National Poisons Information Service for the management of hyperthermia or the serotonin syndrome.

Antimalarials

Overdosage with quinine, chloroquine, or hydroxychloroquine is extremely hazardous and difficult to treat. Urgent advice from the National Poisons Information Service is essential. Life-threatening features include arrhythmias (which can have a very rapid onset) and convulsions (which can be intractable).

Beta-blockers

Therapeutic overdosages with beta-blockers may cause lightheadedness, dizziness, and possibly syncope as a result of bradycardia and hypotension; heart failure may be precipitated or exacerbated. These complications are most likely in patients with conduction system disorders or impaired myocardial function. Bradycardia is the most common arrhythmia caused by beta-blockers, but sotalol may induce ventricular tachyarrhythmias (sometimes of the torsade de pointes type). The effects of massive overdosage can vary from one beta-blocker to another; propranolol overdosage in particular may cause coma and convulsions.

Acute massive overdosage must be managed in hospital and expert advice should be obtained. Maintenance of a clear airway and adequate ventilation is mandatory. An intravenous injection of atropine is required to treat bradycardia and hypotension (3 mg for an adult, 40 micrograms/kg (max. 3 mg) for a child). Cardiogenic shock unresponsive to atropine is probably best treated with an intravenous injection of glucagon 2–10 mg (CHILD 50–150 micrograms/kg) [unlicensed indication and dose] in glucose 5% (with precautions to protect the airway in case of vomiting) followed by an intravenous infusion of 50 micrograms/kg/hour. If glucagon is not available, intravenous isoprenaline [special order only] is an alternative. A cardiac pacemaker can be used to increase the heart rate.

Calcium-channel blockers

Features of calcium-channel blocker poisoning include nausea, vomiting, dizziness, agitation, confusion, and coma in severe poisoning. Metabolic acidosis and hyperglycaemia may occur. Verapamil and diltiazem have a profound cardiac depressant effect causing hypotension and arrhythmias, including complete heart block and asystole. The dihydropyridine calcium-channel blockers cause severe hypotension secondary to profound peripheral vasodilatation.

Activated charcoal is given if the patient presents within 1 hour of overdosage with a calcium-channel blocker; repeated doses of activated charcoal are considered if a modified-release preparation is involved. In patients with significant features of poisoning, calcium chloride or calcium gluconate (section 9.5.1.1) is given by injection; atropine is given to correct symptomatic bradycardia. For the management of hypotension, the choice of inotropic sympathomimetic depends on whether hypotension is secondary to vasodilatation or to myocardial depression and advice should be sought from the National Poisons Information Service.

Hypnotics and anxiolytics

Benzodiazepines Benzodiazepines taken alone cause drowsiness, ataxia, dysarthria, and occasionally minor and short-lived depression of consciousness. Activated charcoal can be given within 1 hour of ingesting a significant quantity of benzodiazepine. Benzodiazepines potentiate the effects of other central nervous system depressants taken concomitantly. Use of the benzodiazepine antagonist flumazenil can be hazardous, particularly in mixed overdoses involving tricyclic antidepressants or in benzodiazepine-dependent patients. Flumazenil should be used on **expert advice** only.

Iron salts

Iron poisoning is commonest in childhood and is usually accidental. The symptoms are nausea, vomiting, abdominal pain, diarrhoea, haematemesis, and rectal bleeding. Hypotension, coma, and hepatocellular necrosis occur later. Mortality is reduced with intensive and specific therapy with **desferrioxamine**, which chelates iron. The stomach should be emptied by gastric lavage (with a wide-bore tube) within 1 hour of ingesting a significant quantity of iron or if radiography reveals tablets in the stomach; whole bowel irrigation may be considered in severe poisoning but advice should be sought from the National Poisons Information Service. The serum-iron concentration is measured as an emergency and intravenous desferrioxamine given to chelate absorbed iron in excess of the expected iron binding capacity. In **severe toxicity** intravenous desferrioxamine should be given *immediately* without waiting for the result of the serum-iron measurement (contact the National Poisons Information Service for advice).

DESFERRIOXAMINE MESILATE
(Deferoxamine Mesilate)

Indications iron poisoning; chronic iron overload (section 9.1.3)

Cautions section 9.1.3

Side-effects section 9.1.3

Dose

- By continuous intravenous infusion, ADULT and CHILD up to 15 mg/kg/hour, reduced after 4–6 hours; max. 80 mg/kg in 24 hours (in severe cases, higher doses on advice from the National Poisons Information Service)

Preparations
Section 9.1.3

Lithium

Most cases of lithium intoxication occur as a complication of long-term therapy and are caused by reduced excretion of the drug due to a variety of factors including dehydration, deterioration of renal function, infections, and co-administration of diuretics or NSAIDs (or other drugs that interact). Acute deliberate overdoses may also occur with delayed onset of symptoms (12 hours or more) owing to slow entry of lithium into the tissues and continuing absorption from modified-release formulations.

The early clinical features are non-specific and may include apathy and restlessness which could be confused with mental changes arising from the patient's depressive illness. Vomiting, diarrhoea, ataxia, weakness, dysarthria, muscle twitching, and tremor may follow. Severe poisoning is associated with convulsions, coma, renal failure, electrolyte imbalance, dehydration, and hypotension.

Therapeutic lithium concentrations are within the range of 0.4–1.0 mmol/litre; concentrations in excess of 2.0 mmol/litre are usually associated with serious toxicity and such cases may need treatment with haemodialysis if neurological symptoms or renal failure are present. In acute overdosage much higher serum-lithium concentrations may be present without features of toxicity and all that is usually necessary is to take measures to increase urine output (e.g. by increasing fluid intake but avoiding diuretics). Otherwise, treatment is supportive with special regard to electrolyte balance, renal function, and control of convulsions. The stomach should be emptied by gastric lavage if it can be performed within 1 hour of ingesting significant quantities of lithium. Whole-bowel irrigation should be considered for significant ingestion, but advice should be sought from the National Poisons Information Service, p. 27.

Phenothiazines and related drugs

Phenothiazines cause less depression of consciousness and respiration than other sedatives. Hypotension, hypothermia, sinus tachycardia, and arrhythmias may complicate poisoning. Dystonic reactions can occur with therapeutic doses (particularly with prochlorperazine and trifluoperazine), and convulsions may occur in severe cases. Arrhythmias may respond to correction of hypoxia, acidosis, and other biochemical abnormalities, but specialist advice should be sought if arrhythmias result from a prolonged QT interval; the use of some anti-arrhythmic drugs can worsen such arrhythmias. Dystonic reactions are rapidly abolished by injection of drugs such as benzatropine or diazepam (section 4.8.2, emulsion preferred).

Stimulants

Amphetamines These cause wakefulness, excessive activity, paranoia, hallucinations, and hypertension followed by exhaustion, convulsions, hyperthermia, and coma. The early stages can be controlled by diazepam or lorazepam; advice should be sought from the National Poisons Information Service (p. 27) on the management of hypertension. Later, tepid sponging, anticonvulsants, and artificial respiration may be needed.

Cocaine Cocaine stimulates the central nervous system, causing agitation, dilated pupils, tachycardia, hypertension, hallucinations, hyperthermia, hypertonia, and hyperreflexia; cardiac effects include chest pain, myocardial infarction, and arrhythmias.

Initial treatment of cocaine poisoning involves intravenous administration of diazepam to control agitation and cooling measures for hyperthermia (see Body temperature, p. 28); hypertension and cardiac effects require specific treatment and expert advice should be sought.

Ecstasy Ecstasy (methylenedioxymethamfetamine, MDMA) may cause severe reactions, even at doses that were previously tolerated. The most serious effects are delirium, coma, convulsions, ventricular arrhythmias, hyperpyrexia, rhabdomyolysis, acute renal failure, acute hepatitis, disseminated intravascular coagulation, adult respiratory distress syndrome, hyperreflexia, hypotension and intracerebral haemorrhage; hyponatraemia has also been associated with ecstasy use.

Treatment of methylenedioxymethamfetamine poisoning is supportive, with diazepam to control severe agitation or persistent convulsions and close monitoring including ECG. Self-induced water intoxication should be considered in patients with ecstasy poisoning.

'Liquid ecstasy' is a term used for sodium oxybate (gamma-hydroxybutyrate, GHB), which is a sedative.

Theophylline

Theophylline and related drugs are often prescribed as modified-release formulations and toxicity can therefore be delayed. They cause vomiting (which may be severe and intractable), agitation, restlessness, dilated pupils, sinus tachycardia, and hyperglycaemia. More serious effects are haematemesis, convulsions, and supraventricular and ventricular arrhythmias. Profound hypokalaemia may develop rapidly.

Repeated doses of activated charcoal can be used to eliminate theophylline even if more than 1 hour has lapsed after ingestion and especially if a modified-release preparation has been taken (see also under Active Elimination Techniques, p. 28). Hypokalaemia is corrected by intravenous infusion of potassium chloride and may be so severe as to require 60 mmol/hour (high doses require ECG monitoring). Convulsions should be controlled by intravenous administration of lorazepam or diazepam (emulsion preferred). Sedation with diazepam may be necessary in agitated patients.

Provided the patient does **not** suffer from asthma, a short-acting beta-blocker (section 2.4) can be administered intravenously to reverse severe tachycardia, hypokalaemia, and hyperglycaemia.

Other poisons

Consult either the National Poisons Information Service day and night or TOXBASE, see p. 27.

> The **National Poisons Information Service** (Tel: 0844 892 0111) will provide specialist advice on all aspects of poisoning day and night

Cyanides

Oxygen should be administered to patients with cyanide poisoning. Mild cyanide poisoning can be treated with sodium thiosulphate alone. Severe confirmed cyanide poisoning should be treated with dicobalt edetate followed by sodium thiosulphate. However, dicobalt edetate itself is toxic and it is associated with anaphylactic reactions; a regimen of sodium nitrite followed by sodium thiosulphate is an alternative. These antidotes are held for emergency use in hospitals as well as in centres where cyanide poisoning is a risk, such as factories and laboratories.

Hydroxocobalamin is an alternative antidote but its use should ideally be discussed with the National Poisons Information Service; the usual dose is hydroxocobalamin 70 mg/kg by intravenous infusion (repeated once or twice according to severity). *Cyanokit*®, which provides hydroxocobalamin 2.5 g/bottle, is available but it is not licensed for use in the UK.

DICOBALT EDETATE

Indications acute poisoning with cyanides

Cautions owing to toxicity to be used only for definite cyanide poisoning when patient tending to lose, or has lost, consciousness; **not** to be used as a precautionary measure

Side-effects hypotension, tachycardia, and vomiting; anaphylactic reactions including facial and laryngeal oedema and cardiac abnormalities

Dose

- By intravenous injection, ADULT 300 mg over 1 minute (5 minutes if condition less serious) followed immediately by 50 mL of glucose intravenous infusion 50%; if response inadequate a second dose of both may be given, but risk of cobalt toxicity; CHILD consult the National Poisons Information Service

[1]**Dicobalt Edetate** (Cambridge) PoM
Injection, dicobalt edetate 15 mg/mL, net price 20-mL (300-mg) amp = £13.75

SODIUM NITRITE

Indications poisoning with cyanides (used in conjunction with sodium thiosulphate)

Side-effects flushing and headache due to vasodilatation

Dose

- By intravenous injection over 5–20 minutes (as sodium nitrite injection 30 mg/mL), 300 mg; CHILD 4–10 mg/kg (max. 300 mg)

[1]**Sodium Nitrite** PoM
Injection, sodium nitrite 3% (30 mg/mL) in water for injections
'Special-order' [unlicensed] product: contact Martindale, or regional hospital manufacturing unit

SODIUM THIOSULPHATE

Indications mild cyanide poisoning; in conjunction with dicobalt edetate or sodium nitrite for severe cyanide poisoning

Dose

- By intravenous injection over 10 minutes (as sodium thiosulphate injection 500 mg/mL), 12.5 g; dose may be repeated in severe cyanide poisoning if dicobalt edetate not available; CHILD 400 mg/kg (max. 12.5 g); dose may be repeated in severe cyanide poisoning if dicobalt edetate not available

[1]**Sodium Thiosulphate** PoM
Injection, sodium thiosulphate 50% (500 mg/mL) in water for injections
'Special-order' [unlicensed] product: contact Martindale, or regional hospital manufacturing unit

Ethylene glycol and methanol

Ethanol (by mouth or by intravenous infusion) is used for the treatment of ethylene glycol or methanol (methyl alcohol) poisoning. Fomepizole (available on a named-patient basis from specialist importing companies, see p. 888) has also been used for the treatment of ethylene glycol or methanol poisoning. Advice on the treatment of ethylene glycol or methanol poisoning should be obtained from the National Poisons Information Service.

1. PoM restriction does not apply where administration is for saving life in emergency

Heavy metals

Heavy metal antidotes include dimercaprol, penicillamine, and sodium calcium edetate. Other antidotes for heavy metal poisoning include succimer (DMSA) and unithiol (DMPS) [both unlicensed]; they can be valuable in certain cases and the advice of the National Poisons Information Service should be sought.

DIMERCAPROL
(BAL)

Indications poisoning by antimony, arsenic, bismuth, gold, mercury, possibly thallium; adjunct (with sodium calcium edetate) in lead poisoning

Cautions hypertension, renal impairment (discontinue or use with extreme caution if impairment develops during treatment), elderly, pregnancy and breast-feeding; **interactions:** Appendix 1 (dimercaprol)

Contra-indications not indicated for iron, cadmium, or selenium poisoning; severe hepatic impairment (unless due to arsenic poisoning)

Side-effects hypertension, tachycardia, malaise, nausea, vomiting, salivation, lacrimation, sweating, burning sensation (mouth, throat, and eyes), feeling of constriction of throat and chest, headache, muscle spasm, abdominal pain, tingling of extremities; pyrexia in children; local pain and abscess at injection site

Dose

- By intramuscular injection, ADULT and CHILD 2.5–3 mg/kg every 4 hours for 2 days, 2–4 times on the third day, then 1–2 times daily for 10 days or until recovery

Dimercaprol (Sovereign) PoM
Injection, dimercaprol 50 mg/mL. Net price 2-mL amp = £42.73
Note Contains arachis (peanut) oil as solvent

PENICILLAMINE

Indications lead poisoning

Cautions see section 10.1.3

Contra-indications see section 10.1.3

Side-effects see section 10.1.3

Dose

- 1–2 g daily in 3 divided doses before food until urinary lead is stabilised at less than 500 micrograms/day; CHILD 20 mg/kg daily in 3 divided doses before food

Preparations
Section 10.1.3

SODIUM CALCIUM EDETATE
(Sodium Calciumedetate)

Indications poisoning by heavy metals, especially lead

Cautions renal impairment

Side-effects nausea, diarrhoea, abdominal pain, pain at site of injection, thrombophlebitis if given too rapidly, renal damage particularly in overdosage; hypotension, lacrimation, myalgia, nasal congestion, sneezing, malaise, thirst, fever, chills, headache also reported

Dose

- By intravenous infusion, ADULT and CHILD 40 mg/kg twice daily for up to 5 days; if necessary, a second course can be given at least 2 days after the first course, a third course can be given at least 5–7 days after the second course

Ledclair® (Durbin) PoM

Injection, sodium calcium edetate 200 mg/mL, net price 5-mL amp = £7.29

Noxious gases

Carbon monoxide Carbon monoxide poisoning is usually due to inhalation of smoke, car exhaust, or fumes caused by blocked flues or incomplete combustion of fuel gases in confined spaces. Its toxic effects are entirely due to hypoxia.

Immediate treatment of carbon monoxide poisoning is essential. The person should be moved to fresh air, the airway cleared, and **oxygen** 100% administered through a tight-fitting mask with an inflated face seal. Artificial respiration should be given as necessary and continued until adequate spontaneous breathing starts, or stopped only after persistent and efficient treatment of cardiac arrest has failed. The patient should be admitted to hospital because complications may arise after a delay of hours or days. Cerebral oedema should be anticipated in severe poisoning and is treated with an intravenous infusion of mannitol (section 2.2.5). Referral for hyperbaric oxygen treatment should be discussed with the National Poisons Information Service if the victim is or has been unconscious, or has psychiatric or neurological features other than a headache, or has myocardial ischaemia or an arrhythmia, or has a blood carboxyhaemoglobin concentration of more than 20%, or is pregnant.

Sulphur dioxide, chlorine, phosgene, ammonia All of these gases can cause upper respiratory tract and conjunctival irritation. Pulmonary oedema, with severe breathlessness and cyanosis may develop suddenly up to 36 hours after exposure. Death may occur. Patients are kept under observation and those who develop pulmonary oedema are given oxygen. Assisted ventilation may be necessary in the most serious cases.

CS Spray

CS spray, which is used for riot control, irritates the eyes (hence 'tear gas') and the respiratory tract; symptoms normally settle spontaneously within 15 minutes. If symptoms persist, the patient should be removed to a well-ventilated area, and the exposed skin washed with soap and water after removal of contaminated clothing. Contact lenses should be removed and rigid ones washed (soft ones should be discarded). Eye symptoms should be treated by irrigating the eyes with physiological saline (or water if saline is not available) and advice sought from an ophthalmologist. Patients with features of severe poisoning, particularly respiratory complications, should be admitted to hospital for symptomatic treatment.

Nerve agents

Treatment of nerve agent poisoning is similar to organophosphorus insecticide poisoning (see below), but advice must be sought from the National Poisons Information Service. The risk of cross-contamination is significant; adequate decontamination and protective clothing for healthcare personnel are essential. In emergencies involving the release of nerve agents, kits ('NAAS pods') containing **pralidoxime** can be obtained through the Ambulance Service from the National Blood Service (or the Welsh Blood Service in South Wales or designated hospital pharmacies in Northern Ireland and Scotland—see TOXBASE for list of designated centres). In the very rare circumstances where the nerve agent is tabun (GA), **obidoxime** will also be supplied as part of the pod.

> The **National Poisons Information Service** (Tel: 0844 892 0111) will provide specialist advice on all aspects of poisoning day and night

Pesticides

Paraquat Concentrated liquid paraquat preparations (e.g. *Gramoxone®*), available to farmers and horticulturists, contain 10–20% paraquat and are extremely toxic. Granular preparations, for garden use, contain only 2.5% paraquat and have caused few deaths.

Paraquat has local and systemic effects. Splashes in the eyes irritate and ulcerate the cornea and conjunctiva. Copious washing of the eye should aid healing but it may be a long process. Skin irritation, blistering, and ulceration can occur from prolonged contact with both the concentrated and dilute forms. Inhalation of spray, mist, or dust containing paraquat may cause nose bleeding and sore throat but not systemic toxicity.

Ingestion of concentrated paraquat solutions is followed by nausea, vomiting, and diarrhoea. Painful ulceration of the tongue, lips, and fauces may appear after 36 to 48 hours together with renal failure. Some days later there may be dyspnoea with pulmonary fibrosis due to proliferative alveolitis and bronchiolitis.

Treatment should be started immediately. The single most useful measure is oral administration of **activated charcoal**. Vomiting can preclude the use of activated charcoal and an anti-emetic may be required. Gastric lavage is of doubtful value. Intravenous fluids and analgesics are given as necessary. Oxygen therapy should be avoided in the early stages of management since this may exacerbate damage to the lungs, but oxygen may be required in the late stages to palliate symptoms. Measures to enhance elimination of absorbed paraquat are probably of no value but should be discussed with the National Poisons Information Service who will also give guidance on predicting the likely outcome based on plasma concentrations. Paraquat absorption can be confirmed by a simple qualitative urine test.

Organophosphorus insecticides Organophosphorus insecticides are usually supplied as powders or dissolved in organic solvents. All are absorbed through the bronchi and intact skin as well as through the gut and inhibit cholinesterase activity, thereby prolonging and intensifying the effects of acetylcholine. Toxicity between different compounds varies considerably, and onset may be delayed after skin exposure.

Anxiety, restlessness, dizziness, headache, miosis, nausea, hypersalivation, vomiting, abdominal colic, diarrhoea, bradycardia, and sweating are common features of organophosphorus poisoning. Muscle weakness and fasciculation may develop and progress to generalised flaccid paralysis, including the ocular and respiratory muscles. Convulsions, coma, pulmonary oedema with copious bronchial secretions, hypoxia, and arrhythmias occur in severe cases. Hyperglycaemia and glycosuria without ketonuria may also be present.

Further absorption of the organophosphorus insecticide should be prevented by moving the patient to fresh air, removing soiled clothing, and washing contaminated skin. In severe poisoning it is vital to ensure a clear airway, frequent removal of bronchial secretions, and adequate ventilation and oxygenation; gastric lavage may be considered provided that the airway is protected. **Atropine** will reverse the muscarinic effects of acetylcholine and is given in a dose of 2 mg (20 micrograms/kg (max. 2 mg) in a child) as atropine sulphate (intramuscularly or intravenously according to the severity of poisoning) every 5 to 10 minutes until the skin becomes flushed and dry, the pupils dilate, and tachycardia develops.

Pralidoxime chloride, a cholinesterase reactivator, is used as an adjunct to atropine in moderate or severe poisoning. It improves muscle tone within 30 minutes of administration. Pralidoxime chloride is continued until the patient has not required atropine for 12 hours. Pralidoxime chloride can be obtained from designated centres, the names of which are held by the National Poisons Information Service (see p. 27).

PRALIDOXIME CHLORIDE

Indications adjunct to atropine in the treatment of poisoning by organophosphorus insecticide or nerve agent

Cautions renal impairment, myasthenia gravis

Contra-indications poisoning due to carbamates and to organophosphorus compounds without anticholinesterase activity

Side-effects drowsiness, dizziness, disturbances of vision, nausea, tachycardia, headache, hyperventilation, and muscular weakness

Dose

- By intravenous infusion, ADULT and CHILD initially 30 mg/kg over 20 minutes, followed by 8 mg/kg/hour

Note The loading dose may be administered by intravenous injection (diluted to a concentration of 50 mg/mL with water for injections) over at least 5 minutes if pulmonary oedema is present or if it is not practical to administer an intravenous infusion; pralidoxime chloride doses in BNF may differ from those in product literature

[1]Pralidoxime chloride (PoM)

Injection, powder for reconstitution, pralidoxime chloride 1 g/vial

Available as *Protopam*® (from designated centres for organophosphorus insecticide poisoning or from the National Blood Service and the Welsh Blood Service for nerve agent poisoning—see TOXBASE for list of designated centres)

1. (PoM) restriction does not apply where administration is for saving life in emergency

Snake bites and animal stings

Snake bites Envenoming from snake bite is uncommon in the UK. Many exotic snakes are kept, some illegally, but the only indigenous venomous snake is the adder (*Vipera berus*). The bite may cause local and systemic effects. Local effects include pain, swelling, bruising, and tender enlargement of regional lymph nodes. Systemic effects include early anaphylactoid symptoms (transient hypotension with syncope, angioedema, urticaria, abdominal colic, diarrhoea, and vomiting), with later persistent or recurrent hypotension, ECG abnormalities, spontaneous systemic bleeding, coagulopathy, adult respiratory distress syndrome, and acute renal failure. Fatal envenoming is rare but the potential for severe envenoming must not be underestimated.

Early anaphylactoid symptoms should be treated with **adrenaline (epinephrine)** (section 3.4.3). Indications for antivenom treatment include systemic envenoming, especially hypotension (see above), ECG abnormalities, vomiting, haemostatic abnormalities, and marked local envenoming such that after bites on the hand or foot, swelling extends beyond the wrist or ankle within 4 hours of the bite. For both **adults** and **children**, the contents of one vial (10 mL) of **European viper venom antiserum** (available from Movianto) is given *by intravenous injection* over 10–15 minutes or *by intravenous infusion* over 30 minutes after diluting in sodium chloride intravenous infusion 0.9% (use 5 mL diluent/kg bodyweight). The dose can be repeated in 1–2 hours if symptoms of **systemic envenoming** persist. Adrenaline (epinephrine) injection must be immediately to hand for treatment of anaphylactic reactions to the antivenom (for the management of anaphylaxis, see section 3.4.3).

Antivenom is available for bites by certain foreign snakes and spiders, stings by scorpions and fish. For information on identification, management, and supply, telephone:

Oxford	(01865) 221 502
Liverpool	(0151) 708 9393
Liverpool (Royal Liverpool University Hospital) (emergency supply only)	(0151) 706 2000
London (emergency supply only)	(020) 7771 5394

Insect stings Stings from ants, wasps, hornets, and bees cause local pain and swelling but seldom cause severe direct toxicity unless many stings are inflicted at the same time. If the sting is in the mouth or on the tongue local swelling may threaten the upper airway. The stings from these insects are usually treated by cleaning the area. Bee stings should be removed as quickly as possible. Anaphylactic reactions require immediate treatment with intramuscular **adrenaline (epinephrine)**; self-administered intramuscular adrenaline (e.g. *EpiPen*®) is the best first-aid treatment for patients with severe hypersensitivity. An inhaled bronchodilator should be used for asthmatic reactions. For the management of anaphylaxis, see section 3.4.3. A short course of an **oral antihistamine** or a **topical corticosteroid** may help to reduce inflammation and relieve itching.

Marine stings The severe pain of weeverfish (*Trachinus vipera*) stings can be relieved by immersing the stung area immediately in uncomfortably hot, but not scalding, water (not more than 45° C). People stung by jellyfish and Portuguese man-o'-war around the UK coast should be removed from the sea as soon as possible. Adherent tentacles should be lifted off carefully (wearing gloves or using tweezers) or washed off with seawater. Alcoholic solutions, including suntan lotions, should **not** be applied because they may cause further discharge of stinging hairs. Ice packs will reduce pain and a slurry of baking soda (sodium bicarbonate), but not vinegar, may be useful for treating stings from UK species.

1 Gastro-intestinal system

1.1 Dyspepsia and gastro-oesophageal reflux disease 37
1.1.1 Antacids and simeticone 38
1.1.2 Compound alginates and proprietary indigestion preparations 40
1.2 Antispasmodics and other drugs altering gut motility 41
1.3 Antisecretory drugs and mucosal protectants 43
1.3.1 H_2-receptor antagonists 44
1.3.2 Selective antimuscarinics 47
1.3.3 Chelates and complexes 47
1.3.4 Prostaglandin analogues 48
1.3.5 Proton pump inhibitors 48
1.4 Acute diarrhoea 50
1.4.1 Adsorbents and bulk-forming drugs 51
1.4.2 Antimotility drugs 51
1.5 Chronic bowel disorders 52
1.6 Laxatives 57
1.6.1 Bulk-forming laxatives 58
1.6.2 Stimulant laxatives 59
1.6.3 Faecal softeners 61
1.6.4 Osmotic laxatives 61
1.6.5 Bowel cleansing solutions 63
1.7 Local preparations for anal and rectal disorders 64
1.7.1 Soothing haemorrhoidal preparations 64
1.7.2 Compound haemorrhoidal preparations with corticosteroids 65
1.7.3 Rectal sclerosants 66
1.7.4 Management of anal fissures 66
1.8 Stoma care 66
1.9 Drugs affecting intestinal secretions 67
1.9.1 Drugs affecting biliary composition and flow 67
1.9.2 Bile acid sequestrants 67
1.9.3 Aprotinin 68
1.9.4 Pancreatin 68

This chapter also includes advice on the drug management of the following:

antibiotic-associated colitis, p. 53
constipation, p. 57
Crohn's disease, p. 52
diverticular disease, p. 53
food allergy, p. 57
Helicobacter pylori infection, p. 43
irritable bowel syndrome, p. 53
NSAID-associated ulcers, p. 44
ulcerative colitis, p. 52

1.1 Dyspepsia and gastro-oesophageal reflux disease

1.1.1 Antacids and simeticone
1.1.2 Compound alginates and proprietary indigestion preparations

Dyspepsia

Dyspepsia covers pain, fullness, early satiety, bloating, and nausea. It can occur with gastric and duodenal ulceration (section 1.3) and gastric cancer but most commonly it is of uncertain origin.

Urgent endoscopic investigation is required if dyspepsia is accompanied by 'alarm features' (e.g. bleeding, dysphagia, recurrent vomiting, or weight loss). Urgent investigation should also be considered for patients over 55 years with unexplained dyspepsia that has not responded to treatment.

Patients with dyspepsia should be advised about lifestyle changes (see Gastro-oesophageal reflux disease, below). Some medications may cause dyspepsia—these should be stopped, if possible. Antacids may provide some symptomatic relief.

If symptoms persist in *uninvestigated dyspepsia*, treatment involves a **proton pump inhibitor** (section 1.3.5) for 4 weeks. A proton pump inhibitor can be used intermittently to control symptoms long-term. Patients with uninvestigated dyspepsia, who do not respond to an initial trial with a proton pump inhibitor, should be tested for *Helicobacter pylori* and given eradication therapy (section 1.3) if *H. pylori* is present. Alternatively, particularly in populations where *H. pylori* infection is more likely, the 'test and treat' strategy for *H. pylori* can be used before a trial with a proton pump inhibitor.

If *H. pylori* is present in patients with *functional (investigated, non-ulcer) dyspepsia*, eradication therapy should be provided. However, most patients with functional dyspepsia do not benefit symptomatically from *H. pylori* eradication. If symptoms persist, treatment with either a **proton pump inhibitor** (section 1.3.5) or a **histamine**

H_2-receptor antagonist (section 1.3.1) can be given for 4 weeks. These antisecretory drugs can be used intermittently to control symptoms long-term.

Gastro-oesophageal reflux disease

Gastro-oesophageal reflux disease (including non-erosive gastro-oesophageal reflux and erosive oesophagitis) is associated with heartburn, acid regurgitation, and sometimes, difficulty in swallowing (dysphagia); oesophageal inflammation (oesophagitis), ulceration, and stricture formation may occur and there is an association with asthma.

The management of gastro-oesophageal reflux disease includes drug treatment, lifestyle changes and, in some cases, surgery. Initial treatment is guided by the severity of symptoms and treatment is then adjusted according to response. The extent of healing depends on the severity of the disease, the treatment chosen, and the duration of therapy.

Patients with gastro-oesophageal reflux disease should be advised about lifestyle changes (avoidance of excess alcohol and of aggravating foods such as fats); other measures include weight reduction, smoking cessation, and raising the head of the bed.

For *mild symptoms* of gastro-oesophageal reflux disease, initial management may include the use of **antacids** and **alginates**. Alginate-containing antacids can form a 'raft' that floats on the surface of the stomach contents to reduce reflux and protect the oesophageal mucosa. **Histamine H_2-receptor antagonists** (section 1.3.1) may relieve symptoms and permit reduction in antacid consumption. However, **proton pump inhibitors** (section 1.3.5) provide more effective relief of symptoms than H_2-receptor antagonists. When symptoms abate, treatment is titrated down to a level which maintains remission (e.g. by giving treatment intermittently).

For *severe symptoms* of gastro-oesophageal reflux disease or for patients with a proven or severe pathology (e.g. *oesophagitis, oesophageal ulceration, oesophagopharyngeal reflux, Barrett's oesophagus*), initial management involves the use of a **proton pump inhibitor** (section 1.3.5); patients need to be reassessed if symptoms persist despite treatment for 4–6 weeks with a proton pump inhibitor. When symptoms abate, treatment is titrated down to a level which maintains remission (e.g. by reducing the dose of the proton pump inhibitor or by giving it intermittently, or by substituting treatment with a histamine H_2-receptor antagonist). However, for endoscopically confirmed *erosive, ulcerative,* or *stricturing* disease, or *Barrett's oesophagus,* treatment with a proton pump inhibitor usually needs to be maintained at the minimum effective dose.

A prokinetic drug such as **metoclopramide** (section 4.6) may improve gastro-oesophageal sphincter function and accelerate gastric emptying.

Children Gastro-oesophageal reflux disease is common in infancy but most symptoms resolve without treatment between 12 and 18 months of age. In infants, mild or moderate reflux without complications can be managed initially by changing the frequency and volume of feed; a feed thickener or thickened formula feed can be used (with advice of a dietitian—see Appendix 7 for suitable products). If necessary, a suitable alginate-containing preparation can be used instead of thickened feeds. For older children, life-style changes similar to those for adults (see above) may be helpful followed if necessary by treatment with an alginate-containing preparation.

Children who do not respond to these measures or who have problems such as respiratory disorders or suspected oesophagitis need to be referred to hospital; an H_2-receptor antagonist (section 1.3.1) may be needed to reduce acid secretion. If the oesophagitis is resistant to H_2-receptor blockade, the proton pump inhibitor omeprazole (section 1.3.5) can be tried.

1.1.1 Antacids and simeticone

Antacids (usually containing aluminium or magnesium compounds) can often relieve symptoms in *ulcer dyspepsia* and in *non-erosive gastro-oesophageal reflux* (see also section 1.1); they are also sometimes used in functional (non-ulcer) dyspepsia but the evidence of benefit is uncertain. Antacids are best given when symptoms occur or are expected, usually between meals and at bedtime, 4 or more times daily; additional doses may be required up to once an hour. Conventional doses e.g. 10 mL 3 or 4 times daily of liquid magnesium–aluminium antacids promote ulcer healing, but less well than antisecretory drugs (section 1.3); proof of a relationship between healing and neutralising capacity is lacking. Liquid preparations are more effective than tablet preparations.

Aluminium- and **magnesium-containing** antacids (e.g. aluminium hydroxide, and magnesium carbonate, hydroxide and trisilicate), being relatively insoluble in water, are long-acting if retained in the stomach. They are suitable for most antacid purposes. Magnesium-containing antacids tend to be laxative whereas aluminium-containing antacids may be constipating; antacids containing both magnesium and aluminium may reduce these colonic side-effects. Aluminium accumulation does not appear to be a risk if renal function is normal (see also Appendix 3).

The acid-neutralising capacity of preparations that contain more than one antacid may be the same as simpler preparations. Complexes such as **hydrotalcite** confer no special advantage.

Sodium bicarbonate should no longer be prescribed alone for the relief of dyspepsia but it is present as an ingredient in many indigestion remedies. However, it retains a place in the management of urinary-tract disorders (section 7.4.3) and acidosis (section 9.2.1.3 and section 9.2.2). Sodium bicarbonate should be avoided in patients on salt-restricted diets.

Bismuth-containing antacids (unless chelates) are not recommended because absorbed bismuth can be neurotoxic, causing encephalopathy; they tend to be constipating. **Calcium-containing** antacids (section 1.1.2) can induce rebound acid secretion: with modest doses the clinical significance is doubtful, but prolonged high doses also cause hypercalcaemia and alkalosis, and can precipitate the milk-alkali syndrome.

Simeticone (activated dimeticone) is added to an antacid as an antifoaming agent to relieve flatulence. These preparations may be useful for the relief of hiccup in palliative care. **Alginates**, added as protectants, may be useful in gastro-oesophageal reflux disease (section 1.1 and section 1.1.2). The amount of additional ingredient or antacid in individual preparations varies widely, as does their sodium content, so that preparations may not be freely interchangeable.

See also section 1.3 for drugs used in the treatment of peptic ulceration.

Interactions Antacids should preferably not be taken at the same time as other drugs since they may impair absorption. Antacids may also damage enteric coatings designed to prevent dissolution in the stomach. See also **Appendix 1** (antacids, calcium salts).

> Low Na^+
> The words low Na^+ added after some preparations indicate a sodium content of less than 1 mmol per tablet or 10-mL dose.

Aluminium- and magnesium-containing antacids

ALUMINIUM HYDROXIDE

Indications dyspepsia; hyperphosphataemia (section 9.5.2.2)

Cautions see notes above; renal impairment (Appendix 3); **interactions:** Appendix 1 (antacids)

Contra-indications hypophosphataemia; neonates and infants

Side-effects see notes above

Aluminium-only preparations

Aluminium Hydroxide (Non-proprietary)
Tablets, dried aluminium hydroxide 500 mg. Net price 20 = 28p
Dose 1–2 tablets chewed 4 times daily and at bedtime or as required

Alu-Cap® (3M)
Capsules, green/red, dried aluminium hydroxide 475 mg (low Na^+). Net price 120-cap pack = £3.75
Dose antacid, 1 capsule 4 times daily and at bedtime; CHILD not recommended for antacid therapy

Co-magaldrox

Co-magaldrox is a mixture of aluminium hydroxide and magnesium hydroxide; the proportions are expressed in the form *x/y* where *x* and *y* are the strengths in milligrams per unit dose of magnesium hydroxide and aluminium hydroxide respectively

Maalox® (Sanofi-Aventis)
Suspension, sugar-free, co-magaldrox 195/220 (magnesium hydroxide 195 mg, dried aluminium hydroxide 220 mg/5 mL (low Na^+)). Net price 500 mL = £2.79
Dose ADULT and CHILD over 14 years, 10–20 mL 20–60 minutes after meals and at bedtime or when required

Mucogel® (Forest)
Suspension, sugar-free, co-magaldrox 195/220 (magnesium hydroxide 195 mg, dried aluminium hydroxide 220 mg/5 mL (low Na^+)). Net price 500 mL = £1.71
Dose ADULT and CHILD over 12 years, 10–20 mL 3 times daily, 20–60 minutes after meals, and at bedtime or when required

MAGNESIUM CARBONATE

Indications dyspepsia

Cautions renal impairment (Appendix 3); see also notes above; **interactions:** Appendix 1 (antacids)

Contra-indications hypophosphataemia

Side-effects diarrhoea; belching due to liberated carbon dioxide

Aromatic Magnesium Carbonate Mixture, BP (Aromatic Magnesium Carbonate Oral Suspension)
Oral suspension, light magnesium carbonate 3%, sodium bicarbonate 5%, in a suitable vehicle containing aromatic cardamom tincture. Contains about 6 mmol Na^+/10 mL. Net price 200 mL = 66p
Dose 10 mL 3 times daily in water
For **preparations** also containing aluminium, see above and section 1.1.2.

MAGNESIUM TRISILICATE

Indications dyspepsia

Cautions see under Magnesium Carbonate

Contra-indications see under Magnesium Carbonate

Side-effects diarrhoea, belching due to liberated carbon dioxide; silica-based renal stones reported on long-term treatment

Magnesium Trisilicate Tablets, Compound, BP
Tablets, magnesium trisilicate 250 mg, dried aluminium hydroxide 120 mg
Dose 1–2 tablets chewed when required

Magnesium Trisilicate Mixture, BP (Magnesium Trisilicate Oral Suspension)
Oral suspension, 5% each of magnesium trisilicate, light magnesium carbonate, and sodium bicarbonate in a suitable vehicle with a peppermint flavour. Contains about 6 mmol Na^+/10 mL
Dose 10 mL 3 times daily in water
For **preparations** also containing aluminium, see above and section 1.1.2.

Aluminium-magnesium complexes

HYDROTALCITE
Aluminium magnesium carbonate hydroxide hydrate

Indications dyspepsia

Cautions see notes above; **interactions:** Appendix 1 (antacids)

Side-effects see notes above

Hydrotalcite (Peckforton)
Suspension, hydrotalcite 500 mg/5 mL (low Na^+). Net price 500-mL pack = £1.96
Dose 10 mL between meals and at bedtime; CHILD 6–12 years 5 mL between meals and at bedtime
Note The brand name *Altacite®* (NHS) is used for hydrotalcite suspension; for *Altacite Plus®* suspension, see below

Antacid preparations containing simeticone

Altacite Plus® (Peckforton)
Suspension, sugar-free, co-simalcite 125/500 (simeticone 125 mg, hydrotalcite 500 mg)/5 mL (low Na^+). Net price 500 mL = £1.96
Dose 10 mL between meals and at bedtime when required; CHILD 8–12 years 5 mL between meals and at bedtime when required

Asilone® (Thornton & Ross)
Suspension, sugar-free, dried aluminium hydroxide 420 mg, simeticone 135 mg, light magnesium oxide 70 mg/5 mL (low Na^+). Net price 500 mL = £1.95
Dose ADULT and CHILD over 12 years, 5–10 mL after meals and at bedtime or when required up to 4 times daily

Maalox Plus® (Sanofi-Aventis)
Suspension, sugar-free, dried aluminium hydroxide 220 mg, simeticone 25 mg, magnesium hydroxide 195 mg/5 mL (low Na^+). Net price 500 mL = £2.79
Dose 5–10 mL 4 times daily (after meals and at bedtime or when required); CHILD under 5 years 5 mL 3 times daily, over 5 years appropriate proportion of adult dose

Simeticone alone

Simeticone (activated dimeticone) is an antifoaming agent. It is licensed for infantile colic but evidence of benefit is uncertain.

Dentinox® (DDD)
Colic drops (= emulsion), simeticone 21 mg/2.5-mL dose. Net price 100 mL = £1.73
Dose colic or wind pains, NEONATE and INFANT 2.5 mL with or after each feed (max. 6 doses in 24 hours); may be added to bottle feed
Note The brand name *Dentinox®* is also used for other preparations including teething gel

Infacol® (Forest)
Liquid, sugar-free, simeticone 40 mg/mL (low Na^+). Net price 50 mL = £2.14 Counselling, use of dropper
Dose colic or wind pains, NEONATE and INFANT 0.5–1 mL before feeds

1.1.2 Compound alginates and proprietary indigestion preparations

Alginate taken in combination with an antacid increases the viscosity of stomach contents and can protect the oesophageal mucosa from acid reflux. Some alginate-containing preparations form a viscous gel ('raft') that floats on the surface of the stomach contents, thereby reducing symptoms of reflux.

Compound alginate preparations

Acidex® (Pinewood)
Liquid, sugar-free, sodium alginate 250 mg, sodium bicarbonate 133.5 mg, calcium carbonate 80 mg/5 mL. Contains about 3 mmol Na^+/5 mL. Net price 500 mL (aniseed- or peppermint-flavour) = £1.70
Dose 10–20 mL after meals and at bedtime; CHILD 6–12 years 5–10 mL after meals and at bedtime

Gastrocote® (Thornton & Ross)
Tablets, alginic acid 200 mg, dried aluminium hydroxide 80 mg, magnesium trisilicate 40 mg, sodium bicarbonate 70 mg. Contains about 1 mmol Na^+/tablet. Net price 100-tab pack = £3.51
Cautions diabetes mellitus (high sugar content)
Dose ADULT and CHILD over 6 years, 1–2 tablets chewed 4 times daily (after meals and at bedtime)

Liquid, sugar-free, peach-coloured, dried aluminium hydroxide 80 mg, magnesium trisilicate 40 mg, sodium alginate 220 mg, sodium bicarbonate 70 mg/5 mL. Contains 1.8 mmol Na^+/5 mL. Net price 500 mL = £2.67
Dose 5–15 mL 4 times daily (after meals and at bedtime)

Gaviscon® Advance (R&C)
Tablets, sugar-free, sodium alginate 500 mg, potassium bicarbonate 100 mg. Contains 2.25 mmol Na^+, 1 mmol K^+/tablet. Net price 60-tab pack (peppermint-flavoured) = £3.24
Excipients include aspartame (section 9.4.1)
Dose ADULT and CHILD over 12 years, 1–2 tablets to be chewed after meals and at bedtime; CHILD 6–12 years, 1 tablet to be chewed after meals and at bedtime (under medical advice only)

Suspension, sugar-free, aniseed- or peppermint flavour, sodium alginate 500 mg, potassium bicarbonate 100 mg/5 mL. Contains 2.3 mmol Na^+, 1 mmol K^+/5 mL, net price 250 mL = £2.70, 500 mL = £5.40
Dose ADULT and CHILD over 12 years, 5–10 mL after meals and at bedtime; CHILD 2–12 years, 2.5–5 mL after meals and at bedtime (under medical advice only)

Gaviscon® Infant (R&C)
Oral powder, sugar-free, sodium alginate 225 mg, magnesium alginate 87.5 mg, with colloidal silica and mannitol/dose (half dual-sachet). Contains 0.92 mmol Na^+/dose. Net price 15 dual-sachets (30 doses) = £2.46
Dose INFANT body-weight under 4.5 kg, 1 'dose' (half dual-sachet) mixed with feeds (or water in breast-fed infants) when required (max. 6 times in 24 hours); body-weight over 4.5 kg, 2 'doses' (1 dual-sachet) mixed with feeds (or water in breast-fed infants) when required (max. 6 times in 24 hours); CHILD 2 'doses' (1 dual-sachet) in water after each meal (max. 6 times in 24 hours)
Note Not to be used in preterm neonates, or where excessive water loss likely (e.g. fever, diarrhoea, vomiting, high room temperature), or if intestinal obstruction. Not to be used with other preparations containing thickening agents
Important Each half of the dual-sachet is identified as 'one dose'. To avoid errors prescribe as 'dual-sachet' with directions in terms of 'dose'

Peptac® (IVAX)
Suspension, sugar-free, sodium bicarbonate 133.5 mg, sodium alginate 250 mg, calcium carbonate 80 mg/5 mL. Contains 3.1 mmol Na^+/5mL. Net price 500 mL (aniseed- or peppermint-flavoured) = £2.16
Dose 10–20 mL after meals and at bedtime; CHILD 6–12 years 5–10 mL after meals and at bedtime

Rennie® Duo (Roche Consumer Health)
Suspension, sugar-free, calcium carbonate 600 mg, magnesium carbonate 70 mg, sodium alginate 150 mg/5 mL. Contains 2.6 mmol Na^+/5 mL. Net price 500 mL (mint flavour) = £2.67
Dose ADULT and CHILD over 12 years, 10 mL after meals and at bedtime; an additional 10 mL may be taken between doses for heartburn if necessary, max. 80 mL daily
Excipients include propylene glycol

Topal® (Fabre)
Tablets, alginic acid 200 mg, dried aluminium hydroxide 30 mg, light magnesium carbonate 40 mg with lactose 220 mg, sucrose 880 mg, sodium bicarbonate 40 mg (low Na^+). Net price 42-tab pack = £1.67
Cautions diabetes mellitus (high sugar content)
Dose 1–3 tablets chewed 4 times daily (after meals and at bedtime); CHILD half adult dose

1.2 Antispasmodics and other drugs altering gut motility

Drugs in this section include antimuscarinic compounds and drugs believed to be direct relaxants of intestinal smooth muscle. The smooth muscle relaxant properties of antimuscarinic and other antispasmodic drugs may be useful in *irritable bowel syndrome* and in *diverticular disease*.

The dopamine-receptor antagonists metoclopramide and domperidone (section 4.6) stimulate transit in the gut.

Antimuscarinics

Antimuscarinics (formerly termed 'anticholinergics') reduce intestinal motility. They are used for the management of *irritable bowel syndrome* and *diverticular disease*. However, their value has not been established and response varies. Other indications for antimuscarinic drugs include arrhythmias (section 2.3.1), asthma and airways disease (section 3.1.2), motion sickness (section 4.6), parkinsonism (section 4.9.2), urinary incontinence (section 7.4.2), mydriasis and cycloplegia (section 11.5), premedication (section 15.1.3) and as an antidote to organophosphorus poisoning (p. 36).

Antimuscarinics that are used for gastro-intestinal smooth muscle spasm include the tertiary amines **atropine sulphate** and **dicycloverine hydrochloride** (dicyclomine hydrochloride) and the quaternary ammonium compounds **propantheline bromide** and **hyoscine butylbromide**. The quaternary ammonium compounds are less lipid soluble than atropine and are less likely to cross the blood–brain barrier; they are also less well absorbed from the gastro-intestinal tract.

Dicycloverine hydrochloride has a much less marked antimuscarinic action than atropine and may also have some direct action on smooth muscle. Hyoscine butylbromide is advocated as a gastro-intestinal antispasmodic, but it is poorly absorbed; the injection is useful in endoscopy and radiology. Atropine and the belladonna alkaloids are outmoded treatments, any clinical virtues being outweighed by atropinic side-effects.

Cautions Antimuscarinics should be used with caution in Down's syndrome, in children and in the elderly; they should also be used with caution in gastro-oesophageal reflux disease, diarrhoea, ulcerative colitis, acute myocardial infarction, hypertension, conditions characterised by tachycardia (including hyperthyroidism, cardiac insufficiency, cardiac surgery), pyrexia, pregnancy (Appendix 4) and breast-feeding (Appendix 5), and in individuals susceptible to angle-closure glaucoma. **Interactions**: Appendix 1 (antimuscarinics).

Contra-indications Antimuscarinics are contra-indicated in myasthenia gravis (but may be used to decrease muscarinic side-effects of anticholinesterases—section 10.2.1), paralytic ileus, pyloric stenosis and prostatic enlargement.

Side-effects Side-effects of antimuscarinics include constipation, transient bradycardia (followed by tachycardia, palpitation and arrhythmias), reduced bronchial secretions, urinary urgency and retention, dilatation of the pupils with loss of accommodation, photophobia, dry mouth, flushing and dryness of the skin. Side-effects that occur occasionally include confusion (particularly in the elderly), nausea, vomiting, and giddiness; very rarely angle-closure glaucoma may occur.

ATROPINE SULPHATE

Indications symptomatic relief of gastro-intestinal disorders characterised by smooth muscle spasm; mydriasis and cycloplegia (section 11.5); pre-medication (section 15.1.3); see also notes above
Cautions see notes above
Contra-indications see notes above
Side-effects see notes above
Dose
- 0.6–1.2 mg at night

Atropine (Non-proprietary) PoM
Tablets, atropine sulphate 600 micrograms. Net price 28-tab pack = £11.41
Available from CP

DICYCLOVERINE HYDROCHLORIDE
(Dicyclomine hydrochloride)

Indications symptomatic relief of gastro-intestinal disorders characterised by smooth muscle spasm
Cautions see notes above
Contra-indications see notes above; infants under 6 months
Side-effects see notes above
Dose
- 10–20 mg 3 times daily; INFANT 6–24 months 5–10 mg up to 3–4 times daily, 15 minutes before feeds; CHILD 2–12 years 10 mg 3 times daily

Merbentyl® (Sanofi-Aventis) PoM
Tablets, dicycloverine hydrochloride 10 mg, net price 20 = £1.01; 20 mg (*Merbentyl 20®*), 84-tab pack = £8.47
Syrup, dicycloverine hydrochloride 10 mg/5 mL, net price 120 mL = £1.84
Note Dicycloverine hydrochloride can be sold to the public provided that max. single dose is 10 mg and max. daily dose is 60 mg

Compound preparations

Kolanticon® (Peckforton)
Gel, sugar-free, dicycloverine hydrochloride 2.5 mg, dried aluminium hydroxide 200 mg, light magnesium oxide 100 mg, simeticone 20 mg/5 mL, net price 200 mL = £2.21, 500 mL = £2.79
Dose ADULT and CHILD over 12 years, 10–20 mL every 4 hours when required

HYOSCINE BUTYLBROMIDE

Indications symptomatic relief of gastro-intestinal or genito-urinary disorders characterised by smooth muscle spasm; bowel colic and excessive respiratory secretions (see Prescribing in Palliative Care, p. 18)

Cautions see notes above

Contra-indications see notes above

Side-effects see notes above

Dose

- By mouth (but poorly absorbed, see notes above), smooth muscle spasm, 20 mg 4 times daily; CHILD 6–12 years, 10 mg 3 times daily

  Irritable bowel syndrome, 10 mg 3 times daily, increased if required up to 20 mg 4 times daily
- By intramuscular *or* slow intravenous injection, acute spasm and spasm in diagnostic procedures, 20 mg repeated after 30 minutes if necessary (may be repeated more frequently in endoscopy), max. 100 mg daily; CHILD 2–18 years, see *BNF for Children*

Buscopan® (Boehringer Ingelheim) PoM

Tablets, coated, hyoscine butylbromide 10 mg. Net price 56-tab pack = £2.59

Note Hyoscine butylbromide tablets can be sold to the public provided single dose does not exceed 20 mg, daily dose does not exceed 80 mg, and pack does not contain a total of more than 240 mg

Injection, hyoscine butylbromide 20 mg/mL. Net price 1-mL amp = 20p

PROPANTHELINE BROMIDE

Indications symptomatic relief of gastro-intestinal disorders characterised by smooth muscle spasm; urinary frequency (section 7.4.2); gustatory sweating (section 6.1.5)

Cautions see notes above; also renal impairment

Contra-indications see notes above

Side-effects see notes above

Dose

- 15 mg 3 times daily at least 1 hour before meals and 30 mg at night, max. 120 mg daily; CHILD not recommended

Pro-Banthine® (Concord) PoM

Tablets, pink, s/c, propantheline bromide 15 mg, net price 112-tab pack = £15.32. Label: 23

Other antispasmodics

Alverine, **mebeverine**, and **peppermint oil** are believed to be direct relaxants of intestinal smooth muscle and may relieve pain in *irritable bowel syndrome* and *diverticular disease*. They have no serious adverse effects but, like all antispasmodics, should be avoided in paralytic ileus. Peppermint oil occasionally causes heartburn.

ALVERINE CITRATE

Indications adjunct in gastro-intestinal disorders characterised by smooth muscle spasm; dysmenorrhoea

Cautions pregnancy; breast-feeding (Appendix 5)

Contra-indications paralytic ileus; when combined with sterculia, intestinal obstruction, faecal impaction, colonic atony

Side-effects nausea; headache, dizziness; pruritus, rash; also reported, hepatitis

Dose

- 60–120 mg 1–3 times daily; CHILD under 12 years not recommended

Spasmonal® (Norgine)

Capsules, alverine citrate 60mg (blue/grey), net price 100-cap pack = £11.95; 120mg (*Spasmonal® Forte*, blue/grey), 60-cap pack = £13.80

MEBEVERINE HYDROCHLORIDE

Indications adjunct in gastro-intestinal disorders characterised by smooth muscle spasm

Cautions pregnancy (Appendix 4); avoid in porphyria (section 9.8.2.)

Contra-indications paralytic ileus

Side-effects rarely allergic reactions (including rash, urticaria, angioedema)

Dose

- ADULT and CHILD over 10 years 135–150 mg 3 times daily preferably 20 minutes before meals; CHILD under 10 years see *BNF for Children*

[1]**Mebeverine Hydrochloride** (Non-proprietary) PoM

Tablets, mebeverine hydrochloride 135 mg, net price 20 = £1.87

Oral suspension, mebeverine hydrochloride (as mebeverine embonate) 50 mg/5 mL, net price 300 mL = £107.00

1. Mebeverine hydrochloride can be sold to the public for symptomatic relief of irritable bowel syndrome provided that max. single dose is 135 mg and max. daily dose is 405 mg; for uses other than symptomatic relief of irritable bowel syndrome provided that max. single dose is 100 mg and max. daily dose is 300 mg

Colofac® (Solvay) PoM

Tablets, s/c, mebeverine hydrochloride 135 mg. Net price 20 = £1.50

Modified release

Colofac® MR (Solvay) PoM

Capsules, m/r, mebeverine hydrochloride 200 mg, net price 60-cap pack = £6.67. Label: 25

Dose irritable bowel syndrome, 1 capsule twice daily preferably 20 minutes before meals; CHILD 12–18 years, see *BNF for Children*

Compound preparations

[1]**Fybogel® Mebeverine** (R&C) PoM

Granules, buff, effervescent, ispaghula husk 3.5 g, mebeverine hydrochloride 135 mg/sachet. Contains 2.5 mmol K^+/sachet, net price 10 sachets = £2.50. Label: 13, 22, counselling, see below

Excipients include aspartame (section 9.4.1)

Dose irritable bowel syndrome, ADULT and CHILD over 12 years, 1 sachet in water, morning and evening 30 minutes before food; an additional sachet may also be taken before the midday meal if necessary

Counselling Preparations that swell in contact with liquid should always be carefully swallowed with water and should not be taken immediately before going to bed

1. 10-sachet pack can be sold to the public

Gastro-intestinal system 1

PEPPERMINT OIL

Indications relief of abdominal colic and distension, particularly in irritable bowel syndrome

Cautions sensitivity to menthol

Side-effects heartburn, perianal irritation; rarely, allergic reactions (including rash, headache, bradycardia, muscle tremor, ataxia)

Local irritation Capsules should not be broken or chewed because peppermint oil may irritate mouth or oesophagus

Dose

- See preparations

Colpermin® (Pharmacia)

Capsules, m/r, e/c, light blue/dark blue, blue band, peppermint oil 0.2 mL. Net price 100-cap pack = £12.05. Label: 5, 22, 25

Excipients include arachis (peanut) oil

Dose ADULT and CHILD over 15 years, 1–2 capsules, swallowed whole with water, 3 times daily for up to 2–3 months if necessary

Mintec® (Shire)

Capsules, e/c, green/ivory, peppermint oil 0.2 mL. Net price 84-cap pack = £7.04. Label: 5, 22, 25

Dose ADULT over 18 years, 1–2 capsules swallowed whole with water, 3 times daily before meals for up to 2–3 months if necessary

Motility stimulants

Metoclopramide and **domperidone** (section 4.6) are dopamine antagonists which stimulate gastric emptying and small intestinal transit, and enhance the strength of oesophageal sphincter contraction. They are used in some patients with *functional dyspepsia* that has not responded to a proton pump inhibitor or a H_2-receptor antagonist. Metoclopramide is also used to speed the transit of barium during intestinal follow-through examination, and as accessory treatment for *gastro-oesophageal reflux disease*. For the management of gastroparesis in patients with diabetes, see section 6.1.5. Metoclopramide and domperidone are useful in non-specific and in cytotoxic-induced nausea and vomiting. Metoclopramide and occasionally domperidone may induce an acute dystonic reaction, particularly in young women and children—for further details of this and other side-effects, see section 4.6.

1.3 Antisecretory drugs and mucosal protectants

1.3.1 H2-receptor antagonists
1.3.2 Selective antimuscarinics
1.3.3 Chelates and complexes
1.3.4 Prostaglandin analogues
1.3.5 Proton pump inhibitors

Peptic ulceration commonly involves the stomach, duodenum, and lower oesophagus; after gastric surgery it involves the gastro-enterostomy stoma.

Healing can be promoted by general measures, stopping smoking and taking antacids and by antisecretory drug treatment, but relapse is common when treatment ceases. Nearly all duodenal ulcers and most gastric ulcers not associated with NSAIDs are caused by *Helicobacter pylori*.

The management of *H. pylori* infection and of NSAID-associated ulcers is discussed below.

Helicobacter pylori infection

Eradication of *Helicobacter pylori* reduces recurrence of gastric and duodenal ulcers and the risk of bleeding associated with these ulcers. The presence of *H. pylori* should be confirmed before starting eradication treatment. Acid inhibition combined with antibacterial treatment is highly effective in the eradication of *H. pylori*; reinfection is rare. Antibiotic-induced colitis is an uncommon risk.

For initial treatment, a one-week triple-therapy regimen that comprises a proton pump inhibitor, clarithromycin, and *either* amoxicillin *or* metronidazole can be used. However, if a patient has been treated with metronidazole for other infections, a regimen containing a proton pump inhibitor, amoxicillin and clarithromycin is preferred for initial therapy. If a patient has been treated with clarithromycin for other infections, a regimen containing a proton pump inhibitor, amoxicillin and metronidazole is preferred for initial therapy. These regimens eradicate *H. pylori* in about 85% of cases. There is usually no need to continue antisecretory treatment (with a proton pump inhibitor or H_2-receptor antagonist) unless the ulcer is large, or complicated by haemorrhage or perforation. Treatment failure usually indicates antibacterial resistance or poor compliance. Resistance to amoxicillin is rare. However, resistance to clarithromycin and metronidazole is common and can develop during treatment.

Two-week triple-therapy regimens offer the possibility of higher eradication rates compared to one-week regimens, but adverse effects are common and poor compliance is likely to offset any possible gain.

Two-week dual-therapy regimens using a proton pump inhibitor and a single antibacterial are licensed, but produce low rates of *H. pylori* eradication and are **not** recommended.

Tinidazole is also used occasionally for *H. pylori* eradication; it should be combined with antisecretory drugs and other antibacterials.

A two-week regimen comprising a proton pump inhibitor *plus* tripotassium dicitratobismuthate (section 1.3.3), *plus* tetracycline 500 mg four times daily, *plus* metronidazole 400 mg three times daily can be used for eradication failure. Alternatively, the patient can be referred for endoscopy and treatment based on the results of culture and sensitivity testing.

For the role of *H. pylori* eradication therapy in patients starting or taking a NSAID, see NSAID-associated Ulcers, p. 44. For *H. pylori* eradication in patients with dyspepsia, see also section 1.1.

1 Gastro-intestinal system

Recommended regimens for *Helicobacter pylori* eradication in adults

Acid suppressant	Antibacterial			Price for 7-day course
	Amoxicillin	Clarithromycin	Metronidazole	
Esomeprazole 20 mg twice daily	1 g twice daily	500 mg twice daily	—	£17.81
	—	250 mg twice daily	400 mg twice daily	£13.61
Lansoprazole 30 mg twice daily	1 g twice daily	500 mg twice daily	—	£10.93
	1 g twice daily	—	400 mg twice daily	£4.41
	—	250 mg twice daily	400 mg twice daily	£6.73
Omeprazole 20 mg twice daily	1 g twice daily	500 mg twice daily	—	£9.58
	500 mg 3 times daily	—	400 mg 3 times daily	£3.00
	—	250 mg twice daily	400 mg twice daily	£5.38
Pantoprazole 40 mg twice daily	1 g twice daily	500 mg twice daily	—	£19.26
	—	250 mg twice daily	400 mg twice daily	£15.06
Rabeprazole 20 mg twice daily	1 g twice daily	500 mg twice daily	—	£19.14
	—	250 mg twice daily	400 mg twice daily	£14.94

Test for *Helicobacter pylori*

^{13}C-Urea breath test kits are available for the diagnosis of gastro-duodenal infection with *Helicobacter pylori*. The test involves collection of breath samples before and after ingestion of an oral solution of ^{13}C-urea; the samples are sent for analysis by an appropriate laboratory. The test should not be performed within 4 weeks of treatment with an antibacterial or within 2 weeks of treatment with an antisecretory drug. A specific ^{13}C-urea breath test kit for children is available (*Helicobacter Test INFAI for children of the age 3–11®*). However, the appropriateness of testing for *H.pylori* infection in children has not been established.

diabact UBT® (MDE) PoM

Tablets, ^{13}C-urea 50 mg, net price 1 kit (including 1 tablet, 4 breath-sample containers, straws) = £18.95 (analysis included), 10-kit pack (hosp. only) = £74.50 (analysis not included)

Helicobacter Test INFAI® (Infai) PoM

Oral powder, ^{13}C-urea 75 mg, net price 1 kit (including 4 breath-sample containers, straws) = £19.20 (spectrometric analysis included), 1 kit (including 2 breath bags) = £14.20 (spectroscopic analysis not included), 50-test set = £855.00 (spectrometric analysis included); 45 mg (*Helicobacter Test INFAI for children of the age 3–11®*), 1 kit (including 4 breath-sample containers, straws) = £19.20 (spectrometric analysis included)

Pylobactell® (Torbet) PoM

Soluble tablets, ^{13}C-urea 100 mg, net price 1 kit (including 6 breath-sample containers, 30-mL mixing and administration vial, straws) = £20.75 (analysis included)

NSAID-associated ulcers

Gastro-intestinal bleeding and ulceration can occur with NSAID use (section 10.1.1). Wherever possible, NSAIDs should be **withdrawn** if an ulcer occurs.

In those at risk of ulceration a proton pump inhibitor, an H_2-receptor antagonist such as ranitidine given at twice the usual dose, or misoprostol may be considered for protection against NSAID-associated gastric and duodenal ulcers; colic and diarrhoea may limit the dose of misoprostol.

NSAID use and *H. pylori* infection are independent risk factors for gastro-intestinal bleeding and ulceration. In patients already taking a NSAID, eradication of *H. pylori* is unlikely to reduce the risk of NSAID-induced bleeding or ulceration. However, in patients about to start long-term NSAID treatment who are *H. pylori* positive and have dyspepsia or a history of gastric or duodenal ulcer, eradication of *H. pylori* may reduce the overall risk of ulceration.

If the *NSAID can be discontinued* in a patient who has developed an ulcer, a proton pump inhibitor usually produces the most rapid healing, but the ulcer can be treated with an H_2-receptor antagonist or misoprostol.

If *NSAID treatment needs to continue*, the following options are suitable:

- Treat ulcer with a proton pump inhibitor and on healing continue the proton pump inhibitor (dose not normally reduced because asymptomatic ulcer recurrence may occur);
- Treat ulcer with a proton pump inhibitor and on healing switch to misoprostol for maintenance therapy (colic and diarrhoea may limit the dose of misoprostol);
- Treat ulcer with a proton pump inhibitor and switch NSAID to a cyclo-oxygenase-2 selective inhibitor, but see NSAIDs and Cardiovascular Events, p. 536; on healing, continuing the proton pump inhibitor in patients with a history of upper gastro-intestinal bleeding provides further protection against recurrence.

1.3.1 H_2-receptor antagonists

Histamine H_2-receptor antagonists heal *gastric and duodenal ulcers* by reducing gastric acid output as a result of histamine H_2-receptor blockade; they are also used to relieve symptoms of *gastro-oesophageal reflux disease* (section 1.1). High doses of H_2-receptor antagonists have been used in *Zollinger–Ellison syndrome*, but a proton pump inhibitor (section 1.3.5) is preferred.

Maintenance treatment with low doses for the prevention of peptic ulcer disease has largely been replaced in *Helicobacter pylori* positive patients by eradication regimens (section 1.3).

H_2-receptor antagonists are used for the treatment of *functional dyspepsia* (section 1.1). Treatment of *uninvestigated dyspepsia* with H_2-receptor antagonists used regularly or on an intermittent basis, may be acceptable in younger patients but care is required in older people because of the possibility of gastric cancer in these patients.

H_2-receptor antagonist therapy can promote healing of *NSAID-associated ulcers* (particularly duodenal) (section 1.3).

Treatment with a H_2-receptor antagonist has not been shown to be beneficial in haematemesis and melaena, but prophylactic use reduces the frequency of bleeding from *gastroduodenal erosions in hepatic coma*, and possibly in other conditions requiring intensive care. H_2-receptor antagonists also reduce the risk of *acid aspiration* in obstetric patients at delivery (Mendelson's syndrome).

Cautions H_2-receptor antagonists should be used with caution in renal impairment (Appendix 3), pregnancy (Appendix 4), and in breast-feeding (Appendix 5). H_2-receptor antagonists might mask symptoms of gastric cancer; particular care is required in those whose symptoms change and in those who are middle-aged or older.

Side-effects Side-effects of the H_2-receptor antagonists include diarrhoea and other gastro-intestinal disturbances, altered liver function tests (rarely liver damage), headache, dizziness, rash, and tiredness. Rare side-effects include acute pancreatitis, bradycardia, AV block, confusion, depression, and hallucinations particularly in the elderly or the very ill, hypersensitivity reactions (including fever, arthralgia, myalgia, anaphylaxis), blood disorders (including agranulocytosis, leucopenia, pancytopenia, thrombocytopenia), and skin reactions (including erythema multiforme and toxic epidermal necrolysis). There have been occasional reports of gynaecomastia and impotence.

Interactions Cimetidine retards oxidative hepatic drug metabolism by binding to microsomal cytochrome P450. It should be avoided in patients stabilised on warfarin, phenytoin, and theophylline (or aminophylline), but other interactions (see **Appendix** 1) may be of less clinical relevance. Famotidine, nizatidine, and ranitidine do not share the drug metabolism inhibitory properties of cimetidine.

CIMETIDINE

Indications benign gastric and duodenal ulceration, stomal ulcer, reflux oesophagitis, Zollinger–Ellison syndrome, other conditions where gastric acid reduction is beneficial (see notes above and section 1.9.4)

Cautions see notes above; also preferably avoid intravenous injection (use intravenous infusion) particularly in high dosage and in cardiovascular impairment (risk of arrhythmias); hepatic impairment (Appendix 2); **interactions:** Appendix 1 (histamine H_2-antagonists) and notes above

Side-effects see notes above; also alopecia; very rarely tachycardia, interstitial nephritis

Dose

- By mouth, 400 mg twice daily (with breakfast and at night) *or* 800 mg at night (benign gastric and duodenal ulceration) for at least 4 weeks (6 weeks in gastric ulceration, 8 weeks in NSAID-associated ulceration); when necessary the dose may be increased to 400 mg 4 times daily; INFANT under 1 year 20 mg/kg daily in divided doses has been used; CHILD 1–12 years, 25–30 mg/kg daily in divided doses; max. 400 mg 4 times daily

  Maintenance, 400 mg at night *or* 400 mg morning and night

  Reflux oesophagitis, 400 mg 4 times daily for 4–8 weeks

  Zollinger–Ellison syndrome (but see notes above), 400 mg 4 times daily or occasionally more (max. 2.4 g daily)

  Prophylaxis of stress ulceration, 200–400 mg every 4–6 hours

  Gastric acid reduction (prophylaxis of acid aspiration; do not use syrup), obstetrics 400 mg at start of labour, then up to 400 mg every 4 hours if required (max. 2.4 g daily); surgical procedures 400 mg 90–120 minutes before induction of general anaesthesia

  Short-bowel syndrome, 400 mg twice daily (with breakfast and at bedtime) adjusted according to response

  To reduce degradation of pancreatic enzyme supplements, 0.8–1.6 g daily in 4 divided doses 1–1½ hours before meals
- By intramuscular injection, 200 mg every 4–6 hours
- By slow intravenous injection (but see Cautions above) over at least 5 minutes, 200 mg; may be repeated every 4–6 hours; if larger dose needed or if cardiovascular impairment, dilute and give injection over at least 10 minutes (infusion preferable); max. 2.4 g daily
- By intravenous infusion, 200–400 mg (may be repeated every 4–6 hours) *or* by continuous intravenous infusion usually at a rate of 50–100 mg/hour over 24 hours, max. 2.4 g daily; INFANT under 1 year, by slow intravenous injection *or* by intravenous infusion, 20 mg/kg daily in divided doses has been used; CHILD 1–12 years, 25–30 mg/kg daily in divided doses

[1]**Cimetidine** (Non-proprietary) PoM

Tablets, cimetidine 200 mg, net price 60-tab pack = £1.26; 400 mg, 60-tab pack = £1.54; 800 mg, 30-tab pack = £1.91

Brands include *Peptimax*®

Oral solution, cimetidine 200 mg/5 mL, net price 300 mL = £14.24

Excipients may include propylene glycol (see Excipients, p. 2)

1. Cimetidine can be sold to the public for adults and children over 16 years (provided packs do not contain more than 2 weeks' supply) for the short-term symptomatic relief of heartburn, dyspepsia, and hyperacidity (max. single dose 200 mg, max. daily dose 800 mg), and for the prophylactic management of nocturnal heartburn (single night-time dose 100 mg)

Tagamet® (Chemidex) PoM
Tablets, all green, f/c, cimetidine 200 mg, net price 120-tab pack = £19.58; 400 mg, 60-tab pack = £22.62; 800 mg, 30-tab pack = £22.62

Syrup, orange, cimetidine 200 mg/5 mL. Net price 600 mL = £28.49
Excipients include propylene glycol 10%, (see Excipients, p. 2)

Tagamet® (GSK) PoM
Injection, cimetidine 100 mg/mL. Net price 2-mL amp = 33p

FAMOTIDINE

Indications see under Dose
Cautions see notes above; **interactions:** Appendix 1 (histamine H_2-antagonists) and notes above
Side-effects see notes above; also very rarely anxiety, anorexia, dry mouth, cholestatic jaundice
Dose
- Benign gastric and duodenal ulceration, treatment, 40 mg at night for 4–8 weeks; maintenance (duodenal ulceration), 20 mg at night
- Reflux oesophagitis, 20–40 mg twice daily for 6–12 weeks; maintenance, 20 mg twice daily
- Zollinger–Ellison syndrome (but see notes above), 20 mg every 6 hours (higher dose in those who have previously been receiving another H_2-receptor antagonist); up to 800 mg daily in divided doses has been used
- CHILD not recommended

[1]Famotidine (Non-proprietary) PoM
Tablets, famotidine 20 mg, net price 28-tab pack = £6.45; 40 mg, 28-tab pack = £7.54

1. Famotidine can be sold to the public for adults and children over 16 years (provided packs do not contain more than 2 weeks' supply) for the short-term symptomatic relief of heartburn, dyspepsia, and hyperacidity, and for the prevention of these symptoms when associated with consumption of food or drink including when they cause sleep disturbance (max. single dose 10 mg, max. daily dose 20 mg)

Pepcid® (MSD) PoM
Tablets, f/c, famotidine 20 mg (beige), net price 28-tab pack = £13.37; 40 mg (brown), 28-tab pack = £25.40

NIZATIDINE

Indications see under Dose
Cautions see notes above; also avoid rapid intravenous injection (risk of arrhythmias and postural hypotension); hepatic impairment (Appendix 2); **interactions:** Appendix 1 (histamine H_2-antagonists) and notes above
Side-effects see notes above; also sweating; rarely hyperuricaemia
Dose
- By mouth, benign gastric, duodenal or NSAID-associated ulceration, treatment, 300 mg in the evening *or* 150 mg twice daily for 4–8 weeks; maintenance, 150 mg at night

  Gastro-oesophageal reflux disease, 150–300 mg twice daily for up to 12 weeks
- By intravenous infusion, for short-term use in peptic ulcer as alternative to oral route (for hospital inpatients), by intermittent intravenous infusion over 15 minutes, 100 mg 3 times daily, *or* by continuous intravenous infusion, 10 mg/hour; max. 480 mg daily
- CHILD not recommended

[1]Nizatidine (Non-proprietary) PoM
Capsules, nizatidine 150 mg, net price 30-cap pack = £5.57; 300 mg, 30-cap pack = £4.91

1. Nizatidine can be sold to the public for the prevention and treatment of symptoms of food-related heartburn and meal-induced indigestion in adults and children over 16 years; max. single dose 75 mg, max. daily dose 150 mg for max. 14 days

Axid® (Flynn) PoM
Capsules, nizatidine 150 mg (pale yellow/dark yellow), net price 28-cap pack (hosp. only) = £6.87, 30-cap pack = £7.97; 300 mg (pale yellow/brown), 30-cap pack = £15.80

Injection, nizatidine 25 mg/mL. For dilution and use as an intravenous infusion. Net price 4-mL amp = £1.14

RANITIDINE

Indications see under Dose, other conditions where reduction of gastric acidity is beneficial (see notes above and section 1.9.4)
Cautions see notes above; also porphyria; **interactions:** Appendix 1 (histamine H_2-antagonists) and notes above
Side-effects see notes above; also *rarely* tachycardia, agitation, visual disturbances, alopecia, vasculitis; *very rarely* interstitial nephritis
Dose
- By mouth, benign gastric and duodenal ulceration, chronic episodic dyspepsia, ADULT and CHILD over 12 years, 150 mg twice daily *or* 300 mg at night for 4–8 weeks in benign gastric and duodenal ulceration, up to 6 weeks in chronic episodic dyspepsia, and up to 8 weeks in NSAID-associated ulceration (in duodenal ulcer 300 mg can be given twice daily for 4 weeks to achieve a higher healing rate); CHILD 3–12 years, (benign gastric and duodenal ulceration) 2–4 mg/kg (max. 150 mg) twice daily for 4–8 weeks

  Prophylaxis of NSAID-associated gastric or duodenal ulcer [unlicensed dose], ADULT and CHILD over 12 years, 300 mg twice daily

  Gastro-oesophageal reflux disease, ADULT and CHILD over 12 years, 150 mg twice daily *or* 300 mg at night for up to 8 weeks or if necessary 12 weeks (moderate to severe, 600 mg daily in 2–4 divided doses for up to 12 weeks); long-term treatment of healed gastro-oesophageal reflux disease, 150 mg twice daily; CHILD 3–12 years, 2.5–5 mg/kg (max. 300 mg) twice daily

  Zollinger–Ellison syndrome (but see notes above), ADULT and CHILD over 12 years, 150 mg 3 times daily; doses up to 6 g daily in divided doses have been used

  Gastric acid reduction (prophylaxis of acid aspiration) in obstetrics, ADULT and CHILD over 12 years, by mouth, 150 mg at onset of labour, then every 6 hours; surgical procedures, by intramuscular *or* slow intravenous injection, 50 mg 45–60 minutes before induction of anaesthesia (intravenous injection diluted to 20 mL and given over at least 2 minutes), or by mouth, 150 mg 2 hours before induction of anaesthesia and also when possible on the preceding evening
- By intramuscular injection, 50 mg every 6–8 hours

1 Gastro-intestinal system

- By slow intravenous injection, ADULT and CHILD over 12 years, 50 mg diluted to 20 mL and given over at least 2 minutes; may be repeated every 6–8 hours
- By intravenous infusion, 25 mg/hour for 2 hours; may be repeated every 6–8 hours

  Prophylaxis of stress ulceration, ADULT and CHILD over 12 years, initial slow intravenous injection of 50 mg (as above) then continuous infusion, 125–250 micrograms/kg/hour (may be followed by 150 mg twice daily by mouth when oral feeding commences)

[1]**Ranitidine** (Non-proprietary) PoM

Tablets, ranitidine (as hydrochloride) 150 mg, net price 60-tab pack = £1.03; 300 mg, 30-tab pack = £1.74

Brands include *Ranitic®*, *Rantec®*,

Effervescent tablets, ranitidine (as hydrochloride) 150 mg, net price 60-tab pack = £18.59; 300 mg, 30-tab pack = £18.28. Label: 13

Excipients may include sodium (check with supplier)

Oral solution, ranitidine (as hydrochloride) 75 mg/5 mL, net price 300 mL = £21.47

Excipients may include alcohol (check with supplier)

1. Ranitidine can be sold to the public for adults and children over 16 years (provided packs do not contain more than 2 weeks' supply) for the short-term symptomatic relief of heartburn, dyspepsia, and hyperacidity, and for the prevention of these symptoms when associated with consumption of food or drink (max. single dose 75 mg, max. daily dose 300 mg)

Zantac® (GSK) PoM

Tablets, f/c, ranitidine (as hydrochloride) 150 mg, net price 60-tab pack = £1.30; 300 mg, 30-tab pack = £1.30

Effervescent tablets, pale yellow, ranitidine (as hydrochloride) 150 mg (contains 14.3 mmol Na^+/tablet), net price 60-tab pack = £25.94; 300 mg (contains 20.8 mmol Na^+/tablet), 30-tab pack = £25.51. Label: 13

Excipients include aspartame (section 9.4.1)

Syrup, sugar-free, ranitidine (as hydrochloride) 75 mg/5 mL. Net price 300 mL = £20.76

Excipients include alcohol 8%

Injection, ranitidine (as hydrochloride) 25 mg/mL. Net price 2-mL amp = 60p

1.3.2 Selective antimuscarinics

Pirenzepine is a selective antimuscarinic drug which was used for the treatment of gastric and duodenal ulcers. It has been discontinued.

1.3.3 Chelates and complexes

Tripotassium dicitratobismuthate is a bismuth chelate effective in healing gastric and duodenal ulcers. For the role of tripotassium dicitratobismuthate in a *Helicobacter pylori* eradication regimen for those who have not responded to first-line regimens, see section 1.3.

The bismuth content of tripotassium dicitratobismuthate is low but absorption has been reported; encephalopathy (described with older high-dose bismuth preparations) has not been reported.

Sucralfate may act by protecting the mucosa from acid-pepsin attack in gastric and duodenal ulcers. It is a complex of aluminium hydroxide and sulphated sucrose but has minimal antacid properties. It should be used with caution in patients under intensive care (**important:** reports of bezoar formation, see CSM advice below)

TRIPOTASSIUM DICITRATOBISMUTHATE

Indications benign gastric and duodenal ulceration; see also *Helicobacter pylori* infection, section 1.3

Cautions see notes above; **interactions:** Appendix 1 (tripotassium dicitratobismuthate)

Contra-indications renal impairment (avoid if creatinine clearance less than 10 mL/minute); pregnancy (Appendix 4)

Side-effects may darken tongue and blacken faeces; nausea, vomiting, diarrhoea, constipation, rash, and pruritus reported

De-Noltab® (Astellas)

Tablets, f/c, tripotassium dicitratobismuthate 120 mg. Contains 2 mmol K^+/tablet. Net price 112-tab pack = £7.27. Counselling, see below

Dose 2 tablets twice daily *or* 1 tablet 4 times daily; taken for 28 days followed by further 28 days if necessary; maintenance not indicated but course may be repeated after interval of 1 month; CHILD not recommended

Counselling To be swallowed with half a glass of water; twice-daily dosage to be taken 30 minutes before breakfast and main evening meal; four-times-daily dosage to be taken as follows: one dose 30 minutes before breakfast, midday meal and main evening meal, and one dose 2 hours after main evening meal; milk should not be drunk by itself during treatment but small quantities may be taken in tea or coffee or on cereal; antacids should not be taken half an hour before or after a dose; may darken tongue and blacken faeces

SUCRALFATE

Indications see under Dose

Cautions renal impairment (Appendix 3); pregnancy and breast-feeding; administration of sucralfate and enteral feeds should be separated by 1 hour; **interactions:** Appendix 1 (sucralfate)

Bezoar formation Following reports of bezoar formation associated with sucralfate, the CSM has advised caution in seriously ill patients, especially those receiving concomitant enteral feeds or those with predisposing conditions such as delayed gastric emptying

Side-effects constipation, *less frequently* diarrhoea, nausea, indigestion, flatulence, gastric discomfort, back pain, dizziness, headache, drowsiness, bezoar formation (see above), dry mouth and rash

Dose

- Benign gastric and duodenal ulceration and chronic gastritis, ADULT and CHILD over 15 years, 2 g twice daily (on rising and at bedtime) *or* 1 g 4 times daily 1 hour before meals and at bedtime, taken for 4–6 weeks or in resistant cases up to 12 weeks; max. 8 g daily
- Prophylaxis of stress ulceration, ADULT and CHILD over 15 years, 1 g 6 times daily; max. 8 g daily
- CHILD under 15 years, see *BNF for Children*

Antepsin® (Chugai) PoM

Tablets, scored, sucralfate 1 g, net price 50-tab pack = £4.81. Label: 5

Note Crushed tablets may be dispersed in water

Suspension, sucralfate, 1 g/5 mL, net price 250 mL (aniseed- and caramel-flavoured) = £4.81. Label: 5

1.3.4 Prostaglandin analogues

Misoprostol, a synthetic prostaglandin analogue has antisecretory and protective properties, promoting healing of *gastric and duodenal ulcers*. It can prevent NSAID-associated ulcers, its use being most appropriate for the frail or very elderly from whom NSAIDs cannot be withdrawn.

For comment on the use of misoprostol to induce abortion or labour [unlicensed indications], see section 7.1.1.

MISOPROSTOL

Indications see notes above and under Dose

Cautions conditions where hypotension might precipitate severe complications (e.g. cerebrovascular disease, cardiovascular disease)

Contra-indications pregnancy or planning pregnancy (Appendix 4), (increases uterine tone)—**important:** women of childbearing age, see also below, and breast-feeding (Appendix 5)

Women of childbearing age Manufacturer advises that misoprostol should not be used in women of childbearing age unless the patient requires non-steroidal anti-inflammatory (NSAID) therapy and is at high risk of complications from NSAID-induced ulceration. In such patients it is advised that misoprostol should only be used if the patient takes *effective contraceptive measures* and has been advised of the *risks of taking misoprostol if pregnant.*

Side-effects diarrhoea (may occasionally be severe and require withdrawal, reduced by giving single doses not exceeding 200 micrograms and by avoiding magnesium-containing antacids); also reported: abdominal pain, dyspepsia, flatulence, nausea and vomiting, abnormal vaginal bleeding (including intermenstrual bleeding, menorrhagia, and postmenopausal bleeding), rashes, dizziness

Dose

- Benign gastric and duodenal ulceration and NSAID-associated ulceration, 800 micrograms daily (in 2–4 divided doses) with breakfast (or main meals) and at bedtime; treatment should be continued for at least 4 weeks and may be continued for up to 8 weeks if required
- Prophylaxis of NSAID-induced gastric and duodenal ulcer, 200 micrograms 2–4 times daily taken with the NSAID
- CHILD not recommended

Cytotec® (Pharmacia) PoM

Tablets, scored, misoprostol 200 micrograms, net price 60-tab pack = £10.03, 140-tab pack = £23.40. Label: 21

With diclofenac or naproxen

Section 10.1.1

1.3.5 Proton pump inhibitors

Proton pump inhibitors inhibit gastric acid secretion by blocking the hydrogen-potassium adenosine triphosphatase enzyme system (the 'proton pump') of the gastric parietal cell. Proton pump inhibitors are effective short-term treatments for *gastric and duodenal ulcers*; they are also used in combination with antibacterials for the eradication of *Helicobacter pylori* (see p. 43 for specific regimens). In patients with peptic ulcer bleeding, treatment with a proton pump inhibitor reduces the risk of rebleeding and the need for surgery. Proton pump inhibitors can be used for the treatment of *dyspepsia* and *gastro-oesophageal reflux disease* (section 1.1).

Proton pump inhibitors are also used in the prevention and treatment of NSAID-associated ulcers (see p. 44). In patients who need to continue NSAID treatment after an ulcer has healed, the dose of proton pump inhibitor should normally not be reduced because asymptomatic ulcer deterioration may occur.

A proton pump inhibitor can be used to control excessive secretion of gastric acid in *Zollinger–Ellison syndrome*; high doses are often required.

Cautions Proton pump inhibitors should be used with caution in patients with liver disease (Appendix 2), in pregnancy (Appendix 4) and in breast-feeding (Appendix 5). Proton pump inhibitors may mask the symptoms of gastric cancer; particular care is required in those presenting with 'alarm features' (see p. 37), in such cases gastric malignancy should be ruled out before treatment.

Side-effects Side-effects of the proton pump inhibitors include gastro-intestinal disturbances (including nausea, vomiting, abdominal pain, flatulence, diarrhoea, constipation), headache, and dizziness. Less frequent side-effects include dry mouth, insomnia, drowsiness, malaise, blurred vision, rash, and pruritus. Other side-effects reported rarely or very rarely include taste disturbance, liver dysfunction, peripheral oedema, hypersensitivity reactions (including urticaria, angioedema, bronchospasm, anaphylaxis), photosensitivity, fever, sweating, depression, interstitial nephritis, blood disorders (including leucopenia, leucocytosis, pancytopenia, thrombocytopenia), arthralgia, myalgia and skin reactions (including Stevens-Johnson syndrome, toxic epidermal necrolysis, bullous eruption). Proton pump inhibitors, by decreasing gastric acidity, may increase the risk of gastro-intestinal infections.

ESOMEPRAZOLE

Indications see under Dose

Cautions see notes above; renal impairment (Appendix 3); **interactions:** Appendix 1 (proton pump inhibitors)

Side-effects see notes above; also reported, dermatitis

Dose

- By mouth duodenal ulcer associated with *Helicobacter pylori*, see eradication regimens on p. 43

  NSAID-associated gastric ulcer, ADULT over 18 years, 20 mg once daily for 4–8 weeks; prophylaxis in patients with an increased risk of gastroduodenal complications who require continued NSAID treatment, 20 mg daily

  Gastro-oesophageal reflux disease, ADULT and CHILD over 12 years, 40 mg once daily for 4 weeks, continued for further 4 weeks if not fully healed or symptoms persist; maintenance 20 mg daily; symptomatic treatment in the absence of oesophagitis, 20 mg daily for up to 4 weeks, then in ADULTS over 18 years 20 mg daily when required

  Zollinger–Ellison syndrome, ADULT over 18 years, initially 40 mg twice daily, adjusted according to response; usual range 80–160 mg daily (above 80 mg in 2 divided doses)

Counselling Do not chew or crush tablets, swallow whole or disperse in water

- By intravenous injection over at least 3 minutes or by intravenous infusion, ADULT over 18 years, gastro-oesophageal reflux disease, 40 mg once daily; symptomatic reflux disease without oesophagitis, treatment of NSAID-associated gastric ulcer, prevention of NSAID-associated gastric or duodenal ulcer, 20 mg daily; continue until oral administration possible

Nexium® (AstraZeneca) PoM

Tablets, f/c, esomeprazole (as magnesium trihydrate) 20 mg (light pink), net price 28-tab pack = £18.50 (also 7-tab pack, hosp. only); 40 mg (pink), 28-tab pack = £25.19 (also 7-tab pack, hosp. only). Counselling, administration

Injection, powder for reconstitution, esomeprazole (as sodium salt), net price 40-mg vial = £5.21

LANSOPRAZOLE

Indications see under Dose

Cautions see notes above; **interactions**: Appendix 1 (proton pump inhibitors)

Side-effects see notes above; also reported, alopecia, paraesthesia, bruising, purpura, petechiae, fatigue, vertigo, hallucinations, confusion; rarely gynaecomastia, impotence

Dose

- Benign gastric ulcer, 30 mg daily in the morning for 8 weeks
- Duodenal ulcer, 30 mg daily in the morning for 4 weeks; maintenance 15 mg daily
- NSAID-associated duodenal or gastric ulcer, 30 mg once daily for 4 weeks, continued for further 4 weeks if not fully healed; prophylaxis, 15–30 mg once daily
- Eradication of *Helicobacter pylori* associated with duodenal ulcer or ulcer-like dyspepsia, see eradication regimens on p. 43
- Zollinger-Ellison syndrome (and other hypersecretory conditions), initially 60 mg once daily adjusted according to response; daily doses of 120 mg or more given in two divided doses
- Gastro-oesophageal reflux disease, 30 mg daily in the morning for 4 weeks, continued for further 4 weeks if not fully healed; maintenance 15–30 mg daily
- Acid-related dyspepsia, 15–30 mg daily in the morning for 2–4 weeks
- CHILD under 18 years, see *BNF for Children*

Note Lansoprazole doses in BNF may differ from those in product literature

Lansoprazole (Non-proprietary) PoM

Capsules, enclosing e/c granules, lansoprazole 15 mg, net price 28-cap pack = £2.51; 30 mg, 28-cap pack = £4.74. Label: 5, 25

Zoton® (Wyeth) PoM

FasTab® (= orodispersible tablet), lansoprazole 15 mg, net price 28-tab pack = £5.97; 30 mg, 7-tab pack = £2.74, 14-tab pack = £5.47, 28-tab pack = £11.00. Label: 5, counselling, administration

Excipients include aspartame (section 9.4.1)

Counselling Tablets should be placed on the tongue, allowed to disperse and swallowed, or may be swallowed whole with a glass of water; tablets should not be crushed or chewed.

OMEPRAZOLE

Indications see under Dose

Cautions see notes above; **interactions**: Appendix 1 (proton pump inhibitors)

Side-effects see notes above; also reported, paraesthesia, vertigo, alopecia, gynaecomastia, impotence, stomatitis, encephalopathy in severe liver disease; hyponatraemia; reversible confusion, agitation, and hallucinations in the severely ill; visual impairment reported with high-dose injection

Dose

- By mouth, benign gastric and duodenal ulcers, 20 mg once daily for 4 weeks in duodenal ulceration or 8 weeks in gastric ulceration; in severe or recurrent cases increase to 40 mg daily; maintenance for recurrent duodenal ulcer, 20 mg once daily; prevention of relapse in duodenal ulcer, 10 mg daily increasing to 20 mg once daily if symptoms return

  NSAID-associated duodenal or gastric ulcer and gastroduodenal erosions, 20 mg once daily for 4 weeks, continued for further 4 weeks if not fully healed; prophylaxis in patients with a history of NSAID-associated duodenal or gastric ulcers, gastroduodenal lesions, or dyspeptic symptoms who require continued NSAID treatment, 20 mg once daily

  Duodenal or benign gastric ulcer associated with *Helicobacter pylori*, see eradication regimens on p. 43

  Zollinger–Ellison syndrome, initially 60 mg once daily; usual range 20–120 mg daily (above 80 mg in 2 divided doses)

  Gastric acid reduction during general anaesthesia (prophylaxis of acid aspiration), 40 mg on the preceding evening then 40 mg 2–6 hours before surgery

  Gastro-oesophageal reflux disease, 20 mg once daily for 4 weeks, continued for further 4–8 weeks if not fully healed; 40 mg once daily has been given for 8 weeks in gastro-oesophageal reflux disease refractory to other treatment; maintenance 20 mg once daily

  Acid reflux disease (long-term management), 10 mg daily increasing to 20 mg once daily if symptoms return

  Acid-related dyspepsia, 10–20 mg once daily for 2–4 weeks according to response

  Severe ulcerating reflux oesophagitis, CHILD over 1 year, body-weight 10–20 kg, 10 mg once daily increased if necessary to 20 mg once daily for 4–12 weeks; body-weight over 20 kg, 20 mg once daily increased if necessary to 40 mg once daily for 4–12 weeks; to be initiated by hospital paediatrician
- By intravenous injection over 5 minutes or by intravenous infusion, prophylaxis of acid aspiration, 40 mg completed 1 hour before surgery

  Benign gastric ulcer, duodenal ulcer and gastro-oesophageal reflux, 40 mg once daily until oral administration possible

Counselling Swallow whole, or disperse *MUPS®* tablets in water, or mix capsule contents or *MUPS®* tablets with fruit juice or yoghurt

Omeprazole (Non-proprietary) PoM

Capsules, enclosing e/c granules, omeprazole 10 mg, net price 28-cap pack = £1.94; 20 mg, 28-cap pack = £2.03; 40 mg, 7-cap pack = £2.14, 28-cap pack = £58.00. Counselling, administration

[1]Tablets, e/c, omeprazole 10 mg, net price 28-tab pack = £8.37; 20 mg, 28-tab pack = £9.94; 40 mg, 7-tab pack = £8.74. Label: 25
Brands include *Mepradec®* (tablet within capsule)

Intravenous infusion, powder for reconstitution, omeprazole (as sodium salt), net price 40-mg vial = £5.21

1. Omeprazole 10 mg tablets can be sold to the public for the short-term relief of reflux-like symptoms (e.g. heartburn) in adults over 18 years, max. daily dose 20 mg for max. 4 weeks, and a pack size of 28 tablets

Losec® (AstraZeneca) PoM

MUPS® (multiple-unit pellet system = dispersible tablets), f/c, omeprazole 10 mg (light pink), net price 28-tab pack = £19.34; 20 mg (pink), 28-tab pack = £29.22; 40 mg (red-brown), 7-tab pack = £14.61. Counselling, administration

Capsules, enclosing e/c granules, omeprazole 10 mg (pink), net price 28-cap pack = £19.34; 20 mg (pink/brown), 28-cap pack = £29.22; 40 mg (brown), 7-cap pack = £14.61. Counselling, administration

Intravenous infusion, powder for reconstitution, omeprazole (as sodium salt), net price 40-mg vial = £5.41

Injection, powder for reconstitution, omeprazole (as sodium salt), net price 40-mg vial (with solvent) = £5.41

PANTOPRAZOLE

Indications see under Dose

Cautions see notes above; also renal impairment (Appendix 3); **interactions:** Appendix 1 (proton pump inhibitors)

Side-effects see notes above; also confusion and hallucinations; *very rarely* raised triglycerides

Dose

- By mouth, benign gastric ulcer, 40 mg daily in the morning for 4 weeks, continued for further 4 weeks if not fully healed
  Gastro-oesophageal reflux disease, 20–40 mg daily in the morning for 4 weeks, continued for further 4 weeks if not fully healed; maintenance 20 mg daily, increased to 40 mg daily if symptoms return
  Duodenal ulcer, 40 mg daily in the morning for 2 weeks, continued for further 2 weeks if not fully healed
  Duodenal ulcer associated with *Helicobacter pylori*, see eradication regimens on p. 43
  Prophylaxis of NSAID-associated gastric or duodenal ulcer in patients with an increased risk of gastroduodenal complications who require continued NSAID treatment, 20 mg daily
  Zollinger–Ellison syndrome (and other hypersecretory conditions), initially 80 mg once daily adjusted according to response (ELDERLY max. 40 mg daily); daily doses above 80 mg given in 2 divided doses
  CHILD not recommended
- By intravenous injection over at least 2 minutes *or* by intravenous infusion, ADULT over 18 years, duodenal ulcer, gastric ulcer, and gastro-oesophageal reflux, 40 mg daily until oral administration can be resumed
  Zollinger–Ellison syndrome (and other hypersecretory conditions), ADULT over 18 years, initially 80 mg (160 mg if rapid acid control required) then 80 mg once daily adjusted according to response; daily doses above 80 mg given in 2 divided doses

Protium® (Altana) PoM

Tablets, yellow, e/c, pantoprazole (as sodium sesquihydrate) 20 mg, net price 28-tab pack = £12.31; 40 mg, 28-tab pack = £21.40. Label: 25

Injection, powder for reconstitution, pantoprazole (as sodium salt), net price 40-mg vial = £5.71

RABEPRAZOLE SODIUM

Indications see under Dose

Cautions see notes above; **interactions:** Appendix 1 (proton pump inhibitors)

Side-effects see notes above; also reported, cough, pharyngitis, rhinitis, asthenia, influenza-like syndrome; *less commonly* chest pain, sinusitis, nervousness, urinary tract infection; rarely stomatitis, encephalopathy in severe liver disease, anorexia, weight gain

Dose

- Benign gastric ulcer, 20 mg daily in the morning for 6 weeks, continued for further 6 weeks if not fully healed
- Duodenal ulcer, 20 mg daily in the morning for 4 weeks, continued for further 4 weeks if not fully healed
- Gastro-oesophageal reflux disease, 20 mg once daily for 4–8 weeks; maintenance 10–20 mg daily; symptomatic treatment in the absence of oesophagitis, 10 mg daily for up to 4 weeks, then 10 mg daily when required
- Duodenal and benign gastric ulcer associated with *Helicobacter pylori*, see eradication regimens on p. 43
- Zollinger–Ellison syndrome, initially 60 mg once daily adjusted according to response (max. 120 mg daily); doses above 100 mg daily given in 2 divided doses
- CHILD not recommended

Pariet® (Janssen-Cilag, Eisai) PoM

Tablets, e/c, rabeprazole sodium 10 mg (pink), net price 28-tab pack = £11.56; 20 mg (yellow), 28-tab pack = £21.16. Label: 25

1.4 Acute diarrhoea

1.4.1 Adsorbents and bulk-forming drugs
1.4.2 Antimotility drugs

The priority in acute diarrhoea, as in gastro-enteritis, is the prevention or reversal of fluid and electrolyte depletion. This is particularly important in infants and in frail and elderly patients. For details of **oral rehydration preparations**, see section 9.2.1.2. Severe depletion of fluid and electrolytes requires immediate admission to hospital and urgent replacement.

Antimotility drugs (section 1.4.2) relieve symptoms of acute diarrhoea. They are used in the management of uncomplicated acute diarrhoea in adults; fluid and electrolyte replacement may be necessary in case of dehydration. However, antimotility drugs are **not** recommended for acute diarrhoea in young children.

Antispasmodics (section 1.2) are occasionally of value in treating abdominal cramp associated with diarrhoea but they should **not** be used for primary treatment. Antispasmodics and antiemetics should be **avoided** in young children with gastro-enteritis because they are rarely effective and have troublesome side-effects.

Antibacterial drugs are generally unnecessary in simple gastro-enteritis because the complaint usually resolves quickly without them, and infective diarrhoeas in the UK often have a viral cause. Systemic bacterial infection does, however, need appropriate systemic treatment, for drugs used in campylobacter enteritis, shigellosis, and salmonellosis, see Table 1, section 5.1. **Ciprofloxacin** is occasionally used for prophylaxis against travellers' diarrhoea, but routine use is **not** recommended. Lactobacillus preparations have not been shown to be effective.

Colestyramine (cholestyramine, section 1.9.2), binds unabsorbed bile salts and provides symptomatic relief of diarrhoea following ileal disease or resection.

1.4.1 Adsorbents and bulk-forming drugs

Adsorbents such as kaolin are **not** recommended for *acute diarrhoeas*. Bulk-forming drugs, such as ispaghula, methylcellulose, and sterculia (section 1.6.1) are useful in controlling diarrhoea associated with diverticular disease.

KAOLIN, LIGHT

Indications diarrhoea but see notes above
Cautions interactions: Appendix 1 (kaolin)

Kaolin Mixture, BP
(Kaolin Oral Suspension)
Oral suspension, light kaolin or light kaolin (natural) 20%, light magnesium carbonate 5%, sodium bicarbonate 5% in a suitable vehicle with a peppermint flavour.
Dose 10–20 mL every 4 hours

1.4.2 Antimotility drugs

Antimotility drugs have a role in the management of uncomplicated *acute diarrhoea* in adults but not in young children; see also section 1.4. However, in severe cases, fluid and electrolyte replacement (section 9.2.1.2) are of primary importance.

For comments on the role of antimotility drugs in *chronic bowel disorders* see section 1.5. For their role in *stoma care* see section 1.8.

CODEINE PHOSPHATE

Indications see notes above; cough suppression (section 3.9.1); pain (section 4.7.2)
Cautions see section 4.7.2; also not recommended for children; tolerance and dependence may occur with prolonged use; **interactions**: Appendix 1 (opioid analgesics)
Contra-indications see section 4.7.2; also conditions where inhibition of peristalsis should be avoided, where abdominal distension develops, or in acute diarrhoeal conditions such as acute ulcerative colitis or antibiotic-associated colitis
Side-effects see section 4.7.2
Dose
- See preparations

Codeine Phosphate (Non-proprietary) PoM
Tablets, codeine phosphate 15 mg, net price 28 = 74p; 30 mg, 28 = 89p; 60 mg, 28 = £2.14. Label: 2
Dose acute diarrhoea, 30 mg 3–4 times daily (range 15–60 mg); CHILD not recommended
Note As for schedule 2 controlled drugs, travellers needing to take codeine phosphate tablets abroad may require a doctor's letter explaining why codeine is necessary.

CO-PHENOTROPE

A mixture of diphenoxylate hydrochloride and atropine sulphate in the mass proportions 100 parts to 1 part respectively

Indications adjunct to rehydration in acute diarrhoea (but see notes above); control of faecal consistency after colostomy or ileostomy (section 1.8)
Cautions see under Codeine Phosphate; also young children are particularly susceptible to **overdosage** and symptoms may be delayed and observation is needed for at least 48 hours after ingestion; presence of subclinical doses of atropine may give rise to atropine side-effects in susceptible individuals or in overdosage; **interactions**: Appendix 1 (opioid analgesics)
Contra-indications see under Codeine Phosphate; jaundice
Side-effects see under Codeine Phosphate, section 4.7.2
Dose
- See preparation

Lomotil® (Goldshield) PoM
Tablets, co-phenotrope 2.5/0.025 (diphenoxylate hydrochloride 2.5 mg, atropine sulphate 25 micrograms), net price 20 = £1.79
Dose initially 4 tablets, followed by 2 tablets every 6 hours until diarrhoea controlled; CHILD under 4 years see *BNF for Children*, 4–9 years 1 tablet 3 times daily, 9–12 years 1 tablet 4 times daily, 12–16 years 2 tablets 3 times daily, but see also notes above
Note Co-phenotrope 2.5/0.025 can be sold to the public for adults and children over 16 years (provided packs do not contain more than 20 tablets) as an adjunct to rehydration in acute diarrhoea (max. daily dose 10 tablets)

LOPERAMIDE HYDROCHLORIDE

Indications symptomatic treatment of acute diarrhoea; adjunct to rehydration in acute diarrhoea in adults and children over 4 years (but see notes above); chronic diarrhoea in adults only
Cautions see notes above; also liver disease; pregnancy (Appendix 4); **interactions**: Appendix 1 (loperamide)
Contra-indications conditions where inhibition of peristalsis should be avoided, where abdominal distension develops, or in conditions such as active ulcerative colitis or antibiotic-associated colitis
Side-effects abdominal cramps, dizziness, drowsiness, and skin reactions including urticaria; paralytic ileus and abdominal bloating also reported
Dose
- Acute diarrhoea, 4 mg initially followed by 2 mg after each loose stool for up to 5 days; usual dose 6–8 mg daily; max. 16 mg daily; CHILD under 4 years not recommended; 4–8 years, 1 mg 3–4 times daily for up to *3 days only*; 8–12 years, 2 mg 4 times daily for up to 5 days
- Chronic diarrhoea in adults, initially, 4–8 mg daily in divided doses, subsequently adjusted according to

response and given in 2 divided doses for maintenance; max. 16 mg daily; CHILD under 18 years see *BNF for Children*

Loperamide (Non-proprietary) PoM
Capsules, loperamide hydrochloride 2 mg, net price 30-cap pack = 57p

Tablets, loperamide hydrochloride 2 mg, net price 30-tab pack = £2.15

Brands include *Norimode®*

Note Loperamide can be sold to the public, for adults and children over 12 years, provided it is licensed and labelled for the treatment of acute diarrhoea

Imodium® (Janssen-Cilag) PoM
Capsules, green/grey, loperamide hydrochloride 2 mg. Net price 30-cap pack = £1.13

Syrup, red, sugar-free, loperamide hydrochloride 1 mg/5 mL. Net price 100 mL = 98p

Compound preparations

Imodium® Plus (J&J MSD)
Tablets (chewable), scored, loperamide hydrochloride 2 mg, simeticone 125 mg, net price 6-tab pack = £1.97, 12-tab pack = £3.40, 18-tab pack = £4.54. Label: 24

Caplets (= tablets), loperamide hydrochloride 2 mg, simeticone 125 mg, net price 6-tab pack = £2.14, 12-tab pack = £3.40

Dose acute diarrhoea with abdominal colic, initially 2 tablets or caplets (CHILD 12–18 years 1 tablet or caplet) then 1 tablet or caplet after each loose stool; max. 4 tablets or caplets daily for up to 2 days; CHILD under 12 years not recommended

MORPHINE

Indications see notes above

Cautions see notes above and under Codeine Phosphate (section 4.7.2)

Contra-indications see notes above and under Codeine Phosphate

Side-effects see notes above and under Codeine Phosphate (section 4.7.2); sedation and the risk of dependence are greater

Dose

- See preparation

Kaolin and Morphine Mixture, BP
(Kaolin and Morphine Oral Suspension)
Oral suspension, light kaolin or light kaolin (natural) 20%, sodium bicarbonate 5%, and chloroform and morphine tincture 4% in a suitable vehicle. Contains anhydrous morphine 550–800 micrograms/10 mL.

Dose 10 mL every 4 hours in water

1.5 Chronic bowel disorders

Once tumours are ruled out individual symptoms of chronic bowel disorders need specific treatment including dietary manipulation as well as drug treatment and the maintenance of a liberal fluid intake.

Inflammatory bowel disease

Chronic inflammatory bowel diseases include *ulcerative colitis* and *Crohn's disease.* Effective management requires drug therapy, attention to nutrition, and in severe or chronic active disease, surgery.

Aminosalicylates (balsalazide, mesalazine, olsalazine, and sulfasalazine), and **corticosteroids** (hydrocortisone, budesonide, and prednisolone) form the basis of drug treatment.

Treatment of acute ulcerative colitis and Crohn's disease Acute mild to moderate disease affecting the rectum (proctitis) or the recto-sigmoid (distal colitis) is treated initially with local application of an aminosalicylate or a corticosteroid; foam preparations and suppositories are especially useful where patients have difficulty retaining liquid enemas.

Diffuse inflammatory bowel disease or disease that does not respond to local therapy requires oral treatment. Mild disease affecting the colon can be treated with an oral aminosalicylate alone; a combination of a local and an oral aminosalicylate can be used in distal colitis. Refractory or moderate inflammatory bowel disease usually requires adjunctive use of an oral corticosteroid such as **prednisolone** (section 6.3.2) for 4–8 weeks. Modified-release **budesonide** is licensed for Crohn's disease affecting the ileum and the ascending colon; it causes fewer systemic side-effects than oral prednisolone but may be less effective. **Beclometasone dipropionate** by mouth is licensed as an adjunct to mesalazine for mild to moderate ulcerative colitis, but it is not known whether it is as effective as other corticosteroids.

Severe inflammatory bowel disease calls for hospital admission and treatment with an intravenous corticosteroid (such as hydrocortisone or methylprednisolone, section 6.3.2); other therapy may include intravenous fluid and electrolyte replacement, blood transfusion, and possibly parenteral nutrition. Specialist supervision is required for patients who fail to respond adequately to these measures. Patients with severe ulcerative colitis that has not responded to intravenous corticosteroids, may benefit from a short course of intravenous **ciclosporin** [unlicensed indication] (section 8.2.2). Patients with unresponsive or chronically active Crohn's disease may benefit from **azathioprine** (section 8.2.1), **mercaptopurine** (see below), or once-weekly **methotrexate** (section 10.1.3) [all unlicensed indications].

Infliximab is licensed for the management of severe active Crohn's disease and moderate to severe ulcerative colitis in patients whose condition has not responded adequately to treatment with a corticosteroid and a conventional immunosuppressant or who are intolerant of them. Infliximab is also licensed for the management of refractory fistulating Crohn's disease. Maintenance therapy with infliximab should be considered for patients who respond to the initial induction course; fixed-interval dosing may be superior to intermittent dosing.

> **NICE guidance**
> **Infliximab for Crohn's disease (April 2002)**
> Infliximab is recommended for the treatment of severe active Crohn's disease (with or without fistulae) when treatment with immunomodulating drugs and corticosteroids has failed or is not tolerated and when surgery is inappropriate. Treatment may be repeated if the condition responded to the initial course but relapsed subsequently. Infliximab should be prescribed only by a gastroenterologist.

Adalimumab is licensed for the treatment of severe active Crohn's disease in patients whose condition has not responded adequately to treatment with a corticosteroid and a conventional immunosuppressant, or who are intolerant of them. For inducing remission, adalimumab should be used in combination with a corticosteroid, but it may be given alone if a corticosteroid is inappropriate or is not tolerated.

Metronidazole (section 5.1.11) may be beneficial for the treatment of active Crohn's disease with perianal involvement, possibly through its antibacterial activity [unlicensed indication]. Metronidazole is used at a dose of 10–20 mg/kg daily in divided doses (usual dose 1–1.5 g daily in divided doses); it is usually given for a month but no longer than 3 months because of concerns about developing peripheral neuropathy. Other antibacterials should be given if specifically indicated (e.g. sepsis associated with fistulas and perianal disease) and for managing bacterial overgrowth in the small bowel.

Maintenance of remission of acute ulcerative colitis and Crohn's disease **Aminosalicylates** are of great value in the maintenance of remission of ulcerative colitis. They are of less value in the maintenance of remission of Crohn's disease; an oral formulation of mesalazine is licensed for the long-term management of ileal disease. Corticosteroids are **not** suitable for maintenance treatment because of side-effects. In resistant or frequently relapsing cases either **azathioprine** (section 8.2.1) 2–2.5 mg/kg daily [unlicensed indication] or **mercaptopurine** (section 8.1.3) 1–1.5 mg/kg daily [unlicensed indication], given under close supervision may be helpful; some patients may respond to lower doses of these drugs. Methotrexate (section 10.1.3) is tried in Crohn's disease if azathioprine or mercaptopurine cannot be used [unlicensed indication]. **Infliximab** is licensed for maintenance therapy in Crohn's disease and ulcerative colitis (but see notes above). **Adalimumab** is licensed for maintenance therapy in Crohn's disease.

Adjunctive treatment of inflammatory bowel disease Due attention should be paid to diet; high-fibre or low-residue diets should be used as appropriate. Irritable bowel syndrome during remission of ulcerative colitis calls for avoidance of a high-fibre diet and possible treatment with an antispasmodic (section 1.2).

Antimotility drugs such as codeine and loperamide, and antispasmodic drugs may precipitate paralytic ileus and megacolon in active ulcerative colitis; treatment of the inflammation is more logical. Laxatives may be required in proctitis. Diarrhoea resulting from the loss of bile-salt absorption (e.g. in terminal ileal disease or bowel resection) may improve with **colestyramine** (section 1.9.2), which binds bile salts.

Antibiotic-associated colitis

Antibiotic-associated colitis (pseudomembranous colitis) is caused by colonisation of the colon with *Clostridium difficile* which may follow antibiotic therapy. It is usually of acute onset, but may run a chronic course; it is a particular hazard of clindamycin but few antibiotics are free of this side-effect. Oral **vancomycin** (see section 5.1.7) or **metronidazole** (see section 5.1.11) are used as specific treatment; vancomycin may be preferred for very sick patients.

Diverticular disease

Diverticular disease is treated with a high-fibre diet, **bran supplements**, and **bulk-forming drugs** (section 1.6.1). **Antispasmodics** may provide symptomatic relief when colic is a problem (section 1.2). **Antibacterials** are used only when the diverticula in the intestinal wall become infected (specialist referral). **Antimotility** drugs which slow intestinal motility, e.g. codeine, diphenoxylate, and loperamide could possibly exacerbate the symptoms of diverticular disease and are **contra-indicated**.

Irritable bowel syndrome

Irritable bowel syndrome can present with pain, constipation, or diarrhoea. In some patients there may be important psychological aggravating factors which respond to reassurance and possibly specific treatment e.g. with an antidepressant. A laxative (section 1.6) may be needed to relieve constipation. Antimotility drugs such as loperamide (section 1.4.2) may relieve diarrhoea and antispasmodic drugs (section 1.2) may relieve pain. Opioids with a central action such as codeine are better avoided because of the risk of dependence.

Malabsorption syndromes

Individual conditions need specific management and also general nutritional consideration. Coeliac disease (gluten enteropathy) usually needs a gluten-free diet and pancreatic insufficiency needs pancreatin supplements (section 1.9.4)

For further information on foods for special diets (ACBS), see Appendix 7.

Aminosalicylates

Sulfasalazine is a combination of 5-aminosalicylic acid ('5-ASA') and sulfapyridine; sulfapyridine acts only as a carrier to the colonic site of action but still causes side-effects. In the newer aminosalicylates, **mesalazine** (5-aminosalicylic acid), **balsalazide** (a prodrug of 5-aminosalicylic acid) and **olsalazine** (a dimer of 5-aminosalicylic acid which cleaves in the lower bowel), the sulphonamide-related side-effects of sulfasalazine are avoided, but 5-aminosalicylic acid alone can still cause side-effects including blood disorders (see recommendation below) and lupus-like syndrome also seen with sulfasalazine.

Cautions Aminosalicylates should be used with caution in renal impairment (Appendix 3), during pregnancy (Appendix 4) and breast-feeding (Appendix 5); blood disorders can occur (see recommendation below).

> **Blood disorders**
> Patients receiving aminosalicylates should be advised to report any unexplained bleeding, bruising, purpura, sore throat, fever or malaise that occurs during treatment. A blood count should be performed and the drug stopped immediately if there is suspicion of a blood dyscrasia.

Contra-indications Aminosalicylates should be avoided in salicylate hypersensitivity.

Side-effects Side-effects of the aminosalicylates include diarrhoea, nausea, vomiting, abdominal pain, exacerbation of symptoms of colitis, headache, hypersensitivity reactions (including rash and urticaria); side-effects that occur rarely include acute pancreatitis, hepatitis, myocarditis, pericarditis, lung disorders (including eosinophilia and fibrosing alveolitis), peripheral neuropathy, blood disorders (including agranulocytosis, aplastic anaemia, leucopenia, methaemoglobinaemia, neutropenia, and thrombocytopenia—see also recommendation above), renal dysfunction (interstitial nephritis, nephrotic syndrome), myalgia, arthralgia, skin reactions (including lupus erythematosus-like syndrome, Stevens-Johnson syndrome), alopecia.

BALSALAZIDE SODIUM

Indications treatment of mild to moderate ulcerative colitis and maintenance of remission

Cautions see notes above; also history of asthma; **interactions:** Appendix 1 (aminosalicylates)

Blood disorders See recommendation above

Contra-indications see notes above; also severe hepatic impairment

Side-effects see notes above; also cholelithiasis

Dose

- Acute attack, 2.25 g 3 times daily until remission occurs or for up to max. 12 weeks
- Maintenance, 1.5 g twice daily, adjusted according to response (max. 6 g daily)
- CHILD under 18 years, see *BNF for Children*

Colazide® (Shire) PoM

Capsules, beige, balsalazide sodium 750 mg. Net price 130-cap pack = £39.00. Label: 21, 25, counselling, blood disorder symptoms (see recommendation above)

MESALAZINE

Indications treatment of mild to moderate ulcerative colitis and maintenance of remission; see also under preparations

Cautions see notes above; elderly; with oral preparations, test renal function initially and every 3 months for first year then every 6 months for next 4 years and annually thereafter (risk of serious renal toxicity); **interactions:** Appendix 1 (aminosalicylates)

Blood disorders See recommendation above

Contra-indications see notes above; also severe hepatic impairment (Appendix 2)

Side-effects see notes above

Dose

- See under preparations, below

Note The delivery characteristics of enteric-coated mesalazine preparations may vary; these preparations should not be considered interchangeable

Asacol® (Procter & Gamble Pharm.) PoM

Foam enema, mesalazine 1 g/metered application, net price 14-application cannister with disposable applicators and plastic bags = £28.37. Counselling, blood disorder symptoms (see recommendation above)

Excipients include disodium edetate, hydroxybenzoates (parabens), polysorbate 20, sodium metabisulphite

Dose acute attack affecting the rectosigmoid region, 1 metered application (mesalazine 1 g) into the rectum daily for 4–6 weeks; acute attack affecting the descending colon, 2 metered applications (mesalazine 2 g) once daily for 4–6 weeks; CHILD 12–18 years, see *BNF for Children*

Suppositories, mesalazine 250 mg, net price 20-suppos pack = £5.12; 500 mg, 10-suppos pack = £5.12. Counselling, blood disorder symptoms (see recommendation above)

Dose by rectum 0.75–1.5 g daily in divided doses, with last dose at bedtime; CHILD 12–18 years, see *BNF for Children*

Asacol® MR (Procter & Gamble Pharm.) PoM

Tablets, red, e/c, mesalazine 400 mg, net price 90-tab pack = £31.22, 120-tab pack = £41.62. Label: 5, 25, counselling, blood disorder symptoms (see recommendation above)

Dose ulcerative colitis, acute attack, 2.4 g daily in divided doses; maintenance of remission of ulcerative colitis and Crohn's ileo-colitis, 1.2–2.4 g daily in divided doses; CHILD 12–18 years, see *BNF for Children*

Note Preparations that lower stool pH (e.g. lactulose) may prevent release of mesalazine

Ipocol® (Sandoz) PoM

Tablets, e/c, mesalazine 400 mg, net price 120-tab pack = £41.62. Label: 5, 25, counselling, blood disorder symptoms (see recommendation above)

Dose acute attack, 2.4 g daily in divided doses; maintenance of remission, 1.2–2.4 g daily in divided doses; CHILD not recommended

Note Preparations that lower stool pH (e.g. lactulose) may prevent release of mesalazine

Mesren® MR (IVAX) PoM

Tablets, red-brown, e/c, mesalazine 400 mg, net price 90-tab pack = £20.29, 120-tab pack = £27.05. Label: 5, 25, counselling, blood disorder symptoms (see recommendation above)

Dose acute attack, 2.4 g daily in divided doses; maintenance of remission, 1.2–2.4 g daily in divided doses; CHILD not recommended

Note Preparations that lower stool pH (e.g. lactulose) may prevent release of mesalazine

Mezavant® XL (Shire) PoM

Tablets, m/r, red-brown, e/c, mesalazine 1.2 g, net price 60-tab pack = £62.44. Label: 5, 21, 25, counselling, blood disorder symptoms (see recommendations above)

Dose ADULT over 18 years, acute attack, 2.4 g once daily, increase if necessary to 4.8 g once daily (review treatment at 8 weeks); maintenance, 2.4 g once daily

Pentasa® (Ferring) PoM

Tablets, m/r, scored, mesalazine 500 mg (grey), net price 100-tab pack = £25.48. Label: 25, counselling, administration, see dose, blood disorder symptoms (see recommendation above)

Dose acute attack, up to 4 g daily in 2–3 divided doses; maintenance, 1.5 g daily in 2–3 divided doses; tablets may be dispersed in water, but should not be chewed; CHILD under 15 years see *BNF for Children*

Granules, m/r, pale brown, mesalazine 1 g/sachet, net price 50-sachet pack = £30.02. Label: 25, counselling, administration, see dose, blood disorder symptoms (see recommendation above)

Dose acute attack, up to 4 g daily in 2–4 divided doses; maintenance, 2 g daily in 2 divided doses; granules should be placed on tongue and washed down with water or orange juice without chewing; CHILD under 12 years see *BNF for Children*

Retention enema, mesalazine 1 g in 100-mL pack. Net price 7 enemas = £18.09. Counselling, blood disorder symptoms (see recommendation above)

Dose by rectum 1 enema at bedtime; CHILD not recommended

Suppositories, mesalazine 1 g. Net price 28-suppos pack = £41.55. Counselling, blood disorder symptoms (see recommendation above)
Dose by rectum ulcerative proctitis, ADULT and CHILD over 15 years, acute attack, 1 g daily for 2–4 weeks; maintenance, 1 g daily; CHILD under 15 years see *BNF for Children*

Salofalk® (Dr Falk) PoM
Tablets, e/c, yellow, mesalazine 250 mg. Net price 100-tab pack = £17.40. Label: 5, 25, counselling, blood disorder symptoms (see recommendation above)
Dose acute attack, 1.5 g daily in 3 divided doses; maintenance, 0.75–1.5 g daily in divided doses; CHILD not recommended

Granules, m/r, grey, mesalazine 500 mg/sachet, net price 100-sachet pack = £29.30; 1 g/sachet, 50-sachet pack = £29.30. Label: 25, counselling, administration, see dose, blood disorder symptoms (see recommendation above)
Excipients include aspartame (section 9.4.1)
Dose acute attack, 0.5–1 g 3 times daily; maintenance, 500 mg 3 times daily; CHILD over 6 years, body-weight under 40 kg half adult dose, body-weight over 40 kg, adult dose; granules should be placed on tongue and washed down with water without chewing
Note Preparations that lower stool pH (e.g. lactulose) may prevent release of mesalazine

Suppositories, mesalazine 500 mg. Net price 30-suppos pack = £15.90. Counselling, blood disorder symptoms (see recommendation above)
Dose acute attack, by rectum, 0.5–1 g 2–3 times daily adjusted according to response; CHILD not recommended

Enema, mesalazine 2 g in 59-mL pack. Net price 7 enemas = £31.20. Counselling, blood disorder symptoms (see recommendation above)
Dose acute attack *or* maintenance, by rectum, 2 g daily at bedtime; CHILD not recommended

Rectal foam, mesalazine 1 g/metered application, net price 14-application cannister with disposable applicators and plastic bags = £31.10. Counselling, blood disorder symptoms (see recommendation above)
Excipients include cetostearyl alcohol, disodium edetate, polysorbate 60, propylene glycol, sodium metabisulphite
Dose mild ulcerative colitis affecting sigmoid colon and rectum, ADULT and CHILD over 12 years, 2 metered applications (mesalazine 2 g) into the rectum at bedtime increased if necessary to 2 metered applications (mesalazine 2 g) twice daily

OLSALAZINE SODIUM

Indications treatment of mild ulcerative colitis and maintenance of remission
Cautions see notes above; **interactions:** Appendix 1 (aminosalicylates)
Blood disorders See recommendation above
Contra-indications see notes above
Side-effects see notes above; also watery diarrhoea
Dose

- ADULT and CHILD over 12 years, acute attack, 1 g daily in divided doses after meals increased if necessary over 1 week to max. 3 g daily (max. single dose 1 g); maintenance, 500 mg twice daily after meals
- CHILD under 12 years see *BNF for Children*

Dipentum® (UCB Pharma) PoM
Capsules, brown, olsalazine sodium 250 mg. Net price 112-cap pack = £20.57. Label: 21, counselling, blood disorder symptoms (see recommendation above)

Tablets, yellow, scored, olsalazine sodium 500 mg. Net price 60-tab pack = £22.04. Label: 21, counselling, blood disorder symptoms (see recommendation above)

SULFASALAZINE
(Sulphasalazine)

Indications treatment of mild to moderate and severe ulcerative colitis and maintenance of remission; active Crohn's disease; rheumatoid arthritis (section 10.1.3)
Cautions see notes above; also history of allergy; hepatic impairment; G6PD deficiency (section 9.1.5); slow acetylator status; risk of haematological and hepatic toxicity (differential white cell, red cell and platelet counts initially and at monthly intervals for first 3 months, liver function tests at monthly intervals for first 3 months); test renal function at regular intervals; upper gastro-intestinal side-effects common over 4 g daily; porphyria (section 9.8.2); **interactions:** Appendix 1 (aminosalicylates)
Blood disorders See recommendation above
Contra-indications see notes above; also sulphonamide hypersensitivity; child under 2 years of age
Side-effects see notes above; also loss of appetite; fever; blood disorders (including Heinz body anaemia, megaloblastic anaemia); hypersensitivity reactions (including exfoliative dermatitis, epidermal necrolysis, pruritus, photosensitisation, anaphylaxis, serum sickness); ocular complications (including periorbital oedema); stomatitis, parotitis; ataxia, aseptic meningitis, vertigo, tinnitus, insomnia, depression, hallucinations; kidney reactions (including proteinuria, crystalluria, haematuria); oligospermia; urine may be coloured orange; some soft contact lenses may be stained
Dose

- By mouth acute attack 1–2 g 4 times daily (but see **cautions**) until remission occurs (if necessary corticosteroids may also be given), reducing to a maintenance dose of 500 mg 4 times daily; CHILD over 2 years acute attack 40–60 mg/kg daily, maintenance dose 20–30 mg/kg daily
- By rectum, in suppositories, alone or in conjunction with oral treatment 0.5–1 g morning and night after a bowel movement. As an enema, 3 g at night, retained for at least 1 hour

Sulfasalazine (Non-proprietary) PoM
Tablets, sulfasalazine 500 mg. Net price 112 = £15.37. Label: 14, counselling, blood disorder symptoms (see recommendation above), contact lenses may be stained

Tablets, e/c, sulfasalazine 500 mg. Net price 112-tab pack = £28.39. Label: 5, 14, 25, counselling, blood disorder symptoms (see recommendation above), contact lenses may be stained
Brands include *Sulazine EC®*

Salazopyrin® (Pharmacia) PoM
Tablets, yellow, scored, sulfasalazine 500 mg. Net price 112-tab pack = £6.97 Label: 14, counselling, blood disorder symptoms (see recommendation above), contact lenses may be stained

EN-Tabs® (= tablets e/c), yellow, f/c, sulfasalazine 500 mg. Net price 112-tab pack = £8.43. Label: 5, 14, 25, counselling, blood disorder symptoms (see recommendation above), contact lenses may be stained

Suspension, yellow, sulfasalazine 250 mg/5 mL. Net price 500 mL = £18.84. Label: 14, counselling, blood disorder symptoms (see recommendation above), contact lenses may be stained

Suppositories, yellow, sulfasalazine 500 mg. Net price 10 = £3.30. Label: 14, counselling, blood disorder symptoms (see recommendation above), contact lenses may be stained

Corticosteroids

BECLOMETASONE DIPROPIONATE

Indications adjunct to mesalazine in acute mild to moderate ulcerative colitis; asthma (section 3.2); allergic and vasomotor rhinitis (section 12.2.1); oral ulceration [unlicensed indication] (section 12.3.1)

Cautions section 6.3.2; **interactions:** Appendix 1 (corticosteroids)

Contra-indications section 6.3.2

Side-effects section 6.3.2; also nausea, constipation, headache, and drowsiness

Dose

- 5 mg in the morning; max. duration of treatment 4 weeks; CHILD safety and efficacy not established

Clipper® (Trinity-Chiesi) ▼ PoM

Tablets, m/r, ivory, beclometasone dipropionate 5 mg, net price 30-tab pack = £60.00. Label: 25

BUDESONIDE

Indications see preparations

Cautions section 6.3.2; **interactions:** Appendix 1 (corticosteroids)

Contra-indications section 6.3.2

Side-effects section 6.3.2

Dose

- See preparations

Budenofalk® (Dr Falk) PoM

Capsules, pink, enclosing e/c pellets, budesonide 3 mg, net price 100-cap pack = £76.70. Label: 5, 10, steroid card, 22, 25

Dose mild to moderate Crohn's disease affecting ileum or ascending colon, chronic diarrhoea due to collagenous colitis, ADULT over 18 years, 3 mg 3 times daily for up to 8 weeks; reduce dose for the last 2 weeks of treatment. See also section 6.3.2

Rectal foam, budesonide 2 mg/metered application, net price 14-application canister with disposable applicators and plastic bags = £58.22

Excipients include cetyl alcohol, disodium edetate, propylene glycol, sorbic acid

Dose ulcerative colitis affecting sigmoid colon and rectum, by rectum, ADULT over 18 years, 1 metered application (budesonide 2 mg) once daily for up to 8 weeks

Entocort® (AstraZeneca) PoM

CR Capsules, grey/pink, enclosing e/c, m/r granules, budesonide 3 mg, net price 100-cap pack = £99.00. Label: 5, 10, steroid card, 25

Note Dispense in original container (contains dessicant)

Dose mild to moderate Crohn's disease affecting the ileum or ascending colon, 9 mg once daily in the morning for up to 8 weeks; reduce dose for the last 2–4 weeks of treatment. See also section 6.3.2

CHILD not recommended

Enema, budesonide 2 mg/100 mL when dispersible tablet reconstituted in isotonic saline vehicle, net price pack of 7 dispersible tablets and bottles of vehicle = £33.00

Dose ulcerative colitis involving rectal and recto-sigmoid disease, by rectum, 1 enema at bedtime for 4 weeks; CHILD not recommended

HYDROCORTISONE

Indications ulcerative colitis, proctitis, proctosigmoiditis

Cautions section 6.3.2; systemic absorption may occur; prolonged use should be avoided

Contra-indications intestinal obstruction, bowel perforation, recent intestinal anastomoses, extensive fistulas; untreated infection

Side-effects section 6.3.2; also local irritation

Dose

- By rectum see preparations

Colifoam® (Meda) PoM

Foam in aerosol pack, hydrocortisone acetate 10%, net price 14-application cannister with applicator = £8.21

Excipients include cetyl alcohol, hydroxybenzoates (parabens), propylene glycol

Dose initially 1 metered application (125 mg hydrocortisone acetate) inserted into the rectum once or twice daily for 2–3 weeks, then once on alternate days

PREDNISOLONE

Indications ulcerative colitis, and Crohn's disease; other indications, see section 6.3.2, see also preparations

Cautions section 6.3.2; systemic absorption may occur with rectal preparations; prolonged use should be avoided

Contra-indications section 6.3.2; intestinal obstruction, bowel perforation, recent intestinal anastomoses, extensive fistulas; untreated infection

Side-effects section 6.3.2

Dose

- By mouth, initially 20–40 mg daily in single or divided doses, until remission occurs, followed by reducing doses
- By rectum, see under preparations

Oral preparations

Section 6.3.2

Rectal preparations

Predenema® (Forest) PoM

Retention enema, prednisolone 20 mg (as sodium metasulphobenzoate) in 100-mL single-dose disposable pack. Net price 1 (standard tube) = 71p, 1 (long tube) = £1.21

Dose ulcerative colitis, by rectum, ADULT and CHILD over 12 years, initially 20 mg at bedtime for 2–4 weeks, continued if good response

Predfoam® (Forest) PoM

Foam in aerosol pack, prednisolone 20 mg (as metasulphobenzoate sodium)/metered application, net price 14-application cannister with disposable applicators = £6.32

Excipients include cetostearyl alcohol, disodium edetate, polysorbate 20, sorbic acid

Dose proctitis and distal ulcerative colitis, 1 metered application (20 mg prednisolone) inserted into the rectum once or twice daily for 2 weeks, continued for further 2 weeks if good response; CHILD not recommended

Predsol® (UCB Pharma) PoM
Retention enema, prednisolone 20 mg (as sodium phosphate) in 100-mL single-dose disposable packs fitted with a nozzle. Net price 7 = £7.50
Dose rectal and rectosigmoidal ulcerative colitis and Crohn's disease, by rectum, initially 20 mg at bedtime for 2–4 weeks, continued if good response; CHILD not recommended

Suppositories, prednisolone 5 mg (as sodium phosphate). Net price 10 = £1.40
Dose ADULT and CHILD proctitis and rectal complications of Crohn's disease, by rectum, 5 mg inserted night and morning after a bowel movement

Cytokine modulators

Infliximab and **adalimumab** are monoclonal antibodies which inhibit the pro-inflammatory cytokine, tumour necrosis factor α. They should be used under specialist supervision. Adequate resuscitation facilities must be available when infliximab is used.

ADALIMUMAB

Indications see under Inflammatory Bowel Disease, p. 52; ankylosing spondylitis, psoriatic arthritis, rheumatoid arthritis (section 10.1.3)
Cautions section 10.1.3
Contra-indications section 10.1.3
Side-effects section 10.1.3
Dose
- By subcutaneous injection, severe active Crohn's disease, ADULT over 18 years, initially 80 mg, then 40 mg 2 weeks after initial dose *or* accelerated regimen, initially 160 mg in 4 divided doses over 1–2 days, then 80 mg 2 weeks after initial dose; maintenance, 40 mg on alternate weeks, increased if necessary to 40 mg weekly; review treatment if no response within 12 weeks

Preparations
Section 10.1.3

INFLIXIMAB

Indications see under Inflammatory Bowel Disease, p. 52; ankylosing spondylitis, psoriasis, rheumatoid arthritis (section 10.1.3)
Cautions see section 10.1.3; also history of dysplasia or colon carcinoma
Hypersensitivity reactions Risk of delayed hypersensitivity if drug-free interval exceeds 16 weeks
Contra-indications see section 10.1.3
Side-effects see section 10.1.3; also hepatosplenic T-cell lymphoma
Dose
- By intravenous infusion, severe active Crohn's disease, ADULT over 18 years, initially 5 mg/kg, then 5 mg/kg 2 weeks after initial dose; then if the condition has responded, maintenance *either* 5 mg/kg 6 weeks after initial dose, then 5 mg/kg every 8 weeks *or* further dose of 5 mg/kg if signs and symptoms recur; CHILD 6–18 years, initially 5 mg/kg, then 5 mg/kg 2 weeks and 6 weeks after initial dose, then 5 mg/kg every 8 weeks; interval between maintenance doses adjusted according to response; discontinue if no response within 10 weeks of initial dose

Fistulating Crohn's disease, ADULT over 18 years, initially 5 mg/kg, then 5 mg/kg 2 weeks and 6 weeks after initial dose, then if condition has responded, consult product literature for guidance on further doses; CHILD under 18 years, see *BNF for Children*

Moderate to severe active ulcerative colitis, ADULT over 18 years, initially 5 mg/kg, then 5 mg/kg 2 weeks and 6 weeks after initial dose, then 5 mg/kg every 8 weeks; discontinue if no response 14 weeks after initial dose; CHILD under 18 years, see *BNF for Children*

Preparations
Section 10.1.3

Food allergy

Allergy with classical symptoms of vomiting, colic and diarrhoea caused by specific foods such as shellfish should be managed by strict avoidance. The condition should be distinguished from symptoms of occasional food intolerance in those with irritable bowel syndrome. **Sodium cromoglicate** (sodium cromoglycate) may be helpful as an adjunct to dietary avoidance.

SODIUM CROMOGLICATE
(Sodium cromoglycate)

Indications food allergy (in conjunction with dietary restriction); asthma (section 3.3); allergic conjunctivitis (section 11.4.2); allergic rhinitis (section 12.2.1)
Side-effects occasional nausea, rashes, and joint pain
Dose
- 200 mg 4 times daily before meals; may be increased if necessary after 2–3 weeks to a max. of 40 mg/kg daily and then reduced according to response; CHILD 2–14 years 100 mg 4 times daily before meals; may be increased if necessary after 2–3 weeks to a max. of 40 mg/kg daily and then reduced according to response

Counselling Capsules may be swallowed whole or the contents dissolved in hot water and diluted with cold water before taking

Nalcrom® (Sanofi-Aventis) PoM
Capsules, sodium cromoglicate 100 mg. Net price 100-cap pack = £62.17. Label: 22, counselling, see dose above

1.6 Laxatives

1.6.1 Bulk-forming laxatives
1.6.2 Stimulant laxatives
1.6.3 Faecal softeners
1.6.4 Osmotic laxatives
1.6.5 Bowel cleansing solutions

Before prescribing laxatives it is important to be sure that the patient *is* constipated and that the constipation is *not* secondary to an underlying undiagnosed complaint.

It is also important for those who complain of constipation to understand that bowel habit can vary considerably in frequency without doing harm. Some people tend to consider themselves constipated if they do not

1 Gastro-intestinal system

have a bowel movement each day. A useful definition of constipation is the passage of hard stools less frequently than the patient's own normal pattern and this can be explained to the patient.

Misconceptions about bowel habits have led to excessive laxative use. Abuse may lead to hypokalaemia.

Thus, laxatives should generally be **avoided** except where straining will exacerbate a condition (such as angina) or increase the risk of rectal bleeding as in haemorrhoids. Laxatives are also of value in *drug-induced constipation*, for the expulsion of *parasites* after anthelmintic treatment, and to clear the alimentary tract before *surgery and radiological procedures.* Prolonged treatment of constipation is sometimes necessary.

Children Laxatives should be prescribed by a healthcare professional experienced in the management of constipation in children. Delays of greater than 3 days between stools may increase the likelihood of pain on passing hard stools leading to anal fissure, anal spasm and eventually to a learned response to avoid defaecation.

If increased fluid and fibre intake is insufficient, an osmotic laxative containing macrogols or lactulose (section 1.6.4) can be used. If there is evidence of minor faecal retention, the addition of a stimulant laxative (section 1.6.2) may overcome withholding but may lead to colic or, in the presence of faecal impaction in the rectum, an increase of faecal overflow.

In children with faecal impaction, an oral preparation containing macrogols is used to clear faecal mass and to establish and maintain soft well-formed stools. Rectal administration of laxatives may be effective but this route is frequently distressing for the child and may lead to persistent withholding. If the impacted mass is not expelled following treatment with macrogols, referral to hospital may be necessary. Enemas may be administered under heavy sedation in hospital or alternatively, a bowel cleansing solution (section 1.6.5) may be tried. In severe cases or where the child is afraid, a manual evacuation under anaesthetic may be appropriate.

Long-term regular use of laxatives is essential to maintain well-formed stools and prevent recurrence of faecal impaction; intermittent use may provoke relapses.

> For children with chronic constipation, it may be necessary to exceed the licensed doses of some laxatives. Parents and carers of children should be advised to adjust the dose of laxative given in order to establish a regular pattern of bowel movements in which stools are soft, well-formed, and passed without discomfort.

Pregnancy If dietary and lifestyle changes fail to control constipation in pregnancy, moderate doses of poorly absorbed laxatives may be used. A bulk-forming laxative should be tried first. An osmotic laxative, such as lactulose, can also be used. Bisacodyl or senna may be suitable, if a stimulant effect is necessary.

> The laxatives that follow have been divided into 5 main groups (sections 1.6.1–1.6.5). This simple classification disguises the fact that some laxatives have a complex action.

1.6.1 Bulk-forming laxatives

Bulk-forming laxatives relieve constipation by increasing faecal mass which stimulates peristalsis; patients should be advised that the full effect may take some days to develop.

Bulk-forming laxatives are of particular value in those with small hard stools, but should not be required unless fibre cannot be increased in the diet. A balanced diet, including adequate fluid intake and fibre is of value in preventing constipation.

Bulk-forming laxatives are useful in the management of patients with *colostomy, ileostomy, haemorrhoids, anal fissure, chronic diarrhoea associated with diverticular disease, irritable bowel syndrome*, and as adjuncts in *ulcerative colitis* (section 1.5). Adequate fluid intake must be maintained to avoid intestinal obstruction. Unprocessed wheat **bran**, taken with food or fruit juice, is a most effective bulk-forming preparation. Finely ground bran, though more palatable, has poorer water-retaining properties, but can be taken as bran bread or biscuits in appropriately increased quantities. Oat bran is also used.

Methylcellulose, ispaghula, and **sterculia** are useful in patients who cannot tolerate bran. Methylcellulose also acts as a faecal softener.

ISPAGHULA HUSK

Indications see notes above

Cautions adequate fluid intake should be maintained to avoid intestinal obstruction—it may be necessary to supervise elderly or debilitated patients or those with intestinal narrowing or decreased motility

Contra-indications difficulty in swallowing, intestinal obstruction, colonic atony, faecal impaction

Side-effects flatulence, abdominal distension, gastro-intestinal obstruction or impaction; hypersensitivity reported

Dose

- See preparations below

Counselling Preparations that swell in contact with liquid should always be carefully swallowed with water and should not be taken immediately before going to bed

Fibrelief® (Manx)

Granules, sugar- and gluten-free, ispaghula husk 3.5 g/sachet (natural or orange flavour), net price 10 sachets = £1.23, 30 sachets = £2.07. Label: 13, counselling, see above

Excipients include aspartame (section 9.4.1)

Dose ADULT and ADOLESCENT over 12 years, 1–6 sachets daily in water in 1–3 divided doses

Fybogel® (R&C)

Granules, buff, effervescent, sugar- and gluten-free, ispaghula husk 3.5 g/sachet (low Na^+), net price 30 sachets (plain, lemon, or orange flavour) = £2.12. Label: 13, counselling, see above

Excipients include aspartame 16 mg/sachet (see section 9.4.1)

Dose 1 sachet or 2 level 5-mL spoonfuls in water twice daily preferably after meals; CHILD (but see section 1.6) 6–12 years ½–1 level 5-mL spoonful in water, twice daily (children under 6 years on doctor's advice only)

Isogel® (Potters)
Granules, brown, sugar- and gluten-free, ispaghula husk 90%. Net price 200 g = £2.67. Label: 13, counselling, see above

Dose constipation, 2 level 5-mL spoonfuls in water once or twice daily, preferably at mealtimes; CHILD (but see section 1.6) 1 level 5-mL spoonful
Diarrhoea (section 1.4.1), 1 level 5-mL spoonful 3 times daily
Note May be difficult to obtain

Ispagel Orange® (LPC)
Granules, beige, effervescent, sugar- and gluten-free, ispaghula husk 3.5 g/sachet, net price 30 sachets = £2.10. Label: 13, counselling, see above
Excipients include aspartame (section 9.4.1)
Dose 1 sachet in water 1–3 times daily; CHILD (but see section 1.6) 6–12 years ½ adult dose (children under 6 years on doctor's advice only)

Regulan® (Procter & Gamble)
Powder, beige, sugar- and gluten-free, ispaghula husk 3.4 g/5.85-g sachet (orange or lemon/lime flavour). Net price 30 sachets = £2.54. Label: 13, counselling, see above
Excipients include aspartame (section 9.4.1)
Dose 1 sachet in 150 mL water 1–3 times daily; CHILD (but see section 1.6) 6–12 years 2.5–5 mL in water 1–3 times daily

METHYLCELLULOSE

Indications see notes above and section 1.6 [unlicensed dose in children]; adjunct in obesity (but see section 4.5.1)
Cautions see under Ispaghula Husk
Contra-indications see under Ispaghula Husk; also infective bowel disease
Side-effects see under Ispaghula Husk
Dose
- See preparations below

Counselling Preparations that swell in contact with liquid should always be carefully swallowed with water and should not be taken immediately before going to bed

Celevac® (Shire)
Tablets, pink, scored, methylcellulose '450' 500 mg. Net price 112-tab pack = £2.69. Counselling, see above and dose
Dose constipation and diarrhoea, 3–6 tablets twice daily. In constipation the dose should be taken with at least 300 mL liquid. In diarrhoea, ileostomy, and colostomy control, minimise liquid intake for 30 minutes before and after dose
Adjunct in obesity (but see section 4.5.1), 3 tablets with at least 300 mL warm liquid 30 minutes before food or when hungry

STERCULIA

Indications see notes above
Cautions see under Ispaghula Husk
Contra-indications see under Ispaghula Husk
Side-effects see under Ispaghula Husk
Dose
- See under preparations below

Counselling Preparations that swell in contact with liquid should always be carefully swallowed with water and should not be taken immediately before going to bed

Normacol® (Norgine)
Granules, coated, gluten-free, sterculia 62%. Net price 500 g = £6.18; 60 × 7-g sachets = £5.19. Label: 25, 27, counselling, see above
Dose 1–2 heaped 5-mL spoonfuls, or the contents of 1–2 sachets, washed down without chewing with plenty of liquid once or twice daily after meals; CHILD (but see section 1.6) 6–12 years half adult dose

Normacol Plus® (Norgine)
Granules, brown, coated, gluten-free, sterculia 62%, frangula (standardised) 8%. Net price 500 g = £6.60; 60 × 7 g sachets = £5.56. Label: 25, 27, counselling, see above
Dose constipation and after haemorrhoidectomy, ADULT and CHILD over 12 years, 1–2 heaped 5-mL spoonfuls or the contents of 1–2 sachets washed down without chewing with plenty of liquid once or twice daily after meals

1.6.2 Stimulant laxatives

Stimulant laxatives include **bisacodyl** and members of the **anthraquinone** group, **senna** and **dantron** (danthron). The indications for dantron are limited (see below) by its potential carcinogenicity (based on *rodent* carcinogenicity studies) and evidence of genotoxicity. Powerful stimulants such as **cascara** (an anthraquinone) and **castor oil** are obsolete. **Docusate sodium** probably acts both as a stimulant and as a softening agent.

Stimulant laxatives increase intestinal motility and often cause abdominal cramp; they should be avoided in intestinal obstruction. Excessive use of stimulant laxatives can cause diarrhoea and related effects such as hypokalaemia; however, prolonged use may be justifiable in some circumstances (see section 1.6 for the use of stimulant laxatives in children).

Glycerol suppositories act as a rectal stimulant by virtue of the mildly irritant action of glycerol.

The **parasympathomimetics** bethanechol, distigmine, neostigmine, and pyridostigmine (see section 7.4.1 and section 10.2.1) enhance parasympathetic activity in the gut and increase intestinal motility. They are rarely used for their gastro-intestinal effects. Organic obstruction of the gut must first be excluded and they should not be used shortly after bowel anastomosis.

BISACODYL

Indications see under Dose
Cautions see notes above; pregnancy, see p. 58
Contra-indications see notes above, acute surgical abdominal conditions, acute inflammatory bowel disease, severe dehydration
Side-effects see notes above; tablets, griping; suppositories, local irritation
Dose
- Constipation, by mouth, 5–10 mg at night; CHILD (but see section 1.6) 4–10 years (on medical advice only) 5 mg at night, over 10 years, adult dose

  By rectum in suppositories, 10 mg in the morning; CHILD (but see section 1.6) under 10 years (on medical advice only) 5 mg, over 10 years, adult dose
- Before radiological procedures and surgery, by mouth, 10–20 mg the night before procedure and by rectum in suppositories, 10 mg the following morning; CHILD 4–10 years by mouth, 5 mg the night before procedure and by rectum in suppositories, 5 mg the following morning; over 10 years, adult dose

Note tablets act in 10–12 hours; suppositories act in 20–60 minutes

Bisacodyl (Non-proprietary)
Tablets, e/c, bisacodyl 5 mg. Net price 20 = 54p. Label: 5, 25

Suppositories, bisacodyl 10 mg. Net price 12 = 77p

Paediatric suppositories, bisacodyl 5 mg. Net price 5 = 94p

Note The brand name *Dulco-lax*® NHS (Boehringer Ingelheim) is used for bisacodyl tablets, net price 10-tab pack = 74p; suppositories (10 mg), 10 = £1.57; paediatric suppositories (5 mg), 5 = 94p

The brand names *Dulco-lax*® *Liquid* and *Dulco-lax*® *Perles* are used for sodium picosulfate preparations

DANTRON
(Danthron)

Indications only for constipation in terminally ill patients of all ages

Cautions see notes above; *rodent* studies indicate potential carcinogenic risk; avoid prolonged contact with skin (as in incontinent patients)—risk of irritation and excoriation; pregnancy (Appendix 4) and breast-feeding (Appendix 5)

Contra-indications see notes above

Side-effects see notes above; urine may be coloured red

Dose

- See under preparations

1 Gastro-intestinal system

With poloxamer '188' (as co-danthramer)

Note Co-danthramer suspension 5 mL = one co-danthramer capsule, **but** strong co-danthramer suspension 5 mL = two strong co-danthramer capsules

Co-danthramer (Non-proprietary) PoM

Capsules, co-danthramer 25/200 (dantron 25 mg, poloxamer '188' 200 mg). Net price 60-cap pack = £12.86. Label: 14, (urine red)

Dose 1–2 capsules at bedtime; CHILD 1 capsule at bedtime (restricted indications, see notes above)

Strong capsules, co-danthramer 37.5/500 (dantron 37.5 mg, poloxamer '188' 500 mg). Net price 60-cap pack = £15.55. Label: 14, (urine red)

Dose ADULT and CHILD over 12 years, 1–2 capsules at bedtime (restricted indications, see notes above)

Suspension, co-danthramer 25/200 in 5 mL (dantron 25 mg, poloxamer '188' 200 mg/5 mL). Net price 300 mL = £11.27, 1 litre = £37.57. Label: 14, (urine red)

Dose 5–10 mL at night; CHILD 2.5–5 mL (restricted indications, see notes above)

Brands include *Codalax*® NHS, *Danlax*®

Strong suspension, co-danthramer 75/1000 in 5 mL (dantron 75 mg, poloxamer '188' 1 g/5 mL). Net price 300 mL = £30.13. Label: 14, (urine red)

Dose ADULT and CHILD over 12 years, 5 mL at night (restricted indications, see notes above)

Brands include *Codalax Forte*® NHS

With docusate sodium (as co-danthrusate)

Co-danthrusate (Non-proprietary) PoM

Capsules, co-danthrusate 50/60 (dantron 50 mg, docusate sodium 60 mg). Net price 63-cap pack = £13.61. Label: 14, (urine red)

Dose 1–3 capsules at night; CHILD 6–12 years 1 capsule at night (restricted indications, see notes above)

Brands include *Capsuvac*®, *Normax*® NHS

Suspension, yellow, co-danthrusate 50/60 (dantron 50 mg, docusate sodium 60 mg/5 mL). Net price 200 mL = £8.75. Label: 14, (urine red)

Dose 5–15 mL at night; CHILD 6–12 years 5 mL at night (restricted indications, see notes above)

Brands include *Normax*®

DOCUSATE SODIUM
(Dioctyl sodium sulphosuccinate)

Indications constipation, adjunct in abdominal radiological procedures

Cautions see notes above; do not give with liquid paraffin; rectal preparations not indicated if haemorrhoids or anal fissure; pregnancy (Appendix 4); breast-feeding (Appendix 5)

Contra-indications see notes above

Side-effects see notes above

Dose

- By mouth, chronic constipation, up to 500 mg daily in divided doses; CHILD (but see section 1.6) 6 months–2 years 12.5 mg 3 times daily, 2–12 years 12.5–25 mg 3 times daily (use paediatric oral solution only)

Note Oral preparations act within 1–2 days

With barium meal, ADULT and CHILD over 12 years, 400 mg

Dioctyl® (UCB Pharma)

Capsules, yellow/white, docusate sodium 100 mg, net price 30-cap pack = £2.40, 100-cap pack = £8.00

Docusol® (Typharm)

Adult oral solution, sugar-free, docusate sodium 50 mg/5 mL, net price 300 mL = £2.48

Paediatric oral solution, sugar-free, docusate sodium 12.5 mg/5 mL, net price 300 mL = £1.63

Rectal preparations

Norgalax Micro-enema® (Norgine)

Enema, docusate sodium 120 mg in 10-g single-dose disposable packs. Net price 10-g unit = 60p

Dose ADULT and CHILD (but see section 1.6) over 12 years, 10-g unit

GLYCEROL
(Glycerin)

Indications constipation

Dose

- See below

Glycerol Suppositories, BP (Glycerin Suppositories)

Suppositories, gelatin 140 mg, glycerol 700 mg, purified water to 1 g. Net price 12 = 90p (infant), 92p (child), £1.29 (adult)

Dose 1 suppository moistened with water before use. The usual sizes are for INFANT under 1 year, small (1-g mould) 1–2 years medium (2-g mould), CHILD medium (2-g mould), ADULT large (4-g mould)

SENNA

Indications constipation

Cautions see notes above; pregnancy, see p. 58

Contra-indications see notes above

Side-effects see notes above

Dose

- See under preparations

Note Acts in 8–12 hours

Senna (Non-proprietary)
Tablets, total sennosides (calculated as sennoside B) 7.5 mg. Net price 60 = £1.57
Dose 2–4 tablets, usually at night; initial dose should be low then gradually increased; CHILD (but see section 1.6) 6–12 years, half adult dose in the morning (on doctor's advice only)
Note Lower dose on packs on sale to the public
Brands include *Senokot®*

Manevac® (Galen)
Granules, coated, senna fruit 12.4%, ispaghula 54.2%, net price 400 g = £7.45. Label: 25, 27, counselling, see Ispaghula Husk
Dose 1–2 level 5-mL spoonfuls with water or warm drink after supper and, if necessary, before breakfast *or* every 6 hours in resistant cases for 1–3 days; CHILD (but see section 1.6) 5–12 years 1 level 5-mL spoonful daily
Counselling Preparations that swell in contact with liquid should always be carefully swallowed with water and should not be taken immediately before going to bed

Senokot® (R&C)
Tablets, see above
Granules, brown, total sennosides (calculated as sennoside B) 15 mg/5 mL or 5.5 mg/g (one 5-mL spoonful = 2.7 g). Net price 100 g = £3.10
Dose 5–10 mL, usually at bedtime; CHILD (but see section 1.6) 6–12 years 2.5–5 mL in the morning
Note Lower dose on packs on sale to the public
Syrup, sugar-free, brown, total sennosides (calculated as sennoside B) 7.5 mg/5 mL. Net price 500 mL = £2.69
Dose 10–20 mL, usually at bedtime; CHILD (but see section 1.6) 2–6 years 2.5–5 mL in the morning (doctor's advice only), 6–12 years 5–10 mL at night or in the morning
Note Lower dose on packs on sale to the public

SODIUM PICOSULFATE
(Sodium picosulphate)

Indications constipation; bowel evacuation before abdominal radiological and endoscopic procedures on the colon, and surgery (section 1.6.5); acts within 6–12 hours
Cautions see notes above; active inflammatory bowel disease (avoid if fulminant); pregnancy, see p. 58; breast-feeding (Appendix 5)
Contra-indications see notes above; severe dehydration
Side-effects see notes above
Dose
- 5–10 mg at night; CHILD (but see section 1.6) 1 month–4 years 250 micrograms/kg (max. 5 mg) at night; 4–10 years 2.5–5 mg at night; over 10 years, adult dose

Sodium Picosulfate (Non-proprietary)
Elixir, sodium picosulfate 5 mg/5 mL, net price 100 mL = £1.85
Note The brand names *Laxoberal®* and *Dulco-lax® Liquid* (both Boehringer Ingelheim) are used for sodium picosulfate elixir 5 mg/5 mL

Dulco-lax® (Boehringer Ingelheim)
Perles® (= capsules), sodium picosulfate 2.5 mg, net price 20-cap pack = £1.93, 50-cap pack = £2.73
Note The brand name *Dulco-lax®* is also used for bisacodyl tablets and suppositories

Bowel cleansing solutions
Section 1.6.5

Other stimulant laxatives

Unstandardised preparations of cascara, frangula, rhubarb, and senna should be **avoided** as their laxative action is unpredictable. Aloes, colocynth, and jalap should be **avoided** as they have a drastic purgative action.

1.6.3 Faecal softeners

Liquid paraffin, the traditional lubricant, has disadvantages (see below). Bulk laxatives (section 1.6.1) and non-ionic surfactant 'wetting' agents e.g. docusate sodium (section 1.6.2) also have softening properties. Such drugs are useful for oral administration in the management of haemorrhoids and anal fissure; glycerol (section 1.6.2) is useful for rectal use.

Enemas containing **arachis oil** (ground-nut oil, peanut oil) lubricate and soften impacted faeces and promote a bowel movement.

ARACHIS OIL

Indications see notes above
Dose
- See below

Fletchers' Arachis Oil Retention Enema® (Forest)
Enema, arachis (peanut) oil in 130-mL single-dose disposable packs. Net price 130 mL = 96p
Dose to soften impacted faeces, 130 mL; the enema should be warmed before use; CHILD (but see section 1.6) under 3 years not recommended; over 3 years reduce adult dose in proportion to body-weight (medical supervision only), see *BNF for Children*

LIQUID PARAFFIN

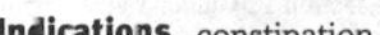

Indications constipation
Cautions avoid prolonged use; contra-indicated in children under 3 years
Side-effects anal seepage of paraffin and consequent anal irritation after prolonged use, granulomatous reactions caused by absorption of small quantities of liquid paraffin (especially from the emulsion), lipoid pneumonia, and interference with the absorption of fat-soluble vitamins
Dose
- See under preparation

Liquid Paraffin Oral Emulsion, BP
Oral emulsion, liquid paraffin 5 mL, vanillin 5 mg, chloroform 0.025 mL, benzoic acid solution 0.2 mL, methylcellulose-20 200 mg, saccharin sodium 500 micrograms, water to 10 mL
Dose 10–30 mL at night when required
Counselling Should not be taken immediately before going to bed

1.6.4 Osmotic laxatives

Osmotic laxatives increase the amount of water in the large bowel, either by drawing fluid from the body into the bowel or by retaining the fluid they were administered with.

Lactulose is a semi-synthetic disaccharide which is not absorbed from the gastro-intestinal tract. It produces an osmotic diarrhoea of low faecal pH, and discourages the proliferation of ammonia-producing organisms. It is therefore useful in the treatment of *hepatic encephalopathy*.

Macrogols are inert polymers of ethylene glycol which sequester fluid in the bowel; giving fluid with macrogols may reduce the dehydrating effect sometimes seen with osmotic laxatives.

Saline purgatives such as **magnesium hydroxide** are commonly abused but are satisfactory for occasional use; adequate fluid intake should be maintained. **Magnesium salts** are useful where rapid bowel evacuation is required. **Sodium salts** should be avoided as they may give rise to sodium and water retention in susceptible individuals. **Phosphate enemas** are useful in bowel clearance before radiology, endoscopy, and surgery.

LACTULOSE

Indications constipation (may take up to 48 hours to act), hepatic encephalopathy (portal systemic encephalopathy)

Cautions lactose intolerance; **interactions:** Appendix 1 (lactulose)

Contra-indications galactosaemia, intestinal obstruction

Side-effects flatulence, cramps, and abdominal discomfort

Dose

- See under preparations below

Lactulose (Non-proprietary)

Solution, lactulose 3.1–3.7 g/5 mL with other ketoses. Net price 300-mL pack = £2.26, 500-mL pack = £2.63

Dose constipation, initially 15 mL twice daily, adjusted according to patient's needs; CHILD (but see section 1.6) under 1 year 2.5 mL twice daily, 1–5 years 5 mL twice daily, 5–10 years 10 mL twice daily

Hepatic encephalopathy, 30–50 mL 3 times daily, subsequently adjusted to produce 2–3 soft stools daily

Brands include *Duphalac®* (NHS), *Lactugal®*, *Regulose®*

MACROGOLS
(Polyethylene glycols)

Indications see preparations below

Cautions pregnancy (Appendix 4); breast-feeding (Appendix 5); discontinue if symptoms of fluid and electrolyte disturbance; see also preparations below

Contra-indications intestinal perforation or obstruction, paralytic ileus, severe inflammatory conditions of the intestinal tract (such as Crohn's disease, ulcerative colitis, and toxic megacolon), see also preparations below

Side-effects abdominal distension and pain, nausea

Dose

- See preparations below

Idrolax® (Ipsen)

Oral powder, macrogol '4000' (polyethylene glycol '4000') 10 g/sachet, net price 20-sachet pack (orange-grapefruit flavour) = £4.84. Label: 13

Dose constipation, 1–2 sachets preferably as a single dose in the morning; content of each sachet dissolved in a glass of water; CHILD over 8 years, as adult dose for max. 3 months

Movicol® (Norgine)

Oral powder, macrogol '3350' (polyethylene glycol '3350') 13.125 g, sodium bicarbonate 178.5 mg, sodium chloride 350.7 mg, potassium chloride 46.6 mg/sachet, net price 20-sachet pack (lime and lemon flavour) = £4.63, 30-sachet pack (lime- and lemon- or plain-flavoured) = £6.95, 50-sachet pack (lime- and lemon- or plain-flavoured) = £11.60. Label: 13

Cautions patients with cardiovascular impairment should not take more than 2 sachets in any 1 hour

Dose chronic constipation, ADULT and CHILD over 12 years, 1–3 sachets daily in divided doses usually for up to 2 weeks; content of each sachet dissolved in half a glass (approx. 125 mL) of water; maintenance, 1–2 sachets daily

Faecal impaction, ADULT and CHILD over 12 years, 8 sachets daily dissolved in 1 litre water and drunk within 6 hours, usually for max. 3 days

After reconstitution the solution should be kept in a refrigerator and discarded if unused after 6 hours

Movicol®-Half (Norgine)

Oral powder, macrogol '3350' (polyethylene glycol '3350') 6.563 g, sodium bicarbonate 89.3 mg, sodium chloride 175.4 mg, potassium chloride 23.3 mg/sachet, net price 20-sachet pack (lime and lemon flavour) = £2.78, 30-sachet pack = £4.17. Label: 13

Cautions patients with cardiovascular impairment should not take more than 4 sachets in any 1 hour

Dose chronic constipation, ADULT and CHILD over 12 years, 2–6 sachets daily in divided doses usually for up to 2 weeks; content of each sachet dissolved in quarter of a glass (approx. 60–65 mL) of water; maintenance, 2–4 sachets daily

Faecal impaction, ADULT and CHILD over 12 years, 16 sachets daily dissolved in 1 litre of water and drunk within 6 hours, usually for max. 3 days

After reconstitution the solution should be kept in a refrigerator and discarded if unused after 6 hours

Movicol® Paediatric Plain (Norgine) PoM

Oral powder, macrogol '3350' (polyethylene glycol '3350') 6.563 g, sodium bicarbonate 89.3 mg, sodium chloride 175.4 mg, potassium chloride 25.1 mg/sachet, net price 30-sachet pack = £4.63. Label: 13

Cautions *with high doses*, impaired gag reflex, reflux oesophagitis, impaired consciousness

Contra-indications cardiovascular impairment; renal impairment

Dose chronic constipation and recurrence of faecal impaction, CHILD 2–6 years 1 sachet daily; 7–11 years 2 sachets daily; adjust according to response, max. 4 sachets daily

Faecal impaction, CHILD (taken in divided doses over 12 hours each day until impaction resolves or for max. 7 days) 5–11 years 4 sachets on first day then increased in steps of 2 sachets daily to 12 sachets daily; content of each sachet dissolved in quarter of a glass (approx. 60–65 mL) of water

After reconstitution the solution should be kept in a refrigerator and discarded if unused after 24 hours

MAGNESIUM SALTS

Indications see under preparations below

Cautions renal impairment (Appendix 3; risk of magnesium accumulation); hepatic impairment (see Appendix 2); elderly and debilitated; see also notes above; **interactions:** Appendix 1 (antacids)

Contra-indications acute gastro-intestinal conditions

Side-effects colic

Dose

- See preparations

▲Magnesium hydroxide

Magnesium Hydroxide Mixture, BP

Aqueous suspension containing about 8% hydrated magnesium oxide. Do not store in cold place

Dose constipation, 30–45 mL with water at bedtime when required; CHILD 3–12 years, 5–10 mL with water at bedtime when required

▲Magnesium hydroxide with liquid paraffin

Liquid Paraffin and Magnesium Hydroxide Oral Emulsion, BP

Oral emulsion, 25% liquid paraffin in aqueous suspension containing 6% hydrated magnesium oxide

Dose constipation, 5–20 mL when required

Note Liquid paraffin and magnesium hydroxide preparations on sale to the public include: *Milpar®* (NHS)

▲Magnesium sulphate

Magnesium Sulphate

Label: 13, 23

Dose rapid bowel evacuation (acts in 2–4 hours) 5–10 g in a glass of water preferably before breakfast

Note Magnesium sulphate is on sale to the public as Epsom Salts

▲Bowel cleansing solutions

Section 1.6.5

PHOSPHATES (RECTAL)

Indications rectal use in constipation; bowel evacuation before abdominal radiological procedures, endoscopy, and surgery

Cautions elderly and debilitated

Contra-indications acute gastro-intestinal conditions

Side-effects local irritation

Dose

- See under preparations

Carbalax® (Forest)

Suppositories, sodium acid phosphate (anhydrous) 1.3 g, sodium bicarbonate 1.08 g, net price 12 = £2.01

Dose constipation, ADULT and CHILD over 12 years, 1 suppository, inserted 30 minutes before evacuation required; moisten with water before use

Fleet® Ready-to-use Enema (De Witt)

Enema, sodium acid phosphate 21.4 g, sodium phosphate 9.4 g/118 mL, net price 133-mL pack (delivers 118 mL dose) with standard tube = 46p

Dose ADULT and CHILD (but see section 1.6) over 12 years, 118 mL; CHILD 3–12 years, on doctor's advice only (under 3 years not recommended)

Fletchers' Phosphate Enema® (Forest)

Enema, sodium acid phosphate 12.8 g, sodium phosphate 10.24 g, purified water, freshly boiled and cooled, to 128 mL (corresponds to Phosphates Enema Formula B). Net price 128 mL with standard tube = 41p, with long rectal tube = 57p

Dose 128 mL; CHILD (but see section 1.6) over 3 years, reduced according to body weight, see *BNF for Children*

SODIUM CITRATE (RECTAL)

Indications rectal use in constipation

Cautions elderly and debilitated; see also notes above

Contra-indications acute gastro-intestinal conditions

Dose

- See under preparations

Micolette Micro-enema® (Pinewood)

Enema, sodium citrate 450 mg, sodium lauryl sulphoacetate 45 mg, glycerol 625 mg, together with citric acid, potassium sorbate, and sorbitol in a viscous solution, in 5-mL single-dose disposable packs with nozzle. Net price 5 mL = 31p

Dose ADULT and CHILD over 3 years, 5–10 mL (but see section 1.6)

Micralax Micro-enema® (UCB Pharma)

Enema, sodium citrate 450 mg, sodium alkylsulphoacetate 45 mg, sorbic acid 5 mg, together with glycerol and sorbitol in a viscous solution in 5-mL single-dose disposable packs with nozzle. Net price 5 mL = 41p

Dose ADULT and CHILD over 3 years, 5 mL (but see section 1.6)

Relaxit Micro-enema® (Crawford)

Enema, sodium citrate 450 mg, sodium lauryl sulphate 75 mg, sorbic acid 5 mg, together with glycerol and sorbitol in a viscous solution in 5-mL single-dose disposable packs with nozzle. Net price 5 mL = 32p

Dose ADULT and CHILD (but see section 1.6) 5 mL (insert only half nozzle length in child under 3 years)

1.6.5 Bowel cleansing solutions

Bowel cleansing solutions are used before colonic surgery, colonoscopy, or radiological examination to ensure the bowel is free of solid contents. They are **not** treatments for constipation.

BOWEL CLEANSING SOLUTIONS

Indications see above

Cautions pregnancy; renal impairment (Appendix 3); heart disease; ulcerative colitis; diabetes mellitus; reflux oesophagitis, impaired gag reflex; unconscious or semiconscious or possibility of regurgitation or aspiration

Contra-indications gastro-intestinal obstruction, gastric retention, gastro-intestinal ulceration, perforated bowel, congestive cardiac failure; toxic colitis, toxic megacolon or ileus

Side-effects nausea, vomiting, abdominal pain (usually transient—reduced by taking more slowly), abdominal distention, anal discomfort; *less frequently* headache, rash, and electrolyte disturbances

Dose

- See under preparations

CitraFleet® (De Witt)

Oral powder, sugar-free, sodium picosulfate 10 mg/sachet, with magnesium citrate, net price 2-sachet pack (lemon-flavoured) = £3.25. Label: 10, patient information leaflet, 13, counselling, see below

Dose bowel evacuation on day before radiological examination, endoscopy, or surgery, ADULT over 18 years, 1 sachet before 8 a.m. then 1 sachet 6–8 hours later

Note Low residue diet recommended on the day before procedure and copious intake of water or other clear fluids recommended during treatment

Counselling One sachet should be reconstituted with 150 mL (approx. half a glass) of cold water; patients should be warned that heat is generated during reconstitution and that the solution should be allowed to cool before drinking

Citramag® (Sanochemia)
Oral powder, sugar-free, effervescent, magnesium carbonate 11.57 g, anhydrous citric acid 17.79 g/sachet, net price 10-sachet pack (lemon and lime flavour) = £14.90. Label: 10, patient information leaflet, 13, counselling, see below

Dose bowel evacuation for surgery, colonoscopy or radiological examination, on day before procedure, 1 sachet at 8 a.m. and 1 sachet between 2 and 4 p.m.; CHILD 5–9 years one-third adult dose; over 10 years and frail ELDERLY one-half adult dose

Counselling The patient information leaflet advises that hot water (200 mL) is needed to make the solution and provides guidance on the timing and procedure for reconstitution; it also mentions need for high fluid, low residue diet beforehand (according to hospital advice), and explains that only clear fluids can be taken after *Citramag®* until procedure completed

Fleet Phospho-soda® (De Witt)
Oral solution, sugar-free, sodium dihydrogen phosphate dihydrate 24.4 g, disodium phosphate dodecahydrate 10.8 g/45 mL. Net price 2 × 45-mL bottles = £4.79. Label: 10, patient information leaflet, counselling

Dose ADULT and CHILD over 15 years, 45 mL diluted with half a glass (120 mL) of cold water, followed by one full glass (240 mL) of cold water

Timing of doses is dependent on the time of the procedure

For morning procedure, first dose should be taken at 7 a.m. and second at 7 p.m. on day before the procedure

For afternoon procedure, first dose should be taken at 7 p.m. on day before and second dose at 7 a.m. on day of the procedure

Solid food must not be taken during dosing period; clear liquids or water should be substituted for meals

Klean-Prep® (Norgine)
Oral powder, sugar-free, macrogol '3350' (polyethylene glycol '3350') 59 g, anhydrous sodium sulphate 5.685 g, sodium bicarbonate 1.685 g, sodium chloride 1.465 g, potassium chloride 743 mg/sachet, net price 4 sachets = £8.56. Label: 10, patient information leaflet, 13, counselling

Excipients include aspartame (section 9.4.1)

Four sachets when reconstituted with water to 4 litres provides an iso-osmotic solution for bowel cleansing before surgery, colonoscopy or radiological procedures

Dose a glass (approx. 250 mL) of reconstituted solution every 10–15 minutes, or by nasogastric tube 20–30 mL/minute, until 4 litres have been consumed or watery stools are free of solid matter; CHILD not recommended

The solution from all 4 sachets should be drunk within 4–6 hours (250 mL drunk rapidly every 10–15 minutes); flavouring such as clear fruit cordials may be added if required; to facilitate gastric emptying domperidone or metoclopramide may be given 30 minutes before starting.

Alternatively the administration may be divided into two, e.g. taking the solutions from 2 sachets on the evening before examination and the remaining 2 on the morning of the examination

After reconstitution the solution should be kept in a refrigerator and discarded if unused after 24 hours

Note Allergic reactions reported

Moviprep® (Norgine)
Oral powder, sugar-free, lemon-flavoured, *Sachet A* (containing macrogol '3350' (polyethylene glycol '3350') 100 g, anhydrous sodium sulphate 7.5 g, sodium chloride 2.691 g, potassium chloride 1.015 g) and *Sachet B* (containing ascorbic acid 4.7 g, sodium ascorbate 5.9 g), net price 4-sachet pack (2 each of sachet A and B) = £10.27. Label: 10, patient information leaflet, 13, counselling, see below

Excipients include aspartame (section 9.4.1)

Contra-indications G6PD deficiency

Dose bowel evacuation for surgery, colonoscopy or radiological examination, ADULT over 18 years, 2 litres of reconstituted solution on the evening before procedure *or* 1 litre of reconstituted solution on the evening before procedure and 1 litre of reconstituted solution early on the morning of procedure; treatment should be completed at least 1 hour before colonoscopy

Counselling One pair of sachets (A and B) should be reconstituted in 1 litre of water and taken over 1–2 hours. Solid food should not be taken during treatment. 1 litre of other clear fluid should also be taken during treatment

Picolax® (Ferring)
Oral powder, sugar-free, sodium picosulfate 10 mg/sachet, with magnesium citrate, net price 2-sachet pack = £3.53. Label: 10, patient information leaflet, 13, counselling, see below

Dose bowel evacuation on day before radiological procedure, endoscopy, or surgery, ADULT and CHILD over 9 years, 1 sachet before 8 a.m. then 1 sachet 6–8 hours later; CHILD 1–2 years, quarter sachet before 8 a.m. then quarter sachet 6–8 hours later; 2–4 years, half sachet before 8 a.m. then half sachet 6–8 hours later; 4–9 years, 1 sachet before 8 a.m. then half sachet 6–8 hours later

Acts within 3 hours of first dose

Note Low residue diet recommended on the day before procedure and copious intake of water or other clear fluids recommended during treatment

Counselling One sachet should be reconstituted with 150 mL (approx. half a glass) of cold water; patients should be warned that heat is generated during reconstitution and that the solution should be allowed to cool before drinking

1.7 Local preparations for anal and rectal disorders

1.7.1 Soothing haemorrhoidal preparations
1.7.2 Compound haemorrhoidal preparations with corticosteroids
1.7.3 Rectal sclerosants
1.7.4 Management of anal fissures

Anal and perianal pruritus, soreness, and excoriation are best treated by application of bland ointments and suppositories (section 1.7.1). These conditions occur commonly in patients suffering from haemorrhoids, fistulas, and proctitis. Cleansing with attention to any minor faecal soiling, adjustment of the diet to avoid hard stools, the use of bulk-forming materials such as bran (section 1.6.1) and a high residue diet are helpful. In proctitis these measures may supplement treatment with corticosteroids or sulfasalazine (see section 1.5).

When necessary topical preparations containing **local anaesthetics** (section 1.7.1) or **corticosteroids** (section 1.7.2) are used provided perianal thrush has been excluded. Perianal thrush is best treated with **nystatin** by mouth and by local application (see section 5.2, section 7.2.2, and section 13.10.2).

For the management of *anal fissures*, see section 1.7.4.

1.7.1 Soothing haemorrhoidal preparations

Soothing preparations containing mild astringents such as bismuth subgallate, zinc oxide, and hamamelis may give symptomatic relief in haemorrhoids. Many proprietary preparations also contain lubricants, vasoconstrictors, or mild antiseptics.

Local anaesthetics are used to relieve pain associated with *haemorrhoids* and *pruritus ani* but good evidence is lacking. Lidocaine (lignocaine) ointment (section 15.2) is used before emptying the bowel to relieve pain associated with *anal fissure*. Alternative local anaesthetics include tetracaine (amethocaine), cinchocaine (dibucaine), and pramocaine (pramoxine), but they are more irritant. Local anaesthetic ointments can be absorbed through the rectal mucosa therefore excessive application should be **avoided**, particularly in infants and children. Preparations containing local anaesthetics should be used for short periods only (no longer than a few days) since they may cause sensitisation of the anal skin.

1.7.2 Compound haemorrhoidal preparations with corticosteroids

Corticosteroids are often combined with local anaesthetics and soothing agents in preparations for haemorrhoids. They are suitable for occasional short-term use after exclusion of infections, such as herpes simplex; prolonged use can cause atrophy of the anal skin. See section 13.4 for general comments on topical corticosteroids and section 1.7.1 for comment on local anaesthetics.

Children Haemorrhoids in children are rare. Treatment is usually symptomatic and the use of a locally applied cream is appropriate for short periods; however, local anaesthetics can cause stinging initially and this may aggravate the child's fear of defaecation.

Anugesic-HC® (Pfizer) PoM

Cream, benzyl benzoate 1.2%, bismuth oxide 0.875%, hydrocortisone acetate 0.5%, Peru balsam 1.85%, pramocaine hydrochloride 1%, zinc oxide 12.35%. Net price 30 g (with rectal nozzle) = £3.71

Dose apply night and morning and after a bowel movement; do not use for longer than 7 days; CHILD not recommended

Suppositories, buff, benzyl benzoate 33 mg, bismuth oxide 24 mg, bismuth subgallate 59 mg, hydrocortisone acetate 5 mg, Peru balsam 49 mg, pramocaine hydrochloride 27 mg, zinc oxide 296 mg, net price 12 = £2.69

Dose insert 1 suppository night and morning and after a bowel movement; do not use for longer than 7 days; CHILD not recommended

Anusol-HC® (Pfizer Consumer) PoM

Ointment, benzyl benzoate 1.25%, bismuth oxide 0.875%, bismuth subgallate 2.25%, hydrocortisone acetate 0.25%, Peru balsam 1.875%, zinc oxide 10.75%. Net price 30 g (with rectal nozzle) = £3.50

Dose apply night and morning and after a bowel movement; do not use for longer than 7 days; CHILD not recommended

Note A proprietary brand (*Anusol Plus HC®* ointment) is on sale to the public

Suppositories, benzyl benzoate 33 mg, bismuth oxide 24 mg, bismuth subgallate 59 mg, hydrocortisone acetate 10 mg, Peru balsam 49 mg, zinc oxide 296 mg. Net price 12 = £2.46

Dose insert 1 suppository night and morning and after a bowel movement; do not use for longer than 7 days; CHILD not recommended

Note A proprietary brand (*Anusol Plus HC®* suppositories) is on sale to the public

Perinal® (Dermal)

Spray application, hydrocortisone 0.2%, lidocaine hydrochloride 1%. Net price 30-mL pack = £6.39

Dose ADULT and CHILD over 14 years, spray once over the affected area up to 3 times daily; do not use for longer than 7 days without medical advice; CHILD under 14 years on medical advice only

Proctofoam HC® (Meda) PoM

Foam in aerosol pack, hydrocortisone acetate 1%, pramocaine hydrochloride 1%. Net price 21.2-g pack (approx. 40 applications) with applicator = £5.06

Dose haemorrhoids and proctitis, 1 applicatorful (4–6 mg hydrocortisone acetate, 4–6 mg pramocaine hydrochloride) by rectum 2–3 times daily and after a bowel movement (max. 4 times daily); do not use for longer than 7 days; CHILD not recommended

Proctosedyl® (Aventis Pharma) PoM

Ointment, cinchocaine (dibucaine) hydrochloride 0.5%, hydrocortisone 0.5%. Net price 30 g = £9.40 (with cannula)

Dose apply morning and night and after a bowel movement, externally or by rectum; do not use for longer than 7 days

Suppositories, cinchocaine (dibucaine) hydrochloride 5 mg, hydrocortisone 5 mg. Net price 12 = £4.24

Dose insert 1 suppository night and morning and after a bowel movement; do not use for longer than 7 days

Scheriproct® (Valeant) PoM

Ointment, cinchocaine (dibucaine) hydrochloride 0.5%, prednisolone hexanoate 0.19%. Net price 30 g = £3.00

Dose apply twice daily for 5–7 days (3–4 times daily on 1st day if necessary), then once daily for a few days after symptoms have cleared

Suppositories, cinchocaine (dibucaine) hydrochloride 1 mg, prednisolone hexanoate 1.3 mg. Net price 12 = £1.41

Dose insert 1 suppository daily after a bowel movement, for 5–7 days (in severe cases initially 2–3 times daily)

Ultraproct® (Meadow) PoM

Ointment, cinchocaine (dibucaine) hydrochloride 0.5%, fluocortolone caproate 0.095%, fluocortolone pivalate 0.092%, net price 30 g (with rectal nozzle) = £4.57

Dose apply twice daily for 5–7 days (3–4 times daily on 1st day if necessary), then once daily for a few days after symptoms have cleared

Suppositories, cinchocaine (dibucaine) hydrochloride 1 mg, fluocortolone caproate 630 micrograms, fluocortolone pivalate 610 micrograms, net price 12 = £2.15

Dose insert 1 suppository daily after a bowel movement, for 5–7 days (in severe cases initially 2–3 times daily) then 1 suppository every other day for 1 week

Uniroid-HC® (Chemidex) PoM

Ointment, cinchocaine (dibucaine) hydrochloride 0.5%, hydrocortisone 0.5%. Net price 30 g (with applicator) = £4.23

Dose ADULT and CHILD over 12 years, apply twice daily and after a bowel movement, externally or by rectum, do not use for longer than 7 days; CHILD under 12 years on medical advice only

Suppositories, cinchocaine (dibucaine) hydrochloride 5 mg, hydrocortisone 5 mg. Net price 12 = £1.91

Dose ADULT and CHILD over 12 years, insert 1 suppository twice daily and after a bowel movement; do not use for longer than 7 days

Xyloproct® (AstraZeneca) PoM
Ointment (water-miscible), aluminium acetate 3.5%, hydrocortisone acetate 0.275%, lidocaine 5%, zinc oxide 18%, net price 20 g (with applicator) = £2.26
Dose apply several times daily; short-term use only

1.7.3 Rectal sclerosants

Oily phenol injection is used to inject haemorrhoids particularly when unprolapsed.

PHENOL

Indications see notes above
Side-effects irritation, tissue necrosis

Oily Phenol Injection, BP PoM
phenol 5% in a suitable fixed oil. Net price 5-mL amp = £5.00
Dose 2–3 mL into the submucosal layer at the base of the pile; several injections may be given at different sites, max. total injected 10 mL at any one time
Available from UCB Pharma

1.7.4 Management of anal fissures

The management of *anal fissures* requires stool softening by increasing dietary fibre in the form of bran or by using a bulk-forming laxative. Short-term use of local anaesthetic preparations may help (section 1.7.1). If these measures are inadequate, the patient should be referred for specialist treatment in hospital. The use of a topical nitrate (e.g. glyceryl trinitrate 0.4% ointment) may be considered. Before considering surgery, topical diltiazem 2% may be used twice daily [unlicensed indication] in patients with chronic anal fissures unresponsive to topical nitrates.

GLYCERYL TRINITRATE

Indications anal fissure; angina, left ventricular failure (section 2.6.1); extravasation (section 10.3)
Cautions section 2.6.1
Contra-indications section 2.6.1
Side-effects section 2.6.1; also diarrhoea, burning, itching, and rectal bleeding
Dose
- See preparations

Rectogesic® (Strakan) ▼ PoM
Rectal ointment, glyceryl trinitrate 0.4%, net price 30 g = £32.80
Excipients include lanolin, propylene glycol
Dose ADULT over 18 years, apply 2.5 cm of ointment to anal canal every 12 hours until pain stops; max. duration of use 8 weeks
Note 2.5 cm of ointment contains glyceryl trinitrate 1.5 mg; discard tube 8 weeks after first opening

1.8 Stoma care

Prescribing for patients with stoma calls for special care. The following is a brief account of some of the main points to be borne in mind.

Enteric-coated and *modified-release* preparations are **unsuitable**, particularly in patients with an ileostomy, as there may not be sufficient release of the active ingredient.

Laxatives. Enemas and washouts should **not** be prescribed for patients with an ileostomy as they may cause rapid and severe loss of water and electrolytes.

Colostomy patients may suffer from constipation and whenever possible should be treated by increasing fluid intake or dietary fibre. **Bulk-forming drugs** (section 1.6.1) should be tried. If they are insufficient, as small a dose as possible of senna (section 1.6.2) should be used.

Antidiarrhoeals. Drugs such as **loperamide**, **codeine phosphate**, or **co-phenotrope** (diphenoxylate with atropine) are effective. Bulk-forming drugs (section 1.6.1) may be tried but it is often difficult to adjust the dose appropriately.

Antibacterials should **not** be given for an episode of acute diarrhoea.

Antacids. The tendency to diarrhoea from magnesium salts or constipation from aluminium salts may be increased in these patients.

Diuretics should be used with caution in patients with an ileostomy as they may become excessively dehydrated and potassium depletion may easily occur. It is usually advisable to use a **potassium-sparing** diuretic (see section 2.2.3).

Digoxin. Patients with a stoma are particularly susceptible to hypokalaemia if on digoxin therapy and potassium supplements or a potassium-sparing diuretic may be advisable (for comment see section 9.2.1.1).

Potassium supplements. Liquid formulations are preferred to modified-release formulations (see above).

Analgesics. Opioid analgesics (see section 4.7.2) may cause troublesome constipation in colostomy patients. When a non-opioid analgesic is required **paracetamol** is usually suitable but anti-inflammatory analgesics may cause gastric irritation and bleeding.

Iron preparations may cause loose stools and sore skin in these patients. If this is troublesome and if iron is definitely indicated an intramuscular iron preparation (see section 9.1.1.2) should be used. Modified-release preparations should be **avoided** for the reasons given above.

Patients are usually given advice about the use of *cleansing agents, protective creams, lotions, deodorants,* or *sealants* whilst in hospital, either by the surgeon or by stoma care nurses. Voluntary organisations offer help and support to patients with stoma.

1.9 Drugs affecting intestinal secretions

1.9.1 Drugs affecting biliary composition and flow
1.9.2 Bile acid sequestrants
1.9.3 Aprotinin
1.9.4 Pancreatin

1.9.1 Drugs affecting biliary composition and flow

The use of laparoscopic cholecystectomy and of endoscopic biliary techniques has limited the place of the bile acid **ursodeoxycholic acid** in gallstone disease. Ursodeoxycholic acid is suitable for patients with unimpaired gall bladder function, small or medium-sized radiolucent stones, and whose mild symptoms are not amenable to other treatment; it should be used cautiously in those with liver disease (but see below). Patients should be given dietary advice (including avoidance of excessive cholesterol and calories) and they require radiological monitoring. Long-term prophylaxis may be needed after complete dissolution of the gallstones has been confirmed because they may recur in up to 25% of patients within one year of stopping treatment.

Ursodeoxycholic acid is also used in primary biliary cirrhosis; liver tests improve in most patients but the effect on overall survival is uncertain. Ursodeoxycholic acid has also been tried in primary sclerosing cholangitis [unlicensed indication].

URSODEOXYCHOLIC ACID

Indications see under Dose and under preparations

Cautions see notes above; **interactions:** Appendix 1 (ursodeoxycholic acid)

Contra-indications radio-opaque stones, pregnancy (Appendix 4), non-functioning gall bladder, inflammatory diseases and other conditions of the small intestine, colon and liver which interfere with enterohepatic circulation of bile salts

Side-effects nausea, vomiting, diarrhoea; gallstone calcification; pruritus

Dose

- Dissolution of gallstones, 8–12 mg/kg daily as a single dose at bedtime *or* in two divided doses, for up to 2 years; treatment is continued for 3–4 months after stones dissolve
- Primary biliary cirrhosis, see under *Ursofalk®*

Ursodeoxycholic Acid (Non-proprietary) PoM
Tablets, ursodeoxycholic acid 150 mg, net price 60-tab pack = £18.51. Label: 21
Capsules, ursodeoxycholic acid 250 mg, net price 60-cap pack = £35.11. Label: 21

Destolit® (Norgine) PoM
Tablets, scored, ursodeoxycholic acid 150 mg, net price 60-tab pack = £18.39. Label: 21

Urdox® (CP) PoM
Tablets, f/c, ursodeoxycholic acid 300 mg, net price 60-tab pack = £26.50. Label: 21

Ursofalk® (Dr Falk) PoM
Capsules, ursodeoxycholic acid 250 mg, net price 60-cap pack = £31.10, 100-cap pack = £32.85. Label: 21
Suspension, sugar-free, ursodeoxycholic acid 250 mg/5 mL, net price 250 mL = £28.50. Label: 21
Dose primary biliary cirrhosis, 10–15 mg/kg daily in 2–4 divided doses
Dissolution of gallstones, see Dose, above

Ursogal® (Galen) PoM
Tablets, scored, ursodeoxycholic acid 150 mg, net price 60-tab pack = £17.05. Label: 21
Capsules, ursodeoxycholic acid 250 mg, net price 60-cap pack = £30.50. Label: 21

Other preparations for biliary disorders

A terpene mixture (*Rowachol®*) raises biliary cholesterol solubility. It is not considered to be a useful adjunct.

Rowachol® (Rowa) PoM
Capsules, green, e/c, borneol 5 mg, camphene 5 mg, cineole 2 mg, menthol 32 mg, menthone 6 mg, pinene 17 mg in olive oil. Net price 50-cap pack = £7.35. Label: 22
Dose 1–2 capsules 3 times daily before food (but see notes above)
Interactions: Appendix 1 (*Rowachol®*)

1.9.2 Bile acid sequestrants

Colestyramine (cholestyramine) is an anion-exchange resin that is not absorbed from the gastro-intestinal tract. It relieves diarrhoea and pruritus by forming an insoluble complex with bile acids in the intestine. Colestyramine can interfere with the absorption of a number of drugs. Colestyramine is also used in hypercholesterolaemia (section 2.12).

COLESTYRAMINE
(Cholestyramine)

Indications pruritus associated with partial biliary obstruction and primary biliary cirrhosis; diarrhoea associated with Crohn's disease, ileal resection, vagotomy, diabetic vagal neuropathy, and radiation; hypercholesterolaemia (section 2.12)

Cautions see section 2.12

Contra-indications see section 2.12

Side-effects see section 2.12

Dose

- Pruritus, 4–8 g daily in a suitable liquid; CHILD 6–12 years, consult product literature
- Diarrhoea, initially 4 g daily increased by 4 g at weekly intervals to 12–24 g daily in a suitable liquid in 1–4 divided doses, then adjusted as required; max. 36 g daily; CHILD 6–12 years, consult product literature

Counselling Other drugs should be taken at least 1 hour before or 4–6 hours after colestyramine to reduce possible interference with absorption

Note The contents of each sachet should be mixed with at least 150 mL of water or other suitable liquid such as fruit juice, skimmed milk, thin soups, and pulpy fruits with a high moisture content

Preparations
Section 2.12

1.9.3 Aprotinin

Aprotinin is no longer used for the treatment of acute pancreatitis.

1.9.4 Pancreatin

Supplements of pancreatin are given by mouth to compensate for reduced or absent exocrine secretion in cystic fibrosis, and following pancreatectomy, gastrectomy, or chronic pancreatitis. They assist the digestion of starch, fat, and protein. Pancreatin may also be necessary if a tumour (e.g. pancreatic cancer) obstructs outflow from the pancreas.

Pancreatin is inactivated by gastric acid therefore pancreatin preparations are best taken with food (or immediately before or after food). Gastric acid secretion may be reduced by giving cimetidine or ranitidine an hour beforehand (section 1.3). Concurrent use of antacids also reduces gastric acidity. Enteric-coated preparations deliver a higher enzyme concentration in the duodenum (provided the capsule contents are swallowed whole without chewing). Higher-strength preparations are also available (**important**: see CSM advice below).

Since pancreatin is also inactivated by heat, excessive heat should be avoided if preparations are mixed with liquids or food; the resulting mixtures should not be kept for more than one hour.

Dosage is adjusted according to size, number, and consistency of stools, so that the patient thrives; extra allowance may be needed if snacks are taken between meals.

Pancreatin can irritate the perioral skin and buccal mucosa if retained in the mouth, and excessive doses can cause perianal irritation. The most frequent side-effects are gastro-intestinal, including nausea, vomiting, and abdominal discomfort; hyperuricaemia and hyperuricosuria have been associated with very high doses. Hypersensitivity reactions occur occasionally and may affect those handling the powder.

PANCREATIN

Indications see above

Cautions see above and (for higher-strength preparations) see below

Side-effects see above and (for higher-strength preparations) see below

Dose

- See preparations

Creon® 10 000 (Solvay)

Capsules, brown/clear, enclosing buff-coloured e/c granules of pancreatin (pork), providing: protease 600 units, lipase 10 000 units, amylase 8000 units. Net price 100-cap pack = £16.66. Counselling, see dose

Dose ADULT and CHILD initially 1–2 capsules with meals either taken whole or contents mixed with fluid or soft food (then swallowed immediately without chewing)

Creon® Micro (Solvay)

Gastro-resistant granules, brown, pancreatin (pork), providing: protease 200 units, lipase 5000 units, amylase 3600 units per 100 mg, net price 20 g = £31.50 Counselling, see dose

Dose ADULT and CHILD initially 100 mg with meals either taken whole or mixed with acidic fluid or soft food (then swallowed immediately without chewing)

Nutrizym 10® (Merck)

Capsules, red/yellow, enclosing e/c minitablets of pancreatin (pork), providing minimum of: protease 500 units, lipase 10 000 units, amylase 9000 units. Net price 100 = £14.47. Counselling, see dose

Dose ADULT and CHILD 1–2 capsules with meals and 1 capsule with snacks, swallowed whole or contents taken with water or sprinkled on soft food (then swallowed immediately without chewing); higher doses may be required according to response

Pancrex® (Paines & Byrne)

Granules, pancreatin (pork), providing minimum of: protease 300 units, lipase 5000 units, amylase 4000 units/g. Net price 300 g = £20.39. Label: 25, counselling, see dose

Dose ADULT and CHILD 5–10 g just before meals washed down or mixed with a little milk or water

Pancrex V® (Paines & Byrne)

Capsules, pancreatin (pork), providing minimum of: protease 430 units, lipase 8000 units, amylase 9000 units. Net price 300-cap pack = £15.80. Counselling, see dose

Dose ADULT and CHILD over 1 year 2–6 capsules with meals, swallowed whole or sprinkled on food; INFANT up to 1 year contents of 1–2 capsules mixed with feeds

Capsules '125', pancreatin (pork), providing minimum of: protease 160 units, lipase 2950 units, amylase 3300 units. Net price 300-cap pack = £9.72. Counselling, see dose

Dose NEONATE contents of 1–2 capsules mixed with feeds

Tablets, e/c, pancreatin (pork), providing minimum of: protease 110 units, lipase 1900 units, amylase 1700 units. Net price 300-tab pack = £4.51. Label: 5, 25, counselling, see dose

Dose ADULT and CHILD 5–15 tablets before meals

Tablets forte, e/c, pancreatin (pork), providing minimum of: protease 330 units, lipase 5600 units, amylase 5000 units. Net price 300-tab pack = £13.74. Label: 5, 25, counselling, see dose

Dose ADULT and CHILD 6–10 tablets before meals

Powder, pancreatin (pork), providing minimum of: protease 1400 units, lipase 25 000 units, amylase 30 000 units/g. Net price 300 g = £24.28. Counselling, see dose

Dose ADULT and CHILD over 1 month, 0.5–2 g with meals washed down or mixed with liquid; NEONATE 250–500 mg with each feed

Higher-strength preparations

The **CSM** has advised of data associating the high-strength pancreatin preparations *Nutrizym 22®* and *Pancreatin HL®* with the development of large bowel strictures (fibrosing colonopathy) in children with cystic fibrosis aged between 2 and 13 years. No association was found with *Creon® 25 000*. The following was recommended:

- *Pancrease HL®*, *Nutrizym 22®*, *Panzytrat® 25 000* [now discontinued] should not be used in children aged 15 years or less with cystic fibrosis;
- the total dose of pancreatic enzyme supplements used in patients with cystic fibrosis should not usually exceed 10 000 units of lipase per kg body-weight daily;
- if a patient on any pancreatin preparation develops new abdominal symptoms (or any change in existing abdominal symptoms) the patient should be reviewed to exclude the possibility of colonic damage.

Possible risk factors are gender (boys at greater risk than girls), more severe cystic fibrosis, and concomitant use of laxatives. The peak age for developing fibrosing colonopathy is between 2 and 8 years.

Counselling It is important to ensure adequate hydration at all times in patients receiving higher-strength pancreatin preparations.

Creon® 25 000 (Solvay) PoM

Capsules, orange/clear, enclosing brown-coloured e/c pellets of pancreatin (pork), providing: protease (total) 1000 units, lipase 25 000 units, amylase 18 000 units, net price 100-cap pack = £30.03. Counselling, see above and under dose

Dose ADULT and CHILD initially 1 capsule with meals either taken whole or contents mixed with fluid or soft food (then swallowed immediately without chewing)

Creon® 40 000 (Solvay) PoM

Capsules, brown/clear, enclosing brown-coloured e/c granules of pancreatin (pork), providing: protease (total) 1600 units, lipase 40 000 units, amylase 25 000 units, net price 100-cap pack = £60.00. Counselling, see above and under dose

Dose ADULT and CHILD initially 1–2 capsules with meals either taken whole or contents mixed with fluid or soft food (then swallowed immediately without chewing)

Nutrizym 22® (Merck) PoM

Capsules, red/yellow, enclosing e/c minitablets of pancreatin (pork), providing minimum of: protease 1100 units, lipase 22 000 units, amylase 19 800 units. Net price 100-cap pack = £33.33. Counselling, see above and under dose

Dose ADULT and CHILD over 15 years, 1–2 capsules with meals and 1 capsule with snacks, swallowed whole or contents taken with water or sprinkled on soft food (then swallowed immediately without chewing)

Pancrease HL® (Janssen-Cilag) PoM

Capsules, enclosing light brown e/c minitablets of pancreatin (pork), providing minimum of: protease 1250 units, lipase 25 000 units, amylase 22 500 units. Net price 100 = £33.65. Counselling, see above and under dose

Dose ADULT and CHILD over 15 years, 1–2 capsules during each meal and 1 capsule with snacks swallowed whole or contents sprinkled on slightly acidic liquid or soft food (then swallowed immediately without chewing)

2 Cardiovascular system

2.1 Positive inotropic drugs **70**
2.1.1 Cardiac glycosides 70
2.1.2 Phosphodiesterase inhibitors 72
2.2 Diuretics **72**
2.2.1 Thiazides and related diuretics 73
2.2.2 Loop diuretics 74
2.2.3 Potassium-sparing diuretics and aldosterone antagonists 76
2.2.4 Potassium-sparing diuretics with other diuretics 77
2.2.5 Osmotic diuretics 78
2.2.6 Mercurial diuretics 78
2.2.7 Carbonic anhydrase inhibitors 78
2.2.8 Diuretics with potassium 78
2.3 Anti-arrhythmic drugs **78**
2.3.1 Management of arrhythmias 78
2.3.2 Drugs for arrhythmias 79
2.4 Beta-adrenoceptor blocking drugs **84**
2.5 Hypertension and heart failure **91**
2.5.1 Vasodilator antihypertensive drugs 93
2.5.2 Centrally acting antihypertensive drugs 95
2.5.3 Adrenergic neurone blocking drugs 96
2.5.4 Alpha-adrenoceptor blocking drugs 97
2.5.5 Drugs affecting the renin-angiotensin system 99
2.5.5.1 Angiotensin-converting enzyme inhibitors 99
2.5.5.2 Angiotensin-II receptor antagonists 105
2.5.5.3 Renin inhibitors 107
2.6 Nitrates, calcium-channel blockers, and other antianginal drugs **107**
2.6.1 Nitrates 108
2.6.2 Calcium-channel blockers 111
2.6.3 Other antianginal drugs 117
2.6.4 Peripheral vasodilators and related drugs 118
2.7 Sympathomimetics **119**
2.7.1 Inotropic sympathomimetics 119
2.7.2 Vasoconstrictor sympathomimetics 120
2.7.3 Cardiopulmonary resuscitation 121
2.8 Anticoagulants and protamine **122**
2.8.1 Parenteral anticoagulants 122
2.8.2 Oral anticoagulants 127
2.8.3 Protamine sulphate 128
2.9 Antiplatelet drugs **129**
2.10 Myocardial infarction and fibrinolysis **132**
2.10.1 Management of myocardial infarction 132
2.10.2 Fibrinolytic drugs 133
2.11 Antifibrinolytic drugs and haemostatics **135**
2.12 Lipid-regulating drugs **137**
2.13 Local sclerosants **144**

This chapter also includes advice on the drug management of the following:

angina, p. 107
arrhythmias, p. 78
cardiovascular disease risk, p. 91 and p. 137
heart failure, p. 99
hypertension, p. 91
myocardial infarction, p. 132
phaeochromocytoma, p. 98

2.1 Positive inotropic drugs

2.1.1 Cardiac glycosides
2.1.2 Phosphodiesterase inhibitors

Positive inotropic drugs increase the force of contraction of the myocardium; for sympathomimetics with inotropic activity see section 2.7.1.

2.1.1 Cardiac glycosides

Cardiac glycosides increase the force of myocardial contraction and reduce conductivity within the atrioventricular (AV) node. Digoxin is the most commonly used cardiac glycoside.

Cardiac glycosides are most useful in the treatment of supraventricular tachycardias, especially for controlling ventricular response in persistent atrial fibrillation (section 2.3.1). For reference to the role of digoxin in heart failure, see section 2.5.5.

For management of atrial fibrillation the maintenance dose of the cardiac glycoside can usually be determined by the ventricular rate at rest, which should not be allowed to fall below 60 beats per minute except in special circumstances, e.g. with the concomitant administration of a beta-blocker.

Digoxin is now rarely used for rapid control of heart rate (see section 2.3 for the management of supraventricular arrhythmias). Even with intravenous administration, response may take many hours; persistence of tachycardia is therefore not an indication for exceeding the recommended dose. The intramuscular route is not recommended.

In patients with mild heart failure a loading dose is not required, and a satisfactory plasma-digoxin concentration can be achieved over a period of about a week, using a dose of digoxin 125 to 250 micrograms twice a day which is then reduced.

Digoxin has a long half-life and maintenance doses need to be given only once daily (although higher doses may be divided to avoid nausea). **Digitoxin** also has a long half-life and maintenance doses need to be given only once daily or on alternate days. Renal function is the most important determinant of digoxin dosage, whereas elimination of digitoxin depends on metabolism by the liver.

Unwanted effects depend both on the concentration of the cardiac glycoside in the plasma and on the sensitivity of the conducting system or of the myocardium, which is often increased in heart disease. It can sometimes be difficult to distinguish between toxic effects and clinical deterioration because symptoms of both are similar. Also, the plasma concentration alone cannot indicate toxicity reliably but the likelihood of toxicity increases progressively through the range 1.5 to 3 micrograms/litre for digoxin. Cardiac glycosides should be used with special care in the elderly who may be particularly susceptible to digitalis toxicity.

Regular monitoring of plasma-digoxin concentration during maintenance treatment is not necessary unless problems are suspected. Hypokalaemia predisposes the patient to digitalis toxicity; it is managed by giving a potassium sparing diuretic or, if necessary, potassium supplementation.

Toxicity can often be managed by discontinuing digoxin; serious manifestations require urgent specialist management. **Digoxin-specific antibody fragments** are available for reversal of life-threatening overdosage (see below).

Children The dose is based on body-weight; children require a relatively larger dose of digoxin than adults.

DIGOXIN

Indications heart failure (see also section 2.5.5), supraventricular arrhythmias (particularly atrial fibrillation and atrial flutter; see also section 2.3.2)

Cautions recent myocardial infarction; sick sinus syndrome; thyroid disease; reduce dose in the elderly; hypokalaemia or hypomagnesaemia (risk of digitalis toxicity); avoid rapid intravenous administration (nausea and risk of arrhythmias); renal impairment (Appendix 3); pregnancy (Appendix 4); **interactions:** Appendix 1 (cardiac glycosides)

Contra-indications intermittent complete heart block, second degree AV block; supraventricular arrhythmias associated with accessory conducting pathways e.g. Wolff-Parkinson-White syndrome; ventricular tachycardia or fibrillation; hypertrophic cardiomyopathy (unless concomitant atrial fibrillation and heart failure—but with caution)

Side-effects usually associated with excessive dosage, include: anorexia, nausea, vomiting, diarrhoea, abdominal pain; visual disturbances, headache, fatigue, drowsiness, confusion, dizziness, delirium, hallucinations, depression; arrhythmias, heart block; rarely rash, intestinal ischaemia; gynaecomastia on long-term use; thrombocytopenia reported; see also notes above

Dose

- Rapid digitalisation, by mouth, 1–1.5 mg in divided doses over 24 hours; less urgent digitalisation, 250–500 micrograms daily (higher dose may be divided)
- Maintenance, by mouth, 62.5–500 micrograms daily (higher dose may be divided) according to renal function and, in atrial fibrillation, on heart-rate response; usual range, 125–250 micrograms daily (lower dose may be appropriate in elderly)
- Emergency loading dose, by intravenous infusion (but rarely necessary), 0.75–1 mg over at least 2 hours (see also Cautions) then maintenance dose by mouth on the following day

Note The above doses may need to be reduced if digoxin (or another cardiac glycoside) has been given in the preceding 2 weeks. Digoxin doses in the BNF may differ from those in product literature. For plasma concentration monitoring, blood should ideally be taken at least 6 hours after a dose

Digoxin (Non-proprietary) PoM

Tablets, digoxin 62.5 micrograms, net price 28 = £1.49; 125 micrograms, 28 = £1.43; 250 micrograms, 28 = £1.34

Injection, digoxin 250 micrograms/mL, net price 2-mL amp = 70p

Available from Antigen

Paediatric injection, digoxin 100 micrograms/mL

'Special order' [unlicensed] product

Lanoxin® (GSK) PoM

Tablets, digoxin 125 micrograms, net price 20 = 32p; 250 micrograms (scored), 20 = 32p

Injection, digoxin 250 micrograms/mL. Net price 2-mL amp = 66p

Lanoxin-PG® (GSK) PoM

Tablets, blue, digoxin 62.5 micrograms. Net price 20 = 32p

Elixir, yellow, digoxin 50 micrograms/mL. Do not dilute, measure with pipette. Net price 60 mL = £5.35. Counselling, use of pipette

DIGITOXIN

Indications heart failure, supraventricular arrhythmias (particularly atrial fibrillation)

Cautions see under Digoxin

Contra-indications see under Digoxin

Side-effects see under Digoxin

Dose

- Maintenance, 100 micrograms daily *or* on alternate days; may be increased to 200 micrograms daily if necessary

Digitoxin (Non-proprietary) PoM

Tablets, digitoxin 100 micrograms, net price 28 = £4.11

2 Cardiovascular system

Digoxin-specific antibody

Digoxin-specific antibody fragments are indicated for the treatment of known or strongly suspected digoxin or digitoxin overdosage, in situations where measures beyond the withdrawal of the cardiac glycoside and correction of any electrolyte abnormalities are felt to be necessary (see also notes above).

Digibind® (GSK) PoM
Injection, powder for preparation of infusion, digoxin-specific antibody fragments (F(ab)) 38 mg. Net price per vial = £93.97 (hosp. and poisons centres only)
Dose consult product literature

2.1.2 Phosphodiesterase inhibitors

Enoximone and **milrinone** are selective phosphodiesterase inhibitors which exert most of their effect on the myocardium. Sustained haemodynamic benefit has been observed after administration, but there is no evidence of any beneficial effect on survival.

ENOXIMONE

Indications congestive heart failure where cardiac output reduced and filling pressures increased

Cautions heart failure associated with hypertrophic cardiomyopathy, stenotic or obstructive valvular disease or other outlet obstruction; monitor blood pressure, heart rate, ECG, central venous pressure, fluid and electrolyte status, renal function, platelet count, hepatic enzymes; avoid extravasation; renal impairment (Appendix 3); pregnancy (Appendix 4); breast-feeding (Appendix 5)

Side-effects ectopic beats; less frequently ventricular tachycardia or supraventricular arrhythmias (more likely in patients with pre-existing arrhythmias); hypotension; also headache, insomnia, nausea and vomiting, diarrhoea; occasionally, chills, oliguria, fever, urinary retention; upper and lower limb pain

Dose

- By slow intravenous injection (rate not exceeding 12.5 mg/minute), diluted before use, initially 0.5–1 mg/kg, then 500 micrograms/kg every 30 minutes until satisfactory response or total of 3 mg/kg given; maintenance, initial dose of up to 3 mg/kg may be repeated every 3–6 hours as required
- By intravenous infusion, initially 90 micrograms/kg/minute over 10–30 minutes, followed by continuous or intermittent infusion of 5–20 micrograms/kg/minute

Total dose over 24 hours should not usually exceed 24 mg/kg

Perfan® (INCA-Pharm) PoM
Injection, enoximone 5 mg/mL. For dilution before use. Net price 20-mL amp = £15.02
Excipients include alcohol, propylene glycol
Note Plastic apparatus should be used; crystal formation if glass used

MILRINONE

Indications short-term treatment of severe congestive heart failure unresponsive to conventional maintenance therapy (not immediately after myocardial infarction); acute heart failure, including low output states, following heart surgery

Cautions see under Enoximone; also correct hypokalaemia, monitor renal function; renal impairment (Appendix 3); pregnancy (Appendix 4); breast-feeding (Appendix 5)

Side-effects see under Enoximone; also chest pain, tremor, bronchospasm, anaphylaxis, and rash reported

Dose

- By intravenous injection over 10 minutes, diluted before use, 50 micrograms/kg followed by intravenous infusion at a rate of 375–750 nanograms/kg/minute, usually for up to 12 hours following surgery or for 48–72 hours in congestive heart failure; max. daily dose 1.13 mg/kg

Primacor® (Sanofi-Synthelabo) PoM
Injection, milrinone (as lactate) 1 mg/mL. For dilution before use. Net price 10-mL amp = £16.61

2.2 Diuretics

2.2.1 Thiazides and related diuretics
2.2.2 Loop diuretics
2.2.3 Potassium-sparing diuretics and aldosterone antagonists
2.2.4 Potassium-sparing diuretics with other diuretics
2.2.5 Osmotic diuretics
2.2.6 Mercurial diuretics
2.2.7 Carbonic anhydrase inhibitors
2.2.8 Diuretics with potassium

Thiazides (section 2.2.1) are used to relieve oedema due to chronic heart failure (section 2.5.5) and, in lower doses, to reduce blood pressure.

Loop diuretics (section 2.2.2) are used in pulmonary oedema due to left ventricular failure and in patients with chronic heart failure (section 2.5.5).

Combination diuretic therapy may be effective in patients with oedema resistant to treatment with one diuretic. Vigorous diuresis, particularly with loop diuretics, may induce acute hypotension; rapid reduction of plasma volume should be avoided.

Elderly Lower initial doses of diuretics should be used in the elderly because they are particularly susceptible to the side-effects. The dose should then be adjusted according to renal function. Diuretics should not be used continuously on a long-term basis to treat simple gravitational oedema (which will usually respond to increased movement, raising the legs, and support stockings).

Potassium loss Hypokalaemia may occur with both thiazide and loop diuretics. The risk of hypokalaemia depends on the duration of action as well as the potency and is thus greater with thiazides than with an equipotent dose of a loop diuretic.

Hypokalaemia is dangerous in severe cardiovascular disease and in patients also being treated with cardiac glycosides. Often the use of potassium-sparing diuretics (section 2.2.3) avoids the need to take potassium supplements.

In hepatic failure, hypokalaemia caused by diuretics can precipitate encephalopathy, particularly in alcoholic cirrhosis; diuretics may also increase the risk of hypomagnesaemia in alcoholic cirrhosis, leading to arrhythmias. Spironolactone, a potassium-sparing diuretic (section 2.2.3), is chosen for oedema arising from cirrhosis of the liver.

Potassium supplements or potassium-sparing diuretics are seldom necessary when thiazides are used in the routine treatment of hypertension (see also section 9.2.1.1).

2.2.1 Thiazides and related diuretics

Thiazides and related compounds are moderately potent diuretics; they inhibit sodium reabsorption at the beginning of the distal convoluted tubule. They act within 1 to 2 hours of oral administration and most have a duration of action of 12 to 24 hours; they are usually administered early in the day so that the diuresis does not interfere with sleep.

In the management of *hypertension* a low dose of a thiazide, e.g. bendroflumethiazide (bendrofluazide) 2.5 mg daily, produces a maximal or near-maximal blood pressure lowering effect, with very little biochemical disturbance. Higher doses cause more marked changes in plasma potassium, sodium, uric acid, glucose, and lipids, with little advantage in blood pressure control. For reference to the use of thiazides in chronic heart failure see section 2.5.5.

Bendroflumethiazide (bendrofluazide) is widely used for mild or moderate heart failure and for hypertension—alone in the treatment of mild hypertension or with other drugs in more severe hypertension.

Chlortalidone (chlorthalidone), a thiazide-related compound, has a longer duration of action than the thiazides and may be given on alternate days to control oedema. It is also useful if acute retention is liable to be precipitated by a more rapid diuresis or if patients dislike the altered pattern of micturition caused by other diuretics.

Other thiazide diuretics (including benzthiazide, clopamide, cyclopenthiazide, hydrochlorothiazide, and hydroflumethiazide) do not offer any significant advantage over bendroflumethiazide or chlortalidone.

Metolazone is particularly effective when combined with a loop diuretic (even in renal failure); profound diuresis can occur and the patient should therefore be monitored carefully.

Xipamide and **indapamide** are chemically related to chlortalidone. Indapamide is claimed to lower blood pressure with less metabolic disturbance, particularly less aggravation of diabetes mellitus.

Cautions See also section 2.2. Thiazides and related diuretics may exacerbate diabetes, gout, and systemic lupus erythematosus. Electrolytes should be monitored particularly with high doses, long-term use, or in renal impairment. Thiazides and related diuretics should also be used with caution in nephrotic syndrome, hyperaldosteronism, malnourishment, hepatic impairment (avoid if severe; Appendix 2), renal impairment (Appendix 3), pregnancy (Appendix 4), and breast-feeding (Appendix 5); **interactions**: Appendix 1 (diuretics)

Contra-indications Thiazides and related diuretics should be avoided in refractory hypokalaemia, hyponatraemia, and hypercalcaemia, symptomatic hyperuricaemia, and Addison's disease.

Side-effects Side-effects of thiazides and related diuretics include mild gastro-intestinal disturbances, postural hypotension, altered plasma lipid concentration, metabolic and electrolyte disturbances including hypokalaemia (see also notes above), hyponatraemia, hypomagnesaemia, hypercalcaemia, hyperglycaemia, hypochloraemic alkalosis, hyperuricaemia, and gout. Less common side-effects include blood disorders such as agranulocytosis, leucopenia, and thrombocytopenia, and impotence. Pancreatitis, intrahepatic cholestasis, cardiac arrhythmias, headache, dizziness, paraesthesia, visual disturbances, and hypersensitivity reactions (including pneumonitis, pulmonary oedema, photosensitivity, and severe skin reactions) have also been reported.

BENDROFLUMETHIAZIDE
(Bendrofluazide)

Indications oedema, hypertension (see also notes above)
Cautions see notes above
Contra-indications see notes above
Side-effects see notes above
Dose
- Oedema, initially 5–10 mg daily in the morning *or* on alternate days; maintenance 5–10 mg 1–3 times weekly
- Hypertension, 2.5 mg daily in the morning; higher doses rarely necessary (see notes above)

Bendroflumethiazide (Non-proprietary) PoM
Tablets, bendroflumethiazide 2.5 mg, net price 28 = 43p; 5 mg, 28 = 66p
Brands include *Aprinox*®, *Neo-NaClex*®

CHLORTALIDONE
(Chlorthalidone)

Indications ascites due to cirrhosis in stable patients (under close supervision), oedema due to nephrotic syndrome, hypertension (see also notes above), mild to moderate chronic heart failure; diabetes insipidus (see section 6.5.2)
Cautions see notes above
Contra-indications see notes above
Side-effects see notes above; also *rarely* jaundice and allergic interstitial nephritis

Dose
- Oedema, up to 50 mg daily
- Hypertension, 25 mg daily in the morning, increased to 50 mg daily if necessary (but see notes above)
- Heart failure, 25–50 mg daily in the morning, increased if necessary to 100–200 mg daily (reduce to lowest effective dose for maintenance)

Hygroton® (Alliance) PoM
Tablets, yellow, scored, chlortalidone 50 mg, net price 28-tab pack = £1.64

CYCLOPENTHIAZIDE

Indications oedema, hypertension (see also notes above); heart failure
Cautions see notes above
Contra-indications see notes above
Side-effects see notes above; also *rarely* depression
Dose
- Heart failure, 250–500 micrograms daily in the morning increased if necessary to 1 mg daily (reduce to lowest effective dose for maintenance)
- Hypertension, initially 250 micrograms daily in the morning, increased if necessary to 500 micrograms daily (but see notes above)
- Oedema, up to 500 micrograms daily for a short period

Navidrex® (Goldshield) PoM
Tablets, scored, cyclopenthiazide 500 micrograms. Net price 28-tab pack = £1.27
Excipients include gluten

INDAPAMIDE

Indications essential hypertension
Cautions see notes above; also porphyria (section 9.8.2)
Contra-indications see notes above
Side-effects see notes above; also palpitation, diuresis with doses above 2.5 mg daily
Dose
- 2.5 mg daily in the morning

Indapamide (Non-proprietary) PoM
Tablets, s/c, indapamide 2.5 mg, net price 28-tab pack = £1.63, 56-tab pack = £2.51

Natrilix® (Servier) PoM
Tablets, f/c, indapamide 2.5 mg. Net price 30-tab pack = £4.50, 60-tab pack = £9.00

Modified release

Natrilix SR® (Servier) PoM
Tablets, m/r, indapamide 1.5 mg. Net price 30-tab pack = £4.50. Label: 25
Dose hypertension, 1 tablet daily, preferably in the morning

METOLAZONE

Indications oedema, hypertension (see also notes above)
Cautions see notes above; also porphyria (section 9.8.2)
Contra-indications see notes above
Side-effects see notes above; also chills, chest pain
Dose
- Oedema, 5–10 mg daily in the morning, increased if necessary to 20 mg daily in resistant oedema, max. 80 mg daily
- Hypertension, initially 5 mg daily in the morning; maintenance 5 mg on alternate days

Metenix 5® (Borg) PoM
Tablets, blue, metolazone 5 mg. Net price 100-tab pack = £18.94

XIPAMIDE

Indications oedema, hypertension (see also notes above)
Cautions see notes above; also porphyria (section 9.8.2)
Contra-indications see notes above
Side-effects see notes above
Dose
- Oedema, initially 40 mg daily in the morning, increased to 80 mg in resistant cases; maintenance 20 mg in the morning
- Hypertension, 20 mg daily in the morning

Diurexan® (Viatris) PoM
Tablets, scored, xipamide 20 mg. Net price 140-tab pack = £19.46

2.2.2 Loop diuretics

Loop diuretics are used in pulmonary oedema due to left ventricular failure; intravenous administration produces relief of breathlessness and reduces pre-load sooner than would be expected from the time of onset of diuresis. Loop diuretics are also used in patients with chronic heart failure. Diuretic-resistant oedema (except lymphoedema and oedema due to peripheral venous stasis or calcium-channel blockers) can be treated with a loop diuretic combined with a thiazide or related diuretic (e.g. bendroflumethiazide 5–10 mg daily or metolazone 5–20 mg daily).

If necessary, a loop diuretic can be added to antihypertensive treatment to achieve better control of blood pressure.

Loop diuretics inhibit reabsorption from the ascending limb of the loop of Henlé in the renal tubule and are powerful diuretics. Hypokalaemia may develop, and care is needed to avoid hypotension. If there is an enlarged prostate, urinary retention may occur; this is less likely if small doses and less potent diuretics are used initially.

Furosemide (frusemide) and **bumetanide** are similar in activity; both act within 1 hour of oral administration and diuresis is complete within 6 hours so that, if necessary, they can be given twice in one day without interfering with sleep. Following intravenous administration they have a peak effect within 30 minutes. The diuresis associated with these drugs is dose related. In patients with impaired renal function very large doses may occasionally be needed; in such doses both drugs can cause deafness and bumetanide can cause myalgia.

Torasemide has properties similar to those of furosemide and bumetanide, and is indicated for oedema and for hypertension.

FUROSEMIDE
(Frusemide)

Indications oedema (see notes above); oliguria in chronic renal impairment

Cautions monitor electrolytes; hypotension; prostatic enlargement; impaired micturition; gout; diabetes; although manufacturer advises that rate of intravenous administration should not exceed 4 mg/minute, single doses of up to 80 mg may be administered more rapidly; hepatorenal syndrome; hepatic impairment (Appendix 2); renal impairment (Appendix 3); pregnancy (Appendix 4); breast-feeding (Appendix 5); **interactions**: Appendix 1 (diuretics)

Contra-indications hypovolaemia, dehydration, severe hypokalaemia, severe hyponatraemia; comatose or precomatose states associated with liver cirrhosis; renal failure due to nephrotoxic or hepatotoxic drugs, anuria

Side-effects mild gastro-intestinal disturbances; hypotension; hyperglycaemia (less common than with thiazides); hyperuricaemia and gout; electrolyte disturbances including hyponatraemia, hypokalaemia (see also section 2.2), hypocalcaemia, and hypomagnesaemia, metabolic alkalosis; *rarely* paraethesia, blood disorders (including thrombocytopenia, leucopenia, agranulocytosis, aplastic anaemia, haemolytic anaemia), bone marrow depression (withdraw treatment), tinnitus and deafness (usually with large parenteral doses and rapid administration, in renal impairment, or in hypoproteinaemia), and hypersensitivity reactions (including rashes, photosensitivity, eosinophilia, exfoliative dermatitis, purpura, and anaphylaxis), pancreatitis, intrahepatic cholestasis; temporary increase in plasma cholesterol and triglyceride concentration also reported

Dose
- By mouth, oedema, initially 40 mg in the morning; maintenance 20–40 mg daily, increased in resistant oedema to 80 mg daily or more; CHILD 1–3 mg/kg daily, max. 40 mg daily
  Oliguria in chronic renal impairment (but rarely used), initially 250 mg, increased if necessary in steps of 250 mg every 4–6 hours; max. 2 g daily
- By intramuscular injection *or* slow intravenous injection (rate of administration, see Cautions above), initially 20–50 mg, increased if necessary in steps of 20 mg not less than every 2 hours; doses greater than 50 mg by intravenous infusion only; max. 1.5 g daily; CHILD 0.5–1.5 mg/kg daily, max. 20 mg daily

Furosemide (Non-proprietary) PoM
Tablets, furosemide 20 mg, net price 28 = 20p; 40 mg, 28 = 23p; 500 mg, 28 = £5.23
Brands include *Froop*®, *Frusid*®, *Rusyde*®
Oral solution, sugar-free, furosemide, net price 20 mg/5 mL, 150 mL = £12.07; 40 mg/5 mL, 150 mL = £15.58; 50 mg/5 mL, 150 mL = £16.84
Brands include *Frusol*® (contains alcohol 10%)
Injection, furosemide 10 mg/mL, net price 2-mL amp = 55p, 5-mL amp = 66p, 25-mL amp = £2.50

Lasix® (Sanofi-Aventis) PoM
Injection, furosemide 10 mg/mL, net price 2-mL amp = 78p
Note Large-volume furosemide injections also available; brands include *Minijet*®

BUMETANIDE

Indications oedema (see notes above)

Cautions see under Furosemide; hepatic impairment (Appendix 2); pregnancy (Appendix 4); breast-feeding (Appendix 5)

Contra-indications see under Furosemide

Side-effects see under Furosemide; also headache, dizziness, fatigue, gynaecomastia, myalgia

Dose
- By mouth, 1 mg in the morning, repeated after 6–8 hours if necessary; severe cases, 5 mg daily increased by 5 mg every 12–24 hours according to response; ELDERLY, 500 micrograms daily may be sufficient
- By intravenous injection, 1–2 mg, repeated after 20 minutes if necessary; ELDERLY, 500 micrograms daily may be sufficient
- By intravenous infusion, 2–5 mg over 30–60 minutes; ELDERLY, 500 micrograms daily may be sufficient
- By intramuscular injection, 1 mg initially then adjusted according to response; ELDERLY, 500 micrograms daily may be sufficient

Bumetanide (Non-proprietary) PoM
Tablets, bumetanide 1 mg, net price 28-tab pack = 89p; 5 mg, 28-tab pack = £2.54
Liquid, bumetanide 1 mg/5 mL, net price 150 mL = £15.22
Injection, bumetanide 500 micrograms/mL, net price 4-mL amp = £1.79

Burinex® (LEO) PoM
Tablets, both scored, bumetanide 1 mg, net price 28-tab pack = £1.52; 5 mg, 28 = £9.67

TORASEMIDE

Indications oedema (see notes above), hypertension

Cautions see under Furosemide; hepatic impairment (Appendix 2); renal impairment (Appendix 3); pregnancy (Appendix 4)

Contra-indications see under Furosemide

Side-effects see under Furosemide; also dry mouth; rarely limb paraesthesia

Dose
- Oedema, 5 mg once daily, preferably in the morning, increased if required to 20 mg once daily; usual max. 40 mg daily
- Hypertension, 2.5 mg daily, increased if necessary to 5 mg once daily

Torasemide (Non-proprietary) PoM
Tablets, torasemide 5 mg, net price 28-tab pack = £5.51; 10 mg, 28-tab pack = £8.02

Torem® (Roche) PoM
Tablets, torasemide 2.5 mg, net price 28-tab pack = £3.78; 5 mg (scored), 28-tab pack = £5.53; 10 mg (scored), 28-tab pack = £8.14

2.2.3 Potassium-sparing diuretics and aldosterone antagonists

Amiloride and **triamterene** on their own are weak diuretics. They cause retention of potassium and are therefore given with thiazide or loop diuretics as a more effective alternative to potassium supplements. See section 2.2.4 for compound preparations with thiazides or loop diuretics.

Potassium supplements must **not** be given with potassium-sparing diuretics. Administration of a potassium-sparing diuretic to a patient receiving an ACE inhibitor or an angiotensin-II receptor antagonist can also cause severe hyperkalaemia.

AMILORIDE HYDROCHLORIDE

Indications oedema, potassium conservation with thiazide and loop diuretics

Cautions diabetes mellitus; elderly; renal impairment (avoid if creatinine clearance less than 20 mL/minute; Appendix 3); pregnancy (Appendix 4); breast-feeding (Appendix 5); **interactions**: Appendix 1 (diuretics)

Contra-indications hyperkalaemia, renal failure

Side-effects include gastro-intestinal disturbances, dry mouth, rashes, confusion, postural hypotension, hyperkalaemia, hyponatraemia

Dose

- Used alone, initially 10 mg daily *or* 5 mg twice daily, adjusted according to response; max. 20 mg daily
- With other diuretics, congestive heart failure and hypertension, initially 5–10 mg daily; cirrhosis with ascites, initially 5 mg daily

Amiloride (Non-proprietary) PoM

Tablets, amiloride hydrochloride 5 mg, net price 28-tab pack = 34p

Oral solution, sugar-free, amiloride hydrochloride 5 mg/5 mL, net price 150 mL = £39.73

Brands include *Amilamont®*

Compound preparations with thiazide or loop diuretics

Section 2.2.4

TRIAMTERENE

Indications oedema, potassium conservation with thiazide and loop diuretics

Cautions see under Amiloride Hydrochloride; may cause blue fluorescence of urine

Contra-indications see under Amiloride Hydrochloride

Side-effects include gastro-intestinal disturbances, dry mouth, rashes; slight decrease in blood pressure, hyperkalaemia, hyponatraemia; photosensitivity and blood disorders also reported; triamterene found in kidney stones

Dose

- Initially 150–250 mg daily, reducing to alternate days after 1 week; taken in divided doses after breakfast and lunch; lower initial dose when given with other diuretics

Counselling Urine may look slightly blue in some lights

Dytac® (Goldshield) PoM

Capsules, maroon, triamterene 50 mg. Net price 30-cap pack = £17.35 Label: 14, (see above), 21

Compound preparations with thiazides or loop diuretics

Section 2.2.4

Aldosterone antagonists

Spironolactone potentiates thiazide or loop diuretics by antagonising aldosterone; it is a potassium-sparing diuretic. Spironolactone is of value in the treatment of oedema and ascites caused by cirrhosis of the liver; furosemide (section 2.2.2) can be used as an adjunct. Low doses of spironolactone are beneficial in severe heart failure, see section 2.5.5.

Spironolactone is also used in primary hyperaldosteronism (Conn's syndrome). It is given before surgery or if surgery is not appropriate, in the lowest effective dose for maintenance.

Eplerenone is licensed for use as an adjunct in left ventricular dysfunction with evidence of heart failure after a myocardial infarction (see also section 2.5.5 and section 2.10.1).

Potassium supplements must **not** be given with aldosterone antagonists.

EPLERENONE

Indications adjunct in stable patients with left ventricular dysfunction with evidence of heart failure, following myocardial infarction (start therapy within 3–14 days of event)

Cautions measure plasma-potassium concentration before treatment, during initiation, and when dose changed; elderly; hepatic impairment (Appendix 2); renal impairment (avoid if creatinine clearance less than 50 mL/minute; Appendix 3); pregnancy; breast-feeding (Appendix 5); **interactions**: Appendix 1 (diuretics)

Contra-indications hyperkalaemia; concomitant use of potassium-sparing diuretics or potassium supplements

Side-effects diarrhoea, nausea; hypotension; dizziness; hyperkalaemia; *less commonly* flatulence, vomiting, atrial fibrillation, postural hypotension, arterial thrombosis, dyslipidaemia, pharyngitis, headache, insomnia, pyelonephritis, hyponatraemia, dehydration, eosinophilia, asthenia, malaise, back pain, leg cramps, impaired renal function, azotaemia, sweating and pruritus

Dose

- Initially 25 mg once daily, increased within 4 weeks to 50 mg once daily; CHILD not recommended

Inspra® (Pfizer) ▼ PoM

Tablets, yellow, f/c, eplerenone 25 mg, net price 28-tab pack = £42.72; 50 mg, 28-tab pack = £42.72

SPIRONOLACTONE

Indications oedema and ascites in cirrhosis of the liver, malignant ascites, nephrotic syndrome, congestive heart failure (section 2.5.5); primary hyperaldosteronism

Cautions potential metabolic products carcinogenic in *rodents*; elderly; monitor electrolytes (discontinue if hyperkalaemia); porphyria (section 9.8.2); hepatic impairment; renal impairment (avoid if creatinine clearance less than 20 mL/minute; Appendix 3); pregnancy (Appendix 4); breast-feeding (Appendix 5); **interactions:** Appendix 1 (diuretics)

Contra-indications hyperkalaemia, hyponatraemia; Addison's disease

Side-effects gastro-intestinal disturbances; impotence, gynaecomastia; menstrual irregularities; lethargy, headache, confusion; rashes; hyperkalaemia (discontinue); hyponatraemia; hepatotoxicity, osteomalacia, and blood disorders reported

Dose

- 100–200 mg daily, increased to 400 mg if required; CHILD initially 3 mg/kg daily in divided doses
- Heart failure, see section 2.5.5

Spironolactone (Non-proprietary) PoM
Tablets, spironolactone 25 mg, net price 28 = £2.11; 50 mg, 28 = £3.46; 100 mg, 28 = £4.91. Label: 21
Oral suspensions, spironolactone 5 mg/5 mL, 10 mg/5 mL, 25 mg/5 mL, 50 mg/5 mL, and 100 mg/5 mL. Label: 21
Available from Rosemont as 'special order' (sugar-free)

Aldactone® (Pharmacia) PoM
Tablets, all f/c, spironolactone 25 mg (buff), net price 100-tab pack = £8.89; 50 mg (off-white), 100-tab pack = £17.78; 100 mg (buff), 28-tab pack = £9.96. Label: 21

◢With thiazides or loop diuretics

Section 2.2.4

2.2.4 Potassium-sparing diuretics with other diuretics

Although it is preferable to prescribe thiazides (section 2.2.1) and potassium-sparing diuretics (section 2.2.3) separately, the use of fixed combinations may be justified if compliance is a problem. Potassium-sparing diuretics are not usually necessary in the routine treatment of hypertension, unless hypokalaemia develops. For **interactions**, see Appendix 1 (diuretics).

◢Amiloride with thiazides

Co-amilozide (Non-proprietary) PoM
Tablets, co-amilozide 2.5/25 (amiloride hydrochloride 2.5 mg, hydrochlorothiazide 25 mg), net price 28-tab pack = £1.96
Brands include *Moduret 25®*
Dose hypertension, initially 1 tablet daily, increased if necessary to max. 2 tablets daily
Congestive heart failure, initially 1 tablet daily, increased if necessary to max. 4 tablets daily
Oedema and ascites in cirrhosis of the liver, initially 2 tablets daily, increased if necessary to max. 4 tablets daily; reduce for maintenance if possible

Tablets, co-amilozide 5/50 (amiloride hydrochloride 5 mg, hydrochlorothiazide 50 mg), net price 28 = 77p
Brands include *Amil-Co®*, *Moduretic®*
Dose hypertension, initially ½ tablet daily, increased if necessary to max. 1 tablet daily
Congestive heart failure, initially ½ tablet daily, increased if necessary to max. 2 tablets daily
Oedema and ascites in cirrhosis of the liver, initially 1 tablet daily, increased if necessary to max. 2 tablets daily; reduce for maintenance if possible

Navispare® (Goldshield) PoM
Tablets, f/c, orange, amiloride hydrochloride 2.5 mg, cyclopenthiazide 250 micrograms. Net price 28-tab pack = £2.70
Excipients include gluten
Dose hypertension, 1–2 tablets in the morning

◢Amiloride with loop diuretics

Co-amilofruse (Non-proprietary) PoM
Tablets, co-amilofruse 2.5/20 (amiloride hydrochloride 2.5 mg, furosemide 20 mg). Net price 28-tab pack = £1.06, 56-tab pack = £1.60
Brands include *Frumil LS®*
Dose oedema, 1 tablet in the morning

Tablets, co-amilofruse 5/40 (amiloride hydrochloride 5 mg, furosemide 40 mg). Net price 28-tab pack = £1.14, 56-tab pack = £1.74
Brands include *Fru-Co®*, *Frumil®*
Dose oedema, 1–2 tablets in the morning

Tablets, co-amilofruse 10/80 (amiloride hydrochloride 10 mg, furosemide 80 mg). Net price 28-tab pack = £7.90, 56-tab pack = £14.86
Brands include *Aridil®*
Dose oedema, 1 tablet in the morning

Burinex A® (LEO) PoM
Tablets, ivory, scored, amiloride hydrochloride 5 mg, bumetanide 1 mg. Net price 28-tab pack = £2.63
Dose oedema, 1–2 tablets daily

◢Triamterene with thiazides

Counselling Urine may look slightly blue in some lights

Co-triamterzide (Non-proprietary) PoM
Tablets, co-triamterzide 50/25 (triamterene 50 mg, hydrochlorothiazide 25 mg), net price 30-tab pack = 95p. Label: 14, (see above), 21
Dose hypertension, 1 tablet daily after breakfast, increased if necessary, max. 4 daily
Oedema, 2 tablets daily (1 after breakfast and 1 after midday meal) increased to 3 daily if necessary (2 after breakfast and 1 after midday meal); usual maintenance in oedema, 1 daily or 2 on alternate days; max. 4 daily
Brands include *Triam-Co®*

Dyazide® (Goldshield) PoM
Tablets, peach, scored, co-triamterzide 50/25 (triamterene 50 mg, hydrochlorothiazide 25 mg). Net price 30-tab pack = 95p. Label: 14, (see above), 21
Dose hypertension, 1 tablet daily after breakfast, increased if necessary, max. 4 daily
Oedema, 2 tablets daily (1 after breakfast and 1 after midday meal) increased to 3 daily if necessary (2 after breakfast and 1 after midday meal); usual maintenance in oedema, 1 daily or 2 on alternate days; max. 4 daily

Dytide® (Goldshield) PoM
Capsules, clear/maroon, triamterene 50 mg, benzthiazide 25 mg. Net price 30-cap pack = £17.35. Label: 14, (see above), 21
Dose oedema, initially 3 capsules daily (2 after breakfast and 1 after midday meal) for 1 week then 1 or 2 on alternate days

Kalspare® (DHP Healthcare) PoM
Tablets, orange, f/c, scored, triamterene 50 mg, chlortalidone 50 mg. Net price 28-tab pack = £3.05. Label: 14, (see above), 21
Dose hypertension, oedema, 1–2 tablets in the morning

Triamterene with loop diuretics
Counselling Urine may look slightly blue in some lights

Frusene® (Orion) PoM
Tablets, yellow, scored, triamterene 50 mg, furosemide 40 mg. Net price 56-tab pack = £4.54. Label: 14, (see above), 21
Dose oedema, ½–2 tablets daily in the morning

Spironolactone with thiazides
Co-flumactone (Non-proprietary) PoM
Tablets, co-flumactone 25/25 (hydroflumethiazide 25 mg, spironolactone 25 mg). Net price 100-tab pack = £20.23
Brands include *Aldactide 25®*
Dose congestive heart failure, initially 4 tablets daily; range 1–8 tablets daily (but not recommended because spironolactone generally given in lower dose)

Tablets, co-flumactone 50/50 (hydroflumethiazide 50 mg, spironolactone 50 mg). Net price 28-tab pack = £10.70
Brands include *Aldactide 50®*
Dose congestive heart failure, initially 2 tablets daily; range 1–4 tablets daily (but not recommended because spironolactone generally given in lower dose)

Spironolactone with loop diuretics
Lasilactone® (Borg) PoM
Capsules, blue/white, spironolactone 50 mg, furosemide 20 mg. Net price 28-cap pack = £8.29
Dose resistant oedema, 1–4 capsules daily

2.2.5 Osmotic diuretics

Mannitol is an osmotic diuretic which can be used to treat cerebral oedema and raised intra-ocular pressure; it is rarely used for diuresis.

MANNITOL

Indications see notes above; glaucoma (section 11.6)
Cautions extravasation causes inflammation and thrombophlebitis
Contra-indications congestive cardiac failure, pulmonary oedema
Side-effects chills, fever
Dose
- Diuresis, by intravenous infusion, 50–200 g over 24 hours, preceded by a test dose of 200 mg/kg by slow intravenous injection
- Cerebral oedema and raised intra-ocular pressure by intravenous infusion over 30–60 minutes, 0.25–2 g/kg as a 15–20% solution

Mannitol (Baxter) PoM
Intravenous infusion, mannitol 10% and 20%

2.2.6 Mercurial diuretics

Mercurial diuretics are effective but are now almost never used because of their nephrotoxicity.

2.2.7 Carbonic anhydrase inhibitors

The carbonic anhydrase inhibitor **acetazolamide** is a weak diuretic and is little used for its diuretic effect. It is used for prophylaxis against mountain sickness [unlicensed indication] but is not a substitute for acclimatisation.

Acetazolamide and eye drops of dorzolamide and brinzolamide inhibit the formation of aqueous humour and are used in glaucoma (section 11.6).

2.2.8 Diuretics with potassium

Many patients on diuretics do not need potassium supplements (section 9.2.1.1). For many of those who do, the amount of potassium in combined preparations may not be enough, and for this reason their use is to be discouraged.

Diuretics with potassium and potassium-sparing diuretics should **not** usually be given together.
Counselling Modified-release potassium tablets should be swallowed whole with plenty of fluid during meals while sitting or standing

Centyl K® (LEO) PoM
Tablets, green, s/c, bendroflumethiazide 2.5 mg, potassium 7.7 mmol for modified release, net price 56-tab pack = £7.50. Label: 25, 27, counselling, see above

Diumide-K Continus® (Teofarma) PoM
Tablets, white/orange, f/c, furosemide 40 mg, potassium 8 mmol for modified release, net price 30-tab pack = £3.00. Label: 25, 27, counselling, see above

Lasikal® (Borg) PoM
Tablets, white/yellow, f/c, furosemide 20 mg, potassium 10 mmol for modified release. Net price 100-tab pack = £15.21. Label: 25, 27, counselling, see above

Neo-NaClex-K® (Goldshield) PoM
Tablets, pink/white, f/c, bendroflumethiazide 2.5 mg, potassium 8.4 mmol for modified release. Net price 100 tab-pack = £8.99. Label: 25, 27, counselling, see above

2.3 Anti-arrhythmic drugs

2.3.1 Management of arrhythmias
2.3.2 Drugs for arrhythmias

2.3.1 Management of arrhythmias

Management of an arrhythmia requires precise diagnosis of the type of arrhythmia, and electrocardiography is essential; underlying causes such as heart failure require appropriate treatment.

Ectopic beats If ectopic beats are spontaneous and the patient has a normal heart, treatment is rarely required and reassurance to the patient will often suffice. If they are particularly troublesome, beta-blockers are sometimes effective and may be safer than other suppressant drugs.

Atrial fibrillation The ventricular rate in atrial fibrillation can be controlled with a beta-blocker (see p. 85), or diltiazem [unlicensed indication], or verapamil. Digoxin is usually effective for controlling the rate at rest; it is also appropriate if atrial fibrillation is accompanied by congestive heart failure. If the rate at rest or during exercise cannot be controlled, diltiazem or verapamil may be combined with digoxin, but care is required if the ventricular function is diminished. In some cases, e.g. acute atrial fibrillation or paroxysmal atrial fibrillation, diltiazem or verapamil or a beta-blocker may be more appropriate than digoxin (see also Paroxysmal Supraventricular Tachycardia and Supraventricular Arrhythmias below). Anticoagulants are indicated especially in valvular or myocardial disease, and in the elderly; in the very elderly the overall benefit and risk needs careful assessment. Younger patients with lone atrial fibrillation in the absence of heart disease probably do not need anticoagulation. Aspirin is less effective than warfarin at preventing emboli but may be appropriate if there are no other risk factors for stroke; aspirin 75 mg may be used.

Atrial flutter The ventricular rate at rest can sometimes be controlled with digoxin. Reversion to sinus rhythm (if indicated) may be achieved by appropriately synchronised d.c. shock. Alternatively, amiodarone may be used to restore sinus rhythm, and amiodarone or sotalol to maintain it. If the arrhythmia is long-standing a period of treatment with anticoagulants should be considered before cardioversion to avoid the complication of emboli.

Paroxysmal supraventricular tachycardia In most patients this remits spontaneously or can be returned to sinus rhythm by reflex vagal stimulation with respiratory manoeuvres, prompt squatting, or pressure over one carotid sinus (**important**: pressure over carotid sinus should be restricted to monitored patients—it can be dangerous in recent ischaemia, digitalis toxicity, or the elderly).

If vagal stimulation fails, intravenous administration of adenosine is usually the treatment of choice. Intravenous administration of verapamil is useful for patients without myocardial or valvular disease (**important**: never in patients recently treated with beta-blockers, see p. 117). For arrhythmias that are poorly tolerated, synchronised d.c. shock usually provides rapid relief.

In cases of paroxysmal supraventricular tachycardia with block, digitalis toxicity should be suspected. In addition to stopping administration of the cardiac glycoside and giving potassium supplements, intravenous administration of a beta-blocker may be useful. Specific digoxin antibody is available if the toxicity is considered life-threatening (section 2.1.1).

Arrhythmias after myocardial infarction In patients with a paroxysmal tachycardia or rapid irregularity of the pulse it is best not to administer an anti-arrhythmic until an ECG record has been obtained. Bradycardia, particularly if complicated by hypotension, should be treated with atropine sulphate, given intravenously in a dose of 0.3–1 mg. If the initial dose is effective it can be repeated if necessary.

Ventricular tachycardia Drug treatment is used both for the treatment of ventricular tachycardia and for prophylaxis of recurrent attacks that merit suppression. Ventricular tachycardia requires treatment most commonly in the acute stage of myocardial infarction, but the likelihood of this and other life-threatening arrhythmias diminishes sharply over the first 24 hours after the attack, especially in patients without heart failure or shock. Lidocaine (lignocaine) is the preferred drug for emergency use. Other drugs are best administered under specialist supervision. Very rapid ventricular tachycardia causes profound circulatory collapse and should be treated urgently with d.c. shock.

Torsade de pointes is a form of ventricular tachycardia associated with a long QT interval (usually drug-induced, but other factors including hypokalaemia, severe bradycardia, and genetic predisposition are also implicated). Episodes are usually self-limiting, but are frequently recurrent and can cause impairment or loss of consciousness. If not controlled, the arrhythmia can progress to ventricular fibrillation and sometimes death. Intravenous infusion of magnesium sulphate (section 9.5.1.3) is usually effective. A beta-blocker (but not sotalol) and atrial (or ventricular) pacing can be considered. Anti-arrhythmics (including lidocaine) can further prolong the QT interval, thus worsening the condition.

2.3.2 Drugs for arrhythmias

Anti-arrhythmic drugs can be classified clinically into those that act on supraventricular arrhythmias (e.g. verapamil), those that act on both supraventricular and ventricular arrhythmias (e.g. disopyramide), and those that act on ventricular arrhythmias (e.g. lidocaine (lignocaine)).

They can also be classified according to their effects on the electrical behaviour of myocardial cells during activity:

- Class I: membrane stabilising drugs (e.g. lidocaine, flecainide)
- Class II: beta-blockers
- Class III: amiodarone and sotalol (also Class II)
- Class IV: calcium-channel blockers (includes verapamil but not dihydropyridines)

This latter classification (the Vaughan Williams classification) is of less clinical significance.

Cautions The negative inotropic effects of anti-arrhythmic drugs tend to be additive. Therefore special care should be taken if two or more are used, especially if myocardial function is impaired. Most or all drugs that are effective in countering arrhythmias can also provoke them in some circumstances; moreover, hypokalaemia enhances the arrhythmogenic (pro-arrhythmic) effect of many drugs.

Supraventricular arrhythmias

Adenosine is usually the treatment of choice for terminating paroxysmal supraventricular tachycardia. As it has a very short duration of action (half-life only about 8 to 10 seconds, but prolonged in those taking dipyridamole), most side-effects are short lived. Unlike verapamil, adenosine may be used after a beta-blocker. Verapamil may be preferable to adenosine in asthma.

Oral administration of a **cardiac glycoside** (such as digoxin, section 2.1.1) slows the ventricular response in cases of atrial fibrillation and atrial flutter. However, intravenous infusion of digoxin is rarely effective for rapid control of ventricular rate. Cardiac glycosides are contra-indicated in supraventricular arrhythmias associated with accessory conducting pathways (e.g. Wolff-Parkinson-White syndrome).

Verapamil (section 2.6.2) is usually effective for supraventricular tachycardias. An initial intravenous dose (**important**: serious beta-blocker interaction hazard, see p. 117) may be followed by oral treatment; hypotension may occur with large doses. It should not be used for tachyarrhythmias where the QRS complex is wide (i.e. broad complex) unless a supraventricular origin has been established beyond reasonable doubt. It is also contra-indicated in atrial fibrillation with pre-excitation (e.g. Wolff-Parkinson-White syndrome). It should not be used in children with arrhythmias without specialist advice; some supraventricular arrhythmias in childhood can be accelerated by verapamil with dangerous consequences.

Intravenous administration of a **beta-blocker** (section 2.4) such as esmolol or propranolol, can achieve rapid control of the ventricular rate.

Drugs for both supraventricular and ventricular arrhythmias include **amiodarone**, **beta-blockers** (see p. 85), **disopyramide**, **flecainide**, **procainamide**, and **propafenone**, see below under Supraventricular and Ventricular Arrhythmias.

ADENOSINE

Indications rapid reversion to sinus rhythm of paroxysmal supraventricular tachycardias, including those associated with accessory conducting pathways (e.g. Wolff-Parkinson-White syndrome); aid to diagnosis of broad or narrow complex supraventricular tachycardias

Cautions atrial fibrillation or flutter with accessory pathway (conduction down anomalous pathway may increase); heart transplant (see below); **interactions**: Appendix 1 (adenosine)

Contra-indications second- or third-degree AV block and sick sinus syndrome (unless pacemaker fitted); asthma

Side-effects include transient facial flush, chest pain, dyspnoea, bronchospasm, choking sensation, nausea, light-headedness; severe bradycardia reported (requiring temporary pacing); ECG may show transient rhythm disturbances

Dose

- By rapid intravenous injection into central or large peripheral vein, 3 mg over 2 seconds with cardiac monitoring; if necessary followed by 6 mg after 1–2 minutes, and then by 12 mg after a further 1–2 minutes; increments should not be given if high level AV block develops at any particular dose

Note 3-mg dose ineffective in a number of patients, therefore higher initial dose sometimes used, but patients with *heart transplant* are **very sensitive** to effects of adenosine, and should **not** receive higher initial dose. Also if essential to give with dipyridamole reduce initial dose to 0.5–1 mg

Adenocor® (Sanofi-Synthelabo) PoM
Injection, adenosine 3 mg/mL in physiological saline. Net price 2-mL vial = £4.45 (hosp. only)

Note Intravenous infusion of adenosine (*Adenoscan®*, Sanofi Winthrop) may be used in conjunction with radionuclide myocardial perfusion imaging in patients who cannot exercise adequately or for whom exercise is inappropriate—consult product literature

Supraventricular and ventricular arrhythmias

Amiodarone is used in the treatment of arrhythmias particularly when other drugs are ineffective or contra-indicated. It may be used for paroxysmal supraventricular, nodal and ventricular tachycardias, atrial fibrillation and flutter, and ventricular fibrillation. It may also be used for tachyarrhythmias associated with Wolff-Parkinson-White syndrome. It should be initiated only under hospital or specialist supervision. Amiodarone may be given by intravenous infusion as well as by mouth, and has the advantage of causing little or no myocardial depression. Unlike oral amiodarone, intravenous amiodarone may act relatively rapidly.

Intravenous injection of amiodarone may be used in cardiopulmonary resuscitation for ventricular fibrillation or pulseless tachycardia unresponsive to other interventions (section 2.7.3).

Amiodarone has a very long half-life (extending to several weeks) and only needs to be given once daily (but high doses may cause nausea unless divided). Many weeks or months may be required to achieve steady-state plasma-amiodarone concentration; this is particularly important when drug interactions are likely (see also Appendix 1).

Most patients taking amiodarone develop corneal microdeposits (reversible on withdrawal of treatment); these rarely interfere with vision, but drivers may be dazzled by headlights at night. However, if vision is impaired or if optic neuritis or optic neuropathy occur, amiodarone must be stopped to prevent blindness and expert advice sought. Because of the possibility of phototoxic reactions, patients should be advised to shield the skin from light during treatment and for several months after discontinuing amiodarone; a wide-spectrum sunscreen (section 13.8.1) to protect against both long-wave ultraviolet and visible light should be used.

Amiodarone contains iodine and can cause disorders of thyroid function; both hypothyroidism and hyperthyroidism may occur. Clinical assessment alone is unreliable, and laboratory tests should be performed before treatment and every 6 months. Thyroxine (T4) may be raised in the absence of hyperthyroidism; therefore tri-iodothyronine (T3), T4, and thyroid-stimulating hormone (thyrotrophin, TSH) should all be measured. A raised T3 and T4 with a very low or undetectable TSH concentration suggests the development of thyrotoxicosis. The thyrotoxicosis may be very refractory, and amiodarone should usually be withdrawn at least temporarily to help achieve control; treatment with carbimazole may be required. Hypothyroidism can be treated with replacement therapy without withdrawing amiodarone if it is essential; careful supervision is required.

Pneumonitis should always be suspected if new or progressive shortness of breath or cough develops in a patient taking amiodarone. Fresh neurological symptoms should raise the possibility of peripheral neuropathy.

Amiodarone is also associated with hepatotoxicity and treatment should be discontinued if severe liver function abnormalities or clinical signs of liver disease develop.

Beta-blockers act as anti-arrhythmic drugs principally by attenuating the effects of the sympathetic system on automaticity and conductivity within the heart, for details see section 2.4. For special reference to the role of **sotalol** in ventricular arrhythmias, see p. 85.

Disopyramide may be given by intravenous injection to control arrhythmias after myocardial infarction (including those not responding to lidocaine (lignocaine)), but it impairs cardiac contractility. Oral administration of disopyramide is useful but it has an antimuscarinic effect which limits its use in patients susceptible to angle-closure glaucoma or prostatic hypertrophy.

Flecainide belongs to the same general class as lidocaine and may be of value in serious symptomatic ventricular arrhythmias. It may also be indicated for junctional re-entry tachycardias and for paroxysmal atrial fibrillation. However, it can precipitate serious arrhythmias in a small minority of patients (including those with otherwise normal hearts).

Procainamide is given by intravenous injection to control ventricular arrhythmias.

Propafenone is used for the prophylaxis and treatment of ventricular arrhythmias and also for some supraventricular arrhythmias. It has complex mechanisms of action, including weak beta-blocking activity (therefore caution is needed in obstructive airways disease—contra-indicated if severe).

Drugs for supraventricular arrhythmias include **adenosine**, **cardiac glycosides**, and **verapamil**; see above under Supraventricular Arrhythmias. Drugs for ventricular arrhythmias include **lidocaine**, **mexiletine**, and **phenytoin**; see below under Ventricular Arrhythmias.

AMIODARONE HYDROCHLORIDE

Indications see notes above (should be initiated in hospital or under specialist supervision)

Cautions liver-function and thyroid-function tests required before treatment and then every 6 months (see notes above for tests of thyroid function); hypokalaemia (measure serum-potassium concentration before treatment); chest x-ray required before treatment; heart failure; elderly; severe bradycardia and conduction disturbances in excessive dosage; intravenous use may cause moderate and transient fall in blood pressure (circulatory collapse precipitated by rapid administration or overdosage) or severe hepatocellular toxicity (monitor transaminases closely); ECG monitoring and resuscitation facilities must be available during intravenous use; porphyria (section 9.8.2); **interactions:** Appendix 1 (amiodarone)

Contra-indications (except in cardiac arrest) sinus bradycardia, sino-atrial heart block; unless pacemaker fitted avoid in severe conduction disturbances or sinus node disease; thyroid dysfunction; iodine sensitivity; avoid *intravenous use* in severe respiratory failure, circulatory collapse, severe arterial hypotension; avoid bolus injection in congestive heart failure or cardiomyopathy; pregnancy (Appendix 4); breast-feeding (Appendix 5)

Side-effects nausea, vomiting, taste disturbances, raised serum transaminases (may require dose reduction or withdrawal if accompanied by acute liver disorders), jaundice; bradycardia (see Cautions); pulmonary toxicity (including pneumonitis and fibrosis); tremor, sleep disorders; hypothyroidism, hyperthyroidism; reversible corneal microdeposits (sometimes with night glare); phototoxicity, persistent slate-grey skin discoloration (see also notes above); *less commonly* onset or worsening of arrhythmia, conduction disturbances (see Cautions), peripheral neuropathy and myopathy (usually reversible on withdrawal); *very rarely* chronic liver disease including cirrhosis, sinus arrest, bronchospasm (in patients with severe respiratory failure), ataxia, benign intracranial hypertension, headache, vertigo, epididymo-orchitis, impotence, haemolytic or aplastic anaemia, thrombocytopenia, rash (including exfoliative dermatitis), hypersensitivity including vasculitis, alopecia, impaired vision due to optic neuritis or optic neuropathy (including blindness), anaphylaxis on rapid injection, also hypotension, respiratory distress syndrome, sweating, and hot flushes

Dose

- By mouth, 200 mg 3 times daily for 1 week reduced to 200 mg twice daily for a further week; maintenance, usually 200 mg daily or the minimum required to control the arrhythmia
- By intravenous infusion via central venous catheter, initially 5 mg/kg over 20–120 minutes with ECG monitoring; subsequent infusion given if necessary according to response up to max. 1.2 g in 24 hours
- Ventricular fibrillation or pulseless ventricular tachycardia refractory to defibrillation, section 2.7.3

Amiodarone (Non-proprietary) PoM

Tablets, amiodarone hydrochloride 100 mg, net price 28-tab pack = £1.17; 200 mg, 28-tab pack = £1.29. Label: 11

Brands include *Amyben®*

Injection, amiodarone hydrochloride 30 mg/mL, net price 10-mL prefilled syringe = £10.25

Excipients may include benzyl alcohol (avoid in neonates, see Excipients, p. 2)

Sterile concentrate, amiodarone hydrochloride 50 mg/mL, net price 3-mL amp = £1.33, 6-mL amp = £2.86. For dilution and use as an infusion

Excipients may include benzyl alcohol (avoid in neonates, see Excipients, p. 2)

Cordarone X® (Sanofi-Synthelabo) PoM

Tablets, both scored, amiodarone hydrochloride 100 mg, net price 28-tab pack = £4.45; 200 mg, 28-tab pack = £7.27. Label: 11

Sterile concentrate, amiodarone hydrochloride 50 mg/mL. Net price 3-mL amp = £1.33. For dilution and use as an infusion

Excipients include benzyl alcohol (avoid in neonates, see Excipients, p. 2)

2 Cardiovascular system

DISOPYRAMIDE

Indications ventricular arrhythmias, especially after myocardial infarction; supraventricular arrhythmias

Cautions monitor for hypotension, hypoglycaemia, ventricular tachycardia, ventricular fibrillation or torsade de pointes (discontinue if occur); atrial flutter or atrial tachycardia with partial block, bundle branch block, heart failure (avoid if severe); prostatic enlargement; susceptibility to angle-closure glaucoma; hepatic impairment (Appendix 2); renal impairment (Appendix 3); pregnancy (Appendix 4); breast-feeding (Appendix 5); **interactions**: Appendix 1 (disopyramide)

Contra-indications second- and third-degree heart block and sinus node dysfunction (unless pacemaker fitted); cardiogenic shock; severe uncompensated heart failure

Side-effects ventricular tachycardia, ventricular fibrillation or torsade de pointes (usually associated with prolongation of QRS complex or QT interval—see Cautions above), myocardial depression, hypotension, AV block; antimuscarinic effects include dry mouth, blurred vision, urinary retention, and very rarely angle-closure glaucoma; gastro-intestinal irritation; psychosis, cholestatic jaundice, hypoglycaemia also reported (see Cautions above)

Dose

- By mouth, 300–800 mg daily in divided doses
- By slow intravenous injection, 2 mg/kg over at least 5 minutes to a max. of 150 mg, with ECG monitoring, followed immediately *either* by 200 mg by mouth, then 200 mg every 8 hours for 24 hours *or* 400 micrograms/kg/hour by intravenous infusion; max. 300 mg in first hour and 800 mg daily

Disopyramide (Non-proprietary) PoM
Capsules, disopyramide (as phosphate) 100 mg, net price 84 = £41.24; 150 mg, 84 = £47.41

Rythmodan® (Borg) PoM
Capsules, disopyramide 100 mg (green/beige), net price 84-cap pack = £14.71; 150 mg, 84-cap pack = £19.52

Injection, disopyramide (as phosphate) 10 mg/mL, net price 5-mL amp = £2.72

Modified release

Rythmodan Retard® (Borg) PoM
Tablets, m/r, scored, f/c, disopyramide (as phosphate) 250 mg. Net price 56-tab pack = £28.85. Label: 25

Dose 250–375 mg every 12 hours

FLECAINIDE ACETATE

Indications *Tablets and injection:* AV nodal reciprocating tachycardia, arrhythmias associated with accessory conducting pathways (e.g. Wolff-Parkinson-White syndrome), disabling symptoms of paroxysmal atrial fibrillation in patients without left ventricular dysfunction (arrhythmias of recent onset will respond more readily)

Tablets only: symptomatic sustained ventricular tachycardia, disabling symptoms of premature ventricular contractions or non-sustained ventricular tachycardia in patients resistant to or intolerant of other therapy

Injection only: ventricular tachyarrhythmias resistant to other treatment

Cautions patients with pacemakers (especially those who may be pacemaker dependent because stimulation threshold may rise appreciably); avoid in sinus node dysfunction, atrial conduction defects, second-degree or greater AV block, bundle branch block or distal block unless pacing rescue available; atrial fibrillation following heart surgery; elderly (accumulation may occur); ECG monitoring and resuscitation facilities must be available during intravenous use; hepatic impairment (Appendix 2); renal impairment (monitor plasma-flecainide concentration, see also Appendix 3); pregnancy (Appendix 4); breast-feeding (Appendix 5); **interactions**: Appendix 1 (flecainide)

Contra-indications heart failure; history of myocardial infarction and either asymptomatic ventricular ectopics or asymptomatic non-sustained ventricular tachycardia; long-standing atrial fibrillation where conversion to sinus rhythm not attempted; haemodynamically significant valvular heart disease

Side-effects nausea, vomiting; pro-arrhythmic effects; dyspnoea; visual disturbances; less commonly gastro-intestinal disturbances, jaundice, hepatic dysfunction, AV block, heart failure, myocardial infarction, hypotension, pneumonitis, hallucinations, depression, convulsions, peripheral neuropathy, paraesthesia, ataxia, dyskinesia, hypoaesthesia, tinnitus, vertigo, reduction in red blood cells, in white blood cells and in platelets, corneal deposits, rashes, alopecia, sweating, urticaria, photosensitivity, increased antinuclear antibodies

Dose

- By mouth (initiated under direction of hospital consultant), ventricular arrhythmias, initially 100 mg twice daily (max. 400 mg daily usually reserved for rapid control or in heavily built patients), reduced after 3–5 days if possible
  Supraventricular arrhythmias, 50 mg twice daily, increased if required to max. 300 mg daily
- By slow intravenous injection (in hospital), 2 mg/kg over 10–30 minutes, max. 150 mg, with ECG monitoring; followed if required by infusion at a rate of 1.5 mg/kg/hour for 1 hour, subsequently reduced to 100–250 micrograms/kg/hour for up to 24 hours; max. cumulative dose in first 24 hours, 600 mg; transfer to *oral* treatment, as above

Note Pre-dose ('trough') plasma-flecainide concentration for optimum response 0.2–1 mg/litre

Flecainide (Non-proprietary) PoM
Tablets, flecainide acetate 50 mg, net price 60-tab pack = £16.77; 100 mg, 60-tab pack = £24.05

Tambocor® (3M) PoM
Tablets, flecainide acetate 50 mg, net price 60-tab pack = £14.46; 100 mg (scored), 60-tab pack = £20.66

Injection, flecainide acetate 10 mg/mL. Net price 15-mL amp = £4.40

PROCAINAMIDE HYDROCHLORIDE

Indications ventricular arrhythmias, especially after myocardial infarction; atrial tachycardia

Cautions elderly; asthma, myasthenia gravis; hepatic impairment (Appendix 2); renal impairment (Appendix 3); pregnancy (Appendix 4); **interactions:** Appendix 1 (procainamide)

Contra-indications heart block, heart failure, hypotension; systemic lupus erythematosus; not indicated for torsade de pointes (can exacerbate); breast-feeding (Appendix 5)

Side-effects nausea, diarrhoea, rashes, fever, myocardial depression, heart failure, lupus erythematosus-like syndrome, agranulocytosis after prolonged treatment; psychosis and angioedema also reported

Dose

- By slow intravenous injection, rate not exceeding 50 mg/minute, 100 mg with ECG monitoring, repeated at 5-minute intervals until arrhythmia controlled; max. 1 g
- By intravenous infusion, 500–600 mg over 25–30 minutes with ECG monitoring, followed by maintenance at rate of 2–6 mg/minute, then if necessary oral anti-arrhythmic treatment starting 3–4 hours after infusion

Note Serum procainamide concentration for optimum response 3–10 mg/litre

Pronestyl® (Squibb) PoM

Injection, procainamide hydrochloride 100 mg/mL. Net price 10-mL vial = £1.90

PROPAFENONE HYDROCHLORIDE

Indications ventricular arrhythmias; paroxysmal supraventricular tachyarrhythmias which include paroxysmal atrial flutter or fibrillation and paroxysmal re-entrant tachycardias involving the AV node or accessory pathway, where standard therapy ineffective or contra-indicated

Cautions heart failure; elderly; pacemaker patients; great caution in obstructive airways disease owing to beta-blocking activity (contra-indicated if severe); hepatic impairment (Appendix 2); renal impairment; pregnancy (Appendix 4); breast-feeding (Appendix 5); **interactions:** Appendix 1 (propafenone)

Contra-indications uncontrolled congestive heart failure, cardiogenic shock (except arrhythmia induced), severe bradycardia, electrolyte disturbances, severe obstructive pulmonary disease, marked hypotension; myasthenia gravis; unless adequately paced avoid in sinus node dysfunction, atrial conduction defects, second degree or greater AV block, bundle branch block or distal block

Side-effects antimuscarinic effects including constipation, blurred vision, and dry mouth; dizziness, nausea and vomiting, fatigue, bitter taste, diarrhoea, headache, and allergic skin reactions reported; postural hypotension, particularly in elderly; bradycardia, sino-atrial, atrioventricular, or intraventricular blocks; arrhythmogenic (pro-arrhythmic) effect; rarely hypersensitivity reactions (cholestasis, blood disorders, lupus syndrome), seizures; myoclonus also reported

Dose

- Body-weight 70 kg and over, initially 150 mg 3 times daily after food under direct hospital supervision with ECG monitoring and blood pressure control (if QRS interval prolonged by more than 20%, reduce dose or discontinue until ECG returns to normal limits); may be increased at intervals of at least 3 days to 300 mg twice daily and, if necessary, to max. 300 mg 3 times daily; body-weight under 70 kg, reduce dose; ELDERLY may respond to lower doses

Arythmol® (Abbott) PoM

Tablets, both f/c, propafenone hydrochloride 150 mg, net price 90-tab pack = £7.37; 300 mg, 60-tab pack = £9.34. Label: 21, 25

Ventricular arrhythmias

Lidocaine (lignocaine) is relatively safe when used by slow intravenous injection and should be considered first for emergency use. Though effective in suppressing ventricular tachycardia and reducing the risk of ventricular fibrillation following myocardial infarction, it has not been shown to reduce mortality when used prophylactically in this condition. In patients with cardiac or hepatic failure doses may need to be reduced to avoid convulsions, depression of the central nervous system, or depression of the cardiovascular system.

Mexiletine may be given as a slow intravenous injection if lidocaine is ineffective; it has a similar action. Adverse cardiovascular and central nervous system effects may limit the dose tolerated; nausea and vomiting may prevent an effective dose being given by mouth.

Moracizine (*Ethmozine®*, Shire) is available on a named-patient basis for the prophylaxis and treatment of serious and life-threatening ventricular arrhythmias for patients already stabilised on moracizine.

Drugs for both supraventricular and ventricular arrhythmias include **amiodarone**, **beta-blockers**, **disopyramide**, **flecainide**, **procainamide**, and **propafenone**, see above under Supraventricular and Ventricular Arrhythmias

LIDOCAINE HYDROCHLORIDE

(Lignocaine hydrochloride)

Indications ventricular arrhythmias, especially after myocardial infarction

Cautions lower doses in congestive cardiac failure and following cardiac surgery; elderly; hepatic impairment (Appendix 2); renal impairment (Appendix 3); pregnancy (Appendix 4); **interactions:** Appendix 1 (lidocaine)

Contra-indications sino-atrial disorders, all grades of atrioventricular block, severe myocardial depression; porphyria (see section 9.8.2)

Side-effects dizziness, paraesthesia, or drowsiness (particularly if injection too rapid); other CNS effects include confusion, respiratory depression and convulsions; hypotension and bradycardia (may lead to cardiac arrest); *rarely* hypersensitivity reactions including anaphylaxis

Dose

- By intravenous injection, in patients without gross circulatory impairment, 100 mg as a bolus over a few minutes (50 mg in lighter patients or those whose circulation is severely impaired), followed immediately by infusion of 4 mg/minute for 30 minutes, 2 mg/minute for 2 hours, then 1 mg/minute; reduce concentration further if infusion continued beyond 24 hours (ECG monitoring and specialist advice for infusion)

Note Following *intravenous injection* lidocaine has a short duration of action (lasting for 15–20 minutes). If an *intravenous infusion* is not immediately available the initial *intravenous injection* of 50–100 mg can be repeated if necessary once or twice at intervals of not less than 10 minutes

Lidocaine (Non-proprietary) PoM
Injection 2%, lidocaine hydrochloride 20 mg/mL, net price 2-mL amp = 28p; 5-mL amp = 26p; 10-mL amp = 60p; 20-mL amp = 61p
Available from Braun

Infusion, lidocaine hydrochloride 0.1% (1 mg/mL) and 0.2% (2 mg/mL) in glucose intravenous infusion 5%. 500-mL containers
Available from Baxter

Minijet® Lignocaine (Celltech) PoM
Injection, lidocaine hydrochloride 1% (10 mg/mL), net price 10-mL disposable syringe = £4.85; 2% (20 mg/mL), 5-mL disposable syringe = £4.73

MEXILETINE HYDROCHLORIDE

Indications life-threatening ventricular arrhythmias
Cautions close monitoring on initiation of therapy (including ECG and blood pressure) particularly in patients with sinus node dysfunction, conduction defects, bradycardia, hypotension, or heart failure; hepatic impairment (Appendix 2); renal impairment (Appendix 3); pregnancy (Appendix 4); **interactions:** Appendix 1 (mexiletine)
Contra-indications cardiogenic shock; second- or third-degree AV block (unless pacemaker fitted)
Side-effects nausea, vomiting, constipation, diarrhoea, taste disturbance, dry mouth, hiccups, dyspepsia; bradycardia, hypotension, atrial fibrillation, palpitation, conduction defects, exacerbation of arrhythmias, torsade de pointes, exacerbation of heart failure; drowsiness, insomnia, dizziness, confusion, convulsions, psychiatric disorders, dysarthria, ataxia, paraesthesia, nystagmus, tremor, visual disturbances; jaundice, hepatitis, rash, Stevens-Johnson syndrome, pulmonary toxicity, and blood disorders reported; see also notes above
Dose
- By mouth, initial dose 400 mg (may be increased to 600 mg after myocardial infarction if opioid analgesics also given), followed after 2 hours by 200–250 mg 3–4 times daily
- By intravenous injection, 100–250 mg at a rate of 25 mg/minute with ECG monitoring followed by infusion of 250 mg as a 0.1% solution over 1 hour, 125 mg/hour for 2 hours, then 500 micrograms/minute

Mexitil® (Boehringer Ingelheim) PoM
Capsules, mexiletine hydrochloride 50 mg (purple/red), net price 100-cap pack = £4.95; 200 mg (red), 100-cap pack = £11.87. Label: 21, 27

Injection, mexiletine hydrochloride 25 mg/mL. Net price 10-mL amp = £1.49

2.4 Beta-adrenoceptor blocking drugs

Beta-adrenoceptor blocking drugs (beta-blockers) block the beta-adrenoreceptors in the heart, peripheral vasculature, bronchi, pancreas, and liver.

Many beta-blockers are now available and in general they are all equally effective. There are, however, differences between them which may affect choice in treating particular diseases or individual patients.

Intrinsic sympathomimetic activity (ISA, partial agonist activity) represents the capacity of beta-blockers to stimulate as well as to block adrenergic receptors. **Oxprenolol**, **pindolol**, **acebutolol** and **celiprolol** have intrinsic sympathomimetic activity; they tend to cause less bradycardia than the other beta-blockers and may also cause less coldness of the extremities.

Some beta-blockers are lipid soluble and some are water soluble. **Atenolol**, **celiprolol**, **nadolol**, and **sotalol** are the most water-soluble; they are less likely to enter the brain, and may therefore cause less sleep disturbance and nightmares. Water-soluble beta-blockers are excreted by the kidneys and dosage reduction is often necessary in renal impairment.

Beta-blockers with a relatively short duration of action have to be given two or three times daily. Many of these are, however, available in modified-release formulations so that administration once daily is adequate for hypertension. For angina twice-daily treatment may sometimes be needed even with a modified-release formulation. Some beta-blockers such as atenolol, bisoprolol, carvedilol, celiprolol, and nadolol have an intrinsically longer duration of action and need to be given only once daily.

Beta-blockers slow the heart and can depress the myocardium; they are contra-indicated in patients with second- or third-degree heart block. Beta-blockers should also be avoided in patients with worsening unstable heart failure; care is required when initiating a beta-blocker in those with stable heart failure (see also section 2.5.5). **Sotalol** may prolong the QT interval, and it occasionally causes life-threatening ventricular arrhythmias (**important:** particular care is required to avoid hypokalaemia in patients taking sotalol).

Labetalol, **celiprolol**, **carvedilol** and **nebivolol** are beta-blockers which have, in addition, an arteriolar vasodilating action, by diverse mechanisms, and thus lower peripheral resistance. There is no evidence that these drugs have important advantages over other beta-blockers in the treatment of hypertension.

Beta-blockers may precipitate asthma and this effect can be dangerous. Beta-blockers should be **avoided** in patients with a history of asthma or bronchospasm; if there is no alternative, a cardioselective beta-blocker may be used with extreme caution under specialist supervision. **Atenolol**, **bisoprolol**, **metoprolol**, **nebivolol** and (to a lesser extent) **acebutolol**, have less effect on the $beta_2$ (bronchial) receptors and are, therefore, relatively *cardioselective*, but they are **not** *cardiospecific*. They have a lesser effect on airways resistance but are **not** free of this side-effect.

Beta-blockers are also associated with fatigue, coldness of the extremities (may be less common with those with ISA, see above), and sleep disturbances with nightmares (may be less common with the water-soluble beta-blockers, see above).

Beta-blockers are not contra-indicated in diabetes; however, they can lead to a small deterioration of glucose tolerance and interfere with metabolic and autonomic responses to hypoglycaemia. Cardioselective beta-blockers (see above) may be preferable and beta-blockers should be avoided altogether in those with frequent episodes of hypoglycaemia. Beta blockers, especially when combined with a thiazide diuretic, should be avoided for the routine treatment of uncomplicated hypertension in patients with diabetes or in those at high risk of developing diabetes.

Hypertension The mode of action of beta-blockers in hypertension is not understood, but they reduce cardiac output, alter baroceptor reflex sensitivity, and block peripheral adrenoceptors. Some beta-blockers depress plasma renin secretion. It is possible that a central effect may also partly explain their mode of action.

Beta-blockers are effective for reducing blood pressure but other antihypertensives (section 2.5) are usually more effective for reducing the incidence of stroke, myocardial infarction, and cardiovascular mortality, especially in the elderly. Other antihypertensives are therefore preferred for routine initial treatment of uncomplicated hypertension.

In general, the dose of a beta-blocker does not have to be high; for example, atenolol is given in a dose of 25–50 mg daily and it is rarely necessary to increase the dose to 100 mg.

Beta-blockers can be used to control the pulse rate in patients with *phaeochromocytoma* (section 2.5.4). However, they should never be used alone as beta-blockade without concurrent alpha-blockade may lead to a hypertensive crisis. For this reason phenoxybenzamine should always be used together with the beta-blocker.

Angina By reducing cardiac work beta-blockers improve exercise tolerance and relieve symptoms in patients with *angina* (for further details on the management of stable and unstable angina see section 2.6). As with hypertension there is no good evidence of the superiority of any one drug, although occasionally a patient will respond better to one beta-blocker than to another. There is some evidence that sudden withdrawal may cause an exacerbation of angina and therefore gradual reduction of dose is preferable when beta-blockers are to be stopped. There is a risk of precipitating heart failure when beta-blockers and verapamil are used together in established ischaemic heart disease (**important**: see p. 117).

Myocardial infarction For advice on the management of ST-segment-elevation myocardial infarction see section 2.10.1; for advice on the management of non-ST-segment-elevation myocardial infarction see section 2.6. Several studies have shown that some beta-blockers can reduce the recurrence rate of *myocardial infarction*. However, uncontrolled heart failure, hypotension, bradyarrhythmias, and obstructive airways disease render beta-blockers unsuitable in some patients following a myocardial infarction. **Atenolol** and **metoprolol** may reduce early mortality after intravenous and subsequent oral administration in the acute phase, while **acebutolol**, **metoprolol**, **propranolol**, and **timolol** have protective value when started in the early convalescent phase. The evidence relating to other beta-blockers is less convincing, some have not been tested in trials of secondary protection. It is possible that sudden cessation may cause a rebound worsening of myocardial ischaemia.

Arrhythmias Beta-blockers act as *anti-arrhythmic drugs* principally by attenuating the effects of the sympathetic system on automaticity and conductivity within the heart. They may be used in conjunction with digoxin to control the ventricular response in atrial fibrillation, especially in patients with thyrotoxicosis. Beta-blockers are also useful in the management of supraventricular tachycardias, and are used to control those following myocardial infarction, see above.

Esmolol is a relatively cardioselective beta-blocker with a very short duration of action, used intravenously for the short-term treatment of supraventricular arrhythmias, sinus tachycardia, or hypertension, particularly in the peri-operative period. It may also be used in other situations, such as acute myocardial infarction, where sustained beta blockade might be hazardous.

Sotalol, a non-cardioselective beta-blocker with additional class III anti-arrhythmic activity, is used for prophylaxis in paroxysmal supraventricular arrhythmias. It also suppresses ventricular ectopic beats and non-sustained ventricular tachycardia. It has been shown to be more effective than lidocaine (lignocaine) in the termination of spontaneous sustained ventricular tachycardia due to coronary disease or cardiomyopathy. However, it may induce torsade de pointes in susceptible patients.

Heart failure Beta-blockers may produce benefit in heart failure by blocking sympathetic activity. **Bisoprolol** and **carvedilol** reduce mortality in any grade of stable heart failure; **nebivolol** is licensed for stable mild to moderate heart failure in patients over 70 years. Treatment should be initiated by those experienced in the management of heart failure (section 2.5.5).

Thyrotoxicosis Beta-blockers are used in pre-operative preparation for thyroidectomy. Administration of propranolol can reverse clinical symptoms of *thyrotoxicosis* within 4 days. Routine tests of increased thyroid function remain unaltered. The thyroid gland is rendered less vascular thus making surgery easier (section 6.2.2).

Other uses Beta-blockers have been used to alleviate some symptoms of *anxiety*; probably patients with palpitation, tremor, and tachycardia respond best (see also section 4.1.2 and section 4.3.3). Beta-blockers are also used in the *prophylaxis of migraine* (section 4.7.4.2). Betaxolol, carteolol, levobunolol, metipranolol and timolol are used topically in *glaucoma* (section 11.6).

PROPRANOLOL HYDROCHLORIDE

Indications see under Dose

Cautions see notes above; also avoid abrupt withdrawal especially in ischaemic heart disease; first-degree AV block; portal hypertension (risk of deterioration in liver function); diabetes; history of obstructive airways disease (introduce cautiously and monitor lung function—see also Bronchospasm below); myasthenia gravis; symptoms of hypoglycaemia and thyrotoxicosis may be masked (also see notes above); history of hypersensitivity—may increase sensitivity to allergens and result in more serious hypersensitivity response, also may reduce response to adrenaline (epinephrine) (see also section 3.4.3); reduce dose of oral propranolol in hepatic impairment; renal impairment (Appendix 3); pregnancy (Appendix 4); breast-feeding (Appendix 5); **interactions**: Appendix 1 (beta-blockers), **important**: verapamil interaction, see also p. 117

Contra-indications asthma (**important**: see Bronchospasm below), uncontrolled heart failure, Prinzmetal's angina, marked bradycardia, hypotension, sick sinus syndrome, second- or third- degree AV block, cardiogenic shock, metabolic acidosis, severe peripheral arterial disease; phaeochromocytoma (apart from specific use with alpha-blockers, see also notes above)

Bronchospasm The CSM has advised that beta-blockers, including those considered to be cardioselective, should not be given to patients with a history of asthma or bronchospasm. However, in rare situations where there is no alternative a cardioselective beta-blocker is given to these patients with extreme caution and under specialist supervision

Side-effects see notes above; also gastro-intestinal disturbances; bradycardia, heart failure, hypotension, conduction disorders, peripheral vasoconstriction (including exacerbation of intermittent claudication and Raynaud's phenomenon); bronchospasm, dyspnoea; headache, fatigue, sleep disturbances, paraesthesia, dizziness, vertigo, psychoses; sexual dysfunction; purpura, thrombocytopenia; visual disturbances; exacerbation of psoriasis, alopecia; *rarely* rashes and dry eyes (reversible on withdrawal); **overdosage**: see Emergency Treatment of Poisoning, p. 32

Dose

- By mouth, hypertension, initially 80 mg twice daily, increased at weekly intervals as required; maintenance 160–320 mg daily

  Portal hypertension, Initially 40 mg twice daily, increased to 80 mg twice daily according to heart-rate; max. 160 mg twice daily

  Phaeochromocytoma (only with an alpha-blocker), 60 mg daily for 3 days before surgery *or* 30 mg daily in patients unsuitable for surgery

  Angina, initially 40 mg 2–3 times daily; maintenance 120–240 mg daily

  Arrhythmias, hypertrophic cardiomyopathy, anxiety tachycardia, and thyrotoxicosis (adjunct), 10–40 mg 3–4 times daily

  Anxiety with symptoms such as palpitation, sweating, tremor, 40 mg once daily, increased to 40 mg 3 times daily if necessary

  Prophylaxis after myocardial infarction, 40 mg 4 times daily for 2–3 days, then 80 mg twice daily, beginning 5 to 21 days after infarction

  Migraine prophylaxis and essential tremor, initially 40 mg 2–3 times daily; maintenance 80–160 mg daily
- By intravenous injection, arrhythmias and thyrotoxic crisis, 1 mg over 1 minute; if necessary repeat at 2-minute intervals; max. 10 mg (5 mg in anaesthesia)

  Note Excessive bradycardia can be countered with intravenous injection of atropine sulphate 0.6–2.4 mg in divided doses of 600 micrograms; for **overdosage** see Emergency Treatment of Poisoning, p. 32

Propranolol (Non-proprietary) PoM

Tablets, propranolol hydrochloride 10 mg, net price 28 = 60p; 40 mg, 28 = 66p; 80 mg, 56 = £2.14; 160 mg, 56 = £4.03. Label: 8

Brands include *Angilol®*

Oral solution, propranolol hydrochloride 5 mg/5 mL, net price 150 mL = £12.50; 10 mg/5 mL, 150 mL = £16.45; 50 mg/5 mL, 150 mL = £19.98. Label: 8

Brands include *Syprol®*

Inderal® (AstraZeneca) PoM

Injection, propranolol hydrochloride 1 mg/mL, net price 1-mL amp = 21p

Modified release

Note Modified-release preparations may be used for once daily administration

Half-Inderal LA® (AstraZeneca) PoM

Capsules, m/r, lavender/pink, propranolol hydrochloride 80 mg. Net price 28-cap pack = £5.40. Label: 8, 25

Note Modified-release capsules containing propranolol hydrochloride 80 mg also available; brands include *Bedranol SR®*, *Half Beta Prograne®*

Inderal-LA® (AstraZeneca) PoM

Capsules, m/r, lavender/pink, propranolol hydrochloride 160 mg. Net price 28-cap pack = £6.67. Label: 8, 25

Note Modified-release capsules containing propranolol hydrochloride 160 mg also available; brands include *Bedranol SR®*, *Beta Prograne®*, *Slo-Pro®*

ACEBUTOLOL

Indications see under Dose

Cautions see under Propranolol Hydrochloride; renal impairment (Appendix 3)

Contra-indications see under Propranolol Hydrochloride

Side-effects see under Propranolol Hydrochloride

Dose

- Hypertension, initially 400 mg once daily *or* 200 mg twice daily, increased after 2 weeks to 400 mg twice daily if necessary
- Angina, initially 400 mg once daily *or* 200 mg twice daily; 300 mg 3 times daily in severe angina; up to 1.2 g daily has been used
- Arrhythmias, 0.4–1.2 g daily in 2–3 divided doses

Sectral® (Sanofi-Aventis) PoM

Capsules, acebutolol (as hydrochloride) 100 mg (buff/white), net price 84-cap pack = £14.97; 200 mg (buff/pink), 56-cap pack = £19.18. Label: 8

Tablets, f/c, acebutolol 400 mg (as hydrochloride). Net price 28-tab pack = £18.62. Label: 8

ATENOLOL

Indications see under Dose

Cautions see under Propranolol Hydrochloride; renal impairment (Appendix 3)

Contra-indications see under Propranolol Hydrochloride

Side-effects see under Propranolol Hydrochloride

Dose

- By mouth, hypertension, 25–50 mg daily (higher doses rarely necessary)

  Angina, 100 mg daily in 1 or 2 doses

  Arrhythmias, 50–100 mg daily
- By intravenous injection, arrhythmias, 2.5 mg at a rate of 1 mg/minute, repeated at 5-minute intervals to a max. of 10 mg

  Note Excessive bradycardia can be countered with intravenous injection of atropine sulphate 0.6–2.4 mg in divided doses of 600 micrograms; for **overdosage** see Emergency Treatment of Poisoning, p. 32
- By intravenous infusion, arrhythmias, 150 micrograms/kg over 20 minutes, repeated every 12 hours if required

Early intervention within 12 hours of myocardial infarction (section 2.10.1), by intravenous injection over 5 minutes, 5 mg, then by mouth, 50 mg after 15 minutes, 50 mg after 12 hours, then 100 mg daily

Atenolol (Non-proprietary) PoM
Tablets, atenolol 25 mg, net price 28-tab pack = 26p; 50 mg, 28-tab pack = 29p; 100 mg, 28-tab pack = 29p. Label: 8
Brands include *Atenix®*

Tenormin® (AstraZeneca) PoM
'25' tablets, f/c, atenolol 25 mg. Net price 28-tab pack = £4.41. Label: 8
LS tablets, orange, f/c, scored, atenolol 50 mg. Net price 28-tab pack = £5.11. Label: 8
Tablets, orange, f/c, scored, atenolol 100 mg. Net price 28-tab pack = £6.50. Label: 8
Syrup, sugar-free, atenolol 25 mg/5mL. Net price 300 mL = £8.55. Label: 8
Injection, atenolol 500 micrograms/mL. Net price 10-mL amp = 96p (hosp. only)

With diuretic

Co-tenidone (Non-proprietary) PoM
Tablets, co-tenidone 50/12.5 (atenolol 50 mg, chlortalidone 12.5 mg), net price 28-tab pack = 86p; co-tenidone 100/25 (atenolol 100 mg, chlortalidone 25 mg), 28-tab pack = £1.11. Label: 8
Brands include *Totaretic®*
Dose hypertension, 1 tablet daily (but see also under Dose above)

Kalten® (BPC 100) PoM
Capsules, red/ivory, atenolol 50 mg, co-amilozide 2.5/25 (anhydrous amiloride hydrochloride 2.5 mg, hydrochlorothiazide 25 mg). Net price 28-cap pack = £10.01. Label: 8
Dose hypertension, 1 capsule daily

Tenoret 50® (AstraZeneca) PoM
Tablets, brown, f/c, co-tenidone 50/12.5 (atenolol 50 mg, chlortalidone 12.5 mg). Net price 28-tab pack = £5.70. Label: 8
Dose hypertension, 1 tablet daily

Tenoretic® (AstraZeneca) PoM
Tablets, brown, f/c, co-tenidone 100/25 (atenolol 100 mg, chlortalidone 25 mg). Net price 28-tab pack = £8.12. Label: 8
Dose hypertension, 1 tablet daily (but see also under Dose above)

With calcium-channel blocker

Note Only indicated when calcium-channel blocker or beta-blocker alone proves inadequate. For cautions, contra-indications, and side-effects of nifedipine see section 2.6.2

Beta-Adalat® (Bayer) PoM
Capsules, reddish-brown, atenolol 50 mg, nifedipine 20 mg (m/r). Net price 28-cap pack = £10.41. Label: 8, 25
Dose hypertension, 1 capsule daily, increased if necessary to twice daily; elderly, 1 daily
Angina, 1 capsule twice daily

Tenif® (AstraZeneca) PoM
Capsules, reddish-brown, atenolol 50 mg, nifedipine 20 mg (m/r). Net price 28-cap pack = £10.63. Label: 8, 25
Dose hypertension, 1 capsule daily, increased if necessary to twice daily; elderly, 1 daily
Angina, 1 capsule twice daily

BISOPROLOL FUMARATE

Indications see under Dose

Cautions see under Propranolol Hydrochloride; in heart failure monitor clinical status for 4 hours after initiation (with low dose) and ensure heart failure not worsening before increasing each dose; psoriasis; hepatic impairment (Appendix 2); renal impairment (Appendix 3)

Contra-indications see under Propranolol Hydrochloride; also acute or decompensated heart failure requiring intravenous inotropes; sino-atrial block

Side-effects see under Propranolol Hydrochloride

Dose

- Hypertension and angina, usually 10 mg once daily (5 mg may be adequate in some patients); max. 20 mg daily
- Adjunct in stable moderate to severe heart failure (section 2.5.5), initially 1.25 mg once daily (in the morning) for 1 week then, if well tolerated, increased to 2.5 mg once daily for 1 week, then 3.75 mg once daily for 1 week, then 5 mg once daily for 4 weeks, then 7.5 mg once daily for 4 weeks, then 10 mg once daily; max. 10 mg daily

Bisoprolol Fumarate (Non-proprietary) PoM
Tablets, bisoprolol fumarate 5 mg, net price 28-tab pack = £2.31; 10 mg, 28-tab pack = £1.60. Label: 8
Brands include *Vivacor®*

Cardicor® (Merck) PoM
Tablets, f/c, bisoprolol fumarate 1.25 mg, net price 28-tab pack = £8.56; 2.5 mg (scored), 28-tab pack = £4.90; 3.75 mg (scored, white-yellow), 28-tab pack = £5.90; 5 mg (scored, light yellow), 28-tab pack = £5.90; 7.5 mg (scored, yellow), 28-tab pack = £5.90; 10 mg (scored, orange), 28-tab pack = £5.90. Label: 8

Emcor® (Merck) PoM
LS Tablets, yellow, f/c, scored, bisoprolol fumarate 5 mg. Net price 28-tab pack = £11.30. Label: 8
Tablets, orange, f/c, scored, bisoprolol fumarate 10 mg. Net price 28-tab pack = £12.68. Label: 8

CARVEDILOL

Indications hypertension; angina; adjunct to diuretics, digoxin, or ACE inhibitors in symptomatic chronic heart failure

Cautions see under Propranolol Hydrochloride; monitor renal function during dose titration in patients with heart failure who also have renal impairment, low blood pressure, ischaemic heart disease or diffuse vascular disease; severe heart failure, avoid in acute or decompensated heart failure requiring intravenous inotropes

Contra-indications see under Propranolol Hydrochloride; severe chronic heart failure; hepatic impairment

Side-effects postural hypotension, dizziness, headache, fatigue, gastro-intestinal disturbances, bradycardia; occasionally diminished peripheral circulation, peripheral oedema and painful extremities, dry mouth, dry eyes, eye irritation or disturbed vision, impotence, disturbances of micturition, influenza-like symptoms; rarely angina, AV block, exacerbation of intermittent claudication or Raynaud's phenomenon; allergic skin reactions, exacerbation of psoriasis, nasal stuffiness, wheezing, depressed mood, sleep disturbances, paraesthesia, heart failure, changes in liver enzymes, thrombocytopenia, leucopenia also reported

Dose

- Hypertension, initially 12.5 mg once daily, increased after 2 days to usual dose of 25 mg once daily; if necessary may be further increased at intervals of at least 2 weeks to max. 50 mg daily in single or divided doses; ELDERLY initial dose of 12.5 mg daily may provide satisfactory control
- Angina, initially 12.5 mg twice daily, increased after 2 days to 25 mg twice daily
- Adjunct in heart failure (section 2.5.5) initially 3.125 mg twice daily (with food), dose increased at intervals of at least 2 weeks to 6.25 mg twice daily, then to 12.5 mg twice daily, then to 25 mg twice daily; increase to highest dose tolerated, max. 25 mg twice daily in patients with severe heart failure or body-weight less than 85 kg and 50 mg twice daily in patients over 85 kg

Carvedilol (Non-proprietary) PoM
Tablets, carvedilol 3.125 mg, net price 28-tab pack = £5.79; 6.25 mg, 28-tab pack = £6.10; 12.5 mg, 28-tab pack = £1.57; 25 mg, 28-tab pack = £2.28. Label: 8

Eucardic® (Roche) PoM
Tablets, all scored, carvedilol 3.125 mg (pink), net price 28-tab pack = £7.57; 6.25 mg (yellow), 28-tab pack = £8.41; 12.5 mg (peach), 28-tab pack = £9.35; 25 mg, 28-tab pack = £11.68. Label: 8

CELIPROLOL HYDROCHLORIDE

Indications mild to moderate hypertension

Cautions see under Propranolol Hydrochloride; renal impairment (avoid if creatinine clearance less than 15 mL/minute; Appendix 3)

Contra-indications see under Propranolol Hydrochloride

Side-effects headache, dizziness, fatigue, nausea and somnolence; also bradycardia, bronchospasm; depression and pneumonitis reported rarely

Dose

- 200 mg once daily in the morning, increased to 400 mg once daily if necessary

Celiprolol (Non-proprietary) PoM
Tablets, celiprolol hydrochloride 200 mg, net price 28-tab pack = £8.63; 400 mg, 28-tab pack = £53.78. Label: 8, 22

Celectol® (Winthrop) PoM
Tablets, both f/c, scored, celiprolol hydrochloride 200 mg (yellow), net price 28-tab pack = £20.63; 400 mg, 28-tab pack = £41.26. Label: 8, 22

ESMOLOL HYDROCHLORIDE

Indications short-term treatment of supraventricular arrhythmias (including atrial fibrillation, atrial flutter, sinus tachycardia); tachycardia and hypertension in peri-operative period

Cautions see under Propranolol Hydrochloride; renal impairment

Contra-indications see under Propranolol Hydrochloride

Side-effects see under Propranolol Hydrochloride; also on infusion venous irritation and thrombophlebitis

Dose

- By intravenous infusion, usually within range 50–200 micrograms/kg/minute (consult product literature for details of dose titration and doses during peri-operative period)

Brevibloc® (Baxter) PoM
Injection, esmolol hydrochloride 10 mg/mL, net price 10-mL vial = £7.79, 250-mL infusion bag = £89.69

LABETALOL HYDROCHLORIDE

Indications hypertension (including hypertension in pregnancy, hypertension with angina, and hypertension following acute myocardial infarction); hypertensive crisis (but see section 2.5); controlled hypotension in anaesthesia

Cautions see under Propranolol Hydrochloride; interferes with laboratory tests for catecholamines; liver damage (see below); renal impairment (Appendix 3)

Liver damage Severe hepatocellular damage reported after both short-term and long-term treatment. Appropriate laboratory testing needed at first symptom of liver dysfunction and if laboratory evidence of damage (or if jaundice) labetalol should be stopped and not restarted

Contra-indications see under Propranolol Hydrochloride

Side-effects postural hypotension (avoid upright position during and for 3 hours after intravenous administration), tiredness, weakness, headache, rashes, scalp tingling, difficulty in micturition, epigastric pain, nausea, vomiting; liver damage (see above); rarely lichenoid rash

Dose

- By mouth, initially 100 mg (50 mg in elderly) twice daily with food, increased at intervals of 14 days to usual dose of 200 mg twice daily; up to 800 mg daily in 2 divided doses (3–4 divided doses if higher); max. 2.4 g daily
- By intravenous injection, 50 mg over at least 1 minute, repeated after 5 minutes if necessary; max. total dose 200 mg

  Note Excessive bradycardia can be countered with intravenous injection of atropine sulphate 0.6–2.4 mg in divided doses of 600 micrograms; for **overdosage** see Emergency Treatment of Poisoning, p. 32
- By intravenous infusion, 2 mg/minute until satisfactory response then discontinue; usual total dose 50–200 mg, (**not** recommended for phaeochromocytoma, see under Phaeochromocytoma, section 2.5.4)

  Hypertension of pregnancy, 20 mg/hour, doubled every 30 minutes; usual max. 160 mg/hour

  Hypertension following myocardial infarction, 15 mg/hour, gradually increased to max. 120 mg/hour

Labetalol Hydrochloride (Non-proprietary) PoM
Tablets, all f/c, labetalol hydrochloride 100 mg, net price, 56 = £10.17; 200 mg, 56 = £16.99; 400 mg, 56 = £26.36. Label: 8, 21

Trandate® (UCB Pharma) PoM
Tablets, all orange, f/c, labetalol hydrochloride 50 mg, net price 56-tab pack = £3.79; 100 mg, 56-tab pack = £4.17; 200 mg, 56-tab pack = £6.77; 400 mg, 56-tab pack = £9.42. Label: 8, 21
Injection, labetalol hydrochloride 5 mg/mL, net price 20-mL amp = £2.12

METOPROLOL TARTRATE

Indications see under Dose

Cautions see under Propranolol Hydrochloride; hepatic impairment (Appendix 2)

Contra-indications see under Propranolol Hydrochloride

Side-effects see under Propranolol Hydrochloride

Dose

- By mouth, hypertension, initially 100 mg daily, increased if necessary to 200 mg daily in 1–2 divided doses; max. 400 mg daily (but high doses rarely necessary)
  Angina, 50–100 mg 2–3 times daily
  Arrhythmias, usually 50 mg 2–3 times daily; up to 300 mg daily in divided doses if necessary
  Migraine prophylaxis, 100–200 mg daily in divided doses
  Hyperthyroidism (adjunct), 50 mg 4 times daily
- By intravenous injection, arrhythmias, up to 5 mg at rate 1–2 mg/minute, repeated after 5 minutes if necessary, total dose 10–15 mg
  Note Excessive bradycardia can be countered with intravenous injection of atropine sulphate 0.6–2.4 mg in divided doses of 600 micrograms; for **overdosage** see Emergency Treatment of Poisoning, p. 32
  In surgery, by slow intravenous injection 2–4 mg at induction or to control arrhythmias developing during anaesthesia; 2-mg doses may be repeated to a max. of 10 mg
  Early intervention within 12 hours of infarction, by intravenous injection 5 mg every 2 minutes to a max. of 15 mg, followed after 15 minutes by 50 mg by mouth every 6 hours for 48 hours; maintenance 200 mg daily in divided doses

Metoprolol Tartrate (Non-proprietary) PoM
Tablets, metoprolol tartrate 50 mg, net price 28 = £1.11, 56 = £1.57; 100 mg, 28 = £2.03, 56 = £2.60. Label: 8

Betaloc® (AstraZeneca) PoM
Injection, metoprolol tartrate 1 mg/mL. Net price 5-mL amp = 42p

Lopresor® (Novartis) PoM
Tablets, both f/c, scored, metoprolol tartrate 50 mg (pink), net price 56-tab pack = £2.57; 100 mg (blue), 56-tab pack = £6.68. Label: 8

Modified release

Betaloc-SA® (AstraZeneca) PoM
Durules® (= tablets, m/r), metoprolol tartrate 200 mg, net price 28-tab pack = £4.56. Label: 8, 25
Dose hypertension, angina, 200 mg daily in the morning, increased to 400 mg daily if necessary; migraine prophylaxis, 200 mg daily

Lopresor SR® (Novartis) PoM
Tablets, m/r, yellow, f/c, metoprolol tartrate 200 mg, net price 28-tab pack = £9.80. Label: 8, 25
Dose hypertension, 200 mg daily; angina, 200-400 mg daily; migraine prophylaxis, 200 mg daily

NADOLOL

Indications see under Dose

Cautions see under Propranolol Hydrochloride; hepatic impairment; renal impairment (Appendix 3)

Contra-indications see under Propranolol Hydrochloride

Side-effects see under Propranolol Hydrochloride

Dose

- Hypertension, initially 80 mg once daily, increased by increments of up to 80 mg at weekly intervals if required; max. 240 mg daily (higher doses rarely necessary)
- Angina, initially 40 mg once daily, increased at weekly intervals if required; usual max. 160 mg daily (rarely up to 240 mg may be required)
- Arrhythmias, initially 40 mg once daily, increased at weekly intervals to 160 mg if required; reduce to 40 mg if bradycardia occurs
- Migraine prophylaxis, initially 40 mg once daily, increased by 40 mg increments at weekly intervals; usual maintenance dose 80–160 mg once daily
- Thyrotoxicosis (adjunct), 80–160 mg once daily

Corgard® (Sanofi-Synthelabo) PoM
Tablets, blue, scored, nadolol 80 mg, net price 28-tab pack = £5.20. Label: 8

NEBIVOLOL

Indications essential hypertension; adjunct in stable mild to moderate heart failure in patients over 70 years

Cautions see under Propranolol Hydrochloride; reduce dose in renal impairment (Appendix 3)

Contra-indications see under Propranolol Hydrochloride; also acute or decompensated heart failure requiring intravenous inotropes; hepatic impairment (Appendix 2)

Side-effects see under Propranolol Hydrochloride; oedema, headache, dizziness, depression, visual disturbances, paraesthesia, impotence

Dose

- Hypertension, 5 mg daily; ELDERLY initially 2.5 mg daily, increased if necessary to 5 mg daily
- Adjunct in heart failure (section 2.5.5), initially 1.25 mg once daily, then if tolerated increased at intervals of 1–2 weeks to 2.5 mg once daily, then to 5 mg once daily, then to max. 10 mg once daily

Nebilet® (Menarini) PoM
Tablets, scored, nebivolol (as hydrochloride) 5 mg, net price 28-tab pack = £9.23. Label: 8

OXPRENOLOL HYDROCHLORIDE

Indications see under Dose

Cautions see under Propranolol Hydrochloride; reduce dose in hepatic impairment

Contra-indications see under Propranolol Hydrochloride

Side-effects see under Propranolol Hydrochloride

Dose

- Hypertension, 80–160 mg daily in 2–3 divided doses, increased as required; max. 320 mg daily
- Angina, 80–160 mg daily in 2–3 divided doses; max. 320 mg daily
- Arrhythmias, 40–240 mg daily in 2–3 divided doses; max. 240 mg daily
- Anxiety symptoms (short-term use), 40–80 mg daily in 1–2 divided doses

Oxprenolol (Non-proprietary) PoM
Tablets, all coated, oxprenolol hydrochloride 20 mg, net price 56 = £1.86; 40 mg, 56 = £3.73; 80 mg, 56 = £6.20; 160 mg, 20 = £2.36. Label: 8

Trasicor® (Amdipharm) PoM
Tablets, all f/c, oxprenolol hydrochloride 20 mg (contain gluten), net price 56-tab pack = £1.86; 40 mg (contain gluten), 56-tab pack = £3.73; 80 mg (yellow), 56-tab pack = £6.20. Label: 8

Modified release

Slow-Trasicor® (Amdipharm) PoM
Tablets, m/r, f/c, oxprenolol hydrochloride 160 mg. Net price 28-tab pack = £6.63. Label: 8, 25
Dose hypertension, angina, initially 160 mg once daily; if necessary may be increased to max. 320 mg daily

With diuretic

Trasidrex® (Goldshield) PoM
Tablets, red, s/c, co-prenozide 160/0.25 (oxprenolol hydrochloride 160 mg (m/r), cyclopenthiazide 250 micrograms). Net price 28-tab pack = £10.66. Label: 8, 25
Dose hypertension, 1 tablet daily, increased if necessary to 2 daily as a single dose

PINDOLOL

Indications see under Dose
Cautions see under Propranolol Hydrochloride
Contra-indications see under Propranolol Hydrochloride; severe renal impairment (Appendix 3)
Side-effects see under Propranolol Hydrochloride
Dose
- Hypertension, initially 5 mg 2–3 times daily *or* 15 mg once daily, increased as required at weekly intervals; usual maintenance 15–30 mg daily; max. 45 mg daily
- Angina, 2.5–5 mg up to 3 times daily

Pindolol (Non-proprietary) PoM
Tablets, pindolol 5 mg, net price 100-tab pack = £7.81. Label: 8

Visken® (Amdipharm) PoM
Tablets, both scored, pindolol 5 mg, net price 56-tab pack = £5.85; 15 mg, 28-tab pack = £8.79. Label: 8

With diuretic

Viskaldix® (Amdipharm) PoM
Tablets, scored, pindolol 10 mg, clopamide 5 mg. Net price 28-tab pack = £6.70. Label: 8
Dose hypertension, 1 tablet daily in the morning, increased if necessary to 2 daily; max. 3 daily

SOTALOL HYDROCHLORIDE

Indications *Tablets and injection:* life-threatening arrhythmias including ventricular tachyarrhythmias, symptomatic non-sustained ventricular tachyarrhythmias

Tablets only: prophylaxis of paroxysmal atrial tachycardia or fibrillation, paroxysmal AV re-entrant tachycardias (both nodal and involving accessory pathways), paroxysmal supraventricular tachycardia after cardiac surgery, maintenance of sinus rhythm following cardioversion of atrial fibrillation or flutter

Injection only: electrophysiological study of inducible ventricular and supraventricular arrhythmias; temporary substitution for tablets

CSM advice. The use of sotalol should be limited to the treatment of ventricular arrhythmias or prophylaxis of supraventricular arrhythmias (see above). It should no longer be used for angina, hypertension, thyrotoxicosis or for secondary prevention after myocardial infarction; when stopping sotalol for these indications, the dose should be reduced gradually

Cautions see under Propranolol Hydrochloride; reduce dose in renal impairment (avoid if creatinine clearance less than 10 ml/minute; Appendix 3); correct hypokalaemia, hypomagnesaemia, or other electrolyte disturbances; severe or prolonged diarrhoea; **interactions:** Appendix 1 (beta-blockers), **important:** verapamil interaction see also p. 117
Contra-indications see under Propranolol Hydrochloride; congenital or acquired long QT syndrome; torsade de pointes; renal failure
Side-effects see under Propranolol Hydrochloride; arrhythmogenic (pro-arrhythmic) effect (torsade de pointes—increased risk in women)
Dose
- By mouth with ECG monitoring and measurement of corrected QT interval, arrhythmias, initially 80 mg daily in 1–2 divided doses increased gradually at intervals of 2–3 days to usual dose of 160–320 mg daily in 2 divided doses; higher doses of 480–640 mg daily for life-threatening ventricular arrhythmias under specialist supervision
- By intravenous injection over 10 minutes, acute arrhythmias, 20–120 mg with ECG monitoring, repeated if necessary with 6-hour intervals between injections

Diagnostic use, see product literature

Note Excessive bradycardia can be countered with intravenous injection of atropine sulphate 0.6–2.4 mg in divided doses of 600 micrograms; for **overdosage** see Emergency Treatment of Poisoning, p. 32

Sotalol (Non-proprietary) PoM
Tablets, sotalol hydrochloride 40 mg, net price 56 = £1.34; 80 mg, 56 = £1.99; 160 mg, 28 = £2.63. Label: 8

Beta-Cardone® (UCB Pharma) PoM
Tablets, all scored, sotalol hydrochloride 40 mg (green), net price 56-tab pack = £1.34; 80 mg (pink), 56-tab pack = £1.99; 200 mg, 28-tab pack = £2.50. Label: 8

Sotacor® (Bristol-Myers Squibb) PoM
Tablets, both scored, sotalol hydrochloride 80 mg, net price 28-tab pack = £3.25; 160 mg, 28-tab pack = £6.41. Label: 8
Injection, sotalol hydrochloride 10 mg/mL. Net price 4-mL amp = £1.76

TIMOLOL MALEATE

Indications see under Dose; glaucoma (section 11.6)
Cautions see under Propranolol Hydrochloride; hepatic impairment (Appendix 2); renal impairment (Appendix 3)
Contra-indications see under Propranolol Hydrochloride
Side-effects see under Propranolol Hydrochloride

Dose

- Hypertension, initially 10 mg daily in 1–2 divided doses; gradually increased if necessary to max. 60 mg daily, usual maintenance dose 10–30 mg daily (doses above 30 mg daily given in divided doses)
- Angina, initially 5 mg twice daily increased if necessary by 10 mg daily every 3–4 days; max. 30 mg twice daily
- Prophylaxis after myocardial infarction, initially 5 mg twice daily, increased after 2 days to 10 mg twice daily if tolerated
- Migraine prophylaxis, 10–20 mg daily in 1–2 divided doses

Betim® (Valeant) PoM
Tablets, scored, timolol maleate 10 mg. Net price 30-tab pack = £2.08. Label: 8

With diuretic

Moducren® (MSD) PoM
Tablets, blue, scored, timolol maleate 10 mg, co-amilozide 2.5/25 (amiloride hydrochloride 2.5 mg, hydrochlorothiazide 25 mg). Net price 28-tab pack = £8.00. Label: 8
Dose hypertension, 1–2 tablets daily as a single dose

Prestim® (Valeant) PoM
Tablets, scored, timolol maleate 10 mg, bendroflumethiazide 2.5 mg. Net price 30-tab pack = £3.49. Label: 8
Dose hypertension, 1–2 tablets daily; max. 4 daily

2.5 Hypertension and heart failure

2.5.1 Vasodilator antihypertensive drugs
2.5.2 Centrally acting antihypertensive drugs
2.5.3 Adrenergic neurone blocking drugs
2.5.4 Alpha-adrenoceptor blocking drugs
2.5.5 Drugs affecting the renin-angiotensin system

Lowering raised blood pressure decreases the risk of stroke, coronary events, heart failure, and renal impairment. Advice on antihypertensive therapy in this section takes into account the recommendations of the Joint British Societies (JBS2: British Societies' guidelines on prevention of cardiovascular disease in clinical practice. *Heart* 2005; 91 (Suppl V): v1–v52).

Possible causes of hypertension (e.g. renal disease, endocrine causes), contributory factors, risk factors, and the presence of any complications of hypertension, such as left ventricular hypertrophy, should be established. Patients should be given advice on lifestyle changes to reduce blood pressure or cardiovascular risk; these include smoking cessation, weight reduction, reduction of excessive intake of alcohol, reduction of dietary salt, reduction of total and saturated fat, increasing exercise, and increasing fruit and vegetable intake.

Thresholds and targets for treatment The following thresholds for treatment[1] are recommended:

- Accelerated (malignant) hypertension (with papilloedema or fundal haemorrhages and exudates) *or* acute cardiovascular complications, admit for **immediate treatment**;
- Where the initial blood pressure is systolic ≥ 220 mmHg *or* diastolic ≥ 120 mmHg, **treat immediately**;
- Where the initial blood pressure is systolic 180–219 mmHg *or* diastolic 110–119 mmHg, confirm over 1–2 weeks then **treat** if these values are sustained;
- Where the initial blood pressure is systolic 160–179 mmHg *or* diastolic 100–109 mmHg, *and* the patient has cardiovascular complications, target-organ damage (e.g. left ventricular hypertrophy, renal impairment) or diabetes mellitus (type 1 or 2), confirm over 3–4 weeks then **treat** if these values are sustained;
- Where the initial blood pressure is systolic 160–179 mmHg *or* diastolic 100–109 mmHg, but the patient has *no* cardiovascular complications, no target-organ damage, or no diabetes, advise lifestyle changes, reassess weekly initially and **treat** if these values are sustained on repeat measurements over 4–12 weeks;
- Where the initial blood pressure is systolic 140–159 mmHg *or* diastolic 90–99 mmHg *and* the patient has cardiovascular complications, target-organ damage or diabetes, confirm within 12 weeks and **treat** if these values are sustained;
- Where the initial blood pressure is systolic 140–159 mmHg *or* diastolic 90–99 mmHg and *no* cardiovascular complications, no target-organ damage, or no diabetes, advise lifestyle changes and **reassess** monthly; **treat** persistent mild hypertension if the 10-year cardiovascular disease risk is 20% or more.[2]

A target systolic blood pressure < 140 mmHg *and* diastolic blood pressure < 90 mmHg is suggested. A lower target systolic blood pressure < 130 mmHg *and* diastolic blood pressure < 80 mmHg should be considered for those with established atherosclerotic cardiovascular disease, diabetes, or chronic renal failure. In some individuals it may not be possible to reduce blood pressure below the suggested targets despite the use of appropriate therapy.

Drug treatment of hypertension The choice of antihypertensive drug will depend on the relevant indications or contra-indications for the individual patient; *some* indications and contra-indications for various antihypertensive drugs are shown below (see also under individual drug entries for details):

- **Thiazides** (section 2.2.1)—particularly indicated for hypertension in the elderly (see below); a contra-indication is gout;

1. Thresholds and targets for treatment based on blood pressure measured in clinic may not apply to ambulatory or home blood-pressure monitoring, which usually give lower values.
2. Cardiovascular disease risk may be determined from the chart issued by the Joint British Societies (*Heart* 2005; 91 (Suppl V): v1–v52)—see inside back cover. The Joint British Societies' 'Cardiac Risk Assessor' computer programme may also be used to determine cardiovascular disease risk.

- **Beta-blockers** (section 2.4)—although no longer preferred for routine initial treatment of uncomplicated hypertension, other indications include myocardial infarction, angina; compelling contra-indications include asthma, heart block;
- **ACE inhibitors** (section 2.5.5.1)—indications include heart failure, left ventricular dysfunction and diabetic nephropathy; contra-indications include renovascular disease (but see section 2.5.5.1) and pregnancy;
- **Angiotensin-II receptor antagonists** (section 2.5.5.2) are alternatives for those who cannot tolerate ACE inhibitors because of persistent dry cough, but they have the same contra-indications as ACE inhibitors;
- **Calcium-channel blockers**. There are important differences between calcium-channel blockers (section 2.6.2). **Dihydropyridine calcium-channel blockers** are valuable in isolated systolic hypertension in the elderly when a low-dose thiazide is contra-indicated or not tolerated (see below). **'Rate-limiting' calcium-channel blockers** (diltiazem and verapamil) can be valuable in angina; contra-indications include heart failure and heart block;
- **Alpha-blockers** (section 2.5.4)—can be used with other antihypertensive drugs in the treatment of resistant hypertension; another possible indication is prostatism; a contra-indication is urinary incontinence.

A single antihypertensive drug is often not adequate and other antihypertensive drugs are usually added in a step-wise manner until control is achieved. Unless it is necessary to lower the blood pressure urgently, an interval of at least 4 weeks should be allowed to determine response.

Response to drug treatment for hypertension may be affected by the patient's age and ethnic background. An ACE inhibitor or an angiotensin-II receptor antagonist may be the most appropriate initial drug in younger Caucasians; however a beta-blocker may be considered if an ACE inhibitor or an angiotensin-II receptor antagonist is not tolerated or is contra-indicated (see also Hypertension in Pregnancy, p. 93). Afro-Caribbean patients and those aged over 55 years respond less well to ACE inhibitors and angiotensin-II receptor antagonists, therefore a thiazide or a calcium-channel blocker may be chosen for initial treatment.

Beta-blockers, especially when combined with a thiazide diuretic, should be avoided for the routine treatment of uncomplicated hypertension in patients with diabetes or in those at high risk of developing diabetes.

Where two antihypertensive drugs are needed, an ACE inhibitor *or* an angiotensin-II receptor antagonist may be combined with *either* a thiazide *or* a calcium-channel blocker.

If control is inadequate with 2 drugs, a thiazide *and* a calcium-channel blocker may be added. The addition of an alpha-blocker, spironolactone, another diuretic or a beta-blocker should be considered in resistant hypertension. In patients with *primary hyperaldosteronism*, spironolactone (section 2.2.3) is effective.

Other measures to reduce cardiovascular risk

Aspirin (section 2.9) in a dose of 75 mg daily reduces the risk of cardiovascular events and myocardial infarction. Unduly high blood pressure must be controlled before aspirin is given. Unless contra-indicated, aspirin is recommended for all patients with established cardiovascular disease or those with a 10-year cardiovascular disease risk[1] of 20% or more and aged over 50 years. Aspirin is also of benefit in those with diabetes (see also section 2.9).

Lipid-regulating drugs can also be of benefit in cardiovascular disease or in those who are at high risk of developing cardiovascular disease (section 2.12).

Hypertension in the elderly Benefit from antihypertensive therapy is evident up to at least 80 years of age, but it is probably inappropriate to apply a strict age limit when deciding on drug therapy. Patients who reach 80 years of age while taking antihypertensive drugs should continue treatment, provided that it continues to be of benefit and does not cause significant side-effects. The thresholds for treatment are diastolic pressure averaging $\geq$ 90 mmHg *or* systolic pressure averaging $\geq$ 160 mmHg over 3 to 6 months' observation (despite appropriate lifestyle interventions). Treatment with a low dose of a thiazide or a dihydropyridine calcium-channel blocker is effective. An ACE inhibitor (or an angiotensin-II receptor antagonist) (section 2.5.5) can be added if necessary.

Isolated systolic hypertension Isolated systolic hypertension (systolic pressure $\geq$ 160 mmHg, diastolic pressure $<$ 90 mmHg) is associated with an increased cardiovascular disease risk, particularly in those aged over 60 years. Systolic blood pressure averaging 160 mmHg or higher over 3 to 6 months (despite appropriate lifestyle interventions) should be lowered in those over 60 years, even if diastolic hypertension is absent. Treatment with a low dose of a thiazide or a dihydropyridine calcium-channel blocker is effective. An ACE inhibitor (or an angiotensin-II receptor antagonist) (section 2.5.5) can be added if necessary. Patients with severe postural hypotension should not receive blood pressure lowering drugs.

Isolated systolic hypertension in younger patients is uncommon but treatment may be indicated in those with a threshold systolic pressure of 160 mmHg (or less if at increased risk of cardiovascular disease, see above).

Hypertension in diabetes For patients with diabetes, the aim should be to maintain systolic pressure $<$ 130 mmHg and diastolic pressure $<$ 80 mmHg. However, in some individuals, it may not be possible to achieve this level of control despite appropriate therapy. Most patients require a combination of antihypertensive drugs.

Hypertension is common in type 2 (non-insulin-dependent) diabetes and antihypertensive treatment prevents macrovascular and microvascular complications. In type 1 (insulin-dependent) diabetes, hypertension usually indicates the presence of diabetic nephropathy. An ACE inhibitor (or an angiotensin-II receptor antagonist) may have a specific role in the management of diabetic nephropathy (section 6.1.5); in patients with type 2 diabetes, an ACE inhibitor (or an angiotensin-II receptor antagonist) can delay progression of microalbuminuria to nephropathy.

1. Cardiovascular disease risk may be determined from the chart issued by the Joint British Societies (*Heart* 2005; 91 (Suppl V): v1–v52)—see inside back cover. The Joint British Societies' 'Cardiac Risk Assessor' computer programme may also be used to determine cardiovascular disease risk.

Hypertension in renal disease The threshold for antihypertensive treatment in patients with renal impairment or persistent proteinuria is a systolic blood pressure ≥ 140 mmHg *or* a diastolic blood pressure ≥ 90 mmHg. Optimal blood pressure is a systolic blood pressure < 130 mmHg and a diastolic pressure < 80 mmHg, or lower if proteinuria exceeds 1 g in 24 hours. An ACE inhibitor (or an angiotensin-II receptor antagonist) should be considered for patients with proteinuria; however, ACE inhibitors should be used with caution in renal impairment (section 2.5.5.1). Thiazide diuretics may be ineffective and high doses of loop diuretics may be required. A dihydropyridine calcium channel blocker can be added.

Hypertension in pregnancy High blood pressure in pregnancy may usually be due to pre-existing essential hypertension or to pre-eclampsia. Methyldopa (section 2.5.2) is safe in pregnancy. Beta-blockers are effective and safe in the third trimester. Modified-release preparations of nifedipine [unlicensed] are also used for hypertension in pregnancy. Intravenous administration of labetalol (section 2.4) can be used to control hypertensive crises; alternatively, hydralazine (section 2.5.1) may be used by the intravenous route. For use of magnesium sulphate in pre-eclampsia and eclampsia, see section 9.5.1.3.

Accelerated or very severe hypertension Accelerated (or malignant) hypertension or very severe hypertension (e.g. diastolic blood pressure > 140 mmHg) requires urgent treatment in hospital, but it is not an indication for parenteral antihypertensive therapy. Normally treatment should be by mouth with a beta-blocker (atenolol or labetalol) or a long-acting calcium-channel blocker (e.g. amlodipine or modified-release nifedipine). Within the first 24 hours the diastolic blood pressure should be reduced to 100–110 mmHg. Over the next 2 or 3 days blood pressure should be further reduced using a calcium-channel blocker, diuretic, ACE inhibitor, beta-blocker, or vasodilator, alone or in combination. Rapid reduction in blood pressure can reduce organ perfusion leading to cerebral infarction and blindness, deterioration in renal function, and myocardial ischaemia. Sodium nitroprusside by infusion is the drug of choice on the rare occasions when parenteral treatment is necessary.

For advice on short-term management of hypertensive episodes in phaeochromocytoma, see under Phaeochromocytoma, section 2.5.4.

2.5.1 Vasodilator antihypertensive drugs

Vasodilators have a potent hypotensive effect, especially when used in combination with a beta-blocker and a thiazide. **Important**: for a warning on the hazards of a very rapid fall in blood pressure, see Accelerated or Very Severe Hypertension, above.

Diazoxide has been used by intravenous injection in hypertensive emergencies.

Hydralazine is given by mouth as an adjunct to other antihypertensives for the treatment of resistant hypertension but is rarely used; when used alone it causes tachycardia and fluid retention. The incidence of side-effects is lower if the dose is kept below 100 mg daily, but systemic lupus erythematosus should be suspected if there is unexplained weight loss, arthritis, or any other unexplained ill health.

Sodium nitroprusside is given by intravenous infusion to control severe hypertensive crises on the rare occasions when parenteral treatment is necessary.

Minoxidil should be reserved for the treatment of severe hypertension resistant to other drugs. Vasodilatation is accompanied by increased cardiac output and tachycardia and the patients develop fluid retention. For this reason the addition of a beta-blocker and a diuretic (usually furosemide, in high dosage) are mandatory. Hypertrichosis is troublesome and renders this drug unsuitable for women.

Prazosin, doxazosin, and terazosin (section 2.5.4) have alpha-blocking and vasodilator properties.

Bosentan, **epoprostenol** (section 2.8.1), **iloprost**, **sildenafil**, and **sitaxentan** are licensed for the treatment of some types of pulmonary hypertension and should be used under specialist supervision. The *Scottish Medicines Consortium* has advised (November 2005) that iloprost is accepted for restricted use in patients in whom bosentan is ineffective or not tolerated.

BOSENTAN

Indications pulmonary arterial hypertension; systemic sclerosis with ongoing digital ulcer disease (to reduce number of new digital ulcers)

Cautions not to be initiated if systemic systolic blood pressure is below 85 mmHg; monitor haemoglobin before and during treatment (monthly for first 4 months, then 3-monthly); avoid abrupt withdrawal; monitor liver function before treatment, at monthly intervals during treatment, and 2 weeks after dose increase (reduce dose or suspend treatment if liver enzymes raised significantly)—discontinue if symptoms of liver impairment; hepatic impairment (Appendix 2); **interactions:** Appendix 1 (bosentan)

Contra-indications porphyria (section 9.8.2) pregnancy (Appendix 4); breast-feeding (Appendix 5)

Side-effects gastro-intestinal disturbances, dry mouth, rectal haemorrhage, hepatic impairment (see Cautions, above); flushing, hypotension, palpitation, oedema, chest pain; dyspnoea; headache, dizziness, fatigue; back pain and pain in extremities; anaemia; hypersensitivity reactions (including rash, pruritus, and anaphylaxis)

Dose

- Pulmonary arterial hypertension, initially 62.5 mg twice daily increased after 4 weeks to 125 mg twice daily; max. 250 mg twice daily CHILD under 12 years see *BNF for Children*
- Systemic sclerosis with ongoing digital ulcer disease, initially 62.5 mg twice daily increased after 4 weeks to 125 mg twice daily

Tracleer® (Actelion) ▼ PoM

Tablets, f/c, orange, bosentan (as monohydrate) 62.5 mg, net price 56-tab pack = £1541.00; 125 mg, 56-tab pack = £1541.00

DIAZOXIDE

Indications hypertensive emergency including severe hypertension associated with renal disease (but see section 2.5); hypoglycaemia (section 6.1.4)

Cautions ischaemic heart disease; renal impairment (Appendix 3); pregnancy and labour (Appendix 4); **interactions**: Appendix 1 (diazoxide)

Side-effects tachycardia, hypotension, hyperglycaemia, sodium and water retention; *rarely* cardiomegaly, hyperosmolar non-ketotic coma, leucopenia, thrombocytopenia, and hirsuitism

Dose

- By rapid intravenous injection (less than 30 seconds), 1–3 mg/kg to max. single dose of 150 mg (see below); may be repeated after 5–15 minutes if required

Note Single doses of 300 mg have been associated with angina and with myocardial and cerebral infarction

Eudemine® (Goldshield) PoM

Injection, diazoxide 15 mg/mL. Net price 20-mL amp = £30.00

Tablets, see section 6.1.4

HYDRALAZINE HYDROCHLORIDE

Indications moderate to severe hypertension (adjunct); heart failure (with long-acting nitrate, but see section 2.5.5); hypertensive crisis (including during pregnancy) (but see section 2.5)

Cautions hepatic impairment (Appendix 2); renal impairment (Appendix 3); coronary artery disease (may provoke angina, avoid after myocardial infarction until stabilised), cerebrovascular disease; occasionally blood pressure reduction too rapid even with low parenteral doses; pregnancy (Appendix 4); breast-feeding (Appendix 5); manufacturer advises test for antinuclear factor and for proteinuria every 6 months and check acetylator status before increasing dose above 100 mg daily, but evidence of clinical value unsatisfactory; **interactions**: Appendix 1 (hydralazine)

Contra-indications idiopathic systemic lupus erythematosus, severe tachycardia, high output heart failure, myocardial insufficiency due to mechanical obstruction, cor pulmonale, dissecting aortic aneurysm; porphyria (section 9.8.2)

Side-effects tachycardia, palpitation, flushing, hypotension, fluid retention, gastro-intestinal disturbances; headache, dizziness; systemic lupus erythematosus-like syndrome after long-term therapy with over 100 mg daily (or less in women and in slow acetylator individuals) (see also notes above); rarely rashes, fever, peripheral neuritis, polyneuritis, paraesthesia, arthralgia, myalgia, increased lacrimation, nasal congestion, dyspnoea, agitation, anxiety, anorexia; blood disorders (including leucopenia, thrombocytopenia, haemolytic anaemia), abnormal liver function, jaundice, raised plasma creatinine, proteinuria and haematuria reported

Dose

- By mouth, hypertension, 25 mg twice daily, increased to usual max. 50 mg twice daily (see notes above)

  Heart failure (initiated in hospital) 25 mg 3–4 times daily, increased every 2 days if necessary; usual maintenance dose 50–75 mg 4 times daily
- By slow intravenous injection, hypertension with renal complications and hypertensive crisis, 5–10 mg diluted with 10 mL sodium chloride 0.9%; may be repeated after 20–30 minutes (see Cautions)
- By intravenous infusion, hypertension with renal complications and hypertensive crisis, initially 200–300 micrograms/minute; maintenance usually 50–150 micrograms/minute

Hydralazine (Non-proprietary) PoM

Tablets, hydralazine hydrochloride 25 mg, net price 56 = £9.45; 50 mg, 56 = £13.94

Apresoline® (Amdipharm) PoM

Tablets, yellow, s/c, hydralazine hydrochloride 25 mg, net price 84-tab pack = £2.82

Excipients include gluten

Injection, powder for reconstitution, hydralazine hydrochloride. Net price 20-mg amp = £1.84

ILOPROST

Indications primary pulmonary hypertension

Cautions unstable pulmonary hypertension with advanced right heart failure; hypotension (do not initiate if systolic blood pressure below 85 mmHg); hepatic impairment (Appendix 2); **interactions**: Appendix 1 (iloprost)

Contra-indications unstable angina; within 6 months of myocardial infarction; decompensated cardiac failure (unless under close medical supervision); severe arrhythmias; congenital or acquired heart-valve defects; within 3 months of cerebrovascular events; pulmonary veno-occlusive disease; conditions which increase risk of bleeding; pregnancy (Appendix 4); breast-feeding (Appendix 5)

Side-effects vasodilatation, hypotension, syncope, cough, headache, throat or jaw pain; nausea and chest pain also reported

Dose

- By inhalation of nebulised solution, initial dose 2.5 micrograms increased to 5 micrograms for second dose, if tolerated maintain at 5 micrograms 6–9 times daily according to response; reduce to 2.5 micrograms 6–9 times daily if higher dose not tolerated; CHILD 8–18 years see *BNF for Children*

Ventavis® (Schering Health) ▼ PoM

Nebuliser solution, iloprost (as trometamol) 10 micrograms/mL, net price 30 × 1-mL (10 microgram) unit-dose vials = £425.00, 168 × 1-mL = £2377.20. For use with *Prodose®* NHS or *Venta-Neb®* NHS nebuliser

MINOXIDIL

Indications severe hypertension, in addition to a diuretic and a beta-blocker

Cautions see notes above; angina; after myocardial infarction (until stabilised); lower doses in dialysis patients; porphyria (section 9.8.2); pregnancy (Appendix 4); **interactions**: Appendix 1 (vasodilator antihypertensives)

Contra-indications phaeochromocytoma

Side-effects sodium and water retention; weight gain, peripheral oedema, tachycardia, hypertrichosis; reversible rise in creatinine and blood urea nitrogen; occasionally, gastro-intestinal disturbances, breast tenderness, rashes

Dose

- Initially 5 mg (elderly, 2.5 mg) daily, in 1–2 divided doses, increased by 5–10 mg every 3 or more days; max. 100 mg daily (seldom necessary to exceed 50 mg daily)

Loniten® (Pharmacia) PoM
Tablets, all scored, minoxidil 2.5 mg, net price 60-tab pack = £8.88; 5 mg, 60-tab pack = £15.83; 10 mg, 60-tab pack = £30.68

SILDENAFIL

Indications pulmonary arterial hypertension; erectile dysfunction (section 7.4.5)

Cautions hypotension (avoid if systolic blood pressure below 90 mmHg); intravascular volume depletion; left ventricular outflow obstruction; cardiovascular disease; autonomic dysfunction; pulmonary veno-occlusive disease; anatomical deformation of the penis, predisposition to priapism; bleeding disorders or active peptic ulceration; consider gradual withdrawal; hepatic impairment (avoid if severe; Appendix 2); renal impairment (Appendix 3); pregnancy (Appendix 4); breast-feeding (Appendix 5); **interactions:** Appendix 1 (sildenafil)

Contra-indications recent history of stroke or myocardial infarction, history of non-arteritic anterior ischaemic optic neuropathy; hereditary degenerative retinal disorders; avoid concomitant use of nitrates

Side-effects gastro-intestinal disturbances, dry mouth; flushing, oedema; bronchitis, cough; headache, migraine, night sweats, paraesthesia, insomnia, anxiety, tremor, vertigo; fever, influenza-like symptoms; anaemia; back and limb pain, myalgia; visual disturbances, retinal haemorrhage, photophobia, painful red eyes; nasal congestion, epistaxis; cellulitis, alopecia; *less commonly* gynaecomastia, priapism; *also reported* rash, retinal vascular occlusion and non-arteritic anterior ischaemic optic neuropathy (discontinue if sudden visual impairment), and sudden hearing loss (seek medical advice)

Dose

- 20 mg 3 times daily; CHILD under 18 years see *BNF for Children*

Revatio® (Pfizer) ▼ PoM
Tablets, f/c, sildenafil (as citrate), 20 mg, net price 90-tab pack = £373.50

Viagra® (Pfizer) PoM NHS
Section 7.4.5 (erectile dysfunction)

SITAXENTAN SODIUM

Indications pulmonary arterial hypertension

Cautions monitor liver function before treatment and at monthly intervals thereafter (discontinue treatment if liver enzymes significantly raised); monitor haemoglobin concentration before treatment, after 1–3 months, then 3-monthly; pregnancy (Appendix 4); **interactions:** Appendix 1 (sitaxentan)

Contra-indications hepatic impairment; breast-feeding (Appendix 5)

Side-effects gastro-intestinal disturbances; peripheral oedema, flushing; headache, insomnia, fatigue, dizziness; decreased haemoglobin, prolonged prothrombin time, increased INR; muscle cramp; nasal congestion, epistaxis

Dose

- ADULT over 18 years 100 mg once daily

Thelin® (Encysive) ▼ PoM
Tablets, f/c, yellow-orange, sitaxentan sodium 100 mg, net price 28-tab pack = £1540.00

SODIUM NITROPRUSSIDE

Indications hypertensive crisis (but see section 2.5); controlled hypotension in anaesthesia; acute or chronic heart failure

Cautions hypothyroidism, hyponatraemia, ischaemic heart disease, impaired cerebral circulation, elderly; hypothermia; monitor blood pressure and blood-cyanide concentration and if treatment exceeds 3 days, also blood-thiocyanate concentration; avoid sudden withdrawal—terminate infusion over 15–30 minutes; hepatic impairment (Appendix 2); renal impairment (Appendix 3); pregnancy (Appendix 4); breast-feeding; **interactions:** Appendix 1 (sodium nitroprusside)

Contra-indications severe vitamin B_{12} deficiency; Leber's optic atrophy; compensatory hypertension

Side-effects associated with over rapid reduction in blood pressure (reduce infusion rate): headache, dizziness, nausea, retching, abdominal pain, perspiration, palpitation, anxiety, retrosternal discomfort; occasionally reduced platelet count, acute transient phlebitis

Cyanide Side-effects caused by excessive plasma concentration of the cyanide metabolite include tachycardia, sweating, hyperventilation, arrhythmias, marked metabolic acidosis (discontinue and give antidote, see p. 33)

Dose

- Hypertensive crisis, by intravenous infusion, initially 0.5–1.5 micrograms/kg/minute, then increased in steps of 500 nanograms/kg/minute every 5 minutes within range 0.5–8 micrograms/kg/minute (lower doses if already receiving other antihypertensives); stop if response unsatisfactory with max. dose in 10 minutes

  Note Lower initial dose of 300 nanograms/kg/minute has been used
- Maintenance of blood pressure at 30–40% lower than pretreatment diastolic blood pressure, 20–400 micrograms/minute (lower doses for patients being treated with other antihypertensives)
- Controlled hypotension in surgery, by intravenous infusion, max. 1.5 micrograms/kg/minute
- Heart failure, by intravenous infusion, initially 10–15 micrograms/minute, increased every 5–10 minutes as necessary; usual range 10–200 micrograms/minute normally for max. 3 days

Sodium Nitroprusside (Mayne) PoM
Intravenous infusion, powder for reconstitution, sodium nitroprusside 10 mg/mL. For dilution and use as an infusion, net price 5-mL vial = £8.00

2.5.2 Centrally acting antihypertensive drugs

Methyldopa is a centrally acting antihypertensive; it may be used for the management of hypertension in pregnancy. Side-effects are minimised if the daily dose is kept below 1 g.

Clonidine has the disadvantage that sudden withdrawal may cause a hypertensive crisis.

Moxonidine, a centrally acting drug, is licensed for mild to moderate essential hypertension. It may have a role when thiazides, calcium-channel blockers, ACE inhibitors, and beta-blockers are not appropriate or have failed to control blood pressure.

CLONIDINE HYDROCHLORIDE

Indications hypertension; migraine (section 4.7.4.2); menopausal flushing (section 6.4.1.1)

Cautions must be withdrawn gradually to avoid hypertensive crisis; Raynaud's syndrome or other occlusive peripheral vascular disease; history of depression; avoid in porphyria (section 9.8.2); pregnancy (Appendix 4); breast-feeding (Appendix 5); **interactions:** Appendix 1 (clonidine)

Driving Drowsiness may affect performance of skilled tasks (e.g. driving); effects of alcohol may be enhanced

Side-effects dry mouth, sedation, depression, fluid retention, bradycardia, Raynaud's phenomenon, headache, dizziness, euphoria, nocturnal unrest, rash, nausea, constipation, rarely impotence

Dose

- By mouth, 50–100 micrograms 3 times daily, increased every second or third day; usual max. dose 1.2 mg daily
- By slow intravenous injection, 150–300 micrograms; max. 750 micrograms in 24 hours

Catapres® (Boehringer Ingelheim) PoM

Tablets, both scored, clonidine hydrochloride 100 micrograms, net price 100-tab pack = £5.60; 300 micrograms, 100-tab pack = £13.04. Label: 3, 8

Injection, clonidine hydrochloride 150 micrograms/mL. Net price 1-mL amp = 29p

Dixarit® PoM

Section 4.7.4.2

METHYLDOPA

Indications hypertension

Cautions monitor blood counts and liver-function before treatment and at intervals during first 6–12 weeks or if unexplained fever occurs; history of depression; positive direct Coombs' test in up to 20% of patients (may affect blood cross-matching); interference with laboratory tests; hepatic impairment (avoid in active liver disease; Appendix 2); renal impairment (Appendix 3); **interactions:** Appendix 1 (methyldopa)

Driving Drowsiness may affect performance of skilled tasks (e.g. driving); effects of alcohol may be enhanced

Contra-indications depression, active liver disease, phaeochromocytoma; porphyria (section 9.8.2)

Side-effects gastro-intestinal disturbances, dry mouth, stomatitis, sialadenitis; bradycardia, exacerbation of angina, postural hypotension, oedema; sedation, headache, dizziness, asthenia, myalgia, arthralgia, paraesthesia, nightmares, mild psychosis, depression, impaired mental acuity, parkinsonism, Bell's palsy; abnormal liver function tests, hepatitis, jaundice; pancreatitis; haemolytic anaemia; bone-marrow depression, leucopenia, thrombocytopenia, eosinophilia; hypersensitivity reactions including lupus erythematosus-like syndrome, drug fever, myocarditis, pericarditis; rashes (including toxic epidermal necrolysis); nasal congestion, failure of ejaculation, impotence, decreased libido, gynaecomastia, hyperprolactinaemia, amenorrhoea

Dose

- Initially 250 mg 2–3 times daily, increased gradually at intervals of at least 2 days, max. 3 g daily; ELDERLY initially 125 mg twice daily, increased gradually, max. 2 g daily

Methyldopa (Non-proprietary) PoM

Tablets, coated, methyldopa (anhydrous) 125 mg, net price 56-tab pack = £9.94; 250 mg, 56-tab pack = £6.83; 500 mg, 56-tab pack = £10.31. Label: 3, 8

Aldomet® (MSD) PoM

Tablets, all yellow, f/c, methyldopa (anhydrous) 250 mg, net price 60 = £1.88; 500 mg, 30 = £1.90. Label: 3, 8

MOXONIDINE

Indications mild to moderate essential hypertension

Cautions avoid abrupt withdrawal (if concomitant treatment with beta-blocker has to be stopped, discontinue beta-blocker first, then moxonidine after a few days); susceptibility to angle-closure glaucoma; renal impairment (avoid if creatinine clearance less than 30 mL/minute; Appendix 3); **interactions:** see Appendix 1 (moxonidine)

Contra-indications history of angioedema; conduction disorders (sick sinus syndrome, sino-atrial block, second- or third-degree AV block); bradycardia; life-threatening arrhythmia; severe heart failure; severe coronary artery disease, unstable angina; severe liver disease or severe renal impairment; also on theoretical grounds: Raynaud's syndrome, intermittent claudication, epilepsy, depression, Parkinson's disease; pregnancy (Appendix 4); breast-feeding (Appendix 5)

Side-effects dry mouth; headache, fatigue, dizziness, nausea, sleep disturbance (rarely sedation), asthenia, vasodilatation; *rarely* skin reactions; *very rarely* angle-closure glaucoma

Dose

- 200 micrograms once daily in the morning, increased if necessary after 3 weeks to 400 micrograms daily in 1–2 divided doses; max. 600 micrograms daily in 2 divided doses (max. single dose 400 micrograms)

Moxonidine (Non-proprietary) PoM

Tablets, all f/c, moxonidine 200 micrograms, net price 28-tab pack = £6.71; 300 micrograms, net price 28-tab pack = £8.10; 400 micrograms, net price 28-tab pack = £8.05. Label: 3

Physiotens® (Solvay) PoM

Tablets, f/c, moxonidine 200 micrograms (pink), net price 28-tab pack = £9.72; 300 micrograms (red), 28-tab pack = £11.49; 400 micrograms (red), 28-tab pack = £13.26. Label: 3

2.5.3 Adrenergic neurone blocking drugs

Adrenergic neurone blocking drugs prevent the release of noradrenaline from postganglionic adrenergic neurones. These drugs do not control supine blood pressure and may cause postural hypotension. For this reason they have largely fallen from use, but may be necessary with other therapy in resistant hypertension.

Guanethidine, which also depletes the nerve endings of noradrenaline, is licensed for the rapid control of blood pressure.

GUANETHIDINE MONOSULPHATE

Indications hypertensive crisis (but see section 2.5)

Cautions coronary or cerebral arteriosclerosis, asthma, history of peptic ulceration; renal impairment (avoid if creatinine clearance less than 40 mL/minute; Appendix 3); pregnancy (Appendix 4); **interactions**: Appendix 1 (adrenergic neurone blockers)

Contra-indications phaeochromocytoma, heart failure

Side-effects postural hypotension, failure of ejaculation, fluid retention, nasal congestion, headache, diarrhoea, drowsiness

Dose

- By intramuscular injection, 10–20 mg, repeated after 3 hours if required

Ismelin® (Amdipharm) PoM
Injection, guanethidine monosulphate 10 mg/mL. Net price 1-mL amp = £1.56

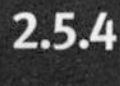

2.5.4 Alpha-adrenoceptor blocking drugs

Prazosin has post-synaptic alpha-blocking and vasodilator properties and rarely causes tachycardia. It may, however, reduce blood pressure rapidly after the first dose and should be introduced with caution. **Doxazosin**, **indoramin**, and **terazosin** have properties similar to those of prazosin.

Alpha-blockers can be used with other antihypertensive drugs in the treatment of resistant hypertension (section 2.5).

Prostatic hyperplasia Alfuzosin, doxazosin, indoramin, prazosin, tamsulosin, and terazosin are indicated for benign prostatic hyperplasia (section 7.4.1).

DOXAZOSIN

Indications hypertension (see notes above); benign prostatic hyperplasia (section 7.4.1)

Cautions care with initial dose (postural hypotension); hepatic impairment (Appendix 2); susceptibility to heart failure; pregnancy (Appendix 4); breast-feeding (Appendix 5); **interactions**: Appendix 1 (alpha-blockers)

Side-effects postural hypotension; dizziness, vertigo, headache, fatigue, asthenia, oedema, sleep disturbance, nausea, rhinitis; less frequently abdominal discomfort, diarrhoea, vomiting, agitation, tremor, rash, pruritus; rarely blurred vision, epistaxis, haematuria, thrombocytopenia, purpura, leucopenia, hepatitis, jaundice, cholestasis, and urinary incontinence; isolated cases of priapism and impotence reported

Dose

- Hypertension, 1 mg daily, increased after 1–2 weeks to 2 mg once daily, and thereafter to 4 mg once daily, if necessary; max. 16 mg daily

Doxazosin (Non-proprietary) PoM
Tablets, doxazosin (as mesilate) 1 mg, net price 28-tab pack = 46p; 2 mg, 28-tab pack = 63p; 4 mg, 28-tab pack = £1.49
Brands include *Doxadura®*

Cardura® (Pfizer) PoM
Tablets, doxazosin (as mesilate) 1 mg, net price 28-tab pack = £10.56; 2 mg, 28-tab pack = £14.08

Modified-release

Doxazosin (Non-proprietary) PoM
Tablets, m/r, doxazosin (as mesilate) 4 mg, net price 28-tab pack = £6.33. Label: 25
Dose hypertension, benign prostatic hyperplasia, 4 mg once daily, increased to 8 mg once daily after 4 weeks if necessary
Brands include *Doxadura® XL, Slocinx® XL*

Cardura® XL (Pfizer) PoM
Tablets, m/r, doxazosin (as mesilate) 4 mg, net price 28-tab pack = £6.33; 8 mg, 28-tab pack = £12.67. Label: 25
Dose hypertension, benign prostatic hyperplasia, 4 mg once daily, increased to 8 mg once daily after 4 weeks if necessary

INDORAMIN

Indications hypertension (see notes above); benign prostatic hyperplasia (section 7.4.1)

Cautions avoid alcohol (enhances rate and extent of absorption); control incipient heart failure with diuretics and digoxin, hepatic or renal impairment; elderly patients; Parkinson's disease; epilepsy (convulsions in *animal* studies); history of depression; **interactions**: Appendix 1 (alpha-blockers)
Driving Drowsiness may affect performance of skilled tasks (e.g. driving); effects of alcohol may be enhanced

Contra-indications established heart failure; patients receiving MAOIs

Side-effects sedation; also dizziness, depression, failure of ejaculation, dry mouth, nasal congestion, weight gain; rarely exacerbation of Parkinson's disease

Dose

- Hypertension, initially 25 mg twice daily, increased by 25–50 mg daily at intervals of 2 weeks; max. daily dose 200 mg in 2–3 divided doses

Baratol® (Shire) PoM
Tablets, blue, f/c, indoramin (as hydrochloride) 25 mg, net price 84-tab pack = £9.00. Label: 2

Doralese® PoM
Section 7.4.1 (prostatic hyperplasia)

PRAZOSIN

Indications hypertension (see notes above); congestive heart failure (but see section 2.5.5); Raynaud's syndrome (see also section 2.6.4); benign prostatic hyperplasia (section 7.4.1)

Cautions first dose may cause collapse due to hypotension (therefore should be taken on retiring to bed); elderly; hepatic impairment (Appendix 2); renal impairment (Appendix 3); pregnancy (Appendix 4);

breast-feeding (Appendix 5); **interactions:** Appendix 1 (alpha-blockers)

Contra-indications not recommended for congestive heart failure due to mechanical obstruction (e.g. aortic stenosis)

Side-effects gastro-intestinal disturbances; postural hypotension, oedema, palpitation; dyspnoea, nasal congestion; drowsiness, headache, depression, nervousness, vertigo; urinary frequency; weakness; blurred vision; *less commonly* tachycardia, insomnia, paraesthesia, sweating, impotence, arthralgia, eye disorders, tinnitus, epistaxis, allergic reactions including rash, pruritus, and urticaria; *rarely* pancreatitis, flushing, vasculitis, bradycardia, hallucinations, worsening of narcolepsy, gynaecomastia, priapism, urinary incontinence, and alopecia

Dose

- Hypertension (see notes above), 500 micrograms 2–3 times daily for 3–7 days, the initial dose on retiring to bed at night (to avoid collapse, see Cautions); increased to 1 mg 2–3 times daily for a further 3–7 days; further increased if necessary to max. 20 mg daily in divided doses
- Congestive heart failure (but see section 2.5.5), 500 micrograms 2–4 times daily (initial dose at bedtime, see above), increasing to 4 mg daily in divided doses; maintenance 4–20 mg daily in divided doses (but rarely used)
- Raynaud's syndrome (but efficacy not established, see section 2.6.4), initially 500 micrograms twice daily (initial dose at bedtime, see above) increased, if necessary, after 3–7 days to usual maintenance 1–2 mg twice daily

Prazosin (Non-proprietary) PoM
Tablets, prazosin (as hydrochloride) 500 micrograms, net price 56-tab pack = £2.51; 1 mg, 56-tab pack = £3.23; 2 mg, 56-tab pack = £4.39; 5 mg, 56-tab pack = £8.75. Label: 3, counselling, initial dose

Hypovase® (Pfizer) PoM
Tablets, prazosin (as hydrochloride) 500 micrograms, net price 60-tab pack = £2.69; 1 mg, scored, 60-tab pack = £3.46. Label: 3, counselling, initial dose

TERAZOSIN

Indications mild to moderate hypertension (see notes above); benign prostatic hyperplasia (section 7.4.1)

Cautions first dose may cause collapse due to hypotension (within 30–90 minutes, therefore should be taken on retiring to bed) (may also occur with rapid dose increase); pregnancy (Appendix 4); **interactions:** Appendix 1 (alpha-blockers)

Side-effects drowsiness, dizziness, lack of energy, peripheral oedema; urinary frequency and priapism reported; see also section 7.4.1

Dose

- Hypertension, 1 mg at bedtime (compliance with bedtime dose important, see Cautions); dose doubled after 7 days if necessary; usual maintenance dose 2–10 mg once daily; more than 20 mg daily rarely improves efficacy

Terazosin (Non-proprietary) PoM
Tablets, terazosin (as hydrochloride) 2 mg, net price 28-tab pack = £3.06; 5 mg, 28-tab pack = £4.51; 10 mg, 28-tab pack = £11.77. Label: 3, counselling, see dose above

Hytrin® (Amdipharm) PoM
Tablets, terazosin (as hydrochloride) 2 mg (yellow), net price 28-tab pack = £4.57; 5 mg (tan), 28-tab pack = £8.57; 10 mg (blue), 28-tab pack = £17.14; starter pack (for hypertension) of 7 × 1-mg tabs with 21 × 2-mg tabs = £13.00. Label: 3, counselling, see dose above

Phaeochromocytoma

Long-term management of phaeochromocytoma involves surgery. Alpha-blockers are used in the short-term management of hypertensive episodes in phaeochromocytoma. Once alpha blockade is established, tachycardia can be controlled by the cautious addition of a beta-blocker (section 2.4); a cardioselective beta-blocker is preferred.

Phenoxybenzamine, a powerful alpha-blocker, is effective in the management of phaeochromocytoma but it has many side-effects. **Phentolamine** is a short-acting alpha-blocker used mainly during surgery of phaeochromocytoma; its use for the diagnosis of phaeochromocytoma has been superseded by measurement of catecholamines in blood and urine.

Metirosine (available from specialist importing companies, see p. 888) inhibits the enzyme tyrosine hydroxylase, and hence the synthesis of catecholamines. It is rarely used in the pre-operative management of phaeochromocytoma, and long term in patients unsuitable for surgery; an alpha-adrenoceptor blocking drug may also be required. Metirosine should **not** be used to treat essential hypertension.

PHENOXYBENZAMINE HYDROCHLORIDE

Indications hypertensive episodes in phaeochromocytoma

Cautions elderly; congestive heart failure; severe heart disease (see also Contra-indications); cerebrovascular disease (avoid if history of cerebrovascular accident); renal impairment; carcinogenic in *animals*; avoid in porphyria (section 9.8.2); avoid infusion in hypovolaemia; avoid extravasation (irritant to tissues); pregnancy (Appendix 4); breast-feeding (Appendix 5)

Contra-indications history of cerebrovascular accident; during recovery period after myocardial infarction (usually 3–4 weeks)

Side-effects postural hypotension with dizziness and marked compensatory tachycardia, lassitude, nasal congestion, miosis, inhibition of ejaculation; rarely gastro-intestinal disturbances; decreased sweating and dry mouth after intravenous infusion; idiosyncratic profound hypotension within few minutes of starting infusion

Dose

- See under preparations

Phenoxybenzamine (Goldshield) PoM
Injection concentrate, phenoxybenzamine hydrochloride 50 mg/mL. To be diluted before use, net price 2-mL amp = £57.14 (hosp. only)

Dose by *intravenous infusion* (preferably through large vein), adjunct in severe shock (but rarely used) and phaeochromocytoma, 1 mg/kg daily over at least 2 hours; do not repeat within 24 hours (intensive care facilities needed)

Caution Owing to risk of contact sensitisation healthcare professionals should avoid contamination of hands

Dibenyline® (Goldshield) PoM

Capsules, red/white, phenoxybenzamine hydrochloride 10 mg. Net price 30-cap pack = £10.84

Dose phaeochromocytoma, 10 mg daily, increased by 10 mg daily; usual dose 1–2 mg/kg daily in 2 divided doses

PHENTOLAMINE MESILATE

Indications hypertensive episodes due to phaeochromocytoma e.g. during surgery; diagnosis of phaeochromocytoma

Cautions monitor blood pressure (avoid in hypotension), heart rate; renal impairment; gastritis, peptic ulcer; elderly; pregnancy (Appendix 4) and breast-feeding (Appendix 5); **interactions**: Appendix 1 (alpha-blockers)

Asthma Presence of sulphites in ampoules may (especially in patients with asthma) lead to hypersensitivity (with bronchospasm and shock)

Contra-indications hypotension; history of myocardial infarction; coronary insufficiency, angina, or other evidence of coronary artery disease

Side-effects postural hypotension, tachycardia, dizziness, flushing; nausea and vomiting, diarrhoea, nasal congestion; also acute or prolonged hypotension, angina, chest pain, arrhythmias

Dose

- Hypertensive episodes, by intravenous injection, 2–5 mg repeated if necessary
- Diagnosis of phaeochromocytoma, consult product literature

Rogitine® (Alliance) PoM

Injection, phentolamine mesilate 10 mg/mL. Net price 1-mL amp = £1.66

2.5.5 Drugs affecting the renin-angiotensin system

2.5.5.1 Angiotensin-converting enzyme inhibitors
2.5.5.2 Angiotensin-II receptor antagonists
2.5.5.3 Renin inhibitors

Heart failure

Drug treatment of heart failure due to left ventricular systolic dysfunction is covered below; optimal management of heart failure with preserved left ventricular function is not established.

The treatment of chronic heart failure aims to relieve symptoms, improve exercise tolerance, reduce the incidence of acute exacerbations, and reduce mortality. An **ACE inhibitor**, titrated to a 'target dose' (or the maximum tolerated dose if lower), and a beta-blocker generally achieves these aims. A diuretic is also necessary in most patients to reduce symptoms of fluid overload.

An ACE inhibitor (section 2.5.5.1) is generally advised for patients with asymptomatic left ventricular dysfunction or symptomatic heart failure. An **angiotensin-II receptor antagonist** (section 2.5.5.2) may be a useful alternative for patients who, because of side-effects such as cough, cannot tolerate ACE inhibitors; a relatively high dose of the angiotensin-II receptor antagonist may be required to produce benefit.

The **beta-blockers** bisoprolol and carvedilol (section 2.4) are of value in any grade of stable heart failure and left-ventricular systolic dysfunction; nebivolol (section 2.4) is licensed for stable mild to moderate heart failure in patients over 70 years. Beta-blocker treatment should be started by those experienced in the management of heart failure, at a very low dose and titrated very slowly over a period of weeks or months. Symptoms may deteriorate initially, calling for adjustment of concomitant therapy.

Patients with fluid overload should also receive either a loop or a thiazide diuretic (with salt or fluid restriction where appropriate). A **thiazide diuretic** (section 2.2.1) may be of benefit in patients with mild heart failure and good renal function; however, thiazide diuretics are ineffective in patients with poor renal function (estimated creatinine clearance less than 30 mL/minute, see Appendix 3) and a **loop diuretic** (section 2.2.2) is preferred. If diuresis with a single diuretic is insufficient, a combination of a loop diuretic and a thiazide diuretic may be tried; addition of metolazone (section 2.2.1) may also be considered but the resulting diuresis may be profound and care is needed to avoid potentially dangerous electrolyte disturbances.

The aldosterone antagonist **spironolactone** (section 2.2.3) may be considered for patients with moderate to severe heart failure who are already receiving an ACE inhibitor and a beta-blocker; low doses of spironolactone (usually 25 mg daily) reduce symptoms and mortality in these patients. If spironolactone cannot be used, eplerenone (section 2.2.3) may be considered for the management of heart failure after an acute myocardial infarction with evidence of left ventricular dysfunction. Close monitoring of serum creatinine and potassium is necessary with any change in treatment or in the patient's condition.

Digoxin (section 2.1.1) improves symptoms of heart failure and exercise tolerance and reduces hospitalisation due to acute exacerbations but it does not reduce mortality. Digoxin is reserved for patients with atrial fibrillation and also for selected patients in sinus rhythm who remain symptomatic despite treatment with an ACE inhibitor, a diuretic, and a beta-blocker.

Patients who cannot tolerate an ACE inhibitor or an angiotensin-II receptor antagonist, or in whom they are contra-indicated, may be given **isosorbide dinitrate** (section 2.6.1) with **hydralazine** (section 2.5.1), but this combination may be poorly tolerated. Afro-Caribbean patients respond less well to ACE inhibitors, therefore the combination of isosorbide dinitrate and hydralazine may be considered in addition to standard therapy if necessary.

2.5.5.1 Angiotensin-converting enzyme inhibitors

Angiotensin-converting enzyme inhibitors (ACE inhibitors) inhibit the conversion of angiotensin I to angiotensin II. They have many uses and are generally well tolerated. The main indications of ACE inhibitors are shown below.

Heart failure ACE inhibitors are used in all grades of heart failure, usually combined with a beta-blocker (section 2.5.5). Potassium supplements and potassium-sparing diuretics should be discontinued before introducing an ACE inhibitor because of the risk of hyperkalaemia. However, a low dose of spironolactone may be beneficial in severe heart failure (section 2.5.5) and can be used with an ACE inhibitor provided serum potassium is monitored carefully. Profound first-dose hypotension may occur when ACE inhibitors are introduced to patients with heart failure who are already taking a high dose of a loop diuretic (e.g. furosemide 80 mg daily or more). Temporary withdrawal of the loop diuretic reduces the risk, but may cause severe rebound pulmonary oedema. Therefore, for patients on high doses of loop diuretics, the ACE inhibitor may need to be initiated under specialist supervision, see below. An ACE inhibitor can be initiated in the community in patients who are receiving a low dose of a diuretic or who are not otherwise at risk of serious hypotension; nevertheless, care is required and a very low dose of the ACE inhibitor is given initially.

Hypertension An ACE inhibitor may be the most appropriate initial drug for hypertension in younger Caucasian patients; Afro-Caribbean patients, those aged over 55 years, and those with primary aldosteronism respond less well (see section 2.5). ACE inhibitors are particularly indicated for hypertension in insulin-dependent diabetics with nephropathy (see also section 6.1.5). They may reduce blood pressure very rapidly in some patients particularly in those receiving diuretic therapy (see Cautions, below); the first dose should preferably be given at bedtime.

Diabetic nephropathy For comment on the role of ACE inhibitors in the management of diabetic nephropathy, see section 6.1.5.

Prophylaxis of cardiovascular events ACE inhibitors are used in the early and long-term management of patients who have had a myocardial infarction, see section 2.10.1. ACE inhibitors may also have a role in preventing cardiovascular events.

Initiation under specialist supervision ACE inhibitors should be initiated under specialist supervision and with careful clinical monitoring in those with severe heart failure or in those:

- receiving multiple or high-dose diuretic therapy (e.g. more than 80 mg of furosemide daily or its equivalent);
- with hypovolaemia;
- with hyponatraemia (plasma-sodium concentration below 130 mmol/litre);
- with hypotension (systolic blood pressure below 90 mmHg);
- with unstable heart failure;
- receiving high-dose vasodilator therapy;
- known renovascular disease.

Renal effects Renal function and electrolytes should be checked before starting ACE inhibitors (or increasing the dose) and monitored during treatment (more frequently if features mentioned below present); hyperkalaemia and other side-effects of ACE inhibitors are more common in those with impaired renal function and the dose may need to be reduced (Appendix 3). Although ACE inhibitors now have a specialised role in some forms of renal disease, including chronic kidney disease, they also occasionally cause impairment of renal function which may progress and become severe in other circumstances (at particular risk are the elderly). A specialist should be involved if renal function is significantly reduced as a result of treatment with an ACE inhibitor.

Concomitant treatment with NSAIDs increases the risk of renal damage, and potassium-sparing diuretics (or potassium-containing salt substitutes) increase the risk of hyperkalaemia.

In patients with severe bilateral renal artery stenosis (or severe stenosis of the artery supplying a single functioning kidney), ACE inhibitors reduce or abolish glomerular filtration and are likely to cause severe and progressive renal failure. They are therefore not recommended in patients known to have these forms of critical renovascular disease.

ACE inhibitor treatment is unlikely to have an adverse effect on overall renal function in patients with severe unilateral renal artery stenosis and a normal contralateral kidney, but glomerular filtration is likely to be reduced (or even abolished) in the affected kidney and the long-term consequences are unknown.

ACE inhibitors are therefore best avoided in patients with known or suspected renovascular disease, unless the blood pressure cannot be controlled by other drugs. If ACE inhibitors are used, they should be initiated only under specialist supervision and renal function should be monitored regularly.

ACE inhibitors should also be used with particular caution in patients who may have undiagnosed and clinically silent renovascular disease. This includes patients with peripheral vascular disease or those with severe generalised atherosclerosis.

Cautions ACE inhibitors need to be initiated with care in patients receiving diuretics (**important:** see Concomitant diuretics, below); first doses may cause hypotension especially in patients taking high doses of diuretics, on a low-sodium diet, on dialysis, dehydrated or with heart failure (see above). They should also be used with caution in peripheral vascular disease or generalised atherosclerosis owing to risk of clinically silent renovascular disease; for use in known renovascular disease, see Renal Effects above. The risk of agranulocytosis is possibly increased in collagen vascular disease (blood counts recommended). ACE inhibitors should be used with care in patients with severe or symptomatic aortic stenosis (risk of hypotension) and in hypertrophic cardiomyopathy. They should also be used with care (or avoided) in those with a history of idiopathic or hereditary angioedema. ACE inhibitors should be used with caution in breast-feeding (Appendix 5). **Interactions:** Appendix 1 (ACE inhibitors).

Anaphylactoid reactions To prevent anaphylactoid reactions, ACE inhibitors should be avoided during dialysis with high-flux polyacrylonitrile membranes and during low-density lipoprotein apheresis with dextran sulphate; they should also be withheld before desensitisation with wasp or bee venom.

Concomitant diuretics ACE inhibitors can cause a very rapid fall in blood pressure in volume-depleted patients; treatment should therefore be initiated with very low doses. If the dose of diuretic is greater than 80 mg furosemide or equivalent, the ACE inhibitor should be initiated under close supervision and in some patients the diuretic dose may need to be reduced or the diuretic discontinued at least 24 hours beforehand (may not be possible in heart failure—risk of pulmonary oedema). If high-dose diuretic therapy cannot be stopped, close observation is recommended after administration of the first dose of ACE inhibitor, for at least 2 hours or until the blood pressure has stabilised.

Contra-indications ACE inhibitors are contra-indicated in patients with hypersensitivity to ACE inhibitors (including angioedema). ACE inhibitors should not be used in pregnancy (Appendix 4).

Side-effects ACE inhibitors can cause profound hypotension (see Cautions) and renal impairment (see Renal effects above), and a persistent dry cough. They can also cause angioedema (onset may be delayed; higher incidence reported in Afro-Caribbean patients), rash (which may be associated with pruritus and urticaria), pancreatitis, and upper respiratory-tract symptoms such as sinusitis, rhinitis, and sore throat. Gastro-intestinal effects reported with ACE inhibitors include nausea, vomiting, dyspepsia, diarrhoea, constipation, and abdominal pain. Altered liver function tests, cholestatic jaundice, and hepatitis have been reported. Hyperkalaemia, hypoglycaemia, and blood disorders including thrombocytopenia, leucopenia, neutropenia, and haemolytic anaemia have also been reported. Other reported side-effects include headache, dizziness, fatigue, malaise, taste disturbance, paraesthesia, bronchospasm, fever, serositis, vasculitis, myalgia, arthralgia, positive antinuclear antibody, raised erythrocyte sedimentation rate, eosinophilia, leucocytosis, and photosensitivity.

Combination products Products incorporating an ACE inhibitor with a thiazide diuretic or a calcium-channel blocker are available for the management of hypertension. Use of these combination products should be reserved for patients whose blood pressure has not responded adequately to a single antihypertensive drug and who have been stabilised on the individual components of the combination in the same proportions.

CAPTOPRIL

Indications mild to moderate essential hypertension alone or with thiazide therapy and severe hypertension resistant to other treatment; congestive heart failure with left ventricular dysfunction (adjunct—see section 2.5.5); following myocardial infarction, see dose; diabetic nephropathy (microalbuminuria greater than 30 mg/day) in insulin-dependent diabetes

Cautions see notes above

Contra-indications see notes above

Side-effects see notes above; tachycardia, serum sickness, weight loss, stomatitis, maculopapular rash, photosensitivity, flushing and acidosis

Dose

- Hypertension, used alone, initially 12.5 mg twice daily; if used in addition to diuretic (see notes above), or in elderly, initially 6.25 mg twice daily (first dose at bedtime); usual maintenance dose 25 mg twice daily; max. 50 mg twice daily (rarely 3 times daily in severe hypertension)
- Heart failure (adjunct), initially 6.25–12.5 mg under close medical supervision (see notes above), increased gradually at intervals of at least 2 weeks up to max. 150 mg daily in divided doses if tolerated
- Prophylaxis after infarction in clinically stable patients with asymptomatic or symptomatic left ventricular dysfunction (radionuclide ventriculography or echocardiography undertaken before initiation), initially 6.25 mg, starting as early as 3 days after infarction, then increased over several weeks to 150 mg daily (if tolerated) in divided doses
- Diabetic nephropathy, 75–100 mg daily in divided doses; if further blood pressure reduction required, other antihypertensives may be used in conjunction with captopril; in severe renal impairment, initially 12.5 mg twice daily (if concomitant diuretic therapy required, loop diuretic rather than thiazide should be chosen)

Captopril (Non-proprietary) PoM

Tablets, captopril 12.5 mg, net price 56-tab pack = 71p; 25 mg, 56-tab pack = 94p; 50 mg, 56-tab pack = £1.37

Brands include *Ecopace®*, *Kaplon®*, *Tensopril®*

Capoten® (Squibb) PoM

Tablets, captopril 12.5 mg (scored), net price 56-tab pack = £9.82; 25 mg, 56-tab pack = £11.19; 50 mg (scored), 56-tab pack = £19.07 (also available as *Acepril®*)

With diuretic

Note For mild to moderate hypertension in patients stabilised on the individual components in the same proportions

Co-zidocapt (Non-proprietary) PoM

Tablets, co-zidocapt 12.5/25 (hydrochlorothiazide 12.5 mg, captopril 25 mg), net price 28-tab pack = £11.00

Brands include *Capto-co®*

Tablets, co-zidocapt 25/50 (hydrochlorothiazide 25 mg, captopril 50 mg), net price 28-tab pack = £14.00

Brands include *Capto-co®*

Capozide® (Squibb) PoM

LS tablets, scored, co-zidocapt 12.5/25 (hydrochlorothiazide 12.5 mg, captopril 25 mg). Net price 28-tab pack = £10.46

Tablets, scored, co-zidocapt 25/50 (hydrochlorothiazide 25 mg, captopril 50 mg). Net price 28-tab pack = £7.45 (also available as *Acezide®*)

CILAZAPRIL

Indications essential hypertension; congestive heart failure (adjunct—see section 2.5.5)

Cautions see notes above; severe hepatic impairment (Appendix 2)

Contra-indications see notes above; ascites

Side-effects see notes above, dyspnoea and bronchitis

Dose

- Hypertension, initially 1 mg once daily (reduced to 500 micrograms daily if used in addition to diuretic (see notes above), in the elderly, and in renal impairment), then adjusted according to response; usual maintenance dose 2.5–5 mg once daily; max. 5 mg daily
- Heart failure (adjunct), initially 500 micrograms once daily under close medical supervision (see notes above), increased gradually to 1–2.5 mg once daily if tolerated; max. 5 mg once daily

Vascace® (Roche) PoM

Tablets, f/c, cilazapril 500 micrograms (white), net price 28-tab pack = £3.65; 1 mg (yellow), 28-tab pack = £6.01; 2.5 mg (pink), 28-tab pack = £7.64; 5 mg (brown), 28-tab pack = £13.28

ENALAPRIL MALEATE

Indications hypertension; symptomatic heart failure (adjunct—see section 2.5.5); prevention of symptomatic heart failure in patients with asymptomatic left ventricular dysfunction

Cautions see notes above; hepatic impairment (Appendix 2)

Contra-indications see notes above

Side-effects see notes above; also dyspnoea; depression, asthenia; blurred vision; *less commonly* dry mouth, peptic ulcer, anorexia, ileus; arrhythmias, palpitation, flushing; confusion, nervousness, drowsiness, insomnia, vertigo; impotence; muscle cramps; tinnitus; alopecia, sweating; hyponatraemia; *rarely* stomatitis, glossitis, hepatic failure, Raynaud's syndrome, pulmonary infiltrates, allergic alveolitis, dream abnormalities, gynaecomastia, Stevens-Johnson syndrome, toxic epidermal necrolysis, exfoliative dermatitis, pemphigus; *very rarely* gastro-intestinal angioedema

Dose

- Hypertension, used alone, initially 5 mg once daily; if used in addition to diuretic (see notes above), or in renal impairment, lower initial doses may be required; usual maintenance dose 20 mg once daily; max. 40 mg once daily
- Heart failure (adjunct), asymptomatic left ventricular dysfunction, initially 2.5 mg daily under close medical supervision (see notes above), increased gradually over 2–4 weeks to 10–20 mg twice daily if tolerated

Enalapril Maleate (Non-proprietary) PoM

Tablets, enalapril maleate 2.5 mg, net price 28-tab pack = 37p; 5 mg, 28-tab pack = 46p; 10 mg, 28-tab pack = 54p; 20 mg, 28-tab pack = 66p
Brands include *Ednyt®*

Innovace® (MSD) PoM

Tablets, enalapril maleate 2.5 mg, net price 28-tab pack = £5.35; 5 mg (scored), 28-tab pack = £7.51; 10 mg (red), 28-tab pack = £10.53; 20 mg (peach), 28-tab pack = £12.51

With diuretic

Note For mild to moderate hypertension in patients stabilised on the individual components in the same proportions

Innozide® (MSD) PoM

Tablets, yellow, scored, enalapril maleate 20 mg, hydrochlorothiazide 12.5 mg. Net price 28-tab pack = £12.82

Note Non-proprietary tablets containing enalapril maleate (20 mg) and hydrochlorothiazide (12.5 mg) are available

FOSINOPRIL SODIUM

Indications hypertension; congestive heart failure (adjunct—see section 2.5.5)

Cautions see notes above; hepatic impairment (Appendix 2)

Contra-indications see notes above

Side-effects see notes above; chest pain; musculoskeletal pain

Dose

- Hypertension, initially 10 mg daily, increased if necessary after 4 weeks; usual dose range 10–40 mg (doses over 40 mg not shown to increase efficacy); if used in addition to diuretic see notes above
- Heart failure (adjunct), initially 10 mg once daily under close medical supervision (see notes above), increased gradually to 40 mg once daily if tolerated

Fosinopril sodium (Non-proprietary) PoM

Tablets, fosinopril sodium 10 mg, net price 28-tab pack = £3.00; 20 mg, 28-tab pack = £3.97

Staril® (Squibb) PoM

Tablets, fosinopril sodium 10 mg, net price 28-tab pack = £11.20; 20 mg, 28-tab pack = £12.09

IMIDAPRIL HYDROCHLORIDE

Indications essential hypertension

Cautions see notes above; hepatic impairment (Appendix 2)

Contra-indications see notes above

Side-effects see notes above; dry mouth, glossitis, ileus; bronchitis, dyspnoea; sleep disturbances, depression, confusion, blurred vision, tinnitus, impotence

Dose

- Initially 5 mg daily before food; if used in addition to diuretic (see notes above), in elderly, in patients with heart failure, angina or cerebrovascular disease, or in renal or hepatic impairment, initially 2.5 mg daily; if necessary increase dose at intervals of at least 3 weeks; usual maintenance dose 10 mg once daily; max. 20 mg daily (elderly, 10 mg daily)

Tanatril® (Trinity) PoM

Tablets, scored, imidapril hydrochloride 5 mg, net price 28-tab pack = £6.78; 10 mg, 28-tab pack = £7.66; 20 mg, 28-tab pack = £9.20

LISINOPRIL

Indications hypertension (but see notes above); symptomatic heart failure (adjunct—see section 2.5.5); short-term treatment following myocardial infarction in haemodynamically stable patients; diabetic nephropathy in normotensive insulin-dependent and hypertensive non-insulin-dependent diabetes mellitus

Cautions see notes above

Contra-indications see notes above

Side-effects see notes above; also *less commonly* tachycardia, palpitation, cerebrovascular accident, myocardial infarction, Raynaud's syndrome, confusion, mood changes, vertigo, sleep disturbances, asthenia, impotence; *rarely* dry mouth, gynaecomastia, alopecia, psoriasis; *very rarely* allergic alveolitis, pulmonary infiltrates, profuse sweating, pemphigus, Stevens-Johnson syndrome, and toxic epidermal necrolysis

Dose

- Hypertension, initially 10 mg once daily; if used in addition to diuretic (see notes above) or in cardiac decompensation or in volume depletion, initially 2.5–5 mg once daily; usual maintenance dose 20 mg once daily; max. 40 mg once daily
- Heart failure (adjunct), initially 2.5 mg once daily under close medical supervision (see notes above); increased in steps no greater than 10 mg at intervals of at least 2 weeks up to max. 35 mg once daily if tolerated
- Prophylaxis after myocardial infarction, systolic blood pressure over 120 mmHg, 5 mg within 24 hours, fol-

lowed by further 5 mg 24 hours later, then 10 mg after a further 24 hours, and continuing with 10 mg once daily for 6 weeks (or continued if heart failure); systolic blood pressure 100–120 mmHg, initially 2.5 mg once daily, increased to maintenance dose of 5 mg once daily

Note Should not be started after myocardial infarction if systolic blood pressure less than 100 mmHg; temporarily reduce maintenance dose to 5 mg and if necessary 2.5 mg daily if systolic blood pressure 100 mmHg or less during treatment; withdraw if prolonged hypotension occurs (systolic blood pressure less than 90 mmHg for more than 1 hour)

- Diabetic nephropathy, initially 2.5 mg once daily adjusted according to response; usual dose range 10–20 mg once daily

Lisinopril (Non-proprietary) PoM
Tablets, lisinopril (as dihydrate) 2.5 mg, net price 28-tab pack = 43p; 5 mg, 28-tab pack = 57p; 10 mg, 28-tab pack = 74p; 20 mg, 28-tab pack = £1.34

Carace® (Bristol-Myers Squibb) PoM
Tablets, lisinopril 5 mg (scored), net price 28-tab pack = £8.51; 10 mg (yellow, scored), 28-tab pack = £10.51; 20 mg (orange, scored), 28-tab pack = £11.89

Zestril® (AstraZeneca) PoM
Tablets, lisinopril (as dihydrate) 2.5 mg, net price 28-tab pack = £6.26; 5 mg (pink, scored), 28-tab pack = £7.86; 10 mg (pink), 28-tab pack = £9.70; 20 mg (pink), 28-tab pack = £10.97

With diuretic

Note For mild to moderate hypertension in patients stabilised on the individual components in the same proportions

Carace Plus® (Bristol-Myers Squibb) PoM
Carace 10 Plus tablets, blue, lisinopril 10 mg, hydrochlorothiazide 12.5 mg. Net price 28-tab pack = £11.88
Carace 20 Plus tablets, yellow, scored, lisinopril 20 mg, hydrochlorothiazide 12.5 mg. Net price 28-tab pack = £13.44

Lisicostad® (Genus) PoM
Lisicostad 10/12.5 mg tablets, scored, lisinopril (as dihydrate) 10 mg, hydrochlorothiazide 12.5 mg, net price 28-tab pack = £10.99
Lisicostad 20/12.5 mg tablets, scored, lisinopril (as dihydrate) 20 mg, hydrochlorothiazide 12.5 mg, net price 28-tab pack = £11.99

Zestoretic® (AstraZeneca) PoM
Zestoretic 10 tablets, peach, lisinopril (as dihydrate) 10 mg, hydrochlorothiazide 12.5 mg. Net price 28-tab pack = £13.01
Zestoretic 20 tablets, lisinopril (as dihydrate) 20 mg, hydrochlorothiazide 12.5 mg. Net price 28-tab pack = £14.72

MOEXIPRIL HYDROCHLORIDE

Indications essential hypertension
Cautions see notes above; hepatic impairment (Appendix 2)
Contra-indications see notes above
Side-effects see notes above; arrhythmias, angina, chest pain, syncope, cerebrovascular accident, myocardial infarction; appetite and weight changes; dry mouth, photosensitivity, flushing, nervousness, mood changes, anxiety, drowsiness, sleep disturbance, tinnitus, influenza-like syndrome, sweating and dyspnoea
Dose
- Used alone, initially 7.5 mg once daily; if used in addition to diuretic (see notes above), with nifedipine, in elderly, in renal or hepatic impairment, initially 3.75 mg once daily; usual range 15–30 mg once daily; doses above 30 mg daily not shown to increase efficacy

Perdix® (UCB Pharma) PoM
Tablets, f/c, both pink, scored, moexipril hydrochloride 7.5 mg, net price 28-tab pack = £7.55; 15 mg, 28-tab pack = £8.70

PERINDOPRIL ERBUMINE

Indications hypertension (but see notes above); symptomatic heart failure (adjunct—see section 2.5.5); prophylaxis of cardiac events following myocardial infarction or revascularisation in stable coronary artery disease
Cautions see notes above; hepatic impairment (Appendix 2)
Contra-indications see notes above
Side-effects see notes above; asthenia, mood and sleep disturbances
Dose
- Hypertension, initially 4 mg once daily in the morning; if used in addition to diuretic (see notes above), in elderly or in renal impairment, initially 2 mg once daily; usual maintenance dose 4 mg once daily; max. 8 mg daily
- Heart failure (adjunct), initially 2 mg once daily in the morning under close medical supervision (see notes above), increased after at least 2 weeks to max. 4 mg once daily if tolerated
- Following myocardial infarction or revascularisation, initially 4 mg once daily in the morning increased after 2 weeks to 8 mg once daily if tolerated; ELDERLY 2 mg once daily for 1 week, then 4 mg once daily for 1 week, thereafter increased to 8 mg once daily if tolerated

Perindopril (Non-proprietary) PoM
Tablets, perindopril erbumine (= *tert*-butylamine) 2 mg, net price 30-tab pack = £11.02; 4 mg, 30-tab pack = £11.02; 8 mg, 30-tab pack = £11.02. Label: 22

Coversyl® (Servier) PoM
Tablets, perindopril erbumine (= *tert*-butylamine) 2 mg (white), net price 30-tab pack = £11.36; 4 mg (light green, scored), 30-tab pack = £11.36; 8 mg (green), 30-tab pack = £11.36. Label: 22

With diuretic

Note For hypertension not adequately controlled by perindopril alone

Coversyl® Plus (Servier) PoM
Tablets, perindopril erbumine (= *tert*-butylamine) 4 mg, indapamide 1.25 mg, net price 30-tab pack = £14.49. Label: 22

QUINAPRIL

Indications essential hypertension; congestive heart failure (adjunct—see section 2.5.5)
Cautions see notes above; hepatic impairment (Appendix 2)
Contra-indications see notes above

Side-effects see notes above; asthenia, chest pain, oedema, flatulence, nervousness, depression, insomnia, blurred vision, impotence, and back pain

Dose

- Hypertension, initially 10 mg once daily; with a diuretic (see notes above), in elderly, or in renal impairment initially 2.5 mg daily; usual maintenance dose 20–40 mg daily in single or 2 divided doses; up to 80 mg daily has been given
- Heart failure (adjunct), initial dose 2.5 mg daily under close medical supervision (see notes above), increased gradually to 10–20 mg daily in 1–2 divided doses if tolerated; max. 40 mg daily

Quinapril (Non-proprietary) PoM

Tablets, quinapril (as hydrochloride) 5 mg, net price 28-tab pack = £1.29; 10 mg, 28-tab pack = £1.71; 20 mg, 28-tab pack = £2.37; 40 mg, 28-tab pack = £3.08

Brands include *Quinil®*

Accupro® (Pfizer) PoM

Tablets, f/c, quinapril (as hydrochloride) 5 mg (brown), net price 28-tab pack = £8.60; 10 mg (brown), 28-tab pack = £8.60; 20 mg (brown), 28-tab pack = £10.79; 40 mg (red-brown), 28-tab pack = £9.75

With diuretic

Note For hypertension in patients stabilised on the individual components in the same proportions

Accuretic® (Pfizer) PoM

Tablets, pink, f/c, scored, quinapril (as hydrochloride) 10 mg, hydrochlorothiazide 12.5 mg. Net price 28-tab pack = £11.75

RAMIPRIL

Indications mild to moderate hypertension; congestive heart failure (adjunct—see section 2.5.5); following myocardial infarction in patients with clinical evidence of heart failure; susceptible patients over 55 years, prevention of myocardial infarction, stroke, cardiovascular death or need of revascularisation procedures (consult product literature)

Cautions see notes above; hepatic impairment (Appendix 2)

Contra-indications see notes above

Side-effects see notes above; arrhythmias, angina, chest pain, syncope, cerebrovascular accident, myocardial infarction, loss of appetite, stomatitis, dry mouth, skin reactions including erythema multiforme and pemphigoid exanthema; precipitation or exacerbation of Raynaud's syndrome; conjunctivitis, onycholysis, confusion, nervousness, depression, anxiety, impotence, decreased libido, alopecia, bronchitis and muscle cramps

Dose

- Hypertension, initially 1.25 mg once daily, increased at intervals of 1–2 weeks; usual range 2.5–5 mg once daily; max. 10 mg once daily; if used in addition to diuretic see notes above
- Heart failure (adjunct), initially 1.25 mg once daily under close medical supervision (see notes above), increased gradually at intervals of 1–2 weeks to max. 10 mg daily if tolerated (daily doses of 2.5 mg or more may be taken in 1–2 divided doses)
- Prophylaxis after myocardial infarction (started in hospital 3 to 10 days after infarction), initially 2.5 mg twice daily, increased after 2 days to 5 mg twice daily; maintenance 2.5–5 mg twice daily

  Note If initial 2.5-mg dose not tolerated, give 1.25 mg twice daily for 2 days before increasing to 2.5 mg twice daily, then 5 mg twice daily
- Prophylaxis of cardiovascular events or stroke, initially 2.5 mg once daily, increased after 1 week to 5 mg once daily, then increased after a further 3 weeks to 10 mg once daily

Ramipril (Non-proprietary) PoM

Capsules, ramipril 1.25 mg, net price 28-cap pack = 60p; 2.5 mg, 28-cap pack = 80p; 5 mg, 28-cap pack = £1.03; 10 mg, 28-cap pack = £1.37

Brands include *Lopace®*

Tablets, ramipril 1.25 mg, net price 28-tab pack = £1.91; 2.5 mg, 28-tab pack = £2.00; 5 mg, 28-tab pack = £2.88; 10 mg, 28-tab pack = £3.46

Tritace® (Aventis Pharma) PoM

Tablets, all scored, ramipril 1.25 mg (white), net price 28-tab pack = £5.30; 2.5 mg (yellow), 28-tab pack = £7.51; 5 mg (red), 28-tab pack = £10.46; 10 mg (white), 28-tab pack = £14.24

Titration pack, capsules, 35-day starter pack of ramipril 7 × 2.5 mg with 21 × 5 mg and 7 × 10 mg, net price = £13.00

With calcium-channel blocker

Note For hypertension in patients stabilised on the individual components in the same proportions. For cautions, contra-indications and side-effects of felodipine, see section 2.6.2

Triapin® (Aventis Pharma) ▼ PoM

Triapin® tablets, f/c, brown, ramipril 5 mg, felodipine 5 mg (m/r), net price 28-tab pack = £32.26. Label: 25

Triapin mite® tablets, f/c, orange, ramipril 2.5 mg, felodipine 2.5 mg (m/r), net price 28-tab pack = £25.55. Label: 25

TRANDOLAPRIL

Indications mild to moderate hypertension; following myocardial infarction in patients with left ventricular dysfunction

Cautions see notes above; hepatic impairment (Appendix 2)

Contra-indications see notes above

Side-effects see notes above; also ileus, dry mouth; tachycardia, palpitation, arrhythmias, angina, transient ischaemic attacks, cerebral haemorrhage, myocardial infarction; dyspnoea, bronchitis; asthenia; alopecia, skin reactions including Stevens-Johnson syndrome, toxic epidermal necrolysis, and psoriasis-like efflorescence

Dose

- Hypertension, initially 500 micrograms once daily, increased at intervals of 2–4 weeks; usual range 1–2 mg once daily; max. 4 mg daily; if used in addition to diuretic see notes above
- Prophylaxis after myocardial infarction (starting as early as 3 days after infarction), initially 500 micrograms once daily, gradually increased to max. 4 mg once daily

  Note If symptomatic hypotension develops during titration, do not increase dose further; if possible, reduce dose of any adjunctive treatment and if this is not effective or feasible, reduce dose of trandolapril

Gopten® (Abbott) PoM
Capsules, trandolapril 500 micrograms (red/yellow), net price 14-cap pack = £1.40; 1 mg (red/orange) 28-cap pack = £12.28; 2 mg (red/red), 28-cap pack = £6.86; 4 mg (red/maroon), 28-cap pack = £11.64

With calcium-channel blocker

Note For hypertension in patients stabilised on the individual components in the same proportions. For cautions, contra-indications and side-effects of verapamil, see section 2.6.2

Tarka® (Abbott) ▼ PoM
Capsules, pink, trandolapril 2 mg, verapamil hydrochloride 180 mg (m/r). Net price 28 cap-pack = £17.85. Label: 25

2.5.5.2 Angiotensin-II receptor antagonists

Candesartan, eprosartan, irbesartan, losartan, olmesartan, telmisartan, and **valsartan** are angiotensin-II receptor antagonists with many properties similar to those of the ACE inhibitors. However, unlike ACE inhibitors, they do not inhibit the breakdown of bradykinin and other kinins, and thus are unlikely to cause the persistent dry cough which commonly complicates ACE inhibitor therapy. They are therefore a useful alternative for patients who have to discontinue an ACE inhibitor because of persistent cough.

An angiotensin-II receptor antagonist may be used as an alternative to an ACE inhibitor in the management of heart failure (section 2.5.5) or diabetic nephropathy (section 6.1.5).

Cautions Angiotensin-II receptor antagonists should be used with caution in renal artery stenosis (see also Renal Effects under ACE Inhibitors, section 2.5.5.1). Monitoring of plasma-potassium concentration is advised, particularly in the elderly and in patients with renal impairment; lower initial doses may be appropriate in these patients. Angiotensin-II receptor antagonists should be used with caution in aortic or mitral valve stenosis and in hypertrophic cardiomyopathy. Those with primary aldosteronism, and Afro-Caribbean patients (particularly those with left ventricular hypertrophy), may not benefit from an angiotensin-II receptor antagonist. **Interactions:** Appendix 1 (angiotensin-II receptor antagonists).

Contra-indications Angiotensin-II receptor antagonists, like the ACE inhibitors, should also be avoided in pregnancy (Appendix 4) and breast-feeding (Appendix 5).

Side-effects Side-effects are usually mild. Symptomatic hypotension including dizziness may occur, particularly in patients with intravascular volume depletion (e.g. those taking high-dose diuretics). Hyperkalaemia occurs occasionally; angioedema has also been reported with some angiotensin-II receptor antagonists.

CANDESARTAN CILEXETIL

Indications hypertension; heart failure with impaired left ventricular systolic function in conjunction with an ACE inhibitor, or when ACE inhibitors are not tolerated (see also section 2.5.5)

Cautions see notes above; hepatic impairment (Appendix 2); renal impairment (Appendix 3)

Contra-indications see notes above; also cholestasis

Side-effects see notes above; also vertigo, headache; *very rarely* nausea, hepatitis, blood disorders, hyponatraemia, back pain, arthralgia, myalgia, rash, urticaria, pruritus

Dose

- Hypertension, initially 8 mg (hepatic impairment 2 mg, renal impairment or intravascular volume depletion 4 mg) once daily, increased if necessary at intervals of 4 weeks to max. 32 mg once daily; usual maintenance dose 8 mg once daily
- Heart failure, initially 4 mg once daily, increased at intervals of at least 2 weeks to 'target' dose of 32 mg once daily or to max. tolerated dose

Amias® (Takeda) PoM
Tablets, candesartan cilexetil 2 mg (white), net price 7-tab pack = £2.99; 4 mg (white, scored), 7-tab pack = £3.24, 28-tab pack = £8.15; 8 mg (pink, scored), 28-tab pack = £9.89; 16 mg (pink, scored), 28-tab pack = £12.72; 32 mg (pink, scored), 28-tab pack = £16.13

EPROSARTAN

Indications hypertension (see also notes above)

Cautions see notes above; also hepatic impairment (Appendix 2); renal impairment (Appendix 3)

Contra-indications see notes above

Side-effects see notes above; also flatulence, hypertriglyceridaemia, arthralgia, rhinitis; *rarely* headache, asthenia, anaemia, hypersensitivity reactions (including rash, pruritus, urticaria); *very rarely* nausea

Dose

- 600 mg once daily (elderly over 75 years, mild to moderate hepatic impairment, renal impairment, initially 300 mg once daily); if necessary increased after 2–3 weeks to 800 mg once daily

Teveten® (Solvay) PoM
Tablets, f/c, eprosartan (as mesilate) 300 mg (white), net price 28-tab pack = £11.63; 400 mg (pink), 56-tab pack = £15.77; 600 mg (white), 28-tab pack = £14.31. Label: 21

IRBESARTAN

Indications hypertension; renal disease in hypertensive type 2 diabetes mellitus (see also notes above)

Cautions see notes above

Contra-indications see notes above

Side-effects see notes above; also nausea, vomiting; fatigue; musculoskeletal pain; *less commonly* diarrhoea, dyspepsia, flushing, tachycardia, chest pain, cough, and sexual dysfunction; *rarely* rash, urticaria; *very rarely* headache, myalgia, arthralgia, tinnitus, taste disturbance, hepatitis, renal dysfunction, and vasculitis

Dose

- Hypertension, initially 150 mg once daily, increased if necessary to 300 mg once daily (in haemodialysis or in ELDERLY over 75 years, initial dose of 75 mg once daily may be used); CHILD not recommended
- Renal disease in hypertensive type 2 diabetes mellitus, initially 150 mg once daily, increased to 300 mg once daily if tolerated (in haemodialysis or in ELDERLY over

2 Cardiovascular system

75 years, consider initial dose of 75 mg once daily); CHILD not recommended

Aprovel® (Bristol-Myers Squibb, Sanofi-Synthelabo) PoM
Tablets, f/c, irbesartan 75 mg, net price 28-tab pack = £10.29; 150 mg, 28-tab pack = £12.57; 300 mg, 28-tab pack = £16.91

With diuretic

Note For hypertension not adequately controlled with irbesartan alone

CoAprovel® (Bristol-Myers Squibb, Sanofi-Synthelabo) PoM
Tablets, f/c, irbesartan 150 mg, hydrochlorothiazide 12.5 mg (peach), net price 28-tab pack = £12.57; irbesartan 300 mg, hydrochlorothiazide 12.5 mg (peach), 28-tab pack = £16.91; irbesartan 300 mg, hydrochlorothiazide 25 mg (pink), 28-tab pack = £16.91

LOSARTAN POTASSIUM

Indications hypertension (including reduction of stroke risk in hypertension with left ventricular hypertrophy); diabetic nephropathy in type 2 diabetes mellitus (see also notes above)

Cautions see notes above; hepatic impairment (Appendix 2); renal impairment (Appendix 3)

Contra-indications see notes above

Side-effects see notes above; diarrhoea, cough, arthralgia, myalgia, asthenia, fatigue, migraine, vertigo, urticaria, pruritus, rash; *rarely* hepatitis, anaemia (in severe renal disease or following renal transplantation), thrombocytopenia, vasculitis (including Henoch-Schönlein purpura), and anaphylaxis

Dose

- Usually 50 mg once daily (intravascular volume depletion, initially 25 mg once daily); if necessary increased after several weeks to 100 mg once daily; ELDERLY over 75 years initially 25 mg daily

Cozaar® (MSD) PoM
Tablets, f/c, losartan potassium 25 mg, net price 28-tab pack = £16.18; 50 mg (scored), 28-tab pack = £12.80; 100 mg, 28-tab pack = £16.18

With diuretic

Note For hypertension not adequately controlled with losartan alone

Cozaar-Comp® (MSD) PoM
Tablets 50/12.5, yellow, f/c, losartan potassium 50 mg, hydrochlorothiazide 12.5 mg, net price 28-tab pack = £12.80

Tablets 100/12.5, white, f/c, losartan potassium 100 mg, hydrochlorothiazide 12.5 mg, net price 28-tab pack = £16.18

Tablets 100/25, yellow, f/c, losartan potassium 100 mg, hydrochlorothiazide 25 mg, net price 28-tab pack = £16.18

OLMESARTAN MEDOXOMIL

Indications hypertension (see also notes above)

Cautions see notes above; hepatic impairment (avoid in severe impairment; Appendix 2); renal impairment (avoid if creatinine clearance less than 20 mL/minute; Appendix 3)

Contra-indications see notes above; biliary obstruction

Side-effects see notes above; also gastro-intestinal disturbances; chest pain, peripheral oedema, hypertriglyceridaemia; fatigue; influenza-like symptoms, cough, pharyngitis, rhinitis; urinary-tract infection; haematuria, hyperuricaemia; arthritis, musculoskeletal pain; *less commonly* angina, vertigo, rash; *very rarely* headache, thrombocytopenia, myalgia, pruritus, urticaria

Dose

- Initially 10 mg once daily; if necessary increased to 20 mg once daily; max. 40 mg daily

Olmetec® (Sankyo) PoM
Tablets, f/c, olmesartan medoxomil 10 mg, net price 28-tab pack = £10.95; 20 mg, 28-tab pack = £12.95; 40 mg, 28-tab pack = £17.50

With diuretic

Note For hypertension not adequately controlled with olmesartan alone

Olmetec Plus® (Sankyo) ▼ PoM
Tablets, f/c, olmesartan medoxomil 20 mg, hydrochlorothiazide 12.5 mg (red-yellow), net price 28-tab pack = £12.95; olmesartan medoxomil 20 mg, hydrochlorothiazide 25 mg (pink), 28-tab pack = £12.95

TELMISARTAN

Indications hypertension (see also notes above)

Cautions see notes above; hepatic impairment (Appendix 2; avoid in severe impairment); renal impairment (Appendix 3)

Contra-indications see notes above; biliary obstruction

Side-effects see notes above; also gastro-intestinal disturbances; chest pain; influenza-like symptoms including pharyngitis and sinusitis, urinary-tract infection; arthralgia, myalgia, back pain, leg cramps; eczema; *less commonly* dry mouth, flatulence, anxiety, vertigo, tendinitis-like symptoms, abnormal vision, increased sweating; *rarely* bradycardia, tachycardia, dyspnoea, insomnia, depression, blood disorders, increase in uric acid, eosinophilia, rash, and pruritus; syncope and asthenia also reported

Dose

- Usually 40 mg once daily (but 20 mg may be sufficient), increased if necessary after at least 4 weeks, to max. 80 mg once daily

Micardis® (Boehringer Ingelheim) PoM
Tablets, telmisartan 20 mg, net price 28-tab pack = £9.25; 40 mg, 28-tab pack = £11.34; 80 mg, 28-tab pack = £14.18

With diuretic

Note For patients with hypertension not adequately controlled by telmisartan alone

Micardis Plus® (Boehringer Ingelheim) PoM
Tablets 40/12.5, red/white, telmisartan 40 mg, hydrochlorothiazide 12.5 mg, net price 28-tab pack = £11.34

Tablets 80/12.5, red/white, telmisartan 80 mg, hydrochlorothiazide 12.5 mg, net price 28-tab pack = £14.18

VALSARTAN

Indications hypertension; myocardial infarction with left ventricular failure or left ventricular systolic dysfunction (adjunct—see section 2.5.5 and section 2.10.1)

Cautions see notes above; hepatic impairment (Appendix 2); renal impairment (Appendix 3)

Contra-indications see notes above, cirrhosis, biliary obstruction

Side-effects see notes above; *rarely* anaemia, neutropenia; *very rarely* diarrhoea, taste disturbance, syncope, fatigue, cough, headache, thrombocytopenia, epistaxis, arthralgia, myalgia, and hypersensitivity reactions (including rash, pruritus, vasculitis, and serum sickness)

Dose

- Hypertension, usually 80 mg once daily (initially 40 mg once daily in intravascular volume depletion); if necessary increased at intervals of 4 weeks up to max. 320 mg daily; ELDERLY over 75 years, initially 40 mg once daily
- Myocardial infarction, initially 20 mg twice daily increased over several weeks to 160 mg twice daily if tolerated

Diovan® (Novartis) PoM

Capsules, valsartan 40 mg (grey), net price 28-cap pack = £16.44; 80 mg (grey/pink), 28-cap pack = £16.44, 98-cap pack = £57.54; 160 mg (dark grey/pink), 28-cap pack = £21.66, 98-cap pack = £75.81

Tablets, f/c, valsartan 40 mg (yellow), scored, net price 7-tab pack = £4.11; 320 mg (dark grey-violet), 28-tab pack = £23.80, 98-tab pack = £83.30

With diuretic

Note For hypertension not adequately controlled by valsartan alone

Co-Diovan® (Novartis) ▼ PoM

Tablets 80/12.5, orange, f/c, valsartan 80 mg, hydrochlorothiazide 12.5 mg, net price 28-tab pack = £16.44

Tablets 160/12.5, red, f/c, valsartan 160 mg, hydrochlorothiazide 12.5 mg, net price 28-tab pack = £21.66

Tablets 160/25, brown-orange, f/c, valsartan 160 mg, hydrochlorothiazide 25 mg, net price 28-tab pack = £21.66

2.5.5.3 Renin inhibitors

Renin inhibitors inhibit renin directly; renin converts angiotensinogen to angiotensin I. **Aliskiren** is licensed for the treatment of hypertension, either alone or in combination with other antihypertensives.

ALISKIREN

Indications essential hypertension

Cautions patients taking concomitant diuretics, on a low-sodium diet, or who are dehydrated (first doses may cause hypotension—initiate with care); renal artery stenosis; renal impairment (Appendix 3); monitor plasma-potassium concentration and renal function in renal impairment, diabetes mellitus, and heart failure; **interactions**: Appendix 1 (aliskiren)

Contra-indications pregnancy (Appendix 4); breast-feeding (Appendix 5)

Side-effects diarrhoea; *less commonly* rash; *rarely* angioedema; anaemia and hyperkalaemia also reported

Dose

- ADULT over 18 years 150 mg once daily, increased if necessary to 300 mg once daily

Rasilez® (Novartis) ▼ PoM

Tablets, f/c, aliskiren 150 mg (pink), net price 28-tab pack = £19.80; 300 mg (red), net price 28-tab pack = £23.80. Label: 21

2.6 Nitrates, calcium-channel blockers, and other antianginal drugs

2.6.1 Nitrates
2.6.2 Calcium-channel blockers
2.6.3 Other antianginal drugs
2.6.4 Peripheral vasodilators and related drugs

Nitrates, calcium-channel blockers, and potassium-channel activators have a vasodilating effect. Vasodilators can act in heart failure by arteriolar dilatation which reduces both peripheral vascular resistance and left ventricular pressure during systole resulting in improved cardiac output. They can also cause venous dilatation which results in dilatation of capacitance vessels, increase of venous pooling, and diminution of venous return to the heart (decreasing left ventricular end-diastolic pressure).

Angina

It is important to distinguish unstable angina from stable angina. *Stable angina* usually results from atherosclerotic plaques in the coronary arteries and is often precipitated by exertion and relieved by rest. *Unstable angina* is usually due to plaque rupture and is often characterised by new onset severe angina or sudden worsening of previously stable angina. Treatment of stable and unstable angina involves management of acute anginal pain, and long-term management to prevent angina attacks and to reduce the risk of cardiovascular events.

Stable angina Acute attacks of stable angina should be managed with sublingual **glyceryl trinitrate**; sublingual glyceryl trinitrate can also be given before performing activities which are known to bring on an attack. If attacks occur more than twice a week, regular drug therapy is required and should be introduced in a stepwise manner according to response.

Patients with mild or moderate stable angina should be given a **beta-blocker** (section 2.4). In those with left-ventricular dysfunction, beta-blocker treatment should be started at a very low dose and titrated very slowly over a period of weeks or months (section 2.5.5).

For those patients in whom beta-blockers are not tolerated or are contra-indicated, a long-acting **nitrate** (section 2.6.1) or a rate-limiting **calcium-channel blocker** (diltiazem or verapamil, section 2.6.2) may be used; in patients with left-ventricular dysfunction diltiazem and verapamil are contra-indicated because heart failure may be precipitated (**important**: see p. 111), however a long-acting dihydropyridine calcium-channel blocker, such as amlodipine or felodipine, is suitable. Nicorandil or ivabradine (section 2.6.3) are alternatives.

When a single drug fails to control symptoms, combination treatment may be used. A calcium-channel blocker may be added to a beta-blocker, although combinations of verapamil and a beta-blocker should be avoided (see p. 117); combinations including diltiazem and a beta-blocker should be used with caution. Long-acting nitrates may also be used with a beta-blocker or a calcium-channel blocker, if appropriate. Combinations that include nicorandil can also be considered.

Patients should be referred to a specialist if a combination of two drugs fails to control symptoms. Revascularisation procedures may be appropriate.

Unstable angina Unstable angina and non-ST-segment elevation myocardial infarction are managed similarly. The aims of management are to provide supportive care and pain relief during the acute attack and to prevent further cardiac events and death. For advice on the management of patients with ST-segment elevation acute myocardial infarction, see section 2.10.1.

Initial management **Aspirin** (chewed or dispersed in water) is given for its antiplatelet effect at a dose of 300 mg (section 2.9). If aspirin is given before arrival at hospital, a note saying that it has been given should be sent with the patient. **Clopidogrel** in a dose of 300 mg (section 2.9) and a **low molecular weight heparin** or **fondaparinux** (section 2.8.1), should also be given.

Nitrates (section 2.6.1) are used to relieve ischaemic pain. If sublingual glyceryl trinitrate is not effective, intravenous or buccal glyceryl trinitrate or intravenous isosorbide dinitrate is given.

Patients without contra-indications should receive **beta-blockers** (section 2.4) which should be continued indefinitely. In patients without left ventricular dysfunction and in whom beta-blockers are inappropriate, **diltiazem** or **verapamil** may be given (section 2.6.2).

The glycoprotein IIb/IIIa inhibitors **eptifibatide** and **tirofiban** (section 2.9) are recommended (with aspirin and heparin) for unstable angina or for non-ST-segment elevation myocardial infarction in patients at a high risk of either myocardial infarction or death.

Abciximab, eptifibatide, or tirofiban may also be used with aspirin and heparin in patients undergoing percutaneous coronary intervention, to reduce the immediate risk of vascular occlusion.

Revascularisation procedures are often appropriate for patients with unstable angina.

Long-term management The need for long-term angina treatment or for coronary angiography should be assessed. If there is continuing ischaemia, standard angina treatment should be continued; if not, anti-anginal treatment may be withdrawn cautiously at least 2 months after the acute attack.

Prevention of cardiovascular events Patients with stable and unstable angina should be given advice and treatments to reduce their cardiovascular risk. The importance of life-style changes, especially stopping smoking, should be emphasised. Patients should receive **aspirin** indefinitely in a dose of 75 mg daily. A combination of aspirin and clopidogrel is given for up to 12 months in those patients with non-ST-segment elevation acute coronary syndromes (section 2.9). An **ACE inhibitor** (section 2.5.5.1) and a **statin** (section 2.12) should also be given.

2.6.1 Nitrates

Nitrates have a useful role in *angina* (for details on the management of stable angina, see section 2.6). Although they are potent coronary vasodilators, their principal benefit follows from a reduction in venous return which reduces left ventricular work. Unwanted effects such as flushing, headache, and postural hypotension may limit therapy, especially when angina is severe or when patients are unusually sensitive to the effects of nitrates.

Sublingual **glyceryl trinitrate** is one of the most effective drugs for providing rapid symptomatic relief of angina, but its effect lasts only for 20 to 30 minutes; the 300-microgram tablet is often appropriate when glyceryl trinitrate is first used. The *aerosol spray* provides an alternative method of rapid relief of symptoms for those who find difficulty in dissolving sublingual preparations. Duration of action may be prolonged by *modified-release* and *transdermal* preparations (but tolerance may develop, see below).

Isosorbide dinitrate is active *sublingually* and is a more stable preparation for those who only require nitrates infrequently. It is also effective by mouth for prophylaxis; although the effect is slower in onset, it may persist for several hours. Duration of action of up to 12 hours is claimed for *modified-release* preparations. The activity of isosorbide dinitrate may depend on the production of active metabolites, the most important of which is isosorbide mononitrate. **Isosorbide mononitrate** itself is also licensed for angina prophylaxis; modified-release formulations (for once daily administration) are available.

Glyceryl trinitrate or isosorbide dinitrate may be tried by *intravenous injection* when the sublingual form is ineffective in patients with chest pain due to myocardial infarction or severe ischaemia. Intravenous injections are also useful in the treatment of acute left ventricular failure.

Tolerance Many patients on long-acting or transdermal nitrates rapidly develop tolerance (with reduced therapeutic effects). Reduction of blood-nitrate concentrations to low levels for 4 to 8 hours each day usually maintains effectiveness in such patients. If tolerance is suspected during the use of transdermal patches they should be left off for several consecutive hours in each 24 hours; in the case of modified-release tablets of isosorbide dinitrate (and conventional formulations of isosorbide mononitrate), the second of the two daily doses should be given after about 8 hours rather than after 12 hours. Conventional formulations of isosorbide mononitrate should not usually be given more than twice daily unless small doses are used; modified-release formulations of isosorbide mononitrate should only be given once daily, and used in this way do not produce tolerance.

GLYCERYL TRINITRATE

Indications prophylaxis and treatment of angina; left ventricular failure; anal fissure (section 1.7.4); extravasation (section 10.3)

Cautions hypothyroidism, malnutrition, hypothermia; head trauma, cerebral haemorrhage; recent history of myocardial infarction; hypoxaemia or other ventilation and perfusion abnormalities; susceptibility to angle-closure glaucoma; metal-containing transdermal systems should be removed before cardioversion or diathermy; avoid abrupt withdrawal; tolerance (see notes above); severe hepatic impairment; severe renal impairment; pregnancy (Appendix 4); breast-feeding (Appendix 5); **interactions:** Appendix 1 (nitrates)

Contra-indications hypersensitivity to nitrates; hypotensive conditions and hypovolaemia; hypertrophic cardiomyopathy, aortic stenosis, cardiac tamponade, constrictive pericarditis, mitral stenosis; marked anaemia

Side-effects postural hypotension, tachycardia (but paradoxical bradycardia also reported); throbbing headache, dizziness; *less commonly* nausea, vomiting, heartburn; flushing; temporary hypoxaemia; rash; application site reactions with transdermal patches; *very rarely* angle-closure glaucoma

Injection Specific side-effects following injection (particularly if given too rapidly) include severe hypotension, diaphoresis, apprehension, restlessness, muscle twitching, retrosternal discomfort, palpitation, abdominal pain, syncope; prolonged administration has been associated with methaemoglobinaemia

Dose

- Sublingually, 0.3–1 mg, repeated as required
- By mouth, see under preparations
- By intravenous infusion, 10–200 micrograms/minute
- By transdermal application, see under preparations

Short-acting tablets and sprays

Glyceryl Trinitrate (Non-proprietary)

Sublingual tablets, glyceryl trinitrate 300 micrograms, net price 100 = £2.71; 500 micrograms, 100 = £5.63; 600 micrograms, 100 = £19.51. Label: 16

Note Glyceryl trinitrate tablets should be supplied in glass containers of not more than 100 tablets, closed with a foil-lined cap, and containing no cotton wool wadding; they should be discarded after 8 weeks in use

Aerosol spray, glyceryl trinitrate 400 micrograms/metered dose. Net price 200-dose unit = £3.13

Dose treatment or prophylaxis of angina, spray 1–2 doses under tongue and then close mouth

Coro-Nitro Pump Spray® (Ayrton Saunders)

Aerosol spray, glyceryl trinitrate 400 micrograms/metered dose. Net price 200-dose unit = £3.13

Dose treatment or prophylaxis of angina, spray 1–2 doses under tongue and then close mouth

Glytrin Spray® (Sanofi-Synthelabo)

Aerosol spray, glyceryl trinitrate 400 micrograms/metered dose. Net price 200-dose unit = £3.49

Dose treatment or prophylaxis of angina, spray 1–2 doses under tongue and then close mouth

Cautions flammable

GTN 300 mcg (Martindale)

Sublingual tablets, glyceryl trinitrate 300 micrograms. Net price 100 = £2.71. Label: 16

Nitrolingual Pumpspray® (Merck)

Aerosol spray, glyceryl trinitrate 400 micrograms/metered dose, net price 200-dose unit = £3.65

Dose treatment or prophylaxis of angina, spray 1–2 doses under tongue and then close mouth

Nitromin® (Egis)

Aerosol spray, glyceryl trinitrate 400 micrograms/metered dose, net price 180-dose unit = £2.63, 200-dose unit = £2.82

Dose treatment or prophylaxis of angina, spray 1–2 doses under tongue and then close mouth

Longer-acting tablets

Suscard® (Forest)

Buccal tablets, m/r, glyceryl trinitrate 2 mg, net price 100-tab pack = £12.70; 3 mg, 100-tab pack = £18.33; 5 mg, 100-tab pack = £24.96. Counselling, see below

Dose treatment of angina, 2 mg as required, increased to 3 mg if necessary; prophylaxis 2–3 mg 3 times daily; 5 mg in severe angina

Unstable angina (adjunct), up to 5 mg with ECG monitoring

Congestive heart failure, 5 mg 3 times daily, increased to 10 mg 3 times daily in severe cases

Acute heart failure, 5 mg repeated until symptoms abate

Counselling Tablets have rapid onset of effect; they are placed between upper lip and gum, and left to dissolve; vary site to reduce risk of dental caries

Parenteral preparations

Note Glass or polyethylene apparatus is preferable; loss of potency will occur if PVC is used

Glyceryl Trinitrate (Non-proprietary) PoM

Injection, glyceryl trinitrate 5 mg/mL. To be diluted before use. Net price 5-mL amp = £6.49; 10-mL amp = £12.98

Excipients may include ethanol, propylene glycol (see Excipients, p. 2)

Nitrocine® (UCB Pharma) PoM

Injection, glyceryl trinitrate 1 mg/mL. To be diluted before use or given undiluted with syringe pump. Net price 10-mL amp = £7.34; 50-mL bottle = £17.21

Excipients include propylene glycol (see Excipients, p. 2)

Nitronal® (Merck) PoM

Injection, glyceryl trinitrate 1 mg/mL. To be diluted before use or given undiluted with syringe pump. Net price 5-mL vial = £1.92; 50-mL vial = £15.67

Transdermal preparations

Deponit® (UCB Pharma)

Patches, self-adhesive, transparent, glyceryl trinitrate, *'5' patch* (releasing approx. 5 mg/24 hours when in contact with skin), net price 28 = £15.96; *'10' patch* (releasing approx. 10 mg/24 hours), 28 = £17.57

Dose prophylaxis of angina, apply one '5' or one '10' patch to lateral chest wall, upper arm, thigh, abdomen, or shoulder; increase to two '10' patches every 24 hours if necessary; replace every 24 hours, siting replacement patch on different area; see also notes above (Tolerance)

Minitran® (3M)

Patches, self-adhesive, transparent, glyceryl trinitrate, *'5' patch* (releasing approx. 5 mg/24 hours when in contact with skin), net price 30 = £11.62; *'10' patch* (releasing approx. 10 mg/24 hours), 30 = £12.87; *'15' patch* (releasing approx. 15 mg/24 hours), 30 = £14.19

Dose prophylaxis of angina, apply one '5' patch to chest or upper arm; replace every 24 hours, siting replacement patch on different area; adjust dose according to response; see also notes above (Tolerance)

Maintenance of venous patency ('5' patch only), consult product literature

Nitro-Dur® (Schering-Plough)
Patches, self-adhesive, buff, glyceryl trinitrate, *'0.2 mg/h' patch* (releasing approx. 5 mg/24 hours when in contact with skin), net price 28 = £11.01; *'0.4 mg/h' patch* (releasing approx. 10 mg/24 hours), 28 = £12.18; *'0.6 mg/h' patch* (releasing approx.15 mg/24 hours), 28 = £13.41
Dose prophylaxis of angina, apply one '0.2 mg/h' patch to chest or outer upper arm; replace every 24 hours, siting replacement patch on different area: adjust dose according to response; see also notes above (Tolerance)

Percutol® (PLIVA)
Ointment, glyceryl trinitrate 2%. Net price 60 g = £9.55. Counselling, see administration below
Excipients include wool fat
Dose prophylaxis of angina, usual dose 1–2 inches of ointment measured on to *Applirule®*, and applied (usually to chest, arm, or thigh) without rubbing in and secured with surgical tape, every 3–4 hours as required; to determine dose, ½ inch on first day then increased by ½ inch/day until headache occurs, then reduced by ½ inch
Note Approx. 800 micrograms/hour absorbed from 1 inch of ointment

Transiderm-Nitro® (Novartis)
Patches, self-adhesive, pink, glyceryl trinitrate, *'5' patch* (releasing approx. 5 mg/24 hours when in contact with skin), net price 28 = £21.31; *'10' patch* (releasing approx. 10 mg/24 hours), 28 = £23.43
Dose prophylaxis of angina, apply one '5' or one '10' patch to lateral chest wall; replace every 24 hours, siting replacement patch on different area; max. two '10' patches daily; see also notes above (Tolerance)
Prophylaxis of phlebitis and extravasation ('5' patch only), consult product literature

Trintek® (Goldshield)
Patches, self-adhesive, glyceryl trinitrate, '5' patch (releasing approx. 5 mg/24 hours when in contact with skin), net price 30 = £11.84; '10' patch (releasing approx. 10 mg/24 hours), net price 30 = £13.10; '15' patch (releasing approx. 15 mg/24 hours), net price 30 = £14.42
Dose prophylaxis of angina, apply one '5' patch to lateral chest wall; replace every 24 hours, siting replacement patch on different area; adjust dose according to response, max one '15' patch daily; see also notes above (Tolerance)

ISOSORBIDE DINITRATE

Indications prophylaxis and treatment of angina; left ventricular failure
Cautions see under Glyceryl Trinitrate
Contra-indications see under Glyceryl Trinitrate
Side-effects see under Glyceryl Trinitrate
Dose
- By mouth, daily in divided doses, angina 30–120 mg, left ventricular failure 40–160 mg, up to 240 mg if required
- By intravenous infusion, 2–10 mg/hour; higher doses up to 20 mg/hour may be required

Short-acting tablets and sprays

Isosorbide Dinitrate (Non-proprietary)
Tablets, isosorbide dinitrate 10 mg, net price 56-tab pack = £8.74; 20 mg, 56-tab pack = £10.91

Angitak® (LPC)
Aerosol spray, isosorbide dinitrate 1.25 mg/metered dose, net price 200-dose unit = £3.95
Dose treatment or prophylaxis of angina, spray 1–3 doses under tongue whilst holding breath; allow 30 second interval between each dose

Modified-release preparations

Cedocard Retard® (Pharmacia)
Retard-20 tablets, m/r, yellow, scored, isosorbide dinitrate 20 mg. Net price 60-tab pack = £6.85. Label: 25
Dose prophylaxis of angina, 1 tablet every 12 hours
Retard-40 tablets, m/r, orange-red, scored, isosorbide dinitrate 40 mg. Net price 60-tab pack = £13.31. Label: 25
Dose prophylaxis of angina, 1–2 tablets every 12 hours

Isoket Retard® (UCB Pharma)
Retard-20 tablets, m/r, scored, isosorbide dinitrate 20 mg, net price 56-tab pack = £3.23. Label: 25
Retard-40 tablets, m/r, scored, isosorbide dinitrate 40 mg, net price 56-tab pack = £7.95. Label: 25
Dose prophylaxis of angina, 40 mg daily in 1–2 divided doses, increased if necessary to 60–80 mg daily in 2–3 divided doses

Parenteral preparations

Isoket® (UCB Pharma) PoM
Injection 0.05%, isosorbide dinitrate 500 micrograms/mL. To be diluted before use or given undiluted with syringe pump. Net price 50-mL bottle = £8.94
Injection 0.1%, isosorbide dinitrate 1 mg/mL. To be diluted before use. Net price 10-mL amp = £3.37; 50-mL bottle = £16.70; 100-mL bottle = £25.98
Note Glass or polyethylene infusion apparatus is preferable; loss of potency if PVC used

ISOSORBIDE MONONITRATE

Indications prophylaxis of angina; adjunct in congestive heart failure
Cautions see under Glyceryl Trinitrate
Contra-indications see under Glyceryl Trinitrate
Side-effects see under Glyceryl Trinitrate
Dose
- Initially 20 mg 2–3 times daily *or* 40 mg twice daily (10 mg twice daily in those who have not previously received nitrates); up to 120 mg daily in divided doses if required

Isosorbide Mononitrate (Non-proprietary)
Tablets, isosorbide mononitrate 10 mg, net price 56 = 60p; 20 mg, 56 = 69p; 40 mg, 56 = £1.37. Label: 25
Brands include *Angeze®*, *Dynamin®*

Elantan® (UCB Pharma)
Elantan 10 tablets, scored, isosorbide mononitrate 10 mg, net price 56-tab pack = £3.31; 84-tab pack = £4.97. Label: 25
Elantan 20 tablets, scored, isosorbide mononitrate 20 mg, net price 56-tab pack = £4.32; 84-tab pack = £6.13. Label: 25
Elantan 40 tablets, scored, isosorbide mononitrate 40 mg, net price 56-tab pack = £7.03; 84-tab pack = £10.56. Label: 25

Ismo® (Roche)
Ismo 10 tablets, isosorbide mononitrate 10 mg. Net price 60-tab pack = £3.01. Label: 25
Ismo 20 tablets, scored, isosorbide mononitrate 20 mg. Net price 60-tab pack = £4.42. Label: 25

Modified release

Chemydur® 60XL (Sovereign) PoM

Tablets, m/r, scored, ivory, isosorbide mononitrate 60 mg, net price 28-tab pack = £5.99. Label: 25

Dose prophylaxis of angina, 1 tablet in the morning (half a tablet for 2–4 days to minimise possibility of headache), increased if necessary to 2 tablets

Elantan LA® (UCB Pharma)

Elantan LA 25 capsules, m/r, brown/white, enclosing white micropellets, isosorbide mononitrate 25 mg, net price 28-cap pack = £6.59. Label: 25

Dose prophylaxis of angina, 1 capsule in the morning, increased if necessary to 2 capsules

Elantan LA 50 capsules, m/r, brown/pink, enclosing white micropellets, isosorbide mononitrate 50 mg, net price 28-cap pack = £10.54. Label: 25

Dose prophylaxis of angina, 1 capsule daily in the morning, increased if necessary to 2 capsules

Imdur® (AstraZeneca)

Durules® (= tablets m/r), yellow, f/c, scored, isosorbide mononitrate 60 mg. Net price 28-tab pack = £11.14. Label: 25

Dose prophylaxis of angina, 1 tablet in the morning (half a tablet if headache occurs), increased to 2 tablets in the morning if required

Isib 60XL® (Ashbourne)

Tablets, m/r, scored, ivory, isosorbide mononitrate 60 mg. Net price 28-tab pack = £8.75. Label: 25

Dose prophylaxis of angina, 1 tablet in the morning (half a tablet for 2–4 days if headache occurs), increased if necessary to 2 tablets

Ismo Retard® (Roche)

Tablets, m/r, s/c, isosorbide mononitrate 40 mg, net price 30-tab pack = £9.75. Label: 25

Dose prophylaxis of angina, 1 tablet daily in morning

Isodur® (Galen)

Isodur 25XL capsules, m/r, brown/white, isosorbide mononitrate 25 mg, net price 28-cap pack = £5.63. Label: 25

Isodur 50XL capsules, m/r, brown/pink, isosorbide mononitrate 50 mg, net price 28-cap pack = £9.07. Label: 25

Dose prophylaxis of angina, 25–50 mg daily in the morning, increased if necessary to 50–100 mg once daily

Isotard® (ProStrakan)

Isotard 25XL tablets, m/r, ivory, isosorbide mononitrate 25 mg, net price 28-tab pack = £5.95. Label: 25

Isotard 40XL tablets, m/r, ivory, isosorbide mononitrate 40 mg, net price 28-tab pack = £6.78. Label: 25

Isotard 50XL tablets, m/r, ivory, isosorbide mononitrate 50 mg, net price 28-tab pack = £6.78. Label: 25

Isotard 60XL tablets, m/r, ivory, isosorbide mononitrate 60 mg, net price 28-tab pack = £6.78. Label: 25

Dose prophylaxis of angina, 25–60 mg daily in the morning (if headache occurs with 60-mg tablet, half a 60-mg tablet may be given for 2–4 days), increased if necessary to 50–120 mg daily

Modisal LA® (Schwarz)

Modisal LA25 capsules, m/r, brown/white, isosorbide mononitrate 25 mg, net price 28-cap pack = £6.22. Label: 25

Modisal LA50 capsules, m/r, brown/peach, isosorbide mononitrate 50 mg, net price 28-cap pack = £10.03. Label: 25

Dose prophylaxis of angina, 25–50 mg daily in the morning, increased if necessary to 100 mg once daily

Modisal XL® (Sandoz)

Tablets, m/r, ivory, isosorbide mononitrate 60 mg. Net price 28-tab pack = £10.36. Label: 25

Dose prophylaxis of angina, 1 tablet daily in the morning (half a tablet for first 2–4 days to minimise possibility of headache), increased if necessary to 2 tablets once daily

Monomax® (Trinity-Chiesi)

Monomax® SR, capsules, m/r, isosorbide mononitrate 40 mg, net price 28-cap pack = £8.31; 60 mg, 28-cap pack = £9.03. Label: 25

Dose prophylaxis of angina, 40–60 mg daily in the morning, increased if necessary to 120 mg daily

Note Also available as *Angeze SR®*

Monomax® XL tablets, m/r, isosorbide mononitrate 60 mg, net price 28-tab pack = £6.75. Label: 25

Dose prophylaxis of angina, 1 tablet in the morning (half a tablet for first 2–4 days to minimise possibility of headache), increased if necessary to 2 tablets

Monomil XL® (IVAX) PoM

Tablets, m/r, isosorbide mononitrate 60 mg, net price 28-tab pack = £4.50. Label: 25

Dose prophylaxis of angina, 1 tablet daily in the morning (half a tablet daily for first 2–4 days to minimise possibility of headache), increased if necessary to 2 tablets once daily

Monosorb XL 60® (Dexcel) PoM

Tablets, m/r, f/c, isosorbide mononitrate 60 mg. Net price 28-tab pack = £16.66. Label: 25

Dose prophylaxis of angina, 1 tablet daily in the morning (half a tablet for first 2–4 days to minimise possibility of headache), increased if necessary to 2 tablets

Note Also available as *Monigen® XL, Trangina® XL, Xismox® XL 60*

Zemon® (Neolab)

Zemon 40XL tablets, m/r, ivory, isosorbide mononitrate 40 mg, net price 28-tab pack = £14.25. Label: 25

Zemon 60XL tablets, scored, m/r, ivory, isosorbide mononitrate 60 mg, net price 28-tab pack = £11.14. Label: 25

Dose prophylaxis of angina, 40–60 mg daily in the morning (half a 60-mg tablet may be given for 2–4 days to minimise possibility of headache), increased if necessary to 80–120 mg once daily

2.6.2 Calcium-channel blockers

Calcium-channel blockers (less correctly called 'calcium-antagonists') interfere with the inward displacement of calcium ions through the slow channels of active cell membranes. They influence the myocardial cells, the cells within the specialised conducting system of the heart, and the cells of vascular smooth muscle. Thus, myocardial contractility may be reduced, the formation and propagation of electrical impulses within the heart may be depressed, and coronary or systemic vascular tone may be diminished.

Calcium-channel blockers differ in their predilection for the various possible sites of action and, therefore, their therapeutic effects are disparate, with much greater variation than those of beta-blockers. There are important differences between verapamil, diltiazem, and the dihydropyridine calcium-channel blockers (amlodipine, felodipine, isradipine, lacidipine, lercanidipine, nicardipine, nifedipine, nimodipine, and nisoldipine). Verapamil and diltiazem should usually be **avoided** in *heart failure* because they may further depress cardiac function and cause clinically significant deterioration.

Verapamil is used for the treatment of *angina* (section 2.6), *hypertension* (section 2.5), and *arrhythmias* (section

2.3.2). It is a highly negatively inotropic calcium channel-blocker and it reduces cardiac output, slows the heart rate, and may impair atrioventricular conduction. It may precipitate heart failure, exacerbate conduction disorders, and cause hypotension at high doses and should **not** be used with beta-blockers (see p. 117). Constipation is the most common side-effect.

Nifedipine relaxes vascular smooth muscle and dilates coronary and peripheral arteries. It has more influence on vessels and less on the myocardium than does verapamil, and unlike verapamil has no anti-arrhythmic activity. It rarely precipitates heart failure because any negative inotropic effect is offset by a reduction in left ventricular work. Short-acting formulations of nifedipine are not recommended for angina or long-term management of hypertension; their use may be associated with large variations in blood pressure and reflex tachycardia. **Nicardipine** has similar effects to those of nifedipine and may produce less reduction of myocardial contractility. **Amlodipine** and **felodipine** also resemble nifedipine and nicardipine in their effects and do not reduce myocardial contractility and they do not produce clinical deterioration in heart failure. They have a longer duration of action and can be given once daily. Nifedipine, nicardipine, amlodipine, and felodipine are used for the treatment of angina (section 2.6) or hypertension. All are valuable in forms of *angina associated with coronary vasospasm*. Side-effects associated with vasodilatation such as flushing and headache (which become less obtrusive after a few days), and ankle swelling (which may respond only partially to diuretics) are common.

Isradipine, **lacidipine**, **lercanidipine** and **nisoldipine** have similar effects to those of nifedipine and nicardipine; isradipine, lacidipine, and lercanidipine are only indicated for *hypertension* whereas nisoldipine is indicated for angina and hypertension.

Nimodipine is related to nifedipine but the smooth muscle relaxant effect preferentially acts on cerebral arteries. Its use is confined to prevention and treatment of *vascular spasm following aneurysmal subarachnoid haemorrhage*.

Diltiazem is effective in most forms of *angina* (section 2.6); the longer-acting formulation is also used for *hypertension*. It may be used in patients for whom beta-blockers are contra-indicated or ineffective. It has a less negative inotropic effect than verapamil and significant myocardial depression occurs rarely. Nevertheless because of the risk of bradycardia it should be used with caution in association with beta-blockers.

Unstable angina Calcium-channel blockers do not reduce the risk of myocardial infarction in unstable angina. The use of diltiazem or verapamil should be reserved for patients resistant to treatment with beta-blockers.

Withdrawal There is some evidence that sudden withdrawal of calcium-channel blockers may be associated with an exacerbation of angina.

AMLODIPINE

Indications hypertension, prophylaxis of angina

Cautions hepatic impairment (Appendix 2); pregnancy (Appendix 4); **interactions:** Appendix 1 (calcium-channel blockers)

Contra-indications cardiogenic shock, unstable angina, significant aortic stenosis; porphyria (section 9.8.2); breast-feeding (Appendix 5)

Side-effects abdominal pain, nausea; palpitation, flushing, oedema; headache, dizziness, sleep disturbances, fatigue; *less commonly* gastro-intestinal disturbances, dry mouth, taste disturbances, hypotension, syncope, chest pain, dyspnoea, rhinitis, mood changes, asthenia, tremor, paraesthesia, urinary disturbances, impotence, gynaecomastia, weight changes, myalgia, muscle cramps, back pain, arthralgia, visual disturbances, tinnitus, pruritus, rashes (including isolated reports of erythema multiforme), sweating, alopecia, purpura, and skin discolouration; *very rarely* gastritis, pancreatitis, hepatitis, jaundice, cholestasis, gingival hyperplasia, myocardial infarction, arrhythmias, tachycardia, vasculitis, coughing, peripheral neuropathy, hyperglycaemia, thrombocytopenia, angioedema, and urticaria

Dose

- Hypertension or angina, initially 5 mg once daily; max. 10 mg once daily

Note Tablets from various suppliers may contain different salts (e.g. amlodipine besilate, amlodipine maleate, and amlodipine mesilate) but the strength is expressed in terms of amlodipine (base); tablets containing different salts are considered interchangeable

Amlodipine (Non-proprietary) PoM

Tablets, amlodipine (as maleate or as mesilate) 5 mg, net price 28-tab pack = £1.43; 10 mg, 28-tab pack = £1.17

Brands include *Amlostin®*

Istin® (Pfizer) PoM

Tablets, amlodipine (as besilate) 5 mg. Net price 28-tab pack = £13.04; 10 mg, 28-tab pack = £19.47

With valsartan

Note For hypertension in patients stabilised on the individual components in the same proportions. For cautions, contra-indications, and side-effects of valsartan, see section 2.5.5.2

Exforge® (Novartis) ▼ PoM

Tablets 5/80, f/c, dark yellow, amlodipine 5 mg, valsartan 80 mg, net price 28-tab pack = £16.44

Tablets 5/160, f/c, dark yellow, amlodipine 5 mg, valsartan 160 mg, net price 28-tab pack = £21.66

Tablets 10/160, f/c, light yellow, amlodipine 10 mg, valsartan 160 mg, net price 28-tab pack = £21.66

DILTIAZEM HYDROCHLORIDE

Indications prophylaxis and treatment of angina; hypertension

Cautions reduce dose in hepatic and renal impairment; heart failure or significantly impaired left ventricular function, bradycardia (avoid if severe), first degree AV block, or prolonged PR interval; **interactions:** Appendix 1 (calcium-channel blockers)

Contra-indications severe bradycardia, left ventricular failure with pulmonary congestion, second- or third-degree AV block (unless pacemaker fitted), sick sinus syndrome; porphyria (but see section 9.8.2); pregnancy; breast-feeding (Appendix 5)

Side-effects bradycardia, sino-atrial block, AV block, palpitation, dizziness, hypotension, malaise, asthenia, headache, hot flushes, gastro-intestinal disturbances, oedema (notably of ankles); rarely rashes (including erythema multiforme and exfoliative dermatitis), photosensitivity; hepatitis, gynaecomastia, gum hyperplasia, extrapyramidal symptoms, depression reported

Dose

- Angina, 60 mg 3 times daily (elderly initially twice daily); increased if necessary to 360 mg daily
- Longer-acting formulations, see under preparations below

Standard formulations

Note These formulations are licensed as generics and there is no requirement for brand name dispensing. Although their means of formulation has called for the strict designation 'modified-release' their duration of action corresponds to that of tablets requiring administration 3 times daily

Diltiazem (Non-proprietary) PoM
Tablets, m/r (but see note above), diltiazem hydrochloride 60 mg, net price 84 = £2.97. Label: 25
Brands include *Optil®*

Tildiem® (Sanofi-Synthelabo) PoM
Tablets, m/r (but see note above), off-white, diltiazem hydrochloride 60 mg. Net price 90-tab pack = £8.28. Label: 25

Longer-acting formulations

Note Different versions of modified-release preparations may not have the same clinical effect. To avoid confusion between these different formulations of diltiazem, prescribers should specify the brand to be dispensed

Adizem-SR® (Napp) PoM
Capsules, m/r, diltiazem hydrochloride 90 mg (white), net price 56-cap pack = £8.98; 120 mg (brown/white), 56-cap pack = £9.98; 180 mg (brown/white), 56-cap pack = £14.95. Label: 25
Tablets, m/r, f/c, scored, diltiazem hydrochloride 120 mg. Net price 56-tab pack = £14.72. Label: 25
Dose mild to moderate hypertension, usually 120 mg twice daily (dose form not appropriate for initial dose titration)
Angina, initially 90 mg twice daily (elderly, dose form not appropriate for initial dose titration); increased to 180 mg twice daily if required

Adizem-XL® (Napp) PoM
Capsules, m/r, diltiazem hydrochloride 120 mg (pink/blue), net price 28-cap pack = £9.66; 180 mg (dark pink/blue), 28-cap pack = £10.96; 200 mg (brown), 28-cap pack = £6.66; 240 mg (red/blue), 28-cap pack = £12.17; 300 mg (maroon/blue), 28-cap pack = £9.66. Label: 25
Dose angina and mild to moderate hypertension, initially 240 mg once daily, increased if necessary to 300 mg once daily; in elderly and in hepatic or renal impairment, initially 120 mg daily

Angitil SR® (Trinity-Chiesi) PoM
Capsules, m/r, diltiazem hydrochloride 90 mg (white), net price 56-cap pack = £7.86; 120 mg (brown), 56-cap pack = £8.73; 180 mg (brown), 56-cap pack = £14.08. Label: 25
Dose angina and mild to moderate hypertension, initially 90 mg twice daily; increased if necessary to 120 mg or 180 mg twice daily
Note Also available as *Disogram®* *SR*

Angitil XL® (Trinity-Chiesi) PoM
Capsules, m/r, diltiazem hydrochloride 240 mg (white), net price 28-cap pack = £9.44; 300 mg (yellow), 28-cap pack = £8.57. Label: 25
Dose angina and mild to moderate hypertension, initially 240 mg once daily (elderly and in hepatic and renal impairment, dose form not appropriate for initial dose titration); increased if necessary to 300 mg once daily
Note Also available as *Disogram®* *SR*

Calcicard CR® (IVAX) PoM
Tablets, m/r, both f/c, diltiazem hydrochloride 90 mg, net price 56-tab pack = £6.33; 120 mg, 56-tab pack = £7.04. Label: 25
Dose mild to moderate hypertension, initially 90 mg or 120 mg twice daily; up to 360 mg daily may be required: ELDERLY and in hepatic and renal impairment, initially 120 mg once daily; up to 240 mg daily may be required
Angina, initially 90 mg or 120 mg twice daily; up to 480 mg daily in divided doses may be required; ELDERLY and in hepatic and renal impairment, dose form not appropriate for initial dose titration; up to 240 mg daily may be required

Dilcardia SR® (Generics) PoM
Capsules, m/r, diltiazem hydrochloride 60 mg (pink/white), net price 56-cap pack = £8.31; 90 mg (pink/yellow), 56-cap pack = £10.33; 120 mg (pink/orange), 56-cap pack = £11.49. Label: 25
Dose angina and mild to moderate hypertension, initially 90 mg twice daily; increased if necessary to 180 mg twice daily; ELDERLY and in hepatic or renal impairment, initially 60 mg twice daily, max. 90 mg twice daily

Dilzem SR® (Zeneus) PoM
Capsules, m/r, all beige, diltiazem hydrochloride 60 mg, net price 56-cap pack = £6.40; 90 mg, 56-cap pack = £9.59; 120 mg, 56-cap pack = £10.95. Label: 25
Dose angina and mild to moderate hypertension, initially 90 mg twice daily (elderly 60 mg twice daily); up to 180 mg twice daily may be required

Dilzem XL® (Zeneus) PoM
Capsules, m/r, diltiazem hydrochloride 120 mg, net price 28-cap pack = £6.61; 180 mg, 28-cap pack = £9.81; 240 mg, 28-cap pack = £11.70. Label: 25
Dose angina and mild to moderate hypertension, initially 180 mg once daily (elderly and in hepatic and renal impairment, 120 mg once daily); if necessary may be increased to 360 mg once daily

Slozem® (Merck) PoM
Capsules, m/r, diltiazem hydrochloride 120 mg (pink/clear), net price 28-cap pack = £7.00; 180 mg (pink/clear), 28-cap pack = £7.80; 240 mg (red/clear), 28-cap pack = £8.20; 300 mg (red/white), 28-cap pack = £8.50. Label: 25
Dose angina and mild to moderate hypertension, initially 240 mg once daily (elderly and in hepatic and renal impairment, 120 mg once daily); if necessary may be increased to 360 mg once daily

Tildiem LA® (Sanofi-Synthelabo) PoM
Capsules, m/r, diltiazem hydrochloride 200 mg (pink/grey, containing white pellets), net price 28-cap pack = £6.66; 300 mg (white/yellow, containing white pellets), 28-cap pack = £7.51. Label: 25
Dose angina and mild to moderate hypertension, initially 200 mg once daily before or with food, increased if necessary to 300–400 mg daily, max. 500 mg daily; ELDERLY and in hepatic or renal impairment, initially 200 mg daily, increased if necessary to 300 mg daily

Tildiem Retard® (Sanofi-Synthelabo) PoM
Tablets, m/r, diltiazem hydrochloride 90 mg, net price 56-tab pack = £8.55; 120 mg, 56-tab pack = £9.53. Label: 25
Counselling Tablet membrane may pass through gastro-intestinal tract unchanged, but being porous has no effect on efficacy
Dose mild to moderate hypertension, initially 90 mg or 120 mg twice daily; increased if necessary to 360 mg daily in divided doses; ELDERLY and in hepatic or renal impairment, initially 120 mg once daily; increased if necessary to 120 mg twice daily
Angina, initially 90 mg or 120 mg twice daily; increased if necessary to 480 mg daily in divided doses; ELDERLY and in hepatic or renal impairment, dose form not appropriate for initial titration; up to 120 mg twice daily may be required

Viazem XL® (Genus) PoM
Capsules, m/r, diltiazem hydrochloride 120 mg (lavender), net price 28-cap pack = £6.60; 180 mg

(white/blue-green), 28-cap pack = £7.36; 240 mg (blue-green/lavender), 28-cap pack = £7.74; 300 mg (white/lavender), 28-cap pack = £8.03; 360 mg (blue-green), 28-cap pack = £14.70. Label: 25

Dose angina and mild to moderate hypertension, initially 180 mg once daily, adjusted according to response to 240 mg once daily; max. 360 mg once daily; ELDERLY and in hepatic or renal impairment, initially 120 mg once daily, adjusted according to response

Zemtard® (Galen) PoM

Zemtard 120XL capsules, m/r, brown/orange, diltiazem hydrochloride 120 mg, net price 28-cap pack = £6.40. Label: 25

Zemtard 180XL capsules, m/r, grey/pink, diltiazem hydrochloride 180 mg, net price 28-cap pack = £6.50 Label: 25

Zemtard 240XL capsules, m/r, blue, diltiazem hydrochloride 240 mg, net price 28-cap pack = £6.60. Label: 25

Zemtard 300XL capsules, m/r, white/blue, diltiazem hydrochloride 300 mg, net price 28-cap pack = £7.45. Label: 25

Dose angina and mild to moderate hypertension, 180–300 mg once daily, increased if necessary to 360 mg once daily in hypertension and to 480 mg once daily in angina; ELDERLY and in hepatic or renal impairment, initially 120 mg once daily

FELODIPINE

Indications hypertension, prophylaxis of angina

Cautions withdraw if ischaemic pain occurs or existing pain worsens shortly after initiating treatment or if cardiogenic shock develops; severe left ventricular dysfunction; avoid grapefruit juice (may affect metabolism); reduce dose in hepatic impairment; breast-feeding (Appendix 5); **interactions**: Appendix 1 (calcium-channel blockers)

Contra-indications unstable angina, uncontrolled heart failure; significant aortic stenosis; within 1 month of myocardial infarction; porphyria (section 9.8.2); pregnancy (Appendix 4)

Side-effects flushing, headache, palpitation, dizziness, fatigue, gravitational oedema; rarely rash, pruritus, cutaneous vasculitis, gum hyperplasia, urinary frequency, impotence, fever

Dose

- Hypertension, initially 5 mg (elderly 2.5 mg) daily in the morning; usual maintenance 5–10 mg once daily; doses above 20 mg daily rarely needed
- Angina, initially 5 mg daily in the morning, increased if necessary to 10 mg once daily

Felodipine (Non-proprietary) PoM

Tablets, m/r, felodipine 2.5 mg, net price 28-tab pack = £6.70; 5 mg, 28-tab pack = £8.93; 10 mg, 28-tab pack = £12.01, 30-tab pack = £12.87. Label: 25

Brands include *Cardioplen XL®*, *Felogen XL®*, *Felotens XL®*, *Keloc SR®*, *Neofel XL®*, *Parmid XL®*, *Vascalpha®*

Plendil® (AstraZeneca) PoM

Tablets, m/r, f/c, felodipine 2.5 mg (yellow), net price 28-tab pack = £6.70; 5 mg (pink), 28-tab pack = £4.47; 10 mg (brown), 28-tab pack = £6.01. Label: 25

ISRADIPINE

Indications hypertension

Cautions sick sinus syndrome (if pacemaker not fitted); avoid grapefruit juice (may affect metabolism); reduce dose in hepatic or renal impairment; pregnancy (Appendix 4); **interactions**: Appendix 1 (calcium-channel blockers)

Contra-indications cardiogenic shock; symptomatic or tight aortic stenosis; within 1 month of myocardial infarction; unstable angina; porphyria (section 9.8.2); breast-feeding (Appendix 5)

Side-effects headache, flushing, dizziness, tachycardia and palpitation, localised peripheral oedema; hypotension uncommon; rarely weight gain, fatigue, abdominal discomfort, rashes

Dose

- 2.5 mg twice daily (1.25 mg twice daily in elderly, hepatic or renal impairment); increased if necessary after 3–4 weeks to 5 mg twice daily (exceptionally up to 10 mg twice daily); maintenance 2.5 or 5 mg once daily may be sufficient

Prescal® (Novartis) PoM

Tablets, yellow, scored, isradipine 2.5 mg. Net price 56-tab pack = £16.54

LACIDIPINE

Indications hypertension

Cautions cardiac conduction abnormalities; poor cardiac reserve; avoid grapefruit juice (may affect metabolism); hepatic impairment (Appendix 2); **interactions**: Appendix 1 (calcium-channel blockers)

Contra-indications cardiogenic shock, unstable angina, aortic stenosis; avoid within 1 month of myocardial infarction; porphyria (section 9.8.2); pregnancy (Appendix 4); breast-feeding (Appendix 5)

Side-effects flushing, palpitation, oedema; headache, dizziness; *rarely* gastro-intestinal disturbances, gum hyperplasia, aggravation of angina, mood disturbances, asthenia, polyuria, muscle cramps, skin rash (including pruritus and erythema)

Dose

- Initially 2 mg as a single daily dose, preferably in the morning; increased after 3–4 weeks to 4 mg daily, then if necessary to 6 mg daily

Motens® (Boehringer Ingelheim) PoM

Tablets, both f/c, lacidipine 2 mg, net price 28-tab pack = £9.92; 4 mg (scored), 28-tab pack = £13.48

LERCANIDIPINE HYDROCHLORIDE

Indications mild to moderate hypertension

Cautions left ventricular dysfunction; sick sinus syndrome (if pacemaker not fitted); avoid grapefruit juice (may affect metabolism); hepatic impairment (Appendix 2); **interactions**: Appendix 1 (calcium-channel blockers)

Contra-indications aortic stenosis; unstable angina, uncontrolled heart failure; within 1 month of myocardial infarction; renal impairment; porphyria (section 9.8.2); pregnancy (Appendix 4); breast-feeding

Side-effects flushing, peripheral oedema, palpitation, tachycardia, headache, dizziness, asthenia; also gastro-intestinal disturbances, hypotension, drowsiness, myalgia, polyuria, rash

Dose

- Initially 10 mg once daily; increased, if necessary, after at least 2 weeks to 20 mg daily

Zanidip® (Recordati) PoM
Tablets, f/c, lercanidipine hydrochloride 10 mg (yellow), net price 28-tab pack = £5.80; 20 mg (pink), 28-tab pack = £11.00. Label: 22

NICARDIPINE HYDROCHLORIDE

Indications prophylaxis of angina; mild to moderate hypertension

Cautions withdraw if ischaemic pain occurs or existing pain worsens within 30 minutes of initiating treatment or increasing dose; congestive heart failure or significantly impaired left ventricular function; elderly; avoid grapefruit juice (may affect metabolism); hepatic impairment (Appendix 2); renal impairment (Appendix 3); pregnancy (Appendix 4); **interactions**: Appendix 1 (calcium-channel blockers)

Contra-indications cardiogenic shock; advanced aortic stenosis; unstable or acute attacks of angina; avoid within 1 month of myocardial infarction; porphyria (section 9.8.2); breast-feeding (Appendix 5)

Side-effects dizziness, headache, peripheral oedema, flushing, palpitation, nausea; also gastro-intestinal disturbances, drowsiness, insomnia, tinnitus, hypotension, rashes, dyspnoea, paraesthesia, frequency of micturition; thrombocytopenia, depression and impotence reported

Dose

- Initially 20 mg 3 times daily, increased, after at least three days, to 30 mg 3 times daily (usual range 60–120 mg daily)

Nicardipine (Non-proprietary) PoM
Capsules, nicardipine hydrochloride 20 mg, net price 56-cap pack = £7.51; 30 mg, 56-cap pack = £8.88

Cardene® (Astellas) PoM
Capsules, nicardipine hydrochloride 20 mg (blue/white), net price 56-cap pack = £8.57; 30 mg (blue/pale blue), 56-cap pack = £9.95

Modified release

Cardene SR® (Astellas) PoM
Capsules, m/r, nicardipine hydrochloride 30 mg, net price 56-cap pack = £10.21; 45 mg (blue), 56-cap pack = £14.86. Label: 25
Dose mild to moderate hypertension, initially 30 mg twice daily; usual effective dose 45 mg twice daily (range 30–60 mg twice daily)

NIFEDIPINE

Indications prophylaxis of angina; hypertension; Raynaud's phenomenon

Cautions see notes above; also withdraw if ischaemic pain occurs or existing pain worsens shortly after initiating treatment; poor cardiac reserve; heart failure or significantly impaired left ventricular function (heart failure deterioration observed); severe hypotension; reduce dose in hepatic impairment (Appendix 2); diabetes mellitus; may inhibit labour; pregnancy (Appendix 4); breast-feeding (Appendix 5); avoid grapefruit juice (may affect metabolism); **interactions**: Appendix 1 (calcium-channel blockers)

Contra-indications cardiogenic shock; advanced aortic stenosis; within 1 month of myocardial infarction; unstable or acute attacks of angina; porphyria (section 9.8.2)

Side-effects headache, flushing, dizziness, lethargy; tachycardia, palpitation; short-acting preparations may induce an exaggerated fall in blood pressure and reflex tachycardia which may lead to myocardial or cerebrovascular ischaemia; gravitational oedema, rash (erythema multiforme reported), pruritus, urticaria, nausea, constipation or diarrhoea, increased frequency of micturition, eye pain, visual disturbances, gum hyperplasia, asthenia, paraesthesia, myalgia, tremor, impotence, gynaecomastia; depression, telangiectasia, cholestasis, jaundice reported

Dose

- See preparations below

Nifedipine (Non-proprietary) PoM
Capsules, nifedipine 5 mg, net price 84-cap pack = £3.94; 10 mg, 84-cap pack = £5.17
Dose angina prophylaxis (but not recommended, see notes above) and Raynaud's phenomenon, initially 5 mg 3 times daily, adjusted according to response to 20 mg 3 times daily
Hypertension, not recommended therefore no dose stated

Adalat® (Bayer) PoM
Capsules, both orange, nifedipine 5 mg, net price 90-cap pack = £6.08; 10 mg, 90-cap pack = £7.74
Dose angina prophylaxis (but not recommended, see notes above) and Raynaud's phenomenon, initially 5 mg 3 times daily, adjusted according to response to 20 mg 3 times daily
Hypertension, not recommended therefore no dose stated

Modified release

Note Different versions of modified-release preparations may not have the same clinical effect. To avoid confusion between these different formulations of nifedipine, prescribers should specify the brand to be dispensed. Modified-release formulations may not be suitable for dose titration in hepatic disease

Adalat® LA (Bayer) PoM
LA 20 tablets, m/r, pink, nifedipine 20 mg, net price 28-tab pack = £5.27. Label: 25
LA 30 tablets, m/r, pink, nifedipine 30 mg, net price 28-tab pack = £7.59. Label: 25
LA 60 tablets, m/r, pink, nifedipine 60 mg, net price 28-tab pack = £9.09. Label: 25
Counselling Tablet membrane may pass through gastro-intestinal tract unchanged, but being porous has no effect on efficacy
Dose hypertension, 20–30 mg once daily, increased if necessary; max. 90 mg once daily
Angina prophylaxis, 30 mg once daily, increased if necessary; max. 90 mg once daily
Cautions dose form not appropriate for use in hepatic impairment or where there is a history of oesophageal or gastro-intestinal obstruction, decreased lumen diameter of the gastro-intestinal tract, or inflammatory bowel disease (including Crohn's disease)

Adalat® Retard (Bayer) PoM
Retard 10 tablets, m/r, grey-pink, nifedipine 10 mg. Net price 56-tab pack = £8.50. Label: 25
Retard 20 tablets, m/r, pink, nifedipine 20 mg. Net price 56-tab pack = £10.20. Label: 25
Dose hypertension and angina prophylaxis, 10 mg twice daily, adjusted according to response to 40 mg twice daily

Adipine® MR (Trinity-Chiesi) PoM
Tablets, m/r, nifedipine 10 mg (apricot), net price 56-tab pack = £5.96; 20 mg (pink), 56-tab pack = £7.43. Label: 21, 25
Dose hypertension and angina prophylaxis, 20 mg twice daily after food (initial titration 10 mg twice daily); max. 40 mg twice daily

Adipine® XL (Trinity-Chiesi) PoM
Tablets, m/r, both red, nifedipine 30 mg, net price 28-tab pack = £5.89; 60 mg, 28-tab pack = £8.84. Label: 25
Dose hypertension and angina prophylaxis, 30 mg once daily, increased if necessary; max. 90 mg once daily

Cardilate MR® (IVAX) PoM
Tablets, m/r, nifedipine 10 mg (pink), net price 56-tab pack = £4.97; 20 mg (brown), net price 100-tab pack = £16.62. Label: 25
Dose hypertension and angina prophylaxis, 20 mg twice daily (initial titration 10 mg twice daily); max. 80 mg daily

Coracten SR® (UCB Pharma) PoM
Capsules, m/r, nifedipine 10 mg (grey/pink, enclosing yellow pellets), net price 60-cap pack = £4.70; 20 mg (pink/brown, enclosing yellow pellets), 60-cap pack = £6.52. Label: 25
Dose hypertension and angina prophylaxis, one 20-mg capsule every 12 hours, adjusted within range 10–40 mg every 12 hours

Coracten XL® (UCB Pharma) PoM
Capsules, m/r, nifedipine 30 mg (brown), net price 28-cap pack = £5.89; 60 mg (orange), 28-cap pack = £8.84. Label: 25
Dose hypertension and angina prophylaxis, 30 mg once daily, increased if necessary; max. 90 mg once daily

Fortipine LA 40® (Goldshield) PoM
Tablets, m/r, red, nifedipine 40 mg, net price 30-tab pack = £9.60. Label: 21, 25
Dose hypertension and angina prophylaxis, 40 mg once daily, increased if necessary to 80 mg daily in 1–2 divided doses

Hypolar® Retard 20 (Sandoz) PoM
Tablets, m/r, red, f/c, nifedipine 20 mg. Net price 56-tab pack = £5.75. Label: 25
Dose hypertension and angina prophylaxis, 20 mg twice daily, increased if necessary to 40 mg twice daily

Nifedipress® MR (Dexcel) PoM
Tablets, m/r, pink, nifedipine 10 mg, net price 56-tab pack = £9.23; 20 mg, 56-tab pack = £10.06. Label: 25
Dose hypertension and angina prophylaxis, initially 10 mg twice daily adjusted according to response to 40 mg twice daily

Nifopress® Retard (Goldshield) PoM
Tablets, m/r, pink, nifedipine 20 mg, net price 56-tab pack = £10.00. Label: 21, 25
Dose mild to moderate hypertension, angina prophylaxis and Raynaud's phenomenon, usually 20 mg twice daily, adjusted according to response to 40 mg twice daily

Tensipine MR® (Genus) PoM
Tablets, m/r, both pink, nifedipine 10 mg, net price 56-tab pack = £3.99; 20 mg, 56-tab pack = £5.49. Label: 21, 25
Dose hypertension and angina prophylaxis, initially 10 mg twice daily adjusted according to response to 40 mg twice daily

With atenolol
Section 2.4

NIMODIPINE

Indications prevention and treatment of ischaemic neurological deficits following aneurysmal subarachnoid haemorrhage

Cautions cerebral oedema or severely raised intracranial pressure; hypotension; avoid concomitant administration of nimodipine tablets and infusion, other calcium-channel blockers, or beta-blockers; concomitant nephrotoxic drugs; avoid grapefruit juice (may affect metabolism); hepatic impairment (Appendix 2); renal impairment (Appendix 3); pregnancy (Appendix 4); **interactions:** Appendix 1 (calcium-channel blockers, alcohol (infusion only))

Contra-indications within 1 month of myocardial infarction; unstable angina; porphyria (section 9.8.2)

Side-effects hypotension, variation in heart-rate, flushing, headache, gastro-intestinal disorders, nausea, sweating and feeling of warmth; thrombocytopenia and ileus reported

Dose
- Prevention, by mouth, 60 mg every 4 hours, starting within 4 days of aneurysmal subarachnoid haemorrhage and continued for 21 days
- Treatment, by intravenous infusion via central catheter, initially 1 mg/hour (up to 500 micrograms/hour if body-weight less than 70 kg or if blood pressure unstable), increased after 2 hours to 2 mg/hour if no severe fall in blood pressure; continue for at least 5 days (max. 14 days); if surgical intervention during treatment, continue for at least 5 days after surgery; max. total duration of nimodipine use 21 days

Nimotop® (Bayer) PoM
Tablets, yellow, f/c, nimodipine 30 mg. Net price 100-tab pack = £38.85
Intravenous infusion, nimodipine 200 micrograms/mL; also contains ethanol 20% and macrogol '400' 17%. Net price 50-mL vial (with polyethylene infusion catheter) = £13.24
Note Polyethylene, polypropylene or glass apparatus should be used; PVC should be avoided

NISOLDIPINE

Indications prophylaxis of angina, mild to moderate hypertension

Cautions elderly; hypotension; avoid grapefruit juice (may affect metabolism); **interactions:** Appendix 1 (calcium-channel blockers)

Contra-indications cardiogenic shock, aortic stenosis, unstable or acute attacks of angina; within 1 week of myocardial infarction; porphyria (section 9.8.2); hepatic impairment (dose form not appropriate); pregnancy (Appendix 4); breast-feeding (Appendix 5)

Side-effects gravitational oedema, headache, flushing, tachycardia, palpitation; dizziness, asthenia, gastro-intestinal disturbances (including nausea, constipation); less frequently paraesthesia, myalgia, tremor, hypotension, weakness, dyspnoea, allergic skin reactions, increased frequency of micturition; rarely exacerbation of angina, visual disturbances, gynaecomastia, gum hyperplasia

Dose
- Initially 10 mg daily, preferably before breakfast; if necessary increase at intervals of at least 1 week (usual maintenance in angina 20–40 mg once daily); max. 40 mg daily

Syscor MR® (Forest) PoM
Tablets, m/r, f/c, yellow, nisoldipine 10 mg, net price 28-tab pack = £8.77. Label: 22, 25

VERAPAMIL HYDROCHLORIDE

Indications see under Dose and preparations

Cautions first-degree AV block; acute phase of myocardial infarction (avoid if bradycardia, hypotension, left ventricular failure); patients taking beta-blockers (**important:** see below); hepatic impairment (Appendix 2); children, specialist advice only (section 2.3.2); pregnancy (Appendix 4) and breast-feeding (Appendix 5); avoid grapefruit juice (may affect metabolism); **interactions:** Appendix 1 (calcium-channel blockers)

Verapamil and beta-blockers Verapamil injection should not be given to patients recently treated with beta-blockers because of the risk of hypotension and asystole. The suggestion that when verapamil injection has been given first, an interval of 30 minutes before giving a beta-blocker is sufficient has not been confirmed.

It may also be hazardous to give verapamil and a beta-blocker together by mouth (should only be contemplated if myocardial function well preserved).

Contra-indications hypotension, bradycardia, second- and third-degree AV block, sick sinus syndrome, cardiogenic shock, sino-atrial block; history of heart failure or significantly impaired left ventricular function, even if controlled by therapy; atrial flutter or fibrillation complicating syndromes associated with accessory conducting pathways (e.g. Wolff-Parkinson-White syndrome); porphyria (section 9.8.2)

Side-effects constipation; less commonly nausea, vomiting, flushing, headache, dizziness, fatigue, ankle oedema; rarely allergic reactions (erythema, pruritus, urticaria, angioedema, Stevens-Johnson syndrome); myalgia, arthralgia, paraesthesia, erythromelalgia; increased prolactin concentration; rarely gynaecomastia and gingival hyperplasia after long-term treatment; after intravenous administration or high doses, hypotension, heart failure, bradycardia, heart block, and asystole

Dose

- By mouth, supraventricular arrhythmias (but see also Contra-indications), 40–120 mg 3 times daily
  Angina, 80–120 mg 3 times daily
  Hypertension, 240–480 mg daily in 2–3 divided doses
- By slow intravenous injection over 2 minutes (3 minutes in elderly), supraventricular arrhythmias (but see also Contra-indications), 5–10 mg (preferably with ECG monitoring); in paroxysmal tachyarrhythmias a further 5 mg after 5–10 minutes if required

Verapamil (Non-proprietary) PoM
Tablets, coated, verapamil hydrochloride 40 mg, net price 84-tab pack = £1.66; 80 mg, 84-tab pack = £1.91; 120 mg, 28-tab pack = £1.51; 160 mg, 56-tab pack = £15.59
Oral solution, verapamil hydrochloride 40 mg/5 mL, net price 150 mL = £36.90
Brands include *Zolvera®*

Cordilox® (Dexcel) PoM
Tablets, all yellow, f/c, verapamil hydrochloride 40 mg, net price 84-tab pack = £1.50; 80 mg, 84-tab pack = £2.05; 120 mg, 28-tab pack = £1.15; 160 mg, 56-tab pack = £2.80
Injection, verapamil hydrochloride 2.5 mg/mL, net price 2-mL amp = £1.11

Securon® (Abbott) PoM
Injection, verapamil hydrochloride 2.5 mg/mL. Net price 2-mL amp = £1.08

Modified release

Half Securon SR® (Abbott) PoM
Tablets, m/r, f/c, verapamil hydrochloride 120 mg, net price 28-tab pack = £7.50. Label: 25
Dose see *Securon SR®*

Securon SR® (Abbott) PoM
Tablets, m/r, pale green, f/c, scored, verapamil hydrochloride 240 mg, net price 28-tab pack = £6.29. Label: 25
Dose hypertension, 240 mg daily (new patients initially 120 mg), increased if necessary to max. 480 mg daily (doses above 240 mg daily as 2 divided doses)
Angina, 240 mg twice daily (may sometimes be reduced to once daily)
Prophylaxis after myocardial infarction where beta-blockers not appropriate (started at least 1 week after infarction), 360 mg daily in divided doses, given as 240 mg in the morning and 120 mg in the evening *or* 120 mg 3 times daily

Univer® (Zeneus) PoM
Capsules, m/r, verapamil hydrochloride 120 mg (yellow/dark blue), net price 28-cap pack = £7.51; 180 mg (yellow), 56-cap pack = £18.15; 240 mg (yellow/dark blue), 28-cap pack = £12.24. Label: 25
Dose hypertension, 240 mg daily, max. 480 mg daily (new patients, initial dose 120 mg); angina, 360 mg daily, max. 480 mg daily

Verapress MR® (Dexcel) PoM
Tablets, m/r, pale green, f/c, verapamil hydrochloride 240 mg, net price 28-tab pack = £9.90. Label: 25
Dose hypertension, 1 tablet daily, increased to twice daily if necessary; angina, 1 tablet twice daily (may sometimes be reduced to once daily)
Note Also available as *Cordilox® MR*

Vertab® SR 240 (Trinity-Chiesi) PoM
Tablets, m/r, pale green, f/c, scored, verapamil hydrochloride 240 mg, net price 28-tab pack = £8.63. Label: 25
Dose mild to moderate hypertension, 240 mg daily, increased to twice daily if necessary; angina, 240 mg twice daily (may sometimes be reduced to once daily)

2.6.3 Other antianginal drugs

Nicorandil, a potassium-channel activator with a nitrate component, has both arterial and venous vasodilating properties and is licensed for the prevention and long-term treatment of angina (section 2.6). Nicorandil has similar efficacy to other antianginal drugs in controlling symptoms; it may produce additional symptomatic benefit in combination with other antianginal drugs [unlicensed indication].

Ivabradine lowers the heart rate by its action on the sinus node. It is licensed for the treatment of angina in patients in normal sinus rhythm when beta-blockers are contra-indicated or not tolerated.

IVABRADINE

Indications treatment of angina in patients in normal sinus rhythm (see notes above)

Cautions mild heart failure including asymptomatic left ventricular dysfunction; monitor for atrial fibrillation or other arrhythmias (treatment ineffective); hypotension (avoid if severe); retinitis pigmentosa; elderly; hepatic impairment (avoid if severe; Appendix 2); renal impairment (Appendix 3); **interactions**: Appendix 1 (ivabradine)

Contra-indications severe bradycardia (not to be initiated if heart rate below 60 beats per minute); cardiogenic shock; acute myocardial infarction; immediately after cerebrovascular accident; sick-sinus syndrome; sino-atrial block; moderate to severe heart failure; patients with pacemaker; unstable angina; second- and third-degree heart block; congenital QT syndrome; pregnancy (Appendix 4); breast-feeding (Appendix 5)

Side-effects bradycardia, first-degree heart block, ventricular extrasystoles; headache, dizziness; visual disturbances including phosphenes and blurred vision; *less commonly* nausea, constipation, diarrhoea, palpitations, supraventricular extrasystoles, dyspnoea, vertigo, muscle cramps, eosinophilia, hyperuricaemia, and raised plasma-creatinine concentration

Dose

- Initially 5 mg twice daily, increased if necessary after 3–4 weeks to 7.5 mg twice daily (if not tolerated reduce dose to 2.5–5 mg twice daily); ELDERLY initially 2.5 mg twice daily

Note Ventricular rate at rest should not be allowed to fall below 50 beats per minute

Procoralan® (Servier) ▼ PoM

Tablets, both pink, f/c, ivabradine (as hydrochloride) 5 mg (scored), net price 56-tab pack = £39.00; 7.5 mg, 56-tab pack = £39.00

NICORANDIL

Indications prophylaxis and treatment of angina

Cautions hypovolaemia; low systolic blood pressure; acute pulmonary oedema; acute myocardial infarction with acute left ventricular failure and low filling pressures; pregnancy (Appendix 4); **interactions:** Appendix 1 (nicorandil)

Driving Patients should be warned not to drive or operate machinery until it is established that their performance is unimpaired

Contra-indications cardiogenic shock; left ventricular failure with low filling pressures; hypotension; breast-feeding

Side-effects headache (especially on initiation, usually transitory); cutaneous vasodilatation with flushing; nausea, vomiting, dizziness, weakness also reported; *rarely* oral ulceration, myalgia, and rash; at high dosage, reduction in blood pressure and/or increase in heart rate; angioedema, hepatic dysfunction, and anal ulceration also reported

Dose

- Initially 10 mg twice daily (if susceptible to headache 5 mg twice daily); usual dose 10–20 mg twice daily; up to 30 mg twice daily may be used

Ikorel® (Rhône-Poulenc Rorer) PoM

Tablets, both scored, nicorandil 10 mg, net price 60-tab pack = £8.18; 20 mg, 60-tab pack = £15.54

2.6.4 Peripheral vasodilators and related drugs

Peripheral vascular disease can be either occlusive (e.g. *intermittent claudication*) where occlusion of the peripheral arteries is caused by atherosclerosis, or vasospastic (e.g. *Raynaud's syndrome*).

Peripheral arterial occlusive disease is associated with an increased risk of cardiovascular events; this risk is reduced by measures such as smoking cessation (section 4.10), effective control of blood pressure (section 2.5), regulating blood lipids (section 2.12), optimising glycaemic control in diabetes (section 6.1), taking aspirin in a dose of 75 mg daily (section 2.9), and possibly weight reduction in obesity (section 4.5). Exercise training, treatment with cilostazol or naftidrofuryl (see below), and possibly statin therapy can improve symptoms of intermittent claudication.

Cilostazol is licensed for use in intermittent claudication to improve walking distance in patients without peripheral tissue necrosis who do not have pain at rest. Patients receiving cilostazol should be assessed for improvement after 3 months. The *Scottish Medicines Consortium* has advised (October 2005) that cilostazol is not recommended for the treatment of intermittent claudication.

Naftidrofuryl can alleviate symptoms of intermittent claudication and improve pain-free walking distance in moderate disease. Patients receiving naftidrofuryl should be assessed for improvement after 3–6 months.

Inositol nicotinate, pentoxifylline (oxpentifylline), and cinnarizine are not established as being effective for the treatment of intermittent claudication.

Management of *Raynaud's syndrome* includes avoidance of exposure to cold and stopping smoking. More severe symptoms may require vasodilator treatment, which is most often successful in primary Raynaud's syndrome. **Nifedipine** (section 2.6.2) is useful for reducing the frequency and severity of vasospastic attacks. Alternatively, **naftidrofuryl** may produce symptomatic improvement; **inositol nicotinate** (a nicotinic acid derivative) may also be considered. Cinnarizine, pentoxifylline, prazosin, and moxisylyte (thymoxamine) are not established as being effective for the treatment of Raynaud's syndrome.

Vasodilator therapy is not established as being effective for *chilblains* (section 13.13).

CILOSTAZOL

Indications intermittent claudication in patients without rest pain and no peripheral tissue necrosis

Cautions atrial or ventricular ectopy, atrial fibrillation, atrial flutter; diabetes mellitus (higher risk of intraocular bleeding); concomitant drugs that increase risk of bleeding; hepatic impairment (Appendix 2); **interactions:** Appendix 1 (cilostazol)

Contra-indications predisposition to bleeding (e.g. active peptic ulcer, haemorrhagic stroke in previous 6 months, surgery in previous 3 months, proliferative diabetic retinopathy, poorly controlled hypertension); history of ventricular tachycardia, of ventricular fibrillation and of multifocal ventricular ectopics, prolongation of QT interval, congestive heart failure; renal impairment (avoid if creatinine clearance less than 25 mL/minute); pregnancy (Appendix 4); breast-feeding (Appendix 5)

Side-effects gastro-intestinal disturbances; tachycardia, palpitation, angina, arrhythmia, chest pain, oedema; rhinitis; dizziness, headache; asthenia; rash, pruritus, ecchymosis; *less commonly* gastritis, congestive heart failure, postural hypotension, dyspnoea, pneumonia, cough, insomnia, abnormal dreams, anxiety, hyperglycaemia, diabetes mellitus, anaemia, haemorrhage, myalgia, hypersensitivity reactions (including Stevens-Johnson syndrome and toxic epidermal necrolysis in rare cases); *rarely* anorexia, hypertension, paresis, increased urinary frequency, bleeding disorders, renal impairment, conjunctivitis, tinnitus, and jaundice

Dose

- 100 mg twice daily (30 minutes before or 2 hours after food)

Pletal® (Otsuka) ▼ PoM
Tablets, cilostazol 50 mg, net price 56-tab pack = £35.31; 100 mg, 56-tab pack = £35.31

INOSITOL NICOTINATE

Indications peripheral vascular disease; hyperlipidaemia (section 2.12)

Cautions cerebrovascular insufficiency, unstable angina

Contra-indications recent myocardial infarction, acute phase of a cerebrovascular accident; pregnancy (Appendix 4)

Side-effects nausea, vomiting, hypotension, flushing, syncope, oedema, headache, dizziness, paraesthesia, rash

Dose

- 3 g daily in 2–3 divided doses; max. 4 g daily

Hexopal® (Genus)
Tablets, scored, inositol nicotinate 500 mg. Net price 20 = £4.10

Tablets forte, scored, inositol nicotinate 750 mg Net price 112-tab pack = £34.02

MOXISYLYTE
(Thymoxamine)

Indications primary Raynaud's syndrome (short-term treatment)

Cautions diabetes mellitus

Contra-indications active liver disease; pregnancy (Appendix 4)

Side-effects nausea, diarrhoea, flushing, headache, dizziness; hepatic reactions including cholestatic jaundice and hepatitis reported to CSM

Dose

- Initially 40 mg 4 times daily, increased to 80 mg 4 times daily if poor initial response; discontinue after 2 weeks if no response

Opilon® (Concord) PoM
Tablets, yellow, f/c, moxisylyte 40 mg (as hydrochloride). Net price 112-tab pack = £79.98. Label: 21

NAFTIDROFURYL OXALATE

Indications see under Dose

Side-effects nausea, epigastric pain, rash, hepatitis, hepatic failure

Dose

- Peripheral vascular disease (see notes above), 100–200 mg 3 times daily
- Cerebral vascular disease, 100 mg 3 times daily

Naftidrofuryl (Non-proprietary) PoM
Capsules, naftidrofuryl oxalate 100 mg. Net price 84-cap pack = £7.60. Label: 25, 27

Praxilene® (Merck) PoM
Capsules, pink, naftidrofuryl oxalate 100 mg. Net price 84-cap pack = £8.60. Label: 25, 27

PENTOXIFYLLINE
(Oxpentifylline)

Indications peripheral vascular disease; venous leg ulcers [unlicensed indication] (Appendix A8.2.5)

Cautions hypotension, coronary artery disease; renal impairment (Appendix 3), severe hepatic impairment; avoid in porphyria (section 9.8.2); **interactions:** Appendix 1 (pentoxifylline)

Contra-indications cerebral haemorrhage, extensive retinal haemorrhage, acute myocardial infarction; pregnancy and breast-feeding

Side-effects gastro-intestinal disturbances, dizziness, agitation, sleep disturbances, headache; rarely flushing, tachycardia, angina, hypotension, thrombocytopenia, intrahepatic cholestasis, hypersensitivity reactions including rash, pruritus and bronchospasm

Dose

- 400 mg 2–3 times daily

Trental® (Aventis Pharma) PoM
Tablets, m/r, pink, s/c, pentoxifylline 400 mg. Net price 90-tab pack = £20.48. Label: 21, 25

Other preparations used in peripheral vascular disease

Rutosides (oxerutins, *Paroven®*) are not vasodilators and are not generally regarded as effective preparations as capillary sealants or for the treatment of cramps; side-effects include headache, flushing, rashes, mild gastro-intestinal disturbances.

Paroven® (Novartis Consumer Health)
Capsules, yellow, oxerutins 250 mg. Net price 120-cap pack = £13.05
Dose relief of symptoms of oedema associated with chronic venous insufficiency, 500 mg twice daily

2.7 Sympathomimetics

2.7.1 Inotropic sympathomimetics
2.7.2 Vasoconstrictor sympathomimetics
2.7.3 Cardiopulmonary resuscitation

The properties of sympathomimetics vary according to whether they act on alpha or on beta adrenergic receptors. Adrenaline (epinephrine) (section 2.7.3) acts on both alpha and beta receptors and increases both heart rate and contractility (beta$_1$ effects); it can cause peripheral vasodilation (a beta$_2$ effect) or vasoconstriction (an alpha effect).

2.7.1 Inotropic sympathomimetics

The cardiac stimulants **dobutamine** and **dopamine** act on beta$_1$ receptors in cardiac muscle, and increase contractility with little effect on rate.

Dopexamine acts on beta$_2$ receptors in cardiac muscle to produce its positive inotropic effect; and on periph-

2 Cardiovascular system

eral dopamine receptors to increase renal perfusion; it is reported not to induce vasoconstriction.

Isoprenaline injection is available on special order only.

Shock Shock is a medical emergency associated with a high mortality. The underlying causes of shock such as haemorrhage, sepsis, or myocardial insufficiency should be corrected. The profound hypotension of shock must be treated promptly to prevent tissue hypoxia and organ failure. Volume replacement is essential to correct the hypovolaemia associated with haemorrhage and sepsis but may be detrimental in cardiogenic shock. Depending on haemodynamic status, cardiac output may be improved by the use of sympathomimetic inotropes such as adrenaline (epinephrine), dobutamine or dopamine (see notes above). In septic shock, when fluid replacement and inotropic support fail to maintain blood pressure, the vasoconstrictor noradrenaline (norepinephrine) (section 2.7.2) may be considered. In cardiogenic shock peripheral resistance is frequently high and to raise it further may worsen myocardial performance and exacerbate tissue ischaemia.

The use of sympathomimetic inotropes and vasoconstrictors should preferably be confined to the intensive care setting and undertaken with invasive haemodynamic monitoring.

For advice on the management of anaphylactic shock, see section 3.4.3.

DOBUTAMINE

Indications inotropic support in infarction, cardiac surgery, cardiomyopathies, septic shock, and cardiogenic shock

Cautions pregnancy; **interactions:** Appendix 1 (sympathomimetics)

Side-effects tachycardia and marked increase in systolic blood pressure indicate overdosage; phlebitis; *rarely* thrombocytopenia

Dose

- By intravenous infusion, 2.5–10 micrograms/kg/minute, adjusted according to response

Dobutamine (Non-proprietary) PoM
Strong sterile solution, dobutamine (as hydrochloride) 12.5 mg/mL. For dilution and use as an intravenous infusion. Net price 20-mL amp = £5.20

DOPAMINE HYDROCHLORIDE

Indications cardiogenic shock in infarction or cardiac surgery

Cautions correct hypovolaemia; low dose in shock due to acute myocardial infarction—see notes above; pregnancy (Appendix 4); **interactions:** Appendix 1 (sympathomimetics)

Contra-indications tachyarrhythmia, phaeochromocytoma

Side-effects nausea and vomiting, peripheral vasoconstriction, hypotension, hypertension, tachycardia

Dose

- By intravenous infusion, 2–5 micrograms/kg/minute initially (see notes above)

Dopamine (Non-proprietary) PoM
Sterile concentrate, dopamine hydrochloride 40 mg/mL, net price 5-mL amp = £3.88; 160 mg/mL, net price 5-mL amp = £14.75. For dilution and use as an intravenous infusion
Intravenous infusion, dopamine hydrochloride 1.6 mg/mL in glucose 5% intravenous infusion, net price 250-mL container (400 mg) = £11.69; 3.2 mg/mL, 250-mL container (800 mg) = £22.93 (both hosp. only)

Select-A-Jet® Dopamine (Celltech) PoM
Strong sterile solution, dopamine hydrochloride 40 mg/mL. Net price 5-mL vial = £5.01; 10-mL vial = £8.05. For dilution and use as an intravenous infusion

DOPEXAMINE HYDROCHLORIDE

Indications inotropic support and vasodilator in exacerbations of chronic heart failure and in heart failure associated with cardiac surgery

Cautions myocardial infarction, recent angina, hypokalaemia, hyperglycaemia; correct hypovolaemia before starting and during treatment, monitor blood pressure, pulse, plasma potassium, and blood glucose; avoid abrupt withdrawal; pregnancy; **interactions:** Appendix 1 (sympathomimetics)

Contra-indications left ventricular outlet obstruction such as hypertrophic cardiomyopathy or aortic stenosis; phaeochromocytoma, thrombocytopenia

Side-effects nausea, vomiting; tachycardia, bradycardia, arrhythmias, angina, myocardial infarction; tremor, headache; dyspnoea; reversible thrombocytopenia; sweating

Dose

- By intravenous infusion into central or large peripheral vein, 500 nanograms/kg/minute, may be increased to 1 microgram/kg/minute and further increased up to 6 micrograms/kg/minute in increments of 0.5–1 microgram/kg/minute at intervals of not less than 15 minutes

Dopacard® (Zeneus) PoM
Strong sterile solution, dopexamine hydrochloride 10 mg/mL (1%). For dilution and use as an intravenous infusion. Net price 5-mL amp = £21.00
Note Contact with metal in infusion apparatus should be minimised

2.7.2 Vasoconstrictor sympathomimetics

Vasoconstrictor sympathomimetics raise blood pressure transiently by acting on alpha-adrenergic receptors to constrict peripheral vessels. They are sometimes used as an emergency method of elevating blood pressure where other measures have failed (see also section 2.7.1).

The danger of vasoconstrictors is that although they raise blood pressure they also reduce perfusion of vital organs such as the kidney.

Spinal and epidural anaesthesia may result in sympathetic block with resultant hypotension. Management may include intravenous fluids (which are usually given prophylactically), oxygen, elevation of the legs, and injection of a pressor drug such as ephedrine. As well as constricting peripheral vessels **ephedrine** also accelerates the heart rate (by acting on beta receptors). Use is made of this dual action of ephedrine to manage associated bradycardia (although intravenous injection of atropine sulphate 400 to 600 micrograms may also be required if bradycardia persists).

EPHEDRINE HYDROCHLORIDE

Indications see under Dose

Cautions hyperthyroidism, diabetes mellitus, ischaemic heart disease, hypertension, susceptibility to angle-closure glaucoma, elderly, pregnancy (Appendix 4); may cause acute urine retention in prostatic hypertrophy; **interactions**: Appendix 1 (sympathomimetics)

Contra-indications breast-feeding (Appendix 5)

Side-effects nausea, vomiting, anorexia; tachycardia (sometimes bradycardia), arrhythmias, anginal pain, vasoconstriction with hypertension, vasodilation with hypotension, dizziness and flushing; dyspnoea; headache, anxiety, restlessness, confusion, psychoses, insomnia, tremor; difficulty in micturition, urine retention; sweating, hypersalivation; changes in blood-glucose concentration; *very rarely* angle-closure glaucoma

Dose

- Reversal of hypotension from spinal or epidural anaesthesia, by slow intravenous injection of a solution containing ephedrine hydrochloride 3 mg/mL, 3–6 mg (max. 9 mg) repeated every 3–4 minutes according to response to max. 30 mg

Ephedrine Hydrochloride (Non-proprietary) PoM
Injection, ephedrine hydrochloride 3 mg/mL, net price 10-mL amp = £2.83; 30 mg/mL, net price 1-mL amp = £1.70

METARAMINOL

Indications acute hypotension (see notes above); priapism (section 7.4.5) [unlicensed indication]

Cautions see under Noradrenaline Acid Tartrate; longer duration of action than noradrenaline (norepinephrine), see below; cirrhosis; pregnancy (Appendix 4); breast-feeding (Appendix 5)

Hypertensive response Metaraminol has a longer duration of action than noradrenaline, and an excessive vasopressor response may cause a prolonged rise in blood pressure

Contra-indications see under Noradrenaline Acid Tartrate

Side-effects see under Noradrenaline Acid Tartrate; tachycardia; fatal ventricular arrhythmia reported in Laennec's cirrhosis

Dose

- By intravenous infusion, 15–100 mg, adjusted according to response
- In emergency, by intravenous injection, 0.5–5 mg then by intravenous infusion, 15–100 mg, adjusted according to response

Metaraminol (Non-proprietary) PoM
Injection, metaraminol 10 mg (as tartrate)/mL.
Available from regional hospital manufacturing unit ('special order')

NORADRENALINE ACID TARTRATE/ NOREPINEPHRINE BITARTRATE

Indications see under dose

Cautions coronary, mesenteric, or peripheral vascular thrombosis; following myocardial infarction, Prinzmetal's variant angina, hyperthyroidism, diabetes mellitus; hypoxia or hypercapnia; uncorrected hypovolaemia; elderly; extravasation at injection site may cause necrosis; **interactions**: Appendix 1 (sympathomimetics)

Contra-indications hypertension (monitor blood pressure and rate of flow frequently); pregnancy (Appendix 4)

Side-effects hypertension, headache, bradycardia, arrhythmias, peripheral ischaemia

Dose

- Acute hypotension, by intravenous infusion, via central venous catheter, of a solution containing noradrenaline acid tartrate 80 micrograms/mL (equivalent to noradrenaline base 40 micrograms/mL) at an initial rate of 0.16–0.33 mL/minute, adjusted according to response
- Cardiac arrest, by rapid intravenous *or* intracardiac injection, 0.5–0.75 mL of a solution containing noradrenaline acid tartrate 200 micrograms/mL (equivalent to noradrenaline base 100 micrograms/mL)

Noradrenaline/Norepinephrine (Non-proprietary) PoM
Injection, noradrenaline acid tartrate 2 mg/mL (equivalent to noradrenaline base 1 mg/mL). For dilution before use. Net price 2-mL amp = £1.01, 4-mL amp = £1.50, 20-mL amp = £6.35

PHENYLEPHRINE HYDROCHLORIDE

Indications acute hypotension (see notes above); priapism (section 7.4.5) [unlicensed indication]

Cautions see under Noradrenaline Acid Tartrate; longer duration of action than noradrenaline (norepinephrine), see below; coronary disease

Hypertensive response Phenylephrine has a longer duration of action than noradrenaline, and an excessive vasopressor response may cause a prolonged rise in blood pressure

Contra-indications see under Noradrenaline Acid Tartrate; severe hyperthyroidism; pregnancy (Appendix 4)

Side-effects see under Noradrenaline Acid Tartrate; tachycardia or reflex bradycardia

Dose

- By subcutaneous *or* intramuscular injection, 2–5 mg, followed if necessary by further doses of 1–10 mg
- By slow intravenous injection of a 1 mg/mL solution, 100–500 micrograms repeated as necessary after at least 15 minutes
- By intravenous infusion, initial rate up to 180 micrograms/minute reduced to 30–60 micrograms/minute according to response

Phenylephrine (Sovereign) PoM
Injection, phenylephrine hydrochloride 10 mg/mL (1%). Net price 1-mL amp = £5.50

2.7.3 Cardiopulmonary resuscitation

The algorithm for cardiopulmonary resuscitation (see inside back cover) reflects the most recent recommendations of the Resuscitation Council (UK). These guidelines are available at www.resus.org.uk.

In cardiac arrest **adrenaline (epinephrine)** 1 in 10 000 (100 micrograms/mL) is recommended in a dose of 10 mL by intravenous injection, preferably through a central line. If injected through a peripheral line, the drug must be flushed with at least 20 mL sodium chloride 0.9% injection (to aid entry into the central circulation). Intravenous injection of **amiodarone** 300 mg *or* 5 mg/kg (from a prefilled syringe *or* diluted in 20 mL Glucose 5%) should be considered after adrenaline to treat ventricular fibrillation or pulseless ventricular tachycardia in cardiac arrest refractory to defibrillation. If ventricular fibrillation persists, an additional dose of amiodarone 150 mg (*or* 2.5 mg/kg) can be given. **Atropine** 3 mg by intravenous injection (section 15.1.3) as a single dose is also used in cardiopulmonary resuscitation to block vagal activity.

For the management of acute anaphylaxis see section 3.4.3.

ADRENALINE/EPINEPHRINE

Indications see notes above

Cautions heart disease, hypertension, arrhythmias, cerebrovascular disease, phaeochromocytoma; diabetes mellitus, hyperthyroidism; susceptibility to angle-closure glaucoma; elderly; **interactions:** Appendix 1 (sympathomimetics)

Side-effects nausea, vomiting; tachycardia, arrhythmias, palpitation, cold extremities, hypertension (risk of cerebral haemorrhage); dyspnoea, pulmonary oedema (on excessive dosage or extreme sensitivity); anxiety, tremor, restlessness, headache, weakness, dizziness; hyperglycaemia; urinary retention; sweating; tissue necrosis at injection site and angle-closure glaucoma also reported

Dose

- See notes above

Adrenaline/Epinephrine 1 in 10 000, Dilute (Non-proprietary) PoM

Injection, adrenaline (as acid tartrate) 100 micrograms/mL. 10-mL amp.

Brands include *Minijet® Adrenaline*

2.8 Anticoagulants and protamine

2.8.1 Parenteral anticoagulants
2.8.2 Oral anticoagulants
2.8.3 Protamine sulphate

The main use of anticoagulants is to prevent thrombus formation or extension of an existing thrombus in the slower-moving venous side of the circulation, where the thrombus consists of a fibrin web enmeshed with platelets and red cells. They are therefore widely used in the prevention and treatment of *deep-vein thrombosis in the legs.*

Anticoagulants are of less use in preventing thrombus formation in arteries, for in faster-flowing vessels thrombi are composed mainly of platelets with little fibrin. They are used to prevent thrombi forming on *prosthetic heart valves.*

2.8.1 Parenteral anticoagulants

Heparin

Heparin initiates anticoagulation rapidly but has a short duration of action. It is often referred to as '**standard**' or '**unfractionated heparin**' to distinguish it from the **low molecular weight heparins** (see p. 123), which have a longer duration of action. Although a low molecular weight heparin is generally preferred for routine use, heparin can be used in those at high risk of bleeding because its effect can be terminated rapidly by stopping the infusion.

Treatment For the initial treatment of deep-vein thrombosis and pulmonary embolism a low molecular weight heparin is used; alternatively, heparin is given as an intravenous loading dose, followed by continuous intravenous infusion (using an infusion pump) or by intermittent subcutaneous injection. Intermittent intravenous injection of heparin is no longer recommended. An oral anticoagulant (usually warfarin, section 2.8.2) is started at the same time as the heparin (the heparin needs to be continued for at least 5 days and until the INR has been in the therapeutic range for 2 consecutive days). Laboratory monitoring, preferably on a daily basis, is essential; determination of the activated partial thromboplastin time (APTT) is the most widely used measure. A low molecular weight heparin is also used in regimens for the management of myocardial infarction (section 2.10.1) and unstable angina (section 2.6).

Prophylaxis In patients undergoing general surgery, a low molecular weight heparin is effective for the prevention of postoperative deep-vein thrombosis and pulmonary embolism in 'high-risk' patients (i.e. those with obesity, malignant disease, history of deep-vein thrombosis or pulmonary embolism, patients over 40 years, or those with an established thrombophilic disorder or who are undergoing major or complicated surgery). Subcutaneous injection of low-dose heparin is an alternative; this regimen does not require laboratory monitoring.

To combat the increased risk in major orthopaedic surgery an adjusted dose regimen of heparin (with monitoring), low molecular weight heparin (p. 123) or fondaparinux (p. 126) can be used—a low molecular weight heparin is probably more effective.

Pregnancy Heparins are used for the management of thromboembolic disease in pregnancy because they do not cross the placenta. Low molecular weight heparins are preferred because they have a lower risk of osteoporosis and of heparin-induced thrombocytopenia. Low molecular weight heparins are eliminated more rapidly in pregnancy, requiring alteration of the dosage regimen for drugs such as dalteparin, enoxaparin, and tinzaparin. Treatment should be stopped at the onset of labour and advice sought from a specialist on continuing therapy after birth.

Extracorporeal circuits Heparin is also used in the maintenance of extracorporeal circuits in cardiopulmonary bypass and haemodialysis.

Haemorrhage If haemorrhage occurs it is usually sufficient to withdraw heparin, but if rapid reversal of the effects of heparin is required, protamine sulphate (section 2.8.3) is a specific antidote (but only partially reverses the effects of low molecular weight heparins).

HEPARIN

Indications see under Dose

Cautions see notes above; also elderly; hepatic impairment (Appendix 2); renal impairment (Appendix 3); pregnancy (Appendix 4); **interactions:** Appendix 1 (heparin)

Heparin-induced thrombocytopenia Clinically important heparin-induced thrombocytopenia is immune-mediated and does not usually develop until after 5–10 days; it can be complicated by thrombosis. Platelet counts should be measured just before treatment with heparin (including low molecular weight heparins) and regular monitoring of platelet counts is recommended if given for longer than 4 days. Signs of heparin-induced thrombocytopenia include a 50% reduction of platelet count, thrombosis, or skin allergy. If heparin-induced thrombocytopenia is strongly suspected or confirmed, heparin should be **stopped** and an alternative anticoagulant, such as lepirudin or danaparoid, should be given. Ensure platelet counts return to normal range in those who require warfarin

Hyperkalaemia Inhibition of aldosterone secretion by heparin (including low molecular weight heparins) can result in hyperkalaemia; patients with diabetes mellitus, chronic renal failure, acidosis, raised plasma potassium or those taking potassium-sparing drugs seem to be more susceptible. The risk appears to increase with duration of therapy and the CSM has recommended that plasma-potassium concentration should be measured in patients at risk of hyperkalaemia before starting heparin and monitored regularly thereafter, particularly if heparin is to be continued for longer than 7 days

Contra-indications haemophilia and other haemorrhagic disorders, thrombocytopenia (including history of heparin-induced thrombocytopenia), recent cerebral haemorrhage, severe hypertension; severe liver disease (including oesophageal varices), peptic ulcer; after major trauma or recent surgery to eye or nervous system; acute bacterial endocarditis; spinal or epidural anaesthesia with treatment doses of heparin; hypersensitivity to heparin or to low molecular weight heparins

Side-effects haemorrhage (see notes above), thrombocytopenia (see Cautions), *rarely* rebound hyperlipidaemia following heparin withdrawal, priapism, hyperkalaemia (see Cautions), osteoporosis (risk lower with low molecular weight heparins), alopecia on prolonged use, injection-site reactions, skin necrosis, and hypersensitivity reactions (including urticaria, angioedema, and anaphylaxis)

Dose

- Treatment of deep-vein thrombosis, pulmonary embolism, unstable angina, and acute peripheral arterial occlusion, by intravenous injection, loading dose of 5000 units *or* 75 units/kg (10 000 units in severe pulmonary embolism), followed by continuous intravenous infusion of 18 units/kg/hour *or* treatment of deep-vein thrombosis, by subcutaneous injection of 15 000 units every 12 hours (laboratory monitoring essential—preferably on a daily basis, and dose adjusted accordingly); CHILD under 18 years *see* BNF for Children
- Prophylaxis in orthopaedic surgery, see notes above
- Prophylaxis in general and gynaecological surgery (see notes above), by subcutaneous injection, 5000 units 2 hours before surgery, then every 8–12 hours for 7–10 days or until patient is ambulant (monitoring not needed); during pregnancy (with monitoring), 5000–10 000 units every 12 hours (**important**: prevention of prosthetic heart-valve thrombosis in pregnancy calls for **specialist management**)
- Myocardial infarction, see notes above
- Prevention of clotting in extracorporeal circuits, consult product literature

> Doses above reflect the guidelines of the British Society for Haematology; for doses of the low molecular weight heparins, see below

Heparin (Non-proprietary) PoM
Injection, heparin sodium 1000 units/mL, net price 1-mL amp = 19p, 5-mL amp = 85p, 5-mL vial = 47p, 10-mL amp = £1.46, 20-mL amp = £2.40; 5000 units/mL, 1-mL amp = 36p, 5-mL amp = £1.00, 5-mL vial = 92p; 25 000 units/mL, 1-mL amp = £1.01, 5-mL vial = £3.68

Monoparin® (CP) PoM
Injection, heparin sodium (mucous) 1000 units/mL, net price 1-mL amp = 28p; 5-mL amp = 52p; 10-mL amp = 69p; 20-mL amp = £1.24; 5000 units/mL, 1-mL amp = 54p; 5-mL amp = 74p; 25 000 units/mL, 0.2-mL amp = 46p, 1-mL amp = £1.52

Monoparin Calcium® (CP) PoM
Injection, heparin calcium 25 000 units/mL, net price 0.2-mL amp = 73p

Multiparin® (CP) PoM
Injection, heparin sodium (mucous) 1000 units/mL, net price 5-mL vial = 70p; 5000 units/mL, 5-mL vial = £1.57; 25 000 units/mL, 5-mL vial = £5.93
Excipients include benzyl alcohol (avoid in neonates, see Excipients, p. 2)

Low molecular weight heparins

Low molecular weight heparins (**bemiparin, dalteparin, enoxaparin,** and **tinzaparin**) are usually preferred over unfractionated heparin in the *prevention* of venous thromboembolism because they are as effective and they have a lower risk of heparin-induced thrombocytopenia. Also, the standard prophylactic regimen does not require monitoring. In orthopaedic practice low molecular weight heparins are probably more effective than unfractionated heparin; fondaparinux (p. 126) can also be used. The duration of action of low molecular weight heparins is longer than that of unfractionated heparin; *once-daily subcutaneous* dosage means that they are convenient to use.

Low molecular weight heparins are also used in the *treatment* of deep-vein thrombosis, pulmonary embolism, unstable coronary artery disease (section 2.6) and for the prevention of clotting in extracorporeal circuits.

Routine monitoring of anti-Factor Xa activity is not usually required during treatment with low molecular weight heparins, but may be necessary in patients at increased risk of bleeding (e.g. in renal impairment and those who are underweight or overweight).

Haemorrhage See under Heparin.

Pregnancy See under Heparin.

BEMIPARIN SODIUM

Indications see notes above and under preparations
Cautions see under Heparin and notes above
Contra-indications see under Heparin; breast-feeding (Appendix 5)
Side-effects see under Heparin
Dose
- See under preparations below

Zibor® (Amdipharm) ▼ PoM
Injection, bemiparin sodium 12 500 units/mL, net price 0.2-mL (2500-unit) prefilled syringe = £3.39; 17 500 units/mL, 0.2-mL (3500-unit) prefilled syringe = £4.52
Dose prophylaxis of deep-vein thrombosis, by subcutaneous injection, moderate risk, 2500 units 2 hours before or 6 hours after surgery then 2500 units every 24 hours for 7–10 days; high risk, 3500 units 2 hours before or 6 hours after surgery then 3500 units every 24 hours for 7–10 days
Prevention of clotting in extracorporeal circuits, consult product literature

Injection, bemiparin sodium 25 000 units/mL, net price 0.2-mL (5000-unit) prefilled syringe = £6.96, 0.3-mL (7500-unit) prefilled syringe = £8.63, 0.4-mL (10 000-unit) prefilled syringe = £12.60
Dose treatment of deep-vein thrombosis (with or without pulmonary embolism), by subcutaneous injection, 115 units/kg every 24 hours for 5–9 days (and until adequate oral anti-coagulation established)

2 Cardiovascular system

DALTEPARIN SODIUM

Indications see notes above and under preparations
Cautions see under Heparin and notes above
Contra-indications see under Heparin
Side-effects see under Heparin
Dose
- See under preparations below

Fragmin® (Pharmacia) PoM
Injection (single-dose syringe), dalteparin sodium 12 500 units/mL, net price 0.2-mL (2500-unit) syringe = £1.86; 25 000 units/mL, 0.2-mL (5000-unit) syringe = £2.82, 0.3-mL (7500-unit) syringe = £4.23, 0.4-mL (10 000-unit) syringe = £5.65, 0.5-mL (12 500-unit) syringe = £7.06, 0.6-mL (15 000-unit) syringe = £8.47, 0.72-mL (18 000-unit) syringe = £10.16
Dose prophylaxis of deep-vein thrombosis, in surgical patients, by subcutaneous injection, moderate risk, 2500 units 1–2 hours before surgery then 2500 units every 24 hours for 5–7 days or longer; high risk, 2500 units 1–2 hours before surgery, then 2500 units 8–12 hours later (*or* 5000 units on the evening before surgery, then 5000 units on the following evening), then 5000 units every 24 hours for 5–7 days or longer (5 weeks in hip replacement)
Prophylaxis of deep-vein thrombosis in medical patients, by subcutaneous injection, 5000 units every 24 hours
Treatment of deep-vein thrombosis and of pulmonary embolism, by subcutaneous injection, as a single daily dose, ADULT body-weight under 46 kg, 7500 units daily; body-weight 46–56 kg, 10 000 units daily; body-weight 57–68 kg, 12 500 units daily; body-weight 69–82 kg, 15 000 units daily; body-weight 83 kg and over, 18 000 units daily, with oral anticoagulant treatment until prothrombin complex concentration in therapeutic range (usually for at least 5 days); monitoring of anti-Factor Xa not usually required; for patients at increased risk of haemorrhage, see below
Treatment of thromboembolic disease in pregnancy [unlicensed indication], by subcutaneous injection, early pregnancy body-weight under 50 kg, 5000 units twice daily; body-weight 50–70 kg, 6000 units twice daily; body-weight 70–90 kg, 8000 units twice daily; body-weight over 90 kg, 10 000 units twice daily

Injection, dalteparin sodium 2500 units/mL (for subcutaneous or intravenous use), net price 4-mL (10 000-unit) amp = £5.12; 10 000-units/mL (for subcutaneous or intravenous use), 1-mL (10 000-unit) amp = £5.12; 25 000 units/mL (for subcutaneous use only), 4-mL (100 000-unit) vial = £48.66
Dose treatment of deep-vein thrombosis and of pulmonary embolism, by subcutaneous injection, 200 units/kg (max. 18 000 units) as a single daily dose (*or* 100 units/kg twice daily if increased risk of haemorrhage) with oral anticoagulant treatment until prothrombin complex concentration in therapeutic range (usually for at least 5 days)
Note For monitoring, blood should be taken 3–4 hours after a dose (recommended plasma concentration of anti-Factor Xa 0.5–1 unit/mL); monitoring not required for once-daily treatment regimen and not generally necessary for twice-daily regimen
Unstable coronary artery disease, by subcutaneous injection, 120 units/kg every 12 hours (max. 10 000 units twice daily) for 5–8 days
Prevention of clotting in extracorporeal circuits, consult product literature

Injection (graduated syringe), dalteparin sodium 10 000 units/mL, net price 1-mL (10 000-unit) syringe = £5.65
Dose unstable coronary artery disease (including non-ST-segment-elevation myocardial infarction), by subcutaneous injection, 120 units/kg every 12 hours (max. 10 000 units twice daily) for up to 8 days; beyond 8 days (if awaiting angiography or revascularisation) women body-weight less than 80 kg and men less than 70 kg, 5000 units every 12 hours, women body-weight greater than 80 kg and men greater than 70 kg, 7500 units every 12 hours, until day of procedure (max. 45 days)

ENOXAPARIN SODIUM

Indications see notes above and under preparations
Cautions see under Heparin and notes above; low body-weight (increased risk of bleeding)
Contra-indications see under Heparin; breast-feeding (Appendix 5)
Side-effects see under Heparin
Dose
- See under preparation below

Clexane® (Rhône-Poulenc Rorer) PoM
Injection, enoxaparin sodium 100 mg/mL, net price 0.2-mL (20-mg, 2000-units) syringe = £3.15, 0.4-mL (40-mg, 4000-units) syringe = £4.20, 0.6-mL (60-mg, 6000-units) syringe = £4.75, 0.8-mL (80-mg, 8000-units) syringe = £5.40, 1-mL (100-mg, 10 000-units) syringe = £6.69; 3-mL (300 mg, 30 000-units) vial (*Clexane® Multidose*) = £22.20; 150 mg/mL (*Clexane® Forte*), 0.8-mL (120-mg, 12 000-units) syringe = £9.77, 1-mL (150-mg, 15 000-units) syringe = £11.10
Dose prophylaxis of deep-vein thrombosis especially in surgical patients, by subcutaneous injection, *moderate risk*, 20 mg (2000 units) approx. 2 hours before surgery then 20 mg (2000 units) every 24 hours for 7–10 days; *high risk* (e.g. orthopaedic surgery), 40 mg (4000 units) 12 hours before surgery then 40 mg (4000 units) every 24 hours for 7–10 days
Prophylaxis of deep-vein thrombosis in medical patients, by subcutaneous injection, 40 mg (4000 units) every 24 hours for at least 6 days and continued until patient ambulant (max. 14 days)
Treatment of deep-vein thrombosis or pulmonary embolism, by subcutaneous injection, 1.5 mg/kg (150 units/kg) every 24 hours, usually for at least 5 days (and until adequate oral anticoagulation established)
Unstable angina and non-ST-segment-elevation myocardial infarction, by subcutaneous injection, 1 mg/kg (100 units/kg) every 12 hours usually for 2–8 days (minimum 2 days)
Prevention of clotting in extracorporeal circuits, consult product literature
Treatment of thromboembolic disease in pregnancy [unlicensed indication], by subcutaneous injection, early pregnancy body-weight under 50 kg, 40 mg (4000 units) twice daily; body-weight 50–70 kg, 60 mg (6000 units) twice daily; body-weight 70–90 kg, 80 mg (8000 units) twice daily; body-weight over 90 kg, 100 mg (10 000 units) twice daily

TINZAPARIN SODIUM

Indications see notes above and under preparations
Cautions see under Heparin and notes above
Contra-indications see under Heparin; breast-feeding (Appendix 5)
Side-effects see under Heparin
Dose
- See under preparations below

Innohep® (LEO) PoM

Injection, tinzaparin sodium 10 000 units/mL, net price 2500-unit (0.25-mL) syringe = £2.13, 3500-unit (0.35-mL) syringe = £2.98, 4500-unit (0.45-mL) syringe = £3.83, 20 000-unit (2-mL) vial = £11.36

Dose prophylaxis of deep-vein thrombosis, by subcutaneous injection, general surgery, 3500 units 2 hours before surgery, then 3500 units every 24 hours for 7–10 days; orthopaedic surgery (high risk), 50 units/kg 2 hours before surgery, then 50 units/kg every 24 hours for 7–10 days *or* 4500 units 12 hours before surgery, then 4500 units every 24 hours for 7–10 days

Prevention of clotting in extracorporeal circuits, consult product literature

Injection, tinzaparin sodium 20 000 units/mL, net price 0.5-mL (10 000-unit) syringe = £9.65, 0.7-mL (14 000-unit) syringe = £13.51, 0.9-mL (18 000-unit) syringe = £17.37, 2-mL (40 000-unit) vial = £36.77

Dose treatment of deep-vein thrombosis and of pulmonary embolism, by subcutaneous injection, 175 units/kg once daily for at least 6 days (and until adequate oral anticoagulation established)

Treatment of thromboembolic disease in pregnancy [unlicensed indication], by subcutaneous injection, 175 units/kg once daily

Note Treatment regimens do not require anticoagulation monitoring

Asthma Presence of sulphites in formulation may (especially in patients with asthma) lead to hypersensitivity (with bronchospasm and shock)

Heparinoids

Danaparoid is a heparinoid used for prophylaxis of deep-vein thrombosis in patients undergoing general or orthopaedic surgery. Providing there is no evidence of cross-reactivity, it also has a role in patients who develop thrombocytopenia in association with heparin.

DANAPAROID SODIUM

Indications prevention of deep-vein thrombosis in general or orthopaedic surgery; thromboembolic disease in patients with history of heparin-induced thrombocytopenia
Cautions recent bleeding or risk of bleeding; antibodies to heparins (risk of antibody-induced thrombocytopenia); body-weight over 90 kg (monitor anti factor Xa activity); hepatic impairment (Appendix 2); renal impairment (Appendix 3); pregnancy (Appendix 4); breast-feeding (Appendix 5)
Contra-indications haemophilia and other haemorrhagic disorders, thrombocytopenia (unless patient has heparin-induced thrombocytopenia), recent cerebral haemorrhage, severe hypertension, active peptic ulcer (unless this is the reason for operation), diabetic retinopathy, acute bacterial endocarditis, spinal or epidural anaesthesia with treatment doses of danaparoid
Side-effects bleeding; hypersensitivity reactions (including rash)
Dose
- Prevention of deep-vein thrombosis, by subcutaneous injection, 750 units twice daily for 7–10 days; initiate treatment before operation (with last pre-operative dose 1–4 hours before surgery)
- Thromboembolic disease in patients with history of heparin-induced thrombocytopenia, by intravenous injection, 2500 units (1250 units if body-weight under 55 kg, 3750 units if over 90 kg), followed by intravenous infusion of 400 units/hour for 2 hours, *then* 300 units/hour for 2 hours, *then* 200 units/hour for 5 days

Orgaran® (Organon) PoM

Injection, danaparoid sodium 1250 units/mL, net price 0.6-mL amp (750 units) = £29.80

Hirudins

Lepirudin, a recombinant hirudin, is licensed for anticoagulation in patients with Type II (immune) heparin-induced thrombocytopenia who require parenteral antithrombotic treatment. The dose of lepirudin is adjusted according to activated partial thromboplastin time (APTT). **Bivalirudin**, a hirudin analogue, is a thrombin inhibitor which is licensed as an anticoagulant for patients undergoing percutaneous coronary intervention. The *Scottish Medicines Consortium* has advised (March 2005) that bivalirudin is accepted for restricted use for patients undergoing percutaneous coronary intervention who would have been considered for treatment with unfractionated heparin combined with a glycoprotein IIb/IIIa inhibitor; it should not be used alone.

BIVALIRUDIN

Indications anticoagulation for patients undergoing percutaneous coronary intervention
Cautions exposure to lepirudin (theoretical risk from lepirudin antibodies); brachytherapy procedures; renal impairment (avoid if creatinine clearance less than 30 mL/minute; Appendix 3); pregnancy (Appendix 4); breast-feeding (Appendix 5)
Contra-indications severe hypertension; subacute bacterial endocarditis; active bleeding; bleeding disorders
Side-effects bleeding (discontinue); *less commonly* nausea, vomiting, tachycardia, bradycardia, hypotension, angina, dyspnoea, allergic reactions (including isolated reports of anaphylaxis), headache, thrombocytopenia, anaemia, back and chest pain, and injection-site reactions; *very rarely* thrombosis
Dose
- Initially by intravenous injection, 750 micrograms/kg then by intravenous infusion 1.75 mg/kg/hour for up to 4 hours after procedure

Angiox® (Nycomed) ▼ PoM

Injection, powder for reconstitution, bivalirudin, net price 250-mg vial = £310.00

LEPIRUDIN

Indications thromboembolic disease requiring parenteral anticoagulation in patients with heparin-induced thrombocytopenia type II

Cautions hepatic impairment (Appendix 2); renal impairment (Appendix 3); recent bleeding or risk of bleeding including recent puncture of large vessels, organ biopsy, recent major surgery, stroke, bleeding disorders, severe hypertension, bacterial endocarditis; determine activated partial thromboplastin time 4 hours after start of treatment (or after infusion rate altered) and at least once daily thereafter

Contra-indications pregnancy and breast-feeding

Side-effects bleeding; reduced haemoglobin concentration without obvious source of bleeding; fever, hypersensitivity reactions (including rash); injection-site reactions

Dose

- Initially by slow intravenous injection (of 5 mg/mL solution), 400 micrograms/kg followed by continuous intravenous infusion of 150 micrograms/kg/hour (max. 16.5 mg/hour), adjusted according to activated partial thromboplastin time, for 2–10 days (longer if necessary)

Refludan® (Pharmion) PoM

Injection, powder for reconstitution, lepirudin. Net price 50-mg vial = £57.00

Heparin flushes

For maintaining patency of peripheral venous catheters, sodium chloride injection 0.9% is as effective as heparin flushes.

Heparin Sodium (Non-proprietary) PoM

Solution, heparin sodium 10 units/mL, net price 5-mL amp = 25p; 100 units/mL, 2-mL amp = 28p

Dose to maintain patency of catheters, cannulas, etc. 10–200 units flushed through every 4–8 hours. Not for therapeutic use

Canusal® (CP) PoM

Solution, heparin sodium 100 units/mL. Net price 2-mL amp = 57p

Dose to maintain patency of catheters, cannulas, etc., 200 units flushed through every 4 hours or as required. Not for therapeutic use

Hepsal® (CP) PoM

Solution, heparin sodium 10 units/mL. Net price 5-mL amp = 54p

Dose to maintain patency of catheters, cannulas, etc., 50 units flushed through every 4 hours or as required. Not for therapeutic use

Epoprostenol

Epoprostenol (prostacyclin) can be given to inhibit platelet aggregation during renal dialysis either alone or with heparin. It is also licensed for the treatment of primary pulmonary hypertension resistant to other treatment, usually with oral anticoagulation. Since its half-life is only about 3 minutes it must be given by continuous intravenous infusion. It is a potent vasodilator and therefore its side-effects include flushing, headache, and hypotension.

EPOPROSTENOL

Indications see notes above

Cautions anticoagulant monitoring required when given with heparin; haemorrhagic diathesis; dose titration for pulmonary hypertension should be in hospital (risk of pulmonary oedema); pregnancy (Appendix 4)

Contra-indications severe left ventricular dysfunction

Side-effects see notes above; also bradycardia, tachycardia, pallor, sweating with higher doses; gastro-intestinal disturbances; lassitude, anxiety, agitation; dry mouth, jaw pain, chest pain; also reported, hyperglycaemia and injection-site reactions

Dose

- See product literature

Flolan® (GSK) PoM

Infusion, powder for reconstitution, epoprostenol (as sodium salt). Net price 500-microgram vial (with diluent) = £64.57; 1.5-mg vial (with diluent) = £130.07

Fondaparinux

Fondaparinux sodium is a synthetic pentasaccharide that inhibits activated factor X.

FONDAPARINUX SODIUM

Indications prophylaxis of venous thromboembolism in medical patients immobilised due to acute illness, and patients undergoing major orthopaedic surgery of the legs or abdominal surgery; treatment of deep-vein thrombosis and of pulmonary embolism; treatment of unstable angina or non-ST-segment elevation myocardial infarction; treatment of ST-segment elevation myocardial infarction

Cautions bleeding disorders, active gastro-intestinal ulcer disease; recent intracranial haemorrhage; brain, spinal, or ophthalmic surgery; spinal or epidural anaesthesia (risk of spinal haematoma—avoid if using treatment doses); risk of catheter thrombus during percutaneous coronary intervention; low body-weight; elderly patients; concomitant use of drugs that increase risk of bleeding; hepatic impairment (Appendix 2); renal impairment (Appendix 3); pregnancy (Appendix 4); breast-feeding (Appendix 5)

Contra-indications active bleeding; bacterial endocarditis

Side-effects bleeding, purpura, anaemia; *less commonly* gastro-intestinal disturbances, oedema, hepatic impairment, chest pain, dyspnoea, thrombocytopenia, thrombocythaemia, rash, pruritus; *rarely* hypotension, flushing, cough, vertigo, dizziness, anxiety, drowsiness, confusion, headache, hypokalaemia, hyperbilirubinaemia, injection-site reactions; also reported atrial fibrillation, tachycardia, and pyrexia

Dose

- See under preparation below

Arixtra® (GSK) ▼ PoM

Injection, fondaparinux sodium 5 mg/mL, net price 0.3-mL (1.5-mg) prefilled syringe = £6.67

Dose prophylaxis of venous thromboembolism after surgery, by subcutaneous injection, 2.5 mg 6 hours after surgery then 2.5 mg once daily for 5–9 days (longer after hip surgery); CHILD under 17 years not recommended

Prophylaxis of venous thromboembolism in medical patients, by subcutaneous injection, 2.5 mg once daily usually for 6–14 days; CHILD under 17 years not recommended

Injection, fondaparinux sodium 5 mg/mL, net price 0.5-mL (2.5-mg) prefilled syringe = £6.66

Dose prophylaxis of venous thromboembolism after surgery, by subcutaneous injection, 2.5 mg 6 hours after surgery then 2.5 mg once daily for 5–9 days (longer after hip surgery); CHILD under 17 years not recommended

Prophylaxis of venous thromboembolism in medical patients, by subcutaneous injection, 2.5 mg once daily usually for 6–14 days; CHILD under 17 years not recommended
Unstable angina and non-ST-segment elevation myocardial infarction, by subcutaneous injection, 2.5 mg once daily for up to 8 days (or until hospital discharge if sooner); CHILD under 17 years not recommended
ST-segment elevation myocardial infarction, initially by intravenous injection or infusion, 2.5 mg for first day, thereafter by subcutaneous injection 2.5 mg once daily for up to 8 days (or until hospital discharge if sooner); CHILD under 17 years not recommended

Injection, fondaparinux sodium 12.5 mg/mL, net price 0.4-mL (5-mg) prefilled syringe = £12.37, 0.6-mL (7.5-mg) prefilled syringe = £12.37, 0.8-mL (10-mg) prefilled syringe = £12.37
Dose treatment of deep-vein thrombosis and of pulmonary embolism, by subcutaneous injection, ADULT body-weight under 50 kg, 5 mg every 24 hours; body-weight 50–100 kg, 7.5 mg every 24 hours; body-weight over 100 kg, 10 mg every 24 hours; usually for at least 5 days (and until adequate oral anticoagulation established); CHILD under 17 years not recommended

2.8.2 Oral anticoagulants

Oral anticoagulants antagonise the effects of vitamin K, and take at least 48 to 72 hours for the anticoagulant effect to develop fully; if an immediate effect is required, heparin must be given concomitantly.

Uses The main indication for an oral anticoagulant is *deep-vein thrombosis.* Patients with *pulmonary embolism* should also be treated, as should those with *atrial fibrillation who are at risk of embolisation* (see also section 2.3.1), and those with *mechanical prosthetic heart valves* (to prevent emboli developing on the valves); an antiplatelet drug may also be useful in these patients but this combination increases the risk of bleeding.

Warfarin is the drug of choice; **acenocoumarol** (nicoumalone) and **phenindione** are seldom required.

Oral anticoagulants should not be used in cerebral artery thrombosis or peripheral artery occlusion as first-line therapy; aspirin (section 2.9) is more appropriate for reduction of risk in transient ischaemic attacks. Heparin or a low molecular weight heparin (section 2.8.1) is usually preferred for the prophylaxis of venous thromboembolism in patients undergoing surgery; alternatively, warfarin can be continued in selected patients currently taking long-term warfarin and who are at high risk of thromboembolism (seek expert advice).

Dose Whenever possible, the base-line prothrombin time should be determined but the initial dose should not be delayed whilst awaiting the result.

For patients who require rapid anticoagulation the usual adult induction dose of warfarin is 10 mg[1] on the first day; subsequent doses depend upon the prothrombin time, reported as INR (international normalised ratio). For patients who do not require rapid anticoagulation, a lower loading dose can be used over 3–4 weeks. The daily maintenance dose of warfarin is usually 3–9 mg (taken at the **same time** each day). The following indications and target INRs[2] take into account recommendations of the British Society for Haematology[3]:

- INR 2.5 for treatment of deep-vein thrombosis and pulmonary embolism (including those associated with antiphospholipid syndrome or for recurrence in patients no longer receiving warfarin), for atrial fibrillation, cardioversion (higher target values, such as an INR of 3, can be used for up to 4 weeks before the procedure to avoid cancellations due to low INR), dilated cardiomyopathy, mural thrombus, symptomatic inherited thrombophilia, coronary artery thrombosis (if anticoagulated), and paroxysmal nocturnal haemoglobinuria;
- INR 3.5 for recurrent deep-vein thrombosis and pulmonary embolism (in patients currently receiving warfarin with INR above 2);
- For mechanical prosthetic heart valves, the recommended target INR depends on the type and location of the valve. Generally, a target INR of 3 is recommended for mechanical aortic valves, and 3.5 for mechanical mitral valves.

Monitoring It is essential that the INR be determined daily or on alternate days in early days of treatment, *then* at longer intervals (depending on response[4]) *then* up to every 12 weeks.

Haemorrhage The main adverse effect of all oral anticoagulants is haemorrhage. Checking the INR and omitting doses when appropriate is essential; if the anticoagulant is stopped but not reversed, the INR should be measured 2–3 days later to ensure that it is falling. The following recommendations (which take into account the recommendations of the British Society for Haematology[3]) are based on the result of the INR and whether there is major or minor bleeding; the recommendations apply to patients taking warfarin:

- Major bleeding—stop warfarin; give phytomenadione (vitamin K_1) 5–10 mg by slow intravenous injection; give prothrombin complex concentrate (factors II, VII, IX, and X) 30–50 units/kg *or* (if no concentrate available) fresh frozen plasma 15 mL/kg
- INR > 8.0, no bleeding or minor bleeding—stop warfarin, restart when INR < 5.0; if there are other risk factors for bleeding give phytomenadione (vitamin K_1) 500 micrograms by slow intravenous injection or 5 mg by mouth (for partial reversal of anticoagulation give smaller oral doses of phytomenadione e.g. 0.5–2.5 mg using the intra-

1. First dose reduced if base-line prothrombin time prolonged, if liver-function tests abnormal, or if patient in cardiac failure, on parenteral feeding, less than average body weight, elderly, or receiving other drugs known to potentiate oral anticoagulants.

2. An INR which is within 0.5 units of the target value is generally satisfactory; larger deviations require dosage adjustment. Target values (rather than ranges) are now recommended.
3. Guidelines on Oral Anticoagulation (warfarin): third edition—2005 update. *Br J Haematol* 2005; **132**: 277–285.
4. Change in patient's clinical condition, particularly associated with liver disease, intercurrent illness, or drug administration, necessitates more frequent testing. See also **interactions**, Appendix 1 (warfarin). Major changes in diet (especially involving salads and vegetables) and in alcohol consumption may also affect warfarin control.

venous preparation orally); repeat dose of phytomenadione if INR still too high after 24 hours

- INR 6.0–8.0, no bleeding or minor bleeding—stop warfarin, restart when INR < 5.0
- INR < 6.0 but more than 0.5 units above target value—reduce dose or stop warfarin, restart when INR < 5.0
- Unexpected bleeding at therapeutic levels—always investigate possibility of underlying cause e.g. unsuspected renal or gastro-intestinal tract pathology

Pregnancy Oral anticoagulants are teratogenic and should not be given in the first trimester of pregnancy. Women of child-bearing age should be warned of this danger since stopping warfarin before the sixth week of gestation may largely avoid the risk of fetal abnormality. Oral anticoagulants cross the placenta with risk of placental or fetal haemorrhage, especially during the last few weeks of pregnancy and at delivery. Therefore, if at all possible, oral anticoagulants should be avoided in pregnancy, especially in the first and third trimesters. Difficult decisions may have to be made, particularly in women with prosthetic heart valves, atrial fibrillation, or with a history of recurrent venous thrombosis or pulmonary embolism.

Treatment booklets Anticoagulant treatment booklets should be issued to patients, and are available for distribution to local healthcare professionals from Health Authorities and from:

England and Wales:
RR Donnelley Global Document Solutions (formerly Astron)
Causeway Distribution Centre
Oldham Broadway Business Park
Chadderton
Oldham OL9 9XD
(0161) 683 2376

Scotland:
Banner Business Supplies
20 South Gyle Crescent
Edinburgh EH12 9EB
(0131) 479 3279

Northern Ireland:
Central Services Agency
25 Adelaide St
Belfast BT2 8FH
(028) 9053 5652

These booklets include advice for patients on anticoagulant treatment. Electronic copies are also available at www.npsa.nhs.uk/health/alerts.

WARFARIN SODIUM

Indications prophylaxis of embolisation in rheumatic heart disease and atrial fibrillation; prophylaxis after insertion of prosthetic heart valve; prophylaxis and treatment of venous thrombosis and pulmonary embolism; transient ischaemic attacks

Cautions see notes above; also recent surgery; bacterial endocarditis (increased risk of bleeding; avoid use to reduce risk of emboli if warfarin not otherwise indicated); hepatic impairment (Appendix 2); breast-feeding (Appendix 5); avoid cranberry juice; **interactions:** Appendix 1 (coumarins)

Contra-indications peptic ulcer, severe hypertension; renal impairment (avoid if creatinine clearance less than 10 mL/minute); pregnancy (see notes above and Appendix 4)

Side-effects haemorrhage—see notes above; other side-effects reported include hypersensitivity, rash, alopecia, diarrhoea, unexplained drop in haematocrit, 'purple toes', skin necrosis, jaundice, hepatic dysfunction; also nausea, vomiting, and pancreatitis

Dose

- See notes above

Warfarin (Non-proprietary) PoM
Tablets, warfarin sodium 0.5 mg (white), net price 28-tab pack = 71p; 1 mg (brown), 28 = 40p; 3 mg (blue), 28 = 46p; 5 mg (pink), 28 = 63p. Label: 10, anticoagulant card
Brands include *Marevan*®

ACENOCOUMAROL
(Nicoumalone)

Indications see under Warfarin Sodium

Cautions see under Warfarin Sodium

Contra-indications see under Warfarin Sodium

Side-effects see under Warfarin Sodium

Dose

- 4–12 mg on first day, 4–8 mg on second day, maintenance dose usually 1–8 mg daily

Sinthrome® (Alliance) PoM
Tablets, acenocoumarol 1 mg. Net price 20 = 92p. Label: 10, anticoagulant card

PHENINDIONE

Indications prophylaxis of embolisation in rheumatic heart disease and atrial fibrillation; prophylaxis after insertion of prosthetic heart valve; prophylaxis and treatment of venous thrombosis and pulmonary embolism

Cautions see under Warfarin Sodium; **interactions:** Appendix 1 (phenindione)

Contra-indications see under Warfarin Sodium; breast-feeding (Appendix 5)

Side-effects see under Warfarin Sodium; also hypersensitivity reactions including rashes, exfoliative dermatitis, exanthema, fever, leucopenia, agranulocytosis, eosinophilia, diarrhoea, renal and hepatic damage; urine coloured pink or orange

Dose

- 200 mg on day 1; 100 mg on day 2; maintenance dose usually 50–150 mg daily

Phenindione (Non-proprietary) PoM
Tablets, phenindione 10 mg, net price 100 = £14.50; 25 mg, 100 = £16.57; 50 mg, 100 = £21.14. Label: 10, anticoagulant card, 14, (urine pink or orange)

2.8.3 Protamine sulphate

Protamine sulphate is used to treat overdosage of heparin, including low molecular weight heparins. The long half-life of low molecular weight heparins should be taken into consideration when estimating the dose of protamine sulphate; the effects of low molecular weight heparins may persist for up to 24 hours after administration. Excessive doses of protamine sulphate can have an anticoagulant effect.

PROTAMINE SULPHATE
(Protamine Sulfate)

Indications see above

Cautions see above; also monitor activated partial thromboplastin time or other appropriate blood clotting parameters; increased risk of allergic reaction to protamine (including previous treatment with protamine or protamine insulin, allergy to fish, men who are infertile or who have had a vasectomy)

Side-effects nausea, vomiting, lassitude, flushing, hypotension, hypertension, bradycardia, dyspnoea, rebound bleeding, back pain; hypersensitivity reactions (including angioedema, anaphylaxis) and pulmonary oedema reported

Dose
- Overdosage with intravenous injection of heparin, by intravenous injection (rate not exceeding 5 mg/ minute), 1 mg neutralises 80–100 units heparin when given within 15 minutes of heparin; if longer than 15 minutes since heparin, less protamine required (consult product literature for details) as heparin rapidly excreted; max. 50 mg
- Overdosage with intravenous infusion of heparin, by intravenous injection (rate not exceeding 5 mg/ minute), 25–50 mg once heparin infusion stopped
- Overdosage with subcutaneous injection of heparin, 1 mg neutralises 100 units heparin; give 25–50 mg by intravenous injection (rate not exceeding 5 mg/ minute) and remainder of dose by intravenous infusion over 8–16 hours
- Overdosage with subcutaneous injection of low molecular weight heparin, by intermittent intravenous injection (rate not exceeding 5 mg/minute) or by continuous intravenous infusion, 1 mg neutralises approx. 100 units low molecular weight heparin (consult product literature of low molecular weight heparin for details); max. 50 mg when given by intermittent intravenous injection

Protamine Sulphate (Non-proprietary) PoM
Injection, protamine sulphate 10 mg /mL, net price 5-mL amp = £1.14, 10-mL amp = £3.96

Prosulf® (CP) PoM
Injection, protamine sulphate 10 mg/mL. Net price 5-mL amp = 96p (glass), £1.20 (polypropylene)

2.9 Antiplatelet drugs

Antiplatelet drugs decrease platelet aggregation and may inhibit thrombus formation in the arterial circulation, where anticoagulants have little effect.

A single dose of aspirin 300 mg is given as soon as possible after an ischaemic event, preferably dispersed in water or chewed. The initial dose is followed by long-term treatment of aspirin 75 mg daily in order to prevent further cardiovascular disease events.

Long-term use of aspirin, in a dose of 75 mg daily, is also of benefit for all patients with established cardiovascular disease, for patients with a 10-year cardiovascular disease risk[1] of 20% or more and aged over 50 years, for patients with diabetes aged over 50 years or who have had diabetes for more than 10 years, and for patients with diabetes who are receiving antihypertensive treatment. Unduly high blood pressure must be controlled before aspirin is given.

Aspirin in a dose of 75 mg daily is also given following coronary bypass surgery. For details on the use of aspirin in atrial fibrillation see section 2.3.1, for stable angina see section 2.6 and for intermittent claudication see section 2.6.4.

If the patient is at a high risk of gastro-intestinal bleeding, a proton pump inhibitor (section 1.3.5) can be added.

Clopidogrel is licensed for the prevention of ischaemic events in patients with a history of symptomatic ischaemic disease. Clopidogrel, in combination with low-dose aspirin, is also licensed for acute coronary syndrome without ST-segment elevation; in these circumstances the combination is usually given for 12 months (there is no evidence of benefit beyond 12 months). Clopidogrel, in combination with low-dose aspirin, is also licensed for acute myocardial infarction with ST-segment elevation; the combination should be continued for at least 4 weeks. Use of clopidogrel with aspirin increases the risk of bleeding. Clopidogrel monotherapy is an alternative when aspirin is contra-indicated, for example in those with aspirin hypersensitivity, or when aspirin is not tolerated despite the addition of a proton pump inhibitor.

The *Scottish Medicines Consortium* has advised (February 2004) that clopidogrel be accepted for restricted use for the treatment of confirmed acute coronary syndrome (without ST-segment elevation), in combination with aspirin. The *Scottish Medicines Consortium* has also advised (July 2007) that clopidogrel be accepted for restricted use for patients with ST-segment elevation acute myocardial infarction in combination with aspirin; treatment with clopidogrel is restricted to 4 weeks only. Clopidogrel should be initiated in hospital inpatients only.

NICE guidance
Clopidogrel in the treatment of non-ST-segment elevation acute coronary syndrome (July 2004)
Clopidogrel in combination with low-dose aspirin is recommended for the management of non-ST-segment elevation acute coronary syndrome in those at moderate to high risk of myocardial infarction or of death.
Clopidogrel in combination with low-dose aspirin may be used for up to 12 months after the last event of non-ST-segment elevation acute coronary syndrome.

Dipyridamole is used by mouth as an adjunct to oral anticoagulation for prophylaxis of thromboembolism associated with prosthetic heart valves. Modified-release preparations are licensed for secondary prevention of ischaemic stroke and transient ischaemic attacks.

1. Cardiovascular disease risk may be determined from the chart issued by the Joint British Societies (*Heart* 2005; 91 (Suppl V): v1–v52)—see inside back cover. The Joint British Societies' 'Cardiac Risk Assessor' computer programme may also be used to determine cardiovascular disease risk.

Dipyridamole is also used in combination with low-dose aspirin; this combination may reduce the risk of recurrent stroke but evidence of long-term benefit on cardiovascular mortality has not been established (but see NICE guidance below).

> **NICE guidance**
> **Clopidogrel and modified-release dipyridamole in the prevention of occlusive vascular events (May 2005)**
> The combination of modified-release dipyridamole and aspirin is recommended to prevent occlusive vascular events in those who have had a transient ischaemic attack or an ischaemic stroke; this combination should be used for 2 years after the last event. Long-term treatment with low-dose aspirin is continued after this period.
> Clopidogrel monotherapy may be used for those who cannot tolerate low-dose aspirin and have had an occlusive vascular event or have symptomatic peripheral arterial disease.

Glycoprotein IIb/IIIa inhibitors Glycoprotein IIb/IIIa inhibitors prevent platelet aggregation by blocking the binding of fibrinogen to receptors on platelets. **Abciximab** is a monoclonal antibody which binds to glycoprotein IIb/IIIa receptors and to other related sites; it is licensed as an adjunct to heparin and aspirin for the prevention of ischaemic complications in high-risk patients undergoing percutaneous transluminal coronary intervention. Abciximab should be used once only (to avoid additional risk of thrombocytopenia). **Eptifibatide** and **tirofiban** also inhibit glycoprotein IIb/IIIa receptors; they are licensed for use with heparin and aspirin to prevent early myocardial infarction in patients with unstable angina (section 2.6) or non-ST-segment-elevation myocardial infarction. Abciximab, eptifibatide and tirofiban should be used by specialists only.

For use of epoprostenol, see section 2.8.1.

> **NICE guidance**
> **Glycoprotein IIb/IIIa inhibitors for acute coronary syndromes (September 2002)**
> A glycoprotein IIb/IIIa inhibitor (abciximab, eptifibatide, and tirofiban) should be considered for the management of unstable angina or non-ST-segment-elevation myocardial infarction.
> A glycoprotein IIb/IIIa inhibitor is recommended for patients at high risk of myocardial infarction or death when early percutaneous coronary intervention is desirable but does not occur immediately; either eptifibatide or tirofiban is recommended in addition to other appropriate drug treatment.
> A glycoprotein IIb/IIIa inhibitor is recommended as an adjunct to percutaneous coronary intervention:
> - when early percutaneous coronary intervention is indicated but it is delayed;
> - in patients with diabetes;
> - if the procedure is complex.
>
> **Note** Only abciximab is licensed as an adjunct to percutaneous coronary intervention

ABCIXIMAB

Indications prevention of ischaemic cardiac complications in patients undergoing percutaneous coronary intervention; short-term prevention of myocardial infarction in patients with unstable angina not responding to conventional treatment and who are scheduled for percutaneous coronary intervention (use under specialist supervision)

Cautions measure baseline prothrombin time, activated clotting time, activated partial thromboplastin time, platelet count, haemoglobin and haematocrit; monitor haemoglobin and haematocrit 12 hours and 24 hours after start of treatment and platelet count 2–4 hours and 24 hours after start of treatment; concomitant use of drugs that increase risk of bleeding; discontinue if uncontrollable serious bleeding occurs or emergency cardiac surgery needed; consult product literature for details of procedures to minimise bleeding; elderly; hepatic impairment (Appendix 2); renal impairment (Appendix 3); pregnancy (Appendix 4)

Contra-indications active internal bleeding; major surgery, intracranial or intraspinal surgery or trauma within last 2 months; stroke within last 2 years; intracranial neoplasm, arteriovenous malformation or aneurysm, severe hypertension, haemorrhagic diathesis, thrombocytopenia, vasculitis, hypertensive retinopathy; breast-feeding (Appendix 5)

Side-effects bleeding manifestations; nausea, vomiting, hypotension, bradycardia, chest pain, back pain, headache, fever, puncture site pain, thrombocytopenia; *rarely* cardiac tamponade, adult respiratory distress, hypersensitivity reactions

Dose

- ADULT initially by intravenous injection over 1 minute, 250 micrograms/kg, then by intravenous infusion, 125 nanograms/kg/minute (max. 10 micrograms/minute); for prevention of ischaemic complications start 10–60 minutes before percutaneous coronary intervention and continue infusion for 12 hours; for unstable angina start up to 24 hours before possible percutaneous coronary intervention and continue infusion for 12 hours after intervention

ReoPro® (Lilly) PoM
Injection, abciximab 2 mg/mL, net price 5-mL vial = £260.40

ASPIRIN (antiplatelet)
(Acetylsalicylic Acid)

Indications prophylaxis of cerebrovascular disease or myocardial infarction (see section 2.10.1 and notes above)

Cautions asthma; uncontrolled hypertension; previous peptic ulceration (but manufacturers may advise avoidance of low-dose aspirin in history of peptic ulceration); hepatic impairment (Appendix 2); renal impairment (avoid if creatinine clearance less than 10 mL/minute; Appendix 3); pregnancy (Appendix 4); **interactions**: Appendix 1 (aspirin)

Contra-indications use other than as an antiplatelet in children and adolescents under 16 years (Reye's syndrome, section 4.7.1); active peptic ulceration; haemophilia and other bleeding disorders; breast-feeding (Appendix 5)

Hypersensitivity Aspirin and other NSAIDs are **contra-indicated** in history of hypersensitivity to aspirin or any other NSAID—which includes those in whom attacks of asthma, angioedema, urticaria, or rhinitis have been precipitated by aspirin or any other NSAID

Side-effects bronchospasm; gastro-intestinal haemorrhage (occasionally major), also other haemorrhage (e.g. subconjunctival)

Dose

- See notes above

2 Cardiovascular system

[1]**Aspirin** (Non-proprietary) PoM
Dispersible tablets, aspirin 75 mg, net price 28 = 29p; 300 mg, see section 4.7.1. Label: 13, 21, 32
Tablets, e/c, aspirin 75 mg, net price 28-tab pack = 51p; 56-tab pack = 86p; 300 mg, see section 4.7.1. Label: 5, 25, 32
Brands include *Gencardia®*, *Micropirin®*

Angettes 75® (Bristol-Myers Squibb)
Tablets, aspirin 75 mg, net price 28-tab pack = 94p. Label: 32

Caprin® (Sinclair) PoM
Tablets, e/c, pink, aspirin 75 mg, net price 28-tab pack = £1.55, 56-tab pack = £3.08, 100-tab pack = £5.24; 300 mg, see section 4.7.1. Label: 5, 25, 32

Nu-Seals® Aspirin (Alliance) PoM
Tablets, e/c, aspirin 75 mg, net price 56-tab pack = £2.60; 300 mg, see section 4.7.1. Label: 5, 25, 32
Note Tablets may be chewed at diagnosis for rapid absorption

CLOPIDOGREL

Indications prevention of atherosclerotic events in peripheral arterial disease, or within 35 days of myocardial infarction, or within 6 months of ischaemic stroke; prevention of artherosclerotic events in acute coronary syndrome without ST-segment elevation (given with aspirin—see notes above) and in acute myocardial infarction with ST-segment elevation (given with aspirin—see notes above)

Cautions patients at risk of increased bleeding from trauma, surgery or other pathological conditions; concomitant use of drugs that increase risk of bleeding; discontinue 7 days before elective surgery if antiplatelet effect not desirable; liver impairment (Appendix 2); renal impairment (Appendix 3); pregnancy (Appendix 4); **interactions**: Appendix 1 (clopidogrel)

Contra-indications active bleeding, breast-feeding (Appendix 5)

Side-effects dyspepsia, abdominal pain, diarrhoea; bleeding disorders (including gastro-intestinal and intracranial); *less commonly* nausea, vomiting, gastritis, flatulence, constipation, gastric and duodenal ulcers, headache, dizziness, paraesthesia, leucopenia, decreased platelets (very rarely severe thrombocytopenia), eosinophilia, rash, and pruritus; *rarely* vertigo; *very rarely* colitis, pancreatitis, hepatitis, acute liver failure, vasculitis, confusion, hallucinations, taste disturbance, stomatitis, bronchospasm, interstitial pneumonitis, blood disorders (including thrombocytopenic purpura, agranulocytosis and pancytopenia), and hypersensitivity-like reactions (including fever, glomerulonephritis, arthralgia, Stevens-Johnson syndrome, toxic epidermal necrolysis, lichen planus)

Dose

- Prevention of artherosclerotic events in peripheral arterial disease or after myocardial infarction or ischaemic stroke, 75 mg once daily
- Acute coronary syndrome (without ST-segment elevation), initially 300 mg then 75 mg daily (with aspirin—see notes above)
- Acute myocardial infarction (with ST-segment elevation), initially 300 mg then 75 mg daily (with aspirin—see notes above); initial dose omitted if patient over 75 years

1. Aspirin tablets 75 mg may be sold to the public in packs of up to 100 tablets; for details relating to other strengths see section 4.7.1 and *Medicines, Ethics and Practice*, No. 31, London, Pharmaceutical Press, 2007 (and subsequent editions as available)

Plavix® (Bristol-Myers Squibb, Sanofi-Synthelabo) PoM
Tablets, pink, f/c, clopidogrel (as hydrogen sulphate) 75 mg, net price 30-tab pack = £37.83

DIPYRIDAMOLE

Indications see notes above and under Dose

Cautions rapidly worsening angina, aortic stenosis, recent myocardial infarction, heart failure; may exacerbate migraine; hypotension; myasthenia gravis (risk of exacerbation); breast-feeding (Appendix 5); **interactions**: Appendix 1 (dipyridamole)

Side-effects gastro-intestinal effects, dizziness, myalgia, throbbing headache, hypotension, hot flushes and tachycardia; worsening symptoms of coronary heart disease; hypersensitivity reactions such as rash, urticaria, severe bronchospasm and angioedema; increased bleeding during or after surgery; thrombocytopenia reported

Dose

- By mouth, 300–600 mg daily in 3–4 divided doses before food
  Modified-release preparations, see under preparation below
- By intravenous injection, diagnostic only, consult product literature

Dipyridamole (Non-proprietary) PoM
Tablets, coated, dipyridamole 25 mg, net price 84 = £4.40; 100 mg, 84 = £4.60. Label: 22
Oral suspension, dipyridamole 50 mg/5 mL, net price 150 mL = £35.47

Persantin® (Boehringer Ingelheim) PoM
Tablets, both s/c, dipyridamole 25 mg (orange), net price 84-tab pack = £1.57; 100 mg, 84-tab pack = £4.38. Label: 22
Injection, dipyridamole 5 mg/mL. Net price 2-mL amp = 11p

Modified release

Persantin® Retard (Boehringer Ingelheim) PoM
Capsules, m/r, red/orange containing yellow pellets, dipyridamole 200 mg. Net price 60-cap pack = £8.38. Label: 21, 25
Dose secondary prevention of ischaemic stroke and transient ischaemic attacks (used alone or with aspirin), adjunct to oral anticoagulation for prophylaxis of thromboembolism associated with prosthetic heart valves, 200 mg twice daily preferably with food
Note Dispense in original container (pack contains a desiccant) and discard any capsules remaining 6 weeks after opening

With aspirin

For cautions, contra-indications and side-effects of aspirin, see under Aspirin, above

Asasantin® Retard (Boehringer Ingelheim) PoM
Capsules, red/ivory, aspirin 25 mg, dipyridamole 200 mg (m/r), net price 60-cap pack = £8.20. Label: 21, 25
Dose secondary prevention of ischaemic stroke and transient ischaemic attacks, 1 capsule twice daily
Note Dispense in original container (pack contains a desiccant) and discard any capsules remaining 6 weeks after opening

EPTIFIBATIDE

Indications prevention of early myocardial infarction in patients with unstable angina or non-ST-segment-elevation myocardial infarction and with last episode of chest pain within 24 hours (use under specialist supervision)

Cautions risk of bleeding, concomitant drugs that increase risk of bleeding—discontinue immediately if uncontrolled serious bleeding; measure baseline prothrombin time, activated partial thromboplastin time, platelet count, haemoglobin, haematocrit and serum creatinine; monitor haemoglobin, haematocrit and platelets within 6 hours after start of treatment then at least once daily; discontinue if thrombolytic therapy, intra-aortic balloon pump or emergency cardiac surgery necessary; hepatic impairment (Appendix 2); renal impairment (avoid if creatinine clearance less than 30 mL/minute; Appendix 3); pregnancy (Appendix 4); breast-feeding (Appendix 5)

Contra-indications abnormal bleeding within 30 days, major surgery or severe trauma within 6 weeks, stroke within last 30 days or any history of haemorrhagic stroke, intracranial disease (aneurysm, neoplasm or arteriovenous malformation), severe hypertension, haemorrhagic diathesis, increased prothrombin time or INR, thrombocytopenia, significant hepatic impairment; breast-feeding

Side-effects bleeding manifestations; *very rarely* anaphylaxis and rash

Dose

- Initially by intravenous injection, 180 micrograms/kg, then by intravenous infusion, 2 micrograms/kg/minute for up to 72 hours (up to 96 hours if percutaneous coronary intervention during treatment)

Integrilin® (GSK) PoM

Injection, eptifibatide 2 mg/mL, net price 10-mL (20-mg) vial = £14.45

Infusion, eptifibatide 750 micrograms/mL, net price 100-mL (75-mg) vial = £45.42

TIROFIBAN

Indications prevention of early myocardial infarction in patients with unstable angina or non-ST-segment-elevation myocardial infarction and with last episode of chest pain within 12 hours (use under specialist supervision)

Cautions hepatic impairment (avoid if severe; Appendix 2); renal impairment (Appendix 3); major surgery or severe trauma within 3 months (avoid if within 6 weeks); traumatic or protracted cardiopulmonary resuscitation, organ biopsy or lithotripsy within last 2 weeks; risk of bleeding including active peptic ulcer within 3 months; acute pericarditis, aortic dissection, haemorrhagic retinopathy, vasculitis, haematuria, faecal occult blood; severe heart failure, cardiogenic shock, anaemia; puncture of non-compressible vessel within 24 hours; concomitant drugs that increase risk of bleeding (including within 48 hours of thrombolytic administration); monitor platelet count, haemoglobin and haematocrit before treatment, 2–6 hours after start of treatment and then at least once daily; discontinue if thrombolytic therapy, intra-aortic balloon pump or emergency cardiac surgery necessary; discontinue immediately if serious bleeding uncontrolled by pressure occurs; pregnancy (Appendix 4)

Contra-indications abnormal bleeding within 30 days, stroke within 30 days or any history of haemorrhagic stroke, intracranial disease (aneurysm, neoplasm or arteriovenous malformation), severe hypertension, haemorrhagic diathesis, increased prothrombin time or INR, thrombocytopenia; breast-feeding (Appendix 5)

Side-effects bleeding manifestations; reversible thrombocytopenia

Dose

- By intravenous infusion, initially 400 nanograms/kg/minute for 30 minutes, then 100 nanograms/kg/minute for at least 48 hours (continue during and for 12–24 hours after percutaneous coronary intervention); max. duration of treatment 108 hours

Aggrastat® (MSD) PoM

Concentrate for intravenous infusion, tirofiban (as hydrochloride) 250 micrograms/mL. For dilution before use, net price 50-mL (12.5-mg) vial = £146.11

Intravenous infusion, tirofiban (as hydrochloride) 50 micrograms/mL, net price 250-mL *Intravia®* bag = £160.72

2.10 Myocardial infarction and fibrinolysis

2.10.1 Management of myocardial infarction
2.10.2 Fibrinolytic drugs

2.10.1 Management of myocardial infarction

Local guidelines for the management of myocardial infarction should be followed where they exist

Myocardial infarction is part of the spectrum of acute coronary syndromes which includes unstable angina, and myocardial infarction with or without ST-segment elevation.

These notes give an overview of the initial and long-term management of myocardial infarction with ST-segment elevation. For advice on the management of non-ST-segment elevation myocardial infarction and unstable angina, see section 2.6. The aims of management of ST-segment elevation myocardial infarction are to provide supportive care and pain relief, to promote reperfusion and to reduce mortality. Oxygen, diamorphine and nitrates can provide initial support and pain relief; aspirin and percutaneous coronary intervention or thrombolytics promote reperfusion; long-term use of aspirin, beta-blockers, ACE inhibitors, and statins help to reduce mortality further.

Initial management **Oxygen** (section 3.6) should be administered if there is evidence of hypoxia, pulmonary oedema, or continuing myocardial ischaemia; hyperoxia should be avoided and particular care is required in patients with chronic obstructive airways disease.

The pain (and anxiety) of myocardial infarction is managed with slow intravenous injection of **diamorphine** (section 4.7.2); an antiemetic such as metoclopramide (or, if left ventricular function is not compromised, cyclizine) by intravenous injection should also be given (section 4.6).

Aspirin (chewed or dispersed in water) is given for its antiplatelet effect (section 2.9); a dose of 300 mg is suitable. If aspirin is given before arrival at hospital, a note saying that it has been given should be sent with the patient. **Clopidogrel**, in a dose of 300 mg, should also be given (section 2.9).

Patency of the occluded artery can be restored by percutaneous coronary intervention or by giving a **thrombolytic drug** (section 2.10.2), unless contra-indicated. Percutaneous coronary intervention is the preferred method and patients should receive a **glycoprotein IIb/IIIa inhibitor** (section 2.9) to reduce the risk of immediate vascular occlusion. In those patients who cannot be provided with percutaneous coronary intervention within 90 minutes of diagnosis, a thrombolytic drug should be administered. A **low molecular weight heparin** or **fondaparinux** (section 2.8.1) should also be given to all patients; anticoagulant treatment should be continued for no longer than 8 days, or until percutaneous coronary intervention, or hospital discharge.

Nitrates (section 2.6.1) are used to relieve ischaemic pain. If sublingual glyceryl trinitrate is not effective, intravenous glyceryl trinitrate or isosorbide dinitrate is given.

Early administration of some **beta-blockers** (section 2.4) has been shown to be of benefit and should be given to patients without contra-indications.

ACE inhibitors (section 2.5.5.1), and angiotensin-II receptor antagonists (section 2.5.5.2) if an ACE inhibitor cannot be used, are also of benefit to patients who have no contra-indications; in hypertensive and normotensive patients treatment with an ACE inhibitor, or an angiotensin-II receptor antagonist, can be started within 24 hours of the myocardial infarction and continued for at least 5–6 weeks (see below for long-term treatment).

All patients should be closely monitored for hyperglycaemia; those with diabetes or raised blood-glucose concentration should receive **insulin**.

Long-term management Long-term management involves the use of several drugs which should ideally be started before the patient is discharged from hospital.

Aspirin (section 2.9) should be given to all patients, unless contra-indicated, at a dose of 75 mg daily. **Warfarin** (with or without aspirin) may confer greater benefit than aspirin alone, but the risk of bleeding is increased. **Clopidogrel**, in combination with aspirin, is licensed for use after myocardial infarction (section 2.9).

Beta-blockers (section 2.4) should be given to all patients in whom they are not contra-indicated. Acebutolol, metoprolol, propranolol and timolol are suitable; for patients with left ventricular dysfunction, carvedilol, bisoprolol or long-acting metoprolol may be appropriate (section 2.5.5).

Verapamil or **diltiazem** (section 2.6.2) can be considered if a beta-blocker cannot be used; however, they are contra-indicated in those with left ventricular dysfunction. Other calcium-channel blockers have no place in routine long-term management after a myocardial infarction.

An **ACE inhibitor** (section 2.5.5.1) should be considered for all patients, especially those with evidence of left ventricular dysfunction. If an ACE inhibitor cannot be used, an angiotensin-II receptor antagonist may be used for patients with heart failure. A relatively high dose of either the ACE inhibitor or angiotensin-II receptor antagonist may be required to produce benefit.

Nitrates (section 2.6.1) are used for patients with angina.

Eplerenone (section 2.2.3) is licensed for use following a myocardial infarction in those with left ventricular dysfunction and evidence of heart failure.

Statins are beneficial in preventing recurrent cardiovascular events (section 2.12).

2.10.2 Fibrinolytic drugs

Fibrinolytic drugs act as thrombolytics by activating plasminogen to form plasmin, which degrades fibrin and so breaks up thrombi.

The value of thrombolytic drugs for the treatment of *myocardial infarction* has been established (section 2.10.1). **Streptokinase** and **alteplase** have been shown to reduce mortality. **Reteplase and tenecteplase** are also licensed for acute myocardial infarction. Thrombolytic drugs are indicated for any patient with acute myocardial infarction for whom the benefit is likely to outweigh the risk of treatment. Trials have shown that the benefit is greatest in those with ECG changes that include ST segment elevation (especially in those with anterior infarction) and in patients with bundle branch block. Patients should not be denied thrombolytic treatment on account of age alone because mortality in the elderly is high and the reduction in mortality is the same as in younger patients.

Alteplase, reteplase and streptokinase need to be given within 12 hours of symptom onset, ideally within 1 hour; use after 12 hours requires specialist advice. Tenecteplase should be given as early as possible and usually within 6 hours of symptom onset. Antibodies to streptokinase appear after 4 days and it should not therefore be used again after this time.

Alteplase, streptokinase, and **urokinase** can be used for other thromboembolic disorders such as deep-vein thrombosis and pulmonary embolism. Alteplase is also used for acute ischaemic stroke. Treatment must be started promptly.

Urokinase is also licensed to restore the patency of occluded intravenous catheters and cannulas blocked with fibrin clots.

> **NICE guidance**
> **Alteplase for the treatment of acute ischaemic stroke (June 2007)**
> Alteplase, used in accordance with the licence for *Actilyse®*, is recommended for the treatment of acute ischaemic stroke.

Cautions Thrombolytic drugs should be used with caution if there is a risk of bleeding including that from venepuncture or invasive procedures. They should also be used with caution in external chest compression, pregnancy (Appendix 4), elderly, hypertension, conditions in which thrombolysis might give rise to embolic complications such as enlarged left atrium with atrial fibrillation (risk of dissolution of clot and subsequent embolisation), diabetic retinopathy (very small risk of retinal bleeding), and recent or concurrent use of drugs that increase the risk of bleeding.

Contra-indications Thrombolytic drugs are contra-indicated in recent haemorrhage, trauma, or surgery (including dental extraction), coagulation defects, bleeding diatheses, aortic dissection, aneurysm, coma, history of cerebrovascular disease especially recent events or with any residual disability, recent symptoms of possible peptic ulceration, heavy vaginal bleeding, severe hypertension, active pulmonary disease with cavitation, acute pancreatitis, pericarditis, bacterial endocarditis, severe liver disease, and oesophageal varices; also in the case of streptokinase, previous allergic reactions to either streptokinase or anistreplase (no longer available).

Prolonged persistence of antibodies to streptokinase and anistreplase (no longer available) can reduce the effectiveness of subsequent treatment; therefore, streptokinase should not be used again beyond 4 days of first administration of either streptokinase or anistreplase.

Side-effects Side-effects of thrombolytics are mainly nausea and vomiting and bleeding. When thrombolytics are used in myocardial infarction, reperfusion arrhythmias and recurrent ischaemia and angina may occur. Reperfusion may also cause cerebral and pulmonary oedema. Hypotension can also occur and can usually be controlled by elevating the patient's legs, or by reducing the rate of infusion or stopping it temporarily. Back pain, fever, and convulsions have been reported. Bleeding is usually limited to the site of injection, but intracerebral haemorrhage or bleeding from other sites can occur. Serious bleeding calls for discontinuation of the thrombolytic and may require administration of coagulation factors and antifibrinolytic drugs (e.g. tranexamic acid). Rarely further embolism may occur (either due to clots that break away from the original thrombus or to cholesterol crystal emboli). Thrombolytics can cause allergic reactions (including rash, flushing and uveitis) and anaphylaxis has been reported (for details of management see Allergic Emergencies, section 3.4.3). Guillain-Barré syndrome has been reported rarely after streptokinase treatment.

ALTEPLASE
(rt-PA, tissue-type plasminogen activator)

Indications acute myocardial infarction (see notes above and section 2.10.1); pulmonary embolism; acute ischaemic stroke (treatment under specialist neurology physician **only**)

Cautions see notes above; *in acute stroke*, monitor for intracranial haemorrhage, monitor blood pressure (antihypertensive recommended if systolic above 180 mmHg or diastolic above 105 mmHg)

Contra-indications see notes above; *in acute stroke*, convulsion accompanying stroke, severe stroke, history of stroke in patients with diabetes, stroke in last 3 months, hypoglycaemia, hyperglycaemia

Side-effects see notes above; also risk of cerebral bleeding increased in acute stroke

Dose

- Myocardial infarction, accelerated regimen (initiated within 6 hours of symptom onset), 15 mg by intravenous injection, followed by intravenous infusion of 50 mg over 30 minutes, then 35 mg over 60 minutes (total dose 100 mg over 90 minutes); in patients less than 65 kg, 15 mg by intravenous injection, followed by intravenous infusion of 0.75 mg/kg over 30 minutes, then 0.5 mg/kg over 60 minutes (max. total dose 100 mg over 90 minutes)
- Myocardial infarction, initiated within 6–12 hours of symptom onset, 10 mg by intravenous injection, followed by intravenous infusion of 50 mg over 60 minutes, then 4 infusions each of 10 mg over 30 minutes (total dose 100 mg over 3 hours; max. 1.5 mg/kg in patients less than 65 kg)
- Pulmonary embolism, 10 mg by intravenous injection over 1–2 minutes, followed by intravenous infusion of 90 mg over 2 hours; max. 1.5 mg/kg in patients less than 65 kg
- Acute stroke (treatment **must** begin within 3 hours of symptom onset), by intravenous administration over 60 minutes, 900 micrograms/kg (max. 90 mg); initial 10% of dose by intravenous injection, remainder by intravenous infusion; ELDERLY over 80 years not recommended

Actilyse® (Boehringer Ingelheim) PoM
Injection, powder for reconstitution, alteplase 10 mg (5.8 million units)/vial, net price per vial (with diluent) = £135.00; 20 mg (11.6 million units)/vial (with diluent and transfer device) = £180.00; 50 mg (29 million-units)/vial (with diluent, transfer device, and infusion bag) = £300.00

RETEPLASE

Indications acute myocardial infarction (see notes above and section 2.10.1)

Cautions see notes above; breast-feeding (Appendix 5)

Contra-indications see notes above

Side-effects see notes above

Dose

- By intravenous injection (initiated within 12 hours of symptom onset), 10 units over not more than 2 minutes, followed after 30 minutes by a further 10 units

Rapilysin® (Roche) PoM
Injection, powder for reconstitution, reteplase 10 units/vial, net price pack of 2 vials (with 2 prefilled syringes of diluent and transfer device) = £666.11

STREPTOKINASE

Indications acute myocardial infarction (see notes above and section 2.10.1); deep-vein thrombosis, pulmonary embolism, acute arterial thromboembolism, and central retinal venous or arterial thrombosis

Cautions see notes above

Contra-indications see notes above

Side-effects see notes above

Dose

- Myocardial infarction (initiated within 12 hours of symptom onset), by intravenous infusion, 1.5 million units over 60 minutes
- Deep-vein thrombosis, pulmonary embolism, acute arterial thromboembolism, central retinal venous or

arterial thrombosis, by intravenous infusion, 250 000 units over 30 minutes, then 100 000 units every hour for up to 12–72 hours according to condition with monitoring of clotting parameters (consult product literature)

Streptokinase (Non-proprietary) PoM
Injection, powder for reconstitution, streptokinase, net price 100 000-unit vial = £10.00; 250 000-unit vial = £14.33; 750 000-unit vial = £38.20; 1.5 million-unit vial = £81.18

Streptase® (CSL Behring) PoM
Injection, powder for reconstitution, streptokinase, net price 250 000-unit vial = £15.91; 750 000-unit vial = £41.72; 1.5 million-unit vial = £83.44 (hosp. only)

TENECTEPLASE

Indications acute myocardial infarction (see notes above and section 2.10.1)

Cautions see notes above; breast-feeding (Appendix 5)

Contra-indications see notes above

Side-effects see notes above

Dose

- By intravenous injection over 10 seconds (initiated within 6 hours of symptom onset), 30–50 mg according to body-weight—consult product literature; max. 50 mg

Metalyse® (Boehringer Ingelheim) PoM
Injection, powder for reconstitution, tenecteplase, net price 40-mg (8000-unit) vial = £612.50; 50-mg (10 000-unit) vial = £612.50 (both with prefilled syringe of water for injection)

UROKINASE

Indications thromboembolic occlusive vascular disease including deep-vein thrombosis, pulmonary embolism, and peripheral vascular occlusion; occluded intravenous catheters and cannulas blocked by fibrin clots

Cautions see notes above

Contra-indications see notes above

Side-effects see notes above

Dose

- Deep-vein thrombosis, by intravenous infusion, initially 4400 units/kg in 15 mL sodium chloride 0.9% over 10 minutes, followed by 4400 units/kg/hour for 12–24 hours
- Pulmonary embolism, by intravenous infusion, initially 4400 units/kg in 15mL sodium chloride 0.9% over 10 minutes, followed by 4400 units/kg/hour for 12 hours *or* by injection into pulmonary artery, initially 15 000 units/kg, subsequent doses adjusted according to response; max. 3 doses in 24 hours
- Peripheral vascular occlusion, consult product literature
- Occluded catheters and cannulas, by injection directly into catheter or cannula, 5000–25 000 units in 2 mL sodium chloride 0.9%; leave for up to 4 hours then aspirate the lysate

Syner-KINASE® (Syner-Med) PoM
Injection, powder for reconstitution, urokinase, net price 25 000 unit vial = £45.95; 100 000 unit vial = £112.95

2.11 Antifibrinolytic drugs and haemostatics

Fibrin dissolution can be impaired by the administration of **tranexamic acid**, which inhibits fibrinolysis. It can be used to prevent bleeding or to treat bleeding associated with excessive fibrinolysis (e.g. in prostatectomy, bladder surgery, in dental extraction in patients with haemophilia, in conisation of the cervix, and in traumatic hyphaema) and in the management of menorrhagia. Tranexamic acid may also be used in hereditary angioedema, epistaxis, and in thrombolytic overdose.

Desmopressin (section 6.5.2) is used in the management of mild to moderate haemophilia and von Willebrand's disease. It is also used for fibrinolytic response testing.

Etamsylate (ethamsylate) reduces capillary bleeding in the presence of a normal number of platelets. It does not act by fibrin stabilisation, but probably by correcting abnormal adhesion.

ETAMSYLATE
(Ethamsylate)

Indications blood loss in menorrhagia

Contra-indications porphyria (see section 9.8.2)

Side-effects nausea, headache, rashes

Dose

- 500 mg 4 times daily during menstruation

Dicynene® (Sanofi-Synthelabo) PoM
Tablets, scored, etamsylate 500 mg, net price 100-tab pack = £8.78

TRANEXAMIC ACID

Indications see notes above

Cautions renal impairment (Appendix 3); massive haematuria (avoid if risk of ureteric obstruction); not for use in disseminated intravascular coagulation; irregular menstrual bleeding (establish cause before initiating therapy); pregnancy (Appendix 4); regular eye examinations and liver function tests in long-term treatment of hereditary angioedema

Note Requirement for regular eye examinations during long-term treatment is based on unsatisfactory evidence

Contra-indications thromboembolic disease

Side-effects nausea, vomiting, diarrhoea (reduce dose); *rarely* disturbances in colour vision (discontinue), thromboembolic events, allergic skin reactions; giddiness and hypotension on rapid intravenous injection

Dose

- By mouth, local fibrinolysis, 15–25 mg/kg 2–3 times daily

  Menorrhagia (initiated when menstruation has started), 1 g 3 times daily for up to 4 days; max. 4 g daily

  Hereditary angioedema, 1–1.5 g 2–3 times daily

  Epistaxis, 1 g 3 times daily for 7 days
- By slow intravenous injection, local fibrinolysis, 0.5–1 g 3 times daily

Tranexamic acid (Non-proprietary) PoM
Tablets, tranexamic acid 500 mg, net price 60-tab pack = £6.77

Cyklokapron® (Meda) PoM
Tablets, f/c, scored, tranexamic acid 500 mg, net price 60-tab pack = £14.30
Injection, tranexamic acid 100 mg/mL, net price 5-mL amp = £1.55

Blood products

ANTITHROMBIN III CONCENTRATE

Dried antithrombin III is prepared from human plasma

Indications congenital deficiency of antithrombin III
Side-effects nausea, flushing, headache, dizziness; *rarely* allergic reactions and fever
Available from BPL (Dried Antithrombin III)
Note Preparation of recombinant human antithrombin (antithrombin alfa) available from LEO (*ATryn®*) indicated for the prophylaxis of venous thromboembolism in surgery in patients with congenital antithrombin deficiency

DROTRECOGIN ALFA (ACTIVATED)

Recombinant activated protein C

Indications adjunctive treatment of severe sepsis with multiple organ failure—start treatment within 24 hours (and no later than 48 hours) after onset of organ failure
Cautions increased risk of bleeding, concomitant use of drugs that increase risk of bleeding; pregnancy (Appendix 4); breast-feeding (Appendix 5); **interactions:** Appendix 1 (drotrecogin alfa)
Contra-indications internal bleeding; intracranial neoplasm or cerebral herniation; chronic severe hepatic disease; thrombocytopenia; not recommended for use in children under 18 years or in single organ failure
Side-effects bleeding; headache; ecchymosis; pain
Available from Lilly (*Xigris®* ▼)

> **NICE guidance**
> **Drotrecogin alfa (activated) for severe sepsis (September 2004)**
> Drotrecogin alfa (activated) should be considered for adults with severe sepsis that has resulted in the failure of two or more major organs and who are receiving optimum intensive care support. Drotrecogin alfa (activated) should be initiated and supervised only by a specialist consultant with intensive care skills and experience in the care of patients with sepsis.

FACTOR VIIa (RECOMBINANT)

Eptacog alfa (activated)

Indications treatment and prophylaxis of haemorrhage in patients with haemophilia A or B with antibodies to factors VIII or IX, acquired haemophilia, factor VII deficiency, or Glanzmann's thrombasthenia
Cautions risk of thrombosis or disseminated intravascular coagulation
Side-effects *very rarely* nausea, thrombotic events (including myocardial infarction and cerebrovascular accident), coagulation disorders, fever, pain, and allergic reactions including rash
Available from Novo Nordisk (*NovoSeven®*)

FACTOR VIII FRACTION, DRIED

(Human Antihaemophilic Fraction, Dried)

Dried factor VIII fraction is prepared from human plasma by a suitable fractionation technique

Indications treatment and prophylaxis of haemorrhage in congenital factor VIII deficiency (haemophilia A), acquired factor VIII deficiency, von Willebrand's disease
Cautions monitor for development of factor VIII inhibitors; intravascular haemolysis after large or frequently repeated doses in patients with blood groups A, B, or AB—less likely with high potency concentrates
Side-effects gastro-intestinal disturbances, taste disturbances; flushing, palpitation; dyspnoea, coughing; headache, dizziness, paraesthesia, drowsiness; blurred vision; allergic reactions including hypotension, chills, fever, urticaria, and anaphylaxis
Available from CSL Behring (*Haemate® P*), BPL (*Optivate®*, High Purity Factor VIII and von Willebrand factor concentrate; *Replenate®*; *8Y®*), Grifols (*Alphanate®*; *Fanhdi®*)
Note Preparation of recombinant human antihaemophilic factor VIII (octocog alfa) available from CSL Behring (*Helixate® NexGen*), Baxter Bioscience (*Advate®*), Bayer (*Kogenate® Bayer*), Wyeth (*ReFacto®*)

FACTOR VIII INHIBITOR BYPASSING FRACTION

Preparations with factor VIII inhibitor bypassing activity are prepared from human plasma

Indications treatment and prophylaxis of haemorrhage in patients with congenital factor VIII deficiency (haemophilia A) and factor VIII inhibitors; treatment of haemorrhage in non-haemophiliac patients with acquired factor VIII inhibitors
Contra-indications disseminated intravascular coagulation
Side-effects paraesthesia; pyrexia; allergic reactions including hypotension, flushing, urticaria, rash, and anaphylaxis
Available from Baxter (*FEIBA®*)
Note A porcine preparation of antihaemophilic factor for patients with inhibitors to human factor VIII is available from Ipsen (*Hyate C®*)

FACTOR IX FRACTION, DRIED

Dried factor IX fraction is prepared from human plasma by a suitable fractionation technique; it may also contain clotting factors II, VII, and X

Indications treatment and prophylaxis of haemorrhage in congenital factor IX deficiency (haemophilia B)
Cautions risk of thrombosis—principally with former low purity products
Contra-indications disseminated intravascular coagulation
Side-effects gastro-intestinal disturbances; headache, dizziness; allergic reactions, including chills, fever
Available from CSL Behring (*Mononine®*), BPL (*Replenine®-VF*, Dried Factor IX Fraction), Grifols (*AlphaNine®*)
Note Preparation of recombinant coagulation factor IX (nonacog alfa) available from Wyeth (*BeneFIX®*)

FACTOR XIII FRACTION, DRIED
(Human Fibrin-stabilising Factor, Dried)

Indications congenital factor XIII deficiency

Side-effects rarely, allergic reactions and fever

Available from CSL Behring (*Fibrogammin® P*)

FRESH FROZEN PLASMA

Fresh frozen plasma is prepared from the supernatant liquid obtained by centrifugation of one donation of whole blood

Indications to replace coagulation factors or other plasma proteins where their concentration or functional activity is critically reduced, e.g. to reverse warfarin effect

Cautions avoid in circulatory overload; need for compatibility

Side-effects allergic reactions including chills, fever, bronchospasm; adult respiratory distress syndrome

Available from Regional Blood Transfusion Services and BPL

Note A preparation of solvent/detergent treated human plasma (frozen) is available from Octapharma (*Octaplas®*)

PROTEIN C CONCENTRATE

Protein C is prepared from human plasma

Indications congenital protein C deficiency

Cautions hypersensitivity to heparin

Side-effects fever, arrhythmia, bleeding and thrombosis reported; *rarely* allergic reactions

Available from Baxter (*Ceprotin®*▼)

2.12 Lipid-regulating drugs

Measures should be taken to prevent cardiovascular disease in those at high risk of atherosclerosis. Individuals at high risk include those who already have atherosclerotic disease, those with diabetes aged over 40 years, or those with familial hypercholesterolaemia.

Measures are also required for other individuals who may also be at high risk of developing atherosclerotic cardiovascular disease; the risk is assessed on the basis of lipid concentration as well as other risk factors such as smoking, blood pressure, impaired glucose tolerance, male sex, age, premature menopause, ethnicity, obesity, triglyceride concentration, chronic kidney disease, and a family history of premature cardiovascular disease. Those with a 10-year risk of cardiovascular disease[1] of 20% or more stand to benefit most from drug treatment.

Lowering the concentration of low-density lipoprotein (LDL) cholesterol and raising high-density lipoprotein (HDL) cholesterol slows the progression of atherosclerosis and may even induce regression. Changes in lifestyle and diet can be of benefit. Lipid-regulating drug treatment must be combined with advice on diet and lifestyle measures, lowering of raised blood pressure (section 2.5), the use of low-dose aspirin (section 2.9), and management of diabetes (section 6.1).

1. Cardiovascular disease risk may be determined from the chart issued by the Joint British Societies (*Heart* 2005; **91** (Suppl V): v1–v52)—see inside back cover. The Joint British Societies' 'Cardiac Risk Assessor' computer programme may also be used to determine cardiovascular disease risk.

A **statin** (see p. 140) is effective for reducing the risk of cardiovascular disease events irrespective of the degree of dyslipidaemia. A statin is the drug of first choice for treating hypercholesterolaemia and moderate hypertriglyceridaemia. Severe hyperlipidaemia not adequately controlled with a maximal dose of a statin may require the use of an additional lipid-regulating drug such as **ezetimibe** or **colestyramine**; such treatment should generally be supervised by a specialist.

A number of conditions, some familial, are characterised by very high LDL-cholesterol concentration, high triglyceride concentration, or both. A **fibrate** is added to statin therapy if triglycerides remain high even after the LDL-cholesterol concentration has been reduced adequately; **nicotinic acid** may also be used to further lower triglyceride or LDL-cholesterol concentration.

Combination of a statin with a fibrate or with nicotinic acid carries an increased risk of side-effects (including rhabdomyolysis—see CSM advice below) and should be used under specialist supervision; monitoring of liver function and creatine kinase should also be considered. The concomitant administration of gemfibrozil with a statin increases the risk of rhabdomyolysis considerably—this combination should **not** be used.

Patients with hypothyroidism should receive adequate thyroid replacement therapy before assessing the requirement for lipid-regulating treatment because correcting hypothyroidism itself may resolve the lipid abnormality. Untreated hypothyroidism increases the risk of myositis with lipid-regulating drugs.

CSM advice (muscle effects)

The CSM has advised that rhabdomyolysis associated with lipid-regulating drugs such as the fibrates and statins appears to be rare (approx. 1 case in every 100 000 treatment years) but may be increased in those with renal impairment and possibly in those with hypothyroidism (see also notes above). Concomitant treatment with drugs that increase plasma-statin concentration increase the risk of muscle toxicity; concomitant treatment with a fibrate and a statin may also be associated with an increased risk of serious muscle toxicity.

Bile acid sequestrants

Colesevelam, **colestipol**, and **colestyramine** (cholestyramine) are anion-exchange resins used in the management of hypercholesterolaemia. They act by binding bile acids, preventing their reabsorption; this promotes hepatic conversion of cholesterol into bile acids; the resultant increased LDL-receptor activity of liver cells increases the clearance of LDL-cholesterol from the plasma. Bile acid sequestrants effectively reduce LDL-cholesterol but can aggravate hypertriglyceridaemia.

Cautions Bile acid sequestrants interfere with the absorption of fat-soluble vitamins; supplements of vitamins A, D and K may be required when treatment is prolonged. **Interactions:** Appendix 1 (bile acid sequestrants)

Side-effects As bile acid sequestrants are not absorbed, gastro-intestinal side-effects predominate. Constipation is common, but diarrhoea has occurred, as have nausea, vomiting, and gastro-intestinal discomfort. Hypertriglyceridaemia may be aggravated. An increased bleeding tendency has been reported due to hypoprothrombinaemia associated with vitamin K deficiency.

Counselling Other drugs should be taken at least 1 hour before or 4–6 hours after bile acid sequestrants to reduce possible interference with absorption. Colesevelam and a statin can be taken at the same time.

COLESEVELAM HYDROCHLORIDE

Indications primary hypercholesterolaemia as an adjunct to dietary measures either alone or with a statin

Cautions see notes above; also gastro-intestinal motility disorders, major gastro-intestinal surgery, inflammatory bowel disease, hepatic impairment; pregnancy (Appendix 4); breast-feeding (Appendix 5)

Contra-indications bowel or biliary obstruction

Side-effects see notes above; also headache; myalgia

Dose

- Monotherapy, 3.75 g daily in 1–2 divided doses; max. 4.375 g daily
- Combination therapy with statin, 2.5–3.75 g daily in 1–2 divided doses

Cholestagel® (Genzyme) ▼ PoM
Tablets, f/c, colesevelam hydrochloride 625 mg, net price 180-cap pack = £92.66. Label: 21, counselling, avoid other drugs at same time (see notes above)

COLESTYRAMINE
(Cholestyramine)

Indications hyperlipidaemias, particularly type IIa, in patients who have not responded adequately to diet and other appropriate measures; primary prevention of coronary heart disease in men aged 35–59 years with primary hypercholesterolaemia who have not responded to diet and other appropriate measures; pruritus associated with partial biliary obstruction and primary biliary cirrhosis (section 1.9.2); diarrhoeal disorders (section 1.9.2)

Cautions see notes above; hepatic impairment (Appendix 2); pregnancy (Appendix 4); breast-feeding (Appendix 5); **interactions**: Appendix 1 (colestyramine)

Contra-indications complete biliary obstruction (not likely to be effective)

Side-effects see notes above; intestinal obstruction reported rarely and hyperchloraemic acidosis reported on prolonged use

Dose

- Lipid reduction, initially 4 g daily increased by 4 g at weekly intervals to 12–24 g daily in a suitable liquid in 1–4 divided doses, then adjusted as required; max. 36 g daily
- Pruritus, see section 1.9.2
- Diarrhoeal disorders, see section 1.9.2
- CHILD 6–12 years, see product literature

Note The contents of each sachet should be mixed with at least 150 mL of water or other suitable liquid such as fruit juice, skimmed milk, thin soups, and pulpy fruits with a high moisture content

Colestyramine (Non-proprietary) PoM
Powder, colestyramine (anhydrous) 4 g/sachet, net price 50-sachet pack = £11.42. Label: 13, counselling, avoid other drugs at same time (see notes above)
Excipients include aspartame (section 9.4.1)

Questran® (Bristol-Myers Squibb) PoM
Powder, colestyramine (anhydrous) 4 g/sachet. Net price 50-sachet pack = £11.42. Label: 13, counselling, avoid other drugs at same time (see notes above)
Excipients include sucrose 3.79g/sachet

Questran Light® (Bristol-Myers Squibb) PoM
Powder, sugar-free, colestyramine (anhydrous) 4 g/sachet, net price 50-sachet pack = £16.99. Label: 13, counselling, avoid other drugs at same time (see notes above)
Excipients include aspartame (section 9.4.1)

COLESTIPOL HYDROCHLORIDE

Indications hyperlipidaemias, particularly type IIa, in patients who have not responded adequately to diet and other appropriate measures

Cautions see notes above; pregnancy (Appendix 4); breast-feeding (Appendix 5); **interactions**: Appendix 1 (colestipol)

Side-effects see notes above

Dose

- Initially 5 g 1–2 times daily in liquid increased if necessary in 5-g increments at intervals of 1 month to max. 30 g daily (in 1–2 divided doses)

Note The contents of each sachet should be mixed with at least 100 mL of water or other suitable liquid such as fruit juice, skimmed milk, thin soups, cereals, yoghurt, and pulpy fruits with a high moisture content

Colestid® (Pharmacia) PoM
Granules, yellow, colestipol hydrochloride 5 g/sachet. Net price 30 sachets = £15.05. Label: 13, counselling, avoid other drugs at same time (see notes above)
Colestid Orange, granules, yellow/orange, colestipol hydrochloride 5 g/sachet, with aspartame. Net price 30 sachets = £15.05. Label: 13, counselling, avoid other drugs at same time (see notes above)

Ezetimibe

Ezetimibe inhibits the intestinal absorption of cholesterol. It is licensed as an adjunct to dietary manipulation in patients with primary hypercholesterolaemia in combination with a statin or alone (if a statin is inappropriate), in patients with homozygous familial hypercholesterolaemia in combination with a statin, and in patients with homozygous familial sitosterolaemia (phytosterolaemia). If ezetimibe is used in combination with a statin, there is an increased risk of rhabdomyolysis (see also CSM advice on p. 137).

NICE guidance
Ezetimibe for the treatment of primary hypercholesterolaemia (November 2007)
Ezetimibe, used in accordance with the licensed indications for *Ezetrol®*, is an option for the treatment of adults with primary hypercholesterolaemia.

EZETIMIBE

Indications adjunct to dietary measures and statin treatment in primary hypercholesterolaemia and homozygous familial hypercholesterolaemia (ezetimibe alone in primary hypercholesterolaemia if statin inappropriate or not tolerated); adjunct to dietary measures in homozygous sitosterolaemia

Cautions hepatic impairment (avoid if moderate or severe; Appendix 2); pregnancy (Appendix 4); breast-feeding (Appendix 5); **interactions**: Appendix 1 (ezetimibe)

Side-effects gastro-intestinal disturbances; headache, fatigue; myalgia; *rarely* arthralgia, hypersensitivity reactions (including rash, angioedema, and anaphylaxis), hepatitis; *very rarely* pancreatitis, cholelithiasis, cholecystitis, thrombocytopenia, raised creatine kinase, myopathy, and rhabdomyolysis

Dose

- ADULT and CHILD over 10 years, 10 mg once daily

Ezetrol® (MSD, Schering-Plough) ▼ PoM
Tablets, ezetimibe 10 mg, net price 28-tab pack = £26.31

With simvastatin
See under Simvastatin

Fibrates

Bezafibrate, **ciprofibrate**, **fenofibrate**, and **gemfibrozil** act mainly by decreasing serum triglycerides; they have variable effects on LDL-cholesterol. Although a fibrate can reduce the risk of coronary heart disease events in those with low HDL-cholesterol or with raised triglycerides, a statin should be used first. Fibrates are first-line therapy only in those whose serum-triglyceride concentration is greater than 10 mmol/litre or in those who cannot tolerate a statin. In type 2 diabetes a fibrate can be added to a statin for those with a serum-triglyceride concentration exceeding 2.3 mmol/litre, despite 6 months of treatment with a statin and optimal glycaemic control.

Fibrates can cause a myositis-like syndrome, especially if renal function is impaired. Also, combination of a fibrate with a statin increases the risk of muscle effects (especially rhabdomyolysis) and should be used with caution (see CSM advice on p. 137) and monitoring of liver function and creatinine kinase should be considered; gemfibrozil and statins should **not** be used concomitantly.

BEZAFIBRATE

Indications hyperlipidaemias of types IIa, IIb, III, IV, and V in patients who have not responded adequately to diet and other appropriate measures; also see notes above

Cautions correct hypothyroidism before initiating treatment (see p. 137); hepatic impairment (Appendix 2); renal impairment (avoid if creatinine clearance less than 15 mL/minute; Appendix 3; see also under Myotoxicity below); **interactions**: Appendix 1 (fibrates)

Myotoxicity Special care needed in patients with renal disease, as progressive increases in serum creatinine concentration or failure to follow dosage guidelines may result in myotoxicity (rhabdomyolysis); discontinue if myotoxicity suspected or creatine kinase concentration increases significantly

Contra-indications severe hepatic and renal impairment, hypoalbuminaemia, primary biliary cirrhosis, gall bladder disease, nephrotic syndrome, pregnancy (Appendix 4); breast-feeding (Appendix 5)

Side-effects gastro-intestinal disturbances, anorexia; *less commonly* cholestasis, weight gain, dizziness, headache, fatigue, drowsiness, renal impairment, raised serum creatinine (unrelated to renal impairment), erectile dysfunction, myotoxicity (with myasthenia or myalgia)—special risk in renal impairment (see Cautions), urticaria, pruritus, photosensitivity reactions; *very rarely* gallstones, hypoglycaemia, anaemia, leucopenia, thrombocytopenia, increased platelet count, alopecia, Stevens-Johnson syndrome, and toxic epidermal necrolysis

Dose

- See preparations below

Bezafibrate (Non-proprietary) PoM
Tablets, bezafibrate 200 mg, net price 100-tab pack = £10.40. Label: 21
Dose 200 mg 3 times daily; CHILD over 10 years, see *BNF for Children*

Bezalip® (Roche) PoM
Tablets, f/c, bezafibrate 200 mg, net price 100-tab pack = £9.15. Label: 21
Dose 200 mg 3 times daily; CHILD over 10 years, see *BNF for Children*

Modified release

Bezafibrate (Non-proprietary) PoM
Tablets, m/r, bezafibrate 400 mg, net price 28-tab pack = £7.68. Label: 21, 25
Dose 400 mg once daily (dose form not appropriate in patients with renal impairment)
Brands include *Fibrazate® XL*, *Zimbacol® XL*

Bezalip® Mono (Roche) PoM
Tablets, m/r, f/c, bezafibrate 400 mg, net price 30-tab pack = £8.09. Label: 21, 25
Dose 400 mg once daily (dose form not appropriate in patients with renal impairment)

CIPROFIBRATE

Indications hyperlipidaemias of types IIa, IIb, III, and IV in patients who have not responded adequately to diet; also see notes above

Cautions see under Bezafibrate; renal impairment (avoid if creatinine clearance less than 10 mL/minute; Appendix 3)

Contra-indications see under Bezafibrate

Side-effects see under Bezafibrate

Dose

- 100 mg daily

Modalim® (Sanofi-Synthelabo) PoM
Tablets, scored, ciprofibrate 100 mg. Net price 28-tab pack = £17.66

FENOFIBRATE

Indications hyperlipidaemias of types IIa, IIb, III, IV, and V in patients who have not responded adequately to diet and other appropriate measures; also see notes above

Cautions see under Bezafibrate; liver function tests recommended every 3 months for first year (discontinue treatment if significantly raised); renal impairment (avoid if creatinine clearance less than 10 mL/minute; Appendix 3)
Contra-indications gall bladder disease; photosensitivity to ketoprofen; severe hepatic impairment (Appendix 2); pregnancy (Appendix 4); breast-feeding (Appendix 5)
Side-effects see under Bezafibrate; also *very rarely* hepatitis, pancreatitis, and interstitial pneumopathies
Dose
- See preparations below

Fenofibrate (Non-proprietary) PoM
Capsules, fenofibrate 200 mg, net price 30-cap pack = £14.75. Label: 21
Dose 1 capsule daily (dose form not appropriate for children or in renal impairment)
Brands include *Fenogal®*

Lipantil® (Solvay) PoM
Lipantil® Micro 67 capsules, yellow, fenofibrate (micronised) 67 mg, net price 90-cap pack = £23.30. Label: 21
Dose initially 3 capsules daily in divided doses; usual range 2–4 capsules daily; CHILD 4–15 years 1 capsule/20 kg daily

Lipantil® Micro 200 capsules, orange, fenofibrate (micronised) 200 mg, net price 28-cap pack = £17.95. Label: 21
Dose initially 1 capsule daily (dose form not appropriate for children or in renal impairment)

Lipantil® Micro 267 capsules, orange/cream, fenofibrate (micronised) 267 mg, net price 28-cap pack = £21.75. Label: 21
Dose severe hyperlipidaemia, 1 capsule daily (dose form not appropriate for children or in renal impairment)
Note For an equivalent therapeutic effect, 100 mg previously available non-micronised fenofibrate ≡ 67 mg micronised fenofibrate

Supralip® 160 (Solvay) PoM
Tablets, f/c, fenofibrate (micronised) 160 mg, net price 28-tab pack = £14.75. Label: 21
Dose 160 mg daily (dose form not appropriate for children or in renal impairment)

GEMFIBROZIL

Indications hyperlipidaemias of types IIa, IIb, III, IV and V in patients who have not responded adequately to diet and other appropriate measures; primary prevention of cardiovascular disease in men with hyperlipidaemias that have not responded to diet and other appropriate measures; also see notes above
Cautions lipid profile, blood counts, and liver-function tests before initiating long-term treatment; preferably avoid use with statins (high risk of rhabdomyolysis); correct hypothyroidism before initiating treatment (see p. 137); elderly; renal impairment (avoid if creatinine clearance less than 30 mL/minute; Appendix 3); **interactions**: Appendix 1 (fibrates)
Contra-indications alcoholism, biliary-tract disease including gallstones; photosensitivity to fibrates; hepatic impairment (Appendix 2); pregnancy (Appendix 4); breast-feeding (Appendix 5)
Side-effects gastro-intestinal disturbances; headache, fatigue, vertigo; eczema, rash; *less commonly* atrial fibrillation; *rarely* pancreatitis, appendicitis, disturbances in liver function including hepatitis and cholestatic jaundice, dizziness, paraesthesia, sexual dysfunction, thrombocytopenia, anaemia, leucopenia, eosinophilia, bone-marrow suppression, myalgia, myopathy, myasthenia, myositis accompanied by increase in creatine kinase (discontinue if raised significantly), blurred vision, exfoliative dermatitis, alopecia, and photosensitivity)
Dose
- 1.2 g daily, usually in 2 divided doses; range 0.9–1.2 g daily; CHILD not recommended

Gemfibrozil (Non-proprietary) PoM
Capsules, gemfibrozil 300 mg, net price 112-cap pack = £43.76. Label: 22
Tablets, gemfibrozil 600 mg, net price 30-tab pack = £19.94, 56-tab pack = £58.84. Label: 22

Lopid® (Pfizer) PoM
'300' capsules, white/maroon, gemfibrozil 300 mg. Net price 112-cap pack = £35.57. Label: 22
'600' tablets, f/c, gemfibrozil 600 mg. Net price 56-tab pack = £35.57. Label: 22

Statins

The statins (**atorvastatin**, **fluvastatin**, **pravastatin**, **rosuvastatin**, and **simvastatin**) competitively inhibit 3-hydroxy-3-methylglutaryl coenzyme A (HMG CoA) reductase, an enzyme involved in cholesterol synthesis, especially in the liver. Statins are more effective than other lipid-regulating drugs at lowering LDL-cholesterol concentration but they are less effective than the fibrates in reducing triglyceride concentration. However, statins reduce cardiovascular disease events and total mortality irrespective of the initial cholesterol concentration.

Statins should be considered for all patients, including the elderly, with symptomatic cardiovascular disease such as those with coronary heart disease (including history of angina or acute myocardial infarction), occlusive arterial disease (including peripheral vascular disease, non-haemorrhagic stroke, or transient ischaemic attacks).

In patients with diabetes mellitus, the risk of developing cardiovascular disease depends on the duration and complications of diabetes, age, and concomitant risk factors. Statin therapy should be considered for *all* patients over 40 years with diabetes mellitus (type 1 and 2). In younger patients with diabetes, treatment with a statin should be considered if there is target-organ damage, poor glycaemic control (HbA_{1c} greater than 9%), low HDL-cholesterol and raised triglyceride concentration, hypertension, or a family history of premature cardiovascular disease.

Statins are also used for the prevention of cardiovascular disease events in asymptomatic individuals who are at increased risk (see p. 137). Individuals with a 10-year cardiovascular disease risk[1] of 20% or more stand to benefit from statin treatment irrespective of the cholesterol concentration, and a statin should be used in combination with lifestyle measures and other interven-

1. Cardiovascular disease risk may be determined from the chart issued by the Joint British Societies (*Heart* 2005; **91** (Suppl V): v1–v52)—see inside back cover. The Joint British Societies' 'Cardiac Risk Assessor' computer programme may also be used to determine cardiovascular disease risk.

tions that reduce cardiovascular risk. Statin treatment should also be considered if the total cholesterol concentration to HDL-cholesterol ratio exceeds 6.

Cautions Statins should be used with caution in those with a history of liver disease or with a high alcohol intake (use should be avoided in active liver disease). Hypothyroidism should be managed adequately before starting treatment with a statin (see p. 137). Liver-function tests should be carried out before and within 1–3 months of starting treatment and thereafter at intervals of 6 months for 1 year, unless indicated sooner by signs or symptoms suggestive of hepatotoxicity. Treatment should be discontinued if serum transaminase concentration rises to, and persists at, 3 times the upper limit of the reference range. Statins should be used with caution in those with risk factors for myopathy or rhabdomyolysis; patients should be advised to report unexplained muscle pain (see Muscle Effects below). Statins should be avoided in porphyria (section 9.8.2) but rosuvastatin is thought to be safe. **Interactions:** Appendix 1 (statins).

Contra-indications Statins are contra-indicated in active liver disease (or persistently abnormal liver function tests), in pregnancy (adequate contraception required during treatment and for 1 month afterwards) and during breast-feeding (see Appendix 4 and Appendix 5).

Side-effects Reversible myositis is a rare but significant side-effect of the statins (see also CSM advice (Muscle Effects), p. 137 and below). The statins also cause headache, altered liver-function tests (rarely, hepatitis), paraesthesia, and gastro-intestinal effects including abdominal pain, flatulence, constipation, diarrhoea, nausea and vomiting. Rash and hypersensitivity reactions (including angioedema and anaphylaxis) have been reported rarely.

Muscle effects Myalgia, myositis, and myopathy have been reported with the statins; if myopathy is suspected and creatine kinase is markedly elevated (more than 5 times upper limit of normal), or muscular symptoms are severe, treatment should be discontinued; in patients at high risk of muscle effects, a statin should not be started if creatine kinase is elevated. Patients at high risk of myopathy include those with a personal or family history of muscular disorders, previous history of muscular toxicity or liver disease, and the elderly (see also CSM advice p. 137). There is also an increased incidence of myopathy if a statin is given at a high dose or given with a fibrate, with lipid-lowering doses of nicotinic acid, or with immunosuppressants such as ciclosporin; close monitoring of liver function and, if symptomatic, of creatine kinase is required in patients receiving these drugs. Rhabdomyolysis with acute renal impairment secondary to myoglobinuria has also been reported.

Counselling Advise patient to report promptly unexplained muscle pain, tenderness, or weakness.

ATORVASTATIN

Indications primary hypercholesterolaemia, heterozygous familial hypercholesterolaemia, homozygous familial hypercholesterolaemia or combined (mixed) hyperlipidaemia in patients who have not responded adequately to diet and other appropriate measures; prevention of cardiovascular events in patients with type 2 diabetes and at least one additional risk factor for cardiovascular disease

Cautions see notes above; also haemorrhagic stroke

Contra-indications see notes above

Side-effects see notes above; also chest pain; fatigue, asthenia, insomnia, dizziness, hypoaesthesia; arthralgia, back pain; *less commonly* anorexia, pancreatitis, malaise, weight gain, amnesia, hypoglycaemia, hyperglycaemia, peripheral neuropathy, impotence, thrombocytopenia, tinnitus, alopecia; *rarely* cholestatic jaundice, peripheral oedema; *very rarely* taste disturbances, gynaecomastia, visual disturbances, hearing loss, Stevens-Johnson Syndrome, and toxic epidermal necrolysis

Dose

- Primary hypercholesterolaemia and combined hyperlipidaemia, usually 10 mg once daily; if necessary, may be increased at intervals of at least 4 weeks to max. 80 mg once daily; CHILD 10–17 years usually 10 mg once daily (limited experience with doses above 20 mg daily)
- Familial hypercholesterolaemia, initially 10 mg daily, increased at intervals of at least 4 weeks to 40 mg once daily; if necessary, further increased to max. 80 mg once daily (or 40 mg once daily combined with anion-exchange resin in heterozygous familial hypercholesterolaemia); CHILD 10–17 years initially 10 mg daily, increased if necessary after at least 4 weeks to 20 mg once daily (limited experience with higher doses)
- Prevention of cardiovascular events in type 2 diabetes, 10 mg once daily

Note Max. 10 mg daily with concomitant ciclosporin; max. 20 mg daily (or temporarily discontinue atorvastatin) with concomitant clarithromycin; max. 40 mg daily (or temporarily discontinue atorvastatin) with concomitant itraconazole

Lipitor® (Pfizer) PoM

Tablets, all f/c, atorvastatin (as calcium trihydrate) 10 mg, net price 28-tab pack = £18.03; 20 mg, 28-tab pack = £24.64; 40 mg 28-tab pack = £28.21; 80 mg, 28-tab pack = £28.21. Counselling, muscle effects, see notes above

FLUVASTATIN

Note The *Scottish Medicines Consortium* has advised (February 2004) that fluvastatin is accepted for restricted use for the secondary prevention of coronary events after percutaneous coronary angioplasty; if the patient has previously been receiving another statin, then there is no need to change the statin

Indications adjunct to diet in primary hypercholesterolaemia or combined (mixed) hyperlipidaemia (types IIa and IIb); adjunct to diet to slow progression of coronary atherosclerosis in primary hypercholesterolaemia and concomitant coronary heart disease; prevention of coronary events after percutaneous coronary intervention

Cautions see notes above

Contra-indications see notes above

Side-effects see notes above; also insomnia; *very rarely* dysaesthesia, hypoesthesia, peripheral neuropathy, thrombocytopenia, vasculitis, eczema, dermatitis, bullous exanthema, and lupus erythematosus-like syndrome

Dose

- Hypercholesterolaemia or combined hyperlipidaemia, initially 20–40 mg daily in the evening, adjusted at intervals of at least 4 weeks; up to 80 mg daily may be required; CHILD and ADOLESCENT under 18 years, not recommended

- Prevention of progression of coronary atherosclerosis, 40 mg daily in the evening
- Following percutaneous coronary intervention, 80 mg daily

Lescol® (Novartis) PoM
Capsules, fluvastatin (as sodium salt) 20 mg (brown/yellow), net price 28-cap pack = £15.26; 40 mg (brown/orange), 28-cap pack = £15.26, 56-cap pack = £30.53. Counselling, muscle effects, see notes above

Modified release

Lescol® XL (Novartis) PoM
Tablets, m/r, yellow, fluvastatin (as sodium salt) 80 mg, net price 28-tab pack = £19.20. Label: 25, counselling, muscle effects, see notes above
Dose 80 mg once daily (dose form not appropriate for initial dose titration in hypercholesterolaemia or combined hyperlipidaemia)

PRAVASTATIN SODIUM

Indications adjunct to diet for primary hypercholesterolaemia or combined (mixed) hyperlipidaemias in patients who have not responded adequately to dietary control; adjunct to diet to prevent cardiovascular events in patients with hypercholesterolaemia; prevention of cardiovascular events in patients with previous myocardial infarction or unstable angina; reduction of hyperlipidaemia in patients receiving immunosuppressive therapy following solid-organ transplantation
Cautions see notes above; renal impairment (Appendix 3)
Contra-indications see notes above
Side-effects see notes above; *less commonly* fatigue, dizziness, sleep disturbances, abnormal urination (including dysuria, nocturia and frequency), sexual dysfunction, visual disturbances, alopecia, *very rarely* pancreatitis, jaundice, fulminant hepatic necrosis, peripheral neuropathy, lupus erythematosus-like syndrome
Dose
- Hypercholesterolaemia or combined hyperlipidaemias, 10–40 mg once daily at night, adjusted at intervals of at least 4 weeks
- Familial hypercholesterolaemia, CHILD 8–14 years 10–20 mg once daily at night, 14–18 years 10–40 mg once daily at night
- Prevention of cardiovascular events, 40 mg once daily at night
- Post-transplantation hyperlipidaemia, initially 20 mg once daily at night, increased if necessary (under close medical supervision) to max. 40 mg once daily at night

Pravastatin (Non-proprietary) PoM
Tablets, pravastatin sodium 10 mg, net price 28-tab pack = £3.40; 20 mg, 28-tab pack = £4.91; 40 mg, 28-tab pack = £7.54. Counselling, muscle effects, see notes above

Lipostat® (Squibb) PoM
Tablets, all yellow, pravastatin sodium 10 mg, net price 28-tab pack = £15.05; 20 mg, 28-tab pack = £27.61; 40 mg, 28-tab pack = £27.61. Counselling, muscle effects, see notes above

ROSUVASTATIN

Indications primary hypercholesterolaemia (type IIa including heterozygous familial hypercholesterolaemia), mixed dyslipidaemia (type IIb), or homozygous familial hypercholesterolaemia in patients who have not responded adequately to diet and other appropriate measures
Cautions see notes above; patients of Asian origin (see under Dose); max. dose 20 mg in patients with risk factors for myopathy or rhabdomyolysis (including personal or family history of muscular disorders or toxicity); renal impairment (avoid if creatinine clearance less than 30 mL/minute; Appendix 3)
Contra-indications see notes above
Side-effects see notes above; also dizziness and asthenia; proteinuria; *rarely* pancreatitis, jaundice, arthralgia, and polyneuropathy; *very rarely* haematuria
Dose
- Initially 5–10 mg once daily increased if necessary at intervals of at least 4 weeks to 20 mg once daily, increased after further 4 weeks to 40 mg daily only in severe hypercholesterolaemia with high cardiovascular risk and under specialist supervision; ELDERLY initially 5 mg once daily; patient of ASIAN origin, initially 5 mg once daily increased if necessary to max. 20 mg daily

Note Initially 5 mg once daily with concomitant fibrate increased if necessary to max. 20 mg daily

Crestor® (AstraZeneca) PoM
Tablets, f/c, rosuvastatin (as calcium salt) 5 mg (yellow), net price 28-tab pack = £18.03; 10 mg (pink), 28-tab pack = £18.03; 20 mg (pink), 28-tab pack = £26.02; 40 mg (pink), 28-tab pack = £29.69. Counselling, muscle effects, see notes above

SIMVASTATIN

Indications primary hypercholesterolaemia, homozygous familial hypercholesterolaemia or combined (mixed) hyperlipidaemia in patients who have not responded adequately to diet and other appropriate measures; prevention of cardiovascular events in patients with atherosclerotic cardiovascular disease or diabetes mellitus
Cautions see notes above; renal impairment (Appendix 3)
Contra-indications see notes above
Side-effects see notes above; also alopecia, anaemia, dizziness, peripheral neuropathy, asthenia, jaundice, pancreatitis
Dose
- Primary hypercholesterolaemia, combined hyperlipidaemia, 10–20 mg daily at night, adjusted at intervals of at least 4 weeks; usual range 10–80 mg once daily at night
- Homozygous familial hypercholesterolaemia, 40 mg daily at night *or* 80 mg daily in 3 divided doses (with largest dose at night)
- Prevention of cardiovascular events, initially 20–40 mg once daily at night, adjusted at intervals of at least 4 weeks; max. 80 mg once daily at night

Note Max. 10 mg daily with concomitant ciclosporin, danazol, fibrate or lipid-lowering dose of nicotinic acid. Max. 20 mg daily with concomitant amiodarone or verapamil. Max. 40 mg daily with diltiazem

[1]Simvastatin (Non-proprietary) PoM
Tablets, simvastatin 10 mg, net price 28-tab pack = 34p, 20 mg, 28-tab pack = 54p; 40 mg, 28-tab pack = £1.31; 80 mg, 28-tab pack = £4.91. Counselling, muscle effects, see notes above
Brands include *Simvador®*

[1]Zocor® (MSD) PoM
Tablets, all f/c, simvastatin 10 mg (peach), net price 28-tab pack = £18.03; 20 mg (tan), 28-tab pack = £29.69; 40 mg (red), 28-tab pack = £29.69; 80 mg (red), 28-tab pack = £29.69. Counselling, muscle effects, see notes above

With ezetimibe

Note For hypercholesterolaemia in patients stabilised on the individual components in the same proportions, or for patients not adequately controlled by statin alone. The *Scottish Medicines Consortium* has advised (June 2005) that Inegy® is accepted for restricted use for patients not adequately controlled with a maximal dose of a statin. For cautions, contra-indications, and side-effects of ezetimibe, see Ezetimibe

Inegy® (MSD, Schering-Plough) ▼ PoM
Tablets, simvastatin 20 mg, ezetimibe 10 mg, net price 28-tab pack = £33.42; simvastatin 40 mg, ezetimibe 10 mg, 28-tab pack = £38.98; simvastatin 80 mg, ezetimibe 10 mg, 28-tab pack = £41.21. Counselling, muscle effects, see notes above

Nicotinic acid group

The value of **nicotinic acid** is limited by its side-effects, especially vasodilatation. In doses of 1.5 to 3 g daily it lowers both cholesterol and triglyceride concentrations by inhibiting synthesis; it also increases HDL-cholesterol. Nicotinic acid is licensed for use with a statin if the statin alone cannot adequately control dyslipidaemia (raised LDL-cholesterol, triglyceridaemia, and low HDL-cholesterol); it can be used alone if the patient is intolerant of statins (for advice on treatment of dyslipidaemia, including use of combination treatment, see p. 137). The *Scottish Medicines Consortium* has advised (January 2006) that *Niaspan®* is not recommended for the treatment of dyslipidaemia.

Acipimox seems to have fewer side-effects than nicotinic acid but may be less effective in its lipid-modulating capabilities.

ACIPIMOX

Indications hyperlipidaemias of types IIb and IV in patients who have not responded adequately to diet and other appropriate measures

Cautions renal impairment (avoid if creatinine clearance less than 30 mL/minute; Appendix 3)

Contra-indications peptic ulcer; pregnancy (Appendix 4); breast-feeding (Appendix 5)

Side-effects vasodilatation, flushing, itching, rashes, urticaria, erythema; heartburn, epigastric pain, nausea, diarrhoea, headache, malaise, dry eyes; rarely angioedema, bronchospasm, anaphylaxis

Dose
- Usually 500–750 mg daily in divided doses

Olbetam® (Pharmacia) PoM
Capsules, brown/pink, acipimox 250 mg. Net price 90-cap pack = £46.33. Label: 21

NICOTINIC ACID

Indications adjunct to statin in dyslipidaemia or used alone if statin not tolerated (see also p. 137)

Cautions unstable angina, acute myocardial infarction, diabetes mellitus, gout, history of peptic ulceration; hepatic impairment (Appendix 2); renal impairment; pregnancy (Appendix 4); **interactions**: Appendix 1 (nicotinic acid)

Contra-indications arterial bleeding; active peptic ulcer disease; breast-feeding

Side-effects diarrhoea, nausea, vomiting, abdominal pain, dyspepsia; flushing; pruritus, rash; *less commonly* tachycardia, palpitation, shortness of breath, peripheral oedema, headache, dizziness, increase in uric acid, hypophosphataemia, prolonged prothrombin time, and reduced platelet count; *rarely* hypotension, syncope, rhinitis, insomnia, reduced glucose tolerance, myalgia, myopathy, and myasthenia; *very rarely* anorexia, rhabdomyolysis

Note Prostaglandin-mediated symptoms (such as flushing) can be reduced by low initial doses taken with meals

Dose
- See under preparation

Modified release

Niaspan® (Merck) PoM
Tablets, m/r, nicotinic acid 500 mg, net price 56-tab pack = £17.25; 750 mg, 56-tab pack = £26.25; 1 g, 56-tab pack = £34.75; 21-day starter pack of 7 × 375-mg tab with 7 × 500-mg tab and 7 × 750-mg tab = £14.00. Label: 21, 25

Dose 375 mg once daily at night (after a low-fat snack) for 1 week, then 500 mg once daily at night for 1 week, then 750 mg once daily at night for 1 week, then 1 g once daily at night for 4 weeks, increased if necessary in steps of 500 mg at intervals of at least 4 weeks to max. 2 g daily; usual maintenance dose 1–2 g once daily at night

Omega-3 fatty acid compounds

The omega-3 fatty acid compounds comprise omega-3-acid ethyl esters (*Omacor®*) and omega-3-marine triglycerides (*Maxepa®*). Omega-3 fatty acid compounds may be used to reduce triglycerides, as an alternative to a fibrate and in addition to a statin, in patients with combined (mixed) hyperlipidaemia not adequately controlled with a statin alone. A triglyceride concentration exceeding 10 mmol/litre is associated with acute pancreatitis and lowering the concentration reduces this risk. The fat content of omega-3 fatty acid compounds (including excipients in the preparations) should be taken into consideration when treating hypertriglyceridaemia. There is little clinical trial evidence that the triglyceride lowering effect decreases the risk of cardiovascular disease.

OMEGA-3-ACID ETHYL ESTERS

Indications adjunct to diet and statin in type IIb or III hypertriglyceridaemia; adjunct to diet in type IV hyp-

1. Simvastatin 10 mg tablets can be sold to the public to reduce risk of first coronary event in individuals at moderate risk of coronary heart disease (approx. 10–15% risk of major event in 10 years), max. daily dose 10 mg and pack size of 28 tablets; treatment should form part of a programme to reduce risk of coronary heart disease; a proprietary brand *Zocor Heart-Pro®* is on sale to the public

ertriglyceridaemia; adjunct in secondary prevention after myocardial infarction

Cautions haemorrhagic disorders, anticoagulant treatment (bleeding time increased); hepatic impairment (Appendix 2); pregnancy (Appendix 4)

Contra-indications breast-feeding (Appendix 5)

Side-effects gastro-intestinal disturbances; *less commonly* taste disturbances, dizziness, and hypersensitivity reactions; *rarely* hepatic disorders, headache, hyperglycaemia, acne, and rash; *very rarely* hypotension, nasal dryness, urticaria, and increased white cell count

Dose

- See under preparation below

Omacor® (Solvay)

Capsules, 1 g of omega-3-acid ethyl esters 90 containing eicosapentaenoic acid 460 mg and docosahexaenoic acid 380 mg, net price 28-cap pack = £13.89, 100-cap pack = £49.60. Label: 21

Dose hypertriglyceridaemia, initially 2 capsules daily with food, increased if necessary to 4 capsules daily

Secondary prevention after myocardial infarction, 1 capsule daily with food

OMEGA-3-MARINE TRIGLYCERIDES

Indications adjunct in the reduction of plasma triglycerides in severe hypertriglyceridaemia

Cautions haemorrhagic disorders, anticoagulant treatment; aspirin-sensitive asthma; type 2 diabetes

Side-effects occasional nausea and belching

Dose

- See under preparations below

Maxepa® (Seven Seas)

Capsules, 1 g (approx. 1.1 mL) concentrated fish oils containing eicosapentaenoic acid 170 mg, docosahexaenoic acid 115 mg. Vitamin A content less than 100 units/g, vitamin D content less than 10 units/g, net price 200-cap pack = £27.28. Label: 21

Dose 5 capsules twice daily with food

Liquid, golden-coloured, concentrated fish oils containing eicosapentaenoic acid 170 mg, docosahexaenoic acid 115 mg/g (1.1 mL). Vitamin A content less than 100 units/g, vitamin D content less than 10 units/g, net price 150 mL = £20.46. Label: 21

Dose 5 mL twice daily with food

2.13 Local sclerosants

Ethanolamine oleate and sodium tetradecyl sulphate are used in sclerotherapy of varicose veins, and phenol is used in haemorrhoids (section 1.7.3).

ETHANOLAMINE OLEATE
(Monoethanolamine Oleate)

Indications sclerotherapy of varicose veins

Cautions extravasation may cause necrosis of tissues

Contra-indications inability to walk, acute phlebitis, oral contraceptive use, obese legs

Side-effects allergic reactions (including anaphylaxis)

Ethanolamine Oleate (UCB Pharma) PoM

Injection, ethanolamine oleate 5%, net price 2-mL amp = £3.19, 5-mL amp = £2.28

Dose by slow injection into empty isolated segment of vein, 2–5 mL divided between 3–4 sites; repeated at weekly intervals

SODIUM TETRADECYL SULPHATE

Indications sclerotherapy of varicose veins

Cautions see under Ethanolamine Oleate

Contra-indications see under Ethanolamine Oleate

Side-effects see under Ethanolamine Oleate

Fibro-Vein® (STD Pharmaceutical) PoM

Injection, sodium tetradecyl sulphate 0.2%, net price 5-mL amp = £5.51; 0.5%, 2-mL amp = £2.87; 1%, 2-mL amp = £3.31; 3%, 2-mL amp = £4.07, 5-mL vial = £10.25

Dose by slow injection into empty isolated segment of vein, 0.1–1 mL according to site and condition being treated (consult product literature)

3 Respiratory system

3.1 Bronchodilators 145
3.1.1 Adrenoceptor agonists 149
3.1.1.1 Selective beta$_2$ agonists 149
3.1.1.2 Other adrenoceptor agonists 153
3.1.2 Antimuscarinic bronchodilators 153
3.1.3 Theophylline 154
3.1.4 Compound bronchodilator preparations 156
3.1.5 Peak flow meters, inhaler devices and nebulisers 156
3.2 Corticosteroids 159
3.3 Cromoglicate and related therapy and leukotriene receptor antagonists 164
3.3.1 Cromoglicate and related therapy 164
3.3.2 Leukotriene receptor antagonists 165
3.4 Antihistamines, hyposensitisation, and allergic emergencies 165
3.4.1 Antihistamines 165
3.4.2 Allergen Immunotherapy 169
3.4.3 Allergic emergencies 170
3.5 Respiratory stimulants and pulmonary surfactants 172
3.5.1 Respiratory stimulants 172
3.5.2 Pulmonary surfactants 173
3.6 Oxygen 173
3.7 Mucolytics 175
3.8 Aromatic inhalations 176
3.9 Cough preparations 176
3.9.1 Cough suppressants 176
3.9.2 Expectorant and demulcent cough preparations 177
3.10 Systemic nasal decongestants 178

This chapter also includes advice on the drug management of the following:

acute severe asthma, p. 148
anaphylaxis, p. 170
angioedema, p. 171
chronic asthma, p. 146
chronic obstructive pulmonary disease, p. 148
croup, p. 148

3.1 Bronchodilators

3.1.1 Adrenoceptor agonists
3.1.2 Antimuscarinic bronchodilators
3.1.3 Theophylline
3.1.4 Compound bronchodilator preparations
3.1.5 Peak flow meters, inhaler devices and nebulisers

Asthma

Drugs used in the management of asthma include beta$_2$ agonists (section 3.1.1), antimuscarinic bronchodilators (section 3.1.2), theophylline (section 3.1.3), corticosteroids (section 3.2), cromoglicate and nedocromil (section 3.3.1), and leukotriene receptor antagonists (section 3.3.2).

For tables outlining the management of chronic asthma and acute severe asthma see p. 146 and p. 147. For advice on the management of medical emergencies in dental practice, see p. 21.

Administration of drugs for asthma

Inhalation This route delivers the drug directly to the airways; the dose required is smaller than when given by mouth and side-effects are reduced. *Pressurised metered-dose inhalers* are an effective and convenient method of administering many drugs used for asthma. A spacer device (section 3.1.5) may improve drug delivery, particularly for children under 15 years and those who have difficulty using a pressurised metered-dose inhaler; spacers also reduce local adverse effects caused by inhaled corticosteroids. Breath-actuated inhalers and dry powder inhalers are also available.

Solutions for nebulisation are available for use in acute severe asthma. They are administered over 5–10 minutes from a nebuliser, usually driven by oxygen in hospital. Electric compressors are best suited to domiciliary use.

Oral The oral route is used when administration by inhalation is not possible. Systemic side-effects occur more frequently when a drug is given orally rather than by inhalation. Drugs given by mouth for the treatment of asthma include beta$_2$ agonists, corticosteroids, theophylline, and leukotriene receptor antagonists.

Parenteral Drugs such as beta$_2$ agonists, corticosteroids, and aminophylline can be given by injection in acute severe asthma when administration by nebulisation is inadequate or inappropriate. If the patient is being treated in the community, urgent transfer to hospital should be arranged.

Management of chronic asthma in adults and children

Start at step most appropriate to initial severity

Chronic asthma: adults and schoolchildren

Step 1: occasional relief bronchodilators

Inhaled short-acting $beta_2$ agonist as required (up to once daily)

NOTE. Move to step 2 if needed more than twice a week, or if night-time symptoms more than once a week, or if exacerbation in the last 2 years requiring systemic corticosteroid or nebulised bronchodilator; check compliance and inhaler technique

Step 2: regular inhaled preventer therapy

Inhaled short-acting $beta_2$ agonist as required

plus

Regular standard-dose[1] inhaled corticosteroid (alternatives[2] are considerably less effective)

Step 3: inhaled corticosteroid + long-acting inhaled $beta_2$ agonist

Inhaled short-acting $beta_2$ agonist as required

plus

Regular standard-dose[1] inhaled corticosteroid

plus

Regular inhaled long-acting $beta_2$ agonist (salmeterol *or* formoterol)

If asthma not controlled

Increase dose of inhaled corticosteroid to upper end of standard dose[1]

and

Either stop long-acting $beta_2$ agonist if of no benefit

Or continue long-acting $beta_2$ agonist if of some benefit

If asthma still not controlled and long-acting $beta_2$ agonist stopped

Add one of

- Leukotriene receptor antagonist
- Modified-release oral theophylline
- Modified-release oral $beta_2$ agonist

Step 4: high-dose inhaled corticosteroid + regular bronchodilators

Inhaled short-acting $beta_2$ agonist as required

with

Regular high-dose[3] inhaled corticosteroid

plus

Inhaled long-acting $beta_2$ agonist

plus

In adults 6-week sequential therapeutic trial of one or more of

- Leukotriene receptor antagonist
- Modified-release oral theophylline
- Modified-release oral $beta_2$ agonist

Step 5: regular corticosteroid tablets

Inhaled short-acting $beta_2$ agonist as required

with

Regular high-dose[3] inhaled corticosteroid

and

One or more long-acting bronchodilators (see step 4)

plus

Regular prednisolone tablets (as single daily dose)

NOTE. In addition to regular prednisolone, continue high-dose inhaled corticosteroid (in exceptional cases may exceed licensed doses); these patients should normally be referred to an asthma clinic

Stepping down

Review treatment every 3 months; if control achieved stepwise reduction may be possible; use lowest possible dose of corticosteroid which controls asthma; reduce dose of *inhaled* corticosteroid slowly (consider reduction every 3 months, decreasing dose by up to 50% each time)

Chronic asthma: children under 5 years[4]

Step 1: occasional relief bronchodilators

Short-acting $beta_2$ agonist as required (not more than once daily)

NOTE. Whenever possible inhaled (less effective and more side-effects when given by mouth); check compliance, technique and that inhaler device is appropriate

Move to step 2 if needed more than twice a week, or if night-time symptoms more than once a week, or if exacerbation in last 2 years

Step 2: regular preventer therapy

Inhaled short-acting $beta_2$ agonist as required

plus

Either regular standard-dose[1] inhaled corticosteroid

Or (if inhaled corticosteroid cannot be used) leukotriene receptor antagonist or theophylline

Step 3: add-on therapy

Children 2–5 years:

Inhaled short-acting $beta_2$ agonist as required

plus

Regular inhaled corticosteroid in standard dose[1]

plus

Leukotriene receptor antagonist

Children under 2 years:

Refer to respiratory paediatrician

Step 4: persistent poor control

Refer to respiratory paediatrician

Stepping down

Regularly review need for treatment

1. Standard-dose inhaled corticosteroids (given through metered dose inhaler) are beclometasone dipropionate or budesonide 100–400 micrograms (CHILD 100–200 micrograms) twice daily *or* fluticasone propionate 50–200 micrograms (CHILD 50–100 micrograms) twice daily *or* mometasone furoate (given through dry powder inhaler) 200 micrograms twice daily; initial dose according to severity of asthma; use large-volume spacer in children under 5 years
2. Alternatives to inhaled corticosteroid are leukotriene receptor antagonist, theophylline, and in adults, regular cromoglicate, and in children over 5 years, regular nedocromil
3. High-dose inhaled corticosteroids (given through metered dose inhaler) are beclometasone dipropionate or budesonide 0.8–2 mg daily (in divided doses) *or* fluticasone propionate 0.4–1 mg daily (in divided doses) *or* mometasone furoate (given through dry powder inhaler) up to 800 micrograms daily (in 2 divided doses); CHILD 5–12 years, beclometasone dipropionate or budesonide up to 400 micrograms twice daily *or* fluticasone propionate up to 200 micrograms twice daily; use a large-volume spacer

   NOTE. Failure to achieve control with these doses is unusual. Before moving beyond step 4 consider whether diagnosis is correct and check compliance, see also Side-effects of Inhaled Corticosteroids, section 3.2
4. Lung-function measurements cannot be used to guide management in those under 5 years

Advice on the management of chronic asthma is based on the recommendations of the British Thoracic Society and Scottish Intercollegiate Guidelines Network (updated July 2007)

Management of acute severe asthma in general practice

MANAGEMENT OF ACUTE SEVERE ASTHMA IN GENERAL PRACTICE

Moderate asthma exacerbation
— Peak flow >50–75% of predicted or best
— No features of acute severe asthma
— Increasing symptoms
Treat at home but response to treatment **must** be assessed before doctor leaves
Treatment:
High-flow oxygen if available
Salbutamol or terbutaline via large-volume spacer (4–6 puffs each inhaled separately; dose repeated every 10–20 minutes if necessary) or nebuliser
Monitor response 15–30 minutes after nebulisation
Give oral prednisolone 40–50 mg daily for at least 5 days and step up usual treatment
Follow up
Monitor symptoms and peak flow
Set up asthma action plan
Review in surgery within 48 hours
Modify treatment at review according to guidelines for chronic asthma (see Management of Chronic Asthma in Adults and Children)

Important: regard each emergency consultation as being for **acute severe asthma** until shown otherwise.

Important: failure to respond adequately **at any time** requires immediate referral to hospital.

Acute severe asthma in adults
— Cannot complete sentences in one breath
— Pulse ≥ 110 beats/minute
— Respiration ≥ 25 breaths/minute
— Peak flow 33–50% of predicted or best
Seriously consider hospital admission if more than one of above features present
Treatment:
High-flow oxygen if available
Salbutamol or terbutaline via large-volume spacer (4–6 puffs each inhaled separately; dose repeated every 10–20 minutes if necessary) or nebuliser (oxygen driven if available)
Oral prednisolone 40–50 mg daily for at least 5 days (or i/v hydrocortisone 400 mg daily in 4 divided doses)
Monitor response 15–30 minutes after nebulisation
If any signs of acute asthma persist:
Arrange hospital admission
While awaiting ambulance repeat nebulised beta$_2$ agonist and give with nebulised ipratropium 500 micrograms
Alternatively if symptoms have improved, respiration and pulse settling, and peak flow >50% of predicted or best:
Step up usual treatment *and* continue prednisolone for at least 5 days
Follow up
Monitor symptoms and peak flow, set up asthma action plan, review in surgery within 24 hours, modify treatment at review (see Management of Chronic Asthma)

Life-threatening asthma in adults
— Silent chest
— Cyanosis
— Feeble respiratory effort
— Bradycardia, exhaustion, arrhythmia, hypotension, confusion, or coma
— Peak flow <33% of predicted or best
— Arterial oxygen saturation <92%
Arrange **immediate** hospital admission
Treatment:
Oral prednisolone 40–50 mg daily for at least 5 days (or i/v hydrocortisone 400 mg daily in 4 divided doses) (immediately)
Oxygen-driven nebuliser in ambulance
Nebulised[1] beta$_2$ agonist with nebulised ipratropium
Stay with patient until ambulance arrives

1. If nebuliser not available give 1 puff of beta$_2$ agonist using large-volume spacer and repeat 10–20 times

Important: patients with severe or life-threatening attacks may not be distressed and may not have all these abnormalities; the presence of any should alert doctor.

Acute episodes or exacerbations of asthma in young children in primary care

Mild/moderate episode in young children
– short-acting beta$_2$ agonist from metered dose inhaler *via* large-volume spacer (and face mask in very young), up to 10 puffs; alternatively give by nebuliser
– if favourable response (respiratory rate reduced, reduced use of accessory muscles, improved 'behaviour' pattern), repeat inhaled beta$_2$ agonist as needed
– start short course of oral prednisolone for 3 days (under 2 years 10 mg; 2–5 years 20 mg; over 5 years 30–40 mg daily; those already on prednisolone tablets 2 mg/kg up to max. 60 mg)
– consider i/v hydrocortisone in those who are unable to retain oral prednisolone

If unresponsive or relapse within 3–4 hours:
– immediately refer to hospital
– give nebulised beta$_2$ agonist with nebulised ipratropium 250 micrograms every 20–30 minutes
– give high-flow oxygen *via* face mask

Signs of acute asthma in children

Acute severe asthma:
– too breathless to talk
– too breathless to feed
– respiration >50 breaths/minute (> 30/minute in children over 5 years)
– pulse >130 beats/minute (>120 beats/minute in children over 5 years)
– in younger children, use of accessory muscles of breathing
– in older children, peak flow ≤50% of predicted or best

Life-threatening features:
– cyanosis, silent chest, or poor respiratory effort
– exhaustion
– agitation, hypotension, confusion, reduced level of consciousness, or coma
– in older children, peak flow <33% of predicted or best

Advice on the management of acute asthma is based on the recommendations of the British Thoracic Society and Scottish Intercollegiate Guidelines Network (updated July 2007)

Pregnancy and breast-feeding

It is particularly important that asthma should be well controlled during pregnancy; when this is achieved asthma has no important effects on pregnancy, labour, or on the fetus. Drugs for asthma should preferably be administered by inhalation to minimise exposure of the fetus. Women planning to become pregnant should be counselled about the importance of taking their asthma medication regularly to maintain good control.

Severe exacerbations of asthma can have an adverse effect on pregnancy and should be treated promptly with conventional therapy, including oral or parenteral administration of a corticosteroid and nebulisation of a beta$_2$ agonist; prednisolone is the preferred corticosteroid for oral administration since very little of the drug reaches the fetus. Oxygen should be given immediately to maintain arterial oxygen saturation above 95% and prevent maternal and fetal hypoxia.

Inhaled drugs, theophylline, and prednisolone can be taken as normal during pregnancy and breast-feeding.

Acute severe asthma

Acute severe asthma can be fatal and **must** be treated promptly and energetically. Patients should be given **oxygen** (if available), inhaled **salbutamol** or **terbutaline** via a large-volume spacer or nebuliser (if there are life-threatening features, a nebuliser should be used), and a systemic **corticosteroid** (section 6.3.2). For adults, prednisolone 40–50 mg by mouth or hydrocortisone 100 mg (preferably as sodium succinate) intravenously should be given. For children, prednisolone 1–2 mg/kg by mouth (max. 40 mg) or intravenous hydrocortisone (under 1 year 25 mg, 1–5 years 50 mg, 6–12 years 100 mg) (preferably as sodium succinate) are used. In case of vomiting, the parenteral route may be used for the first dose. In life-threatening asthma, initial treatment with **ipratropium** by nebuliser (section 3.1.2) should also be considered.

Most patients do not require and do not benefit from the addition of intravenous aminophylline or of intravenous beta$_2$ agonist; both cause more adverse effects than nebulised beta$_2$ agonists. Nevertheless, an occasional patient who has not been taking theophylline may benefit from aminophylline infusion. Patients with severe asthma may be helped by **magnesium sulphate** [unlicensed indication] 1.2–2 g given by intravenous infusion over 20 minutes, but evidence of benefit is limited.

Treatment of acute severe asthma is safer in hospital where resuscitation facilities are immediately available. Treatment should **never** be delayed for investigations, patients should **never** be sedated, and the possibility of a pneumothorax should be considered.

If the patient's condition deteriorates despite pharmacological treatment, intermittent positive pressure ventilation may be needed.

For a table outlining the management of acute severe asthma, see p. 147.

Chronic obstructive pulmonary disease

Smoking cessation (section 4.10) reduces the progressive decline in lung function in chronic obstructive pulmonary disease (COPD, chronic bronchitis, or emphysema). Infection can complicate chronic obstructive pulmonary disease and may be prevented by vaccination (pneumococcal vaccine and influenza vaccine, section 14.4).

A trial of a high-dose inhaled corticosteroid *or* an oral corticosteroid is recommended for patients with moderate airflow obstruction to ensure that asthma has not been overlooked.

Symptoms of chronic obstructive pulmonary disease may be alleviated by an inhaled **short-acting beta$_2$ agonist** (section 3.1.1.1) or a **short-acting antimuscarinic bronchodilator** (section 3.1.2) used as required.

When the airways obstruction is more severe, an inhaled **antimuscarinic bronchodilator** (section 3.1.2) given regularly should be added. In those who remain symptomatic or have two or more exacerbations in a year, a **long-acting beta$_2$ agonist** or a **long-acting antimuscarinic bronchodilator** given regularly should be added. A short-acting antimuscarinic bronchodilator should be discontinued when a long-acting antimuscarinic bronchodilator is started. If symptoms persist or if the patient is unable to use an inhaler, oral modified-release **aminophylline** or **theophylline** (section 3.1.3) can be used.

In moderate or severe chronic obstructive pulmonary disease, either a combination of a long-acting beta$_2$ agonist with an **inhaled corticosteroid** (section 3.2) or a long-acting antimuscarinic bronchodilator should be tried.

A mucolytic drug (section 3.7) may be considered for a patient with a chronic productive cough.

Long-term **oxygen** therapy (section 3.6) prolongs survival in patients with severe chronic obstructive pulmonary disease and hypoxaemia.

During an exacerbation of chronic obstructive pulmonary disease, bronchodilator therapy can be administered through a nebuliser if necessary and oxygen given if appropriate. **Aminophylline** can be given intravenously if response to nebulised bronchodilators is poor. A short course of **oral corticosteroid** (section 6.3.2), such as prednisolone 30 mg daily for 7–14 days, should be given if increased breathlessness interferes with daily activities. **Antibacterial** treatment (Table 1, section 5.1) is required when sputum becomes purulent or if there are other signs of infection.

Croup

Mild croup is largely self-limiting, but treatment with a single dose of a corticosteroid (e.g. dexamethasone 150 micrograms/kg) by mouth may be of benefit. More severe croup (or mild croup that might cause complications) calls for hospital admission; a single dose of a corticosteroid (e.g. dexamethasone 150 micrograms/kg by mouth, section 6.3.2) should be administered before transfer to hospital. In hospital, dexamethasone 150 micrograms/kg (by mouth or by injection) or budesonide 2 mg (by nebulisation, section 3.2) will often reduce symptoms; the dose may need to be repeated after 12 hours if necessary. For severe croup not effectively controlled with corticosteroid treatment, nebulised adrenaline solution 1 in 1000 (1 mg/mL) should be given with close clinical monitoring in a dose of 400 micrograms/kg (max. 5 mg) repeated after 30 minutes if necessary; the effects of nebulised adrenaline last 2–3 hours and the child needs to be monitored carefully for recurrence of the obstruction.

3.1.1 Adrenoceptor agonists (Sympathomimetics)

3.1.1.1 Selective beta$_2$ agonists
3.1.1.2 Other adrenoceptor agonists

The selective beta$_2$ agonists (selective beta$_2$-adrenoceptor agonists, selective beta$_2$ stimulants) (section 3.1.1.1) such as salbutamol or terbutaline are the safest and most effective short-acting beta$_2$ agonists for asthma. Less selective beta$_2$ agonists such as orciprenaline (section 3.1.1.2) should be avoided whenever possible.

Adrenaline (epinephrine) (which has both alpha- and beta-adrenoceptor agonist properties) is used in the emergency management of allergic and anaphylactic reactions (section 3.4.3) and in the management of croup (see above).

3.1.1.1 Selective beta$_2$ agonists

Selective beta$_2$ agonists produce bronchodilation. A short-acting beta$_2$ agonist is used for immediate relief of asthma symptoms while a long-acting beta$_2$ agonist is added to an inhaled corticosteroid in patients requiring prophylactic treatment.

Chronic Asthma table, see p. 146
Acute Severe Asthma table, see p. 147

Short-acting beta$_2$ agonists Mild to moderate symptoms of asthma respond rapidly to the inhalation of a selective short-acting beta$_2$ agonist such as **salbutamol** or **terbutaline**. If beta$_2$ agonist inhalation is needed more often than once daily, prophylactic treatment should be considered, using a stepped approach as outlined in the Management of Chronic Asthma table, p. 146. Regular treatment with an inhaled short-acting beta$_2$ agonist is less effective than 'as required' inhalation and is not appropriate prophylactic treatment.

A short-acting beta$_2$ agonist inhaled immediately before exertion reduces *exercise-induced asthma*; however, frequent exercise-induced asthma probably reflects poor overall control and calls for reassessment of asthma treatment.

Long-acting beta$_2$ agonists **Formoterol** (eformoterol) and **salmeterol** are longer-acting beta$_2$ agonists which are administered by inhalation. Added to regular inhaled corticosteroid treatment, they have a role in the long-term control of chronic asthma (see Chronic Asthma table, p. 146) and they can be useful in nocturnal asthma. Salmeterol should not be used for the relief of an asthma attack; it has a slower onset of action than salbutamol or terbutaline. Formoterol is licensed for short-term symptom relief and for the prevention of exercise-induced bronchospasm; its speed of onset of action is similar to that of salbutamol.

> **CHM advice**
> To ensure safe use, the CHM has advised that for the management of chronic asthma, long-acting beta$_2$ agonists (formoterol and salmeterol) should:
> - be added only if regular use of standard-dose inhaled corticosteroids has failed to control asthma adequately;
> - not be initiated in patients with rapidly deteriorating asthma;
> - be introduced at a low dose and the effect properly monitored before considering dose increase;
> - be discontinued in the absence of benefit;
> - be reviewed as clinically appropriate: stepping down therapy should be considered when good long-term asthma control has been achieved.
>
> Patients should be advised to report any deterioration in symptoms following initiation of treatment with a long-acting beta$_2$ agonist, see Management of Chronic Asthma table, p. 146.

Inhalation *Pressurised-metered dose inhalers* are an effective and convenient method of drug administration in mild to moderate asthma. A spacer device (section 3.1.5) may improve drug delivery. At recommended inhaled doses the duration of action of salbutamol, terbutaline and fenoterol is about 3 to 5 hours and for salmeterol and formoterol 12 hours. The **dose**, the frequency, and the maximum number of inhalations in 24 hours of the beta$_2$ agonist should be **stated explicitly** to the patient. The patient should be advised to seek medical advice when the prescribed dose of beta$_2$ agonist fails to provide the usual degree of symptomatic relief because this usually indicates a worsening of the asthma and the patient may require a prophylactic drug such as an inhaled corticosteroid (see Chronic Asthma table, p. 146).

Nebuliser (or respirator) solutions of salbutamol and terbutaline are used for the treatment of severe acute asthma in hospital or in general practice. Patients with a severe attack of asthma should preferably have oxygen during nebulisation since beta$_2$ agonists can increase arterial hypoxaemia. For the use of nebulisers in chronic obstructive pulmonary disease, see section 3.1.5. The dose given by nebuliser is substantially higher than that given by inhaler. Patients should therefore be warned that it is dangerous to exceed the prescribed dose and they should seek medical advice if they fail to respond to the usual dose of the respirator solution. See also guidelines in section 3.1.5.

CFC-free inhalers Chlorofluorocarbon (CFC) propellants in pressurised metered-dose inhalers are being replaced by hydrofluoroalkane (HFA) propellants. Patients receiving CFC-free inhalers should be reassured about the efficacy of the new inhalers and counselled that the aerosol may feel and taste different; any difficulty with the new inhaler should be discussed with the doctor or pharmacist.

Oral Oral preparations of beta$_2$ agonists may be used by patients who cannot manage the inhaled route. They are sometimes used for children and the elderly, but inhaled beta$_2$ agonists are more effective and have fewer side-effects. The longer-acting oral preparations, including bambuterol, may be of value in nocturnal asthma but they have a limited role and inhaled long-acting beta$_2$ agonists are usually preferred.

Parenteral Salbutamol or terbutaline are given by intravenous infusion for severe asthma. The regular use of beta$_2$ agonists by the subcutaneous route is not recommended since the evidence of benefit is uncertain and it may be difficult to withdraw such treatment once started. Patients supplied with a selective beta$_2$ agonist injection for severe attacks should be advised to attend hospital immediately after using the injection, for further assessment. Beta$_2$ agonists may also be given by intramuscular injection.

Children Selective beta$_2$ agonists are useful even in children under the age of 18 months. They are most effective by the inhaled route; a pressurised metered-dose inhaler should be used with a spacer device in children under 5 years (see NICE guidance, section 3.1.5). A beta$_2$ agonist may also be given by mouth but administration by inhalation is preferred; a long-acting inhaled beta$_2$ agonist may be used where appropriate (see Chronic Asthma table, p. 146). In severe attacks nebulisation using a selective beta$_2$ agonist or ipratropium is advisable (see also Asthma tables, p. 146 and p. 147).

Cautions Beta$_2$ agonists should be used with caution in hyperthyroidism, cardiovascular disease, arrhythmias, susceptibility to QT-interval prolongation, and hypertension. If high doses are needed during pregnancy they should be given by inhalation because a parenteral beta$_2$ agonist can affect the myometrium (section 7.1.3) and possibly cause cardiac problems; see also Pregnancy and Breast-feeding, section 3.1. Beta$_2$ agonists should be used with caution in diabetes—monitor blood glucose (risk of ketoacidosis, especially when beta$_2$ agonist given intravenously). **Interactions**: Appendix 1 (sympathomimetics, beta$_2$).

Hypokalaemia The CSM has advised that potentially serious hypokalaemia may result from beta$_2$ agonist therapy. Particular caution is required in severe asthma, because this effect may be potentiated by concomitant treatment with theophylline and its derivatives, corticosteroids, and diuretics, and by hypoxia. Plasma-potassium concentration should therefore be monitored in severe asthma.

Side-effects Side-effects of the beta$_2$ agonists include fine tremor (particularly in the hands), nervous tension, headache, muscle cramps, and palpitation. Other side-effects include tachycardia, arrhythmias, peripheral vasodilation, myocardial ischaemia, and disturbances of sleep and behaviour. Paradoxical bronchospasm, urticaria, angioedema, hypotension, and collapse have also been reported. High doses of beta$_2$ agonists are associated with hypokalaemia (for CSM advice, see under Hypokalaemia above).

BAMBUTEROL HYDROCHLORIDE

Note Bambuterol is a pro-drug of terbutaline

Indications asthma and other conditions associated with reversible airways obstruction

Cautions see notes above; renal impairment (Appendix 3); hepatic impairment (avoid if severe); manufacturer advises avoid in pregnancy

Side-effects see notes above

Dose

- 20 mg once daily at bedtime if patient has previously tolerated beta$_2$ agonists; other patients, initially 10 mg once daily at bedtime, increased if necessary after 1–2 weeks to 20 mg once daily; CHILD not recommended

Bambec® (AstraZeneca) PoM
Tablets, both scored, bambuterol hydrochloride 10 mg, net price 28-tab pack = £12.05; 20 mg, 28-tab pack = £13.14

FENOTEROL HYDROBROMIDE

Indications reversible airways obstruction

Cautions see notes above

Side-effects see notes above

Compound preparations
For **compound preparation** containing fenoterol, see section 3.1.4

FORMOTEROL FUMARATE
(Eformoterol fumarate)

Indications reversible airways obstruction (including nocturnal asthma and prevention of exercise-induced bronchospasm) in patients requiring long-term regular bronchodilator therapy, see also Chronic Asthma table, p. 146; chronic obstructive pulmonary disease

Cautions see notes above; liver disease (Appendix 2); pregnancy (Appendix 4 and notes above); breast-feeding (Appendix 5)

Side-effects see notes above; taste disturbances, nausea, dizziness, rash, and pruritus also reported

Dose

- See under preparations below

Counselling Advise patients not to exceed prescribed dose, and to follow manufacturer's directions; if a previously effective dose of inhaled formoterol fails to provide adequate relief, a doctor's advice should be obtained as soon as possible

Formoterol (Non-proprietary) PoM
Dry powder for inhalation, formoterol fumarate 12 micrograms/metered inhalation, net price 120-dose unit = £24.80. Counselling, dose
Brands include *Easyhaler® Formoterol*
Dose by inhalation of powder, asthma, ADULT and CHILD over 6 years, 12 micrograms twice daily, increased to 24 micrograms twice daily in more severe airways obstruction
Chronic obstructive pulmonary disease, 12 micrograms twice daily

Atimos Modulite® (Trinity-Chiesi) ▼ PoM
Aerosol inhalation, formoterol fumarate 12 micrograms/metered inhalation, net price 100-dose unit = £31.28. Counselling, dose
Dose by aerosol inhalation, asthma, ADULT and CHILD over 12 years, 12 micrograms twice daily, increased to max. 24 micrograms twice daily in more severe airways obstruction
Chronic obstructive pulmonary disease, ADULT over 18 years, 12 micrograms twice daily; for symptom relief additional doses may be taken to total max. 48 micrograms daily (max. single dose 24 micrograms)
Note Each metered inhalation of *Atimos Modulite®* delivers 10.1 micrograms formoterol fumarate

Foradil® (Novartis) PoM
Dry powder for inhalation, formoterol fumarate 12 micrograms/capsule, net price 60-cap pack (with inhaler device) = £29.23. Counselling, dose
Dose by inhalation of powder, asthma, ADULT and CHILD over 5 years, 12 micrograms twice daily, increased to 24 micrograms twice daily in more severe airways obstruction
Chronic obstructive pulmonary disease, 12 micrograms twice daily

Oxis® (AstraZeneca) PoM
Turbohaler® (= dry powder inhaler), formoterol fumarate 6 micrograms/metered inhalation, net price

60-dose unit = £24.80; 12 micrograms/metered inhalation, 60-dose unit = £24.80. Counselling, dose

Dose by inhalation of powder, chronic asthma, 6–12 micrograms 1–2 times daily, increased up to 24 micrograms twice daily if necessary; occasionally up to 72 micrograms daily may be needed (max. single dose 36 micrograms); reassess treatment if additional doses required on more than 2 days a week; CHILD 6–18 years, 6–12 micrograms 1–2 times daily; occasionally up to 48 micrograms daily may be needed (max. single dose 12 micrograms)

Relief of bronchospasm, ADULT and CHILD over 6 years, 6–12 micrograms

Prevention of exercise-induced bronchospasm, 12 micrograms before exercise; CHILD 6–18 years, 6–12 micrograms before exercise

Chronic obstructive pulmonary disease, 12 micrograms 1–2 times daily; for symptom relief additional doses may be taken to total max. 48 micrograms daily (max. single dose 24 micrograms)

Note Each metered inhalation of *Oxis 6 Turbohaler®* delivers 4.5 micrograms formoterol fumarate; each metered inhalation of *Oxis 12 Turbohaler®* delivers 9 micrograms formoterol fumarate

Compound preparations

For **compound preparations** containing formoterol, see section 3.2

SALBUTAMOL

(Albuterol)

Indications asthma and other conditions associated with reversible airways obstruction; premature labour (section 7.1.3)

Cautions see notes above

Side-effects see notes above

Dose

- By mouth (but use by inhalation preferred), 4 mg (elderly and sensitive patients initially 2 mg) 3–4 times daily; max. single dose 8 mg (but unlikely to provide much extra benefit or to be tolerated); CHILD under 2 years 100 micrograms/kg 4 times daily [unlicensed]; 2–6 years 1–2 mg 3–4 times daily, 6–12 years 2 mg 3–4 times daily
- By subcutaneous *or* intramuscular injection, 500 micrograms, repeated every 4 hours if necessary
- By slow intravenous injection (dilute to a concentration of 50 micrograms/mL), 250 micrograms, repeated if necessary; CHILD 1 month–2 years 5 micrograms/kg as a single dose [unlicensed]; 2–18 years 15 micrograms/kg (max. 250 micrograms) as a single dose [unlicensed]
- By intravenous infusion, initially 5 micrograms/minute, adjusted according to response and heart-rate usually in range 3–20 micrograms/minute, or more if necessary; CHILD 1 month–18 years initially 1–5 micrograms/kg/minute, adjusted according to response and heart rate (doses above 2 micrograms/kg/minute in intensive care setting) [unlicensed]
- By aerosol inhalation, 100–200 micrograms (1–2 puffs); for persistent symptoms up to 4 times daily (but see also Chronic Asthma table); CHILD 100 micrograms (1 puff), increased to 200 micrograms (2 puffs) if necessary; for persistent symptoms up to 4 times daily (but see also Chronic Asthma table)

  Prophylaxis in exercise-induced bronchospasm, 200 micrograms (2 puffs); CHILD 100 micrograms (1 puff), increased to 200 micrograms (2 puffs) if necessary
- By inhalation of powder (for *Ventolin Accuhaler®* and *Asmasal®* dose see under preparation), 200–400 micrograms; for persistent symptoms up to 4 times daily (but see also Chronic Asthma table); CHILD 200 micrograms; for persistent symptoms up to 4 times daily (but see also Chronic Asthma table)

  Prophylaxis in exercise-induced bronchospasm, 400 micrograms; CHILD 200 micrograms
- By inhalation of nebulised solution, chronic bronchospasm unresponsive to conventional therapy and severe acute asthma, ADULT and CHILD over 18 months 2.5–5 mg, repeated up to 4 times daily; more frequently in severe cases; max. 40 mg daily; CHILD under 18 months, [unlicensed] (transient hypoxaemia may occur—consider supplemental oxygen), 2.5 mg up to 4 times daily or more frequently in severe cases

Oral

Salbutamol (Non-proprietary) PoM

Tablets, salbutamol (as sulphate) 2 mg, net price 28-tab pack = £9.20; 4 mg, 28-tab pack = £9.83

Oral solution, salbutamol (as sulphate) 2 mg/5 mL, net price 150 mL = £1.06

Brands include *Salapin®* (sugar-free)

Ventmax® SR (Trinity) PoM

Capsules, m/r, salbutamol (as sulphate) 4 mg (green/grey), net price 56-cap pack = £8.57; 8 mg (white), 56-cap pack = £10.28. Label: 25

Dose 8 mg twice daily; CHILD 3–12 years 4 mg twice daily

Ventolin® (A&H) PoM

Syrup, sugar-free, salbutamol (as sulphate) 2 mg/5 mL, net price 150 mL = 60p

Volmax® (A&H) PoM

Tablets, m/r salbutamol (as sulphate) 4 mg, net price 56-tab pack = £9.81; 8 mg, 56-tab pack = £11.77. Label: 25

Dose 8 mg twice daily; CHILD 3–12 years 4 mg twice daily

Parenteral

Ventolin® (A&H) PoM

Injection, salbutamol (as sulphate) 500 micrograms/mL, net price 1-mL amp = 40p

Solution for intravenous infusion, salbutamol (as sulphate) 1 mg/mL. Dilute before use. Net price 5-mL amp = £2.58

Inhalation

Counselling Advise patients not to exceed prescribed dose and to follow manufacturer's directions; if a previously effective dose of inhaled salbutamol fails to provide at least 3 hours relief, a doctor's advice should be obtained as soon as possible.

Patients receiving CFC-free inhalers should be reassured about their efficacy and counselled that aerosol may feel and taste different

Salbutamol (Non-proprietary) PoM

Aerosol inhalation, salbutamol 100 micrograms/metered inhalation, net price 200-dose unit = £2.88. Counselling, dose

Excipients include CFC propellants

Aerosol inhalation, salbutamol (as sulphate) 100 micrograms/metered inhalation, net price 200-dose unit = £2.99. Counselling, dose, change to CFC-free inhaler

Excipients include HFA-134a (a non-CFC propellant), alcohol

Brands include *Salamol®*

Note Can be supplied against a generic prescription but if CFC-free not specified will be reimbursed at price for CFC-containing inhaler

Dry powder for inhalation, salbutamol 100 micrograms/metered inhalation, net price 200-dose unit = £3.46; 200 micrograms/metered inhalation, 100-dose unit = £5.05, 200-dose unit = £6.92. Counselling, dose
Brands include *Easyhaler® Salbutamol*, *Pulvinal® Salbutamol*

Inhalation powder, *hard capsule* (for use with *Cyclohaler®* device), salbutamol 200 micrograms, net price 120-cap pack = £8.99; 400 micrograms, 120-cap pack = £12.99. Counselling, dose
Brands include *Salbutamol Cyclocaps®*

Nebuliser solution, salbutamol (as sulphate) 1 mg/mL, net price 20 × 2.5 mL (2.5 mg) = £1.99; 2 mg/mL, 20 × 2.5 mL (5 mg) = £3.98. May be diluted with sterile sodium chloride 0.9%
Brands include *Salamol Steri-Neb®*

Airomir® (IVAX) PoM

Aerosol inhalation, salbutamol (as sulphate) 100 micrograms/metered inhalation, net price 200-dose unit = £1.97. Counselling, dose, change to CFC-free inhaler
Excipients include HFA-134a (a non-CFC propellant), alcohol
Note Can be supplied against a generic prescription but if 'CFC-free' not specified will be reimbursed at price for CFC-containing inhaler

Autohaler (breath-actuated aerosol inhalation), salbutamol (as sulphate) 100 micrograms/metered inhalation, net price 200-dose unit = £6.02. Counselling, dose, change to CFC-free inhaler
Excipients include HFA-134a (a non-CFC propellant), alcohol

Asmasal Clickhaler® (UCB Pharma) PoM

Dry powder for inhalation, salbutamol (as sulphate) 95 micrograms/metered inhalation, net price 200-dose unit = £5.88. Counselling, dose
Dose acute bronchospasm 1–2 puffs
Persistent symptoms, 2 puffs 3–4 times daily
Prophylaxis in exercise-induced bronchospasm, 2 puffs

Salamol Easi-Breathe® (IVAX) PoM

Aerosol inhalation, salbutamol 100 micrograms/metered inhalation, net price 200-dose breath-actuated unit = £1.58. Counselling, dose
Excipients include HFA-134a (a non-CFC propellant), alcohol

Ventolin® (A&H) PoM

Accuhaler® (dry powder for inhalation), disk containing 60 blisters of salbutamol (as sulphate) 200 micrograms/blister with *Accuhaler®* device, net price = £5.12. Counselling, dose
Dose by inhalation of powder, ADULT and CHILD 200 micrograms; for persistent symptoms up to 4 times daily (but see also Chronic Asthma table)
Prophylaxis in allergen- or exercise-induced bronchospasm, 200 micrograms

Evohaler® (aerosol inhalation), salbutamol (as sulphate) 100 micrograms/metered inhalation, net price 200-dose unit = £1.50. Counselling, dose, change to CFC-free inhaler
Excipients include HFA-134a (a non-CFC propellant)
Note Can be supplied against a generic prescription but if CFC-free not specified will be reimbursed at price for CFC-containing inhaler

Nebules® (for use with nebuliser), salbutamol (as sulphate) 1 mg/mL, net price 20 × 2.5 mL (2.5 mg) = £1.75; 2 mg/mL, 20 × 2.5 mL (5 mg) = £2.95. May be diluted with sterile sodium chloride 0.9% if administration time in excess of 10 minutes is required

Respirator solution (for use with a nebuliser or ventilator), salbutamol (as sulphate) 5 mg/mL. Net price 20 mL = £2.27 (hosp. only). May be diluted with sterile sodium chloride 0.9%

Compound preparations

For **compound preparations** containing salbutamol, see section 3.1.4

Chronic Asthma table, see p. 146
Acute Severe Asthma table, see p. 147

SALMETEROL

Indications reversible airways obstruction (including nocturnal asthma and prevention of exercise-induced bronchospasm) in patients requiring long-term regular bronchodilator therapy, see also Chronic Asthma table, p. 146; chronic obstructive pulmonary disease
Note Not for immediate relief of acute asthma attacks; existing corticosteroid therapy should not be reduced or withdrawn

Cautions see notes above

Side-effects see notes above; nausea, dizziness, arthralgia, and rash also reported

Dose

- By inhalation, asthma, 50 micrograms (2 puffs or 1 blister) twice daily; up to 100 micrograms (4 puffs or 2 blisters) twice daily in more severe airways obstruction; CHILD over 4 years, 50 micrograms (2 puffs or 1 blister) twice daily

  Chronic obstructive pulmonary disease 50 micrograms (2 puffs or 1 blister) twice daily

Counselling Advise patients that salmeterol should **not** be used for relief of acute attacks, not to exceed prescribed dose, and to follow manufacturer's directions; if a previously effective dose of inhaled salmeterol fails to provide adequate relief, a doctor's advice should be obtained as soon as possible

Serevent® (A&H) PoM

Accuhaler® (dry powder for inhalation), disk containing 60 blisters of salmeterol (as xinafoate) 50 micrograms/blister with *Accuhaler®* device, net price = £29.26. Counselling, dose

Evohaler® aerosol inhalation, salmeterol (as xinafoate) 25 micrograms/metered inhalation, net price 120-dose unit = £29.26. Counselling, dose, change to CFC-free inhaler
Excipients include HFA-134a (a non-CFC propellant)

Diskhaler® (dry powder for inhalation), disks containing 4 blisters of salmeterol (as xinafoate) 50 micrograms/blister, net price 15 disks with *Diskhaler®* device = £35.79, 15-disk refill = £35.15. Counselling, dose

Compound preparations

For **compound preparations** containing salmeterol, see section 3.2

TERBUTALINE SULPHATE

Indications asthma and other conditions associated with reversible airways obstruction; premature labour (section 7.1.3)

Cautions see notes above

Side-effects see notes above

Dose

- By mouth (but use by inhalation preferred), initially 2.5 mg 3 times daily for 1–2 weeks, then up to 5 mg 3 times daily; CHILD 1 month–7 years 75 micrograms/kg 3 times daily; 7–15 years 2.5 mg 2–3 times daily

- By subcutaneous *or* slow intravenous injection, 250–500 micrograms up to 4 times daily; CHILD 2–15 years 10 micrograms/kg to a max. of 300 micrograms
- By continuous intravenous infusion as a solution containing 3–5 micrograms/mL, 90–300 micrograms/hour for 8–10 hours; CHILD 1 month–18 years, initially 2–4 micrograms/kg as a loading dose, then 1–10 micrograms/kg/hour according to response and heart rate (max. 300 micrograms/hour); high doses with close monitoring
- By inhalation of powder (*Turbohaler®*), 500 micrograms (1 inhalation); for persistent symptoms up to 4 times daily (but see also Chronic Asthma table); CHILD under 5 years not recommended
- By inhalation of nebulised solution, 5–10 mg 2–4 times daily; additional doses may be necessary in severe acute asthma; CHILD, up to 3 years 2 mg, 3–6 years 3 mg; 6–8 years 4 mg, over 8 years 5 mg, 2–4 times daily

Oral and parenteral

Bricanyl® (AstraZeneca) PoM

Tablets, scored, terbutaline sulphate 5 mg, net price 20 = 82p

Syrup, sugar-free, terbutaline sulphate 1.5 mg/5 mL, net price 100 mL = £2.00

Injection, terbutaline sulphate 500 micrograms/mL, net price 1-mL amp = 30p; 5-mL amp = £1.40

Inhalation

Counselling Advise patients not to exceed prescribed dose and to follow manufacturer's directions; if a previously effective dose of inhaled terbutaline fails to provide at least 3 hours relief, a doctor's advice should be obtained as soon as possible

Bricanyl® (AstraZeneca) PoM

Turbohaler® (= dry powder inhaler), terbutaline sulphate 500 micrograms/metered inhalation, net price 100-dose unit = £6.92. Counselling, dose

Respules® (= single-dose units for nebulisation), terbutaline sulphate 2.5 mg/mL, net price 20 × 2-mL units (5-mg) = £4.04

3.1.1.2 Other adrenoceptor agonists

Ephedrine and the partially selective beta agonist, orciprenaline, are less suitable and less safe for use as bronchodilators than the selective $beta_2$ agonists, because they are more likely to cause arrhythmias and other side-effects. They should be avoided whenever possible.

Adrenaline (epinephrine) injection (1 in 1000) is used in the emergency treatment of acute allergic and anaphylactic reactions (section 3.4.3), in angioedema (section 3.4.3), and in cardiopulmonary resuscitation (section 2.7.3). Adrenaline solution (1 in 1000) is used by nebulisation in the management of severe croup (section 3.1).

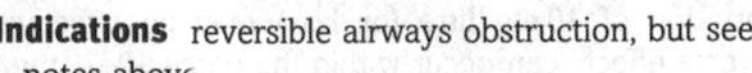

EPHEDRINE HYDROCHLORIDE

Indications reversible airways obstruction, but see notes above

Cautions hyperthyroidism, diabetes mellitus, ischaemic heart disease, hypertension, renal impairment, elderly; prostatic hypertrophy (risk of acute retention); interaction with MAOIs a disadvantage; **interactions:** Appendix 1 (sympathomimetics)

Side-effects tachycardia, anxiety, restlessness, insomnia common; also tremor, arrhythmias, dry mouth, cold extremities

Dose

- 15–60 mg 3 times daily; CHILD up to 1 year 7.5 mg 3 times daily, 1–5 years 15 mg 3 times daily, 6–12 years 30 mg 3 times daily

[1]**Ephedrine Hydrochloride** (Non-proprietary) PoM

Tablets, ephedrine hydrochloride 15 mg, net price 28 = £3.69; 30 mg, 28 = £4.82

1. For exemptions see *Medicines, Ethics and Practice*, No. 31, London, Pharmaceutical Press, 2007 (and subsequent editions as available)

ORCIPRENALINE SULPHATE 

Indications reversible airways obstruction, but see notes above

Cautions see section 3.1.1.1 and notes above; **interactions:** Appendix 1 (sympathomimetics)

Side-effects see section 3.1.1.1 and notes above

Dose

- 20 mg 4 times daily; CHILD up to 1 year 5–10 mg 3 times daily, 1–3 years 5–10 mg 4 times daily, 3–12 years 40–60 mg daily in divided doses

Alupent® (Boehringer Ingelheim) PoM

Syrup, sugar-free, orciprenaline sulphate 10 mg/5 mL, net price 300 mL = £6.75

3.1.2 Antimuscarinic bronchodilators

Ipratropium can provide short-term relief in chronic asthma, but short-acting $beta_2$ agonists act more quickly and are preferred. Ipratropium by nebulisation can be added to other standard treatment in life-threatening asthma or if acute asthma fails to improve with standard therapy (see Acute Severe Asthma table, p. 147).

The aerosol inhalation of ipratropium can be used for short-term relief in mild chronic obstructive pulmonary disease in patients who are not using a long-acting antimuscarinic drug. Its maximal effect occurs 30–60 minutes after use; its duration of action is 3 to 6 hours and bronchodilation can usually be maintained with treatment 3 times a day.

Tiotropium, a long-acting antimuscarinic bronchodilator, is effective for the management of chronic obstructive pulmonary disease; it is not suitable for the relief of acute bronchospasm.

Cautions Antimuscarinic bronchodilators should be used with caution in patients with prostatic hyperplasia, bladder outflow obstruction, and those susceptible to angle-closure glaucoma (see below); **interactions:** Appendix 1 (antimuscarinics)

Glaucoma *Acute angle-closure glaucoma* reported with nebulised ipratropium, particularly when given with nebulised salbutamol (and possibly other $beta_2$ agonists); care needed to protect patient's eyes from nebulised drug or from drug powder.

Side-effects Dry mouth is the most common side-effect of antimuscarinic bronchodilators; less commonly nausea and headache occur. Constipation, tachycardia, palpitation, paradoxical bronchospasm, urinary retention, blurred vision, angle-closure glaucoma, and hypersensitivity reactions including rash, urticaria, and angioedema occur rarely.

IPRATROPIUM BROMIDE

Indications reversible airways obstruction, particularly in chronic obstructive pulmonary disease; rhinitis (section 12.2.2)

Cautions see notes above

Side-effects see notes above

Dose

- By aerosol inhalation, 20–40 micrograms, 3–4 times daily; CHILD up to 6 years 20 micrograms 3 times daily, 6–12 years 20–40 micrograms 3 times daily
- By inhalation of powder, ADULT and CHILD over 12 years, 40 micrograms 3–4 times daily (may be doubled in less responsive patients)
- By inhalation of nebulised solution, reversible airways obstruction in chronic obstructive pulmonary disease, 250–500 micrograms 3–4 times daily

Acute bronchospasm (see also Acute Asthma table, p. 147), 500 micrograms repeated as necessary; CHILD under 5 years 125–250 micrograms, max. 1 mg daily; 6–12 years 250 micrograms, max. 1 mg daily

Counselling Advise patient not to exceed prescribed dose and to follow manufacturer's directions

Ipratropium Bromide (Non-proprietary) PoM

Nebuliser solution, ipratropium bromide 250 micrograms/mL, net price 20 × 1-mL (250-microgram) unit-dose vials = £6.75, 60 × 1-mL = £21.78; 20 × 2-mL (500-microgram) = £7.43, 60 × 2-mL = £26.97. If dilution is necessary use only sterile sodium chloride 0.9%

Atrovent® (Boehringer Ingelheim) PoM

Aerocaps® (dry powder for inhalation; for use with *Atrovent Aerohaler®*), green, ipratropium bromide 40 micrograms, net price pack of 100 caps with *Aerohaler®* = £14.53; 100 caps = £10.53. Counselling, dose

Note One *Atrovent Aerocap®* is equivalent to 2 puffs of *Atrovent®* metered aerosol inhalation

Aerosol inhalation▼, ipratropium bromide 20 micrograms/metered inhalation, net price 200-dose unit = £4.21. Counselling, dose, change to CFC-free inhaler

Excipients include HFA-134a (a non-CFC propellant), alcohol

Nebuliser solution, isotonic, ipratropium bromide 250 micrograms/mL, net price 20 × 1-mL unit-dose vials = £5.18, 60 × 1-mL vials = £15.55; 20 × 2-mL vials = £6.08, 60 × 2-mL vials = £18.24. If dilution is necessary use only sterile sodium chloride 0.9%

Ipratropium Steri-Neb® (IVAX) PoM

Nebuliser solution, isotonic, ipratropium bromide 250 micrograms/mL, net price 20 × 1-mL (250-microgram) unit-dose vials = £8.72; 20 × 2-mL (500-microgram) = £9.94. If dilution is necessary use only sterile sodium chloride 0.9%

Respontin® (A&H) PoM

Nebuliser solution, isotonic, ipratropium bromide 250 micrograms/mL, net price 20 × 1-mL (250-microgram) unit-dose vials = £5.07; 20 × 2-mL (500-microgram) = £5.95. If dilution is necessary use only sterile sodium chloride 0.9%

Compound ipratropium preparations

Section 3.1.4

TIOTROPIUM

Indications maintenance treatment of chronic obstructive pulmonary disease

Cautions see notes above; renal impairment (Appendix 3); pregnancy (Appendix 4); breast-feeding (Appendix 5)

Side-effects see notes above; *less commonly* taste disturbance and dizziness; *rarely* epistaxis

Dose

- See under preparations below

Spiriva® (Boehringer Ingelheim) PoM

Inhalation powder, hard capsule (for use with *HandiHaler®* device), green, tiotropium (as tiotropium bromide monohydrate) 18 micrograms, net price 30-cap pack with *HandiHaler®* device = £37.62, 30-cap refill = £34.40

Dose by inhalation of powder, ADULT over 18 years, 18 micrograms once daily

Note Each *Spiriva®* 18 microgram capsule delivers 10 micrograms of tiotropium

Respimat® (solution for inhalation)▼, tiotropium (as tiotropium bromide monohydrate) 2.5 micrograms/metered inhalation, net price 60-dose unit = £37.62

Dose by inhalation, ADULT over 18 years, 5 micrograms (2 puffs) once daily

Note The *Scottish Medicines Consortium* has advised (November 2007) that *Spiriva Respimat®* is restricted for use in chronic obstructive pulmonary disease in patients who have poor manual dexterity and difficulty using the *Handihaler®* device

3.1.3 Theophylline

Theophylline is a bronchodilator used for *asthma* and stable *chronic obstructive pulmonary disease*; it is not generally effective in exacerbations of chronic obstructive pulmonary disease. It may have an additive effect when used in conjunction with small doses of beta$_2$ agonists; the combination may increase the risk of side-effects, including hypokalaemia (for CSM advice see p. 150).

Theophylline is metabolised in the liver; there is considerable variation in plasma-theophylline concentration particularly in smokers, in patients with hepatic impairment or heart failure, or if certain drugs are taken concurrently. The plasma-theophylline concentration is *increased* in heart failure, cirrhosis, viral infections, in the elderly, and by drugs that inhibit its metabolism. The plasma-theophylline concentration is *decreased* in smokers and in chronic alcoholism and by drugs that induce liver metabolism. For other interactions of theophylline see Appendix 1.

Differences in the half-life of theophylline are important because its toxic dose is close to the therapeutic dose; particular care is required when introducing or withdrawing drugs that interact with theophylline. In most individuals a plasma-theophylline concentration of between 10–20 mg/litre is required for satisfactory bronchodilation, although a plasma-theophylline concentration of 10 mg/litre (or less) may be effective. Adverse effects can occur within the range 10–20 mg/litre and both the frequency and severity increase at concentrations above 20 mg/litre.

Theophylline is given by injection as **aminophylline**, a mixture of theophylline with ethylenediamine, which is 20 times more soluble than theophylline alone. Aminophylline injection is needed rarely for severe attacks of asthma. It must be given by **very slow** intravenous injection (over at least 20 minutes); it is too irritant for intramuscular use. Measurement of plasma theophylline concentration may be helpful, and is **essential** if aminophylline is to be given to patients who have been taking theophylline, because serious side-effects such as convulsions and arrhythmias can occasionally precede other symptoms of toxicity.

THEOPHYLLINE

Indications reversible airways obstruction, acute severe asthma; for guidelines see also Asthma tables (p. 146 and p. 147)

Cautions cardiac disease, hypertension, hyperthyroidism; peptic ulcer; epilepsy; elderly; fever; **CSM** advice on hypokalaemia risk, p. 150; avoid in porphyria (section 9.8.2); hepatic impairment (Appendix 2); pregnancy (Appendix 4); breast-feeding (Appendix 5); **interactions:** Appendix 1 (theophylline) and notes above

Side-effects tachycardia, palpitation, nausea and other gastro-intestinal disturbances, headache, CNS stimulation, insomnia, arrhythmias, and convulsions especially if given rapidly by intravenous injection; **overdosage:** see Emergency Treatment of Poisoning, p. 33

Dose

- See below

Note Plasma-theophylline concentration for optimum response 10–20 mg/litre (55–110 micromol/litre); 4–6 hours after a dose and at least 5 days after starting treatment; narrow margin between therapeutic and toxic dose, see also notes above

Modified release

Note The rate of absorption from modified-release preparations can vary between brands. The Council of the Royal Pharmaceutical Society of Great Britain advises pharmacists that if a general practitioner prescribes a modified-release oral theophylline preparation without specifying a brand name, the pharmacist should contact the prescriber and agree the brand to be dispensed. Additionally, it is essential that a patient discharged from hospital should be maintained on the brand on which that patient was stabilised as an in-patient.

Nuelin SA® (3M)

SA tablets, m/r, theophylline 175 mg. Net price 60-tab pack = £3.19. Label: 21, 25

Dose 175–350 mg every 12 hours; CHILD over 6 years 175 mg every 12 hours

SA 250 tablets, m/r, scored, theophylline 250 mg. Net price 60-tab pack = £4.46. Label: 21, 25

Dose 250–500 mg every 12 hours; CHILD over 6 years 125–250 mg every 12 hours

Slo-Phyllin® (Merck)

Capsules, all m/r, theophylline 60 mg (white/clear, enclosing white pellets), net price 56-cap pack = £2.76; 125 mg (brown/clear, enclosing white pellets), 56-cap pack = £3.48; 250 mg (blue/clear, enclosing white pellets), 56-cap pack = £4.34. Label: 25, or counselling, see below

Dose 250–500 mg every 12 hours; CHILD, every 12 hours, 2–6 years 60–120 mg, 7–12 years 125–250 mg

Counselling Swallow whole with fluid *or* swallow enclosed granules with soft food (e.g. yoghurt)

Uniphyllin Continus® (Napp)

Tablets, m/r, all scored, theophylline 200 mg, net price 56-tab pack = £3.13; 300 mg, 56-tab pack = £4.77; 400 mg, 56-tab pack = £5.65. Label: 25

Dose 200 mg every 12 hours increased according to response to 400 mg every 12 hours

May be appropriate to give larger evening or morning dose to achieve optimum therapeutic effect when symptoms most severe; in patients whose night or daytime symptoms persist despite other therapy, who are not currently receiving theophylline, total daily requirement may be added as single evening or morning dose

CHILD 9 mg/kg twice daily; some children with chronic asthma may require 10–16 mg/kg every 12 hours

AMINOPHYLLINE

Note Aminophylline is a stable mixture or combination of theophylline and ethylenediamine; the ethylenediamine confers greater solubility in water

Indications reversible airways obstruction, acute severe asthma

Cautions see under Theophylline

Side-effects see under Theophylline; also allergy to ethylenediamine can cause urticaria, erythema, and exfoliative dermatitis

Dose

- See under preparations, below

Note Plasma-theophylline concentration for optimum response 10–20 mg/litre (55–110 micromol/litre); measure plasma-theophylline concentration 4–6 hours after dose by mouth and at least 5 days after starting oral treatment; measure plasma-theophylline concentration 4–6 hours after the start of intravenous infusion; narrow margin between therapeutic and toxic dose, see also notes above

> To avoid excessive dosage in obese patients, dose should be calculated on the basis of ideal weight for height

Aminophylline (Non-proprietary) PoM

Injection, aminophylline 25 mg/mL, net price 10-mL amp = 72p

Brands include *Minijet® Aminophylline*

Dose acute severe asthma or acute exacerbation of chronic obstructive pulmonary disease **not** previously treated with theophylline, by slow intravenous injection over at least 20 minutes (with close monitoring), 250–500 mg (5 mg/kg), then see below; CHILD 5 mg/kg, then see below

Acute severe asthma or acute exacerbation of chronic obstructive pulmonary disease, by intravenous infusion (with close monitoring), 500 micrograms/kg/hour, adjusted according to plasma-theophylline concentration; CHILD 6 months–9 years 1 mg/kg/hour, 10–16 years 800 micrograms/kg/hour, adjusted according to plasma-theophylline concentration

Note Patients taking oral theophylline or aminophylline should not normally receive intravenous aminophylline unless plasma-theophylline concentration is available to guide dosage

Modified release

Note Advice about modified-release theophylline preparations on p. 155 also applies to modified-release aminophylline preparations

Phyllocontin Continus® (Napp)

Tablets, m/r, yellow, f/c, aminophylline hydrate 225 mg, net price 56-tab pack = £2.54. Label: 25

Dose ADULT and CHILD body-weight over 40 kg initially 1 tablet twice daily, increased after 1 week to 2 tablets twice daily according to plasma-theophylline concentration

Note Brands of modified-release tablets containing aminophylline 225 mg include *Norphyllin® SR*

Forte tablets, m/r, yellow, f/c, aminophylline hydrate 350 mg, net price 56-tab pack = £4.22. Label: 25

Dose initially 1 tablet twice daily, increased after 1 week to 2 tablets twice daily if necessary

Note *Phyllocontin Continus® Forte* tablets are for smokers and other patients with shorter theophylline half-life (see notes above)

3.1.4 Compound bronchodilator preparations

In general, patients are best treated with single-ingredient preparations, such as a selective $beta_2$ agonist (section 3.1.1.1) or ipratropium bromide (section 3.1.2), so that the dose of each drug can be adjusted. This flexibility is lost with compound bronchodilator preparations. However, a combination product may be appropriate for patients stabilised on individual components in the same proportion.

For **cautions, contra-indications** and **side-effects** see under individual drugs.

Combivent® (Boehringer Ingelheim) PoM

Nebuliser solution, isotonic, ipratropium bromide 500 micrograms, salbutamol (as sulphate) 2.5 mg/2.5-mL vial, net price 60 unit-dose vials = £25.08

Dose bronchospasm in chronic obstructive pulmonary disease, by inhalation of nebulised solution, 1 vial 3–4 times daily; CHILD under 12 years not recommended

Glaucoma In addition to other potential side-effects acute angle-closure glaucoma has been reported with nebulised ipratropium—for details, see p. 153

Duovent® (Boehringer Ingelheim) PoM

Nebuliser solution, isotonic, fenoterol hydrobromide 1.25 mg, ipratropium bromide 500 micrograms/4-mL vial, net price 20 unit-dose vials = £11.00

Dose acute severe asthma or acute exacerbation of chronic asthma, by inhalation of nebulised solution, 1 vial (4 mL); may be repeated up to max. 4 vials in 24 hours; CHILD under 14 years, not recommended

Glaucoma In addition to other potential side-effects acute angle-closure glaucoma has been reported with nebulised ipratropium—for details, see p. 153

3.1.5 Peak flow meters, inhaler devices and nebulisers

Peak flow meters

Measurement of peak flow is particularly helpful for patients who are 'poor perceivers'and hence slow to detect deterioration in their asthma, and for those with moderate or severe asthma.

Standard-range peak flow meters are suitable for both adults and children; low-range peak flow meters are appropriate for severely restricted airflow in adults and children. Patients must be given clear guidelines as to the action they should take if their peak flow falls below a certain level. Patients can be encouraged to adjust some of their own treatment (within specified limits) according to changes in peak flow rate.

Standard Range Peak Flow Meter

Conforms to standard EN 13826

MicroPeak®, range 60–800 litres/minute, net price = £6.50, replacement mouthpiece = 38p (Micro Medical)

Mini-Wright®, range 60–800 litres/minute, net price = £6.86, replacement mouthpiece = 38p (Clement Clarke)

Piko-1®, range 15–999 litres/minute, net price = £9.50, replacement mouthpiece = 38p (Ferraris)

Pocketpeak®, range 60–800 litres/minute, net price = £6.53, replacement mouthpiece = 38p (Ferraris)

Vitalograph®, range 50–800 litres/minute, net price = £4.50 (children's coloured version also available), replacement mouthpiece = 40p (Vitalograph)

Note Readings from new peak flow meters are often lower than those obtained from old Wright-scale peak flow meters and the correct recording chart should be used

Low Range Peak Flow Meter

Compliant to standard EN 13826 except for scale range

Mini-Wright®, range 30–400 litres/minute, net price = £6.90, replacement mouthpiece = 38p (Clement Clarke)

Pocketpeak®, range 50–400 litres/minute, net price = £6.53, replacement mouthpiece = 38p (Ferraris)

Note Readings from new peak flow meters are often lower than those obtained from old Wright-scale peak flow meters and the correct recording chart should be used

Drug delivery devices

Inhaler devices These include *pressurised metered-dose inhalers, breath-actuated inhalers* and *dry powder inhalers.* Many patients can be taught to use a pressurised metered-dose inhaler effectively but some patients, particularly the elderly and children, find them difficult to use. *Spacer devices* (see below) can help such patients because they remove the need to coordinate actuation with inhalation and are effective particularly for children under 15 years. Alternatively, breath-actuated inhalers or dry powder inhalers (which are activated by patient's inhalation) may be used but they are less suitable for young children. On changing from a pressurised metered-dose inhaler to a dry powder inhaler patients may notice a lack of sensation in the mouth and throat previously associated with each actuation. Coughing may also occur.

The patient should be instructed carefully on the use of the inhaler and it is important to check that the inhaler continues to be used correctly because inadequate inhalation technique may be mistaken for a lack of response to the drug.

NICE guidance

Inhaler devices for children with chronic asthma (children under 5 years, August 2000; children 6–15 years, March 2002)

A child's needs, ability to develop and maintain effective technique, and likelihood of good compliance should govern the choice of inhaler and spacer device; only then should cost be considered.

For children aged under 5 years:

- corticosteroid and bronchodilator therapy should be delivered by pressurised metered-dose inhaler and spacer device, with a facemask if necessary;
- if this is not effective, and depending on the child's condition, nebulised therapy may be considered and, in children over 3 years, a dry powder inhaler may also be considered [but see notes above].

For children aged 5–15 years:

- corticosteroid therapy should be routinely delivered by a pressurised metered-dose inhaler and spacer device;
- children and their carers should be trained in the use of the chosen device; suitability of the device should be reviewed at least annually. Inhaler technique and compliance should be monitored.

3 Respiratory system

Spacer devices Spacer devices remove the need for co-ordination between actuation of a pressurised metered-dose inhaler and inhalation. The spacer device reduces the velocity of the aerosol and subsequent impaction on the oropharynx. In addition the device allows more time for evaporation of the propellant so that a larger proportion of the particles can be inhaled and deposited in the lungs. The size of the spacer is important, the larger spacers with a one-way valve (*Nebuhaler®*, *Volumatic®*) being most effective. Spacer devices are particularly useful for patients with poor inhalation technique, for children, for patients requiring higher doses, for nocturnal asthma, and for patients prone to candidiasis with inhaled corticosteroids. It is important to prescribe a spacer device that is compatible with the metered-dose inhaler.

Use and care of spacer devices Patients should inhale from the spacer device as soon as possible after actuation because the drug aerosol is very short-lived; single-dose actuation is recommended. Tidal breathing is as effective as single breaths. The device should be cleansed once a month by washing in mild detergent and then allowed to dry in air; the mouthpiece should be wiped clean of detergent before use. More frequent cleaning should be avoided since any electrostatic charge may affect drug delivery. Spacer devices should be replaced every 6–12 months.

Able Spacer® (Clement Clarke)
Spacer device, small-volume device. For use with pressurised (aerosol) inhalers, net price standard device = £4.20; with infant, child or adult mask = £6.86

AeroChamber® Plus (GSK)
Spacer device, medium-volume device. For use with *Airomir®*, *Alvesco®*, *Atrovent®*, *Duovent®*, and *Qvar®* inhalers, net price standard device (blue) = £4.43, with mask (blue) = £7.40; infant device (orange) with mask = £7.40; child device (yellow) with mask = £7.40

Babyhaler® (A&H) NHS
Spacer device, for paediatric use with *Ventolin® Evohaler*, net price = £11.34

Haleraid® (A&H) NHS
Inhalation aid, device to place over standard inhalers to aid when strength in hands is impaired (e.g. in arthritis). Available as *Haleraid®-120* for 120-dose inhalers and *Haleraid®-200* for 200-dose inhalers. Net price = 80p

Nebuchamber® (AstraZeneca)
Spacer device, for use with *Pulmicort®* aerosol inhalation. Free of charge from manufacturer

Nebuhaler® (AstraZeneca)
Spacer device, large-volume device. For use with *Pulmicort®* inhalers, with paediatric mask = £4.28

PARI Vortex Spacer® (Pari) NHS
Spacer device, medium-volume device. For use with a pressurised (aerosol) inhaler, net price with mouthpiece = £6.07; with mask for infant or child = £7.91; with adult mask = £9.97

Pocket Chamber® (Ferraris)
Spacer device, small-volume device. For use with a pressurised (aerosol) inhaler, net price = £4.18; with infant, small, medium, or large mask = £9.75

Spinhaler® (Rhône-Poulenc Rorer)
Inhalation device, for use with *Intal Spincaps®*. Net price = £1.92

Volumatic® (A&H)
Spacer inhaler, large-volume device. For use with *Clenil Modulite®*, *Flixotide®*, *Seretide®*, *Serevent®*, and *Ventolin®* inhalers, net price = £2.75; with paediatric mask = £2.75

Nebulisers

In England and Wales nebulisers and compressors are not available on the NHS (but they are free of VAT); some nebulisers (but not compressors) are available on form GP10A in Scotland (for details consult Scottish Drug Tariff).

A nebuliser converts a solution of a drug into an aerosol for inhalation. It is used to deliver higher doses of drug to the airways than is usual with standard inhalers. The main indications for use of a nebuliser are:

- to deliver a beta$_2$ agonist or ipratropium to a patient with an *acute exacerbation* of asthma or of chronic obstructive pulmonary disease;
- to deliver a beta$_2$ agonist or ipratropium on a *regular basis* to a patient with severe asthma or reversible airways obstruction who has been shown to benefit from regular treatment with higher doses;
- to deliver *prophylactic medication* such as a corticosteroid to a patient unable to use other inhalational devices (particularly to a young child);
- to deliver an antibiotic (such as colistin) to a patient with chronic purulent infection (as in cystic fibrosis or bronchiectasis);
- to deliver budesonide to a child with severe croup;
- to deliver pentamidine for the prophylaxis and treatment of pneumocystis pneumonia.

The proportion of a nebuliser solution that reaches the lungs depends on the type of nebuliser and although it can be as high as 30%, it is more frequently close to 10% and sometimes below 10%. The remaining solution is left in the nebuliser as residual volume or it is deposited in the mouthpiece and tubing. The extent to which the nebulised solution is deposited in the airways or alveoli depends on particle size. Particles with a mass median diameter of 1–5 microns are deposited in the airways and are therefore appropriate for asthma whereas a particle size of 1–2 microns is needed for alveolar deposition of pentamidine to combat pneumocystis infection. The type of nebuliser is therefore chosen according to the deposition required and according to the viscosity of the solution (antibiotic solutions usually being more viscous).

Some jet nebulisers are able to increase drug output during inspiration and hence increase efficiency.

The patient should be aware that the dose of a bronchodilator given by nebulisation is usually **much higher** than that from an aerosol inhaler.

The British Thoracic Society has advised that nebulised bronchodilators are appropriate for patients with chronic persistent asthma or those with severe acute asthma. In chronic persistent asthma, nebulised bronchodilators should only be used to relieve persistent daily wheeze (see Chronic Asthma table p. 146). The British Thoracic Society has recommended that the use of nebulisers in chronic persistent asthma should be considered only:

- after a review of the diagnosis;
- if the airflow obstruction is significantly reversible by bronchodilators without unacceptable side-effects;
- after the patient has been using the usual hand-held inhaler correctly;

- after a larger dose of bronchodilator from a hand-held inhaler (with a spacer if necessary) has been tried for at least 2 weeks;
- if the patient is complying with the prescribed dose and frequency of anti-inflammatory treatment including regular use of high-dose inhaled corticosteroid.

Before prescribing a nebuliser, a home trial should preferably be undertaken to monitor peak flow for up to 2 weeks on standard treatment and up to 2 weeks on nebulised treatment. If prescribed, patients must:

- have clear instructions from doctor, specialist nurse or pharmacist on the use of the nebuliser and on peak-flow monitoring;
- be instructed not to treat acute attacks at home without also seeking help;
- receive an education program;
- have regular follow up including peak-flow monitoring and be seen by doctor, specialist nurse or physiotherapist.

Jet nebulisers

Jet nebulisers are more widely used than ultrasonic nebulisers. Most jet nebulisers require an optimum gas flow rate of 6–8 litres/minute and in hospital can be driven by piped air or oxygen; in acute asthma the nebuliser should be driven by oxygen. Domiciliary oxygen cylinders do not provide an adequate flow rate therefore an electrical compressor is required for domiciliary use.

For patients with *chronic obstructive pulmonary disease and hypercapnia*, oxygen can be dangerous and the nebuliser should be driven by air (see also p. 149). In exacerbations of chronic obstructive pulmonary disease, the nebuliser should be driven by compressed air in hypercapnia or acidosis. If oxygen is required, it should be given simultaneously by nasal cannula.

> **Important**: the Department of Health has reminded users of the need to use the correct grade of tubing when connecting a nebuliser to a medical gas supply or compressor.

Medix Lifecare Nebuliser Chamber® (Medix) NHS
Jet nebuliser, disposable; for use with bronchodilators, antimuscarinics, corticosteroids, and antibacterials, replacement recommended every 2–3 months if used 4 times a day. Compatible with *AC 2000 Hi Flo®* NHS, *World Traveller Hi Flo®* NHS, and *Econoneb®* NHS, net price = £1.00

Medix Lifecare Nebuliser System® (Medix) NHS
Jet nebuliser, consisting of mouthpiece, tubing, and nebuliser chamber, net price = £2.00; mask kits with tubing and nebuliser chamber also available, net price (adult) = £2.00; (child) = £2.10

PARI LC® SPRINT (Pari) NHS
Jet nebuliser, non-disposable, for hospital or home use; for use with bronchodilators, antibacterials, and corticosteroids, replacement recommended yearly if used 4 times a day. Compatible with *PARI TurboBOY® S* NHS, *PARI JuniorBOY® S* NHS, *PARI BOY® Mobile S* NHS, and *PARI WALK BOY®* NHS compressors, net price = £16.05

PARI LC® SPRINT BABY (Pari) NHS
Jet nebuliser, non-disposable, for hospital or home use; for use with bronchodilators, antibacterials and corticosteroids; replacement recommended yearly if used 4 times a day. Compatible with *PARI TurboBOY® S* NHS, *PARI JuniorBOY® S* NHS, *PARI BOY® Mobile S* NHS, *PARI WALK BOY®* NHS compressors. Available separately for children aged less than 1 year, 1–4 years or 4–7 years, net price (with mask and connection tube) = £32.15

Sidestream Durable® (Profile Respiratory) NHS
Jet nebuliser, non-disposable, for home use; for use with bronchodilators; yearly replacement recommended if 4 six-minute treatments used per day. Compatible with *Freeway Freedom®* NHS and *Porta-Neb®* NHS, net price year pack = £20.40 (*Porta-Neb®*), £29.00 (*Freeway Freedom®*). *Disposable Sidestream®* NHS nebuliser also available

Ventstream® (Profile Respiratory) NHS
Jet nebuliser, closed-system, for use with low flow compressors, compatible with *Porta-Neb®* NHS, and *Freeway Freedom®* NHS compressors; for use with antibacterials, bronchodilators, and corticosteroids, replacement recommended yearly if used 3 times a day, net price year pack with filter = £39.00 (*Porta-Neb®*), £41.00 (*Freeway Freedom®*)

Home compressors with nebulisers

AC 2000 HI FLO® (Medix) NHS
Home and hospital use, containing 1 *Jet Nebuliser®* NHS set with mouthpiece, 1 adult and 1 child mask,1 spare inlet filter, filter spanner. Mains operated. Nebulises bronchodilators, corticosteroids, and antibacterials, net price = £117.00; carrying case available

AC 4000® (Medix) NHS
Home and hospital use, containing 1 *Jet Nebuliser®* NHS set with mouthpiece, 1 adult and 1 child face mask, 1 spare inlet filter, filter spanner. Mains operated. Nebulises bronchodilators, corticosteroids, and antibacterials, net price = £80.10

Aquilon® (Henleys) NHS
Portable, home use, with 1 adult or 1 child mask and tubing. Mains operated; for use with bronchodilators, corticosteroids and antibacterials, net price = £82.50

Econoneb® (Medix) NHS
Home, clinic and hospital use, used with 1 *Jet Nebuliser®* NHS set with mouthpiece, 1 adult and 1 child mask, 1 spare inlet filter, filter spanner. Nebulises bronchodilators, corticosteroids, and antibacterials. Mains operated, net price = £99.00

Freeway Freedom® (Profile Respiratory) NHS
Portable, containing *Sidestream Durable®* NHS nebuliser, 1 adult mask, 1 child mask, 1 angled mouthpiece, 1 coiled *Duratube®*, 4 inlet filters, charger and power lead, net price = £203.20; with *Ventstream®* NHS nebuliser, 1 straight mouthpiece, 1 coiled *Duratube®*, 4 inlet filters, 1 aerosol hose, charger and power lead, net price = £203.20

PARI JuniorBOY® S (Pari) NHS
Portable, for hospital or home use, containing *PARI LC® SPRINT Junior* NHS nebuliser with child mouthpiece, mask, connection tube, and mains cable. Filter replacement recommended every 12 months. Compatible with *PARI LC® SPRINT* NHS, and *PARI LC® SPRINT BABY* NHS nebulisers, net price = £70.00

PARI TurboBOY® S (Pari) NHS
Portable, for hospital or home use, containing *PARI® SPRINT* NHS nebuliser with adult mouthpiece, mask, connection tube and mains cable. Filter replacement recommended every 12 months. Compatible with *PARI LC® SPRINT* NHS, and *PARI LC® SPRINT BABY* NHS nebulisers, net price = £65.00

PARI BOY® Mobile S (Pari) NHS
Portable, containing *PARI LC® SPRINT* NHS nebuliser with connection tube, mains cable, rechargeable battery, car battery adaptor, and carrying case. Compatible with *PARI LC® SPRINT BABY* NHS nebuliser. Nebulises bronchodilators, corticosteroids, and antibacterials, net price = £180.00

Porta-Neb® (Profile Respiratory) NHS
Portable, containing *Sidestream Durable®* NHS nebuliser, 1 adult mask, 1 child mask, 1 angled mouthpiece, 1 coiled *Duratube®*, 4 inlet filters. Mains operated, net price = £94.00; with *Ventstream®* NHS nebuliser, 1 straight mouthpiece, 1 coiled *Duratube®*, 4 inlet filters, aerosol hose. Mains operated, net price = £104.80

De Vilbiss 5650® (De Vilbiss) NHS
Home, clinic use, containing disposable nebuliser set, mouthpiece, mask, mains lead, tubing, thumb-valve. For use with bronchodilators, net price = £142.14

De Vilbiss 4650® (De Vilbiss) NHS
Home, clinic and hospital use, with mouthpiece. Mains operated, net price = £93.95

Tourer® (Henleys) NHS
Portable, home use, mains/car battery operated; for use with bronchodilators, corticosteroids and antibacterials, net price = £101.25

Ultima® (Henleys) NHS
Portable, home use, rechargable or mains/car battery operated. Nebulises bronchodilators and corticosteroids, net price = £156.00 (includes case)

World Traveller HI FLO® (Medix) NHS
Portable, containing 1 *Jet Nebuliser®* NHS set with mouthpiece, 1 adult and 1 child mask, 1 spare inlet filter, filter spanner. Battery, car, and mains operated; rechargeable battery pack available. Nebulises bronchodilators, corticosteroids, and antibacterials, net price excluding battery = £166.00; with battery = £216.00; carrying case available

Compressors

Omron CX3® (Omron) NHS
Home and hospital use, mains operated, net price = £48.75

Omron compAIR CX^Pro® (Omron) NHS
Home and hospital use, mains operated, net price = £56.78 (includes 1 adult mask, child mask, 5 spare filters, and carrying case)

System 22 CR60® (Profile Respiratory) NHS
Hospital use, high flow compressor. Mains operated, net price = £199.90. Also compatible with *System 22 Antibiotic Tee®* NHS for nebulisation of high viscosity drugs such as antibacterials

Turboneb® (Medix) NHS
Hospital use, high flow compressor. Nebulises bronchodilators, corticosteroids, antibacterials, and pentamidine. Mains operated, net price = £125.00

Ultrasonic nebulisers

Ultrasonic nebulisers produce an aerosol by ultrasonic vibration of the drug solution and therefore do not require a gas flow

F16 Wave® (Parkside) NHS
Portable, adjustable delivery rate. Mains/car battery operated or rechargeable battery pack (supplied), net price = £130.00

Liberty® (Medix) NHS
Portable, home and clinic use, containing disposable mouthpiece and chamber cover. Mains and car battery operated. Nebulises bronchodilators and antibacterials, net price £112.49

Omron MicroAIR® (Omron) NHS
Portable, battery operated, net price = £149.96 (includes 1 adult mask, 1 child mask, and carrying case; mains adaptor also available)

Omron NE-U17® (Omron) NHS
Clinic and hospital use, mains operated, net price = £650.17

Ultra Neb 2000® (De Vilbiss) NHS
Hospital, clinic, and home use, delivery rate adjustable. Supplied with stand, net price = £1205.00

Nebuliser diluent

Nebulisation may be carried out using an undiluted nebuliser solution or it may require dilution beforehand. The usual diluent is sterile sodium chloride 0.9% (physiological saline).

Sodium Chloride (Non-proprietary) PoM
Nebuliser solution, sodium chloride 0.9%, net price 20 × 2.5 mL = £5.49
Brands include *Saline Steripoule®*, *Saline Steri-Neb®*

3.2 Corticosteroids

Corticosteroids are used for the management of reversible and irreversible airways disease. An inhaled corticosteroid used for 3–4 weeks may help to distinguish asthma from chronic obstructive pulmonary disease; clear improvement over 3–4 weeks suggests asthma.

Doses for CFC-free corticosteroid inhalers may be different from those that contain CFCs.

CFC-free inhalers Chlorofluorocarbon (CFC) propellants in pressurised aerosol inhalers are being replaced by hydrofluoralkane (HFA) propellants. Patients receiving CFC-free inhalers should be reassured about the efficacy of the new inhalers and counselled that the aerosol may feel and taste different; any difficulty with the new inhaler should be discussed with the doctor or pharmacist.

If the inhaled corticosteroid causes coughing, the use of a beta$_2$ agonist beforehand may help.

Asthma Corticosteroids are effective in *asthma*; they reduce airway inflammation (and hence reduce oedema and secretion of mucus into the airway).

An inhaled corticosteroid is used regularly for prophylaxis of asthma when patients require a beta$_2$ agonist more than twice a week, or if symptoms disturb sleep more than once a week, or if the patient has suffered exacerbations in the last 2 years requiring a systemic corticosteroid or a nebulised bronchodilator (see Chronic Asthma table, p. 146). *Regular use* of inhaled corticosteroids reduces the risk of exacerbation of asthma.

Current and previous smoking reduces the effectiveness of inhaled corticosteroids and higher doses may be necessary.

Corticosteroid inhalers must be used regularly for maximum benefit; alleviation of symptoms usually occurs 3 to 7 days after initiation. **Beclometasone dipropionate** (beclomethasone dipropionate), **budesonide**, **fluticasone propionate**, and **mometasone furoate** appear to be equally effective. Preparations that combine a corticosteroid with a long-acting beta$_2$ agonist may be helpful for patients stabilised on the individual components in the same proportion.

Patients taking long-term oral corticosteroids for asthma can often be transferred to an inhaled corticosteroid but the transfer must be slow, with gradual reduction in the dose of the oral corticosteroid, and at a time when the asthma is well controlled.

High doses of inhaled corticosteroid can be prescribed for patients who respond only partially to standard doses with a long-acting beta$_2$ agonist or another long-acting bronchodilator (see Chronic Asthma table, p. 146). High doses should be continued only if there is clear benefit over the lower dose. The recommended maximum dose of an inhaled corticosteroid should not generally be exceeded. However, if a higher dose is required, then it should be initiated and supervised by a specialist. The use of high doses of inhaled corticosteroid can minimise the requirement for an oral corticosteroid.

Systemic corticosteroid therapy may be necessary during episodes of infection or if the asthma is worsening, when higher doses are needed and access of inhaled drug to small airways may be reduced; patients may need a reserve supply of tablets.

Chronic obstructive pulmonary disease In *chronic obstructive pulmonary disease* inhaled corticosteroid treatment may reduce exacerbations. An inhaled corticosteroid [unlicensed indication] should be considered (in addition to bronchodilator treatment) if the forced expiratory volume in 1 second (FEV_1) is less than 50% of the predicted value and if the patient has had 2 or more exacerbations in a year which require antibacterial treatment or an oral corticosteroid.

Cautions of inhaled corticosteroids Systemic therapy may be required during periods of stress or when either airways obstruction or mucus prevent drug access to smaller airways; **interactions:** Appendix 1 (corticosteroids)

Paradoxical bronchospasm The potential for paradoxical bronchospasm (calling for discontinuation and alternative therapy) should be borne in mind—mild bronchospasm may be prevented by inhalation of a short-acting $beta_2$ agonist (or by transfer from an aerosol inhalation to a dry powder inhalation).

Side-effects of inhaled corticosteroids Inhaled corticosteroids have considerably fewer systemic effects than oral corticosteroids (section 6.3.2), but adverse effects have been reported.

High doses of inhaled corticosteroids (see Chronic Asthma table, p. 146) used for prolonged periods can induce adrenal suppression (section 6.3.2) and patients using high doses should be given a 'steroid card'; such patients may need corticosteroid cover during an episode of stress (e.g. an operation). Inhaled corticosteroids have been associated with adrenal crisis and coma in children; excessive doses should be **avoided**, particularly of fluticasone, which should be given in a dose of 50–100 micrograms twice daily and should not exceed 200 micrograms twice daily.

High doses of inhaled corticosteroid have been associated with lower respiratory tract infections, including pneumonia, in older patients with chronic obstructive pulmonary disease.

Bone mineral density may be reduced following long-term inhalation of higher doses of corticosteroids, predisposing patients to osteoporosis (section 6.6). It is therefore sensible to ensure that the dose of an inhaled corticosteroid is no higher than necessary to keep a patient's asthma under good control. Treatment with an inhaled corticosteroid can usually be stopped after a mild exacerbation as long as the patient knows that it is necessary to reinstate it should the asthma deteriorate or the peak flow rate fall.

In children, growth restriction associated with systemic corticosteroid therapy does not seem to occur with recommended doses of inhaled therapy; although initial growth velocity may be reduced, there appears to be no effect on achieving normal adult height. However, the CSM has recommended that the height of children receiving prolonged treatment of inhaled corticosteroid is monitored; if growth is slowed, referral to a paediatrician should be considered. Large-volume spacer devices should be used for administering inhaled corticosteroids in children under 5 years (see NICE guidance, section 3.1.5); they are also useful in older children and adults, particularly if high doses are required. Spacer devices increase airway deposition and reduce oropharyngeal deposition.

A small risk of glaucoma with prolonged high doses of inhaled corticosteroids has been reported; cataracts have also been reported with inhaled corticosteroids. Hoarseness and candidiasis of the mouth or throat have been reported, usually only with large doses (see also below). Hypersensitivity reactions (including rash and angioedema) have been reported rarely. Other side-effects that have been reported very rarely include paradoxical bronchospasm, anxiety, depression, sleep disturbances, and behavioural changes including hyperactivity and irritability.

Candidiasis The risk of oral candidiasis can be reduced by using a spacer device with the corticosteroid inhaler; rinsing the mouth with water (or cleaning child's teeth) after inhalation of a dose may also be helpful. Antifungal lozenges (section 12.3.2) can be used to treat oral candidiasis without discontinuing therapy.

Oral An acute attack of asthma should be treated with a short course of an oral corticosteroid starting with a high dose, e.g. prednisolone 40–50 mg daily for a few days. Patients whose asthma has deteriorated rapidly usually respond quickly to corticosteroids. The dose can usually be stopped abruptly in a mild exacerbation of asthma (see also Withdrawal of Corticosteroids, section 6.3.2) but it should be reduced gradually in those with poorer asthma control, to reduce the possibility of serious relapse. For use of corticosteroids in the emergency treatment of acute severe asthma see table on p. 147.

In chronic continuing asthma, when the response to other drugs has been inadequate, longer term administration of an oral corticosteroid may be necessary; in such cases high doses of an inhaled corticosteroid should be continued to minimise oral corticosteroid requirements. In chronic obstructive pulmonary disease prednisolone 30 mg daily should be given for 7–14 days; treatment can be stopped abruptly. Prolonged treatment with oral prednisolone is of no benefit and maintenance treatment is not normally recommended.

An oral corticosteroid should normally be taken as a single dose in the morning to reduce the disturbance to circadian cortisol secretion. Dosage should always be titrated to the lowest dose that controls symptoms. Regular peak-flow measurements help to optimise the dose.

Parenteral For the use of hydrocortisone injection in the emergency treatment of acute severe asthma, see Acute Severe Asthma table, p. 147.

BECLOMETASONE DIPROPIONATE
(Beclomethasone Dipropionate)

Indications prophylaxis of asthma (see also Chronic Asthma table, p. 146)

Cautions see notes above

Side-effects see notes above

Dose

- Standard-dose inhalers

  By aerosol inhalation (for *Qvar*® dose see under preparation), 200 micrograms twice daily *or* 100 micrograms 3–4 times daily (in more severe cases initially 600–800 micrograms daily); CHILD 50–100 micrograms 2–4 times daily

  By inhalation of powder (for *Asmabec*® dose see under preparation), 400 micrograms twice daily *or*

200 micrograms 3–4 times daily; CHILD 100 micrograms 2–4 times daily *or* 200 micrograms twice daily

- High-dose inhalers

By aerosol inhalation (for *Qvar*® dose see under preparation), 500 micrograms twice daily *or* 250 micrograms 4 times daily; if necessary may be increased to 500 micrograms 4 times daily; CHILD not recommended

By inhalation of powder (for *Asmabec*® dose see under preparation), 400 micrograms twice daily; if necessary may be increased to 800 micrograms twice daily; CHILD not recommended

Standard-dose inhalers

Beclometasone (Non-proprietary) PoM

Aerosol inhalation, beclometasone dipropionate 50 micrograms/metered inhalation, net price 200-dose unit = £5.94; 100 micrograms/metered inhalation, 200-dose unit = £9.65; 200 micrograms/metered inhalation, 200-dose unit = £17.25. Label: 8, counselling, dose

Excipients include CFC propellants

Brands include *Beclazone*®, *Filair*®

Dental prescribing on NHS Beclometasone Dipropionate Aerosol Inhalation 50 micrograms/metered dose may be prescribed

Dry powder for inhalation, beclometasone dipropionate 100 micrograms/metered inhalation, net price 100-dose unit = £5.58; 200 micrograms/metered inhalation, 100-dose unit = £10.29, 200-dose unit = £15.60. Label: 8, counselling, dose

Brands include *Pulvinal*® *Beclometasone Dipropionate, Easyhaler*® *Beclometasone Dipropionate*

Inhalation powder, hard capsule (for use with *Cyclohaler*® device), beclometasone dipropionate 100 micrograms, net price 120-cap pack = £15.99; 200 micrograms, 120-cap pack = £25.00. Label: 8, counselling, dose

Brands include *Beclometasone Cyclocaps*®

AeroBec® (3M) PoM

AeroBec 50 Autohaler® (breath-actuated aerosol inhalation), beclometasone dipropionate 50 micrograms/metered inhalation, net price 200-dose unit = £4.04. Label: 8, counselling, dose

Excipients include CFC propellants

AeroBec 100 Autohaler® (breath-actuated aerosol inhalation), beclometasone dipropionate 100 micrograms/metered inhalation, net price 200-dose unit = £7.66. Label: 8, counselling, dose

Excipients include CFC propellants

Asmabec Clickhaler® (UCB Pharma) PoM

Dry powder for inhalation, beclometasone dipropionate 50 micrograms/metered inhalation, net price 200-dose unit = £6.68; 100 micrograms/metered inhalation, 200-dose unit = £9.81. Label: 8, counselling, dose

Dose by inhalation of powder, 200–400 micrograms daily, in 2–4 divided doses (in more severe cases initially 0.8–1.6 mg daily, in 2–4 divided doses—see also High-dose inhalers); CHILD 50–100 micrograms 2–4 times daily

Beclazone Easi-Breathe® (IVAX) PoM

Aerosol inhalation, beclometasone dipropionate 50 micrograms/metered inhalation, net price 200-dose breath-actuated unit = £3.26; 100 micrograms/metered inhalation, 200-dose breath-actuated unit = £10.30. Label: 8, counselling, dose

Excipients include CFC propellants

Becodisks® (A&H) PoM

Dry powder for inhalation, disks containing 8 blisters of beclometasone dipropionate 100 micrograms/blister, net price 15 disks with *Diskhaler*® device = £12.00, 15-disk refill = £11.42; 200 micrograms/blister, 15 disks with *Diskhaler*® device = £22.87, 15-disk refill = £22.28. Label: 8, counselling, dose

Clenil Modulite® (Trinity-Chiesi) ▼ PoM

Aerosol inhalation, beclometasone dipropionate 50 micrograms/metered inhalation, net price 200-dose unit = £3.85; 100 micrograms/metered inhalation = £7.72; 200 micrograms/metered inhalation = £16.83; 250 micrograms/metered inhalation = £16.95. Label: 8, counselling, dose; 250-microgram strength also label 10, steroid card

Excipients include HFA-134a (a non-CFC propellant)

Note *Clenil Modulite*® is not interchangeable with other CFC-free beclometasone dipropionate inhalers; the MHRA has advised (August 2006) that CFC-free beclometasone dipropionate inhalers should be prescribed by brand name

Qvar® (IVAX) PoM

Qvar® aerosol inhalation, beclometasone dipropionate 50 micrograms/metered inhalation, net price 200-dose unit = £7.87; 100 micrograms/metered inhalation, 200-dose unit = £17.21. Label: 8, counselling, dose, 100-microgram strength also label 10, steroid card

Qvar Autohaler® (breath-actuated aerosol inhalation), beclometasone dipropionate 50 micrograms/metered inhalation, net price 200-dose unit = £7.87; 100 micrograms/metered inhalation, 200-dose unit = £17.21. Label: 8, counselling, dose; 100-microgram strength also label 10, steroid card

Excipients include HFA-134a (a non-CFC propellant)

Qvar Easi-Breathe® (breath-actuated aerosol inhalation), beclometasone dipropionate 50 micrograms/metered inhalation, net price 200-dose = £7.74; 100 micrograms/metered inhalation, 200-dose = £16.95. Label: 8, counselling, dose; 100-microgram strength also label 10, steroid card

Excipients include HFA-134a (a non-CFC propellant)

Dose by aerosol inhalation, ADULT and CHILD over 12 years, 50–200 micrograms twice daily, if necessary may be increased to max. 400 micrograms twice daily

When switching a patient with well-controlled asthma from another corticosteroid inhaler, initially a 100-microgram metered dose of *Qvar*® should be prescribed for:

- 200–250 micrograms of beclometasone dipropionate or budesonide
- 100 micrograms of fluticasone propionate

When switching a patient with poorly controlled asthma from another corticosteroid inhaler, initially a 100-microgram metered dose of *Qvar*® should be prescribed for 100 micrograms of beclometasone dipropionate, budesonide, or fluticasone propionate; the dose of *Qvar*® should be adjusted according to response

Note The MHRA has advised (August 2006) that beclometasone dipropionate CFC-free inhalers should be prescribed by brand name

High-dose inhalers

Note High-dose inhalers not indicated for children

Chronic Asthma table, see p. 146
Acute Severe Asthma table, see p. 147

Beclometasone (Non-proprietary) PoM

Aerosol inhalation, beclometasone dipropionate 250 micrograms/metered inhalation, net price 200-

dose unit = £25.28. Label: 8, counselling, dose, 10, steroid card
Excipients include CFC propellants
Brands include *Beclazone®*, *Filair Forte®*

Dry powder for inhalation, beclometasone dipropionate 400 micrograms/metered inhalation, net price 100-dose unit = £20.41. Label: 8, counselling, dose, 10, steroid card
Brands include *Pulvinal® Beclometasone Dipropionate*

Inhalation powder, hard capsule (for use with *Cyclohaler®* device), beclometasone dipropionate 400 micrograms, net price 120-cap pack = £32.25. Label: 8, counselling, dose, 10, steroid card
Brands include *Beclometasone 400 Cyclocaps®*

AeroBec Forte® (3M) PoM
Aerosol inhalation, beclometasone dipropionate 250 micrograms/metered inhalation, net price 200-inhalation breath-actuated unit (*Autohaler®*) = £16.76. Label: 8, counselling, dose, 10, steroid card
Excipients include CFC propellants

Asmabec Clickhaler® (UCB Pharma) PoM
Dry powder for inhalation, beclometasone dipropionate 250 micrograms/metered inhalation, net price 100-dose unit = £12.31. Label: 8, counselling, dose, 10, steroid card
Dose by inhalation of powder, 500 micrograms twice daily *or* 250 micrograms 4 times daily; if necessary may be increased to 500 micrograms 4 times daily; CHILD not recommended

Beclazone Easi-Breathe® (IVAX) PoM
Aerosol inhalation, beclometasone dipropionate 250 micrograms/metered inhalation, net price 200-dose breath-actuated unit = £20.25. Label: 8, counselling, dose, 10, steroid card
Excipients include CFC propellants

Becodisks® (A&H) PoM
Dry powder for inhalation, disks containing 8 blisters of beclometasone dipropionate 400 micrograms/blister, 15 disks with *Diskhaler®* device = £45.14, 15-disk refill = £44.57. Label: 8, counselling, dose, 10, steroid card

Clenil Modulite® (Trinity-Chiesi) ▼ PoM
See under Standard-dose inhalers above

Qvar® (IVAX) PoM
See under Standard-dose inhalers above

Compound preparations

Fostair® (Trinity-Chiesi) ▼ PoM
Aerosol inhalation, beclometasone dipropionate 100 micrograms, formoterol fumarate 6 micrograms/metered inhalation, net price 120-dose unit = £29.32. Label: 8, counselling, dose, 10, steroid card
Excipients include HFA-134a (a non-CFC propellant)
Dose by aerosol inhalation, asthma, ADULT over 18 years, 1–2 puffs twice daily; max. 4 puffs daily
Note Each metered inhalation of *Fostair® 100/6* delivers 86 micrograms beclometasone dipropionate and 5 micrograms formoterol fumarate

BUDESONIDE

Indications prophylaxis of asthma (see also Chronic Asthma table, p. 146); croup
Cautions see notes above
Side-effects see notes above
Dose
- See preparations below

Budesonide (Non-proprietary) PoM
Dry powder for inhalation, budesonide 100 micrograms/metered inhalation, net price 200-dose unit = £9.25; 200 micrograms/metered inhalation, 200-dose unit = £18.50; 400 micrograms/metered inhalation, 100-dose unit = £18.50. Label: 8, counselling, dose, 10, steroid card
Brands include *Easyhaler® Budesonide*
Dose by inhalation of powder, ADULT and CHILD over 12 years, 100–800 micrograms twice daily, adjusted as necessary; alternatively, in mild to moderate asthma, 200–400 micrograms (max. 800 micrograms if stabilised on equivalent daily dose given in divided doses) as a single dose each evening; CHILD 6–12 years, 100–400 micrograms twice daily; alternatively, in mild to moderate asthma, 200–400 micrograms as a single dose each evening

Inhalation powder, hard capsule (for use with *Cyclohaler®* device), budesonide 200 micrograms, net price 100-cap pack = £15.48; 400 micrograms, 50-cap pack = £15.48. Label: 8, counselling, dose, 10, steroid card
Brands include *Budesonide Cyclocaps®*
Dose 0.2–1.6 mg daily in divided doses adjusted as necessary; CHILD over 6 years 200–400 micrograms daily in divided doses adjusted as necessary (max. 800 micrograms daily)

Novolizer® (Viatris) ▼ PoM
Dry powder for inhalation, budesonide 200 micrograms, net price refillable inhaler device and 100-dose cartridge = £14.86; 100-dose refill cartridge = £9.59. Label: 8, counselling, dose, 10, steroid card
Dose 0.2–1.6 mg daily in divided doses, adjusted as necessary; alternatively, in mild to moderate asthma (if stabilised on equivalent daily dose given in divided doses) as a single daily dose each evening; CHILD 6–12 years 200–400 micrograms daily in divided doses adjusted as necessary (max. 800 micrograms daily)

Pulmicort® (AstraZeneca) PoM
LS aerosol inhalation, budesonide 50 micrograms/metered inhalation. Net price 200-dose unit = £7.33. Label: 8, counselling, dose
Excipients include CFC propellants

Aerosol inhalation, budesonide 200 micrograms/metered inhalation. Net price 200-dose unit = £20.90; 100-dose unit = £7.60 (hosp. only; may be difficult to obtain). Label: 8, counselling, dose, 10, steroid card
Excipients include CFC propellants
Dose by aerosol inhalation, 200 micrograms twice daily; may be reduced in well-controlled asthma to 200 micrograms daily; in severe asthma dose may be increased to 1.6 mg daily; CHILD 50–400 micrograms twice daily

Turbohaler® (= dry powder inhaler), budesonide 100 micrograms/metered inhalation, net price 200-dose unit = £18.50; 200 micrograms/metered inhalation, 100-dose unit = £18.50; 400 micrograms/metered inhalation, 50-dose unit = £18.50. Label: 8, counselling, dose, 10, steroid card
Dose by inhalation of powder, when starting treatment, during periods of severe asthma, and while reducing or discontinuing oral corticosteroid, 0.2–1.6 mg daily in 2 divided doses; in less severe cases 200–400 micrograms once daily (each evening); patients already controlled on inhaled beclometasone dipropionate or budesonide administered twice daily may be transferred to once-daily dosing (each evening) at the same equivalent total daily dose (up to 800 micrograms once daily); CHILD under 12 years 200–800 micrograms daily in 2 divided doses (800 micrograms daily in severe asthma) *or* 200–400 micrograms once daily (each evening)

Respules® (= single-dose units for nebulisation), budesonide 250 micrograms/mL, net price 20 × 2-mL (500-microgram) unit = £32.00; 500 micrograms/mL, 20 × 2-mL (1-mg) unit = £44.64. May be diluted with sterile sodium chloride 0.9%. Label: 8, counselling, dose, 10, steroid card
Dose by inhalation of nebulised suspension, when starting treatment, during periods of severe asthma, and while reducing or discontinuing oral corticosteroids, 1–2 mg twice daily (may be

increased further in very severe asthma); CHILD 3 months–12 years, 0.5–1 mg twice daily
Maintenance, usually half above doses
Croup, 2 mg as a single dose (*or* as two 1-mg doses separated by 30 minutes)

Compound preparations

Symbicort® (AstraZeneca) PoM

Symbicort 100/6 Turbohaler® (= dry powder inhaler), budesonide 100 micrograms, formoterol fumarate 6 micrograms/metered inhalation, net price 120-dose unit = £33.00. Label: 8, counselling, dose

Dose by inhalation of powder, asthma maintenance therapy, 1–2 puffs twice daily increased if necessary to max. 4 puffs twice daily, reduced to 1 puff once daily if control maintained; CHILD 6–12 years, 2 puffs twice daily reduced to 1 puff once daily if control maintained; 12–17 years, 1–2 puffs twice daily reduced to 1 puff once daily if control maintained
Asthma, maintenance and reliever therapy, ADULT over 18 years, 2 puffs daily in 1–2 divided doses; for relief of symptoms, 1 puff as needed up to max. 6 puffs at a time; max. 8 puffs daily; up to 12 puffs can be used for a limited time but medical assessment should be considered

Note Each metered inhalation of *Symbicort® 100/6* delivers 80 micrograms budesonide and 4.5 micrograms formoterol fumarate

Symbicort 200/6 Turbohaler® (= dry powder inhaler), budesonide 200 micrograms, formoterol fumarate 6 micrograms/metered inhalation, net price 120-dose unit = £38.00. Label: 8, counselling, dose, 10, steroid card

Dose by inhalation of powder, asthma maintenance therapy, 1–2 puffs twice daily increased if necessary to max. 4 puffs twice daily, reduced to 1 puff once daily if control maintained; CHILD 12–17 years 1–2 puffs twice daily reduced to 1 puff once daily if control maintained
Asthma, maintenance and reliever therapy, ADULT over 18 years, 2 puffs daily in 1–2 divided doses, increased if necessary to 2 puffs twice daily; for relief of symptoms, 1 puff as needed up to max. 6 puffs at a time; max. 8 puffs daily; up to 12 puffs can be used for a limited time but medical assessment should be considered
Chronic obstructive pulmonary disease, 2 puffs twice daily

Note Each metered inhalation of *Symbicort® 200/6* delivers 160 micrograms budesonide and 4.5 micrograms formoterol fumarate

Symbicort 400/12 Turbohaler® (= dry powder inhaler), budesonide 400 micrograms, formoterol fumarate 12 micrograms/metered inhalation, net price 60-dose unit = £38.00. Label: 8, counselling, dose, 10, steroid card

Dose by inhalation of powder, asthma maintenance therapy, 1 puff twice daily increased if necessary to max. 2 puffs twice daily, reduced to 1 puff once daily if control maintained; CHILD 12–17 years 1 puff twice daily reduced to 1 puff once daily if control maintained
Chronic obstructive pulmonary disease, 1 puff twice daily

Note Each metered inhalation of *Symbicort® 400/12* delivers 320 micrograms budesonide and 9 micrograms formoterol fumarate

CICLESONIDE

Indications prophylaxis of asthma
Cautions see notes above
Side-effects see notes above
Dose

- By aerosol inhalation, ADULT and CHILD over 12 years, 160 micrograms daily as a single dose reduced to 80 micrograms daily if control maintained

Alvesco® (Altana) ▼ PoM

Aerosol inhalation, ciclesonide 80 micrograms/metered inhalation, net price 120-dose unit = £28.56; 160 micrograms/metered inhalation, 60-dose unit = £16.80, 120-dose unit = £33.60. Label: 8, counselling, dose

Excipients include HFA-134a (a non-CFC propellant), ethanol

FLUTICASONE PROPIONATE

Indications prophylaxis of asthma (see also Chronic Asthma table, p. 146)
Cautions see notes above
Side-effects see notes above; also *very rarely* dyspepsia, hyperglycaemia, and arthralgia
Dose

- See preparations below

Flixotide® (A&H) PoM

Accuhaler® (dry powder for inhalation), disk containing 60 blisters of fluticasone propionate 50 micrograms/blister with *Accuhaler®* device, net price = £6.38; 100 micrograms/blister with *Accuhaler®* device = £8.93; 250 micrograms/blister with *Accuhaler®* device = £21.26; 500 micrograms/blister with *Accuhaler®* device = £36.14. Label: 8, counselling, dose; 250- and 500-microgram strengths also label 10, steroid card

Note *Flixotide Accuhaler®* 250 micrograms and 500 micrograms are not indicated for children

Dose by inhalation of powder, ADULT and CHILD over 16 years, 100–250 micrograms twice daily, increased according to severity of asthma to 1 mg twice daily; CHILD 4–16 years, 50–100 micrograms twice daily adjusted as necessary; max. 200 micrograms twice daily

Diskhaler® (dry powder for inhalation), fluticasone propionate 50 micrograms/blister, net price 15 disks of 4 blisters with *Diskhaler®* device = £8.17, 15-disk refill = £7.64; 100 micrograms/blister, 15 disks of 4 blisters with *Diskhaler®* device = £12.71, 15-disk refill = £12.18; 250 micrograms/blister, 15 disks of 4 blisters with *Diskhaler®* device = £24.11, 15-disk refill = £23.58; 500 micrograms/blister, 15 disks of 4 blisters with *Diskhaler®* device = £40.05, 15-disk refill = £39.52. Label: 8, counselling, dose; 250- and 500-microgram strengths also label 10, steroid card

Note *Flixotide Diskhaler®* 250 micrograms and 500 micrograms are not indicated for children

Dose by inhalation of powder, ADULT and CHILD over 16 years, 100–250 micrograms twice daily, increased according to severity of asthma to 1 mg twice daily; CHILD 4–16 years, 50–100 micrograms twice daily adjusted as necessary; max. 200 micrograms twice daily

Evohaler® *aerosol inhalation*, fluticasone propionate 50 micrograms/metered inhalation, net price 120-dose unit = £5.44; 125 micrograms/metered inhalation, 120-dose unit = £21.26, 250 micrograms/metered inhalation, 120-dose unit = £36.14. Label: 8, counselling, dose, change to CFC-free inhaler, 250-microgram strength also label 10, steroid card

Excipients include HFA-134a (a non-CFC propellant)

Note *Flixotide Evohaler®* 125 micrograms and 250 micrograms not indicated for children

Dose by aerosol inhalation, ADULT and CHILD over 16 years, 100–250 micrograms twice daily, increased according to severity of asthma to 1 mg twice daily; CHILD 4–16 years, 50–100 micrograms twice daily adjusted as necessary; max. 200 micrograms twice daily

Nebules® (= single-dose units for nebulisation) fluticasone propionate 250 micrograms/mL, net price 10 × 2-mL (500-microgram) unit = £9.34; 1 mg/mL, 10 × 2-mL (2-mg) unit = £37.35. May be diluted with sterile sodium chloride 0.9%. Label: 8, counselling, dose, 10, steroid card

Dose by inhalation of nebulised suspension, ADULT and CHILD over 16 years, 0.5–2 mg twice daily; CHILD 4–16 years, 1 mg twice daily

Compound preparations

Seretide® (A&H) PoM

Seretide 100 Accuhaler® (dry powder for inhalation), disk containing 60 blisters of fluticasone propionate 100 micrograms, salmeterol (as xinafoate) 50 micrograms/blister with *Accuhaler®* device, net price = £31.19. Label: 8, counselling, dose

Dose by inhalation of powder, asthma, ADULT and CHILD over 4 years, 1 blister twice daily, reduced to 1 blister once daily if control maintained

Seretide 250 Accuhaler® (dry powder for inhalation), disk containing 60 blisters of fluticasone propionate 250 micrograms, salmeterol (as xinafoate) 50 micrograms/blister with *Accuhaler®* device, net price = £36.65. Label: 8, counselling, dose, 10, steroid card

Dose by inhalation of powder, asthma, ADULT and CHILD over 12 years, 1 blister twice daily

Seretide 500 Accuhaler® (dry powder for inhalation), disk containing 60 blisters of fluticasone propionate 500 micrograms, salmeterol (as xinafoate) 50 micrograms/blister with *Accuhaler®* device, net price = £40.92. Label: 8, counselling, dose, 10, steroid card

Dose by inhalation of powder, asthma, ADULT and CHILD over 12 years, 1 blister twice daily

Chronic obstructive pulmonary disease, ADULT 1 blister twice daily

Seretide 50 Evohaler® (aerosol inhalation), fluticasone propionate 50 micrograms, salmeterol (as xinafoate) 25 micrograms/metered inhalation, net price 120-dose unit = £18.14. Label: 8, counselling, dose, change to CFC-free inhaler

Excipients include HFA-134a (a non-CFC propellant)

Dose by aerosol inhalation, asthma, ADULT and CHILD over 4 years, 2 puffs twice daily, reduced to 2 puffs once daily if control maintained

Seretide 125 Evohaler® (aerosol inhalation), fluticasone propionate 125 micrograms, salmeterol (as xinafoate) 25 micrograms/metered inhalation, net price 120-dose unit = £36.65. Label: 8, counselling, dose, change to CFC-free inhaler, 10, steroid card

Excipients include HFA-134a (a non-CFC propellant)

Dose by aerosol inhalation, asthma, ADULT and CHILD over 12 years, 2 puffs twice daily

Seretide 250 Evohaler® (aerosol inhalation), fluticasone propionate 250 micrograms, salmeterol (as xinafoate) 25 micrograms/metered inhalation, net price 120-dose unit = £62.29. Label: 8, counselling, dose, change to CFC-free inhaler, 10, steroid card

Excipients include HFA-134a (a non-CFC propellant)

Dose by aerosol inhalation, asthma, ADULT and CHILD over 12 years, 2 puffs twice daily

MOMETASONE FUROATE

Indications prophylaxis of asthma (see also Chronic Asthma table, p. 146)

Cautions see notes above

Side-effects see notes above; also pharyngitis, headache; *less commonly* palpitation

Dose

- By inhalation of powder, 200–400 micrograms as a single dose in the evening or in 2 divided doses; dose increased to 400 micrograms twice daily if necessary; CHILD not recommended

Asmanex® (Schering-Plough) ▼ PoM

Twisthaler (= dry powder inhaler), mometasone furoate 200 micrograms/metered inhalation, net price 30-dose unit = £16.00, 60-dose unit = £24.00; 400 micrograms/metered inhalation, 30-dose unit = £22.20, 60-dose unit = £36.75. Label: 8, counselling, dose, 10, steroid card

Note The *Scottish Medicines Consortium* has advised (November 2003) that *Asmanex®* is restricted for use following failure of first-line inhaled corticosteroids

3.3 Cromoglicate and related therapy and leukotriene receptor antagonists

3.3.1 Cromoglicate and related therapy
3.3.2 Leukotriene receptor antagonists

3.3.1 Cromoglicate and related therapy

The mode of action of **sodium cromoglicate** and **nedocromil** is not completely understood. They may be of value in asthma with an allergic basis, but, in practice, it is difficult to predict who will benefit; they could probably be given for 4 to 6 weeks to assess response. Dose frequency is adjusted according to response but is usually 3 to 4 times a day initially; this may subsequently be reduced.

In general, *prophylaxis* with sodium cromoglicate is less effective than prophylaxis with corticosteroid inhalations (see Chronic Asthma table, p. 146). There is evidence of efficacy of nedocromil in children aged 5–12 years. Sodium cromoglicate is of no value in the treatment of acute attacks of asthma.

Sodium cromoglicate can prevent exercise-induced asthma. However, exercise-induced asthma may reflect poor overall control and the patient should be assessed.

If inhalation of the dry powder form of sodium cromoglicate causes bronchospasm a selective $beta_2$-adrenoceptor stimulant such as salbutamol or terbutaline should be inhaled a few minutes beforehand. The nebuliser solution is an alternative means of delivery for children who cannot manage the dry powder inhaler or the aerosol.

SODIUM CROMOGLICATE
(Sodium Cromoglycate)

Indications prophylaxis of asthma; food allergy (section 1.5); allergic conjunctivitis (section 11.4.2); allergic rhinitis (section 12.2.1)

Side-effects coughing, transient bronchospasm, and throat irritation due to inhalation of powder (see also notes above)

Dose

- By inhalation of powder (*Spincaps®*), ADULT and CHILD, 20 mg 4 times daily, increased in severe cases to 8 times daily; additional doses may also be taken before exercise

Intal® (Rhône-Poulenc Rorer) PoM

Spincaps®, yellow/clear, sodium cromoglicate 20 mg. Net price 112-cap pack = £15.44. Label: 8

Spinhaler insufflator® (for use with *Intal Spincaps*). Net price = £1.92

NEDOCROMIL SODIUM

Indications prophylaxis of asthma

Side-effects see under Sodium Cromoglicate; also headache, nausea, vomiting, dyspepsia and abdominal pain; bitter taste (masked by mint flavour)

Dose

- By aerosol inhalation, ADULT and CHILD over 6 years 4 mg (2 puffs) 4 times daily, when control achieved may be possible to reduce to twice daily

Counselling Regular use is necessary

Tilade CFC-free Inhaler® (Sanofi-Aventis) ▼ PoM

Aerosol inhalation, mint-flavoured, nedocromil sodium 2 mg/metered inhalation. Net price 112-dose unit = £39.94. Label: 8, counselling, change to CFC-free inhaler

Excipients include HFA-227 (a non-CFC propellant)

3.3.2 Leukotriene receptor antagonists

The leukotriene receptor antagonists, **montelukast** and **zafirlukast**, block the effects of cysteinyl leukotrienes in the airways. They are effective in asthma when used alone or with an inhaled corticosteroid (see Chronic Asthma table, p. 146). Montelukast has not been shown to be more effective than a standard dose of inhaled corticosteroid but the two drugs appear to have an additive effect. The leukotriene receptor antagonists may be of benefit in exercise-induced asthma and in those with concomitant rhinitis but they are less effective in those with severe asthma who are also receiving high doses of other drugs.

Churg-Strauss syndrome has occurred very rarely in association with the use of leukotriene receptor antagonists; in many of the reported cases the reaction followed the reduction or withdrawal of oral corticosteroid therapy. The CSM has advised that prescribers should be alert to the development of eosinophilia, vasculitic rash, worsening pulmonary symptoms, cardiac complications, or peripheral neuropathy.

MONTELUKAST

Indications prophylaxis of asthma, see notes above and Chronic Asthma table, p. 146; symptomatic relief of seasonal allergic rhinitis in patients with asthma

Cautions pregnancy (Appendix 4); breast-feeding (Appendix 5); **interactions:** Appendix 1 (leukotriene antagonists)

Side-effects abdominal pain, thirst; hyperkinesia (in young children), headache; *very rarely* Churg-Strauss syndrome (see notes above); dry mouth, diarrhoea, dyspepsia, nausea, vomiting, hepatic disorders, palpitation, oedema, increased bleeding, depression, tremor, asthenia, dizziness, hallucinations, paraesthesia, hypoaesthesia, sleep disturbances, abnormal dreams, agitation, aggression, seizures, arthralgia, myalgia, pruritus, and rash also reported

Dose

- Prophylaxis of asthma, ADULT and CHILD over 15 years, 10 mg once daily in the evening; CHILD 6 months–6 years 4 mg once daily in the evening, 6–15 years 5 mg once daily in the evening
- Seasonal allergic rhinitis, ADULT and CHILD over 15 years, 10 mg once daily in the evening

Singulair® (MSD) PoM

Chewable tablets, pink, cherry-flavoured, montelukast (as sodium salt) 4 mg, net price 28-tab pack = £25.69; 5 mg, 28-tab pack = £25.69. Label: 23, 24

Excipients include aspartame equivalent to phenylalanine 674 micrograms/4-mg tablet and 842 micrograms/5-mg tablet (section 9.4.1)

Granules, montelukast (as sodium salt) 4 mg, net price 28-sachet pack = £25.69. Counselling, administration

Counselling Granules may be swallowed or mixed with cold food (but not fluid) and taken immediately

Tablets, beige, f/c, montelukast (as sodium salt) 10 mg, net price 28-tab pack = £26.97

Note The *Scottish Medicines Consortium* has advised (June 2007) that *Singulair®* chewable tablets and granules are restricted for use as an alternative to low-dose inhaled corticosteroids for children 2-14 years with mild persistent asthma who have not recently had serious asthma attacks that required oral corticosteroid use and who are not capable of using inhaled corticosteroids; *Singulair®* chewable tablets and granules should be initiated by a specialist in paediatric asthma

ZAFIRLUKAST

Indications prophylaxis of asthma, see notes above and Chronic Asthma table, p. 146

Cautions elderly, renal impairment (Appendix 3); pregnancy (Appendix 4); **interactions:** Appendix 1 (leukotriene antagonists)

Hepatic disorders Patients or their carers should be told how to recognise development of liver disorder and advised to seek medical attention if symptoms or signs such as persistent nausea, vomiting, malaise, or jaundice develop

Contra-indications hepatic impairment; breast-feeding (Appendix 5)

Side-effects gastro-intestinal disturbances, headache, insomnia, malaise; *rarely* bleeding disorders, hypersensitivity reactions including angioedema and skin reactions, arthralgia, myalgia, hepatitis, hyperbilirubinaemia, thrombocytopenia; *very rarely* Churg-Strauss syndrome (see notes above), agranulocytosis

Dose

- ADULT and CHILD over 12 years, 20 mg twice daily

Accolate® (AstraZeneca) PoM

Tablets, f/c, zafirlukast 20 mg, net price 56-tab pack = £28.26. Label: 23

3.4 Antihistamines, hyposensitisation, and allergic emergencies

3.4.1 Antihistamines

3.4.2 Allergen Immunotherapy

3.4.3 Allergic emergencies

3.4.1 Antihistamines

All antihistamines are of potential value in the treatment of nasal allergies, particularly seasonal allergic rhinitis (hay fever), and they may be of some value in vasomotor rhinitis. They reduce rhinorrhoea and sneezing but are usually less effective for nasal congestion. Antihistamines are used topically in the eye (section 11.4.2), in the nose (section 12.2.1), and on the skin (section 13.3).

Oral antihistamines are also of some value in preventing urticaria and are used to treat urticarial rashes, pruritus, and insect bites and stings; they are also used in drug allergies. Injections of chlorphenamine (chlorphenir-amine) or promethazine are used as an adjunct to adrenaline (epinephrine) in the emergency treatment of anaphylaxis and angioedema (section 3.4.3). For the use of antihistamines (including cinnarizine, cyclizine, and promethazine teoclate) in nausea and vomiting, see section 4.6. Buclizine is included as an anti-emetic in a preparation for migraine (section 4.7.4.1). For reference to the use of antihistamines for occasional insomnia, see section 4.1.1.

All older antihistamines cause sedation but **alimemazine** (trimeprazine) and **promethazine** may be more sedating whereas **chlorphenamine** and **cyclizine** (section 4.6) may be less so. This sedating activity is sometimes used to manage the pruritus associated with some allergies. There is little evidence that any one of the older, 'sedating' antihistamines is superior to another and patients vary widely in their response.

Non-sedating antihistamines such as **cetirizine**, **desloratadine** (an active metabolite of loratadine), **fexofenadine** (an active metabolite of terfenadine), **levocetirizine** (an isomer of cetirizine), **loratadine**, and **mizolastine** cause less sedation and psychomotor impairment than the older antihistamines because they penetrate the blood brain barrier only to a slight extent.

Dental surgery Antihistamines are used widely as anti-emetics (section 4.6) but diazepam is likely to be more effective in patients with an overactive gag reflex. See also Anaphylaxis under Medical Emergencies in Dental Practice, p. 21.

Cautions and contra-indications Sedating antihistamines have significant antimuscarinic activity and they should therefore be used with caution in prostatic hypertrophy, urinary retention, susceptibility to angle-closure glaucoma, and pyloroduodenal obstruction. Antihistamines should be used with caution in hepatic disease (Appendix 2). Caution may be required in epilepsy. Children and the elderly are more susceptible to side-effects. Many antihistamines should be avoided in porphyria although some (e.g. chlorphenamine and cetirizine) are thought to be safe (section 9.8.2). **Interactions**: Appendix 1 (antihistamines).

Side-effects Drowsiness is a significant side-effect with most of the older antihistamines although paradoxical stimulation may occur rarely, especially with high doses or in children and the elderly. Drowsiness may diminish after a few days of treatment and is considerably less of a problem with the newer antihistamines (see also notes above). Side-effects that are more common with the older antihistamines include headache, psychomotor impairment, and antimuscarinic effects such as urinary retention, dry mouth, blurred vision, and gastro-intestinal disturbances.

Other rare side-effects of antihistamines include hypotension, extrapyramidal effects, dizziness, confusion, depression, sleep disturbances, tremor, convulsions, palpitation, arrhythmias, hypersensitivity reactions (including bronchospasm, angioedema, and anaphylaxis, rashes, and photosensitivity reactions), blood disorders, liver dysfunction, and angle-closure glaucoma.

Non-sedating antihistamines

Driving Although drowsiness is rare, nevertheless patients should be advised that it can occur and may affect performance of skilled tasks (e.g. driving); excess alcohol should be avoided.

CETIRIZINE HYDROCHLORIDE

Indications symptomatic relief of allergy such as hay fever, chronic idiopahtic urticaria

Cautions see notes above; also renal impairment (Appendix 3)

Contra-indications see notes above; also pregnancy (Appendix 4); breast-feeding (Appendix 5)

Side-effects see notes above

Dose

- ADULT and CHILD over 6 years, 10 mg once daily *or* 5 mg twice daily; CHILD 1–2 years see *BNF for Children*, 2–6 years, hay fever, 5 mg once daily *or* 2.5 mg twice daily

Cetirizine (Non-proprietary)

Tablets, cetirizine hydrochloride 10 mg, net price 30-tab pack = 46p. Counselling, driving

Oral solution, cetirizine hydrochloride 5 mg/5 mL, net price 200 mL = £3.03. Counselling, driving

DESLORATADINE

Note Desloratadine is a metabolite of loratadine

Indications symptomatic relief of allergy such as hay fever, chronic idiopathic urticaria

Cautions see notes above; also renal impairment (Appendix 3)

Contra-indications see notes above; also hypersensitivity to loratadine; pregnancy (Appendix 4) and breast-feeding (Appendix 5)

Side-effects see notes above; *rarely* myalgia; *very rarely* hallucinations

Dose

- 5 mg once daily; CHILD 1–6 years 1.25 mg once daily, 6–12 years 2.5 mg once daily

Neoclarityn® (Schering-Plough) PoM

Tablets, blue, f/c, desloratadine 5 mg, net price 30-tab pack = £7.04. Counselling, driving

Syrup, desloratadine 2.5 mg/5 mL, net price 100 mL (bubblegum-flavour) = £7.04. Counselling, driving

FEXOFENADINE HYDROCHLORIDE

Note Fexofenadine is a metabolite of terfenadine

Indications see under Dose

Cautions see notes above; also pregnancy (Appendix 4)

Contra-indications see notes above; also breast-feeding (Appendix 5)

Side-effects see notes above

Dose

- Seasonal allergic rhinitis, 120 mg once daily; CHILD 6–12 years, 30 mg twice daily
- Chronic idiopathic urticaria, ADULT and CHILD over 12 years, 180 mg once daily

Telfast® (Aventis Pharma) PoM

Tablets, f/c, peach, fexofenadine hydrochloride 30 mg, net price 60-tab pack = £5.68; 120 mg, 30-tab pack = £6.23; 180 mg, 30-tab pack = £7.89. Counselling, driving

LEVOCETIRIZINE HYDROCHLORIDE

Note Levocetirizine is an isomer of cetirizine

Indications symptomatic relief of allergy such as hay fever, urticaria

Cautions see notes above; also renal impairment (avoid if creatinine clearance less than 10 mL/minute; Appendix 3); pregnancy (Appendix 4) and breast-feeding (Appendix 5)

Contra-indications see notes above

Side-effects see notes above; *very rarely* weight gain

Dose

- ADULT and CHILD over 6 years, 5 mg once daily; CHILD 2–6 years 1.25 mg twice daily

Xyzal® (UCB Pharma) PoM

Tablets, f/c, levocetirizine hydrochloride 5 mg, net price 30-tab pack = £5.20. Counselling, driving

Oral solution, levocetirizine hydrochloride 2.5 mg/5 mL, net price 200 mL = £6.00. Counselling, driving

LORATADINE

Indications symptomatic relief of allergy such as hay fever, chronic idiopathic urticaria

Cautions see notes above

Contra-indications see notes above; also pregnancy (Appendix 4) and breast-feeding (Appendix 5)

Side-effects see notes above

Dose

- ADULT and CHILD over 6 years 10 mg once daily; CHILD 2–6 years 5 mg once daily

Loratadine (Non-proprietary)

Tablets, loratadine 10 mg, net price 30-tab pack = £1.06. Counselling, driving

Syrup, loratadine 5 mg/5 mL, net price 100 mL = £5.18. Counselling, driving

MIZOLASTINE

Indications symptomatic relief of allergy such as hay fever, urticaria

Cautions see notes above

Contra-indications see notes above; also susceptibility to QT-interval prolongation (including cardiac disease and hypokalaemia); significant hepatic impairment; pregnancy (Appendix 4) and breast-feeding (Appendix 5)

Side-effects see notes above; weight gain; anxiety, asthenia; *less commonly* arthralgia and myalgia

Dose

- ADULT and CHILD over 12 years, 10 mg once daily

Mizollen® (Sanofi-Aventis) PoM

Tablets, m/r, f/c, scored, mizolastine 10 mg, net price 30-tab pack = £5.77. Label: 25, Counselling, driving

Sedating antihistamines

Driving Drowsiness may affect performance of skilled tasks (e.g. driving); sedating effects enhanced by alcohol.

ALIMEMAZINE TARTRATE

(Trimeprazine tartrate)

Indications urticaria and pruritus, premedication

Cautions see notes above; pregnancy (Appendix 4); see also section 4.2.1

Contra-indications see notes above; also renal impairment; breast-feeding (Appendix 5); see also section 4.2.1

Side-effects see notes above; see also section 4.2.1

Dose

- Urticaria and pruritus, 10 mg 2–3 times daily, in severe cases up to max. 100 mg daily has been used; ELDERLY 10 mg 1–2 times daily; CHILD over 2 years 2.5–5 mg 3–4 times daily
- Premedication, CHILD 2–7 years up to 2 mg/kg 1–2 hours before operation

Vallergan® (Sanofi-Aventis) PoM

Tablets, blue, f/c, alimemazine tartrate 10 mg, net price 28-tab pack = £3.89. Label: 2

Syrup, straw-coloured, alimemazine tartrate 7.5 mg/5 mL, net price 100 mL = £4.44. Label: 2

Syrup forte, alimemazine tartrate 30 mg/5 mL, net price 100 mL = £6.86. Label: 2

CHLORPHENAMINE MALEATE

(Chlorpheniramine maleate)

Indications symptomatic relief of allergy such as hay fever, urticaria; emergency treatment of anaphylactic reactions (section 3.4.3)

Cautions see notes above; also pregnancy (Appendix 4) and breast-feeding (Appendix 5)

Contra-indications see notes above

Side-effects see notes above; also exfoliative dermatitis and tinnitus reported; injections may cause transient hypotension or CNS stimulation and may be irritant

Dose

- By mouth, 4 mg every 4–6 hours, max. 24 mg daily; CHILD under 1 year see *BNF for Children*, 1–2 years 1 mg twice daily; 2–6 years 1 mg every 4–6 hours, max. 6 mg daily; 6–12 years 2 mg every 4–6 hours, max. 12 mg daily
- By subcutaneous *or* intramuscular injection *or* by intravenous injection over 1 minute, 10–20 mg, repeated if required up to 4 times in 24 hours; max. 40 mg in 24 hours; CHILD 1 month–1 year 250 micrograms/kg, repeated if required up to 4 times in 24 hours; 1–12 years 200 micrograms/kg *or* 1–6 years 2.5–5 mg, repeated if required up to 4 times in 24 hours; 6–12 years 5–10 mg, repeated if required up to 4 times in 24 hours

Chlorphenamine (Non-proprietary)

Tablets, chlorphenamine maleate 4 mg, net price 28 = 69p. Label: 2

Dental prescribing on NHS Chlorphenamine tablets may be prescribed

Oral solution, chlorphenamine maleate 2 mg/5 mL, net price 150 mL = £2.21. Label: 2

Injection PoM[1], chlorphenamine maleate 10 mg/mL, net price 1-mL amp = £1.62

1. PoM restriction does not apply where administration is for saving life in emergency

3 Respiratory system

Piriton® (GSK Consumer Healthcare)
Tablets, yellow, scored, chlorphenamine maleate 4 mg, net price 28 = £1.62. Label: 2
Syrup, chlorphenamine maleate 2 mg/5 mL, net price 150 mL = £2.16. Label: 2

CLEMASTINE

Indications symptomatic relief of allergy such as hay fever, urticaria
Cautions see notes above; also pregnancy (Appendix 4) and breast-feeding (Appendix 5)
Contra-indications see notes above
Side-effects see notes above
Dose
- 1 mg twice daily, increased up to 6 mg daily if required; INFANT under 1 year not recommended, CHILD 1–3 years 250–500 micrograms twice daily; 3–6 years 500 micrograms twice daily; 6–12 years 0.5–1 mg twice daily

Tavegil® (Novartis Consumer Health)
Tablets, scored, clemastine (as hydrogen fumarate) 1 mg. Net price 60-tab pack = £2.35. Label: 2

CYPROHEPTADINE HYDROCHLORIDE

Indications symptomatic relief of allergy such as hay fever, urticaria; migraine (section 4.7.4.2)
Cautions see notes above; also pregnancy (Appendix 4)
Contra-indications see notes above; also breast-feeding (Appendix 5)
Side-effects see notes above
Dose
- Allergy, usual dose 4 mg 3–4 times daily; usual range 4–20 mg daily, max. 32 mg daily; INFANT under 2 years not recommended, CHILD 2–6 years 2 mg 2–3 times daily, max. 12 mg daily; 7–14 years 4 mg 2–3 times daily, max. 16 mg daily
- Migraine, 4 mg with a further 4 mg after 30 minutes if necessary; maintenance, 4 mg every 4–6 hours

Periactin® (MSD)
Tablets, scored, cyproheptadine hydrochloride 4 mg, net price 30-tab pack = 86p. Label: 2

HYDROXYZINE HYDROCHLORIDE

Indications pruritus, anxiety (short-term) (section 4.1.2)
Cautions see notes above
Contra-indications see notes above; also pregnancy (Appendix 4) and breast-feeding (Appendix 5)
Side-effects see notes above
Dose
- Pruritus, initially 25 mg at night increased if necessary to 25 mg 3–4 times daily; CHILD 6 months–6 years initially 5–15 mg daily increased if necessary to 50 mg daily in divided doses; over 6 years initially 15–25 mg daily increased if necessary to 50–100 mg daily in divided doses
- Anxiety (adults only), 50–100 mg 4 times daily

Atarax® (Alliance) PoM
Tablets, both s/c, hydroxyzine hydrochloride 10 mg (orange), net price 84-tab pack = £1.82; 25 mg (green), 28-tab pack = £1.22. Label: 2

Ucerax® (UCB Pharma) PoM
Tablets NHS, f/c, scored, hydroxyzine hydrochloride 25 mg, net price 25-tab pack = 85p. Label: 2
Syrup, hydroxyzine hydrochloride 10 mg/5 mL. Net price 200-mL pack = £1.78. Label: 2

KETOTIFEN

Indications allergic rhinitis
Cautions see notes above
Contra-indications pregnancy (Appendix 4); breast-feeding (Appendix 5)
Side-effects see notes above; also excitation, irritability, nervousness; *less commonly* cystitis; *rarely* weight gain; *very rarely* Stevens-Johnson syndrome
Dose
- 1 mg twice daily with food increased if necessary to 2 mg twice daily; initial treatment in readily sedated patients 0.5–1 mg at night; CHILD 3 years and over, 1 mg twice daily

Zaditen® (Novartis) PoM
Tablets, scored, ketotifen (as hydrogen fumarate) 1 mg, net price 60-tab pack = £10.75. Label: 2, 21
Elixir, ketotifen (as hydrogen fumarate), 1 mg/5 mL, net price 300 mL (strawberry-flavoured) = £12.73. Label: 2, 21

PROMETHAZINE HYDROCHLORIDE

Indications symptomatic relief of allergy such as hay fever, urticaria; premedication; emergency treatment of anaphylactic reactions (section 3.4.3); sedation (section 4.1.1); motion sickness (section 4.6)
Cautions see notes above; severe coronary artery disease; pregnancy (Appendix 4); breast-feeding (Appendix 5)
Contra-indications see notes above
Side-effects see notes above; also restlessness; intramuscular injection may be painful
Dose
- By mouth, 25 mg at night increased to 25 mg twice daily if necessary *or* 10–20 mg 2–3 times daily; CHILD under 2 years not recommended, 2–5 years 5–15 mg daily in 1–2 divided doses, 5–10 years 10–25 mg daily in 1–2 divided doses

  Premedication, CHILD under 2 years not recommended, 2–5 years 15–20 mg, 5–10 years 20–25 mg
- By deep intramuscular injection, 25–50 mg; max. 100 mg; CHILD 5–10 years 6.25–12.5 mg

  Premedication, 25–50 mg 1 hour before operation; CHILD 5–10 years, 6.25–12.5 mg
- By slow intravenous injection in emergencies, 25–50 mg as a solution containing 2.5 mg/mL in water for injections; max. 100 mg

Phenergan® (Rhône-Poulenc Rorer)
Tablets, both blue, f/c, promethazine hydrochloride 10 mg, net price 56-tab pack = £2.05; 25 mg, 56-tab pack = £3.06. Label: 2
Dental prescribing on NHS May be prescribed as Promethazine Hydrochloride Tablets 10 mg or 25 mg
Elixir, golden, promethazine hydrochloride 5 mg/5 mL, net price 100 mL = £1.93. Label: 2
Dental prescribing on NHS May be prescribed as Promethazine Hydrochloride Oral Solution 5 mg/5 mL

Injection [PoM][1], promethazine hydrochloride 25 mg/mL, net price 1-mL amp = 70p
Promethazine hydrochloride injection 25 mg/mL (1-mL and 2-mL ampoules) also available from Antigen

1. [PoM] restriction does not apply where administration is for saving life in emergency

3.4.2 Allergen Immunotherapy

Immunotherapy using allergen vaccines containing house dust mite, animal dander (cat or dog), or extracts of grass and tree pollen can reduce symptoms of asthma and allergic rhinoconjunctivitis. A vaccine containing extracts of wasp and bee venom is used to reduce the risk of severe anaphylaxis and systemic reactions in individuals with hypersensitivity to wasp and bee stings. Those requiring immunotherapy must be referred to a hospital specialist for accurate diagnosis, assessment, and treatment.

> In view of concerns about the safety of desensitising vaccines, it is recommended that they are used by specialists and only for the following indications:
> - seasonal allergic hay fever (caused by pollen) that has not responded to anti-allergic drugs;
> - hypersensitivity to wasp and bee venoms.
>
> Desensitising vaccines should generally be avoided or used with particular care in patients with asthma.

Desensitising vaccines should be avoided in pregnant women, in children under five years old, and in those taking beta-blockers (adrenaline may be ineffective in case of a hypersensitivity reaction), or ACE inhibitors (risk of severe anaphylactoid reactions).

Hypersensitivity reactions to immunotherapy (especially to wasp and bee venom extracts) can be life-threatening; bronchospasm usually develops within 1 hour and anaphylaxis within 30 minutes of injection. Therefore patients need to be monitored for 1 hour after injection. If symptoms or signs of hypersensitivity develop (e.g. rash, urticaria, bronchospasm, faintness), **even when mild**, the patient should be observed until these have **resolved completely**.

For details of the management of anaphylactic shock, see section 3.4.3.

Each set of allergen extracts usually contains vials for the administration of graded amounts of allergen to patients undergoing hyposensitisation. Maintenance sets containing vials at the highest strength are also available. Product literature must be consulted for details of allergens, vial strengths, and administration.

BEE AND WASP ALLERGEN EXTRACTS

Indications hypersensitivity to wasp or bee venom (see notes above)

Cautions see notes above and consult product literature

CSM advice The CSM has advised that facilities for cardiopulmonary resuscitation must be immediately available and patients monitored closely for one hour after each injection

Contra-indications see notes above and consult product literature

Side-effects consult product literature

Dose

- By subcutaneous injection, consult product literature

Pharmalgen® (ALK-Abelló) [PoM]

Bee venom extract (*Apis mellifera*) or wasp venom extract (*Vespula* spp.), net price initial treatment set = £59.77 (bee), £73.28 (wasp); maintenance treatment set = £69.54 (bee), £89.45 (wasp)

GRASS AND TREE POLLEN EXTRACTS

Indications treatment of seasonal allergic hay fever due to grass or tree pollen in patients who have failed to respond to anti-allergy drugs (see notes above)

Cautions see notes above and consult product literature

CSM advice The CSM has advised that facilities for cardiopulmonary resuscitation must be immediately available and patients monitored closely for one hour after each injection

Contra-indications see notes above and consult product literature

Side-effects see notes above and consult product literature

Dose

- See under preparations, below

Pollinex® (Allergy) [PoM]

Grasses and rye or tree pollen extract, net price initial treatment set (3 vials) and extension course treatment (1 vial) = £320.00

Dose By subcutaneous injection, consult product literature

▲Grass pollen extract

Grazax® (ALK-Abelló) ▼ [PoM]

Oral lyophilisates (= freeze-dried tablets), grass pollen extract 75 000 units, net price 30-tab pack = £67.50. Counselling, administration

Dose ADULT over 18 years, 1 tablet daily during pollen season; start treatment at least 4 months before start of pollen season

Counselling Tablets should be placed under the tongue and allowed to disperse

Omalizumab

Omalizumab is a monoclonal antibody that binds to immunoglobulin E (IgE). It is licensed for use as additional therapy in individuals with proven IgE-mediated sensitivity to inhaled allergens, whose severe persistent allergic asthma cannot be controlled adequately with high-dose inhaled corticosteroid together with a long-acting beta$_2$ agonist. Omalizumab should be initiated by physicians experienced in the treatment of severe persistent asthma.

Churg-Strauss syndrome has occurred rarely in patients given omalizumab; the reaction is usually associated with the reduction of oral corticosteroid therapy. Churg-Strauss syndrome can present as eosinophilia, vasculitic rash, cardiac complications, worsening pulmonary symptoms, or peripheral neuropathy. Hypersensitivity reactions can also occur immediately following treatment with omalizumab or sometimes more than 24 hours after the first injection.

For details on the management of anaphylactic shock, see section 3.4.3.

> **NICE guidance**
> **Omalizumab for severe persistent allergic asthma (November 2007)**
> Omalizumab is recommended as additional therapy for the prophylaxis of severe persistent allergic asthma in adults and children over 12 years, who cannot be controlled adequately with high-dose inhaled corticosteroids and long-acting $beta_2$ agonists in addition to leukotriene receptor antagonists, theophylline, oral corticosteroids, oral $beta_2$ agonists, and smoking cessation where clinically appropriate. The following conditions apply:
> - confirmation of IgE-mediated allergy to a perennial allergen by clinical history and allergy skin testing;
> - either 2 or more severe exacerbations of asthma requiring hospital admission within the previous year, or 3 or more severe exacerbations of asthma within the previous year, at least one of which required hospital admission, and a further 2 which required treatment or monitoring in excess of the patient's usual regimen, in an accident and emergency unit.
>
> Omalizumab should be initiated and monitored by a physician experienced in both allergy and respiratory medicine in a specialist centre, and discontinued at 16 weeks in patients who have not shown an adequate response to therapy.

3 Respiratory system

OMALIZUMAB

Indications prophylaxis of allergic asthma (see notes above)

Cautions autoimmune disease; susceptibility to helminth infection—discontinue if infection does not respond to anthelmintic; hepatic impairment; renal impairment; pregnancy (Appendix 4)

Contra-indications breast-feeding (Appendix 5)

Side-effects headache; injection-site reactions; *less commonly* nausea, diarrhoea, dyspepsia, flushing, fatigue, dizziness, drowsiness, paraesthesia, weight gain, influenza-like symptoms, photosensitivity, hypersensitivity reactions (including hypotension, bronchospasm, laryngoedema, rash, pruritus, and anaphylaxis); Churg-Strauss syndrome (see notes above), thrombocytopenia, arthralgia, myalgia, and alopecia also reported

Dose

- By subcutaneous injection, ADULT and CHILD over 12 years, according to immunoglobulin E concentration and body-weight, consult product literature

Xolair® (Novartis) ▼ PoM
Injection, powder for reconstitution, omalizumab, net price 150-mg vial = £256.15 (with solvent)
Excipients include sucrose 108 mg/vial

3.4.3 Allergic emergencies

Adrenaline (epinephrine) provides physiological reversal of the immediate symptoms (such as laryngeal oedema, bronchospasm, and hypotension) associated with hypersensitivity reactions such as *anaphylaxis* and *angioedema*.

Anaphylaxis

Anaphylactic shock requires prompt treatment of *laryngeal oedema, bronchospasm,* and *hypotension.* Atopic individuals are particularly susceptible. Insect stings are a recognised risk (in particular wasp and bee stings). Certain foods, including eggs, fish, cow's milk protein, peanuts, and tree nuts may also precipitate anaphylaxis. Medicinal products particularly associated with anaphylaxis include blood products, vaccines, hyposensitising (allergen) preparations, antibacterials, aspirin and other NSAIDs, heparin, and neuromuscular blocking drugs. In the case of drugs, anaphylaxis is more likely after parenteral administration; resuscitation facilities must always be available for injections associated with special risk. Anaphylactic reactions may also be associated with *additives and excipients* in foods and medicines. Refined arachis (peanut) oil, which may be present in some medicinal products, is unlikely to cause an allergic reaction—nevertheless it is wise to check the full formula of preparations which may contain allergenic fats or oils.

First-line treatment of anaphylaxis includes securing the airway, restoration of blood pressure (laying the patient flat and raising the legs, or in the recovery position if unconscious or nauseated and at risk of vomiting) and administration of **adrenaline** (epinephrine) injection. Adrenaline is given **intramuscularly** in a dose of 500 micrograms (0.5 mL adrenaline injection 1 in 1000); a dose of 300 micrograms (0.3 mL adrenaline injection 1 in 1000) may be appropriate for *immediate self-administration.* The dose is repeated if necessary at 5-minute intervals according to blood pressure, pulse, and respiratory function (**important:** possible need for *intravenous route* using *dilute solution,* see below). High-flow **oxygen** administration and intravenous fluids (section 9.2.2) are also of primary importance. An antihistamine (e.g. **chlorphenamine**, given by slow intravenous injection in a dose of 10 mg, see p. 167) is a useful adjunctive treatment, given after adrenaline injection and continued for 24 to 48 hours to prevent relapse. Patients receiving beta-blockers require special consideration (see under Adrenaline, p. 171).

Continuing respiratory deterioration requires further treatment with **bronchodilators** including inhaled or intravenous salbutamol (see p. 151), inhaled ipratropium (see p. 154), intravenous aminophylline (see p. 155), or intravenous magnesium sulphate [unlicensed indication] (see under Acute Severe Asthma, p. 148); in addition to oxygen, assisted respiration and possibly emergency tracheotomy may be necessary.

An intravenous corticosteroid e.g. **hydrocortisone** (as sodium succinate) in a dose of 200 mg (section 6.3.2) is of secondary value in the initial management of anaphylactic shock because the onset of action is delayed for several hours, but should be given to prevent further deterioration in severely affected patients.

When a patient is so ill that there is doubt about the adequacy of the circulation, the initial injection of adrenaline may need to be given as a *dilute solution by the intravenous route*; for details of cautions, dose, and strength, see under Intravenous Adrenaline (Epinephrine), below.

Cardiopulmonary arrest may follow an anaphylactic reaction; resuscitation should be started immediately (see p. 121).

For advice on the management of medical emergencies in dental practice, see p. 21.

Patients who are suspected of having had an anaphylactic reaction should be referred to a specialist for specific allergy diagnosis; avoidance of the allergen is the principal treatment.

Angioedema

Angioedema is dangerous if *laryngeal oedema* is present. In this circumstance adrenaline (epinephrine) injection and oxygen should be given as described under Anaphylaxis (see above); antihistamines and corticosteroids should also be given (see again above). Tracheal intubation may be necessary.

Hereditary angioedema The administration of C_1 esterase inhibitor (in fresh frozen plasma or in partially purified form) can terminate acute attacks of *hereditary angioedema*, but is not practical for long-term prophylaxis. **Tranexamic acid** (section 2.11) and **danazol** (section 6.7.2) [unlicensed indication] are used for short-term and long-term prophylaxis of hereditary angioedema. Short-term prophylaxis is started several days before planned procedures (e.g. dental work) and continued for 2–5 days afterwards. Danazol should be avoided in children because of its androgenic effects.

Intramuscular adrenaline (epinephrine)

The *intramuscular route* is the *first choice route* for the administration of adrenaline (epinephrine) in the management of anaphylactic shock. Adrenaline has a rapid onset of action after intramuscular administration and in the shocked patient its absorption from the intramuscular site is faster and more reliable than from the subcutaneous site (the intravenous route should be reserved for extreme emergency when there is doubt about the adequacy of the circulation; for details of cautions, dose and strength see under Intravenous Adrenaline (Epinephrine), below).

Patients with severe allergy should ideally be instructed in the self-administration of adrenaline by intramuscular injection (for details see under Self-administration of Adrenaline (Epinephrine), below).

Prompt injection of adrenaline is of paramount importance. The following adrenaline doses are based on the revised recommendations of the Working Group of the Resuscitation Council (UK).

Dose of *intramuscular* injection of adrenaline (epinephrine) for anaphylactic shock

Age	Dose	Volume of adrenaline **1 in 1000** (1 mg/mL)
Child under 6 years	150 micrograms	0.15 mL[1]
Child 6–12 years	300 micrograms	0.3 mL
Adult and child 12–18 years	500 micrograms	0.5 mL

These doses may be repeated several times if necessary at 5-minute intervals according to blood pressure, pulse, and respiratory function.

1. Use suitable syringe for measuring small volume

Intravenous adrenaline (epinephrine)

When the patient is severely ill and there is real doubt about the adequacy of the circulation and absorption after intramuscular injection, adrenaline (epinephrine) can be given by **slow** *intravenous injection* in a dose of 50 micrograms (0.5 mL of the dilute 1 in 10 000 adrenaline injection) repeated according to response; if multiple doses are required, adrenaline should be given as a **slow** intravenous infusion *stopping when a response has been obtained*; children may respond to as little as 1 microgram/kg (0.01 mL/kg of the dilute 1 in 10 000 adrenaline injection) by **slow** *intravenous injection* over several minutes.

Intravenous adrenaline should be given only by those experienced in its use, in a setting where patients can be carefully monitored; it should only be given to children when intravenous access is already available.

Great vigilance is needed to ensure that the *correct strength* is used; anaphylactic shock kits need to make a *very clear distinction* between the 1 in 10 000 strength and the 1 in 1000 strength. It is also important that, where intramuscular injection might still succeed, time should not be wasted seeking intravenous access.

For reference to the use of the intravenous route for *cardiac resuscitation*, see section 2.7.3.

Self-administration of adrenaline (epinephrine)

Individuals at considerable risk of anaphylaxis need to carry adrenaline (epinephrine) at all times and need to be *instructed in advance* how to inject it. In addition, the packs need to be labelled so that in the case of rapid collapse someone else is able to administer the adrenaline. It is important to ensure that an adequate supply is provided to treat symptoms until medical assistance is available.

Some patients may best cope with a pre-assembled syringe fitted with a needle suitable for very rapid administration (if necessary by a bystander). *Anapen®* and *EpiPen®* consist of a fully assembled syringe and needle delivering a dose of 300 micrograms of adrenaline by *intramuscular injection*; 150-microgram versions (*Anapen® Junior, EpiPen® Jr*) are also available for use in children.

ADRENALINE/EPINEPHRINE

Indications emergency treatment of acute anaphylaxis; angioedema; cardiopulmonary resuscitation (section 2.7.3); priapism [unlicensed indication] (section 7.4.5)

Cautions heart disease, hypertension, arrhythmias, cerebrovascular disease, phaeochromocytoma; diabetes mellitus, hyperthyroidism; susceptibility to angle-closure glaucoma; elderly

Interactions Severe anaphylaxis in patients taking non-cardioselective beta-blockers may not respond to adrenaline, calling for intravenous salbutamol (see p. 151); adrenaline can cause severe hypertension and bradycardia in those taking non-cardioselective beta-blockers. Other **interactions**, see Appendix 1 (sympathomimetics).

Side-effects nausea, vomiting; tachycardia, arrhythmias, palpitation, cold extremities, hypertension (risk of cerebral haemorrhage); dyspnoea, pulmonary oedema (on excessive dosage or extreme sensitivity); anxiety, tremor, restlessness, headache, weakness, dizziness; hyperglycaemia; urinary retention; sweating; tissue necrosis at injection site and angle-closure glaucoma also reported

Dose

- Acute anaphylaxis, by intramuscular injection (preferably midpoint in anterolateral thigh) of 1 in 1000 (1 mg/mL) solution, see notes and table above
- Acute anaphylaxis when there is doubt as to the adequacy of the circulation, by slow intravenous injection of 1 in 10 000 (100 micrograms/mL) solution (extreme caution—specialist use only), see notes above

Important Intravenous route should be used with **extreme care** by specialist only, see notes above

Intramuscular or subcutaneous

[1]**Adrenaline/Epinephrine 1 in 1000** (Non-proprietary) PoM

Injection, adrenaline (as acid tartrate) 1 mg/mL, net price 0.5-mL amp = 50p; 1-mL amp = 46p

[1]**Minijet® Adrenaline 1 in 1000** (UCB Pharma) PoM

Injection, adrenaline (as hydrochloride) 1 in 1000 (1 mg/mL), net price 1 mL (with 25 gauge × 0.25 inch needle for subcutaneous injection) = £9.81, 1 mL (with 21 gauge × 1.5 inch needle for intramuscular injection) = £5.78 (both disposable syringes)

Excipients include sulphites

Intravenous

Extreme caution, see notes above

Adrenaline/Epinephrine 1 in 10 000, Dilute (Non-proprietary) PoM

Injection, adrenaline (as acid tartrate) 100 micrograms/mL, 10-mL amp, 1-mL and 10-mL prefilled syringe

Minijet® Adrenaline 1 in 10 000 (UCB Pharma) PoM

Injection, adrenaline (as hydrochloride) 1 in 10 000 (100 micrograms/mL), net price 3-mL prefilled syringe = £5.70; 10-mL prefilled syringe = £5.30

Excipients include sulphites

Intramuscular injection for self-administration

Adrenaline/Epinephrine 1 in 1000 (Non-proprietary) PoM

[1]Auto-injector (delivering a single dose of adrenaline 500 micrograms), adrenaline (as acid tartrate) 1 mg/mL, net price 1-mL auto-injector = £25.24

Note 0.5 mL of the solution remains in the auto-injector after use

Dose by intramuscular injection, ADULT and CHILD over 12 years 500 micrograms repeated after 10 minutes as necessary

Anapen® (Lincoln Medical) PoM

[1]Anapen® 0.3 mg solution for injection (delivering a single dose of adrenaline 300 micrograms), adrenaline 1 mg/mL (1 in 1000), net price 1.05-mL auto-injector device = £30.67

Excipients include sulphites

Note 0.75 mL of the solution remains in the auto-injector device after use

Dose by intramuscular injection, ADULT and CHILD over 30 kg, 300 micrograms repeated after 10–15 minutes as necessary

Anapen® Junior 0.15 mg solution for injection (delivering a single dose of adrenaline 150 micrograms), adrenaline 500 micrograms/mL (1 in 2000), net price 1.05-mL auto-injector device = £30.67

Excipients include sulphites

Note 0.75 mL of the solution remains in the auto-injector device after use

Dose by intramuscular injection, CHILD 15–30 kg, 150 micrograms repeated after 10–15 minutes as necessary

EpiPen® (ALK-Abelló) PoM

[1]EpiPen® Auto-injector 0.3 mg (delivering a single dose of adrenaline 300 micrograms), adrenaline 1 mg/mL (1 in 1000), net price 2-mL auto-injector = £28.05

Excipients include sulphites

Note 1.7 mL of the solution remains in the *Auto-injector* after use

Dose by intramuscular injection, ADULT and CHILD over 30 kg, 300 micrograms repeated after 15 minutes as necessary

Epipen® Jr Auto-injector 0.15 mg (delivering a single dose of adrenaline 150 micrograms), adrenaline 500 micrograms/mL (1 in 2000), net price 2-mL auto-injector = £28.05

Excipients include sulphites

Note 1.7 mL of the solution remains in the *Auto-injector* after use

Dose by intramuscular injection, CHILD 15–30 kg, 150 micrograms (but on the basis of a dose of 10 micrograms/kg, 300 micrograms may be more appropriate for some children) repeated after 15 minutes as necessary

1. PoM restriction does not apply to adrenaline injection 1 mg/mL where administration is for saving life in emergency

3.5 Respiratory stimulants and pulmonary surfactants

3.5.1 Respiratory stimulants
3.5.2 Pulmonary surfactants

3.5.1 Respiratory stimulants

Respiratory stimulants (analeptic drugs) have a limited place in the treatment of ventilatory failure in patients with chronic obstructive pulmonary disease. They are effective only when given by intravenous injection or infusion and have a short duration of action. Their use has largely been replaced by ventilatory support including nasal intermittent positive pressure ventilation. However, occasionally when ventilatory support is contra-indicated and in patients with hypercapnic respiratory failure who are becoming drowsy or comatose, respiratory stimulants in the short term may arouse patients sufficiently to co-operate and clear their secretions.

Respiratory stimulants can also be harmful in respiratory failure since they stimulate non-respiratory as well as respiratory muscles. They should only be given under **expert supervision** in hospital and must be combined with active physiotherapy. There is at present no oral respiratory stimulant available for long-term use in chronic respiratory failure.

Doxapram is given by continuous intravenous infusion. Frequent arterial blood gas and pH measurements are necessary during treatment to ensure correct dosage.

DOXAPRAM HYDROCHLORIDE

Indications see under Dose

Cautions give with oxygen in severe irreversible airways obstruction or severely decreased lung compliance (because of increased work load of breathing); give with beta$_2$ agonist in bronchoconstriction; hypertension (avoid if severe), impaired cardiac reserve; hepatic impairment, pregnancy (compelling reasons only); **interactions**: Appendix 1 (doxapram)

Contra-indications severe hypertension, status asthmaticus, coronary artery disease, thyrotoxicosis, epilepsy, physical obstruction of respiratory tract

Side-effects perineal warmth, dizziness, sweating, moderate increase in blood pressure and heart rate; side-effects reported in postoperative period (causal effect not established) include muscle fasciculation, hyperactivity, confusion, hallucinations, cough, dyspnoea, laryngospasm, bronchospasm, sinus tachycardia, bradycardia, extrasystoles, nausea, vomiting and salivation

Dose

- Postoperative respiratory depression, by intravenous injection over at least 30 seconds, 1–1.5 mg/kg repeated if necessary after intervals of 1 hour *or* alternatively by intravenous infusion, 2–3 mg/minute adjusted according to response; CHILD not recommended
- Acute respiratory failure, by intravenous infusion, 1.5–4 mg/minute adjusted according to response (given concurrently with oxygen and whenever possible monitor with frequent measurement of blood gas tensions); CHILD not recommended
- Neonatal apnoea, see *BNF for Children*

Dopram® (Anpharm) PoM
Injection, doxapram hydrochloride 20 mg/mL. Net price 5-mL amp = £2.24
Intravenous infusion, doxapram hydrochloride 2 mg/mL in glucose 5%. Net price 500-mL bottle = £21.33

3.5.2 Pulmonary surfactants

Pulmonary surfactants are used in the management of respiratory distress syndrome (hyaline membrane disease) in neonates and preterm neonates. They may also be given prophylactically to those considered at risk of developing the syndrome.

Cautions Continuous monitoring is required to avoid hyperoxaemia caused by rapid improvement in arterial oxygen concentration.

Side-effects Pulmonary haemorrhage has been rarely associated with therapy especially in more preterm neonates; obstruction of the endotracheal tube by mucous secretions has also been reported.

BERACTANT

Indications treatment of respiratory distress syndrome in preterm neonates over 700 g; prophylaxis of respiratory distress syndrome in preterm neonates less than 32 weeks post-menstrual age

Cautions see notes above

Side-effects see notes above

Dose

- By endotracheal tube, phospholipid 100 mg/kg equivalent to a volume of 4 mL/kg, preferably within 8 hours of birth; may be repeated within 48 hours at intervals of at least 6 hours for up to 4 doses

Survanta® (Abbott) PoM
Suspension, beractant (bovine lung extract) providing phospholipid 25 mg/mL, with lipids and proteins, net price 8-mL vial = £306.43

PORACTANT ALFA

Indications treatment of respiratory distress syndrome or hyaline membrane disease in neonates over 700 g; prophylaxis of respiratory distress syndrome in preterm neonates

Cautions see notes above

Side-effects see notes above

Dose

- By endotracheal tube, treatment, 100–200 mg/kg; further doses of 100 mg/kg may be repeated 12 hours later and after further 12 hours if still intubated; max. total dose 300–400 mg/kg; prophylaxis, 100–200 mg/kg soon after birth (preferably within 15 minutes); further doses of 100 mg/kg may be repeated 6–12 hours later and after further 12 hours if still intubated; max. total dose 300–400 mg/kg

Curosurf® (Trinity) PoM
Suspension, poractant alfa (porcine lung phospholipid fraction) 80 mg/mL, net price 1.5-mL vial = £298.74; 3-mL vial = £580.64

3.6 Oxygen

Oxygen should be regarded as a drug. It is prescribed for hypoxaemic patients to increase alveolar oxygen tension and decrease the work of breathing. The concentration depends on the condition being treated; the administration of an inappropriate concentration of oxygen can have serious or even fatal consequences.

High concentration oxygen therapy, with concentrations of up to 60%, is safe in uncomplicated cases of conditions such as pneumonia, pulmonary thromboembolism, and fibrosing alveolitis. In such conditions low arterial oxygen (P_aO_2) is usually associated with low or normal arterial carbon dioxide (P_aCO_2), and therefore there is little risk of hypoventilation and carbon dioxide retention.

In acute severe asthma, the arterial carbon dioxide (P_aCO_2) is usually subnormal but as asthma deteriorates it may rise steeply (particularly in children). These patients usually require high concentrations of oxygen and if the arterial carbon dioxide (P_aCO_2) remains high despite other treatment, intermittent positive-pressure ventilation needs to be considered urgently. Where facilities for blood gas measurement are not immediately available, for example while transferring the patient to hospital, 40 to 60% oxygen delivered through a high-flow mask is recommended.

Low concentration oxygen therapy (controlled oxygen therapy) is reserved for patients with ventilatory failure due to chronic obstructive pulmonary disease or other

3 Respiratory system

causes. The concentration of oxygen administered should not exceed 28% and in some patients a concentration above 24% may be excessive. The aim is to provide the patient with enough oxygen to achieve an acceptable arterial oxygen tension without worsening carbon dioxide retention and respiratory acidosis. Treatment should be initiated in hospital because repeated blood gas measurements are required to determine the correct concentration.

Domiciliary oxygen Oxygen should only be prescribed for use in the home after careful evaluation in hospital by respiratory experts.

Patients should be advised of the risks of continuing to smoke when receiving oxygen therapy, including the risk of fire. Smoking cessation techniques (section 4.10) should be tried before home oxygen prescription.

Air travel Some patients with arterial hypoxaemia require supplementary oxygen for air travel. The patient's requirement should be discussed with the airline before travel.

Long-term oxygen therapy

Long-term administration of oxygen (usually at least 15 hours daily) prolongs survival in some patients with chronic obstructive pulmonary disease.

Assessment for long-term oxygen therapy requires measurement of arterial blood gas tensions. Measurements should be taken on 2 occasions at least 3 weeks apart to demonstrate clinical stability, and not sooner than 4 weeks after an acute exacerbation of the disease. Long-term oxygen therapy should be considered for patients with:

- chronic obstructive pulmonary disease with $P_aO_2 < 7.3$ kPa when breathing air during a period of clinical stability;
- chronic obstructive pulmonary disease with P_aO_2 7.3–8 kPa in the presence of secondary polycythaemia, nocturnal hypoxaemia, peripheral oedema, or evidence of pulmonary hypertension;
- severe chronic asthma with $P_aO_2 < 7.3$ kPa or persistent disabling breathlessness;
- interstitial lung disease with $P_aO_2 < 8$ kPa and in patients with $P_aO_2 > 8$ kPa with disabling dyspnoea;
- cystic fibrosis when $P_aO_2 < 7.3$ kPa *or* if P_aO_2 7.3–8 kPa in the presence of secondary polycythaemia, nocturnal hypoxaemia, pulmonary hypertension, or peripheral oedema;
- pulmonary hypertension, without parenchymal lung involvement when $P_aO_2 < 8$ kPa;
- neuromuscular or skeletal disorders, after specialist assessment;
- obstructive sleep apnoea despite continuous positive airways pressure therapy, after specialist assessment;
- pulmonary malignancy or other terminal disease with disabling dyspnoea;
- heart failure with daytime $P_aO_2 < 7.3$ kPa when breathing air or with nocturnal hypoxaemia;
- paediatric respiratory disease, after specialist assessment.

Increased respiratory depression is seldom a problem in patients with stable respiratory failure treated with low concentrations of oxygen although it may occur during exacerbations; patients and relatives should be warned to call for medical help if drowsiness or confusion occur.

Short-burst oxygen therapy

Oxygen is occasionally prescribed for short-burst (intermittent) use for episodes of breathlessness not relieved by other treatment in patients with severe chronic obstructive pulmonary disease, interstitial lung disease, heart failure, and in palliative care. It is important, however, that the patient does not rely on oxygen instead of obtaining medical help or taking more specific treatment. Short-burst oxygen therapy can be used to improve exercise capacity and recovery. Short-burst oxygen should only be continued if there is proven improvement in breathlessness or exercise tolerance.

Ambulatory oxygen therapy

Ambulatory oxygen is prescribed for patients on long-term oxygen therapy who need to be away from home on a regular basis. Patients who are not on long-term oxygen therapy can be considered for ambulatory oxygen therapy if there is evidence of exercise-induced oxygen desaturation and of improvement in blood oxygen saturation and exercise capacity with oxygen. Ambulatory oxygen therapy is not recommended for patients with heart failure or those who smoke.

Oxygen therapy equipment

Under the NHS oxygen may be supplied as **oxygen cylinders**. Oxygen flow can be adjusted as the cylinders are equipped with an oxygen flow meter with 'medium' (2 litres/minute) and 'high' (4 litres/minute) settings.

Oxygen concentrators are more economical for patients who require oxygen for long periods, and in England and Wales can be ordered on the NHS on a regional tendering basis (see below). A concentrator is recommended for a patient who requires oxygen for more than 8 hours a day (or 21 cylinders per month). Exceptionally, if a higher concentration of oxygen is required the output of 2 oxygen concentrators can be combined using a 'Y' connection.

A nasal cannula is usually preferred for long-term oxygen therapy from an oxygen concentrator. It can, however, produce dermatitis and mucosal drying in sensitive individuals.

Giving oxygen by nasal cannula allows the patient to talk, eat, and drink, but the concentration of oxygen is not controlled; this may not be appropriate for acute respiratory failure. When oxygen is given through a nasal cannula at a rate of 1–2 litres/minute the inspiratory oxygen concentration is usually low, but it varies with ventilation and can be high if the patient is underventilating.

Arrangements for supplying oxygen

The following oxygen services may be ordered in England and Wales:

- emergency oxygen;
- short-burst (intermittent) oxygen therapy;
- long-term oxygen therapy;
- ambulatory oxygen.

The type of oxygen service (or combination of services) should be ordered on a Home Oxygen Order Form (HOOF); the amount of oxygen required (hours per day) and flow rate should be specified. The supplier will determine the appropriate equipment to be provided. Special needs or preferences should be specified on the HOOF.

The clinician should obtain the patient's consent to pass on the patient's details to the supplier and the fire brigade. The supplier will contact the patient to make arrangements for delivery, installation, and maintenance of the equipment. The supplier will also train the patient to use the equipment.

The clinician should send order forms to the supplier by facsimile (see below); a copy of the HOOF should be sent to the Primary Care Trust or Local Health Board. The supplier will continue to provide the service until a revised order is received, or until notified that the patient no longer requires the home oxygen service.

Region	Supplier
Eastern South West	BOC Medical *to order*: Tel: 0800 136 603 Fax: 0800 169 9989
South East London Kent, Surrey and Sussex South West London Thames Valley, Hampshire and Isle of Wight	Allied Respiratory *to order*: Tel: 0500 823 773 Fax: 0800 781 4610
North West Yorkshire and Humberside East Midlands West Midlands North London Wales	Air Products *to order*: Tel: 0800 373 580 Fax: 0800 214 709
North East	Air Liquide *to order*: Tel: 0808 202 0999 Fax: 0191 497 4340

In **Scotland** refer the patient for assessment by a respiratory consultant. If the need for a concentrator is confirmed the consultant will arrange for the provision of a concentrator through the Common Services Agency. In **Northern Ireland** oxygen concentrators and cylinders should be prescribed on form HS21; oxygen concentrators are supplied by a local contractor. In **Scotland** and **Northern Ireland** prescriptions for oxygen cylinders and accessories can be dispensed by pharmacists contracted to provide domiciliary oxygen services.

3.7 Mucolytics

Mucolytics are prescribed to facilitate expectoration by reducing sputum viscosity. In some patients with chronic obstructive pulmonary disease and a chronic productive cough, mucolytics can reduce exacerbations; mucolytic therapy should be stopped if there is no benefit after a 4-week trial. Steam inhalation with postural drainage is effective in bronchiectasis and in some cases of chronic bronchitis.

Mucolytics should be used with caution in those with a history of peptic ulceration because they may disrupt the gastric mucosal barrier.

For reference to dornase alfa, see below.

CARBOCISTEINE

Indications reduction of sputum viscosity
Cautions see notes above; pregnancy (Appendix 4)
Contra-indications active peptic ulceration
Side-effects *rarely* gastro-intestinal bleeding, rashes
Dose

- initially 2.25 g daily in divided doses, then 1.5 g daily in divided doses as condition improves; CHILD 2–5 years 62.5–125 mg 4 times daily, 5–12 years 250 mg 3 times daily

Carbocisteine (Sanofi-Aventis) PoM

Capsules, carbocisteine 375 mg, net price 120-cap pack = £16.68
Brands include *Mucodyne®*

Oral liquid, carbocisteine 125 mg/5 mL, net price 300 mL = £4.57; 250 mg/5 mL, 300 mL = £5.84
Brands include *Mucodyne® Paediatric* 125 mg/5 mL (cherry- and raspberry-flavoured) and *Mucodyne®* 250 mg/5 mL (cinnamon- and rum-flavoured)

ERDOSTEINE

Indications symptomatic treatment of acute exacerbations of chronic bronchitis
Cautions see notes above; hepatic impairment (avoid if severe—Appendix 2); renal impairment (Appendix 3); pregnancy (Appendix 4)
Contra-indications breast-feeding (Appendix 5)
Side-effects *very rarely* nausea, vomiting, diarrhoea, abdominal pain, taste disturbance, headache, rash, and urticaria
Dose

- ADULT over 18 years, 300 mg twice daily for up to 10 days

Erdotin® (KoGEN) ▼ PoM

Capsules, yellow/green, erdosteine 300 mg, net price 20-cap pack = £5.00
Note The *Scottish Medicines Consortium* (October 2007) has advised that erdosteine (*Erdotin®*) is not recommended for the symptomatic treatment of acute exacerbations of chronic bronchitis

MECYSTEINE HYDROCHLORIDE
(Methyl Cysteine Hydrochloride)

Indications reduction of sputum viscosity
Cautions see notes above
Contra-indications pregnancy; breast-feeding
Side-effects nausea, heartburn
Dose

- 200 mg 4 times daily for 2 days, then 200 mg 3 times daily for 6 weeks, then 200 mg twice daily; CHILD 5–12 years 100 mg 3 times daily

Visclair® (Ranbaxy)

Tablets, yellow, s/c, e/c, mecysteine hydrochloride 100 mg, net price 20 = £3.66. Label: 5, 22, 25

Dornase alfa

Dornase alfa is a genetically engineered version of a naturally occurring human enzyme which cleaves extracellular deoxyribonucleic acid (DNA). It is used in cystic fibrosis and is administered by inhalation using a jet nebuliser (section 3.1.5).

DORNASE ALFA
Phosphorylated glycosylated recombinant human deoxyribonuclease 1 (rhDNase)

Indications management of cystic fibrosis patients with a forced vital capacity (FVC) of greater than 40% of predicted to improve pulmonary function

Cautions pregnancy (Appendix 4); breast-feeding (Appendix 5)

Side-effects pharyngitis, voice changes, chest pain; occasionally laryngitis, rashes, urticaria, conjunctivitis

Dose

- By inhalation of nebulised solution (by jet nebuliser), 2500 units (2.5 mg) once daily (patients over 21 years may benefit from twice daily dosage); CHILD under 5 years not recommended

Pulmozyme® (Roche) PoM

Nebuliser solution, dornase alfa 1000 units (1 mg)/mL. Net price 2.5-mL (2500 units) vial = £17.57

Note For use undiluted with jet nebulisers only; ultrasonic nebulisers are unsuitable

3.8 Aromatic inhalations

Inhalations containing volatile substances such as eucalyptus oil are traditionally used and although the vapour may contain little of the additive it encourages deliberate inspiration of warm moist air which is often comforting in bronchitis; boiling water should not be used owing to the risk of scalding. Inhalations are also used for the relief of nasal obstruction in acute rhinitis or sinusitis. Menthol and eucalyptus inhalation is used to relieve sinusitis affecting the maxillary antrum (section 12.2.2)

Children The use of strong aromatic decongestants (applied as rubs or to pillows) is not advised for infants under the age of 3 months. Carers of young infants in whom nasal obstruction with mucus is a problem can readily be taught appropriate techniques of suction aspiration but sodium chloride 0.9% given as nasal drops is preferred.

Benzoin Tincture, Compound, BP (Friars' Balsam)

Tincture, balsamic acids approx. 4.5%. Label: 15

Dose add one teaspoonful to a pint of hot, **not** boiling, water and inhale the vapour

Menthol and Eucalyptus Inhalation, BP 1980

Inhalation, racementhol or levomenthol 2 g, eucalyptus oil 10 mL, light magnesium carbonate 7 g, water to 100 mL

Dose add one teaspoonful to a pint of hot, **not** boiling, water and inhale the vapour

Dental prescribing on the NHS Menthol and Eucalyptus Inhalation BP, 1980 may be prescribed

Karvol® (Crookes) NHS

Inhalation capsules, levomenthol 35.55 mg, with chlorobutanol, pine oils, terpineol, and thymol, net price 10-cap pack = £2.25; 20-cap pack = £4.06

Inhalation solution, levomenthol 7.9%, with chlorobutanol, pine oils, terpineol, and thymol, net price 12-mL dropper bottle = £1.90

Dose express into handkerchief or add to a pint of hot, **not** boiling, water the contents of 1 capsule or 6 drops of solution; avoid in infants under 3 months

3.9 Cough preparations

3.9.1 Cough suppressants
3.9.2 Expectorant and demulcent cough preparations

3.9.1 Cough suppressants

Cough may be a symptom of an underlying disorder, such as asthma (section 3.1.1), gastro-oesophageal reflux disease (section 1.1), or rhinitis (section 12.2.1), which should be addressed before prescribing cough suppressants. Cough may be a side-effect of another drug, such as an ACE inhibitor (section 2.5.5.1), or it can be associated with smoking or environmental pollutants. Cough can also have a significant habit component. When there is no identifiable cause, cough suppressants may be useful, for example if sleep is disturbed. They may cause sputum retention and this may be harmful in patients with chronic bronchitis and bronchiectasis.

Codeine may be effective but it is constipating and can cause dependence; **dextromethorphan** and **pholcodine** have fewer side-effects.

Sedating antihistamines are used as the cough suppressant component of many compound cough preparations on sale to the public; all tend to cause drowsiness which may reflect their main mode of action.

Children The use of cough suppressants containing codeine or similar opioid analgesics is not generally recommended in children and should be avoided altogether in those under 1 year of age.

CODEINE PHOSPHATE

Indications dry or painful cough; diarrhoea (section 1.4.2); pain (section 4.7.2)

Cautions asthma; hepatic impairment; renal impairment (Appendix 3); history of drug abuse; see also notes above and section 4.7.2; **interactions**: Appendix 1 (opioid analgesics)

Contra-indications liver disease, ventilatory failure

Side-effects constipation, respiratory depression in sensitive patients or if given large doses

3 Respiratory system

Codeine Linctus, BP[1] PoM

Linctus (= oral solution), codeine phosphate 15 mg/ 5 mL. Net price 100 mL = 58p (diabetic, 73p)

Brands include *Galcodine®*

Dose 5–10 mL 3–4 times daily; CHILD (but not generally recommended) 5–12 years, 2.5–5 mL

Note BP directs that when Diabetic Codeine Linctus is prescribed, Codeine Linctus formulated with a vehicle appropriate for administration to diabetics, whether or not labelled 'Diabetic Codeine Linctus', shall be dispensed or supplied

1. Can be sold to the public provided the maximum single dose does not exceed 5 mL

Codeine Linctus, Paediatric, BP

Linctus (= oral solution), codeine phosphate 3 mg/ 5 mL. Net price 100 mL = 18p

Brands include *Galcodine® Paediatric* (sugar-free)

Dose CHILD (but not generally recommended) 1–5 years 5 mL 3–4 times daily

Note BP directs that Paediatric Codeine Linctus may be prepared extemporaneously by diluting Codeine Linctus with a suitable vehicle in accordance with the manufacturer's instructions

Other preparations

Tablets, syrup, and injection section 4.7.2

PHOLCODINE

Indications dry or painful cough
Cautions see under Codeine Phosphate
Contra-indications see under Codeine Phosphate
Side-effects see under Codeine Phosphate

Pholcodine Linctus, BP

Linctus (= oral solution), pholcodine 5 mg/5 mL in a suitable flavoured vehicle, containing citric acid monohydrate 1%. Net price 100 mL = 42p

Brands include *Pavacol-D®* (sugar-free), *Galenphol®* (sugar-free)

Dose 5–10 mL 3–4 times daily; CHILD (but not generally recommended, see notes above) 5–12 years 2.5–5 mL

Pholcodine Linctus, Strong, BP

Linctus (= oral solution), pholcodine 10 mg/5 mL in a suitable flavoured vehicle, containing citric acid monohydrate 2%. Net price 100 mL = 33p

Dose 5 mL 3–4 times daily

Brands include *Galenphol®*

Galenphol® (Thornton & Ross)

Paediatric linctus (= oral solution), orange, sugar-free, pholcodine 2 mg/5 mL. Net price 90-mL pack = £1.11

Dose CHILD (but not generally recommended, see notes above) 1–5 years 5–10 mL 3 times daily; 6–12 years 10 mL 3 times daily

Palliative care

Diamorphine and methadone have been used to control distressing cough in terminal lung cancer although morphine is now preferred (see p. 16). In other circumstances they are contra-indicated because they induce sputum retention and ventilatory failure as well as causing opioid dependence. Methadone linctus should be avoided because it has a long duration of action and tends to accumulate.

METHADONE HYDROCHLORIDE

Indications cough in terminal disease
Cautions see notes in section 4.7.2
Contra-indications see notes in section 4.7.2
Side-effects see notes in section 4.7.2; longer-acting than morphine therefore effects may be cumulative
Dose

- See below

Methadone Linctus CD

Linctus (= oral solution), methadone hydrochloride 2 mg/5 mL in a suitable vehicle with a tolu flavour. Label: 2

Dose 2.5–5 mL every 4–6 hours, reduced to twice daily on prolonged use

MORPHINE HYDROCHLORIDE

Indications cough in terminal disease (see also Prescribing in Palliative Care p. 16)
Cautions see notes in section 4.7.2
Contra-indications see notes in section 4.7.2
Side-effects see notes in section 4.7.2
Dose

- Initially 5 mg every 4 hours

Preparation

Section 4.7.2

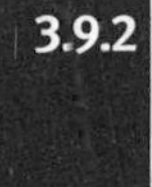

3.9.2 Expectorant and demulcent cough preparations

Expectorants are claimed to promote expulsion of bronchial secretions but there is no evidence that any drug can specifically facilitate expectoration. The assumption that sub-emetic doses of expectorants, such as ammonium chloride, ipecacuanha, and squill promote expectoration is a myth. However, a simple expectorant mixture may serve a useful placebo function and has the advantage of being inexpensive.

Demulcent cough preparations contain soothing substances such as syrup or glycerol and some patients believe that such preparations relieve a dry irritating cough. Preparations such as **simple linctus** have the advantage of being harmless and inexpensive; **paediatric simple linctus** is particularly useful in children.

Compound preparations are on sale to the public for the treatment of cough and colds; the rationale for some is dubious.

Ammonia and Ipecacuanha Mixture, BP

Mixture, ammonium bicarbonate 200 mg, liquorice liquid extract 0.5 mL, ipecacuanha tincture 0.3 mL, concentrated camphor water 0.1 mL, concentrated anise water 0.05 mL, double-strength chloroform water 5 mL, water to 10 mL. It should be recently prepared

Dose 10–20 mL 3–4 times daily

Simple Linctus, BP

Linctus (= oral solution), citric acid monohydrate 2.5% in a suitable vehicle with an anise flavour. Net price 200 mL = 34p

Dose ADULT and CHILD over 12 years 5 mL 3–4 times daily

A sugar-free version is also available

Simple Linctus, Paediatric, BP
Linctus (= oral solution), citric acid monohydrate 0.625% in a suitable vehicle with an anise flavour. Net price 200 mL = 69p
Dose CHILD 1 month–12 years 5–10 mL 3–4 times daily
A sugar-free version is also available

3.10 Systemic nasal decongestants

Nasal decongestants for administration by mouth may not be as effective as preparations for local application (section 12.2.2) but they do not give rise to rebound nasal congestion on withdrawal. **Pseudoephedrine** is available over the counter; it has few sympathomimetic effects.

Systemic decongestants should be used with **caution** in diabetes, hypertension, hyperthyroidism, susceptibility to angle-closure glaucoma, prostatic hypertrophy, renal impairment (Appendix 3), pregnancy (Appendix 4), and ischaemic heart disease, and should be **avoided** in patients taking monoamine oxidase inhibitors; **interactions**: Appendix 1 (sympathomimetics).

PSEUDOEPHEDRINE HYDROCHLORIDE

Indications see notes above
Cautions see notes above
Side-effects tachycardia, anxiety, restlessness, insomnia; *rarely* hallucinations, rash; *very rarely* angle-closure glaucoma; urinary retention also reported
Dose
- 60 mg 3–4 times daily; CHILD 2–6 years 15 mg 3–4 times daily, 6–12 years 30 mg 3–4 times daily

Galpseud® (Thornton & Ross)
Tablets, pseudoephedrine hydrochloride 60 mg, net price 20 = 91p
Linctus, orange, sugar-free, pseudoephedrine hydrochloride 30 mg/5 mL, net price 100 mL = 69p

Sudafed® (Pfizer Consumer)
Tablets, red, f/c, pseudoephedrine hydrochloride 60 mg, net price 24 = £2.12
Elixir, red, pseudoephedrine hydrochloride 30 mg/5 mL, net price 100 mL = £1.48

4 Central nervous system

4.1 Hypnotics and anxiolytics 179
4.1.1 Hypnotics 180
4.1.2 Anxiolytics 184
4.1.3 Barbiturates 187
4.2 Drugs used in psychoses and related disorders 187
4.2.1 Antipsychotic drugs 187
4.2.2 Antipsychotic depot injections 197
4.2.3 Antimanic drugs 199
4.3 Antidepressant drugs 201
4.3.1 Tricyclic and related antidepressant drugs 203
4.3.2 Monoamine-oxidase inhibitors 206
4.3.3 Selective serotonin re-uptake inhibitors 208
4.3.4 Other antidepressant drugs 211
4.4 CNS stimulants and drugs used for attention deficit hyperactivity disorder 213
4.5 Drugs used in the treatment of obesity 215
4.5.1 Anti-obesity drugs acting on the gastro-intestinal tract 216
4.5.2 Centrally acting appetite suppressants 216
4.6 Drugs used in nausea and vertigo 217
4.7 Analgesics 224
4.7.1 Non-opioid analgesics 225
4.7.2 Opioid analgesics 229
4.7.3 Neuropathic pain 238
4.7.4 Antimigraine drugs 238
4.7.4.1 Treatment of acute migraine 238
4.7.4.2 Prophylaxis of migraine 242
4.7.4.3 Cluster headache 243
4.8 Antiepileptics 243
4.8.1 Control of epilepsy 243
4.8.2 Drugs used in status epilepticus 255
4.8.3 Febrile convulsions 258
4.9 Drugs used in parkinsonism and related disorders 258
4.9.1 Dopaminergic drugs used in parkinsonism 259
4.9.2 Antimuscarinic drugs used in parkinsonism 266
4.9.3 Drugs used in essential tremor, chorea, tics, and related disorders 267
4.10 Drugs used in substance dependence 269
4.11 Drugs for dementia 274

4.1 Hypnotics and anxiolytics

4.1.1 Hypnotics
4.1.2 Anxiolytics
4.1.3 Barbiturates

Most anxiolytics ('sedatives') will induce sleep when given at night and most hypnotics will sedate when given during the day. Prescribing of these drugs is widespread but dependence (both physical and psychological) and tolerance occurs. This may lead to difficulty in withdrawing the drug after the patient has been taking it regularly for more than a few weeks (see Dependence and Withdrawal, below). Hypnotics and anxiolytics should therefore be reserved for short courses to alleviate acute conditions after causal factors have been established.

Benzodiazepines are the most commonly used anxiolytics and hypnotics; they act at benzodiazepine receptors which are associated with gamma-aminobutyric acid (GABA) receptors. Older drugs such as meprobamate and barbiturates (section 4.1.3) are **not** recommended—they have more side-effects and interactions than benzodiazepines and are much more dangerous in overdosage.

Paradoxical effects A paradoxical increase in hostility and aggression may be reported by patients taking benzodiazepines. The effects range from talkativeness and excitement, to aggressive and antisocial acts. Adjustment of the dose (up or down) sometimes attenuates the impulses. Increased anxiety and perceptual disorders are other paradoxical effects. Increased hostility and aggression after barbiturates and alcohol usually indicates intoxication.

Driving Hypnotics and anxiolytics may impair judgement and increase reaction time, and so affect ability to drive or operate machinery; they increase the effects of alcohol. Moreover the hangover effects of a night dose may impair driving on the following day. See also Drugs and Driving under General Guidance, p. 2.

Dependence and withdrawal Withdrawal of a benzodiazepine should be gradual because abrupt withdrawal may produce confusion, toxic psychosis, convulsions, or a condition resembling delirium tremens. Abrupt withdrawal of a barbiturate (section 4.1.3) is even more likely to have serious effects.

The benzodiazepine withdrawal syndrome may develop at any time up to 3 weeks after stopping a long-acting benzodiazepine, but may occur within a day in the case of a short-acting one. It is characterised by insomnia, anxiety, loss of appetite and of body-weight, tremor, perspiration, tinnitus, and perceptual disturbances. Some symptoms may be similar to the original complaint and encourage further prescribing; some symptoms may continue for weeks or months after stopping benzodiazepines.

A benzodiazepine can be withdrawn in steps of about one-eighth (range one-tenth to one-quarter) of the daily dose every fortnight. A suggested withdrawal protocol for patients who have difficulty is as follows:

1. Transfer patient to equivalent daily dose of diazepam[1] preferably taken at night
2. Reduce diazepam dose every 2–3 weeks in steps of 2 or 2.5 mg; if withdrawal symptoms occur, maintain this dose until symptoms improve
3. Reduce dose further, if necessary in smaller steps;[2] it is better to reduce too slowly rather than too quickly
4. Stop completely; time needed for withdrawal can vary from about 4 weeks to a year or more

Counselling may help; beta-blockers should **only** be tried if other measures fail; antidepressants should be used **only** where depression or panic disorder co-exist or emerge; **avoid** antipsychotics (which may aggravate withdrawal symptoms).

CSM advice

1. Benzodiazepines are indicated for the short-term relief (two to four weeks only) of anxiety that is severe, disabling or subjecting the individual to unacceptable distress, occurring alone or in association with insomnia or short-term psychosomatic, organic, or psychotic illness.
2. The use of benzodiazepines to treat short-term 'mild' anxiety is inappropriate and unsuitable.
3. Benzodiazepines should be used to treat insomnia only when it is severe, disabling, or subjecting the individual to extreme distress.

4.1.1 Hypnotics

Before a hypnotic is prescribed the cause of the insomnia should be established and, where possible, underlying factors should be treated. However, it should be noted that some patients have unrealistic sleep expectations, and others understate their alcohol consumption which is often the cause of the insomnia.

Transient insomnia may occur in those who normally sleep well and may be due to extraneous factors such as noise, shift work, and jet lag. If a hypnotic is indicated one that is rapidly eliminated should be chosen, and only one or two doses should be given.

Short-term insomnia is usually related to an emotional problem or serious medical illness. It may last for a few weeks and may recur; a hypnotic can be useful but should not be given for more than three weeks (preferably only one week). Intermittent use is desirable with omission of some doses. A rapidly eliminated drug is generally appropriate.

Chronic insomnia is rarely benefited by hypnotics and is sometimes due to mild dependence caused by injudicious prescribing of hypnotics. Psychiatric disorders such as anxiety, depression, and abuse of drugs and alcohol are common causes. Sleep disturbance is very common in depressive illness and early wakening is often a useful pointer. The underlying psychiatric complaint should be treated, adapting the drug regimen to alleviate insomnia. For example, clomipramine or mirtazapine prescribed for depression will also help to promote sleep if taken at night. Other causes of insomnia include daytime cat-napping and physical causes such as pain, pruritus, and dyspnoea.

Hypnotics should **not** be prescribed indiscriminately and routine prescribing is undesirable. They should be reserved for short courses in the acutely distressed. Tolerance to their effects develops within 3 to 14 days of continuous use and long-term efficacy cannot be assured. A major drawback of long-term use is that withdrawal can cause rebound insomnia and a withdrawal syndrome (section 4.1).

Where prolonged administration is unavoidable hypnotics should be discontinued as soon as feasible and the patient warned that sleep may be disturbed for a few days before normal rhythm is re-established; broken sleep with vivid dreams may persist for several weeks.

Children The prescribing of hypnotics to children, except for occasional use such as for night terrors and somnambulism (sleep-walking), is not justified.

Elderly Hypnotics should be avoided in the elderly, because the elderly are at greater risk of becoming ataxic and confused and so liable to fall and injure themselves.

Dental procedures Some anxious patients may benefit from the use of a hypnotic for 1 to 3 nights before the dental appointment. Hypnotics do not relieve pain, and if pain interferes with sleep an appropriate analgesic should be given. **Diazepam** (section 4.1.2), **nitrazepam** or **temazepam** are used at night for dental patients. Temazepam is preferred when it is important to minimise any residual effect the following day. For information on anxiolytics for dental procedures, see section 15.1.4.1.

Benzodiazepines

Benzodiazepines used as hypnotics include **nitrazepam** and **flurazepam** which have a prolonged action and may give rise to residual effects on the following day; repeated doses tend to be cumulative.

Loprazolam, **lormetazepam**, and **temazepam** act for a shorter time and they have little or no hangover effect.

1. Approximate equivalent doses, diazepam 5 mg
≡chlordiazepoxide 15 mg
≡loprazolam 0.5–1 mg
≡lorazepam 500 micrograms
≡lormetazepam 0.5–1 mg
≡nitrazepam 5 mg
≡oxazepam 15 mg
≡temazepam 10 mg
2. Steps may be adjusted according to initial dose and duration of treatment and can range from diazepam 500 micrograms (one-quarter of a 2-mg tablet) to 2.5 mg

Withdrawal phenomena are more common with the short-acting benzodiazepines.

If insomnia is associated with daytime anxiety then the use of a long-acting benzodiazepine anxiolytic such as **diazepam** given as a single dose at night may effectively treat both symptoms.

For general guidelines on benzodiazepine prescribing see section 4.1.2 and for benzodiazepine withdrawal see section 4.1.

NITRAZEPAM

Indications insomnia (short-term use; see CSM advice, p. 180)

Cautions respiratory disease, muscle weakness and myasthenia gravis, history of drug or alcohol abuse, marked personality disorder, pregnancy (Appendix 4), breast-feeding (Appendix 5); reduce dose in elderly and debilitated, and in hepatic impairment (avoid if severe; Appendix 2) and renal impairment (Appendix 3); avoid prolonged use (and abrupt withdrawal thereafter); porphyria (section 9.8.2); **interactions**: Appendix 1 (anxiolytics and hypnotics)

Driving Drowsiness may persist the next day and affect performance of skilled tasks (e.g. driving); effects of alcohol enhanced

Contra-indications respiratory depression; marked neuromuscular respiratory weakness including unstable myasthenia gravis; acute pulmonary insufficiency; severe hepatic impairment; sleep apnoea syndrome; not for use alone to treat depression (or anxiety associated with depression) or chronic psychosis

Side-effects drowsiness and lightheadedness the next day; confusion and ataxia (especially in the elderly); amnesia may occur; dependence; see also under Diazepam (section 4.1.2); **overdosage**: see Emergency Treatment of Poisoning, p. 32

Dose

- 5–10 mg at bedtime; ELDERLY (or debilitated) 2.5–5 mg; CHILD see *BNF for Children*

Nitrazepam (Non-proprietary) PoM

Tablets, nitrazepam 5 mg, net price 28 = 77p. Label: 19
Brands include *Mogadon*® NHS, *Remnos*® NHS

Dental prescribing on NHS Nitrazepam Tablets may be prescribed

Oral suspension, nitrazepam 2.5 mg/5 mL. Net price 150 mL = £5.30. Label: 19
Brands include *Somnite*® NHS

FLURAZEPAM

Indications insomnia (short-term use; see CSM advice, p. 180)

Cautions see under Nitrazepam

Contra-indications see under Nitrazepam

Side-effects see under Nitrazepam

Dose

- 15–30 mg at bedtime; ELDERLY (or debilitated) 15 mg; CHILD not recommended

Dalmane® (Valeant) PoM NHS

Capsules, flurazepam (as hydrochloride), 15 mg (grey/yellow), net price 30-cap pack = £5.44; 30 mg (black/grey), 30-cap pack = £6.98. Label: 19

LOPRAZOLAM

Indications insomnia (short-term use; see CSM advice, p. 180)

Cautions see under Nitrazepam

Contra-indications see under Nitrazepam

Side-effects see under Nitrazepam; shorter acting

Dose

- 1 mg at bedtime, increased to 1.5 or 2 mg if required; ELDERLY (or debilitated) 0.5 or 1 mg; CHILD not recommended

Loprazolam (Non-proprietary) PoM

Tablets, loprazolam 1 mg (as mesilate). Net price 28-tab pack = £9.00. Label: 19

LORMETAZEPAM

Indications insomnia (short-term use; see CSM advice, p. 180)

Cautions see under Nitrazepam

Contra-indications see under Nitrazepam

Side-effects see under Nitrazepam; shorter acting

Dose

- 0.5–1.5 mg at bedtime; ELDERLY (or debilitated) 500 micrograms; CHILD not recommended

Lormetazepam (Non-proprietary) PoM

Tablets, lormetazepam 500 micrograms, net price 30-tab pack = £67.41; 1 mg, 30-tab pack = £86.71. Label: 19

TEMAZEPAM

Indications insomnia (short-term use; see CSM advice, p. 180); see also section 15.1.4.1 for peri-operative use

Cautions see under Nitrazepam

Contra-indications see under Nitrazepam

Side-effects see under Nitrazepam; shorter acting

Dose

- 10–20 mg at bedtime, exceptional circumstances 30–40 mg; ELDERLY (or debilitated) 10 mg at bedtime, exceptional circumstances 20 mg; CHILD not recommended

Temazepam (Non-proprietary) CD

Tablets, temazepam 10 mg, net price 28-tab pack = £2.94; 20 mg, 28-tab pack = £1.41. Label: 19

Oral solution, temazepam 10 mg/5 mL, net price 300 mL = £9.53. Label: 19

Note Sugar-free versions are available and can be ordered by specifying 'sugar-free' on the prescription

Dental prescribing on NHS Temazepam Tablets or Oral Solution may be prescribed

Zaleplon, zolpidem, and zopiclone

Zaleplon, zolpidem and **zopiclone** are non-benzodiazepine hypnotics, but they act at the benzodiazepine receptor. Zolpidem and zopiclone have a short duration of action; zaleplon is very short acting. All three drugs are not licensed for long-term use; dependence has been reported in a small number of patients.

ZALEPLON

Indications insomnia (short-term use—up to 2 weeks)

Cautions respiratory insufficiency (avoid if severe); muscle weakness and myasthenia gravis, history of drug or alcohol abuse; depression (risk of suicidal ideation); avoid prolonged use (risk of tolerance and withdrawal symptoms); hepatic impairment (avoid if severe; Appendix 2); pregnancy (Appendix 4); breast-feeding (Appendix 5); **interactions**: Appendix 1 (anxiolytics and hypnotics)

Contra-indications sleep apnoea syndrome, marked neuromuscular respiratory weakness including unstable myasthenia gravis

Side-effects amnesia, paraesthesia, drowsiness; dysmenorrhea; *less commonly* nausea, anorexia, asthenia, incoordination, confusion, impaired concentration, depression, depersonalisation, dizziness, hallucinations, disturbances of smell, hearing, speech, and vision; photosensitivity; paradoxical effects (see p. 179) and dependence also reported

Dose

- 10 mg at bedtime or after going to bed if difficulty falling asleep; ELDERLY 5 mg; CHILD under 18 years not recommended

Note Patients should be advised not to take a second dose during a single night

Sonata® (Wyeth) PoM
Capsules, zaleplon 5 mg (white/light brown), net price 14-cap pack = £3.12; 10 mg (white), 14-cap pack = £3.76. Label: 2

ZOLPIDEM TARTRATE

Indications insomnia (short-term use—up to 4 weeks)

Cautions depression, muscle weakness and myasthenia gravis, history of drug or alcohol abuse, hepatic impairment (avoid if severe; Appendix 2); renal impairment; elderly; avoid prolonged use (and abrupt withdrawal thereafter); **interactions**: Appendix 1 (anxiolytics and hypnotics)

Driving Drowsiness may persist the next day and affect performance of skilled tasks (e.g. driving); effects of alcohol enhanced

Contra-indications obstructive sleep apnoea, acute or severe respiratory depression, marked neuromuscular respiratory weakness including unstable myasthenia gravis, severe hepatic impairment, psychotic illness, pregnancy, breast-feeding (Appendix 5)

Side-effects diarrhoea, nausea, vomiting, vertigo, dizziness, headache, drowsiness, asthenia, amnesia; dependence, memory disturbances, nightmares, nocturnal restlessness, depression, confusion, perceptual disturbances or diplopia, tremor, ataxia, falls, skin reactions, changes in libido; paradoxical effects (see p. 179)

Dose

- 10 mg at bedtime; ELDERLY (or debilitated) 5 mg; CHILD not recommended

Zolpidem (Non-proprietary) PoM
Tablets, zolpidem tartrate 5 mg, net price 28-tab pack = £1.80; 10 mg, 28-tab pack = £2.51. Label: 19

Stilnoct® (Sanofi-Synthelabo) PoM
Tablets, both f/c, zolpidem tartrate 5 mg, net price 28-tab pack = £3.08; 10 mg, 28-tab pack = £4.48. Label: 19

ZOPICLONE

Indications insomnia (short-term use—up to 4 weeks)

Cautions elderly; muscle weakness and myasthenia gravis, history of drug abuse, psychiatric illness; avoid prolonged use (risk of tolerance and withdrawal symptoms); hepatic impairment (avoid if severe; Appendix 2); renal impairment (Appendix 3); pregnancy (Appendix 4); **interactions**: Appendix 1 (anxiolytics and hypnotics)

Driving Drowsiness may persist the next day and affect performance of skilled tasks (e.g. driving); effects of alcohol enhanced

Contra-indications marked neuromuscular respiratory weakness including unstable myasthenia gravis, respiratory failure, severe sleep apnoea syndrome; breast-feeding (Appendix 5)

Side-effects taste disturbance; *less commonly* gastro-intestinal disturbances (including nausea and vomiting), dry mouth, dizziness, drowsiness, headache; *rarely* lightheadedness, and incoordination; irritability, aggression, confusion, depression, hallucinations, nightmares, and amnesia reported

Dose

- 7.5 mg at bedtime; ELDERLY initially 3.75 mg at bedtime increased if necessary; CHILD not recommended

Zopiclone (Non-proprietary) PoM
Tablets, zopiclone 3.75 mg, net price 28-tab pack = £1.91; 7.5 mg, 28-tab pack = £1.77. Label: 19

Zimovane® (Rhône-Poulenc Rorer) PoM
Tablets, f/c, zopiclone 3.75 mg (*Zimovane® LS*), net price 28-tab pack = £2.33; 7.5 mg (scored), 28-tab pack = £3.39. Label: 19

Chloral and derivatives

Chloral hydrate and derivatives were formerly popular hypnotics for children (but the use of hypnotics in children is not usually justified). There is no convincing evidence that they are particularly useful in the elderly and their role as hypnotics is now very limited. **Triclofos** causes fewer gastro-intestinal disturbances than chloral hydrate.

CHLORAL HYDRATE

Indications insomnia (short-term use)

Cautions respiratory disease, history of drug or alcohol abuse, marked personality disorder; reduce dose in elderly and debilitated; avoid prolonged use (and abrupt withdrawal thereafter); avoid contact with skin and mucous membranes; hepatic impairment (avoid if severe—Appendix 2); **interactions**: Appendix 1 (anxiolytics and hypnotics)

Driving Drowsiness may persist the next day and affect performance of skilled tasks (e.g. driving); effects of alcohol enhanced

Contra-indications severe cardiac disease, gastritis, severe hepatic impairment, renal impairment (avoid if creatinine clearance less than 10 mL/minute); pregnancy; breast-feeding (Appendix 5); porphyria (section 9.8.2)

Side-effects gastric irritation (nausea and vomiting reported), abdominal distention and flatulence; also ataxia, confusion, rashes, headache, lightheadedness, ketonuria, excitement, nightmares, delirium (especially on abrupt withdrawal); dependence (may be associated with gastritis and renal damage) on prolonged use

Dose

- See under preparations below

Chloral Mixture, BP 2000 PoM

(Chloral Oral Solution)

Mixture, chloral hydrate 500 mg/5 mL in a suitable vehicle. Extemporaneous preparations should be recently prepared according to the following formula: chloral hydrate 1 g, syrup 2 mL, water to 10 mL. Net price 100 mL = 53p. Label: 19, 27

Dose 5–20 mL; CHILD 1–5 years 2.5–5 mL, 6–12 years 5–10 mL, taken well diluted with water at bedtime

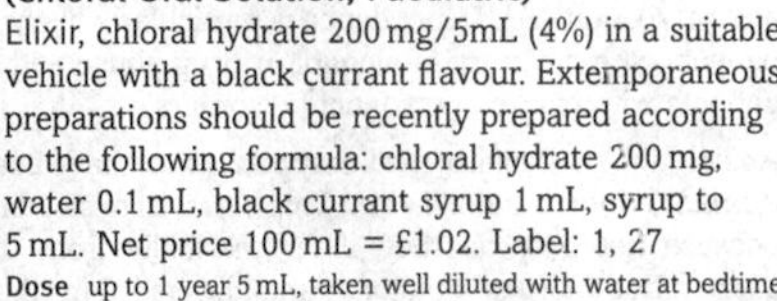

Chloral Elixir, Paediatric, BP 2000 PoM

(Chloral Oral Solution, Paediatric)

Elixir, chloral hydrate 200 mg/5mL (4%) in a suitable vehicle with a black currant flavour. Extemporaneous preparations should be recently prepared according to the following formula: chloral hydrate 200 mg, water 0.1 mL, black currant syrup 1 mL, syrup to 5 mL. Net price 100 mL = £1.02. Label: 1, 27

Dose up to 1 year 5 mL, taken well diluted with water at bedtime

Cloral betaine

Welldorm® (Alphashow) PoM

Tablets, blue-purple, f/c, cloral betaine 707 mg (≡ chloral hydrate 414 mg). Net price 30-tab pack = £7.90. Label: 19, 27

Dose ADULT and CHILD over 12 years, 1–2 tablets with water or milk at bedtime, max. 5 tablets (chloral hydrate 2 g) daily

Elixir, red, chloral hydrate 143.3 mg/5 mL. Net price 150-mL pack = £6.67. Label: 19, 27

Dose 15–45 mL (chloral hydrate 0.4–1.3 g) with water or milk at bedtime, max. 70 mL (chloral hydrate 2 g) daily; CHILD under 12 years, 1–1.75 mL/kg (chloral hydrate 30–50 mg/kg), max. 35 mL (chloral hydrate 1 g) daily

TRICLOFOS SODIUM 

Indications insomnia (short-term use)

Cautions see Chloral Hydrate

Contra-indications see Chloral Hydrate

Side-effects see Chloral Hydrate but less gastric irritation

Dose

- See under preparation below

Triclofos Oral Solution, BP PoM

(Triclofos Elixir)

Oral solution, triclofos sodium 500 mg/5 mL. Net price 300 mL = £28.23. Label: 19

Dose 10–20 mL (1–2 g triclofos sodium) at bedtime; CHILD up to 1 year 25–30 mg/kg, 1–5 years 2.5–5 mL (250–500 mg triclofos sodium), 6–12 years 5–10 mL (0.5–1 g triclofos sodium)

Clomethiazole

Clomethiazole (chlormethiazole) may be a useful hypnotic for elderly patients because of its freedom from hangover but, as with all hypnotics, routine administration is undesirable and dependence occurs. It is licensed for use as a hypnotic only in the elderly (and for *very short-term use* in younger adults to attenuate alcohol withdrawal symptoms, see section 4.10).

CLOMETHIAZOLE

(Chlormethiazole)

Indications see under Dose; alcohol withdrawal (section 4.10)

Cautions cardiac and respiratory disease (confusional state may indicate hypoxia); history of drug abuse; marked personality disorder; elderly; excessive sedation may occur (particularly with higher doses); hepatic impairment (especially if severe because sedation can mask hepatic coma; Appendix 2); renal impairment (Appendix 3); avoid prolonged use (and abrupt withdrawal thereafter); **interactions:** Appendix 1 (anxiolytics and hypnotics)

Driving Drowsiness may persist the next day and affect performance of skilled tasks (e.g. driving); effects of alcohol enhanced

Contra-indications acute pulmonary insufficiency; alcohol-dependent patients who continue to drink

Side-effects nasal congestion and irritation (increased nasopharyngeal and bronchial secretions), conjunctival irritation, headache; rarely, paradoxical excitement, confusion, dependence, gastro-intestinal disturbances, rash, urticaria, bullous eruption, anaphylaxis, alterations in liver enzymes

Dose

- Severe insomnia in the elderly (short-term use), 1–2 capsules (*or* 5–10 mL syrup) at bedtime; CHILD not recommended
- Restlessness and agitation in the elderly, 1 capsule (*or* 5 mL syrup) 3 times daily
- Alcohol withdrawal, initially 2–4 capsules, if necessary repeated after some hours; day 1 (first 24 hours), 9–12 capsules in 3–4 divided doses; day 2, 6–8 capsules in 3–4 divided doses; day 3, 4–6 capsules in 3–4 divided doses; then gradually reduced over days 4–6; total treatment for not more than 9 days

Heminevrin® (AstraZeneca) PoM

Capsules, grey-brown, clomethiazole base 192 mg in an oily basis. Net price 60-cap pack = £4.78. Label: 19

Syrup, sugar-free, clomethiazole edisilate 250 mg/5 mL. Net price 300-mL pack = £4.00. Label: 19

Note For an equivalent therapeutic effect 1 capsule ≡ 5 mL syrup

Antihistamines

Some **antihistamines** (section 3.4.1) such as promethazine are on sale to the public for occasional insomnia; their prolonged duration of action can often cause drowsiness the following day. The sedative effect of antihistamines may diminish after a few days of continued treatment; antihistamines are associated with headache, psychomotor impairment and antimuscarinic effects.

Promethazine is also popular for use in children, but the use of hypnotics in children is not usually justified.

PROMETHAZINE HYDROCHLORIDE

Indications night sedation and insomnia (short-term use); other indications (section 3.4.1, section 4.6)

Cautions section 3.4.1

Contra-indications section 3.4.1

Side-effects section 3.4.1

Dose

- By mouth, 25 mg at bedtime increased to 50 mg if necessary; CHILD under 2 years not recommended, 2–5 years 15–20 mg, 5–10 years 20–25 mg, at bedtime

Preparations
Section 3.4.1

Alcohol

Alcohol is a poor hypnotic because the diuretic action interferes with sleep during the latter part of the night. Alcohol also disturbs sleep patterns, and so can worsen sleep disorders; **interactions:** Appendix 1 (alcohol).

Sodium oxybate

Sodium oxybate is a central nervous system depressant that is licensed for the treatment of narcolepsy with cataplexy.

SODIUM OXYBATE

Indications narcolepsy with cataplexy (under specialist supervision)

Cautions history of drug abuse or depression; epilepsy; elderly; respiratory disorders; heart failure and hypertension (high sodium content); risk of discontinuation effects including rebound cataplexy and withdrawal symptoms; porphyria; hepatic impairment (Appendix 2); renal impairment (Appendix 3); breast-feeding (Appendix 5); **interactions:** Appendix 1 (sodium oxybate)

Contra-indications pregnancy (Appendix 4)

Side-effects nausea, vomiting, diarrhoea, abdominal pain, anorexia; hypertension, peripheral oedema; dyspnoea; sleep disorders, confusion, disorientation, impaired attention, depression, drowsiness, anxiety, dizziness, headache, tremor, asthenia, fatigue; urinary incontinence, nocturnal enuresis; arthralgia, muscle cramps; blurred vision; sweating; *less commonly* faecal incontinence, myoclonus, psychosis, paranoia, hallucination, agitation, amnesia, and rash; *rarely* dependence; respiratory depression, seizures, and urticaria also reported

Dose

- Initially 2.25 g on retiring and repeated 2.5–4 hours later, increased according to response in steps of 1.5 g daily in 2 divided doses at intervals of 1–2 weeks; max. 9 g daily in two divided doses; CHILD and ADOLESCENT under 18 years not recommended

Note Dose titration should be repeated if restarting after interval of more than 14 days

Counselling Dilute each dose with 60 mL water; prepare both doses before retiring. Observe the same time interval (2–3 hours) each night between the last meal and the first dose

Xyrem® (UCB Pharma) ▼ PoM
Oral solution, sugar-free, sodium oxybate 500 mg/mL, net price 180 mL = £360.00. Label: 13, 19, counselling, administration
Electrolytes Na^+ 3.62 mmol/mL

4.1.2 Anxiolytics

Benzodiazepine anxiolytics can be effective in alleviating anxiety states. Although these drugs are often prescribed to almost anyone with stress-related symptoms, unhappiness, or minor physical disease, their use in many situations is unjustified. In particular, they are not appropriate for treating depression or chronic psychosis. In bereavement, psychological adjustment may be inhibited by benzodiazepines. In children anxiolytic treatment should be used only to relieve acute anxiety (and related insomnia) caused by fear (e.g. before surgery).

Anxiolytic treatment should be limited to the lowest possible dose for the shortest possible time (see CSM advice, section 4.1). Dependence is particularly likely in patients with a history of alcohol or drug abuse and in patients with marked personality disorders.

Anxiolytics, particularly the benzodiazepines, have been termed 'minor tranquillisers'. This term is misleading because not only do they differ markedly from the antipsychotic drugs ('major tranquillisers') but their use is by no means minor. Antipsychotics, in low doses, are also sometimes used in severe anxiety for their sedative action but long-term use should be avoided in view of a possible risk of tardive dyskinesia (section 4.2.1).

Some antidepressants (section 4.3) are licensed for use in anxiety and related disorders; see section 4.3 for a comment on their role in chronic anxiety, generalised anxiety disorder, and panic disorders. The use of antihistamines (e.g. hydroxyzine, section 3.4.1) for their sedative effect in anxiety is not considered to be appropriate.

Benzodiazepines

Benzodiazepines are indicated for the *short-term relief of severe anxiety* but long-term use should be avoided (see CSM advice, p. 180). Diazepam, alprazolam, chlordiazepoxide, and clobazam have a sustained action. Shorter-acting compounds such as **lorazepam** and **oxazepam** may be preferred in patients with hepatic impairment but they carry a greater risk of withdrawal symptoms.

In *panic disorders* (with or without agoraphobia) resistant to antidepressant therapy (section 4.3), a benzodiazepine (lorazepam 3–5 mg daily or clonazepam 1–2 mg daily (section 4.8.1) [both unlicensed]) may be used; alternatively, a benzodiazepine may be used as short-term adjunctive therapy at the start of antidepressant treatment to prevent the initial worsening of symptoms.

Diazepam or lorazepam are very occasionally administered intravenously for the *control of panic attacks.* This route is the most rapid but the procedure is not without risk (section 4.8.2) and should be used only when alternative measures have failed. The intramuscular route has no advantage over the oral route.

For guidelines on benzodiazepine withdrawal, see p. 179.

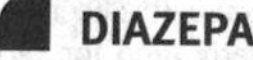

DIAZEPAM

Indications short-term use in anxiety or insomnia (see CSM advice, p. 180), adjunct in acute alcohol withdrawal; status epilepticus (section 4.8.2); febrile convulsions (section 4.8.3); muscle spasm (section 10.2.2); peri-operative use (section 15.1.4.1)

Cautions respiratory disease, muscle weakness and myasthenia gravis, history of drug or alcohol abuse, marked personality disorder, pregnancy (Appendix 4), breast-feeding (Appendix 5); reduce dose in elderly and debilitated, and in hepatic impairment (avoid if severe; Appendix 2), renal impairment (Appendix 3); avoid prolonged use (and abrupt withdrawal thereafter); special precautions for intravenous injection (section 4.8.2); porphyria (section 9.8.2); when given parenterally, close observation required until full recovery from sedation; **interactions:** Appendix 1 (anxiolytics and hypnotics)

Driving Drowsiness may affect performance of skilled tasks (e.g. driving); effects of alcohol enhanced

Contra-indications respiratory depression; marked neuromuscular respiratory weakness including unstable myasthenia gravis; acute pulmonary insufficiency; sleep apnoea syndrome; severe hepatic impairment; not for chronic psychosis; should not be used alone in depression or in anxiety with depression; avoid injections containing benzyl alcohol in neonates (see under preparations below)

Side-effects drowsiness and lightheadedness the next day; confusion and ataxia (especially in the elderly); amnesia; dependence; paradoxical increase in aggression (see also section 4.1); muscle weakness; *occasionally:* headache, vertigo, hypotension, salivation changes, gastro-intestinal disturbances, visual disturbances, dysarthria, tremor, changes in libido, incontinence, urinary retention; blood disorders and jaundice reported; skin reactions; on intravenous injection, pain, thrombophlebitis, and rarely apnoea; **overdosage:** see Emergency Treatment of Poisoning, p. 32

Dose

- By mouth, anxiety, 2 mg 3 times daily increased if necessary to 15–30 mg daily in divided doses; ELDERLY (or debilitated) half adult dose

  Insomnia associated with anxiety, 5–15 mg at bedtime
- By intramuscular injection *or* slow intravenous injection (into a large vein, at a rate of not more than 5 mg/minute), for severe acute anxiety, control of acute panic attacks, and acute alcohol withdrawal, 10 mg, repeated if necessary after not less than 4 hours

  Note Only use intramuscular route when oral and intravenous routes not possible; special precautions for intravenous injection see section 4.8.2
- By rectum as rectal solution, acute anxiety and agitation, 500 micrograms/kg repeated after 12 hours as required; ELDERLY 250 micrograms/kg; CHILD not recommended

  As suppositories, anxiety when oral route not appropriate, 10–30 mg (higher dose divided); dose form not appropriate for less than 10 mg

Diazepam (Non-proprietary) PoM

Tablets, diazepam 2 mg, net price 28 = 54p; 5 mg, 28 = 63p; 10 mg, 28 = 71p. Label: 2 or 19

Brands include *Rimapam*® NHS, *Tensium*® NHS

Oral solution, diazepam 2 mg/5 mL, net price 100 mL = £6.75. Label: 2 or 19

Brands include *Dialar*® NHS

Strong oral solution, diazepam 5 mg/5 mL, net price 100-mL pack = £6.38. Label: 2 or 19 NHS

Brands include *Dialar*® NHS

Injection (solution), diazepam 5 mg/mL. Do not dilute (except for intravenous infusion, see Appendix 6). Net price 2-mL amp = 35p

Excipients may include benzyl alcohol (avoid in neonates, see Excipients, p. 2), ethanol, propylene glycol

Injection (emulsion), diazepam 5 mg/mL. For intravenous injection or infusion, see Appendix 6. Net price 2-mL amp = 84p

Brands include *Diazemuls*®

Rectal tubes (= rectal solution), diazepam 2 mg/mL, net price 1.25-mL (2.5-mg) tube = 90p, 2.5-mL (5-mg) tube = £1.27; 4 mg/mL, 2.5-mL (10-mg) tube = £1.59

Brands include *Diazepam Rectubes*®, *Stesolid*®

Suppositories, diazepam 10 mg, net price 6 = £10.20. Label: 2 or 19

Brands include *Valclair*®

Dental prescribing on NHS Diazepam Tablets or Diazepam Oral Solution 2 mg/5 mL may be prescribed

ALPRAZOLAM

Indications anxiety (short-term use; see CSM advice, p. 180)

Cautions see under Diazepam

Contra-indications see under Diazepam

Side-effects see under Diazepam

Dose

- 250–500 micrograms 3 times daily (ELDERLY or debilitated 250 micrograms 2–3 times daily), increased if necessary to a total of 3 mg daily; CHILD not recommended

Alprazolam (Non-proprietary) PoM NHS

Tablets, alprazolam 250 micrograms, net price 60-tab pack = £2.97, 500 micrograms, 60-tab pack = £5.69. Label: 2

Brands include *Xanax*® NHS

CHLORDIAZEPOXIDE HYDROCHLORIDE

Indications anxiety (short-term use; see CSM advice, p. 180); adjunct in acute alcohol withdrawal (section 4.10)

Cautions see under Diazepam

Contra-indications see under Diazepam

Side-effects see under Diazepam

Dose

- Anxiety, 10 mg 3 times daily increased if necessary to 60–100 mg daily in divided doses; ELDERLY (or debilitated) half adult dose; CHILD not recommended

Chlordiazepoxide (Non-proprietary) PoM

Capsules, chlordiazepoxide hydrochloride 5 mg, net price 20 = 74p; 10 mg, 20 = £2.04. Label: 2

Brands include *Librium*® NHS, *Tropium*® NHS

Chlordiazepoxide Hydrochloride (Non-proprietary) PoM

Tablets, chlordiazepoxide hydrochloride 5 mg, net price 20 = 26p; 10 mg, 20 = £1.78. Label: 2

LORAZEPAM

Indications short-term use in anxiety or insomnia (see CSM advice, p. 180); status epilepticus (section 4.8.2); peri-operative (section 15.1.4.1)

Cautions see under Diazepam; short acting; when given parenterally, facilities for managing respiratory depression with mechanical ventilation must be at hand

Contra-indications see under Diazepam
Side-effects see under Diazepam
Dose
- By mouth, anxiety, 1–4 mg daily in divided doses; ELDERLY (or debilitated) half adult dose
  Insomnia associated with anxiety, 1–2 mg at bedtime; CHILD not recommended
- By intramuscular *or* slow intravenous injection (into a large vein), acute panic attacks, 25–30 micrograms/kg (usual range 1.5–2.5 mg), repeated every 6 hours if necessary; CHILD not recommended
  Note Only use intramuscular route when oral and intravenous routes not possible

Lorazepam (Non-proprietary) PoM
Tablets, lorazepam 1 mg, net price 28-tab pack = £10.97; 2.5 mg, 28-tab pack = £19.71. Label: 2 or 19
Injection, lorazepam 4 mg/mL. Net price 1-mL amp = 37p
Excipients include benzyl alcohol, propylene glycol (see Excipients, p. 2)
Brands include *Ativan®* NHS
Note For intramuscular injection it should be diluted with an equal volume of water for injections or physiological saline (but only use when oral and intravenous routes not possible)

OXAZEPAM

Indications anxiety (short-term use; see CSM advice, p. 180)
Cautions see under Diazepam; short acting
Contra-indications see under Diazepam
Side-effects see under Diazepam
Dose
- Anxiety, 15–30 mg (elderly or debilitated 10–20 mg) 3–4 times daily; CHILD not recommended
- Insomnia associated with anxiety, 15–25 mg (max. 50 mg) at bedtime; CHILD not recommended

Oxazepam (Non-proprietary) PoM
Tablets, oxazepam 10 mg, net price 28-tab pack = £4.66; 15 mg, 28-tab pack = £5.00. Label: 2

Buspirone

Buspirone is thought to act at specific serotonin ($5HT_{1A}$) receptors. Response to treatment may take up to 2 weeks. It does not alleviate the symptoms of benzodiazepine withdrawal. Therefore a patient taking a benzodiazepine still needs to have the benzodiazepine withdrawn gradually; it is advisable to do this before starting buspirone. The dependence and abuse potential of buspirone is low; it is, however, licensed for short-term use only (but specialists occasionally use it for several months).

BUSPIRONE HYDROCHLORIDE

Indications anxiety (short-term use)
Cautions does not alleviate benzodiazepine withdrawal (see notes above); hepatic impairment (Appendix 2); renal impairment (avoid if creatinine clearance less than 20 mL/minute; Appendix 3); **interactions:** Appendix 1 (anxiolytics and hypnotics)
Driving May affect performance of skilled tasks (e.g. driving); effects of alcohol may be enhanced
Contra-indications epilepsy; porphyria (section 9.8.2); pregnancy (Appendix 4); breast-feeding (Appendix 5)
Side-effects nausea; dizziness, headache, nervousness, excitement; *rarely* dry mouth, tachycardia, palpitation, chest pain, drowsiness, confusion, seizures, fatigue, and sweating
Dose
- ADULT and CHILD over 18 years, 5 mg 2–3 times daily, increased as necessary every 2–3 days; usual range 15–30 mg daily in divided doses; max. 45 mg daily

Buspirone Hydrochloride (Non-proprietary) PoM
Tablets, buspirone hydrochloride 5 mg, net price 30-tab pack = £29.62; 10 mg, 30-tab pack = £35.96. Counselling, driving

Buspar® (Bristol-Myers Squibb) PoM
Tablets, buspirone hydrochloride 5 mg, net price 90-tab pack = £28.08; 10 mg, 90-tab pack = £42.12. Counselling, driving

Beta-blockers

Beta-blockers (e.g. propranolol, oxprenolol) (section 2.4) do not affect psychological symptoms, such as worry, tension, and fear, but they do reduce autonomic symptoms, such as palpitation and tremor; they do not reduce non-autonomic symptoms, such as muscle tension. Beta-blockers are therefore indicated for patients with predominantly somatic symptoms; this, in turn, may prevent the onset of worry and fear. Patients with predominantly psychological symptoms may obtain no benefit.

Meprobamate

Meprobamate is **less effective** than the benzodiazepines, more hazardous in overdosage, and can also induce dependence. It is **not** recommended.

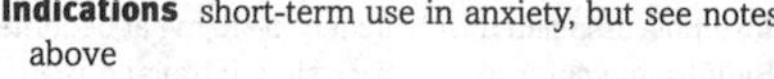

MEPROBAMATE

Indications short-term use in anxiety, but see notes above
Cautions respiratory disease, muscle weakness, epilepsy (may induce seizures), history of drug or alcohol abuse, marked personality disorder, pregnancy (Appendix 4); elderly and debilitated; hepatic impairment (Appendix 2), renal impairment (Appendix 3); avoid prolonged use, abrupt withdrawal may precipitate convulsions; **interactions:** Appendix 1 (anxiolytics and hypnotics)
Driving Drowsiness may affect performance of skilled tasks (e.g. driving); effects of alcohol enhanced
Contra-indications acute pulmonary insufficiency; respiratory depression; porphyria (section 9.8.2); breast-feeding (Appendix 5)
Side-effects see under Diazepam, but incidence greater and drowsiness most common side-effect; also gastro-intestinal disturbances, hypotension, paraesthesia, weakness, CNS effects including headache, paradoxical excitement, disturbances of vision; rarely agranulocytosis and rashes
Dose
- 400 mg 3–4 times daily; elderly patients half adult dose or less; CHILD not recommended

Meprobamate (Non-proprietary) CD
Tablets, scored, meprobamate 400 mg. Net price 84-tab pack = £19.95. Label: 2

4.1.3 Barbiturates

The intermediate-acting **barbiturates** have a place only in the treatment of severe intractable insomnia in patients **already taking** barbiturates; they should be **avoided** in the elderly. The long-acting barbiturate phenobarbital is still sometimes of value in epilepsy (section 4.8.1) but its use as a sedative is unjustified. The very short-acting barbiturate thiopental is used in anaesthesia (section 15.1.1).

BARBITURATES

Indications severe intractable insomnia **only** in patients already taking barbiturates; see also notes above

Cautions avoid use where possible; dependence and tolerance readily occur; abrupt withdrawal may precipitate serious withdrawal syndrome (rebound insomnia, anxiety, tremor, dizziness, nausea, convulsions, delirium, and death); repeated doses are cumulative and may lead to excessive sedation; depression and suicidal ideation; shock; respiratory disease (avoid if dyspnoea or obstruction present); hepatic impairment (avoid if severe; Appendix 2); renal impairment (Appendix 3); **interactions:** Appendix 1 (barbiturates)

Driving Drowsiness may persist the next day and affect performance of skilled tasks (e.g. driving); effects of alcohol enhanced

Contra-indications insomnia caused by pain; porphyria (section 9.8.2); children, young adults, elderly and debilitated patients, also patients with history of drug or alcohol abuse; pregnancy (Appendix 4); breast-feeding (Appendix 5)

Side-effects drowsiness, incoordination; *less commonly* nausea, vomiting, constipation, liver damage, bradycardia, hypotension, syncope, hypoventilation, apnoea, respiratory depression, agitation, confusion, hyperkinesia, ataxia, CNS depression, sleep disorders, hallucinations, anxiety, dizziness, headache, paradoxical excitement, impaired memory, fever, and megaloblastic anaemia

Dose

- See under preparations below

Sodium Amytal® (Flynn) CD

Capsules, blue, amobarbital (amylobarbitone) sodium 60 mg, net price 20 = £3.43. Label: 19

Dose 60–200 mg at bedtime (**important:** but see also contra-indications)

Soneryl® (Concord) CD

Tablets, pink, scored, butobarbital (butobarbitone) 100 mg. Net price 56-tab pack = £10.65. Label: 19

Dose 100–200 mg at bedtime (**important:** but see also contra-indications)

Preparations containing secobarbital (quinalbarbitone)

Seconal Sodium® (Flynn) CD

Capsules, orange, secobarbital (quinalbarbitone) sodium 100 mg, 20 = £6.96. Label: 19

Dose 100 mg at bedtime (**important:** but see also contra-indications)

Tuinal® (Flynn) CD

Capsules, orange/blue, a mixture of amobarbital (amylobarbitone) sodium 50 mg, secobarbital (quinalbarbitone) sodium 50 mg. Net price 20 = £3.88. Label: 19

Dose 1–2 capsules at bedtime (**important:** but see also contra-indications)

Note Prescriptions need only specify 'Tuinal capsules'

4.2 Drugs used in psychoses and related disorders

4.2.1 Antipsychotic drugs
4.2.2 Antipsychotic depot injections
4.2.3 Antimanic drugs

Advice of Royal College of Psychiatrists on doses above BNF upper limit. Unless otherwise stated, doses in the BNF are licensed doses—any higher dose is therefore **unlicensed** (for an explanation of the significance of this, see p. 1).

1. Consider alternative approaches including adjuvant therapy and newer or atypical neuroleptics such as clozapine.
2. Bear in mind risk factors, including obesity—particular caution is indicated in older patients especially those over 70.
3. Consider potential for drug interactions—see **interactions**: Appendix 1 (antipsychotics).
4. Carry out ECG to exclude untoward abnormalities such as prolonged QT interval; repeat ECG periodically and reduce dose if prolonged QT interval or other adverse abnormality develops.
5. Increase dose slowly and not more often than once weekly.
6. Carry out regular pulse, blood pressure, and temperature checks; ensure that patient maintains adequate fluid intake
7. Consider high-dose therapy to be for limited period and review regularly; abandon if no improvement after 3 months (return to standard dosage).

Important When prescribing an antipsychotic for administration on an emergency basis, the intramuscular dose should be **lower** than the corresponding oral dose (owing to absence of first-pass effect), particularly if the patient is very active (increased blood flow to muscle considerably increases the rate of absorption). The prescription should specify the dose for **each route** and should **not** imply that the same dose can be given by mouth or by intramuscular injection. The dose of antipsychotic for emergency use should be reviewed at least **daily**.

4.2.1 Antipsychotic drugs

Antipsychotic drugs are also known as 'neuroleptics' and (misleadingly) as 'major tranquillisers'. Antipsychotic drugs generally tranquillise without impairing consciousness and without causing paradoxical excitement but they should not be regarded merely as tranquillisers. For conditions such as schizophrenia the tranquillising effect is of secondary importance.

In the short term they are used to quieten disturbed patients whatever the underlying psychopathology, which may be schizophrenia, brain damage, mania, toxic delirium, or agitated depression. Antipsychotic drugs are used to alleviate severe anxiety but this too should be a short-term measure.

Schizophrenia Antipsychotic drugs relieve florid psychotic symptoms such as thought disorder, hallucinations, and delusions, and prevent relapse. Although they are usually less effective in apathetic withdrawn patients, they sometimes appear to have an activating influence. Patients with acute schizophrenia generally respond better than those with chronic symptoms.

Long-term treatment of a patient with a definite diagnosis of schizophrenia may be necessary even after the first episode of illness in order to prevent the manifest illness from becoming chronic. Withdrawal of drug treatment requires careful surveillance because the patient who appears well on medication may suffer a disastrous relapse if treatment is withdrawn inappropriately. In addition the need for continuation of treatment may not become immediately evident because relapse is often delayed for several weeks after cessation of treatment.

Antipsychotic drugs are considered to act by interfering with dopaminergic transmission in the brain by blocking dopamine D_2 receptors, which may give rise to the extrapyramidal effects described below, and also to hyperprolactinaemia. Antipsychotic drugs may also affect cholinergic, alpha-adrenergic, histaminergic, and serotonergic receptors.

Cautions and contra-indications Antipsychotics should be used with **caution** in patients with hepatic impairment (Appendix 2), renal impairment (Appendix 3), cardiovascular disease, Parkinson's disease (may be exacerbated by antipsychotics), epilepsy (and conditions predisposing to epilepsy), depression, myasthenia gravis, prostatic hypertrophy, or a susceptibility to angle-closure glaucoma. Caution is also required in severe respiratory disease and in patients with a history of jaundice or who have blood dyscrasias (perform blood counts if unexplained infection or fever develops). Antipsychotics should be used with caution in the elderly, who are particularly susceptible to postural hypotension and to hyper- or hypothermia in very hot or cold weather. Serious consideration should be given before prescribing these drugs for elderly patients. As photosensitisation may occur with higher dosages, patients should avoid direct sunlight.

Antipsychotic drugs may be **contra-indicated** in comatose states, CNS depression, and phaeochromocytoma. Most antipsychotics are best avoided during pregnancy, unless essential (Appendix 4) and it is advisable to discontinue breast-feeding during treatment (Appendix 5); **interactions:** Appendix 1 (antipsychotics).

Driving Drowsiness may affect performance of skilled tasks (e.g. driving or operating machinery), especially at start of treatment; effects of alcohol are enhanced.

Withdrawal Withdrawal of antipsychotic drugs after long-term therapy should always be gradual and closely monitored to avoid the risk of acute withdrawal syndromes or rapid relapse.

Side-effects Extrapyramidal symptoms are the most troublesome. They occur most frequently with the piperazine phenothiazines (fluphenazine, perphenazine, prochlorperazine, and trifluoperazine), the butyrophenones (benperidol and haloperidol), and the depot preparations. They are easy to recognise but cannot be predicted accurately because they depend on the dose, the type of drug, and on individual susceptibility.

Extrapyramidal symptoms consist of:

- *parkinsonian symptoms* (including tremor), which may occur more commonly in adults or the elderly and may appear gradually;
- *dystonia* (abnormal face and body movements) and *dyskinesia*, which occur more commonly in children or young adults and appear after only a few doses;
- *akathisia* (restlessness), which characteristically occurs after large initial doses and may resemble an exacerbation of the condition being treated; and
- *tardive dyskinesia* (rhythmic, involuntary movements of tongue, face, and jaw), which usually develops on long-term therapy or with high dosage, but it may develop on short-term treatment with low doses—short-lived tardive dyskinesia may occur after withdrawal of the drug.

Parkinsonian symptoms remit if the drug is withdrawn and may be suppressed by the administration of **antimuscarinic** drugs (section 4.9.2). However, routine administration of such drugs is not justified because not all patients are affected and because they may unmask or worsen tardive dyskinesia.

Tardive dyskinesia is of particular concern because it may be irreversible on withdrawing therapy and treatment is usually ineffective. However, some manufacturers suggest that drug withdrawal at the earliest signs of tardive dyskinesia (fine vermicular movements of the tongue) may halt its full development. Tardive dyskinesia occurs fairly frequently, especially in the elderly, and treatment must be carefully and regularly reviewed.

Hypotension and interference with temperature regulation are dose-related side-effects and are liable to cause dangerous falls and hypothermia or hyperthermia in the elderly.

Neuroleptic malignant syndrome (hyperthermia, fluctuating level of consciousness, muscle rigidity, and autonomic dysfunction with pallor, tachycardia, labile blood pressure, sweating, and urinary incontinence) is a rare but potentially fatal side-effect of some drugs. Discontinuation of the antipsychotic is essential because there is no proven effective treatment, but cooling, bromocriptine, and dantrolene have been used. The syndrome, which usually lasts for 5–7 days after drug discontinuation, may be unduly prolonged if depot preparations have been used.

Other side-effects include: drowsiness; apathy; agitation, excitement and insomnia; convulsions; dizziness; headache; confusion; gastro-intestinal disturbances; nasal congestion; antimuscarinic symptoms (such as dry mouth, constipation, difficulty with micturition, and blurred vision; *very rarely*, precipitation of angle-closure glaucoma); cardiovascular symptoms (such as hypotension, tachycardia, and arrhythmias); ECG changes (cases of sudden death have occurred); endocrine effects such as menstrual disturbances, galactorrhoea, gynaecomastia, impotence, and weight gain; blood dyscrasias (such as agranulocytosis and leucopenia), photosensitisation, contact sensitisation and rashes, and jaundice (including cholestatic); corneal and lens opacities, and purplish pigmentation of the skin, cornea, conjunctiva, and retina.

Overdosage: for poisoning with phenothiazines and related compounds, see Emergency Treatment of Poisoning, p. 33.

Classification of antipsychotics The **phenothiazine** derivatives can be divided into 3 main groups.

Group 1: chlorpromazine, levomepromazine (methotrimeprazine), and promazine, generally characterised by pronounced sedative effects and moderate antimuscarinic and extrapyramidal side-effects.

Group 2: pericyazine and pipotiazine, generally characterised by moderate sedative effects, marked antimuscarinic effects, but fewer extrapyramidal side-effects than groups 1 or 3.

Group 3: fluphenazine, perphenazine, prochlorperazine, and trifluoperazine, generally characterised by fewer sedative effects, fewer antimuscarinic effects, but more pronounced extrapyramidal side-effects than groups 1 and 2.

Drugs of other chemical groups tend to resemble the phenothiazines of *group 3*. They include the **butyrophenones** (benperidol and haloperidol); **diphenylbutylpiperidines** (pimozide); **thioxanthenes** (flupentixol and zuclopenthixol); and the **substituted benzamides** (sulpiride).

For details of the newer antipsychotic drugs amisulpride, clozapine, olanzapine, quetiapine, risperidone, sertindole, and zotepine, see under Atypical Antipsychotics, p. 193.

Choice As indicated above, the various drugs differ somewhat in predominant actions and side-effects. Selection is influenced by the degree of sedation required and the patient's susceptibility to extrapyramidal side-effects. However, the differences between antipsychotic drugs are less important than the great variability in patient response; moreover, tolerance to secondary effects such as sedation usually develops. The atypical antipsychotics may be appropriate if extrapyramidal side-effects are a particular concern (see under Atypical Antipsychotics, below). Clozapine is used for schizophrenia when other antipsychotics are ineffective or not tolerated.

Prescribing of more than one antipsychotic at the same time is **not** recommended; it may constitute a hazard and there is no significant evidence that side-effects are minimised.

Chlorpromazine is still widely used despite the wide range of adverse effects associated with it. It has a marked sedating effect and is useful for treating violent patients without causing stupor. Agitated states in the elderly can be controlled without confusion, a dose of 10 to 25 mg once or twice daily usually being adequate.

Flupentixol (flupenthixol) and **pimozide** (see CSM advice p. 192) are less sedating than chlorpromazine.

Sulpiride in high doses controls florid positive symptoms, but in lower doses it has an alerting effect on apathetic withdrawn schizophrenics.

Fluphenazine, **haloperidol**, and **trifluoperazine** are also of value but their use is limited by the high incidence of extrapyramidal symptoms. Haloperidol may be preferred for the rapid control of hyperactive psychotic states; it causes less hypotension than chlorpromazine and is therefore also popular for agitation and restlessness in the elderly, despite the high incidence of extrapyramidal side-effects.

Promazine is not sufficiently active by mouth to be used as an antipsychotic drug; it has been used to treat agitation and restlessness in the elderly (see Other uses, below).

Other uses Nausea and vomiting (section 4.6), choreas, motor tics (section 4.9.3), and intractable hiccup (see under Chlorpromazine Hydrochloride and under Haloperidol). **Benperidol** is used in deviant antisocial sexual behaviour but its value is not established; see also section 6.4.2 for the role of cyproterone acetate.

Psychomotor agitation and, in the elderly, agitation and restlessness, should be investigated for an underlying cause; they can be managed with low doses of chlorpromazine or haloperidol used for short periods. The use of promazine for agitation and restlessness in the elderly has declined. **Olanzapine** and **risperidone** may be effective for agitation and restlessness in the elderly [both unlicensed].

Equivalent doses of oral antipsychotics

These equivalences are intended **only** as an approximate guide; individual dosage instructions should **also** be checked; patients should be carefully monitored after **any** change in medication

Antipsychotic drug	Daily dose
Chlorpromazine	100 mg
Clozapine	50 mg
Haloperidol	2–3 mg
Pimozide	2 mg
Risperidone	0.5–1 mg
Sulpiride	200 mg
Trifluoperazine	5 mg

Important These equivalences must **not** be extrapolated beyond the max. dose for the drug. Higher doses require careful titration in specialist units and the equivalences shown here may not be appropriate

Dosage
After an initial period of stabilisation, in most patients, the total daily oral dose can be given as a single dose. For the advice of The Royal College of Psychiatrists on doses above the BNF upper limit, see p. 187.

BENPERIDOL

Indications control of deviant antisocial sexual behaviour (but see notes above)

Cautions see notes above; also manufacturer advises regular blood counts and liver function tests during long-term treatment

Contra-indications see notes above

Side-effects see notes above

Dose

- 0.25–1.5 mg daily in divided doses, adjusted according to response; ELDERLY (or debilitated) initially half adult dose; CHILD not recommended

4 Central nervous system

Anquil® (Concord) PoM
Tablets, scored, benperidol 250 micrograms, net price 112-tab pack = £104.00. Label: 2
Note The proprietary name *Benquil®* has been used for benperidol tablets

CHLORPROMAZINE HYDROCHLORIDE

Warning Owing to the risk of contact sensitisation, pharmacists, nurses, and other health workers should avoid direct contact with chlorpromazine; tablets should not be crushed and solutions should be handled with care

Indications see under Dose; antiemetic in palliative care (section 4.6)

Cautions see notes above; also patients should remain supine and the blood pressure monitored for 30 minutes after intramuscular injection

Contra-indications see notes above

Side-effects see notes above; also intramuscular injection may be painful, cause hypotension and tachycardia, and give rise to nodule formation

Dose

- By mouth, schizophrenia and other psychoses, mania, short-term adjunctive management of severe anxiety, psychomotor agitation, excitement, and violent or dangerously impulsive behaviour initially 25 mg 3 times daily (*or* 75 mg at night), adjusted according to response, to usual maintenance dose of 75–300 mg daily (but up to 1 g daily may be required in psychoses); ELDERLY (or debilitated) third to half adult dose; CHILD (childhood schizophrenia and autism) 1–5 years 500 micrograms/kg every 4–6 hours (max. 40 mg daily); 6–12 years 10 mg 3 times daily (max. 75 mg daily)
  Intractable hiccup, 25–50 mg 3–4 times daily
- By deep intramuscular injection, (for relief of acute symptoms but see also Cautions and Side-effects), 25–50 mg every 6–8 hours; CHILD, 1–5 years 500 micrograms/kg every 6–8 hours (max. 40 mg daily); 6–12 years 500 micrograms/kg every 6–8 hours (max. 75 mg daily)
  Induction of hypothermia (to prevent shivering), 25–50 mg every 6–8 hours; CHILD 1–12 years, initially 0.5–1 mg/kg, followed by maintenance 500 micrograms/kg every 4–6 hours
- By rectum in suppositories as chlorpromazine base 100 mg every 6–8 hours [unlicensed]
  Note For equivalent therapeutic effect 100 mg chlorpromazine base given *rectally* as a suppository ≡ 20–25 mg chlorpromazine hydrochloride *by intramuscular injection* ≡ 40–50 mg of chlorpromazine base or hydrochloride *by mouth*

Chlorpromazine (Non-proprietary) PoM
Tablets, coated, chlorpromazine hydrochloride 25 mg, 28-tab pack = £4.06; 50 mg, 28-tab pack = £3.80; 100 mg, 28-tab pack = £4.11. Label: 2, 11
Brands include *Chloractil®*
Oral solution, chlorpromazine hydrochloride 25 mg/5 mL, net price 150 mL = £1.35, 100 mg/5 mL, 150 mL = £3.57. Label: 2, 11
Injection, chlorpromazine hydrochloride 25 mg/mL, net price 1-mL amp = 60p; 2-mL amp = 63p
Suppositories, chlorpromazine 25 mg and 100 mg. Label: 2, 11
'Special order' [unlicensed] product; contact Martindale or regional hospital manufacturing unit

Largactil® (Sanofi-Aventis) PoM
Injection, chlorpromazine hydrochloride 25 mg/mL. Net price 2-mL amp = 63p

FLUPENTIXOL
(Flupenthixol)

Indications schizophrenia and other psychoses, particularly with apathy and withdrawal but not mania or psychomotor hyperactivity; depression (section 4.3.4)

Cautions see notes above; avoid in porphyria (section 9.8.2)

Contra-indications see notes above; also excitable and overactive patients

Side-effects see notes above; less sedating but extrapyramidal symptoms frequent

Dose

- Psychosis, initially 3–9 mg twice daily adjusted according to the response; max. 18 mg daily; ELDERLY (or debilitated) initially quarter to half adult dose; CHILD not recommended

Depixol® (Lundbeck) PoM
Tablets, yellow, s/c, flupentixol 3 mg (as dihydrochloride). Net price 20 = £2.78. Label: 2

Depot preparation
Section 4.2.2

HALOPERIDOL

Indications see under Dose; motor tics (section 4.9.3)

Cautions see notes above; also subarachnoid haemorrhage and metabolic disturbances such as hypokalaemia, hypocalcaemia, or hypomagnesaemia

Contra-indications see notes above

Side-effects see notes above, but less sedating and fewer antimuscarinic or hypotensive symptoms; pigmentation and photosensitivity reactions rare; extrapyramidal symptoms, particularly dystonic reactions and akathisia especially in thyrotoxic patients; rarely weight loss; hypoglycaemia; inappropriate antidiuretic hormone secretion

Dose

- Schizophrenia and other psychoses, mania, short-term adjunctive management of psychomotor agitation, excitement, and violent or dangerously impulsive behaviour, by mouth, initially 1.5–3 mg 2–3 times daily *or* 3–5 mg 2–3 times daily in severely affected or resistant patients; in resistant schizophrenia up to 30 mg daily may be needed; adjusted according to response to lowest effective maintenance dose (as low as 5–10 mg daily); ELDERLY (or debilitated) initially half adult dose; CHILD initially 25–50 micrograms/kg daily (in 2 divided doses) to max. 10 mg
  By intramuscular *or* by intravenous injection, initially 2–10 mg, then every 4–8 hours according to response to total max. 18 mg daily; severely disturbed patients may require initial dose of up to 18 mg; ELDERLY (or debilitated) initially half adult dose; CHILD not recommended
- Agitation and restlessness in the elderly, by mouth, initially 0.5–1.5 mg once or twice daily
- Short-term adjunctive management of severe anxiety, by mouth, 500 micrograms twice daily; CHILD not recommended

- Intractable hiccup, by mouth, 1.5 mg 3 times daily adjusted according to response; CHILD not recommended
- Nausea and vomiting, by mouth, 1 mg daily (see also Prescribing in Palliative Care, p. 17)

  By intramuscular *or* intravenous injection, 0.5–2 mg

Haloperidol (Non-proprietary) PoM

Tablets, haloperidol 500 micrograms, net price 28-tab pack = 91p; 1.5 mg, 28 = £1.83; 5 mg, 28 = £4.80; 10 mg, 28 = £5.86; 20 mg, 28 = £10.80. Label: 2

Dozic® (Rosemont) PoM

Oral liquid, sugar-free, haloperidol 1 mg/mL. Net price 100-mL pack = £6.86. Label: 2

Haldol® (Janssen-Cilag) PoM

Tablets, both scored, haloperidol 5 mg (blue), net price 20 = £1.53; 10 mg (yellow), 20 = £2.99. Label: 2

Oral liquid, sugar-free, haloperidol 2 mg/mL. Net price 100-mL pack (with pipette) = £4.72. Label: 2

Injection, haloperidol 5 mg/mL. Net price 1-mL amp = 30p

Serenace® (IVAX) PoM

Capsules, green, haloperidol 500 micrograms, net price 30-cap pack = 98p. Label: 2

Tablets, haloperidol 1.5 mg, net price 30-tab pack = £1.73; 5 mg (pink), 30-tab pack = £4.90; 10 mg (pale pink), 30-tab pack = £8.81. Label: 2

Oral liquid, sugar-free, haloperidol 2 mg/mL, net price 500-mL pack = £43.83. Label: 2

Depot preparation

Section 4.2.2

LEVOMEPROMAZINE
(Methotrimeprazine)

Indications see under Dose

Cautions see notes above; patients receiving large initial doses should remain supine

Elderly Risk of postural hypotension; not recommended for ambulant patients over 50 years unless risk of hypotensive reaction assessed

Contra-indications see notes above

Side-effects see notes above; occasionally raised erythrocyte sedimentation rate occurs

Dose

- Schizophrenia, by mouth initially 25–50 mg daily in divided doses increased as necessary; bedpatients initially 100–200 mg daily usually in 3 divided doses, increased if necessary to 1 g daily; ELDERLY, see Cautions
- Adjunctive treatment in Palliative care (including management of pain and associated restlessness, distress, or vomiting), by mouth, 12.5–50 mg every 4–8 hours, but see also Prescribing in Palliative Care, p. 16 and p. 17

  By intramuscular injection *or* by intravenous injection (by intravenous injection after dilution with an equal volume of sodium chloride 0.9% injection), 12.5–25 mg (severe agitation up to 50 mg) every 6–8 hours if necessary

  By continuous subcutaneous infusion (via syringe driver), diluted in a suitable volume of sodium chloride 0.9% injection, see Prescribing in Palliative Care, p. 18; CHILD (experience limited), 0.35–3 mg/kg daily

Nozinan® (Link) PoM

Tablets, scored, levomepromazine maleate 25 mg, net price 84-tab pack = £20.26. Label: 2

Injection, levomepromazine hydrochloride 25 mg/mL, net price 1-mL amp = £2.01

PERICYAZINE
(Periciazine)

Indications see under Dose

Cautions see notes above

Contra-indications see notes above; renal impairment

Side-effects see notes above; more sedating; hypotension common when treatment initiated; respiratory depression

Dose

- Schizophrenia and other psychoses, initially 75 mg daily in divided doses increased at weekly intervals by steps of 25 mg according to response; usual max. 300 mg daily (elderly initially 15–30 mg daily); CHILD and INFANT over 1 year (schizophrenia or behavioural disorders only), initially, 500 micrograms daily for 10-kg child, increased by 1 mg for each additional 5 kg body-weight to max. total daily dose of 10 mg; dose may be gradually increased according to response but maintenance should not exceed twice initial dose
- Short-term adjunctive management of severe anxiety, psychomotor agitation, and violent or dangerously impulsive behaviour, initially 15–30 mg (elderly 5–10 mg) daily divided into 2 doses, taking the larger dose at bedtime, adjusted according to response; CHILD not recommended

Neulactil® (Sanofi-Aventis) PoM

Tablets, all yellow, scored, pericyazine 2.5 mg, net price 84-tab pack = £9.23; 10 mg, 84-tab pack = £24.95. Label: 2

Syrup forte, brown, pericyazine 10 mg/5 mL. Net price 100-mL pack = £12.08. Label: 2

PERPHENAZINE

Indications see under Dose, antiemetic (section 4.6)

Cautions see notes above

Contra-indications see notes above; also agitation and restlessness in the elderly

Side-effects see notes above; less sedating; extrapyramidal symptoms, especially dystonia, more frequent, particularly at high dosage; rarely systemic lupus erythematosus

Dose

- Schizophrenia and other psychoses, mania, short-term adjunctive management of anxiety, severe psychomotor agitation, excitement, and violent or dangerously impulsive behaviour, initially 4 mg 3 times daily adjusted according to the response; max. 24 mg daily; ELDERLY quarter to half adult dose (but see Cautions); CHILD under 14 years not recommended

Fentazin® (Goldshield) PoM

Tablets, both s/c, perphenazine 2 mg, net price 20 = £4.48; 4 mg, 20 = £5.27. Label: 2

PIMOZIDE

Indications see under Dose

Cautions see notes above

CSM warning Following reports of sudden unexplained death, the CSM recommends ECG before treatment. The CSM also recommends that patients on pimozide should have an annual ECG (if the QT interval is prolonged, treatment should be reviewed and either withdrawn or dose reduced under close supervision) and that pimozide should **not** be given with other antipsychotic drugs (including depot preparations), tricyclic antidepressants or other drugs which prolong the QT interval, such as certain antimalarials, anti-arrhythmic drugs and certain antihistamines and should **not** be given with drugs which cause electrolyte disturbances (especially diuretics)

Contra-indications see notes above; history of arrhythmias or congenital QT prolongation

Side-effects see notes above; less sedating; serious arrhythmias reported; glycosuria and, rarely, hyponatraemia reported

Dose

- Schizophrenia, ADULT and CHILD over 12 years, initially 2 mg daily, increased according to response in steps of 2–4 mg at intervals of not less than 1 week; usual dose range 2–20 mg daily; ELDERLY half usual starting dose
- Monosymptomatic hypochondriacal psychosis, paranoid psychosis, ADULT and CHILD over 12 years, initially 4 mg daily, increased according to response in steps of 2–4 mg at intervals of not less than 1 week; max. 16 mg daily; ELDERLY half usual starting dose

Orap® (Janssen-Cilag) PoM

Tablets, scored, green, pimozide 4 mg, net price 20 = £5.70. Label: 2

PROCHLORPERAZINE

Indications see under Dose; antiemetic (section 4.6)

Cautions see notes above; also hypotension more likely after intramuscular injection

Contra-indications see notes above; children, but see section 4.6 for use as antiemetic

Side-effects see notes above; less sedating; extrapyramidal symptoms, particularly dystonias, more frequent; respiratory depression may occur in susceptible patients

Dose

- By mouth, schizophrenia and other psychoses, mania, prochlorperazine maleate or mesilate, 12.5 mg twice daily for 7 days adjusted at intervals of 4–7 days to usual dose of 75–100 mg daily according to response; CHILD not recommended
  Short-term adjunctive management of severe anxiety, 15–20 mg daily in divided doses; max. 40 mg daily; CHILD not recommended
- By deep intramuscular injection, psychoses, mania, prochlorperazine mesilate 12.5–25 mg 2–3 times daily; CHILD not recommended

Preparations

Section 4.6

PROMAZINE HYDROCHLORIDE

Indications see under Dose

Cautions see notes above; also cerebral arteriosclerosis

Contra-indications see notes above

Side-effects see notes above; also haemolytic anaemia

Dose

- Short-term adjunctive management of psychomotor agitation, 100–200 mg 4 times daily; CHILD not recommended
- Agitation and restlessness in elderly, 25–50 mg 4 times daily

Promazine (Non-proprietary) PoM

Tablets, coated, promazine hydrochloride 25 mg, net price 20 = £1.14; 50 mg, 20 = £3.48. Label: 2

Oral solution, promazine hydrochloride 25 mg/5 mL, net price 150 mL = £3.70; 50 mg/5 mL, 150 mL = £3.80. Label: 2

SULPIRIDE

Indications schizophrenia

Cautions see notes above; also excited, agitated, or aggressive patients (even low doses may aggravate symptoms); renal impairment (avoid if creatinine clearance less than 10 mL/minute)

Contra-indications see notes above; also porphyria (section 9.8.2)

Side-effects see notes above; also hepatitis

Dose

- 200–400 mg twice daily; max. 800 mg daily in predominantly negative symptoms, and 2.4 g daily in mainly positive symptoms; ELDERLY, lower initial dose, increased gradually according to response; CHILD under 14 years not recommended

Sulpiride (Non-proprietary) PoM

Tablets, sulpiride 200 mg, net price 30-tab pack = £7.11, 56-tab pack = £6.23; 400 mg, 30-tab pack = £10.89. Label: 2

Dolmatil® (Sanofi-Synthelabo) PoM

Tablets, both scored, sulpiride 200 mg, net price 100-tab pack = £13.85; 400 mg (f/c), 100-tab pack = £36.29. Label: 2

Sulpor® (Rosemont) PoM

Oral solution, sugar-free, lemon- and aniseed-flavoured, sulpiride 200 mg/5 mL, net price 150 mL = £25.38. Label: 2

TRIFLUOPERAZINE

Indications see under Dose; antiemetic (section 4.6)

Cautions see notes above

Contra-indications see notes above

Side-effects see notes above; extrapyramidal symptoms more frequent, especially at doses exceeding 6 mg daily; pancytopenia; thrombocytopenia; hyperpyrexia; anorexia

Dose

- Schizophrenia and other psychoses, short-term adjunctive management of psychomotor agitation, excitement, and violent or dangerously impulsive behaviour, initially 5 mg twice daily, increased by 5 mg after 1 week, then at intervals of 3 days, according to the response; CHILD up to 12 years, initially up to 5 mg daily in divided doses, adjusted according to response, age, and body-weight; ELDERLY reduce initial dose by at least half

- Short-term adjunctive management of severe anxiety, 2–4 mg daily in divided doses, increased if necessary to 6 mg daily; CHILD 3–5 years up to 1 mg daily, 6–12 years up to 4 mg daily; ELDERLY reduce initial dose by at least half

Trifluoperazine (Non-proprietary) PoM
Tablets, coated, trifluoperazine (as hydrochloride) 1 mg, net price 20 = 98p; 5 mg, 20 = 93p. Label: 2
Oral solution, trifluoperazine (as hydrochloride) 5 mg/5 mL. Net price 150-mL = £8.80. Label: 2

Stelazine® (Goldshield) PoM
Tablets, both blue, f/c, trifluoperazine (as hydrochloride) 1 mg, net price 20 = 61p; 5 mg, 20 = 87p. Label: 2
Syrup, sugar-free, yellow, trifluoperazine (as hydrochloride) 1 mg/5 mL, net price 200-mL pack = £2.95. Label: 2

ZUCLOPENTHIXOL ACETATE

Indications short-term management of acute psychosis, mania, or exacerbations of chronic psychosis
Cautions see notes above; avoid in porphyria (section 9.8.2)
Contra-indications see notes above
Side-effects see notes above
Dose
- By deep intramuscular injection into the gluteal muscle or lateral thigh, 50–150 mg (ELDERLY 50–100 mg), if necessary repeated after 2–3 days (1 additional dose may be needed 1–2 days after the first injection); max. cumulative dose 400 mg per course and max. 4 injections; max. duration of treatment 2 weeks—if maintenance treatment necessary change to an oral antipsychotic 2–3 days after last injection, *or* to a longer acting antipsychotic depot injection given concomitantly with last injection of zuclopenthixol acetate; CHILD not recommended

Clopixol Acuphase® (Lundbeck) PoM
Injection (oily), zuclopenthixol acetate 50 mg/mL. Net price 1-mL amp = £4.84; 2-mL amp = £9.33

Depot preparation
Section 4.2.2

ZUCLOPENTHIXOL

Indications schizophrenia and other psychoses, particularly when associated with agitated, aggressive, or hostile behaviour
Cautions see notes above; avoid in porphyria (section 9.8.2)
Contra-indications see notes above; apathetic or withdrawn states
Side-effects see notes above; urinary frequency or incontinence; weight loss (less common than weight gain)
Dose
- By mouth, initially 20–30 mg daily in divided doses, increasing to a max. of 150 mg daily if necessary; usual maintenance dose 20–50 mg daily; ELDERLY (or debilitated) initially quarter to half adult dose; CHILD not recommended

Clopixol® (Lundbeck) PoM
Tablets, all f/c, pink, zuclopenthixol (as dihydrochloride) 2 mg, net price 20 = 60p; 10 mg, 20 = £1.61; 25 mg, 20 = £3.22. Label: 2

Depot preparation
Section 4.2.2

Atypical antipsychotics

The 'atypical antipsychotics' **amisulpride, aripiprazole, clozapine, olanzapine, paliperidone, quetiapine, risperidone**, and **zotepine** may be better tolerated than other antipsychotics; extrapyramidal symptoms may be less frequent than with older antipsychotics.

Aripiprazole, clozapine, olanzapine, quetiapine, and sertindole cause little or no elevation of prolactin concentration; when changing from other antipsychotics, a reduction in prolactin may increase fertility.

Clozapine is licensed for the treatment of schizophrenia only in patients unresponsive to, or intolerant of, conventional antipsychotic drugs. It can cause agranulocytosis and its use is restricted to patients registered with a clozapine patient monitoring service (see under preparations, below).

Sertindole has been reintroduced following an earlier suspension of the drug because of concerns about arrhythmias; its use is restricted to patients who are enrolled in clinical studies and who are intolerant of at least one other antipsychotic.

> NICE guidance
> Atypical antipsychotics for schizophrenia (June 2002)
> NICE has recommended that:
> - the atypical antipsychotics (amisulpride, olanzapine, quetiapine, risperidone, and zotepine) should be considered when choosing first-line treatment of *newly diagnosed schizophrenia*;
> - an atypical antipsychotic is considered the treatment option of choice for managing an *acute schizophrenic episode* when discussion with the individual is not possible;
> - an atypical antipsychotic should be considered for an individual who is suffering unacceptable side-effects from a conventional antipsychotic;
> - an atypical antipsychotic should be considered for an individual in relapse whose symptoms were previously inadequately controlled;
> - changing to an atypical antipsychotic is not necessary if a conventional antipsychotic controls symptoms adequately and the individual does not suffer unacceptable side-effects;
> - clozapine should be introduced if schizophrenia is inadequately controlled despite the sequential use of two or more antipsychotics (one of which should be an atypical antipsychotic) each for at least 6–8 weeks

Cautions and contra-indications While atypical antipsychotics have not generally been associated with clinically significant prolongation of the QT interval, they should be used with care if prescribed with other drugs that increase the QT interval. Atypical antipsychotics should be used with caution in patients with cardiovascular disease, or a history of epilepsy; they should be used with caution in the elderly; **interactions**: Appendix 1 (antipsychotics).

Atypical antipsychotics and stroke

Olanzapine and risperidone are associated with an increased risk of stroke in elderly patients with dementia. The CSM has advised:

- risperidone or olanzapine should **not** be used for treating behavioural symptoms of dementia;
- for acute psychotic conditions in elderly patients with dementia, risperidone should be limited to short-term use under specialist advice; olanzapine is not licensed for acute psychoses;
- the possibility of cerebrovascular events should be considered carefully before treating any patient with a history of stroke or transient ischaemic attack; risk factors for cerebrovascular disease (e.g. hypertension, diabetes, smoking, and atrial fibrillation) should also be considered.

Driving Atypical antipsychotics may affect performance of skilled tasks (e.g. driving); effects of alcohol are enhanced.

Withdrawal Withdrawal of antipsychotic drugs after long-term therapy should always be gradual and closely monitored to avoid the risk of acute withdrawal syndromes or rapid relapse.

Side-effects Side-effects of the atypical antipsychotics include weight gain, dizziness, postural hypotension (especially during initial dose titration) which may be associated with syncope or reflex tachycardia in some patients, extrapyramidal symptoms (usually mild and transient and which respond to dose reduction or to an antimuscarinic drug), and occasionally tardive dyskinesia on long-term administration (discontinue drug on appearance of early signs). Hyperglycaemia and sometimes diabetes can occur, particularly with clozapine and olanzapine; monitoring weight and plasma glucose may identify the development of hyperglycaemia. Neuroleptic malignant syndrome has been reported rarely.

AMISULPRIDE

Indications schizophrenia

Cautions see notes above; also Parkinson's disease; renal impairment (Appendix 3)

Contra-indications see notes above; also phaeochromocytoma, prolactin-dependent tumours; pregnancy (Appendix 4); breast-feeding (Appendix 5)

Side-effects see notes above; also insomnia, anxiety, agitation, drowsiness, gastro-intestinal disorders such as constipation, nausea, vomiting, and dry mouth; hyperprolactinaemia; *occasionally* bradycardia; *rarely* seizures

Dose

- Acute psychotic episode, 400–800 mg daily in 2 divided doses, adjusted according to response; max. 1.2 g daily; CHILD under 15 years not recommended
- Predominantly negative symptoms, 50–300 mg daily; CHILD under 15 years not recommended

Amisulpride (Non-proprietary) PoM

Tablets, amisulpride 50 mg, net price 60-tab pack = £33.42; 100 mg, 60-tab pack = £36.72; 200 mg, 60-tab pack = £61.38; 400 mg, 60-tab pack = £122.76. Label: 2

Solian® (Sanofi-Synthelabo) PoM

Tablets, scored, amisulpride 50 mg, net price 60-tab pack = £23.69; 100 mg, 60-tab pack = £36.72; 200 mg, 60-tab pack = £61.38; 400 mg, 60-tab pack = £122.76. Label: 2

Solution, 100 mg/mL, net price 60 mL (caramel flavour) = £30.69. Label: 2

ARIPIPRAZOLE

Indications schizophrenia

Cautions see notes above; cerebrovascular disease; elderly (reduce initial dose); hepatic impairment (Appendix 2); pregnancy (Appendix 4)

Contra-indications see notes above; breast-feeding (Appendix 5)

Side-effects see notes above; nausea, vomiting, dyspepsia, constipation; insomnia, akathisia, drowsiness, restlessness, tremor, headache, asthenia, blurred vision; *less commonly* tachycardia; *very rarely* abdominal pain, anorexia, dysphagia, oropharyngeal spasm, laryngospasm, hepatitis, jaundice, hypersalivation, pancreatitis, oedema, thromboembolism, arrhythmias, bradycardia, hypertension, chest pain, agitation, anxiety, speech disorder, suicidal ideation, seizures, hyponatraemia, stiffness, myalgia, rhabdomyolysis, priapism, urinary retention and incontinence, blood disorders, sweating, alopecia, photosensitivity reactions, rash, weight loss, and impaired temperature regulation

Dose

- ADULT over 18 years 10–15 mg once daily, usual maintenance 15 mg once daily; max. 30 mg once daily

Abilify® (Bristol-Myers Squibb) PoM

Tablets, aripiprazole 5 mg (blue), net price 28-tab pack = £101.63; 10 mg (pink), 28-tab pack = £101.63; 15 mg (yellow), 28-tab pack = £101.63; 30 mg (pink), 28-tab pack = £203.26. Label: 2

Orodispersible tablets, aripiprazole 10 mg (pink), net price 28-tab pack = £101.63; 15 mg (yellow), 28-tab pack = £101.63. Label: 2

Excipients include aspartame (section 9.4.1)

Oral solution, aripiprazole 1 mg/mL, net price 150 mL with measuring cup = £108.89. Label: 2

CLOZAPINE

Indications schizophrenia (including psychosis in Parkinson's disease) in patients unresponsive to, or intolerant of, conventional antipsychotic drugs

Cautions see notes above; elderly; monitor leucocyte and differential blood counts (see Agranulocytosis, below); prostatic hypertrophy, susceptibility to angle-closure glaucoma; taper off other antipsychotics before starting; close medical supervision during initiation (risk of collapse because of hypotension); hepatic impairment (Appendix 2); pregnancy (Appendix 4)

Withdrawal On planned withdrawal reduce dose over 1–2 weeks to avoid risk of rebound psychosis. If abrupt withdrawal necessary observe patient carefully

Agranulocytosis Neutropenia and potentially fatal agranulocytosis reported. Leucocyte and differential blood counts must be normal before starting; monitor counts every week for 18 weeks then at least every 2 weeks and if clozapine continued and blood count stable after 1 year at least every 4 weeks (and 4 weeks after discontinuation); if leucocyte count below 3000/mm³ or if absolute neutrophil count below 1500/mm³ discontinue permanently and refer to haematologist. Avoid drugs which depress leucopoiesis; patients should report immediately symptoms of infection, especially influenza-like illness

Myocarditis and cardiomyopathy Fatal myocarditis (most commonly in first 2 months) and cardiomyopathy reported. The CSM has advised:

- physical examination and medical history before starting clozapine;
- specialist examination if cardiac abnormalities or history of heart disease found—clozapine initiated only in absence of severe heart disease and if benefit outweighs risk;
- persistent tachycardia especially in first 2 months should prompt observation for other indicators for myocarditis or cardiomyopathy;
- if myocarditis or cardiomyopathy suspected clozapine should be stopped and patient evaluated urgently by cardiologist;
- discontinue permanently in clozapine-induced myocarditis or cardiomyopathy

Gastro-intestinal obstruction Reactions resembling gastro-intestinal obstruction reported. Clozapine should be used cautiously with drugs which cause constipation (e.g. antimuscarinic drugs) or in history of colonic disease or bowel surgery. Monitor for constipation and prescribe laxative if required

Contra-indications severe cardiac disorders (e.g. myocarditis; see Myocarditis and Cardiomyopathy, above); renal impairment (avoid if creatinine clearance less than 10 mL/minute); history of neutropenia or agranulocytosis (see Agranulocytosis, above); bone-marrow disorders; paralytic ileus (see Gastro-intestinal Obstruction, above); alcoholic and toxic psychoses; history of circulatory collapse; drug intoxication; coma or severe CNS depression; uncontrolled epilepsy; breast-feeding (Appendix 5)

Side-effects see notes above; also constipation (see Gastro-intestinal Obstruction, above), hypersalivation, dry mouth, nausea, vomiting, anorexia; tachycardia, ECG changes, hypertension; drowsiness, headache, tremor, seizures, fatigue, impaired temperature regulation; urinary incontinence and retention; leucopenia, eosinophilia, leucocytosis; blurred vision; sweating; *less commonly* agranulocytosis (**important**: see Agranulocytosis, above); *rarely* dysphagia, hepatitis, cholestatic jaundice, pancreatitis, circulatory collapse, arrhythmia, myocarditis (**important**: see Myocarditis, above), pericarditis, thromboembolism, agitation, confusion, delirium, anaemia; *very rarely* parotid gland enlargement, intestinal obstruction (see Gastro-intestinal Obstruction, above), cardiomyopathy, myocardial infarction, respiratory depression, priapism, interstitial nephritis, thrombocytopenia, thrombocythaemia, hyperlipidaemia, angle-closure glaucoma, fulminant hepatic necrosis, and skin reactions

Dose

- Schizophrenia, ADULT over 16 years, 12.5 mg once or twice (ELDERLY 12.5 mg once) on first day then 25–50 mg (ELDERLY 25–37.5 mg) on second day then increased gradually (if well tolerated) in steps of 25–50 mg daily (ELDERLY max. increment 25 mg daily) over 14–21 days up to 300 mg daily in divided doses (larger dose at night, up to 200 mg daily may be taken as a single dose at bedtime); if necessary may be further increased in steps of 50–100 mg once (preferably) or twice weekly; usual dose 200–450 mg daily (max. 900 mg daily)

  Note *Restarting* after *interval of more than 2 days,* 12.5 mg once or twice on first day (but may be feasible to increase more quickly than on initiation)—extreme caution if previous respiratory or cardiac arrest with initial dosing

- Psychosis in Parkinson's disease, ADULT over 16 years, 12.5 mg at bedtime then increased according to response in steps of 12.5 mg up to twice weekly; usual dose range 25–37.5 mg at bedtime, usual max. 50 mg daily; exceptionally, dose may be increased further in steps of 12.5 mg weekly to max. 100 mg daily in 1–2 divided doses

Clozaril® (Novartis) PoM

Tablets, both yellow, clozapine 25 mg (scored), net price 28-tab pack = £6.17, 84-tab pack (hosp. only) = £18.49; 100 mg, 28-tab pack = £24.64, 84-tab pack (hosp. only) = £73.92. Label: 2, 10, patient information leaflet

Note Patient, prescriber, and supplying pharmacist must be registered with the Clozaril Patient Monitoring Service—takes several days to do this

Denzapine® (Merz) PoM

Tablets, both yellow, scored, clozapine 25 mg, net price 28-tab pack = £6.17, 84-tab pack = £18.49; 100 mg, 28-tab pack = £24.64, 84-tab pack = £73.92. Label: 2, 10, patient information leaflet

Note Patient, prescriber, and supplying pharmacist must be registered with the Denzapine Patient Monitoring Service—takes several days to do this

Zaponex® (IVAX) PoM

Tablets, both yellow, scored, clozapine 25 mg, net price 84-tab pack = £22.17; 100 mg, 84-tab pack = £50.00. Label: 2, 10, patient information leaflet

Note Patient, prescriber, and supplying pharmacist must be registered with the Zaponex Treatment Access System—takes several days to do this

OLANZAPINE

Indications see under Dose

Cautions see notes above (including advice on atypical antipsychotics and stroke); also prostatic hypertrophy, susceptibility to angle-closure glaucoma, paralytic ileus, diabetes mellitus (risk of exacerbation or ketoacidosis), low leucocyte or neutrophil count, bone-marrow depression, hypereosinophilic disorders, myeloproliferative disease, Parkinson's disease; hepatic impairment (Appendix 2); renal impairment (Appendix 3); pregnancy (Appendix 4)

CNS and respiratory depression Blood pressure, pulse and respiratory rate should be monitored for at least 4 hours after intramuscular injection, particularly in those also receiving another antipsychotic or benzodiazepine

Contra-indications breast-feeding (Appendix 5); *for injection*, acute myocardial infarction, unstable angina, severe hypotension or bradycardia, sick sinus syndrome, recent heart surgery

Side-effects see notes above; also mild, transient antimuscarinic effects (*very rarely* precipitation of angle-closure glaucoma); drowsiness, speech difficulty, exacerbation of Parkinson's disease, abnormal gait, hallucinations, akathisia, asthenia, increased appetite, increased body temperature, raised triglyceride concentration, oedema, hyperprolactinaemia (but clinical manifestations rare), urinary incontinence; eosinophilia; *less commonly* hypotension, bradycardia, QT interval prolongation, photosensitivity; *rarely* seizures, leucopenia, rash; *very rarely* thromboembolism, hypercholesterolaemia, hypothermia, urinary retention, priapism, thrombocytopenia, neutropenia, rhabdomyolysis, hepatitis, pancreatitis and alopecia; *with injection*, injection-site reactions, sinus pause, hypoventilation

Dose

- Schizophrenia, combination therapy for mania, preventing recurrence in bipolar disorder, by mouth, ADULT over 18 years, 10 mg daily adjusted to usual range of 5–20 mg daily; doses greater than 10 mg daily only after reassessment; max. 20 mg daily; CHILD 12–18 years, see *BNF for Children*
- Monotherapy for mania, by mouth, ADULT over 18 years, 15 mg daily adjusted to usual range of 5–20 mg daily; doses greater than 15 mg only after reassessment; max. 20 mg daily; CHILD 12–18 years, see *BNF for Children*
- Control of agitation and disturbed behaviour in schizophrenia or mania, by intramuscular injection, ADULT over 18 years, initially 5–10 mg (usual dose 10 mg) as a single dose followed by 5–10 mg after 2 hours if necessary; ELDERLY initially 2.5–5 mg as a single dose followed by 2.5–5 mg after 2 hours if necessary; max. 3 injections daily for 3 days; max. daily combined oral and parenteral dose 20 mg

Note When one or more factors present that might result in slower metabolism (e.g. female gender, elderly, non-smoker) consider lower initial dose and more gradual dose increase

Zyprexa® (Lilly) PoM

Tablets, f/c, olanzapine 2.5 mg, net price 28-tab pack = £33.29; 5 mg, 28-tab pack = £48.78; 7.5 mg, 56-tab pack = £146.34; 10 mg, 28-tab pack = £79.45, 15 mg (blue), 28-tab pack = £119.18; 20 mg (pink), 28-tab pack = £158.90. Label: 2

Orodispersible tablet (*Velotab®*), yellow, olanzapine 5 mg, net price 28-tab pack = £48.78; 10 mg, 28-tab pack = £79.45; 15 mg, 28-tab pack = £119.18; 20 mg, 28-tab pack = £158.90. Label: 2, counselling, administration

Excipients include aspartame (section 9.4.1)

Counselling *Velotab®* may be placed on the tongue and allowed to dissolve or dispersed in water, orange juice, apple juice, milk, or coffee

Injection ▼, powder for reconstitution, olanzapine 5 mg/mL, net price 10-mg vial = £3.48

PALIPERIDONE

Note Paliperidone is a metabolite of risperidone

Indications schizophrenia

Cautions see notes above; predisposition to gastro-intestinal obstruction; elderly patients with dementia and risk factors for stroke; Parkinson's disease; severe hepatic impairment; renal impairment (avoid if creatinine clearance less than 10 mL/minute; Appendix 3); pregnancy (Appendix 4)

Contra-indications breast-feeding (Appendix 5)

Side-effects see notes above; also abdominal pain, dry mouth, hypersalivation, vomiting; tachycardia, bradycardia, first-degree AV block, bundle branch block; drowsiness, headache, asthenia; *less commonly* palpitation, arrhythmias, ischaemia, oedema, seizures, nightmare, syncope, menstrual disturbances, erectile dysfunction, galactorrhoea, and gynaecomastia

Dose

- ADULT over 18 years, 6 mg once daily in the morning, adjusted if necessary; usual range 3–12 mg daily

Counselling Always take with breakfast or always take on an empty stomach

Invega® (Janssen-Cilag) ▼ PoM

Tablets, m/r, paliperidone 3 mg (white), net price 28-tab pack = £97.28; 6 mg (beige), 28-tab pack = £97.28; 9 mg (pink), 28-tab pack = £145.92. Label: 2, 25, counselling, administration

QUETIAPINE

Indications schizophrenia; treatment of episodes of mania either alone or with mood stabilisers

Cautions see notes above; also pregnancy (Appendix 4), hepatic impairment (Appendix 2), renal impairment (Appendix 3), cerebrovascular disease

Contra-indications breast-feeding (Appendix 5)

Side-effects see notes above; also drowsiness, dyspepsia, constipation, dry mouth, mild asthenia, rhinitis, tachycardia; leucopenia, neutropenia and occasionally eosinophilia reported; elevated plasma-triglyceride and cholesterol concentrations, reduced plasma-thyroid hormone concentrations; possible QT interval prolongation; rarely oedema; very rarely priapism

Dose

- Schizophrenia 25 mg twice daily on day 1, 50 mg twice daily on day 2, 100 mg twice daily on day 3, 150 mg twice daily on day 4, then adjusted according to response, usual range 300–450 mg daily in 2 divided doses; max. 750 mg daily; ELDERLY initially 25 mg daily as a single dose, increased in steps of 25–50 mg daily in 2 divided doses; CHILD 12–18 years, see *BNF for Children*
- Mania, 50 mg twice daily on day 1, 100 mg twice daily on day 2, 150 mg twice daily on day 3, 200 mg twice daily on day 4, then adjusted according to response in steps of up to 200 mg daily to max. 800 mg daily; usual range 400–800 mg daily in 2 divided doses; ELDERLY initially 25 mg daily as a single dose, increased in steps of 25–50 mg daily in 2 divided doses; CHILD under 18 years, not recommended

Seroquel® (AstraZeneca) PoM

Tablets, f/c, quetiapine (as fumarate) 25 mg (peach), net price 60-tab pack = £33.83; 100 mg (yellow), 60-tab pack = £113.10; 150 mg (pale yellow), 60-tab pack = £113.10; 200 mg (white), 60-tab pack = £113.10; 300 mg (white), 60-tab pack = £170.00. Label: 2

RISPERIDONE

Indications acute and chronic psychoses, mania

Cautions see notes above (including advice on atypical antipsychotics and stroke); Parkinson's disease; hepatic impairment (Appendix 2); renal impairment (Appendix 3); pregnancy (Appendix 4)

Contra-indications breast-feeding (Appendix 5)

Side-effects see notes above; also sleep disturbances, agitation, anxiety, and headache; *less commonly* constipation, nausea and vomiting, dyspepsia, abdominal pain, hypertension, drowsiness, impaired concentration, dizziness, fatigue, hyperprolactinaemia (with galactorrhoea, menstrual disturbances, gynaecomastia), sexual dysfunction, priapism, urinary incontinence, abnormal vision, and rash; *rarely* seizures, hyponatraemia, abnormal temperature regulation, and epistaxis; *very rarely* benign prostatic adenoma; oedema, and blood disorders also reported

Dose

- Psychoses, 2 mg in 1–2 divided doses on first day then 4 mg in 1–2 divided doses on second day (slower titration appropriate in some patients); usual dose range 4–6 mg daily; doses above 10 mg daily only if benefit considered to outweigh risk (max. 16 mg daily); ELDERLY initially 500 micrograms twice daily increased in steps of 500 micrograms twice daily to 1–2 mg twice daily; CHILD 12–15 years see *BNF for Children*
- Mania, initially 2 mg once daily, increased if necessary in steps of 1 mg daily; usual dose range 1–6 mg daily; ELDERLY initially 500 micrograms twice daily increased in steps of 500 micrograms twice daily to 1–2 mg twice daily

Risperdal® (Janssen-Cilag) PoM

Tablets, f/c, scored, risperidone 500 micrograms (brown-red), net price 20-tab pack = £7.06; 1 mg (white), 20-tab pack = £11.61, 60-tab pack = £34.84; 2 mg (orange), 60-tab pack = £68.69; 3 mg (yellow), 60-tab pack = £101.01; 4 mg (green), 60-tab pack = £133.34; 6 mg (yellow), 28-tab pack = £94.28. Label: 2

Orodispersible tablets (*Quicklet®*), pink, risperidone 500 micrograms, net price 28-tab pack = £11.43; 1 mg, 28-tab pack = £18.39; 2 mg, 28-tab pack = £34.66; 3 mg, 28-tab pack = £50.34; 4 mg, 28-tab pack = £64.84. Label: 2, counselling, administration

Excipients include aspartame (section 9.4.1)

Counselling Tablets should be placed on the tongue, allowed to dissolve and swallowed

Liquid, risperidone 1 mg/mL, net price 100 mL = £56.12. Label: 2

Note Liquid may be diluted with mineral water, orange juice or black coffee (should be taken immediately)

Depot preparation

Section 4.2.2

SERTINDOLE

Indications schizophrenia, see also notes above

Cautions see notes above; hepatic impairment (Appendix 2); correct hypokalaemia or hypomagnesaemia before treatment; monitor ECG during treatment; monitor blood pressure during dose titration and early maintenance therapy (risk of postural hypotension)

Contra-indications see notes above; pregnancy (Appendix 4), breast-feeding (Appendix 5), severe hepatic impairment, QT interval prolongation (ECG required before and during treatment—consult product literature); concomitant administration of drugs which prolong QT interval (see interactions); uncorrected hypokalaemia or hypomagnesaemia

Side-effects see notes above; prolonged QT interval, peripheral oedema, dry mouth, rhinitis, nasal congestion, dyspnoea, paraesthesia, abnormal ejaculation (decreased volume); rarely seizures, hyperglycaemia

Dose

- Initially 4 mg daily increased in steps of 4 mg at intervals of 4–5 days to usual maintenance of 12–20 mg as a single daily dose; max. 24 mg daily; ELDERLY consider slower dose titration and lower maintenance dose; CHILD and ADOLESCENT not recommended

Serdolect® (Lundbeck) ▼ PoM

Tablets, f/c, sertindole 4 mg, 30-tab pack; 12 mg 28-tab pack; 16 mg, 28-tab pack; 20 mg 28-tab pack

Available only on named-patient basis (see notes above)

ZOTEPINE

Indications schizophrenia

Cautions see notes above; personal or close family history of epilepsy; withdrawal of concomitantly prescribed CNS depressants; QT interval prolongation—ECG required (before treatment and at each dose increase) in patients at risk of arrhythmias; monitor plasma electrolytes particularly before treatment and at each dose increase; hepatic impairment (Appendix 2); renal impairment (Appendix 3); prostatic hypertrophy, urinary retention, susceptibility to angle-closure glaucoma, paralytic ileus, pregnancy (Appendix 4)

Contra-indications acute intoxication with CNS depressants; high doses of concomitantly prescribed antipsychotics; acute gout (avoid for 3 weeks after episode resolves), history of nephrolithiasis; breast-feeding (Appendix 5)

Side-effects see notes above; constipation, dyspepsia, dry mouth, tachycardia, QT interval prolongation, rhinitis, agitation, anxiety, depression, asthenia, headache, EEG abnormalities, insomnia, drowsiness, hyperthermia or hypothermia, increased salivation, blood dyscrasias (including leucocytosis, leucopenia), raised erythrocyte sedimentation rate, blurred vision, sweating; less frequently anorexia, diarrhoea, nausea and vomiting, abdominal pain, hypertension, influenza-like syndrome, cough, dyspnoea, confusion, convulsions, decreased libido, speech disorder, vertigo, hyperprolactinaemia, anaemia, thrombocythaemia, increased serum creatinine, hypoglycaemia and hyperglycaemia, hyperlipidaemia, hypouricaemia, oedema, thirst, impotence, urinary incontinence, arthralgia, myalgia, conjunctivitis, acne, dry skin, rash; rarely bradycardia, epistaxis, abdominal enlargement, amnesia, ataxia, coma, delirium, hypaesthesia, myoclonus, thrombocytopenia, abnormal ejaculation, urinary retention, menstrual irregularities, myasthenia, alopecia, photosensitivity; *very rarely* angle-closure glaucoma

Dose

- Initially 25 mg 3 times daily increased according to response at intervals of 4 days to max. 100 mg 3 times daily; ELDERLY initially 25 mg twice daily increased according to response to max. 75 mg twice daily; CHILD and ADOLESCENT under 18 years not recommended

Zoleptil® (Orion) PoM

Tablets, s/c, zotepine 25 mg (white), net price 30-tab pack = £21.50, 90-tab pack = £42.98; 50 mg (yellow), 30-tab pack = £28.65, 90-tab pack = £57.30; 100 mg (pink), 30-tab pack = £47.28, 90-tab pack = £94.55. Label: 2

4.2.2 Antipsychotic depot injections

Long-acting depot injections are used for maintenance therapy especially when compliance with oral treatment is unreliable. However, depot injections of conventional antipsychotics may give rise to a higher incidence of extrapyramidal reactions than oral preparations; extrapyramidal reactions occur less frequently with atypical antipsychotics such as risperidone.

Administration Depot antipsychotics are administered by deep intramuscular injection at intervals of 1 to 4 weeks. When initiating therapy with sustained-release preparations of conventional antipsychotics, patients should first be given a small test-dose as undesirable side-effects are prolonged. In general not more than 2–3 mL of oily injection should be administered at any one site; correct injection technique (including the use of z-track technique) and rotation of injection sites are essential. If the dose needs to be reduced to alleviate side-effects, it is important to recognise that the plasma-drug concentration may not fall for some time after reducing the dose, therefore it may be a month or longer before side-effects subside.

> **Dosage** Individual responses to neuroleptic drugs are very variable and to achieve optimum effect, dosage and dosage interval must be titrated according to the patient's response. For the advice of The Royal College of Psychiatrists on doses above the BNF upper limit, see p. 187.

Equivalent doses of depot antipsychotics

These equivalences are intended **only** as an approximate guide; individual dosage instructions should **also** be checked; patients should be carefully monitored after **any** change in medication

Antipsychotic drug	Dose (mg)	Interval
Flupentixol decanoate	40	2 weeks
Fluphenazine decanoate	25	2 weeks
Haloperidol (as decanoate)	100	4 weeks
Pipotiazine palmitate	50	4 weeks
Zuclopenthixol decanoate	200	2 weeks

Important These equivalences must **not** be extrapolated beyond the max. dose for the drug

Choice There is no clear-cut division in the use of the conventional antipsychotics, but **zuclopenthixol** may be suitable for the treatment of agitated or aggressive patients whereas **flupentixol** can cause over-excitement in such patients. The incidence of extrapyramidal reactions is similar for the conventional antipsychotics.

Cautions See section 4.2.1. Treatment requires careful monitoring for optimum effect. When transferring from oral to depot therapy, dosage by mouth should be reduced gradually.

Contra-indications See section 4.2.1. Do not use in children.

Side-effects See section 4.2.1. Pain may occur at injection site and occasionally erythema, swelling, and nodules. For side-effects of specific antipsychotics see under the relevant drug.

FLUPENTIXOL DECANOATE
(Flupenthixol Decanoate)

Indications maintenance in schizophrenia and other psychoses

Cautions see notes on p. 188 and also under Flupentixol (section 4.2.1) and notes above; an alternative antipsychotic may be necessary if symptoms such as aggression or agitation appear

Contra-indications see notes on p. 188 and also under Flupentixol (section 4.2.1) and notes above

Side-effects see notes on p. 188 and also under Flupentixol (section 4.2.1) and notes above, but may have a mood elevating effect

Dose

- By deep intramuscular injection into the gluteal muscle, test dose 20 mg, then after at least 7 days 20–40 mg repeated at intervals of 2–4 weeks, adjusted according to response; max. 400 mg weekly; usual maintenance dose 50 mg every 4 weeks to 300 mg every 2 weeks; ELDERLY initially quarter to half adult dose; CHILD not recommended

Depixol® (Lundbeck) PoM
Injection (oily), flupentixol decanoate 20 mg/mL. Net price 1-mL amp = £1.52; 2-mL amp = £2.54

Depixol Conc.® (Lundbeck) PoM
Injection (oily), flupentixol decanoate 100 mg/mL. Net price 0.5-mL amp = £3.42; 1-mL amp = £6.25

Depixol Low Volume® (Lundbeck) PoM
Injection (oily), flupentixol decanoate 200 mg/mL. Net price 1-mL amp = £19.52

FLUPHENAZINE DECANOATE

Indications maintenance in schizophrenia and other psychoses

Cautions see notes on p. 188 and also notes above

Contra-indications see notes on p. 188 and also notes above

Side-effects see notes on p. 188 and notes above; less sedating and fewer antimuscarinic or hypotensive symptoms, but extrapyramidal symptoms, particularly dystonic reactions and akathisia, more frequent; systemic lupus erythematosus, inappropriate antidiuretic hormone secretion, oedema, also reported; extrapyramidal symptoms usually appear a few hours after injection and continue for about 2 days but may be delayed

Dose

- By deep intramuscular injection into the gluteal muscle, test dose 12.5 mg (6.25 mg in elderly), then after 4–7 days 12.5–100 mg repeated at intervals of 14–35 days, adjusted according to response; CHILD not recommended

Fluphenazine decanoate (Non-proprietary) PoM
Injection (oily), fluphenazine decanoate 25 mg/mL, net price 1-mL amp = £2.35; 100 mg/mL, 0.5-mL amp = £4.50, 1-mL amp = £8.79
Excipients include sesame oil

Modecate® (Sanofi-Synthelabo) PoM
Injection (oily), fluphenazine decanoate 25 mg/mL. Net price 0.5-mL amp = £1.35, 1-mL amp = £2.35, 2-mL amp = £4.62
Excipients include sesame oil

Modecate Concentrate® (Sanofi-Synthelabo) PoM
Injection (oily), fluphenazine decanoate 100 mg/mL. Net price 0.5-mL amp = £4.66, 1-mL amp = £9.10
Excipients include sesame oil

HALOPERIDOL

Indications maintenance in schizophrenia and other psychoses

Cautions see notes on p. 188 and also under Haloperidol (section 4.2.1) and notes above

Contra-indications see notes on p. 188 and also under Haloperidol (section 4.2.1) and notes above

Side-effects see notes on p. 188 and also under Haloperidol (section 4.2.1) and notes above

Dose

- By deep intramuscular injection into the gluteal muscle, initially 50 mg every 4 weeks, if necessary increasing by 50-mg increments to 300 mg every 4 weeks; higher doses may be needed in some patients; ELDERLY, initially 12.5–25 mg every 4 weeks; CHILD not recommended

Note If 2-weekly administration preferred, doses should be halved

Haldol Decanoate® (Janssen-Cilag) PoM
Injection (oily), haloperidol (as decanoate) 50 mg/mL, net price 1-mL amp = £4.05; 100 mg/mL, 1-mL amp = £5.36
Excipients include sesame oil

PIPOTIAZINE PALMITATE
(Pipothiazine Palmitate)

Indications maintenance in schizophrenia and other psychoses

Cautions see notes on p. 188 and notes above

Contra-indications see notes on p. 188 and notes above

Side-effects see notes on p. 188 and notes above

Dose

- By deep intramuscular injection into the gluteal muscle, test dose 25 mg, then a further 25–50 mg after 4–7 days, then adjusted according to response at intervals of 4 weeks; usual maintenance range 50–100 mg (max. 200 mg) every 4 weeks; ELDERLY initially 5–10 mg; CHILD not recommended

Piportil Depot® (Sanofi-Aventis) PoM
Injection (oily), pipotiazine palmitate 50 mg/mL. Net price 1-mL amp = £13.57; 2-mL amp = £22.21
Excipients include sesame oil

RISPERIDONE

Indications schizophrenia and other psychoses in patients tolerant to risperidone by mouth

Cautions see under Risperidone (section 4.2.1) and notes above

Contra-indications see under Risperidone (section 4.2.1)

Side-effects see under Risperidone (section 4.2.1); also depression, *less commonly* apathy, weight loss, and pruritus

Dose

- By deep intramuscular injection into the gluteal muscle, patients taking oral risperidone up to 4 mg daily, initially 25 mg every 2 weeks; patients taking oral risperidone over 4 mg daily, initially 37.5 mg every 2 weeks; dose adjusted at intervals of at least 4 weeks in steps of 12.5 mg to max. 50 mg (ELDERLY 25 mg) every 2 weeks; CHILD and ADOLESCENT under 18 years not recommended

Note During initiation risperidone by mouth may need to be continued for 4–6 weeks; risperidone by mouth may also be used during dose adjustment of depot injection

Risperdal Consta® (Janssen-Cilag) ▼ PoM
Injection, powder for reconstitution, risperidone 25-mg vial, net price = £82.92; 37.5-mg vial = £115.84; 50-mg vial = £148.55 (all with diluent)

ZUCLOPENTHIXOL DECANOATE

Indications maintenance in schizophrenia and other psychoses, particularly with aggression and agitation

Cautions see notes on p. 188 and notes above; avoid in porphyria (section 9.8.2)

Contra-indications see notes on p. 188 and notes above

Side-effects see notes on p. 188 and notes above

Dose

- By deep intramuscular injection into the gluteal muscle, test dose 100 mg, followed after at least 7 days by 200–500 mg or more, repeated at intervals of 1–4 weeks, adjusted according to response; max. 600 mg weekly; ELDERLY quarter to half usual starting dose; CHILD not recommended

Clopixol® (Lundbeck) PoM
Injection (oily), zuclopenthixol decanoate 200 mg/mL. Net price 1-mL amp = £3.15

Clopixol Conc.® (Lundbeck) PoM
Injection (oily), zuclopenthixol decanoate 500 mg/mL. Net price 1-mL amp = £7.44

4.2.3 Antimanic drugs

Drugs are used in mania to control acute attacks and to prevent their recurrence.

Benzodiazepines

Use of benzodiazepines (section 4.1) may be helpful in the initial stages of treatment until lithium achieves its full effect; they should not be used for long periods because of the risk of dependence.

Antipsychotic drugs

In an acute attack of mania, treatment with an antipsychotic drug (section 4.2.1) is usually required because it may take a few days for lithium to exert its antimanic effect. Lithium may be given concurrently with the antipsychotic drug, and treatment with the antipsychotic gradually tailed off as lithium becomes effective. Alternatively, lithium therapy may be commenced once the patient's mood has been stabilised with the antipsychotic. The adjunctive use of atypical antipsychotics such as olanzapine (section 4.2.1) and risperidone with either lithium or valproic acid may also be of benefit.

High doses of haloperidol or flupentixol may be hazardous when used with lithium; irreversible toxic encephalopathy has been reported.

Carbamazepine

Carbamazepine (section 4.8.1) may be used for the prophylaxis of bipolar disorder (manic-depressive disorder) in patients unresponsive to lithium; it seems to be particularly effective in patients with rapid-cycling manic-depressive illness (4 or more affective episodes per year).

Valproic acid

Valproic acid (as the semisodium salt) is licensed for the treatment of manic episodes associated with bipolar disorder. It may be useful in patients unresponsive to lithium. Sodium valproate (section 4.8.1) has also been used, but it is unlicensed for this indication.

VALPROIC ACID

Indications treatment of manic episodes associated with bipolar disorder

Cautions see Sodium Valproate (section 4.8.1); monitor closely if dose greater than 45 mg/kg daily

Contra-indications see Sodium Valproate (section 4.8.1)

Side-effects see Sodium Valproate (section 4.8.1)

Dose

- Initially 750 mg daily in 2–3 divided doses, increased according to response, usual dose 1–2 g daily; CHILD and ADOLESCENT under 18 years not recommended

Depakote® (Sanofi-Synthelabo) PoM

Tablets, e/c, valproic acid (as semisodium valproate) 250 mg, net price 90-tab pack = £12.17; 500 mg, 90-tab pack = £24.29. Label: 25

Note Semisodium valproate comprises equimolar amounts of sodium valproate and valproic acid.

Lithium

Lithium salts are used in the prophylaxis and treatment of mania, in the prophylaxis of bipolar disorder (manic-depressive disorder) and in the prophylaxis of recurrent depression (unipolar illness or unipolar depression). Lithium is unsuitable for children.

The decision to give prophylactic lithium usually requires *specialist advice*, and must be based on careful consideration of the likelihood of recurrence in the individual patient, and the benefit weighed against the risks. In long-term use lithium has been associated with thyroid disorders and mild cognitive and memory impairment. Long-term treatment should therefore be undertaken only with careful assessment of risk and benefit, and with regular monitoring of thyroid function. The need for continued therapy should be assessed regularly and patients should be maintained on lithium after 3–5 years only if benefit persists.

Serum concentrations Lithium salts have a narrow therapeutic/toxic ratio and should therefore not be prescribed unless facilities for monitoring serum-lithium concentrations are available. There seem few if any reasons for preferring one or other of the salts of lithium available. Doses are adjusted to achieve serum-lithium concentration of 0.4–1 mmol/litre (lower end of the range for maintenance therapy and elderly patients) on samples taken 12 hours after the preceding dose. It is important to determine the optimum range for each individual patient.

Overdosage, usually with serum-lithium concentration of over 1.5 mmol/litre, may be fatal and toxic effects include tremor, ataxia, dysarthria, nystagmus, renal impairment, and convulsions. If these potentially hazardous signs occur, treatment should be stopped, serum-lithium concentrations redetermined, and steps taken to reverse lithium toxicity. In mild cases withdrawal of lithium and administration of generous amounts of sodium salts and fluid will reverse the toxicity. Serum-lithium concentration in excess of 2 mmol/litre require urgent treatment as indicated under Emergency Treatment of Poisoning, p. 32.

Interactions Lithium toxicity is made worse by sodium depletion, therefore concurrent use of diuretics (particularly thiazides) is hazardous and should be avoided. For other **interactions** with lithium, see Appendix 1 (lithium).

Withdrawal While there is no clear evidence of withdrawal or rebound psychosis, abrupt discontinuation of lithium increases the risk of relapse. If lithium is to be discontinued, the dose should be reduced gradually over a period of a few weeks and patients should be warned of possible relapse if it is discontinued abruptly.

Lithium cards

A lithium treatment card available from pharmacies tells patients how to take lithium preparations, what to do if a dose is missed, and what side-effects to expect. It also explains why regular blood tests are important and warns that some medicines and illnesses can change serum-lithium concentration.
Cards may be purchased from the National Pharmacy Association.
Tel: (01727) 858 687
sales@npa.co.uk

LITHIUM CARBONATE

Indications treatment and prophylaxis of mania, bipolar disorder, and recurrent depression (see also notes above); aggressive or self-mutilating behaviour

Cautions measure serum-lithium concentration regularly (every 3 months on stabilised regimens), measure renal function and thyroid function every 6–12 months on stabilised regimens and advise patient to seek attention if symptoms of hypothyroidism develop (women at greater risk) e.g. lethargy, feeling cold; maintain adequate sodium and fluid intake; test renal function before initiating and if evidence of toxicity, avoid in renal impairment (Appendix 3), cardiac disease, and conditions with sodium imbalance such as Addison's disease; reduce dose or discontinue in diarrhoea, vomiting and intercurrent infection (especially if sweating profusely); psoriasis (risk of exacerbation); pregnancy (Appendix 4), breast-feeding (Appendix 5), elderly (reduce dose), diuretic treatment, myasthenia gravis; surgery (section 15.1); avoid abrupt withdrawal (see notes above); **interactions**: Appendix 1 (lithium)

Counselling Patients should maintain adequate fluid intake and avoid dietary changes which reduce or increase sodium intake; lithium treatment cards are available from pharmacies (see above)

Side-effects gastro-intestinal disturbances, fine tremor, renal impairment (particularly impaired urinary concentration and polyuria), polydipsia, leucocytosis; also weight gain and oedema (may respond to dose reduction); hyperparathyroidism and hypercalcaemia reported; signs of intoxication are blurred vision, increasing gastro-intestinal disturbances (anorexia, vomiting, diarrhoea), muscle weakness, increased CNS disturbances (mild drowsiness and sluggishness increasing to giddiness with ataxia, coarse tremor, lack of co-ordination, dysarthria), and require withdrawal of treatment; with severe **overdosage** (serum-lithium concentration above 2 mmol/litre) hyperreflexia and hyperextension of limbs, convulsions, toxic psychoses, syncope, renal failure, circulatory failure, coma, and occasionally, death; goitre, raised antidiuretic hormone concentration, hypothyroidism, hypokalaemia, ECG changes, and kidney changes may also occur; see also Emergency Treatment of Poisoning, p. 32

Dose

- See under preparations below, adjusted to achieve a serum-lithium concentration of 0.4–1 mmol/litre 12 hours after a dose on days 4–7 of treatment, then every week until dosage has remained constant for 4 weeks and every 3 months thereafter; doses are initially divided throughout the day, but once daily administration is preferred when serum-lithium concentration stabilised

Note Preparations vary widely in bioavailability; changing the preparation requires the same precautions as initiation of treatment

Note Lithium carbonate 200 mg ≡ lithium citrate 509 mg

Camcolit® (Norgine) PoM

Camcolit 250® tablets, f/c, scored, lithium carbonate 250 mg (Li^+ 6.8 mmol), net price 20 = 64p. Label: 10, lithium card, counselling, see above

Camcolit 400® tablets, m/r, f/c, scored, lithium carbonate 400 mg (Li^+ 10.8 mmol), net price 20 = 86p. Label: 10, lithium card, 25, counselling, see above

Dose (see Dose above for advice on bioavailability and serum monitoring):

ADULT and CHILD over 12 years, treatment, initially 1–1.5 g daily; prophylaxis, initially 300–400 mg daily

Note *Camcolit 400®* also available as *Lithonate®* (TEVA UK)

Liskonum® (GSK) PoM

Tablets, m/r, f/c, scored, lithium carbonate 450 mg (Li^+ 12.2 mmol), net price 60-tab pack = £2.88. Label: 10, lithium card, 25, counselling, see above

Dose (see Dose above for advice on bioavailability and serum monitoring):

ADULT and CHILD over 12 years, treatment, initially 450–675 mg twice daily (elderly initially 225 mg twice daily); prophylaxis, initially 450 mg twice daily (elderly 225 mg twice daily)

Priadel® (Sanofi-Synthelabo) PoM

Tablets, m/r, both scored, lithium carbonate 200 mg (Li^+ 5.4 mmol), net price 20 = 48p; 400 mg (Li^+ 10.8 mmol), 20 = 70p. Label: 10, lithium card, 25, counselling, see above

Dose (see Dose above for advice on bioavailability and serum monitoring):

Treatment and prophylaxis, initially 0.4–1.2 g daily as a single dose or in 2 divided doses (elderly or patients less than 50 kg, 400 mg daily); CHILD not recommended

Liquid, see under Lithium Citrate below

LITHIUM CITRATE

Indications see under Lithium Carbonate and notes above

Cautions see under Lithium Carbonate and notes above

Counselling Patients should maintain an adequate fluid intake and should avoid dietary changes which might reduce or increase sodium intake; lithium treatment cards are available from pharmacies (see above)

Side-effects see under Lithium Carbonate and notes above

Dose

- See under preparations below, adjusted to achieve serum-lithium concentration of 0.4–1 mmol/litre as described under Lithium Carbonate

Note Preparations vary widely in bioavailability; changing the preparation requires the same precautions as initiation of treatment

Note Lithium carbonate 200 mg ≡ lithium citrate 509 mg

Li-Liquid® (Rosemont) PoM

Oral solution, lithium citrate 509 mg/5 mL (Li^+ 5.4 mmol/5 mL), yellow, net price 150-mL pack = £5.79; 1.018 g/5 mL (Li^+ 10.8 mmol/5 mL), orange, 150-mL pack = £11.58. Label: 10, lithium card, counselling, see above

Dose (see Dose above for advice on bioavailability and serum monitoring):

Treatment and prophylaxis, initially 1.018–3.054 g daily in 2 divided doses (elderly or patients less than 50 kg, initially 509 mg twice daily); CHILD not recommended

Priadel® (Sanofi-Synthelabo) PoM

Tablets, see under Lithium Carbonate, above

Liquid, sugar-free, lithium citrate 520 mg/5 mL (approx. Li^+ 5.4 mmol/5 mL), net price 150-mL pack = £5.84. Label: 10, lithium card, counselling, see above

Dose (see Dose above for advice on bioavailability and serum monitoring, see above).

Treatment and prophylaxis, initially 1.04–3.12 g daily in 2 divided doses (elderly or patients less than 50 kg, 520 mg twice daily); CHILD not recommended

4.3 Antidepressant drugs

4.3.1 Tricyclic and related antidepressant drugs
4.3.2 Monoamine-oxidase inhibitors
4.3.3 Selective serotonin re-uptake inhibitors
4.3.4 Other antidepressant drugs

Antidepressant drugs are effective for treating moderate to severe depression associated with psychomotor and physiological changes such as loss of appetite and sleep disturbance; improvement in sleep is usually the first benefit of therapy. They are also effective for dysthymia (lower grade chronic depression). Antidepressant drugs are not generally effective in mild depression, and cognitive behavioural therapy should be considered initially; however, a trial of antidepressant therapy may be considered in cases refractory to psychological treatments or those associated with psychosocial or medical problems. Drug treatment of mild depression may also be considered in patients with a history of moderate or severe depression.

Choice The major classes of antidepressants include the tricyclics and related antidepressants, the selective serotonin re-uptake inhibitors (SSRIs), and the monoamine oxidase inhibitors (MAOIs). A number of antidepressants cannot be accommodated easily into this classification; these are included in section 4.3.4.

There is little to choose between the different classes of antidepressants in terms of efficacy, so choice should be based on the individual patient's requirements, including the presence of concomitant disease, existing therapy, suicide risk, and previous response to antidepressant therapy. Since there may be an interval of 2 weeks before the antidepressant action takes place electroconvulsive treatment may be required in severe depression when delay is hazardous or intolerable.

SSRIs are better tolerated and are safer in overdose than other classes of antidepressants and should be considered first-line for treating depression. In patients with unstable angina or who have had a recent myocardial infarction, sertraline has been shown to be safe.

Tricyclic antidepressants show similar efficacy to SSRIs but are more likely to be discontinued because of side-effects; toxicity in overdosage is also a problem. See section 4.3.1 for more details.

MAOIs have dangerous interactions with some foods and drugs, and should be reserved for use by specialists.

Although anxiety is often present in depressive illness (and may be the presenting symptom), the use of an antipsychotic or an anxiolytic may mask the true diagnosis. Anxiolytics (section 4.1.2) or antipsychotics (section 4.2.1) should therefore be used with caution in depression but they are useful adjuncts in agitated patients.

See also section 4.2.3 for references to the management of bipolar disorders.

St John's wort (*Hypericum perforatum*) is a popular unlicensed herbal remedy for treating mild depression. However, preparations of St John's wort can induce drug metabolising enzymes and a number of important interactions with conventional drugs have been identified, see Appendix 1 (St John's wort). The amount of active ingredient can vary between different preparations of St John's wort and switching from one to another can change the degree of enzyme induction. Furthermore, when a patient stops taking St John's wort, concentrations of interacting drugs may increase, leading to toxicity. Antidepressants should **not** be used with St John's wort because of the potential for interaction.

Hyponatraemia and antidepressant therapy

Hyponatraemia (usually in the elderly and possibly due to inappropriate secretion of antidiuretic hormone) has been associated with all types of antidepressants; however, it has been reported more frequently with SSRIs than with other antidepressants. The CSM has advised that hyponatraemia should be considered in all patients who develop drowsiness, confusion, or convulsions while taking an antidepressant.

Suicidal behaviour and antidepressant therapy

The use of antidepressants has been linked with suicidal thoughts and behaviour. Where necessary patients should be monitored for suicidal behaviour, self-harm, or hostility, particularly at the beginning of treatment or if the dose is changed.

Management Patients should be reviewed every 1–2 weeks at the start of antidepressant treatment. Treatment should be continued for at least 4 weeks (6 weeks in the elderly) before considering whether to switch antidepressant due to lack of efficacy. In cases of partial response, continue for a further 2 weeks (elderly patients may take longer to respond).

Following remission, antidepressant treatment should be continued at the same dose for at least 6 months (about 12 months in the elderly). Patients with a history of recurrent depression should continue to receive maintenance treatment for at least 2 years.

Failure to respond Failure to respond to initial treatment with an SSRI may require an increase in the dose, or switching to a different SSRI or mirtazapine; in patients with atypical depression, an MAOI such as phenelzine may be effective. Other second-line choices include lofepramine, moclobemide, and reboxetine. Other tricyclic antidepressants and venlafaxine should be considered for more severe forms of depression; dosulepin (dothiepin) and irreversible MAOIs should be prescribed by specialists only. Failure to respond to a second antidepressant may require the addition of another antidepressant of a different class, or an augmenting agent such as lithium, but such adjunctive treatment should be initiated only by doctors with special experience of these combinations. Electroconvulsive therapy may be initiated in severe refractory depression.

Withdrawal Gastro-intestinal symptoms of nausea, vomiting, and anorexia, accompanied by headache, giddiness, 'chills', and insomnia, and sometimes by hypomania, panic-anxiety, and extreme motor restlessness may occur if an antidepressant (particularly an MAOI) is stopped suddenly after regular administration for 8 weeks or more. The dose should preferably be reduced gradually over about 4 weeks, or longer if withdrawal symptoms emerge (6 months in patients who have been on long-term maintenance treatment). SSRIs have been associated with a specific withdrawal syndrome (section 4.3.3).

Anxiety disorders and obsessive compulsive disorder Management of acute anxiety generally involves the use of a benzodiazepine or buspirone (section 4.1.2). For chronic anxiety (of longer than 4 weeks' duration), it may be appropriate to use an antidepressant. Combined therapy with a benzodiazepine may be required until the antidepressant takes effect. *Generalised anxiety disorder*, a form of chronic anxiety, is treated with an SSRI such as escitalopram or paroxetine; pregabalin and venlafaxine are also licensed for the treatment of generalised anxiety disorder.

Panic disorder, obsessive compulsive disorder, post-traumatic stress disorder, and phobic states such as *social anxiety disorder* are treated with SSRIs. Clomipramine or imipramine can be used second-line in panic disorder [unlicensed]; clomipramine can also be used second-line for obsessive compulsive disorder. Moclobemide is licensed for the treatment of social anxiety disorder.

4.3.1 Tricyclic and related antidepressant drugs

This section covers tricyclic antidepressants and also 1-, 2-, and 4-ring structured drugs with broadly similar properties.

Some tricyclic antidepressants are used in the management of *panic disorder* (section 4.3). For reference to the role of some tricyclic antidepressants in some forms of *neuralgia*, see section 4.7.3, and in *nocturnal enuresis* in children, see section 7.4.2.

Dosage About 10 to 20% of patients fail to respond to tricyclic and related antidepressant drugs and inadequate dosage may account for some of these failures. It is important to use doses that are sufficiently high for effective treatment but not so high as to cause toxic effects. Low doses should be used for initial treatment in the **elderly** (see under Side-effects, below).

In most patients the long half-life of tricyclic antidepressant drugs allows **once-daily** administration, usually at night; the use of modified-release preparations is therefore unnecessary.

Choice Tricyclic and related antidepressants block the re-uptake of both serotonin and noradrenaline, although to different extents. For example, clomipramine is more selective for serotonergic transmission, and imipramine is more selective for noradrenergic transmission. Tricyclic and related antidepressant drugs can be roughly divided into those with additional sedative properties and those which are less sedating. Agitated and anxious patients tend to respond best to the sedative compounds whereas withdrawn and apathetic patients will often obtain most benefit from the less sedating ones. Those with **sedative** properties include amitriptyline, clomipramine, dosulepin (dothiepin), doxepin, mianserin, trazodone, and trimipramine. Those with **less sedative** properties include imipramine, lofepramine, and nortriptyline.

Tricyclic and related antidepressants also show varying degrees of antimuscarinic side-effects and cardiotoxicity in overdosage, which may be important in individual patients. **Lofepramine** has a lower incidence of side-effects and is less dangerous in overdosage, so should be considered when a tricyclic antidepressant is indicated; however, lofepramine is infrequently associated with hepatic toxicity. **Imipramine** is also well established, but has more marked antimuscarinic side-effects compared to other tricyclic and related antidepressants. **Amitriptyline** and **dosulepin** (dothiepin) are effective but they are particularly dangerous in overdosage (see Overdosage, below) and are not recommended for the treatment of depression; dosulepin (dothiepin) should be prescribed by specialists only.

Children and adolescents Evidence of the efficacy of tricyclic antidepressants for depression in children has not been established; see also CSM advice, p. 208.

Side-effects *Arrhythmias* and *heart block* occasionally follow the use of tricyclic antidepressants, particularly amitriptyline, and may be a factor in the sudden death of patients with cardiac disease. They are also sometimes associated with *convulsions* (and should be prescribed with special caution in epilepsy as they lower the convulsive threshold). *Hepatic* and *haematological* reactions may occur and have been particularly associated with mianserin.

Other side-effects of tricyclic and related antidepressants include *drowsiness, dry mouth, blurred vision* (very rarely *precipitation of angle-closure glaucoma*), *constipation*, and *urinary retention* (all attributed to antimuscarinic activity), and sweating. The patient should be encouraged to persist with treatment as some tolerance to these side-effects seems to develop. They are reduced if low doses are given initially and then gradually increased, but this must be balanced against the need to obtain a full therapeutic effect as soon as possible. Gradual introduction of treatment is particularly important in the elderly, who, because of the hypotensive effects of these drugs, are prone to attacks of *dizziness* or even *syncope*. Another side-effect to which the elderly are particularly susceptible is *hyponatraemia* (see Hyponatraemia and Antidepressant Therapy on p. 202).

Neuroleptic malignant syndrome (section 4.2.1) may, very rarely, arise in the course of antidepressant treatment.

Suicidal behaviour has been linked with antidepressants (see p. 202).

Overdosage Limited quantities of tricyclic antidepressants should be prescribed at any one time because their cardiovascular effects are dangerous in overdosage. In particular, overdosage with dosulepin (dothiepin) and amitriptyline is associated with a relatively high rate of fatality. For advice on **overdosage** see Emergency Treatment of Poisoning, p. 31.

Withdrawal If possible tricyclic and related antidepressants should be withdrawn slowly (see also section 4.3).

Interactions A tricyclic or related antidepressant (or an SSRI or related antidepressant) should not be started until 2 weeks after stopping an MAOI (3 weeks if starting clomipramine or imipramine). Conversely, an MAOI should not be started until at least 7–14 days after a tricyclic or related antidepressant (3 weeks in the case of clomipramine or imipramine) has been stopped. For guidance relating to the reversible monoamine oxidase inhibitor, moclobemide, see p. 207. For other tricyclic antidepressant **interactions**, see Appendix 1 (antidepressants, tricyclic and antidepressants, tricyclic (related)).

Tricyclic antidepressants

AMITRIPTYLINE HYDROCHLORIDE

Indications depressive illness (but not recommended, see notes above); nocturnal enuresis in children (section 7.4.2); neuropathic pain [unlicensed] (section 4.7.3); migraine prophylaxis [unlicensed] (section 4.7.4.2)

Cautions cardiac disease (particularly with arrhythmias, see Contra-indications below), history of epilepsy, pregnancy (Appendix 4), breast-feeding (Appendix 5), elderly, hepatic impairment (avoid if severe; Appendix 2), thyroid disease, phaeochromocytoma, history of mania, psychoses (may aggravate psychotic symptoms), susceptibility to angle-closure glaucoma, history of urinary retention, concurrent electroconvulsive therapy; if possible avoid abrupt withdrawal; anaesthesia (increased risk of arrhythmias and hypotension, see surgery section 15.1); porphyria (section 9.8.2); see section 7.4.2 for additional nocturnal enuresis warnings; **interactions:** Appendix 1 (antidepressants, tricyclic)

Driving Drowsiness may affect performance of skilled tasks (e.g. driving); effects of alcohol enhanced

Contra-indications recent myocardial infarction, arrhythmias (particularly heart block), not indicated in manic phase, severe liver disease

Side-effects dry mouth, sedation, blurred vision (disturbance of accommodation, increased intra-ocular pressure), constipation, nausea, difficulty with micturition; cardiovascular side-effects (such as ECG changes, arrhythmias, postural hypotension, tachycardia, syncope, particularly with high doses); sweating, tremor, rashes and hypersensitivity reactions (including urticaria, photosensitivity), behavioural disturbances (particularly children), hypomania or mania, confusion or delirium (particularly elderly), headache, interference with sexual function, blood sugar changes; increased appetite and weight gain (occasionally weight loss); endocrine side-effects such as testicular enlargement, gynaecomastia, galactorrhoea; also convulsions (see also Cautions), movement disorders and dyskinesias, dysarthria, paraesthesia, taste disturbances, tinnitus, fever, agranulocytosis, leucopenia, eosinophilia, purpura, thrombocytopenia, hyponatraemia (see Hyponatraemia and Antidepressant Therapy, p. 202), abnormal liver function tests (jaundice); for a general outline of side-effects see also notes above; **overdosage:** see Emergency Treatment of Poisoning, p. 31 (high rate of fatality—see notes above)

Dose

- Depression (but not recommended, see notes above), initially 75 mg (elderly and adolescents 30–75 mg) daily in divided doses *or* as a single dose at bedtime increased gradually as necessary to 150–200 mg; CHILD under 16 years not recommended for depression
- Nocturnal enuresis, CHILD 7–10 years 10–20 mg, 11–16 years 25–50 mg at night; max. period of treatment (including gradual withdrawal) 3 months—full physical examination before further course
- Neuropathic pain [unlicensed indication], initially 10–25 mg daily at night, increased if necessary to 75 mg daily; higher doses under specialist supervision
- Migraine prophylaxis [unlicensed indication], initially 10 mg at night, increased if necessary to maintenance of 50–75 mg at night

Amitriptyline (Non-proprietary) PoM

Tablets, coated, amitriptyline hydrochloride 10 mg, net price 28 = 69p; 25 mg, 28 = 69p; 50 mg, 28 = 94p. Label: 2

Oral solution, amitriptyline hydrochloride 25 mg/5 mL, net price 150 mL = £12.40; 50 mg/5 mL, 150 mL = £13.50. Label: 2

Compound preparations

Triptafen® (Goldshield) PoM

Tablets, pink, s/c, amitriptyline hydrochloride 25 mg, perphenazine 2 mg. Net price 20 = £5.10. Label: 2

Triptafen-M® (Goldshield) PoM

Tablets, pink, s/c, amitriptyline hydrochloride 10 mg, perphenazine 2 mg. Net price 20 = £4.56. Label: 2

CLOMIPRAMINE HYDROCHLORIDE

Indications depressive illness, phobic and obsessional states; adjunctive treatment of cataplexy associated with narcolepsy

Cautions see under Amitriptyline Hydrochloride

Contra-indications see under Amitriptyline Hydrochloride

Side-effects see under Amitriptyline Hydrochloride; also diarrhoea; hair loss reported

Dose

- Depressive illness, initially 10 mg daily, increased gradually as necessary to 30–150 mg daily in divided doses *or* as a single dose at bedtime; max. 250 mg daily; ELDERLY initially 10 mg daily increased carefully over approx. 10 days to 30–75 mg daily; CHILD and ADOLESCENT under 18 years not recommended
- Phobic and obsessional states, initially 25 mg daily (ELDERLY 10 mg daily) increased over 2 weeks to 100–150 mg daily; max. 250 mg daily; CHILD and ADOLESCENT under 18 years not recommended
- Adjunctive treatment of cataplexy associated with narcolepsy, initially 10 mg daily, gradually increased until satisfactory response (range 10–75 mg daily); CHILD and ADOLESCENT under 18 years not recommended

Clomipramine (Non-proprietary) PoM

Capsules, clomipramine hydrochloride 10 mg, net price 28-cap pack = £2.14; 25 mg, 28-cap pack = £2.14; 50 mg, 28-cap pack = £4.00. Label: 2

Anafranil® (Novartis) PoM

Capsules, clomipramine hydrochloride 10 mg (yellow/caramel), net price 84-cap pack = £3.23; 25 mg (orange/caramel), 84-cap pack = £6.35; 50 mg (grey/caramel), 56-cap pack = £8.06. Label: 2

Modified release

Anafranil SR® (Novartis) PoM

Tablets, m/r, grey-red, f/c, clomipramine hydrochloride 75 mg. Net price 28-tab pack = £8.83. Label: 2, 25

DOSULEPIN HYDROCHLORIDE

(Dothiepin hydrochloride)

Indications depressive illness, particularly where sedation is required

Cautions see under Amitriptyline Hydrochloride

Contra-indications see under Amitriptyline Hydrochloride

Side-effects see under Amitriptyline Hydrochloride (high rate of fatality—see notes above)

Dose

- Initially 75 mg (ELDERLY 50–75 mg) daily in divided doses *or* as a single dose at bedtime, increased gradually as necessary to 150 mg daily (ELDERLY 75 mg may be sufficient); up to 225 mg daily in some circumstances (e.g. hospital use); CHILD not recommended

Dosulepin (Non-proprietary) PoM
Capsules, dosulepin hydrochloride 25 mg, net price 28-cap pack = 89p. Label: 2
Brands include *Prepadine*®

Tablets, dosulepin hydrochloride 75 mg, net price 28-tab pack = £2.11. Label: 2
Brands include *Prepadine*®

Prothiaden® (Abbott) PoM
Capsules, red/red-brown, dosulepin hydrochloride 25 mg. Net price 28-cap pack = £1.70. Label: 2

Tablets, red, s/c, dosulepin hydrochloride 75 mg. Net price 28-tab pack = £2.97. Label: 2

DOXEPIN

Indications depressive illness, particularly where sedation is required; pruritus in eczema (section 13.3)
Cautions see under Amitriptyline Hydrochloride
Contra-indications see under Amitriptyline Hydrochloride; breast-feeding (Appendix 5)
Side-effects see under Amitriptyline Hydrochloride
Dose
- ADULT and CHILD over 12 years, initially 75 mg daily in divided doses *or* as a single dose at bedtime, adjusted according to response; usual maintenance 30–300 mg daily (doses above 100 mg given in 3 divided doses); ELDERLY initially 10–50 mg daily adjusted according to response (usual maintenance 30–50 mg daily)

Sinepin® (Marlborough) PoM
Capsules, doxepin (as hydrochloride) 25 mg, net price 28-cap pack = £3.77; 50 mg, 28-cap pack = £5.71. Label: 2

IMIPRAMINE HYDROCHLORIDE

Indications depressive illness; nocturnal enuresis in children (see section 7.4.2)
Cautions see under Amitriptyline Hydrochloride
Contra-indications see under Amitriptyline Hydrochloride
Side-effects see under Amitriptyline Hydrochloride, but less sedating
Dose
- Depression, initially up to 75 mg daily in divided doses increased gradually to 150–200 mg (up to 300 mg in hospital patients); up to 150 mg may be given as a single dose at bedtime; ELDERLY initially 10 mg daily, increased gradually to 30–50 mg daily; CHILD not recommended for depression
- Nocturnal enuresis, CHILD 7–8 years 25 mg, 8–11 years 25–50 mg, over 11 years 50–75 mg at bedtime; max. period of treatment (including gradual withdrawal) 3 months—full physical examination before further course

Imipramine (Non-proprietary) PoM
Tablets, coated, imipramine hydrochloride 10 mg, net price 28-tab pack = £1.00; 25 mg, 28-tab pack = 89p. Label: 2

LOFEPRAMINE

Indications depressive illness
Cautions see under Amitriptyline Hydrochloride
Contra-indications see under Amitriptyline Hydrochloride; hepatic and severe renal impairment
Side-effects see under Amitriptyline Hydrochloride, but less sedating, lower incidence of antimuscarinic effects and less dangerous in overdosage; hepatic disorders reported
Dose
- 140–210 mg daily in divided doses; ELDERLY may respond to lower doses; CHILD not recommended

Lofepramine (Non-proprietary) PoM
Tablets, lofepramine 70 mg (as hydrochloride). Net price 56-tab pack = £41.19. Label: 2
Brands include *Feprapax*®

Oral suspension, lofepramine 70 mg/5 mL (as hydrochloride). Net price 150 mL = £22.22. Label: 2
Brands include *Lomont*® (sugar-free)

NORTRIPTYLINE

Indications depressive illness; nocturnal enuresis in children (section 7.4.2); neuropathic pain (section 4.7.3)
Cautions see under Amitriptyline Hydrochloride; manufacturer advises plasma-nortriptyline concentration monitoring if dose above 100 mg daily, but evidence of practical value uncertain
Contra-indications see under Amitriptyline Hydrochloride
Side-effects see under Amitriptyline Hydrochloride, but less sedating
Dose
- Depression, low dose initially increased as necessary to 75–100 mg daily in divided doses *or* as a single dose (max. 150 mg daily); ADOLESCENT and ELDERLY 30–50 mg daily in divided doses; CHILD not recommended for depression
- Nocturnal enuresis, CHILD 7 years 10 mg, 8–11 years 10–20 mg, over 11 years 25–35 mg, at night; max period of treatment (including gradual withdrawal) 3 months—full physical examination and ECG before further course
- Neuropathic pain [unlicensed], initially 10–25 mg daily at night, increased if necessary to 75 mg daily; higher doses under specialist supervision

Allegron® (King) PoM
Tablets, nortriptyline (as hydrochloride) 10 mg, net price 20 = £2.48; 25 mg (orange, scored), 20 = £4.80. Label: 2

TRIMIPRAMINE

Indications depressive illness, particularly where sedation required
Cautions see under Amitriptyline Hydrochloride
Contra-indications see under Amitriptyline Hydrochloride
Side-effects see under Amitriptyline Hydrochloride
Dose
- Initially 50–75 mg daily in divided doses *or* as a single dose at bedtime, increased as necessary to 150–300 mg daily; ELDERLY initially 10–25 mg 3 times daily, maintenance half adult dose may be sufficient; CHILD not recommended

Surmontil® (Aventis Pharma) PoM

Capsules, green/white, trimipramine 50 mg (as maleate). Net price 28-cap pack = £7.91. Label: 2

Tablets, trimipramine (as maleate) 10 mg, net price 28-tab pack = £3.57, 84-tab pack = £10.69; 25 mg, 28-tab pack = £4.71, 84-tab pack = £14.10. Label: 2

Related antidepressants

Tricyclic-related drugs have a lower incidence of antimuscarinic side-effects compared with older tricyclics. The tricyclic-related drugs may also be associated with a lower risk of cardiotoxicity in overdosage.

MIANSERIN HYDROCHLORIDE

Indications depressive illness, particularly where sedation is required

Cautions see under Amitriptyline Hydrochloride; **interactions:** Appendix 1 (antidepressants, tricyclic (related))

Blood counts A full **blood count** is recommended every 4 weeks during the first 3 months of treatment; clinical monitoring should continue subsequently and treatment should be stopped and a full blood count obtained if *fever, sore throat, stomatitis,* or other signs of infection develop.

Contra-indications see under Amitriptyline Hydrochloride

Side-effects see under Amitriptyline Hydrochloride, fewer and milder antimuscarinic and cardiovascular effects; leucopenia, agranulocytosis and aplastic anaemia (particularly in the elderly); jaundice; arthritis, arthralgia

Dose

- Initially 30–40 mg (elderly 30 mg) daily in divided doses *or* as a single dose at bedtime, increased gradually as necessary; usual dose range 30–90 mg; CHILD not recommended

Mianserin (Non-proprietary) PoM

Tablets, mianserin hydrochloride 10 mg, net price 28-tab pack = £8.05; 20 mg, 28-tab pack = £4.12; 30 mg, 28-tab pack = £12.94. Label: 2, 25

TRAZODONE HYDROCHLORIDE

Indications depressive illness, particularly where sedation is required; anxiety

Cautions see under Amitriptyline Hydrochloride; **interactions:** Appendix 1 (antidepressants, tricyclic (related))

Contra-indications see under Amitriptyline Hydrochloride

Side-effects see under Amitriptyline Hydrochloride but fewer antimuscarinic and cardiovascular effects; rarely priapism (discontinue immediately)

Dose

- Depression, initially 150 mg (elderly 100 mg) daily in divided doses after food *or* as a single dose at bedtime; may be increased to 300 mg daily; hospital patients up to max. 600 mg daily in divided doses; CHILD not recommended
- Anxiety, 75 mg daily, increasing if necessary to 300 mg daily; CHILD not recommended

Trazodone (Non-proprietary) PoM

Capsules, trazodone hydrochloride 50 mg, net price 84-cap pack = £18.91; 100 mg, 56-cap pack = £19.02. Label: 2, 21

Tablets, trazodone hydrochloride 150 mg, net price 28-tab pack = £13.57. Label: 2, 21

Molipaxin® (Hoechst Marion Roussel) PoM

Capsules, trazodone hydrochloride 50 mg (violet/green), net price 84-cap pack = £20.74; 100 mg (violet/fawn), 56-cap pack = £24.40. Label: 2, 21

Tablets, pink, f/c, trazodone hydrochloride 150 mg. Net price 28-tab pack = £13.94. Label: 2, 21

Liquid, sugar-free, trazodone hydrochloride 50 mg/5 mL, net price 120 mL = £11.14. Label: 2, 21

4.3.2 Monoamine-oxidase inhibitors (MAOIs)

Monoamine-oxidase inhibitors are used much less frequently than tricyclic and related antidepressants, or SSRIs and related antidepressants because of the dangers of dietary and drug interactions and the fact that it is easier to prescribe MAOIs when tricyclic antidepressants have been unsuccessful than vice versa. **Tranylcypromine** is the most **hazardous** of the MAOIs because of its stimulant action. The drugs of choice are **phenelzine** or **isocarboxazid** which are less stimulant and therefore safer.

Phobic patients and depressed patients with atypical, hypochondriacal, or hysterical features are said to respond best to MAOIs. However, MAOIs should be tried in any patients who are refractory to treatment with other antidepressants as there is occasionally a dramatic response. Response to treatment may be delayed for 3 weeks or more and may take an additional 1 or 2 weeks to become maximal.

Withdrawal If possible MAOIs should be withdrawn slowly (see also section 4.3).

Interactions MAOIs inhibit monoamine oxidase, thereby causing an accumulation of amine neurotransmitters. The metabolism of some amine drugs such as *indirect-acting sympathomimetics* (present in many cough and decongestant preparations, see section 3.10) is also inhibited and their pressor action may be potentiated; the pressor effect of tyramine (in some foods, such as mature cheese, pickled herring, broad bean pods, and *Bovril®*, *Oxo®*, *Marmite®* or any similar meat or yeast extract or fermented soya bean extract) may also be dangerously potentiated. These interactions may cause a dangerous rise in blood pressure. An early warning symptom may be a throbbing headache. Patients should be advised to eat only fresh foods and avoid food that is suspected of being stale or 'going off'. This is especially important with meat, fish, poultry or offal; game should be avoided. The danger of interaction persists for up to 2 weeks after treatment with MAOIs is discontinued. Patients should also avoid alcoholic drinks or de-alcoholised (low alcohol) drinks.

Other antidepressants should **not** be started for 2 weeks after treatment with MAOIs has been stopped (3 weeks if starting clomipramine or imipramine). Some psychiatrists use selected tricyclics in conjunction with MAOIs but this is hazardous, indeed potentially lethal, except in experienced hands and there is no evidence that the combination is more effective than when either constituent is used alone. The combination of tranylcypromine with clomipramine is particularly **dangerous.**

Conversely, an MAOI should not be started until at least 7–14 days after a tricyclic or related antidepressant (3 weeks in the case of clomipramine or imipramine) has been stopped.

In addition, an MAOI should not be started for at least 2 weeks after a previous MAOI has been stopped (then started at a reduced dose).

For other interactions with MAOIs including those with opioid analgesics (notably pethidine), see Appendix 1 (MAOIs). For guidance on interactions relating to the reversible monoamine oxidase inhibitor, moclobemide, see below; for guidance on interactions relating to SSRIs, see p. 208.

PHENELZINE 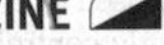

Indications depressive illness

Cautions diabetes mellitus, cardiovascular disease, epilepsy, blood disorders, concurrent electroconvulsive therapy; elderly (great caution); monitor blood pressure (risk of postural hypotension and hypertensive responses—discontinue if palpitations or frequent headaches); if possible avoid abrupt withdrawal; severe hypertensive reactions to certain drugs and foods; avoid in agitated patients; porphyria (section 9.8.2); pregnancy (Appendix 4) and breast-feeding; surgery (section 15.1); **interactions:** Appendix 1 (MAOIs)

Driving Drowsiness may affect performance of skilled tasks (e.g. driving)

Contra-indications hepatic impairment or abnormal liver function tests (Appendix 2), cerebrovascular disease, phaeochromocytoma; not indicated in manic phase

Side-effects commonly postural hypotension (especially in elderly) and dizziness; less common side-effects include drowsiness, insomnia, headache, weakness and fatigue, dry mouth, constipation and other gastro-intestinal disturbances, oedema, myoclonic movement, hyperreflexia, elevated liver enzymes; agitation and tremors, nervousness, euphoria, arrhythmias, blurred vision, nystagmus, difficulty in micturition, sweating, convulsions, rashes, purpura, leucopenia, sexual disturbances, and weight gain with inappropriate appetite may also occur; psychotic episodes with hypomanic behaviour, confusion, and hallucinations may be induced in susceptible persons; suicidal behaviour (see p. 202); jaundice has been reported and, on rare occasions, fatal progressive hepatocellular necrosis; paraesthesia, peripheral neuritis, peripheral neuropathy may be due to pyridoxine deficiency; hyponatraemia (see Hyponatraemia and Antidepressant Therapy, p. 202)

Dose

- 15 mg 3 times daily, increased if necessary to 4 times daily after 2 weeks (hospital patients, max. 30 mg 3 times daily), then reduced gradually to lowest possible maintenance dose (15 mg on alternate days may be adequate); CHILD not recommended

Nardil® (Concord) PoM

Tablets, orange, f/c, phenelzine (as sulphate) 15 mg, net price 20 = £3.99. Label: 3, 10, patient information leaflet

ISOCARBOXAZID

Indications depressive illness

Cautions see under Phenelzine

Contra-indications see under Phenelzine

Side-effects see under Phenelzine

Dose

- Initially 30 mg daily in single or divided doses until improvement occurs (increased after 4 weeks if necessary to max. 60 mg daily for 4–6 weeks under close supervision), then reduced to usual maintenance dose 10–20 mg daily (but up to 40 mg daily may be required); ELDERLY 5–10 mg daily; CHILD not recommended

Isocarboxazid (Non-proprietary) PoM

Tablets, pink, scored, isocarboxazid 10 mg. Net price 56-tab pack = £45.50. Label: 3, 10, patient information leaflet

TRANYLCYPROMINE 

Indications depressive illness

Cautions see under Phenelzine

Contra-indications see under Phenelzine; hyperthyroidism

Side-effects see under Phenelzine; insomnia if given in evening; hypertensive crises with throbbing headache requiring discontinuation of treatment more frequent than with other MAOIs; liver damage less frequent than with phenelzine

Dose

- Initially 10 mg twice daily not later than 3 p.m., increasing the second daily dose to 20 mg after 1 week if necessary; doses above 30 mg daily under close supervision only; usual maintenance dose 10 mg daily; CHILD not recommended

Tranylcypromine (Non-proprietary) PoM

Tablets, tranylcypromine (as sulphate) 10 mg. Net price 28-tab pack = £19.99. Label: 3, 10, patient information leaflet

Reversible MAOIs

Moclobemide is indicated for major depression and social anxiety disorder; it is reported to act by reversible inhibition of monoamine oxidase type A (it is therefore termed a RIMA). It should be reserved as a second-line treatment.

Interactions Moclobemide is claimed to cause less potentiation of the pressor effect of tyramine than the traditional (irreversible) MAOIs, but patients should avoid consuming large amounts of tyramine-rich food (such as mature cheese, yeast extracts and fermented soya bean products).

The risk of drug interactions is also claimed to be less but patients still need to avoid sympathomimetics such as ephedrine and pseudoephedrine. In addition, moclobemide should not be given with another antidepressant. Owing to its short duration of action no treatment-free period is required after it has been stopped but it should not be started until at least a week after a tricyclic or related antidepressant or an SSRI or related antidepressant has been stopped (2 weeks in the case of sertraline, and at least 5 weeks in the case of fluoxetine), or for at least a week after an MAOI has been stopped. For other interactions, see Appendix 1 (moclobemide).

MOCLOBEMIDE

Indications depressive illness; social anxiety disorder

Cautions avoid in agitated or excited patients (or give with sedative for up to 2–3 weeks), thyrotoxicosis, hepatic impairment (Appendix 2), may provoke manic episodes in bipolar disorders, pregnancy (Appendix 4) and breast-feeding (Appendix 5—patient information leaflet advises avoid); **interactions:** see notes above and Appendix 1 (moclobemide)

Contra-indications acute confusional states, phaeochromocytoma

Side-effects sleep disturbances, dizziness, gastro-intestinal disorders, headache, restlessness, agitation; paraesthesia, dry mouth, visual disturbances, oedema, skin reactions, confusional states reported; *rarely* raised liver enzymes, galactorrhoea; hyponatraemia (see Hyponatraemia and Antidepressant Therapy, p. 202)

Dose

- Depression, initially 300 mg daily usually in divided doses after food, adjusted according to response; usual range 150–600 mg daily; CHILD not recommended
- Social anxiety disorder, initially 300 mg daily increased on fourth day to 600 mg daily in 2 divided doses, continued for 8–12 weeks to assess efficacy; CHILD not recommended

Moclobemide (Non-proprietary) PoM
Tablets, moclobemide 150 mg, net price 30-tab pack = £3.20; 300 mg, 30-tab pack = £5.51. Label: 10, patient information leaflet, 21

Manerix® (Roche) PoM
Tablets, yellow, f/c, scored, moclobemide 150 mg, net price 30-tab pack = £9.33; 300 mg, 30-tab pack = £13.99. Label: 10, patient information leaflet, 21

4.3.3 Selective serotonin re-uptake inhibitors

Citalopram, **escitalopram**, **fluoxetine**, **fluvoxamine**, **paroxetine**, and **sertraline** selectively inhibit the re-uptake of serotonin (5-hydroxytryptamine, 5-HT); they are termed selective serotonin re-uptake inhibitors (SSRIs). For a general comment on the management of depression and on the comparison between *tricyclic and related antidepressants* and the *SSRIs and related antidepressants*, see section 4.3.

CSM advice (depressive illness in children and adolescents)

The CSM has advised that the balance of risks and benefits for the treatment of depressive illness in individuals under 18 years is considered unfavourable for the SSRIs citalopram, escitalopram, paroxetine, and sertraline, and for mirtazapine and venlafaxine. Clinical trials have failed to show efficacy and have shown an increase in harmful outcomes. However, it is recognised that specialists may sometimes decide to use these drugs in response to individual clinical need; children and adolescents should be monitored carefully for suicidal behaviour, self-harm or hostility, particularly at the beginning of treatment.

Only fluoxetine has been shown in clinical trials to be effective for treating depressive illness in children and adolescents. However, it is possible that, in common with the other SSRIs, it is associated with a small risk of self-harm and suicidal thoughts. Overall, the balance of risks and benefits for fluoxetine in the treatment of depressive illness in individuals under 18 years is considered favourable, but children and adolescents must be carefully monitored as above.

Cautions SSRIs should be used with caution in patients with epilepsy (avoid if poorly controlled, discontinue if convulsions develop), cardiac disease, diabetes mellitus, susceptibility to angle-closure glaucoma, a history of mania or bleeding disorders (especially gastro-intestinal bleeding), and if used with other drugs that increase the risk of bleeding, hepatic impairment (Appendix 2), renal impairment (Appendix 3), pregnancy (Appendix 4), and breast-feeding (Appendix 5). They should also be used with caution in those receiving concurrent electroconvulsive therapy (prolonged seizures reported with fluoxetine). The risk of suicidal behaviour is possibly higher in young adults, calling for close monitoring of those receiving SSRIs (see also CSM advice, above). SSRIs may also impair performance of skilled tasks (e.g. driving). **Interactions**: see below and Appendix 1 (antidepressants, SSRI).

Withdrawal Gastro-intestinal disturbances, headache, anxiety, dizziness, paraesthesia, sleep disturbances, fatigue, influenza-like symptoms, and sweating are the most common features of abrupt withdrawal of an SSRI or marked reduction of the dose; the dose should be tapered over a few weeks to avoid these effects.

Interactions An SSRI or related antidepressant should not be started until 2 weeks after stopping an MAOI. Conversely, an MAOI should not be started until at least a week after an SSRI or related antidepressant has been stopped (2 weeks in the case of sertraline, at least 5 weeks in the case of fluoxetine). For guidance relating to the reversible monoamine oxidase inhibitor, moclobemide, see above. For other SSRI antidepressant interactions, see Appendix 1 (antidepressants, SSRI).

Contra-indications SSRIs should not be used if the patient enters a manic phase.

Side-effects SSRIs are less sedating and have fewer antimuscarinic and cardiotoxic effects than tricyclic antidepressants (section 4.3). Side-effects of the SSRIs include gastro-intestinal effects (dose-related and fairly common—include nausea, vomiting, dyspepsia, abdominal pain, diarrhoea, constipation), anorexia with weight loss (increased appetite and weight gain also reported) and hypersensitivity reactions including rash (consider discontinuation—may be sign of impending serious systemic reaction, possibly associated with vasculitis), urticaria, angioedema, anaphylaxis, arthralgia, myalgia and photosensitivity; other side-effects include dry mouth, nervousness, anxiety, headache, insomnia, tremor, dizziness, asthenia, hallucinations, drowsiness, convulsions (see Cautions above), galactorrhoea, sexual dysfunction, urinary retention, sweating, hypomania or mania (see Cautions above), movement disorders and dyskinesias, visual disturbances, hyponatraemia (see Hyponatraemia and Antidepressant Therapy, p. 202), and bleeding disorders including ecchymoses and purpura. Suicidal behaviour has been linked with antidepressants (see p. 202). Angle-closure glaucoma may very rarely be precipitated by treatment with SSRIs.

CITALOPRAM

Indications depressive illness, panic disorder

Cautions see notes above

Contra-indications see notes above

Side-effects see notes above; also palpitation, tachycardia, postural hypotension, coughing, yawning, confusion, impaired concentration, malaise, amnesia, migraine, paraesthesia, abnormal dreams, taste disturbance, increased salivation, rhinitis, tinnitus, polyuria, micturition disorders, euphoria; paradoxical increased anxiety during initial treatment of panic disorder (reduce dose)

Dose

- Depressive illness, 20 mg once daily increased if necessary in steps of 20 mg daily at intervals of 3–4 weeks; max. 60 mg daily (ELDERLY over 65 years, max. 40 mg daily); CHILD under 18 years, see *BNF for Children* and CSM advice, p. 208
- Panic disorder, initially 10 mg daily increased gradually if necessary in steps of 10 mg daily, usual dose 20–30 mg daily; max. 60 mg daily (ELDERLY over 65 years, max. 40 mg daily); CHILD under 18 years, not recommended

Note 8 mg (4 drops) *Cipramil®* oral drops is equivalent in therapeutic effect to 10-mg citalopram tablet

Citalopram (Non-proprietary) PoM

Tablets, citalopram (as hydrobromide) 10 mg, net price 28-tab pack = £1.03; 20 mg, 28-tab pack = £1.29; 40 mg, 28-tab pack = £2.00. Counselling, driving

Cipramil® (Lundbeck) PoM

Tablets, f/c, citalopram (as hydrobromide) 10 mg, net price 28-tab pack = £8.97; 20 mg (scored), 28-tab pack = £14.91; 40 mg, 28-tab pack = £25.20. Counselling, driving

Oral drops, sugar-free, citalopram (as hydrochloride) 40 mg/mL, net price 15 mL = £20.16. Counselling, driving, administration

Dose depressive illness, 16 mg daily as a single dose increased if necessary in steps of 16 mg daily at intervals of 3–4 weeks; max. 48 mg daily (ELDERLY over 65 years, max. 32 mg daily); CHILD under 18 years, see *BNF for Children* and CSM advice, p. 208

Panic disorder, initially 8 mg daily as a single dose increased gradually if necessary in steps of 8 mg, usual dose 16–24 mg daily; max. 48 mg daily; (ELDERLY over 65 years, max. 32 mg daily); CHILD under 18 years not recommended

Excipients include alcohol

Note 8 mg (4 drops) *Cipramil®* oral drops may be considered to be equivalent in therapeutic effect to 10-mg citalopram tablet

Mix with water, orange juice, or apple juice before taking

ESCITALOPRAM

Note Escitalopram is the active enantiomer of citalopram

Indications see under Dose

Cautions see notes above

Contra-indications see notes above

Side-effects see notes above; also sinusitis, yawning; fatigue, restlessness, abnormal dreams, paraesthesia; pyrexia; *less commonly* taste disturbance, bruxism, syncope, tachycardia, oedema, confusion, menstrual disturbances, epistaxis, mydriasis, tinnitus, pruritus, and alopecia; *rarely* bradycardia, aggression, and depersonalisation; hepatitis, postural hypotension, QT interval prolongation and thrombocytopenia also reported; paradoxical increased anxiety during initial treatment of panic disorder (reduce dose)

Dose

- ADULT over 18 years, depressive illness, generalised anxiety disorder, and obsessive-compulsive disorder, 10 mg once daily increased if necessary to max. 20 mg daily. ELDERLY initially half adult dose, lower maintenance dose may be sufficient; CHILD not recommended (see CSM advice, p. 208)
- ADULT over 18 years, panic disorder, initially 5 mg once daily increased to 10 mg daily after 7 days; max. 20 mg daily; ELDERLY initially half adult dose, lower maintenance dose may be sufficient
- ADULT over 18 years, social anxiety disorder, initially 10 mg once daily adjusted after 2–4 weeks; usual dose 5–20 mg daily

Cipralex® (Lundbeck) PoM

Tablets, f/c, escitalopram (as oxalate) 5 mg, net price 28-tab pack = £8.97; 10 mg (scored), 28-tab pack = £14.91; 20 mg (scored), 28-tab pack = £25.20. Counselling, driving

Oral drops, sugar-free, escitalopram (as oxalate) 10 mg/mL, net price 28 mL = £18.82. Counselling, driving, administration

Note Can be mixed with water, orange juice, or apple juice before taking

FLUOXETINE

Indications see under Dose

Cautions see notes above

Contra-indications see notes above

Side-effects see notes above; also vasodilatation, postural hypotension, pharyngitis, dyspnoea, chills, taste disturbances, sleep disturbances, euphoria, confusion, yawning, impaired concentration, changes in blood sugar, alopecia, urinary frequency; *rarely* pulmonary inflammation and fibrosis; *very rarely* hepatitis, toxic epidermal necrolysis, and neuroleptic malignant syndrome-like event

Dose

- Major depression, 20 mg once daily increased after 3–4 weeks if necessary, and at appropriate intervals thereafter; max. 60 mg once daily (ELDERLY usual max. 40 mg once daily but 60 mg can be used); CHILD and ADOLESCENT under 18 years, see *BNF for Children*
- Bulimia nervosa, 60 mg once daily; CHILD and ADOLESCENT under 18 years not recommended
- Obsessive-compulsive disorder, 20 mg once daily; if inadequate response after 2 weeks increase gradually to max. 60 mg once daily (ELDERLY usual max. 40 mg

once daily but 60 mg can be used); CHILD and ADOLESCENT under 18 years not recommended

Long duration of action Consider the long half-life of fluoxetine when adjusting dosage (or in overdosage)

Fluoxetine (Non-proprietary) PoM

Capsules, fluoxetine (as hydrochloride) 20 mg, net price 30-cap pack = 69p; 60 mg, 30-cap pack = £49.83. Counselling, driving

Brands include *Oxactin®*

Liquid, fluoxetine (as hydrochloride) 20 mg/5 mL, net price 70 mL = £13.02. Counselling, driving

Brands include *Prozep®*

Prozac® (Lilly) PoM

Capsules, fluoxetine (as hydrochloride) 20 mg (green/yellow), net price 30-cap pack = £14.21. Counselling, driving

Liquid, fluoxetine (as hydrochloride) 20 mg/5 mL, net price 70 mL = £13.26. Counselling, driving

FLUVOXAMINE MALEATE

Indications depressive illness, obsessive-compulsive disorder

Cautions see notes above

CSM advice The CSM has advised that concomitant use of fluvoxamine and theophylline or aminophylline should usually be avoided; see also **interactions**: Appendix 1 (antidepressants, SSRIs)

Contra-indications see notes above

Side-effects see notes above; palpitation, tachycardia (may also cause bradycardia); *rarely* postural hypotension, confusion, ataxia, paraesthesia, malaise, taste disturbance, neuroleptic malignant syndrome-like event, abnormal liver function tests, usually symptomatic (discontinue treatment)

Dose

- Depression, initially 50–100 mg daily in the evening, increased gradually if necessary to max. 300 mg daily (over 150 mg in divided doses); usual maintenance dose 100 mg daily; CHILD and ADOLESCENT under 18 years not recommended
- Obsessive-compulsive disorder, initially 50 mg in the evening increased gradually if necessary after some weeks to max. 300 mg daily (over 150 mg in divided doses); usual maintenance dose 100–300 mg daily; CHILD over 8 years initially 25 mg daily increased if necessary in steps of 25 mg every 4–7 days to max. 200 mg daily (over 50 mg in 2 divided doses)

Note If no improvement in obsessive-compulsive disorder within 10 weeks, treatment should be reconsidered

Fluvoxamine (Non-proprietary) PoM

Tablets, fluvoxamine maleate 50 mg, net price 60-tab pack = £8.48; 100 mg, 30-tab pack = £13.42. Counselling, driving

Faverin® (Solvay) PoM

Tablets, f/c, scored, fluvoxamine maleate 50 mg, net price 60-tab pack = £17.10; 100 mg, 30-tab pack = £17.10. Counselling, driving

PAROXETINE

Indications major depression, obsessive-compulsive disorder, panic disorder; social anxiety disorder; post-traumatic stress disorder; generalised anxiety disorder

Cautions see notes above; also achlorhydria or high gastric pH (reduced absorption of oral suspension)

CSM advice Extrapyramidal reactions (including orofacial dystonias) and withdrawal syndrome are reported to the CSM more commonly with paroxetine than with other SSRIs

Contra-indications see notes above

Side-effects see notes above; also yawning; raised cholesterol; *less commonly* arrhythmias, transient changes in blood pressure, confusion, urinary incontinence; *rarely* panic attacks and paradoxical increased anxiety during initial treatment of panic disorder (reduce dose), depersonalisation, and neuroleptic malignant syndrome-like event; *very rarely* peripheral oedema, acute glaucoma, hepatic disorders (e.g. hepatitis), and priapism

Dose

- Major depression, social anxiety disorder, post-traumatic stress disorder, generalised anxiety disorder, usually 20 mg each morning, higher doses on specialist advice only (see also CSM advice, below); max. 50 mg daily (ELDERLY 40 mg daily); CHILD and ADOLESCENT under 18 years not recommended (see CSM advice, p. 208)
- Obsessive-compulsive disorder, initially 20 mg each morning, increased gradually in steps of 10 mg to usual dose of 40 mg daily, higher doses on specialist advice only (see also CSM advice, below); max. 60 mg daily (ELDERLY 40 mg daily); CHILD and ADOLESCENT under 18 years not recommended
- Panic disorder, initially 10 mg each morning, increased gradually in steps of 10 mg to usual dose of 40 mg daily, higher doses on specialist advice only (see also CSM advice, below); max. 60 mg daily (ELDERLY 40 mg daily); CHILD and ADOLESCENT under 18 years not recommended

CSM advice The recommended dose for the treatment of depression, social anxiety disorder, generalised anxiety disorder, and post-traumatic stress disorder is 20 mg daily and for obsessive-compulsive disorder and panic disorder it is 40 mg daily. There is no evidence that higher doses are more effective.

Paroxetine (Non-proprietary) PoM

Tablets, paroxetine (as hydrochloride) 20 mg, net price 30-tab pack = £4.68; 30 mg, 30-tab pack = £7.45. Label: 21, counselling, driving

Seroxat® (GSK) PoM

Tablets, f/c, scored, paroxetine (as hydrochloride) 10 mg, net price 28-tab pack = £12.32; 20 mg, 30-tab pack = £13.21; 30 mg (blue), 30-tab pack = £23.18. Label: 21, counselling, driving

Oral suspension, orange, sugar-free, paroxetine (as hydrochloride) 10 mg/5 mL. Net price 150-mL pack = £9.49. Label: 5, 21, counselling, driving

SERTRALINE

Indications depressive illness, obsessive-compulsive disorder (under specialist supervision in children), post-traumatic stress disorder in women

Cautions see notes above

Contra-indications see notes above

Side-effects see notes above; pancreatitis, hepatitis, jaundice, liver failure, tachycardia, postural hypotension, amnesia, paraesthesia, aggression, urinary incontinence, and menstrual irregularities also reported

Dose

- Depressive illness, initially 50 mg daily, increased if necessary by increments of 50 mg over several weeks to max. 200 mg daily; usual maintenance dose 50 mg daily; CHILD and ADOLESCENT under 18 years, see *BNF for Children* and CSM advice, p. 208
- Obsessive-compulsive disorder, ADULT and CHILD over 12 years initially 50 mg daily, increased if necessary in steps of 50 mg over several weeks; usual dose range 50–200 mg daily; CHILD 6–12 years initially 25 mg daily, increased to 50 mg daily after 1 week, further increased if necessary in steps of 50 mg at intervals of at least 1 week (max. 200 mg daily)
- Post-traumatic stress disorder, initially 25 mg daily, increased after 1 week to 50 mg daily; if response is partial and if drug tolerated, dose increased in steps of 50 mg over several weeks to max. 200 mg daily; CHILD and ADOLESCENT under 18 years not recommended

Sertraline (Non-proprietary) PoM

Tablets, sertraline (as hydrochloride) 50 mg, net price 28-tab pack = £1.31; 100 mg, 28-tab pack = £2.17. Counselling, driving

Lustral® (Pfizer) PoM

Tablets, f/c, sertraline (as hydrochloride) 50 mg (scored), net price 28-tab pack = £17.82; 100 mg, 28-tab pack = £29.16. Counselling, driving

4.3.4 Other antidepressant drugs

Duloxetine inhibits the re-uptake of both serotonin and noradrenaline and is licensed to treat major depressive disorder.

The thioxanthene **flupentixol** (*Fluanxol®*) has antidepressant properties, and low doses (1 to 3 mg daily) are given by mouth for this purpose. Flupentixol is also used for the treatment of psychoses (section 4.2.1 and section 4.2.2)

Mirtazapine, a presynaptic alpha$_2$-adrenoreceptor antagonist, increases central noradrenergic and serotonergic neurotransmission. It has few antimuscarinic effects, but causes sedation during initial treatment.

Reboxetine, a selective inhibitor of noradrenaline re-uptake, has been introduced for the treatment of depressive illness.

Tryptophan is licensed as adjunctive therapy for depression resistant to standard antidepressants; it has been associated with eosinophilia-myalgia syndrome. Tryptophan should be initiated under specialist supervision.

Venlafaxine is a serotonin and noradrenaline re-uptake inhibitor (SNRI); it lacks the sedative and antimuscarinic effects of the tricyclic antidepressants.

DULOXETINE

Indications major depressive disorder; diabetic neuropathy (section 6.1.5); stress urinary incontinence (section 7.4.2)

Cautions see section 7.4.2; pregnancy (Appendix 4)

Contra-indications see section 7.4.2

Side-effects see section 7.4.2

Dose

- Major depression *or* diabetic neuropathy, 60 mg once daily; CHILD and ADOLESCENT under 18 years not recommended

Note In diabetic neuropathy, discontinue if inadequate response after 2 months; review treatment at least every 3 months

Cymbalta® (Lilly) ▼ PoM

Capsules, duloxetine (as hydrochloride) 30 mg (white/blue), net price 28-cap pack = £22.40; 60 mg (green/blue), 28-cap pack = £27.72. Label: 2

Note The *Scottish Medicines Consortium* has advised (September 2006) that duloxetine (*Cymbalta®*) should be restricted for use by specialists when other treatments for diabetic peripheral neuropathic pain are unsuitable or inadequate

Yentreve® (Lilly) ▼ PoM

Section 7.4.2 (stress urinary incontinence)

FLUPENTIXOL
(Flupenthixol)

Indications depressive illness; psychoses (section 4.2.1)

Cautions cardiovascular disease (including cardiac disorders and cerebral arteriosclerosis), senile confusional states, parkinsonism, hepatic impairment (Appendix 2), renal impairment (Appendix 3); avoid in excitable and overactive patients; porphyria (section 9.8.2); see also section 4.2.1; **interactions**: Appendix 1 (antipsychotics)

Side-effects restlessness, insomnia; hypomania reported; rarely dizziness, tremor, visual disturbances, headache, hyperprolactinaemia, extrapyramidal symptoms; suicidal behaviour (see p. 202)

Dose

- Initially 1 mg (elderly 500 micrograms) in the morning, increased after 1 week to 2 mg (elderly 1 mg) if necessary; max. 3 mg (elderly 2 mg) daily, doses above 2 mg (elderly 1 mg) being divided in 2 portions, second dose not after 4 p.m. Discontinue if no response after 1 week at max. dosage; CHILD and ADOLESCENT under 18 years not recommended

Counselling Although drowsiness may occur, can also have an alerting effect so should not be taken in the evening

Fluanxol® (Lundbeck) PoM

Tablets, both red, s/c, flupentixol (as dihydrochloride) 500 micrograms, net price 60-tab pack = £2.88; 1 mg, 60-tab pack = £4.86. Label: 2, counselling, administration

MIRTAZAPINE

Indications major depression

Cautions cardiac disorders, hypotension, history of urinary retention, susceptibility to angle-closure glaucoma, diabetes mellitus, psychoses (may aggravate psychotic symptoms), history of seizures or bipolar depression; hepatic impairment; renal impairment; pregnancy (Appendix 4); breast-feeding (Appendix 5); **interactions**: Appendix 1 (mirtazapine)

Blood disorders Patients should be advised to report any fever, sore throat, stomatitis or other signs of infection during treatment. Blood count should be performed and the drug stopped immediately if blood dyscrasia suspected

Withdrawal Nausea, vomiting, dizziness, agitation, anxiety, and headache are most common features of withdrawal if treatment stopped abruptly or if dose reduced markedly; dose should be reduced over several weeks

Side-effects increased appetite and weight gain, oedema, sedation; *less commonly* dizziness, headache; *rarely* postural hypotension, abnormal dreams, mania, suicidal behaviour (see p. 202), seizures, tremor, myoclonus, paraesthesia, arthralgia, myalgia, akathisia, rash, and blood disorders including reversible agranulocytosis (see Cautions above); *very rarely* angle-closure glaucoma

Dose

- Initially 15 mg daily at bedtime increased within 2–4 weeks according to response; max. 45 mg daily as a single dose at bedtime or in 2 divided doses; CHILD and ADOLESCENT under 18 years not recommended (see CSM advice, p. 208)

Mirtazapine (Non-proprietary) PoM
Tablets, mirtazapine 15 mg, net price 28-tab pack = £18.37; 30 mg, 28-tab pack = £10.05; 45 mg, 28-tab pack = £14.92. Label: 2, 25

Orodispersible tablets, mirtazapine 15 mg, net price 30-tab pack = £17.25; 30 mg, 30-tab pack = £17.25; 45 mg, 30-tab pack = £17.25. Label: 2, counselling, administration

Oral solution, mirtazapine 15 mg/mL, net price 66 mL = £47.00. Label: 2

Zispin SolTab® (Organon) PoM
Orodispersible tablets, mirtazapine 15 mg, net price 6-tab pack = £3.84, 30-tab pack = £19.19; 30 mg, 30-tab pack = £19.19; 45 mg, 30-tab pack = £19.19. Label: 2, counselling, administration
Excipients include aspartame (section 9.4.1)
Counselling *Zispin SolTab®* should be placed on the tongue, allowed to disperse and swallowed

REBOXETINE

Indications major depression

Cautions history of cardiovascular disease and epilepsy; bipolar disorder; urinary retention; prostatic hypertrophy; susceptibility to angle-closure glaucoma; avoid abrupt withdrawal; hepatic impairment (Appendix 2); renal impairment (Appendix 3); **interactions:** Appendix 1 (reboxetine)

Contra-indications pregnancy (Appendix 4); breast-feeding (Appendix 5)

Side-effects nausea, dry mouth, constipation, anorexia; tachycardia, palpitation, vasodilation, postural hypotension; headache, insomnia, dizziness; chills; impotence; urinary retention; impaired visual accommodation; sweating; lowering of plasma-potassium concentration on prolonged administration in the elderly; *very rarely* angle-closure glaucoma; *also reported* vomiting, hypertension, paraesthesia, agitation, anxiety, irritability, hallucinations, aggression, cold extremities, and rash; suicidal behaviour (see p. 202)

Dose

- 4 mg twice daily increased if necessary after 3–4 weeks to 10 mg daily in divided doses, max. 12 mg daily; CHILD under 18 years and ELDERLY not recommended

Edronax® (Pharmacia) PoM
Tablets, scored, reboxetine (as mesilate) 4 mg, net price 60-tab pack = £18.91. Counselling, driving

TRYPTOPHAN
(L-Tryptophan)

Indications see notes above

Cautions eosinophilia-myalgia syndrome has been reported—close monitoring required (withhold treatment if increased eosinophil count, myalgia, arthralgia, fever, dyspnoea, neuropathy, oedema or skin lesions develop until possibility of eosinophilia-myalgia syndrome excluded); pregnancy and breast-feeding; **interactions:** Appendix 1 (tryptophan)

Contra-indications history of eosinophilia-myalgia syndrome following use of tryptophan

Side-effects drowsiness, nausea, headache, light-headedness, suicidal behaviour (see p. 202); eosinophilia-myalgia syndrome, see Cautions

Dose

- 1 g 3 times daily; max. 6 g daily; ELDERLY lower dose may be appropriate especially where renal or hepatic impairment; CHILD not recommended

Optimax® (Merck) PoM
Tablets, scored, tryptophan 500 mg. Net price 84-tab pack = £23.47. Label: 3

VENLAFAXINE

Indications major depression, generalised anxiety disorder

Cautions heart disease (monitor blood pressure); history of epilepsy; susceptibility to angle-closure glaucoma; concomitant use of drugs that increase risk of bleeding, history of bleeding disorders; hepatic impairment (avoid if severe—Appendix 2); renal impairment (avoid if severe—Appendix 3); breast-feeding (Appendix 5); **interactions:** Appendix 1 (venlafaxine)
Driving May affect performance of skilled tasks (e.g. driving)
Withdrawal Gastro-intestinal disturbances, headache, anxiety, dizziness, paraesthesia, tremor, sleep disturbances, and sweating are most common features of withdrawal if treatment stopped abruptly or if dose reduced markedly; dose should be reduced over several weeks

Contra-indications conditions associated with high risk of cardiac arrhythmia, uncontrolled hypertension; pregnancy (Appendix 4)

Side-effects constipation, nausea, anorexia, weight changes, diarrhoea, dyspepsia, vomiting, abdominal pain; hypertension, palpitation, vasodilatation, changes in serum cholesterol; chills, pyrexia, dyspnoea, yawning; dizziness, dry mouth, insomnia, nervousness, drowsiness, asthenia, headache, abnormal dreams, agitation, anxiety, confusion, hypertonia, paraesthesia, tremor; urinary frequency, sexual dysfunction, menstrual disturbances; arthralgia, myalgia; visual disturbances, mydriasis (very rarely angle-closure glaucoma); tinnitus; sweating, pruritus, rash; *less commonly* bruxism, taste disturbance, hypotension and postural hypotension, arrhythmias, syndrome of inappropriate anti-diuretic hormone secretion (see Hyponatraemia and Antidepressant Therapy, p. 202), apathy, hallucinations, myoclonus, urinary retention, bleeding disorders (including ecchymosis and rarely haemorrhage), alopecia, hypersensitivity reactions including angioedema, urticaria, photosensitivity; *rarely* hepatitis, ataxia, incoordination, speech disorder, mania and hypomania, seizures, and neuroleptic malignant syndrome, Stevens-Johnson syndrome; *very rarely* pancreatitis, QT interval prolongation, aggression, delirium, extrapyramidal symptoms including akathesia, hyperprolactinaemia, blood dyscrasias, rhabdomyolysis; suicidal behaviour (doses over 300 mg under specialist supervision; see also p. 202)

Dose

- Depression, ADULT over 18 years, initially 75 mg daily in 2 divided doses increased if necessary after at least 3–4 weeks to 150 mg daily in 2 divided doses; severely depressed or hospitalised patients, increased further if necessary in steps of up to 75 mg every 2–3 days; max. 375 mg daily; CHILD under 18 years not recommended (see CSM advice, p. 208)
- Generalised anxiety disorder and social anxiety disorder, see under preparations below

Efexor® (Wyeth) PoM
Tablets, peach, venlafaxine (as hydrochloride) 37.5 mg, net price 28-tab pack = £11.71, 56-tab pack = £23.41; 75 mg, 28-tab pack = £19.51, 56-tab pack = £39.03. Label: 3, counselling, driving

Modified release

Efexor® XL (Wyeth) PoM
Capsules, m/r, venlafaxine (as hydrochloride) 75 mg (peach), net price 14-cap pack = £11.71, 28-cap pack = £23.41; 150 mg (orange) 14-cap pack = £19.52, 28-cap pack = £39.03. Label: 3, 25, counselling, driving

Dose depression, ADULT over 18 years, 75 mg daily as a single dose, increased if necessary after at least 2 weeks to 150 mg once daily; max. 225 mg once daily; CHILD under 18 years not recommended (see CSM advice, p. 208)

Generalised anxiety disorder, ADULT over 18 years, 75 mg daily as a single dose; discontinue if no response after 8 weeks

Social anxiety disorder, ADULT over 18 years, 75 mg daily as a single dose; discontinue if no response after 12 weeks

4.4 CNS stimulants and drugs used for attention deficit hyperactivity disorder

Central nervous system stimulants include the **amphetamines** (notably dexamfetamine) **and related drugs** (e.g. methylphenidate). They have very few indications and in particular, should **not** be used to treat depression, obesity, senility, debility, or for relief of fatigue.

Methylphenidate and **atomoxetine** are used for the management of attention deficit hyperactivity disorder (ADHD) in children and adolescents as part of a comprehensive treatment programme. Growth is not generally affected but it is advisable to monitor growth during treatment. **Dexamfetamine** (dexamphetamine) is an alternative in children who do not respond to other drugs. Drug treatment of attention deficit hyperactivity disorder should be initiated by a specialist in ADHD but may be continued by general practitioners, under a shared-care arrangement. Treatment often needs to be continued into adolescence, and may need to be continued into adulthood.

> **NICE guidance**
> **Methylphenidate, atomoxetine, and dexamfetamine for attention deficit hyperactivity disorder (March 2006)**
> Methylphenidate, atomoxetine, and dexamfetamine are options for the treatment of ADHD in children and adolescents as part of a comprehensive treatment programme. Choice of drug should take into consideration:
> - co-morbid conditions (such as tic disorders, Tourette syndrome, and epilepsy);
> - different adverse effects of the drugs;
> - potential for drug misuse;
> - preferences of the child and carers.

Modafinil is used for the treatment of daytime sleepiness associated with narcolepsy or obstructive sleep apnoea syndrome; dependence with long-term use cannot be excluded and it should therefore be used with caution.

Dexamfetamine and methylphenidate [unlicensed indication] are also used to treat narcolepsy.

ATOMOXETINE

Indications attention deficit hyperactivity disorder (initiated by a specialist physician experienced in managing the condition)

Cautions cardiovascular disease including hypertension and tachycardia; monitor growth in children; QT interval prolongation (avoid concomitant administration of drugs that prolong QT interval); history of seizures; susceptibility to angle-closure glaucoma; hepatic impairment (see Hepatic Disorders below; Appendix 2); pregnancy (Appendix 4); breast-feeding (Appendix 5); **interactions:** Appendix 1 (atomoxetine)

Hepatic disorders Following rare reports of hepatic disorders, the CSM has advised that patients and carers should be advised of the risk and be told how to recognise symptoms; prompt medical attention should be sought in case of abdominal pain, unexplained nausea, malaise, darkening of the urine or jaundice

Suicidal ideation Following reports of suicidal thoughts and behaviour, the CSM has advised that patients and their carers should be informed about the risk and told to report clinical worsening, suicidal thoughts or behaviour, irritability, agitation, or depression

Side-effects anorexia, dry mouth, nausea, vomiting, abdominal pain, constipation, dyspepsia, flatulence; palpitation, tachycardia, increased blood pressure, postural hypotension, hot flushes; sleep disturbance, dizziness, headache, fatigue, lethargy, depression, anxiety, irritability, tremor, rigors; urinary retention, enuresis, prostatitis, sexual dysfunction, menstrual disturbances; mydriasis, conjunctivitis; dermatitis, pruritus, rash, sweating, weight changes; *less commonly* suicidal ideation (see Suicidal Ideation, above), cold extremities; *very rarely* hepatic disorders (see Hepatic Disorders above), seizures, angle-closure glaucoma, and Raynaud's phenomenon

Dose

- ADOLESCENT body-weight over 70 kg, initially 40 mg daily for 7 days then increased according to response to usual maintenance dose 80 mg daily; max. 100 mg daily; CHILD over 6 years and ADOLESCENT body-weight up to 70 kg, initially 500 micrograms/kg daily for 7 days then increased according to response to usual maintenance dose 1.2 mg/kg daily (higher dose unlikely to be beneficial)

Note Total daily dose may be given *either* as a single dose in the morning *or* in 2 divided doses with last dose no later than early evening

Strattera® (Lilly) ▼ PoM

Capsules, atomoxetine (as hydrochloride) 10 mg (white), net price 7-cap pack = £15.02, 28-cap pack = £60.06; 18 mg (gold/white), 7-cap pack = £15.02, 28-cap pack = £60.06; 25 mg (blue/white), 7-cap pack = £15.02, 28-cap pack = £60.06; 40 mg (blue), 7-cap pack = £15.02, 28-cap pack = £60.06; 60 mg (blue/gold), 28-cap pack = £60.06. Label: 3

DEXAMFETAMINE SULPHATE

(Dexamphetamine sulphate)

Indications narcolepsy, refractory attention deficit hyperactivity disorder (under specialist supervision)

Cautions mild hypertension (contra-indicated if moderate or severe)—monitor blood pressure; history of epilepsy (discontinue if convulsions occur); tics and Tourette syndrome (use with caution)—discontinue if tics occur; monitor growth in children (see also below); susceptibility to angle-closure glaucoma; avoid abrupt withdrawal; data on safety and efficacy of long-term use not complete; porphyria (see section 9.8.2); **interactions:** Appendix 1 (sympathomimetics)

Special cautions in children Monitor height and weight as growth restriction may occur during prolonged therapy (drug-free periods may allow catch-up in growth but withdraw slowly to avoid inducing depression or renewed hyperactivity). In psychotic children may exacerbate behavioural disturbances and thought disorder

Driving May affect performance of skilled tasks (e.g. driving); effects of alcohol unpredictable

Contra-indications cardiovascular disease including moderate to severe hypertension, hyperexcitability or agitated states, hyperthyroidism, history of drug or alcohol abuse; pregnancy (Appendix 4); breast-feeding (Appendix 5)

Side-effects insomnia, restlessness, irritability and excitability, nervousness, night terrors, euphoria, tremor, dizziness, headache; convulsions (see also Cautions); dependence and tolerance, sometimes psychosis; anorexia, gastro-intestinal symptoms, growth restriction in children (see also under Cautions); dry mouth, sweating, tachycardia (and anginal pain), palpitation, increased blood pressure; visual disturbances; cardiomyopathy reported with chronic use; central stimulants have provoked choreoathetoid movements, tics and Tourette syndrome in predisposed individuals (see also Cautions above); *very rarely* angle-closure glaucoma; **overdosage:** see Emergency Treatment of Poisoning, p. 33

Dose

- Narcolepsy, 10 mg (ELDERLY, 5 mg) daily in divided doses increased by 10 mg (ELDERLY, 5 mg) daily at intervals of 1 week to a max. of 60 mg daily
- Refractory attention deficit hyperactivity disorder, CHILD 4–6 years, 2.5 mg daily, increased if necessary by 2.5 mg daily at intervals of 1 week; CHILD over 6 years 5–10 mg daily, increased if necessary by 5 mg daily at intervals of 1 week; usual max. 20 mg daily (older children have received max. 40 mg daily); maintenance dose given in 2–3 divided doses

Dexedrine® (Celltech) CD

Tablets, scored, dexamfetamine sulphate 5 mg. Net price 28-tab pack = £3.00. Counselling, driving

METHYLPHENIDATE HYDROCHLORIDE

Indications attention deficit hyperactivity disorder (under specialist supervision); narcolepsy [unlicensed indication]

Cautions monitor growth (if prolonged treatment), blood pressure and full blood count; epilepsy (discontinue if increased seizure frequency); susceptibility to angle-closure glaucoma; avoid abrupt withdrawal; pregnancy (Appendix 4); **interactions:** Appendix 1 (sympathomimetics)

Contra-indications anxiety or agitation; severe depression, suicidal ideation; tics or a family history of Tourette syndrome; drug or alcohol dependence; psychosis; hyperthyroidism; cardiovascular disease; breast-feeding (Appendix 5)

Side-effects abdominal pain, nausea, vomiting, dyspepsia, dry mouth, anorexia, reduced weight gain; tachycardia, palpitation, arrhythmias, changes in blood pressure; tics (*very rarely* Tourette Syndrome), insomnia, nervousness, asthenia, depression, irritability, aggression, headache, drowsiness, dizziness, movement disorders; fever; arthralgia; rash, pruritus, alopecia; *less commonly* diarrhoea, abnormal dreams, confusion, suicidal ideation, urinary frequency, haematuria, muscle cramps, epistaxis; *rarely* angina, growth restriction, visual disturbances; *very rarely* hepatic dysfunction, myocardial infarction, cerebral arteritis, psychosis, neuroleptic malignant syndrome, tolerance and dependence, blood disorders including leucopenia and thrombocytopenia, angle-closure glaucoma, exfoliative dermatitis, erythema multiforme

Dose

- Attention deficit hyperactivity disorder, CHILD 4–6 years [unlicensed], 2.5 mg twice daily increased if necessary at weekly intervals by 2.5 mg daily to max. 1.4 mg/kg daily in divided doses; CHILD over 6 years, initially 5 mg 1–2 times daily, increased if necessary at weekly intervals by 5–10 mg daily to max. 60 mg daily in divided doses; discontinue if no response after 1 month, also suspend every 1–2 years to assess child's condition

  Evening dose If effect wears off in evening (with rebound hyperactivity) a dose at bedtime may be appropriate (establish need with trial bedtime dose)
- Narcolepsy [unlicensed indication], 10–60 mg (usually 20–30 mg) daily in divided doses before meals

Methylphenidate Hydrochloride (Non-proprietary) CD

Tablets, methylphenidate hydrochloride 5 mg, net price 30-tab pack = £2.78; 10 mg, 30-tab pack = £5.83; 20 mg, 30-tab pack = £9.98

Brands include *Equasym®*, *Medikinet®*

Ritalin® (Novartis) CD

Tablets, scored, methylphenidate hydrochloride 10 mg, net price 30-tab pack = £5.57

Modified release

Concerta® XL (Janssen-Cilag) CD

Tablets, m/r, methylphenidate hydrochloride 18 mg (yellow), net price 30-tab pack = £29.70; 27 mg (grey), 30-tab pack = £35.06; 36 mg (white), 30-tab pack = £40.43. Label: 25

Counselling Tablet membrane may pass through gastro-intestinal tract unchanged

Cautions dose form not appropriate for use in dysphagia or where gastro-intestinal lumen restricted
Dose CHILD over 6 years, initially 18 mg once daily (in the morning), increased if necessary in weekly steps of 18 mg according to response, max. 54 mg once daily; discontinue if no response after 1 month; suspend every 1–2 years to assess condition
Note Total daily dose of 15 mg of standard-release formulation is considered equivalent to *Concerta*® *XL* 18 mg once daily

Equasym XL® (UCB Pharma) CD
Capsules, m/r, methylphenidate hydrochloride 10 mg (white/green), net price 30-cap pack = £25.00; 20 mg (white/blue), 30-cap pack = £30.00; 30 mg (white/brown), 30-cap pack = £35.00. Label: 25
Dose CHILD over 6 years, initially 10 mg once daily in the morning before breakfast, increased gradually if necessary to max. 60 mg daily; discontinue if no response after 1 month; suspend every 1–2 years to assess condition
Note Contents of capsule can be sprinkled on a tablespoon of apple sauce (then swallowed immediately without chewing)

Medikinet XL® (Flynn) CD
Capsules, m/r, methylphenidate hydrochloride 10 mg (lilac/white), net price 28-cap pack = £21.00; 20 mg (lilac), 28-cap pack = £28.00; 30 mg (purple/light grey), 28-cap pack = £33.72; 40 mg (purple/grey), 28-cap pack = £44.95. Label: 25
Dose CHILD over 6 years, 10 mg once daily in the morning with breakfast, adjusted according to response, max. 60 mg daily; discontinue if no response after 1 month; suspend every 1–2 years to assess condition
Note Contents of capsule can be sprinkled on a tablespoon of apple sauce (then swallowed immediately without chewing)

MODAFINIL

Indications daytime sleepiness associated with narcolepsy, obstructive sleep apnoea syndrome, and chronic shift work
Cautions monitor blood pressure and heart rate in hypertensive patients (but see Contra-indications); possibility of dependence; hepatic impairment (Appendix 2); renal impairment (Appendix 3); **interactions**: Appendix 1 (modafinil)
Contra-indications moderate to severe uncontrolled hypertension, arrhythmia; history of left ventricular hypertrophy, cor pulmonale, or of clinically significant signs of CNS stimulant-induced mitral valve prolapse (including ischaemic ECG changes, chest pain and arrhythmias); pregnancy (Appendix 4); breast-feeding (Appendix 5)
Side-effects dry mouth, appetite changes, gastro-intestinal disturbances (including nausea, diarrhoea, constipation, and dyspepsia), abdominal pain; tachycardia, vasodilation, chest pain, palpitation; headache (uncommonly migraine), anxiety, sleep disturbances, dizziness, depression, confusion, paraesthesia, agitation, asthenia; visual disturbances; *less commonly* mouth ulcers, glossitis, pharyngitis, dysphagia, taste disturbance, hypertension, hypotension, bradycardia, arrhythmia, peripheral oedema, hypercholesterolaemia rhinitis, dyspnoea, dyskinesia, amnesia, emotional lability, abnormal dreams, tremor, decreased libido, weight changes, hyperglycaemia, urinary frequency, menstrual disturbances, eosinophilia, leucopenia, myasthenia, muscle cramps, dry eye, sinusitis, epistaxis, myalgia, arthralgia, acne, sweating, rash, and pruritus; *very rarely* psychosis and mania
Dose
- Narcolepsy and obstructive sleep apnoea syndrome, initially 200 mg daily, *either* in 2 divided doses morning and at noon *or* as a single dose in the morning, dose adjusted according to response to 200–400 mg daily in 2 divided doses or as a single dose; ELDERLY initiate at 100 mg daily; CHILD not recommended
- Chronic shift work sleep disorder, 200 mg taken 1 hour before the start of the work shift

Provigil® (Cephalon) ▼ PoM
Tablets, modafinil 100 mg, net price 30-tab pack = £55.80; 200 mg, 30 tab-pack = £111.60

Cocaine

Cocaine is a drug of addiction which causes central nervous stimulation. Its clinical use is mainly as a topical local anaesthetic (section 15.2). It has been included in analgesic elixirs for the relief of pain in palliative care but this use is obsolete. For management of cocaine poisoning, see p. 33.

4.5 Drugs used in the treatment of obesity

4.5.1 Anti-obesity drugs acting on the gastro-intestinal tract
4.5.2 Centrally acting appetite suppressants

Obesity is associated with many health problems including cardiovascular disease, diabetes mellitus, gallstones and osteoarthritis. Factors that aggravate obesity may include depression, other psychosocial problems, and some drugs.

The main treatment of the obese individual is a suitable diet, carefully explained to the individual, with appropriate support and encouragement; the individual should also be advised to increase physical activity. Smoking cessation (while maintaining body weight) may be worthwhile before attempting supervised weight loss since cigarette smoking may be more harmful than obesity. Attendance at groups (e.g 'weight-watchers') helps some individuals.

Severe obesity should be managed in an appropriate setting by staff who have been trained in the management of obesity; the individual should receive advice on diet and lifestyle modification and be monitored for changes in weight as well as in blood pressure, blood lipids and other associated conditions.

An anti-obesity drug should be considered only for those with a body mass index (BMI, individual's body-weight divided by the square of the individual's height) of 30 kg/m^2 or greater in whom at least 3 months of managed care involving supervised diet, exercise and behaviour modification fails to achieve a realistic reduction in weight. In the presence of risk factors (such as diabetes, coronary heart disease, hypertension, and obstructive sleep apnoea), it may be appropriate to prescribe a drug to individuals with a BMI of 27 kg/m^2 or greater, provided that such use is permitted by the drug's marketing authorisation. Drugs should **never** be used as the sole element of treatment. The individual should be monitored on a regular basis; drug treatment should be discontinued if the individual regains weight at any time whilst receiving drug treatment.

Drugs specifically licensed for the management of obesity are **orlistat** (section 4.5.1), **sibutramine** and **rimonabant** (both section 4.5.2). There is little evidence to guide selection between these drugs, but it may be appropriate to choose orlistat for those who have a high intake of fats whereas sibutramine or rimonabant may be chosen for those who cannot control their eating.

Combination therapy involving more than one anti-obesity drug is **contra-indicated** until further information about efficacy and long-term safety is available.

Thyroid hormones have **no** place in the treatment of obesity except in biochemically proven hypothyroid patients. The use of diuretics, chorionic gonadotrophin, or amphetamines is **not** appropriate for weight reduction.

4.5.1 Anti-obesity drugs acting on the gastro-intestinal tract

Orlistat, a lipase inhibitor, reduces the absorption of dietary fat. It is used in conjunction with a mildly hypocaloric diet in individuals with a body mass index (BMI) of 30 kg/m^2 or more *or* in individuals with a BMI of 28 kg/m^2 in the presence of other risk factors such as type 2 diabetes, hypertension, or hypercholesterolaemia.

Orlistat should be used in conjunction with other lifestyle measures to manage obesity (section 4.5); treatment should only be continued beyond 12 months after discussing potential benefits and risks with the patient. On stopping orlistat, there may be a gradual reversal of weight loss.

Some of the weight loss in those taking orlistat probably results from individuals reducing their fat intake to avoid severe gastro-intestinal effects including steatorrhoea. Vitamin supplementation (especially of vitamin D) may be considered if there is concern about deficiency of fat-soluble vitamins.

The most commonly used bulk-forming drug is **methylcellulose** (section 1.6.1). It is claimed to reduce intake by producing a feeling of satiety but there is little evidence to support its use in the management of obesity.

ORLISTAT

Indications adjunct in obesity (see notes above)

Cautions may impair absorption of fat-soluble vitamins; pregnancy (Appendix 4); **interactions**: Appendix 1 (orlistat)

Multivitamins If a multivitamin supplement is required, it should be taken at least 2 hours after orlistat dose or at bedtime

Contra-indications chronic malabsorption syndrome; cholestasis; breast-feeding (Appendix 5)

Side-effects oily leakage from rectum, flatulence, faecal urgency, liquid or oily stools, faecal incontinence, abdominal distension and pain (gastro-intestinal effects minimised by reduced fat intake), tooth and gingival disorders; respiratory infections; fatigue, anxiety, headache; menstrual disturbances, urinary-tract infection; hypoglycaemia; *rarely* rectal bleeding; *very rarely* diverticulitis, cholelithiasis, hepatitis, and bullous eruptions

Dose

- ADULT over 18 years, 120 mg taken immediately before, during, or up to 1 hour after each main meal (up to max. 360 mg daily); continue treatment beyond 12 weeks only if weight loss since start of treatment exceeds 5% (target for initial weight loss may be lower in patients with type 2 diabetes); CHILD over 12 years, initiated by specialist only [unlicensed use]

Note If a meal is missed or contains no fat, the dose of orlistat should be omitted

Xenical® (Roche) PoM
Capsules, turquoise, orlistat 120 mg, net price 84-cap pack = £33.58

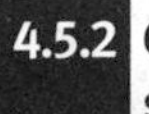

4.5.2 Centrally acting appetite suppressants

Sibutramine inhibits the re-uptake of noradrenaline and serotonin. It is used in the adjunctive management of obesity in individuals with a body mass index (BMI) of 30 kg/m^2 or more (and no associated co-morbidity) or in individuals with a BMI of 27 kg/m^2 or more in the presence of other risk factors such as type 2 diabetes or dyslipidaemia. Sibutramine is not licensed for use for longer than 1 year; on stopping sibutramine, there may be a gradual reversal of weight loss.

Rimonabant is a cannabinoid receptor antagonist for the adjunctive management of obesity in individuals with a BMI of 30 kg/m^2 or more, or in individuals with a BMI above 27 kg/m^2 in the presence of other risk factors such as type 2 diabetes or dyslipidaemia. On stopping rimonabant, there may be a gradual reversal of weight loss.

Dexfenfluramine, fenfluramine, and phentermine have been associated with valvular heart disease and the rare but serious risk of pulmonary hypertension.

RIMONABANT

Indications adjunct in obesity (see notes above)

Cautions epilepsy; history of suicidal ideation or of depressive disorder (avoid unless no alternative); elderly over 75 years; hepatic impairment (avoid if severe—Appendix 2); **interactions**: Appendix 1 (rimonabant)

Contra-indications major depressive illness, concomitant treatment with antidepressant; uncontrolled psychiatric illness; severe renal impairment; pregnancy (Appendix 4); breast-feeding (Appendix 5)

Depression Patients and carers should be informed of the risk of depression and advised to stop treatment and seek medical attention if symptoms occur

Side-effects nausea, vomiting, diarrhoea, dry mouth, anorexia; depression (see above), anxiety, irritability, nervousness, sleep disorders, impaired memory, dizziness, paraesthesia, hypoaesthesia, sciatica, hot flush, asthenia, impaired attention; tendonitis, muscle cramp; pruritus, hyperhidrosis; *less commonly* hiccups, anger, aggression, suicidal ideation; *rarely* hallucinations

Dose

- ADULT over 18 years 20 mg daily before breakfast

Acomplia® (Sanofi-Aventis) ▼ PoM
Tablets, f/c, rimonabant 20 mg, net price 28-tab pack = £44.00. Counselling, depression (see above)

SIBUTRAMINE HYDROCHLORIDE

Indications adjunct in obesity (see notes above)

Cautions monitor blood pressure and pulse rate (every 2 weeks for first 3 months *then* monthly for 3 months *then* at least every 3 months)—discontinue if blood pressure exceeds 145/90 mmHg or if systolic or diastolic pressure raised by more than 10 mmHg or if pulse rate raised by 10 beats per minute at 2 consecutive visits; sleep apnoea syndrome (increased risk of hypertension); epilepsy; open-angle glaucoma, susceptibility to angle-closure glaucoma, history of ocular hypertension; monitor for pulmonary hypertension; family history of motor or vocal tics, history of depression; predisposition to bleeding, concomitant use of drugs that increase risk of bleeding; hepatic impairment (avoid if severe; Appendix 2); renal impairment (avoid if creatinine clearance less than 30 mL/minute; Appendix 3); **interactions**: Appendix 1 (sibutramine)

Contra-indications history of major eating disorders; psychiatric illness, Tourette syndrome; history of coronary artery disease, congestive heart failure, tachycardia, peripheral arterial occlusive disease, arrhythmias, and of cerebrovascular disease; uncontrolled hypertension; hyperthyroidism; prostatic hypertrophy; phaeochromocytoma; history of drug or alcohol abuse; pregnancy (Appendix 4); breast-feeding (Appendix 5)

Side-effects constipation, dry mouth, nausea, taste disturbances, diarrhoea, vomiting, gastro-intestinal haemorrhage, haemorrhoid aggravation; tachycardia, palpitation, arrhythmias, hypertension, flushing; insomnia, lightheadedness, paraesthesia, headache, anxiety, depression, seizures, transient memory disturbance; sexual dysfunction, menstrual disturbances, urinary retention; thrombocytopenia; blurred vision; sweating, alopecia, cutaneous bleeding disorders, hypersensitivity reactions including Henoch-Shönlein purpura, rash, urticaria, angioedema and anaphylaxis; interstitial nephritis, glomerulonephritis; *rarely* headache and increased appetite on withdrawal; *very rarely* angle-closure glaucoma

Dose

- Initially 10 mg daily in the morning, increased if weight loss less than 2 kg after 4 weeks to 15 mg daily; discontinue if weight loss less than 2 kg after 4 weeks at higher dose (see also Discontinuation of Treatment below); max. period of treatment 1 year; CHILD over 12 years, initiated by specialist only [unlicensed use]; ELDERLY over 65 years not recommended

Discontinuation of treatment Discontinue treatment if:

- weight loss after 3 months less than 5% of initial body-weight;
- weight loss stabilises at less than 5% of initial body-weight;
- individuals regain 3 kg or more after previous weight loss

In individuals with co-morbid conditions, treatment should be continued only if weight loss is associated with other clinical benefits

Reductil® (Abbott) PoM
Capsules, sibutramine hydrochloride 10 mg (blue/yellow), net price 28-cap pack = £36.90; 15 mg (blue/white), 28-cap pack = £43.65

4.6 Drugs used in nausea and vertigo

Antiemetics should be prescribed only when the cause of vomiting is known because otherwise they may delay diagnosis, particularly in children. Antiemetics are unnecessary and sometimes harmful when the cause can be treated, such as in diabetic ketoacidosis, or in digoxin or antiepileptic overdose.

If antiemetic drug treatment is indicated, the drug is chosen according to the aetiology of vomiting.

Antihistamines are effective against nausea and vomiting resulting from many underlying conditions. There is no evidence that any one antihistamine is superior to another but their duration of action and incidence of adverse effects (drowsiness and antimuscarinic effects) differ.

The **phenothiazines** are dopamine antagonists and act centrally by blocking the chemoreceptor trigger zone. They are of considerable value for the prophylaxis and treatment of nausea and vomiting associated with diffuse neoplastic disease, radiation sickness, and the emesis caused by drugs such as opioids, general anaesthetics, and cytotoxics. **Prochlorperazine**, **perphenazine**, and **trifluoperazine** are less sedating than **chlorpromazine**; severe dystonic reactions sometimes occur with phenothiazines, especially in children. Other antipsychotic drugs including **haloperidol** and **levomepromazine** (**methotrimeprazine**) (section 4.2.1) are also used for the relief of nausea. Some phenothiazines are available as rectal suppositories, which can be useful in patients with persistent vomiting or with severe nausea; prochlorperazine can also be administered as a buccal tablet which is placed between the upper lip and the gum.

Metoclopramide is an effective antiemetic and its activity closely resembles that of the phenothiazines. Metoclopramide also acts directly on the gastro-intestinal tract and it may be superior to the phenothiazines for emesis associated with gastroduodenal, hepatic, and biliary disease. In postoperative nausea and vomiting, metoclopramide in a dose of 10 mg has limited efficacy. High-dose metoclopramide injection is now less commonly used for cytotoxic-induced nausea and vomiting. As with the phenothiazines, metoclopramide can induce acute dystonic reactions involving facial and skeletal muscle spasms and oculogyric crises. These dystonic effects are more common in the young (especially girls and young women) and the very old; they usually occur shortly after starting treatment with metoclopramide and subside within 24 hours of stopping it. Injection of an antiparkinsonian drug such as procyclidine (section 4.9.2) will abort dystonic attacks.

Domperidone acts at the chemoreceptor trigger zone; it is used for the relief of nausea and vomiting, especially when associated with cytotoxic therapy. It has the advantage over metoclopramide and the phenothiazines of being less likely to cause central effects such as sedation and dystonic reactions because it does not readily cross the blood-brain barrier. In Parkinson's disease, it is used to prevent nausea and vomiting during treatment with apomorphine and also to treat nausea caused by other dopaminergic drugs (section 4.9.1). Domperidone is also used to treat vomiting due to emergency hormonal contraception (section 7.3.5).

Dolasetron, **granisetron**, **ondansetron**, and **tropisetron** are specific $5HT_3$ antagonists which block $5HT_3$ receptors in the gastro-intestinal tract and in the CNS. They are of value in the management of nausea and vomiting in patients receiving cytotoxics and in postoperative nausea and vomiting. **Palonosetron** is licensed for prevention of nausea and vomiting associated with moderately or highly emetogenic cytotoxic chemotherapy.

Dexamethasone (section 6.3.2) has antiemetic effects and it is used in vomiting associated with cancer chemotherapy. It can be used alone or with metoclopramide, prochlorperazine, lorazepam, or a $5HT_3$ antagonist (see also section 8.1).

Aprepitant, a neurokinin 1 receptor antagonist, is licensed for the prevention of acute and delayed nausea and vomiting associated with cisplatin-based cytotoxic chemotherapy; it is given with dexamethasone and a $5HT_3$ antagonist.

Nabilone is a synthetic cannabinoid with antiemetic properties. It may be used for nausea and vomiting caused by cytotoxic chemotherapy that is unresponsive to conventional antiemetics. Side-effects such as drowsiness and dizziness occur frequently with standard doses.

Vomiting during pregnancy

Nausea in the first trimester of pregnancy is generally mild and does not require drug therapy. On rare occasions if vomiting is severe, short-term treatment with an antihistamine, such as **promethazine**, may be required. **Prochlorperazine** or **metoclopramide** may be considered as second-line treatments. If symptoms do not settle in 24 to 48 hours then specialist opinion should be sought. Hyperemesis gravidarum is a more serious condition, which requires intravenous fluid and electrolyte replacement and sometimes nutritional support. Supplementation with thiamine must be considered in order to reduce the risk of Wernicke's encephalopathy.

Postoperative nausea and vomiting

The incidence of postoperative nausea and vomiting depends on many factors including the anaesthetic used, the type and duration of surgery, and the patient's sex. The aim is to prevent postoperative nausea and vomiting from occurring. Drugs used include some **phenothiazines** (e.g. prochlorperazine), **metoclopramide** (but 10-mg dose has limited efficacy and higher parenteral doses associated with greater side-effects), **$5HT_3$ antagonists**, **antihistamines** (such as cyclizine), and **dexamethasone**. A combination of two antiemetic drugs acting at different sites may be needed in resistant postoperative nausea and vomiting.

Motion sickness

Antiemetics should be given to prevent motion sickness rather than after nausea or vomiting develop. The most effective drug for the prevention of motion sickness is **hyoscine**. A transdermal hyoscine patch provides prolonged activity but it needs to be applied several hours before travelling. The sedating antihistamines are slightly less effective against motion sickness, but are generally better tolerated than hyoscine. If a sedative effect is desired **promethazine** is useful, but generally a slightly less sedating antihistamine such as **cyclizine** or **cinnarizine** is preferred. The $5HT_3$ antagonists, domperidone, metoclopramide, and the phenothiazines (except the antihistamine phenothiazine promethazine) are **ineffective** in motion sickness.

Other vestibular disorders

Management of vestibular diseases is aimed at treating the underlying cause as well as treating symptoms of the balance disturbance and associated nausea and vomiting. Vertigo and nausea associated with Ménière's disease and middle-ear surgery can be difficult to treat.

Betahistine is an analogue of histamine and is claimed to reduce endolymphatic pressure by improving the microcirculation. Betahistine is licensed for vertigo, tinnitus, and hearing loss associated with Ménière's disease.

A **diuretic** alone or combined with salt restriction may provide some benefit in vertigo associated with Ménière's disease; **antihistamines** (such as cinnarizine), and **phenothiazines** (such as prochlorperazine) are also used.

For advice to avoid the inappropriate prescribing of drugs (notably phenothiazines) for dizziness in the elderly, see Prescribing for the Elderly, p. 19.

Cytotoxic chemotherapy

For the management of nausea and vomiting induced by cytotoxic chemotherapy, see section 8.1.

Palliative care

For the management of nausea and vomiting in palliative care, see p. 17 and p. 18.

Migraine

For the management of nausea and vomiting associated with migraine, see p. 242.

Antihistamines

CINNARIZINE

Indications vestibular disorders, such as vertigo, tinnitus, nausea, and vomiting in Ménière's disease; motion sickness

Cautions see section 3.4.1; pregnancy (Appendix 4); breast-feeding (Appendix 5)

Contra-indications see section 3.4.1

Side-effects see section 3.4.1; also *rarely* weight gain, sweating, lichen planus, and lupus-like skin reactions

Dose

- Vestibular disorders, 30 mg 3 times daily; CHILD 5–12 years 15 mg 3 times daily
- Motion sickness, 30 mg 2 hours before travel then 15 mg every 8 hours during journey if necessary; CHILD 5–12 years, 15 mg 2 hours before travel then 7.5 mg every 8 hours during journey if necessary

Cinnarizine (Non-proprietary)
Tablets, cinnarizine 15 mg, net price 84-tab pack = £11.40. Label: 2

Stugeron® (Janssen-Cilag)
Tablets, scored, cinnarizine 15 mg, net price 15-tab pack = £1.48, 100-tab pack = £3.49. Label: 2

With dimenhydrinate

Arlevert® (Ashbourne) PoM
Tablets, cinnarizine 20 mg, dimenhydrinate 40 mg, net price 100-tab pack = £14.21. Label: 2
Dose ADULT over 18 years, 1 tablet 3 times daily

CYCLIZINE

Indications nausea, vomiting, vertigo, motion sickness, labyrinthine disorders

Cautions see section 3.4.1; severe heart failure; may counteract haemodynamic benefits of opioids; **interactions**: Appendix 1 (antihistamines)

Contra-indications see section 3.4.1

Side-effects see section 3.4.1

Dose
- By mouth, cyclizine hydrochloride 50 mg up to 3 times daily; CHILD 6–12 years 25 mg up to 3 times daily
- By intramuscular *or* intravenous injection, cyclizine lactate 50 mg 3 times daily

Valoid® (Amdipharm)
Tablets, scored, cyclizine hydrochloride 50 mg. Net price 20 = £1.48. Label: 2
Injection PoM, cyclizine lactate 50 mg/mL. Net price 1-mL amp = 49p

PROMETHAZINE HYDROCHLORIDE

Indications nausea, vomiting, vertigo, labyrinthine disorders, motion sickness; other indications (section 3.4.1, section 4.1.1, section 15.1.4.1)

Cautions see section 3.4.1; also pregnancy (Appendix 4) and breast-feeding (Appendix 5)

Contra-indications see section 3.4.1

Side-effects see section 3.4.1 but more sedating; intramuscular injection may be painful

Dose
- Motion sickness prevention, 20–25 mg at bedtime on night before travel, repeat following morning if necessary; CHILD under 2 years not recommended, 2–5 years 5 mg at night and following morning if necessary, 5–10 years 10 mg at night and following morning if necessary

Preparations
Section 3.4.1

PROMETHAZINE TEOCLATE

Indications nausea, vertigo, labyrinthine disorders, motion sickness (acts longer than the hydrochloride)

Cautions see section 3.4.1; also pregnancy (Appendix 4) and breast-feeding (Appendix 5)

Contra-indications see section 3.4.1

Side-effects see section 3.4.1

Dose
- 25–75 mg, max. 100 mg, daily; CHILD 5–10 years, 12.5–37.5 mg daily
- Motion sickness prevention, ADULT and CHILD over 10 years, 25 mg at bedtime on night before travel *or* 25 mg 1–2 hours before travel; CHILD 5–10 years, 12.5 mg at bedtime on night before travel *or* 12.5 mg 1–2 hours before travel
- Severe vomiting in pregnancy [unlicensed], 25 mg at bedtime, increased if necessary to max. 100 mg daily (but see also Vomiting During Pregnancy in notes above)

Avomine® (Manx)
Tablets, scored, promethazine teoclate 25 mg. Net price 10-tab pack = £1.13; 28-tab pack = £3.13. Label: 2

Phenothiazines and related drugs

CHLORPROMAZINE HYDROCHLORIDE

Indications nausea and vomiting of terminal illness (where other drugs have failed or are not available); other indications (section 4.2.1 and section 15.1.4.1)

Cautions see Chlorpromazine Hydrochloride, section 4.2.1

Contra-indications see Chlorpromazine Hydrochloride, section 4.2.1

Side-effects see Chlorpromazine Hydrochloride, section 4.2.1

Dose
- By mouth, 10–25 mg every 4–6 hours; CHILD 500 micrograms/kg every 4–6 hours (1–5 years max. 40 mg daily, 6–12 years max. 75 mg daily)
- By deep intramuscular injection initially 25 mg then 25–50 mg every 3–4 hours until vomiting stops; CHILD 500 micrograms/kg every 6–8 hours (1–5 years max. 40 mg daily, 6–12 years max. 75 mg daily)
- By rectum in suppositories, chlorpromazine 100 mg every 6–8 hours [unlicensed]

Preparations
Section 4.2.1

PERPHENAZINE

Indications severe nausea, vomiting (see notes above); other indications (section 4.2.1)

Cautions see Perphenazine (section 4.2.1)

Contra-indications see Perphenazine (section 4.2.1)

Side-effects see Perphenazine (section 4.2.1); extrapyramidal symptoms particularly in young adults, elderly, and debilitated

Dose
- 4 mg 3 times daily, adjusted according to response; max. 24 mg daily (chemotherapy-induced); ELDERLY quarter to half adult dose; CHILD under 14 years not recommended

Preparations
Section 4.2.1

PROCHLORPERAZINE

Indications severe nausea, vomiting, vertigo, labyrinthine disorders (see notes above); other indications section 4.2.1

Cautions see under Prochlorperazine (section 4.2.1); oral route only for children (avoid if under 10 kg); elderly (see notes above)

Contra-indications see under Prochlorperazine (section 4.2.1)

Side-effects see under Prochlorperazine (section 4.2.1); extrapyramidal symptoms, particularly in children, elderly, and debilitated

Dose

Note Doses are expressed as prochlorperazine maleate or mesilate; 1 mg prochlorperazine maleate ≡ 1 mg prochlorperazine mesilate

- By mouth, nausea and vomiting, acute attack, 20 mg initially then 10 mg after 2 hours; prevention 5–10 mg 2–3 times daily; CHILD (over 10 kg only) 250 micrograms/kg 2–3 times daily

  Labyrinthine disorders, 5 mg 3 times daily, gradually increased if necessary to 30 mg daily in divided doses, then reduced after several weeks to 5–10 mg daily; CHILD not recommended
- By deep intramuscular injection, nausea and vomiting, 12.5 mg when required followed if necessary after 6 hours by an oral dose, as above; CHILD and ADOLESCENT under 18 years, see *BNF for Children*

Prochlorperazine (Non-proprietary) PoM
Tablets, prochlorperazine maleate 5 mg, net price 28 = £1.49, 84 = £4.37. Label: 2

Stemetil® (Castlemead) PoM
Tablets, prochlorperazine maleate 5 mg (off-white), net price 84-tab pack = £6.18. Label: 2

Syrup, straw-coloured, prochlorperazine mesilate 5 mg/5 mL. Net price 100-mL pack = £3.48. Label: 2

Injection, prochlorperazine mesilate 12.5 mg/mL. Net price 1-mL amp = 54p

Buccal preparation

[1]**Buccastem®** (R&C) PoM
Tablets (buccal), pale yellow, prochlorperazine maleate 3 mg. Net price 5 × 10-tab pack = £5.75. Label: 2, counselling, administration, see under Dose below

Dose ADULT and CHILD over 12 years, 1–2 tablets twice daily; tablets are placed high between upper lip and gum and left to dissolve

1. Prochlorperazine maleate can be sold to the public for adults over 18 years (provided packs do not contain more than 24 mg) for the treatment of nausea and vomiting in previously diagnosed migraine only (max. daily dose 12 mg)

TRIFLUOPERAZINE

Indications severe nausea and vomiting (see notes above); other indications (section 4.2.1)

Cautions see section 4.2.1

Contra-indications see section 4.2.1

Side-effects see section 4.2.1; extrapyramidal symptoms, particularly in children, elderly, and debilitated

Dose

- 2–4 mg daily in divided doses *or* as a single dose of a modified-release preparation; max. 6 mg daily; CHILD 3–5 years up to 1 mg daily, 6–12 years up to 4 mg daily

Preparations
Section 4.2.1

Domperidone and metoclopramide

DOMPERIDONE

Indications nausea and vomiting, dyspepsia, gastro-oesophageal reflux

Cautions children; renal impairment (Appendix 3); breast-feeding (Appendix 5); **interactions**: Appendix 1 (domperidone)

Contra-indications prolactinoma, hepatic impairment; where increased gastro-intestinal motility harmful; pregnancy (Appendix 4)

Side-effects *rarely* gastro-intestinal disturbances (including cramps) and hyperprolactinaemia; *very rarely* extrapyramidal effects and rashes

Dose

- By mouth, ADULT and CHILD body-weight over 35 kg, 10–20 mg 3–4 times daily; max. 80 mg daily; CHILD body-weight up to 35 kg (nausea and vomiting only), 250–500 micrograms/kg 3–4 times daily; max. 2.4 mg/kg daily
- By rectum in suppositories, ADULT and CHILD body-weight over 35 kg, 60 mg twice daily; CHILD 15–35 kg (nausea and vomiting only), 30 mg twice daily; CHILD body-weight under 15 kg, not recommended

[1]**Domperidone** (Non-proprietary) PoM
Tablets, 10 mg (as maleate), net price 30-tab pack = £1.26; 100-tab pack = £3.34

1. Domperidone can be sold to the public (provided packs do not contain more than 200 mg) for the relief of postprandial symptoms of excessive fullness, nausea, epigastric bloating and belching occasionally accompanied by epigastric discomfort and heartburn (max. single dose 10 mg, max. daily dose 40 mg)

Motilium® (Sanofi-Synthelabo) PoM
Tablets, f/c, domperidone 10 mg (as maleate). Net price 30-tab pack = £2.82; 100-tab pack = £9.41

Suspension, sugar-free, domperidone 5 mg/5 mL. Net price 200-mL pack = £2.16

Suppositories domperidone 30 mg. Net price 10 = £3.18

METOCLOPRAMIDE HYDROCHLORIDE

Indications adults, nausea and vomiting, particularly in gastro-intestinal disorders (section 1.2) and treatment with cytotoxics or radiotherapy; migraine (section 4.7.4.1)

Patients under 20 years Use restricted to severe intractable vomiting of known cause, vomiting of radiotherapy and cytotoxics, aid to gastro-intestinal intubation, pre-medication; also, dose should be determined on the basis of body-weight

Cautions hepatic impairment (Appendix 2), renal impairment (Appendix 3); elderly, young adults, and children (measure dose accurately, preferably with a pipette); may mask underlying disorders such as cerebral irritation; epilepsy; pregnancy (Appendix 4); porphyria (section 9.8.2); **interactions**: Appendix 1 (metoclopramide)

Contra-indications gastro-intestinal obstruction, perforation or haemorrhage; 3–4 days after gastro-intestinal surgery; phaeochromocytoma; breast-feeding (Appendix 5)

Side-effects extrapyramidal effects (especially in children and young adults—see p. 217), hyperprolactinaemia, occasionally tardive dyskinesia on prolonged administration; also reported, drowsiness, restlessness, diarrhoea, depression, neuroleptic malignant syndrome, rashes, pruritus, oedema; cardiac conduction abnormalities reported following intravenous administration; rarely methaemoglobinaemia (more severe in G6PD deficiency)

Dose

- By mouth *or* by intramuscular injection *or* by intravenous injection over 1–2 minutes, nausea and vomiting, 10 mg (5 mg in young adults 15–19 years under 60 kg) 3 times daily; CHILD up to 1 year (up to 10 kg) 1 mg twice daily, 1–3 years (10–14 kg) 1 mg 2–3 times daily, 3–5 years (15–19 kg) 2 mg 2–3 times daily, 5–9 years (20–29 kg) 2.5 mg 3 times daily, 9–14 years (30 kg and over) 5 mg 3 times daily

Note Daily dose of metoclopramide should not normally exceed 500 micrograms/kg, particularly for children and young adults (restricted use, see above)

For diagnostic procedures, as a single dose 5–10 minutes before examination, 10–20 mg (10 mg in young adults 15–19 years); CHILD under 3 years 1 mg, 3–5 years 2 mg, 5–9 years 2.5 mg, 9–14 years 5 mg

Metoclopramide (Non-proprietary) PoM

Tablets, metoclopramide hydrochloride 10 mg, net price 28-tab pack = 40p

Oral solution, metoclopramide hydrochloride 5 mg/5 mL, net price 200-mL pack = £3.83

Note Sugar-free versions are available and can be ordered by specifying 'sugar-free' on the prescription

Injection, metoclopramide hydrochloride 5 mg/mL, net price 2-mL amp = 26p

Maxolon® (Shire) PoM

Tablets, scored, metoclopramide hydrochloride 10 mg, net price 84-tab pack = £5.24

Syrup, sugar-free, metoclopramide hydrochloride 5 mg/5 mL. Net price 200-mL pack = £3.83

Paediatric liquid, sugar-free, metoclopramide hydrochloride 1 mg/mL. Net price 15-mL pack with pipette = £1.51. Counselling, use of pipette

Injection, metoclopramide hydrochloride 5 mg/mL. Net price 2-mL amp = 27p

High-dose (with cytotoxic chemotherapy only)

Maxolon High Dose® (Shire) PoM

Injection, metoclopramide hydrochloride 5 mg/mL. Net price 20-mL amp = £2.67.

For dilution and use as an intravenous infusion in nausea and vomiting associated with cytotoxic chemotherapy only

Dose by continuous intravenous infusion (preferred method), initially (before starting chemotherapy), 2–4 mg/kg over 15–20 minutes, then 3–5 mg/kg over 8–12 hours; max. in 24 hours, 10 mg/kg

By intermittent intravenous infusion, initially (before starting chemotherapy), up to 2 mg/kg over at least 15 minutes then up to 2 mg/kg over at least 15 minutes every 2 hours; max. in 24 hours, 10 mg/kg

Modified release

Maxolon SR® (Shire) PoM

Capsules, m/r, clear, enclosing white granules, metoclopramide hydrochloride 15 mg. Net price 56-cap pack = £7.01. Label: 25

Dose patients over 20 years, 1 capsule twice daily

Compound preparations (for migraine)

Section 4.7.4.1

5HT$_3$ antagonists

DOLASETRON MESILATE

Indications see under Dose

Cautions concomitant administration of drugs that prolong QT interval, congestive heart failure; pregnancy (Appendix 4); breast-feeding (Appendix 5); **interactions**: Appendix 1 (dolasetron)

Contra-indications prolonged QT interval, cardiac conduction disorders

Side-effects diarrhoea, constipation, dyspepsia, abdominal pain, flatulence, anorexia, taste disturbance, tachycardia, bradycardia, ECG changes, flushing; fever, shivering; headache, sleep disorder, fatigue, dizziness, drowsiness, hypersensitivity reactions including rash, *rarely* intestinal obstruction, pancreatitis, jaundice, oedema, cardiac arrhythmia, bronchospasm, seizures, *very rarely* severe hypotension following intravenous injection

Dose

- Prevention of nausea and vomiting induced by cytotoxic chemotherapy, by mouth, ADULT over 18 years, 200 mg one hour before treatment *or* by intravenous injection (over 30 seconds) *or* by intravenous infusion, 100 mg 30 minutes before treatment
- Prevention of delayed nausea and vomiting after chemotherapy cycle, by mouth, ADULT over 18 years, 200 mg once daily for up to 4 consecutive days each cycle
- Prevention of postoperative nausea and vomiting, by mouth, ADULT over 18 years, 50 mg before induction of anaesthesia *or* by intravenous injection (over 30 seconds) *or* by intravenous infusion, 12.5 mg at cessation of anaesthesia
- Treatment of postoperative nausea and vomiting, by intravenous injection (over 30 seconds) *or* by intravenous infusion, ADULT over 18 years, 12.5 mg

Anzemet® (Amdipharm) ▼ PoM

Tablets, f/c, pink, dolasetron mesilate 50 mg, net price 3-tab pack = £13.50; 200 mg, 3-tab pack = £42.00, 6-tab pack = £84.00

Injection, dolasetron mesilate 20 mg/mL, net price 0.625-mL (12.5-mg) amp = £4.00, 5-mL (100-mg) amp = £13.00

GRANISETRON

Indications see under Dose

Cautions pregnancy (Appendix 4) and breast-feeding (Appendix 5)

Side-effects constipation, headache, rash; hypersensitivity reactions reported; *rarely* movement disorders

Dose
- Nausea and vomiting induced by cytotoxic chemotherapy or radiotherapy, by mouth, 1–2 mg within 1 hour before start of treatment, then 2 mg daily in 1–2 divided doses during treatment; when intravenous infusion also used, max. combined total 9 mg in 24 hours; CHILD 20 micrograms/kg (max. 1 mg) within 1 hour before start of treatment, then 20 micrograms/kg (max. 1 mg) twice daily for up to 5 days during treatment

  By intravenous injection (diluted in 15 mL sodium chloride 0.9% and given over not less than 30 seconds) *or* by intravenous infusion (over 5 minutes), prevention, 3 mg before start of cytotoxic therapy (up to 2 additional 3-mg doses may be given within 24 hours); treatment, as for prevention (the two additional doses must not be given less than 10 minutes apart); max. 9 mg in 24 hours; CHILD, by intravenous infusion, (over 5 minutes), prevention, 40 micrograms/kg (max. 3 mg) before start of cytotoxic therapy; treatment, as for prevention—one additional dose of 40 micrograms/kg (max. 3 mg) may be given within 24 hours (not less than 10 minutes after initial dose)
- Postoperative nausea and vomiting, by intravenous injection (diluted to 5 mL and given over 30 seconds), prevention, 1 mg before induction of anaesthesia; treatment, 1 mg, given as for prevention; max. 2 mg in one day; CHILD not recommended

Kytril® (Roche) PoM
Tablets, f/c, granisetron (as hydrochloride) 1 mg, net price 10-tab pack = £65.49; 2 mg, 5-tab pack = £65.49
Sterile solution, granisetron (as hydrochloride) 1 mg/mL, for dilution and use as injection or infusion, net price 1-mL amp = £8.60, 3-mL amp = £25.79

ONDANSETRON

Indications see under Dose
Cautions QT interval prolongation (avoid concomitant administration of drugs that prolong QT interval); hepatic impairment (Appendix 2); pregnancy (Appendix 4); breast-feeding (Appendix 5); **interactions:** Appendix 1 (ondansetron)
Side-effects constipation; headache; flushing; injection site-reactions; *less commonly* hiccups, hypotension, bradycardia, chest pain, arrhythmias, movement disorders, seizures; *on intravenous administration, rarely* dizziness, transient visual disturbances (*very rarely* transient blindness); suppositories may cause rectal irritation

Dose
- Moderately emetogenic chemotherapy or radiotherapy, by mouth, 8 mg 1–2 hours before treatment *or* by rectum, 16 mg 1–2 hours before treatment *or* by intramuscular injection *or* slow intravenous injection, 8 mg immediately before treatment

  then by mouth, 8 mg every 12 hours for up to 5 days *or* by rectum, 16 mg daily for up to 5 days; CHILD, by slow intravenous injection *or* by intravenous infusion over 15 minutes, 5 mg/m^2 immediately before chemotherapy then 4 mg by mouth every 12 hours for up to 5 days
- Severely emetogenic chemotherapy, by intramuscular injection *or* slow intravenous injection, 8 mg immediately before treatment, where necessary followed by 2 further doses of 8 mg at intervals of 2–4 hours (*or* followed by 1 mg/hour by continuous intravenous infusion for up to 24 hours)

  then by mouth, 8 mg every 12 hours for up to 5 days *or* by rectum, 16 mg daily for up to 5 days;

  alternatively, by intravenous infusion over at least 15 minutes, 32 mg immediately before treatment *or* by rectum, 16 mg 1–2 hours before treatment

  then by mouth, 8 mg every 12 hours for up to 5 days *or* by rectum, 16 mg daily for up to 5 days; CHILD, by slow intravenous injection, 5 mg/m^2 immediately before chemotherapy then 4 mg by mouth every 12 hours for up to 5 days
- Prevention of postoperative nausea and vomiting, by mouth, 16 mg 1 hour before anaesthesia *or* 8 mg 1 hour before anaesthesia followed by 8 mg at intervals of 8 hours for 2 further doses

  alternatively, by intramuscular *or* slow intravenous injection, 4 mg at induction of anaesthesia; CHILD over 2 years, by slow intravenous injection, 100 micrograms/kg (max. 4 mg) before, during, or after induction of anaesthesia
- Treatment of postoperative nausea and vomiting, by intramuscular *or* slow intravenous injection, 4 mg; CHILD over 2 years, by slow intravenous injection, 100 micrograms/kg (max. 4 mg)

Ondansetron (Non-proprietary) PoM
Tablets, ondansetron (as hydrochloride) 4 mg, net price 30-tab pack = £94.19; 8 mg, 10-tab pack = £62.81
Brands include *Ondemet®*
Injection, ondansetron (as hydrochloride) 2 mg/mL, net price 2-mL amp = £5.39, 4-mL amp = £11.99
Brands include *Ondemet®*

Zofran® (GSK) PoM
Tablets, yellow, f/c, ondansetron (as hydrochloride) 4 mg, net price 30-tab pack = £107.91; 8 mg, 10-tab pack = £71.94
Oral lyophilisates (*Zofran Melt®*), ondansetron 4 mg, net price 10-tab pack = £35.97; 8 mg, 10-tab pack = £71.94. Counselling, administration
Excipients include aspartame (section 9.4.1)
Counselling Tablets should be placed on the tongue, allowed to disperse and swallowed
Syrup, sugar-free, strawberry-flavoured, ondansetron (as hydrochloride) 4 mg/5 mL, net price 50-mL pack = £35.97
Injection, ondansetron (as hydrochloride) 2 mg/mL, net price 2-mL amp = £5.99; 4-mL amp = £11.99
Suppositories, ondansetron 16 mg, net price 1 = £14.39

PALONOSETRON

Indications prevention of nausea and vomiting induced by moderately and severely emetogenic chemotherapy
Cautions history of constipation; intestinal obstruction; concomitant administration of drugs that prolong QT interval; pregnancy (Appendix 4); breast-feeding (Appendix 5)
Driving Dizziness or drowsiness may affect performance of skilled tasks (e.g. driving)
Side-effects diarrhoea, constipation; headache, dizziness; *less commonly* dyspepsia, abdominal pain, dry mouth, flatulence, changes in blood pressure, tachycardia, bradycardia, arrhythmia, myocardial ischaemia, hiccups, drowsiness, asthenia, insomnia, anxiety,

euphoria, paraesthesia, peripheral neuropathy, anorexia, motion sickness, influenza-like symptoms, urinary retention, glycosuria, hyperglycaemia, electrolyte disturbance, arthralgia, eye irritation, amblyopia, tinnitus, rash, pruritus

Dose

- By intravenous injection (over 30 seconds), 250 micrograms as a single dose 30 minutes before treatment; do not repeat dose within 7 days; CHILD and ADOLESCENT under 18 years not recommended

Aloxi® (Maelor) ▼ PoM

Injection, palonosetron (as hydrochloride) 50 micrograms/mL, net price 5-mL amp = £55.89

TROPISETRON

Indications see under Dose

Cautions uncontrolled hypertension (do not exceed recommended doses); cardiac conduction disorders; arrhythmias, concomitant administration of drugs that prolong QT interval; pregnancy (Appendix 4); breast-feeding; **interactions**: Appendix 1 (tropisetron)

Driving Dizziness or drowsiness may affect performance of skilled tasks (e.g. driving)

Side-effects constipation, diarrhoea, abdominal pain; headache, dizziness, fatigue; collapse, syncope, bradycardia, cardiovascular collapse also reported

Dose

- Prevention of nausea and vomiting induced by cytotoxic chemotherapy, by slow intravenous injection *or* by intravenous infusion, 5 mg shortly before chemotherapy, then 5 mg by mouth every morning at least 1 hour before food for 5 days; CHILD over 2 years, by intravenous injection over at least 1 minute *or* by intravenous infusion, 200 micrograms/kg (max. 5 mg) shortly before chemotherapy, then 200 micrograms/kg daily for 4 days; CHILD 25 kg and over, by intravenous injection over at least 1 minute *or* by intravenous infusion, 5 mg shortly before chemotherapy, then by mouth (preferably) *or* by intravenous injection over at least 1 minute *or* by intravenous infusion, 5 mg daily for 5 days
- Postoperative nausea and vomiting, by slow intravenous injection *or* by intravenous infusion, prevention, 2 mg shortly before induction of anaesthesia; treatment, 2 mg within 2 hours of the end of anaesthesia

Navoban® (Novartis) PoM

Capsules, white/yellow, tropisetron (as hydrochloride) 5 mg, net price 5-cap pack = £53.86; 50-cap pack = £538.60. Label: 23

Injection, tropisetron (as hydrochloride), 1 mg/mL, net price 2-mL amp = £4.86, 5-mL amp = £12.16

Neurokinin receptor antagonist

APREPITANT

Indications adjunct to dexamethasone and a $5HT_3$ antagonist in preventing nausea and vomiting associated with moderately and highly emetogenic chemotherapy

Cautions hepatic impairment (Appendix 2); pregnancy (Appendix 4); **interactions**: Appendix 1 (aprepitant)

Contra-indications breast-feeding (Appendix 5)

Side-effects hiccups, dyspepsia, diarrhoea, constipation, anorexia; asthenia, headache, dizziness; *less commonly* weight changes, dry mouth, colitis, flatulence, stomatitis, abdominal pain, gastro-oesophageal reflux, duodenal ulcer, oedema, bradycardia, cough, disorientation, euphoria, anxiety, confusion, thirst, abnormal dreams, hyperglycaemia, polyuria, anaemia, dysuria, haematuria, myalgia, conjunctivitis, pharyngitis, sneezing, tinnitus, sweating, oily skin, pruritus, rash, acne, photosensitivity, flushing, hyponatraemia

Dose

- ADULT over 18 years 125 mg 1 hour before chemotherapy, then 80 mg daily as a single dose for the next 2 days; consult product literature for dose of concomitant corticosteroid and $5HT_3$ antagonist

Emend® (MSD) ▼ PoM

Capsules, aprepitant 80 mg (white), net price 2-cap pack = £31.61; 125 mg (white/pink), 5-cap pack = £79.03; 3-day pack of one 125-mg capsule and two 80-mg capsules = £47.42

Cannabinoid

NABILONE

Indications nausea and vomiting caused by cytotoxic chemotherapy, unresponsive to conventional antiemetics (under close observation, preferably in hospital setting)

Cautions history of psychiatric disorder; elderly; hypertension; heart disease; adverse effects on mental state can persist for 48–72 hours after stopping; pregnancy (Appendix 4); **interactions**: Appendix 1 (nabilone)

Driving Drowsiness may affect performance of skilled tasks (e.g. driving); effects of alcohol enhanced

Contra-indications severe hepatic impairment; breast-feeding (Appendix 5)

Side-effects drowsiness, vertigo, euphoria, dry mouth, ataxia, visual disturbance, concentration difficulties, sleep disturbance, dysphoria, hypotension, headache and nausea, also confusion, disorientation, hallucinations, psychosis, depression, decreased coordination, tremors, tachycardia, decreased appetite, and abdominal pain

Behavioural effects Patients should be made aware of possible changes of mood and other adverse behavioural effects

Dose

- Initially 1 mg twice daily, increased if necessary to 2 mg twice daily, throughout each cycle of cytotoxic therapy and, if necessary, for 48 hours after the last dose of each cycle; max. 6 mg daily given in 3 divided doses. The first dose should be taken the night before initiation of cytotoxic treatment and the second dose 1–3 hours before the first dose of cytotoxic drug; ADOLESCENT and CHILD under 18 years consult local treatment protocol [unlicensed use]

Nabilone (Valeant) PoM

Capsules, blue/white, nabilone 1 mg. Net price 20-cap pack = £125.84. Label: 2, counselling, behavioural effects

Hyoscine

HYOSCINE HYDROBROMIDE
(Scopolamine Hydrobromide)

Indications motion sickness; premedication (section 15.1.3)

Cautions elderly, urinary retention, cardiovascular disease, susceptibility to angle-closure glaucoma, gastro-intestinal obstruction, hepatic or renal impairment; pregnancy (Appendix 4) and breast-feeding (Appendix 5); **interactions**: Appendix 1 (antimuscarinics)

Driving Drowsiness may affect performance of skilled tasks (e.g. driving) and may persist for up to 24 hours or longer after removal of patch: effects of alcohol enhanced

Side-effects drowsiness, dry mouth, dizziness, blurred vision, difficulty with micturition; *very rarely* angle-closure glaucoma

Dose
- See under preparation below

Scopoderm TTS® (Novartis Consumer Health) PoM
Patch, self-adhesive, pink, releasing hyoscine approx. 1 mg/72 hours when in contact with skin. Net price 2 = £4.30. Label: 19, counselling, see below

Dose motion sickness prevention, apply 1 patch to hairless area of skin behind ear 5–6 hours before journey; replace if necessary after 72 hours, siting replacement patch behind other ear; CHILD under 10 years not recommended

Counselling Explain accompanying instructions to patient and in particular emphasise advice to wash hands after handling and to wash application site after removing, and to use one patch at a time

Parenteral preparations
Section 15.1.3

Other drugs for Ménière's disease

Betahistine has been promoted as a specific treatment for Ménière's disease.

BETAHISTINE DIHYDROCHLORIDE

Indications vertigo, tinnitus and hearing loss associated with Ménière's disease

Cautions asthma, history of peptic ulcer; pregnancy and breast-feeding; **interactions**: Appendix 1 (betahistine)

Contra-indications phaeochromocytoma

Side-effects gastro-intestinal disturbances; headache, rashes and pruritus reported

Dose
- Initially 16 mg 3 times daily, preferably with food; maintenance 24–48 mg daily; CHILD not recommended

Betahistine Dihydrochloride (Non-proprietary) PoM
Tablets, betahistine dihydrochloride 8 mg, net price 84-tab pack = £3.71, 120-tab pack = £2.26; 16 mg, 84-tab pack = £3.28. Label: 21

Serc® (Solvay) PoM
Tablets, betahistine dihydrochloride 8 mg (*Serc®-8*), net price 120-tab pack = £9.04; 16 mg (*Serc®-16*) (scored), 84-tab pack = £12.65. Label: 21

4.7 Analgesics

4.7.1 Non-opioid analgesics
4.7.2 Opioid analgesics
4.7.3 Neuropathic pain
4.7.4 Antimigraine drugs

The non-opioid drugs (section 4.7.1), paracetamol and aspirin (and other NSAIDs), are particularly suitable for pain in musculoskeletal conditions, whereas the opioid analgesics (section 4.7.2) are more suitable for moderate to severe pain, particularly of visceral origin.

Pain in palliative care For advice on pain relief in palliative care, see p. 15.

Pain in sickle-cell disease The pain of mild sickle-cell crises is managed with paracetamol, an NSAID, codeine, or dihydrocodeine. Severe crises may require the use of morphine or diamorphine; concomitant use of an NSAID may potentiate analgesia and allow lower doses of the opioid to be used. Pethidine should be avoided if possible because accumulation of a neurotoxic metabolite can precipitate seizures; the relatively short half-life of pethidine necessitates frequent injections.

Dental and orofacial pain Analgesics should be used judiciously in dental care as a **temporary** measure until the cause of the pain has been dealt with.

Dental pain of inflammatory origin, such as that associated with pulpitis, apical infection, localised osteitis (dry socket) or pericoronitis is usually best managed by treating the infection, providing drainage, restorative procedures, and other local measures. Analgesics provide temporary relief of pain (usually for about 1 to 7 days) until the causative factors have been brought under control. In the case of pulpitis, intra-osseous infection or abscess, reliance on analgesics alone is usually inappropriate.

Similarly the pain and discomfort associated with acute problems of the oral mucosa (e.g. acute herpetic gingivostomatitis, erythema multiforme) may be relieved by **benzydamine** mouthwash or spray (see p. 591) until the cause of the mucosal disorder has been dealt with. However, where a patient is febrile, the antipyretic action of **paracetamol** (see p. 226) or **ibuprofen** (see p. 540) is often helpful.

The *choice* of an analgesic for dental purposes should be based on its suitability for the patient. Most dental pain is relieved effectively by non-steroidal anti-inflammatory drugs (NSAIDs). NSAIDs that are used for dental pain include **ibuprofen**, **diclofenac**, and **aspirin**; for further details see section 4.7.1 and section 10.1.1. **Paracetamol** has analgesic and antipyretic effects but no anti-inflammatory effect.

Opioid analgesics (section 4.7.2) such as **dihydrocodeine** and **pethidine** act on the central nervous system and are traditionally used for *moderate to severe pain*. However, opioid analgesics are relatively ineffective in dental pain and their side-effects can be unpleasant. Paracetamol, ibuprofen, or aspirin are adequate for most cases of dental pain and an opioid is rarely required.

Combining a non-opioid with an opioid analgesic can provide greater relief of pain than a non-opioid analgesic given alone. However, this applies only when an appropriate dose combination is used. Most combination analgesic preparations have not been shown to provide greater relief of pain than an adequate dose of the non-opioid component given alone. Moreover, combination preparations have the disadvantage of an increased number of side-effects.

Any analgesic given before a dental procedure should have a low risk of increasing postoperative bleeding. In the case of pain after the dental procedure, taking an analgesic before the effect of the local anaesthetic has worn off can improve control. Postoperative analgesia with ibuprofen or aspirin is usually continued for about 24 to 72 hours.

Temporomandibular dysfunction can be related to anxiety in some patients who may clench or grind their teeth (bruxism) during the day or night. The muscle spasm (which appears to be the main source of pain) may be treated empirically with an overlay appliance which provides a free sliding occlusion and may also interfere with grinding. In addition, **diazepam** (section 4.1.2), which has muscle relaxant as well as anxiolytic properties, may be helpful but it should only be prescribed on a short-term basis during the acute phase. Analgesics such as aspirin (section 4.7.1) or ibuprofen (section 10.1.1) may also be required.

For the management of neuropathic pain, persistent idiopathic facial pain, and trigeminal neuralgia, see section 4.7.3.

Dysmenorrhoea Use of an oral contraceptive prevents the pain of dysmenorrhoea which is generally associated with ovulatory cycles. If treatment is necessary paracetamol or an NSAID (section 10.1.1) will generally provide adequate relief of pain. The vomiting and severe pain associated with dysmenorrhoea in women with endometriosis may call for an antiemetic (in addition to an analgesic). Antispasmodics (such as alverine citrate, section 1.2) have been advocated for dysmenorrhoea but the antispasmodic action does not generally provide significant relief.

4.7.1 Non-opioid analgesics

Aspirin is indicated for headache, transient musculoskeletal pain, dysmenorrhoea and pyrexia. In inflammatory conditions, most physicians prefer anti-inflammatory treatment with another NSAID which may be better tolerated and more convenient for the patient. Aspirin is used increasingly for its antiplatelet properties (section 2.9). Aspirin tablets or dispersible aspirin tablets are adequate for most purposes as they act rapidly.

Gastric irritation may be a problem; it is minimised by taking the dose after food. Enteric-coated preparations are available, but have a slow onset of action and are therefore unsuitable for single-dose analgesic use (though their prolonged action may be useful for night pain).

Aspirin interacts significantly with a number of other drugs and its interaction with warfarin is a **special hazard**, see **interactions:** Appendix 1 (aspirin).

Paracetamol is similar in efficacy to aspirin, but has no demonstrable anti-inflammatory activity; it is less irritant to the stomach and for that reason is now generally preferred to aspirin, particularly in the elderly. **Overdosage** with paracetamol is particularly dangerous as it may cause hepatic damage which is sometimes not apparent for 4 to 6 days (see Emergency Treatment of Poisoning, p. 29).

Nefopam may have a place in the relief of persistent pain unresponsive to other non-opioid analgesics. It causes little or no respiratory depression, but sympathomimetic and antimuscarinic side-effects may be troublesome.

Non-steroidal anti-inflammatory analgesics (NSAIDs, section 10.1.1) are particularly useful for the treatment of patients with chronic disease accompanied by pain and inflammation. Some of them are also used in the short-term treatment of mild to moderate pain including transient musculoskeletal pain but paracetamol is now often preferred, particularly in the elderly (see also p. 20). They are also suitable for the relief of pain in *dysmenorrhoea* and to treat pain caused by *secondary bone tumours*, many of which produce lysis of bone and release prostaglandins (see Prescribing in Palliative Care, p. 15). Selective inhibitors of cyclo-oxygenase-2 may be used in preference to non-selective NSAIDs for patients at high risk of developing serious gastro-intestinal side-effects. NSAIDs including ketorolac are also used for peri-operative analgesia (section 15.1.4.2).

A non-opioid analgesic administered by intrathecal infusion (**ziconotide** (*Prialt*® ▼), available from Eisai Ltd) is licensed for the treatment of chronic severe pain; ziconotide can be used as an adjunct to opioid analgesics.

Dental and orofacial pain Most dental pain is relieved effectively by NSAIDs (section 10.1.1). **Aspirin** (p. 226) is effective against mild to moderate dental pain; dispersible tablets provide a rapidly absorbed form of aspirin suitable for most purposes.

The analgesic effect of **paracetamol** in mild to moderate dental pain is probably less than that of aspirin, but it does not affect bleeding time or interact significantly with warfarin. Moreover, it is less irritant to the stomach. Paracetamol is a suitable analgesic for children; sugar-free versions can be requested by specifying 'sugar-free' on the prescription.

For further information on the management of dental and orofacial pain, see p. 224.

Compound analgesic preparations

Compound analgesic preparations that contain a simple analgesic (such as aspirin or paracetamol) with an opioid component reduce the scope for effective titration of the individual components in the management of pain of varying intensity.

Compound analgesic preparations containing paracetamol or aspirin with a *low dose* of an opioid analgesic (e.g. 8 mg of codeine phosphate per compound tablet) are commonly used, but the advantages have not been substantiated. The low dose of the opioid may be enough to cause opioid side-effects (in particular constipation) and can complicate the treatment of **over-**

dosage (see p. 31) yet may not provide significant additional relief of pain.

A *full dose* of the opioid component (e.g. 60 mg codeine phosphate) in compound analgesic preparations effectively augments the analgesic activity but is associated with the full range of opioid side-effects (including nausea, vomiting, severe constipation, drowsiness, respiratory depression, and risk of dependence on long-term administration). For details of the **side-effects** of opioid analgesics, see p. 229 (**important**: the elderly are particularly susceptible to opioid side-effects and should receive lower doses).

In general, when assessing pain, it is necessary to weigh up carefully whether there is a need for a non-opioid and an opioid analgesic to be taken simultaneously.

For information on the use of combination analgesic preparations in dental and orofacial pain, see p. 224.

Caffeine is a weak stimulant that is often included, in small doses, in analgesic preparations. It is claimed that the addition of caffeine may enhance the analgesic effect, but the alerting effect, mild habit-forming effect and possible provocation of headache may not always be desirable. Moreover, in excessive dosage or on withdrawal caffeine may itself induce headache.

Co-proxamol tablets (dextropropoxyphene in combination with paracetamol) are no longer licensed because of safety concerns, particularly toxicity in overdose. Co-proxamol tablets [unlicensed] may still be prescribed for patients who find it difficult to change, because, for example, alternatives are not effective or suitable.

ASPIRIN

(Acetylsalicylic Acid)

Indications mild to moderate pain, pyrexia; antiplatelet (section 2.9)

Cautions asthma, allergic disease, hepatic impairment (Appendix 2), renal impairment (Appendix 3), dehydration; preferably avoid during fever or viral infection in children (risk of Reye's syndrome, see below); pregnancy (Appendix 4); elderly; G6PD-deficiency (section 9.1.5); **interactions:** Appendix 1 (aspirin)

Contra-indications children under 16 years and in breast-feeding (Reye's syndrome, see below; Appendix 5); previous or active peptic ulceration, haemophilia; not for treatment of gout

Hypersensitivity Aspirin and other NSAIDs are **contra-indicated** in patients with a history of hypersensitivity to aspirin or any other NSAID—*which includes those* in whom attacks of *asthma, angioedema, urticaria or rhinitis* have been precipitated by aspirin or any other NSAID

Reye's syndrome Owing to an association with Reye's syndrome, the CSM has advised that aspirin-containing preparations should not be given to children under 16 years, unless specifically indicated, e.g. for Kawasaki syndrome.

Side-effects generally mild and infrequent but high incidence of gastro-intestinal irritation with slight asymptomatic blood loss, increased bleeding time, bronchospasm and skin reactions in hypersensitive patients. Prolonged administration, see section 10.1.1. **Overdosage:** see Emergency Treatment of Poisoning, p. 29

Dose

- By mouth, 300–900 mg every 4–6 hours when necessary; max. 4 g daily; CHILD under 16 years not recommended (see Reye's syndrome above)
- By rectum, 450–900 mg every 4 hours (max. 3.6 g daily); CHILD under 16 years not recommended (see Contra-indications above)

Aspirin (Non-proprietary)
Tablets PoM[1], aspirin 300 mg. Net price 32-tab pack = 31p. Label: 21, 32
Tablets PoM[1], e/c, aspirin 300 mg, net price 100-tab pack = £4.83; 75 mg, see section 2.9. Label: 5, 25, 32
Dispersible tablets PoM[1], aspirin 300 mg, net price 100-tab pack = £3.08; 75 mg, see section 2.9. Label: 13, 21, 32

Note BP directs that when no strength is stated the 300-mg strength should be dispensed, and that when soluble aspirin tablets are prescribed, dispersible aspirin tablets shall be dispensed.

Dental prescribing on NHS Aspirin Dispersible Tablets 300 mg may be prescribed

Suppositories PoM, aspirin 150 mg, net price 10 = £9.52; 300 mg, 12 = £59.28. Label: 32
Brands include *Resprin®*

Caprin® (Pinewood)
Tablets PoM[1], e/c, f/c, pink, aspirin 300 mg, net price 100-tab pack = £4.89; 75 mg, see section 2.9. Label: 5, 25, 32

Nu-Seals® Aspirin (Alliance)
Tablets PoM[1], e/c, aspirin 300 mg, net price 100-tab pack = £3.46; 75 mg, see section 2.9. Label: 5, 25, 32

With codeine phosphate 8 mg

[1]**Co-codaprin** (Non-proprietary) PoM
Dispersible tablets, co-codaprin 8/400 (codeine phosphate 8 mg, aspirin 400 mg). Net price 100-tab pack = £23.76. Label: 13, 21, 32

Dose 1–2 tablets in water every 4–6 hours; max. 8 tablets daily

When co-codaprin tablets or dispersible tablets are prescribed and no strength is stated, tablets or dispersible tablets, respectively, containing codeine phosphate 8 mg and aspirin 400 mg should be dispensed

Other compound preparations

Aspav® (Alpharma) PoM
Dispersible tablets, aspirin 500 mg, papaveretum 7.71 mg (providing the equivalent of 5 mg of anhydrous morphine). Net price 30-tab pack = £5.98. Label: 2, 13, 21, 32

Dose 1–2 tablets in water every 4–6 hours if necessary; max. 8 tablets daily

PARACETAMOL

(Acetaminophen)

Indications mild to moderate pain, pyrexia

Cautions hepatic impairment (Appendix 2); renal impairment (Appendix 3), alcohol dependence; **interactions:** Appendix 1 (paracetamol)

Side-effects side-effects rare, but rashes, blood disorders (including thrombocytopenia, leucopenia, neutropenia) reported; hypotension also reported on infusion; **important:** liver damage (and less frequently renal damage) following **overdosage**, see Emergency Treatment of Poisoning, p. 29

1. Can be sold to the public provided packs contain no more than 32 capsules or tablets; pharmacists can sell multiple packs up to a total quantity of 100 capsules or tablets in justifiable circumstances; for details see *Medicines, Ethics and Practice*, No. 31, London, Pharmaceutical Press, 2007 (and subsequent editions as available)

Dose

- By mouth, 0.5–1 g every 4–6 hours to a max. of 4 g daily; CHILD 2 months 60 mg for post-immunisation pyrexia, repeated once after 6 hours if necessary; otherwise under 3 months, see *BNF for Children*; 3 months–1 year 60–120 mg, 1–5 years 120–250 mg, 6–12 years 250–500 mg; these doses may be repeated every 4–6 hours when necessary (max. of 4 doses in 24 hours)
- By intravenous infusion over 15 minutes, ADULT and CHILD over 50 kg, 1 g every 4–6 hours, max. 4 g daily; ADULT and CHILD 10–50 kg, 15 mg/kg every 4–6 hours, max. 60 mg/kg daily; NEONATE and CHILD less than 10 kg, 7.5 mg/kg every 4–6 hours, max. 30 mg/kg daily
- By rectum, see preparations

Note For full Joint Committee on Vaccination and Immunisation recommendation on post-immunisation pyrexia, see section 14.1

Paracetamol (Non-proprietary)

Tablets PoM[1], paracetamol 500 mg. Net price 16 = 17p, 32 = 51p, 100 = £1.97. Label: 29, 30

Brands include *Panadol®* NHS

Soluble tablets (= Dispersible tablets) PoM[2], paracetamol 500 mg. Net price 60-tab pack = £4.66. Label: 13, 29, 30

Brands include *Panadol Soluble®* NHS (contains Na^+ 18.6 mmol/tablet)

Paediatric soluble tablets (= Paediatric dispersible tablets), paracetamol 120 mg. Net price 16-tab pack = 91p. Label: 13, 30

Brands include *Disprol® Soluble Paracetamol* NHS

Oral suspension 120 mg/5 mL (= Paediatric Mixture), paracetamol 120 mg/5 mL. Net price 100 mL = 42p. Label: 30

Note BP directs that when Paediatric Paracetamol Oral Suspension or Paediatric Paracetamol Mixture is prescribed Paracetamol Oral Suspension 120 mg/5 mL should be dispensed; sugar-free versions can be ordered by specifying 'sugar-free'on the prescription

Brands include *Calpol® Paediatric*, *Calpol® Paediatric* sugar-free, *Disprol® Paediatric*, *Medinol® Paediatric* sugar-free, *Paldesic®*, *Panadol®* sugar-free

Oral suspension 250 mg/5 mL (= Mixture), paracetamol 250 mg/5 mL. Net price 100 mL = 73p. Label: 30

Brands include *Calpol® 6 Plus* NHS, *Medinol® Over 6* NHS, *Paldesic®*

Suppositories, paracetamol 60 mg, net price 10 = £9.96; 125 mg, 10 = £11.50; 250 mg, 10 = £23.00; 500 mg, 10 = £9.90. Label: 30

Dose by rectum, ADULT and CHILD over 12 years 0.5–1 g up to 4 times daily, CHILD 1–5 years 125–250 mg, 6–12 years 250–500 mg

Brands include *Alvedon®*

Dental prescribing on NHS Paracetamol Tablets, Paracetamol Soluble Tablets 500 mg, and Paracetamol Oral Suspension may be prescribed

Perfalgan® (Bristol-Myers Squibb) ▼ PoM

Intravenous infusion, paracetamol 10 mg/mL, net price 50-mL vial = £1.50, 100-mL vial = £1.50

1. Can be sold to the public provided packs contain no more than 32 capsules or tablets; pharmacists can sell multiple packs up to a total quantity of 100 capsules or tablets in justifiable circumstances; for details see *Medicines, Ethics and Practice*, No. 31, London, Pharmaceutical Press, 2007 (and subsequent editions as available)
2. Can be sold to the public in certain circumstances; for exemptions see *Medicines, Ethics and Practice*, No. 31, London, Pharmaceutical Press, 2007 (and subsequent editions as available)

Co-codamol 8/500

When co-codamol tablets, dispersible (or effervescent) tablets, or capsules are prescribed and **no strength is stated**, tablets, dispersible (or effervescent) tablets, or capsules, respectively, containing codeine phosphate **8 mg** and paracetamol **500 mg** should be dispensed.

[2] **Co-codamol 8/500** (Non-proprietary) PoM

Tablets, co-codamol 8/500 (codeine phosphate 8 mg, paracetamol 500 mg), net price 30-tab pack = £2.19. Label: 29, 30

Brands include *Panadeine®* NHS

Dose 1–2 tablets every 4–6 hours; max. 8 tablets daily; CHILD 6–12 years ½–1 tablet, max. 4 daily

Effervescent *or* dispersible tablets, co-codamol 8/500 (codeine phosphate 8 mg, paracetamol 500 mg). Net price 100-tab pack = £6.77. Label: 13, 29, 30

Brands include *Paracodol®* NHS

Note The Drug Tariff allows tablets of co-codamol labelled 'dispersible' to be dispensed against an order for 'effervescent' and *vice versa*

Dose 1–2 tablets in water every 4–6 hours, max. 8 tablets daily; CHILD 6–12 years ½–1 tablet, max. 4 daily

Capsules, co-codamol 8/500 (codeine phosphate 8 mg, paracetamol 500 mg). Net price 10-cap pack = £1.10, 20-cap pack = £1.66. Label: 29, 30

Brands include *Paracodol®* NHS

Dose 1–2 capsules every 4 hours; max. 8 capsules daily

Co-codamol 15/500

When co-codamol tablets, dispersible (or effervescent) tablets, or capsules are prescribed and **no strength is stated**, tablets, dispersible (or effervescent) tablets, or capsules, respectively, containing codeine phosphate **8 mg** and paracetamol **500 mg** should be dispensed (see preparations above).

See warnings and notes on p. 225 (**important**: special care in elderly—reduce dose)

Codipar (Goldshield) PoM

Caplets (= tablets) co-codamol 15/500 (codeine phosphate 15 mg, paracetamol 500 mg). Net price 100-tab pack = £8.25. Label: 2, 29, 30

Dose 1–2 tablets every 4 hours; max. 8 daily; CHILD not recommended

Co-codamol 30/500

When co-codamol tablets, dispersible (or effervescent) tablets, or capsules are prescribed and **no strength is stated**, tablets, dispersible (or effervescent) tablets, or capsules, respectively, containing codeine phosphate **8 mg** and on paracetamol **500 mg** should be dispensed (see preparations above).

See warnings and notes on p. 225 (**important**: special care in elderly—reduce dose)

Co-codamol 30/500 (Non-proprietary) PoM

Tablets, co-codamol 30/500 (codeine phosphate 30 mg, paracetamol 500 mg), net price 100-tab pack = £4.77. Label: 2, 29, 30

Dose 1–2 tablets every 4 hours; max. 8 tablets daily; CHILD not recommended

Capsules, co-codamol 30/500 (codeine phosphate 30 mg, paracetamol 500 mg), net price 100-cap pack = £7.45. Label: 2, 29, 30

Brands include *Medocodene®*, *Zapain®*

Dose 1–2 capsules every 4 hours; max. 8 capsules daily; CHILD not recommended

Effervescent tablets, co-codamol 30/500 (codeine phosphate 30 mg, paracetamol 500 mg), net price 100-tab pack = £12.74. Label: 2, 13, 29, 30
Brands include *Medocodene® Effervescent* (contains Na^+ 13.6 mmol/tablet)
Dose 1–2 tablets in water every 4 hours; max. 8 tablets daily; CHILD not recommended

Kapake® (Galen) PoM
Tablets, scored, co-codamol 30/500 (codeine phosphate 30 mg, paracetamol 500 mg). Net price 30-tab pack = £2.26 (hosp. only), 100-tab pack = £7.10. Label: 2, 29, 30
Dose 1–2 tablets every 4 hours; max. 8 tablets daily; CHILD not recommended
Capsules, co-codamol 30/500 (codeine phosphate 30 mg, paracetamol 500 mg), net price 100-cap pack = £7.10. Label: 2, 29, 30
Dose 1–2 capsules every 4 hours; max. 8 capsules daily; CHILD not recommended
Effervescent tablets, co-codamol 30/500 (codeine phosphate 30 mg, paracetamol 500 mg). Contains Na^+ 16.9 mmol/tablet; avoid in *renal impairment*, net price 100-tab pack = £8.30. Label: 2, 13, 29, 30
Dose 2 tablets in water every 4 hours; max. 8 daily; CHILD not recommended

Solpadol® (Sanofi-Synthelabo) PoM
Caplets(= tablets), co-codamol 30/500 (codeine phosphate 30 mg, paracetamol 500 mg). Net price 100-tab pack = £7.54. Label: 2, 29, 30
Dose 2 tablets every 4 hours; max. 8 daily; CHILD not recommended
Capsules, grey/purple, co-codamol 30/500 (codeine phosphate 30 mg, paracetamol 500 mg). Net price 100-cap pack = £7.54. Label: 2, 29, 30
Dose 1–2 capsules every 4 hours; max. 8 capsules daily; CHILD not recommended
Effervescent tablets, co-codamol 30/500 (codeine phosphate 30 mg, paracetamol 500 mg). Contains Na^+ 16.9 mmol/tablet; avoid in *renal impairment*. Net price 32-tab pack = £2.69, 100-tab pack = £9.05. Label: 2, 13, 29, 30
Dose 2 tablets in water every 4 hours; max. 8 daily; CHILD not recommended

Tylex® (UCB Pharma) PoM
Capsules, co-codamol 30/500 (codeine phosphate 30 mg, paracetamol 500 mg). Net price 100-cap pack = £8.01. Label: 2, 29, 30
Dose 1–2 capsules every 4 hours; max. 8 capsules daily; CHILD not recommended
Effervescent tablets, co-codamol 30/500 (codeine phosphate 30 mg, paracetamol 500 mg). Contains Na^+ 13.6 mmol/tablet; avoid in *renal impairment*. Net price 90-tab pack = £7.94. Label: 2, 13, 29, 30
Excipients include aspartame 25 mg/tablet (see section 9.4.1)
Dose 1–2 tablets in water every 4 hours; max. 8 tablets daily; CHILD not recommended

With methionine (co-methiamol)

A mixture of methionine and paracetamol; methionine has no analgesic activity but may prevent paracetamol-induced liver toxicity if overdose taken

Paradote® (Penn)
Tablets, f/c, co-methiamol 100/500 (DL-methionine 100 mg, paracetamol 500 mg). Net price 24-tab pack = £1.05, 96-tab pack = £2.77. Label: 29, 30
Dose 2 tablets every 4 hours; max. 8 tablets daily; CHILD 12 years and under, not recommended

With dihydrocodeine tartrate 10 mg

See notes on p. 225

Co-dydramol (Non-proprietary) PoM
Tablets, scored, co-dydramol 10/500 (dihydrocodeine tartrate 10 mg, paracetamol 500 mg). Net price 30-tab pack = 80p. Label: 21, 29, 30
Dose 1–2 tablets every 4–6 hours; max. 8 tablets daily; CHILD not recommended
When co-dydramol tablets are prescribed and no strength is stated tablets containing dihydrocodeine tartrate 10 mg and paracetamol 500 mg should be dispensed.
Note Tablets containing paracetamol 500 mg and dihydrocodeine 7.46 mg (*Paramol®* NHS) are on sale to the public. The name *Paramol®* was formerly applied to a brand of co-dydramol tablets

With dihydrocodeine tartrate 20 or 30 mg

See warnings and notes on p. 225 (**important**: special care in elderly—reduce dose)

Remedeine® (Napp) PoM
Tablets, paracetamol 500 mg, dihydrocodeine tartrate 20 mg. Net price 112-tab pack = £11.23. Label: 2, 21, 29, 30
Dose 1–2 tablets every 4–6 hours; max. 8 tablets daily; CHILD not recommended
Forte tablets, paracetamol 500 mg, dihydrocodeine tartrate 30 mg. Net price 56-tab pack = £6.94. Label: 2, 21, 29, 30
Dose 1–2 tablets every 4–6 hours; max. 8 tablets daily; CHILD not recommended

With isometheptene mucate

Isometheptene mucate (in combination with paracetamol) is licensed for the treatment of acute attacks of migraine; other more effective treatments are available.

[1]Midrid® (Manx) PoM
Capsules, red, isometheptene mucate 65 mg, paracetamol 325 mg. Net price 30-cap pack = £5.50. Label: 30, counselling, dosage
Dose migraine, 2 capsules at onset of attack, followed by 1 capsule every hour if necessary; max. 5 capsules in 12 hours; CHILD not recommended

1. A pack containing 15 capsules may be sold to the public

NEFOPAM HYDROCHLORIDE

Indications moderate pain
Cautions hepatic or renal disease, elderly, urinary retention; pregnancy (Appendix 4) and breast-feeding; **interactions**: Appendix 1 (nefopam)
Contra-indications convulsive disorders; not indicated for myocardial infarction
Side-effects nausea, nervousness, urinary retention, dry mouth, lightheadedness; less frequently vomiting, blurred vision, drowsiness, sweating, insomnia, tachycardia, headache; confusion and hallucinations also reported; may colour urine (pink)
Dose
- By mouth, initially 60 mg (elderly, 30 mg) 3 times daily, adjusted according to response; usual range 30–90 mg 3 times daily; CHILD not recommended

Acupan® (3M) PoM
Tablets, f/c, nefopam hydrochloride 30 mg. Net price 90-tab pack = £11.18. Label: 2, 14

4.7.2 Opioid analgesics

Opioid analgesics are usually used to relieve moderate to severe pain particularly of visceral origin. Repeated administration may cause dependence and tolerance but this is no deterrent in the control of pain in terminal illness, for guidelines see Prescribing in Palliative Care, p. 15. Regular use of a potent opioid may be appropriate for certain cases of chronic non-malignant pain; treatment should be supervised by a specialist and the patient should be assessed at regular intervals.

Cautions Opioids should be used with caution in patients with impaired respiratory function (avoid in chronic obstructive pulmonary disease) and asthma (avoid during an acute attack), hypotension, shock, prostatic hypertrophy, obstructive or inflammatory bowel disorders, diseases of the biliary tract, and convulsive disorders. A reduced dose is recommended in elderly or debilitated patients, in hepatic impairment (avoid if severe; Appendix 2) and renal impairment (avoid if severe; Appendix 3), in hypothyroidism, and in adrenocortical insufficiency. Repeated use of opioid analgesics is associated with the development of psychological and physical dependence; although this is rarely a problem with therapeutic use, caution is advised if prescribing for patients with a history of drug dependence. Avoid abrupt withdrawal after long-term treatment. For prescribing in pregnancy and breast-feeding, see Appendix 4 and Appendix 5, respectively.

Palliative care In the control of pain in terminal illness, the cautions listed above should not necessarily be a deterrent to the use of opioid analgesics.

Contra-indications Opioid analgesics should be avoided in patients with acute respiratory depression, and when there is a risk of paralytic ileus. They are also contra-indicated in conditions associated with raised intracranial pressure, and in head injury (opioid analgesics interfere with pupillary responses vital for neurological assessment). Comatose patients should not be treated with opioid analgesics.

Side-effects Opioid analgesics share many side-effects, although qualitative and quantitative differences exist. The most common side-effects include nausea and vomiting (particularly in initial stages), constipation, dry mouth and biliary spasm; larger doses produce muscle rigidity, hypotension and respiratory depression (for reversal of opioid-induced respiratory depression, see section 15.1.7). Other common side-effects of opioid analgesics include bradycardia, tachycardia, palpitation, oedema, postural hypotension, hallucinations, vertigo, euphoria, dysphoria, mood changes, dependence, dizziness, confusion, drowsiness, sleep disturbances, headache, sexual dysfunction, difficulty with micturition, urinary retention ureteric spasm, miosis, visual disturbances, sweating, flushing, rash, urticaria, and pruritus.
Overdosage: see Emergency Treatment of Poisoning, p. 31.

Interactions See Appendix 1 (opioid analgesics) (**important:** special hazard with *pethidine and possibly other opioids* and MAOIs).

Driving Drowsiness may affect performance of skilled tasks (e.g. driving); effects of alcohol enhanced.

Choice **Morphine** remains the most valuable opioid analgesic for severe pain although it frequently causes nausea and vomiting. It is the standard against which other opioid analgesics are compared. In addition to relief of pain, morphine also confers a state of euphoria and mental detachment.

Morphine is the opioid of choice for the oral treatment of *severe pain in palliative care.* It is given regularly every 4 hours (or every 12 or 24 hours as modified-release preparations). For guidelines on dosage adjustment in palliative care, see p. 15.

Buprenorphine has both opioid agonist and antagonist properties and may precipitate withdrawal symptoms, including pain, in patients dependent on other opioids. It has abuse potential and may itself cause dependence. It has a much longer duration of action than morphine and sublingually is an effective analgesic for 6 to 8 hours. Unlike most opioid analgesics, the effects of buprenorphine are only partially reversed by naloxone.

Codeine is effective for the relief of mild to moderate pain but is too constipating for long-term use.

Diphenoxylate (in combination with atropine, as co-phenotrope) is used in acute diarrhoea (see section 1.4.2).

Dipipanone used alone is less sedating than morphine but the only preparation available contains an anti-emetic and is therefore not suitable for regular regimens in palliative care.

Diamorphine (heroin) is a powerful opioid analgesic. It may cause less nausea and hypotension than morphine. In *palliative care* the greater solubility of diamorphine allows effective doses to be injected in smaller volumes and this is important in the emaciated patient.

Dihydrocodeine has an analgesic efficacy similar to that of codeine. The dose of dihydrocodeine by mouth is usually 30 mg every 4 hours; doubling the dose to 60 mg may provide some additional pain relief but this may be at the cost of more nausea and vomiting. A 40-mg tablet is now also available.

Alfentanil, **fentanyl** and **remifentanil** are used by injection for intra-operative analgesia (section 15.1.4.3); fentanyl is available in a transdermal drug delivery system as a self-adhesive patch which is changed every 72 hours.

Meptazinol is claimed to have a low incidence of respiratory depression. It has a reported length of action of 2 to 7 hours with onset within 15 minutes.

Methadone is less sedating than morphine and acts for longer periods. In prolonged use, methadone should not be administered more often than twice daily to avoid the risk of accumulation and opioid overdosage. Methadone may be used instead of morphine in the occasional patient who experiences excitation (or exacerbation of pain) with morphine.

Oxycodone has an efficacy and side-effect profile similar to that of morphine. It is used primarily for control of *pain in palliative care.*

Papaveretum is rarely used; morphine is easier to prescribe and less prone to error with regard to the strength and dose.

Pentazocine has both agonist and antagonist properties and precipitates withdrawal symptoms, including pain in patients dependent on other opioids. By injection it is more potent than dihydrocodeine or codeine, but hallucinations and thought disturbances may occur. It is not recommended and, in particular, should be avoided after myocardial infarction as it may increase pulmonary and aortic blood pressure as well as cardiac work.

Pethidine produces prompt but short-lasting analgesia; it is less constipating than morphine, but even in high doses is a less potent analgesic. It is not suitable for severe continuing pain. It is used for analgesia in labour; however, other opioids, such as morphine or diamorphine, are often preferred for obstetric pain.

Tramadol produces analgesia by two mechanisms: an opioid effect and an enhancement of serotonergic and adrenergic pathways. It has fewer of the typical opioid side-effects (notably, less respiratory depression, less constipation and less addiction potential); psychiatric reactions have been reported.

Dose The dose of opioids in the BNF may need to be **adjusted individually** according to the degree of analgesia and side-effects; patients' response to opioids varies widely.

Postoperative analgesia The use of intra-operative opioids affects the prescribing of postoperative analgesics and in many cases delays the need for a postoperative analgesic. A postoperative opioid analgesic should be given with care since it may potentiate any residual respiratory depression (for the treatment of opioid-induced respiratory depression, see section 15.1.7). Non-opioid analgesics are also used for postoperative pain (section 15.1.4.2).

Morphine is used most widely. **Tramadol** is not as effective in severe pain as other opioid analgesics. **Buprenorphine** may antagonise the analgesic effect of previously administered opioids and is generally not recommended. **Pethidine** is metabolised to norpethidine which may accumulate, particularly in renal impairment; norpethidine stimulates the central nervous system and may cause convulsions.

Opioids are also given epidurally [unlicensed route] in the postoperative period but are associated with side-effects such as pruritus, urinary retention, nausea and vomiting; respiratory depression can be delayed, particularly with morphine.

For details of patient-controlled analgesia (PCA) to relieve postoperative pain, consult hospital protocols. Formulations specifically designed for PCA are available (*Pharma-Ject® Morphine Sulphate*).

Dental and orofacial pain Opioid analgesics are **relatively ineffective** in dental pain. Like other opioids, **dihydrocodeine** often causes nausea and vomiting which limits its value in dental pain; if taken for more than a few doses it is also liable to cause constipation. Dihydrocodeine is not very effective in postoperative dental pain.

Pethidine can be taken by mouth, but for optimal effect, it needs to be given by injection. Its efficacy in postoperative dental pain is not proven and its use in dentistry is likely to be minimal. The side-effects of pethidine are similar to those of dihydrocodeine and, apart from constipation, pethidine is also more likely to cause them. Dependence is unlikely if very few tablets are prescribed on very few occasions; nevertheless, dental surgeons need to be aware of the possibility that addicts may seek to acquire supplies.

For the management of dental and orofacial pain, see p. 224.

Addicts Although caution is necessary, addicts (and ex-addicts) may be treated with analgesics in the same way as other people when there is a real clinical need. Doctors do not require a special licence to prescribe opioid analgesics for addicts for relief of pain due to organic disease or injury.

BUPRENORPHINE

Indications see under Dose and under Patches; opioid dependence (section 4.10)

Cautions see notes above; also impaired consciousness; effects only partially reversed by naloxone

Fever or external heat Monitor patients using patches for increased side-effects if fever present (increased absorption possible); avoid exposing application site to external heat (may also increase absorption)

Contra-indications see notes above; also myasthenia gravis

Side-effects see notes above; can induce mild withdrawal symptoms in patients dependent on opioids; also diarrhoea, abdominal pain, anorexia, dyspepsia; vasodilation; dyspnoea; paraesthesia, asthenia, fatigue, agitation, anxiety; *less commonly* flatulence, taste disturbance, angina, hypertension, syncope, hypoxia, wheezing, cough, restlessness, depersonalisation, dysarthria, impaired memory, hypoaesthesia, tremor, influenza-like symptoms, pyrexia, rhinitis, rigors, muscle cramp, myalgia, tinnitus, dry eye, and dry skin; *rarely* paralytic ileus, dysphagia, diverticulitis, impaired concentration, and psychosis; *very rarely* retching, hyperventilation, hiccups, and muscle fasciculation

Dose

- Moderate to severe pain, by sublingual administration, 200–400 micrograms every 6–8 hours; CHILD over 6 years, 16–25 kg, 100 micrograms every 6–8 hours; 25–37.5 kg, 100–200 micrograms every 6–8 hours; 37.5–50 kg, 200–300 micrograms every 6–8 hours

  By intramuscular *or* slow intravenous injection, 300–600 micrograms every 6–8 hours; CHILD over 6 months 3–6 micrograms/kg every 6–8 hours (max. 9 micrograms/kg)
- Premedication, by sublingual administration, 400 micrograms

  By intramuscular injection, 300 micrograms
- Intra-operative analgesia, by slow intravenous injection, 300–450 micrograms

Temgesic® (Schering-Plough) CD

Tablets (sublingual), buprenorphine (as hydrochloride), 200 micrograms, net price 50-tab pack = £5.33; 400 micrograms, 50-tab pack = £10.66. Label: 2, 26

Injection, buprenorphine (as hydrochloride) 300 micrograms/mL, net price 1-mL amp = 49p

Patches

BuTrans® (Napp) CD

Patches, self-adhesive, beige, buprenorphine, '5' patch (releasing 5 micrograms/hour for 7 days), net price 2 = £9.16; '10' patch (releasing 10 micrograms/

hour for 7 days), 4 = £33.32; '20' patch (releasing 20 micrograms/hour for 7 days), 4 = £60.68. Label: 2

Dose severe pain unresponsive to non-opioid analgesics, ADULT over 18 years, initially one '5 micrograms/hour' patch; apply to dry, non-irritated, non-hairy skin on upper torso, removing after 7 days and siting replacement patch on a different area (avoid same area for at least 3 weeks)

Dose adjustment When starting, analgesic effect should **not** be evaluated until the system has been worn for **72 hours** (to allow for gradual increase in plasma-buprenorphine concentration)—if necessary, dose should be adjusted at 3-day intervals using a patch of the next strength or 2 patches of the same strength (applied at *same time* to avoid confusion). Max. 2 patches can be used at any one time

Transtec® (Napp) CD

Patches, self-adhesive, skin-coloured, buprenorphine, '35' patch (releasing 35 micrograms/hour for 96 hours), net price 4 = £18.54; '52.5' patch (releasing 52.5 micrograms/hour for 96 hours), 4 = £27.82; '70' patch (releasing 70 micrograms/hour for 96 hours), 4 = £37.08. Label: 2

Dose moderate to severe cancer pain and severe pain unresponsive to non-opioid analgesics, ADULT over 18 years, apply to dry, non-irritated, non-hairy skin on upper torso, removing after no longer than 96 hours and siting replacement patch on a different area (avoid same area for at least 6 days). Patients who have not previously received strong opioid analgesic, initially, one '35 micrograms/hour' patch replaced after no longer than 96 hours; patients who have received strong opioid analgesic, initial dose based on previous 24-hour opioid requirement, consult product literature

Dose adjustment When starting, analgesic effect should **not** be evaluated until the system has been worn for **24 hours** (to allow for gradual increase in plasma-buprenorphine concentration)—if necessary, dose should be adjusted at intervals of no longer than 96 hours using a patch of the next strength *or* using 2 patches of the same strength (applied at *same time* to avoid confusion). Max. 2 patches can be used at any one time. For breakthrough pain, consider 200–400 micrograms buprenorphine sublingually.

Important: it may take approx. 30 hours for the plasma-buprenorphine concentration to decrease by 50% after patch is removed

Long duration of action In view of the long duration of action, patients who have severe side-effects should be monitored for up to 30 hours after removing patch

CODEINE PHOSPHATE

Indications mild to moderate pain; diarrhoea (section 1.4.2); cough suppression (section 3.9.1)

Cautions see notes above; also cardiac arrhythmias; myasthenia gravis; acute abdomen; gallstones

Variation in metabolism The capacity to metabolise codeine can vary considerably and lead to either reduced therapeutic effect or marked increase in side-effects

Contra-indications see notes above

Side-effects see notes above; also abdominal pain, anorexia, seizures, malaise, hypothermia, and muscle fasciculation; pancreatitis also reported

Dose

- By mouth, 30–60 mg every 4 hours when necessary, to a max. of 240 mg daily; CHILD 1–12 years, 3 mg/kg daily in divided doses
- By intramuscular injection, 30–60 mg every 4 hours when necessary

Codeine Phosphate (Non-proprietary)

Tablets PoM, codeine phosphate 15 mg, net price 28 = £2.10; 30 mg, 28 = £2.29; 60 mg, 28 = £4.29. Label: 2

Syrup PoM, codeine phosphate 25 mg/5 mL. Net price 100 mL = 90p. Label: 2

Injection CD, codeine phosphate 60 mg/mL. Net price 1-mL amp = £2.37

Linctus

Section 3.9.1

DIAMORPHINE HYDROCHLORIDE

(Heroin Hydrochloride)

Indications see under Dose; acute pulmonary oedema

Cautions see notes above; also severe diarrhoea; toxic psychosis, CNS depression; severe cor pulmonale

Contra-indications see notes above; also delayed gastric emptying; phaeochromocytoma

Side-effects see notes above; also anorexia, taste disturbance; syncope; asthenia, raised intracranial pressure; myocardial infarction also reported

Dose

- Acute pain, by subcutaneous *or* intramuscular injection, 5 mg repeated every 4 hours if necessary (up to 10 mg for heavier well-muscled patients); by slow intravenous injection, quarter to half corresponding intramuscular dose
- Myocardial infarction, by slow intravenous injection (1 mg/minute), 5 mg followed by a further 2.5–5 mg if necessary; elderly or frail patients, reduce dose by half
- Acute pulmonary oedema, by slow intravenous injection (1 mg/minute) 2.5–5 mg
- Chronic pain, by mouth *or* by subcutaneous *or* intramuscular injection, 5–10 mg regularly every 4 hours; dose may be increased according to needs; intramuscular dose should be approx. half corresponding oral dose, and approx. one third corresponding oral *morphine* dose—see also Prescribing in Palliative Care, p. 15; by subcutaneous infusion (using syringe driver), see Prescribing in Palliative Care, p. 18

Diamorphine (Non-proprietary) CD

Tablets, diamorphine hydrochloride 10 mg. Net price 100-tab pack = £12.30. Label: 2

Injection, powder for reconstitution, diamorphine hydrochloride. Net price 5-mg amp = £1.77, 10-mg amp = £3.09, 30-mg amp = £3.34, 100-mg amp = £6.75, 500-mg amp = £31.03

DIHYDROCODEINE TARTRATE

Indications moderate to severe pain

Cautions see notes above; also pancreatitis; severe cor pulmonale

Contra-indications see notes above

Side-effects see notes above; also paralytic ileus, abdominal pain, and paraesthesia

Dose

- By mouth, 30 mg every 4–6 hours when necessary (see also notes above); CHILD over 4 years 0.5–1 mg/kg every 4–6 hours
- By deep subcutaneous *or* intramuscular injection, up to 50 mg repeated every 4–6 hours if necessary; CHILD over 4 years 0.5–1 mg/kg every 4–6 hours

Dihydrocodeine (Non-proprietary)

Tablets PoM, dihydrocodeine tartrate 30 mg. Net price 28 = £2.40. Label: 2, 21

Dental prescribing on NHS Dihydrocodeine Tablets 30 mg may be prescribed

Oral solution PoM, dihydrocodeine tartrate 10 mg/5 mL. Net price 150 mL = £3.08. Label: 2, 21

Injection CD, dihydrocodeine tartrate 50 mg/mL. Net price 1-mL amp = £2.29

DF 118 Forte® (Martindale) PoM
Tablets, dihydrocodeine tartrate 40 mg. Net price 100-tab pack = £11.51. Label: 2, 21
Dose ADULT and CHILD over 12 years, severe pain, 40–80 mg 3 times daily; max. 240 mg daily

Modified release

DHC Continus® (Napp) PoM
Tablets, m/r, dihydrocodeine tartrate 60 mg, net price 56-tab pack = £5.50; 90 mg, 56-tab pack = £8.66; 120 mg, 56-tab pack = £11.57. Label: 2, 25
Dose ADULT and CHILD over 12 years, chronic severe pain, 60–120 mg every 12 hours
Note Dihydrocodeine is an ingredient of some compound analgesic preparations, see section 4.7.1

DIPIPANONE HYDROCHLORIDE

Indications moderate to severe pain
Cautions see notes above; also diabetes mellitus; phaeochromocytoma
Contra-indications see notes above
Side-effects see notes above; also psychosis, restlessness, raised intracranial pressure
Dose
- See preparation below

Diconal® (Amdipharm) CD
Tablets, pink, scored, dipipanone hydrochloride 10 mg, cyclizine hydrochloride 30 mg. Net price 50-tab pack = £8.70. Label: 2
Dose *acute pain*, 1 tablet gradually increased to 3 tablets every 6 hours; CHILD not recommended
Caution Not recommended in palliative care, see Nausea and Vomiting, p. 18

FENTANYL

Indications see under preparations; parenteral indications (section 15.1.4.3)
Cautions see notes above; also diabetes mellitus, impaired consciousness, cerebral tumour, myasthenia gravis
Fever or external heat Monitor patients using patches for increased side-effects if fever present (increased absorption possible); avoid exposing application site to external heat (may also increase absorption)
Contra-indications see notes above
Side-effects see notes above; also abdominal pain, anorexia, dyspepsia, mouth ulcer, taste disturbance, dry mouth; vasodilation; apnoea; anxiety; myoclonus; *less commonly* flatulence, diarrhoea, laryngospasm, dyspnoea, hypoventilation, depersonalisation, dysarthria, amnesia, incoordination, paraesthesia, malaise, agitation, tremor, and muscle weakness; *rarely* hiccups and arrhythmia; *very rarely* paralytic ileus, haemoptysis, psychosis, and seizures; shock, asystole, pyrexia, ataxia, and muscle fasciculation also reported; *with patches*, local reactions such as rash, erythema, and itching reported
Dose
- See under preparations

Conversion (from oral morphine to transdermal fentanyl), see Prescribing in Palliative Care, p. 16

Lozenges

Actiq® (Cephalon) CD
Lozenge, (with oromucosal applicator), fentanyl (as citrate) 200 micrograms, net price 3 = £18.58, 30 = £185.80; 400 micrograms, 3 = £18.58, 30 = £185.80; 600 micrograms, 3 = £18.58, 30 = £185.80; 800 micrograms, 3 = £18.58, 30 = £185.80; 1.2 mg, 3 = £18.58, 30 = £185.80; 1.6 mg, 3 = £18.58, 30 = £185.80. Label: 2
Dose breakthrough pain in patients receiving opioid therapy for chronic cancer pain, initially 200 micrograms (over 15 minutes) repeated if necessary 15 minutes after first dose (no more than 2 dose units for each pain episode); adjust dose according to response; max. 4 dose units daily
Note If more than 4 episodes of breakthrough pain each day, adjust dose of background analgesic

Patches

Prescriptions Prescriptions for fentanyl patches can be written to show the strength in terms of the release rate and it is acceptable to write '*Fentanyl 25 patches*' to prescribe patches that release fentanyl 25 micrograms per hour. The dosage should be expressed in terms of the interval between applying a patch and replacing it with a new one, e.g. '*one patch to be applied every 72 hours*'. The total quantity of patches should be written in words and figures.

Fentanyl (Non-proprietary) CD
Patches, self-adhesive, fentanyl, '12' patch (releasing approx. 12 micrograms/hour for 72 hours), net price 5 = £18.85; '25' patch (releasing approx. 25 micrograms/hour for 72 hours), 5 = £26.94; '50' patch (releasing approx. 50 micrograms/hour for 72 hours), 5 = £50.32; '75' patch (releasing approx. 75 micrograms/hour for 72 hours), 5 = £70.15; '100' patch (releasing approx. 100 micrograms/hour for 72 hours), 5 = £86.46. Label: 2
Brands include *Tilofyl®*, *Matrifen®* ▼
Dose severe chronic pain, apply to dry, non-irritated, non-irradiated, non-hairy skin on torso or upper arm, removing after 72 hours and siting replacement patch on a different area (avoid using the same area for at least 7 days). ADULT not previously treated with strong opioid analgesic, initial dose one '12' [unlicensed] or '25 micrograms/hour' patch replaced after 72 hours; ADULT previously treated with strong opioid analgesic, initial dose based on previous 24-hour opioid requirement (consult product literature)
Dose adjustment When starting, evaluation of the analgesic effect should **not** be made before the system has been worn for **24 hours** (to allow for the gradual increase in plasma-fentanyl concentration)—previous analgesic therapy should be phased out gradually from time of first patch application; if necessary dose should be adjusted at 72-hour intervals in steps of 12–25 micrograms/hour. More than one patch may be used at a time for doses greater than 100 micrograms/hour (but applied at *same time* to avoid confusion)—consider additional or alternative analgesic therapy if dose required exceeds 300 micrograms/hour (**important:** it may take up to 25 hours for the plasma-fentanyl concentration to decrease by 50%—replacement opioid therapy should be initiated at a low dose and increased gradually).
Long duration of action In view of the long duration of action, patients who have had severe side-effects should be monitored for up to 24 hours after patch removal

Durogesic DTrans® (Janssen-Cilag) CD
Patches, self-adhesive, transparent, fentanyl, '12' patch (releasing approx. 12 micrograms/hour for 72 hours), net price 5 = £18.85; '25' patch (releasing approx. 25 micrograms/hour for 72 hours), 5 = £26.94; '50' patch (releasing approx. 50 micrograms/hour for 72 hours), 5 = £50.32; '75' patch (releasing approx. 75 micrograms/hour for 72 hours), 5 = £70.15; '100' patch (releasing approx. 100 micrograms/hour for 72 hours), 5 = £88.32. Label: 2
Dose chronic intractable pain, apply to dry, non-irritated, non-irradiated, non-hairy skin on torso or upper arm, removing after 72 hours and siting replacement patch on a different area (avoid using the same area for several days). ADULT over 16 years not previously treated with strong opioid analgesic, initial dose, one '12' [unlicensed] or '25 micrograms/hour' patch replaced after 72 hours; ADULT and CHILD over 2 years previously treated with

strong opioid analgesic, initial dose based on previous 24-hour opioid requirement (consult product literature)

Dose adjustment When starting, evaluation of the analgesic effect should **not** be made before the system has been worn for **24 hours** (to allow for the gradual increase in plasma-fentanyl concentration)—previous analgesic therapy should be phased out gradually from time of first patch application; if necessary dose should be adjusted at 72-hour intervals in steps of 12–25 micrograms/hour. More than one patch may be used at a time for doses greater than 100 micrograms/hour (but applied at *same time* to avoid confusion)—consider additional or alternative analgesic therapy if dose required exceeds 300 micrograms/hour (**important:** it may take up to 25 hours for the plasma-fentanyl concentration to decrease by 50%—replacement opioid therapy should be initiated at a low dose and increased gradually).

Long duration of action In view of the long duration of action, patients who have had severe side-effects should be monitored for up to 24 hours after patch removal

HYDROMORPHONE HYDROCHLORIDE

Indications severe pain in cancer

Cautions see notes above; also pancreatitis; toxic psychosis

Contra-indications see notes above; also acute abdomen

Side-effects see notes above; also paralytic ileus, seizures, asthenia, agitation, and myoclonus

Dose

- See under preparations below

Palladone® (Napp) CD

Capsules, hydromorphone hydrochloride 1.3 mg (orange/clear), net price 56-cap pack = £8.82; 2.6 mg (red/clear), 56-cap pack = £17.64. Label: 2, counselling, see below

Dose 1.3 mg every 4 hours, increased if necessary according to severity of pain; CHILD under 12 years not recommended

Counselling Swallow whole or open capsule and sprinkle contents on soft food

Modified release

Palladone® SR (Napp) CD

Capsules, m/r, hydromorphone hydrochloride 2 mg (yellow/clear), net price 56-cap pack = £20.98; 4 mg (pale blue/clear), 56-cap pack = £28.75; 8 mg (pink/clear), 56-cap pack = £56.08; 16 mg (brown/clear), 56-cap pack = £106.53; 24 mg (dark blue/clear), 56-cap pack = £159.82. Label: 2, counselling, see below

Dose 4 mg every 12 hours, increased if necessary according to severity of pain; CHILD under 12 years not recommended

Counselling Swallow whole or open capsule and sprinkle contents on soft food

MEPTAZINOL

Indications moderate to severe pain, including post-operative and obstetric pain and renal colic; peri-operative analgesia, see section 15.1.4.3

Cautions see notes above; effects only partially reversed by naloxone

Contra-indications see notes above; also myocardial infarction; phaeochromocytoma

Side-effects see notes above; can induce withdrawal symptoms in patients dependent on opioids; also diarrhoea, abdominal pain, dyspepsia, and hypothermia

Dose

- By mouth, 200 mg every 3–6 hours as required; CHILD not recommended
- By intramuscular injection, 75–100 mg every 2–4 hours if necessary; obstetric analgesia, 100–150 mg according to patient's weight (2 mg/kg); CHILD not recommended
- By slow intravenous injection, 50–100 mg every 2–4 hours if necessary; CHILD not recommended

Meptid® (Shire) PoM

Tablets, orange, f/c, meptazinol 200 mg, net price 112-tab pack = £22.11. Label: 2

Injection, meptazinol 100 mg (as hydrochloride)/mL, net price 1-mL amp = £1.92

METHADONE HYDROCHLORIDE

Indications severe pain, see notes above; cough in terminal disease (section 3.9.1); adjunct in treatment of opioid dependence (section 4.10)

Cautions see notes above; also myasthenia gravis; history of cardiac conduction abnormalities, family history of sudden death (ECG monitoring recommended; see also QT Interval Prolongation, below)

QT interval prolongation The CHM has recommended that patients with the following risk factors for QT interval prolongation are carefully monitored while taking methadone: heart or liver disease, electrolyte abnormalities, or concomitant treatment with drugs that can prolong QT interval; patients requiring more than 100 mg daily should also be monitored

Contra-indications see notes above; also phaeochromocytoma

Side-effects see notes above; also QT interval prolongation, torsade de pointes, hypothermia, restlessness, raised intracranial pressure, dysmenorrhoea, dry eye, and hyperprolactinaemia

Dose

- By mouth or by subcutaneous or intramuscular injection, 5–10 mg every 6–8 hours, adjusted according to response; on prolonged use not to be given more frequently than every 12 hours; CHILD not recommended

Methadone (Non-proprietary) CD

Tablets, methadone hydrochloride 5 mg. Net price 50 = £2.97. Label: 2

Brands include *Physeptone®*

Injection▼, methadone hydrochloride, 10 mg/mL, net price 1-mL amp = 86p, 2-mL amp = £1.45, 3.5-mL amp = £1.78, 5-mL amp = £1.92

Brands include *Physeptone®*, *Synastone®*

Linctus

Section 3.9.1

Oral solution and oral concentrate

Section 4.10

MORPHINE SALTS

Indications see notes above and under Dose; acute diarrhoea (section 1.4.2); cough in terminal care (section 3.9.1)

Cautions see notes above; also pancreatitis, myasthenia gravis, cardiac arrhythmias, severe cor pulmonale

Contra-indications see notes above; also delayed gastric emptying, acute abdomen; heart failure secondary to chronic lung disease; phaeochromocytoma

Side-effects see notes above; also paralytic ileus, abdominal pain, anorexia, dyspepsia, exacerbation of pancreatitis, taste disturbance, hypertension, hypothermia, syncope, bronchospasm, inhibition of cough reflex, restlessness, seizures, paraesthesia, asthenia, malaise, disorientation, excitation, agitation, delirium, raised intracranial pressure, amenorrhoea, myoclonus, muscle fasciculation, and rhabdomyolysis

Dose

The patient should be closely monitored for pain relief as well as for side-effects especially respiratory depression. See also notes above.

- Acute pain, by subcutaneous injection (not suitable for oedematous patients) *or* by intramuscular injection, initially 10 mg (ELDERLY or frail 5 mg) every 4 hours (or more frequently during titration), adjusted according to response; NEONATE initially 100 micrograms/kg every 6 hours, adjusted according to response; CHILD 1–6 months initially 100–200 micrograms/kg every 6 hours, adjusted according to response; CHILD 6 months–2 years initially 100–200 micrograms/kg every 4 hours, adjusted according to response; CHILD 2–12 years initially 200 micrograms/kg every 4 hours, adjusted according to response; CHILD 12–18 years initially 2.5–10 mg every 4 hours, adjusted according to response

  By slow intravenous injection, initially 2.5 mg (reduce dose in ELDERLY or frail) every 4 hours (or more frequently during titration), adjusted according to response; NEONATE initially 40–100 micrograms/kg every 6 hours, adjusted according to response; CHILD 1–6 months initially 100–200 micrograms/kg every 6 hours, adjusted according to response; CHILD 6 months–12 years initially 100–200 micrograms/kg every 4 hours, adjusted according to response
- Premedication, by subcutaneous *or* intramuscular injection, up to 10 mg 60–90 minutes before operation; CHILD, by intramuscular injection, 150 micrograms/kg
- Patient controlled analgesia (PCA), consult hospital protocols
- Myocardial infarction, by slow intravenous injection (2 mg/minute), 10 mg followed by a further 5–10 mg if necessary; elderly or frail patients, reduce dose by half
- Acute pulmonary oedema, by slow intravenous injection (2 mg/minute) 5–10 mg
- Chronic pain, by mouth *or* by subcutaneous injection (not suitable for oedematous patients) *or* by intramuscular injection, initially 5–20 mg every 4 hours, adjusted according to response; see also Prescribing in Palliative Care, p. 15

  By rectum, initially 15–30 mg every 4 hours, adjusted according to response

  Note The doses stated above refer equally to morphine hydrochloride, sulphate, and tartrate; see below for doses of **modified-release** preparations

Oral solutions

Note For advice on transfer from oral solutions of morphine to modified-release preparations of morphine, see Prescribing in Palliative Care, p. 15

Morphine Oral Solutions

PoM or CD

Oral solutions of morphine can be prescribed by writing the formula:

Morphine hydrochloride 5 mg
Chloroform water to 5 mL

Note The proportion of morphine hydrochloride may be altered when specified by the prescriber; if above 13 mg per 5 mL the solution becomes CD. For sample prescription see Controlled Drugs and Drug Dependence, p. 8. It is usual to adjust the strength so that the dose volume is 5 or 10 mL.

Oramorph® (Boehringer Ingelheim)

Oramorph® oral solution PoM, morphine sulphate 10 mg/5 mL. Net price 100-mL pack = £1.87; 300-mL pack = £5.21; 500-mL pack = £7.86. Label: 2

Oramorph® Unit Dose Vials 10 mg PoM (oral vials), sugar-free, morphine sulphate 10 mg/5-mL vial, net price 20 vials = £2.65. Label: 2

Oramorph® Unit Dose Vials 30 mg CD (oral vials), sugar-free, morphine sulphate 30 mg/5-mL vial, net price 20 vials = £7.44. Label: 2

Oramorph® Unit Dose Vials 100 mg CD (oral vials), sugar-free, morphine sulphate 100 mg/5-mL vial, net price 20 vials = £24.80. Label: 2

Oramorph® concentrated oral solution CD, sugar-free, morphine sulphate 100 mg/5 mL. Net price 30-mL pack = £5.24; 120-mL pack = £19.57 (both with calibrated dropper). Label: 2

Tablets

Sevredol® (Napp) CD

Tablets, f/c, scored, morphine sulphate 10 mg (blue), net price 56-tab pack = £5.61; 20 mg (pink), 56-tab pack = £11.21; 50 mg (pale green), 56-tab pack = £28.02. Label: 2

Modified-release oral preparations

Morphgesic® SR (Amdipharm) CD

Tablets, m/r, f/c, morphine sulphate 10 mg (buff), net price 60-tab pack = £4.09; 30 mg (violet), 60-tab pack = £9.81; 60 mg (orange), 60-tab pack = £19.15; 100 mg (grey), 60-tab pack = £30.30. Label: 2, 25

Dose every 12 hours, dose adjusted according to daily morphine requirements; for further advice on determining dose, see Prescribing in Palliative Care, p. 15; dosage requirements should be reviewed if the brand is altered

Note Prescriptions must also specify 'tablets' (i.e. Morphgesic SR tablets)

MST Continus® (Napp) CD

Tablets, m/r, f/c, morphine sulphate 5 mg (white), net price 60-tab pack = £3.29; 10 mg (brown), 60-tab pack = £5.48; 15 mg (green), 60-tab pack = £9.61; 30 mg (purple), 60-tab pack = £13.17; 60 mg (orange), 60-tab pack = £25.69; 100 mg (grey), 60-tab pack = £40.66; 200 mg (green), 60-tab pack = £81.34. Label: 2, 25

Suspension (= sachet of granules to mix with water), m/r, pink, morphine sulphate 20 mg/sachet, net price 30-sachet pack = £24.58; 30 mg/sachet, 30-sachet pack = £25.54; 60 mg/sachet, 30-sachet pack = £51.09; 100 mg/sachet, 30-sachet pack = £85.15; 200 mg/sachet pack, 30-sachet pack = £170.30. Label: 2, 13

Dose every 12 hours, dose adjusted according to daily morphine requirements; for further advice on determining dose, see Prescribing in Palliative Care, p. 15; dosage requirements should be reviewed if the brand is altered

Note Prescriptions must also specify 'tablets' or 'suspension' (i.e. 'MST Continus tablets' or 'MST Continus suspension')

MXL® (Napp) CD

Capsules, m/r, morphine sulphate 30 mg (light blue), net price 28-cap pack = £10.91; 60 mg (brown), 28-cap pack = £14.95; 90 mg (pink), 28-cap pack = £22.04; 120 mg (green), 28-cap pack = £29.15; 150 mg (blue),

28-cap pack = £36.43; 200 mg (red-brown), 28-cap pack = £46.15. Label: 2, counselling, see below

Dose every 24 hours, dose adjusted according to daily morphine requirements; for further advice on determining dose, see Prescribing in Palliative Care, p. 15; dosage requirements should be reviewed if the brand is altered

Counselling Swallow whole or open capsule and sprinkle contents on soft food

Note Prescriptions must also specify 'capsules' (i.e. 'MXL capsules')

Zomorph® (Link) CD

Capsules, m/r, morphine sulphate 10 mg (yellow/clear enclosing pale yellow pellets), net price 60-cap pack = £4.08; 30 mg (pink/clear enclosing pale yellow pellets), 60-cap pack = £9.77; 60 mg (orange/clear enclosing pale yellow pellets), 60-cap pack = £19.06; 100 mg (white/clear enclosing pale yellow pellets), 60-cap pack = £30.18; 200 mg (clear enclosing pale yellow pellets), 60-cap pack = £60.35. Label: 2, counselling, see below

Dose every 12 hours, dose adjusted according to daily morphine requirements; for further advice on determining doses, see Prescribing in Palliative Care, p. 15; dosage requirements should be reviewed if the brand is altered

Counselling Swallow whole or open capsule and sprinkle contents on soft food

Note Prescriptions must also specify 'capsules' (i.e. 'Zomorph capsules')

Suppositories

Morphine (Non-proprietary) CD

Suppositories, morphine hydrochloride or sulphate 10 mg, net price 12 = £7.24; 15 mg, 12 = £7.14; 20 mg, 12 = £8.92; 30 mg, 12 = £10.38. Label: 2

Available from Aurum, Martindale

Note Both the strength of the suppositories and the morphine salt contained in them must be specified by the prescriber

Injections

Morphine Sulphate (Non-proprietary) CD

Injection, morphine sulphate 10, 15, 20, and 30 mg/mL, net price 1- and 2-mL amp (all) = 72p–£1.09; 10 mg/mL, 1-mL prefilled syringe = £5.00

Intravenous infusion, morphine sulphate 1 mg/mL, net price 50-mL vial = £5.00; 2 mg/mL, 50-mL vial = £5.10

Minijet® Morphine Sulphate (Celltech) CD

Injection, morphine sulphate 1 mg/mL, net price 10-mL disposable syringe = £7.36

Injection with antiemetic

Caution In myocardial infarction cyclizine may aggravate severe heart failure and counteract the haemodynamic benefits of opioids, see section 4.6. **Not recommended** in palliative care, see Nausea and Vomiting, p. 17

Cyclimorph® (Amdipharm) CD

Cyclimorph-10® Injection, morphine tartrate 10 mg, cyclizine tartrate 50 mg/mL. Net price 1-mL amp = £1.34

Dose ADULT and CHILD over 12 years, moderate to severe pain (short-term use only) by subcutaneous, intramuscular, or intravenous injection, 1 mL, repeated not more often than every 4 hours; max. 3 doses in any 24-hour period

Cyclimorph-15® Injection, morphine tartrate 15 mg, cyclizine tartrate 50 mg/mL. Net price 1-mL amp = £1.39

Dose ADULT and CHILD over 12 years, moderate to severe pain (short-term use only) by subcutaneous, intramuscular, or intravenous injection, 1 mL, repeated not more often than every 4 hours; max. 3 doses in any 24-hour period

OXYCODONE HYDROCHLORIDE

Indications moderate to severe pain in patients with cancer; postoperative pain; severe pain

Cautions see notes above; also toxic psychosis; pancreatitis

Contra-indications see notes above; also acute abdomen; delayed gastric emptying; chronic constipation; cor pulmonale; porphyria (section 9.8.2)

Side-effects see notes above; also diarrhoea, abdominal pain, anorexia, dyspepsia; bronchospasm, dyspnoea, impaired cough reflex; asthenia, anxiety; chills; muscle fasciculation; *less commonly* paralytic ileus, gastritis, flatulence, dysphagia, taste disturbance, belching, hiccups, vasodilation, supraventricular tachycardia, syncope, amnesia, hypoaesthesia, restlessness, seizures, pyrexia, amenorrhoea, hypotonia, paraesthesia, disorientation, malaise, agitation, speech disorder, tremor, and dry skin

Dose

- By mouth, initially, 5 mg every 4–6 hours, increased if necessary according to severity of pain, usual max. 400 mg daily, but some patients may require higher doses; CHILD under 18 years, see *BNF for Children*
- By slow intravenous injection, 1–10 mg every 4 hours when necessary; CHILD under 18 years, not recommended
- By intravenous infusion, initially 2 mg/hour, adjusted according to response; CHILD under 18 years not recommended
- By subcutaneous injection, initially 5 mg every 4 hours when necessary; CHILD under 18 years, not recommended
- By subcutaneous infusion, initially 7.5 mg/24 hours adjusted according to response; CHILD under 18 years, not recommended
- Patient controlled analgesia (PCA), consult hospital protocols

Note 2 mg oral oxycodone is approximately equivalent to 1 mg parenteral oxycodone

OxyNorm® (Napp) CD

Capsules, oxycodone hydrochloride 5 mg (orange/beige), net price 56-cap pack = £12.07; 10 mg (white/beige), 56-cap pack = £24.14; 20 mg (pink/beige), 56-cap pack = £48.27. Label: 2

Liquid (= oral solution), sugar-free, oxycodone hydrochloride 5 mg/5 mL, net price 250 mL = £10.26. Label: 2

Concentrate (= concentrated oral solution), sugar-free, oxycodone hydrochloride 10 mg/mL, net price 120 mL = £49.25. Label: 2

Injection, oxycodone hydrochloride 10 mg/mL, net price 1-mL amp = £1.60, 2-mL amp = £3.20

Note The *Scottish Medicines Consortium* has advised (October 2004) that *OxyNorm®* injection is used only in patients with cancer who have difficulty in tolerating morphine or diamorphine

Modified release

OxyContin® (Napp) CD

Tablets, f/c, m/r, oxycodone hydrochloride 5 mg (blue), net price 28-tab pack = £13.23; 10 mg (white), 56-tab pack = £26.45; 20 mg (pink), 56-tab pack =

4 Central nervous system

£52.89; 40 mg (yellow), 56-tab pack = £105.80; 80 mg (green), 56-tab pack = £211.61. Label: 2, 25

Dose initially, 10 mg every 12 hours, increased if necessary according to severity of pain, usual max. 200 mg every 12 hours, but some patients may require higher doses; CHILD under 18 years, see *BNF for Children*

PAPAVERETUM

Important Do **not** confuse with papaverine (section 7.4.5)

A mixture of 253 parts of morphine hydrochloride, 23 parts of papaverine hydrochloride and 20 parts of codeine hydrochloride

The CSM has advised that to avoid confusion the figures of 7.7 mg/ml or 15.4 mg/ml should be used for prescribing purposes

Indications premedication; enhancement of anaesthesia (but see section 15.1.4.3); postoperative analgesia; severe chronic pain

Cautions see notes above; supraventricular tachycardia

Contra-indications see notes above; heart failure secondary to chronic lung disease; phaeochromocytoma

Side-effects see notes above; also hypothermia

Dose

- By subcutaneous, intramuscular, *or* intravenous injection, 7.7–15.4 mg repeated every 4 hours if necessary (ELDERLY initially 7.7 mg); CHILD up to 1 month 115 micrograms/kg, 1–12 months 154 micrograms/kg, 1–5 years 1.93–3.85 mg, 6–12 years, 3.85–7.7 mg

  Intravenous dose In general the intravenous dose should be 25–50% of the corresponding subcutaneous or intramuscular dose

Papaveretum (Non-proprietary) CD

Injection, papaveretum 15.4 mg/mL (providing the equivalent of 10 mg of anhydrous morphine/mL), net price 1-mL amp = £1.43

Note The name *Omnopon®* was formerly used for papaveretum preparations

With hyoscine

Papaveretum and Hyoscine Injection (Non-proprietary) CD

Injection, papaveretum 15.4 mg (providing the equivalent of 10 mg of anhydrous morphine), hyoscine hydrobromide 400 micrograms/mL. Net price 1-mL amp = £2.60

Dose premedication, by subcutaneous or intramuscular injection, 0.5–1 mL

With aspirin

Section 4.7.1

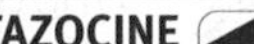

PENTAZOCINE

Indications moderate to severe pain, but see notes above

Cautions see notes above; also pancreatitis, arterial or pulmonary hypertension, cardiac arrhythmias, myocardial infarction, phaeochromocytoma; effects only partially reversed by naloxone

Contra-indications see notes above; patients dependent on opioids (can precipitate withdrawal); heart failure secondary to chronic lung disease; porphyria (section 9.8.2)

Side-effects see notes above; also abdominal pain, hypertension, syncope, seizures, paraesthesia, tremor, raised intracranial pressure, disorientation, hypothermia, chills, blood disorders, myalgia, and toxic epidermal necrolysis

Dose

- By mouth, pentazocine hydrochloride 50 mg every 3–4 hours preferably after food (range 25–100 mg); max. 600 mg daily; CHILD 6–12 years 25 mg
- By subcutaneous, intramuscular, or intravenous injection, moderate pain, pentazocine 30 mg, severe pain 45–60 mg every 3–4 hours when necessary; CHILD over 1 year, by subcutaneous *or* intramuscular injection, up to 1 mg/kg, by intravenous injection up to 500 micrograms/kg
- By rectum in suppositories, pentazocine 50 mg up to 4 times daily; CHILD not recommended

Pentazocine (Non-proprietary) CD

Capsules, pentazocine hydrochloride 50 mg. Net price 28-cap pack = £10.40. Label: 2, 21

Brands include *Fortral®* NHS

Tablets, pentazocine hydrochloride 25 mg. Net price 28-tab pack = £7.80. Label: 2, 21

Brands include *Fortral®* NHS

Injection, pentazocine 30 mg (as lactate)/mL. Net price 1-mL amp = £1.67; 2-mL amp = £3.21

Brands include *Fortral®* NHS

PETHIDINE HYDROCHLORIDE

Indications moderate to severe pain, obstetric analgesia; peri-operative analgesia

Cautions see notes above; not suitable for severe continuing pain; accumulation of metabolites may result in neurotoxicity; myasthenia gravis; cardiac arrhythmias, severe cor pulmonale

Contra-indications see notes above; phaeochromocytoma

Side-effects see notes above; also restlessness and hypothermia; convulsions reported in **overdosage**

Dose

- Acute pain, by mouth, 50–150 mg every 4 hours; CHILD 0.5–2 mg/kg

  By subcutaneous *or* intramuscular injection, 25–100 mg, repeated after 4 hours; CHILD, by intramuscular injection, 0.5–2 mg/kg

  By slow intravenous injection, 25–50 mg, repeated after 4 hours
- Obstetric analgesia, by subcutaneous *or* intramuscular injection, 50–100 mg, repeated 1–3 hours later if necessary; max. 400 mg in 24 hours
- Premedication, by intramuscular injection, 25–100 mg 1 hour before operation; CHILD 0.5–2 mg/kg
- Postoperative pain, by subcutaneous *or* intramuscular injection, 25–100 mg, every 2–3 hours if necessary; CHILD, by intramuscular injection, 0.5–2 mg/kg

  Note In the postoperative period, the patient should be closely monitored for pain relief as well as for side-effects especially respiratory depression

Pethidine (Non-proprietary) CD

Tablets, pethidine hydrochloride 50 mg, net price 20 = £1.97. Label: 2

Dental prescribing on NHS Pethidine Tablets may be prescribed

Injection, pethidine hydrochloride 50 mg/mL, net price 1-mL amp = 53p, 2-mL amp = 56p; 10 mg/mL, 5-mL amp = £2.06, 10-mL amp = £2.18

Pamergan P100® (Martindale) CD ◢

Injection, pethidine hydrochloride 50 mg, promethazine hydrochloride 25 mg/mL. Net price 2-mL amp = £1.44

Dose by intramuscular injection, premedication, 2 mL 60–90 minutes before operation; CHILD 8–12 years 0.75 mL, 13–16 years 1 mL

Obstetric analgesia, 1–2 mL every 4 hours if necessary

Severe pain, 1–2 mL every 4–6 hours if necessary

Note Although usually given intramuscularly, may be given intravenously after dilution to at least 10 mL with water for injections

TRAMADOL HYDROCHLORIDE

Indications moderate to severe pain

Cautions see notes above; impaired consciousness; excessive bronchial secretions; not suitable as substitute in opioid-dependent patients

General anaesthesia Not recommended for analgesia during potentially light planes of general anaesthesia (possibly increased intra-operative recall reported)

Contra-indications see notes above; uncontrolled epilepsy; porphyria (section 9.8.2)

Side-effects see notes above; also diarrhoea; fatigue; *less commonly* retching, gastritis, and flatulence; *rarely* anorexia, syncope, hypertension, bronchospasm, dyspnoea, wheezing, seizures, paraesthesia, and muscle weakness; blood disorders also reported

Dose

- ADULT and CHILD over 12 years, by mouth, 50–100 mg not more often than every 4 hours; total of more than 400 mg daily not usually required
- ADULT and CHILD over 12 years, by intramuscular injection *or* by intravenous injection (over 2–3 minutes) *or* by intravenous infusion, 50–100 mg every 4–6 hours

  Postoperative pain, 100 mg initially then 50 mg every 10–20 minutes if necessary during first hour to total max. 250 mg (including initial dose) in first hour, *then* 50–100 mg every 4–6 hours; max. 600 mg daily

Tramadol Hydrochloride (Non-proprietary) PoM

Capsules, tramadol hydrochloride 50 mg. Net price 30-cap pack = £1.23, 100-cap pack = £3.17. Label: 2

Brands include *Tramake®*

Injection, tramadol hydrochloride 50 mg/mL. Net price 2-mL amp = £1.15

Zamadol® (Viatris) PoM

Capsules, tramadol hydrochloride 50 mg, net price 100-cap pack = £8.00. Label: 2

Orodispersible tablets (*Zamadol Melt®*), tramadol hydrochloride 50 mg, net price 60-tab pack = £7.12. Label: 2, counselling, administration

Excipients include aspartame (section 9.4.1)

Counselling *Zamadol Melt®* should be sucked and then swallowed. May also be dispersed in water

Injection, tramadol hydrochloride 50 mg/mL, net price 2-mL amp = £1.10

Zydol® (Grünenthal) PoM

Capsules, green/yellow, tramadol hydrochloride 50 mg, net price 30-cap pack = £3.35, 100-cap pack = £16.91. Label: 2

Soluble tablets, tramadol hydrochloride 50 mg, net price 20-tab pack = £3.95, 100-tab pack = £17.27. Label: 2, 13

Injection, tramadol hydrochloride 50 mg/mL. Net price 2-mL amp = £1.24

◢Modified release

Dromadol® SR (IVAX) PoM

Tablets, m/r, tramadol hydrochloride 100 mg (white), net price 60-tab pack = £12.78; 150 mg (beige), 60-tab pack = £19.17; 200 mg (orange), 60-tab pack = £25.56. Label: 2, 25

Dose ADULT and CHILD over 12 years, initially 100 mg twice daily increased if necessary; usual max. 200 mg twice daily

Larapam® SR (Sandoz) PoM

Tablets, m/r, tramadol hydrochloride 100 mg, net price 60-tab pack = £18.25; 150 mg, 60-tab pack = £27.35; 200 mg, 60-tab pack = £36.50. Label: 2, 25

Dose ADULT and CHILD over 12 years, initially 100 mg twice daily increased if necessary; usual max. 200 mg twice daily

Maxtron® (Morningside) PoM

Tablets, m/r, tramadol hydrochloride 100 mg, net price 60-tab pack = £15.00; 150 mg, 60-tab pack = £22.50; 200 mg, 60-tab pack = £30.00. Label: 2, 25

Dose ADULT and CHILD over 12 years, 100 mg twice daily increased if necessary; usual max. 200 mg twice daily

Tradorec XL® (Recordati) PoM

Tablets, m/r, tramadol hydrochloride 100 mg, net price 30-tab pack = £14.10; 200 mg, 30-tab pack = £14.98; 300 mg, 30-tab pack = £22.47. Label: 2, 25

Dose ADULT and CHILD over 12 years, initially 100 mg once daily, increased if necessary; usual max. 400 mg once daily

Zamadol® 24hr (Viatris) PoM

Tablets, all f/c, all m/r, tramadol hydrochloride 150 mg, net price 28-tab pack = £10.70; 200 mg, 28-tab pack = £14.26; 300 mg, 28-tab pack = £21.39; 400 mg, 28-tab pack = £28.51. Label: 2, 25

Dose ADULT and CHILD over 12 years, 150 mg once daily increased if necessary; max. 400 mg once daily

Zamadol® SR (Viatris) PoM

Capsules, m/r, tramadol hydrochloride 50 mg (green), net price 60-cap pack = £7.64; 100 mg, 60-cap pack = £15.28; 150 mg (dark green), 60-cap pack = £22.92; 200 mg (yellow), 60-cap pack = £30.55. Label: 2, 25

Dose ADULT and CHILD over 12 years, 50–100 mg twice daily increased if necessary to 150–200 mg twice daily; total of more than 400 mg daily not usually required

Counselling Swallow whole or open capsule and swallow contents immediately without chewing

Zydol SR® (Grünenthal) PoM

Tablets, m/r, f/c, tramadol hydrochloride 100 mg, net price 60-tab pack = £18.26; 150 mg (beige), 60-tab pack = £27.39; 200 mg (orange), 60-tab pack = £36.52. Label: 2, 25

Dose ADULT and CHILD over 12 years, 100 mg twice daily increased if necessary to 150–200 mg twice daily; total of more than 400 mg daily not usually required

Zydol XL® (Grünenthal) PoM

Tablets, m/r, f/c, tramadol hydrochloride 150 mg, net price 30-tab pack = £15.22; 200 mg, 30-tab pack = £20.29; 300 mg, 30-tab pack = £30.44; 400 mg, 30-tab pack = £40.59. Label: 2, 25

Dose ADULT and CHILD over 12 years, 150 mg daily increased if necessary; more than 400 mg once daily not usually required

◢With paracetamol

Tramacet® (Janssen-Cilag) PoM

Tablets, f/c, yellow, tramadol hydrochloride 37.5 mg, paracetamol 325 mg, net price 60-tab pack = £10.07. Label: 2, 25, 29, 30

Dose 2 tablets not more than every 6 hours; max. 8 tablets daily; CHILD under 12 years not recommended

4.7.3 Neuropathic pain

Neuropathic pain, which occurs as a result of damage to neural tissue, includes *postherpetic neuralgia* (see below), *phantom limb pain, complex regional pain syndrome* (reflex sympathetic dystrophy, causalgia) *compression neuropathies, peripheral neuropathies* (e.g. due to diabetes, haematological malignancies, rheumatoid arthritis, alcoholism, drug misuse), *trauma, central pain* (e.g. pain following stroke, spinal cord injury and syringomyelia) and *idiopathic neuropathy*. The pain occurs in an area of sensory deficit and may be described as burning, shooting or scalding and is often accompanied by pain that is evoked by a non-noxious stimulus (allodynia).

Trigeminal neuralgia is also caused by dysfunction of neural tissue, but its management (see below) is distinct from other forms of neuropathic pain.

Neuropathic pain is generally managed with a tricyclic antidepressant and certain antiepileptic drugs. Neuropathic pain may respond only partially to opioid analgesics. Of the opioids, methadone, tramadol, and oxycodone are probably the most effective for neuropathic pain and they may be considered when other measures fail. Nerve blocks, transcutaneous electrical nerve stimulation (TENS) and, in selected cases, central electrical stimulation may help. Many patients with chronic neuropathic pain require multidisciplinary management, including physiotherapy and psychological support.

Gabapentin (p. 247) and **pregabalin** (p. 248) are effective for the treatment of neuropathic pain. **Amitriptyline** (p. 203) is also prescribed frequently [unlicensed indication]; **nortriptyline** [unlicensed indication] (p. 205) may be better tolerated than amitriptyline.

Capsaicin (section 10.3.2) is licensed for neuropathic pain (but the intense burning sensation during initial treatment may limit use). **Ketamine** (section 15.1.1), an NMDA antagonist, or **lidocaine (lignocaine)** by intravenous infusion may also be useful in some forms of neuropathic pain [both unlicensed indication; specialist use only].

A **corticosteroid** may help to relieve pressure in compression neuropathy and thereby reduce pain. The management of trigeminal neuralgia and postherpetic neuralgia are outlined below; for the management of neuropathic pain in *palliative care* see p. 16; for the management of diabetic neuropathy, see section 6.1.5.

Trigeminal neuralgia

Surgery may be the treatment of choice in many patients; a neurological assessment will identify those who stand to benefit. **Carbamazepine** (section 4.8.1) taken during the acute stages of trigeminal neuralgia, reduces the frequency and severity of attacks. It is very effective for the severe pain associated with trigeminal neuralgia and (less commonly) glossopharyngeal neuralgia. Blood counts and electrolytes should be monitored when high doses are given. Small doses should be used initially to reduce the incidence of side-effects e.g. dizziness. **Oxcarbazepine** [unlicensed indication] is an alternative to carbamazepine. **Gabapentin** and **lamotrigine** [unlicensed indication] are also used in trigeminal neuralgia. Some cases respond to **phenytoin** (section 4.8.1); the drug may be given by intravenous infusion (possibly as fosphenytoin) in a crisis (specialist use only).

Postherpetic neuralgia

Postherpetic neuralgia can follow acute herpes zoster infection (shingles), particularly in the elderly. If **amitriptyline** [unlicensed indication] fails to manage the pain adequately, **gabapentin** may improve control. A topical analgesic preparation containing **capsaicin** 0.075% (section 10.3.2) is licensed for use in postherpetic neuralgia. Application of topical local anaesthetic preparations such as lidocaine medicated plasters (section 15.2) may be helpful in some patients.

Chronic facial pain

Chronic oral and facial pain including persistent idiopathic facial pain (also termed 'atypical facial pain') and temporomandibular dysfunction (previously termed temporomandibular joint pain dysfunction syndrome) may call for prolonged use of analgesics or for other drugs. Tricyclic antidepressants (section 4.3.1) may be useful for facial pain [unlicensed indication], but are not on the Dental Practitioners' List. Disorders of this type require specialist referral and psychological support to accompany drug treatment. Patients on long-term therapy need to be monitored both for progress and for side-effects.

4.7.4 Antimigraine drugs

4.7.4.1 Treatment of acute migraine
4.7.4.2 Prophylaxis of migraine
4.7.4.3 Cluster headache

4.7.4.1 Treatment of acute migraine

Treatment of a migraine attack should be guided by response to previous treatment and the severity of the attacks. A **simple analgesic** such as aspirin, paracetamol (preferably in a soluble or dispersible form) or an NSAID is often effective; concomitant **antiemetic** treatment may be required. If treatment with an analgesic is inadequate, an attack may be treated with a specific antimigraine compound such as a **5HT$_1$ agonist** ('triptan'). **Ergot alkaloids** are rarely required now; oral and rectal preparations are associated with many side-effects and they should be avoided in cerebrovascular or cardiovascular disease.

Excessive use of acute treatments for migraine (opioid and non-opioid analgesics, 5HT$_1$ agonists, and ergotamine) is associated with medication-overuse headache (analgesic-induced headache); therefore, increasing consumption of these medicines needs careful management.

Analgesics

Most migraine headaches respond to analgesics such as **aspirin** or **paracetamol** (section 4.7.1) but because peristalsis is often reduced during migraine attacks the medication may not be sufficiently well absorbed to be effective; dispersible or effervescent preparations are therefore preferred.

The NSAID **tolfenamic acid** is licensed specifically for the treatment of an acute attack of migraine; **diclofenac**

Please attach additional pages if necessary

Please list other drugs taken in the last 3 months prior to the reaction (including self-medication & herbal remedies)

Was the patient on any other medication? Yes / No If *yes*, please give the following information if known:

Drug (Brand, if known)	Route	Dosage	Date started	Date stopped	Prescribed for

Additional relevant information e.g. medical history, test results, known allergies, rechallenge (if performed), suspected drug interactions. For congenital abnormalities please state all other drugs taken during pregnancy and the date of the last menstrual period.

REPORTER DETAILS

Name and Professional Address: __________

Post code: __________ Tel No: __________

Speciality: __________

Signature: Date:

CLINICIAN (if not the reporter)

Name and Professional Address: __________

Post code: __________

Tel No: __________ Speciality: __________

If you would like information about other adverse reactions associated with the suspected drug, please tick this box ☐

If you report from an area served by a Yellow Card Centre (YCC), MHRA may ask the Centre to communicate with you, on its behalf, about your report. See BNF (page 11) for further details on YCCs. If you want only MHRA to contact you, please tick this box. ☐

Send to **Medicines and Healthcare products Regulatory Agency, CHM FREEPOST, LONDON SW8 5BR**

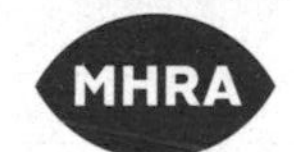

Yellowcard

COMMISSION ON HUMAN MEDICINES

In Confidence

SUSPECTED ADVERSE DRUG REACTIONS

If you suspect that an adverse reaction may be related to a drug, or a combination of drugs, you should complete this Yellow Card or complete a report on the website at www.yellowcard.gov.uk. For *intensively monitored medicines* (identified by ▼) report **all** suspected reactions (including any considered not to be serious). For *established drugs* and *herbal remedies* report **all serious** adverse reactions in adults; report **all serious and minor** adverse reactions in **children** (under 18 years). You do not have to be certain about causality: if in doubt, please report. Do not be put off reporting just because some details are not known. See BNF (page 11) or the MHRA website (www.yellowcard.gov.uk) for additional advice.

PATIENT DETAILS Patient Initials: ____________ Sex: M / F Weight if known (kg): ____________

Age (at time of reaction): ____________ Identification (Your Practice / Hospital Ref.)*: ____________

SUSPECTED DRUG(S)

Give brand name of drug and batch number if known	Route	Dosage	Date started	Date stopped	Prescribed for

SUSPECTED REACTION(S)

Please describe the reaction(s) and any treatment given:

Outcome

Recovered ☐

Recovering ☐

Continuing ☐

Other ☐

Date reaction(s) started: ____________ Date reaction(s) stopped: ____________

Do you consider the reaction to be serious? Yes / No

If *yes*, please indicate why the reaction is considered to be serious (please tick all that apply):

Patient died due to reaction ☐ Involved or prolonged inpatient hospitalisation ☐

Life threatening ☐ Involved persistent or significant disability or incapacity ☐

Congenital abnormality ☐ Medically significant; please give details:

* This is to enable you to identify the patient in any future correspondence concerning this report

potassium, **flurbiprofen**, **ibuprofen**, and **naproxen sodium** (section 10.1.1) are also licensed for use in migraine.

ANALGESICS

Aspirin
Section 4.7.1

Paracetamol
Section 4.7.1

Non-steroidal anti-inflammatory drugs (NSAIDs)
Section 10.1.1

With antiemetics

Migraleve® (Pfizer Consumer)

Tablets, all f/c, *pink tablets*, buclizine hydrochloride 6.25 mg, paracetamol 500 mg, codeine phosphate 8 mg; *yellow tablets*, paracetamol 500 mg, codeine phosphate 8 mg. Net price 48-tab *Migraleve* PoM (32 pink + 16 yellow) = £5.10; 48 pink (*Migraleve Pink*) = £5.56; 48 yellow (*Migraleve Yellow*) = £4.70. Label: 2, (*Migraleve Pink*), 17, 30

Dose 2 pink tablets at onset of attack, or if it is imminent, then 2 yellow tablets every 4 hours if necessary; max. in 24 hours 2 pink and 6 yellow; CHILD under 10 years, only under close medical supervision; 10–14 years, half adult dose

MigraMax® (Zeneus) PoM

Oral powder, aspirin (as lysine acetylsalicylate) 900 mg, metoclopramide hydrochloride 10 mg/sachet, net price 6-sachet pack = £7.00, 20-sachet pack = £23.33. Label: 13, 21, 32

Dose ADULT over 20 years 1 sachet in water at onset of attack, repeated after 2 hours if necessary (max. 3 sachets in 24 hours); YOUNG ADULT (under 20 years) and CHILD not recommended

Important Metoclopramide can cause **severe extrapyramidal effects**, particularly in children and young adults (for further details, see p. 217)

Excipients include aspartame (section 9.4.1)

Paramax® (Sanofi-Synthelabo) PoM

Tablets, scored, paracetamol 500 mg, metoclopramide hydrochloride 5 mg. Net price 42-tab pack = £8.03. Label: 17, 30

Sachets, effervescent powder, sugar-free, the contents of 1 sachet = 1 tablet; to be dissolved in ¼ tumblerful of liquid before administration. Net price 42-sachet pack = £10.43. Label: 13, 17, 30

Dose (tablets or sachets): 2 at onset of attack then every 4 hours when necessary to max. of 6 in 24 hours; YOUNG ADULT 12–19 years, 1 at onset of attack then 1 every 4 hours when necessary to max. of 3 in 24 hours (max. dose of metoclopramide 500 micrograms/kg daily)

Important Metoclopramide can cause **severe extrapyramidal effects**, particularly in children and young adults (for further details, see p. 217)

TOLFENAMIC ACID

Indications treatment of acute migraine

Cautions see NSAIDs, section 10.1.1

Contra-indications see NSAIDs, section 10.1.1

Side-effects see NSAIDs, section 10.1.1; also dysuria (most commonly in men), tremor, euphoria, and fatigue reported

Dose

- 200 mg at onset repeated once after 1–2 hours if necessary

Clotam® (KoGEN) PoM

Rapid Tablets, tolfenamic acid 200 mg. Net price 10-tab pack = £15.00

$5HT_1$ agonists

A $5HT_1$ agonist is of considerable value in the treatment of an acute migraine attack. The $5HT_1$ agonists ('triptans') act on the 5HT (serotonin) 1B/1D receptors and they are therefore sometimes referred to as $5HT_{1B/1D}$-receptor agonists. A $5HT_1$ agonist may be used during the established headache phase of an attack and is the preferred treatment in those who fail to respond to conventional analgesics.

The $5HT_1$ agonists available for treating migraine are **almotriptan**, **eletriptan**, **frovatriptan**, **naratriptan**, **rizatriptan**, **sumatriptan**, and **zolmitriptan**. Sumatriptan is also of value in cluster headache (section 4.7.4.3).

Cautions $5HT_1$ agonists should be used with caution in conditions which predispose to coronary artery disease (pre-existing cardiac disease, see Contra-indications below); hepatic impairment (see Appendix 2); pregnancy (see Appendix 4) and breast-feeding (see Appendix 5). $5HT_1$ agonists are recommended as monotherapy and should not be taken concurrently with other therapies for acute migraine; see also **interactions**: Appendix 1 ($5HT_1$ agonists). Little information is available on the use of these drugs in the elderly (over 65 years).

Contra-indications $5HT_1$ agonists are contra-indicated in ischaemic heart disease, previous myocardial infarction, coronary vasospasm (including Prinzmetal's angina), and uncontrolled or severe hypertension.

Side-effects Side-effects of the $5HT_1$ agonists include sensations of tingling, heat, heaviness, pressure, or tightness of any part of the body (including throat and chest—discontinue if intense, may be due to coronary vasoconstriction or to anaphylaxis; see also CSM advice under Sumatriptan); flushing, dizziness, feeling of weakness; fatigue; nausea and vomiting also reported.

ALMOTRIPTAN

Indications treatment of acute migraine

Cautions see under $5HT_1$ agonists above; sensitivity to sulphonamides; hepatic impairment (avoid if severe—Appendix 2); renal impairment (Appendix 3); **interactions**: Appendix 1 ($5HT_1$ agonists)

Contra-indications see under $5HT_1$ agonists above; previous cerebrovascular accident or transient ischaemic attack; peripheral vascular disease

Side-effects see under $5HT_1$ agonists above; also transient increase in blood pressure, drowsiness; *less commonly* diarrhoea, dyspepsia, dry mouth, chest pain, palpitation, paraesthesia, headache, myalgia, bone pain, tinnitus; *very rarely* myocardial infarction and tachycardia

Dose

- 12.5 mg as soon as possible after onset repeated after 2 hours if migraine recurs (patient not responding should not take second dose for same attack); max. 25 mg in 24 hours; CHILD and ADOLESCENT under 18 years not recommended

Almogran® (Organon) PoM
Tablets, f/c, almotriptan (as hydrogen malate) 12.5 mg, net price 3-tab pack = £9.07; 6-tab pack = £18.14; 9-tab pack = £27.20. Label: 3

ELETRIPTAN

Indications treatment of acute migraine
Cautions see under $5HT_1$ agonists above; renal impairment (avoid if severe—Appendix 3); **interactions**: Appendix 1 ($5HT_1$ agonists)
Contra-indications see under $5HT_1$ agonists above; previous cerebrovascular accident or transient ischaemic attack; arrhythmias; heart failure; peripheral vascular disease; severe hepatic impairment
Side-effects see under $5HT_1$ agonists above; also abdominal pain, dry mouth, dyspepsia; tachycardia, palpitation; drowsiness, headache; pharyngitis, rhinitis, chills; myasthenia, myalgia; sweating; *less commonly* diarrhoea, glossitis, thirst, anorexia, taste disturbance; dyspnoea, yawning, oedema, agitation, confusion, euphoria, depression, insomnia, depersonalisation, tremor, dysarthria, stupor, movement disorders, hypertonia, urinary frequency, arthralgia, photophobia, visual disturbances, tinnitus, rash, and pruritus; *rarely* constipation, oesophagitis, bradycardia, asthma, syncope, lymphadenopathy, and menorrhagia; ischaemic colitis and hypertension also reported
Dose
- ADULT over 18 years, 40 mg repeated after 2 hours if migraine recurs (patient not responding to initial dose should not take second dose for same attack); increase to 80 mg for subsequent attacks if 40-mg dose inadequate; max. 80 mg in 24 hours

Relpax® (Pfizer) ▼ PoM
Tablets, f/c, orange, eletriptan (as hydrobromide) 20 mg, net price 6-tab pack = £22.50; 40 mg, 6-tab pack = £22.50. Label: 3

FROVATRIPTAN

Indications treatment of acute migraine
Cautions see under $5HT_1$ agonists above; **interactions**: Appendix 1 ($5HT_1$ agonists)
Contra-indications see under $5HT_1$ agonists above; severe hepatic impairment; previous cerebrovascular attack or transient ischaemic attack; peripheral vascular disease
Side-effects see under $5HT_1$ agonists above; also dry mouth, dyspepsia, abdominal pain, palpitation, paraesthesia, drowsiness, visual disturbances, sweating; *less commonly* diarrhoea, constipation, dysphagia, flatulence, tachycardia, hypertension, rhinitis, pharyngitis, sinusitis, laryngitis, tremor, anxiety, insomnia, confusion, nervousness, impaired concentration, euphoria, depression, depersonalisation, taste disturbances, fever, micturition disorders, thirst, arthralgia, muscle weakness, tinnitus, pruritus; *rarely* gastro-oesophageal reflux, hiccup, peptic ulcer, stomatitis, bradycardia, syncope, hyperventilation, amnesia, abnormal dreams, hypertonia, hypotonia, hypocalcaemia, hypoglycaemia, bilirubinaemia, epistaxis, urticaria, and purpura
Dose
- 2.5 mg as soon as possible after onset repeated after 2 hours if migraine recurs (patient not responding should not take second dose for same attack); max. 5 mg in 24 hours; CHILD and ADOLESCENT under 18 years not recommended

Migard® (Menarini) PoM
Tablets, f/c, frovatriptan (as succinate) 2.5 mg, net price 6-tab pack = £16.67. Label: 3

NARATRIPTAN

Indications treatment of acute migraine
Cautions see under $5HT_1$ agonists above; sensitivity to sulphonamides; renal impairment (avoid if creatinine clearance less than 15 mL/minute; Appendix 3); **interactions**: Appendix 1 ($5HT_1$ agonists)
Driving Drowsiness may affect performance of skilled tasks (e.g. driving)
Contra-indications see under $5HT_1$ agonists above; previous cerebrovascular accident or transient ischaemic attack; peripheral vascular disease
Side-effects see under $5HT_1$ agonists above; also *less commonly* bradycardia, tachycardia, palpitation, and visual disturbance; *rarely* ischaemic colitis
Dose
- 2.5 mg, repeated after at least 4 hours if migraine recurs (patient not responding should not take second dose for same attack); max. 5 mg in 24 hours; CHILD and ADOLESCENT under 18 years not recommended

Naramig® (GSK) PoM
Tablets, f/c, green, naratriptan (as hydrochloride) 2.5 mg, net price 6-tab pack = £24.55, 12-tab pack = £49.10. Label: 3

RIZATRIPTAN

Indications treatment of acute migraine
Cautions see under $5HT_1$ agonists above; renal impairment (avoid if creatinine clearance less than 10 mL/minute; Appendix 3); **interactions**: Appendix 1 ($5HT_1$ agonists)
Driving Drowsiness may affect performance of skilled tasks (e.g. driving)
Contra-indications see under $5HT_1$ agonists above; previous cerebrovascular accident or transient ischaemic attack; peripheral vascular disease
Side-effects see under $5HT_1$ agonists above; drowsiness, palpitation, tachycardia, dry mouth, diarrhoea, dyspepsia, thirst, pharyngeal discomfort, dyspnoea, headache, paraesthesia, decreased alertness, insomnia, tremor, ataxia, nervousness, vertigo, confusion, myalgia and muscle weakness, sweating, urticaria, pruritus, blurred vision; rarely syncope, hypertension; hypersensitivity reactions (including rash, angioedema, and toxic epidermal necrolysis) and taste disturbance reported
Dose
- 10 mg as soon as possible after onset repeated after 2 hours if migraine recurs (patient not responding should not take second dose for same attack); max. 20 mg in 24 hours; CHILD and ADOLESCENT under 18 years not recommended

Maxalt® (MSD) PoM
Tablets, pink, rizatriptan (as benzoate) 5 mg, net price 6-tab pack = £26.74; 10 mg, 3-tab pack = £13.37, 6-tab pack = £26.74. Label: 3

Oral lyophilisate (*Maxalt® Melt Wafers*), rizatriptan (as benzoate) 10 mg, net price 3-wafer pack = £13.37,

6-wafer pack = £26.74. Label: 3, counselling, administration
Counselling *Maxalt® Melt* wafers should be placed on the tongue and allowed to dissolve
Excipients include aspartame equivalent to phenylalanine 2.1 mg (section 9.4.1)

SUMATRIPTAN

Indications treatment of acute migraine; cluster headache (subcutaneous injection only)

Cautions see under $5HT_1$ agonists above; history of seizures; renal impairment; sensitivity to sulphonamides; **interactions:** Appendix 1 ($5HT_1$ agonists)
Driving Drowsiness may affect performance of skilled tasks (e.g. driving)

Contra-indications see under $5HT_1$ agonists above; previous cerebrovascular accident or transient ischaemic attack; peripheral vascular disease; moderate and severe hypertension

Side-effects see under $5HT_1$ agonists above; also drowsiness, transient increase in blood pressure; *very rarely* ischaemic colitis, hypotension, bradycardia or tachycardia, palpitation, arrhythmias, myocardial infarction, Raynaud's syndrome, seizures, tremor, dystonia, nystagmus, and visual disturbances; erythema at injection site; nasal irritation and epistaxis with nasal spray
CSM advice Following reports of chest pain and tightness (coronary vasoconstriction) CSM has emphasised that sumatriptan should **not** be used in ischaemic heart disease or Prinzmetal's angina, and that use with ergotamine should be **avoided** (see also Cautions).

Dose
- By mouth, 50 mg (some patients may require 100 mg); dose may be repeated after at least 2 hours if migraine recurs; max. 300 mg in 24 hours; CHILD and ADOLESCENT under 18 years, see *BNF for Children*
- By subcutaneous injection using auto-injector, 6 mg; dose may be repeated once after at least 1 hour if migraine recurs; max. 12 mg in 24 hours; CHILD and ADOLESCENT under 18 years not recommended
Important Not for intravenous injection which may cause coronary vasospasm and angina
- Intranasally, 10–20 mg (ADOLESCENT 12–17 years 10 mg) into one nostril; dose may be repeated once after at least 2 hours if migraine recurs; max. 40 mg (ADOLESCENT 12–17 years 20 mg) in 24 hours

Note Patient not responding to initial dose should not take second dose for same attack

[1]Sumatriptan (Non-proprietary) PoM
Tablets, sumatriptan (as succinate) 50 mg, net price 6-tab pack = £12.69; 100 mg, 6-tab pack = £19.89. Label: 3, 10, patient information leaflet

1. Sumatriptan 50 mg tablets can be sold to the public to treat previously diagnosed migraine; max. daily dose 100 mg

Imigran® (GSK) PoM
Tablets, sumatriptan (as succinate) 50 mg, net price 6-tab pack = £27.62, 12-tab pack = £52.48; 100 mg, 6-tab pack = £44.64, 12-tab pack = £89.28. Label: 3, 10, patient information leaflet

Injection, sumatriptan (as succinate) 12 mg/mL (= 6 mg/0.5-mL syringe), net price, treatment pack (2 × 0.5-mL prefilled syringes and auto-injector) = £44.19; refill pack 2 × 0.5-mL prefilled cartridges = £42.05. Label: 3, 10, patient information leaflet

Nasal spray, sumatriptan 10 mg/0.1-mL actuation, net price 2 unit-dose spray device = £12.28; 20 mg/0.1-mL actuation, 2 unit-dose spray device = £12.28, 6 unit-dose spray device = £36.83. Label: 3, 10, patient information leaflet

Imigran® RADIS (GSK) PoM
Tablets, f/c, sumatriptan (as succinate) 50 mg (pink), net price 6-tab pack = £24.87, 12-tab pack = £49.77; 100 mg (white), 6-tab pack = £44.64, 12-tab pack = £89.28. Label: 3, 10, patient information leaflet

ZOLMITRIPTAN

Indications treatment of acute migraine

Cautions see under $5HT_1$ agonists above; should not be taken within 12 hours of any other $5HT_1$ agonist; **interactions:** Appendix 1 ($5HT_1$ agonists)

Contra-indications see under $5HT_1$ agonists above; Wolff-Parkinson-White syndrome or arrhythmias associated with accessory cardiac conduction pathways; previous cerebrovascular accident or transient ischaemic attack

Side-effects see under $5HT_1$ agonists above; also dry mouth, drowsiness, paraesthesia, myalgia, muscle weakness; *rarely* palpitation, tachycardia, angioedema, headache, urticaria; *very rarely* abdominal pain, gastro-intestinal and splenic infarction, ischaemic colitis, angina, myocardial infarction, polyuria, transient increase in blood pressure; taste disturbance and nasal discomfort with nasal spray

Dose
- By mouth, 2.5 mg repeated after not less than 2 hours if migraine persists or recurs (increase to 5 mg for subsequent attacks in patients not achieving satisfactory relief with 2.5-mg dose); max. 10 mg in 24 hours; CHILD not recommended
- Intranasally, 5 mg (1 spray) into one nostril as soon as possible after onset repeated after not less than 2 hours if migraine persists or recurs; max. 10 mg in 24 hours; CHILD not recommended

Zomig® (AstraZeneca) PoM
Tablets, f/c, yellow, zolmitriptan 2.5 mg, net price 6-tab pack = £24.00, 12-tab pack = £48.00

Orodispersible tablets (*Zomig Rapimelt®*), zolmitriptan 2.5 mg, net price 6-tab pack = £24.00; 5 mg, 6-tab pack = £26.16 Counselling, administration
Counselling *Zomig Rapimelt®* should be placed on the tongue, allowed to disperse and swallowed
Excipients include aspartame equivalent to phenylalanine 2.81 mg/tablet (section 9.4.1)

Nasal spray, zolmitriptan 5 mg/0.1-mL unit-dose spray device, net price 6 unit-dose sprays = £40.50

Ergot alkaloids

The value of **ergotamine** for migraine is limited by difficulties in absorption and by its side-effects, particularly nausea, vomiting, abdominal pain, and *muscular cramps*; it is best avoided. The recommended doses of ergotamine preparations should **not** be exceeded and treatment should **not** be repeated at intervals of less than 4 days.

To avoid habituation the frequency of administration of ergotamine should be limited to **no more than** twice a month. It should **never** be prescribed prophylactically but in the management of cluster headache a low dose (e.g. ergotamine 1 mg at night for 6 nights in 7) is occasionally given for 1 to 2 weeks [unlicensed indication].

ERGOTAMINE TARTRATE

Indications treatment of acute migraine and migraine variants unresponsive to analgesics

Cautions risk of peripheral vasospasm (see advice below); elderly; dependence (see Ergot alkaloids above), should not be used for migraine prophylaxis; **interactions:** Appendix 1 (ergot alkaloids) and under Sumatriptan (Cautions), below

Peripheral vasospasm Warn patient to stop treatment immediately if numbness or tingling of extremities develops and to contact doctor.

Contra-indications peripheral vascular disease, coronary heart disease, obliterative vascular disease and Raynaud's syndrome, temporal arteritis, hepatic impairment (Appendix 2), renal impairment (Appendix 3), sepsis, severe or inadequately controlled hypertension, hyperthyroidism, pregnancy (Appendix 4), breast-feeding (Appendix 5), porphyria (section 9.8.2)

Side-effects nausea, vomiting, vertigo, abdominal pain, diarrhoea, muscle cramps, and occasionally headache provoked (usually because of prolonged excessive dosage or abrupt withdrawal); precordial pain, myocardial and intestinal ischaemia, rarely myocardial infarction; repeated high dosage may cause ergotism with gangrene and confusion; pleural, peritoneal and heart-valve fibrosis may occur with excessive use; rectal or anal stricture or ulceration and rectovaginal fistula reported with prolonged use of suppositories

Dose

- See under preparations below

Cafergot® (Alliance) PoM

Tablets, ergotamine tartrate 1 mg, caffeine 100 mg. Net price 30-tab pack = £5.02. Label: 18, counselling, dosage

Dose 1–2 tablets at onset; max. 4 tablets in 24 hours; not to be repeated at intervals of less than 4 days; max. 8 tablets in one week (but see also notes above); CHILD not recommended

Suppositories, ergotamine tartrate 2 mg, caffeine 100 mg. Net price 30 = £10.13. Label: 18, counselling, dosage

Dose 1 suppository at onset; max. 2 in 24 hours; not to be repeated at intervals of less than 4 days; max. 4 suppositories in one week (but see also notes above); CHILD not recommended

Migril® (CP) PoM

Tablets, scored, ergotamine tartrate 2 mg, cyclizine hydrochloride 50 mg, caffeine hydrate 100 mg. Net price 20 = £10.20. Label: 2, 18, counselling, dosage

Dose 1 tablet at onset, followed after 30 minutes by ½–1 tablet, repeated every 30 minutes if necessary; max. 4 tablets per attack and 6 tablets in one week (but see also notes above); CHILD not recommended

Antiemetics

Antiemetics (section 4.6), such as **metoclopramide** or **domperidone**, or phenothiazine and antihistamine antiemetics, relieve the nausea associated with migraine attacks. Antiemetics may be given by intramuscular injection or rectally if vomiting is a problem. Metoclopramide and domperidone have the added advantage of promoting gastric emptying and normal peristalsis; a single dose should be given at the onset of symptoms. Oral analgesic preparations containing metoclopramide are a convenient alternative (**important:** for warnings relating to extrapyramidal effects of metoclopramide particularly in children and young adults, see p. 217).

4.7.4.2 Prophylaxis of migraine

Where migraine attacks are frequent, possible provoking factors such as stress, irregular life-style (e.g. lack of sleep), or chemical triggers (e.g. alcohol and nitrates) should be sought; combined oral contraceptives may also provoke migraine, see section 7.3.1 for advice.

Preventive treatment for migraine should be considered for patients who:

- suffer at least two attacks a month;
- suffer an increasing frequency of headaches;
- suffer significant disability despite suitable treatment for migraine attacks;
- cannot take suitable treatment for migraine attacks.

Prophylaxis is also necessary in some rare migraine subtypes and those at risk of migrainous infarction.

The **beta-blockers** propranolol, metoprolol, nadolol, and timolol (section 2.4) are all effective. Propranolol is the most commonly used.

Pizotifen is an antihistamine and serotonin antagonist structurally related to the tricyclic antidepressants. It affords good prophylaxis but may cause weight gain. To avoid undue drowsiness treatment may be started at a low dose and gradually increased.

Sodium valproate (section 4.8.1) may be effective for migraine prophylaxis [unlicensed indication] in a starting dose of 300 mg twice daily, increased if necessary to 1.2 g daily in divided doses. **Valproic acid** (as semisodium valproate) (section 4.2.3) is similarly effective [unlicensed indication] in a starting dose of 250 mg twice daily, increased if necessary to 1 g daily in divided doses.

Topiramate (section 4.8.1) is effective for migraine prophylaxis. Treatment should be supervised by a specialist.

Tricyclic antidepressants (section 4.3.1) (e.g. **amitriptyline**) are also used for preventing migraine [unlicensed indication].

Cyproheptadine (section 3.4.1), an antihistamine with serotonin-antagonist and calcium channel-blocking properties, may also be tried in refractory cases.

Clonidine (*Dixarit®*) is **not** recommended and may aggravate depression or produce insomnia. **Methysergide**, a semi-synthetic ergot alkaloid, has dangerous side-effects (retroperitoneal fibrosis and fibrosis of the heart valves and pleura); **important:** it should only be administered under hospital supervision.

PIZOTIFEN

Indications prevention of vascular headache including classical migraine, common migraine, and cluster headache

Cautions urinary retention; susceptibility to angle-closure glaucoma; renal impairment; pregnancy;

breast-feeding (Appendix 5); **interactions:** Appendix 1 (pizotifen)

Driving Drowsiness may affect performance of skilled tasks (e.g. driving); effects of alcohol enhanced

Side-effects antimuscarinic effects (*very rarely* angle-closure glaucoma), drowsiness, increased appetite and weight gain; occasionally nausea, dizziness; *rarely* anxiety, aggression, and depression; CNS stimulation may occur in children

Dose

- Initially 500 micrograms at night increased gradually to usual dose of 1.5 mg at night *or* in 3 divided doses; may be further increased up to max. daily dose 4.5 mg (but rarely necessary), max. single dose 3 mg; CHILD over 2 years, up to 1.5 mg daily in divided doses; max. single dose at night 1 mg

Pizotifen (Non-proprietary) PoM
Tablets, pizotifen (as hydrogen malate), 500 micrograms, net price 28-tab pack = £1.23; 1.5 mg, 28-tab pack = £3.94. Label: 2

Sanomigran® (Novartis) PoM
Tablets, both ivory-yellow, s/c, pizotifen (as hydrogen malate), 500 micrograms, net price 60-tab pack = £2.57; 1.5 mg, 28-tab pack = £4.28. Label: 2

Elixir, pizotifen (as hydrogen malate) 250 micrograms/5 mL, net price 300 mL = £4.51. Label: 2

CLONIDINE HYDROCHLORIDE

Indications prevention of recurrent migraine (but see notes above), vascular headache, menopausal flushing; hypertension (section 2.5.2)

Cautions depressive illness, concurrent antihypertensive therapy; porphyria (section 9.8.2); **interactions:** Appendix 1 (alpha$_2$-adrenoceptor stimulant)

Side-effects dry mouth, sedation, dizziness, nausea, nocturnal restlessness; occasionally rashes

Dose

- 50 micrograms twice daily, increased after 2 weeks to 75 micrograms twice daily if necessary; CHILD not recommended

Clonidine (Non-proprietary) PoM
Tablets, clonidine hydrochloride 25 micrograms. Net price 112-tab pack = £14.91

Dixarit® (Boehringer Ingelheim) PoM
Tablets, blue, s/c, clonidine hydrochloride 25 micrograms. Net price 112-tab pack = £7.11

Catapres® PoM
Section 2.5.2 (hypertension)

METHYSERGIDE

Indications prevention of severe recurrent migraine, cluster headache and other vascular headaches in patients who are refractory to other treatment and whose lives are seriously disrupted (**important:** hospital supervision only, see notes above); diarrhoea associated with carcinoid syndrome

Cautions history of peptic ulceration; avoid abrupt withdrawal of treatment; after 6 months withdraw (gradually over 2 to 3 weeks) for reassessment for at least 1 month (see also notes above); **interactions:** Appendix 1 (ergot alkaloids)

Contra-indications renal, hepatic, pulmonary, and cardiovascular disease, severe hypertension, collagen disease, cellulitis, urinary-tract disorders, cachectic or septic conditions, pregnancy, breast-feeding

Side-effects nausea, vomiting, heartburn, abdominal discomfort, drowsiness, and dizziness occur frequently in initial treatment; mental and behavioural disturbances, insomnia, oedema, weight gain, rashes, loss of scalp hair, cramps, arterial spasm (including coronary artery spasm with angina and possible myocardial infarction), paraesthesias of extremities, postural hypotension, and tachycardia also occur; retroperitoneal and other abnormal fibrotic reactions may occur on prolonged administration, requiring immediate withdrawal of treatment

Dose

- Initially 1 mg at bedtime, increased gradually over about 2 weeks to 1–2 mg 3 times daily with food (see notes above); CHILD not recommended
- Diarrhoea associated with carcinoid syndrome, usual range, 12–20 mg daily (hospital supervision); CHILD not recommended

Deseril® (Alliance) PoM
Tablets, s/c, methysergide (as maleate) 1 mg, net price 60-tab pack = £13.46. Label: 2, 21

4.7.4.3 Cluster headache

Cluster headache rarely responds to standard analgesics. **Sumatriptan** given by subcutaneous injection is the drug of choice for the *treatment* of cluster headache. Alternatively, 100% **oxygen** at a rate of 7–12 litres/minute is useful in aborting an attack.

Prophylaxis of cluster headache is considered if the attacks are frequent, or last over 3 weeks, or if the attacks cannot be treated effectively. **Verapamil** or **lithium** [both unlicensed use] are used for prophylaxis. **Ergotamine**, used on an intermittent basis is an alternative for patients with short bouts, but it should **not** be used for prolonged periods. **Methysergide** is effective but must be used with extreme caution (see section 4.7.4.2) and only if other drugs cannot be used or if they are not effective.

4.8 Antiepileptics

4.8.1 Control of epilepsy
4.8.2 Drugs used in status epilepticus
4.8.3 Febrile convulsions

4.8.1 Control of epilepsy

The object of treatment is to prevent the occurrence of seizures by maintaining an effective dose of one or more antiepileptic drugs. Careful adjustment of doses is necessary, starting with low doses and increasing gradually until seizures are controlled or there are significant adverse effects.

When choosing an antiepileptic drug to use, the seizure type, concomitant medication, age, and sex should be taken into account. For women of child-bearing age, see Pregnancy and Breast-feeding, p. 245.

The dose frequency is often determined by the plasma-drug half-life, and should be kept as low as possible to encourage compliance with the prescribed regimen. Most antiepileptics, when used in the usual dosage, may be given twice daily. Lamotrigine, phenobarbital, and phenytoin, which have long half-lives, can be given once daily at bedtime. However, with large doses, some antiepileptics may need to be given more frequently to avoid adverse effects associated with high peak plasma concentration. Young children metabolise antiepileptics more rapidly than adults and therefore require more frequent doses and a higher dose in proportion to their body-weight.

Combination therapy Therapy with two or more antiepileptic drugs concurrently may be necessary; it should preferably only be used when monotherapy with two first-line antiepileptic drugs fails or when a well-tolerated first-line antiepileptic significantly improves seizure control but the patient is not seizure-free when taking the maximum tolerated dose. Combination therapy enhances toxicity and drug interactions may occur between antiepileptics (see below).

Interactions Interactions between antiepileptics are complex and may enhance toxicity without a corresponding increase in antiepileptic effect. Interactions are usually caused by *hepatic enzyme induction* or *hepatic enzyme inhibition*; *displacement from protein binding sites* is not usually a problem. These interactions are highly variable and unpredictable.

Significant interactions that occur **between antiepileptics** themselves are as follows:

> **Note** Check under each drug for possible interactions when two or more antiepileptic drugs are used

Carbamazepine
often lowers plasma concentration of clobazam, clonazepam, lamotrigine, an active metabolite of oxcarbazepine, and of phenytoin (but may also raise phenytoin concentration), tiagabine, topiramate, valproate, and zonisamide
sometimes lowers plasma concentration of ethosuximide, and primidone (but tendency for corresponding increase in phenobarbital level)

Ethosuximide
sometimes raises plasma concentration of phenytoin

Gabapentin
no interactions with gabapentin reported

Lamotrigine
sometimes raises plasma concentration of an active metabolite of carbamazepine (but evidence is conflicting)

Levetiracetam
no interactions with levetiracetam reported

Oxcarbazepine
sometimes lowers plasma concentration of carbamazepine (but may raise concentration of an active metabolite of carbamazepine)
sometimes raises plasma concentration of phenytoin
often raises plasma concentration of phenobarbital

Phenobarbital *or* **Primidone**
often lowers plasma concentration of carbamazepine, clonazepam, lamotrigine, and of phenytoin (but may also raise phenytoin concentration), tiagabine, valproate, and zonisamide
sometimes lowers plasma concentration of ethosuximide

Phenytoin
often lowers plasma concentration of clonazepam, carbamazepine, lamotrigine, an active metabolite of oxcarbazepine, and of tiagabine, topiramate, valproate, and zonisamide
often raises plasma concentration of phenobarbital
sometimes lowers plasma concentration of ethosuximide, and primidone (by increasing conversion to phenobarbital)

Pregabalin
no interactions with pregabalin reported

Rufinamide
sometimes raises plasma concentration of phenytoin

Topiramate
sometimes raises plasma concentration of phenytoin

Valproate
sometimes lowers plasma concentration of an active metabolite of oxcarbazepine
often raises plasma concentration of an active metabolite of carbamazepine, and of lamotrigine, primidone, phenobarbital, and phenytoin (but may also lower)
sometimes raises plasma concentration of ethosuximide, primidone, (and tendency for significant increase in phenobarbital level), and rufinamide

Vigabatrin
often lowers plasma concentration of phenytoin
sometimes lowers plasma concentration of phenobarbital, and primidone

For other important interactions see **Appendix** 1; for advice on hormonal contraception and enzyme-inducing drugs (including antiepileptics), see section 7.3.1 and section 7.3.2.

Withdrawal Antiepileptics should be withdrawn under specialist supervision. Abrupt withdrawal, particularly of the barbiturates and benzodiazepines, should be avoided, as this may precipitate severe rebound seizures. Reduction in dosage should be gradual and, in the case of barbiturates, withdrawal of the drug may take months. The changeover from one antiepileptic drug to another should also be cautious, withdrawing the first drug only when the new regimen has been largely established.

The decision to withdraw antiepileptics from a seizure-free patient, and its timing, is often difficult and depends on individual circumstances. Even in patients who have been seizure-free for several years, there is a significant risk of seizure recurrence on drug withdrawal.

In patients receiving several antiepileptic drugs, only one drug should be withdrawn at a time.

Driving Patients suffering from epilepsy may drive a motor vehicle (but not a heavy goods or public service vehicle) provided that they have had a seizure-free period of one year or, if subject to attacks only while asleep, have established a 3-year period of asleep attacks without awake attacks. Patients affected by drowsiness should not drive or operate machinery.

Guidance issued by the Drivers Medical Unit of the Driver and Vehicle Licensing Agency (DVLA) recommends that patients should be advised not to drive during withdrawal of antiepileptic drugs, or for 6 months afterwards (see also Drugs and Driving under General Guidance, p. 2).

Pregnancy and breast-feeding There is an increased risk of teratogenicity associated with the use of antiepileptic drugs (reduced if treatment is limited to a single drug). In view of the increased risk of neural tube and other defects associated, in particular, with **carbamazepine**, **lamotrigine**, **oxcarbazepine**, **phenytoin**, and **valproate**, women taking antiepileptic drugs who *may become pregnant* should be **informed of the possible consequences**. Those who *wish to become pregnant* should be referred to an appropriate specialist for advice. Women who become pregnant should be **counselled** and offered **antenatal screening** (alpha-fetoprotein measurement and a second trimester ultrasound scan).

To counteract the risk of neural tube defects, adequate folate supplements are advised for women before and during pregnancy (section 9.1.2).

The concentration of antiepileptic drugs in the blood can change during pregnancy, particularly in the later stages. The dose of antiepileptics should be monitored carefully during pregnancy and after birth, and adjustments made on a clinical basis.

Routine injection of vitamin K (section 9.6.6) at birth effectively counteracts any antiepileptic-associated risk of neonatal haemorrhage.

Breast-feeding is acceptable with all antiepileptic drugs, taken in normal doses, with the possible exception of the barbiturates, and also some of the more recently introduced ones, see Appendix 5.

Partial seizures with or without secondary generalisation

Carbamazepine, **lamotrigine**, **oxcarbazepine**, **sodium valproate**, and **topiramate** are the drugs of choice for partial (focal) seizures; second-line drugs include clobazam, gabapentin, levetiracetam, pregabalin, tiagabine, and zonisamide.

Generalised seizures

Tonic-clonic seizures (grand mal) The drugs of choice for tonic-clonic seizures are **carbamazepine**, **lamotrigine**, **sodium valproate**, and **topiramate**. Clobazam, levetiracetam, and oxcarbazepine are second-line drugs.

Absence seizures (petit mal) **Ethosuximide** and **sodium valproate** are the drugs of choice in typical absence seizures; alternatives include clonazepam and lamotrigine. Sodium valproate is also highly effective in treating the generalised tonic-clonic seizures which can co-exist with absence seizures in idiopathic primary generalised epilepsy.

Myoclonic seizures Myoclonic seizures (myoclonic jerks) occur in a variety of syndromes, and response to treatment varies considerably. **Sodium valproate** is the drug of choice; **clonazepam** and **levetiracetam** can also be used. Alternatives include lamotrigine and topiramate, but lamotrigine may occasionally exacerbate myoclonic seizures. For reference to the adjunctive use of piracetam, see section 4.9.3.

Sodium valproate and levetiracetam are effective in treating the generalised tonic-clonic seizures that co-exist with myoclonic seizures in idiopathic generalised epilepsy.

Atypical absence, atonic, and tonic seizures Atypical absence, atonic, and tonic seizures are usually seen in childhood, in specific epilepsy syndromes, or associated with cerebral damage or mental retardation. They may respond poorly to the traditional drugs. **Sodium valproate**, **lamotrigine**, and **clonazepam** can be tried. Second-line drugs that are occasionally helpful include clobazam, levetiracetam, and topiramate.

Carbamazepine and oxcarbazepine

Carbamazepine is a drug of choice for simple and complex partial seizures and for tonic-clonic seizures secondary to a focal discharge. It is essential to initiate carbamazepine therapy at a low dose and build this up slowly with increments of 100–200 mg every two weeks. The side-effects of carbamazepine may be reduced by altering the timing of medication; use of modified-release tablets also significantly lessens the incidence of dose-related side-effects.

Oxcarbazepine is licensed for the treatment of partial seizures with or without secondarily generalised tonic-clonic seizures. Oxcarbazepine induces hepatic enzymes to a lesser extent than carbamazepine.

CARBAMAZEPINE

Indications partial and secondary generalised tonic-clonic seizures, primary generalised tonic-clonic seizures; trigeminal neuralgia; prophylaxis of bipolar disorder unresponsive to lithium

Cautions hepatic impairment (Appendix 2) or renal impairment; cardiac disease (see also Contra-indications), skin reactions (see also Blood, hepatic or skin disorders below and under Side-effects), history of haematological reactions to other drugs; manufacturer recommends blood counts and hepatic and renal function tests (but evidence of practical value unsatisfactory); may exacerbate absence and myoclonic seizures; susceptibility to angle-closure glaucoma; pregnancy (**important**: see p. 245 and Appendix 4 (neural tube screening)), breast-feeding (see p. 245 and Appendix 5); avoid abrupt withdrawal; **interactions**: see p. 244 and Appendix 1 (carbamazepine)

Blood, hepatic or skin disorders Patients or their carers should be told how to recognise signs of blood, liver, or skin disorders, and advised to seek immediate medical attention if symptoms such as fever, sore throat, rash, mouth ulcers, bruising, or bleeding develop. Leucopenia which is severe, progressive or associated with clinical symptoms requires withdrawal (if necessary under cover of suitable alternative).

Contra-indications AV conduction abnormalities (unless paced); history of bone marrow depression, porphyria (section 9.8.2)

Side-effects nausea and vomiting, dizziness, drowsiness, headache, ataxia, confusion and agitation (elderly), visual disturbances (especially diplopia and often associated with peak plasma concentrations); constipation or diarrhoea, anorexia; mild transient generalised erythematous rash may occur in a large number of patients (withdraw if worsens or is accompanied by other symptoms); leucopenia and other blood disorders (including thrombocytopenia, agranulocytosis and aplastic anaemia); other side-effects include cholestatic jaundice, hepatitis and acute renal failure, Stevens-Johnson syndrome, toxic epidermal necrolysis, alopecia, thromboembolism, arthralgia, fever, proteinuria, lymph node enlargement, cardiac conduction disturbances (sometimes arrhythmias), dyskinesias, paraesthesia, depression, impotence (and impaired fertility), gynaecomastia, galactorrhoea, aggression, activation of psychosis; *very rarely* angle-closure glaucoma; photosensitivity, pulmonary hypersensitivity (with dyspnoea and pneumonitis), hyponatraemia, oedema, and disturbances of bone metabolism (with osteomalacia) also reported; suppositories may cause occasional rectal irritation

Dose

Note Different preparations may vary in bioavailability; to avoid reduced effect or excessive side-effects, it may be prudent to avoid changing the formulation (see also notes above on how side-effects may be reduced)

- By mouth, epilepsy, initially, 100–200 mg 1–2 times daily, increased slowly (see notes above) to usual dose of 0.4–1.2 g daily in divided doses; in some cases 1.6–2 g daily may be needed; ELDERLY reduce initial dose; CHILD daily in divided doses, up to 1 year 100–200 mg, 1–5 years 200–400 mg, 5–10 years 400–600 mg, 10–15 years 0.4–1 g

  Trigeminal neuralgia, initially 100 mg 1–2 times daily (but some patients may require higher initial dose), increased gradually according to response; usual dose 200 mg 3–4 times daily, up to 1.6 g daily in some patients

  Prophylaxis of bipolar disorder unresponsive to lithium (see also section 4.2.3), initially 400 mg daily in divided doses increased until symptoms controlled; usual range 400–600 mg daily; max. 1.6 g daily
- By rectum, as suppositories, see below

  Note Plasma concentration for optimum response 4–12 mg/litre (20–50 micromol/litre)

Carbamazepine (Non-proprietary) PoM

Tablets, carbamazepine 100 mg, net price 28 = £3.55; 200 mg, 28 = £3.02; 400 mg, 28 = £6.59. Label: 3, 8, counselling, blood, hepatic or skin disorder symptoms (see above), driving (see notes above)

Brands include *Epimaz®*

Dental prescribing on NHS Carbamazepine Tablets may be prescribed

Tegretol® (Novartis) PoM

Tablets, all scored, carbamazepine 100 mg, net price 84-tab pack = £2.43; 200 mg, 84-tab pack = £4.50; 400 mg, 56-tab pack = £5.90. Label: 3, 8, counselling, blood, hepatic or skin disorder symptoms (see above), driving (see notes above)

Chewtabs, orange, carbamazepine 100 mg, net price 56-tab pack = £3.72; 200 mg, 56-tab pack = £6.92. Label: 3, 8, 21, 24, counselling, blood, hepatic or skin disorder symptoms (see above), driving (see notes above)

Liquid, sugar-free, carbamazepine 100 mg/5 mL. Net price 300-mL pack = £7.20. Label: 3, 8, counselling, blood, hepatic or skin disorder symptoms (see above), driving (see notes above)

Suppositories, carbamazepine 125 mg, net price 5 = £9.45; 250 mg, 5 = £12.60. Label: 3, 8, counselling, blood, hepatic or skin disorder symptoms (see above), driving (see notes above)

Dose epilepsy, for short-term use (max. 7 days) when oral therapy temporarily not possible; suppositories of 125 mg may be considered to be approximately equivalent in therapeutic effect to tablets of 100 mg but final adjustment should always depend on clinical response (plasma concentration monitoring recommended); max. by rectum 1 g daily in 4 divided doses

Modified release

Carbagen® SR (Generics) PoM

Tablets, m/r, f/c, both scored, carbamazepine 200 mg, net price 56-tab pack = £4.88; 400 mg, 56-tab pack = £9.63. Label: 3, 8, 25, counselling, blood, hepatic or skin disorder symptoms (see above), driving (see notes above)

Dose epilepsy (ADULT and CHILD over 5 years), as above; trigeminal neuralgia, as above; total daily dose given in 1–2 divided doses; bipolar disorder, as above

Tegretol® Retard (Novartis) PoM

Tablets, m/r, both scored, carbamazepine 200 mg (beige-orange), net price 56-tab pack = £5.52; 400 mg (brown-orange), 56-tab pack = £10.86. Label: 3, 8, 25, counselling, blood, hepatic or skin disorder symptoms (see above), driving (see notes above)

Dose epilepsy (ADULT and CHILD over 5 years), as above; trigeminal neuralgia, as above; total daily dose given in 2 divided doses

OXCARBAZEPINE

Indications monotherapy and adjunctive treatment of partial seizures with or without secondarily generalised tonic-clonic seizures; trigeminal neuralgia [unlicensed indication] (section 4.7.3)

Cautions hypersensitivity to carbamazepine; avoid abrupt withdrawal; hyponatraemia (monitor plasma-sodium concentration in patients at risk), heart failure (monitor body-weight), cardiac conduction disorders; avoid in porphyria (section 9.8.2); hepatic impairment (Appendix 2); renal impairment (Appendix 3); pregnancy (see p. 245 and Appendix 4); breast-feeding (Appendix 5); **interactions:** Appendix 1 (oxcarbazepine)

Blood, hepatic or skin disorders Patients or their carers should be told how to recognise signs of blood, liver, or skin disorders, and advised to seek immediate medical attention if symptoms such as lethargy, confusion, muscular twitching, fever, sore throat, rash, blistering, mouth ulcers, bruising, or bleeding develop

Side-effects nausea, vomiting, constipation, diarrhoea, abdominal pain; dizziness, headache, drowsiness, agitation, amnesia, asthenia, ataxia, confusion, impaired concentration, depression, tremor; hyponatraemia; acne, alopecia, rash, nystagmus, visual disorders including diplopia; *less commonly* urticaria, leucopenia; *very rarely* hepatitis, pancreatitis, arrhythmias, hypersensitivity reactions, thrombocytopenia, systemic lupus erythematosus, Stevens-Johnson syndrome, and toxic epidermal necrolysis

Dose

- Initially 300 mg twice daily increased according to response in steps of up to 600 mg daily at weekly intervals; usual dose range 0.6–2.4 g daily in divided doses; CHILD 6–18 years, 8–10 mg/kg daily in 2 divided doses increased according to response in steps of up to 10 mg/kg daily at weekly intervals (in adjunctive therapy, maintenance dose approx. 30 mg/kg daily); max. 46 mg/kg daily in divided doses

Note In adjunctive therapy, the dose of concomitant anti-epileptics may need to be reduced when using high doses of oxcarbazepine

Trileptal® (Novartis) PoM

Tablets, f/c, scored, oxcarbazepine 150 mg (green), net price 50-tab pack = £10.00; 300 mg (yellow), 50-tab pack = £20.00; 600 mg (pink), 50-tab pack = £40.00. Label: 3, 8, counselling, blood, hepatic or skin disorders (see above), driving (see notes above)

Oral suspension, sugar-free, oxcarbazepine 300 mg/5 mL, net price 250 mL (with oral syringe) = £40.00. Label: 3, 8, counselling, blood, hepatic or skin disorders (see above), driving (see notes above)

Excipients include propylene glycol (see Excipients, p. 2)

Ethosuximide

Ethosuximide is used in typical absence seizures; it may also be used in atypical absence seizures. Ethosuximide is rarely used for myoclonic or tonic seizures.

ETHOSUXIMIDE

Indications see notes above

Cautions avoid abrupt withdrawal; hepatic impairment; renal impairment; pregnancy (see p. 245 and Appendix 4); breast-feeding (Appendix 5); avoid in porphyria (section 9.8.2); **interactions:** Appendix 1 (ethosuximide)

Blood disorders Patients or their carers should be told how to recognise signs of blood disorders, and advised to seek immediate medical attention if symptoms such as fever, sore throat, mouth ulcers, bruising, or bleeding develop

Side-effects gastro-intestinal disturbances (including nausea, vomiting, diarrhoea, abdominal pain, anorexia, weight loss); *less frequently* headache, fatigue, drowsiness, dizziness, hiccup, ataxia, mild euphoria, irritability, aggression, impaired concentration; *rarely* tongue swelling, sleep disturbances, night terrors, depression, psychosis, photophobia, dyskinesia, increased libido, vaginal bleeding, myopia, gingival hypertrophy, and rash; also reported, hyperactivity, increase in seizure frequency, blood disorders such as leucopenia, agranulocytosis, pancytopenia, and aplastic anaemia (blood counts required if features of infection), systemic lupus erythematosus, and Stevens-Johnson syndrome

Dose

- ADULT and CHILD over 6 years initially, 500 mg daily, increased by 250 mg at intervals of 4–7 days to usual dose of 1–1.5 g daily; occasionally up to 2 g daily may be needed; CHILD up to 6 years initially 250 mg daily, increased gradually to usual dose of 20 mg/kg daily; max. 1 g daily

Ethosuximide (Non-proprietary) PoM

Capsules, ethosuximide 250 mg, net price 56-cap pack = £38.23. Label: 8, counselling, blood disorders (see above), driving (see notes above)

Emeside® (Chemidex) PoM

Syrup, black currant, ethosuximide 250 mg/5 mL, net price 200-mL pack = £6.60. Label: 8, counselling, blood disorders (see above), driving (see notes above)

Zarontin® (Pfizer) PoM

Syrup, yellow, ethosuximide 250 mg/5 mL, net price 200-mL pack = £4.48. Label: 8, counselling, blood disorders (see above), driving (see notes above)

Gabapentin and pregabalin

Gabapentin and **pregabalin** are used for the treatment of partial seizures with or without secondary generalisation. They are also licensed for the treatment of neuropathic pain (p. 238). Pregabalin is licensed for the treatment of generalised anxiety disorder (p. 202).

GABAPENTIN

Indications monotherapy and adjunctive treatment of partial seizures with or without secondary generalisation; peripheral neuropathic pain (section 4.7.3); trigeminal neuralgia [unlicensed indication] (section 4.7.3)

Cautions avoid abrupt withdrawal (may cause anxiety, insomnia, nausea, pain, and sweating—taper off over at least 1 week); elderly; renal impairment (Appendix 3); diabetes mellitus; pregnancy (see p. 245 and Appendix 4); breast-feeding (see p. 245 and Appendix 5); **interactions:** Appendix 1 (gabapentin)

Side-effects diarrhoea, dry mouth, dyspepsia, nausea, vomiting, constipation, abdominal pain, flatulence, appetite changes, gingivitis, weight gain; hypertension, vasodilation, oedema; dyspnoea, cough, rhinitis; confusion, depression, hostility, insomnia, headache, fatigue, impaired coordination; dizziness, drowsiness, anxiety, amnesia, ataxia, nystagmus, tremor, asthenia, paraesthesia, emotional lability, hyperkinesia; influenza-like symptoms; impotence, urinary incontinence; leucopenia; myalgia, arthralgia; diplopia, amblyopia; rash, purpura, pruritus, acne; *rarely* pancreatitis, hepatitis, jaundice, palpitation, hallucinations, movement disorders, false-positive readings with some urinary protein tests, thrombocytopenia, blood-glucose fluctuations in patients with diabetes, tinnitus, acute renal failure, Stevens-Johnson syndrome, and alopecia

Dose

- Epilepsy, 300 mg on day 1, then 300 mg twice daily on day 2, then 300 mg 3 times daily on day 3 *or* initially 300 mg 3 times daily on day 1, then increased according to response in steps of 300 mg daily (in 3 divided doses) every 2–3 days; usual dose 0.9–3.6 g daily in 3 divided doses (approx. every 8 hours); CHILD 6–12 years (adjunctive therapy only) 10–15 mg/kg daily in 3 divided doses, increased according to response over 3 days, usual dose 25–35 mg/kg daily (in 3 divided doses approx. every 8 hours)
- Neuropathic pain, ADULT over 18 years, 300 mg on day 1, then 300 mg twice daily on day 2, then 300 mg 3 times daily (approx. every 8 hours) on day 3 *or* initially 300 mg 3 times daily on day 1, then increased according to response in steps of 300 mg daily (in 3 divided doses) every 2–3 days to max. 3.6 g daily

Gabapentin (Non-proprietary) PoM

Capsules, gabapentin 100 mg, net price 100-cap pack = £16.68; 300 mg, 100-cap pack = £32.16; 400 mg, 100-cap pack = £26.96. Label: 3, 5, 8, counselling, driving (see notes above)

Tablets, gabapentin 600 mg, net price 100-tab pack = £106.00; 800 mg, 100-tab pack = £205.07. Label: 3, 5, 8, counselling, driving (see notes above)

Neurontin® (Pfizer) PoM

Capsules, gabapentin 100 mg (white), net price 100-cap pack = £22.86; 300 mg (yellow), 100-cap pack = £53.00; 400 mg (orange), 100-cap pack = £61.33. Label: 3, 5, 8, counselling, driving (see notes above)

Tablets, f/c, gabapentin 600 mg, net price 100-tab pack = £106.00; 800 mg, 100-tab pack = £122.66. Label: 3, 5, 8, counselling, driving (see notes above)

PREGABALIN

Indications peripheral and central neuropathic pain; adjunctive therapy for partial seizures with or without secondary generalisation; generalised anxiety disorder

Cautions avoid abrupt withdrawal (taper over at least 1 week); severe congestive heart failure; renal impairment (Appendix 3); pregnancy (Appendix 4)

Contra-indications breast-feeding (Appendix 5)

Side-effects dry mouth, constipation, nausea, vomiting, flatulence; oedema; dizziness, drowsiness, irritability, attention disturbance, disturbances in muscle control and movement, memory impairment, paraesthesia, euphoria, confusion, fatigue, appetite changes, weight gain; changes in sexual function; visual disturbances and ocular disorders (including blurred vision, diplopia, eye strain and eye irritation); *less commonly* abdominal distension, increased salivation, gastro-oesophageal reflux disease, taste disturbance, thirst, hot flushes, tachycardia, syncope, dyspnoea, chest tightness, nasal dryness, stupor, depersonalisation, depression, insomnia, abnormal dreams, hallucinations, agitation, mood swings, panic attacks, asthenia, speech disorder, dysuria, urinary incontinence, thrombocytopenia, joint swelling, muscle cramp, myalgia, arthralgia, sweating, and rash; *rarely* ascites, dysphagia, pancreatitis, hypotension, hypertension, cold extremities, first-degree AV block, arrhythmia, bradycardia, nasopharyngitis, cough, epistaxis, rhinitis, parosmia, pyrexia, rigors, disinhibition, weight loss, hypoglycaemia or hyperglycaemia, renal failure, menstrual disturbances, breast pain, breast discharge, breast hypertrophy, neutropenia, rhabdomyolysis, hyperacusis, hypokalaemia, and leucocytosis; diarrhoea, swollen tongue, congestive heart failure, loss of consciousness, headache, and pruritus also reported

Dose

- Neuropathic pain, ADULT over 18 years, initially 150 mg daily in 2–3 divided doses, increased if necessary after 3–7 days to 300 mg daily in 2–3 divided doses, increased further if necessary after 7 days to max. 600 mg daily in 2–3 divided doses
- Epilepsy, ADULT over 18 years, initially 25 mg twice daily, increased at 7-day intervals in steps of 50 mg daily to 300 mg daily in 2–3 divided doses, increased further if necessary after 7 days to max. 600 mg daily in 2–3 divided doses
- Generalised anxiety disorder, ADULT over 18 years, initially 150 mg daily in 2–3 divided doses, increased if necessary at 7-day intervals in steps of 150 mg daily; max. 600 mg daily in 2–3 divided doses

Lyrica® (Pfizer) ▼ PoM

Capsules, pregabalin 25 mg (white), net price 56-cap pack = £64.40, 84-cap pack = £96.60; 50 mg (white), 84-cap pack = £96.60; 75 mg (white/orange), 56-cap pack = £64.40; 100 mg (orange), 84-cap pack = £96.60; 150 mg (white), 56-cap pack = £64.40; 200 mg (orange), 84-cap pack = £96.60; 300 mg (white/orange), 56-cap pack = £64.40. Label: 3, 8, counselling, driving (see notes above)

Note The *Scottish Medicines Consortium* has advised (July 2007) that *Lyrica®* is not recommended for the treatment of central neuropathic pain

Lamotrigine

Lamotrigine is an antiepileptic for partial seizures and primary and secondarily generalised tonic-clonic seizures. Lamotrigine may cause serious skin rash especially in children; dose recommendations should be adhered to closely.

Lamotrigine is used either as sole treatment or as an adjunct to treatment with other antiepileptic drugs. Valproate increases plasma-lamotrigine concentration whereas the enzyme inducing antiepileptics reduce it; care is therefore required in choosing the appropriate initial dose and subsequent titration. Where the potential for interaction is not known, treatment should be initiated with lower doses such as those used with valproate.

LAMOTRIGINE

Indications monotherapy and adjunctive treatment of partial seizures and primary and secondarily generalised tonic-clonic seizures; seizures associated with Lennox-Gastaut syndrome; trigeminal neuralgia [unlicensed indication] (section 4.7.3)

Cautions closely monitor and consider withdrawal if rash, fever, or other signs of hypersensitivity syndrome develop; avoid abrupt withdrawal (taper off over 2 weeks or longer) unless serious skin reaction occurs; hepatic impairment (Appendix 2); renal impairment (Appendix 3); pregnancy (see p. 245 and Appendix 4); breast-feeding (Appendix 5); **interactions:** see p. 244 and Appendix 1 (lamotrigine)

Blood disorders The CSM has advised prescribers to be alert for symptoms and signs suggestive of bone-marrow failure such as anaemia, bruising, or infection. Aplastic anaemia, bone-marrow depression and pancytopenia have been associated rarely with lamotrigine.

Side-effects rash (see Skin Reactions, below); hypersensitivity syndrome (possibly including rash, fever, lymphadenopathy, hepatic dysfunction, blood disorders, disseminated intravascular coagulation and multi-organ dysfunction); nausea, vomiting, diarrhoea, hepatic dysfunction; headache, fatigue, dizziness, sleep disturbances, tremor, movement disorders, agitation, confusion, hallucinations, occasional increase in seizure frequency; blood disorders (including leucopenia, thrombocytopenia, pancytopenia—see Blood Disorders, above); arthralgia; lupus erythematosus-like effect; photosensitivity; nystagmus, diplopia, blurred vision, conjunctivitis

Skin reactions Serious skin reactions including Stevens-Johnson syndrome and toxic epidermal necrolysis (rarely with fatalities) have developed especially in children; most rashes occur in the first 8 weeks. Rash is sometimes associated with hypersensitivity syndrome (see Side-effects, above) and is more common in patients with history of allergy or rash from other antiepileptic drugs. Consider

4 Central nervous system

withdrawal if rash or signs of hypersensitivity syndrome develop. The CSM has advised that factors associated with increased risk of serious skin reactions include concomitant use of valproate, initial lamotrigine dosing higher than recommended, and more rapid dose escalation than recommended.

Counselling Warn patients to see their doctor immediately if rash or signs or symptoms of hypersensitivity syndrome develop

Dose

Important Do not confuse the different combinations; see also notes above

Note Dose titration should be repeated if restarting after an interval of more than 5 days

- *Monotherapy*, ADULT and CHILD over 12 years, initially 25 mg once daily for 14 days, increased to 50 mg once daily for further 14 days, then increased by max. 50–100 mg daily every 7–14 days; usual maintenance 100–200 mg daily in 1–2 divided doses (up to 500 mg daily has been required)
- Adjunctive therapy *with valproate*, initially 25 mg every other day for 14 days then 25 mg once daily for further 14 days, thereafter increased by max. 25–50 mg daily every 7–14 days; usual maintenance, 100–200 mg daily in 1–2 divided doses; CHILD 2–12 years initially 150 micrograms/kg once daily for 14 days (those weighing under 13 kg may receive 2 mg on alternate days for first 14 days) then 300 micrograms/kg once daily for further 14 days, thereafter increased by max. 300 micrograms/kg daily every 7–14 days; usual maintenance 1–5 mg/kg daily in 1–2 divided doses (max. single dose 100 mg)
- Adjunctive therapy (with enzyme inducing drugs) *without valproate*, initially 50 mg once daily for 14 days then 50 mg twice daily for further 14 days, thereafter increased by max. 100 mg daily every 7–14 days; usual maintenance 200–400 mg daily in 2 divided doses (up to 700 mg daily has been required); CHILD 2–12 years initially 600 micrograms/kg daily in 2 divided doses for 14 days then 1.2 mg/kg daily in 2 divided doses for further 14 days, thereafter increased by max. 1.2 mg/kg daily every 7–14 days; usual maintenance 5–15 mg/kg daily in 2 divided doses (max. single dose 200 mg)
- Adjunctive therapy *with oxcarbazepine*, initially 25 mg once daily for 14 days, increased to 50 mg once daily for further 14 days, then increased by max. 50–100 mg daily every 7–14 days; usual maintenance 100–200 mg daily in 1–2 divided doses; CHILD 2–12 years initially 300 micrograms/kg daily in 1–2 divided doses for 14 days then 600 micrograms/kg daily in 1–2 divided doses for further 14 days, thereafter increased by max. 600 micrograms/kg daily every 7–14 days; usual maintenance 1–10 mg/kg daily in 1–2 divided doses; max. 200 mg daily

Lamotrigine (Non-proprietary) PoM

Tablets, lamotrigine 25 mg, net price 56-tab pack = £2.91; 50 mg, 56-tab pack = £4.11; 100 mg, 56-tab pack = £5.60; 200 mg, 30-tab pack = £27.53, 56-tab pack = £12.68. Label: 8, counselling, driving (see notes above), skin reactions

Dispersible tablets, lamotrigine 5 mg, net price 28-tab pack = £3.74; 25 mg, 56-tab pack = £6.54; 100 mg, 56-tab pack = £18.61. Label: 8, 13, counselling, driving (see notes above), skin reactions

Lamictal® (GSK) PoM

Tablets, yellow, lamotrigine 25 mg, net price 21-tab pack (*'Valproate Add-on therapy' Starter Pack*) = £7.65, 42-tab pack (*'Monotherapy' Starter Pack*) = £15.30, 56-tab pack = £20.41; 50 mg, 42-tab pack (*'Non-valproate Add-on therapy' Starter Pack*) = £26.02, 56-tab pack = £34.70; 100 mg, 56-tab pack = £59.86; 200 mg, 56-tab pack = £101.76. Label: 8, counselling, driving (see notes above), skin reactions

Dispersible tablets, chewable, lamotrigine 2 mg, net price 30-tab pack = £8.71; 5 mg, 28-tab pack = £8.14; 25 mg, 56-tab pack = £20.41; 100 mg, 56-tab pack = £59.86. Label: 8, 13, counselling, driving (see notes above), skin reactions

Levetiracetam

Levetiracetam is licensed for monotherapy and adjunctive treatment of partial seizures with or without secondary generalisation, and for adjunctive therapy of myoclonic seizures and primarily generalised tonic-clonic seizures.

LEVETIRACETAM

Indications see notes above

Cautions avoid abrupt withdrawal; hepatic impairment (Appendix 2); renal impairment (Appendix 3); pregnancy (see p. 245 and Appendix 4); breast-feeding (Appendix 5)

Side-effects nausea, vomiting, dyspepsia, diarrhoea, abdominal pain, anorexia, weight changes; cough; drowsiness, asthenia, amnesia, ataxia, seizures, dizziness, headache, tremor, hyperkinesia, depression, emotional lability, insomnia, anxiety, impaired attention, aggression, irritability; thrombocytopenia; myalgia; visual disturbances; pruritus, rash; *also reported* pancreatitis, hepatic dysfunction, confusion, psychosis, hallucinations, suicidal ideation, paraesthesia, leucopenia, pancytopenia, and alopecia

Dose

- Monotherapy of partial seizures with or without secondary generalisation, by mouth *or* by intravenous infusion, ADULT and CHILD over 16 years, initially 250 mg twice daily increased according to response in steps of 250 mg twice daily every 2 weeks; max. 1.5 g twice daily
- Adjunctive therapy of partial seizures with or without secondary generalisation, myoclonic seizures, and primarily generalised tonic-clonic seizures, by mouth *or* by intravenous infusion, ADULT and CHILD over 12 years, body-weight over 50 kg, initially 500 mg twice daily, adjusted in steps of 500 mg twice daily every 2 to 4 weeks; max. 1.5 g twice daily; CHILD 4–18 years (12–18 years for myoclonic and tonic-clonic seizures), body-weight under 50 kg, initially 10 mg/kg twice daily, adjusted in steps not exceeding 10 mg/kg twice daily every 2 weeks; max. 30 mg/kg twice daily

Keppra® (UCB Pharma) PoM

Tablets, f/c, levetiracetam 250 mg (blue), net price 60-tab pack = £29.70; 500 mg (yellow), 60-tab pack = £52.30; 750 mg (orange) 60-tab pack = £89.10; 1 g (white), 60-tab pack = £101.10. Label: 8

Oral solution, sugar-free, levetiracetam 100 mg/mL, net price 300 mL = £71.00. Label: 8

Concentrate for intravenous infusion, levetiracetam 100 mg/mL. For dilution before use. Net price 5-mL vial = £13.50
Electrolytes Na^+ <0.5 mmol/vial

Phenobarbital and other barbiturates

Phenobarbital (phenobarbitone) is effective for tonic-clonic and partial seizures but may be sedative in adults and cause behavioural disturbances and hyperkinesia in children. It may be tried for atypical absence, atonic, and tonic seizures. Rebound seizures may be a problem on withdrawal. Monitoring plasma concentrations is less useful than with other drugs because tolerance occurs.

Primidone is largely converted to phenobarbital and this is probably responsible for its antiepileptic action. A small starting dose of primidone (125 mg) is essential, and the drug should be introduced over several weeks.

PHENOBARBITAL
(Phenobarbitone)

Indications all forms of epilepsy except absence seizures; status epilepticus (section 4.8.2)

Cautions see notes above; elderly; debilitated; children; respiratory depression (avoid if severe); avoid abrupt withdrawal (dependence with prolonged use); history of drug or alcohol abuse; avoid in porphyria (section 9.8.2); hepatic impairment (avoid if severe—Appendix 2); renal impairment; pregnancy (see p. 245 and Appendix 4); breast-feeding (see p. 245 and Appendix 5); **interactions:** see p. 244 and Appendix 1 (barbiturates)

Side-effects hepatitis, cholestasis; hypotension; respiratory depression; behavioural disturbances, nystagmus, irritability, drowsiness, lethargy, depression, ataxia, paradoxical excitement, hallucinations, impaired memory and cognition, hyperactivity particularly in the elderly and in children; osteomalacia; megaloblastic anaemia (may be treated with folic acid), agranulocytosis, thrombocytopenia; allergic skin reactions; *very rarely* Stevens-Johnson syndrome and toxic epidermal necrolysis; **overdosage:** see Emergency Treatment of Poisoning, p. 28

Dose

- By mouth, 60–180 mg at night; CHILD 5–8 mg/kg daily

Note For therapeutic purposes phenobarbital and phenobarbital sodium may be considered equivalent in effect. Plasma-phenobarbital concentration for optimum response 15–40 mg/litre (60–180 micromol/litre)

Phenobarbital (Non-proprietary) CD

Tablets, phenobarbital 15 mg, net price 28-tab pack = 81p; 30 mg, 28-tab pack = 60p; 60 mg, 28-tab pack = 71p. Label: 2, 8, counselling, driving (see notes above)

Elixir, phenobarbital 15 mg/5 mL in a suitable flavoured vehicle, containing alcohol 38%, net price 100 mL = 77p. Label: 2, 8, counselling, driving (see notes above)

Note Some hospitals supply **alcohol-free** formulations of varying phenobarbital strengths

Injection
Section 4.8.2

PRIMIDONE

Indications all forms of epilepsy except absence seizures; essential tremor (also section 4.9.3)

Cautions see under Phenobarbital; **interactions:** see p. 244 and Appendix 1 (primidone)

Side-effects see under Phenobarbital; also nausea and visual disturbances; *less commonly* vomiting, headache, and dizziness; *rarely* arthralgia

Dose

- Epilepsy, ADULT and CHILD over 9 years, initially 125 mg daily at bedtime, increased by 125 mg every 3 days to 500 mg daily in 2 divided doses, then increased according to response by 250 mg every 3 days to usual maintenance 0.75–1.5 g daily in 2 divided doses; CHILD under 9 years, initially 125 mg daily at bedtime, increased by 125 mg every 3 days according to response; usual maintenance, CHILD under 2 years, 250–500 mg daily in 2 divided doses; 2–5 years, 500–750 mg daily in 2 divided doses; 5–9 years 0.75–1 g daily in 2 divided doses
- Essential tremor, initially 62.5 mg daily increased gradually over 2–3 weeks according to response; max. 750 mg daily

Note Monitor plasma concentrations of derived phenobarbital. Optimum range as for phenobarbital. Primidone doses in BNF may differ from those in product literature

Mysoline® (Acorus) PoM

Tablets, scored, primidone 250 mg, net price 100-tab pack = £12.60. Label: 2, 8, counselling, driving (see notes above)

Phenytoin

Phenytoin is effective in tonic-clonic and partial seizures. It has a narrow therapeutic index and the relationship between dose and plasma concentration is non-linear; small dosage increases in some patients may produce large rises in plasma concentrations with acute toxic side-effects. Monitoring of plasma concentration greatly assists dosage adjustment. A few missed doses or a small change in drug absorption may result in a marked change in plasma concentration.

Phenytoin may cause coarse facies, acne, hirsutism, and gingival hyperplasia and so may be particularly undesirable in adolescent patients.

When only parenteral administration is possible, **fosphenytoin** (section 4.8.2), a pro-drug of phenytoin, may be convenient to give. Whereas phenytoin can be given intravenously only, fosphenytoin may also be given by intramuscular injection.

PHENYTOIN

Indications all forms of epilepsy except absence seizures; status epilepticus (section 4.8.2); trigeminal neuralgia if carbamazepine inappropriate (see also section 4.7.3)

Cautions avoid abrupt withdrawal; manufacturer recommends blood counts (but evidence of practical value unsatisfactory); avoid in porphyria (section 9.8.2); hepatic impairment (Appendix 2); pregnancy (**important:** see notes above and Appendix 4); breast-feeding (see notes above and Appendix 5); **interactions:** see p. 244 and Appendix 1 (phenytoin)

Blood or skin disorders Patients or their carers should be told how to recognise signs of blood or skin disorders, and advised to seek immediate medical attention if symptoms such as fever, sore throat, rash, mouth ulcers, bruising, or bleeding develop. Leucopenia which is severe, progressive, or associated with clinical symptoms requires withdrawal (if necessary under cover of suitable alternative)

Side-effects nausea, vomiting, constipation, insomnia, transient nervousness, tremor, paraesthesia, dizziness, headache, anorexia; gingival hypertrophy and tenderness; rash (discontinue; if mild re-introduce cautiously but discontinue immediately if recurrence), acne, hirsutism, coarse facies; *rarely* hepatotoxicity, peripheral neuropathy, dyskinesia, lymphadenopathy, osteomalacia, blood disorders (including megaloblastic anaemia (may be treated with folic acid), leucopenia, thrombocytopenia, and aplastic anaemia), polyarteritis nodosa, lupus erythematosus, Stevens-Johnson syndrome, and toxic epidermal necrolysis; also reported pneumonitis and interstitial nephritis; *with excessive dosage* nystagmus, diplopia, slurred speech, ataxia, confusion, and hyperglycaemia

Dose

- By mouth, initially 3–4 mg/kg daily *or* 150–300 mg daily (as a single dose *or* in 2 divided doses) increased gradually as necessary (with plasma-phenytoin concentration monitoring); usual dose 200–500 mg daily (exceptionally, higher doses may be used); CHILD initially 5 mg/kg daily in 2 divided doses, usual dose range 4–8 mg/kg daily (max. 300 mg daily)

Note Plasma concentration for optimum response 10–20 mg/litre (40–80 micromol/litre)

Counselling Take preferably with or after food

Phenytoin (Non-proprietary) PoM

Tablets, coated, phenytoin sodium 100 mg, net price 28-tab pack = £113.62. Label: 8, counselling, administration, blood or skin disorder symptoms (see above), driving (see notes above)

Note On the basis of single dose tests there are no clinically relevant differences in bioavailability between available phenytoin sodium tablets and capsules but there may be a pharmacokinetic basis for maintaining the same brand of phenytoin in some patients

Epanutin® (Pfizer) PoM

Capsules, phenytoin sodium 25 mg (white/purple), net price 28-cap pack = 66p; 50 mg (white/pink), 28-cap pack = 67p; 100 mg (white/orange), 84-cap pack = £2.83; 300 mg (white/green), 28-cap pack = £2.83. Label: 8, counselling, administration, blood or skin disorder symptoms (see above), driving (see notes above)

Infatabs® (= chewable tablets), yellow, scored, phenytoin 50 mg, net price 112 = £7.38. Label: 8, 24, counselling, blood or skin disorder symptoms (see above), driving (see notes above)

Note Contain phenytoin 50 mg (as against phenytoin sodium) therefore care is needed on changing to capsules or tablets containing phenytoin sodium

Suspension, red, phenytoin 30 mg/5 mL, net price 500 mL = £4.27. Label: 8, counselling, administration, blood or skin disorder symptoms (see above), driving (see notes above)

Note Suspension of phenytoin 90 mg in 15 mL may be considered to be approximately equivalent in therapeutic effect to capsules or tablets containing phenytoin sodium 100 mg, but nevertheless care is needed in making changes

Rufinamide

Rufinamide is licensed for the adjunctive treatment of seizures in Lennox-Gastaut syndrome.

RUFINAMIDE

Indications adjunctive treatment of seizures in Lennox-Gastaut syndrome

Cautions closely monitor and consider withdrawal if rash, fever, or other signs of hypersensitivity syndrome develop; avoid abrupt withdrawal; hepatic impairment (avoid if severe; Appendix 2); pregnancy (see p. 245 and Appendix 4); **interactions:** see p. 244 and Appendix 1 (rufinamide)

Contra-indications breast-feeding (Appendix 5)

Side-effects nausea, vomiting, constipation, diarrhoea, dyspepsia, abdominal pain, weight loss, anorexia; rhinitis, epistaxis; dizziness, headache, drowsiness, insomnia, anxiety, fatigue, increase in seizure frequency, impaired coordination, hyperactivity, tremor, gait disturbances; influenza-like symptoms; oligomenorrhoea; back pain; nystagmus, diplopia, blurred vision; rash and acne; hypersensitivity syndrome (possibly including rash, fever, lymphadenopathy, hepatic dysfunction, haematuria, and multi-organ dysfunction) also reported

Hypersensitivity syndrome Serious hypersensitivity syndrome (see Side-effects) has developed especially in children and upon initiation of therapy, consider withdrawal if rash or signs or symptoms of hypersensitivity syndrome develop

Counselling Warn patients to seek immediate medical attention if signs or symptoms of hypersensitivity develop

Dose

- ADULT and CHILD over 4 years body-weight over 30 kg, initially 200 mg twice daily increased according to response in steps of 200 mg twice daily at intervals not less than 2 days; body-weight 30–50 kg max. 900 mg twice daily; body-weight 50–70 kg max. 1.2 g twice daily; body-weight over 70 kg max. 1.6 g twice daily; CHILD over 4 years body-weight less than 30 kg, initially 100 mg twice daily increased according to response in steps of 100 mg twice daily at intervals not less than 2 days; max. 500 mg twice daily (max. 200 mg twice daily when adjunctive therapy *with valproate*)

Inovelon® (Eisai) ▼ PoM

Tablets, pink, f/c, scored, rufinamide 100 mg, net price10-tab pack = £8.58; 200 mg, 60-tab pack = £51.48; 400 mg, 60-tab pack = £85.80. Label: 21, counselling, driving (see notes above), hypersensitivity syndrome

Tiagabine

Tiagabine is used as adjunctive treatment for partial seizures, with or without secondary generalisation.

TIAGABINE

Indications adjunctive treatment for partial seizures with or without secondary generalisation not satisfactorily controlled with other antiepileptics

Cautions avoid in porphyria (section 9.8.2); hepatic impairment (Appendix 2); avoid abrupt withdrawal; **interactions:** Appendix 1 (tiagabine)

Driving May impair performance of skilled tasks (e.g. driving)

Side-effects diarrhoea; dizziness, tiredness, nervousness, tremor, impaired concentration, emotional lability, speech impairment; *rarely* confusion, depression, drowsiness, psychosis, non-convulsive status epilepticus, bruising, and visual disturbances; leucopenia also reported

Dose

- Adjunctive therapy, ADULT and CHILD over 12 years, with *enzyme-inducing* drugs, 5 mg twice daily for 1 week, then increased at weekly intervals in steps of 5–10 mg daily; usual maintenance dose 30–45 mg daily (doses above 30 mg given in 3 divided doses); in patients receiving *non-enzyme-inducing* drugs, initial maintenance dose 15–30 mg daily

Gabitril® (Cephalon) PoM

Tablets, f/c, scored, tiagabine (as hydrochloride) 5 mg, net price 100-tab pack = £43.37; 10 mg, 100-tab pack = £86.74; 15 mg, 100-tab pack = £130.11. Label: 21

Topiramate

Topiramate can be given alone or as adjunctive treatment in generalised tonic-clonic seizures or partial seizures with or without secondary generalisation. It can be used as adjunctive treatment for seizures associated with Lennox-Gastaut syndrome. Topiramate is also licensed for prophylaxis of migraine (section 4.7.4.2).

TOPIRAMATE

Indications monotherapy and adjunctive treatment of generalised tonic-clonic seizures or partial seizures with or without secondary generalisation; adjunctive treatment of seizures in Lennox-Gastaut syndrome; migraine prophylaxis (under specialist supervision)

Cautions avoid abrupt withdrawal; ensure adequate hydration (especially if predisposition to nephrolithiasis or in strenuous activity or warm environment); avoid in porphyria (section 9.8.2); hepatic impairment (Appendix 2); renal impairment (Appendix 3); pregnancy (see notes above and Appendix 4); **interactions:** see p. 245 and Appendix 1 (topiramate)

CSM advice Topiramate has been associated with acute myopia with secondary angle-closure glaucoma, typically occurring within 1 month of starting treatment. Choroidal effusions resulting in anterior displacement of the lens and iris have also been reported. The CSM advises that if raised intra-ocular pressure occurs:

- seek specialist ophthalmological advice;
- use appropriate measures to reduce intra-ocular pressure;
- stop topiramate as rapidly as feasible

Contra-indications breast-feeding (Appendix 5)

Side-effects nausea, abdominal pain, dyspepsia, diarrhoea, dry mouth, taste disturbance, weight loss, anorexia; paraesthesia, hypoaesthesia, headache, fatigue, dizziness, speech disorder, drowsiness, insomnia, impaired memory and concentration, anxiety, depression; visual disturbances; *less commonly* suicidal ideation; *rarely* reduced sweating mainly in children, metabolic acidosis, and alopecia; *very rarely* leucopenia, thrombocytopenia, and serious skin reactions

Dose

- Monotherapy, initially 25 mg at night for 1 week *then* increased in steps of 25–50 mg daily at intervals of 1–2 weeks taken in 2 divided doses; usual dose 100 mg daily in 2 divided doses; max. 400 mg daily; CHILD 6–16 years, initially 0.5–1 mg/kg at night for 1 week *then* increased in steps of 0.5–1 mg/kg daily at intervals of 1–2 weeks taken in 2 divided doses; usual dose 3–6 mg/kg daily in 2 divided doses; max. 15 mg/kg daily
- Adjunctive therapy, initially 25 mg at night for 1 week *then* increased in steps of 25–50 mg daily at intervals of 1–2 weeks taken in 2 divided doses; usual dose 200–400 mg daily in 2 divided doses; max. 800 mg daily; CHILD 2–16 years, initially 25 mg at night for one week *then* increased in steps of 1–3 mg/kg daily at intervals of 1–2 weeks taken in 2 divided doses; recommended dose range 5–9 mg/kg daily in 2 divided doses; max. 15 mg/kg daily
- Migraine prophylaxis ADULT and CHILD over 16 years, initially 25 mg daily at night for 1 week *then* increased in steps of 25 mg daily at intervals of 1 week; usual dose 50–100 mg daily in 2 divided doses

Note If patient cannot tolerate titration regimens recommended above then smaller steps or longer interval between steps may be used

Topamax® (Janssen-Cilag) ▼ PoM

Tablets, f/c, topiramate 25 mg, net price 60-tab pack = £19.08; 50 mg (light yellow), 60-tab pack = £32.12; 100 mg (yellow), 60-tab pack = £55.31; 200 mg (salmon), 60-tab pack = £102.80. Label: 3, 8, counselling, driving (see notes above)

Sprinkle capsules, topiramate 15 mg, net price 60-cap pack = £15.70; 25 mg, 60-cap pack = £23.55; 50 mg, 60-cap pack = £35.57. Label: 3, 8, counselling, administration, driving (see notes above)

Counselling Swallow whole or open capsule and sprinkle contents on soft food

Valproate

Sodium valproate is effective in controlling tonic-clonic seizures, particularly in primary generalised epilepsy. It is a drug of choice in primary generalised epilepsy, generalised absences and myoclonic seizures, and can be tried in atypical absence, atonic, and tonic seizures. Plasma-valproate concentrations are not a useful index of efficacy, therefore routine monitoring is unhelpful. The drug has widespread metabolic effects, and may have dose-related side-effects.

Valproic acid (as semisodium valproate) (section 4.2.3) is licensed for acute mania associated with bipolar disorder.

SODIUM VALPROATE

Indications all forms of epilepsy

Cautions monitor liver function before therapy and during first 6 months especially in patients most at risk (see also below); measure full blood count and ensure no undue potential for bleeding before starting and before surgery; systemic lupus erythematosus; false-positive urine tests for ketones; avoid abrupt withdrawal; renal impairment (Appendix 3); pregnancy (**important** see notes above and Appendix 4); breast-feeding (Appendix 5); **interactions:** see p. 244 and Appendix 1 (valproate)

Liver toxicity Liver dysfunction (including fatal hepatic failure) has occurred in association with valproate (especially in children under 3 years and in those with metabolic or degenerative disorders, organic brain disease or severe seizure disorders associated with mental retardation) usually in first 6 months and usually involving multiple antiepileptic therapy. Raised liver enzymes during valproate treatment are usually transient but patients should be reassessed clinically and liver function (including prothrombin time) monitored until return to normal—discontinue if abnormally prolonged prothrombin time (particularly in association with other relevant abnormalities).

Blood or hepatic disorders Patients or their carers should be told how to recognise signs and symptoms of blood or liver disorders and advised to seek immediate medical attention if symptoms develop

Pancreatitis Patients or their carers should be told how to recognise signs and symptoms of pancreatitis and advised to seek immediate medical attention if symptoms such as abdominal pain, nausea and vomiting develop; discontinue if pancreatitis is diagnosed

Contra-indications active liver disease, family history of severe hepatic dysfunction; porphyria (section 9.8.2)

Side-effects nausea, gastric irritation, diarrhoea; weight gain; hyperammonaemia, thrombocytopenia; transient hair loss (regrowth may be curly); *less frequently* increased alertness, aggression, hyperactivity, behavioural disturbances, ataxia, tremor, and vasculitis; *rarely* hepatic dysfunction (see under Cautions; withdraw treatment immediately if persistent vomiting and abdominal pain, anorexia, jaundice, oedema, malaise, drowsiness, or loss of seizure control), lethargy, drowsiness, confusion, stupor, hallucinations, menstrual disturbances, anaemia, leucopenia, pancytopenia, hearing loss, and rash; *very rarely* pancreatitis (see under Cautions), peripheral oedema, increase in bleeding time, extrapyramidal symptoms, dementia, encephalopathy, coma, gynaecomastia, Fanconi's syndrome, hirsutism, acne, enuresis, hyponatraemia, toxic epidermal necrolysis, and Stevens-Johnson syndrome

Dose

- By mouth, initially 600 mg daily in 2 divided doses, preferably after food, increased by 200 mg daily every 3 days to max. 2.5 g daily, usual maintenance dose 1–2 g daily (20–30 mg/kg daily); CHILD bodyweight up to 20 kg, initially 20 mg/kg daily in divided doses, may be increased provided plasma concentration monitored (dose above 40 mg/kg daily also monitor clinical chemistry and haematological parameters); CHILD under 12 years bodyweight over 20 kg, initially 400 mg daily in divided doses increased according to response (usual range 20–30 mg/kg daily); max. 35 mg/kg daily
- By intravenous injection (over 3–5 minutes) *or* by intravenous infusion, continuation of valproate treatment, same as current dose by oral route

  Initiation of valproate therapy, by intravenous injection (over 3–5 minutes), 400–800 mg (up to 10 mg/kg) followed by intravenous infusion up to max. 2.5 g daily; CHILD under 12 years, usually 20–30 mg/kg daily, may be increased provided plasma concentration monitored (dose above 40 mg/kg daily also monitor clinical chemistry and haematological parameters)

◢Oral

Sodium Valproate (Non-proprietary) PoM

Tablets (crushable), scored, sodium valproate 100 mg, net price 100-tab pack = £4.67. Label: 8, counselling, blood or hepatic disorder symptoms (see above), driving (see notes above)

Tablets, e/c, sodium valproate 200 mg, net price 100-tab pack = £8.54; 500 mg, 100-tab pack = £19.54. Label: 5, 8, 25, counselling, blood or hepatic disorder symptoms (see above), driving (see notes above)

Brands include *Orlept®*

Oral solution, sodium valproate 200 mg/5 mL, net price 300 mL = £8.71. Label: 8, counselling, blood or hepatic disorder symptoms (see above), driving (see notes above)

Brands include *Orlept®* sugar-free

Epilim® (Sanofi-Synthelabo) PoM

Tablets (crushable), scored, sodium valproate 100 mg, net price 100 = £4.67. Label: 8, counselling, blood or hepatic disorder symptoms (see above), driving (see notes above)

Tablets, both e/c, lilac, sodium valproate 200 mg, net price 100 = £7.70; 500 mg, 100 = £19.25. Label: 5, 8, 25, counselling, blood or hepatic disorder symptoms (see above), driving (see notes above)

Liquid, red, sugar-free, sodium valproate 200 mg/5 mL, net price 300-mL pack = £7.78. Label: 8, counselling, blood or hepatic disorder symptoms (see above), driving (see notes above)

Syrup, red, sodium valproate 200 mg/5 mL, net price 300-mL pack = £7.78. Label: 8, counselling, blood or hepatic disorder symptoms (see above), driving (see notes above)

◢Modified release

Epilim Chrono® (Sanofi-Synthelabo) PoM

Tablets, m/r, lilac, sodium valproate 200 mg (as sodium valproate and valproic acid), net price 100-tab pack = £9.71; 300 mg, 100-tab pack = £14.56; 500 mg, 100-tab pack = £24.25. Label: 8, 25, counselling, blood or hepatic disorder symptoms (see above), driving (see notes above)

Dose ADULT and CHILD over 20 kg, as above, total daily dose given in 1–2 divided doses

Episenta® (Beacon) PoM

Capsules, m/r, sodium valproate 150 mg, net price 100-cap pack = £5.70; 300 mg, 100-cap pack = £10.90. Label: 8, 25, counselling, administration, blood or hepatic disorder symptoms (see above), driving (see notes above)

Dose ADULT and CHILD, as above, total daily dose given in 1–2 divided doses

Counselling Contents of capsule may be mixed with cold food or drink and swallowed immediately without chewing

Granules, m/r, sodium valproate 500 mg, net price 100-sachet pack = £18.00; 1 g, 100-sachet pack = £35.50. Label: 8, 25, counselling, administration, blood or hepatic disorder symptoms (see above), driving (see notes above)

Dose ADULT and CHILD, as above, total daily dose given in 1–2 divided doses

Counselling Granules may be mixed with cold food or drink and swallowed immediately without chewing

◢Parenteral

Epilim® Intravenous (Sanofi-Synthelabo) PoM

Injection, powder for reconstitution, sodium valproate, net price 400-mg vial (with 4-mL amp water for injections) = £11.58

Episenta® (Beacon) PoM

Injection, sodium valproate 100 mg/mL, net price 3-mL amp = £7.00

▲Valproic acid

Convulex® (Pharmacia) PoM

Capsules, e/c, valproic acid 150 mg, net price 100-cap pack = £3.68; 300 mg, 100-cap pack = £7.35; 500 mg, 100-cap pack = £12.25. Label: 8, 25, counselling, blood or hepatic disorder symptoms (see above), driving (see notes above)

Dose ADULT and CHILD as for sodium valproate, total daily dose given in 2–4 divided doses

Equivalence to sodium valproate Manufacturer advises that *Convulex®* has a 1:1 dose relationship with products containing sodium valproate, but nevertheless care is needed in making changes.

Vigabatrin

For partial epilepsy with or without secondary generalisation, **vigabatrin** is given in combination with other antiepileptic treatment; its use is restricted to patients in whom all other combinations are inadequate or are not tolerated. It can be used as sole therapy in the management of infantile spasms in West's syndrome.

About one-third of patients treated with vigabatrin have suffered visual field defects; counselling and **careful monitoring** for this side-effect are required (see also Visual Field Defects under Cautions below). Vigabatrin has prominent behavioural side-effects in some patients.

VIGABATRIN

Indications initiated and supervised by appropriate specialist, adjunctive treatment of partial seizures with or without secondary generalisation not satisfactorily controlled with other antiepileptics; monotherapy for management of infantile spasms (West's syndrome)

Cautions renal impairment (Appendix 3); elderly; closely monitor neurological function; avoid sudden withdrawal (taper off over 2–4 weeks); history of psychosis, depression or behavioural problems; pregnancy (see p. 245 and Appendix 4) and breast-feeding (Appendix 5); absence seizures (may be exacerbated); **interactions**: see p. 244 and Appendix 1 (vigabatrin)

Visual field defects Vigabatrin is associated with visual field defects. The CSM has advised that onset of symptoms varies from 1 month to several years after starting. In most cases, visual field defects have persisted despite discontinuation. Product literature advises visual field testing before treatment and at 6-month intervals; a procedure for testing visual fields in those with a developmental age of less than 9 years is available from the manufacturers. Patients should be warned to report any new visual symptoms that develop and those with symptoms should be referred for an urgent ophthalmological opinion. Gradual withdrawal of vigabatrin should be considered.

Contra-indications visual field defects

Side-effects drowsiness (rarely, encephalopathic symptoms consisting of marked sedation, stupor, and confusion with non-specific slow wave EEG—reduce dose or withdraw), fatigue, visual field defects (see also under Cautions), dizziness, nervousness, irritability, behavioural effects such as excitation and agitation especially in children; depression, abnormal thinking, headache, nystagmus, ataxia, tremor, paraesthesia, impaired concentration; less commonly confusion, aggression, psychosis, mania, memory disturbance, visual disturbance (e.g. diplopia); also weight gain, oedema, gastro-intestinal disturbances, alopecia, rash; less commonly, urticaria, occasional increase in seizure frequency (especially if myoclonic), decrease in liver enzymes, slight decrease in haemoglobin; photophobia and retinal disorders (e.g. peripheral retinal atrophy); optic neuritis, optic atrophy, hallucinations also reported

Dose

- With current antiepileptic therapy, initially 1 g daily in single or 2 divided doses then increased according to response in steps of 500 mg at weekly intervals; usual range 2–3 g daily (max. 3 g daily); CHILD initially 40 mg/kg daily in single or 2 divided doses then adjusted according to body-weight 10–15 kg, 0.5–1 g daily; body-weight 15–30 kg, 1–1.5 g daily; body-weight 30–50 kg, 1.5–3 g daily; body-weight over 50 kg, 2–3 g daily
- Infantile spasms (West's syndrome), *monotherapy*, 50 mg/kg daily, adjusted according to response over 7 days; up to 150 mg/kg daily used with good tolerability

Sabril® (Aventis Pharma) PoM

Tablets, f/c, scored, vigabatrin 500 mg, net price 100-tab pack = £30.84. Label: 3, 8, counselling, driving (see notes above)

Powder, sugar-free, vigabatrin 500 mg/sachet. Net price 50-sachet pack = £17.08. Label: 3, 8, 13, counselling, driving (see notes above)

Note The contents of a sachet should be dissolved in water or a soft drink immediately before taking

Zonisamide

Zonisamide can be used as adjunctive treatment for refractory partial seizures with or without secondary generalisation.

ZONISAMIDE

Indications adjunctive therapy for refractory partial seizures with or without secondary generalisation

Cautions elderly; ensure adequate hydration (especially if predisposition to nephrolithiasis or in strenuous activity or warm environment); concomitant use of drugs that increase risk of hyperthermia or nephrolithiasis; avoid abrupt withdrawal; hepatic impairment (avoid if severe—Appendix 2); renal impairment (Appendix 3); pregnancy (Appendix 4); **interactions**: see p. 244 and Appendix 1 (zonisamide)

Contra-indications hypersensitivity to sulphonamides; breast-feeding (Appendix 5)

Side-effects nausea, diarrhoea, abdominal pain, anorexia, weight loss; drowsiness, dizziness, confusion, agitation, irritability, depression, ataxia, speech disorder, impaired memory and attention, pyrexia; diplopia; rash (consider withdrawal); *less commonly* vomiting, cholelithiasis, cholecystitis, aggression, suicidal ideation, convulsions, psychosis, urinary calculus, hypokalaemia; *very rarely* hepatitis, pancreatitis, dyspnoea, hallucinations, insomnia, amnesia, coma, myasthenic syndrome, neuroleptic malignant syndrome, heat stroke, hydronephrosis, renal impairment, metabolic acidosis, blood disorders, rhabdomyolysis, impaired sweating, pruritus, and Stevens-Johnson syndrome

Dose

- ADULT over 18 years, initially 50 mg daily in 2 divided doses, increased after 7 days to 100 mg daily in 2 divided doses; then increase if necessary by 100 mg every 7 days; usual maintenance 300–500 mg daily in 1–2 divided doses

Zonegran® (Eisai) ▼ PoM
Capsules, zonisamide 25 mg (white), net price 14-cap pack = £8.82; 50 mg (white/grey), 56-cap pack = £47.04; 100 mg (white/red), 56-cap pack = £62.72. Label: 3

Benzodiazepines

Clonazepam is occasionally used in tonic-clonic or partial seizures, but its sedative side-effects may be prominent. **Clobazam** may be used as adjunctive therapy in the treatment of epilepsy (section 4.1.2), but the effectiveness of these and other **benzodiazepines** may wane considerably after weeks or months of continuous therapy.

CLOBAZAM

Indications adjunct in epilepsy; anxiety (short-term use)
Cautions see under Diazepam (section 4.1.2)
Contra-indications see under Diazepam (section 4.1.2)
Side-effects see under Diazepam (section 4.1.2)
Dose

- Epilepsy, 20–30 mg daily; max. 60 mg daily; CHILD over 3 years, not more than half adult dose
- Anxiety, 20–30 mg daily in divided doses or as a single dose at bedtime, increased in severe anxiety (in hospital patients) to a max. of 60 mg daily in divided doses; ELDERLY (or debilitated) 10–20 mg daily

[1]**Clobazam** (Non-proprietary) PoM NHS
Tablets, clobazam 10 mg. Net price 30-tab pack = £9.74. Label: 2 or 19, 8, counselling, driving (see notes above)
Brands include *Frisium®* NHS

1. NHS except for epilepsy and endorsed 'SLS'

CLONAZEPAM

Indications all forms of epilepsy; myoclonus; status epilepticus (section 4.8.2)
Cautions see notes above; elderly and debilitated, respiratory disease, spinal or cerebellar ataxia; history of alcohol or drug abuse, depression or suicidal ideation; avoid sudden withdrawal; myasthenia gravis (avoid if unstable); porphyria (section 9.8.2); hepatic impairment (avoid if severe; Appendix 2); renal impairment; pregnancy (see notes above and Appendix 4); breast-feeding (see notes above and Appendix 5); **interactions:** Appendix 1 (anxiolytics and hypnotics)
Driving Drowsiness may affect performance of skilled tasks (e.g. driving); effects of alcohol enhanced
Contra-indications respiratory depression; acute pulmonary insufficiency; sleep apnoea syndrome; marked neuromuscular respiratory weakness including unstable myasthenia gravis
Side-effects drowsiness, fatigue, dizziness, muscle hypotonia, co-ordination disturbances; also poor concentration, restlessness, confusion, amnesia, dependence, and withdrawal; salivary or bronchial hypersecretion in infants and small children; *rarely* gastro-intestinal symptoms, respiratory depression, headache, paradoxical effects including aggression and anxiety, sexual dysfunction, urinary incontinence, urticaria, pruritus, reversible hair loss, skin pigmentation changes; dysarthria, and visual disturbances on long-term treatment; blood disorders reported; **overdosage:** see Emergency Treatment of Poisoning, p. 32
Dose

- 1 mg (ELDERLY 500 micrograms) initially at night for 4 nights, increased according to response over 2–4 weeks to usual maintenance dose of 4–8 mg usually at night (may be given in 3–4 divided doses if necessary); CHILD up to 1 year, initially 250 micrograms increased as above to usual maintenance dose of 0.5–1 mg, 1–5 years, initially 250 micrograms increased as above to 1–3 mg, 5–12 years, initially 500 micrograms increased as above to 3–6 mg
Note Clonazepam doses in BNF may differ from those in product literature

Rivotril® (Roche) PoM
Tablets, both scored, clonazepam 500 micrograms (beige), net price 100 = £3.92; 2 mg (white), 100 = £5.23. Label: 2, 8, counselling, driving (see notes above)
Injection, section 4.8.2

Other drugs

Acetazolamide (section 11.6), a carbonic anhydrase inhibitor, has a specific role in treating epilepsy associated with menstruation. It can also be used with other antiepileptics for tonic-clonic and partial seizures. It is occasionally helpful in atypical absence, atonic, and tonic seizures.

Piracetam (section 4.9.3) is used as adjunctive treatment for cortical myoclonus.

4.8.2 Drugs used in status epilepticus

Immediate measures to manage status epilepticus include positioning the patient to avoid injury, supporting respiration including the provision of oxygen, maintaining blood pressure, and the correction of any hypoglycaemia. Parenteral **thiamine** should be considered if alcohol abuse is suspected; **pyridoxine** (section 9.6.2) should be given if the status epilepticus is caused by pyridoxine deficiency.

Major status epilepticus should be treated urgently with intravenous **lorazepam**, repeated once after 10 minutes if seizures recur. Intravenous diazepam is effective but it is associated with a high risk of thrombophlebitis (reduced by using an emulsion formulation). Absorption of diazepam from intramuscular injection or from suppositories is too slow for treatment of status epilepticus. **Clonazepam** can also be used as an alternative.

Where facilities for resuscitation are not immediately available, **diazepam** can be administered as a rectal solution or **midazolam** [unlicensed use] can be given into the buccal cavity.

> **Important**
> If seizures recur or fail to respond within 30 minutes, phenytoin sodium, fosphenytoin, or phenobarbital sodium should be used.
> If these measures fail to control seizure within 60 minutes, anaesthesia with thiopental (section 15.1.1), midazolam (section 15.1.4), or in adults, a non-barbiturate anaesthetic such as propofol [unlicensed indication] (section 15.1.1), should be instituted with full intensive care support.

Phenytoin sodium may be given by slow intravenous injection, with ECG monitoring, followed by the maintenance dosage. Intramuscular use of phenytoin is not recommended (absorption is slow and erratic).

Alternatively, **fosphenytoin**, a pro-drug of phenytoin, can be given more rapidly and when given intravenously causes fewer injection-site reactions than phenytoin. Intravenous administration requires ECG monitoring. Although it can also be given intramuscularly, absorption is too slow by this route for treatment of status epilepticus. Doses of fosphenytoin should be expressed in terms of phenytoin sodium.

Paraldehyde also remains a valuable drug. Given rectally it causes little respiratory depression and is therefore useful where facilities for resuscitation are poor.

For advice on the management of epileptic seizures in dental practice, see p. 22

Non-convulsive status epilepticus The urgency to treat non-convulsive status epilepticus depends upon the severity of the patient's condition. If there is incomplete loss of awareness, usual oral antiepileptic therapy should be continued or restarted. Patients who fail to respond to oral antiepileptic therapy or have complete lack of awareness can be treated in the same way as for convulsive status epilepticus, although anaesthesia is rarely needed.

CLONAZEPAM

Indications status epilepticus; other forms of epilepsy, and myoclonus (section 4.8.1)

Cautions see section 4.8.1; facilities for reversing respiratory depression with mechanical ventilation must be at hand (but see also notes above)

Intavenous infusion Intravenous infusion of clonazepam is potentially hazardous (especially if prolonged), calling for close and constant observation and best carried out in specialist centres with intensive care facilities. Prolonged infusion may lead to accumulation and delay recovery

Contra-indications see section 4.8.1; avoid injections containing benzyl alcohol in neonates (see under preparations below)

Side-effects see section 4.8.1; hypotension and apnoea

Dose

- By intravenous injection into a large vein (over at least 2 minutes) *or* by intravenous infusion, 1 mg, repeated if necessary; CHILD all ages, 500 micrograms

Rivotril® (Roche) PoM

Injection, clonazepam 1 mg/mL in solvent, for dilution with 1 mL water for injections immediately before injection or as described in Appendix 6. Net price 1-mL amp (with 1 mL water for injections) = 63p

Excipients include benzyl alcohol (avoid in neonates, see Excipients, p. 2), ethanol, propylene glycol

Oral preparations

Section 4.8.1

DIAZEPAM

Indications status epilepticus; febrile convulsions; convulsions due to poisoning (see p. 28); other indications (section 4.1.2, section 10.2.2, and section 15.1.4.1)

Cautions see section 4.1.2; when given intravenously facilities for reversing respiratory depression with mechanical ventilation must be at hand (but see also notes above)

Contra-indications see section 4.1.2

Side-effects see section 4.1.2; hypotension and apnoea

Dose

- Status epilepticus (but see notes above), febrile convulsions, and convulsions due to poisoning, by intravenous injection, 10 mg at a rate of 1 mL (5 mg) per minute, repeated if necessary after 10 minutes; CHILD under 12 years, 300–400 micrograms/kg [unlicensed dose], repeated after 10 minutes if necessary

  By rectum as rectal solution, ADULT and CHILD over 10 kg, 500 micrograms/kg, up to max. 30 mg (ELDERLY 250 micrograms/kg, up to max. 15 mg); repeated after 15 minutes if necessary

Diazepam (Non-proprietary) PoM

Injection (solution), diazepam 5 mg/mL. See Appendix 6. Net price 2-mL amp = 35p

Excipients may include benzyl alcohol (avoid in neonates, see Excipients, p. 2), ethanol, propylene glycol

Injection (emulsion), diazepam 5 mg/mL (0.5%). See Appendix 6. Net price 2-mL amp = 84p

Brands include *Diazemuls®*

Rectal tubes (= rectal solution), diazepam 2 mg/mL, net price 1.25-mL (2.5-mg) tube = 90p, 2.5-mL (5-mg) tube = £1.27; 4 mg/mL, 2.5-mL (10-mg) tube = £1.59

Brands include *Diazepam Rectubes®*, *Stesolid®*

Oral preparations

Section 4.1.2

FOSPHENYTOIN SODIUM

Note Fosphenytoin is a pro-drug of phenytoin

Indications status epilepticus; seizures associated with neurosurgery or head injury; when phenytoin by mouth not possible

Cautions see Phenytoin Sodium; liver impairment (Appendix 2); renal impairment (Appendix 3); resuscitation facilities must be available; **interactions:** see p. 244 and Appendix 1 (phenytoin)

Contra-indications see Phenytoin Sodium

Side-effects see Phenytoin Sodium

CSM advice Intravenous infusion of fosphenytoin has been associated with severe cardiovascular reactions including asystole, ventricular fibrillation, and cardiac arrest. Hypotension, bradycardia, and heart block have also been reported. The CSM advises:

- monitor heart rate, blood pressure, and respiratory function for duration of infusion
- observe patient for at least 30 minutes after infusion
- if hypotension occurs, reduce infusion rate or discontinue
- reduce dose or infusion rate in elderly, and in renal or hepatic impairment.

Dose

> **Note** Prescriptions for fosphenytoin sodium should state the dose in terms of phenytoin sodium equivalent (PE); fosphenytoin sodium 1.5 mg ≡ phenytoin sodium 1 mg

- Status epilepticus, by intravenous infusion (at a rate of 100–150 mg(PE)/minute), initially 20 mg(PE)/kg then by intravenous infusion (at a rate of 50–100 mg(PE)/minute), 4–5 mg(PE)/kg daily in 1–2 divided doses, dose adjusted according to response and trough plasma-phenytoin concentration
  CHILD 5 years and over, by intravenous infusion (at a rate of 2–3 mg(PE)/kg/minute), initially 20 mg(PE)/kg then by intravenous infusion (at a rate of 1–2 mg(PE)/kg/minute), 4–5 mg(PE)/kg daily in 1–4 divided doses, dose adjusted according to response and trough plasma-phenytoin concentration
- Prophylaxis or treatment of seizures associated with neurosurgery or head injury, by intramuscular injection *or* by intravenous infusion (at a rate of 50–100 mg(PE)/minute), initially 10–15 mg(PE)/kg then by intramuscular injection *or* by intravenous infusion (at a rate of 50–100 mg(PE)/minute), 4–5 mg(PE)/kg daily (in 1–2 divided doses), dose adjusted according to response and trough plasma-phenytoin concentration
  CHILD 5 years and over, by intravenous infusion (at a rate of 1–2 mg(PE)/kg/minute), initially 10–15 mg(PE)/kg then 4–5 mg(PE)/kg daily in 1–4 divided doses, dose adjusted according to response and trough plasma-phenytoin concentration
- Temporary substitution for oral phenytoin, by intramuscular injection *or* by intravenous infusion (at a rate of 50–100 mg(PE)/minute), same dose and dosing frequency as oral phenytoin therapy; CHILD 5 years and over, by intravenous infusion (at a rate of 1–2 mg(PE)/kg/minute), same dose and dosing frequency as oral phenytoin therapy

Note ELDERLY consider 10–25% reduction in dose or infusion rate

Note Fosphenytoin sodium doses in BNF may differ from those in product literature

Pro-Epanutin® (Pfizer) PoM
Injection, fosphenytoin sodium 75 mg/mL (equivalent to phenytoin sodium 50 mg/mL), net price 10-mL vial = £40.00
Electrolytes phosphate 3.7 micromol/mg fosphenytoin sodium (phosphate 5.6 micromol/mg phenytoin sodium)

LORAZEPAM

Indications status epilepticus; other indications (section 4.1.2)
Cautions see section 4.1.2
Contra-indications see under Diazepam (section 4.1.2)
Side-effects see under Diazepam (section 4.1.2)
Dose

- By intravenous injection (into large vein), 4 mg repeated once after 10 minutes if seizures recur; CHILD 100 micrograms/kg (max. 4 mg) repeated once after 10 minutes if seizures recur

Preparations
Section 4.1.2

MIDAZOLAM

Indications status epilepticus [unlicensed indication]; other indications (section 15.1.4)
Cautions section 15.1.4
Contra-indications section 15.1.4
Side-effects section 15.1.4
Dose

- By buccal administration, ADULT and CHILD over 10 years, 10 mg repeated once if necessary; CHILD up to 6 months, 300 micrograms/kg (max. 2.5 mg); 6 months–1 year, 2.5 mg; 1–5 years, 5 mg; 5–10 years, 7.5 mg
  Note Midazolam injection solution may be given by buccal administration

Midazolam (Non-proprietary) CD
Buccal liquid, midazolam 10 mg/mL
'Special order' [unlicensed] product; brands include *Epistatus®*

Injection
Section 15.1.4

PARALDEHYDE

Indications status epilepticus
Cautions bronchopulmonary disease, hepatic impairment; pregnancy (Appendix 4) and breast-feeding (Appendix 5); **interactions**: Appendix 1 (paraldehyde)
Contra-indications gastric disorders; rectal administration in colitis
Side-effects rashes; rectal irritation after enema
Dose

- By rectum, ADULT and CHILD over 12 years, 20 mL; CHILD up to 3 months 0.5 mL, 3–6 months 1 mL, 6–12 months 1.5 mL, 1–2 years 2 mL, 3–5 years 3–4 mL, 6–12 years 5–10 mL
  Administration Administer as an enema containing 1 part paraldehyde diluted with 9 parts physiological saline (some centres mix paraldehyde with an equal volume of arachis (peanut) oil instead)
  Note Do not use paraldehyde if it has a brownish colour or an odour of acetic acid. Avoid contact with rubber and plastics.

Paraldehyde (Non-proprietary) PoM
Injection, sterile paraldehyde, net price 5-mL amp = £9.49

PHENOBARBITAL SODIUM
(Phenobarbitone sodium)

Indications status epilepticus; other forms of epilepsy except absence seizures (section 4.8.1)
Cautions see under Phenobarbital (section 4.8.1)
Side-effects see under Phenobarbital (section 4.8.1)

Dose

- Status epilepticus, by intravenous injection (dilute injection 1 in 10 with water for injections), 10 mg/kg at a rate of not more than 100 mg/minute; max. 1 g

Note For therapeutic purposes phenobarbital and phenobarbital sodium may be considered equivalent in effect

Phenobarbital (Non-proprietary) CD
Injection, phenobarbital sodium 200 mg/mL, net price 1-mL amp = £1.82
Excipients include propylene glycol 90% (see Excipients, p. 2)
Note Must be diluted before intravenous administration (see under Dose)

Oral preparations
Section 4.8.1

PHENYTOIN SODIUM

Indications status epilepticus; seizures in neurosurgery; arrhythmias, but now obsolete (section 2.3.2)

Cautions hypotension and heart failure; resuscitation facilities must be available; injection solutions alkaline (irritant to tissues); see also p. 250 ; **interactions**: see p. 244 and Appendix 1 (phenytoin)

Contra-indications sinus bradycardia, sino-atrial block, and second- and third-degree heart block; Stokes-Adams syndrome; porphyria (section 9.8.2)

Side-effects intravenous injection may cause cardiovascular and CNS depression (particularly if injection too rapid) with arrhythmias, hypotension, and cardiovascular collapse; alterations in respiratory function (including respiratory arrest); injection site reactions; see also p. 250

Dose

- By slow intravenous injection *or* infusion (with blood pressure and ECG monitoring), status epilepticus, 18 mg/kg at a rate not exceeding 50 mg per minute, as a loading dose (see also notes above); maintenance doses of about 100 mg should be given thereafter at intervals of every 6–8 hours, monitored by measurement of plasma concentrations; rate and dose reduced according to weight; CHILD 18 mg/kg as a loading dose (NEONATE 15–20 mg/kg at rate of 1–3 mg/kg/minute)

  Ventricular arrhythmias (but use now obsolete), by intravenous injection via caval catheter, 3.5–5 mg/kg at a rate not exceeding 50 mg/minute, with blood pressure and ECG monitoring; repeated once if necessary

  Note To avoid local venous irritation each injection or infusion should be preceded and followed by an injection of sterile physiological saline through the same needle or catheter
- By intramuscular injection, not recommended (see notes above)

Note Phenytoin sodium doses in BNF may differ from those in product literature

Phenytoin (Non-proprietary) PoM
Injection, phenytoin sodium 50 mg/mL with propylene glycol 40% and alcohol 10% in water for injections, net price 5-mL amp = £3.40

Epanutin® Ready-Mixed Parenteral (Pfizer) PoM
Injection, phenytoin sodium 50 mg/mL with propylene glycol 40% and alcohol 10% in water for injections, net price 5-mL amp = £4.88
Electrolytes 1.1 mmol Na^+ per 5 mL ampoule

Oral preparations
Section 4.8.1

4.8.3 Febrile convulsions

Brief febrile convulsions need only simple treatment such as antipyretic medication, e.g. **paracetamol** (section 4.7.1). *Prolonged febrile convulsions* (those lasting 15 minutes or longer), *recurrent convulsions*, or those occurring in a child at known risk must be treated more actively, as there is the possibility of resulting brain damage. **Diazepam** is the drug of choice given either by slow intravenous injection or preferably rectally in solution (section 4.8.2). The rectal route is preferred as satisfactory absorption is achieved within minutes and administration is much easier. Suppositories are not suitable because absorption is too slow.

Intermittent prophylaxis (i.e. the anticonvulsant administered at the onset of fever) is possible in only a small proportion of children. Again **diazepam** is the treatment of choice, orally or rectally.

Long-term anticonvulsant prophylaxis for febrile convulsions is rarely indicated. Anticonvulsant treatment needs to be considered only for a child at risk from prolonged or complex febrile convulsions, including those whose first seizure occurred at under 14 months or who have neurological abnormalities or who have had previous prolonged or focal convulsions.

4.9 Drugs used in parkinsonism and related disorders

4.9.1 Dopaminergic drugs used in parkinsonism
4.9.2 Antimuscarinic drugs used in parkinsonism
4.9.3 Drugs used in essential tremor, chorea, tics, and related disorders

In idiopathic Parkinson's disease, the progressive degeneration of pigmented neurones in the substantia nigra leads to a deficiency of the neurotransmitter dopamine. The resulting neurochemical imbalance in the basal ganglia causes the characteristic signs and symptoms of the illness. Drug therapy does not prevent disease progression, but it improves most patients' quality of life.

Patients with suspected Parkinson's disease should be referred to a specialist to confirm the diagnosis; the diagnosis should be reviewed every 6–12 months.

Features resembling those of Parkinson's disease can occur in diseases such as progressive supranuclear palsy and multiple system atrophy, but they do not normally show a sustained response to the drugs used in the treatment of idiopathic Parkinson's disease.

When initiating treatment, patients should be advised about its limitations and possible side-effects. About 5–10% of patients with Parkinson's disease respond poorly to treatment.

Treatment is usually not started until symptoms cause significant disruption of daily activities. Therapy with two or more antiparkinsonian drugs may be necessary as the disease progresses. Most patients eventually require **levodopa** and subsequently develop motor complications.

Antiparkinsonian drug therapy should never be stopped abruptly as this carries a small risk of neuroleptic malignant syndrome.

Elderly Antiparkinsonian drugs can cause confusion in the elderly. It is particularly important to initiate treatment with low doses and to increase the dose gradually.

4.9.1 Dopaminergic drugs used in parkinsonism

Dopamine receptor agonists

The dopamine receptor agonists, **bromocriptine**, **cabergoline**, **pergolide**, **pramipexole**, **ropinirole**, and **rotigotine** have a direct action on dopamine receptors. The treatment of new patients is often started with dopamine receptor agonists. They are also used with levodopa in more advanced disease. Rotigotine is licensed for use as monotherapy in early-stage Parkinson's disease.

When used alone, dopamine receptor agonists cause fewer motor complications in long-term treatment compared with levodopa treatment but the overall motor performance improves slightly less. The dopamine receptor agonists are associated with more neuropsychiatric side-effects than levodopa. The ergot-derived dopamine receptor agonists, bromocriptine, cabergoline, and pergolide, have been associated with fibrotic reactions (see notes below). In most cases, non-ergot-derived dopamine agonists are preferred over ergot-derived dopamine agonists.

Dopamine receptor agonists can cause excessive daytime sleepiness and sudden onset of sleep, see Sudden Onset of Sleep, p. 262.

Hypotensive reactions can occur in some patients taking dopamine agonists; these can be particularly problematic during the first few days of treatment and care should be exercised when driving or operating machinery.

Doses of dopamine receptor agonists should be increased slowly according to response and tolerability. Treatment with dopamine receptor agonists should not be withdrawn abruptly.

Fibrotic reactions

The CSM has advised that ergot-derived dopamine receptor agonists, bromocriptine, cabergoline, lisuride [discontinued], and pergolide, have been associated with pulmonary, retroperitoneal, and pericardial fibrotic reactions. Before starting treatment with these ergot derivatives it may be appropriate to measure the erythrocyte sedimentation rate and serum creatinine and to obtain a chest X-ray. Patients should be monitored for dyspnoea, persistent cough, chest pain, cardiac failure, and abdominal pain or tenderness. If long-term treatment is expected, then lung-function tests may also be helpful.

Apomorphine is a potent dopamine agonist that is sometimes helpful in advanced disease for patients experiencing unpredictable 'off' periods with levodopa treatment. Apomorphine is highly emetogenic; patients must receive domperidone for at least 2 days before starting treatment. Specialist supervision is advisable throughout apomorphine treatment.

APOMORPHINE HYDROCHLORIDE

Indications refractory motor fluctuations in Parkinson's disease ('off' episodes) inadequately controlled by levodopa with dopa-decarboxylase inhibitor or other dopaminergics (for capable and motivated patients under specialist supervision)

Cautions see notes above; pulmonary or cardiovascular disease, history of postural hypotension (special care on initiation); neuropsychiatric problems or dementia; hepatic, haemopoietic, renal, and cardiovascular monitoring; *on administration with levodopa* test initially and every 6 months for haemolytic anaemia (development calls for specialist haematological care with dose reduction and possible discontinuation); renal impairment; pregnancy; **interactions:** Appendix 1 (apomorphine)

Contra-indications respiratory depression, hypersensitivity to opioids; not suitable if 'on' response to levodopa marred by severe dyskinesia, hypotonia or psychiatric effects; hepatic impairment; breast-feeding; not for intravenous administration

Side-effects nausea, vomiting (see below under Dose); drowsiness (including sudden onset of sleep), confusion, hallucinations, injection-site reactions (including nodule formation and ulceration)—change injection sites in rotation; *less commonly* postural hypotension, breathing difficulties, dykinesias during 'on' periods (may require discontinuation), haemolytic anaemia with levodopa (see Cautions), and rash; *rarely* eosinophilia; pathological gambling, increased libido, and hypersexuality also reported

Dose

- By subcutaneous injection, usual range (after initiation as below) 3–30 mg daily in divided doses; subcutaneous infusion may be preferable in those requiring division of injections into more than 10 doses daily; max. single dose 10 mg; CHILD and ADOLESCENT under 18 years not recommended
- By continuous subcutaneous infusion (those requiring division into more than 10 injections daily) initially 1 mg/hour daily increased according to response (not more often than every 4 hours) in max. steps of 500 micrograms/hour, to usual rate of 1–4 mg/hour (14–60 micrograms/kg/hour); change infusion site every 12 hours and give during waking hours only (24-hour infusions not advised unless severe night-time symptoms)—intermittent bolus boosts also usually needed; CHILD and ADOLESCENT under 18 years not recommended

Note Total daily dose by either route (or combined routes) max. 100 mg

Requirements for initiation *Hospital admission* and at least 2 days of pretreatment with domperidone for nausea and vomiting, *after at least 3 days* withhold existing antiparkinsonian medication overnight to provoke 'off' episode, *determine* threshold dose, *re-establish* other antiparkinsonian drugs, *determine* effective apomorphine regimen, *teach* to administer by subcutaneous injection into lower abdomen or outer thigh at first sign of 'off' episode, *discharge* from hospital, *monitor* frequently and *adjust* dosage regimen as appropriate (domperidone may normally be withdrawn over several weeks or longer)—for full details of initiation requirements, consult product literature

APO-go® (Britannia) PoM

Injection, apomorphine hydrochloride 10 mg/mL, net price 2-mL amp = £7.59, 5-mL amp = £14.62

Excipients include sulphites

Injection (APO-go® Pen), apomorphine hydrochloride 10 mg/mL, net price 3-mL pen injector = £24.78

Excipients include sulphites

Injection (APO-go® PFS), apomorphine hydrochloride 5 mg/mL, net price 10-mL prefilled syringe = £14.62

Excipients include sulphites

BROMOCRIPTINE

Indications parkinsonism (but not drug-induced extrapyramidal symptoms); endocrine disorders (section 6.7.1)

Cautions see section 6.7.1 and notes above

Contra-indications section 6.7.1

Side-effects section 6.7.1

Dose

- First week 1–1.25 mg at night, second week 2–2.5 mg at night, third week 2.5 mg twice daily, fourth week 2.5 mg 3 times daily then increasing by 2.5 mg every 3–14 days according to response to a usual range of 10–40 mg daily; taken with food

Preparations

Section 6.7.1

CABERGOLINE

Indications alone or as adjunct to levodopa with dopa-decarboxylase inhibitor in Parkinson's disease where dopamine receptor agonists other than ergot derivative not appropriate; endocrine disorders (section 6.7.1)

Cautions see section 6.7.1 and notes above

Contra-indications section 6.7.1

Side-effects section 6.7.1

Dose

- Initially 1 mg daily, increased by increments of 0.5–1 mg at 7 or 14 day intervals; usual range 2–6 mg daily

Note Concurrent dose of levodopa may be decreased gradually while dose of cabergoline is increased

Cabergoline (Non-proprietary) PoM

Tablets, scored, cabergoline 1 mg, net price 20-tab pack = £53.20; 2 mg, 20-tab pack = £64.02; 4 mg, 16-tab pack = £65.72. Label: 21, counselling, hypotensive reactions, driving, see notes above

Note Dispense in original container (contains dessicant)

Cabaser® (Pharmacia) PoM

Tablets, scored, cabergoline 1 mg, net price 20-tab pack = £83.00; 2 mg, 20-tab pack = £83.00; 4 mg, 16-tab pack = £75.84. Label: 21, counselling, hypotensive reactions, driving, see notes above

Note Dispense in original container (contains desiccant)

PERGOLIDE

Indications alone or as adjunct to levodopa with dopa-decarboxylase inhibitor in Parkinson's disease where dopamine receptor agonists other than ergot derivative not appropriate

Cautions see notes above; arrhythmias or underlying cardiac disease; history of confusion, psychosis, or hallucinations, dyskinesia (may exacerbate); porphyria (section 9.8.2); pregnancy (Appendix 4); breast-feeding (Appendix 5); **interactions**: Appendix 1 (pergolide)

Contra-indications history of fibrotic disorders; cardiac valve disease

Side-effects see notes above; also nausea, vomiting, dyspepsia, abdominal pain; dyspnoea, rhinitis; hallucinations, dyskinesia, drowsiness (including sudden onset of sleep); diplopia; also reported constipation, diarrhoea, tachycardia, atrial premature contractions, palpitation, hypotension, syncope, Raynaud's phenomenon, cardiac valvulopathy, pericarditis, pericarditis, pericardial effusion, pleuritis, pleural effusion, pleural fibrosis, insomnia, confusion, dizziness, pathological gambling, neuroleptic malignant syndrome, fever, increased libido, hypersexuality, and rash

Dose

- Monotherapy, 50 micrograms at night on day 1, then 50 micrograms twice daily on days 2–4, then increased by 100–250 micrograms daily every 3–4 days (given in 3 divided doses) up to a daily dose of 1.5 mg at day 28; after day 30, further increases of up to 250 micrograms twice a week; usual maintenance dose approx. 2–2.5 mg daily; max. 5 mg daily
- Adjunctive therapy with levodopa, 50 micrograms daily for 2 days, increased gradually by 100–150 micrograms every 3 days over next 12 days, usually given in 3 divided doses; further increases of 250 micrograms every 3 days; usual maintenance dose 3 mg daily; max. 5 mg daily; during pergolide titration levodopa dose may be reduced cautiously

Pergolide (Non-proprietary) PoM

Tablets, pergolide (as mesilate) 50 micrograms, net price 100-tab pack = £12.34; 250 micrograms, 100-tab pack = £10.57; 1 mg, 100-tab pack = £26.68. Counselling, hypotensive reactions, driving, see notes above

Celance® (Lilly) PoM

Tablets, all scored, pergolide (as mesilate) 50 micrograms (ivory), net price 100-tab pack = £32.44; 250 micrograms (green), 100-tab pack = £48.92; 1 mg (pink), 100-tab pack = £176.58. Counselling, hypotensive reactions, driving, see notes above

PRAMIPEXOLE

Indications Parkinson's disease, used alone or as an adjunct to levodopa with dopa-decarboxylase inhibitor; moderate to severe restless legs syndrome

Cautions see notes above; psychotic disorders; ophthalmological testing recommended (risk of visual disorders); severe cardiovascular disease; renal impairment (Appendix 3); pregnancy (Appendix 4); **interactions**: Appendix 1 (pramipexole)

Contra-indications breast-feeding (Appendix 5)

Side-effects see notes above; also nausea, constipation; postural hypotension, hypotension, headache, confusion, drowsiness (including sudden onset of sleep), fatigue, insomnia, dizziness, hallucinations (mostly visual), dyskinesia, peripheral oedema; hyperkinesia, delusions, abnormal dreams, paradoxical worsening of restless legs syndrome, and behavioural changes including pathological gambling, binge eating, hypersexuality, and changes in libido also reported

Dose

Important Doses and strengths are stated in terms of pramipexole (base); equivalent strengths in terms of pramipexole dihydrochloride monohydrate (salt) are as follows:
88 micrograms base ≡ 125 micrograms salt;
180 micrograms base ≡ 250 micrograms salt;
700 micrograms base ≡ 1 mg salt

- Parkinson's disease, initially 88 micrograms 3 times daily, dose doubled every 5–7 days if tolerated to 350 micrograms 3 times daily; further increased if necessary by 180 micrograms 3 times daily at weekly intervals; max. 3.3 mg daily in 3 divided doses
  Note During pramipexole dose titration and maintenance, levodopa dose may be reduced
- Restless legs syndrome, initially 88 micrograms once daily 2–3 hours before bedtime, dose doubled every 4–7 days if necessary to 350 micrograms daily; max. 540 micrograms daily; CHILD and ADOLESCENT under 18 years not recommended

Mirapexin® (Boehringer Ingelheim) ▼ PoM
Tablets, pramipexole (as hydrochloride) 88 micrograms, net price 30-tab pack = £9.55; 180 micrograms (scored), 30-tab pack = £19.10, 100-tab pack = £63.67; 700 micrograms (scored), 30-tab pack = £76.40, 100-tab pack = £254.69. Counselling, hypotensive reactions, driving, see notes above

ROPINIROLE

Indications Parkinson's disease, either used alone or as an adjunct to levodopa with a dopa-decarboxylase inhibitor; moderate to severe restless legs syndrome

Cautions see notes above; severe cardiovascular disease, major psychotic disorders; hepatic impairment (Appendix 2); renal impairment (Appendix 3); **interactions**: Appendix 1 (ropinirole)

Contra-indications pregnancy (Appendix 4); breast-feeding (Appendix 5)

Side-effects see notes above; also nausea, vomiting, abdominal pain, dyspepsia; hypotension, syncope, leg oedema; drowsiness (including sudden onset of sleep), dizziness, nervousness, fatigue, dyskinesia, hallucinations, confusion; *less commonly* psychosis, pathological gambling, hypersexuality, and increased libido; *very rarely* hepatic disorders; *also reported* paradoxical worsening of restless legs syndrome

Dose

- See under preparations

Adartrel® (GSK) ▼ PoM
Tablets, f/c, ropinirole (as hydrochloride) 250 micrograms (white), net price 12-tab pack = £3.94; 500 micrograms (yellow), 28-tab pack = £15.75, 84-tab pack = £47.26; 2 mg (pink), 28-tab pack = £31.51, 84-tab pack = £94.53. Label: 21, counselling, driving, see notes above

Dose restless legs syndrome, initially 250 micrograms at night for 2 days, increased if tolerated to 500 micrograms at night for 5 days and then to 1 mg at night for 7 days; further increased at weekly intervals in steps of 500 micrograms daily according to response; usual dose 2 mg once daily at night; max. 4 mg once daily; CHILD under 18 years not recommended

Note Repeat dose titration if restarting after interval of more than a few days

The *Scottish Medicines Consortium* has advised (June 2006) that *Adartrel®* should be restricted for use in patients with a baseline score of 24 points or more on the International Restless Legs Scale

Requip® (GSK) PoM
Tablets, f/c, ropinirole (as hydrochloride) 1 mg (green), net price 84-tab pack = £47.26; 2 mg (pink), 84-tab pack = £94.53; 5 mg (blue), 84-tab pack = £163.27; 28-day starter pack of 42 × 250-microgram (white) tablets, 42 × 500-microgram (yellow) tablets, and 21 × 1-mg (green) tablets = £40.10; 28-day follow-on pack of 42 × 500-microgram (yellow) tablets, 42 × 1-mg (green) tablets, and 63 × 2-mg (pink) tablets = £74.40. Label: 21, counselling, driving, see notes above

Dose Parkinson's disease, initially 750 micrograms daily in 3 divided doses, increased by increments of 750 micrograms at weekly intervals to 3 mg daily; further increased by increments of up to 3 mg at weekly intervals according to response; usual range 9–16 mg daily (but higher doses may be required if used with levodopa); max. 24 mg daily

Note When administered as adjunct to levodopa, concurrent dose of levodopa may be reduced by approx. 20%; ropinirole doses in the BNF may differ from those in product literature

ROTIGOTINE

Indications Parkinson's disease, either used alone or as an adjunct to levodopa with dopa-decarboxylase inhibitor

Cautions see notes above; ophthalmic testing recommended; avoid exposure of patch to heat; hepatic impairment (Appendix 2); **interactions**: Appendix 1 (rotigotine)

Contra-indications pregnancy (Appendix 4); breast-feeding (Appendix 5); remove patch (aluminium-containing) before magnetic resonance imaging or cardioversion

Side-effects nausea, vomiting, constipation, dry mouth, diarrhoea, dyspepsia, weight changes; postural hypotension, peripheral oedema; confusion, drowsiness (including sudden onset of sleep), sleep disorders, dizziness, headache, dyskinesia, asthenia, hallucinations; hyperhydrosis, rash (including local reactions to patch), and pruritus; *less commonly* abdominal pain, anorexia, taste disturbance, palpitation, tachycardia, hypotension, hypertension, atrial fibrillation, syncope, dyspnoea, cough, hiccup, tremor, psychosis, pathological gambling, anxiety, impaired attention, dystonia, paraesthesia, impaired memory, erectile dysfunction, increased libido, arthralgia, and visual disturbances; *rarely* convulsions and loss of consciousness

Dose

- Monotherapy, apply '2 mg/24 hours' patch to dry, non-irritated skin on torso, thigh, or upper arm, removing after 24 hours and siting replacement patch on a different area (avoid using the same area for 14 days); increased in steps of 2 mg/24 hours at weekly intervals if required; max. 8 mg/24 hours
- Adjunctive therapy with levodopa, apply '4 mg/24 hours' patch to dry, non-irritated skin on torso, thigh, or upper arm, removing after 24 hours and siting replacement patch on a different area (avoid using the same site for 14 days); increased in steps of 2 mg/24 hours at weekly intervals if required; max. 16 mg/24 hours

Neupro® (UCB Pharma) ▼ PoM
Patches, self-adhesive, beige, rotigotine 2 mg/24 hours, net price 28 = £77.24; 4 mg/24 hours, 28 = £88.28; 6 mg/24 hours, 28 = £110.34; 8 mg/24 hours, 28 = £142.79; 28-day starter pack of 7 × 2 mg/24

hours, 7 × 4 mg/24 hours, 7 × 6 mg/24 hours, and 7 × 8 mg/24 hours patches = £110.34. Counselling, hypotensive reactions, driving, see notes above

Note The *Scottish Medicines Consortium* has advised that *Neupro®* is accepted as monotherapy for the treatment of early-stage idiopathic Parkinson's disease (June 2007) and for restricted use for the treatment of advanced Parkinson's disease in combination with levodopa where the transdermal route would facilitate treatment (July 2007)

Levodopa

Levodopa, the amino-acid precursor of dopamine, acts by replenishing depleted striatal dopamine; it is given with an extracerebral **dopa-decarboxylase inhibitor** that reduces the peripheral conversion of levodopa to dopamine, thereby limiting side-effects such as nausea, vomiting and cardiovascular effects. Additionally, effective brain-dopamine concentrations can be achieved with lower doses of levodopa. The extracerebral dopa-decarboxylase inhibitors used with levodopa are benserazide (in **co-beneldopa**) and carbidopa (in **co-careldopa**).

Levodopa, in combination with a dopa-decarboxylase inhibitor, is useful in the elderly or frail, in patients with other significant illnesses, and in those with more severe symptoms. It is effective and well tolerated in the majority of patients.

Levodopa therapy should be initiated at a low dose and increased in small steps; the final dose should be as low as possible. Intervals between doses should be chosen to suit the needs of the individual patient.

Note When co-careldopa is used, the total daily dose of carbidopa should be at least 70 mg. A lower dose may not achieve full inhibition of extracerebral dopa-decarboxylase, with a resultant increase in side-effects.

Nausea and vomiting with co-beneldopa or co-careldopa are rarely dose-limiting but domperidone (section 4.6) may be useful in controlling these effects.

Levodopa treatment is associated with the development of potentially troublesome motor complications including response fluctuations and dyskinesias. Response fluctuations are characterised by large variations in motor performance, with normal function during the 'on' period, and weakness and restricted mobility during the 'off' period. 'End-of-dose' deterioration also occurs, where the duration of benefit after each dose becomes progressively shorter. Modified-release preparations may help with 'end-of-dose' deterioration or nocturnal immobility and rigidity. Motor complications are particularly problematic in young patients treated with levodopa.

Cautions Levodopa should be used with caution in severe cardiovascular or pulmonary disease, psychiatric illness (avoid if severe), endocrine disorders (including hyperthyroidism, Cushing's syndrome, diabetes mellitus, osteomalacia, and phaeochromocytoma), and in those with a history of convulsions, malignant melanoma, or peptic ulcer. Levodopa should be used with caution in open-angle glaucoma and patients susceptibile to angle-closure glaucoma, and in hepatic or renal impairment. Patients should be advised to avoid abrupt withdrawal (risk of neuroleptic malignant syndrome and rhabdomyolysis), and to be aware of the potential for excessive drowsiness and sudden onset of sleep (see Sudden Onset of Sleep, below). Levodopa should be used with caution in pregnancy (Appendix 4); **interactions:** Appendix 1 (levodopa).

Contra-indications Levodopa should be avoided in breast-feeding (Appendix 5).

Side-effects Side-effects of levodopa include nausea, vomiting, taste disturbances, dry mouth, anorexia, arrhythmias, postural hypotension, syncope, drowsiness (including sudden onset of sleep), fatigue, dementia, psychoses, hallucinations, confusion, euphoria, abnormal dreams, insomnia, depression (very rarely with suicidal ideation), anxiety, dizziness, dystonia, dyskinesia, and chorea.

Less commonly weight loss or gain, constipation, diarrhoea, hypersalivation, dysphagia, flatulence, hypertension, chest pain, oedema, hoarseness, ataxia, increased hand tremor, malaise, muscle cramps, and reddish discoloration of the urine and other body fluids may occur. *Rare* side-effects include abdominal pain, gastro-intestinal bleeding, dyspepsia, phlebitis, dyspnoea, agitation, paraesthesia, bruxism, trismus, hiccups, neuroleptic malignant syndrome (associated with abrupt withdrawal), convulsions, reduced mental acuity, disorientation, headache, urinary retention, urinary incontinence, priapism, activation of malignant melanoma, leucopenia, haemolytic and non-haemolytic anaemia, thrombocytopenia, agranulocytosis, blurred vision, blepharopasm, diplopia, activation of Horner's syndrome, pupil dilatation, oculogyric crisis, angioedema, rash, urticaria, pruritus, flushing, alopecia, exanthema, Henoch-Schönlein purpura, and increased sweating. *Very rarely* angle-closure glaucoma may occur; pathological gambling, increased libido, hypersexuality, and false positive tests for urinary ketones have also been reported.

> **Sudden onset of sleep**
> Excessive daytime sleepiness and sudden onset of sleep can occur with co-careldopa, co-beneldopa, and dopamine receptor agonists.
> Patients starting treatment with these drugs should be warned of the possibility of these effects and of the need to exercise caution when driving or operating machinery.
> Patients who have suffered excessive sedation or sudden onset of sleep, should refrain from driving or operating machines until those effects have stopped recurring.

CO-BENELDOPA

A mixture of benserazide hydrochloride and levodopa in mass proportions corresponding to 1 part of benserazide and 4 parts of levodopa

Indications parkinsonism (but not drug-induced extrapyramidal symptoms), see notes above
Cautions see notes above
Contra-indications see notes above
Side-effects see notes above
Dose

- See preparations

Madopar® (Roche) PoM
Capsules 62.5, blue/grey, co-beneldopa 12.5/50 (benserazide 12.5 mg (as hydrochloride), levodopa 50 mg). Net price 100-cap pack = £6.20. Label: 14, counselling, driving, see notes above

4 Central nervous system

Capsules 125, blue/pink, co-beneldopa 25/100 (benserazide 25 mg (as hydrochloride), levodopa 100 mg). Net price 100-cap pack = £8.64. Label: 14, counselling, driving, see notes above

Capsules 250, blue/caramel, co-beneldopa 50/200 (benserazide 50 mg (as hydrochloride), levodopa 200 mg). Net price 100-cap pack = £14.73. Label: 14, counselling, driving, see notes above

Dispersible tablets 62.5, scored, co-beneldopa 12.5/50 (benserazide 12.5 mg (as hydrochloride), levodopa 50 mg). Net price 100-tab pack = £7.37. Label: 14, counselling, administration, see below, driving, see notes above

Dispersible tablets 125, scored, co-beneldopa 25/100 (benserazide 25 mg (as hydrochloride) levodopa 100 mg). Net price 100-tab pack = £13.06. Label: 14, counselling, administration, see below, driving, see notes above

Note The tablets can be dispersed in water or orange squash (not orange juice) or swallowed whole

Dose expressed as levodopa, initially 50 mg 3–4 times daily (100 mg 3 times daily in advanced disease), increased by 100 mg daily once or twice weekly according to response; usual maintenance dose 400–800 mg daily in divided doses; ELDERLY initially 50 mg once or twice daily, increased by 50 mg daily every 3–4 days according to response

Note When transferring patients from another levodopa/dopa-decarboxylase inhibitor preparation, the previous preparation should be discontinued 12 hours before (although interval can be shorter)

Modified release

Madopar® CR (Roche) PoM

Capsules 125, m/r, dark green/light blue, co-beneldopa 25/100 (benserazide 25 mg (as hydrochloride), levodopa 100 mg). Net price 100-cap pack = £15.96. Label: 5, 14, 25, counselling, driving, see notes above

Dose Patients not taking levodopa/dopa-decarboxylase inhibitor therapy, initially 1 capsule 3 times daily (max. initial dose 6 capsules daily)

Patients transferring from immediate-release levodopa/dopa-decarboxylase inhibitor preparations, initially 1 capsule substituted for every 100 mg of levodopa and given at same dosage frequency, increased every 2–3 days according to response; average increase of 50% needed over previous levodopa dose and titration may take up to 4 weeks

Supplementary dose of immediate-release *Madopar®* may be needed with first morning dose; if response still poor to total daily dose of *Madopar® CR* plus *Madopar®* corresponding to 1.2 g levodopa, consider alternative therapy

CO-CARELDOPA

A mixture of carbidopa and levodopa; the proportions are expressed in the form *x/y* where *x* and *y* are the strengths in milligrams of carbidopa and levodopa respectively

Indications parkinsonism (but not drug-induced extrapyramidal symptoms), see notes above

Cautions see notes above

Contra-indications see notes above

Side-effects see notes above

Dose

- See preparations

Note At least 70 mg carbidopa daily is necessary to achieve full inhibition of peripheral dopa-decarboxylase

Sinemet® (Bristol-Myers Squibb) PoM

Sinemet-62.5 tablets, yellow, scored, co-careldopa 12.5/50 (carbidopa 12.5 mg (as monohydrate), levodopa 50 mg), net price 90-tab pack = £6.54. Label: 14, counselling, driving, see notes above

Note 2 tablets *Sinemet-62.5®* ≡ 1 tablet *Sinemet Plus®*

Sinemet-110 tablets, blue, scored, co-careldopa 10/100 (carbidopa 10 mg (as monohydrate), levodopa 100 mg), net price 90-tab pack = £6.84. Label: 14, counselling, driving, see notes above

Sinemet-Plus tablets, yellow, scored, co-careldopa 25/100 (carbidopa 25 mg (as monohydrate), levodopa 100 mg), net price 90-tab pack = £10.05. Label: 14, counselling, driving, see notes above

Note Co-careldopa 25/100 provides an adequate dose of carbidopa when low doses of levodopa are needed

Sinemet-275 tablets, blue, scored, co-careldopa 25/250 (carbidopa 25 mg (as monohydrate), levodopa 250 mg), net price 90-tab pack = £14.28. Label: 14, counselling, driving, see notes above

Dose Expressed as levodopa, initially 100 mg (with carbidopa 25 mg, as *Sinemet-Plus®*) 3 times daily, increased by 50–100 mg (with carbidopa 12.5–25 mg, as *Sinemet-62.5®* or *Sinemet-Plus®*) daily or on alternate days according to response, up to 800 mg (with carbidopa 200 mg) daily in divided doses

Alternatively, initially 50–100 mg (with carbidopa 10–12.5 mg, as *Sinemet-62.5®* or *Sinemet-110®*) 3–4 times daily, increased by 50–100 mg daily or on alternate days according to response, up to 800 mg (with carbidopa 80–100 mg) daily in divided doses

Alternatively, initially 125 mg (with carbidopa 12.5 mg, as ½ tablet of *Sinemet-275®*) 1–2 times daily, increased by 125 mg (with carbidopa 12.5 mg) daily or on alternate days according to response

Note When transferring patients from another levodopa/dopa-decarboxylase inhibitor preparation, the previous preparation should be discontinued at least 12 hours before

For use with enteral tube

Duodopa® (Solvay) ▼ PoM

Intestinal gel, co-careldopa 5/20 (carbidopa 5mg as monohydrate, levodopa 20mg)/mL, net price 100 mL cassette (for use with *Duodopa®* portable pump) = £77.00. Label: 14, counselling, driving, see notes above

Dose Severe Parkinson's disease inadequately controlled by other preparations, consult product literature

Modified release

Caramet® CR (Teva) PoM

Tablets, m/r, orange-brown, co-careldopa 25/100 (carbidopa 25 mg (as monohydrate), levodopa 100 mg), net price 60-tab pack = £11.47; co-careldopa 50/200 (carbidopa 50 mg (as monohydrate), levodopa 200 mg), 60-tab pack = £11.47. Label: 14, 25, counselling, driving, see notes above

Dose patients not receiving levodopa/dopa-decarboxylase inhibitor preparations, expressed as levodopa, initially 100–200 mg twice daily (at least 6 hours between doses); dose adjusted according to response at intervals of at least 2 days

Patients transferring from immediate-release levodopa/dopa-decarboxylase inhibitor preparations, discontinue previous preparation at least 12 hours before first dose of *Caramet® CR*; substitute *Caramet® CR* to provide a similar amount of levodopa daily and extend dosing interval by 30–50%; dose then adjusted according to response at intervals of at least 2 days

Half Sinemet® CR (Bristol-Myers Squibb) PoM

Tablets, m/r, pink, co-careldopa 25/100 (carbidopa 25 mg (as monohydrate), levodopa 100 mg), net price 60-tab pack = £12.07. Label: 14, 25, counselling, driving, see notes above

Dose For fine adjustment of *Sinemet® CR* dose (see below)

Sinemet® CR (Bristol-Myers Squibb) PoM

Tablets, m/r, peach, scored, co-careldopa 50/200 (carbidopa 50 mg (as monohydrate), levodopa 200 mg), net price 60-tab pack = £12.07. Label: 14, 25, counselling, driving, see notes above

Dose Patients not receiving levodopa/dopa-decarboxylase inhibitor therapy, initially, 1 *Sinemet® CR* tablet twice daily; both dose and interval then adjusted according to response at intervals of not less than 3 days

Patients transferring from immediate-release levodopa/dopa-decarboxylase inhibitor preparations, 1 *Sinemet*® *CR* tablet twice daily can be substituted for a daily dose of levodopa 300–400 mg in immediate-release *Sinemet*® tablets (substitute *Sinemet*® *CR* to provide approx. 10% more levodopa per day and extend dosing interval by 30–50%); dose and interval then adjusted according to response at intervals of not less than 3 days

With entacapone

Note For Parkinson's disease and end-of-dose motor fluctuations not adequately controlled with levodopa and dopa-decarboxylase inhibitor treatment

Stalevo® (Orion) ▼ PoM

Stalevo 50 mg/12.5 mg/200 mg tablets, f/c, brown, levodopa 50 mg, carbidopa 12.5 mg, entacapone 200 mg, net price 30-tab pack = £21.72, 100-tab pack = £72.40. Label: 14 (urine reddish-brown), 25, counselling, driving, see notes above, avoid iron-containing preparations at the same time of day

Stalevo 100 mg/25 mg/200 mg tablets, f/c, brown, levodopa 100 mg, carbidopa 25 mg, entacapone 200 mg, net price 30-tab pack = £21.72, 100-tab pack = £72.40. Label: 14 (urine reddish-brown), 25, counselling, driving, see notes above, avoid iron-containing preparations at the same time of day

Stalevo 150 mg/37.5 mg/200 mg tablets, f/c, brown, levodopa 150 mg, carbidopa 37.5 mg, entacapone 200 mg, net price 30-tab pack = £21.72, 100-tab pack = £72.40. Label: 14 (urine reddish-brown), 25, counselling, driving, see notes above, avoid iron-containing preparations at the same time of day

Dose only 1 tablet of *Stalevo*® to be taken for each dose; max. 10 tablets daily

Patients receiving standard-release co-careldopa or co-beneldopa alone, initiate *Stalevo*® at a dose that provides similar (or slightly lower) amount of levodopa

Patients with dyskinesia or receiving more than 800 mg levodopa daily, introduce entacapone before transferring to *Stalevo*® (levodopa dose may need to be reduced by 10–30% initially)

Patients receiving entacapone and standard-release co-careldopa or co-beneldopa, initiate *Stalevo*® at a dose that provides similar (or slightly higher) amount of levodopa

Monoamine-oxidase-B inhibitors

Rasagiline, a monoamine-oxidase-B inhibitor, is licensed for the management of Parkinson's disease used alone or as an adjunct to levodopa for 'end-of-dose' fluctuations.

Selegiline is a monoamine-oxidase-B inhibitor used in conjunction with levodopa to reduce 'end-of-dose' deterioration in advanced Parkinson's disease. Early treatment with selegiline alone can delay the need for levodopa therapy. When combined with levodopa, selegiline should be avoided or used with great caution in postural hypotension.

RASAGILINE

Indications Parkinson's disease, used alone or as adjunct to levodopa with dopa-decarboxylase inhibitor

Cautions avoid abrupt withdrawal; hepatic impairment (Appendix 2); pregnancy (Appendix 4); breast-feeding (Appendix 5); **interactions**: Appendix 1 (rasagiline)

Side-effects dry mouth, dyspepsia, constipation; angina; headache, depression, anorexia, weight loss, abnormal dreams, vertigo, hallucinations; influenza-like symptoms; urinary urgency; leucopenia; arthralgia; conjunctivitis; rash; *less commonly* myocardial infarction, and cerebrovascular accident

Dose

- 1 mg daily

Azilect® (Teva) PoM

Tablets, rasagiline (as mesilate) 1 mg, net price 28-tab pack = £70.72

SELEGILINE HYDROCHLORIDE

Indications Parkinson's disease, used alone or as adjunct to levodopa with dopa-decarboxylase inhibitor

Cautions avoid abrupt withdrawal; gastric and duodenal ulceration (avoid in active ulceration), uncontrolled hypertension, arrhythmias, angina, psychosis, side-effects of levodopa may be increased, concurrent levodopa dosage can be reduced by 10–20%; **interactions**: Appendix 1 (selegiline)

Contra-indications pregnancy (Appendix 4); breast-feeding (Appendix 5)

Side-effects nausea, constipation, diarrhoea, dry mouth; postural hypotension; dyskinesia, vertigo, sleeping disorders, confusion, hallucinations; arthralgia, myalgia; mouth ulcers with oral lyophilisate; *rarely* arrhythmias, agitation, headache, micturition difficulties, skin reactions; also reported chest pain

Dose

- 10 mg in the morning, or 5 mg at breakfast and mid-day; ELDERLY see below

Elderly To avoid initial confusion and agitation, it may be appropriate to start treatment with a dose of 2.5 mg daily, particularly in the elderly

Selegiline Hydrochloride (Non-proprietary) PoM

Tablets, selegiline hydrochloride 5 mg, net price 56-tab pack = £4.99; 10 mg, 30-tab pack = £11.08

Eldepryl® (Orion) PoM

Tablets, both scored, selegiline hydrochloride 5 mg, net price 60-tab pack = £10.35; 10 mg, 30-tab pack = £10.10

Oral liquid, selegiline hydrochloride 10 mg/5 mL, net price 200 mL = £18.72

Oral lyophilisate

Zelapar® (Zeneus) PoM

Oral lyophilisates (= freeze-dried tablets), yellow, selegiline hydrochloride 1.25 mg, net price 30-tab pack = £59.95. Counselling, administration

Excipients include aspartame (section 9.4.1)

Dose initially 1.25 mg daily before breakfast

Counselling Tablets should be placed on the tongue and allowed to dissolve. Advise patient not to drink, rinse, or wash mouth out for 5 minutes after taking the tablet

Note Patients receiving 10 mg conventional selegiline hydrochloride tablets can be switched to *Zelapar*® 1.25 mg

Catechol-*O*-methyltransferase inhibitors

Entacapone and **tolcapone** prevent the peripheral breakdown of levodopa, by inhibiting catechol-*O*-methyltransferase, allowing more levodopa to reach the brain. They are licensed for use as an adjunct to co-beneldopa or co-careldopa for patients with Parkinson's disease who experience 'end-of-dose' deterioration and cannot be stabilised on these combinations. Due to the risk of hepatotoxicity, tolcapone should be prescribed under specialist supervision only, when other catechol-*O*-methyltransferase inhibitors combined with co-beneldopa or co-careldopa are ineffective.

ENTACAPONE

Indications adjunct to levodopa with dopa-decarboxylase inhibitor in Parkinson's disease and 'end-of-dose' motor fluctuations

Cautions avoid abrupt withdrawal; concurrent levodopa dose may need to be reduced by about 10–30%; **interactions:** Appendix 1 (entacapone)

Contra-indications pregnancy (Appendix 4); breast-feeding (Appendix 5); hepatic impairment; phaeochromocytoma; history of neuroleptic malignant syndrome or non-traumatic rhabdomyolysis

Side-effects nausea, vomiting, abdominal pain, constipation, diarrhoea, urine may be coloured reddish-brown, dry mouth; confusion, dizziness, abnormal dreams, fatigue, insomnia, dystonia, dyskinesia, hallucinations; increased sweating; *rarely* hepatic dysfunction and rash; *very rarely* anorexia, weight loss, agitation, and urticaria; also reported colitis, neuroleptic malignant syndrome, rhabdomyolysis, and skin, hair, and nail discoloration

Dose

- 200 mg with each dose of levodopa with dopa-decarboxylase inhibitor; max. 2 g daily

Comtess® (Orion) PoM
Tablets, f/c, brown/orange, entacapone 200 mg, net price 30-tab pack = £18.00, 100-tab pack = £60.00. Label: 14, (urine reddish-brown), counselling, driving, see notes above, avoid iron-containing products at the same time of day

TOLCAPONE

Indications adjunct to levodopa with dopa-decarboxylase inhibitor in Parkinson's disease and 'end-of-dose' motor fluctuations if another inhibitor of peripheral catechol-*O*-methyltransferase inappropriate (under specialist supervision)

Cautions avoid abrupt withdrawal; most patients receiving more than 600 mg levodopa daily require reduction of levodopa dose by about 30%; renal impairment (Appendix 3); pregnancy (Appendix 4); **interactions:** Appendix 1 (tolcapone)

Hepatotoxicity Potentially life-threatening hepatotoxicity including fulminant hepatitis reported rarely, usually in females and during the first 6 months, but late-onset liver injury has also been reported; test liver function before treatment, and monitor every 2 weeks for first year, every 4 weeks for next 6 months and every 8 weeks thereafter (restart monitoring schedule if dose increased); discontinue if abnormal liver function tests or symptoms of liver disorder (counselling, see below); do not re-introduce tolcapone once discontinued

Counselling Patients should be told how to recognise signs of liver disorder and advised to seek immediate medical attention if symptoms such as anorexia, nausea, vomiting, fatigue, abdominal pain, dark urine, or pruritus develop

Contra-indications hepatic impairment or raised liver enzymes (see Hepatotoxicity above), severe dyskinesia, phaeochromocytoma, previous history of neuroleptic malignant syndrome, rhabdomyolysis, or hyperthermia; breast-feeding (Appendix 5)

Side-effects diarrhoea, constipation, dyspepsia, abdominal pain, nausea, vomiting, anorexia, xerostomia, hepatotoxicity (see above); chest pain; confusion, dystonia, dyskinesia, drowsiness, headache, dizziness, sleep disturbances, excessive dreaming, hallucinations; syncope; urine discoloration; sweating; neuroleptic malignant syndrome and rhabdomyolysis reported on dose reduction or withdrawal

Dose

- 100 mg 3 times daily, leave 6 hours between each dose; max. 200 mg 3 times daily in exceptional circumstances; first daily dose should be taken at the same time as levodopa with dopa-decarboxylase inhibitor

Note Continue beyond 3 weeks **only** if substantial improvement

Tasmar® (Valeant) ▼ PoM
Tablets, f/c, yellow, tolcapone 100 mg, net price 100-tab pack = £95.20. Label: 14, 25

Amantadine

Amantadine is a weak dopamine agonist with modest antiparkinsonian effects. It improves mild bradykinetic disabilities as well as tremor and rigidity. It may also be useful for dyskinesias in more advanced disease. Tolerance to its effects may develop and confusion and hallucinations may occasionally occur. Withdrawal of amantadine should be gradual irrespective of the patient's response to treatment.

AMANTADINE HYDROCHLORIDE

Indications Parkinson's disease (but not drug-induced extrapyramidal symptoms); antiviral (section 5.3.4)

Cautions hepatic impairment; renal impairment (avoid if creatinine clearance less than 15 mL/minute; Appendix 3), congestive heart disease (may exacerbate oedema), confused or hallucinatory states, elderly; avoid abrupt withdrawal in Parkinson's disease; **interactions:** Appendix 1 (amantadine)

Driving May affect performance of skilled tasks (e.g. driving)

Contra-indications epilepsy; history of gastric ulceration; pregnancy (Appendix 4), breast-feeding (Appendix 5)

Side-effects anorexia, nausea, nervousness, inability to concentrate, insomnia, dizziness, convulsions, hallucinations or feelings of detachment, blurred vision, gastro-intestinal disturbances, livedo reticularis and peripheral oedema; rarely leucopenia, rashes

Dose

- Parkinson's disease, 100 mg daily increased after one week to 100 mg twice daily, usually in conjunction with other treatment; some patients may require higher doses, max. 400 mg daily; ELDERLY 65 years and over, 100 mg daily adjusted according to response
- Post-herpetic neuralgia, 100 mg twice daily for 14 days, continued for a further 14 days if necessary

Symmetrel® (Alliance) PoM
Capsules, red-brown, amantadine hydrochloride 100 mg. Net price 56-cap pack = £16.88. Counselling, driving

Syrup, amantadine hydrochloride 50 mg/5 mL. Net price 150-mL pack = £5.55. Counselling, driving

Lysovir® (Alliance) PoM
See p. 342

4.9.2 Antimuscarinic drugs used in parkinsonism

Antimuscarinic drugs exert their antiparkinsonian action by reducing the effects of the relative central cholinergic excess that occurs as a result of dopamine deficiency. Antimuscarinic drugs can be useful in drug-induced parkinsonism, but they are generally not used in idiopathic Parkinson's disease because they are less effective than dopaminergic drugs and they are associated with cognitive impairment.

The antimuscarinic drugs, **benzatropine**, **orphenadrine**, **procyclidine**, and **trihexyphenidyl** (benzhexol), reduce the symptoms of parkinsonism induced by antipsychotic drugs, but there is no justification for giving them routinely in the absence of parkinsonian side-effects. Tardive dyskinesia is not improved by antimuscarinic drugs and may be made worse.

In idiopathic Parkinson's disease, antimuscarinic drugs reduce tremor and rigidity but they have little effect on bradykinesia. They may be useful in reducing sialorrhoea.

No important differences exist between the antimuscarinic drugs, but some patients tolerate one better than another.

Benzatropine may be given parenterally and it is effective emergency treatment for acute drug-induced dystonic reactions.

Cautions Antimuscarinics should be used with caution in cardiovascular disease, hypertension, psychotic disorders, prostatic hypertrophy, pyrexia, in those susceptible to angle-closure glaucoma, and in the elderly. Antimuscarinics should not be withdrawn abruptly in patients receiving long-term treatment. Antimuscarinics are liable to abuse. They should also be used with caution in hepatic impairment, renal impairment, pregnancy (Appendix 4), and breast-feeding (Appendix 5). **Interactions:** Appendix 1 (Antimuscarinics)

Driving May affect performance of skilled tasks (e.g. driving)

Contra-indications Antimuscarinics should be avoided in gastro-intestinal obstruction and myasthenia gravis.

Side-effects Side-effects of antimuscarinics include constipation, dry mouth, nausea, vomiting, tachycardia, dizziness, confusion, euphoria, hallucinations, impaired memory, anxiety, restlessness, urinary retention, blurred vision, and rash. Angle-closure glaucoma may occur very rarely

BENZATROPINE MESILATE
(Benztropine mesylate)

Indications acute dystonic reactions; drug-induced extrapyramidal symptoms (but not tardive dyskinesia, see notes above)

Cautions see notes above

Contra-indications see notes above; avoid in children under 3 years

Side-effects see notes above, but causes sedation rather than stimulation; also reported depression and hyperthermia

Dose

- By intramuscular *or* intravenous injection, 1–2 mg, repeated if symptoms reappear; max. 6 mg daily; ELDERLY preferably lower end of range

Benzatropine Mesilate (Non-proprietary) PoM

Injection, benzatropine mesilate 1 mg/mL, net price 2-mL amp = £4.46

Available on a named-patient basis from specialist importing companies, see p. 888

ORPHENADRINE HYDROCHLORIDE

Indications parkinsonism; drug-induced extrapyramidal symptoms (but not tardive dyskinesia, see notes above)

Cautions see notes above

Contra-indications see notes above; also porphyria (section 9.8.2)

Side-effects see notes above; *less commonly* insomnia and impaired coordination

Dose

- Initially 150 mg daily in divided doses, increased gradually in steps of 50 mg every 2–3 days according to response; usual dose range 150–300 mg daily in divided doses; max. 400 mg daily; ELDERLY preferably lower end of range

Orphenadrine Hydrochloride (Non-proprietary) PoM

Tablets, orphenadrine hydrochloride 50 mg, net price 20 = £9.51. Counselling, driving

Oral solution, orphenadrine hydrochloride 50 mg/5 mL, net price 200 mL = £9.47. Counselling, driving

Biorphen® (Alliance) PoM

Elixir, sugar-free, orphenadrine hydrochloride 25 mg/5 mL, net price 200 mL = £7.07. Counselling, driving

Disipal® (Astellas) PoM

Tablets, yellow, s/c, orphenadrine hydrochloride 50 mg, net price 20 = 69p. Counselling, driving

Excipients include tartrazine

PROCYCLIDINE HYDROCHLORIDE

Indications parkinsonism; drug-induced extrapyramidal symptoms (but not tardive dyskinesia, see notes above)

Cautions see notes above

Contra-indications see notes above

Side-effects see notes above, but causes sedation rather than stimulation; also gingivitis

Dose

- By mouth, 2.5 mg 3 times daily, increased gradually in steps of 2.5–5 mg daily every 2–3 days if necessary; usual max. 30 mg daily in 2–4 divided doses (60 mg daily in exceptional circumstances); ELDERLY preferably lower end of range
- By intramuscular *or* intravenous injection, acute dystonia, 5–10 mg (occasionally more than 10 mg), usually effective in 5–10 minutes but may need 30 minutes for relief; ELDERLY preferably lower end of range

Procyclidine (Non-proprietary) PoM
Tablets, procyclidine hydrochloride 5 mg, net price 28-tab pack = £2.57. Counselling, driving

Arpicolin® (Rosemont) PoM
Syrup, sugar-free, procyclidine hydrochloride 2.5 mg/5 mL, net price 150 mL = £4.22; 5 mg/5 mL, 150 mL pack = £7.54. Counselling, driving

Kemadrin® (GSK) PoM
Tablets, scored, procyclidine hydrochloride 5 mg, net price 20 = 94p. Counselling, driving

Kemadrin® (Auden Mckenzie) PoM
Injection, procyclidine hydrochloride 5 mg/mL, net price 2-mL amp = £1.49

TRIHEXYPHENIDYL HYDROCHLORIDE
(Benzhexol hydrochloride)

Indications parkinsonism; drug-induced extrapyramidal symptoms (but not tardive dyskinesia, see notes above)
Cautions see notes above
Contra-indications see notes above
Side-effects see notes above
Dose
- 1 mg daily, increased gradually; usual maintenance dose 5–15 mg daily in 3–4 divided doses (max. 20 mg daily); ELDERLY preferably lower end of range

Trihexyphenidyl (Non-proprietary) PoM
Tablets, trihexyphenidyl hydrochloride 2 mg, net price 84-tab pack = £9.45; 5 mg, 100-tab pack = £7.40. Counselling, with or after food, driving

Broflex® (Alliance) PoM
Syrup, pink, black currant, trihexyphenidyl hydrochloride 5 mg/5 mL, net price 200 mL = £6.20. Counselling, driving

4.9.3 Drugs used in essential tremor, chorea, tics, and related disorders

Tetrabenazine is mainly used to control movement disorders in Huntington's chorea and related disorders. It may act by depleting nerve endings of dopamine. It has useful action in only a proportion of patients and its use may be limited by the development of depression.

Haloperidol may be useful in improving motor tics and symptoms of Tourette syndrome and related choreas. **Pimozide** [unlicensed indication] (see section 4.2.1 for CSM warning), **clonidine** [unlicensed indication] (section 4.7.4.2), and **sulpiride** [unlicensed indication] (section 4.2.1) are also used in Tourette syndrome. **Trihexyphenidyl (benzhexol)** (section 4.9.2) in high dosage can also improve some movement disorders; it is sometimes necessary to build the dose up over many weeks, to 20 to 30 mg daily or higher. **Chlorpromazine** and **haloperidol** are used to relieve intractable hiccup (section 4.2.1).

Propranolol or another beta-adrenoceptor blocking drug (section 2.4) may be useful in treating essential tremor or tremors associated with anxiety or thyrotoxicosis. Propranolol is given in a dosage of 40 mg 2 or 3 times daily, increased if necessary; 80 to 160 mg daily is usually required for maintenance.

Primidone (section 4.8.1) in some cases provides relief from benign essential tremor; the dose is increased slowly to reduce side-effects.

Piracetam is used as an adjunctive treatment for myoclonus of cortical origin.

Riluzole is used to extend life or the time to mechanical ventilation in patients with motor neurone disease who have amyotrophic lateral sclerosis.

> **NICE guidance**
> **Riluzole for motor neurone disease (January 2001)**
> Riluzole is recommended for treating the amyotrophic lateral sclerosis (ALS) form of motor neurone disease (MND). Treatment should be initiated by a specialist in MND but it can then be supervised under a shared-care arrangement involving the general practitioner.

HALOPERIDOL

Indications motor tics, adjunctive treatment in choreas and Tourette syndrome; other indications, section 4.2.1
Cautions section 4.2.1
Contra-indications section 4.2.1
Side-effects section 4.2.1
Dose
- By mouth, 0.5–1.5 mg 3 times daily adjusted according to the response; 10 mg daily or more may occasionally be necessary in Tourette syndrome; CHILD Tourette syndrome, up to 10 mg daily

Preparations
Section 4.2.1

PIRACETAM

Indications adjunctive treatment of cortical myoclonus
Cautions avoid abrupt withdrawal; elderly; haemostasis, major surgery, or severe haemorrhage; renal impairment (avoid if creatinine clearance less than 20 mL/minute; Appendix 3)
Contra-indications cerebral haemorrhage; hepatic impairment; pregnancy; breast-feeding
Side-effects weight gain, nervousness, hyperkinesia; *less commonly* drowsiness, depression, asthenia,; *also reported* abdominal pain, nausea, vomiting, diarrhoea, headache, anxiety, confusion, hallucination, vertigo, ataxia, insomnia, and rash

Dose

- Initially 7.2 g daily in 2–3 divided doses, increased according to response by 4.8 g daily every 3–4 days to max. 20 g daily (subsequently, attempts should be made to reduce dose of concurrent therapy); CHILD under 16 years not recommended

Oral solution Follow the oral solution with a glass of water (or soft drink) to reduce bitter taste.

Nootropil® (UCB Pharma) PoM
Tablets, f/c, scored, piracetam 800 mg, net price 90-tab pack = £14.69; 1.2 g, 60-tab pack = £13.71. Label: 3
Oral solution, piracetam, 333.3 mg/mL, net price 300-mL pack = £20.39. Label: 3

RILUZOLE

Indications to extend life or the time to mechanical ventilation for patients with amyotrophic lateral sclerosis, initiated by specialists experienced in the management of motor neurone disease

Cautions history of abnormal hepatic function (consult product literature for details)

Blood disorders Patients or their carers should be told how to recognise signs of neutropenia and advised to seek immediate medical attention if symptoms such as fever occur; white blood cell counts should be determined in febrile illness; neutropenia requires discontinuation of riluzole

Driving Dizziness or vertigo may affect performance of skilled tasks (e.g. driving)

Contra-indications hepatic impairment; renal impairment (Appendix 3); pregnancy (Appendix 4); breast-feeding (Appendix 5)

Side-effects nausea, vomiting, diarrhoea, abdominal pain; tachycardia; asthenia, headache, dizziness, drowsiness, oral paraesthesia; *less commonly* pancreatitis and anaemia; *rarely* neutropenia; *very rarely* hepatitis

Dose

- 50 mg twice daily; CHILD not recommended

Rilutek® (Aventis Pharma) PoM
Tablets, f/c, riluzole 50 mg. Net price 56-tab pack = £242.39. Counselling, blood disorders, driving

TETRABENAZINE

Indications see under Dose

Cautions pregnancy (Appendix 4); avoid in breast-feeding; **interactions**: Appendix 1 (tetrabenazine)

Driving May affect performance of skilled tasks (e.g. driving)

Side-effects drowsiness, gastro-intestinal disturbances, depression, extrapyramidal dysfunction, hypotension; rarely parkinsonism; neuroleptic malignant syndrome reported

Dose

- Movement disorders due to Huntington's chorea, hemiballismus, senile chorea, and related neurological conditions, initially 12.5 mg twice daily (elderly 12.5 mg daily) gradually increased to 12.5–25 mg 3 times daily; max. 200 mg daily
- Moderate to severe tardive dyskinesia, initially 12.5 mg daily, gradually increased according to response

Xenazine® 25 (Cambridge) PoM
Tablets, yellow, scored, tetrabenazine 25 mg. Net price 112-tab pack = £100.00. Label: 2

Torsion dystonias and other involuntary movements

BOTULINUM TOXIN TYPE A

Indications focal spasticity, including arm symptoms in conjunction with physiotherapy, dynamic equinus foot deformity caused by spasticity in ambulant paediatric cerebral palsy patients over 2 years, and hand and wrist disability associated with stroke; blepharospasm; hemifacial spasm; spasmodic torticollis; severe hyperhidrosis of axillae; temporary improvement of moderate to severe wrinkles between the eyebrows (all specialist use only)

Cautions history of dysphagia or aspiration; neurological disorders (can lead to increased sensitivity and exaggerated muscle weakness); pregnancy (Appendix 4); breast-feeding (Appendix 5)

Specific cautions for blepharospasm or hemifacial spasm Caution if risk of angle-closure glaucoma; reduced blinking can lead to corneal exposure, persistent epithelial defect and corneal ulceration (especially in those with VIIth nerve disorders)—careful testing of corneal sensation in previously operated eyes, avoidance of injection in lower lid area to avoid ectropion, and vigorous treatment of epithelial defect needed

Contra-indications generalised disorders of muscle activity (e.g. myasthenia gravis)

Side-effects increased electrophysiologic jitter in some distant muscles; misplaced injections may paralyse nearby muscle groups and excessive doses may paralyse distant muscles; influenza-like symptoms; *rarely* arrhythmias, myocardial infarction, seizures, hypersensitivity reactions including rash, pruritus and anaphylaxis, antibody formation (substantial deterioration in response), and injection-site reactions; *very rarely* exaggerated muscle weakness, dysphagia, and aspiration (seek medical attention if swallowing, speech, or respiratory disorders)

Specific side-effects for blepharospasm or hemifacial spasm Ptosis; keratitis, lagophthalmos, dry eye, irritation, photophobia, lacrimation; facial oedema; *less commonly* facial weakness (including drooping), dizziness, tiredness, ectropion, entropion, diplopia, visual disturbances; *rarely* eyelid bruising and swelling (minimised by applying gentle pressure at injection site immediately after injection); *very rarely* angle-closure glaucoma, corneal ulceration

Specific side-effects in paediatric cerebral palsy Drowsiness, paraesthesia, urinary incontinence, myalgia

Specific side-effects for temporary improvement of moderate to severe wrinkles between the eyebrows Headache; ptosis; *less commonly* nausea, dry mouth, facial oedema, dizziness, asthenia, anxiety, paraesthesia, visual disturbances, blepharitis, photosensitivity reactions, and dry skin

Specific side-effects in torticollis Dysphagia and pooling of saliva (occurs most frequently after injection into sternomastoid muscle), nausea, dry mouth, rhinitis, drowsiness, headache, dizziness, hypertonia, stiffness; *less commonly* dyspnoea, voice alteration, diplopia, and ptosis

Specific side-effects in axillary hyperhidrosis Non-axillary sweating, hot flushes; *less commonly* myalgia and joint pain

Specific side-effects in focal upper-limb spasticity associated with stroke Dysphagia; hypertonia; *less commonly* arthralgia and bursitis

Dose

- Consult product literature (**important**: specific to **each individual preparation and not interchangeable**)

Botox® (Allergan) PoM
Injection, powder for reconstitution, botulinum toxin type A complex, net price 100-unit vial = £128.93

Dysport® (Ipsen) PoM
Injection, powder for reconstitution, botulinum toxin-haemagglutinin complex type A , net price 500-unit vial = £164.50

Vistabel® (Allergan) PoM
Injection, powder for reconstitution, botulinum toxin type A, net price 50-unit vial = £85.00

BOTULINUM TOXIN TYPE B

Indications spasmodic torticollis (cervical dystonia)—specialist use only

Cautions history of dysphagia or aspiration; inadvertent injection into a blood vessel; tolerance may occur

Contra-indications neuromuscular or neuromuscular junctional disorders; pregnancy (Appendix 4) and breast-feeding (Appendix 5)

Side-effects increased electrophysiologic jitter in some distant muscles; dry mouth, dyspepsia, worsening torticollis, neck pain, myasthenia, voice changes, taste disturbances; *very rarely* exaggerated muscle weakness, dysphagia, and aspiration (seek medical attention if swallowing, speech, or respiratory disorders)

Dose

- By intramuscular injection, initially 5000–10 000 units divided between 2–4 most affected muscles; adjust dose and frequency according to response; **important: not** interchangeable with other botulinum toxin preparations

NeuroBloc® (Zeneus) PoM
Injection, botulinum toxin type B 5000 units/mL, net price 0.5-mL vial = £111.20; 1-mL vial = £148.27; 2-mL vial = £197.69
Note May be diluted with sodium chloride 0.9%

4.10 Drugs used in substance dependence

This section includes drugs used in alcohol dependence, cigarette smoking, and opioid dependence.

The health departments of the UK have produced a report, *Drug Misuse and Dependence* which contains guidelines on clinical management.

Drug Misuse and Dependence, London, The Stationery Office, 1999 can be obtained from:

The Publications Centre
PO Box 276
London, SW8 5DT
Tel: (087) 0600 5522
Fax: (087) 0600 5533

or from The Stationery Office bookshops and through all good booksellers.

It is **important** to be aware that *people who misuse drugs* may be at risk not only from the intrinsic toxicity of the drug itself but also from the practice of injecting preparations intended for administration by mouth. Excipients used in the production of oral dose forms are usually insoluble and may lead to *abscess formation at the site of injection*, or even to *necrosis and gangrene*; moreover, deposits in the heart or lungs may lead to *severe cardiac or pulmonary toxicity*. Additional hazards include *infection* following the use of a dirty needle or an unsterilised diluent.

Alcohol dependence

Disulfiram is used as an adjunct to the treatment of alcohol dependence. It gives rise to extremely unpleasant systemic reactions after the ingestion of even a small amount of alcohol because it leads to accumulation of acetaldehyde in the body. Reactions include flushing of the face, throbbing headache, palpitation, tachycardia, nausea, vomiting, and, with large doses of alcohol, arrhythmias, hypotension, and collapse. Small amounts of alcohol included in many oral medicines may be sufficient to precipitate a reaction (even toiletries and mouthwashes that contain alcohol should be avoided). It may be advisable for patients to carry a card warning of the danger of administration of alcohol.

Long-acting **benzodiazepines** (section 4.1) are used to attenuate withdrawal symptoms but they also have a dependence potential. To minimise the risk of dependence, administration should be for a limited period only (e.g. **chlordiazepoxide** 10–50 mg 4 times daily, gradually reducing over 7–14 days). Benzodiazepines should not be prescribed if the patient is likely to continue drinking alcohol.

Clomethiazole (chlormethiazole) (section 4.1.1) should be used for the management of withdrawal in an **in-patient setting only**. It is associated with a risk of dependence and should not be prescribed if the patient is likely to continue drinking alcohol.

Acamprosate, in combination with counselling, may be helpful in maintaining abstinence in alcohol-dependent patients. It should be initiated as soon as possible *after* abstinence has been achieved and should be maintained if the patient relapses. Continued alcohol abuse, however, negates the therapeutic benefit of acamprosate.

ACAMPROSATE CALCIUM

Indications maintenance of abstinence in alcohol dependence

Cautions continued alcohol abuse (risk of treatment failure)

Contra-indications severe hepatic impairment; renal impairment (avoid if serum creatinine greater than 120 micromol/litre; Appendix 3); pregnancy; breast-feeding

Side-effects diarrhoea, nausea, vomiting, abdominal pain; fluctuation in libido; pruritus, maculopapular rash; *rarely* bullous skin reactions

Dose

- ADULT 18–65 years, body-weight 60 kg and over, 666 mg 3 times daily; body-weight less than 60 kg, 666 mg at breakfast, 333 mg at midday and 333 mg at night

Treatment course Treatment should be initiated as soon as possible after alcohol withdrawal period and maintained if patient relapses; recommended treatment period 1 year

Campral EC® (Merck) PoM
Tablet, e/c, acamprosate calcium 333 mg, net price 168-tab pack = £28.92. Label: 21, 25
Electrolytes Ca^{2+} 0.8 mmol/tablet

DISULFIRAM

Indications adjunct in the treatment of chronic alcohol dependence (under specialist supervision)

Cautions ensure that alcohol not consumed for at least 24 hours before initiating treatment; see also notes above; alcohol challenge **not** recommended on routine basis (if considered essential—specialist units only with resuscitation facilities); hepatic or renal impairment, respiratory disease, diabetes mellitus, epilepsy; **interactions:** Appendix 1 (disulfiram)
Alcohol reaction Patients should be warned of unpredictable and occasionally severe nature of disulfiram-alcohol interactions. Reactions can occur within 10 minutes and last several hours (may require intensive supportive therapy—oxygen should be available). Patients should not ingest alcohol at all and should be warned of possible presence of alcohol in liquid medicines, remedies, tonics, foods and even in toiletries (alcohol should also be avoided for at least 1 week after stopping)

Contra-indications cardiac failure, coronary artery disease, history of cerebrovascular accident, hypertension, psychosis, severe personality disorder, suicide risk, pregnancy (Appendix 4), breast-feeding (Appendix 5)

Side-effects initially drowsiness and fatigue; nausea, vomiting, halitosis, reduced libido; rarely psychotic reactions (depression, paranoia, schizophrenia, mania), allergic dermatitis, peripheral neuritis, hepatic cell damage

Dose
- 800 mg as a single dose on first day, reducing over 5 days to 100–200 mg daily; should not be continued for longer than 6 months without review; CHILD not recommended

Antabuse® (Alpharma) PoM
Tablets, scored, disulfiram 200 mg. Net price 50-tab pack = £26.28. Label: 2, counselling, alcohol reaction

Cigarette smoking

Smoking cessation interventions are a cost-effective way of reducing ill health and prolonging life. Smokers should be advised to stop and offered help if interested in doing so, with follow-up when appropriate.

When possible, smokers should have access to a smoking cessation clinic for behavioural support. **Nicotine replacement therapy** and **bupropion** are effective aids to smoking cessation for those smoking more than 10 cigarettes a day. **Bupropion** has been used as an antidepressant but its mode of action in smoking cessation is not clear and may involve an effect on noradrenaline and dopamine neurotransmission. **Varenicline** is a selective nicotine receptor partial agonist used as an aid for smoking cessation. Nicotine replacement therapy is regarded as the pharmacological treatment of choice in the management of smoking cessation.

Cigarette smoking should stop completely before starting nicotine replacement therapy. If complete smoking cessation is not possible some nicotine preparations are licensed for use as part of a programme to reduce smoking before stopping completely; the smoking cessation regimen can be followed during a quit attempt.

NICE guidance
Nicotine replacement therapy and bupropion for smoking cessation (March 2002)
Nicotine replacement therapy or bupropion should be prescribed only for a smoker who commits to a target stop date. The smoker should be offered advice and encouragement to aid smoking cessation.
Therapy to aid smoking cessation is chosen according to the smoker's likely compliance, availability of counselling and support, previous experience of smoking-cessation aids, contra-indications and adverse effects of the products, and the smoker's preferences.
Initial supply of the prescribed smoking-cessation therapy should be sufficient to last only 2 weeks after the target stop date; normally this will be 2 weeks of nicotine replacement therapy or 3–4 weeks of bupropion. A second prescription should be issued only if the smoker demonstrates a continuing attempt to stop smoking.
If an attempt to stop smoking is unsuccessful, the NHS should not normally fund a further attempt within 6 months.
There is currently insufficient evidence to recommend the combined use of nicotine replacement therapy and bupropion.

NICE guidance
Varenicline for smoking cessation (July 2007)
Varenicline is recommended as an adjunct to smoking cessation for smokers who have expressed a desire to quit smoking; it should normally be prescribed only as a part of a programme of behavioural support.

CSM advice (bupropion)
The CSM has issued a reminder that bupropion is contra-indicated in patients with a history of seizures or of eating disorders, a CNS tumour, or who are experiencing acute symptoms of alcohol or benzodiazepine withdrawal. Bupropion should not be prescribed to patients with other risk factors for seizures unless the potential benefit of smoking cessation clearly outweighs the risk. Factors that increase the risk of seizures include concomitant administration of drugs that can lower the seizure threshold (e.g. antidepressants, antimalarials [such as mefloquine and chloroquine], antipsychotics, quinolones, sedating antihistamines, systemic corticosteroids, theophylline, tramadol), alcohol abuse, history of head trauma, diabetes, and use of stimulants and anorectics.

BUPROPION HYDROCHLORIDE
(Amfebutamone hydrochloride)

Indications see notes above

Cautions elderly; predisposition to seizures (see CSM advice above); measure blood pressure before and during treatment (monitor weekly if used with nicotine products); hepatic impairment (Appendix 2), renal impairment (Appendix 3); **interactions**: Appendix 1 (bupropion)
Driving May impair performance of skilled tasks (e.g. driving)

Contra-indications see CSM advice above; history of bipolar disorder; pregnancy (Appendix 4); breast-feeding (Appendix 5)

Side-effects dry mouth, gastro-intestinal disturbances, taste disturbance; insomnia (reduced by avoiding dose at bedtime), tremor, impaired concentration, headache, dizziness, depression, agitation, anxiety; fever; rash, pruritus, sweating; *less commonly* chest pain, tachycardia, hypertension, flushing, confusion, tinnitus, asthenia, and visual disturbances; *rarely* jaundice, hepatitis, palpitation, postural hypotension, hallucinations, depersonalisation, seizures, dystonia, ataxia, abnormal dreams, memory impairment, paraesthesia, blood-glucose disturbances, urinary retention, urinary frequency, Stevens-Johnson syndrome, and exacerbation of psoriasis; *very rarely* delusions, and aggression

Dose

- ADULT over 18 years, start 1–2 weeks before target stop date, initially 150 mg daily for 6 days then 150 mg twice daily (max. single dose 150 mg, max. daily dose 300 mg; minimum 8 hours between doses); period of treatment 7–9 weeks; discontinue if abstinence not achieved at 7 weeks; consider max. 150 mg daily in patients with risk factors for seizures (see CSM advice above); ELDERLY max. 150 mg daily

Zyban® (GSK) PoM

Tablets, m/r, f/c, bupropion hydrochloride 150 mg, net price 60-tab pack = £39.85. Label: 25, counselling, driving, see above

NICOTINE

Indications see notes above

Cautions severe or unstable cardiovascular disease (including hospitalisation for severe arrhythmias, recent myocardial infarction, or recent cerebrovascular accident)—initiate under medical supervision; uncontrolled hyperthyroidism; diabetes mellitus (monitor blood-glucose concentration closely when initiating treatment); phaeochromocytoma; *oral preparations*, oesophagitis, gastritis, peptic ulcers; *patches*, skin disorders (patches should not be placed on broken skin); hepatic impairment (Appendix 2); renal impairment (Appendix 3); pregnancy (Appendix 4); breast-feeding (Appendix 5)

Note Most warnings under Cautions also apply to continuation of cigarette smoking

Side-effects gastro-intestinal disturbances (including nausea, vomiting, dyspepsia); headache, dizziness; influenza-like symptoms; dry mouth; rash; *less frequently* palpitation; *rarely* atrial fibrillation; *with nasal spray* sneezing, epistaxis, watering eyes, ear sensations; *with lozenges*, thirst, paraesthesia of mouth, taste disturbances; *with patches*, skin reactions (discontinue if severe)—vasculitis also reported, blood pressure changes *with patches* or *lozenges*, sleep disturbances, nightmares, chest pain; *with gum* or *lozenges*, mouth ulceration, increased salivation; *with gum, lozenge, sublingual tablets*, or *inhalator*, hiccups, throat irritation

Dose

- See under preparations, below

Nicorette® (Pharmacia)

Microtab (sublingual), nicotine (as a cyclodextrin complex) 2 mg, net price starter pack of 2 × 15-tablet discs with dispenser = £3.99; refill pack of 7 × 15-tablet discs = £11.12. Label: 26

Dose smoking cessation, individuals smoking *20 cigarettes or less daily*, sublingually, 2 mg each hour; for patients who fail to stop smoking or have significant withdrawal symptoms, consider increasing to 4 mg each hour; individuals smoking *more than 20 cigarettes daily*, sublingually, 4 mg each hour; max. 80 mg daily; treatment continued for at least 3 months followed by a gradual reduction in dose; review treatment if abstinence not achieved within 9 months; CHILD 12–18 years, treatment continued for up to 8 weeks followed by gradual reduction over 4 weeks; review treatment if abstinence not achieved within 3 months

Chewing gum, sugar-free, nicotine (as resin) 2 mg, net price pack of 15 = £1.71, pack of 30 = £3.25, pack of 105 = £8.89; 4 mg, net price pack of 15 = £2.11, pack of 30 = £3.99, pack of 105 = £10.83

Note Also available in mint, freshfruit, and freshmint flavours

Dose smoking cessation, individuals smoking *20 cigarettes or less daily*, initially chew one 2-mg piece slowly (chew gum until taste becomes strong, then rest gum between cheek and gum, when taste fades start chewing again) for approx. 30 minutes when urge to smoke occurs; individuals smoking *more than 20 cigarettes daily* or needing more than 15 pieces of 2-mg gum daily should use the 4-mg strength; max. 15 pieces of 4-mg strength daily; withdraw gradually after 3 months; review treatment if abstinence not achieved within 9 months; CHILD 12–18 years, treatment continued for up to 8 weeks followed by gradual reduction over 4 weeks; review treatment if abstinence not achieved within 3 months

Smoking reduction, chew 1 piece when urge to smoke occurs between smoking episodes; reduce smoking within 6 weeks and attempt smoking cessation within 6 months; review treatment if abstinence not achieved within 9 months

Note Children under 18 years should consult a healthcare professional before starting smoking-reduction regimen

Patches, self-adhesive, beige, nicotine, *'5 mg' patch* (releasing approx 5 mg/16 hours), net price 7 = £9.07; *'10 mg' patch* (releasing approx. 10 mg/16 hours), 7 = £9.07; *'15 mg' patch* (releasing approx. 15 mg/16 hours), 2 = £2.85, 7 = £9.07

Dose smoking cessation, ADULT and CHILD over 12 years, apply on waking to dry, non-hairy skin on hip, chest or upper arm, removing after approx. 16 hours, usually when retiring to bed; site next patch on different area (avoid using same area on consecutive days); initially '15-mg' patch for 16 hours daily for 8 weeks then if abstinence achieved '10-mg' patch for 16 hours daily for 2 weeks then '5-mg' patch for 16 hours daily for 2 weeks; review treatment if abstinence not achieved within 3 months—further courses may be given if considered beneficial

Nasal spray, nicotine 500 micrograms/metered spray, net price 200-spray unit = £12.26

Dose smoking cessation, ADULT and CHILD over 12 years, apply 1 spray into each nostril as required to max. twice an hour for 16 hours daily (max. 64 sprays daily) for 8 weeks, then reduce gradually over next 4 weeks (reduce by half at end of first 2 weeks, stop altogether at end of next 2 weeks); review treatment if abstinence not achieved within 3 months

Inhalator (nicotine-impregnated plug for use in inhalator mouthpiece), nicotine 10 mg/cartridge, net price 6-cartridge (starter) pack = £3.99, 42-cartridge (refill) pack = £12.82

Dose smoking cessation, ADULT and CHILD over 12 years, inhale when urge to smoke occurs; initially use between 6 and 12 cartridges daily for up to 8 weeks, then reduce number of cartridges used by half over next 2 weeks and then stop altogether at end of further 2 weeks; review treatment if abstinence not achieved within 3 months

Smoking reduction, ADULT and CHILD over 12 years, inhale when urge to smoke occurs between smoking episodes; reduce smoking within 6 weeks and attempt smoking cessation within 6 months; review treatment if abstinence not achieved within 9 months

Note Children under 18 years should consult a healthcare professional before starting a smoking-reduction regimen

Nicotinell® (Novartis Consumer Health)

Chewing gum, sugar-free, nicotine (as polacrilin complex) 2 mg, net price pack of 12 = £1.71, pack of 24 = £3.01, pack of 96 = £8.26; 4 mg, pack of 12 = £1.70, pack of 24 = £3.30, pack of 96 = £10.26

Note Also available in fruit, liquorice and mint flavours

Dose smoking cessation, individuals smoking *20 cigarettes or less daily*, initially chew one 2-mg piece slowly (chew gum until taste becomes strong, then rest gum between cheek and gum, when taste fades start chewing again) for approx. 30 minutes, when urge to smoke occurs; individuals smoking *more than 20 cigarettes daily* should use the 4-mg strength; max. 60 mg daily; withdraw gradually after 3 months; max. period of treatment should not usually exceed 6 months; CHILD 12–18 years, withdraw gradually and review treatment if abstinence not achieved within 3 months

Mint lozenge, sugar-free, nicotine (as bitartrate) 1 mg, net price pack of 12 = £1.71, pack of 36 = £4.27, pack of 96 = £9.12; 2 mg, net price pack of 12 = £1.99, pack of 36 = £4.95, pack of 96 = £10.60.

Excipients include aspartame (section 9.4.1)

Dose smoking cessation, individuals smoking *30 cigarettes or less daily*, initially suck one 1-mg lozenge every 1–2 hours, when urge to smoke occurs; individuals smoking *more than 30 cigarettes daily* should use the 2-mg strength; max. 30 mg daily; withdraw gradually after 3 months; max. period of treatment should not usually exceed 6 months; CHILD 12–18 years, withdraw gradually and review treatment if abstinence not achieved within 3 months

TTS Patches, self-adhesive, all yellowish-ochre, nicotine, *'10' patch* (releasing approx. 7 mg/24 hours), net price 7 = £9.12; *'20' patch* (releasing approx. 14 mg/24 hours), net price 2 = £2.57, 7 = £9.40; *'30' patch* (releasing approx. 21 mg/24 hours), net price 2 = £2.85, 7 = £9.97, 21 = £24.51

Dose smoking cessation, ADULT and CHILD over 12 years, apply to dry, non-hairy skin on trunk or upper arm, removing after 24 hours and siting replacement patch on a different area (avoid using the same area for several days); individuals smoking *less than 20 cigarettes daily*, initially '20' patch daily; individuals smoking *20 or more cigarettes daily*, initially '30' patch daily; withdraw gradually, reducing dose every 3–4 weeks; review treatment if abstinence not achieved within 3 months

NiQuitin® (GSK Consumer Healthcare)

Chewing gum, sugar-free, mint-flavour, nicotine 2 mg (white), net price pack of 12 = £1.71, pack of 24 = £2.85, pack of 96 = £8.55; 4 mg (yellow), net price pack of 12 = £1.71, pack of 24 = £2.85, pack of 96 = £8.55

Dose smoking cessation, initially chew 1 piece slowly (chew gum until taste becomes strong, then rest gum between cheek and gum, when taste fades start chewing again) for approx. 30 minutes, when urge to smoke occurs; max. 15 pieces daily; withdraw gradually after 3 months; review treatment if abstinence not achieved within 9 months; CHILD 12–18 years, withdraw gradually and review treatment if abstinence not achieved within 3 months

Smoking reduction, chew 1 piece when urge to smoke occurs between smoking episodes (max. 15 pieces daily); reduce smoking within 6 weeks and attempt cessation within 6 months; review treatment if abstinence not achieved within 9 months

Note Children under 18 years should consult a healthcare professional before starting smoking-reduction regimen

Temporary abstinence, chew 1 piece when urge to smoke occurs between smoking episodes (max. 15 pieces daily); review treatment if unable to undertake permanent quit attempt within 6 months

Lozenges, sugar-free, nicotine (as polacrilex) 2 mg, net price pack of 36 = £5.12, pack of 72 = £9.97; 4 mg, pack of 36 = £5.12, pack of 72 = £9.97. Contains 0.65 mmol Na^+/lozenge

Excipients include aspartame (section 9.4.1)

Dose smoking cessation, initially suck 1 lozenge every 1–2 hours when urge to smoke occurs (max. 15 lozenges daily) for 6 weeks, then 1 lozenge every 2–4 hours for 3 weeks, then 1 lozenge every 4–8 hours for 3 weeks; withdraw gradually after 3 months; review treatment if abstinence not achieved within 9 months; CHILD 12–18 years, withdraw gradually and review treatment if abstinence not achieved within 3 months

Smoking reduction, suck 1 lozenge when urge to smoke occurs between smoking episodes (max. 15 lozenges daily); reduce smoking within 6 weeks and attempt cessation within 6 months; review treatment if abstinence not achieved within 9 months

Note Children under 18 years should consult a healthcare professional before starting smoking-reduction regimen

Temporary abstinence, suck 1 lozenge every 1-2 hours when urge to smoke occurs between smoking episodes (max. 15 lozenges daily); review treatment if unable to undertake permanent quit attempt within 6 months

Patches, self-adhesive, pink/beige, nicotine *'7 mg' patch* (releasing approx. 7 mg/24 hours), net price 7 = £9.97; *'14 mg' patch* (releasing approx. 14 mg/24 hours), 7 = £9.97; *'21 mg' patch* (releasing approx. 21 mg/24 hours), 7 = £9.97, 14 = £18.79

Note Also available as a clear patch

Dose smoking cessation, apply on waking to dry, non-hairy skin site, removing after 24 hours and siting replacement patch on different area (avoid using same area for 7 days); individuals smoking *10 or more cigarettes daily*, initially '21-mg' patch daily for 6 weeks then '14-mg' patch daily for 2 weeks then '7-mg' patch daily for 2 weeks; individuals smoking *less than 10 cigarettes daily*, initially '14-mg' patch daily for 6 weeks then '7-mg' patch daily for 2 weeks; review treatment if abstinence not achieved within 9 months; CHILD 12–18 years, withdraw gradually and review if abstinence not achieved within 3 months

Note Patients using the '21-mg' patch who experience excessive side-effects, which do not resolve within a few days, should change to '14-mg' patch for the remainder of the initial 6 weeks before switching to the '7-mg' patch for the final 2 weeks

VARENICLINE

Indications see notes above

Cautions avoid abrupt withdrawal (risk of relapse, irritability, depression, insomnia); history of psychiatric illness (may exacerbate underlying illness including depression); renal impairment (Appendix 3); breast-feeding (Appendix 5)

Contra-indications pregnancy (Appendix 4)

Side-effects gastro-intestinal disturbances, appetite changes, dry mouth, taste disturbance; headache, drowsiness, dizziness, sleep disorders, abnormal dreams; *less commonly* thirst, weight gain, aphthous stomatitis, gingival pain, chest pain, hypertension, tachycardia, atrial fibrillation, palpitation, panic attack, abnormal thinking, mood swings, dysarthria, asthenia, tremor, incoordination, hypertonia, restlessness, hypoaesthesia, impaired temperature regulation, menorrhagia, vaginal discharge, sexual dysfunction, dysuria, arthralgia, muscle spasm, visual disturbances, eye pain, lacrimation, tinnitus, acne, sweating, rash, and pruritus; myocardial infarction, depression, and suicidal ideation also reported

Dose

- ADULT over 18 years, start 1–2 weeks before target stop date, initially 500 micrograms once daily for 3 days, increased to 500 micrograms twice daily for 4 days, then 1 mg twice daily for 11 weeks (reduce to 500 micrograms twice daily if not tolerated); treatment can be repeated in abstinent individuals to reduce risk of relapse

Champix® (Pfizer) ▼ PoM

Tablets, f/c, varenicline (as tartrate) 500 micrograms (white), net price 56-tab pack = £54.60; 1 mg (blue) 28-tab pack = £27.30, 56-tab pack = £54.60; starter pack of 11 × 500-microgram tabs with 14 × 1-mg tabs = £27.30

Opioid dependence

The management of opioid dependence requires medical, social, and psychological treatment; access to a multidisciplinary team is valuable. Treatment with opioid substitutes or with naltrexone is best initiated under the supervision of an appropriately qualified physician.

Methadone, an opioid *agonist*, can be substituted for opioids such as diamorphine, preventing the onset of withdrawal symptoms; it is itself addictive and should only be prescribed for those who are physically dependent on opioids. It is administered in a single daily dose usually as methadone oral solution 1 mg/mL. The dose is adjusted according to the degree of dependence.

Buprenorphine is an opioid partial agonist. Because of its abuse and dependence potential it should be prescribed only for those who are already physically dependent on opioids. It can be used as substitution therapy for patients with moderate opioid dependence. In patients dependent on high doses of opioids, buprenorphine may precipitate withdrawal due to its partial antagonist properties; in these patients, the daily opioid dose should be reduced gradually before initiating therapy with buprenorphine.

Naltrexone, an opioid *antagonist*, blocks the action of opioids and precipitates withdrawal symptoms in opioid-dependent subjects. Because the euphoric action of opioid agonists is blocked by naltrexone it is given to former addicts as an aid to prevent relapse.

Lofexidine is used for the alleviation of symptoms in individuals whose opioid use is well controlled and are undergoing opioid withdrawal. Like clonidine it is an alpha-adrenergic agonist and appears to act centrally to produce a reduction in sympathetic tone, but reduction in blood pressure is less marked.

> **NICE guidance**
> **Methadone and buprenorphine for the management of opioid dependence (January 2007)**
> Oral methadone and buprenorphine are recommended for maintenance therapy in the management of opioid dependence. Patients should be committed to a supportive care programme including a flexible dosing regimen administered under supervision for at least 3 months, until compliance is assured. Selection of methadone or buprenorphine should be made on a case-by-case basis, but methadone should be prescribed if both drugs are equally suitable.

> **NICE guidance**
> **Naltrexone for the management of opioid dependence (January 2007)**
> Naltrexone is recommended for the prevention of relapse in detoxified formerly opioid-dependent patients who are motivated to remain in a supportive care abstinence programme. Naltrexone should be administered under supervision and its effectiveness in preventing opioid misuse reviewed regularly.

BUPRENORPHINE

Indications adjunct in the treatment of opioid dependence; premedication, peri-operative analgesia, analgesia in other situations (section 4.7.2)

Cautions see section 4.7.2 and notes above; effects only partially reversed by naloxone

Contra-indications see section 4.7.2; breast-feeding (Appendix 5)

Side-effects see section 4.7.2

Dose

- By sublingual administration, initially, 0.8–4 mg as a single daily dose, adjusted according to response; max. 32 mg daily; withdraw gradually; CHILD under 16 years not recommended

Note In patients who have not undergone opioid withdrawal, buprenorphine should be given at least 4 hours after last use of opioid or when signs of withdrawal appear
In patients receiving methadone, dose of methadone should be reduced to max. 30 mg daily before starting buprenorphine

Subutex® (Schering-Plough) CD
Tablets (sublingual), buprenorphine (as hydrochloride) 400 micrograms, net price 7-tab pack = £1.60; 2 mg, 7-tab pack = £6.72; 8 mg, 7-tab pack = £20.16. Label: 2, 26

With naloxone

Suboxone® (Schering-Plough) ▼ CD
Suboxone 2 mg/500 micrograms tablets (sublingual), buprenorphine (as hydrochloride) 2 mg, naloxone (as hydrochloride) 500 micrograms, net price 28-tab pack = £26.88. Label: 2, 26
Suboxone 8mg/2mg tablets (sublingual), buprenorphine (as hydrochloride) 8 mg, naloxone (as hydrochloride) 2 mg, net price 28-tab pack = £80.64. Label: 2, 26

Dose expressed as buprenorphine, ADULT and CHILD over 15 years, initially 2–8 mg once daily, increased in steps of 2–8 mg according to response; max. 24 mg daily; total weekly dose may be divided and given on alternate days or 3 times weekly (but max. daily dose 24 mg)

Note In patients who have not undergone opioid withdrawal, *Suboxone®* should be given when signs of withdrawal appear, at least 6 hours after last use of opioid
In patients receiving methadone, dose of methadone should be reduced to max. 30 mg daily before starting *Suboxone®*; first dose of *Suboxone®* should be given when signs of withdrawal appear, at least 24 hours after last dose of methadone

Note The *Scottish Medicines Consortium* has advised (February 2007) that *Suboxone®* should be restricted for use in patients in whom methadone is not suitable

LOFEXIDINE HYDROCHLORIDE

Indications management of symptoms of opioid withdrawal

Cautions severe coronary insufficiency, recent myocardial infarction, cerebrovascular disease, marked bradycardia (monitor pulse rate); history of QT prolongation, concomitant administration of drugs that prolong QT interval; withdraw gradually over 2–4 days (or longer) to minimise risk of rebound hypertension and associated symptoms; renal impairment (Appendix 3); pregnancy (Appendix 4); breast-feeding (Appendix 5); **interactions**: Appendix 1 (lofexidine)

Side-effects dry mucous membranes, hypotension, bradycardia, rebound hypertension on withdrawal, drowsiness

Dose

- Initially, 800 micrograms daily in divided doses, increased as necessary in steps of 400–800 micrograms daily to max. 2.4 mg daily in divided doses; max. single dose 800 micrograms; recommended duration of treatment 7–10 days if no opioid use (but longer may be required); CHILD and ADOLESCENT under 18 years not recommended

BritLofex® (Britannia) PoM

Tablets, peach, f/c, lofexidine hydrochloride 200 micrograms, net price 60-tab pack = £61.79. Label: 2

METHADONE HYDROCHLORIDE

Indications adjunct in treatment of opioid dependence, see notes above; analgesia (section 4.7.2); cough in terminal disease (section 3.9.1)

Cautions section 4.7.2

Contra-indications section 4.7.2

Side-effects section 4.7.2; **overdosage:** see Emergency Treatment of Poisoning, p. 31

Important Methadone, even in low doses is a **special hazard** for children; non-dependent adults are also at risk of toxicity; dependent adults are at risk if tolerance is incorrectly assessed during induction

Incompatibility Syrup preserved with hydroxybenzoate (parabens) esters may be incompatible with methadone hydrochloride.

Dose

- Initially 10–40 mg daily, increased by up to 10 mg daily (max. weekly increase 30 mg) until no signs of withdrawal or intoxication; usual dose range 60–120 mg daily; CHILD not recommended (see also important note above)

Note Methadone hydrochloride doses in the BNF may differ from those in the product literature

Methadone (Non-proprietary) CD

Oral solution 1 mg/mL, methadone hydrochloride 1 mg/mL, net price 30 mL = 44p, 50 mL = 73p, 100 mL = £1.45, 500 mL = £9.60. Label: 2

Brands include *Metharose®* (sugar-free), *Physeptone* (also as sugar-free)

Important This preparation is 2½ times the strength of Methadone Linctus (section 3.9.1); many preparations of this strength are licensed for opioid drug addiction only but some are also licensed for analgesia in severe pain

Injection, methadone hydrochloride 25 mg/mL, net price 2-mL amp = £2.05; 50 mg/mL, 1-mL amp = £2.05

Brands include *Synastone®*

Methadose® (Rosemont) CD

Oral concentrate, methadone hydrochloride 10 mg/mL (blue), net price 150 mL = £12.01; 20 mg/mL (brown), 150 mL = £24.02. Label: 2

Note The final strength of the methadone mixture to be dispensed to the patient must be specified on the prescription

Important Care is required in prescribing and dispensing the **correct strength** since any confusion could lead to an overdose; this preparation should be dispensed only **after dilution** as appropriate with *Methadose® Diluent* (life of diluted solution 3 months) and is for drug dependent persons (see also p. 8)

NALTREXONE HYDROCHLORIDE

Indications adjunct to prevent relapse in detoxified formerly opioid-dependent patients (who have remained opioid-free for at least 7–10 days)

Cautions liver function tests needed before and during treatment; test for opioid dependence with naloxone before treatment; avoid concomitant use of opioids but increased dose of opioid analgesic may be required for pain (monitor for opioid intoxication); hepatic impairment (Appendix 2); renal impairment (Appendix 3); pregnancy (Appendix 4); breast-feeding (Appendix 5)

Note Patients should be warned that an attempt to overcome the blockade of opioid receptors by overdosing could result in acute opioid intoxication

Contra-indications patients currently dependent on opioids

Side-effects nausea, vomiting, abdominal pain, diarrhoea, constipation, reduced appetite, increased thirst; chest pain; anxiety, sleep disorders, headache, reduced energy, increased energy, irritability, emotional lability, dizziness; chills; urinary retention; delayed ejaculation, decreased potency; arthralgia, myalgia; increased lacrimation; rash, and increased sweating; *rarely* hepatic dysfunction, suicidal ideation, and speech disorders; *very rarely* hallucinations, tremor, and idiopathic thrombocytopenia

Dose

- ADULTS over 18 years (initiate in specialist clinics only) 25 mg initially then 50 mg daily; total weekly dose (350 mg) may be divided and given on 3 days of the week for improved compliance (e.g. 100 mg on Monday and Wednesday, and 150 mg on Friday)

Nalorex® (Bristol-Myers Squibb) PoM

Tablets, yellow, f/c, scored, naltrexone hydrochloride 50 mg, net price 28-tab pack = £23.72

Opizone® (Britannia) PoM

Tablets, beige, f/c, scored, naltrexone hydrochloride 50 mg, net price 28-tab pack = £23.00

4.11 Drugs for dementia

Acetylcholinesterase inhibiting drugs are used in the treatment of Alzheimer's disease, specifically for mild to moderate disease. Rivastigmine is also licensed for mild to moderate dementia associated with Parkinson's disease. The evidence to support the use of these drugs relates to their cognitive enhancement.

Treatment with drugs for dementia should be initiated and supervised only by a specialist experienced in the management of dementia.

Benefit is assessed by repeating the cognitive assessment at around 3 months. Such assessment cannot demonstrate how the disease may have progressed in the absence of treatment but it can give a good guide to response. Up to half the patients given these drugs will show a slower rate of cognitive decline. Drugs for dementia should be discontinued in those thought not to be responding. Many specialists repeat the cognitive assessment 4 to 6 weeks after discontinuation to assess deterioration; if significant deterioration occurs during this short period, consideration should be given to restarting therapy.

Donepezil is a reversible inhibitor of acetylcholinesterase. **Galantamine** is a reversible inhibitor of acetylcholinesterase and it also has nicotinic receptor agonist properties. **Rivastigmine** is a reversible non-competitive inhibitor of acetylcholinesterases; it is also licensed for treating mild to moderate dementia in Parkinson's disease.

Acetylcholinesterase inhibitors can cause unwanted dose-related cholinergic effects and should be started at a low dose and the dose increased according to response and tolerability.

Memantine is a NMDA-receptor antagonist that affects glutamate transmission; it is licensed for treating moderate to severe Alzheimer's disease.

> **NICE guidance**
> **Donepezil, galantamine, rivastigmine, and memantime for Alzheimer's disease (September 2007)**
> Donepezil, galantamine, and rivastigmine are recommended for the adjunctive treatment of moderate Alzheimer's disease in those whose mini mental-state examination (MMSE) score is 10–20 points under the following conditions:
> - Alzheimer's disease must be diagnosed in a specialist clinic; the clinic should also assess cognitive, global, and behavioural functioning, activities of daily living, and the likelihood of compliance with treatment;
> - treatment should be initiated by specialists but can be continued by general practitioners under a shared-care protocol;
> - the carers' views of the condition should be sought before and during drug treatment;
> - the patient should be assessed every 6 months and drug treatment should normally continue only if the MMSE score remains at or above 10 points and if treatment is considered to have a worthwhile effect on the global, functional, and behavioural condition.
> - Patients receiving acetylcholinesterase inhibitors for mild Alzheimer's disease can continue treatment until they, their carers, or their specialist consider it appropriate to stop.
>
> Healthcare professionals should not rely solely on the MMSE score to assess the severity of Alzheimer's disease when the patient has learning or other disabilities, or other communication difficulties.
> NICE does not recommend memantine for moderately severe to severe Alzheimer's disease except as part of well designed clinical studies; patients already receiving memantine can continue treatment until they, their carers, or their specialist consider it appropriate to stop.

DONEPEZIL HYDROCHLORIDE

Indications mild to moderate dementia in Alzheimer's disease

Cautions sick sinus syndrome or other supraventricular conduction abnormalities; susceptibility to peptic ulcers; asthma, chronic obstructive pulmonary disease, hepatic impairment (Appendix 2); pregnancy (Appendix 4); **interactions:** Appendix 1 (parasympathomimetics)

Contra-indications breast-feeding

Side-effects nausea, vomiting, anorexia, diarrhoea; fatigue, insomnia, headache, dizziness, syncope, hallucinations, agitation, aggression; muscle cramps; urinary incontinence; rash, pruritus; *less commonly* gastric and duodenal ulcers, gastro-intestinal haemorrhage, bradycardia, seizures; *rarely* sino-atrial block, AV block, hepatitis, extrapyramidal symptoms; potential for bladder outflow obstruction

Dose

- Initially 5 mg once daily at bedtime, increased if necessary after one month to max. 10 mg daily

Aricept® (Pfizer, Eisai) PoM
Tablets, f/c, donepezil hydrochloride 5 mg (white), net price 28-tab pack = £63.54; 10 mg (yellow), 28-tab pack = £89.06.

Aricept Evess® (Pfizer, Eisai) PoM
Orodispersible tablets, donepezil hydrochloride 5 mg (white), net price 28-tab pack = £63.54; 10 mg (yellow), 28-tab pack = £89.06. Counselling, administration
Counselling *Aricept Evess®* should be placed on the tongue, allowed to disperse, and swallowed

GALANTAMINE

Indications mild to moderate dementia in Alzheimer's disease

Cautions cardiac disease (including sick sinus syndrome or other supraventricular conduction abnormalities, unstable angina, congestive heart failure); electrolyte disturbances; susceptibility to peptic ulcers; asthma, chronic obstructive pulmonary disease, pulmonary infection; avoid in urinary retention and gastro-intestinal obstruction; hepatic impairment (Appendix 2—avoid if severe); pregnancy (Appendix 4); **interactions**. Appendix 1 (parasympathomimetics)

Contra-indications renal impairment (avoid if creatinine clearance less than 9 mL/minute; Appendix 3); breast-feeding (Appendix 5)

Side-effects nausea, vomiting, diarrhoea, abdominal pain, dyspepsia; syncope; rhinitis; sleep disturbances, dizziness, confusion depression, headache, fatigue, anorexia, tremor; fever, weight loss; *less commonly* arrythmias, palpitation, myocardial infarction, cerebrovascular disease, paraesthesia, tinnitus, and leg cramps; *rarely* bradycardia, seizures, hallucinations, agitation, aggression, dehydration, hypokalaemia, and rash; *very rarely* gastrointestinal bleeding, dysphagia, hypotension, exacerbation of Parkinson's disease, and sweating

Dose

- Initially 4 mg twice daily for 4 weeks increased to 8 mg twice daily for 4 weeks; maintenance 8–12 mg twice daily

Reminyl® (Shire) PoM
Tablets, all f/c, galantamine (as hydrobromide) 8 mg (pink), net price 56-tab pack = £68.32; 12 mg (orange-brown), 56-tab pack = £84.00 Label: 3, 21
Oral solution, galantamine (as hydrobromide) 4 mg/mL, net price 100 mL with pipette = £120.00. Label: 3, 21

Modified release

Reminyl® XL (Shire) PoM
Capsules, m/r, galantamine (as hydrobromide) 8 mg (white), net price 28-cap pack = £54.60; 16 mg (pink),

28-cap pack = £68.32; 24 mg (beige), 28-cap pack = £84.00. Label: 3, 21, 25

Dose initially 8 mg once daily for 4 weeks increased to 16 mg once daily for 4 weeks; maintenance 16–24 mg daily

MEMANTINE HYDROCHLORIDE

Indications moderate to severe dementia in Alzheimer's disease

Cautions history of convulsions; renal impairment (avoid if creatinine clearance less than 5 mL/minute; Appendix 3); pregnancy (Appendix 4); **interactions:** Appendix 1 (memantine)

Contra-indications breast-feeding

Side-effects constipation; hypertension; headache, dizziness, drowsiness; *less commonly* vomiting, thrombosis, confusion, fatigue, hallucinations, and abnormal gait; *very rarely* seizures; pancreatitis, psychosis, depression, and suicidal ideation also reported

Dose

- Initially 5 mg in the morning, increased in steps of 5 mg at weekly intervals, up to max. 10 mg twice daily; doses over 5 mg given in 2 divided doses

Ebixa® (Lundbeck) PoM

Tablets, f/c, scored, memantine hydrochloride 10 mg, net price 28-tab pack = £34.50, 56-tab pack = £69.01, 112-tab pack = £138.01

Oral drops, memantine hydrochloride 10 mg/g, net price 50 g = £61.61, 100 g = £123.23

Note 5 mg ≡ 10 drops of memantine hydrochloride oral drops

Note The *Scottish Medicines Consortium* has advised (January 2004) that *Ebixa®* is not recommended for the treatment of Alzheimer's disease

RIVASTIGMINE

Indications mild to moderate dementia in Alzheimer's disease or in Parkinson's disease

Cautions gastric or duodenal ulcers (or susceptibility to ulcers); monitor body-weight; sick sinus syndrome, conduction abnormalities; history of asthma or chronic obstructive pulmonary disease; history of seizures; bladder outflow obstruction; hepatic impairment (avoid if severe—Appendix 2); renal impairment (Appendix 3); pregnancy (Appendix 4); **interactions:** Appendix 1 (parasympathomimetics)

Note If treatment interrupted for more than several days, re-introduce with initial dose and increase gradually (see Dose)

Contra-indications breast-feeding (Appendix 5)

Side-effects nausea, vomiting, diarrhoea, dyspepsia, anorexia, abdominal pain; dizziness, headache, drowsiness, tremor, asthenia, malaise, agitation, confusion; sweating; weight loss; *less commonly* gastric or duodenal ulceration, bradycardia, syncope, depression, insomnia; *rarely* angina pectoris, seizures; *very rarely* gastro-intestinal haemorrhage, pancreatitis, cardiac arrhythmias, hypertension, hallucinations, extrapyramidal symptoms (including worsening of Parkinson's disease), and rash; *with patches* application-site reactions

Note Gastro-intestinal side-effects more common in women

Dose

- See under preparations below

Exelon® (Novartis) ▼ PoM

Capsules, rivastigmine (as hydrogen tartrate) 1.5 mg (yellow), net price 28-cap pack = £39.12, 56-cap pack = £78.25; 3 mg (orange), 28-cap pack = £39.12, 56-cap pack = £78.25; 4.5 mg (red), 28-cap pack = £39.12, 56-cap pack = £78.25; 6 mg (red/orange), 28-cap pack = £39.12, 56-cap pack = £78.25. Label: 21, 25

Oral solution, rivastigmine (as hydrogen tartrate) 2 mg/mL, net price 120 mL (with oral syringe) = £116.64. Label: 21

Dose initially 1.5 mg twice daily, increased in steps of 1.5 mg twice daily at intervals of at least 2 weeks according to response and tolerance; usual range 3–6 mg twice daily; max. 6 mg twice daily

Patches, self-adhesive, beige, rivastigmine 4.6 mg/24 hours, net price 30 = £83.84; 9.5 mg/24 hours, 30 = £83.84

Dose initially apply 4.6 mg/24 hours patch to clean, dry, non-hairy, non-irritated skin on back, upper arm, or chest, removing after 24 hours and siting a replacement patch on a different area (avoid using the same area for 14 days); if well tolerated increase to 9.5 mg/24 hours patch daily after no less than 4 weeks; if patch not applied for more than several days, treatment should be restarted with 4.6 mg/24 hours patch

Note When switching a patient from oral to transdermal therapy, patients taking 3-6 mg daily should be prescribed the 4.6 mg/24 hours patch; patients taking 9 mg daily who do not tolerate the dose well should be prescribed the 4.6 mg/24 hours patch, while those taking 9 mg daily who tolerate the dose well should be prescribed the 9.5 mg/24 hours patch; patients taking 12 mg daily should be prescribed the 9.5 mg/24 hours patch. The first patch should be applied on the day following the last oral dose

Note The *Scottish Medicines Consortium* has advised (October 2007) that *Exelon®* patches should be restricted for use in patients with moderately severe Alzheimer's disease under the conditions of the NICE guidance (September 2007) and when a transdermal patch is an appropriate choice of formulation

5 Infections

5.1	**Antibacterial drugs**	**277**
5.1.1	Penicillins	284
5.1.1.1	Benzylpenicillin and phenoxymethylpenicillin	284
5.1.1.2	Penicillinase-resistant penicillins	285
5.1.1.3	Broad-spectrum penicillins	287
5.1.1.4	Antipseudomonal penicillins	290
5.1.1.5	Mecillinams	290
5.1.2	Cephalosporins and other beta-lactams	291
5.1.3	Tetracyclines	296
5.1.4	Aminoglycosides	299
5.1.5	Macrolides	301
5.1.6	Clindamycin	303
5.1.7	Some other antibacterials	304
5.1.8	Sulphonamides and trimethoprim	308
5.1.9	Antituberculosis drugs	310
5.1.10	Antileprotic drugs	314
5.1.11	Metronidazole and tinidazole	315
5.1.12	Quinolones	316
5.1.13	Urinary-tract infections	319
5.2	**Antifungal drugs**	**320**
5.3	**Antiviral drugs**	**327**
5.3.1	HIV infection	327
5.3.2	Herpesvirus infections	335
5.3.2.1	Herpes simplex and varicella–zoster infection	335
5.3.2.2	Cytomegalovirus infection	338
5.3.3	Viral hepatitis	339
5.3.4	Influenza	341
5.3.5	Respiratory syncytial virus	342
5.4	**Antiprotozoal drugs**	**344**
5.4.1	Antimalarials	344
5.4.2	Amoebicides	352
5.4.3	Trichomonacides	353
5.4.4	Antigiardial drugs	353
5.4.5	Leishmaniacides	353
5.4.6	Trypanocides	354
5.4.7	Drugs for toxoplasmosis	354
5.4.8	Drugs for pneumocystis pneumonia	354
5.5	**Anthelmintics**	**355**
5.5.1	Drugs for threadworms	355
5.5.2	Ascaricides	356
5.5.3	Drugs for tapeworm infections	356
5.5.4	Drugs for hookworms	357
5.5.5	Schistosomicides	357
5.5.6	Filaricides	357
5.5.7	Drugs for cutaneous larva migrans	357
5.5.8	Drugs for strongyloidiasis	357

This chapter also includes advice on the drug management of the following:

- anthrax, p. 316
- antibiotic-associated colitis, p. 279
- bacterial infections (summary of treatment and prophylaxis), p. 279–p. 283
- Lyme disease, p. 287
- MRSA infections, p. 286
- oral infections, p. 278, p. 281, p. 321

Notifiable diseases

Doctors must notify the Proper Officer of the local authority (usually the consultant in communicable disease control) when attending a patient suspected of suffering from any of the diseases listed below; a form is available from the Proper Officer.

Anthrax	Ophthalmia neonatorum
Cholera	Paratyphoid fever
Diphtheria	Plague
Dysentery (amoebic or bacillary)	Poliomyelitis, acute
Encephalitis, acute	Rabies
Food poisoning	Relapsing fever
Haemorrhagic fever (viral)	Rubella
Hepatitis, viral	Scarlet fever
Leprosy	Smallpox
Leptospirosis	Tetanus
Malaria	Tuberculosis
Measles	Typhoid fever
Meningitis	Typhus
Meningococcal septicaemia (without meningitis)	Whooping cough
Mumps	Yellow fever

Note It is good practice for doctors to also inform the consultant in communicable disease control of instances of other infections (e.g. psittacosis) where there could be a public health risk.

5.1 Antibacterial drugs

Choice of a suitable drug Before selecting an antibacterial the clinician must first consider two factors—the patient and the known or likely causative organism. Factors related to the patient which must be considered include history of allergy, renal and hepatic function, susceptibility to infection (i.e. whether immunocompromised), ability to tolerate drugs by mouth, severity of illness, ethnic origin, age, whether taking other medication and, if female, whether pregnant, breast-feeding or taking an oral contraceptive.

The known or likely organism and its antibacterial sensitivity, in association with the above factors, will suggest one or more antibacterials, the final choice depending on the microbiological, pharmacological, and toxicological properties.

An example of a rational approach to the selection of an antibacterial is treatment of a urinary-tract infection in a patient complaining of nausea in early pregnancy. The organism is reported as being resistant to ampicillin but sensitive to nitrofurantoin (can cause nausea), gentamicin (can be given only by injection and best avoided in pregnancy), tetracycline (causes dental discoloration) and trimethoprim (folate antagonist therefore theoretical teratogenic risk), and cefalexin. The safest antibiotics in pregnancy are the penicillins and cephalosporins; therefore, cefalexin would be indicated for this patient.

The principles involved in selection of an antibacterial must allow for a number of variables including changing renal and hepatic function, increasing bacterial resistance, and new information on side-effects. Duration of therapy, dosage, and route of administration depend on site, type and severity of infection and response.

Antibacterial policies Local policies often limit the antibacterials that may be used to achieve reasonable economy consistent with adequate cover, and to reduce the development of resistant organisms. A policy may indicate a range of drugs for general use, and permit other drugs only on the advice of the microbiologist or physician responsible for the control of infectious diseases.

Before starting therapy The following precepts should be considered before starting:

- Viral infections should not be treated with antibacterials. However, antibacterials are occasionally helpful in controlling secondary bacterial infection (e.g. acute necrotising ulcerative gingivitis secondary to herpes simplex infection);
- Samples should be taken for culture and sensitivity testing; **'blind'** antibacterial prescribing for unexplained pyrexia usually leads to further difficulty in establishing the diagnosis;
- Knowledge of **prevalent organisms** and their current sensitivity is of great help in choosing an antibacterial before bacteriological confirmation is available;
- The **dose** of an antibacterial varies according to a number of factors including age, weight, hepatic function, renal function, and severity of infection. The prescribing of the so-called 'standard' dose in serious infections may result in failure of treatment or even death of the patient; therefore it is important to prescribe a dose appropriate to the condition. An inadequate dose may also increase the likelihood of antibacterial resistance. On the other hand, for an antibacterial with a narrow margin between the toxic and therapeutic dose (e.g. an aminoglycoside) it is also important to avoid an excessive dose and the concentration of the drug in the plasma may need to be monitored;
- The **route** of administration of an antibacterial often depends on the severity of the infection. Life-threatening infections require intravenous therapy. Antibacterials that are well absorbed may be given by mouth even for some serious infections. Parenteral administration is also appropriate when the oral route cannot be used (e.g. because of vomiting) or if absorption is inadequate. Whenever possible, painful intramuscular injections should be avoided in children;
- **Duration** of therapy depends on the nature of the infection and the response to treatment. Courses should not be unduly prolonged because they encourage resistance, they may lead to side-effects and they are costly. However, in certain infections such as tuberculosis or chronic osteomyelitis it is necessary to treat for prolonged periods. Conversely a single dose of an antibacterial may cure uncomplicated urinary-tract infections.

Oral bacterial infections Antibacterial drugs should only be prescribed for the *treatment* of oral infections on the basis of defined need. They may be used in conjunction with (but not as an alternative to) other appropriate measures, such as providing drainage or extracting a tooth.

The 'blind' prescribing of an antibacterial for unexplained pyrexia, cervical lymphadenopathy, or facial swelling can lead to difficulty in establishing the diagnosis. In severe oral infections, a sample should always be taken for bacteriology.

Oral infections which require antibacterial treatment include acute suppurative pulpitis, acute periapical or periodontal abscess, cellulitis, oral-antral fistula (and acute sinusitis), severe pericoronitis, localised osteitis, acute necrotising ulcerative gingivitis, and destructive forms of chronic periodontal disease. Most of these infections are readily resolved by the early establishment of drainage and removal of the cause (typically an infected necrotic pulp). Antibacterials may be indicated if treatment has to be delayed and they are essential in immunocompromised patients or in those with conditions such as diabetes or Paget's disease. Certain rarer infections including bacterial sialadenitis, osteomyelitis, actinomycosis, and infections involving fascial spaces such as Ludwig's angina, require antibiotics and specialist hospital care.

Antibacterial drugs may also be useful after dental surgery in some cases of spreading infection. Infection may spread to involve local lymph nodes, to fascial spaces (where it can cause airway obstruction), or into the bloodstream (where it can lead to cavernous sinus thrombosis and other serious complications). Extension of an infection can also lead to maxillary sinusitis; osteomyelitis is a complication, which usually arises when host resistance is reduced.

If the oral infection fails to respond to antibacterial treatment within 48 hours the antibacterial should be changed, preferably on the basis of bacteriological investigation. Failure to respond may also suggest an incorrect diagnosis, lack of essential additional measures (such as drainage), poor host resistance, or poor patient compliance.

Combination of a penicillin (or erythromycin) with metronidazole may sometimes be helpful for the treatment of severe oral infections or oral infections that have not responded to initial antibacterial treatment.

See also **Penicillins** (section 5.1.1), **Cephalosporins** (section 5.1.2), **Tetracyclines** (section 5.1.3), **Macrolides** (section 5.1.5), **Clindamycin** (section 5.1.6), **Metronidazole** (section 5.1.11), **Fusidic acid** (section 13.10.1.2) .

Superinfection In general, broad-spectrum antibacterial drugs such as the cephalosporins are more likely to be associated with adverse reactions related to the selection of resistant organisms e.g. *fungal infections* or *antibiotic-associated colitis* (pseudomembranous colitis); other problems associated with superinfection include vaginitis and pruritus ani.

Therapy Suggested treatment is shown in table 1. When the pathogen has been isolated treatment may be changed to a more appropriate antibacterial if necessary. If no bacterium is cultured the antibacterial can be continued or stopped on clinical grounds. Infections for which prophylaxis is useful are listed in table 2.

Table 1. Summary of antibacterial therapy

> If treating a patient suspected of suffering from a notifiable disease, the consultant in communicable disease control should be informed (see p. 277)

Gastro-intestinal system

Gastro-enteritis
Antibacterial not usually indicated
Frequently self-limiting and may not be bacterial

Campylobacter enteritis
Ciprofloxacin *or* erythromycin
Frequently self-limiting: treat severe infection

Invasive salmonellosis
Ciprofloxacin *or* cefotaxime
Includes severe infections which may be invasive

Shigellosis
Ciprofloxacin *or* azithromycin [unlicensed indication]
Amoxicillin or trimethoprim can be used if organism sensitive. Antibacterial not indicated for mild cases.

Typhoid fever
Ciprofloxacin *or* cefotaxime
Infections from Indian subcontinent, Middle-East, and South-East Asia may be multiple-antibacterial-resistant and sensitivity should be tested; azithromycin [unlicensed indication] may be an option in mild or moderate disease caused by multiple antibacterial-resistant organisms

Antibiotic-associated colitis (pseudomembranous colitis)
Oral metronidazole *or* oral vancomycin
Give metronidazole by intravenous infusion if oral treatment inappropriate

Biliary-tract infection
Ciprofloxacin *or* gentamicin *or* a cephalosporin

Peritonitis
A cephalosporin (*or* gentamicin) + metronidazole (*or* clindamycin)

Peritoneal dialysis-associated peritonitis
Either vancomycin[1] + ceftazidime added to dialysis fluid *or* vancomycin added to dialysis fluid + ciprofloxacin by mouth
Treat for 14 days or longer

1. Where vancomycin is suggested teicoplanin may be used.

Cardiovascular system

Endocarditis: initial 'blind' therapy
Flucloxacillin (*or* benzylpenicillin if symptoms less severe) + gentamicin
Substitute flucloxacillin (or benzylpenicillin) with vancomycin + rifampicin if cardiac prostheses present, or if penicillin-allergic, or if meticillin-resistant *Staphylococcus aureus* suspected

Endocarditis caused by staphylococci
Flucloxacillin (*or* vancomycin + rifampicin if penicillin-allergic or if meticillin-resistant *Staphylococcus aureus*)
Treat for at least 4 weeks; treat prosthetic valve endocarditis for at least 6 weeks and if using flucloxacillin add rifampicin for at least 2 weeks

Endocarditis caused by streptococci (e.g. viridans streptococci)
Benzylpenicillin (*or* vancomycin[1] if penicillin- allergic or highly penicillin-resistant) + gentamicin
Treat endocarditis caused by fully sensitive streptococci with benzylpenicillin or vancomycin alone for 4 weeks *or* (if no cardiac or embolic complications) with benzylpenicillin + gentamicin for 2 weeks. Treat more resistant organisms for 4–6 weeks (stopping gentamicin after 2 weeks for organisms moderately sensitive to penicillin); if aminoglycoside cannot be used and if streptococci moderately sensitive to penicillin, treat with benzylpenicillin alone for 4 weeks. Treat prosthetic valve endocarditis for at least 6 weeks (stopping gentamicin after 2 weeks if organisms fully sensitive to penicillin)

Endocarditis caused by enterococci (e.g. *Enterococcus faecalis*)
Amoxicillin[2] (*or* vancomycin[1] if penicillin-allergic or penicillin-resistant) + gentamicin
Treat for at least 4 weeks (at least 6 weeks for prosthetic valve endocarditis); if gentamicin-resistant, substitute gentamicin with streptomycin

Endocarditis caused by haemophilus, actinobacillus, cardiobacterium, eikenella, and kingella species ('HACEK' organisms)
Amoxicillin[2] (*or* ceftriazone if amoxicillin-resistant) + low-dose gentamicin
Treat for 4 weeks (6 weeks for prosthetic valve endocarditis); stop gentamicin after 2 weeks

Respiratory system

***Haemophilus influenzae* epiglottitis**
Cefotaxime *or* chloramphenicol
Give intravenously

Exacerbations of chronic bronchitis
Amoxicillin[2] *or* tetracycline (*or* erythromycin[3])
Some pneumococci and *Haemophilus influenzae* strains tetracycline-resistant; 15% *H. influenzae* strains amoxicillin-resistant

Uncomplicated community-acquired pneumonia
Amoxicillin[2] (*or* benzylpenicillin if previously healthy chest *or* erythromycin[3] if penicillin-allergic)
Add flucloxacillin if staphylococci suspected, e.g. in influenza or measles (or vancomycin[1] if meticillin-resistant *Staphylococcus aureus* suspected); treat for 7 days (14–21 days for infections caused by staphylococci); pneumococci with decreased penicillin sensitivity being isolated but not yet common in UK; add erythromycin[3] if atypical pathogens suspected

2. Where amoxicillin is suggested ampicillin may be used.
3. Where erythromycin is suggested another macrolide (e.g. azithromycin or clarithromycin) may be used.

Severe community-acquired pneumonia of unknown aetiology
Cefuroxime (or cefotaxime) + erythromycin[1]
Add flucloxacillin if staphylococci suspected (or vancomycin[2] if meticillin-resistant *Staphylococcus aureus* suspected); treat for 10 days (14–21 days if staphylococci, legionella, or Gram-negative enteric bacilli suspected)

Pneumonia possibly caused by atypical pathogens
Erythromycin[1]
Severe Legionella infections may require addition of rifampicin; tetracycline is an alternative for chlamydial and mycoplasma infections; treat for at least 14 days (14–21 days for legionella)

Hospital-acquired pneumonia
A broad-spectrum cephalosporin (e.g. cefotaxime or ceftazidime) *or* an antipseudomonal penicillin or another antipseudomonal beta-lactam *or* a quinolone (e.g. ciprofloxacin)
An aminoglycoside may be added in severe illness

Central nervous system

Meningitis: initial 'blind' therapy

- Transfer patient urgently to hospital.
- If bacterial meningitis and especially if *meningococcal disease* suspected, general practitioners should give benzylpenicillin (see p. 285 for dose) before urgent transfer to hospital; cefotaxime (section 5.1.2) may be an alternative in penicillin allergy; chloramphenicol (section 5.1.7) may be used if history of immediate hypersensitivity reaction to penicillin or to cephalosporins
- Consider adjunctive treatment with dexamethasone (particularly if pneumococcal meningitis suspected in adults; section 6.3.2) starting before or with first dose of antibacterial; avoid dexamethasone in septic shock, meningococcal disease, or if immunocompromised, or in meningitis following surgery

Meningitis caused by meningococci
Benzylpenicillin *or* cefotaxime
Treat for at least 5 days; substitute chloramphenicol if history of anaphylaxis to penicillin or to cephalosporins. To eliminate nasopharyngeal carriage give rifampicin for 2 days

Meningitis caused by pneumococci
Cefotaxime
Treat for 10–14 days; substitute benzylpenicillin if organism penicillin-sensitive; if organism highly penicillin- and cephalosporin-resistant, add vancomycin and if necessary rifampicin. Consider adjunctive treatment with dexamethasone (section 6.3.2) starting before or with first dose of antibacterial (but may reduce penetration of vancomycin into cerebrospinal fluid)

Meningitis caused by *Haemophilus influenzae*
Cefotaxime
Treat for at least 10 days; substitute chloramphenicol if history of anaphylaxis to penicillin or to cephalosporins or if organism resistant to cefotaxime. Consider adjunctive treatment with dexamethasone (section 6.3.2) starting before or with first dose of antibacterial. For *H. influenzae* type b give rifampicin for 4 days before hospital discharge

Meningitis caused by Listeria
Amoxicillin[3] + gentamicin
Treat for 10–14 days

Urinary tract

Acute pyelonephritis
A broad-spectrum cephalosporin *or* a quinolone
Treat for 10–14 days; longer treatment may be necessary in complicated pyelonephritis

1. Where erythromycin is suggested another macrolide (e.g. azithromycin or clarithromycin) may be used.
2. Where vancomycin is suggested teicoplanin may be used.
3. Where amoxicillin is suggested ampicillin may be used.

Acute prostatitis
A quinolone *or* trimethoprim
Treat for 28 days; in severe infection, start treatment with a high dose broad-spectrum cephalosporin (e.g. cefuroxime or cefotaxime) + gentamicin

'Lower' urinary-tract infection
Trimethoprim *or* nitrofurantoin *or* amoxicillin[3] *or* oral cephalosporin
Treat for 7 days but a short course (e.g. 3 days) of trimethoprim or nitrofurantoin is usually adequate for uncomplicated urinary-tract infections in women. See also section 5.1.13

Genital system

Syphilis
Benzathine benzylpenicillin [unlicensed] *or* doxycycline *or* erythromycin
Treat early syphilis with benzathine benzylpenicillin as a single dose (repeat dose after 7 days for women in the third trimester of pregnancy) or with doxycycline or erythromycin for 14 days. Treat late latent syphilis (asymptomatic infection of more than 2 years) with doxycycline for 28 days or with benzathine benzylpenicillin once weekly for 2 weeks. Treat asymptomatic contacts of patients with infectious syphilis with doxycycline for 14 days. Contact tracing recommended.

Uncomplicated gonorrhoea
Cefixime [unlicensed indication] *or* ciprofloxacin
Single-dose treatment in uncomplicated infection. Choice depends on locality where infection acquired. Pharyngeal infection requires treatment with ceftriaxone. Use ciprofloxacin only if organism sensitive. Contact-tracing recommended; remember chlamydia

Uncomplicated genital chlamydial infection, non-gonococcal urethritis and non-specific genital infection
Doxycycline *or* azithromycin
Treat with doxycycline for 7 days or with azithromycin as a single dose; alternatively, treat with erythromycin for 14 days. Contact tracing recommended

Pelvic inflammatory disease
Doxycycline + metronidazole + i/m ceftriaxone *or* ofloxacin + metronidazole
Treat for at least 14 days (use i/m ceftriaxone as a single dose). In severely ill patients initial treatment with doxycycline + i/v ceftriaxone (as a single dose) + i/v metronidazole, then switch to oral treatment with doxycycline + metronidazole to complete 14 days' treatment. Contact tracing recommended

Bacterial vaginosis
Oral or topical metronidazole *or* topical clindamycin
Oral treatment for 5–7 days (or with high-dose metronidazole as a single dose); topical treatment for 5 days (7 days with clindamycin)

Blood

Community-acquired septicaemia
A broad-spectrum antipseudomonal penicillin (e.g. *Tazocin®*, *Timentin®*) *or* a broad-spectrum cephalosporin (e.g. ceftazidime, cefotaxime)
Add aminoglycoside if pseudomonas suspected, or if severe sepsis, or if patient recently discharged from hospital. Add vancomycin[2] if meticillin-resistant *Staphylococcus aureus* suspected. Add metronidazole to broad-spectrum cephalosporin if anaerobic infection suspected

Hospital-acquired septicaemia
A broad-spectrum antipseudomonal beta-lactam antibacterial (e.g. *Tazocin®*, *Timentin®*, ceftazidime, imipenem (with cilastatin as *Primaxin®*) *or* meropenem)
Add aminoglycoside if pseudomonas suspected, or if multiple-resistant organisms suspected, or if severe sepsis. Add vancomycin[2] if meticillin-resistant *Staphylococcus aureus* suspected. Add metronidazole to broad-spectrum cephalosporin if anaerobic infection suspected

Septicaemia related to vascular catheter

Vancomycin[1]

Add an aminoglycoside + a broad-spectrum antipseudomonal beta-lactam if Gram-negative sepsis suspected, especially in the immunocompromised. Consider removing vascular catheter, particularly if infection caused by *Staphylococcus aureus*, pseudomonas, or candida

Meningococcal septicaemia

Benzylpenicillin *or* cefotaxime

If meningococcal disease suspected, general practitioners advised to give a single dose of benzylpenicillin (see p. 285 for dose) before urgent transfer to hospital; cefotaxime (section 5.1.2) may be an alternative in penicillin allergy; chloramphenicol may be used if history of anaphylaxis to penicillin or to cephalosporins. To eliminate nasopharyngeal carriage give rifampicin for 2 days

Musculoskeletal system

Osteomyelitis

Flucloxacillin *or* clindamycin if penicillin-allergic (*or* vancomycin[1] if resistant *Staphylococcus epidermidis* or meticillin-resistant *Staph. aureus*)

Treat acute infection for 4–6 weeks and chronic infection for at least 12 weeks. Combine vancomycin[1] with either fusidic acid or rifampicin if prostheses present or if life-threatening condition

Septic arthritis

Flucloxacillin + fusidic acid *or* clindamycin alone if penicillin-allergic (*or* vancomycin[1] if resistant *Staphylococcus epidermidis* or meticillin-resistant *Staph. aureus*) (*or* cefotaxime if gonococcal arthritis or Gram-negative infection)

Treat usually for 6 weeks (longer if infection complicated or if prosthesis present; treat for 2 weeks if gonococcal infection). Combine vancomycin[1] with either fusidic acid or rifampicin if prostheses present or if life-threatening condition

Eye

Purulent conjunctivitis

Chloramphenicol *or* gentamicin eye-drops

Ear, nose, and oropharynx

Pericoronitis

Metronidazole *or* amoxicillin

Antibacterial required only in presence of systemic features of infection or of trismus or persistent swelling despite local treatment; treat for 3 days or until symptoms resolve

Acute necrotising ulcerative gingivitis

Metronidazole *or* amoxicillin

Antibacterial required only if systemic features of infection; treat for 3 days or until symptoms resolve

Periapical or periodontal abscess

Amoxicillin *or* metronidazole

Antibacterial required only in severe disease with cellulitis or if systemic features of infection; treat for 5 days

Periodontitis

Metronidazole *or* doxycycline

Antibacterial required for severe disease or disease unresponsive to local treatment

Throat infections

Phenoxymethylpenicillin (*or* erythromycin[2] if penicillin-allergic)

Most throat infections are caused by viruses and many do not require antibiotic therapy. Consider antibacterial, if history of valvular heart disease, if marked systemic upset, if peritonsillar cellulitis or if at increased risk from acute infection (e.g. in immunosuppression, diabetes); prescribe antibacterial for beta-haemolytic streptococcal pharyngitis; treat for 10 days. **Avoid** amoxicillin if possibility of glandular fever, see section 5.1.1.3. Initial parenteral therapy (in severe infection) with benzylpenicillin, then oral therapy with phenoxymethylpenicillin *or* amoxicillin[3]

Sinusitis

Amoxicillin[3] *or* doxycycline *or* erythromycin[2]

Antibacterial should usually be used only for persistent symptoms and purulent discharge lasting at least 7 days or if severe symptoms; treat for 7 days

Otitis externa

Flucloxacillin (*or* erythromycin[2] if penicillin-allergic)

Consider systemic antibacterial if spreading cellulitis or patient systemically unwell. Use ciprofloxacin (or an aminoglycoside) if pseudomonas suspected. For topical preparations see section 12.1.1

Otitis media

Amoxicillin[3] (*or* erythromycin[2] if penicillin-allergic)

Many infections caused by viruses. Most uncomplicated cases resolve without antibacterial treatment. In children without systemic features, antibacterial treatment may be started after 72 hours if no improvement (earlier in immunocompromised patients, children under 2 years, or if deterioration). Treat for 5 days (longer if severely ill); initial parenteral therapy in severe infections; consider co-amoxiclav or ceftriaxone if no improvement after 24–48 hours

Skin

Impetigo

Topical fusidic acid (*or* mupirocin if meticillin-resistant *Staphylococcus aureus*); oral flucloxacillin *or* erythromycin[2] if widespread

Topical treatment for 7 days usually adequate; max. duration of topical treatment 10 days; seek local microbiology advice before using topical treatment in hospital; oral treatment for 7 days; add phenoxymethylpenicillin to flucloxacillin if streptococcal infection suspected

Erysipelas

Phenoxymethylpenicillin (*or* erythromycin[2] if penicillin-allergic)

Treat for at least 7 days; add flucloxacillin to phenoxymethylpenicillin if staphylococcus suspected; substitute benzylpenicillin for phenoxymethylpenicillin if parenteral treatment required

Cellulitis

Benzylpenicillin + flucloxacillin (*or* erythromycin[2] alone if penicillin-allergic)

Substitute phenoxymethylpenicillin for benzylpenicillin if oral treatment appropriate. Discontinue flucloxacillin if streptococcal infection confirmed. Substitute treatment with broad-spectrum antibacterials if Gram-negative bacteria or anaerobes suspected

Animal and human bites

Co-amoxiclav alone (*or* doxycycline + metronidazole if penicillin-allergic)

Cleanse wound thoroughly. For tetanus-prone wound, give human tetanus immunoglobulin (with a tetanus-containing vaccine if necessary, according to immunisation history and risk of infection), see under Tetanus Vaccines, section 14.4. Consider rabies prophylaxis (section 14.4) for bites from animals in endemic countries; assess risk of blood-borne viruses

Acne

See section 13.6

1. Where vancomycin is suggested teicoplanin may be used.
2. Where erythromycin is suggested another macrolide (e.g. azithromycin or clarithromycin) may be used.
3. Where amoxicillin is suggested ampicillin may be used.

Table 2. Summary of antibacterial prophylaxis

Prevention of recurrence of *rheumatic fever*

Phenoxymethylpenicillin 250 mg twice daily *or* sulfadiazine 1 g daily (500 mg daily for patients under 30 kg)

Prevention of secondary case of group A *streptococcal infection*[1]

Phenoxymethylpenicillin 250–500 mg every 6 hours for 10 days; CHILD under 1 year 62.5 mg every 6 hours, 1–5 years 125 mg every 6 hours, 6–12 years 250 mg every 6 hours

Patients who are penicillin allergic,

either erythromycin ADULT and CHILD over 8 years, 250–500 mg every 6 hours for 10 days; CHILD under 2 years 125 mg every 6 hours, 2–8 years 250 mg every 6 hours

or azithromycin [unlicensed indication] 500 mg once daily for 5 days; CHILD over 6 months, 12 mg/kg (max. 500 mg) once daily

Prevention of secondary case of *meningococcal meningitis*[2]

Rifampicin 600 mg every 12 hours for 2 days; CHILD 10 mg/kg (under 1 year, 5 mg/kg) every 12 hours for 2 days

or ciprofloxacin [unlicensed indication] 500 mg as a single dose; CHILD 2–5 years 125 mg; 5–12 years 250 mg

or i/m ceftriaxone [unlicensed indication] 250 mg as a single dose; CHILD under 12 years 125 mg

Prevention of secondary case of *Haemophilus influenzae type b disease*[2]

Rifampicin 600 mg once daily for 4 days (regimen of choice for adults); CHILD 1–3 months 10 mg/kg once daily for 4 days, over 3 months 20 mg/kg once daily for 4 days (max. 600 mg daily)

Prevention of secondary case of *diphtheria* in non-immune patient

Erythromycin 500 mg every 6 hours for 7 days; CHILD up to 2 years 125 mg every 6 hours, 2–8 years 250 mg every 6 hours

Treat for further 10 days if nasopharyngeal swabs positive after first 7 days' treatment

1. Prophylaxis is recommended for mother and baby if either develops invasive group A streptococcal disease in the neonatal period, for close contacts (of a case of group A streptococcal disease) who have symptoms of localised group A streptococcal infection, and for a household with 2 or more cases of invasive group A streptococcal disease within 30 days
2. For details of those who should receive chemoprophylaxis contact a consultant in communicable disease control (or a consultant in infectious diseases or the local Health Protection Agency laboratory). Unless there has been direct exposure of the mouth or nose to infectious droplets from a patient with meningococcal disease who has received less than 24 hours of antibacterial treatment, healthcare workers do not generally require chemoprophylaxis.
3. Where erythromycin is suggested another macrolide (e.g. azithromycin or clarithromycin) may be used.

Prevention of secondary case of *pertussis* in non-immune patient or partially immune patient

Erythromycin[3] ADULT and CHILD over 8 years, 250–500 mg every 6 hours for 7 days; CHILD under 2 years 125 mg every 6 hours, 2–8 years 250 mg every 6 hours

Prevention of *pneumococcal infection* in asplenia or in patients with sickle cell disease

Phenoxymethylpenicillin 500 mg every 12 hours; CHILD under 5 years 125 mg every 12 hours, 6–12 years 250 mg every 12 hours—if cover also needed for *H. influenzae* in CHILD give amoxicillin instead (under 5 years 125 mg every 12 hours, over 5 years 250 mg every 12 hours)

Note Antibiotic prophylaxis is not fully reliable; for vaccines in asplenia see p. 642

Prevention of *gas-gangrene* in high lower-limb amputations or following major trauma

Benzylpenicillin 300–600 mg every 6 hours for 5 days *or* if penicillin-allergic metronidazole 400–500 mg every 8 hours

Prevention of *tuberculosis* in susceptible close contacts or those who have become tuberculin positive[4]

Isoniazid 300 mg daily for 6 months; CHILD 5 mg/kg daily (max. 300 mg daily)

or isoniazid 300 mg daily + rifampicin 600 mg daily (450 mg if less than 50 kg) for 3 months; CHILD isoniazid 5 mg/kg daily (max. 300 mg daily) + rifampicin 10 mg/kg daily (max. 450 mg daily if body-weight less than 50 kg; max. 600 mg daily if body-weight over 50 kg)

or (if isoniazid-resistant tuberculosis in patients under 35 years) rifampicin 600 mg daily (450 mg if less than 50 kg) for 6 months; CHILD 10 mg/kg daily (max. 450 mg daily if body-weight less than 50 kg; max. 600 mg daily if body-weight over 50 kg)

Prevention of infection in *gastro-intestinal* procedures

Operations on stomach or oesophagus for carcinoma

Single dose[5] of i/v gentamicin *or* i/v cefuroxime

Open biliary surgery

Single dose[5] of i/v cefuroxime + i/v metronidazole[6] *or* i/v gentamicin + i/v metronidazole[6]

4. For details of those who should receive chemoprophylaxis contact the lead clinician for local tuberculosis services (or a consultant in communicable disease control). See also section 5.1.9, for advice on immunocompromised patients and on prevention of tuberculosis
5. Additional intra-operative or postoperative doses of antibacterial may be given for prolonged procedures or if there is major blood loss
6. Metronidazole may alternatively be given by suppository but to allow adequate absorption, it should be given 2 hours before surgery

Resections of colon and rectum for carcinoma, and resections in inflammatory bowel disease, and appendicectomy

Single dose[1] of i/v gentamicin + i/v metronidazole[2] *or* i/v cefuroxime + i/v metronidazole[2] *or* i/v co-amoxiclav alone

Endoscopic retrograde cholangiopancreatography

Single dose of i/v gentamicin *or* oral or i/v ciprofloxacin

Prophylaxis particularly recommended if bile stasis, pancreatic pseudocyst, previous cholangitis or neutropenia

Prevention of infection in *orthopaedic* surgery

Joint replacement including hip and knee and management of fractures

Single dose[1] of i/v cefuroxime or i/v flucloxacillin

Substitute i/v vancomycin if history of allergy to penicillins or to cephalosporins or if high risk of meticillin-resistant *Staphylococcus aureus*; use cefuroxime + metronidazole for complex open fractures with extensive soft-tissue damage; prophylaxis continued for 24 hours in open fractures (longer if complex open fractures)

Prevention of infection in *urological* procedures

Transrectal prostate biopsy

Single dose[1] of oral ciprofloxacin + oral metronidazole *or* i/v gentamicin + i/v metronidazole[2]

Transurethral resection of prostate

Single dose[1] of oral ciprofloxacin *or* i/v gentamicin *or* i/v cefuroxime

Prevention of infection in *obstetric* and *gynaecological* surgery

Caesarean section

Single dose[1] of i/v cefuroxime

Administer immediately after umbilical cord is clamped; substitute i/v clindamycin if history of allergy to penicillins or cephalosporins

Hysterectomy

Single dose[1] of i/v cefuroxime + i/v metronidazole[2] *or* i/v gentamicin + i/v metronidazole[2] *or* i/v co-amoxiclav alone

Termination of pregnancy

Single dose[1] of oral metronidazole

If genital chlamydial infection cannot be ruled out, give doxycycline (section 5.1.3) postoperatively

Prevention of infection in *vascular* surgery

Reconstructive arterial surgery of abdomen, pelvis or legs

Single dose[1] of i/v cefuroxime *or* i/v ciprofloxacin

Add i/v metronidazole for patients at risk from anaerobic infections including those with diabetes, gangrene, or undergoing amputation; add i/v vancomycin if high risk of meticillin-resistant *Staphylococcus aureus*

Prevention of *endocarditis*

NICE guidance

Antimicrobial prophylaxis against infective endocarditis in adults and children undergoing interventional procedures (March 2008)

Antibacterial prophylaxis and chlorhexidine mouthwash are **not** recommended for the prevention of endocarditis in patients undergoing dental procedures.

Antibacterial prophylaxis is **not** recommended for the prevention of endocarditis in patients undergoing procedures of the:

- upper and lower respiratory tract (including ear, nose, and throat procedures and bronchoscopy);
- genito-urinary tract (including urological, gynaecological, and obstetric procedures);
- upper and lower gastro-intestinal tract.

Whilst these procedures can cause bacteraemia, there is no clear association with the development of infective endocarditis. Prophylaxis may expose patients to the adverse effects of antimicrobials when the evidence of benefit has not been proven.

Any infection in patients at risk of endocarditis[3] should be investigated promptly and treated appropriately to reduce the risk of endocarditis.

If patients at risk of endocarditis[3] are undergoing a gastro-intestinal or genito-urinary tract procedure at a site where infection is suspected, they should receive appropriate antibacterial therapy that includes cover against organisms that cause endocarditis.

Patients at risk of endocarditis[3] should be:

- advised to maintain good oral hygiene;
- told how to recognise signs of infective endocarditis, and advised when to seek expert advice.

Dermatological procedures

Advice of a Working Party of the British Society for Antimicrobial Chemotherapy is that patients who undergo dermatological procedures[4] do not require antibacterial prophylaxis against endocarditis.

1. Additional intra-operative or postoperative doses of antibacterial may be given for prolonged procedures or if there is major blood loss
2. Metronidazole may alternatively be given by suppository but to allow adequate absorption, it should be given 2 hours before surgery
3. Patients at risk of endocarditis include those with valve replacement, acquired valvular heart disease with stenosis or regurgitation, structural congenital heart disease (including surgically corrected or palliated structural conditions, but excluding isolated atrial septal defect, fully repaired ventricular septal defect, fully repaired patent ductus arteriosus, and closure devices considered to be endothelialised), hypertrophic cardiomyopathy, or a previous episode of infective endocarditis.
4. The British Association of Dermatologists Therapy Guidelines and Audit Subcommittee advise that such dermatological procedures include skin biopsies and excision of moles or of malignant lesions

Joint prostheses and dental treatment

Advice of a Working Party of the British Society for Antimicrobial Chemotherapy is that patients with prosthetic joint implants (including total hip replacements) do not require antibiotic prophylaxis for dental treatment. The Working Party considers that it is unacceptable to expose patients to the adverse effects of antibiotics when there is no evidence that such prophylaxis is of any benefit, but that those who develop any intercurrent infection require prompt treatment with antibiotics to which the infecting organisms are sensitive.

The Working Party has commented that joint infections have rarely been shown to follow dental procedures and are even more rarely caused by oral streptococci.

Immunosuppression and indwelling intraperitoneal catheters

Advice of a Working Party of the British Society for Antimicrobial Chemotherapy is that patients who are immunosuppressed (including transplant patients) and patients with indwelling intraperitoneal catheters do not require antibiotic prophylaxis for dental treatment provided there is no other indication for prophylaxis.

The Working Party has commented that there is little evidence that dental treatment is followed by infection in immunosuppressed and immunodeficient patients nor is there evidence that dental treatment is followed by infection in patients with indwelling intraperitoneal catheters.

5.1.1 Penicillins

5.1.1.1 Benzylpenicillin and phenoxymethylpenicillin
5.1.1.2 Penicillinase-resistant penicillins
5.1.1.3 Broad-spectrum penicillins
5.1.1.4 Antipseudomonal penicillins
5.1.1.5 Mecillinams

The penicillins are bactericidal and act by interfering with bacterial cell wall synthesis. They diffuse well into body tissues and fluids, but penetration into the cerebrospinal fluid is poor except when the meninges are inflamed. They are excreted in the urine in therapeutic concentrations.

Hypersensitivity reactions The most important side-effect of the penicillins is hypersensitivity which causes rashes and anaphylaxis and can be fatal. Allergic reactions to penicillins occur in 1–10% of exposed individuals; anaphylactic reactions occur in fewer than 0.05% of treated patients. Patients with a history of atopic allergy (e.g. asthma, eczema, hay fever) are at a higher risk of anaphylactic reactions to penicillins. Individuals with a history of anaphylaxis, urticaria, or rash immediately after penicillin administration are at risk of immediate hypersensitivity to a penicillin; these individuals should not receive a penicillin. Patients who are allergic to one penicillin will be allergic to all because the hypersensitivity is related to the basic penicillin structure. As patients with a history of immediate hypersensitivity to penicillins may also react to the cephalosporins and other beta-lactam antibiotics, they should not receive these antibiotics; aztreonam may be less likely to cause hypersensitivity in penicillin-sensitive patients and can be used with caution. If a penicillin (or another beta-lactam antibiotic) is essential in an individual with immediate hypersensitivity to penicillin then specialist advice should be sought on hypersensitivity testing.

Individuals with a history of a minor rash (i.e. non-confluent, non-pruritic rash restricted to a small area of the body) or a rash that occurs more than 72 hours after penicillin administration are probably not allergic to penicillin and in these individuals a penicillin should not be withheld unnecessarily for serious infections; the possibility of an allergic reaction should, however, be borne in mind. Other beta-lactam antibiotics (including cephalosporins) can be used in these patients.

A rare but serious toxic effect of the penicillins is encephalopathy due to cerebral irritation. This may result from excessively high doses or in patients with severe renal failure. The penicillins should **not** be given by intrathecal injection because they can cause encephalopathy which may be fatal.

Another problem relating to high doses of penicillin, or normal doses given to patients with renal failure, is the accumulation of electrolyte since most injectable penicillins contain either sodium or potassium.

Diarrhoea frequently occurs during oral penicillin therapy. It is most common with broad-spectrum penicillins, which can also cause antibiotic-associated colitis.

5.1.1.1 Benzylpenicillin and phenoxymethylpenicillin

Benzylpenicillin (Penicillin G) remains an important and useful antibiotic but is inactivated by bacterial beta-lactamases. It is effective for many streptococcal (including pneumococcal), gonococcal, and meningococcal infections and also for anthrax (section 5.1.12), diphtheria, gas-gangrene, leptospirosis, and treatment of Lyme disease (section 5.1.1.3). Pneumococci, meningococci, and gonococci which have decreased sensitivity to penicillin have been isolated; benzylpenicillin is no longer the drug of first choice for pneumococcal meningitis. Although benzylpenicillin is effective in the treatment of tetanus, metronidazole (section 5.1.11) is preferred. Benzylpenicillin is inactivated by gastric acid and absorption from the gut is low; therefore it is best given by injection.

Benzathine benzylpenicillin (available on a named-patient basis from specialist importing companies, see p. 888) is used for the treatment of early syphilis and late latent syphilis; it is given by intramuscular injection.

Phenoxymethylpenicillin (Penicillin V) has a similar antibacterial spectrum to benzylpenicillin, but is less active. It is gastric acid-stable, so is suitable for oral administration. It should not be used for serious infections because absorption can be unpredictable and plasma concentrations variable. It is indicated principally for respiratory-tract infections in children, for streptococcal tonsillitis, and for continuing treatment after one or more injections of benzylpenicillin when clinical response has begun. It should not be used for meningococcal or gonococcal infections. Phenoxymethylpenicillin is used for prophylaxis against streptococcal infections following rheumatic fever and against pneumococcal infections following splenectomy or in sickle-cell disease.

Oral infections Phenoxymethylpenicillin is effective for dentoalveolar abscess.

BENZYLPENICILLIN
(Penicillin G)

Indications throat infections, otitis media, endocarditis, meningococcal disease, pneumonia, cellulitis (Table 1, section 5.1); anthrax; prophylaxis in limb amputation (Table 2, section 5.1); see also notes above

Cautions history of allergy; false-positive urinary glucose (if tested for reducing substances); renal impairment (Appendix 3); **interactions:** Appendix 1 (penicillins)

Contra-indications penicillin hypersensitivity

Side-effects hypersensitivity reactions including urticaria, fever, joint pains, rashes, angioedema, anaphylaxis, serum sickness-like reaction; *rarely* CNS toxicity including convulsions (especially with high doses or in severe renal impairment), interstitial nephritis, haemolytic anaemia, leucopenia, thrombocytopenia, and coagulation disorders; also reported diarrhoea (including antibiotic-associated colitis)

Dose

- By intramuscular *or* by slow intravenous injection *or* by infusion, 2.4–4.8 g daily in 4 divided doses, increased if necessary in more serious infections (single doses over 1.2 g intravenous route only; see also below); PRETERM NEONATE and NEONATE under 1 week, 50 mg/kg daily in 2 divided doses; NEONATE 1–4 weeks, 75 mg/kg daily in 3 divided doses; CHILD 1 month–12 years, 100 mg/kg daily in 4 divided doses (higher doses may be required, see also below); intravenous route recommended in neonates and infants
- Endocarditis (in combination with another antibacterial if necessary, see Table 1, section 5.1), by slow intravenous injection *or* by infusion, 7.2 g daily in 6 divided doses, increased if necessary (e.g. in enterococcal endocarditis or if benzylpenicillin used alone) to 14.4 g daily in 6 divided doses
- Anthrax (in combination with other antibacterials, see also section 5.1.12), by slow intravenous injection *or* by infusion, 2.4 g every 4 hours; CHILD 150 mg/kg daily in 4 divided doses
- Intrapartum prophylaxis against group B streptococcal infection, by slow intravenous injection *or* by infusion, initially 3 g then 1.5 g every 4 hours until delivery
- Meningitis, meningococcal disease, by slow intravenous injection *or* by infusion, 2.4 g every 4 hours; PRETERM NEONATE and NEONATE, 225 mg/kg daily in 3 divided doses; CHILD 1 month–12 years, 180–300 mg/kg daily in 4–6 divided doses

Important. If bacterial meningitis and especially if meningococcal disease is suspected general practitioners are advised to give a single injection of benzylpenicillin by intravenous injection (or by intramuscular injection) before transferring the patient urgently to hospital. Suitable doses are: ADULT 1.2 g; INFANT under 1 year 300 mg; CHILD 1–9 years 600 mg, 10 years and over as for adult. In **penicillin allergy**, cefotaxime (section 5.1.2) may be an alternative; chloramphenicol may be used if there is a history of anaphylaxis to penicillins

- By intrathecal injection, **not** recommended

Note Benzylpenicillin doses in BNF may differ from those in product literature

Crystapen® (Britannia) PoM
Injection, powder for reconstitution, benzylpenicillin sodium (unbuffered), net price 600-mg vial = 46p, 2-vial 'GP pack' = £1.90; 1.2-g vial = 92p
Electrolytes Na^+ 1.68 mmol/600-mg vial; 3.36 mmol/1.2-g vial

PHENOXYMETHYLPENICILLIN
(Penicillin V)

Indications oral infections (see notes above); tonsillitis, otitis media, erysipelas, cellulitis; group A streptococcal infection, rheumatic fever and pneumococcal infection prophylaxis (Table 2, section 5.1)

Cautions see under Benzylpenicillin; **interactions:** Appendix 1 (penicillins)

Contra-indications see under Benzylpenicillin

Side-effects see under Benzylpenicillin

Dose

- 500 mg every 6 hours increased up to 1 g every 6 hours in severe infections; CHILD up to 1 year 62.5 mg every 6 hours, increased up to 12.5 mg/kg every 6 hours in severe infections; 1–6 years, 125 mg every 6 hours, increased up to 12.5 mg/kg every 6 hours in severe infections; 6–12 years, 250 mg every 6 hours, increased up to 12.5 mg/kg every 6 hours in severe infections

Note Phenoxymethylpenicillin doses in the BNF may differ from those in product literature

Phenoxymethylpenicillin (Non-proprietary) PoM
Tablets, phenoxymethylpenicillin (as potassium salt) 250 mg, net price 28-tab pack = £3.26. Label: 9, 23
Oral solution, phenoxymethylpenicillin (as potassium salt) for reconstitution with water, net price 125 mg/5 mL, 100 mL = £1.90; 250 mg/5 mL, 100 mL = £2.55. Label: 9, 23

Dental prescribing on NHS Phenoxymethylpenicillin Tablets and Oral Solution may be prescribed

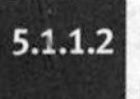

5.1.1.2 Penicillinase-resistant penicillins

Most staphylococci are now resistant to benzylpenicillin because they produce penicillinases. **Flucloxacillin**, however, is not inactivated by these enzymes and is thus effective in infections caused by penicillin-resistant staphylococci, which is the sole indication for its use. Flucloxacillin is acid-stable and can, therefore, be given by mouth as well as by injection.

Flucloxacillin is well absorbed from the gut. For CSM warning on hepatic disorders see under Flucloxacillin.

Temocillin is active against Gram-negative bacteria and is stable against a wide range of beta-lactamases. It should be reserved for the treatment of infections caused by beta-lactamase-producing strains of Gram-negative bacteria, including those resistant to third-generation cephalosporins. Temocillin is not active against *Pseudomonas aeruginosa* or *Acinetobacter* spp.

MRSA Infection from *Staphylococcus aureus* strains resistant to meticillin [now discontinued] (meticillin-resistant *Staph. aureus*, MRSA) and to flucloxacillin can be difficult to manage. Treatment is guided by the sensitivity of the infecting strain.

A **tetracycline** can be used for *skin* and *soft-tissue infections* caused by MRSA; **clindamycin** is an alternative. A **glycopeptide** (e.g. vancomycin, section 5.1.7) can be used for severe skin and soft-tissue infections associated with MRSA; if a glycopeptide is unsuitable, **linezolid** (section 5.1.7) can be used on expert advice. As linezolid is **not** active against Gram-negative organisms, it can be used for mixed skin and soft-tissue infections only when other treatments are not available; linezolid must be given with other antibacterials if the infection also involves Gram-negative organisms. **Rifampicin** or **sodium fusidate** should **not** be used alone because resistance may develop rapidly. A combination of a glycopeptide and sodium fusidate *or* a glycopeptide and rifampicin *or* rifampicin and sodium fusidate can be considered for skin and soft-tissue infections that have failed to respond to a single antibacterial.

The combination of the streptogramin antibiotics **quinupristin** and **dalfopristin** (section 5.1.7) should be reserved for skin and soft-tissue infections that have not responded to other antibacterials or for patients who cannot tolerate other antibacterials. **Tigecycline** (section 5.1.3) and **daptomycin** (section 5.1.7) are licensed for the treatment of complicated skin and soft-tissue infections; they may have a limited role in infections caused by MRSA.

A **tetracycline** or **clindamycin** can be used for *bronchiectasis* caused by MRSA. A **glycopeptide** can be used for *pneumonia* associated with MRSA; if a glycopeptide is unsuitable, **linezolid** can be used on expert advice. Linezolid must be given with other antibacterials if the infection also involves Gram-negative organisms. **Quinupristin** and **dalfopristin** should be reserved for hospital acquired pneumonia that has not responded to other antibacterials or for patients who cannot tolerate other antibacterials.

A **tetracycline** can be used for *urinary-tract infections* caused by MRSA; **trimethoprim** or **nitrofurantoin** are alternatives. A **glycopeptide** can be used for urinary-tract infections that are severe or resistant to other antibacterials.

A **glycopeptide** can be used for *septicaemia* associated with MRSA.

For the management of *endocarditis, osteomyelitis*, or *septic arthritis* associated with MRSA, see Table 1, section 5.1.

Prophylaxis with vancomycin or teicoplanin (alone or in combination with another antibacterial active against other pathogens) is appropriate for patients undergoing surgery if:

- there is a history of MRSA colonisation or infection without documented eradication;
- there is a risk that the patient's MRSA carriage has recurred;
- the patient comes from an area with a high prevalence of MRSA

For eradication of nasal carriage of MRSA, see section 12.2.3.

FLUCLOXACILLIN

Indications infections due to beta-lactamase-producing staphylococci including otitis externa; adjunct in pneumonia, impetigo, cellulitis, osteomyelitis and in staphylococcal endocarditis (Table 1, section 5.1)

Cautions see under Benzylpenicillin (section 5.1.1.1); also hepatic impairment (see CSM advice below); risk of kernicterus in jaundiced neonates when high doses given parenterally

CSM advice (hepatic disorders)

CSM has advised that very rarely cholestatic jaundice and hepatitis may occur up to several weeks after treatment with flucloxacillin has been stopped. Administration for more than 2 weeks and increasing age are risk factors. CSM has reminded that:

- flucloxacillin should not be used in patients with a history of hepatic dysfunction associated with flucloxacillin;
- flucloxacillin should be used with caution in patients with hepatic impairment;
- careful enquiry should be made about hypersensitivity reactions to beta-lactam antibacterials.

Contra-indications see under Benzylpenicillin (section 5.1.1.1)

Side-effects see under Benzylpenicillin (section 5.1.1.1); also gastro-intestinal disturbances; *very rarely* hepatitis and cholestatic jaundice (see also CSM advice above)

Dose

- By mouth, 250–500 mg every 6 hours, at least 30 minutes before food; CHILD under 2 years quarter adult dose; 2–10 years half adult dose
- By intramuscular injection, 250–500 mg every 6 hours; CHILD under 2 years quarter adult dose; 2–10 years half adult dose
- By slow intravenous injection *or* by intravenous infusion, 0.25–2 g every 6 hours; CHILD under 2 years quarter adult dose; 2–10 years half adult dose

  Endocarditis (in combination with another antibacterial, see Table 1, section 5.1), body-weight under 85 kg, 8 g daily in 4 divided doses; body-weight over 85 kg, 12 g daily in 6 divided doses

  Osteomyelitis (see Table 1, section 5.1), up to 8 g daily in 3–4 divided doses
- Surgical prophylaxis, by slow intravenous injection *or* by intravenous infusion, 1–2 g at induction; up to 4 further doses of 500 mg may be given every 6 hours by mouth, *or* by intramuscular injection, *or* by slow intravenous injection *or* by intravenous infusion for high risk procedures

Note Flucloxacillin doses in BNF may differ from those in product literature

Flucloxacillin (Non-proprietary) PoM

Capsules, flucloxacillin (as sodium salt) 250 mg, net price 28 = £2.06; 500 mg, 28 = £4.91. Label: 9, 23
Brands include *Floxapen®*, *Fluclomix®*, *Ladropen®*

Oral solution (= elixir or syrup), flucloxacillin (as sodium salt) for reconstitution with water, 125 mg/5 mL, net price 100 mL = £3.57; 250 mg/5 mL, 100 mL = £6.81. Label: 9, 23
Brands include *Ladropen®*

Injection, powder for reconstitution, flucloxacillin (as sodium salt). Net price 250-mg vial = 91p; 500-mg vial = £1.81; 1-g vial = £3.63

Floxapen® (GSK) PoM

Suspension (= syrup), flucloxacillin (as magnesium salt) for reconstitution with water, 125 mg/5 mL, net price 100 mL = £3.25; 250 mg/5 mL, 100 mL = £6.48. Label: 9, 23

TEMOCILLIN

Indications septicaemia, urinary-tract infections, lower respiratory-tract infections caused by susceptible Gram-negative bacteria

Cautions see under Benzylpenicillin (section 5.1.1.1); renal impairment (Appendix 3); pregnancy (Appendix 4); breast-feeding (Appendix 5)

Contra-indications see under Benzylpenicillin (section 5.1.1.1)

Side-effects see under Benzylpenicillin (section 5.1.1.1)

Dose

- By intramuscular injection *or* by intravenous injection over 3–4 minutes, *or* by intravenous infusion, ADULT and CHILD over 12 years (body-weight over 45 kg), 1–2 g every 12 hours

  Uncomplicated urinary-tract infections, ADULT and CHILD over 12 years (body-weight over 45 kg), 1 g daily as a single daily dose or in divided doses

Negaban® (Eumedica) PoM

Injection, powder for reconstitution, temocillin (as sodium salt), net price 1-g vial = £25.45

Electrolytes Na^+ 4.35 mmol/g

5.1.1.3 Broad-spectrum penicillins

Ampicillin is active against certain Gram-positive and Gram-negative organisms but is inactivated by penicillinases including those produced by *Staphylococcus aureus* and by common Gram-negative bacilli such as *Escherichia coli*. Almost all staphylococci, 50% of *E. coli* strains and 15% of *Haemophilus influenzae* strains are now resistant. The likelihood of resistance should therefore be considered before using ampicillin for the 'blind' treatment of infections; in particular, it should not be used for hospital patients without checking sensitivity.

Ampicillin is well excreted in the bile and urine. It is principally indicated for the treatment of exacerbations of chronic bronchitis and middle ear infections, both of which may be due to *Streptococcus pneumoniae* and *H. influenzae*, and for urinary-tract infections (section 5.1.13).

Ampicillin can be given by mouth but less than half the dose is absorbed, and absorption is further decreased by the presence of food in the gut.

Maculopapular rashes commonly occur with ampicillin (and amoxicillin) but are not usually related to true penicillin allergy. They almost always occur in patients with glandular fever; broad-spectrum penicillins should not therefore be used for 'blind' treatment of a sore throat. Rashes are also common in patients with acute or chronic lymphocytic leukaemia or in cytomegalovirus infection.

Amoxicillin (amoxycillin) is a derivative of ampicillin and has a similar antibacterial spectrum. It is better absorbed than ampicillin when given by mouth, producing higher plasma and tissue concentrations; unlike ampicillin, absorption is not affected by the presence of food in the stomach. Amoxicillin is used for endocarditis prophylaxis (section 5.1, table 2); it may also be used for the treatment of Lyme disease [not licensed], see below.

Co-amoxiclav consists of amoxicillin with the beta-lactamase inhibitor clavulanic acid. Clavulanic acid itself has no significant antibacterial activity but, by inactivating beta-lactamases, it makes the combination active against beta-lactamase-producing bacteria that are resistant to amoxicillin. These include resistant strains of *Staph. aureus*, *E. coli*, and *H. influenzae*, as well as many *Bacteroides* and *Klebsiella* spp. Co-amoxiclav should be reserved for infections likely, or known, to be caused by amoxicillin-resistant beta-lactamase-producing strains; for CSM warning on cholestatic jaundice see under Co-amoxiclav.

A combination of ampicillin with flucloxacillin (as co-fluampicil) is available to treat infections involving either streptococci or staphylococci (e.g. cellulitis).

Lyme disease Lyme disease should generally be treated by those experienced in its management. **Doxycycline** (p. 297), **amoxicillin** [unlicensed indication] or **cefuroxime axetil** are the antibacterials of choice for *early Lyme disease* or *Lyme arthritis*. If these antibacterials are contra-indicated, a **macrolide** (e.g. erythromycin) can be used for early Lyme disease. Intravenous administration of **ceftriaxone**, **cefotaxime** (section 5.1.2), or **benzylpenicillin** (p. 285) is recommended for Lyme disease associated with cardiac or neurological complications. The duration of treatment is usually 2–4 weeks; Lyme arthritis may require further treatment.

Oral infections Amoxicillin or ampicillin are as effective as phenoxymethylpenicillin (section 5.1.1.1) but they are better absorbed; however, they may encourage emergence of resistant organisms. Like phenoxymethylpenicillin, amoxicillin and ampicillin are ineffective against bacteria that produce beta-lactamases. Amoxicillin may be useful for short-course oral regimens.

AMOXICILLIN
(Amoxycillin)

Indications see under Ampicillin; oral infections (see notes above); also endocarditis treatment (Table 1, section 5.1); anthrax (section 5.1.12); adjunct in listerial meningitis (Table 1, section 5.1); *Helicobacter pylori* eradication (section 1.3)

Cautions see under Ampicillin; maintain adequate hydration with high doses (particularly during parenteral therapy)

Contra-indications see under Ampicillin

Side-effects see under Ampicillin

Dose

- By mouth, 250 mg every 8 hours, doubled in severe infections; CHILD up to 10 years, 125 mg every 8 hours, doubled in severe infections

  Otitis media, 1 g every 8 hours; CHILD 40 mg/kg daily in 3 divided doses (max. 3 g daily)

  Pneumonia, 0.5–1 g every 8 hours

  Anthrax (treatment and post-exposure prophylaxis—see also section 5.1.12), 500 mg every 8 hours; CHILD body-weight under 20 kg, 80 mg/kg daily in 3 divided doses, body-weight over 20 kg, adult dose

- *Short-course oral therapy*

  Dental abscess, 3 g repeated after 8 hours

  Urinary-tract infections, 3 g repeated after 10–12 hours

- By intramuscular injection, 500 mg every 8 hours; CHILD, 50–100 mg/kg daily in divided doses
- By intravenous injection *or* infusion, 500 mg every 8 hours increased to 1 g every 6 hours in severe infections; CHILD, 50–100 mg/kg daily in divided doses
- Listerial meningitis (in combination with another antibiotic, see Table 1, section 5.1), by intravenous infusion, 2 g every 4 hours for 10–14 days
- Endocarditis (in combination with another antibiotic if necessary, see Table 1, section 5.1), by intravenous infusion, 2 g every 6 hours, increased to 2 g every 4 hours e.g. in enterococcal endocarditis or if amoxicillin used alone

Note Amoxicillin doses in BNF may differ from those in product literature

Amoxicillin (Non-proprietary) PoM

Capsules, amoxicillin (as trihydrate) 250 mg, net price 21 = 69p; 500 mg, 21 = £1.09. Label: 9
Brands include *Amix®*, *Amoram®*, *Amoxident®*, *Galenamox®*, *Rimoxallin®*

Oral suspension, amoxicillin (as trihydrate) for reconstitution with water, 125 mg/5 mL, net price 100 mL = 83p; 250 mg/5 mL, 100 mL = £1.06. Label: 9
Note Sugar-free versions are available and can be ordered by specifying 'sugar-free' on the prescription
Brands include *Amoram®*, *Galenamox®*, *Rimoxallin®*

Sachets, sugar-free, amoxicillin (as trihydrate) 3 g/sachet, net price 2-sachet pack = £4.83, 14-sachet pack = £31.94. Label: 9, 13

Injection, powder for reconstitution, amoxicillin (as sodium salt), net price 250-mg vial = 32p; 500-mg vial = 66p; 1-g vial = £1.16

Dental prescribing on NHS Amoxicillin Capsules and Oral Suspension may be prescribed. Amoxicillin Sachets may be prescribed as Amoxicillin Oral Powder

Amoxil® (GSK) PoM

Capsules, both maroon/gold, amoxicillin (as trihydrate), 250 mg, net price 21-cap pack = £3.59; 500 mg, 21-cap pack = £7.19. Label: 9

Paediatric suspension, amoxicillin 125 mg (as trihydrate)/1.25 mL when reconstituted with water, net price 20 mL (peach- strawberry- and lemon-flavoured) = £3.38. Label: 9, counselling , use of pipette
Excipients include sucrose 600 mg/1.25 mL

Sachets SF, powder, sugar-free, amoxicillin (as trihydrate) 3 g/sachet, 2-sachet pack (peach- strawberry- and lemon-flavoured) = £2.99. Label: 9, 13

Injection, powder for reconstitution, amoxicillin (as sodium salt), net price 500-mg vial = 58p; 1-g vial = £1.16
Electrolytes Na^+ 3.3 mmol/g

AMPICILLIN

Indications urinary-tract infections, otitis media, sinusitis, oral infections (see notes above), bronchitis, uncomplicated community-acquired pneumonia (Table 1, section 5.1), *Haemophilus influenzae* infections, invasive salmonellosis; listerial meningitis (Table 1, section 5.1)

Cautions history of allergy; renal impairment (Appendix 3); erythematous rashes common in glandular fever, cytomegalovirus infection, and acute or chronic lymphocytic leukaemia (see notes above); **interactions**: Appendix 1 (penicillins)

Contra-indications penicillin hypersensitivity

Side-effects nausea, vomiting, diarrhoea; rashes (discontinue treatment); rarely, antibiotic-associated colitis; see also under Benzylpenicillin (section 5.1.1.1)

Dose
- By mouth, 0.25–1 g every 6 hours, at least 30 minutes before food; CHILD under 10 years, half adult dose
  Urinary-tract infections, 500 mg every 8 hours; CHILD under 10 years, half adult dose
- By intramuscular injection *or* intravenous injection *or* infusion, 500 mg every 4–6 hours; CHILD under 10 years, half adult dose
- Endocarditis (in combination with another antibiotic if necessary), by intravenous infusion, 2 g every 6 hours, increased to 2 g every 4 hours e.g. in enterococcal endocarditis or if ampicillin used alone
- Listerial meningitis (in combination with another antibiotic), by intravenous infusion, 2 g every 4 hours for 10–14 days; NEONATE 50 mg/kg every 6 hours; INFANT 1–3 months, 50–100 mg/kg every 6 hours; CHILD 3 months–12 years, 100 mg/kg every 6 hours (max. 12 g daily)

Note Ampicillin doses in BNF may differ from those in product literature

Ampicillin (Non-proprietary) PoM

Capsules, ampicillin 250 mg, net price 28 = £3.74; 500 mg, 28 = £18.99. Label: 9, 23
Brands include *Rimacillin®*

Oral suspension, ampicillin 125 mg/5 mL when reconstituted with water, net price 100 mL = £3.26; 250 mg/5 mL, 100 mL = £6.38. Label: 9, 23
Brands include *Rimacillin®*

Injection, powder for reconstitution, ampicillin (as sodium salt), net price 500-mg vial = £7.83

Dental prescribing on NHS Ampicillin Capsules and Oral Suspension may be prescribed

Penbritin® (Chemidex) PoM

Capsules, grey/red, ampicillin (as trihydrate) 250 mg, net price 28-cap pack = £2.10; 500 mg, 28-cap pack = £5.28. Label: 9, 23

Syrup, apricot- caramel- and peppermint-flavoured, ampicillin (as trihydrate) for reconstitution with water, 125 mg/5 mL, net price 100 mL = £3.78; 250 mg/5 mL, 100 mL = £7.39. Label: 9, 23
Excipients include sucrose 3.6 g/5 mL

With flucloxacillin

See Co-fluampicil

CO-AMOXICLAV

A mixture of amoxicillin (as the trihydrate or as the sodium salt) and clavulanic acid (as potassium clavulanate); the proportions are expressed in the form x/y where x and y are the strengths in milligrams of amoxicillin and clavulanic acid respectively

Indications infections due to beta-lactamase-producing strains (where amoxicillin alone not appropriate) including respiratory-tract infections, genito-urinary and abdominal infections, cellulitis, animal bites, severe dental infection with spreading cellulitis

Cautions see under Ampicillin and notes above; also caution in hepatic impairment (monitor hepatic function), pregnancy; maintain adequate hydration with high doses (particularly during parenteral therapy)

Cholestatic jaundice CSM has advised that cholestatic jaundice can occur either during or shortly after the use of

5 Infections

co-amoxiclav. An epidemiological study has shown that the risk of acute liver toxicity was about 6 times greater with co-amoxiclav than with amoxicillin. Cholestatic jaundice is more common in patients above the age of 65 years and in men; these reactions have only rarely been reported in children. Jaundice is usually self-limiting and very rarely fatal. The duration of treatment should be appropriate to the indication and should not usually exceed 14 days

Contra-indications penicillin hypersensitivity, history of co-amoxiclav-associated or penicillin-associated jaundice or hepatic dysfunction

Side-effects see under Ampicillin; hepatitis, cholestatic jaundice (see above); Stevens-Johnson syndrome, toxic epidermal necrolysis, exfoliative dermatitis, vasculitis reported; rarely prolongation of bleeding time, dizziness, headache, convulsions (particularly with high doses or in renal impairment); superficial staining of teeth with suspension, phlebitis at injection site

Dose

- By mouth, expressed as amoxicillin, 250 mg every 8 hours, dose doubled in severe infections; CHILD see under preparations below (under 6 years *Augmentin® '125/31 SF'* suspension; 6–12 years *Augmentin® '250/62 SF'* suspension *or* for short-term treatment with twice daily dosage in CHILD 2 months–12 years *Augmentin-Duo® 400/57* suspension)

  Severe dental infections (but not generally first-line, see notes above), expressed as amoxicillin, 250 mg every 8 hours for 5 days
- By intravenous injection over 3–4 minutes or by intravenous infusion, expressed as amoxicillin, 1 g every 8 hours increased to 1 g every 6 hours in more serious infections; INFANTS up to 3 months 25 mg/kg every 8 hours (every 12 hours in the perinatal period and in premature infants); CHILD 3 months–12 years, 25 mg/kg every 8 hours increased to 25 mg/kg every 6 hours in more serious infections

  Surgical prophylaxis, expressed as amoxicillin, 1 g at induction; for high risk procedures (e.g. colorectal surgery) up to 2–3 further doses of 1 g may be given every 8 hours

Co-amoxiclav (Non-proprietary) PoM

Tablets, co-amoxiclav 250/125 (amoxicillin 250 mg as trihydrate, clavulanic acid 125 mg as potassium salt), net price 21-tab pack = £4.20. Label: 9

Tablets, co-amoxiclav 500/125 (amoxicillin 500 mg as trihydrate, clavulanic acid 125 mg as potassium salt), net price 21-tab pack = £9.97. Label: 9

Oral suspension, co-amoxiclav 125/31 (amoxicillin 125 mg as trihydrate, clavulanic acid 31.25 mg as potassium salt)/5 mL when reconstituted with water, net price 100 mL = £4.37. Label: 9

Oral suspension, co-amoxiclav 250/62 (amoxicillin 250 mg as trihydrate, clavulanic acid 62.5 mg as potassium salt)/5 mL when reconstituted with water, net price 100 mL = £5.34. Label: 9

Injection 500/100, powder for reconstitution, co-amoxiclav 500/100 (amoxicillin 500 mg as sodium salt, clavulanic acid 100 mg as potassium salt), net price per vial = £1.21

Injection 1000/200, powder for reconstitution, co-amoxiclav 1000/200 (amoxicillin 1 g as sodium salt, clavulanic acid 200 mg as potassium salt), net price per vial = £2.42

Augmentin® (GSK) PoM

Tablets 375 mg, f/c, co-amoxiclav 250/125 (amoxicillin 250 mg as trihydrate, clavulanic acid 125 mg as potassium salt), net price 21-tab pack = £4.45. Label: 9

Tablets 625 mg, f/c, co-amoxiclav 500/125 (amoxicillin 500 mg as trihydrate, clavulanic acid 125 mg as potassium salt). Net price 21-tab pack = £8.49. Label: 9

Dispersible tablets, sugar-free, co-amoxiclav 250/125 (amoxicillin 250 mg as trihydrate, clavulanic acid 125 mg as potassium salt). Net price 21-tab pack = £10.22. Label: 9, 13

Suspension '125/31 SF', sugar-free, co-amoxiclav 125/31 (amoxicillin 125 mg as trihydrate, clavulanic acid 31 mg as potassium salt)/5 mL when reconstituted with water. Net price 100 mL (raspberry-and orange-flavoured) = £4.25. Label: 9

Excipients include aspartame 12.5 mg/5 mL (section 9.4.1)

Dose CHILD 1–6 years (10–18 kg) 5 mL every 8 hours *or* INFANT and CHILD up to 6 years 0.8 mL/kg daily in 3 divided doses; in severe infections dose increased to 1.6 mL/kg daily in 3 divided doses

Suspension '250/62 SF', sugar-free, co-amoxiclav 250/62 (amoxicillin 250 mg as trihydrate, clavulanic acid 62 mg as potassium salt)/5 mL when reconstituted with water. Net price 100 mL (raspberry-and orange-flavoured) = £5.97. Label: 9

Excipients include aspartame 12.5 mg/5 mL (section 9.4.1)

Dose CHILD 6–12 years (18–40 kg) 5 mL every 8 hours *or* 0.4 mL/kg daily in 3 divided doses; in severe infections dose increased to 0.8 mL/kg daily in 3 divided doses

Injection 600 mg, powder for reconstitution, co-amoxiclav 500/100 (amoxicillin 500 mg as sodium salt, clavulanic acid 100 mg as potassium salt). Net price per vial = £1.38

Electrolytes Na^+ 1.35 mmol, K^+ 0.5 mmol/600-mg vial

Injection 1.2 g, powder for reconstitution, co-amoxiclav 1000/200 (amoxicillin 1 g as sodium salt, clavulanic acid 200 mg as potassium salt). Net price per vial = £2.76

Electrolytes Na^+ 2.7 mmol, K^+ 1 mmol/1.2-g vial

Augmentin-Duo® (GSK) PoM

Suspension '400/57', sugar-free, strawberry-flavoured, co-amoxiclav 400/57 (amoxicillin 400 mg as trihydrate, clavulanic acid 57 mg as potassium salt)/5 mL when reconstituted with water. Net price 35 mL = £4.38, 70 mL = £6.15. Label: 9

Excipients include aspartame 12.5 mg/5 mL (section 9.4.1)

Dose CHILD 2 months–2 years 0.15 mL/kg twice daily, 2–6 years (13–21 kg) 2.5 mL twice daily, 7–12 years (22–40 kg) 5 mL twice daily, doubled in severe infections

CO-FLUAMPICIL

A mixture of equal parts by mass of flucloxacillin and ampicillin

Indications mixed infections involving beta-lactamase-producing staphylococci

Cautions see under Ampicillin and Flucloxacillin

Contra-indications see under Ampicillin and Flucloxacillin

Side-effects see under Ampicillin and Flucloxacillin

Dose

- By mouth, co-fluampicil, 250/250 every 6 hours, dose doubled in severe infections; CHILD under 10 years half adult dose, dose doubled in severe infections

- By intramuscular *or* slow intravenous injection *or* by intravenous infusion, co-fluampicil 250/250 every 6 hours, dose doubled in severe infections; CHILD under 2 years quarter adult dose, 2–10 years half adult dose, dose doubled in severe infections

Co-fluampicil (Non-proprietary) PoM

Capsules, co-fluampicil 250/250 (flucloxacillin 250 mg as sodium salt, ampicillin 250 mg as trihydrate), net price 28-cap pack = £10.25. Label: 9, 22

Brands include *Flu-Amp®*

Magnapen® (CP) PoM

Capsules, black/turquoise, co-fluampicil 250/250 (flucloxacillin 250 mg as sodium salt, ampicillin 250 mg as trihydrate), net price 20-cap pack = £4.00. Label: 9, 22

Syrup, co-fluampicil 125/125 (flucloxacillin 125 mg as magnesium salt, ampicillin 125 mg as trihydrate)/ 5 mL when reconstituted with water, net price 100 mL = £4.99. Label: 9, 22

Excipients include sucrose 3.14 g/5 mL

Injection 500 mg, powder for reconstitution, co-fluampicil 250/250 (flucloxacillin 250 mg as sodium salt, ampicillin 250 mg as sodium salt), net price per vial = £1.33

Electrolytes Na^+ 1.3 mmol/vial

5.1.1.4 Antipseudomonal penicillins

The carboxypenicillin, **ticarcillin**, is principally indicated for serious infections caused by *Pseudomonas aeruginosa* although it also has activity against certain other Gram-negative bacilli including *Proteus* spp. and *Bacteroides fragilis*.

Ticarcillin is now available only in combination with clavulanic acid (section 5.1.1.3); the combination (*Timentin®*) is active against beta-lactamase-producing bacteria resistant to ticarcillin.

Tazocin® contains the ureidopenicillin **piperacillin** with the beta-lactamase inhibitor tazobactam. Piperacillin is more active than ticarcillin against *Ps. aeruginosa*. The spectrum of activity of *Tazocin®* is comparable to that of the carbapenems, imipenem and meropenem (section 5.1.2).

For pseudomonas septicaemias (especially in neutropenia or endocarditis) these antipseudomonal penicillins should be given with an aminoglycoside (e.g. gentamicin section 5.1.4) since they have a synergistic effect. Penicillins and aminoglycosides must not, however, be mixed in the same syringe or infusion.

Owing to the sodium content of many of these antibiotics, high doses may lead to hypernatraemia.

PIPERACILLIN

Indications see preparations

Cautions see under Benzylpenicillin (section 5.1.1.1); renal impairment (Appendix 3); pregnancy (Appendix 4); breast-feeding (Appendix 5)

Contra-indications see under Benzylpenicillin (section 5.1.1.1)

Side-effects see under Benzylpenicillin (section 5.1.1.1); also nausea, vomiting, diarrhoea; *less commonly* stomatitis, dyspepsia, constipation, jaundice, hypotension, headache, insomnia, and injection-site reactions; *rarely* abdominal pain, hepatitis, oedema, fatigue, and eosinophilia; *very rarely* hypoglycaemia, hypokalaemia, pancytopenia, Stevens-Johnson syndrome, and toxic epidermal necrolysis

Dose

- See preparations

With tazobactam

Tazocin® (Lederle) PoM

Injection 2.25 g, powder for reconstitution, piperacillin 2 g (as sodium salt), tazobactam 250 mg (as sodium salt). Net price per vial = £7.96

Electrolytes Na^+ 4.69 mmol/2.25-g vial

Injection 4.5 g, powder for reconstitution, piperacillin 4 g (as sodium salt), tazobactam 500 mg (as sodium salt). Net price per vial = £15.79

Electrolytes Na^+ 9.37 mmol/4.5-g vial

Dose lower respiratory-tract, urinary-tract, intra-abdominal and skin infections, and septicaemia, ADULT and CHILD over 12 years, by intravenous injection over 3–5 minutes *or* by intravenous infusion, 2.25–4.5 g every 6–8 hours, usually 4.5 g every 8 hours

Complicated appendicitis, by intravenous injection over 3–5 minutes or by intravenous infusion, CHILD 2–12 years, 112.5 mg/kg every 8 hours (max. 4.5 g every 8 hours) for 5–14 days; CHILD under 2 years, not recommended

Infections in neutropenic patients (in combination with an aminoglycoside), by intravenous injection over 3–5 minutes *or* by intravenous infusion, ADULT and CHILD over 50 kg, 4.5 g every 6 hours; CHILD less than 50 kg, 90 mg/kg every 6 hours

TICARCILLIN

Indications infections due to *Pseudomonas* and *Proteus* spp, see notes above

Cautions see under Benzylpenicillin (section 5.1.1.1)

Contra-indications see under Benzylpenicillin (section 5.1.1.1)

Side-effects see under Benzylpenicillin (section 5.1.1.1); also nausea, vomiting, coagulation disorders, haemorrhagic cystitis (more frequent in children), injection-site reactions, Stevens-Johnson syndrome, toxic epidermal necrolysis, hypokalaemia, eosinophilia

Dose

- See under preparation

With clavulanic acid

Note For a CSM warning on cholestatic jaundice possibly associated with clavulanic acid, see under Co-amoxiclav p. 288.

Timentin (GSK) PoM

Injection 3.2 g, powder for reconstitution, ticarcillin 3 g (as sodium salt), clavulanic acid 200 mg (as potassium salt). Net price per vial = £5.66

Electrolytes Na^+ 16 mmol, K^+ 1 mmol/3.2-g vial

Dose by intravenous infusion, 3.2 g every 6–8 hours increased to every 4 hours in more severe infections; CHILD 80 mg/kg every 6–8 hours (every 12 hours in neonates)

5.1.1.5 Mecillinams

Pivmecillinam has significant activity against many Gram-negative bacteria including *Escherichia coli*, klebsiella, enterobacter, and salmonellae. It is not active against *Pseudomonas aeruginosa* or enterococci. Pivmecillinam is hydrolysed to mecillinam, which is the active drug.

PIVMECILLINAM HYDROCHLORIDE

Indications see under Dose below

Cautions see under Benzylpenicillin (section 5.1.1.1); also liver and renal function tests required in long-term use; avoid in porphyria (section 9.8.2); pregnancy; **interactions:** Appendix 1 (penicillins)

Contra-indications see under Benzylpenicillin (section 5.1.1.1); also carnitine deficiency, oesophageal strictures, gastro-intestinal obstruction, infants under 3 months

Side-effects see under Benzylpenicillin (section 5.1.1.1); nausea, vomiting, dyspepsia; also reduced serum and total body carnitine (especially with long-term or repeated use)

Dose

- Acute uncomplicated cystitis, ADULT and CHILD over 40 kg, initially 400 mg then 200 mg every 8 hours for 3 days
- Chronic or recurrent bacteriuria, ADULT and CHILD over 40 kg, 400 mg every 6–8 hours
- Urinary-tract infections, CHILD under 40 kg, 20–40 mg/kg daily in 3–4 divided doses
- Salmonellosis, not recommended therefore no dose stated

Counselling Tablets should be swallowed whole with plenty of fluid during meals while sitting or standing

Selexid® (LEO) PoM
Tablets, f/c, pivmecillinam hydrochloride 200 mg, net price 10-tab pack = £4.50. Label 9, 21, 27, counselling, posture (see Dose above)

5.1.2 Cephalosporins and other beta-lactams

Antibiotics in this section include the **cephalosporins**, such as cefotaxime, ceftazidime, cefuroxime, cefalexin and cefradine, the **monobactam**, aztreonam, and the **carbapenems**, imipenem (a thienamycin derivative) and meropenem.

Cephalosporins

The cephalosporins are broad-spectrum antibiotics which are used for the treatment of septicaemia, pneumonia, meningitis, biliary-tract infections, peritonitis, and urinary-tract infections. The pharmacology of the cephalosporins is similar to that of the penicillins, excretion being principally renal. Cephalosporins penetrate the cerebrospinal fluid poorly unless the meninges are inflamed; cefotaxime is a suitable cephalosporin for infections of the CNS (e.g meningitis).

The principal side-effect of the cephalosporins is hypersensitivity and about 10% of penicillin-sensitive patients will also be allergic to the cephalosporins.

Antibiotic-associated colitis may occur with the use of broad-spectrum cephalosporins.

Cefradine (cephradine) has generally been replaced by the newer cephalosporins.

Cefuroxime is a 'second generation' cephalosporin that is less susceptible than the earlier cephalosporins to inactivation by beta-lactamases. It is, therefore, active against certain bacteria which are resistant to the other drugs and has greater activity against *Haemophilus influenzae* and *Neisseria gonorrhoeae.*

Cefotaxime, **ceftazidime** and **ceftriaxone** are 'third generation' cephalosporins with greater activity than the 'second generation' cephalosporins against certain Gram-negative bacteria. However, they are less active than cefuroxime against Gram-positive bacteria, most notably *Staphylococcus aureus*. Their broad antibacterial spectrum may encourage superinfection with resistant bacteria or fungi.

Ceftazidime has good activity against pseudomonas. It is also active against other Gram-negative bacteria.

Ceftriaxone has a longer half-life and therefore needs to be given only once daily. Indications include serious infections such as septicaemia, pneumonia, and meningitis. The calcium salt of ceftriaxone forms a precipitate in the gall bladder which may rarely cause symptoms but these usually resolve when the antibiotic is stopped.

Orally active cephalosporins The orally active 'first generation' cephalosporins, **cefalexin** (cephalexin), **cefradine**, and **cefadroxil** and the 'second generation' cephalosporin, **cefaclor**, have a similar antimicrobial spectrum. They are useful for urinary-tract infections which do not respond to other drugs or which occur in pregnancy, respiratory-tract infections, otitis media, sinusitis, and skin and soft-tissue infections. Cefaclor has good activity against *H. influenzae*, but it is associated with protracted skin reactions especially in children. Cefadroxil has a long duration of action and can be given twice daily; it has poor activity against *H. influenzae*. **Cefuroxime axetil**, an ester of the 'second generation' cephalosporin cefuroxime, has the same antibacterial spectrum as the parent compound; it is poorly absorbed.

Cefixime has a longer duration of action than the other cephalosporins that are active by mouth. It is only licensed for acute infections.

Cefpodoxime proxetil is more active than the other oral cephalosporins against respiratory bacterial pathogens and it is licensed for upper and lower respiratory-tract infections.

For treatment of Lyme disease, see section 5.1.1.3.

Oral infections The cephalosporins offer little advantage over the penicillins in dental infections, often being less active against anaerobes. Infections due to oral streptococci (often termed viridans streptococci) which become resistant to penicillin are usually also resistant to cephalosporins. This is of importance in the case of patients who have had rheumatic fever and are on long-term penicillin therapy. Cefalexin and cefradine have been used in the treatment of oral infections.

CEFACLOR

Indications infections due to sensitive Gram-positive and Gram-negative bacteria, but see notes above

Cautions sensitivity to beta-lactam antibacterials (avoid if history of immediate hypersensitivity reaction, see also p. 284); renal impairment (Appendix 3); pregnancy and breast-feeding (but appropriate to use); false positive urinary glucose (if tested for reducing substances) and false positive Coombs' test; **interactions:** Appendix 1 (cephalosporins)

Contra-indications cephalosporin hypersensitivity

Side-effects diarrhoea and rarely antibiotic-associated colitis (CSM has warned both more likely with higher doses), nausea and vomiting, abdominal discomfort, headache; allergic reactions including rashes, pruritus, urticaria, serum sickness-like reactions with rashes, fever and arthralgia, and anaphylaxis; Stevens-Johnson syndrome, toxic epidermal necrolysis reported; disturbances in liver enzymes, transient hepatitis and cholestatic jaundice; other side-effects reported include eosinophilia and blood disorders (including thrombocytopenia, leucopenia, agranulocytosis, aplastic anaemia and haemolytic anaemia); reversible interstitial nephritis, hyperactivity, nervousness, sleep disturbances, hallucinations, confusion, hypertonia, and dizziness

Dose

- 250 mg every 8 hours, doubled for severe infections; max. 4 g daily; CHILD over 1 month, 20 mg/kg daily in 3 divided doses, doubled for severe infections, max. 1 g daily; *or* 1 month–1 year, 62.5 mg every 8 hours; 1–5 years, 125 mg; over 5 years, 250 mg; doses doubled for severe infections

Cefaclor (Non-proprietary) PoM

Capsules, cefaclor (as monohydrate) 250 mg, net price 21-cap pack = £8.74; 500 mg, 50-cap pack = £44.21. Label: 9

Brands include *Keftid®*

Suspension, cefaclor (as monohydrate) for reconstitution with water, 125 mg/5 mL, net price 100 mL = £8.33; 250 mg/5 mL, 100 mL = £9.33. Label: 9

Note Sugar-free versions are available and can be ordered by specifying 'sugar-free' on the prescription

Brands include *Keftid®*

Distaclor® (Flynn) PoM

Capsules, cefaclor (as monohydrate) 500 mg (violet/grey), net price 20 = £17.33. Label: 9

Suspension, both pink, cefaclor (as monohydrate) for reconstitution with water, 125 mg/5 mL, net price 100 mL = £4.13; 250 mg/5 mL, 100 mL = £8.26. Label: 9

Distaclor MR® (Flynn) PoM

Tablets, m/r, both blue, cefaclor (as monohydrate) 375 mg. Net price 14-tab pack = £6.93. Label: 9, 21, 25

Dose 375 mg every 12 hours with food, dose doubled for pneumonia

Lower urinary-tract infections, 375 mg every 12 hours with food

CEFADROXIL

Indications see under Cefaclor; see also notes above

Cautions see under Cefaclor

Contra-indications see under Cefaclor

Side-effects see under Cefaclor

Dose

- Patients over 40 kg, 0.5–1 g twice daily; skin, soft tissue, and simple urinary-tract infections, 1 g daily; CHILD under 1 year, 25 mg/kg daily in divided doses; 1–6 years, 250 mg twice daily; over 6 years, 500 mg twice daily

Cefadroxil (Non-proprietary) PoM

Capsules, cefadroxil (as monohydrate) 500 mg, net price 20-cap pack = £5.25. Label: 9

Baxan® (Bristol-Myers Squibb) PoM

Capsules, cefadroxil (as monohydrate) 500 mg, net price 20-cap pack = £5.64. Label: 9

Suspension, cefadroxil (as monohydrate) for reconstitution with water, 125 mg/5 mL, net price 60 mL = £1.63; 250 mg/5 mL, 60 mL = £3.24; 500 mg/5 mL, 60 mL = £4.85. Label: 9

CEFALEXIN
(Cephalexin)

Indications see under Cefaclor

Cautions see under Cefaclor

Contra-indications see under Cefaclor

Side-effects see under Cefaclor

Dose

- 250 mg every 6 hours *or* 500 mg every 8–12 hours increased to 1–1.5 g every 6–8 hours for severe infections; CHILD 25 mg/kg daily in divided doses, doubled for severe infections, max. 100 mg/kg daily; *or* under 1 year 125 mg every 12 hours, 1–5 years 125 mg every 8 hours, 5–12 years 250 mg every 8 hours
- Prophylaxis of recurrent urinary-tract infection, ADULT 125 mg at night

Cefalexin (Non-proprietary) PoM

Capsules, cefalexin 250 mg, net price 28-cap pack = £2.23; 500 mg, 21-cap pack = £2.83. Label: 9

Tablets, cefalexin 250 mg, net price 28-tab pack = £2.80; 500 mg, 21-tab pack = £3.57. Label: 9

Oral suspension, cefalexin for reconstitution with water, 125 mg/5 mL, net price 100 mL = £2.20; 250 mg/5 mL, 100 mL = £2.57. Label: 9

Dental prescribing on NHS Cefalexin Capsules, Tablets, and Oral Suspension may be prescribed

Ceporex® (Galen) PoM

Capsules, both caramel/grey, cefalexin 250 mg, net price 28-cap pack = £4.02; 500 mg, 28-cap pack = £7.85. Label: 9

Tablets, all pink, f/c, cefalexin 250 mg, net price 28-tab pack = £4.02; 500 mg, 28-tab pack = £7.85. Label: 9

Syrup, all orange, cefalexin for reconstitution with water, 125 mg/5 mL, net price 100 mL = £1.43; 250 mg/5 mL, 100 mL = £2.87; 500 mg/5 mL, 100 mL = £5.57. Label: 9

Keflex® (Flynn) PoM

Capsules, cefalexin 250 mg (green/white), net price 28-cap pack = £1.76; 500 mg (pale green/dark green), 21-cap pack = £2.66. Label: 9

Tablets, both peach, cefalexin 250 mg, net price 28-tab pack = £2.09; 500 mg (scored), 21-tab pack = £2.47. Label: 9

Suspension, cefalexin for reconstitution with water, 125 mg/5 mL, net price 100 mL = 88p; 250 mg/5 mL, 100 mL = £1.51. Label: 9

CEFIXIME

Indications see under Cefaclor (acute infections only); gonorrhoea [unlicensed indication] (Table 1, section 5.1)

Cautions see under Cefaclor

Contra-indications see under Cefaclor

Side-effects see under Cefaclor

Dose

- ADULT and CHILD over 10 years, 200–400 mg daily in 1–2 divided doses; CHILD over 6 months 8 mg/kg daily in

1–2 divided doses *or* 6 months–1 year 75 mg daily; 1–4 years 100 mg daily; 5–10 years 200 mg daily

- Gonorrhoea [unlicensed indication], 400 mg as a single dose

Suprax® (Rhône-Poulenc Rorer) PoM
Tablets, f/c, scored, cefixime 200 mg. Net price 7-tab pack = £13.23. Label: 9
Paediatric oral suspension, cefixime 100 mg/5 mL when reconstituted with water, net price 50 mL (with double-ended spoon for measuring 3.75 mL or 5 mL since dilution not recommended) = £10.53, 100 mL = £18.91. Label: 9

CEFOTAXIME

Indications see under Cefaclor; gonorrhoea; surgical prophylaxis; Haemophilus epiglottitis and meningitis (Table 1, section 5.1); see also notes above
Cautions see under Cefaclor
Contra-indications see under Cefaclor
Side-effects see under Cefaclor; rarely arrhythmias following rapid injection reported
Dose

- By intramuscular *or* intravenous injection *or* by intravenous infusion, 1 g every 12 hours increased in severe infections (e.g. meningitis) to 8 g daily in 4 divided doses; higher doses (up to 12 g daily in 3–4 divided doses) may be required; NEONATE 50 mg/kg daily in 2–4 divided doses increased to 150–200 mg/kg daily in severe infections; CHILD 100–150 mg/kg daily in 2–4 divided doses increased up to 200 mg/kg daily in very severe infections
Gonorrhoea, 500 mg as a single dose

Important. If bacterial meningitis and especially if meningococcal disease is suspected the patient should be transferred urgently to hospital. If benzylpenicillin cannot be given (e.g. because of an allergy), a single dose of cefotaxime may be given (if available) before urgent transfer to hospital. Suitable doses of cefotaxime by intravenous injection (or by intramuscular injection) are ADULT and CHILD over 12 years 1 g; CHILD under 12 years 50 mg/kg; chloramphenicol (section 5.1.7) may be used if there is a history of anaphylaxis to penicillins or cephalosporins

Cefotaxime (Non-proprietary) PoM
Injection, powder for reconstitution, cefotaxime (as sodium salt), net price 500-mg vial = £2.14; 1-g vial = £4.31; 2-g vial = £8.57

Claforan® (Aventis Pharma) PoM
Injection, powder for reconstitution, cefotaxime (as sodium salt), net price 500-mg vial = £2.14; 1-g vial (with or without infusion connector) = £4.31; 2-g vial (with or without infusion connector) = £8.57
Electrolytes Na^+ 2.09 mmol/g

CEFPODOXIME

Indications see under Dose
Cautions see under Cefaclor
Contra-indications see under Cefaclor
Side-effects see under Cefaclor
Dose

- Upper respiratory-tract infections (but in pharyngitis and tonsillitis reserved for infections which are recurrent, chronic, or resistant to other antibacterials), 100 mg twice daily (200 mg twice daily in sinusitis); CHILD 15 days–6 months 4 mg/kg every 12 hours, 6 months–2 years 40 mg every 12 hours, 3–8 years 80 mg every 12 hours, over 9 years 100 mg every 12 hours
- Lower respiratory-tract infections (including bronchitis and pneumonia), 100–200 mg twice daily; CHILD 15 days–6 months 4 mg/kg every 12 hours, 6 months–2 years 40 mg every 12 hours, 3–8 years 80 mg every 12 hours, over 9 years 100 mg every 12 hours
- Skin and soft-tissue infections, 200 mg twice daily; CHILD 15 days–6 months 4 mg/kg every 12 hours, 6 months–2 years 40 mg every 12 hours, 3–8 years 80 mg every 12 hours, over 9 years 100 mg every 12 hours
- Uncomplicated urinary-tract infections, 100 mg twice daily (200 mg twice daily in uncomplicated upper urinary-tract infections); CHILD 15 days–6 months 4 mg/kg every 12 hours, 6 months–2 years 40 mg every 12 hours, 3–8 years 80 mg every 12 hours, over 9 years 100 mg every 12 hours
- Uncomplicated gonorrhoea, 200 mg as a single dose

Orelox® (Hoechst Marion Roussel) PoM
Tablets, f/c, cefpodoxime 100 mg (as proxetil), net price 10-tab pack = £10.18. Label: 5, 9, 21
Oral suspension, cefpodoxime (as proxetil) for reconstitution with water, 40 mg/5 mL, net price 100 mL = £11.97. Label: 5, 9, 21
Excipients include aspartame (section 9.4.1)

CEFRADINE
(Cephradine)

Indications see under Cefaclor; surgical prophylaxis
Cautions see under Cefaclor
Contra-indications see under Cefaclor
Side-effects see under Cefaclor
Dose

- By mouth, 250–500 mg every 6 hours *or* 0.5–1 g every 12 hours; up to 1 g every 6 hours in severe infections; CHILD, 25–50 mg/kg daily in 2–4 divided doses
- By deep intramuscular injection *or* by intravenous injection over 3–5 minutes *or* by intravenous infusion, 0.5–1 g every 6 hours, increased to 8 g daily in severe infections; CHILD 50–100 mg/kg daily in 4 divided doses
- Surgical prophylaxis, by deep intramuscular injection *or* by intravenous injection over 3–5 minutes, 1–2 g at induction

Cefradine (Non-proprietary) PoM
Capsules, cefradine 250 mg, net price 20-cap pack = £5.28; 500 mg, 20-cap pack = £10.80. Label: 9
Brands include *Nicef®*
Dental prescribing on NHS Cefradine Capsules may be prescribed

Velosef® (Squibb) PoM
Capsules, cefradine 250 mg (orange/blue), net price 20-cap pack = £3.55; 500 mg (blue), 20-cap pack = £7.00. Label: 9
Syrup, cefradine 250 mg/5 mL when reconstituted with water. Net price 100 mL = £4.22. Label: 9
Dental prescribing on NHS *Velosef®* syrup may be prescribed as Cefradine Oral Solution
Injection, powder for reconstitution, cefradine. Net price 500-mg vial = 99p; 1-g vial = £1.95

CEFTAZIDIME

Indications see under Cefaclor; see also notes above
Cautions see under Cefaclor
Contra-indications see under Cefaclor
Side-effects see under Cefaclor
Dose
- By deep intramuscular injection *or* intravenous injection *or* infusion, 1 g every 8 hours *or* 2 g every 12 hours; 2 g every 8–12 hours *or* 3 g every 12 hours in severe infections; single doses over 1 g intravenous route only; ELDERLY usual max. 3 g daily; CHILD, up to 2 months 25–60 mg/kg daily in 2 divided doses, over 2 months 30–100 mg/kg daily in 2–3 divided doses; up to 150 mg/kg daily (max. 6 g daily) in 3 divided doses if immunocompromised or meningitis; intravenous route recommended for children

  Urinary-tract and less serious infections, 0.5–1 g every 12 hours

  Pseudomonal lung infection in cystic fibrosis, ADULT 100–150 mg/kg daily in 3 divided doses; CHILD up to 150 mg/kg daily (max. 6 g daily) in 3 divided doses; intravenous route recommended for children

  Surgical prophylaxis, prostatic surgery, 1 g at induction of anaesthesia repeated if necessary when catheter removed

Ceftazidime (Non-proprietary) PoM
Injection, powder for reconstitution, ceftazidime (as pentahydrate), with sodium carbonate, net price 1-g vial = £8.50; 2-g vial = £17.90

Fortum® (GSK) PoM
Injection, powder for reconstitution, ceftazidime (as pentahydrate), with sodium carbonate, net price 250-mg vial = £2.20, 500-mg vial = £4.40, 1-g vial = £8.79, 2-g vial = £17.59, 3-g vial = £25.76; *Monovial*, 2 g vial (with transfer needle) = £17.59
Electrolytes Na^+ 2.3 mmol/g

Kefadim® (Flynn) PoM
Injection, powder for reconstitution, ceftazidime (as pentahydrate), with sodium carbonate, net price 1-g vial = £7.92; 2-g vial = £15.84
Electrolytes Na^+ 2.3 mmol/g

CEFTRIAXONE

Indications see under Cefaclor and notes above; surgical prophylaxis; prophylaxis of meningococcal meningitis [unlicensed indication] (Table 2, section 5.1)
Cautions see under Cefaclor; severe renal impairment (Appendix 3); hepatic impairment if accompanied by renal impairment (Appendix 2); premature neonates; may displace bilirubin from serum albumin, administer over 60 minutes in neonates (see also Contra-indications); treatment longer than 14 days, renal failure, dehydration—risk of ceftriaxone precipitation in gall bladder
Contra-indications see under Cefaclor; neonates with jaundice, hypoalbuminaemia, acidosis or impaired bilirubin binding; concomitant treatment with calcium in neonates—risk of precipitation in urine and lungs
Side-effects see under Cefaclor; calcium ceftriaxone precipitates in urine (particularly in very young, dehydrated or those who are immobilised) or in gall bladder—consider discontinuation if symptomatic; rarely prolongation of prothrombin time, pancreatitis
Dose
- By deep intramuscular injection, *or* by intravenous injection over at least 2–4 minutes, *or* by intravenous infusion, 1 g daily; 2–4 g daily in severe infections; intramuscular doses over 1 g divided between more than one site; single intravenous doses above 1 g by intravenous infusion only
  NEONATE by intravenous infusion over 60 minutes, 20–50 mg/kg daily (max. 50 mg/kg daily) INFANT and CHILD under 50 kg, by deep intramuscular injection, *or* by intravenous injection over 2–4 minutes, *or* by intravenous infusion, 20–50 mg/kg daily; up to 80 mg/kg daily in severe infections; doses of 50 mg/kg and over by intravenous infusion only; 50 kg and over, adult dose
- Endocarditis caused by haemophilus, actinobacillus, cardiobacterium, eikenella, and kingella species ('HACEK organisms') (in combination with another antibacterial, see Table 1, section 5.1; [unlicensed indication]), by intravenous infusion, 2–4 g daily
- Early syphilis [unlicensed indication], by deep intramuscular injection, 500 mg daily for 10 days
- Uncomplicated gonorrhoea, by deep intramuscular injection, 250 mg as a single dose
- Surgical prophylaxis, by deep intramuscular injection *or* by intravenous injection over at least 2–4 minutes, 1 g at induction; colorectal surgery, by deep intramuscular injection *or* by intravenous infusion, 2 g at induction; intramuscular doses over 1 g divided between more than one site

Ceftriaxone (Non-proprietary) PoM
Injection, powder for reconstitution, ceftriaxone (as sodium salt), net price 1-g vial = £10.17; 2-g vial = £20.36

Rocephin® (Roche) PoM
Injection, powder for reconstitution, ceftriaxone (as sodium salt), net price 250-mg vial = £2.55; 1-g vial = £10.17; 2-g vial = £20.36
Electrolytes Na^+ 3.6 mmol/g

CEFUROXIME

Indications see under Cefaclor; surgical prophylaxis; more active against *Haemophilus influenzae* and *Neisseria gonorrhoeae*; Lyme disease
Cautions see under Cefaclor
Contra-indications see under Cefaclor
Side-effects see under Cefaclor
Dose
- By mouth (as cefuroxime axetil), 250 mg twice daily in most infections including mild to moderate lower respiratory-tract infections (e.g. bronchitis); doubled for more severe lower respiratory-tract infections or if pneumonia suspected

  Urinary-tract infection, 125 mg twice daily, doubled in pyelonephritis

  Gonorrhoea, 1 g as a single dose

  CHILD over 3 months, 125 mg twice daily, if necessary doubled in child over 2 years with otitis media

  Lyme disease, ADULT and CHILD over 12 years, 500 mg twice daily for 20 days
- By intramuscular injection *or* intravenous injection *or* infusion, 750 mg every 6–8 hours; 1.5 g every 6–8 hours in severe infections; single doses over 750 mg intravenous route only

5 Infections

CHILD usual dose 60 mg/kg daily (range 30–100 mg/kg daily) in 3–4 divided doses (2–3 divided doses in neonates)

- Gonorrhoea, 1.5 g as a single dose by intramuscular injection (divided between 2 sites)
- Surgical prophylaxis, 1.5 g by intravenous injection at induction; up to 3 further doses of 750 mg may be given by intramuscular *or* intravenous injection every 8 hours for high-risk procedures
- Meningitis, 3 g intravenously every 8 hours; CHILD, 200–240 mg/kg daily (in 3–4 divided doses) reduced to 100 mg/kg daily after 3 days or on clinical improvement; NEONATE, 100 mg/kg daily reduced to 50 mg/kg daily

Cefuroxime (Non-proprietary) PoM
Tablets, cefuroxime (as axetil) 250 mg, net price 14-tab pack = £9.04. Label: 9, 21, 25

Zinacef® (GSK) PoM
Injection, powder for reconstitution, cefuroxime (as sodium salt). Net price 250-mg vial = 94p; 750-mg vial = £2.34; 1.5-g vial = £4.70
Electrolytes Na^+ 1.8 mmol/750-mg vial

Zinnat® (GSK) PoM
Tablets, both f/c, cefuroxime (as axetil) 125 mg, net price 14-tab pack = £4.84; 250 mg, 14-tab pack = £9.67. Label: 9, 21, 25
Suspension, cefuroxime (as axetil) 125 mg/5 mL when reconstituted with water, net price 70 mL (tutti-frutti-flavoured) = £5.52. Label: 9, 21
Excipients include aspartame (section 9.4.1), sucrose 3.1 g/5mL

Other beta-lactam antibiotics

Aztreonam is a monocyclic beta-lactam ('monobactam') antibiotic with an antibacterial spectrum limited to Gram-negative aerobic bacteria including *Pseudomonas aeruginosa*, *Neisseria meningitidis*, and *Haemophilus influenzae*; it should not be used alone for 'blind' treatment since it is not active against Gram-positive organisms. Aztreonam is also effective against *Neisseria gonorrhoeae* (but not against concurrent chlamydial infection). Side-effects are similar to those of the other beta-lactams although aztreonam may be less likely to cause hypersensitivity in penicillin-sensitive patients.

Imipenem, a carbapenem, has a broad spectrum of activity which includes many aerobic and anaerobic Gram-positive and Gram-negative bacteria. Imipenem is partially inactivated in the kidney by enzymatic activity and is therefore administered in combination with **cilastatin**, a specific enzyme inhibitor, which blocks its renal metabolism. Side-effects are similar to those of other beta-lactam antibiotics; neurotoxicity has been observed at very high dosage or in renal failure.

Meropenem is similar to imipenem but is stable to the renal enzyme which inactivates imipenem and therefore can be given without cilastatin. Meropenem has less seizure-inducing potential and can be used to treat central nervous system infection.

Ertapenem has a broad spectrum of activity that covers Gram-positive and Gram-negative organisms and anaerobes. It is licensed for treating abdominal and gynaecological infections and for community-acquired pneumonia, but it is not active against atypical respiratory pathogens and it has limited activity against penicillin-resistant pneumococci. It is also licensed for treating foot infections of the skin and soft tissue in patients with diabetes. Unlike imipenem and meropenem, ertapenem is not active against *Pseudomonas* or against *Acinetobacter* spp.

AZTREONAM

Indications Gram-negative infections including *Pseudomonas aeruginosa, Haemophilus influenzae*, and *Neisseria meningitidis*

Cautions hypersensitivity to beta-lactam antibiotics; hepatic impairment; renal impairment (Appendix 3); breast-feeding (Appendix 5); **interactions:** Appendix 1 (aztreonam)

Contra-indications aztreonam hypersensitivity; pregnancy (Appendix 4)

Side-effects nausea, vomiting, diarrhoea, abdominal cramps; mouth ulcers, altered taste; jaundice and hepatitis; flushing; hypersensitivity reactions; blood disorders (including thrombocytopenia and neutropenia); rashes, injection-site reactions; rarely hypotension, seizures, asthenia, confusion, dizziness, headache, halitosis, and breast tenderness; very rarely antibiotic-associated colitis, gastro-intestinal bleeding, and toxic epidermal necrolysis

Dose

- By deep intramuscular injection *or* by intravenous injection over 3–5 minutes *or* by intravenous infusion, 1 g every 8 hours *or* 2 g every 12 hours; 2 g every 6–8 hours for severe infections (including systemic *Pseudomonas aeruginosa* and lung infections in cystic fibrosis); single doses over 1 g intravenous route only
  Urinary-tract infections, 0.5–1 g every 8–12 hours
- CHILD over 1 week, by intravenous injection *or* infusion, 30 mg/kg every 6–8 hours increased in severe infections for child of 2 years or older to 50 mg/kg every 6–8 hours; max. 8 g daily
- Gonorrhoea, cystitis, by intramuscular injection, 1 g as a single dose

Azactam® (Squibb) PoM
Injection, powder for reconstitution, aztreonam. Net price 500-mg vial = £5.00; 1-g vial = £9.98; 2-g vial = £19.98

ERTAPENEM

Indications abdominal infections; acute gynaecological infections; community-acquired pneumonia; diabetic foot infections of the skin and soft-tissue; prophylaxis for colorectal surgery

Cautions sensitivity to beta-lactam antibacterials (avoid if history of immediate hypersensitivity reaction, see also p. 284); elderly, renal impairment (Appendix 3), CNS disorders—risk of seizures; pregnancy (Appendix 4); **interactions:** Appendix 1 (ertapenem)

Contra-indications breast-feeding (Appendix 5)

Side-effects diarrhoea, nausea, vomiting, headache, injection-site reactions, rash, pruritus, raised platelet count; *less commonly* dry mouth, taste disturbances, dyspepsia, abdominal pain, anorexia, constipation, melaena, antibiotic-associated colitis, bradycardia, hypotension, chest pain, oedema, pharyngeal discomfort, dyspnoea, dizziness, sleep disturbances, confusion, asthenia, seizures, vaginitis, raised glucose, petechiae; *rarely* dysphagia, cholecystitis, liver disorder (including jaundice), arrhythmia, increase in blood pressure, syncope, nasal congestion, cough, wheezing, anxiety, depression, agitation, tremor, pelvic peritonitis, renal impairment, muscle cramp, scleral disorder, blood disorders (including neutropenia, thrombocytopenia, haemorrhage), hypoglycaemia, electrolyte disturbances; *very rarely* hallucinations

Dose

- By intravenous infusion, ADULT and ADOLESCENT over 13 years, 1 g once daily; CHILD 3 months–13 years, 15 mg/kg every 12 hours (max. 1 g daily)
  Surgical prophylaxis, colorectal surgery, ADULT over 18 years, 1 g completed within 1 hour before surgery

Invanz® (MSD) ▼ PoM

Intravenous infusion, powder for reconstitution, ertapenem (as sodium salt), net price 1-g vial = £31.65
Electrolytes Na^+ 6 mmol/1-g vial

IMIPENEM WITH CILASTATIN

Indications aerobic and anaerobic Gram-positive and Gram-negative infections; surgical prophylaxis; hospital-acquired septicaemia (Table 1, section 5.1); not indicated for CNS infections

Cautions sensitivity to beta-lactam antibacterials (avoid if history of immediate hypersensitivity reaction, see also p. 284); renal impairment (Appendix 3); CNS disorders (e.g. epilepsy); pregnancy (Appendix 4); breast-feeding (Appendix 5); **interactions:** Appendix 1 (imipenem with cilastatin)

Side-effects nausea, vomiting, diarrhoea (antibiotic-associated colitis reported), taste disturbances, tooth or tongue discoloration, hearing loss; blood disorders, positive Coombs' test; allergic reactions (with rash, pruritus, urticaria, Stevens-Johnson syndrome, fever, anaphylactic reactions, rarely toxic epidermal necrolysis, exfoliative dermatitis); myoclonic activity, convulsions, confusion and mental disturbances reported; slight increases in liver enzymes and bilirubin reported, rarely hepatitis; increases in serum creatinine and blood urea; red coloration of urine in children reported; local reactions: erythema, pain and induration, and thrombophlebitis

Dose

- By deep intramuscular injection, mild to moderate infections, in terms of imipenem, 500–750 mg every 12 hours
- By intravenous infusion, in terms of imipenem, 1–2 g daily (in 3–4 divided doses); less sensitive organisms, up to 50 mg/kg daily (max. 4 g daily) in 3–4 divided doses; CHILD 3 months and older, 60 mg/kg (up to max. of 2 g) daily in 4 divided doses; over 40 kg, adult dose
- Surgical prophylaxis, by intravenous infusion, 1 g at induction repeated after 3 hours, supplemented in high risk (e.g. colorectal) surgery by doses of 500 mg 8 and 16 hours after induction

Primaxin® (MSD) PoM

Intramuscular injection, powder for reconstitution, imipenem (as monohydrate) 500 mg with cilastatin (as sodium salt) 500 mg, net price per vial = £12.00
Electrolytes Na^+ 1.47 mmol/vial

Intravenous infusion, powder for reconstitution, imipenem (as monohydrate) 500 mg with cilastatin (as sodium salt) 500 mg, net price per vial = £12.00; *Monovial* (vial with transfer needle) = £12.00
Electrolytes Na^+ 1.72 mmol/vial

MEROPENEM

Indications aerobic and anaerobic Gram-positive and Gram-negative infections

Cautions sensitivity to beta-lactam antibacterials (avoid if history of immediate hypersensitivity reaction, see also p. 284); hepatic impairment (monitor liver function; Appendix 2); renal impairment (Appendix 3); pregnancy (Appendix 4); breast-feeding (Appendix 5); **interactions:** Appendix 1 (meropenem)

Side-effects nausea, vomiting, diarrhoea (antibiotic-associated colitis reported), abdominal pain, disturbances in liver function tests; headache; thrombocythaemia, positive Coombs' test; rash, pruritus, injection-site reactions; *less commonly* eosinophilia, thrombocytopenia; *rarely* convulsions; also reported paraesthesia, leucopenia, haemolytic anaemia, reduction in partial thromboplastin time, Stevens-Johnson syndrome, and toxic epidermal necrolysis

Dose

- By intravenous injection over 5 minutes *or* by intravenous infusion, 500 mg every 8 hours, dose doubled in hospital-acquired pneumonia, peritonitis, septicaemia and infections in neutropenic patients; CHILD 3 months–12 years [not licensed for infection in neutropenia] 10–20 mg/kg every 8 hours, over 50 kg body weight adult dose
  Meningitis, 2 g every 8 hours; CHILD 3 months–12 years 40 mg/kg every 8 hours, over 50 kg body weight adult dose
  Exacerbations of chronic lower respiratory-tract infection in cystic fibrosis, up to 2 g every 8 hours; CHILD 4–18 years 25–40 mg/kg every 8 hours

Meronem® (AstraZeneca) PoM

Injection, powder for reconstitution, meropenem (as trihydrate), net price 500-mg vial = £14.33; 1-g vial = £28.65
Electrolytes Na^+ 3.9 mmol/g

5.1.3 Tetracyclines

The tetracyclines are broad-spectrum antibiotics whose value has decreased owing to increasing bacterial resistance. They remain, however, the treatment of choice for infections caused by chlamydia (trachoma, psittacosis, salpingitis, urethritis, and lymphogranuloma venereum), rickettsia (including Q-fever), brucella (doxycycline with either streptomycin or rifampicin), and the spirochaete, *Borrelia burgdorferi* (Lyme disease—see section 5.1.1.3). They are also used in respiratory and genital mycoplasma infections, in acne, in destructive (refractory) periodontal disease, in exacerbations of chronic bronchitis (because of their activity against *Haemophilus influenzae*), and for leptospirosis in penicillin hypersensitivity (as an alternative to erythromycin).

For the role of tetracyclines in the management of meticillin-resistant *Staphylococcus aureus* (MRSA) infection, see p. 296.

Microbiologically, there is little to choose between the various tetracyclines, the only exception being **minocycline** which has a broader spectrum; it is active against *Neisseria meningitidis* and has been used for meningococcal prophylaxis but is no longer recommended because of side-effects including dizziness

5 Infections

and vertigo (see section 5.1, table 2 for current recommendations).

Oral infections In adults, tetracyclines can be effective against oral anaerobes but the development of resistance (especially by oral streptococci) has reduced their usefulness for the treatment of acute oral infections; they may still have a role in the treatment of destructive (refractory) forms of periodontal disease. Doxycycline has a longer duration of action than tetracycline or oxytetracycline and need only be given once daily; it is reported to be more active against anaerobes than some other tetracyclines.

For the use of doxycycline in the treatment of recurrent aphthous ulceration, oral herpes, or as an adjunct to gingival scaling and root planing for periodontitis, see section 12.3.1 and section 12.3.2.

Cautions Tetracyclines should be used with caution in patients with hepatic impairment (Appendix 2) or those receiving potentially hepatotoxic drugs. Tetracyclines may increase muscle weakness in patients with myasthenia gravis, and exacerbate systemic lupus erythematosus. Antacids, and aluminium, calcium, iron, magnesium and zinc salts decrease the absorption of tetracyclines; milk also reduces the absorption of demeclocycline, oxytetracycline, and tetracycline. Other **interactions:** Appendix 1 (tetracyclines).

Contra-indications Deposition of tetracyclines in growing bone and teeth (by binding to calcium) causes staining and occasionally dental hypoplasia, and they should **not** be given to children under 12 years, or to pregnant (Appendixes 4) or breast-feeding women (Appendix 5). However, doxycycline may be used in children for treatment and post-exposure prophylaxis of anthrax when an alternative antibacterial cannot be given [unlicensed indication]. With the exception of **doxycycline** and **minocycline**, the tetracyclines may exacerbate renal failure and should **not** be given to patients with kidney disease (Appendix 3). Tetracyclines should not be given to patients with porphyria (section 9.8.2).

Side-effects Side-effects of the tetracyclines include nausea, vomiting, diarrhoea (antibiotic-associated colitis reported occasionally), dysphagia, and oesophageal irritation. Other rare side-effects include hepatotoxicity, pancreatitis, blood disorders, photosensitivity (particularly with demeclocycline), and hypersensitivity reactions (including rash, exfoliative dermatitis, Stevens-Johnson syndrome, urticaria, angioedema, anaphylaxis, pericarditis). Headache and visual disturbances may indicate benign intracranial hypertension (discontinue treatment); bulging fontanelles have been reported in infants.

TETRACYCLINE

Indications see notes above; acne vulgaris, rosacea (section 13.6)

Cautions see notes above

Contra-indications see notes above

Side-effects see notes above; also acute renal failure, skin discoloration

Dose

- 250 mg every 6 hours, increased in severe infections to 500 mg every 6–8 hours
- Acne, see section 13.6.2
- Non-gonococcal urethritis, 500 mg every 6 hours for 7–14 days (21 days if failure or relapse after first course)

Counselling Tablets should be swallowed whole with plenty of fluid while sitting or standing

Tetracycline (Non-proprietary) PoM

Tablets, coated, tetracycline hydrochloride 250 mg, net price 28-tab pack = £8.63. Label: 7, 9, 23, counselling, posture

Dental prescribing on NHS Tetracycline Tablets may be prescribed

DEMECLOCYCLINE HYDROCHLORIDE

Indications see notes above; also inappropriate secretion of antidiuretic hormone, section 6.5.2

Cautions see notes above, but photosensitivity more common (avoid exposure to sunlight or sun lamps)

Contra-indications see notes above

Side-effects see notes above; also reversible nephrogenic diabetes insipidus, acute renal failure

Dose

- 150 mg every 6 hours *or* 300 mg every 12 hours

Ledermycin® (Goldshield) PoM

Capsules, red, demeclocycline hydrochloride 150 mg, net price 28-cap pack = £6.94. Label: 7, 9, 11, 23

DOXYCYCLINE

Indications see notes above; chronic prostatitis; sinusitis, syphilis, pelvic inflammatory disease (Table 1, section 5.1); treatment and prophylaxis of anthrax [unlicensed indication]; malaria treatment and prophylaxis (section 5.4.1); recurrent aphthous ulceration, adjunct to gingival scaling and root planing for periodontitis (section 12.3.1); oral herpes simplex (section 12.3.2); rosacea [unlicensed indication], acne vulgaris (section 13.6)

Cautions see notes above, but may be used in renal impairment; alcohol dependence; photosensitivity reported (avoid exposure to sunlight or sun lamps); avoid in porphyria (section 9.8.2)

Contra-indications see notes above

Side-effects see notes above; also anorexia, flushing, and tinnitus

Dose

- 200 mg on first day, then 100 mg daily; severe infections (including refractory urinary-tract infections), 200 mg daily
- Early syphilis, 100 mg twice daily for 14 days; late latent syphilis 200 mg twice daily for 28 days
- Uncomplicated genital chlamydia, non-gonococcal urethritis, 100 mg twice daily for 7 days (14 days in pelvic inflammatory disease, see also Table 1, section 5.1)
- Anthrax (treatment or post-exposure prophylaxis; see also section 5.1.12), 100 mg twice daily; CHILD (only if alternative antibacterial cannot be given) [unlicensed dose] 5 mg/kg daily in 2 divided doses (max. 200 mg daily)

Counselling Capsules should be swallowed whole with plenty of fluid during meals while sitting or standing

Note Doxycycline doses in BNF may differ from those in product literature

5 Infections

Doxycycline (Non-proprietary) PoM
Capsules, doxycycline (as hyclate) 50 mg, net price 28-cap pack = £2.40; 100 mg, 8-cap pack = 91p. Label: 6, 9, 11, 27, counselling, posture
Brands include *Doxylar®*
Dental prescribing on NHS Doxycycline Capsules 100 mg may be prescribed

Vibramycin® (Pfizer) PoM
Capsules, doxycycline (as hyclate) 50 mg (green/ivory), net price 28-cap pack = £7.74. Label: 6, 9, 11, 27, counselling, posture

Vibramycin-D® (Pfizer) PoM
Dispersible tablets, yellow, scored, doxycycline 100 mg, net price 8-tab pack = £4.91. Label: 6, 9, 11, 13

LYMECYCLINE

Indications see notes above
Cautions see notes above
Contra-indications see notes above
Side-effects see notes above
Dose
- 408 mg every 12 hours, increased to 1.224–1.632 g daily in severe infections
- Acne, 408 mg daily for at least 8 weeks

Tetralysal 300® (Galderma) PoM
Capsules, red/yellow, lymecycline 408 mg (= tetracycline 300 mg), net price 28-cap pack = £7.16, 56-cap pack = £14.26. Label: 6, 9

MINOCYCLINE

Indications see notes above; meningococcal carrier state; acne vulgaris (section 13.6.2)
Cautions see notes above, but may be used in renal impairment; if treatment continued for longer than 6 months, monitor every 3 months for hepatotoxicity, pigmentation and for systemic lupus erythematosus—discontinue if these develop or if pre-existing systemic lupus erythematosus worsens
Contra-indications see notes above
Side-effects see notes above; also dizziness and vertigo (more common in women); *rarely* anorexia, tinnitus, impaired hearing, hyperaesthesia, paraesthesia, acute renal failure, pigmentation (sometimes irreversible), and alopecia; *very rarely* systemic lupus erythematosus, discoloration of conjunctiva, tears, and sweat
Dose
- 100 mg twice daily
- Acne, see section 13.6.2 and under preparations, below
- Prophylaxis of asymptomatic meningococcal carrier state (but no longer recommended, see notes above), 100 mg twice daily for 5 days usually followed by rifampicin

Counselling Tablets or capsules should be swallowed whole with plenty of fluid while sitting or standing

Minocycline (Non-proprietary) PoM
Capsules, minocycline (as hydrochloride) 50 mg, net price 56-cap pack = £15.27; 100 mg, 28-cap pack = £13.09. Label: 6, 9, counselling, posture
Brands include *Aknemin®*
Tablets, minocycline (as hydrochloride) 50 mg, net price 28-tab pack = £6.14, 100 mg, 28-tab pack = £12.60. Label: 6, 9, counselling, posture

Modified release

Acnamino® MR (Dexcel) PoM
Capsules, m/r, buff/brown (enclosing pink and peach tablets), minocycline (as hydrochloride) 100 mg, net price 56-cap pack = £21.14. Label: 6, 25
Dose acne, 1 capsule daily

Minocin MR® (Meda) PoM
Capsules, m/r, orange/brown (enclosing yellow and white pellets), minocycline (as hydrochloride) 100 mg. Net price 56-cap pack = £21.14. Label: 6, 25
Dose acne, 1 capsule daily

Sebomin MR® (Actavis) PoM
Capsules, m/r, orange, minocycline (as hydrochloride) 100 mg, net price 56-cap pack = £21.14. Label: 6, 25
Dose acne, 1 capsule daily

OXYTETRACYCLINE

Indications see notes above; acne vulgaris, rosacea (section 13.6)
Cautions see notes above; porphyria (section 9.8.2)
Contra-indications see notes above
Side-effects see notes above
Dose
- 250–500 mg every 6 hours
- Acne, see section 13.6.2

Oxytetracycline (Non-proprietary) PoM
Tablets, coated, oxytetracycline dihydrate 250 mg, net price 28-tab pack = 54p. Label: 7, 9, 23
Brands include *Oxymycin®*
Dental prescribing on NHS Oxtetracycline Tablets may be prescribed

Tigecycline

Tigecycline is a glycylcycline antibacterial structurally related to the tetracyclines; side-effects similar to those of the tetracyclines can potentially occur. Tigecycline is active against Gram-positive and Gram-negative bacteria, including tetracycline-resistant organisms, and some anaerobes. It is also active against meticillin-resistant *Staphylococcus aureus* and vancomycin-resistant enterococci, however, many strains of *Proteus spp.* or *Pseudomonas aeruginosa* are resistant to tigecycline. Tigecycline should be reserved for the treatment of complicated skin and soft-tissue infections and complicated abdominal infections caused by multiple-antibacterial resistant organisms.

TIGECYCLINE

Indications complicated intra-abdominal infections; complicated skin and soft-tissue infections
Cautions cholestasis, hepatic impairment (Appendix 2); breast-feeding (Appendix 5); **interactions:** Appendix 1 (tigecycline)
Contra-indications hypersensitivity to tetracyclines; pregnancy (Appendix 4)
Side-effects see notes above; also nausea, vomiting, abdominal pain, dyspepsia, diarrhoea, anorexia, bilirubinaemia, dizziness, headache, prolonged

prothrombin time, prolonged activated partial thromboplastin time, rash, pruritus, and injection-site reactions; *less commonly* pancreatitis and hypoproteinaemia; also reported, antibiotic-associated colitis

Dose

- By intravenous infusion, ADULT over 18 years, initially 100 mg, then 50 mg every 12 hours for 5–14 days

Tygacil® (Wyeth) ▼ PoM
Intravenous infusion, powder for reconstitution, tigecycline, net price 50-mg vial = £32.31

5.1.4 Aminoglycosides

These include amikacin, gentamicin, neomycin, streptomycin, and tobramycin. All are bactericidal and active against some Gram-positive and many Gram-negative organisms. Amikacin, gentamicin, and tobramycin are also active against *Pseudomonas aeruginosa*; streptomycin is active against *Mycobacterium tuberculosis* and is now almost entirely reserved for tuberculosis (section 5.1.9).

The aminoglycosides are not absorbed from the gut (although there is a risk of absorption in inflammatory bowel disease and liver failure) and must therefore be given by injection for systemic infections.

Excretion is principally via the kidney and accumulation occurs in renal impairment.

Most side-effects of this group of antibiotics are dose-related therefore care must be taken with dosage and whenever possible treatment should not exceed 7 days. The important side-effects are ototoxicity, and nephrotoxicity; they occur most commonly in the elderly and in patients with renal failure.

If there is impairment of renal function (or high pre-dose serum concentrations) the interval between doses must be increased; if the renal impairment is severe the dose itself should be reduced as well.

Aminoglycosides may impair neuromuscular transmission and should not be given to patients with myasthenia gravis; large doses given during surgery have been responsible for a transient myasthenic syndrome in patients with normal neuromuscular function.

Aminoglycosides should preferably not be given with potentially ototoxic diuretics (e.g. furosemide (frusemide)); if concurrent use is unavoidable administration of the aminoglycoside and of the diuretic should be separated by as long a period as practicable.

Once daily dosage Although aminoglycosides are given in 2–3 divided doses during the 24 hours, *once daily administration* is more convenient (while ensuring adequate serum concentration) but local guidelines on dosage and serum concentrations should be consulted. A once-daily, high-dose regimen of an aminoglycoside should be avoided in patients with endocarditis, extensive burns, or creatinine clearance less than 20 mL/minute.

Serum concentrations Serum concentration monitoring avoids both excessive and subtherapeutic concentrations thus preventing toxicity and ensuring efficacy. In patients with normal renal function, aminoglycoside concentrations should be measured after 3 or 4 doses of a multiple daily dose regimen; patients with renal impairment may require earlier and more frequent measurement of aminoglycoside concentration.

For multiple daily dose regimens, blood samples should be taken approximately 1 hour after intramuscular or intravenous administration ('peak' concentration) and also just before the next dose ('trough' concentration). For once daily dose regimens, consult local guidelines on serum concentration monitoring.

Serum-aminoglycoside concentrations should be measured in all patients and **must** be determined in infants, in the elderly, in obesity, and in cystic fibrosis, *or* if high doses are being given, *or* if there is renal impairment.

Endocarditis **Gentamicin** is used in combination with other antibiotics for the treatment of bacterial endocarditis (Table 1, section 5.1). Serum-gentamicin concentration should be determined twice each week (more often in renal impairment). **Streptomycin** may be used as an alternative in gentamicin-resistant enterococcal endocarditis.

Gentamicin is the aminoglycoside of choice in the UK and is used widely for the treatment of serious infections. It has a broad spectrum but is inactive against anaerobes and has poor activity against haemolytic streptococci and pneumococci. When used for the 'blind' therapy of undiagnosed serious infections it is usually given in conjunction with a penicillin or metronidazole (or both). Gentamicin is used together with another antibiotic for the treatment of endocarditis (see above and Table 1, section 5.1).

Loading and maintenance doses of gentamicin may be calculated on the basis of the patient's weight and renal function (e.g. using a nomogram); adjustments are then made according to serum-gentamicin concentrations. High doses are occasionally indicated for serious infections, especially in the neonate, in the patient with cystic fibrosis, or in the immunocompromised patient. Whenever possible treatment should not exceed 7 days.

Amikacin is more stable than gentamicin to enzyme inactivation. Amikacin is used in the treatment of serious infections caused by gentamicin-resistant Gram-negative bacilli.

Tobramycin has similar activity to gentamicin. It is slightly more active against *Ps. aeruginosa* but shows less activity against certain other Gram-negative bacteria. Tobramycin may be administered by nebuliser on a cyclical basis (28 days of tobramycin followed by a 28-day tobramycin-free interval) for the treatment of chronic pulmonary *Ps. aeruginosa* infection in cystic fibrosis; however, resistance may develop and some patients do not respond to treatment.

Neomycin is too toxic for parenteral administration and can only be used for infections of the skin or mucous membranes or to reduce the bacterial population of the colon prior to bowel surgery or in hepatic failure. Oral administration may lead to malabsorption. Small amounts of neomycin may be absorbed from the gut in patients with hepatic failure and, as these patients may also be uraemic, cumulation may occur with resultant ototoxicity.

GENTAMICIN

Indications septicaemia and neonatal sepsis; meningitis and other CNS infections; biliary-tract infection, acute pyelonephritis or prostatitis, endocarditis (see notes above); pneumonia in hospital patients, adjunct in listerial meningitis (Table 1, section 5.1); eye (section 11.3.1); ear (section 12.1.1)

Cautions pregnancy (Appendix 4), renal impairment, neonates, infants and elderly (adjust dose and monitor renal, auditory and vestibular function together with serum gentamicin concentrations); avoid prolonged use; conditions characterised by muscular weakness; obesity (use ideal weight for height to calculate dose and monitor serum-gentamicin concentration closely); see also notes above; **interactions**: Appendix 1 (aminoglycosides)

Contra-indications myasthenia gravis

Side-effects vestibular and auditory damage, nephrotoxicity; rarely, hypomagnesaemia on prolonged therapy, antibiotic-associated colitis, stomatitis; also reported, nausea, vomiting, rash, blood disorders; see also notes above

Dose

- Multiple daily dose regimen, by intramuscular *or* by slow intravenous injection over at least 3 minutes *or* by intravenous infusion, 3–5 mg/kg daily (in divided doses every 8 hours), see also notes above; NEONATE up to 2 weeks, 3 mg/kg every 12 hours; CHILD 2 weeks–12 years, 2 mg/kg every 8 hours

  Endocarditis (in combination with other antibacterials, see Table 1, section 5.1), ADULT 1 mg/kg every 8 hours
- Once daily dose regimen (see notes above and also consult local guidelines), by intravenous infusion, initially 5–7 mg/kg, then adjust according to serum-gentamicin concentration
- By intrathecal injection, seek specialist advice, 1 mg daily (increased if necessary to 5 mg daily)

Note For multiple daily dose regimen, one-hour ('peak') serum concentration should be 5–10 mg/litre (3–5 mg/litre for endocarditis); pre-dose ('trough') concentration should be less than 2 mg/litre (less than 1 mg/litre for endocarditis). For once-daily dose regimen, consult local guidelines on monitoring serum-gentamicin concentration

Gentamicin (Non-proprietary) PoM

Injection, gentamicin (as sulphate), net price 40 mg/mL, 1-mL amp = £1.40, 2-mL amp = £1.54, 2-mL vial = £1.48

Paediatric injection, gentamicin (as sulphate) 10 mg/mL, net price 2-mL vial = £1.80

Intrathecal injection, gentamicin (as sulphate) 5 mg/mL, net price 1-mL amp = 74p

Cidomycin® (Beacon) PoM

Injection, gentamicin (as sulphate) 40 mg/mL. Net price 2-mL amp or vial = £1.48

Genticin® (Roche) PoM

Injection, gentamicin (as sulphate) 40 mg/mL. Net price 2-mL amp = £1.40

Isotonic Gentamicin Injection (Baxter) PoM

Intravenous infusion, gentamicin (as sulphate) 800 micrograms/mL in sodium chloride intravenous infusion 0.9%. Net price 100-mL (80-mg) *Viaflex®* bag = £1.61

Electrolytes Na^+ 15.4 mmol/100-mL bag

AMIKACIN

Indications serious Gram-negative infections resistant to gentamicin

Cautions see under Gentamicin

Contra-indications see under Gentamicin

Side-effects see under Gentamicin

Dose

- By intramuscular *or* by slow intravenous injection *or* by infusion, 15 mg/kg daily in 2 divided doses, increased to 22.5 mg/kg daily in 3 divided doses in severe infections; max. 1.5 g daily for up to 10 days (max. cumulative dose 15 g); CHILD 15 mg/kg daily in 2 divided doses; NEONATE loading dose of 10 mg/kg then 15 mg/kg daily in 2 divided doses

  Note One-hour ('peak') serum concentration should not exceed 30 mg/litre; pre-dose ('trough') concentration should be less than 10 mg/litre

Amikacin (Non-proprietary) PoM

Injection, amikacin (as sulphate) 250 mg/mL. Net price 2-mL vial = £10.14

Electrolytes Na^+ 0.56 mmol/500-mg vial

Amikin® (Bristol-Myers Squibb) PoM

Injection, amikacin (as sulphate) 250 mg/mL. Net price 2-mL vial = £10.14

Electrolytes $Na^+ < 0.5$ mmol/vial

Paediatric injection, amikacin (as sulphate) 50 mg/mL. Net price 2-mL vial = £2.36

Electrolytes $Na^+ < 0.5$ mmol/vial

NEOMYCIN SULPHATE

Indications bowel sterilisation before surgery, see also notes above

Cautions see under Gentamicin but too toxic for systemic use, see notes above

Contra-indications see under Gentamicin; intestinal obstruction; renal impairment (Appendix 3)

Side-effects see under Gentamicin but poorly absorbed on oral administration; increased salivation, stomatitis, impaired intestinal absorption with steatorrhoea and diarrhoea

Dose

- By mouth, pre-operative bowel sterilisation, 1 g every hour for 4 hours, then 1 g every 4 hours for 2–3 days

  Hepatic coma, up to 4 g daily in divided doses usually for max. 14 days

Neomycin (Non-proprietary) PoM

Tablets, neomycin sulphate 500 mg. Net price 20 = £4.13

Brands include *Nivemycin®*

TOBRAMYCIN

Indications see under Gentamicin and notes above

Cautions see under Gentamicin

Specific cautions for inhaled treatment Other inhaled drugs should be administered before tobramycin; monitor for bronchospasm with initial dose, measure peak flow before and after nebulisation—if bronchospasm occurs, repeat test using bronchodilator; monitor renal function before treatment and then annually; severe haemoptysis

Contra-indications see under Gentamicin

Side-effects see under Gentamicin; *on inhalation*, mouth ulcers, voice alteration, cough, bronchospasm (see Cautions)

5 Infections

Dose

- By intramuscular injection *or* by slow intravenous injection *or* by intravenous infusion, 3 mg/kg daily in divided doses every 8 hours, see also notes above; in severe infections up to 5 mg/kg daily in divided doses every 6–8 hours (reduced to 3 mg/kg as soon as clinically indicated); NEONATE 2 mg/kg every 12 hours; CHILD over 1 week 2–2.5 mg/kg every 8 hours
- Urinary-tract infection, by intramuscular injection, 2–3 mg/kg daily as a single dose

Note One-hour ('peak') serum concentration should not exceed 10 mg/litre; pre-dose ('trough') concentration should be less than 2 mg/litre

Tobramycin (Non-proprietary) PoM

Injection, tobramycin (as sulphate) 40 mg/mL, net price 1-mL (40-mg) vial = £4.00, 2-mL (80-mg) vial = £6.40, 6-mL (240-mg) vial = £19.20

Tobi® (Chiron) PoM

Nebuliser solution, tobramycin 60 mg/mL, net price 56 × 5-mL (300-mg) unit = £1484.00

Dose chronic pulmonary *Pseudomonas aeruginosa* infection in cystic fibrosis patients, by inhalation of nebulised solution, ADULT and CHILD over 6 years, 300 mg every 12 hours for 28 days, courses repeated after 28-day interval

5.1.5 Macrolides

Erythromycin has an antibacterial spectrum that is similar but not identical to that of penicillin; it is thus an alternative in penicillin-allergic patients.

Indications for erythromycin include respiratory infections, whooping cough, legionnaires' disease, and campylobacter enteritis. It is active against many penicillin-resistant staphylococci but some are now also resistant to erythromycin; it has poor activity against *Haemophilus influenzae*. Erythromycin is also active against chlamydia and mycoplasmas.

Erythromycin causes nausea, vomiting, and diarrhoea in some patients; in mild to moderate infections this can be avoided by giving a lower dose (250 mg 4 times daily) but if a more serious infection, such as Legionella pneumonia, is suspected higher doses are needed.

Azithromycin is a macrolide with slightly less activity than erythromycin against Gram-positive bacteria but enhanced activity against some Gram-negative organisms including *H. influenzae*. Plasma concentrations are very low but tissue concentrations are much higher. It has a long tissue half-life and once daily dosage is recommended. For treatment of Lyme disease, see section 5.1.1.3. Azithromycin is also used in the treatment of trachoma [unlicensed indication] (section 11.3.1).

Clarithromycin is an erythromycin derivative with slightly greater activity than the parent compound. Tissue concentrations are higher than with erythromycin. It is given twice daily.

Azithromycin and clarithromycin cause fewer gastro-intestinal side-effects than erythromycin.

Spiramycin is also a macrolide (section 5.4.7).

The ketolide **telithromycin** is a derivative of erythromycin. The antibacterial spectrum of telithromycin is similar to that of macrolides and it is also active against penicillin- and erythromycin-resistant *Streptococcus pneumoniae*. Telithromycin should only be used to treat beta-haemolytic streptococcal pharyngitis and tonsillitis, sinusitis, community-acquired pneumonia, and exacerbations of chronic bronchitis if caused by organisms resistant to beta-lactam antibacterials and other macrolides, or if conventional treatment is contra-indicated.

Oral infections Erythromycin is an alternative for oral infections in penicillin-allergic patients or where a beta-lactamase producing organism is involved. However, many organisms are now resistant to erythromycin or rapidly develop resistance; its use should therefore be limited to short courses. Metronidazole (section 5.1.11) may be preferred as an alternative to a penicillin.

ERYTHROMYCIN

Indications susceptible infections in patients with penicillin hypersensitivity; oral infections (see notes above); campylobacter enteritis, syphilis, non-gonococcal urethritis, respiratory-tract infections (including Legionnaires' disease), skin infections (Table 1, section 5.1); chronic prostatitis; prophylaxis of diphtheria, group A streptococcal infection, and whooping cough (Table 2, section 5.1); acne vulgaris and rosacea (section 13.6)

Cautions neonate under 2 weeks (risk of hypertrophic pyloric stenosis); predisposition to QT interval prolongation (including electrolyte disturbances, concomitant use of drugs that prolong QT interval); avoid in porphyria (section 9.8.2); hepatic impairment (Appendix 2); renal impairment (Appendix 3); pregnancy (not known to be harmful) and breast-feeding (only small amounts in milk); **interactions:** Appendix 1 (macrolides)

Side-effects nausea, vomiting, abdominal discomfort, diarrhoea (antibiotic-associated colitis reported); less frequently urticaria, rashes and other allergic reactions; reversible hearing loss reported after large doses; cholestatic jaundice, pancreatitis, cardiac effects (including chest pain and arrhythmias), myasthenia-like syndrome, Stevens-Johnson syndrome, and toxic epidermal necrolysis also reported

Dose

- By mouth, ADULT and CHILD over 8 years, 250–500 mg every 6 hours *or* 0.5–1 g every 12 hours (see notes above); up to 4 g daily in severe infections; NEONATE 12.5 mg/kg every 6 hours; CHILD 1 month–2 years 125 mg every 6 hours; 2–8 years 250 mg every 6 hours, doses doubled for severe infections

  Early syphilis, 500 mg 4 times daily for 14 days

  Uncomplicated genital chlamydia, non-gonococcal urethritis, 500 mg twice daily for 14 days
- By intravenous infusion, ADULT and CHILD severe infections, 50 mg/kg daily by continuous infusion *or* in divided doses every 6 hours; mild infections (oral treatment not possible), 25 mg/kg daily; NEONATE 30–45 mg/kg daily in 3 divided doses

Erythromycin (Non-proprietary) PoM

Capsules, enclosing e/c microgranules, erythromycin 250 mg, net price 28-cap pack = £5.95. Label: 5, 9, 25

Brands include *Tiloryth®*

Tablets, e/c, erythromycin 250 mg, net price 28 = £3.06. Label: 5, 9, 25

Dental prescribing on NHS Erythromycin Tablets e/c may be prescribed

5 Infections

Erythromycin Ethyl Succinate (Non-proprietary) PoM
Oral suspension, erythromycin (as ethyl succinate) for reconstitution with water 125 mg/5 mL, net price 100 mL = £1.63; 250 mg/5 mL, 100 mL = £2.66; 500 mg/5 mL, 100 mL = £4.88. Label: 9
Note Sugar-free versions are available and can be ordered by specifying 'sugar-free' on the prescription
Brands include *Primacine*®
Dental prescribing on NHS Erythromycin Ethyl Succinate Oral Suspension may be prescribed

Erythromycin Lactobionate (Non-proprietary) PoM
Intravenous infusion, powder for reconstitution, erythromycin (as lactobionate), net price 1-g vial = £9.98

Erymax® (Zeneus) PoM
Capsules, opaque orange/clear orange, enclosing orange and white e/c pellets, erythromycin 250 mg, net price 28-cap pack = £5.95, 112-cap pack = £23.80. Label: 5, 9, 25
Dose 1 capsule every 6 hours *or* 2 capsules every 12 hours; acne, 1 capsule twice daily for 1 month then 1 capsule daily

Erythrocin® (Abbott) PoM
Tablets, both f/c, erythromycin (as stearate), 250 mg, net price 20 = £3.64; 500 mg, 20 = £7.28. Label: 9
Dental prescribing on NHS May be prescribed as Erythromycin Stearate Tablets

Erythroped® (Abbott) PoM
Suspension SF, sugar-free, banana-flavoured, erythromycin (as ethyl succinate) for reconstitution with water, 125 mg/5 mL (*Suspension PI SF*), net price 140 mL = £3.18; 250 mg/5 mL, 140 mL = £6.20; 500 mg/5 mL (*Suspension SF Forte*), 140 mL = £10.99. Label: 9

Erythroped A® (Abbott) PoM
Tablets, yellow, f/c, erythromycin 500 mg (as ethyl succinate). Net price 28-tab pack = £10.78. Label: 9
Dental prescribing on NHS May be prescribed as Erythromycin Ethyl Succinate Tablets

AZITHROMYCIN

Indications respiratory-tract infections; otitis media; skin and soft-tissue infections; uncomplicated genital chlamydial infections and non-gonococcal urethritis (Table 1, section 5.1); mild or moderate typhoid due to multiple-antibacterial-resistant organisms [unlicensed indication]; prophylaxis of group A streptococcal infection (Table 2, section 5.1)

Cautions see under Erythromycin; pregnancy (Appendix 4) and breast-feeding (Appendix 5); **interactions**: Appendix 1 (macrolides)

Contra-indications severe hepatic impairment (Appendix 2)

Side-effects see under Erythromycin; also anorexia, dyspepsia, flatulence, dizziness, headache, drowsiness, convulsions, arthralgia, and disturbances in taste and smell; *rarely* constipation, hepatitis, hepatic failure, syncope, insomnia, agitation, anxiety, asthenia, paraesthesia, hyperactivity, thrombocytopenia, haemolytic anaemia, interstitial nephritis, acute renal failure, photosensitivity, tooth and tongue discoloration

Dose
- 500 mg once daily for 3 days *or* 500 mg on first day then 250 mg once daily for 4 days; CHILD over 6 months 10 mg/kg once daily for 3 days; *or* body-weight 15–25 kg, 200 mg once daily for 3 days; body-weight 26–35 kg, 300 mg once daily for 3 days; body-weight 36–45 kg, 400 mg once daily for 3 days
- Uncomplicated genital chlamydial infections and non-gonococcal urethritis, 1 g as a single dose
- Typhoid [unlicensed indication], 500 mg once daily for 7 days

Azithromycin (Non-proprietary) PoM
Tablets, azithromycin (as monohydrate hemi-ethanolate) 250 mg, net price 4-tab pack = £8.19; 500 mg, 3-tab pack = £10.32. Label: 5, 9

Zithromax® (Pfizer) PoM
Capsules, azithromycin (as dihydrate) 250 mg, net price 4-cap pack = £8.95, 6-cap pack = £13.43. Label: 5, 9, 23
Oral suspension, cherry/banana-flavoured, azithromycin (as dihydrate) 200 mg/5 mL when reconstituted with water. Net price 15-mL pack = £5.08, 22.5-mL pack = £7.62, 30-mL pack = £13.80. Label: 5, 9
Dental prescribing on NHS May be prescribed as Azithromycin Oral Suspension 200 mg/5 mL

CLARITHROMYCIN

Indications respiratory-tract infections, mild to moderate skin and soft tissue infections, otitis media; *Helicobacter pylori* eradication (section 1.3)

Cautions see under Erythromycin; renal impairment (Appendix 3); pregnancy (Appendix 4); breast-feeding (Appendix 5); **interactions**: Appendix 1 (macrolides)

Side-effects see under Erythromycin; also dyspepsia, tooth and tongue discoloration, smell and taste disturbances, stomatitis, glossitis, and headache; *less commonly* hepatitis, arthralgia, and myalgia; *rarely* tinnitus; *very rarely* pancreatitis, dizziness, insomnia, nightmares, anxiety, confusion, psychosis, paraesthesia, convulsions, hypoglycaemia, renal failure, leucopenia, and thrombocytopenia; on intravenous infusion, local tenderness, phlebitis

Dose
- By mouth, 250 mg every 12 hours for 7 days, increased in severe infections to 500 mg every 12 hours for up to 14 days; CHILD body-weight under 8 kg, 7.5 mg/kg twice daily; 8–11 kg (1–2 years), 62.5 mg twice daily; 12–19 kg (3–6 years), 125 mg twice daily; 20–29 kg (7–9 years), 187.5 mg twice daily; 30–40 kg (10–12 years), 250 mg twice daily
- By intravenous infusion into larger proximal vein, 500 mg twice daily; CHILD under 12 years see *BNF for Children*

Clarithromycin (Non-proprietary) PoM
Tablets, clarithromycin 250 mg, net price 14-tab pack = £3.77; 500 mg, 14-tab pack = £7.11. Label: 9

Clarosip® (Grünenthal) PoM
Granules, clarithromycin 125 mg/straw, net price 14-straw pack = £6.70; 187.5 mg/straw, 14-straw pack = £9.70; 250 mg/straw, 14-straw pack = £12.70. Label: 9, counselling, administration
Counselling Place straw in cold or warm drink such as water, carbonated drink, or tea (but **not** full fat milk, milk-shake, or drink with solid particles) and sip drink through straw; several sips may be required to obtain full dose

Klaricid® (Abbott) PoM
Tablets, both yellow, f/c, clarithromycin 250 mg, net price 14-tab pack = £7.43; 500 mg, 14-tab pack = £12.00, 20-tab pack = £17.14. Label: 9

Fucidin® (LEO) PoM

Tablets, f/c, sodium fusidate 250 mg, net price 10-tab pack = £6.02. Label: 9

Dose as sodium fusidate, 500 mg every 8 hours, doubled for severe infections

Skin infection, as sodium fusidate, 250 mg every 12 hours for 5–10 days

Suspension, off-white, banana- and orange-flavoured, fusidic acid 250 mg/5 mL, net price 50 mL = £6.73. Label: 9, 21

Dose as fusidic acid, ADULT 750 mg every 8 hours; CHILD up to 1 year 50 mg/kg daily (in 3 divided doses), 1–5 years 250 mg every 8 hours, 5–12 years 500 mg every 8 hours

Note Fusidic acid is incompletely absorbed and doses recommended for suspension are proportionately higher than those for sodium fusidate tablets

Vancomycin and teicoplanin

The glycopeptide antibiotics vancomycin and teicoplanin have bactericidal activity against aerobic and anaerobic Gram-positive bacteria including multi-resistant staphylococci. However, there are reports of *Staphylococcus aureus* with reduced susceptibility to glycopeptides. There are increasing reports of glycopeptide-resistant enterococci.

Vancomycin is used *by the intravenous route* in the prophylaxis and treatment of endocarditis and other serious infections caused by Gram-positive cocci. It has a relatively long duration of action and can therefore be given every 12 hours. Vancomycin (added to dialysis fluid) is also used in the treatment of peritonitis associated with peritoneal dialysis [unlicensed route] (Table 1 section 5.1).

Vancomycin given *by mouth* is effective in the treatment of antibiotic-associated colitis (pseudomembranous colitis, see also section 1.5); a dose of 125 mg every 6 hours for 7 to 10 days is considered adequate (higher dose may be considered if the infection fails to respond or if it is severe). Vancomycin should **not** be given by mouth for systemic infections since it is not significantly absorbed.

Teicoplanin is very similar to vancomycin but has a significantly longer duration of action allowing once-daily administration. Unlike vancomycin, teicoplanin can be given by intramuscular as well as by intravenous injection; it is not given by mouth.

VANCOMYCIN

Indications see notes above

Cautions avoid rapid infusion (risk of anaphylactoid reactions, see Side-effects); rotate infusion sites; renal impairment (Appendix 3); elderly; avoid if history of deafness; all patients require plasma-vancomycin measurement (after 3 or 4 doses if renal function normal, earlier if renal impairment), blood counts, urinalysis, and renal function tests; monitor auditory function in elderly or if renal impairment; pregnancy (Appendix 4) and breast-feeding (Appendix 5); systemic absorption may follow oral administration especially in inflammatory bowel disorders or following multiple doses; **interactions**: Appendix 1 (vancomycin)

Side-effects after parenteral administration: nephrotoxicity including renal failure and interstitial nephritis; ototoxicity (discontinue if tinnitus occurs); blood disorders including neutropenia (usually after 1 week or cumulative dose of 25 g), rarely agranulocytosis and thrombocytopenia; nausea; chills, fever; eosinophilia, anaphylaxis, rashes (including exfoliative dermatitis, Stevens-Johnson syndrome, toxic epidermal necrolysis, and vasculitis); phlebitis (irritant to tissue); on rapid infusion, severe hypotension (including shock and cardiac arrest), wheezing, dyspnoea, urticaria, pruritus, flushing of the upper body ('red man' syndrome), pain and muscle spasm of back and chest

Dose

- By mouth, antibiotic-associated colitis, 125 mg every 6 hours for 7–10 days, see notes above; CHILD 5 mg/kg every 6 hours, over 5 years, half adult dose

  Note Oral paediatric dose is lower than that on product literature but is adequate
- By intravenous infusion, 1 g every 12 hours; ELDERLY over 65 years, 500 mg every 12 hours *or* 1 g once daily; CHILD over 1 month, 15 mg/kg every 8 hours (max. 2 g daily)

  Note Plasma concentration monitoring required (see Cautions above); pre-dose ('trough') concentration should be 10–15 mg/litre (15–20 mg/litre for less sensitive strains of meticillin-resistant *Staphylococcus aureus*); vancomycin doses in BNF may differ from those in product literature

Vancomycin (Non-proprietary) PoM

Capsules, vancomycin (as hydrochloride) 125 mg, net price 28-cap pack = £66.23; 250 mg, 28-cap pack = £132.47. Label: 9

Injection, powder for reconstitution, vancomycin (as hydrochloride), for use as an infusion, net price 500-mg vial = £8.05; 1-g vial = £16.11

Note Can be used to prepare solution for oral administration

Vancocin® (Flynn) PoM

Matrigel capsules, vancomycin (as hydrochloride) 125 mg, net price 28-cap pack = £88.31. Label: 9

Injection powder for reconstitution, vancomycin (as hydrochloride), for use as an infusion, net price 500-mg vial = £8.05; 1-g vial = £16.11

Note Can be used to prepare solution for oral administration

TEICOPLANIN

Indications potentially serious Gram-positive infections including endocarditis, dialysis-associated peritonitis, and serious infections due to *Staphylococcus aureus*; prophylaxis in orthopaedic surgery at risk of infection with Gram-positive organisms

Cautions vancomycin sensitivity; blood counts and liver and kidney function tests required; monitor plasma-teicoplanin concentration if severe sepsis or burns, deep-seated staphylococcal infection (including bone and joint infection), endocarditis, renal impairment, in elderly, and in intravenous drug abusers; monitor renal and auditory function during prolonged treatment in renal impairment (Appendix 3) or if other nephrotoxic or neurotoxic drugs given; pregnancy (Appendix 4) and breast-feeding; **interactions**: Appendix 1 (teicoplanin)

Side-effects nausea, vomiting, diarrhoea; rash, pruritus, fever, bronchospasm, rigors, urticaria, angioedema, anaphylaxis; dizziness, headache; blood disorders including eosinophilia, leucopenia, neutropenia, and thrombocytopenia; disturbances in liver enzymes, transient increase of serum creatinine, renal failure; tinnitus, mild hearing loss, and vestibular disorders also reported; rarely exfoliative dermatitis, Stevens-Johnson syndrome, toxic epidermal necrolysis; local reactions include erythema, pain, thrombophlebitis, injection site abscess and rarely flushing with infusion

Dose

- By intramuscular injection *or* by intravenous injection *or* infusion, initially 400 mg (for severe infections, by intravenous injection *or* infusion, initially 400 mg every 12 hours for 3 doses), then 200 mg once daily (400 mg once daily for severe infections); higher doses may be required in patients over 85 kg and in severe burns, or meticillin-resistant *Staphylococcus aureus* infection (consult product literature)
- CHILD over 2 months by intravenous injection *or* infusion, initially 10 mg/kg every 12 hours for 3 doses, subsequently 6 mg/kg once daily (severe infections or in neutropenia, 10 mg/kg once daily); subsequent doses can be given by intramuscular injection (but intravenous administration preferred in children); NEONATE by intravenous infusion, initially a single dose of 16 mg/kg, subsequently 8 mg/kg once daily
- Streptococcal endocarditis, by intravenous injection *or* infusion, ADULT initially 6 mg/kg every 12 hours for 3 doses, then 6 mg/kg once daily
- Enterococcal endocarditis, by intravenous injection *or* infusion, ADULT initially 10 mg/kg every 12 hours for 3 doses, then 10 mg/kg once daily
- Orthopaedic surgery prophylaxis, by intravenous injection, 400 mg at induction of anaesthesia

Note Plasma-teicoplanin concentration is not measured routinely because a relationship between plasma concentration and toxicity has not been established. However, the plasma-teicoplanin concentration can be used to optimise treatment in some patients (see Cautions). Pre-dose ('trough') concentrations should be greater than 10 mg/litre (greater than 15–20 mg/litre in endocarditis) but less than 60 mg/litre

Targocid® (Aventis Pharma) PoM
Injection, powder for reconstitution, teicoplanin, net price 200-mg vial (with diluent) = £17.58; 400-mg vial (with diluent) = £35.62
Electrolytes $Na^+ < 0.5$ mmol/200- and 400-mg vial

Daptomycin

Daptomycin is a lipopeptide antibacterial with a spectrum of activity similar to vancomycin but its efficacy against enterococci has not been established. Daptomycin should be reserved for complicated skin and soft-tissue infections caused by resistant Gram-positive bacteria including meticillin-resistant *Staphylococcus aureus* (MRSA). It needs to be given with other antibacterials for mixed infections involving Gram-negative bacteria and some anaerobes.

DAPTOMYCIN

Indications see under Dose

Cautions interference with assay for prothrombin time and INR—take blood sample immediately before daptomycin dose; hepatic impairment (Appendix 2); renal impairment (Appendix 3); pregnancy (Appendix 4); **interactions:** Appendix 1 (daptomycin)

Muscle effects Myalgia, muscle weakness, and myositis may occur uncommonly; rhabdomyolysis is very rare. Monitor creatine kinase before treatment and then weekly during treatment (more frequently if creatine kinase elevated more than 5 times upper limit of normal before treatment, or if receiving another drug known to cause myopathy (preferably avoid concomitant use), or if creatinine clearance less than 30 mL/minute). If unexplained muscle pain, tenderness, weakness, or cramps develop during treatment, measure creatine kinase every 2 days; discontinue if unexplained muscular symptoms and creatine kinase elevated markedly

Contra-indications breast-feeding (Appendix 5)

Side-effects nausea, vomiting, diarrhoea; headache; rash, injection-site reactions; *less commonly* constipation, abdominal pain, dyspepsia, anorexia, taste disturbance, jaundice, hypertension, hypotension, flushing, arrhythmias, anxiety, insomnia, dizziness, fatigue, paraesthesia, hyperglycaemia, vaginitis, renal insufficiency, anaemia, eosinophilia, thrombocythaemia, electrolyte disturbances, muscle effects (see Cautions), arthralgia, glossitis, and pruritus; *very rarely* wheezing

Dose

- By intravenous infusion, complicated skin and soft-tissue infections caused by Gram-positive bacteria, ADULT over 18 years, 4 mg/kg once daily; increased to 6 mg/kg once daily if associated with *Staphylococcus aureus* bacteraemia
  Right-sided endocarditis caused by *Staphylococcus aureus*, ADULT over 18 years, 6 mg/kg once daily

Cubicin® (Novartis) ▼ PoM
Intravenous infusion, powder for reconstitution, daptomycin, net price 350-mg vial = £62.00; 500-mg vial = £88.57

Linezolid

Linezolid, an oxazolidinone antibacterial, is active against Gram-positive bacteria including meticillin-resistant *Staphylococcus aureus* (MRSA), and vancomycin-resistant enterococci. Resistance to linezolid can develop with prolonged treatment or if the dose is less than that recommended. Linezolid is an option if a glycopeptide, such as vancomycin, cannot be used to treat pneumonia or severe skin and soft-tissue infections caused by MRSA. Linezolid is **not** active against Gram-negative organisms and must be given with other antibacterials if the infection also involves Gram-negative organisms (the combination should be used for mixed skin and soft tissue infections only when other treatments are not available). A higher incidence of blood disorders and optic neuropathy have been reported in patients receiving linezolid for more than the maximum recommended duration of 28 days.

LINEZOLID

Indications pneumonia, complicated skin and soft-tissue infections caused by Gram-positive bacteria (initiated under expert supervision)

Cautions monitor full blood count (including platelet count) weekly (see also CSM Advice below); history of seizures; unless close observation and blood-pressure monitoring possible, avoid in uncontrolled hypertension, phaeochromocytoma, carcinoid tumour, thyrotoxicosis, bipolar depression, schizophrenia, or acute confusional states; hepatic impairment (Appendix 2); renal impairment (Appendix 3); pregnancy (Appendix 4); **interactions:** Appendix 1 (MAOIs)

CSM advice (blood disorders)

Haematopoietic disorders (including thrombocytopenia, anaemia, leucopenia, and pancytopenia) have been reported in patients receiving linezolid. It is recommended that full blood counts are monitored weekly. Close monitoring is recommended in patients who:

- receive treatment for more than 10–14 days;
- have pre-existing myelosuppression;
- are receiving drugs that may have adverse effects on haemoglobin, blood counts, or platelet function;
- have severe renal impairment.

If significant myelosuppression occurs, treatment should be stopped unless it is considered essential, in which case intensive monitoring of blood counts and appropriate management should be implemented.

CHM advice (optic neuropathy)

Severe optic neuropathy may occur rarely, particularly if linezolid is used for longer than 28 days. The CHM recommends that:

- patients should be warned to report symptoms of visual impairment (including blurred vision, visual field defect, changes in visual acuity and colour vision) immediately;
- patients experiencing new visual symptoms (regardless of treatment duration) should be evaluated promptly, and referred to an ophthalmologist if necessary;
- visual function should be monitored regularly if treatment is required for longer than 28 days.

Monoamine oxidase inhibition Linezolid is a reversible, non-selective monoamine oxidase inhibitor (MAOI). Patients should avoid consuming large amounts of tyramine-rich foods (such as mature cheese, yeast extracts, undistilled alcoholic beverages, and fermented soya bean products). In addition, linezolid should not be given with another MAOI or within 2 weeks of stopping another MAOI. Unless close observation and blood-pressure monitoring is possible, avoid in those receiving SSRIs, $5HT_1$ agonists ('triptans'), tricyclic antidepressants, sympathomimetics, dopaminergics, buspirone, pethidine and possibly other opioid analgesics. For other interactions see Appendix 1 (MAOIs)

Contra-indications breast-feeding (Appendix 5); see also Monoamine oxidase inhibition above

Side-effects diarrhoea (antibiotic-associated colitis reported), nausea, vomiting, taste disturbances; headache; *less commonly* thirst, dry mouth, glossitis, stomatitis, tongue discoloration, abdominal pain, dyspepsia, gastritis, constipation, pancreatitis, hypertension, fever, fatigue, dizziness, insomnia, hypoaesthesia, paraesthesia, tinnitus, polyuria, anaemia, leucopenia, thrombocytopenia, eosinophilia, electrolyte disturbances, blurred vision, rash, pruritus, diaphoresis, and injection-site reactions; *very rarely* transient ischaemic attacks, renal failure, pancytopenia and Stevens-Johnson syndrome; also reported convulsions, lactic acidosis; peripheral and optic neuropathy reported on prolonged therapy (see also CHM advice above)

Dose

- By mouth, 600 mg every 12 hours usually for 10–14 days (max. duration of treatment 28 days); CHILD [unlicensed] 1 week–12 years, 10 mg/kg every 8 hours; 12–18 years, adult dose
- By intravenous infusion over 30–120 minutes, 600 mg every 12 hours; CHILD [unlicensed] 1 week–12 years, 10 mg/kg every 8 hours; 12–18 years, adult dose

Zyvox® (Pharmacia) ▼ PoM

Tablets, f/c, linezolid 600 mg, net price 10-tab pack = £445.00. Label: 9, 10, patient information leaflet

Suspension, yellow, linezolid 100 mg/5 mL when reconstituted with water, net price 150 mL (orange-flavoured) = £222.50. Label: 9, 10 patient information leaflet

Excipients include aspartame 20 mg/5 mL (section 9.4.1)

Intravenous infusion, linezolid 2 mg/mL, net price 300-mL *Excel®* bag = £44.50

Excipients include Na^+ 5 mmol/300-mL bag, glucose 13.71 g/300-mL bag

Quinupristin and dalfopristin

A combination of the streptogramin antibiotics, **quinupristin** and **dalfopristin** (as *Synercid®*) is licensed for infections due to Gram-positive bacteria. The combination should be reserved for treating infections which have failed to respond to other antibacterials (e.g. meticillin-resistant *Staphylococcus aureus*, MRSA) or for patients who cannot be treated with other antibacterials. Quinupristin and dalfopristin are not active against *Enterococcus faecalis* and they need to be given in combination with other antibacterials for mixed infections which also involve Gram-negative organisms.

QUINUPRISTIN WITH DALFOPRISTIN

A mixture of quinupristin and dalfopristin (both as mesilate salts) in the proportions 3 parts to 7 parts

Indications serious Gram-positive infections where no alternative antibacterial is suitable including hospital-acquired pneumonia, skin and soft-tissue infections, infections due to vancomycin-resistant *Enterococcus faecium*

Cautions hepatic impairment (avoid if severe; Appendix 2); pregnancy (Appendix 4); predisposition to cardiac arrhythmias (including congenital QT syndrome, concomitant use of drugs that prolong QT interval, cardiac hypertrophy, dilated cardiomyopathy, hypokalaemia, hypomagnesaemia, bradycardia); **interactions**: Appendix 1 (quinupristin with dalfopristin)

Contra-indications plasma-bilirubin concentration greater than 3 times upper limit of reference range; breast-feeding (Appendix 5)

Side-effects nausea, vomiting, diarrhoea; headache, asthenia; anaemia, leucopenia, eosinophilia, raised urea and creatinine; arthralgia, myalgia; rash, pruritus; injection-site reactions on peripheral venous administration; *less commonly* stomatitis, constipation, abdominal pain, antibiotic-associated colitis, hepatitis, jaundice, pancreatitis, anorexia, peripheral oedema, hypotension, chest pain, arrhythmias, dyspnoea, insomnia, anxiety, confusion, dizziness, paraesthesia, hypertonia, myasthenia, and gout; *rarely* electrolyte disturbances; *very rarely* thrombocytopenia and pancytopenia

Dose

Note Expressed as a combination of quinupristin and dalfopristin (in a ratio of 3:7)

- ADULT over 18 years, by intravenous infusion into central vein, 7.5 mg/kg every 8 hours for 7 days in skin and soft-tissue infections; for 10 days in hospital-acquired pneumonia; duration of treatment in *E. faecium* infection depends on site of infection

Note In emergency, first dose may be administered *via* peripheral line until central venous catheter in place

5 Infections

Synercid® (Aventis Pharma) PoM
Intravenous infusion, powder for reconstitution, quinupristin (as mesilate) 150 mg, dalfopristin (as mesilate) 350 mg, net price 500-mg vial = £37.00
Electrolytes Na^+ approx. 16 mmol/500-mg vial

Polymyxins

The polymyxin antibiotic, **colistin**, is active against Gram-negative organisms including *Pseudomonas aeruginosa, Acinetobacter baumanii,* and *Klebsiella pneumoniae.* It is **not** absorbed by mouth and thus needs to be given by injection for a systemic effect. Intravenous administration of colistin should be reserved for Gram-negative infections resistant to other antibacterials; its major adverse effects are dose-related neurotoxicity and nephrotoxicity.

Colistin is used by mouth in bowel sterilisation regimens in neutropenic patients (usually with nystatin); it is **not** recommended for gastro-intestinal infections. It is also given by inhalation of a nebulised solution as an adjunct to standard antibacterial therapy in patients with cystic fibrosis.

Both colistin and polymyxin B are included in some preparations for topical application.

COLISTIN

Indications see notes above

Cautions renal impairment (Appendix 3); porphyria (section 9.8.2); risk of bronchospasm on inhalation—may be prevented or treated with a selective $beta_2$ agonist; **interactions:** Appendix 1 (polymyxins)

Contra-indications myasthenia gravis; pregnancy (Appendix 4); breast-feeding (Appendix 5)

Side-effects neurotoxicity reported especially with excessive doses (including apnoea, perioral and peripheral paraesthesia, vertigo; rarely vasomotor instability, slurred speech, confusion, psychosis, visual disturbances); nephrotoxicity; hypersensitivity reactions including rash; injection-site reactions; inhalation may cause sore throat, sore mouth, cough, bronchospasm

Dose

- By mouth, bowel sterilisation, 1.5–3 million units every 8 hours
- By slow intravenous injection into a totally implantable venous access device, *or* by intravenous infusion (but see notes above), ADULT and CHILD body-weight under 60 kg, 50 000–75 000 units/kg daily in 3 divided doses; body-weight over 60 kg, 1–2 million units every 8 hours
  Note Plasma concentration monitoring required in neonates, renal impairment, and in cystic fibrosis; recommended 'peak' plasma-colistin concentration (approx. 30 minutes after intravenous injection or infusion) 10–15 mg/litre (125–200 units/mL)
- By inhalation of nebulised solution, ADULT and CHILD over 2 years, 1–2 million units every 12 hours; CHILD under 2 years, 0.5–1 million units every 12 hours

Colomycin® (Forest) PoM
Tablets, scored, colistin sulphate 1.5 million units. Net price 50 = £58.28
Syrup, colistin sulphate 250 000 units/5 mL when reconstituted with water. Net price 80 mL = £3.48
Injection, powder for reconstitution, colistimethate sodium (colistin sulphomethate sodium). Net price 500 000-unit vial = £1.14; 1 million-unit vial = £1.68; 2 million-unit vial = £3.09
Electrolytes (before reconstitution) Na^+ < 0.5 mmol/500 000-unit, 1 million-unit, and 2 million-unit vial
Note *Colomycin®* Injection (dissolved in physiological saline) may be used for nebulisation

Promixin® (Profile) PoM
Powder for nebuliser solution, colistimethate sodium (colistin sulphomethate sodium), net price 1 million-unit vial = £4.60
Injection, powder for reconstitution, colistimethate sodium (colistin sulphomethate sodium), net price 1 million unit-vial = £2.30
Electrolytes (before reconstitution) Na^+ < 0.5 mmol/1 million-unit vial

5.1.8 Sulphonamides and trimethoprim

The importance of the sulphonamides has decreased as a result of increasing bacterial resistance and their replacement by antibacterials which are generally more active and less toxic.

Sulfamethoxazole (sulphamethoxazole) and trimethoprim are used in combination (as **co-trimoxazole**) because of their synergistic activity. However, co-trimoxazole is associated with rare but serious side-effects (e.g. Stevens-Johnson syndrome and blood dyscrasias, notably bone marrow depression and agranulocytosis) especially in the elderly (see CSM recommendations below).

> **CSM recommendations.** Co-trimoxazole should be limited to the role of drug of choice in *Pneumocystis jiroveci* (*Pneumocystis carinii*) pneumonia; it is also indicated for *toxoplasmosis* and *nocardiasis.* It should now only be considered for use in *acute exacerbations of chronic bronchitis* and *infections of the urinary tract* when there is good bacteriological evidence of sensitivity to co-trimoxazole and good reason to prefer this combination to a single antibacterial; similarly it should only be used in *acute otitis media in children* when there is good reason to prefer it.

Trimethoprim can be used alone for urinary- and respiratory-tract infections and for prostatitis, shigellosis, and invasive salmonella infections. Trimethoprim has side-effects similar to co-trimoxazole but they are less severe and occur less frequently.

For *topical preparations* of sulphonamides used in the treatment of burns see section 13.10.1.1.

CO-TRIMOXAZOLE

A mixture of trimethoprim and sulfamethoxazole in the proportions of 1 part to 5 parts

Indications see CSM recommendations above

Cautions maintain adequate fluid intake; avoid in blood disorders (unless under specialist supervision); monitor blood counts on prolonged treatment; discontinue immediately if blood disorders or rash develop; predisposition to folate deficiency or hyperkalaemia; elderly (see CSM recommendations above); asthma; G6PD deficiency (section 9.1.5); avoid in infants under 6 weeks (except for treatment or prophylaxis of pneumocystis pneumonia); hepatic impairment (avoid if severe); renal impairment (avoid if creatinine clearance less than 15 mL/minute; Appendix 3); pregnancy (Appendix 4); breast-feeding (Appendix 5); **interactions**: Appendix 1 (trimethoprim, sulfamethoxazole)

Contra-indications porphyria (section 9.8.2)

Side-effects nausea, diarrhoea; headache; hyperkalaemia; rash (very rarely including Stevens-Johnson syndrome, toxic epidermal necrolysis, photosensitivity)—discontinue immediately; *less commonly* vomiting; *very rarely* glossitis, stomatitis, anorexia, liver damage (including jaundice and hepatic necrosis), pancreatitis, antibiotic-associated colitis, myocarditis, cough and shortness of breath, pulmonary infiltrates, aseptic meningitis, depression, convulsions, peripheral neuropathy, ataxia, tinnitus, vertigo, hallucinations, hypoglycaemia, blood disorders (including leucopenia, thrombocytopenia, megaloblastic anaemia, eosinophilia), hyponatraemia, renal disorders including interstitial nephritis, arthralgia, myalgia, vasculitis, and systemic lupus erythematosus

Dose

- By mouth, 960 mg every 12 hours; CHILD, every 12 hours, 6 weeks–5 months, 120 mg; 6 months–5 years, 240 mg; 6–12 years, 480 mg
- By intravenous infusion, 960 mg every 12 hours increased to 1.44 g every 12 hours in severe infections; CHILD 36 mg/kg daily in 2 divided doses increased to 54 mg/kg daily in severe infections
- Treatment of *Pneumocystis jiroveci* (*Pneumocystis carinii*) infections (undertaken where facilities for appropriate monitoring available—consult microbiologist and product literature), by mouth *or* by intravenous infusion, ADULT and CHILD over 4 weeks, 120 mg/kg daily in 2–4 divided doses for 14 days
- Prophylaxis of *Pneumocystis jiroveci* (*Pneumocystis carinii*) infections, by mouth, 960 mg once daily (may be reduced to 480 mg once daily to improve tolerance) *or* 960 mg on alternate days (3 times a week) *or* 960 mg twice daily on alternate days (3 times a week); CHILD 6 weeks–5 months, 120 mg twice daily on 3 consecutive or alternate days per week *or* on 7 days per week; 6 months–5 years, 240 mg; 6–12 years, 480 mg

Note 480 mg of co-trimoxazole consists of sulfamethoxazole 400 mg and trimethoprim 80 mg

Co-trimoxazole (Non-proprietary) PoM

Tablets, co-trimoxazole 480 mg, net price 28-tab pack = £13.17, 960 mg, 20 = £4.69. Label: 9
Brands include *Fectrim*®, *Fectrim® Forte*

Paediatric oral suspension, co-trimoxazole 240 mg/5 mL, net price 100 mL = £1.12. Label: 9

Oral suspension, co-trimoxazole 480 mg/5 mL. Net price 100 mL = £4.41. Label: 9

Strong sterile solution, co-trimoxazole 96 mg/mL. For dilution and use as an intravenous infusion. Net price 5-mL amp = £1.58, 10-mL amp = £3.06

Septrin® (GSK) PoM

Tablets, co-trimoxazole 480 mg. Net price 20 = £3.10. Label: 9

Forte tablets, scored, co-trimoxazole 960 mg. Net price 20 = £4.69. Label: 9

Adult suspension, co-trimoxazole 480 mg/5 mL. Net price 100 mL (vanilla-flavoured) = £4.41. Label: 9

Paediatric suspension, sugar-free, co-trimoxazole 240 mg/5 mL. Net price 100 mL (banana- and vanilla-flavoured) = £2.45. Label: 9

Intravenous infusion, co-trimoxazole 96 mg/mL. To be diluted before use. Net price 5-mL amp = £1.48
Excipients include propylene glycol, sulphites

SULFADIAZINE
(Sulphadiazine)

Indications prevention of rheumatic fever recurrence, toxoplasmosis [unlicensed]—see section 5.4.7

Cautions see under Co-trimoxazole; renal impairment (avoid if severe; Appendix 3); pregnancy (Appendix 4); breast-feeding (Appendix 5); **interactions**: Appendix 1 (sulphonamides)

Contra-indications see under Co-trimoxazole

Side-effects see under Co-trimoxazole

Dose

- Prevention of rheumatic fever, *by mouth*, 1 g daily (500 mg daily for patients less than 30 kg)

Sulfadiazine (Non-proprietary) PoM

Tablets, sulfadiazine 500 mg, net price 56-tab pack = £37.50. Label: 9, 27

TRIMETHOPRIM

Indications urinary-tract infections, acute and chronic bronchitis; pneumocystis pneumonia (section 5.4.8)

Cautions renal impairment (Appendix 3); pregnancy (Appendix 4); breast-feeding (Appendix 5); predisposition to folate deficiency; elderly; manufacturer recommends blood counts on long-term therapy (but evidence of practical value unsatisfactory); neonates (specialist supervision required); porphyria (section 9.8.2) **interactions**: Appendix 1 (trimethoprim)

Blood disorders On long-term treatment, patients and their carers should be told how to recognise signs of blood disorders and advised to seek immediate medical attention if symptoms such as fever, sore throat, rash, mouth ulcers, purpura, bruising or bleeding develop

Contra-indications blood dyscrasias

Side-effects gastro-intestinal disturbances including nausea and vomiting, pruritus, rashes, hyperkalaemia, depression of haematopoiesis; rarely erythema multiforme, toxic epidermal necrolysis, photosensitivity and other allergic reactions including angioedema and anaphylaxis; aseptic meningitis and uveitis reported

Dose

- Acute infections, 200 mg every 12 hours; CHILD 1 month–12 years, 4 mg/kg (max. 200 mg) every 12 hours; *or* 6 weeks–6 months 25 mg every 12 hours, 6 months–6 years 50 mg every 12 hours, 6–12 years 100 mg every 12 hours
- Chronic infections and prophylaxis, 100 mg at night; CHILD 1–2 mg/kg at night

Trimethoprim (Non-proprietary) PoM

Tablets, trimethoprim 100 mg, net price 28 = 43p; 200 mg, 14-tab pack = 34p. Label: 9
Brands include *Trimopan*®

Suspension, trimethoprim 50 mg/5 mL, net price 100 mL = £1.62. Label: 9

5.1.9 Antituberculosis drugs

Tuberculosis is treated in two phases—an *initial phase* using 4 drugs and a *continuation phase* using 2 drugs in fully sensitive cases. Treatment requires specialised knowledge, particularly where the disease involves resistant organisms or non-respiratory organs.

The regimens given below are recommended for the treatment of tuberculosis in the UK; variations occur in other countries. Either the unsupervised regimen or the supervised regimen described below should be used; the two regimens should **not** be used concurrently.

Initial phase The concurrent use of 4 drugs during the initial phase is designed to reduce the bacterial population as rapidly as possible and to prevent the emergence of drug-resistant bacteria. The drugs are best given as combination preparations unless one of the components cannot be given because of resistance or intolerance. The treatment of choice for the initial phase is the daily use of isoniazid, rifampicin, pyrazinamide and ethambutol. Treatment should be started without waiting for culture results if clinical features or histology results are consistent with tuberculosis; treatment should be continued even if initial culture results are negative. The initial phase drugs should be continued for 2 months. Where a positive culture for *M. tuberculosis* has been obtained, but susceptibility results are not available after 2 months, treatment with rifampicin, isoniazid, pyrazinamide and ethambutol should be continued until full susceptibility is confirmed, even if this is for longer than 2 months.

Streptomycin is rarely used in the UK but it may be used in the initial phase of treatment if resistance to isoniazid has been established before therapy is commenced.

Continuation phase After the initial phase, treatment is continued for a further 4 months with isoniazid and rifampicin (preferably given as a combination preparation). Longer treatment is necessary for meningitis, direct spinal cord involvement, and for resistant organisms which may also require modification of the regimen.

Unsupervised treatment The following regimen should be used for patients who are likely to take antituberculous drugs reliably **without supervision**. Patients who are unlikely to comply with daily administration of antituberculous drugs should be treated with the regimen described under Supervised Treatment.

Recommended dosage for standard unsupervised 6-month treatment

Rifater® [rifampicin, isoniazid, and pyrazinamide] (for 2-month initial phase only)
ADULT under 40 kg 3 tablets daily, 40–49 kg 4 tablets daily, 50–64 kg 5 tablets daily, over 65 kg 6 tablets daily

Ethambutol (for 2-month initial phase only)
ADULT AND CHILD 15 mg/kg daily

Rifinah® [rifampicin and isoniazid] (for 4-month continuation phase following initial treatment with *Rifater®*)
ADULT under 50 kg 3 tablets daily of *Rifinah®-150*, 50 kg and over, 2 tablets daily of *Rifinah®-300*

or (if combination preparations not appropriate):

Isoniazid (for 2-month initial and 4-month continuation phases)
ADULT 300 mg daily; CHILD 5–10 mg/kg (max. 300 mg) daily

Rifampicin (for 2-month initial and 4-month continuation phases)
ADULT under 50 kg 450 mg daily, 50 kg and over 600 mg daily; CHILD 10 mg/kg (max. 600 mg) daily

Pyrazinamide (for 2-month initial phase only)
ADULT under 50 kg 1.5 g daily, 50 kg and over 2 g daily; CHILD 35 mg/kg daily

Ethambutol (for 2-month initial phase only)
ADULT AND CHILD 15 mg/kg daily

Pregnancy and breast-feeding The standard regimen (above) may be used during pregnancy and breast-feeding. Streptomycin should not be given in pregnancy.

Children Children are given isoniazid, rifampicin, pyrazinamide, and ethambutol for the first 2 months followed by isoniazid and rifampicin during the next 4 months. However, care is needed in young children receiving ethambutol because of the difficulty in testing eyesight and in obtaining reports of visual symptoms (see below).

Supervised treatment Drug administration needs to be **fully supervised** (directly observed therapy, DOT) in patients who cannot comply reliably with the treatment regimen. These patients are given isoniazid, rifampicin, pyrazinamide and ethambutol (or streptomycin) 3 times a week under supervision for the first 2 months followed by isoniazid and rifampicin 3 times a week for a further 4 months.

Recommended dosage for intermittent supervised 6-month treatment

Isoniazid (for 2-month initial and 4-month continuation phases)
ADULT AND CHILD 15 mg/kg (max. 900 mg) 3 times a week

Rifampicin (for 2-month initial and 4-month continuation phases)
ADULT 600–900 mg 3 times a week; CHILD 15 mg/kg (max. 900 mg) 3 times a week

Pyrazinamide (for 2-month initial phase only)
ADULT under 50 kg 2 g 3 times a week, 50 kg and over 2.5 g 3 times a week; CHILD 50 mg/kg 3 times a week

Ethambutol (for 2-month initial phase only)
ADULT AND CHILD 30 mg/kg 3 times a week

Immunocompromised patients Multi-resistant *Mycobacterium tuberculosis* may be present in immunocompromised patients. The organism should always be cultured to confirm its type and drug sensitivity. Confirmed *M. tuberculosis* infection sensitive to first-line drugs should be treated with a standard 6-month regimen; after completing treatment, patients should be closely monitored. The regimen may need to be modified if infection is caused by resistant organisms, and specialist advice is needed.

Specialist advice should be sought about tuberculosis treatment or chemoprophylaxis in a HIV-positive individual; care is required in choosing the regimen and in avoiding potentially hazardous interactions. Starting antiretroviral treatment in the first 2 months of antituberculosis treatment increases the risk of immune reconstitution syndrome.

Infection may also be caused by other mycobacteria e.g. *M. avium* complex in which case specialist advice on management is needed.

Corticosteroids In meningeal or pericardial tuberculosis, a corticosteroid should be started at the same time as antituberculosis therapy.

Prevention of tuberculosis Some individuals may develop tuberculosis owing to reactivation of previously latent disease. Chemoprophylaxis may be required in those who have evidence of latent tuberculosis and are receiving treatment with immunosuppressants (including cytotoxics and possibly long-term treatment with systemic corticosteroids). In these cases, chemoprophylaxis involves use of either isoniazid alone for 6 months or of isoniazid and rifampicin for 3 months, see Table 2, section 5.1; longer chemoprophylaxis is not recommended.

For prevention of tuberculosis in susceptible close contacts or those who have become tuberculin-positive, see Table 2, section 5.1. For advice on immunisation against tuberculosis, see section 14.4

Monitoring Since isoniazid, rifampicin and pyrazinamide are associated with liver toxicity (see Appendix 2), *hepatic function* should be checked before treatment with these drugs. Those with pre-existing liver disease or alcohol dependence should have frequent checks particularly in the first 2 months. If there is no evidence of liver disease (and pre-treatment liver function is normal), further checks are only necessary if the patient develops fever, malaise, vomiting, jaundice or unexplained deterioration during treatment. In view of the need to comply fully with antituberculous treatment on the one hand and to guard against serious liver damage on the other, patients and their carers should be informed carefully how to recognise signs of liver disorders and advised to discontinue treatment and seek **immediate** medical attention should symptoms of liver disease occur.

Renal function should be checked before treatment with antituberculous drugs and appropriate dosage adjustments made. Streptomycin or ethambutol should preferably be avoided in patients with renal impairment, but if used, the dose should be reduced and the plasma-drug concentration monitored.

Visual acuity should be tested before ethambutol is used (see below).

> Major causes of treatment failure are incorrect prescribing by the physician and inadequate compliance by the patient. Monthly tablet counts and urine examination (rifampicin imparts an orange-red coloration) may be useful indicators of compliance with treatment. Avoid both excessive and inadequate dosage. Treatment should be supervised by a specialist physician.

Isoniazid is cheap and highly effective. Like rifampicin it should always be included in any antituberculous regimen unless there is a specific contra-indication. Its only common side-effect is peripheral neuropathy which is more likely to occur where there are pre-existing risk factors such as diabetes, alcohol dependence, chronic renal failure, malnutrition and HIV infection. In these circumstances pyridoxine 10 mg daily (or 20 mg daily if suitable product not available) (section 9.6.2) should be given prophylactically from the start of treatment. Other side-effects such as hepatitis (important: see Monitoring above) and psychosis are rare.

Rifampicin, a rifamycin, is a key component of any antituberculous regimen. Like isoniazid it should always be included unless there is a specific contra-indication.

During the first two months ('initial phase') of rifampicin administration transient disturbance of liver function with elevated serum transaminases is common but generally does not require interruption of treatment. Occasionally more serious liver toxicity requires a change of treatment particularly in those with pre-existing liver disease (important: see Monitoring above).

On intermittent treatment six toxicity syndromes have been recognised—influenza-like, abdominal, and respiratory symptoms, shock, renal failure, and thrombocytopenic purpura—and can occur in 20 to 30% of patients.

Rifampicin induces hepatic enzymes which accelerate the metabolism of several drugs including oestrogens, corticosteroids, phenytoin, sulphonylureas, and anticoagulants; **interactions:** Appendix 1 (rifamycins). **Important:** the effectiveness of hormonal contraceptives is reduced and alternative family planning advice should be offered (section 7.3.1).

Rifabutin, a newly introduced rifamycin, is indicated for *prophylaxis* against *M. avium* complex infections in patients with a low CD4 count; it is also licensed for the *treatment* of non-tuberculous mycobacterial disease and pulmonary tuberculosis. **Important:** as with rifampicin it induces hepatic enzymes and the effectiveness of hormonal contraceptives is reduced requiring alternative family planning methods.

Pyrazinamide [unlicensed] is a bactericidal drug only active against intracellular dividing forms of *Mycobacterium tuberculosis*; it exerts its main effect only in the first two or three months. It is particularly useful in tuberculous meningitis because of good meningeal penetration. It is not active against *M. bovis*. Serious liver toxicity may occasionally occur (important: see Monitoring above).

Ethambutol is included in a treatment regimen if isoniazid resistance is suspected; it can be omitted if the risk of resistance is low.

Side-effects of ethambutol are largely confined to visual disturbances in the form of loss of acuity, colour blindness, and restriction of visual fields. These toxic effects are more common where excessive dosage is used or if the patient's renal function is impaired. The earliest features of ocular toxicity are subjective and patients should be advised to discontinue therapy immediately if they develop deterioration in vision and promptly seek further advice. Early discontinuation of the drug is almost always followed by recovery of eyesight. Patients who cannot understand warnings about visual side-effects should, if possible, be given an alternative drug. In particular, ethambutol should be used with caution in children until they are at least 5 years old and capable of reporting symptomatic visual changes accurately.

Visual acuity should be tested by Snellen chart before treatment with ethambutol.

Streptomycin [unlicensed] is now rarely used in the UK except for resistant organisms. It is given intramuscularly in a dose of 15 mg/kg (max. 1 g) daily; the dose is reduced in those under 50 kg, those over 40 years or those with renal impairment. Plasma-drug concentration should be measured in patients with impaired renal function in whom streptomycin must be used with great care. Side-effects increase after a cumulative dose of 100 g, which should only be exceeded in exceptional circumstances.

Drug-resistant tuberculosis should be treated by a specialist physician with experience in such cases, and where appropriate facilities for infection-control exist. Second-line drugs available for infections caused by resistant organisms, or when first-line drugs cause unacceptable side-effects, include amikacin, capreomycin, cycloserine, newer macrolides (e.g. azithromycin and clarithromycin), moxifloxacin and protionamide (prothionamide; no longer on UK market).

CAPREOMYCIN

Indications in combination with other drugs, tuberculosis resistant to first-line drugs

Cautions hepatic impairment; renal impairment (Appendix 3); auditory impairment; monitor renal, hepatic, auditory, and vestibular function and electrolytes; pregnancy (teratogenic in *animals*; Appendix 4) and breast-feeding (Appendix 5); **interactions:** Appendix 1 (capreomycin)

Side-effects hypersensitivity reactions including urticaria and rashes; leucocytosis or leucopenia, rarely thrombocytopenia; changes in liver function tests; nephrotoxicity, electrolyte disturbances; hearing loss with tinnitus and vertigo; neuromuscular block after large doses, pain and induration at injection site

Dose

- By deep intramuscular injection, 1 g daily (not more than 20 mg/kg) for 2–4 months, then 1 g 2–3 times each week

Capastat® (King) PoM
Injection, powder for reconstitution, capreomycin sulphate 1 million units (= capreomycin approx. 1 g). Net price per vial = £16.01

CYCLOSERINE

Indications in combination with other drugs, tuberculosis resistant to first-line drugs

Cautions reduce dose in renal impairment (avoid if creatinine clearance less than 10 mL/minute); monitor haematological, renal, and hepatic function; pregnancy (Appendix 4); breast-feeding (Appendix 5); **interactions:** Appendix 1 (cycloserine)

Contra-indications severe renal impairment, epilepsy, depression, severe anxiety, psychotic states, alcohol dependence, porphyria (section 9.8.2)

Side-effects mainly neurological, including headache, dizziness, vertigo, drowsiness, tremor, convulsions, confusion, psychosis, depression (discontinue or reduce dose if symptoms of CNS toxicity); rashes, allergic dermatitis (discontinue or reduce dose); megaloblastic anaemia; changes in liver function tests; heart failure at high doses reported

Dose

- Initially 250 mg every 12 hours for 2 weeks increased according to blood concentration and response to max. 500 mg every 12 hours; CHILD initially 10 mg/kg daily adjusted according to blood concentration and response

Note Blood concentration monitoring required especially in renal impairment or if dose exceeds 500 mg daily or if signs of toxicity; blood concentration should not exceed 30 mg/litre

Cycloserine (King) PoM
Capsules, red/grey cycloserine 250 mg, net price 100-cap pack = £303.45. Label: 2, 8

ETHAMBUTOL HYDROCHLORIDE

Indications tuberculosis, in combination with other drugs

Cautions reduce dose in renal impairment and if creatinine clearance less than 30 mL/minute, also monitor plasma-ethambutol concentration (Appendix 3); elderly; pregnancy; test visual acuity before treatment and warn patients to report visual changes—see notes above; young children (see notes above)—routine ophthalmological monitoring recommended

Contra-indications optic neuritis, poor vision

Side-effects optic neuritis, red/green colour blindness, peripheral neuritis, rarely rash, pruritus, urticaria, thrombocytopenia

Dose

- See notes above

Note 'Peak' concentration (2–2.5 hours after dose) should be 2–6 mg/litre (7–22 micromol/litre); 'trough' (pre-dose) concentration should be less than 1 mg/litre (4 micromol/litre); see Cautions above; for advice on laboratory assay of ethambutol contact the Poisons Unit at New Cross Hospital (Tel (020) 7771 5360)

Ethambutol (Non-proprietary) PoM
Tablets, ethambutol hydrochloride 100 mg (yellow), net price 56-tab pack = £11.56; 400 mg (grey), 56-tab pack = £42.80. Label: 8

ISONIAZID

Indications tuberculosis, in combination with other drugs; prophylaxis—Table 2, section 5.1

Cautions hepatic impairment (Appendix 2; see also below); renal impairment (Appendix 3); slow acetylator status (increased risk of side-effects); epilepsy; history of psychosis; alcohol dependence, malnutrition, diabetes mellitus, HIV infection (risk of peripheral neuritis); pregnancy (Appendix 4) and breast-feeding (Appendix 5); porphyria (section 9.8.2); **interactions:** Appendix 1 (isoniazid)

Hepatic disorders Patients or their carers should be told how to recognise signs of liver disorder, and advised to discontinue treatment and seek immediate medical attention if symptoms such as persistent nausea, vomiting, malaise or jaundice develop

Contra-indications drug-induced liver disease

Side-effects nausea, vomiting, constipation, dry mouth; peripheral neuritis with high doses (pyridoxine prophylaxis, see notes above), optic neuritis, convulsions, psychotic episodes, vertigo; hypersensitivity reactions including fever, erythema multiforme, purpura; blood disorders including agranulocytosis, haemolytic anaemia, aplastic anaemia; hepatitis (especially over age of 35 years); systemic lupus erythematosus-like syndrome, pellagra, hyperreflexia, difficulty with micturition, hyperglycaemia, and gynaecomastia reported

Dose

- By mouth *or* by intramuscular *or* intravenous injection, see notes above

Isoniazid (Non-proprietary) PoM
Tablets, isoniazid 50 mg, net price 56-tab pack = £8.34; 100 mg, 28-tab pack = £8.29. Label: 8, 22

Elixir (BPC), isoniazid 50 mg, citric acid monohydrate 12.5 mg, sodium citrate 60 mg, concentrated anise water 0.05 mL, compound tartrazine solution 0.05 mL, glycerol 1 mL, double-strength chloroform water 2 mL, water to 5 mL. Label: 8, 22

'Special order' [unlicensed] product; contact Martindale, Rosemont, or regional hospital manufacturing unit

Injection, isoniazid 25 mg/mL, net price 2-mL amp = £9.20

PYRAZINAMIDE

Indications tuberculosis in combination with other drugs

Cautions pregnancy (Appendix 4); hepatic impairment (monitor hepatic function, see also below and Appendix 2); diabetes; gout (avoid in acute attack); **interactions:** Appendix 1 (pyrazinamide)

Hepatic disorders Patients or their carers should be told how to recognise signs of liver disorder, and advised to discontinue treatment and seek immediate medical attention if symptoms such as persistent nausea, vomiting, malaise or jaundice develop

Contra-indications porphyria (section 9.8.2)

Side-effects hepatotoxicity including fever, anorexia, hepatomegaly, splenomegaly, jaundice, liver failure; nausea, vomiting, flushing, dysuria, arthralgia, sideroblastic anaemia, rash and occasionally photosensitivity

Dose

- See notes above

Pyrazinamide (Non-proprietary) PoM
Tablets, scored, pyrazinamide 500 mg. Label: 8
Available on named-patient basis from specialist importing companies, see p. 888

RIFABUTIN

Indications see under Dose

Cautions see under Rifampicin; hepatic impairment (Appendix 2); renal impairment (Appendix 3); pregnancy (Appendix 4); breast-feeding (Appendix 5); porphyria (section 9.8.2)

Side-effects nausea, vomiting; leucopenia, thrombocytopenia, anaemia, rarely haemolysis; raised liver enzymes, jaundice, rarely hepatitis; uveitis following high doses or administration with drugs which raise plasma concentration—see also **interactions:** Appendix 1 (rifamycins); arthralgia, myalgia, influenza-like syndrome, dyspnoea; also hypersensitivity reactions including fever, rash, eosinophilia, bronchospasm, shock; skin, urine, saliva and other body secretions coloured orange-red; asymptomatic corneal opacities reported with long-term use

Dose

- Prophylaxis of *Mycobacterium avium* complex infections in immunosuppressed patients with low CD4 count (see product literature), 300 mg daily as a single dose
- Treatment of non-tuberculous mycobacterial disease, in combination with other drugs, 450–600 mg daily as a single dose for up to 6 months after cultures negative
- Treatment of pulmonary tuberculosis, in combination with other drugs, 150–450 mg daily as a single dose for at least 6 months
- CHILD not recommended

Mycobutin® (Pharmacia) PoM
Capsules, red-brown, rifabutin 150 mg. Net price 30-cap pack = £90.38. Label: 8, 14, counselling, lenses, see under Rifampicin

RIFAMPICIN

Indications see under Dose

Cautions hepatic impairment (Appendix 2; liver function tests and blood counts in hepatic disorders, alcohol dependence, and on prolonged therapy, see also below); renal impairment (if above 600 mg daily); pregnancy and breast-feeding (see notes above and Appendix 4 and Appendix 5); porphyria (section 9.8.2); **important:** advise patients on hormonal contraceptives to use additional means (see also section 7.3.1); discolours soft contact lenses; see also notes above; **interactions:** Appendix 1 (rifamycins)

Note If treatment interrupted re-introduce with low dosage and increase gradually; discontinue permanently if serious side-effects develop

Hepatic disorders Patients or their carers should be told how to recognise signs of liver disorder, and advised to discontinue treatment and seek immediate medical attention if symptoms such as persistent nausea, vomiting, malaise or jaundice develop

Contra-indications jaundice

Side-effects gastro-intestinal symptoms including anorexia, nausea, vomiting, diarrhoea (antibiotic-associated colitis reported); headache, drowsiness; those occurring mainly on intermittent therapy include influenza-like symptoms (with chills, fever, dizziness, bone pain), respiratory symptoms (including shortness of breath), collapse and shock, haemolytic anaemia, acute renal failure, and thrombocytopenic purpura; alterations of liver function, jaundice; flushing, urticaria, and rashes; other side-effects reported include oedema, muscular weakness and myopathy, exfoliative dermatitis, toxic epidermal necrolysis, pemphigoid reactions, leucopenia, eosinophilia, menstrual disturbances; urine, saliva, and other body secretions coloured orange-red; thrombophlebitis reported if infusion used for prolonged period

Dose

- Brucellosis, legionnaires' disease, endocarditis and serious staphylococcal infections, in combination with other drugs, by mouth *or* by intravenous infusion, 0.6–1.2 g daily (in 2–4 divided doses)
- Tuberculosis, in combination with other drugs, see notes above
- Leprosy, section 5.1.10
- Prophylaxis of meningococcal meningitis and *Haemophilus influenzae* (type b) infection, section 5.1, table 2

Rifampicin (Non-proprietary) PoM
Capsules, rifampicin 150 mg, net price 20 = £7.65; 300 mg, 20 = £20.32. Label: 8, 14, 22, counselling, see lenses above

Rifadin® (Aventis Pharma) PoM
Capsules, rifampicin 150 mg (blue/red), net price 20 = £3.81; 300 mg (red), 20 = £7.62. Label: 8, 14, 22, counselling, see lenses above

Syrup, red, rifampicin 100 mg/5 mL (raspberry-flavoured). Net price 120 mL = £3.70. Label: 8, 14, 22, counselling, see lenses above

Intravenous infusion, powder for reconstitution, rifampicin. Net price 600-mg vial (with solvent) = £7.98
Electrolytes Na^+ < 0.5 mmol/vial

Rimactane® (Sandoz) PoM
Capsules, rifampicin 150 mg (red), net price 60-cap pack = £11.35; 300 mg (red/brown), 60-cap pack = £22.69. Label: 8, 14, 22, counselling, see lenses above

Combined preparations

Rifater® (Aventis Pharma) PoM
Tablets, pink, s/c, rifampicin 120 mg, isoniazid 50 mg, pyrazinamide 300 mg. Net price 20 = £4.39. Label: 8, 14, 22, counselling, see lenses above
Dose initial treatment of pulmonary tuberculosis, patients up to 40 kg 3 tablets daily preferably before breakfast, 40–49 kg 4 tablets daily, 50–64 kg 5 tablets daily, 65 kg or more, 6 tablets daily; not suitable for use in children

Rifinah 150® (Aventis Pharma) PoM
Tablets, pink, s/c, rifampicin 150 mg, isoniazid 100 mg, net price 84-tab pack = £16.55. Label: 8, 14, 22, counselling, see lenses above
Dose ADULT under 50 kg, 3 tablets daily, preferably before breakfast

Rifinah 300® (Aventis Pharma) PoM
Tablets, orange, s/c, rifampicin 300 mg, isoniazid 150 mg, net price 56-tab pack = £21.87. Label: 8, 14, 22, counselling, see lenses above
Dose ADULT 50 kg and over, 2 tablets daily, preferably before breakfast

STREPTOMYCIN

Indications tuberculosis, in combination with other drugs; adjunct to doxycycline in brucellosis; enterococcal endocarditis (Table 1, section 5.1)

Cautions see under Aminoglycosides, section 5.1.4; **interactions:** Appendix 1 (aminoglycosides)

Contra-indications see under Aminoglycosides, section 5.1.4

Side-effects see under Aminoglycosides, section 5.1.4; also hypersensitivity reactions, paraesthesia of mouth

Dose

- By deep intramuscular injection, tuberculosis, see notes above; brucellosis, expert advice essential

Note One-hour ('peak') concentration should be 15–40 mg/litre; pre-dose ('trough') concentration should be less than 5 mg/litre (less than 1 mg/litre in renal impairment or in those over 50 years)

Streptomycin Sulphate (Non-proprietary) PoM
Injection, powder for reconstitution, streptomycin (as sulphate), net price 1-g vial = £8.25
Available on named-patient basis from Celltech

5.1.10 Antileprotic drugs

Advice from a member of the Panel of Leprosy Opinion is essential for the treatment of leprosy (Hansen's disease). Details of the Panel can be obtained from the Department of Health telephone (020) 7972 4480.

The World Health Organization has made recommendations to overcome the problem of dapsone resistance and to prevent the emergence of resistance to other antileprotic drugs. Drugs recommended are **dapsone**, **rifampicin** (section 5.1.9), and **clofazimine**. Other drugs with significant activity against *Mycobacterium leprae* include ofloxacin, minocycline and clarithromycin, but none of these are as active as rifampicin; at present they should be reserved as second-line drugs for leprosy.

A three-drug regimen is recommended for *multibacillary leprosy* (lepromatous, borderline-lepromatous, and borderline leprosy) and a two-drug regimen for *paucibacillary leprosy* (borderline-tuberculoid, tuberculoid, and indeterminate). The following regimens are widely used throughout the world (with minor local variations):

Multibacillary leprosy (3-drug regimen)

Rifampicin	600 mg once-monthly, supervised (450 mg for adults weighing less than 35 kg)
Dapsone	100 mg daily, self-administered (50 mg daily or 1–2 mg/kg daily for adults weighing less than 35 kg)
Clofazimine	300 mg once-monthly, supervised, *and* 50 mg daily (or 100 mg on alternate days), self-administered

Multibacillary leprosy should be treated for at least 2 years. Treatment should be continued unchanged during both type I (reversal) or type II (erythema nodosum leprosum) reactions. During reversal reactions neuritic pain or weakness can herald the rapid onset of permanent nerve damage. Treatment with prednisolone (initially 40–60 mg daily) should be instituted at once. Mild type II reactions may respond to aspirin. Severe type II reactions may require corticosteroids; thalidomide [unlicensed] is also useful in men and post-menopausal women who have become corticosteroid dependent, but it should be used under **specialist supervision** and it should **never** be used in women of child-bearing potential (significant teratogenic risk—for CSM guidance on prescribing, see *Current Problems in Pharmacovigilance* 1994; **20**, 8). Increased doses of clofazimine 100 mg 3 times daily for the first month with subsequent reductions, are also useful but may take 4–6 weeks to attain full effect.

Paucibacillary leprosy (2-drug regimen)

Rifampicin	600 mg once-monthly, supervised (450 mg for those weighing less than 35 kg)
Dapsone	100 mg daily, self-administered (50 mg daily or 1–2 mg/kg daily for adults weighing less than 35 kg)

Paucibacillary leprosy should be treated for 6 months. If treatment is interrupted the regimen should be recommenced where it was left off to complete the full course.

Neither the multibacillary nor the paucibacillary antileprosy regimen is sufficient to treat tuberculosis.

DAPSONE

Indications leprosy, dermatitis herpetiformis; *Pneumocystis jiroveci* (*Pneumocystis carinii*) pneumonia (section 5.4.8)

Cautions cardiac or pulmonary disease; anaemia (treat severe anaemia before starting); susceptibility to haemolysis including G6PD deficiency (section 9.1.5)—susceptible breast-feeding infants also at risk (Appendix 5); pregnancy (Appendix 4); avoid in porphyria (section 9.8.2); **interactions**: Appendix 1 (dapsone)

Blood disorders On long-term treatment, patients and their carers should be told how to recognise signs of blood disorders and advised to seek immediate medical attention if symptoms such as fever, sore throat, rash, mouth ulcers, purpura, bruising or bleeding develop

Side-effects (dose-related and uncommon at doses used for leprosy), haemolysis, methaemoglobinaemia, neuropathy, allergic dermatitis (rarely including toxic epidermal necrolysis and Stevens-Johnson syndrome), anorexia, nausea, vomiting, tachycardia, headache, insomnia, psychosis, hepatitis, agranulocytosis; dapsone syndrome (rash with fever and eosinophilia)—discontinue immediately (may progress to exfoliative dermatitis, hepatitis, hypoalbuminaemia, psychosis and death)

Dose

- Leprosy, 1–2 mg/kg daily, see notes above
- Dermatitis herpetiformis, see specialist literature

Dapsone (Non-proprietary) PoM

Tablets, dapsone 50 mg, net price 28-tab pack = £17.25; 100 mg, 28-tab pack = £25.88. Label: 8

CLOFAZIMINE

Indications leprosy

Cautions hepatic and renal impairment; pregnancy and breast-feeding; may discolour soft contact lenses; avoid if persistent abdominal pain and diarrhoea

Side-effects nausea, vomiting (hospitalise if persistent), abdominal pain; headache, tiredness; brownish-black discoloration of lesions and skin including areas exposed to light; reversible hair discoloration; dry skin; red discoloration of faeces, urine and other body fluids; also rash, pruritus, photosensitivity, acne-like eruptions, anorexia, eosinophilic enteropathy, bowel obstruction, dry eyes, dimmed vision, macular and subepithelial corneal pigmentation; elevation of blood sugar, weight loss, splenic infarction, lymphadenopathy

Dose

- Leprosy, see notes above
- Lepromatous lepra reactions, dosage increased to 300 mg daily for max. of 3 months

Clofazimine (Non-proprietary) PoM

Capsules, clofazimine 100 mg. Label: 8, 14, 21

Available on named-patient basis

5.1.11 Metronidazole and tinidazole

Metronidazole is an antimicrobial drug with high activity against anaerobic bacteria and protozoa; indications include trichomonal vaginitis (section 5.4.3), bacterial vaginosis (notably *Gardnerella vaginalis* infections), and *Entamoeba histolytica* and *Giardia lamblia* infections (section 5.4.2). It is also used for surgical and gynaecological sepsis in which its activity against colonic anaerobes, especially *Bacteroides fragilis*, is important. Metronidazole is also effective in the treatment of antibiotic-associated colitis (pseudomembranous colitis, see also section 1.5). Metronidazole by the rectal route is an effective alternative to the intravenous route when oral administration is not possible. Intravenous metronidazole is used for the treatment of established cases of tetanus; diazepam (section 10.2.2) and tetanus immunoglobulin (section 14.5) are also used.

Topical metronidazole (section 13.10.1.2) reduces the odour produced by anaerobic bacteria in fungating tumours; it is also used in the management of rosacea (section 13.6).

Tinidazole is similar to metronidazole but has a longer duration of action.

Oral infections Metronidazole is an alternative to a penicillin for the treatment of many oral infections where the patient is allergic to penicillin or the infection is due to beta-lactamase-producing anaerobes (Table 1, section 5.1). It is the drug of first choice for the treatment of acute necrotising ulcerative gingivitis (Vincent's infection) and pericoronitis; suitable alternatives are amoxicillin (section 5.1 1.3) and erythromycin (section 5.1.5). For these purposes metronidazole in a dose of 200 mg 3 times daily for 3 days is sufficient, but the duration of treatment may need to be longer in pericoronitis. Tinidazole is licensed for the treatment of acute ulcerative gingivitis.

METRONIDAZOLE

Indications anaerobic infections (including dental), see under Dose below; protozoal infections (section 5.4.2); *Helicobacter pylori* eradication (section 1.3); skin (section 13.10.1.2)

Cautions disulfiram-like reaction with alcohol, hepatic impairment and hepatic encephalopathy (Appendix 2); pregnancy (Appendix 4) and breast-feeding (Appendix 5); avoid in porphyria (section 9.8.2); clinical and laboratory monitoring advised if treatment exceeds 10 days; **interactions**: Appendix 1 (metronidazole)

Side-effects gastro-intestinal disturbances (including nausea and vomiting), taste disturbances, furred tongue, oral mucositis, anorexia; *very rarely* hepatitis, jaundice, pancreatitis, drowsiness, dizziness, headache, ataxia, psychotic disorders, darkening of urine, thrombocytopenia, pancytopenia, myalgia, arthralgia, visual disturbances, rash, pruritus, and erythema multiforme; on prolonged or intensive therapy peripheral neuropathy, transient epileptiform seizures, and leucopenia

Dose

- Anaerobic infections (usually treated for 7 days and for 10 days in antibiotic-associated colitis), by mouth, *either* 800 mg initially then 400 mg every 8 hours *or* 500 mg every 8 hours, CHILD 7.5 mg/kg every 8 hours; by rectum, 1 g every 8 hours for 3 days, then 1 g every 12 hours, CHILD every 8 hours for 3 days, then every 12 hours, age up to 1 year 125 mg, 1–5 years 250 mg, 5–10 years 500 mg, over 10 years, adult dose; by intravenous infusion over 20 minutes, 500 mg every 8 hours; CHILD 7.5 mg/kg every 8 hours
- Leg ulcers and pressure sores, by mouth, 400 mg every 8 hours for 7 days
- Bacterial vaginosis, by mouth, 400–500 mg twice daily for 5–7 days *or* 2 g as a single dose
- Pelvic inflammatory disease (see also Table 1, section 5.1), by mouth, 400 mg twice daily for 14 days

5 Infections

- Acute ulcerative gingivitis, by mouth, 200–250 mg every 8 hours for 3 days; CHILD 1–3 years 50 mg every 8 hours for 3 days; 3–7 years 100 mg every 12 hours; 7–10 years 100 mg every 8 hours
- Acute oral infections, by mouth, 200 mg every 8 hours for 3–7 days (see also notes above); CHILD 1–3 years 50 mg every 8 hours for 3–7 days; 3–7 years 100 mg every 12 hours; 7–10 years 100 mg every 8 hours
- Surgical prophylaxis, by mouth, 400–500 mg 2 hours before surgery; up to 3 further doses of 400–500 mg may be given every 8 hours for high-risk procedures; CHILD 7.5 mg/kg 2 hours before surgery; up to 3 further doses of 7.5 mg/kg may be given every 8 hours for high-risk procedures

  By rectum, 1 g 2 hours before surgery; up to 3 further doses of 1 g may be given every 8 hours for high-risk procedures; CHILD 5–10 years 500 mg 2 hours before surgery; up to 3 further doses of 500 mg may be given every 8 hours for high-risk procedures

  By intravenous infusion (if rectal administration inappropriate), 500 mg at induction; up to 3 further doses of 500 mg may be given every 8 hours for high-risk procedures; CHILD 7.5 mg/kg at induction; up to 3 further doses of 7.5 mg/kg may be given every 8 hours for high-risk procedures

Note Metronidazole doses in BNF may differ from those in product literature

Metronidazole (Non-proprietary) PoM
Tablets, metronidazole 200 mg, net price 21-tab pack = £1.00; 400 mg, 21-tab pack = 89p. Label: 4, 9, 21, 25, 27
Brands include *Vaginyl®*

Tablets, metronidazole 500 mg, net price 21-tab pack = £24.42. Label: 4, 9, 21, 25, 27

Suspension, metronidazole (as benzoate) 200 mg/5 mL. Net price 100 mL = £8.46. Label: 4, 9, 23
Brands include *Norzol®*

Intravenous infusion, metronidazole 5 mg/mL. Net price 20-mL amp = £1.56, 100-mL container = £3.41

Dental prescribing on NHS Metronidazole Tablets and Oral Suspension may be prescribed

Flagyl® (Winthrop) PoM
Tablets, both f/c, ivory, metronidazole 200 mg, net price 21-tab pack = £4.67; 400 mg, 14-tab pack = £6.60. Label: 4, 9, 21, 25, 27

Suppositories, metronidazole 500 mg, net price 10 = £15.80; 1 g, 10 = £24.00. Label: 4, 9

Flagyl® (Aventis Pharma) PoM
Intravenous infusion, metronidazole 5 mg/mL, net price 100-mL *Viaflex®* bag = £3.41
Electrolytes Na^+ 13.6 mmol/100-mL bag

Flagyl S® (Winthrop) PoM
Suspension, orange- and lemon-flavoured, metronidazole (as benzoate) 200 mg/5 mL. Net price 100 mL = £11.63. Label: 4, 9, 23

Metrolyl® (Sandoz) PoM
Intravenous infusion, metronidazole 5 mg/mL, net price 100-mL Steriflex® bag = £1.22
Electrolytes Na^+ 14.53 mmol/100-mL bag

Suppositories, metronidazole 500 mg, net price 10 = £12.34; 1 g, 10 = £18.34. Label: 4, 9

TINIDAZOLE

Indications anaerobic infections, see under Dose below; protozoal infections (section 5.4.2); *Helicobacter pylori* eradication (section 1.3)

Cautions see under Metronidazole; pregnancy (manufacturer advises avoid in first trimester); avoid in porphyria (section 9.8.2); **interactions:** Appendix 1 (tinidazole)

Side-effects see under Metronidazole

Dose
- Anaerobic infections, 2 g initially, followed by 1 g daily *or* 500 mg twice daily, usually for 5–6 days
- Bacterial vaginosis and acute ulcerative gingivitis, a single 2-g dose
- Abdominal surgery prophylaxis, a single 2-g dose approximately 12 hours before surgery

Fasigyn® (Pfizer) PoM
Tablets, f/c, tinidazole 500 mg. Net price 20-tab pack = £13.80. Label: 4, 9, 21, 25

5.1.12 Quinolones

Nalidixic acid and **norfloxacin** are effective in uncomplicated urinary-tract infections.

Ciprofloxacin is active against both Gram-positive and Gram-negative bacteria. It is particularly active against Gram-negative bacteria, including salmonella, shigella, campylobacter, neisseria, and pseudomonas. Ciprofloxacin has only moderate activity against Gram-positive bacteria such as *Streptococcus pneumoniae* and *Enterococcus faecalis*; it should not be used for pneumococcal pneumonia. It is active against chlamydia and some mycobacteria. Most anaerobic organisms are not susceptible. Ciprofloxacin can be used for respiratory tract infections (but not for pneumococcal pneumonia), urinary-tract infections, infections of the gastro-intestinal system (including typhoid fever), bone and joint infections, gonorrhoea and septicaemia caused by sensitive organisms.

Ofloxacin is used for urinary-tract infections, lower respiratory-tract infections, gonorrhoea, and non-gonococcal urethritis and cervicitis.

Levofloxacin is active against Gram-positive and Gram-negative organisms. It has greater activity against pneumococci than ciprofloxacin. Levofloxacin is licensed for community-acquired pneumonia but it is considered to be **second-line treatment** for this indication.

Although ciprofloxacin, levofloxacin and ofloxacin are licensed for skin and soft-tissue infections, many staphylococci are resistant to the quinolones and their use should be avoided in MRSA infections.

Moxifloxacin should be used for treating acute exacerbations of chronic bronchitis **only** if conventional treatment has failed or is contra-indicated, and for **second-line treatment** of community-acquired pneumonia. Moxifloxacin is active against Gram-positive and Gram-negative organisms. It has greater activity against Gram-positive organisms including pneumococci than ciprofloxacin. Moxifloxacin is not active against *Pseudomonas aeruginosa* or meticillin-resistant *Staphylococcus aureus* (MRSA).

Anthrax *Inhalation* or *gastro-intestinal anthrax* should be treated initially with either **ciprofloxacin** or **doxycy-**

cline [unlicensed indication] (section 5.1.3) combined with one or two other antibacterials (such as amoxicillin, benzylpenicillin, chloramphenicol, clarithromycin, clindamycin, imipenem with cilastatin, rifampicin [unlicensed indication], and vancomycin). When the condition improves and the sensitivity of the *Bacillus anthracis* strain is known, treatment may be switched to a single antibacterial. Treatment should continue for 60 days because germination may be delayed.

Cutaneous anthrax should be treated with either ciprofloxacin [unlicensed indication] or doxycycline [unlicensed indication] (section 5.1.3) for 7 days. Treatment may be switched to amoxicillin (section 5.1.1.3) if the infecting strain is susceptible. Treatment may need to be extended to 60 days if exposure is due to aerosol. A combination of antibacterials for 14 days is recommended for cutaneous anthrax with systemic features, extensive oedema, or lesions of the head or neck.

Ciprofloxacin or doxycycline may be given for *post-exposure prophylaxis*. If exposure is confirmed, antibacterial prophylaxis should continue for 60 days. Antibacterial prophylaxis may be switched to amoxicillin after 10–14 days if the strain of *B. anthracis* is susceptible. Vaccination against anthrax (section 14.4) may allow the duration of antibacterial prophylaxis to be shortened.

Cautions Quinolones should be used with caution in patients with a history of epilepsy or conditions that predispose to seizures, in G6PD deficiency (section 9.1.5), myasthenia gravis (risk of exacerbation), in renal impairment (Appendix 3); pregnancy (Appendix 4), during breast-feeding (Appendix 5), and in children or adolescents (arthropathy has developed in weight-bearing joints in young *animals*—see below). Exposure to excessive sunlight should be avoided (discontinue if photosensitivity occurs). The CSM has warned that quinolones may induce **convulsions** in patients with or without a history of convulsions; taking NSAIDs at the same time may also induce them. Other **interactions:** Appendix 1 (quinolones).

Use in children Quinolones cause arthropathy in the weight-bearing joints of immature *animals* and are therefore generally not recommended in children and growing adolescents. However, the significance of this effect in humans is uncertain and in some specific circumstances short-term use of a quinolone in children may be justified. Nalidixic acid is used for urinary-tract infections in children over 3 months of age. Ciprofloxacin is licensed for pseudomonal infections in cystic fibrosis (for children above 5 years of age), and for treatment and prophylaxis of inhalational anthrax.

CSM advice (tendon damage)

Tendon damage (including rupture) has been reported rarely in patients receiving quinolones. Tendon rupture may occur within 48 hours of starting treatment. The CSM has reminded that:

- quinolones are contra-indicated in patients with a history of tendon disorders related to quinolone use;
- elderly patients are more prone to tendinitis;
- the risk of tendon rupture is increased by the concomitant use of corticosteroids;
- if tendinitis is suspected, the quinolone should be discontinued immediately.

Side-effects Side-effects of the quinolones include nausea, vomiting, dyspepsia, abdominal pain, diarrhoea (rarely antibiotic-associated colitis), headache, dizziness, rash (very rarely Stevens-Johnson syndrome and toxic epidermal necrolysis). Less frequent side-effects include anorexia, sleep disturbances, asthenia, confusion, anxiety, depression, hallucinations, tremor, blood disorders (including eosinophilia, leucopenia, thrombocytopenia), arthralgia, myalgia, disturbances in vision and taste. Other side-effects reported rarely or very rarely include hepatic dysfunction (including jaundice and hepatitis), hypotension, vasculitis, dyspnoea (more frequent with moxifloxacin), convulsions, psychoses, paraesthesia, renal failure, interstitial nephritis, tendon inflammation and damage (see also CSM advice above), photosensitivity, disturbances in hearing and smell. The drug should be **discontinued** if psychiatric, neurological or hypersensitivity reactions (including severe rash) occur.

CIPROFLOXACIN

Indications see notes above and under Dose; eye infections (section 11.3.1)

Cautions see notes above; avoid excessive alkalinity of urine and ensure adequate fluid intake (risk of crystalluria); **interactions**: Appendix 1 (quinolones)

Driving May impair performance of skilled tasks (e.g. driving); effects enhanced by alcohol

Side-effects see notes above; also flatulence, pain and phlebitis at injection site; *rarely* dysphagia, pancreatitis, chest pain, tachycardia, syncope, oedema, hot flushes, abnormal dreams, sweating, hyperglycaemia, and erythema nodosum; *very rarely* movement disorders, tinnitus, and tenosynovitis

Dose

- By mouth, respiratory-tract infections, 250–750 mg twice daily

  Urinary-tract infections, 250–500 mg twice daily (100 mg twice daily for 3 days in acute uncomplicated cystitis in women)

  Chronic prostatitis, 500 mg twice daily for 28 days

  Gonorrhoea, 500 mg as a single dose

  Pseudomonal lower respiratory-tract infection in cystic fibrosis, 750 mg twice daily; CHILD 5–17 years (see Cautions above), up to 20 mg/kg (max. 750 mg) twice daily

  Most other infections, 500–750 mg twice daily

  Surgical prophylaxis, 750 mg 60–90 minutes before procedure

  Prophylaxis of meningococcal meningitis [not licensed], Table 2, section 5.1
- By intravenous infusion (over 30–60 minutes; 400 mg over 60 minutes), 200–400 mg twice daily

  Pseudomonal lower respiratory-tract infection in cystic fibrosis, 400 mg twice daily; CHILD 5–17 years (see Cautions above), up to 10 mg/kg (max. 400 mg) 3 times daily

  Urinary-tract infections, 100 mg twice daily

  Gonorrhoea, 100 mg as a single dose
- CHILD and ADOLESCENT not recommended (see Cautions above) but where benefit outweighs risk, by mouth, 5–15 mg/kg (max. 750 mg) twice daily *or* by intravenous infusion, 4–8 mg/kg (max. 400 mg) twice daily
- Anthrax (treatment and post-exposure prophylaxis, see notes above), by mouth, 500 mg twice daily; CHILD and ADOLESCENT 15 mg/kg (max. 500 mg) twice daily

  By intravenous infusion, 400 mg twice daily; CHILD and ADOLESCENT 10 mg/kg (max. 400 mg) twice daily

Ciprofloxacin (Non-proprietary) PoM
Tablets, ciprofloxacin (as hydrochloride) 100 mg, net price 6-tab pack = £1.46; 250 mg, 10-tab pack = 86p, 20-tab pack = 83p; 500 mg, 10-tab pack = 89p, 20-tab pack = 97p; 750 mg, 10-tab pack = £1.46. Label: 7, 9, 25, counselling, driving

Intravenous infusion, ciprofloxacin (as lactate) 2 mg/mL, net price 50-mL bottle = £8.00, 100-mL bottle = £15.00, 200-mL bottle = £22.00

Ciproxin® (Bayer) PoM
Tablets, all f/c, ciprofloxacin (as hydrochloride) 100 mg, net price 6-tab pack = £2.80; 250 mg (scored), 10-tab pack = £7.50, 20-tab pack = £15.00; 500 mg (scored), 10-tab pack = £14.20, 20-tab pack = £28.40; 750 mg, 10-tab pack = £20.00. Label: 7, 9, 25, counselling, driving

Suspension, strawberry-flavoured, ciprofloxacin for reconstitution with diluent provided, 250 mg/5 mL, net price 100 mL = £16.50. Label: 7, 9, 25, counselling, driving

Intravenous infusion, ciprofloxacin (as lactate) 2 mg/mL, in sodium chloride 0.9%, net price 50-mL bottle = £8.65, 100-mL bottle = £16.89, 200-mL bottle = £25.70
Electrolytes Na^+ 15.4 mmol/100-mL bottle

LEVOFLOXACIN

Indications see under Dose

Cautions see notes above; **interactions:** Appendix 1 (quinolones)
Driving May impair performance of skilled tasks (e.g. driving)

Side-effects see notes above; also tachycardia; *very rarely* pneumonitis, hypoglycaemia, and rhabdomyolysis; local reactions and transient hypotension reported with infusion

Dose
- By mouth, acute sinusitis, 500 mg daily for 10–14 days

  Exacerbation of chronic bronchitis, 250–500 mg daily for 7–10 days

  Community-acquired pneumonia, 500 mg once or twice daily for 7–14 days

  Urinary-tract infections, 250 mg daily for 7–10 days (for 3 days in uncomplicated infection)

  Chronic prostatitis, 500 mg once daily for 28 days

  Skin and soft tissue infections, 250 mg daily *or* 500 mg once or twice daily for 7–14 days
- By intravenous infusion (over at least 60 minutes for 500 mg), community-acquired pneumonia, 500 mg once or twice daily

  Complicated urinary-tract infections, 250 mg daily, increased in severe infections

  Skin and soft tissue infections, 500 mg twice daily

Tavanic® (Hoechst Marion Roussel) PoM
Tablets, yellow-red, f/c, scored, levofloxacin 250 mg, net price 5-tab pack = £7.23, 10-tab pack = £14.45; 500 mg, 5-tab pack = £12.93, 10-tab pack = £25.85. Label: 6, 9, 25, counselling, driving

Intravenous infusion, levofloxacin 5 mg/mL, net price 100-mL bottle = £26.40
Electrolytes Na^+ 15.4 mmol/100-mL bottle

MOXIFLOXACIN

Indications community-acquired pneumonia; exacerbation of chronic bronchitis; sinusitis

Cautions see notes above; conditions pre-disposing to arrhythmias, including myocardial ischaemia; **interactions:** Appendix 1 (quinolones)
Driving May impair performance of skilled tasks (e.g. driving)

Contra-indications see notes above; severe hepatic impairment; history of QT-interval prolongation, bradycardia, history of symptomatic arrhythmias, heart failure with reduced left ventricular ejection fraction, electrolyte disturbances, concomitant use with other drugs known to prolong QT-interval

Side-effects see notes above; also gastritis, flatulence, constipation, arrhythmias, palpitation, angina, vasodilatation, hyperlipidaemia, and sweating; *rarely* oedema, hypertension, syncope, dysphagia, abnormal dreams, incoordination, amnesia, hyperglycaemia, hyperuricaemia, and stomatitis; *very rarely* potentially life-threatening hepatic failure

Dose
- 400 mg once daily for 10 days in community-acquired pneumonia, for 5–10 days in exacerbation of chronic bronchitis, for 7 days in sinusitis

Avelox® (Bayer) ▼ PoM
Tablets, red, f/c, moxifloxacin (as hydrochloride) 400 mg, net price 5-tab pack = £11.95. Label: 6, 9, counselling, driving

NALIDIXIC ACID

Indications urinary-tract infections

Cautions see notes above; avoid in porphyria (section 9.8.2); liver disease; false positive urinary glucose (if tested for reducing substances); monitor blood counts, renal and liver function if treatment exceeds 2 weeks; **interactions:** Appendix 1 (quinolones)

Side-effects see notes above; also reported toxic psychosis, increased intracranial pressure, cranial nerve palsy, metabolic acidosis

Dose
- 900 mg every 6 hours for 7 days, reduced in chronic infections to 600 mg every 6 hours; CHILD over 3 months max. 50 mg/kg daily in divided doses; reduced in prolonged therapy to 30 mg/kg daily

Uriben® (Rosemont) PoM
Suspension, pink, nalidixic acid 300 mg/5 mL, net price 150 mL (raspberry- and strawberry-flavoured) = £11.42. Label: 9, 11
Excipients include sucrose 450 mg/5mL

NORFLOXACIN

Indications see under Dose

Cautions see notes above; **interactions:** Appendix 1 (quinolones)
Driving May impair performance of skilled tasks (e.g. driving)

Side-effects see notes above; also tinnitus, epiphora; *rarely* pancreatitis; *very rarely* arrhythmias; also reported, polyneuropathy and exfoliative dermatitis

Dose
- Urinary-tract infections, 400 mg twice daily for 7–10 days (for 3 days in uncomplicated lower urinary-tract infections)

- Chronic relapsing urinary-tract infections, 400 mg twice daily for up to 12 weeks; may be reduced to 400 mg once daily if adequate suppression within first 4 weeks
- Chronic prostatitis, 400 mg twice daily for 28 days

Norfloxacin (Non-proprietary) PoM
Tablets, norfloxacin 400 mg, net price 6-tab pack = £2.68, 14-tab pack = £4.06. Label: 7, 9, 23, counselling, driving

Utinor® (MSD) PoM
Tablets, scored, norfloxacin 400 mg. Net price 7-tab pack = £2.56, 14-tab pack = £5.11. Label: 7, 9, 23, counselling, driving

OFLOXACIN

Indications see under Dose

Cautions see notes above; hepatic impairment (Appendix 2); history of psychiatric illness; **interactions:** Appendix 1 (quinolones)
Driving May affect performance of skilled tasks (e.g. driving); effects enhanced by alcohol

Side-effects see notes above; also tachycardia; *rarely* abnormal dreams, unsteady gait, neuropathy, and extrapyramidal symptoms; *very rarely* changes in blood sugar; isolated cases of pneumonitis and rhabdomyolysis; on intravenous infusion, hypotension and local reactions (including thrombophlebitis)

Dose

- By mouth, urinary-tract infections, 200–400 mg daily preferably in the morning, increased if necessary in upper urinary-tract infections to 400 mg twice daily
  Chronic prostatitis, 200 mg twice daily for 28 days
  Lower respiratory-tract infections, 400 mg daily preferably in the morning, increased if necessary to 400 mg twice daily
  Skin and soft-tissue infections, 400 mg twice daily
  Uncomplicated gonorrhoea, 400 mg as a single dose
  Uncomplicated genital chlamydial infection, non-gonococcal urethritis, 400 mg daily in single or divided doses for 7 days
  Pelvic inflammatory disease (see also section 5.1, table 1), 400 mg twice daily for 14 days
- By intravenous infusion (over at least 30 minutes for each 200 mg), complicated urinary-tract infection, 200 mg daily
  Lower respiratory-tract infection, 200 mg twice daily
  Septicaemia, 200 mg twice daily
  Skin and soft-tissue infections, 400 mg twice daily
  Severe or complicated infections, dose may be increased to 400 mg twice daily

Ofloxacin (Non-proprietary) PoM
Tablets, ofloxacin 200 mg, net price 10-tab pack = £5.91; 400 mg, 5-tab pack = £6.17, 10-tab pack = £8.63. Label: 6, 9, 11, counselling, driving

Tarivid® (Aventis Pharma) PoM
Tablets, f/c, scored, ofloxacin 200 mg, net price 10-tab pack = £7.84, 20-tab pack = £15.66; 400 mg (yellow), 5-tab pack = £7.82, 10-tab pack = £15.60. Label: 6, 9, 11, counselling, driving

Intravenous infusion, ofloxacin (as hydrochloride) 2 mg/mL, net price 100-mL bottle = £16.82 (hosp. only)

5.1.13 Urinary-tract infections

Urinary-tract infection is more common in women than in men; when it occurs in men there is frequently an underlying abnormality of the renal tract. Recurrent episodes of infection are an indication for radiological investigation especially in children in whom untreated pyelonephritis may lead to permanent kidney damage.

Escherichia coli is the most common cause of urinary-tract infection; *Staphylococcus saprophyticus* is also common in sexually active young women. Less common causes include Proteus and Klebsiella spp. *Pseudomonas aeruginosa* infections usually occur in the hospital setting and may be associated with functional or anatomical abnormalities of the renal tract. *Staphylococcus epidermidis* and *Enterococcus faecalis* infection may complicate catheterisation or instrumentation.

> Whenever possible a specimen of urine should be collected for culture and sensitivity testing before starting antibacterial therapy. The antibacterial chosen should reflect current local bacterial sensitivity to antibacterials.

Uncomplicated lower urinary-tract infections often respond to trimethoprim, nitrofurantoin, amoxicillin, or nalidixic acid given for 7 days (3 days of trimethoprim or nitrofurantoin may be adequate for infections in women); those caused by fully sensitive bacteria respond to two 3-g doses of amoxicillin (section 5.1.1.3). Widespread bacterial resistance, especially to ampicillin, amoxicillin, and trimethoprim has increased the importance of urine culture before therapy. Alternatives for resistant organisms include co-amoxiclav (amoxicillin with clavulanic acid), an oral cephalosporin, pivmecillinam, or a quinolone.

Long-term low dose therapy may be required in selected patients to prevent *recurrence of infection*; indications include frequent relapses and significant kidney damage. Trimethoprim, nitrofurantoin and cefalexin have been recommended for long-term therapy.

Methenamine (hexamine) should **not** generally be used because it requires an acidic urine for its antimicrobial activity and it is ineffective for upper urinary-tract infections; it may, however, have a role in the prophylaxis and treatment of chronic or recurrent uncomplicated lower urinary-tract infections and asymptomatic bacteruria.

Acute pyelonephritis can lead to septicaemia and is treated initially by injection of a broad-spectrum antibacterial such as cefuroxime or a quinolone if the patient is severely ill; gentamicin can also be used.

Prostatitis can be difficult to cure and requires treatment for several weeks with an antibacterial which penetrates prostatic tissue such as trimethoprim, or some quinolones.

Where infection is localised and associated with an indwelling *catheter* a bladder instillation is often effective (section 7.4.4).

Urinary-tract infection in *pregnancy* may be asymptomatic and requires prompt treatment to prevent progression to acute pyelonephritis. Penicillins and cephalosporins are suitable for treating urinary-tract infection during pregnancy. Nitrofurantoin may also be used but it should be avoided at term. Sulphonamides, quinolones, and tetracyclines should be avoided during pregnancy; trimethoprim should also preferably be avoided particularly in the first trimester.

In *renal failure* antibacterials normally excreted by the kidney accumulate with resultant toxicity unless the dose is reduced. This applies especially to the aminoglycosides which should be used with great caution; tetracyclines, methenamine, and nitrofurantoin should be avoided altogether.

Children Urinary-tract infections in children require prompt antibacterial treatment to minimise the risk of renal scarring. Uncomplicated 'lower' urinary-tract infections in *children over 3 months of age* can be treated with trimethoprim, nitrofurantoin, a first generation cephalosporin, or co-amoxiclav for 3 days; children should be reassessed if they continue to be unwell 24–48 hours after the initial assessment.

Acute pyelonephritis in children over 3 months of age can be treated with a cephalosporin or co-amoxiclav for 7–10 days. If the patient is severely ill, then the infection is best treated initially by injection of a broad-spectrum antibacterial such as cefotaxime or co-amoxiclav; gentamicin is an alternative.

Children under 3 months of age should be transferred to hospital and treated initially with intravenous antibacterial drugs such as ampicillin with gentamicin, or cefotaxime alone, until the infection responds; full doses of oral antibacterials are then given for a further period.

Recurrent episodes of infection are an indication for radiological investigation. *Antibacterial prophylaxis* with low doses of trimethoprim or nitrofurantoin may be considered for children with recurrent infection, significant urinary-tract anomalies, or significant kidney damage.

NITROFURANTOIN

Indications urinary-tract infections

Cautions anaemia; diabetes mellitus; electrolyte imbalance; vitamin B and folate deficiency; pulmonary disease; hepatic impairment; monitor lung and liver function on long-term therapy, especially in the elderly (discontinue if deterioration in lung function); susceptibility to peripheral neuropathy; false positive urinary glucose (if tested for reducing substances); urine may be coloured yellow or brown; **interactions:** Appendix 1 (nitrofurantoin)

Contra-indications renal impairment (Appendix 3); infants less than 3 months old, G6PD deficiency (including pregnancy at term, and breast-feeding of affected infants, see section 9.1.5 and Appendix 4 and Appendix 5), porphyria (section 9.8.2)

Side-effects anorexia, nausea, vomiting, and diarrhoea; acute and chronic pulmonary reactions (pulmonary fibrosis reported; possible association with lupus erythematosus-like syndrome); peripheral neuropathy; also reported, hypersensitivity reactions (including angioedema, anaphylaxis, sialadenitis, urticaria, rash and pruritus); rarely, cholestatic jaundice, hepatitis, exfoliative dermatitis, erythema multiforme, pancreatitis, arthralgia, blood disorders (including agranulocytosis, thrombocytopenia, and aplastic anaemia), benign intracranial hypertension, and transient alopecia

Dose

- Acute uncomplicated infection, 50 mg every 6 hours with food for 7 days; CHILD over 3 months, 3 mg/kg daily in 4 divided doses
- Severe chronic recurrent infection, 100 mg every 6 hours with food for 7 days (dose reduced or discontinued if severe nausea)
- Prophylaxis (but see Cautions), 50–100 mg at night; CHILD over 3 months, 1 mg/kg at night

Nitrofurantoin (Non-proprietary) PoM

Tablets, nitrofurantoin 50 mg, net price 28-tab pack = £1.84; 100 mg, 28-tab pack = £4.26. Label: 9, 14, 21

Oral suspension, nitrofurantoin 25 mg/5 mL, net price 300 mL = £65.00. Label: 9, 14, 21

Furadantin® (Goldshield) PoM

Tablets, all yellow, scored, nitrofurantoin 50 mg, net price 20 = £1.96; 100 mg, 20 = £3.62. Label: 9, 14, 21

Macrobid® (Goldshield) PoM

Capsules, m/r, blue/yellow, nitrofurantoin 100 mg (as nitrofurantoin macrocrystals and nitrofurantoin monohydrate). Net price 14-cap pack = £4.89. Label: 9, 14, 21, 25

Dose uncomplicated urinary-tract infection, 1 capsule twice daily with food

Genito-urinary surgical prophylaxis, 1 capsule twice daily on day of procedure and for 3 days after

Macrodantin® (Goldshield) PoM

Capsules, nitrofurantoin 50 mg (yellow/white), net price 30-cap pack = £3.05; 100 mg (yellow/white), 20 = £3.84. Label: 9, 14, 21

METHENAMINE HIPPURATE

(Hexamine hippurate)

Indications prophylaxis and long-term treatment of chronic or recurrent lower urinary-tract infections

Cautions pregnancy; avoid concurrent administration with sulphonamides (risk of crystalluria) or urinary alkalinising agents; **interactions:** Appendix 1 (methenamine)

Contra-indications hepatic impairment, renal impairment (avoid if creatinine clearance less than 10 mL/minute; Appendix 3), severe dehydration, gout, metabolic acidosis

Side-effects gastro-intestinal disturbances, bladder irritation, rash

Dose

- 1 g every 12 hours (may be increased in patients with catheters to 1 g every 8 hours); CHILD 6–12 years 500 mg every 12 hours

Hiprex® (3M)

Tablets, scored, methenamine hippurate 1 g. Net price 60-tab pack = £6.58. Label: 9

5.2 Antifungal drugs

Treatment of fungal infections

The systemic treatment of common fungal infections is outlined below; specialist treatment is required in most forms of systemic or disseminated fungal infections. For local treatment of fungal infections, see section 7.2.2 (genital), section 7.4.4 (bladder), section 11.3.2 (eye), section 12.1.1 (ear), section 12.3.2 (oropharynx), and section 13.10.2 (skin).

Aspergillosis Aspergillosis most commonly affects the respiratory tract but in severely immunocompromised patients, invasive forms can affect the sinuses, heart, brain, and skin. **Amphotericin** (liposomal formulation preferred if toxicity or renal impairment are concerns) or **voriconazole** can be used for the treatment of aspergillosis. **Caspofungin** or **itraconazole** are alternatives in patients who are refractory to, or intolerant of amphotericin. Itraconazole is also used as an adjunct for the treatment of allergic bronchopulmonary aspergillosis [unlicensed indication]. The *Scottish Medicines Consortium* (March 2003) does not recommend the use of caspofungin because of a lack of robust data on efficacy and safety in the treatment of invasive aspergillosis.

Candidiasis Many superficial candidal infections including infections of the skin (section 13.10.2) are treated locally; widespread or intractable infection requires systemic antifungal treatment. Vaginal candidiasis (section 7.2.2) may be treated with locally acting antifungals or with fluconazole given by mouth; for resistant organisms, itraconazole can be given by mouth.

Oropharyngeal candidiasis generally responds to topical therapy (section 12.3.2); fluconazole is given by mouth for unresponsive infections; it is effective and is reliably absorbed. Itraconazole may be used for fluconazole-resistant infections. Topical therapy may not be adequate in immunocompromised patients and an oral triazole antifungal is preferred.

For *deep and disseminated candidiasis*, **amphotericin** can be given by intravenous infusion. **Fluconazole** is an alternative for *Candida albicans* infection in clinically stable patients who have not received an azole antifungal recently. **Caspofungin** or **voriconazole** can be used for infections caused by fluconazole-resistant *Candida* spp. that have not responded to amphotericin, or in patients intolerant of amphotericin. In refractory cases, **flucytosine** can be used with intravenous amphotericin.

Cryptococcosis Cryptococcosis is uncommon but infection in the immunocompromised, especially in AIDS patients, can be life-threatening; cryptococcal meningitis is the most common form of fungal meningitis. The treatment of choice in cryptococcal meningitis is **amphotericin** by intravenous infusion and **flucytosine** by intravenous infusion for 2 weeks, followed by **fluconazole** by mouth for 8 weeks or until cultures are negative. In cryptococcosis, **fluconazole** is sometimes given alone as an alternative in AIDS patients with mild, localised infections or in those who cannot tolerate amphotericin. Following successful treatment, fluconazole can be used for prophylaxis against relapse until immunity recovers.

Histoplasmosis Histoplasmosis is rare in temperate climates; it can be life-threatening, particularly in HIV-infected persons. **Itraconazole** can be used for the treatment of immunocompetent patients with indolent non-meningeal infection including chronic pulmonary histoplasmosis; **ketoconazole** is an alternative in immunocompetent patients. **Amphotericin** by intravenous infusion is preferred in patients with fulminant or severe infections. Following successful treatment, itraconazole can be used for prophylaxis against relapse.

Skin and nail infections Mild localised fungal infections of the skin (including tinea corporis, tinea cruris, and tinea pedis) respond to topical therapy (section 13.10.2). Systemic therapy is appropriate if topical therapy fails, if many areas are affected, or if the site of infection is difficult to treat such as in infections of the nails (onychomycosis) and of the scalp (tinea capitis). Oral imidazole or triazole antifungals (particularly **itraconazole**) and **terbinafine** are used more frequently than griseofulvin because they have a broader spectrum of activity and require a shorter duration of treatment.

Tinea capitis is treated systemically; additional topical application of an antifungal (section 13.10.2) may reduce transmission. **Griseofulvin** is used for tinea capitis in adults and children; it is effective against infections caused by *Trichophyton tonsurans* and *Microsporum* spp. **Terbinafine** is used for tinea capitis caused by *T. tonsurans* [unlicensed indication]. The role of terbinafine in the management of *Microsporum* infections is uncertain.

Pityriasis versicolor (section 13.10.2) may be treated with **itraconazole** by mouth if topical therapy is ineffective; **fluconazole** by mouth is an alternative. Oral **terbinafine is not** effective for pityriasis versicolor.

Terbinafine and **itraconazole** have largely replaced griseofulvin for the systemic treatment of *onychomycosis*, particularly of the toenail; terbinafine is considered to be the drug of choice. Itraconazole can be administered as intermittent 'pulse' therapy.

Immunocompromised patients Immunocompromised patients are at particular risk of fungal infections and may receive antifungal drugs prophylactically; oral imidazole or triazole antifungals are the drugs of choice for prophylaxis. **Fluconazole** is more reliably absorbed than itraconazole and ketoconazole and is considered less toxic than ketoconazole for long-term use.

Amphotericin by intravenous infusion is used for the empirical *treatment* of serious fungal infections. Fluconazole is used for treating *Candida albicans* infection. Caspofungin is licensed for the empirical treatment of systemic fungal infections (such as those involving *Candida* spp. or *Aspergillus* spp.) in patients with neutropenia.

Drugs used in fungal infections

Polyene antifungals The polyene antifungals include amphotericin and nystatin; neither drug is absorbed when given by mouth. They are used for oral, oropharyngeal, and perioral infections by local application in the mouth (section 12.3.2).

Amphotericin by intravenous infusion is used for the treatment of systemic fungal infections and is active against most fungi and yeasts. It is highly protein bound and penetrates poorly into body fluids and tissues. When given parenterally amphotericin is toxic and side-effects are common. Lipid formulations of amphotericin (*Abelcet*®, *AmBisome*®, and *Amphocil*®) are significantly less toxic and are recommended when the conventional formulation of amphotericin is contra-indicated because of toxicity, especially nephrotoxicity or when response to conventional amphotericin is inadequate; lipid formulations are more expensive.

Nystatin is used principally for *Candida albicans* infections of the skin and mucous membranes, including oesophageal and intestinal candidiasis.

Imidazole antifungals The imidazole antifungals include clotrimazole, econazole, ketoconazole, sulconazole, and tioconazole. They are used for the local treatment of vaginal candidiasis (section 7.2.2) and for dermatophyte infections (section 13.10.2).

Ketoconazole is better absorbed by mouth than other imidazoles. It has been associated with fatal hepatotoxicity; the CSM has advised that prescribers should weigh the potential benefits of ketoconazole treatment against the risk of liver damage and should carefully monitor patients both clinically and biochemically. It should not be used by mouth for superficial fungal infections.

Miconazole (section 12.3.2) can be used locally for oral infections; it is also effective in intestinal infections. Systemic absorption may follow use of miconazole oral gel and may result in significant drug interactions.

Triazole antifungals **Fluconazole** is very well absorbed after oral administration. It also achieves good penetration into the cerebrospinal fluid to treat fungal meningitis.

Itraconazole is active against a wide range of dermatophytes. Itraconazole capsules require an acid environment in the stomach for optimal absorption.

Itraconazole has been associated with liver damage and should be avoided or used with caution in patients with liver disease; fluconazole is less frequently associated with hepatotoxicity.

Posaconazole is licensed for the treatment of invasive fungal infections unresponsive to conventional treatment.

Voriconazole is a broad-spectrum antifungal drug which is licensed for use in life-threatening infections.

Echinocandin antifungals **Caspofungin** is active against *Aspergillus* spp. and *Candida* spp. **Anidulafungin** is licensed for the treatment of invasive candidiasis.

Other antifungals **Flucytosine** is used with amphotericin in a synergistic combination. Bone marrow depression can occur which limits its use, particularly in AIDS patients; weekly blood counts are necessary during prolonged therapy. Resistance to flucytosine can develop during therapy and sensitivity testing is essential before and during treatment.

Griseofulvin is effective for widespread or intractable dermatophyte infections but has been superseded by newer antifungals, particularly for nail infections. It is the drug of choice for trichophyton infections in children. Duration of therapy is dependent on the site of the infection and may extend to a number of months.

Terbinafine is the drug of choice for fungal nail infections and is also used for ringworm infections where oral treatment is considered appropriate.

5 Infections

AMPHOTERICIN
(Amphotericin B)

Indications See under Dose

Cautions when given parenterally, toxicity common (close supervision necessary and test dose required; see Anaphylaxis below); renal impairment (Appendix 3); hepatic and renal function tests, blood counts, and plasma electrolyte (including plasma-potassium and magnesium concentration) monitoring required; corticosteroids (avoid except to control reactions); pregnancy (Appendix 4); breast-feeding (Appendix 5); avoid rapid infusion (risk of arrhythmias); **interactions:** Appendix 1 (amphotericin)

Anaphylaxis The CSM has advised that anaphylaxis occurs rarely with any intravenous amphotericin product and a test dose is advisable before the first infusion; the patient should be carefully observed for at least 30 minutes after the test dose. Prophylactic antipyretics or hydrocortisone should only be used in patients who have previously experienced acute adverse reactions (in whom continued treatment with amphotericin is essential)

Side-effects when given parenterally, anorexia nausea and vomiting, diarrhoea, epigastric pain; febrile reactions, headache, muscle and joint pain; anaemia; disturbances in renal function (including hypokalaemia and hypomagnesaemia) and renal toxicity; also cardiovascular toxicity (including arrhythmias, blood pressure changes), blood disorders, neurological disorders (including hearing loss, diplopia, convulsions, peripheral neuropathy, encephalopathy), abnormal liver function (discontinue treatment), rash, anaphylactoid reactions (see Anaphylaxis, above); pain and thrombophlebitis at injection site

Dose
- Oral and perioral infections, see section 12.3.2
- By intravenous infusion, see preparations

Note Different preparations of intravenous amphotericin vary in their pharmacodynamics, pharmacokinetics, dosage, and administration; these preparations should **not** be considered interchangeable. To avoid confusion, prescribers should specify the brand to be dispensed.

Fungizone® (Squibb) PoM

Intravenous infusion, powder for reconstitution, amphotericin (as sodium deoxycholate complex). Net price 50-mg vial = £4.12

Electrolytes $Na^+ < 0.5$ mmol/vial

Dose by intravenous infusion, systemic fungal infections, initial test dose of 1 mg over 20–30 minutes then 250 micrograms/kg daily, gradually increased over 2–4 days, if tolerated, to 1 mg/kg daily; max. (severe infection) 1.5 mg/kg daily or on alternate days

Note Prolonged treatment usually necessary; if interrupted for longer than 7 days recommence at 250 micrograms/kg daily and increase gradually

Lipid formulations

Abelcet® (Zeneus) PoM

Intravenous infusion, amphotericin 5 mg/mL as lipid complex with L-α-dimyristoylphosphatidylcholine and L-α-dimyristoylphosphatidylglycerol. Net price 20-mL vial = £82.13 (hosp. only)

Dose by intravenous infusion, severe invasive candidiasis; severe systemic fungal infections in patients not responding to conventional amphotericin or to other antifungal drugs or where toxicity or renal impairment precludes conventional amphotericin, including invasive aspergillosis, cryptococcal meningitis and disseminated cryptococcosis in HIV patients, ADULT and CHILD, initial test dose 1 mg over 15 minutes then 5 mg/kg once daily for at least 14 days

AmBisome® (Gilead) PoM

Intravenous infusion, powder for reconstitution, amphotericin 50 mg encapsulated in liposomes. Net price 50-mg vial = £96.69

Electrolytes Na^+ < 0.5 mmol/vial

Excipients include sucrose 900 mg/vial

Dose by intravenous infusion, severe systemic or deep mycoses where toxicity (particularly nephrotoxicity) precludes use of conventional amphotericin, ADULT and CHILD initial test dose 1 mg over 10 minutes then 1 mg/kg once daily increased gradually if necessary to 3 mg/kg once daily; max. 5 mg/kg once daily [unlicensed dose]

Suspected or proven infection in febrile neutropenic patients unresponsive to broad-spectrum antibacterials, ADULT and CHILD, initial test dose 1 mg over 10 minutes then 3 mg/kg once daily until afebrile for 3 consecutive days; max. period of treatment 42 days; max. 5 mg/kg once daily [unlicensed dose]

Visceral leishmaniasis, see section 5.4.5 and product literature

Amphocil® (Beacon) PoM

Intravenous infusion, powder for reconstitution, amphotericin as a complex with sodium cholesteryl sulphate. Net price 50-mg vial = £104.10, 100-mg vial = £190.05

Electrolytes Na^+ < 0.5 mmol/vial

Dose by intravenous infusion, severe systemic or deep mycoses where toxicity or renal failure preclude use of conventional amphotericin, ADULT and CHILD initial test dose 2 mg over 10 minutes then 1 mg/kg once daily increased gradually if necessary to 3–4 mg/kg once daily; max. 6 mg/kg daily

ANIDULAFUNGIN

Indications invasive candidiasis

Cautions pregnancy (Appendix 4); breast-feeding (Appendix 5)

Side-effects diarrhoea, nausea, vomiting; flushing; convulsion, headache; coagulopathy, hypokalaemia, raised serum creatinine; rash, pruritus; *less commonly* abdominal pain, cholestasis, hypertension, hyperglycaemia, urticaria, and injection-site pain; also reported, hepatitis

Dose

- By intravenous infusion, ADULT over 18 years, 200 mg on first day then 100 mg once daily

Ecalta® (Pfizer) ▼ PoM

Intravenous infusion, powder for reconstitution, anidulafungin, net-price 100-mg vial = £299.99 (with solvent)

Excipients include alcohol 24%

CASPOFUNGIN

Indications invasive aspergillosis either unresponsive to amphotericin or itraconazole or in patients intolerant of amphotericin or itraconazole; invasive candidiasis (see notes above); empirical treatment of systemic fungal infections in patients with neutropenia

Cautions hepatic impairment (Appendix 2); pregnancy (Appendix 4); **interactions:** Appendix 1 (caspofungin)

Contra-indications breast-feeding (Appendix 5)

Side-effects nausea, vomiting, abdominal pain, diarrhoea; tachycardia, flushing; dyspnoea; fever, headache; anaemia, decrease in serum potassium, hypomagnesaemia; rash, pruritus, sweating; injection-site reactions; *less commonly* hypercalcaemia; also reported, hepatic dysfunction, oedema, adult respiratory distress syndrome, hypersensitivity reactions (including anaphylaxis)

Dose

- By intravenous infusion, ADULT over 18 years, 70 mg on first day then 50 mg once daily (70 mg once daily if body-weight over 80 kg)

Cancidas® (MSD) PoM

Intravenous infusion, powder for reconstitution, caspofungin (as acetate), net price 50-mg vial = £327.67; 70-mg vial = £416.78

FLUCONAZOLE

Indications see under Dose

Cautions renal impairment (Appendix 3); pregnancy (Appendix 4) and breast-feeding (Appendix 5); concomitant use with hepatotoxic drugs monitor liver function with high doses or extended courses—discontinue if signs or symptoms of hepatic disease (risk of hepatic necrosis); susceptibility to QT interval prolongation; **interactions:** Appendix 1 (antifungals, triazole)

Contra-indications porphyria (section 9.8.2)

Side-effects nausea, abdominal discomfort, diarrhoea, flatulence, headache, rash (discontinue treatment or monitor closely if infection invasive or systemic); less frequently dyspepsia, vomiting, taste disturbance, hepatic disorders, hypersensitivity reactions, anaphylaxis, dizziness, seizures, alopecia, pruritus, toxic epidermal necrolysis, Stevens-Johnson syndrome (severe cutaneous reactions more likely in AIDS patients), hyperlipidaemia, leucopenia, thrombocytopenia, and hypokalaemia reported

Dose

- Vaginal candidiasis (see also Recurrent Vulvovaginal Candidiasis, section 7.2.2) and candidal balanitis, by mouth, a single dose of 150 mg
- Mucosal candidiasis (except genital), by mouth, 50 mg daily (100 mg daily in unusually difficult infections) given for 7–14 days in oropharyngeal candidiasis (max. 14 days except in severely immunocompromised patients); for 14 days in atrophic oral candidiasis associated with dentures; for 14–30 days in other mucosal infections (e.g. oesophagitis, candiduria, non-invasive bronchopulmonary infections); CHILD by mouth or by intravenous infusion, 3–6 mg/kg on first day then 3 mg/kg daily (every 72 hours in NEONATE up to 2 weeks old, every 48 hours in neonate 2–4 weeks old)
- Tinea pedis, corporis, cruris, pityriasis versicolor, and dermal candidiasis, by mouth, 50 mg daily for 2–4 weeks (for up to 6 weeks in tinea pedis); max. duration of treatment 6 weeks
- Invasive candidal infections (including candidaemia and disseminated candidiasis) and cryptococcal infections (including meningitis), by mouth *or* intravenous infusion, 400 mg on first day then 200–400 mg daily; max. 800 mg daily in severe infections [unlicensed dose]; treatment continued according to response (at least 8 weeks for cryptococcal meningitis); CHILD 6–12 mg/kg daily (every 72 hours in NEONATE up to 2 weeks old, every 48 hours in NEONATE 2–4 weeks old); max. 400 mg daily
- Prevention of relapse of cryptococcal meningitis in AIDS patients after completion of primary therapy, by mouth *or* by intravenous infusion, 200 mg daily

- Prevention of fungal infections in immunocompromised patients, by mouth *or* by intravenous infusion, 50–400 mg daily adjusted according to risk; 400 mg daily if high risk of systemic infections e.g. following bone-marrow transplantation; commence treatment before anticipated onset of neutropenia and continue for 7 days after neutrophil count in desirable range; CHILD according to extent and duration of neutropenia, 3–12 mg/kg daily (every 72 hours in NEONATE up to 2 weeks old, every 48 hours in NEONATE 2–4 weeks old); max. 400 mg daily

Fluconazole (Non-proprietary) PoM

[1]Capsules, fluconazole 50 mg, net price 7-cap pack = 51p; 150 mg, single-capsule pack = 46p; 200 mg, 7-cap pack = £2.57. Label: 9, (50 and 200 mg)

Dental prescribing on NHS Fluconazole Capsules 50 mg may be prescribed

Intravenous infusion, fluconazole 2 mg/mL, net price 25-mL bottle = £7.32; 100-mL bottle = £29.28

Diflucan® (Pfizer) PoM

[1]Capsules, fluconazole 50 mg (blue/white), net price 7-cap pack = £16.61; 150 mg (blue), single-capsule pack = £7.12; 200 mg (purple/white), 7-cap pack = £66.42. Label: 9, (50 and 200 mg)

Oral suspension, orange-flavoured, fluconazole for reconstitution with water, 50 mg/5 mL, net price 35 mL = £16.61; 200 mg/5 mL, 35 mL = £66.42. Label: 9

Dental prescribing on NHS May be prescribed as Fluconazole Oral Suspension 50 mg/5 mL

Intravenous infusion, fluconazole 2 mg/mL in sodium chloride intravenous infusion 0.9%, net price 25-mL bottle = £7.32; 100-mL bottle = £29.28

Electrolytes Na^+ 15 mmol/100-mL bottle

FLUCYTOSINE

Indications systemic yeast and fungal infections; adjunct to amphotericin in cryptococcal meningitis (see Cryptococcosis, p. 321), adjunct to amphotericin in severe systemic candidiasis and in other severe or long-standing infections

Cautions renal impairment (Appendix 3); elderly; blood disorders; liver- and kidney-function tests and blood counts required (weekly in renal impairment or blood disorders); pregnancy (Appendix 4), breast-feeding (Appendix 5); **interactions:** Appendix 1 (flucytosine)

Side-effects nausea, vomiting, diarrhoea, rashes; less frequently cardiotoxicity, confusion, hallucinations, convulsions, headache, sedation, vertigo, alterations in liver function tests (hepatitis and hepatic necrosis reported), and toxic epidermal necrolysis; blood disorders including thrombocytopenia, leucopenia, and aplastic anaemia reported

Dose

- By intravenous infusion over 20–40 minutes, ADULT and CHILD, 200 mg/kg daily in 4 divided doses usually for not more than 7 days; extremely sensitive organisms, 100–150 mg/kg daily may be sufficient

Cryptococcal meningitis (adjunct to amphotericin, see Cryptococcosis, p. 321) 100 mg/kg daily in 4 divided doses for 2 weeks [unlicensed duration]

Note For plasma concentration monitoring, blood should be taken shortly before starting the next infusion; plasma concentration for optimum response 25–50 mg/litre (200–400 micromol/litre)—should not be allowed to exceed 80 mg/litre (620 micromol/litre)

Ancotil® (Valeant) PoM

Intravenous infusion, flucytosine 10 mg/mL. Net price 250-mL infusion bottle = £30.33 (hosp. only)

Electrolytes Na^+ 34.5 mmol/250-mL bottle

Note Flucytosine tablets may be available on a named-patient basis from Bell and Croyden

GRISEOFULVIN

Indications dermatophyte infections of the skin, scalp, hair and nails where topical therapy has failed or is inappropriate

Cautions **interactions:** Appendix 1 (griseofulvin)

Driving May impair performance of skilled tasks (e.g. driving); effects of alcohol enhanced

Contra-indications severe liver disease; systemic lupus erythematosus (risk of exacerbation); porphyria (section 9.8.2); pregnancy (**avoid** pregnancy **during** and for 1 **month after** treatment (Appendix 4); men should not father children within 6 months of treatment); breast-feeding (Appendix 5)

Side-effects nausea, vomiting, diarrhoea; headache; less frequently hepatotoxicity, dizziness, confusion, fatigue, sleep disturbances, impaired co-ordination, peripheral neuropathy, leucopenia, systemic lupus erythematosus, rash (including rarely erythema multiforme, toxic epidermal necrolysis), and photosensitivity

Dose

- Dermatophyte infections, 500 mg once daily or in divided doses; in severe infection dose may be doubled, reducing when response occurs; CHILD under 50 kg, 10 mg/kg once daily or in divided doses
- Tinea capitis caused by *Trichophyton tonsurans*, 1 g once daily or in divided doses; CHILD under 50 kg, 15–20 mg/kg once daily or in divided doses

Note Griseofulvin doses in BNF may differ from those in product literature

Griseofulvin (Non-proprietary) PoM

Tablets, griseofulvin 125 mg, net price 20 = £6.76; 500 mg, 20 = £17.52. Label: 9, 21, counselling, driving

ITRACONAZOLE

Indications see under Dose

Cautions absorption reduced in AIDS and neutropenia (monitor plasma-itraconazole concentration and increase dose if necessary); susceptibility to congestive heart failure (see also CSM advice, below); renal impairment (Appendix 3); pregnancy (Appendix 4) and breast-feeding (Appendix 5); **interactions:** Appendix 1 (antifungals, triazole)

Hepatotoxicity Potentially life-threatening hepatotoxicity reported very rarely. Monitor liver function—discontinue if signs of hepatitis develop; avoid or use with caution if history of hepatotoxicity with other drugs or in active liver disease (Appendix 2); use with caution in patients receiving other hepatotoxic drugs

Counselling Patients should be told how to recognise signs of liver disorder and advised to seek prompt medical atten-

1. Capsules can be sold to the public for vaginal candidiasis and associated candidal balanitis in those aged 16–60 years, in a container or packaging containing not more than 150 mg and labelled to show a max. dose of 150 mg

5 Infections

tion if symptoms such as anorexia, nausea, vomiting, fatigue, abdominal pain or dark urine develop

CSM advice (heart failure)
Following rare reports of heart failure, the CSM has advised caution when prescribing itraconazole to patients at high risk of heart failure. Those at risk include:

- patients receiving high doses and longer treatment courses;
- older patients and those with cardiac disease;
- patients receiving treatment with negative inotropic drugs, e.g. calcium channel blockers.

Contra-indications porphyria (section 9.8.2)

Side-effects *very rarely* nausea, vomiting, dyspepsia, abdominal pain, diarrhoea, constipation, jaundice, hepatitis (see also Hepatotoxicity above), heart failure (see CSM advice above), pulmonary oedema, headache, dizziness, peripheral neuropathy (discontinue treatment), menstrual disorder, hypokalaemia, rash, pruritus, Stevens-Johnson syndrome, and alopecia; *with intravenous injection, very rarely* hypertension and hyperglycaemia

Dose

- By mouth, oropharyngeal candidiasis, 100 mg once daily (200 mg once daily in AIDS or neutropenia) for 15 days; see also under *Sporanox®* oral liquid below
  Vulvovaginal candidiasis, 200 mg twice daily for 1 day
  Pityriasis versicolor, 200 mg once daily for 7 days
  Tinea corporis and tinea cruris, *either* 100 mg once daily for 15 days *or* 200 mg once daily for 7 days
  Tinea pedis and tinea manuum, *either* 100 mg once daily for 30 days *or* 200 mg twice daily for 7 days
  Onychomycosis, *either* 200 mg once daily for 3 months *or* course ('pulse') of 200 mg twice daily for 7 days, subsequent courses repeated after 21-day interval; fingernails 2 courses, toenails 3 courses
  Histoplasmosis, 200 mg 1–2 times daily
  Systemic aspergillosis, candidiasis and cryptococcosis including cryptococcal meningitis where other antifungal drugs inappropriate or ineffective, 200 mg once daily (candidiasis 100–200 mg once daily) increased in invasive or disseminated disease and in cryptococcal meningitis to 200 mg twice daily
  Maintenance in AIDS patients to prevent relapse of underlying fungal infection and prophylaxis in neutropenia when standard therapy inappropriate, 200 mg once daily, increased to 200 mg twice daily if low plasma-itraconazole concentration (see Cautions)
  Prophylaxis in patients with haematological malignancy or undergoing bone-marrow transplant, see under *Sporanox®* oral liquid below
- By intravenous infusion, systemic aspergillosis, candidiasis and cryptococcosis including cryptococcal meningitis where other antifungal drugs inappropriate or ineffective, histoplasmosis, 200 mg every 12 hours for 2 days, then 200 mg once daily for max. 12 days
- CHILD and ELDERLY safety and efficacy not established

Sporanox® (Janssen-Cilag) PoM
Capsules, blue/pink, enclosing coated beads, itraconazole 100 mg, net price 4-cap pack = £3.90; 15-cap pack = £20.96; 28-cap pack (*Sporanox®-Pulse*) = £27.30; 60-cap pack = £58.49. Label: 5, 9, 21, 25, counselling, hepatotoxicity

Oral liquid, sugar-free, cherry-flavoured, itraconazole 10 mg/mL, net price 150 mL (with 10-mL measuring cup) = £48.62. Label: 9, 23, counselling, administration, hepatotoxicity

Dose oral or oesophageal candidiasis in HIV-positive or other immunocompromised patients, 20 mL (2 measuring cups) daily in 1–2 divided doses for 1 week (continue for another week if no response)

Fluconazole-resistant oral or oesophageal candidiasis, 10–20 mL (1–2 measuring cups) twice daily for 2 weeks (continue for another 2 weeks if no response; the higher dose should not be used for longer than 2 weeks if no signs of improvement)

Prophylaxis of deep fungal infections (when standard therapy is inappropriate) in patients with haematological malignancy or undergoing bone-marrow transplantation who are expected to become neutropenic, 5 mg/kg daily in 2 divided doses; starting before transplantation or before chemotherapy (taking care to avoid interaction with cytotoxic drugs) and continued until neutrophil count recovers; CHILD and ELDERLY safety and efficacy not established

Counselling Do not take with food; swish around mouth and swallow, do not rinse afterwards

Concentrate for intravenous infusion, itraconazole 10 mg/mL. For dilution before use. Net price 25-mL amp (with infusion bag and filter) = £66.43

Excipients include propylene glycol

KETOCONAZOLE

Indications see CSM recommendations, p. 322; skin, hair, and mucosal mycoses that cannot be treated with other antifungals (including dermatophytoses, pityrosporum folliculitis, cutaneous candidiasis, chronic mucocutaneous candidiasis, oropharyngeal and oesophageal candidiasis, chronic recurrent vaginal candidiasis); systemic mycoses that cannot be treated with other antifungals (including histoplasmosis, blastomycosis, coccidioidomycosis, paracoccidioidomycosis)

Cautions predisposition to adrenocortical insufficiency; avoid in porphyria (section 9.8.2); pregnancy (Appendix 4); **interactions**: Appendix 1 (antifungals, imidazole)

Hepatotoxicity Potentially life-threatening hepatotoxicity reported very rarely; risk of hepatotoxicity greater if given for longer than 14 days. Monitor liver function before treatment, then on weeks 2 and 4 of treatment, then every month. Avoid or use with caution if abnormal liver function tests (avoid in active liver disease) or if history of hepatotoxicity with other drugs. For CSM advice see p. 322

Counselling Patients should be told how to recognise signs of liver disorder and advised to seek prompt medical attention if symptoms such as anorexia, nausea, vomiting, fatigue, abdominal pain, jaundice, or dark urine develop

Contra-indications porphyria (section 9.8.2); hepatic impairment; breast-feeding

Side-effects nausea, vomiting, abdominal pain; pruritus; *less commonly* diarrhoea, headache, dizziness, drowsiness, and rash; *very rarely* fatal liver damage (see Hepatotoxicity above), dyspepsia, raised intracranial pressure, adrenocortical insufficiency, erectile dysfunction, menstrual disorders, azoospermia (with high doses), gynaecomastia, thrombocytopenia, photophobia, and alopecia

Dose

- 200 mg once daily, increased if response inadequate to 400 mg once daily; continued until symptoms have cleared and cultures negative (usually for 4 weeks in dermatophytoses, 2–3 weeks for oral and cutaneous candidiasis, 1–2 months for hair infections); CHILD body-weight 15–30 kg, 100 mg once daily; body-weight over 30 kg, adult dose
- Chronic, recurrent vaginal candidiasis, 400 mg once daily for 5 days

Nizoral® (Janssen-Cilag) PoM
Tablets, scored, ketoconazole 200 mg. Net price 30-tab pack = £14.59. Label: 5, 9, 21, counselling, hepatotoxicity

NYSTATIN

Indications candidiasis; vaginal infection (section 7.2.2); oral infection (section 12.3.2); skin infection (section 13.10.2)

Side-effects nausea, vomiting, diarrhoea at high doses; oral irritation and sensitisation; rash (including urticaria) and rarely Stevens-Johnson syndrome reported

Dose
- By mouth, intestinal candidiasis 500 000 units every 6 hours, doubled in severe infection; NEONATE 100 000 units 4 times daily; CHILD 1 month–12 years, 100 000 units 4 times daily; immunocompromised children may require higher doses (e.g. 500 000 units 4 times daily)

Note Unlicensed for treatment of candidiasis in NEONATE. Nystatin doses in BNF may differ from those in product literature

Nystan® (Squibb) PoM
Tablets, brown, s/c, nystatin 500 000 units, net price 56-tab pack = £4.37. Label: 9
Suspension, yellow, nystatin 100 000 units/mL, net price 30 mL with pipette = £1.91. Label: 9, counselling, use of pipette

POSACONAZOLE

Indications invasive aspergillosis either unresponsive to, or in patients intolerant of, amphotericin or itraconazole; fusariosis either unresponsive to, or in patients intolerant of, amphotericin; chromoblastomycosis and mycetoma either unresponsive to, or in patients intolerant of, itraconazole; coccidioidomycosis either unresponsive to, or in patients intolerant of, amphotericin, itraconazole, or fluconazole; see also under Dose

Cautions cardiomyopathy, bradycardia, symptomatic arrhythmias, history of QT interval prolongation, concomitant use with other drugs known to cause QT-interval prolongation; monitor electrolytes (including potassium, magnesium, and calcium) before and during therapy, monitor liver function—consider discontinuing if impairment suspected (Appendix 2); pregnancy (ensure effective contraception during treatment; Appendix 4); **interactions**: Appendix 1 (antifungals, triazole)

Contra-indications porphyria (section 9.8.2); breast-feeding (Appendix 5)

Side-effects gastro-intestinal disturbances (including nausea, vomiting, abdominal pain, diarrhoea, dyspepsia, and flatulence); dizziness, headache, paraesthesia, drowsiness, fatigue, fever, anorexia; blood disorders (including anaemia, neutropenia, and thrombocytopenia), electrolyte disturbances; dry mouth; rash; *less commonly* pancreatitis, hepatic disorders, arrhythmias, palpitation, changes in blood pressure, oedema, convulsions, neuropathy, tremor, hyperglycaemia, menstrual disorders, renal failure, musculoskeletal pain, visual disturbances, mouth ulcers, and alopecia; *rarely* ileus, cardiac failure, myocardial infarction, stroke, thrombosis, syncope, pneumonitis, psychosis, depression, encephalopathy, adrenal insufficiency, breast pain, hearing impairment, and Stevens-Johnson syndrome

Dose
- 400 mg twice daily with food *or* if food not tolerated, 200 mg 4 times daily
- Oropharyngeal candidiasis (severe infection or in immunocompromised patients only), 200 mg with food on first day, then 100 mg once daily with food for 13 days
- Prophylaxis of invasive fungal infections in patients undergoing bone-marrow transplantation or receiving chemotherapy for acute myeloid leukaemia and myelodysplastic syndrome who are expected to become neutropenic, and who are intolerant of fluconazole and itraconazole, 200 mg 3 times daily with food, starting before transplantation or before chemotherapy and continued until neutrophil count recovers
- CHILD under 18 years not recommended

Noxafil (Schering-Plough) ▼ PoM
Suspension, posaconazole 200 mg/5 mL, net price 105 mL (cherry-flavoured) = £500.69. Label: 9, 21

TERBINAFINE

Indications dermatophyte infections of the nails, ringworm infections (including tinea pedis, cruris, and corporis) where oral therapy appropriate (due to site, severity or extent)

Cautions psoriasis (risk of exacerbation); autoimmune disease (risk of lupus-erythematosus-like effect); hepatic impairment (Appendix 2); renal impairment (Appendix 3); pregnancy (Appendix 4); breast-feeding (Appendix 5); **interactions**: Appendix 1 (terbinafine)

Side-effects abdominal discomfort, anorexia, nausea, diarrhoea; headache; rash and urticaria occasionally with arthralgia or myalgia; *less commonly* taste disturbance; *rarely* liver toxicity (including jaundice, cholestasis and hepatitis)—discontinue treatment, angioedema, dizziness, malaise, paraesthesia, hypoaesthesia, photosensitivity, serious skin reactions (including Stevens-Johnson syndrome and toxic epidermal necrolysis)—discontinue treatment if progressive skin rash; *very rarely* psychiatric disturbances, blood disorders (including leucopenia and thrombocytopenia), lupus erythematosus-like effect, and exacerbation of psoriasis

Dose
- By mouth, 250 mg daily usually for 2–6 weeks in tinea pedis, 2–4 weeks in tinea cruris, 4 weeks in tinea corporis, 6 weeks–3 months in nail infections (occasionally longer in toenail infections); CHILD [unlicensed] usually for 4 weeks, tinea capitis, over 1 year, body-weight 10–20 kg, 62.5 mg once daily; body-weight 20–40 kg, 125 mg once daily; body-weight over 40 kg, 250 mg once daily

Terbinafine (Non-proprietary) PoM
Tablets, terbinafine (as hydrochloride) 250 mg, net price 14-tab pack = £4.23, 28-tab pack = £3.68. Label: 9

Lamisil® (Novartis) PoM
Tablets, off-white, scored, terbinafine (as hydrochloride) 250 mg, net price 14-tab pack = £23.16, 28-tab pack = £44.66. Label: 9

VORICONAZOLE

Indications invasive aspergillosis; serious infections caused by *Scedosporium* spp., *Fusarium* spp., or invasive fluconazole-resistant *Candida* spp. (including *C. krusei*)

Cautions electrolyte disturbances, cardiomyopathy, bradycardia, symptomatic arrhythmias, history of QT interval prolongation, concomitant use with other drugs that prolong QT interval; avoid exposure to sunlight; patients at risk of pancreatitis; monitor liver function before treatment and during treatment; haematological malignancy (increased risk of hepatic reactions); hepatic impairment (Appendix 2); monitor renal function; renal impairment (Appendix 3); pregnancy (ensure effective contraception during treatment—Appendix 4); **interactions**: Appendix 1 (antifungals, triazole)

Contra-indications porphyria (section 9.8.2); breast-feeding (Appendix 5)

Side-effects gastro-intestinal disturbances (including nausea, vomiting, abdominal pain, diarrhoea), jaundice; oedema, hypotension, chest pain; respiratory distress syndrome, sinusitis; headache, dizziness, asthenia, anxiety, depression, confusion, agitation, hallucinations, paraesthesia, tremor; influenza-like symptoms; hypoglycaemia; haematuria; blood disorders (including anaemia, thrombocytopenia, leucopenia, pancytopenia), acute renal failure, hypokalaemia; visual disturbances including altered perception, blurred vision, and photophobia; rash, pruritus, photosensitivity, alopecia, cheilitis; injection-site reactions; *less commonly* cholecystitis, pancreatitis, hepatitis, constipation, arrhythmias (including QT interval prolongation), syncope, raised serum cholesterol, hypersensitivity reactions (including flushing), ataxia, nystagmus, hypoaesthesia, adrenocortical insufficiency, arthritis, blepharitis, optic neuritis, scleritis, glossitis, gingivitis, psoriasis, and Stevens-Johnson syndrome; *rarely* pseudomembranous colitis, convulsions, sleep disturbances, tinnitus, hearing disturbances, extrapyramidal effects, hypertonia, hypothyroidism, hyperthyroidism, discoid lupus erythematosus, toxic epidermal necrolysis, retinal haemorrhage, optic atrophy, and taste disturbances

Dose

- By mouth, ADULT and ADOLESCENT over 12 years, body-weight over 40 kg, 400 mg every 12 hours for 2 doses then 200 mg every 12 hours, increased if necessary to 300 mg every 12 hours; body-weight under 40 kg, 200 mg every 12 hours for 2 doses then 100 mg every 12 hours, increased if necessary to 150 mg every 12 hours; CHILD 2–12 years, (oral suspension recommended) 200 mg every 12 hours
- By intravenous infusion, 6 mg/kg every 12 hours for 2 doses, then 4 mg/kg every 12 hours (reduced to 3 mg/kg every 12 hours if not tolerated) for max. 6 months; CHILD 2–12 years, 7 mg/kg every 12 hours (reduced to 4 mg/kg every 12 hours if not tolerated) for max. 6 months

Vfend® (Pfizer) PoM

Tablets, f/c, voriconazole 50 mg, net price 28-tablet pack = £275.68; 200 mg, 28-tab pack = £1102.74. Label: 9, 11, 23

Oral suspension, voriconazole 200 mg/5 mL when reconstituted with water, net price 75 mL (orange-flavoured) = £551.37. Label: 9, 11, 23

Intravenous infusion, powder for reconstitution, voriconazole, net price 200-mg vial = £77.14

Excipients include sulphobutylether beta cyclodextrin sodium (risk of accumulation in renal impairment)

Electrolytes Na^+ 9.47 mmol/vial

5.3 Antiviral drugs

5.3.1 HIV infection
5.3.2 Herpesvirus infections
5.3.3 Viral hepatitis
5.3.4 Influenza
5.3.5 Respiratory syncytial virus

The majority of virus infections resolve spontaneously in immunocompetent subjects. A number of specific treatments for viral infections are available, particularly for the immunocompromised. This section includes notes on herpes simplex and varicella-zoster, human immunodeficiency virus, cytomegalovirus, respiratory syncytial virus, viral hepatitis and influenza.

5.3.1 HIV infection

There is no cure for infection caused by the human immunodeficiency virus (HIV) but a number of drugs slow or halt disease progression. Drugs for HIV infection (antiretrovirals) increase life expectancy considerably but they are toxic. Treatment should be undertaken only by those experienced in their use.

Principles of treatment Treatment is aimed at reducing the plasma viral load as much as possible and for as long as possible; it should be started before the immune system is irreversibly damaged. The need for early drug treatment should, however, be balanced against the risk of toxicity. Commitment to treatment and strict adherence over many years are required; the regimen chosen should take into account convenience and patient tolerance. The development of drug resistance is reduced by using a combination of drugs; such combinations should have synergistic or additive activity while ensuring that their toxicity is not additive. It is recommended that viral sensitivity to antiretroviral drugs is established before starting treatment or before switching drugs if the infection is not responding.

Initiation of treatment The optimum time for initiating antiretroviral treatment depends primarily on the CD4 cell count; the plasma viral load and clinical symptoms may also help. The timing and choice of treatment should also take account of the possible effects of antiretroviral drugs on factors such as the risk of cardiovascular events. Initiating treatment with a combination of drugs ('highly active antiretroviral therapy' which includes 2 nucleoside reverse transcriptase inhibitors with *either* a non-nucleoside reverse transcriptase inhibitor *or* a boosted protease inhibitor) is recommended. Patients who require treatment for both HIV and chronic hepatitis B should be treated with antivirals active against both diseases (section 5.3.3).

Switching therapy Deterioration of the condition (including clinical and virological changes) may require either switching therapy or adding another antiretroviral drug. The choice of an alternative regimen depends on factors such as the response to previous treatment, tolerance and the possibility of cross-resistance.

Pregnancy and breast-feeding Treatment of HIV infection in pregnancy aims to reduce the risk of toxicity to the fetus (although the teratogenic potential of most antiretroviral drugs is unknown), to minimise the viral load and disease progression in the mother, and to prevent transmission of infection to the neonate. **All treatment options require careful assessment by a specialist**. Zidovudine monotherapy reduces transmission of infection to the neonate. However, combination antiretroviral therapy maximises the chance of preventing transmission and represents optimal therapy for the mother.

Breast-feeding by HIV-positive mothers may cause HIV infection in the infant and should be avoided.

Children HIV disease in children has a different natural progression to adults. Children infected with HIV should be managed within a formal paediatric HIV clinical network by specialists with access to guidelines and information on antiretroviral drugs for children.

Post-exposure prophylaxis Prophylaxis with antiretroviral drugs [unlicensed indication] may be appropriate following exposure to HIV-contaminated material. Immediate expert advice should be sought in such cases; national guidelines on post-exposure prophylaxis for healthcare workers have been developed (by the Chief Medical Officer's Expert Advisory Group on AIDS, www.dh.gov.uk) and local ones may also be available. Antiretrovirals for prophylaxis are chosen on the basis of efficacy and potential for toxicity. Prompt prophylaxis with antiretroviral drugs [unlicensed indication] is also appropriate following potential sexual exposure to HIV; recommendations have been developed by the British Association for Sexual Health and HIV, www.bashh.org

Drugs for HIV infection **Zidovudine**, a nucleoside reverse transcriptase inhibitor (or 'nucleoside analogue'), was the first anti-HIV drug to be introduced. Other nucleoside reverse transcriptase inhibitors include **abacavir**, **didanosine**, **emtricitabine**, **lamivudine**, **stavudine**, and **tenofovir**.

The protease inhibitors include **amprenavir**, **atazanavir**, **darunavir**, **fosamprenavir** (a pro-drug of amprenavir), **indinavir**, **lopinavir**, **nelfinavir**, **ritonavir**, **saquinavir**, and **tipranavir**. Ritonavir in low doses boosts the activity of amprenavir, atazanavir, darunavir, indinavir, lopinavir, saquinavir, and tipranavir increasing the persistence of plasma concentrations of these drugs; at such a low dose, ritonavir has no intrinsic antiviral activity. A combination of lopinavir with low-dose ritonavir is available. The protease inhibitors are metabolised by cytochrome P450 enzyme systems and therefore have a significant potential for drug interactions. Protease inhibitors are associated with lipodystrophy and metabolic effects (see below).

The non-nucleoside reverse transcriptase inhibitors **efavirenz** and **nevirapine** are active against the subtype HIV-1 but not HIV-2, a subtype prevalent mainly in Africa. These drugs may interact with a number of drugs metabolised in the liver. Nevirapine is associated with a high incidence of rash (including Stevens-Johnson syndrome) and occasionally fatal hepatitis. Rash is also associated with efavirenz but it is usually milder. Efavirenz treatment has also been associated with an increased plasma cholesterol concentration.

Enfuvirtide, which inhibits HIV from fusing to the host cell, is licensed for managing infection that has failed to respond to a regimen of other antiretroviral drugs; enfuvirtide should be combined with other potentially active antiretroviral drugs.

Maraviroc is an antagonist of the CCR5 chemokine receptor. It is licensed for patients exclusively infected with CCR5-tropic HIV.

Immune reconstitution syndrome Improvement in immune function as a result of antiretroviral treatment may provoke a marked inflammatory reaction against residual opportunistic organisms.

Lipodystrophy syndrome Metabolic effects associated with antiretroviral treatment include *fat redistribution*, *insulin resistance* and *dyslipidaemia*; collectively these have been termed *lipodystrophy syndrome*.

Fat redistribution (with loss of subcutaneous fat, increased abdominal fat, 'buffalo hump' and breast enlargement) is associated with regimens containing protease inhibitors and nucleoside reverse transcriptase inhibitors. Stavudine (especially in combination with didanosine), and to a lesser extent zidovudine, are associated with a higher risk of lipoatrophy and should be used only if alternative regimens are not suitable.

Dyslipidaemia (with adverse effects on body lipids) is associated with antiretroviral treatment, particularly with protease inhibitors. Protease inhibitors are associated with insulin resistance and hyperglycaemia. Plasma lipids, blood glucose and the usual risk factors for atherosclerotic disease should be taken into account before prescribing regimens containing a protease inhibitor; patients receiving protease inhibitors should be monitored for changes in plasma lipids and blood glucose.

Osteonecrosis Osteonecrosis has been reported in patients with advanced HIV disease or following long-term exposure to combination antiretroviral therapy.

Nucleoside reverse transcriptase inhibitors

Cautions Nucleoside reverse transcriptase inhibitors should be used with caution in patients with chronic hepatitis B or C (greater risk of hepatic side-effects), in hepatic impairment (see also Lactic Acidosis below and Appendix 2), in renal impairment (Appendix 3), and in pregnancy (see also above and Appendix 4).

Lactic acidosis Life-threatening lactic acidosis associated with hepatomegaly and hepatic steatosis has been reported with nucleoside reverse transcriptase inhibitors. They should be used with caution in patients (particularly obese women) with hepatomegaly, hepatitis (especially hepatitis C treated with interferon alfa and ribavirin), liver-enzyme abnormalities and with other risk factors for liver disease and hepatic steatosis (including alcohol abuse). Treatment with the nucleoside reverse transcriptase inhibitor should be **discontinued** in case of symptomatic hyperlactataemia, lactic acidosis, progressive hepatomegaly or rapid deterioration of liver function. Stavudine, especially with didanosine, is associated with a higher risk of lactic acidosis and should be used only if alternative regimens are not suitable.

Side-effects Side-effects of the nucleoside reverse transcriptase inhibitors include gastro-intestinal disturbances (such as nausea, vomiting, abdominal pain, flatulence and diarrhoea), anorexia, pancreatitis, liver damage (see also Lactic Acidosis, above), dyspnoea, cough, headache, insomnia, dizziness, fatigue, blood disorders (including anaemia, neutropenia, and thrombocytopenia), myalgia, arthralgia, rash, urticaria, and fever. See notes above for metabolic effects and lipodystrophy (Lipodystrophy Syndrome), and Osteonecrosis.

ABACAVIR

Indications HIV infection in combination with other antiretroviral drugs

Cautions see notes above; **interactions:** Appendix 1 (abacavir)

Hypersensitivity reactions Life-threatening hypersensitivity reactions reported—characterised by fever or rash and possibly nausea, vomiting, diarrhoea, abdominal pain, dyspnoea, cough, lethargy, malaise, headache, and myalgia; less frequently mouth ulceration, oedema, hypotension, sore throat, acute respiratory distress syndrome, anaphylaxis, paraesthesia, arthralgia, conjunctivitis, lymphadenopathy, lymphocytopenia and renal failure (CSM has identified hypersensitivity reactions presenting as sore throat, influenza-like illness, cough, and breathlessness); rarely myolysis; laboratory abnormalities may include raised liver function tests (see Lactic Acidosis p. 328) and creatine kinase; symptoms usually appear in the first 6 weeks, but may occur at any time; monitor for symptoms every 2 weeks for 2 months; discontinue immediately if any symptom of hypersensitivity develops and do not rechallenge (risk of more severe hypersensitivity reaction); discontinue if hypersensitivity cannot be ruled out, even when other diagnoses possible—if rechallenge necessary it must be carried out in hospital setting; if abacavir is stopped for any reason other than hypersensitivity, exclude hypersensitivity reaction as the cause and rechallenge only if medical assistance is readily available; care needed with concomitant use of drugs which cause skin toxicity

Counselling Patients should be told the importance of regular dosing (intermittent therapy may increase the risk of sensitisation), how to recognise signs of hypersensitivity, and advised to seek immediate medical attention if symptoms develop or before re-starting treatment; patients should be advised to keep Alert Card with them at all times

Contra-indications breast-feeding (Appendix 5)

Side-effects see notes above; also hypersensitivity reactions (see above); *very rarely* Stevens-Johnson syndrome and toxic epidermal necrolysis; rash and gastro-intestinal disturbances more common in children

Dose

- 600 mg daily in 1–2 divided doses; CHILD 3 months–12 years, 8 mg/kg every 12 hours (max. 600 mg daily)

Ziagen® (GSK) PoM

Tablets, yellow, f/c, abacavir (as sulphate) 300 mg, net price 60-tab pack = £221.81. Counselling, hypersensitivity reactions

Oral solution, sugar-free, banana and strawberry flavoured, abacavir (as sulphate) 20 mg/mL, net price 240-mL = £59.15. Counselling, hypersensitivity reactions

With lamivudine

For **cautions**, **contra-indications** and **side-effects** see under individual drugs

Kivexa (GSK) ▼ PoM

Tablets, orange, f/c, abacavir (as sulphate) 600 mg, lamivudine 300 mg, net price 30-tab pack = £373.94. Counselling, hypersensitivity reactions

Dose ADULT and CHILD over 12 years, body-weight over 40 kg, 1 tablet once daily

With lamivudine and zidovudine

Note For patients stabilised (for 6–8 weeks) on the individual components in the same proportions. For **cautions, contra-indications** and **side-effects** see under individual drugs

Trizivir® (GSK) PoM

Tablets, blue-green, f/c, abacavir (as sulphate) 300 mg, lamivudine 150 mg, zidovudine 300 mg, net price 60-tab pack = £540.40. Counselling, hypersensitivity reactions

Dose ADULT over 18 years, 1 tablet twice daily

DIDANOSINE
(ddI, DDI)

Indications HIV infection in combination with other antiretroviral drugs

Cautions see notes above; also history of pancreatitis (preferably avoid, otherwise extreme caution, see also below); peripheral neuropathy or hyperuricaemia (see under Side-effects); dilated retinal examinations recommended (especially in children) every 6 months, or if visual changes occur; **interactions:** Appendix 1 (didanosine)

Pancreatitis Suspend treatment if serum lipase raised (even if asymptomatic) or if symptoms of pancreatitis develop; discontinue if pancreatitis confirmed. Whenever possible avoid concomitant treatment with other drugs known to cause pancreatic toxicity (e.g. intravenous pentamidine isetionate); monitor closely if concomitant therapy unavoidable. Since significant elevations of triglycerides cause pancreatitis monitor closely if elevated

Contra-indications breast-feeding (Appendix 5)

Side-effects see notes above; also pancreatitis (see also under cautions), liver failure, anaphylactic reactions, peripheral neuropathy—suspend (reduced dose may be tolerated when symptoms resolve), diabetes mellitus, hypoglycaemia, acute renal failure, rhabdomyolysis, dry eyes, retinal and optic nerve changes (especially in children), dry mouth, parotid gland enlargement, sialadenitis, alopecia, hyperuricaemia (suspend if raised significantly)

Dose

- ADULT under 60 kg 250 mg daily in 1–2 divided doses, 60 kg and over 400 mg daily in 1–2 divided doses; CHILD over 3 months (under 6 years *Videx®* tablets only), 240 mg/m² daily (180 mg/m² daily in combination with zidovudine) in 1–2 divided doses

Videx® (Bristol-Myers Squibb) PoM

Tablets, with calcium and magnesium antacids, didanosine 25 mg, net price 60-tab pack = £26.60. Label: 23, counselling, administration, see below

Excipients include aspartame equivalent to phenylalanine 36.5 mg per tablet (section 9.4.1)

Note Antacids in formulation may affect absorption of other drugs—see **interactions:** Appendix 1 (antacids)

Counselling To ensure sufficient antacid, each dose to be taken as at least 2 tablets (CHILD under 1 year 1 tablet) chewed thoroughly, crushed or dispersed in water; clear apple juice may be added for flavouring; tablets to be taken 2 hours after atazanavir with ritonavir or lopinavir with ritonavir

Videx® EC capsules, enclosing e/c granules, didanosine 125 mg, net price 30-cap pack = £51.15; 200 mg, 30-cap pack = £81.84; 250 mg, 30-cap pack = £102.30; 400 mg, 30-cap pack = £163.68. Label: 25, counselling, administration, see below

Counselling Capsules to be taken at least 2 hours before or 2 hours after food

EMTRICITABINE

Indications HIV infection in combination with other antiretroviral drugs

Cautions see notes above; also on discontinuation, monitor patients with hepatitis B (risk of exacerbation of hepatitis); **interactions:** Appendix 1 (emtricitabine)

Contra-indications breast-feeding (Appendix 5)

Side-effects see notes above; also abnormal dreams, pruritus, and hyperpigmentation

Dose

- See preparations

Emtriva® (Gilead) PoM

Capsules, white/blue, emtricitabine 200 mg, net price 30-cap pack = £163.50

Dose ADULT and CHILD body-weight over 33 kg, 200 mg once daily

Oral solution, orange, emtricitabine 10 mg/mL, net price 170-mL pack (candy-flavoured) = £46.50

Dose ADULT and CHILD body-weight over 33 kg, 240 mg once daily; CHILD 4 months–18 years, body-weight under 33 kg, 6 mg/kg once daily

Electrolytes Na^+ 460 micromol/mL

Note 240 mg oral solution ≡ 200 mg capsule; where appropriate the capsule may be used instead of the oral solution

With tenofovir

See under Tenofovir

LAMIVUDINE
(3TC)

Indications see preparations below

Cautions see notes above; **interactions:** Appendix 1 (lamivudine)

Chronic Hepatitis B Recurrent hepatitis in patients with chronic hepatitis B may occur on discontinuation of lamivudine. When treating chronic hepatitis B with lamivudine, monitor liver function tests every 3 months, and viral and serological markers of hepatitis B every 3–6 months, more frequently in patients with advanced liver disease or following transplantation (monitoring to continue after discontinuation)—consult product literature

Contra-indications breast-feeding (Appendix 5)

Side-effects see notes above; also peripheral neuropathy, muscle disorders including rhabdomyolysis, nasal symptoms, alopecia

Dose

- See preparations below

Epivir® (GSK) PoM

Tablets, f/c, lamivudine 150 mg (scored, white), net price 60-tab pack = £152.14; 300 mg (grey), 30-tab pack = £167.21

Oral solution, banana- and strawberry-flavoured, lamivudine 50 mg/5 mL, net price 240-mL pack = £41.41

Excipients include sucrose 1 g/5 mL

Dose HIV infection in combination with other antiretroviral drugs, 150 mg every 12 hours *or* 300 mg once daily; CHILD 3 months–12 years, 4 mg/kg (max. 150 mg) every 12 hours *or* body-weight 14–21 kg, 75 mg twice daily; body-weight 21–30 kg, 75 mg in the morning and 150 mg in the evening; body-weight over 30 kg, 150 mg twice daily

Zeffix® (GSK) PoM

Tablets, brown, f/c, lamivudine 100 mg, net price 28-tab pack = £78.09

Oral solution, banana and strawberry flavoured, lamivudine 25 mg/5 mL, net price 240-mL pack = £22.79

Excipients include sucrose 1 g/5 mL

Dose chronic hepatitis B infection with *either* compensated liver disease (with evidence of viral replication and histology of active liver inflammation or fibrosis), *or* decompensated liver disease, 100 mg daily; CHILD [unlicensed indication] 2–11 years, 3 mg/kg once daily (max. 100 mg daily); 12–17 years, adult dose

Note Patients receiving lamivudine for concomitant HIV infection should continue to receive lamivudine in a dose appropriate for HIV infection

With abacavir

See under Abacavir

With zidovudine

See under Zidovudine

With abacavir and zidovudine

See under Abacavir

STAVUDINE
(d4T)

Indications HIV infection in combination with other antiretroviral drugs

Cautions see notes above; also history of peripheral neuropathy (see under Side-effects); history of pancreatitis or concomitant use with other drugs associated with pancreatitis; **interactions:** Appendix 1 (stavudine)

Contra-indications breast-feeding (Appendix 5)

Side-effects see notes above; also peripheral neuropathy (switch to another antiretroviral if peripheral neuropathy develops), abnormal dreams, cognitive dysfunction, drowsiness, depression, pruritus; *less commonly* anxiety, gynaecomastia

Dose

- ADULT under 60 kg, 30 mg every 12 hours preferably at least 1 hour before food; 60 kg and over, 40 mg every 12 hours; NEONATE under 2 weeks, 500 micrograms/kg every 12 hours; CHILD over 2 weeks, body-weight under 30 kg, 1 mg/kg every 12 hours; body-weight 30 kg and over, adult dose

Zerit® (Bristol-Myers Squibb) PoM

Capsules, stavudine 20 mg (brown), net price 56-cap pack = £148.05; 30 mg (light orange/dark orange), 56-cap pack = £155.25; 40 mg (dark orange), 56-cap pack = £159.94 (all hosp. only)

Oral solution, cherry-flavoured, stavudine for reconstitution with water, 1 mg/mL, net price 200 mL = £24.35

TENOFOVIR DISOPROXIL

Indications HIV infection in combination with other antiretroviral drugs

Cautions see notes above; also test renal function and serum phosphate before treatment, then every 4 weeks (more frequently if at increased risk of renal impairment) for 1 year and then every 3 months, interrupt treatment if renal function deteriorates or serum phosphate decreases; concomitant or recent use of nephrotoxic drugs; on discontinuation, monitor patients with hepatitis B (risk of exacerbation of hepatitis); **interactions:** Appendix 1 (tenofovir)

Contra-indications breast-feeding (Appendix 5)

Side-effects see notes above; also hypophosphataemia, reduced bone density, nephrogenic diabetes insipidus, and renal failure

Dose

- ADULT over 18 years, 245 mg once daily

Viread® (Gilead) PoM

Tablets, f/c, blue, tenofovir disoproxil (as fumarate) 245 mg, net price 30-tab pack = £255.00. Label: 21, counselling, administration

Counselling Patients with swallowing difficulties may disperse tablet in half a glass of water, orange juice, or grape juice (but bitter taste)

With emtricitabine

For **cautions, contra-indications** and **side-effects** see under individual drugs

Truvada® (Gilead) PoM

Tablets, blue, f/c, tenofovir disoproxil (as fumarate) 245 mg, emtricitabine 200 mg, net price 30-tab pack = £418.50. Label: 21, counselling, administration

Counselling Patients with swallowing difficulties may disperse tablet in half a glass of water, orange juice, or grape juice (but bitter taste)

Dose ADULT over 18 years, 1 tablet once daily

ZIDOVUDINE

(Azidothymidine, AZT)

Note The abbreviation AZT which is sometimes used for zidovudine has also been used for another drug

Indications HIV infection in combination with other antiretroviral drugs; prevention of maternal-fetal HIV transmission (see notes above under Pregnancy and Breast-feeding)

Cautions see notes above; also haematological toxicity particularly with high dose and advanced disease—monitor full blood count on week 4 of treatment, then every 3 months; vitamin B_{12} deficiency (increased risk of neutropenia); if anaemia or myelosuppression, reduce dose or interrupt treatment according to product literature, or consider other treatment; elderly; **interactions:** Appendix 1 (zidovudine)

Contra-indications abnormally low neutrophil counts or haemoglobin values (consult product literature); neonates with hyperbilirubinaemia requiring treatment other than phototherapy, or with raised transaminase (consult product literature); porphyria (section 9.8.2); breast-feeding (Appendix 5)

Side-effects see notes above; also anaemia (may require transfusion), taste disturbance, chest pain, influenza-like symptoms, paraesthesia, neuropathy, convulsions, dizziness, drowsiness, anxiety, depression, loss of mental acuity, myopathy, gynaecomastia, urinary frequency, sweating, pruritus, pigmentation of nails, skin and oral mucosa

Dose

- By mouth, 500–600 mg daily in 2–3 divided doses; CHILD 3 months–12 years, 360–480 mg/m² daily in 3–4 divided doses; max. 200 mg every 6 hours
- Prevention of maternal-fetal HIV transmission, seek specialist advice (combination therapy preferred)
- Patients temporarily unable to take zidovudine by mouth, by intravenous infusion over 1 hour, 1–2 mg/kg every 4 hours (approximating to 1.5–3 mg/kg every 4 hours by mouth) usually for not more than 2 weeks; CHILD 3 months–12 years, 80–160 mg/m² every 6 hours (120 mg/m² every 6 hours approximates to 180 mg/m² every 6 hours by mouth)

Retrovir® (GSK) PoM

Capsules, zidovudine 100 mg (white/blue band), net price 100-cap pack = £110.98; 250 mg (blue/white/dark blue band), 40-cap pack = £110.98

Oral solution, sugar-free, strawberry-flavoured, zidovudine 50 mg/5 mL, net price 200-mL pack with 10-mL oral syringe = £22.20

Injection, zidovudine 10 mg/mL. For dilution and use as an intravenous infusion. Net price 20-mL vial = £11.14

With lamivudine

For **cautions, contra-indications,** and **side-effects** see under individual drugs

Combivir® (GSK) PoM

Tablets, f/c, scored, zidovudine 300 mg, lamivudine 150 mg, net price 60-tab pack = £318.60

Dose ADULT and CHILD body-weight over 30 kg, 1 tablet twice daily; CHILD body-weight 14–21 kg, half a tablet twice daily; body-weight 21–30 kg, half a tablet in the morning and one tablet in the evening

With abacavir and lamivudine

See under Abacavir

Protease inhibitors

Cautions Protease inhibitors are associated with hyperglycaemia and should be used with caution in diabetes (see Lipodystrophy Syndrome, p. 328). Caution is also needed in patients with haemophilia who may be at increased risk of bleeding. Protease inhibitors should be used with caution in hepatic impairment (Appendix 2); the risk of hepatic side-effects is increased in patients with chronic hepatitis B or C. Atazanavir, darunavir, fosamprenavir, and tipranavir may be used at usual doses in patients with renal impairment, but other protease inhibitors should be used with caution in renal impairment (Appendix 3). Protease inhibitors should also be used with caution during pregnancy (Appendix 4).

Contra-indications Protease inhibitors should not be given to patients with porphyria (section 9.8.2). Protease inhibitors should not be given to women who are breast-feeding (Appendix 5).

Side-effects Side-effects of the protease inhibitors include gastro-intestinal disturbances (including diarrhoea, nausea, vomiting, abdominal pain, flatulence), anorexia, hepatic dysfunction, pancreatitis; blood disorders including anaemia, neutropenia, and thrombocytopenia; sleep disturbances, fatigue, headache, dizziness, paraesthesia, myalgia, myositis, rhabdomyolysis; taste disturbances; rash, pruritus, Stevens-Johnson syndrome, hypersensitivity reactions including anaphylaxis; see also notes above for lipodystrophy and metabolic effects (Lipodystrophy Syndrome), and Osteonecrosis.

AMPRENAVIR

Indications HIV infection in combination with other antiretroviral drugs in patients previously treated with other protease inhibitors

Cautions see notes above; **interactions**: Appendix 1 (amprenavir)

Rash Rash may occur, usually in the second week of therapy; discontinue permanently if severe rash with systemic or allergic symptoms or, mucosal involvement; if rash mild or moderate, may continue without interruption—rash usually resolves within 2 weeks and may respond to antihistamines

Side-effects see notes above; also reported, rash including rarely Stevens-Johnson syndrome (see also above); tremors, oral or perioral paraesthesia, mood disorders including depression

Dose

- See preparations below

Agenerase® (GSK) PoM

Capsules, ivory, amprenavir 50 mg, net price 480-cap pack = £139.50. Label: 5

Excipients include vitamin E 36 units/50 mg amprenavir (avoid vitamin E supplements)

Dose ADULT and ADOLESCENT over 12 years, body-weight over 50 kg, 1.2 g every 12 hours; ADULT and ADOLESCENT over 12 years, body-weight under 50 kg and CHILD 4–12 years, 20 mg/kg every 12 hours (max. 2.4 g daily)

With low-dose ritonavir, ADULT and ADOLESCENT over 12 years, body-weight over 50 kg, amprenavir 600 mg every 12 hours with ritonavir 100 mg every 12 hours

Oral solution, grape-bubblegum- and peppermint-flavoured, amprenavir 15 mg/mL, net price 240-mL pack = £33.48. Label: 4, 5

Excipients include vitamin E 46 units/mL (avoid vitamin E supplements), propylene glycol 550 mg/mL (see Excipients, p. 2)

Electrolytes K^+ 26 micromol/mL, Na^+ 174 micromol/mL

Dose ADULT and CHILD over 4 years, 17 mg/kg every 8 hours (max. 2.8 g daily); CHILD under 4 years not recommended

Note The bioavailability of *Agenerase®* oral solution is lower than that of capsules; the two formulations are **not** interchangeable on a milligram-for-milligram basis

ATAZANAVIR

Indications HIV infection in combination with other antiretroviral drugs in patients previously treated with antiretrovirals

Cautions see notes above; also concomitant use with drugs that prolong PR interval; cardiac conduction disorders; predisposition to QT interval prolongation (including electrolyte disturbances, concomitant use of drugs that prolong QT interval); **interactions**: Appendix 1 (atazanavir)

Side-effects see notes above; also peripheral neurological symptoms; *less commonly* mouth ulcers, hypertension, syncope, chest pain, dyspnoea, abnormal dreams, amnesia, depression, anxiety, weight changes, increased appetite, gynaecomastia, nephrolithiasis, urinary frequency, haematuria, proteinuria, arthralgia, and alopecia; *rarely* hepatosplenomegaly, oedema, palpitation, and abnormal gait

Dose

- With low-dose ritonavir and food, ADULT over 18 years, 300 mg once daily with ritonavir 100 mg once daily

Reyataz® (Bristol-Myers Squibb) ▼ PoM

Capsules, atazanavir (as sulphate) 100 mg (dark blue/white), net price 60-cap pack = £315.69; 150 mg (dark blue/light blue), 60-cap pack = £315.69; 200 mg (dark blue), 60-cap pack = £315.69. Label: 5, 21

DARUNAVIR

Indications HIV infection (that has not responded to treatment with other protease inhibitors) in combination with other antiretroviral drugs

Cautions see notes above; also sulphonamide sensitivity

Side-effects see notes above; also myocardial infarction, transient ischaemic attack, syncope, tachycardia, hypertension, flushing, peripheral oedema, dyspnoea, cough, hiccups, peripheral neuropathy, anxiety, confusion, memory impairment, mood changes, abnormal coordination, weight gain, hyperthermia, hypothyroidism, osteoporosis, gynaecomastia, erectile dysfunction, dysuria, polyuria, nephrolithiasis, renal failure, hyponatraemia, arthralgia, keratoconjuntivitis sicca, salivation changes, mouth ulcers, increased sweating, and alopecia

Dose

- With low-dose ritonavir, ADULT over 18 years, 600 mg twice daily

Missed dose If a dose is more than 6 hours late, the missed dose should not be taken and the next dose should be taken at the normal time

Prezista® (Janssen-Cilag) ▼ PoM

Tablets, orange, f/c, darunavir (as ethanolate) 300 mg, net price 120-tab pack = £446.70. Label: 21

FOSAMPRENAVIR

Note Fosamprenavir is a pro-drug of amprenavir

Indications HIV infection in combination with other antiretroviral drugs

Cautions see notes above and under Amprenavir

Side-effects see notes above and under Amprenavir

Dose

- With low-dose ritonavir, ADULT and CHILD over 6 years, body-weight over 39 kg, 700 mg twice daily; CHILD over 6 years, body-weight 25–39 kg, 18 mg/kg twice daily

Note 700 mg fosamprenavir is equivalent to approx. 600 mg amprenavir

Telzir® (GSK) ▼ PoM

Tablets, f/c, pink, fosamprenavir (as calcium) 700 mg, net price 60-tab pack = £274.92

Oral suspension, fosamprenavir (as calcium) 50 mg/mL, net price 225-mL pack (grape-bubblegum-and peppermint-flavoured) (with 10-mL oral syringe) = £73.31. Label: 23

INDINAVIR

Indications HIV infection in combination with nucleoside reverse transcriptase inhibitors

Cautions see notes above; also ensure adequate hydration (risk of nephrolithiasis especially in children); patients at risk of nephrolithiasis (monitor for nephrolithiasis); avoid in porphyria (section 9.8.2); **interactions**: Appendix 1 (indinavir)

Side-effects see notes above; also reported, dry mouth, hypoaesthesia, dry skin, hyperpigmentation, alopecia, paronychia, interstitial nephritis (with medullary calcification and cortical atrophy in asymptomatic severe leucocyturia), nephrolithiasis (may require interruption or discontinuation, more frequent in children), dysuria, haematuria, crystalluria, proteinuria, pyuria (in children), pyelonephritis; haemolytic anaemia

Dose

- 800 mg every 8 hours; CHILD and ADOLESCENT 4–17 years, 500 mg/m² every 8 hours (max. 800 mg every 8 hours); CHILD under 4 years, safety and efficacy not established

Crixivan® (MSD) PoM

Capsules, indinavir (as sulphate), 200 mg, net price 360-cap pack = £226.28; 400 mg, 90-cap pack = £113.15, 180-cap pack = £226.28. Label: 27, counselling, administration

Counselling Administer 1 hour before or 2 hours after a meal; may be administered with a low-fat light meal; in combination with didanosine tablets, allow 1 hour between each drug (antacids in didanosine tablets reduce absorption of indinavir); in combination with low-dose ritonavir, give with food

Note Dispense in original container (contains dessicant)

LOPINAVIR WITH RITONAVIR

Indications HIV infection in combination with other antiretroviral drugs

Cautions see notes above; concomitant use with drugs that prolong QT interval; pancreatitis (see below); **interactions:** Appendix 1 (lopinavir, ritonavir)

Pancreatitis Signs and symptoms suggestive of pancreatitis (including raised serum lipase) should be evaluated—discontinue if pancreatitis diagnosed

Side-effects see notes and Cautions above; also electrolyte disturbances in children; *less commonly* dysphagia, appetite changes, weight changes, cholecystitis, hypertension, myocardial infarction, palpitation, thrombophlebitis, vasculitis, chest pain, oedema, dyspnoea, cough, agitation, anxiety, amnesia, ataxia, hypertonia, confusion, depression, abnormal dreams, extrapyramidal effects, neuropathy, influenza-like syndrome, Cushing's syndrome, hypothyroidism, menorrhagia, amenorrhoea, sexual dysfunction, breast enlargement, dehydration, nephritis, hypercalciuria, lactic acidosis, arthralgia, hyperuricaemia, abnormal vision, otitis media, tinnitus, dry mouth, sialadenitis, mouth ulceration, periodontitis, acne, alopecia, dry skin, sweating, skin discoloration, nail disorders, *rarely* prolonged PR interval

Dose

- See preparations below

Kaletra® (Abbott) PoM

Capsules, orange, lopinavir 133.3 mg, ritonavir 33.3 mg, net price 180-cap pack = £307.39. Label: 21

Dose ADULT and CHILD over 2 years with body surface area of 1.4 m² or greater, 3 capsules twice daily with food; CHILD over 2 years with body surface area less than 1.4 m², oral solution preferred; if oral solution inappropriate and body surface area 0.4–0.75 m², 1 capsule twice daily, body surface area 0.8–1.3 m², 2 capsules twice daily

Tablets, yellow, f/c, lopinavir 200 mg, ritonavir 50 mg, net price 120-tab pack = £307.39. Label: 25

Dose ADULT and CHILD with body surface area greater than 1.3 m² or body-weight 40 kg and over, 2 tablets twice daily

Oral solution, lopinavir 400 mg, ritonavir 100 mg/5 mL, net price 5×60-mL packs = £307.39. Label: 21

Excipients include propylene glycol 153 mg/mL (see Excipients, p. 2), alcohol 42%

Dose ADULT and ADOLESCENT, 5 mL twice daily with food; CHILD over 2 years 2.9 mL/m² twice daily with food, max. 5 mL twice daily; CHILD under 2 years, safety and efficacy not established

Note 5 mL oral solution ≡ 3 capsules ≡ 2 tablets; where appropriate, capsules may be used instead of oral solution

NELFINAVIR

Indications HIV infection in combination with other antiretroviral drugs

Cautions see notes above; **interactions:** Appendix 1 (nelfinavir)

Side-effects see notes above; also reported, fever

Dose

- 1.25 g twice daily *or* 750 mg 3 times daily; CHILD 3–13 years, initially 50–55 mg/kg twice daily (max. 1.25 g twice daily) *or* 25–30 mg/kg 3 times daily (max. 750 mg 3 times daily)

Viracept® (Roche) PoM

Tablets, blue, f/c, nelfinavir (as mesilate) 250 mg, net price 300-tab pack = £273.16. Label: 21

Oral powder, nelfinavir (as mesilate) 50 mg/g. Net price 144 g (with 1-g and 5-g scoop) = £28.72. Label: 21, counselling, administration

Excipients include aspartame (section 9.4.1)

Counselling Powder may be mixed with water, milk, formula feeds or pudding; it should **not** be mixed with acidic foods or juices owing to its taste

RITONAVIR

Indications HIV infection in combination with nucleoside reverse transcriptase inhibitors; low doses used to increase effect of some protease inhibitors

Cautions see notes above; avoid in porphyria (section 9.8.2); pancreatitis (see below); **interactions:** Appendix 1 (ritonavir)

Pancreatitis Signs and symptoms suggestive of pancreatitis (including raised serum lipase) should be evaluated—discontinue if pancreatitis diagnosed

Side-effects see notes and Cautions above; also diarrhoea (may impair absorption—close monitoring required), vasodilatation, cough, throat irritation, anxiety, perioral and peripheral paraesthesia, hyperaesthesia, fever, decreased blood thyroxine concentration, electrolyte disturbances, raised uric acid, dry mouth, mouth ulcers, and sweating; *less commonly* increased prothrombin time and dehydration; syncope, postural hypotension, seizures, menorrhagia, and renal failure also reported

Dose

- Initially 300 mg every 12 hours for 3 days, increased in steps of 100 mg every 12 hours over not longer than 14 days to 600 mg every 12 hours; CHILD over 2 years initially 250 mg/m² every 12 hours, increased by 50 mg/m² at intervals of 2–3 days to 350 mg/m² every 12 hours (max. 600 mg every 12 hours)
- Low-dose booster to increase effect of other protease inhibitors, 100–200 mg once or twice daily

Norvir® (Abbott) PoM

Capsules, ritonavir 100 mg, net price 84-cap pack = £94.35. Label 21

Excipients include alcohol 12%

Oral solution, sugar-free, ritonavir 400 mg/5 mL, net price 5 × 90-mL packs (with measuring cup) = £403.20. Label: 21, counselling, administration

Counselling Oral solution contains 43% alcohol; bitter taste can be masked by mixing with chocolate milk; do not mix with water, measuring cup must be dry

With lopinavir

See under Lopinavir with ritonavir

SAQUINAVIR

Indications HIV infection in combination with other antiretroviral drugs

Cautions see notes above; concomitant use of garlic (avoid garlic capsules—reduces plasma-saquinavir concentration); **interactions:** Appendix 1 (saquinavir)

Side-effects see notes above; also dyspnoea, increased appetite, peripheral neuropathy, convulsions, changes in libido, renal impairment, dry mouth, and alopecia

Dose

- With low-dose ritonavir, ADULT and ADOLESCENT over 16 years, 1 g every 12 hours

Invirase® (Roche) PoM

Capsules, brown/green, saquinavir (as mesilate) 200 mg, net price 270-cap pack = £240.06. Label: 21

Tablets, orange, f/c, saquinavir (as mesilate) 500 mg, net price 120-tab pack = £266.73. Label: 21

TIPRANAVIR

Indications HIV infection resistant to other protease inhibitors, in combination with other antiretroviral drugs in patients previously treated with antiretrovirals

Cautions see notes above; also patients at risk of increased bleeding from trauma, surgery or other pathological conditions; concomitant use of drugs that increase risk of bleeding; **interactions:** Appendix 1 (tipranavir)

Hepatotoxicity Potentially life-threatening hepatotoxicity reported; monitor liver function before treatment then on weeks 2 and 4 of treatment, then monthly for 5 months, then every 2–3 months (every 2 weeks for first 3 months, then monthly for 9 months, then every 2–3 months in those with hepatic impairment (Appendix 2)). Discontinue if signs or symptoms of hepatitis develop or if liver-function abnormality develops (consult product literature)

Side-effects see notes above; also dyspnoea, anorexia, peripheral neuropathy, influenza-like symptoms, renal impairment and photosensitivity; *rarely* dehydration

Dose

- With low-dose ritonavir, 500 mg twice daily; CHILD safety and efficacy not established

Aptivus® (Boehringer Ingelheim) ▼ PoM

Capsules, pink, tipranavir 250 mg, net price 120–cap pack = £490.00. Label: 5, 21

Excipients include ethanol 100 mg per capsule

Non-nucleoside reverse transcriptase inhibitors

EFAVIRENZ

Indications HIV infection in combination with other antiretroviral drugs

Cautions chronic hepatitis B or C (greater risk of hepatic side-effects), hepatic impairment (avoid if severe; Appendix 2); severe renal impairment (Appendix 3); pregnancy (Appendix 4); elderly; history of mental illness or seizures; **interactions:** Appendix 1 (efavirenz)

Rash Rash, usually in the first 2 weeks, is the most common side-effect; discontinue if severe rash with blistering, desquamation, mucosal involvement or fever; if rash mild or moderate, may continue without interruption—rash usually resolves within 1 month

Psychiatric disorders Patients or their carers should be advised to seek immediate medical attention if symptoms such as severe depression, psychosis or suicidal ideation occur

Contra-indications porphyria (section 9.8.2); breast-feeding (Appendix 5)

Side-effects rash including Stevens-Johnson syndrome (see Rash above); abdominal pain, diarrhoea, nausea, vomiting; anxiety, depression, sleep disturbances, abnormal dreams, dizziness, headache, fatigue, impaired concentration (administration at bedtime especially in first 2–4 weeks reduces CNS effects); pruritus; *less commonly* pancreatitis, hepatitis, psychosis, mania, suicidal ideation, amnesia, ataxia, convulsions, and blurred vision; also reported hepatic failure, raised serum cholesterol (see Lipodystrophy Syndrome, p. 328), gynaecomastia, photosensitivity

Dose

- See preparations below

Sustiva (Bristol-Myers Squibb) PoM

Capsules, efavirenz 50 mg (yellow/white), net price 30-cap pack = £17.41; 200 mg (yellow), 90-cap pack = £208.40. Label: 23

Dose ADULT and CHILD over 3 years, body-weight 13–14 kg, 200 mg once daily; body-weight 15–19 kg, 250 mg once daily; body-weight 20–24 kg, 300 mg once daily; body-weight 25–32.4 kg, 350 mg once daily; body-weight 32.5–39 kg, 400 mg once daily; body-weight 40 kg and over, 600 mg once daily

Tablets, f/c, yellow, efavirenz 600 mg, net price 30-tab pack = £208.40. Label: 23

Dose ADULT and ADOLESCENT over 12 years, body-weight over 40 kg, 600 mg once daily

Oral solution, sugar-free, strawberry and mint flavour, efavirenz 30 mg/mL, net price 180-mL pack = £56.02

Dose ADULT and CHILD over 5 years, body-weight 13–14 kg, 270 mg once daily; body-weight 15–19 kg, 300 mg once daily; body-weight 20–24 kg, 360 mg once daily; body-weight 25–32.4 kg, 450 mg once daily; body-weight 32.5–39 kg, 510 mg once daily; body-weight 40 kg and over, 720 mg once daily; CHILD 3–4 years, body-weight 13–14 kg, 360 mg once daily; body-weight 15–19 kg, 390 mg once daily; body-weight 20–24 kg, 450 mg once daily; body-weight 25–32.4 kg, 510 mg once daily

Note The bioavailability of *Sustiva®* oral solution is lower than that of the capsules and tablets; the oral solution is **not** interchangeable with either capsules or tablets on a milligram-for-milligram basis

NEVIRAPINE

Indications progressive or advanced HIV infection, in combination with at least two other antiretroviral drugs

Cautions hepatic impairment (see below and Appendix 2); chronic hepatitis B or C, high CD4 cell count, and women (all at greater risk of hepatic side-effects—manufacturer advises avoid in women with CD4 cell count greater than 250 cells/mm^3 or in men with CD4 cell count greater than 400 cells/mm^3 unless potential benefit outweighs risk); pregnancy (Appendix 4); **interactions:** Appendix 1 (nevirapine)

Hepatic disease Potentially life-threatening hepatotoxicity including fatal fulminant hepatitis reported usually in first 6 weeks; close monitoring required during first 18 weeks; monitor liver function before treatment then every 2 weeks for 2 months then after 1 month and then regularly; discontinue permanently if abnormalities in liver function tests accompanied by hypersensitivity reaction (rash, fever, arthralgia, myalgia, lymphadenopathy, hepatitis, renal impairment, eosinophilia, granulocytopenia); suspend if severe abnormalities in liver function tests but no hypersensitivity reaction—discontinue permanently if significant liver function abnormalities recur; monitor patient closely if mild to moderate abnormalities in liver function tests with no hypersensitivity reaction

Rash Rash, usually in first 6 weeks, is most common side-effect; incidence reduced if introduced at low dose and dose increased gradually; monitor closely for skin reactions during first 18 weeks; discontinue permanently if severe rash or if rash accompanied by blistering, oral lesions, conjunctivitis, facial oedema, general malaise or hypersensitivity reactions; if rash mild or moderate may continue without interruption but dose should not be increased until rash resolves

Counselling Patients should be told how to recognise hypersensitivity reactions and advised to discontinue treatment and seek immediate medical attention if severe skin reaction, hypersensitivity reactions, or symptoms of hepatitis develop

Contra-indications porphyria (section 9.8.2); breast-feeding (Appendix 5); severe hepatic impairment; post-exposure prophylaxis

Side-effects rash including Stevens-Johnson syndrome and rarely, toxic epidermal necrolysis (see also Cautions above); nausea, hepatitis (see also Hepatic Disease above), headache; *less commonly* vomiting, abdominal pain, fatigue, fever, and myalgia; *rarely* diarrhoea, angioedema, anaphylaxis, hypersensitivity reactions (may involve hepatic reactions and rash, see Hepatic Disease above), arthralgia, anaemia, and granulocytopenia (more frequent in children); *very rarely* neuropsychiatric reactions

Dose

- ADULT and CHILD over 16 years, 200 mg once daily for first 14 days then (if no rash present) 200 mg twice daily; NEONATE and CHILD under 8 years, 150 mg/m² (max. 200 mg) once daily for first 14 days, then (if no rash present) 150 mg/m² (max. 200 mg) twice daily *or* 4 mg/kg (max. 200 mg) once daily for first 14 days then (if no rash present) 7 mg/kg (max. 200 mg) twice daily; CHILD 8–16 years, 150 mg/m² (max. 200 mg) once daily for first 14 days then (if no rash present) 150 mg/m² (max. 200 mg) twice daily *or* 4 mg/kg (max. 200 mg) once daily for first 14 days then (if no rash present) 4 mg/kg (max. 200 mg) twice daily

Note Dose titration should be repeated if treatment interrupted for more than 7 days

Viramune® (Boehringer Ingelheim) PoM

Tablets, nevirapine 200 mg, net price 60-tab pack = £160.00. Counselling, hypersensitivity reactions

Suspension, nevirapine 50 mg/5 mL, net price 240-mL pack = £50.40. Counselling, hypersensitivity reactions

Other antiretrovirals

ENFUVIRTIDE

Indications HIV infection in combination with other antiretroviral drugs for resistant infection or for patients intolerant to other antiretroviral regimens

Cautions chronic hepatitis B or C (possibly greater risk of hepatic side-effects); hepatic impairment (Appendix 2); renal impairment (Appendix 3); pregnancy (Appendix 4)

Hypersensitivity reactions Hypersensitivity reactions including rash, fever, nausea, vomiting, chills, rigors, low blood pressure, respiratory distress, glomerulonephritis, and raised liver enzymes reported; discontinue immediately if any signs or symptoms of systemic hypersensitivity develop and do not rechallenge

Counselling Patients should be told how to recognise signs of hypersensitivity, and advised to discontinue treatment and seek immediate medical attention if symptoms develop

Contra-indications breast-feeding (Appendix 5)

Side-effects injection-site reactions; pancreatitis, gastro-oesophageal reflux disease, anorexia, weight loss; hypertriglyceridaemia; peripheral neuropathy, asthenia, tremor, anxiety, nightmares, irritability, impaired concentration, vertigo; pneumonia, sinusitis, influenza-like illness; diabetes mellitus; haematuria; renal calculi, lymphadenopathy; myalgia; conjunctivitis; dry skin, acne, erythema, skin papilloma; *less commonly* hypersensitivity reactions (see Cautions)

Dose

- By subcutaneous injection, ADULT and ADOLESCENT over 16 years, 90 mg twice daily; CHILD 6–15 years, 2 mg/kg twice daily (max. 90 mg twice daily)

Fuzeon® (Roche) ▼ PoM

Injection, powder for reconstitution, enfuvirtide 108 mg (= enfuvirtide 90 mg/mL when reconstituted with 1.1 mL Water for Injections), net price 108-mg vial = £19.13 (with solvent, syringe, and alcohol swabs). Counselling, hypersensitivity reactions

MARAVIROC

Indications CCR5-tropic HIV infection in combination with other antiretroviral drugs in patients previously treated with antiretrovirals

Cautions cardiovascular disease; chronic hepatitis B or C; hepatic impairment (Appendix 2); renal impairment (Appendix 3); pregnancy (Appendix 4); **interactions:** Appendix 1 (maraviroc)

Contra-indications breast-feeding (Appendix 5)

Side-effects nausea, vomiting, abdominal pain, dyspepsia, constipation, diarrhoea; cough; dizziness, paraesthesia, asthenia, sleep disturbances, headache, weight loss; muscle spasms, back pain; taste disturbances; rash, pruritus; *less commonly* pancreatitis, hepatic cirrhosis, rectal bleeding, myocardial infarction, myocardial ischaemia, bronchospasm, seizures, hallucinations, loss of consciousness, polyneuropathy, pancytopenia, neutropenia, lymphadenopathy, renal failure, polyuria, and myositis; see also Osteonecrosis, p. 328

Dose

- ADULT over 18 years, 300 mg twice daily

Celsentri® (Pfizer) ▼ PoM

Tablets, blue, f/c, maraviroc, 150 mg, net price 60-tab pack = £551.10; 300 mg, 60-tab pack = £551.10

5.3.2 Herpesvirus infections

5.3.2.1 Herpes simplex and varicella–zoster infection

The two most important herpesvirus pathogens are herpes simplex virus (herpesvirus hominis) and varicella–zoster virus.

Herpes simplex infections Herpes infection of the mouth and lips and in the eye is generally associated with herpes simplex virus serotype 1 (HSV-1); other areas of the skin may also be infected, especially in immunodeficiency. Genital infection is most often associated with HSV-2 and also HSV-1. Treatment of herpes simplex infection should start as early as possible and usually within 5 days of the appearance of the infection.

In individuals with good immune function, mild infection of the eye (ocular herpes, section 11.3.3) and of the lips (herpes labialis or cold sores, section 13.10.3) is treated with a topical antiviral drug. Primary herpetic gingivostomatitis is managed by changes to diet and with analgesics (section 12.3.2). Severe infection, neonatal herpes infection or infection in immunocompromised individuals requires treatment with a systemic antiviral drug. Primary or recurrent genital herpes simplex infection is treated with an antiviral drug given by mouth. Persistence of a lesion or recurrence in an immunocompromised patient may signal the development of resistance.

Specialist advice should be sought for systemic treatment of herpes simplex infection in pregnancy.

Varicella-zoster infections Regardless of immune function and the use of any immunoglobulins, neonates with *chickenpox* should be treated with a parenteral antiviral to reduce the risk of severe disease. Chickenpox in otherwise healthy children between 1 month and 12 years is usually mild and antiviral treatment is not usually required.

Chickenpox is more severe in adolescents and adults than in children; antiviral treatment started within 24 hours of the onset of rash may reduce the duration and severity of symptoms in otherwise healthy adults and adolescents. Antiviral treatment is generally recommended in immunocompromised patients and those at special risk (e.g. because of severe cardiovascular or respiratory disease or chronic skin disorder); in such cases, an antiviral is given for 10 days with at least 7 days of parenteral treatment.

Pregnant women who develop severe chickenpox may be at risk of complications, especially varicella pneumonia. Specialist advice should be sought for the treatment of chickenpox during pregnancy.

Those who have been exposed to chickenpox and are at special risk of complications may require prophylaxis with varicella-zoster immunoglobulin (see under Specific Immunoglobulins, section 14.5).

In *herpes zoster* (shingles) systemic antiviral treatment can reduce the severity and duration of pain, reduce complications, and reduce viral shedding. Treatment with the antiviral should be started within 72 hours of the onset of rash and is usually continued for 7–10 days. Immunocompromised patients at high risk of disseminated or severe infection should be treated with a parenteral antiviral drug.

Chronic pain which persists after the rash has healed (postherpetic neuralgia) requires specific management (section 4.7.3).

Choice **Aciclovir** is active against herpesviruses but does not eradicate them. Uses of aciclovir include systemic treatment of varicella–zoster and the systemic and topical treatment of herpes simplex infections of the skin (section 13.10.3) and mucous membranes (section 7.2.2). It is used by mouth for severe herpetic stomatitis (see also p. 593). Aciclovir eye ointment (section 11.3.3) is used for herpes simplex infections of the eye; it is combined with systemic treatment for ophthalmic zoster.

Famciclovir, a prodrug of penciclovir, is similar to aciclovir and is licensed for use in herpes zoster and genital herpes. Penciclovir itself is used as a cream for herpes simplex labialis (section 13.10.3).

Valaciclovir is an ester of aciclovir, licensed for herpes zoster and herpes simplex infections of the skin and mucous membranes (including genital herpes); it is also licensed for preventing cytomegalovirus disease following renal transplantation. Famciclovir or valaciclovir are suitable alternatives to aciclovir for oral lesions associated with herpes zoster. Valaciclovir once daily may reduce the risk of transmitting genital herpes to heterosexual partners—specialist advice should be sought.

Idoxuridine (section 13.10.3) has been used topically for treating herpes simplex infections of the skin and external genitalia with variable results. Its value in the treatment of shingles is unclear.

Inosine pranobex has been used by mouth for herpes simplex infections; its effectiveness remains unproven.

ACICLOVIR
(Acyclovir)

Indications herpes simplex and varicella–zoster (see also under Dose)

Cautions maintain adequate hydration (especially with infusion or high doses); renal impairment (Appendix 3); pregnancy (Appendix 4); breast-feeding (Appendix 5); **interactions:** Appendix 1 (aciclovir)

Side-effects nausea, vomiting, abdominal pain, diarrhoea, headache, fatigue, rash, urticaria, pruritus, photosensitivity; *very rarely* hepatitis, jaundice, dyspnoea, neurological reactions (including dizziness, confusion, hallucinations, convulsions and drowsiness), acute renal failure, anaemia, thrombocytopenia and leucopenia; on *intravenous infusion*, severe local inflammation (sometimes leading to ulceration), and *very rarely* agitation, tremors, psychosis and fever

Dose

- By mouth, herpes simplex, treatment, 200 mg (400 mg in the immunocompromised or if absorption impaired) 5 times daily, usually for 5 days (longer if new lesions appear during treatment or if healing incomplete; increase dose to 800 mg 5 times daily for genital herpes in the immunocompromised); CHILD under 2 years, half adult dose, over 2 years, adult dose

  Herpes simplex, prevention of recurrence, 200 mg 4 times daily *or* 400 mg twice daily possibly reduced to 200 mg 2 or 3 times daily and interrupted every 6–12 months

  Herpes simplex, prophylaxis in the immunocompromised, 200–400 mg 4 times daily; CHILD under 2 years, half adult dose, over 2 years, adult dose

  Varicella and herpes zoster, treatment, 800 mg 5 times daily for 7 days; CHILD, varicella, 20 mg/kg (max. 800 mg) 4 times daily for 5 days *or* under 2 years 200 mg 4 times daily, 2–5 years 400 mg 4 times daily, over 6 years 800 mg 4 times daily

  Attenuation of chickenpox (if varicella–zoster immunoglobulin not indicated) [unlicensed use], ADULT and CHILD 40 mg/kg daily in 4 divided doses for 7 days starting 1 week after exposure
- By intravenous infusion, treatment of herpes simplex in the immunocompromised, severe initial genital herpes, and varicella–zoster, 5 mg/kg every 8 hours usually for 5 days, doubled to 10 mg/kg

every 8 hours in varicella–zoster in the immunocompromised and in simplex encephalitis (usually given for at least 10 days in encephalitis, possibly for 14–21 days); prophylaxis of herpes simplex in the immunocompromised, 5 mg/kg every 8 hours

Note To avoid excessive dosage in obese patients, parenteral dose should be calculated on the basis of ideal weight for height

NEONATE and INFANT up to 3 months, with disseminated herpes simplex, 20 mg/kg every 8 hours for 14 days (21 days if CNS involvement); varicella–zoster [unlicensed use] 10–20 mg/kg every 8 hours for at least 7 days; CHILD 3 months–12 years, herpes simplex or varicella–zoster, 250 mg/m² every 8 hours usually for 5 days, doubled to 500 mg/m² every 8 hours for varicella–zoster in the immunocompromised and in simplex encephalitis (usually given for at least 10 days in encephalitis, possibly for 14–21 days)

- By topical application, see section 13.10.3 (skin) and section 11.3.3 (eye)

Note Aciclovir doses in BNF may differ from those in product literature

Aciclovir (Non-proprietary) PoM

Tablets, aciclovir 200 mg, net price 25-tab pack = £4.01; 400 mg, 56-tab pack = £7.31; 800 mg, 35-tab pack = £9.21. Label: 9

Brands include *Virovir®*

Dental prescribing on NHS Aciclovir Tablets 200 mg or 800 mg may be prescribed

Dispersible tablets, aciclovir 200 mg, net price 25-tab pack = £2.26; 400 mg, 56-tab pack = £7.68; 800 mg, 35-tab pack = £8.80. Label: 9

Intravenous infusion, powder for reconstitution, aciclovir (as sodium salt). Net price 250-mg vial = £10.91; 500-mg vial = £20.22

Electrolytes Na^+ 1.1 mmol/250-mg vial

Intravenous infusion, aciclovir (as sodium salt), 25 mg/mL, net price 10-mL (250-mg) vial = £10.37; 20-mL (500-mg) vial = £19.21; 40-mL (1-g) vial = £40.44

Electrolytes Na^+ 1.16 mmol/250-mg vial

Zovirax® (GSK) PoM

Tablets, all dispersible, f/c, aciclovir 200 mg, net price 25-tab pack = £18.80; 400 mg, 56-tab pack = £68.98; 800 mg (scored, *Shingles Treatment Pack*), 35-tab pack = £69.85. Label: 9

Suspension, both off-white, sugar-free, aciclovir 200 mg/5 mL (banana-flavoured), net price 125 mL = £29.53; 400 mg/5 mL (*Double Strength Suspension*, orange-flavoured) 100 mL = £33.01. Label: 9

Dental prescribing on NHS May be prescribed as Aciclovir 200 mg/5 mL oral Suspension

Intravenous infusion, powder for reconstitution, aciclovir (as sodium salt). Net price 250-mg vial = £10.15; 500-mg vial = £18.81

Electrolytes Na^+ 1.1 mmol/250-mg vial

FAMCICLOVIR

Note Famciclovir is a pro-drug of penciclovir

Indications treatment of herpes zoster, acute genital herpes simplex and suppression of recurrent genital herpes

Cautions hepatic impairment (Appendix 2); renal impairment (Appendix 3); pregnancy (Appendix 4) and breast-feeding (Appendix 5); **interactions**: Appendix 1 (famciclovir)

Side-effects *rarely* nausea, headache, confusion; *very rarely* vomiting, jaundice, dizziness, drowsiness, hallucinations, rash, and pruritus; abdominal pain and fever have been reported in immunocompromised patients

Dose

- Herpes zoster, 250 mg 3 times daily for 7 days *or* 750 mg once daily for 7 days (in immunocompromised, 500 mg 3 times daily for 10 days)
- Genital herpes, first episode, 250 mg 3 times daily for 5 days (longer if new lesions appear during treatment or if healing incomplete); recurrent infection, 125 mg twice daily for 5 days (in immunocompromised, all episodes, 500 mg twice daily for 7 days)
- Genital herpes, suppression, 250 mg twice daily (in HIV patients, 500 mg twice daily) interrupted every 6–12 months
- CHILD not recommended

Famvir® (Novartis) PoM

Tablets, all f/c, famciclovir 125 mg, net price 10-tab pack = £37.12; 250 mg, 15-tab pack = £111.35, 21-tab pack = £155.87; 56-tab pack = £415.67; 500 mg, 14-tab pack = £207.86, 30-tab pack = £445.28, 56-tab pack = £831.46; 750 mg, 7-tab pack = £148.79. Label: 9

INOSINE PRANOBEX 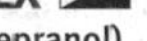

(Inosine acedoben dimepranol)

Indications see under Dose

Cautions renal impairment (Appendix 3); history of gout or hyperuricaemia

Contra-indications pregnancy

Side-effects reversible increase in serum and urinary uric acid; *less commonly* nausea, vomiting, epigastric discomfort, headache, vertigo, fatigue, arthralgia, rashes and itching; *rarely* diarrhoea, constipation, anxiety, sleep disturbances, and polyuria

Dose

- Mucocutaneous herpes simplex, 1 g 4 times daily for 7–14 days
- Adjunctive treatment of genital warts, 1 g 3 times daily for 14–28 days
- Subacute sclerosing panencephalitis, 50–100 mg/kg daily in 6 divided doses

Imunovir® (Ardern) PoM ▲

Tablets, scored, inosine pranobex 500 mg. Net price 100-tab pack = £39.50. Label: 9

VALACICLOVIR

Note Valaciclovir is a pro-drug of aciclovir

Indications treatment of herpes zoster; treatment of initial and suppression of recurrent herpes simplex infections of skin and mucous membranes including initial and recurrent genital herpes; reduction of transmission of genital herpes; prevention of cytomegalovirus disease following renal transplantation

Cautions see under Aciclovir; hepatic impairment (Appendix 2); renal impairment (Appendix 3)

Side-effects see under Aciclovir but neurological reactions more frequent with high doses

Dose

- Herpes zoster, 1 g 3 times daily for 7 days
- Herpes simplex, first episode, 500 mg twice daily for 5 days (longer if new lesions appear during treatment or if healing incomplete); recurrent infection, 500 mg twice daily for 5 days

- Herpes simplex, suppression, 500 mg daily in 1–2 divided doses (in immunocompromised, 500 mg twice daily)
- Reduction of transmission of genital herpes, seek specialist advice, 500 mg once daily to be taken by the infected partner
- Prevention of cytomegalovirus disease following renal transplantation (preferably starting within 72 hours of transplantation), 2 g 4 times daily usually for 90 days
- CHILD not recommended

Valtrex® (GSK) PoM
Tablets, f/c, valaciclovir (as hydrochloride) 250 mg, net price 60-tab pack = £130.87; 500 mg, 10-tab pack = £21.86, 42-tab pack = £91.61. Label: 9

5.3.2.2 Cytomegalovirus infection

Recommendations for the optimum maintenance therapy of cytomegalovirus (CMV) infections and the duration of treatment are subject to rapid change.

Ganciclovir is related to aciclovir but it is more active against cytomegalovirus; it is also much more toxic than aciclovir and should therefore be prescribed only when the potential benefit outweighs the risks. Ganciclovir is administered by intravenous infusion for the *initial treatment* of CMV retinitis. Ganciclovir causes profound myelosuppression when given with zidovudine; the two should not normally be given together particularly during initial ganciclovir therapy. The likelihood of ganciclovir resistance increases in patients with a high viral load or in those who receive the drug over a long duration; cross-resistance to cidofovir is common.

Valaciclovir (see p. 337) is licensed for prevention of cytomegalovirus disease following renal transplantation.

Valganciclovir is an ester of ganciclovir which is licensed for the *initial treatment* and *maintenance treatment* of CMV retinitis in AIDS patients. Valganciclovir is also licensed for preventing CMV disease following solid organ transplantation from a cytomegalovirus-positive donor.

Foscarnet is also active against cytomegalovirus; it is toxic and can cause renal impairment.

Cidofovir is given in combination with probenecid for CMV retinitis in AIDS patients when ganciclovir and foscarnet are contra-indicated. Cidofovir is nephrotoxic.

For local treatment of CMV retinitis, see section 11.3.3.

CIDOFOVIR

Indications cytomegalovirus retinitis in AIDS patients for whom other drugs are inappropriate

Cautions monitor renal function (serum creatinine and urinary protein) and neutrophil count within 24 hours before each dose; co-treatment with probenecid and prior hydration with intravenous fluids necessary to minimise potential nephrotoxicity (see below); diabetes mellitus (increased risk of ocular hypotony); **interactions:** Appendix 1 (cidofovir)

Nephrotoxicity Do not initiate treatment in renal impairment (assess creatinine clearance and proteinuria—consult product literature); discontinue treatment and give intravenous fluids if renal function deteriorates—consult product literature

Ocular disorders Regular ophthalmological examinations recommended; iritis and uveitis have been reported which may respond to a topical corticosteroid with or without a cycloplegic drug—discontinue cidofovir if no response to topical corticosteroid or if condition worsens, or if iritis or uveitis recurs after successful treatment

Contra-indications renal impairment (creatinine clearance 55 mL/minute or less); concomitant administration of potentially nephrotoxic drugs (discontinue potentially nephrotoxic drugs at least 7 days before starting cidofovir); pregnancy (avoid pregnancy during and for 1 month after treatment, men should not father a child during or within 3 months of treatment; Appendix 4), breast-feeding (Appendix 5)

Side-effects nephrotoxicity (see Cautions above); neutropenia, fever, asthenia, alopecia, nausea, vomiting, hypotony, decreased intra-ocular pressure, iritis, uveitis (see Cautions above)

Dose

- Initial (induction) treatment, ADULT over 18 years, by intravenous infusion over 1 hour, 5 mg/kg once weekly for 2 weeks (give probenecid and intravenous fluids with each dose, see below)
- Maintenance treatment, beginning 2 weeks after completion of induction, ADULT over 18 years, by intravenous infusion over 1 hour, 5 mg/kg once every 2 weeks (give probenecid and intravenous fluids with each dose, see below)

Probenecid co-treatment By mouth (preferably after food), probenecid 2 g 3 hours before cidofovir infusion followed by probenecid 1 g at 2 hours and 1 g at 8 hours after the end of cidofovir infusion (total probenecid 4 g); for cautions, contra-indications and side-effects of probenecid see section 10.1.4

Prior hydration Sodium chloride 0.9%, by intravenous infusion, 1 litre over 1 hour immediately before cidofovir infusion (if tolerated an additional 1 litre may be given over 1–3 hours, starting at the same time as the cidofovir infusion or immediately afterwards)

Vistide® (Pharmacia) PoM
Intravenous infusion, cidofovir 75 mg/mL, net price 5-mL vial = £653.22

Caution in handling Cidofovir is toxic and personnel should be adequately protected during handling and administration; if solution comes into contact with skin or mucosa, wash off immediately with water

GANCICLOVIR

Indications life-threatening or sight-threatening cytomegalovirus infections in immunocompromised patients only; prevention of cytomegalovirus disease during immunosuppressive therapy following organ transplantation; local treatment of CMV retinitis (section 11.3.3)

Cautions close monitoring of full blood count (severe deterioration may require correction and possibly treatment interruption); history of cytopenia; low platelet count; potential carcinogen and teratogen; renal impairment (Appendix 3); radiotherapy; ensure adequate hydration during intravenous administration; vesicant—infuse into vein with adequate flow preferably using plastic cannula; children (possible risk of long-term carcinogenic or reproductive toxicity—not for neonatal or congenital cytomegalovirus disease); **interactions:** Appendix 1 (ganciclovir)

Contra-indications pregnancy (ensure effective contraception during treatment and barrier contraception for men during and for at least 90 days after treatment; Appendix 4); breast-feeding; hypersensitivity to ganciclovir or aciclovir; abnormally low haemoglobin, neutrophil, or platelet counts (consult product literature)

Side-effects diarrhoea, nausea, vomiting, dyspepsia, abdominal pain, constipation, flatulence, dysphagia, hepatic dysfunction; dyspnoea, chest pain, cough; headache, insomnia, convulsions, dizziness, neuropathy, depression, anxiety, confusion, abnormal thinking, fatigue, weight loss, anorexia; infection, fever, night sweats; anaemia, leucopenia, thrombocytopenia, pancytopenia, renal impairment; myalgia, arthralgia; macular oedema, retinal detachment, vitreous floaters, eye pain; ear pain, taste disturbance; dermatitis, pruritus; injection-site reactions; *less commonly* mouth ulcers, pancreatitis, arrhythmias, hypotension, anaphylactic reactions, psychosis, tremor, male infertility, haematuria, disturbances in hearing and vision, and alopecia

Dose

- By intravenous infusion, initially (induction) 5 mg/kg every 12 hours for 14–21 days for treatment or for 7–14 days for prevention; maintenance (for patients at risk of relapse of retinitis) 6 mg/kg daily on 5 days per week *or* 5 mg/kg daily until adequate recovery of immunity; if retinitis progresses initial induction treatment may be repeated

Cymevene® (Roche) PoM
Intravenous infusion, powder for reconstitution, ganciclovir (as sodium salt). Net price 500-mg vial = £31.60
Electrolytes Na^+ 2 mmol/500-mg vial
Caution in handling Ganciclovir is toxic and personnel should be adequately protected during handling and administration; if solution comes into contact with skin or mucosa, wash off immediately with soap and water

FOSCARNET SODIUM

Indications cytomegalovirus retinitis in AIDS patients; mucocutaneous herpes simplex virus infections unresponsive to aciclovir in immunocompromised patients

Cautions renal impairment (reduce dose; consult product literature); monitor electrolytes, particularly calcium and magnesium; monitor serum creatinine every second day during induction and every week during maintenance; ensure adequate hydration; avoid rapid infusion; **interactions:** Appendix 1 (foscarnet)

Contra-indications pregnancy; breast-feeding (Appendix 5)

Side-effects nausea, vomiting, diarrhoea (occasionally constipation and dyspepsia), abdominal pain, anorexia; changes in blood pressure and ECG; headache, fatigue, mood disturbances (including psychosis), asthenia, paraesthesia, convulsions, tremor, dizziness, and other neurological disorders; rash; impairment of renal function including acute renal failure; hypocalcaemia (sometimes symptomatic) and other electrolyte disturbances; abnormal liver function tests; decreased haemoglobin concentration, leucopenia, granulocytopenia, thrombocytopenia; thrombophlebitis if given undiluted by peripheral vein; genital irritation and ulceration (due to high concentrations excreted in urine); isolated reports of pancreatitis

Dose

- CMV retinitis, by intravenous infusion, induction 60 mg/kg every 8 hours for 2–3 weeks then maintenance, 60 mg/kg daily, increased to 90–120 mg/kg if tolerated; if retinitis progresses on maintenance dose, repeat induction regimen
- Mucocutaneous herpes simplex infection, by intravenous infusion, 40 mg/kg every 8 hours for 2–3 weeks or until lesions heal

Foscavir® (AstraZeneca) PoM
Intravenous infusion, foscarnet sodium hexahydrate 24 mg/mL, net price 250-mL bottle = £34.49

VALGANCICLOVIR

Note Valganciclovir is a pro-drug of ganciclovir

Indications induction and maintenance treatment of cytomegalovirus retinitis in AIDS patients; prevention of cytomegalovirus disease following solid organ transplantation from a cytomegalovirus-positive donor.

Cautions see under Ganciclovir

Side-effects see under Ganciclovir

Dose

- CMV retinitis, induction, 900 mg twice daily for 21 days then 900 mg once daily; induction regimen may be repeated if retinitis progresses
- Prevention of cytomegalovirus disease following solid organ transplantation (starting within 10 days of transplantation), 900 mg once daily for 100 days
- CHILD under 18 years not recommended

Note Oral valganciclovir 900 mg twice daily is equivalent to intravenous ganciclovir 5 mg/kg twice daily

Valcyte® (Roche) PoM
Tablets, pink, f/c, valganciclovir (as hydrochloride) 450 mg, net price 60-tab pack = £1148.05. Label: 21
Caution in handling Valganciclovir is a potential teratogen and carcinogen and caution is advised for handling of broken tablets; if broken tablets come into contact with skin or mucosa, wash off immediately with water

5.3.3 Viral hepatitis

Treatment for viral hepatitis should be initiated by a specialist. The management of uncomplicated acute viral hepatitis is largely symptomatic. Early treatment of acute hepatitis C with interferon alfa [unlicensed indication] may reduce the risk of chronic infection. Hepatitis B and hepatitis C viruses are major causes of chronic hepatitis. For details on immunisation against hepatitis A and B infections, see section 14.4 (active immunisation) and section 14.5 (passive immunisation).

Chronic Hepatitis B **Peginterferon alfa-2a** (section 8.2.4) is an option for the initial treatment of chronic hepatitis B (see NICE guidance below) and may be preferable to **interferon alfa**. The use of peginterferon alfa-2a and interferon alfa is limited by a response rate of less than 50% and relapse is frequent. Treatment should be discontinued if no improvement occurs after 3–4 months. The manufacturers of peginterferon alfa-2a and interferon alfa contraindicate use in decompensated liver disease but low doses can be used with great caution in these patients. Although interferon alfa is contra-indicated in patients receiving immunosuppressant treatment (or who have received it recently), cautious use of peginterferon alfa-2a may be justified in some cases.

Lamivudine (see p. 330) is an option for the initial treatment of chronic hepatitis B. It can also be used in patients with decompensated liver disease. Hepatitis B viruses with reduced susceptibility to lamivudine have emerged following extended therapy.

Adefovir dipivoxil is licensed for the treatment of chronic hepatitis B (see NICE guidance below). It is effective in lamivudine-resistant chronic hepatitis B. It can be used in patients with decompensated liver disease.

Entecavir is licensed for the treatment of chronic hepatitis B. It is effective in patients not previously treated with nucleoside analogues and in those resistant to lamivudine.

Telbivudine is licensed for the treatment of chronic hepatitis B. It should not be used in lamivudine-resistant chronic hepatitis B because cross-resistance may occur.

Treatment with lamivudine, adefovir, entecavir, or telbivudine should be continued if there is no toxicity or loss of efficacy, until adequate seroconversion has occurred (consult product literature). Treatment with lamivudine or adefovir is continued long-term in patients with decompensated liver disease.

Tenofovir, or a combination of tenofovir with either emtricitabine or lamivudine may be used with other antiretrovirals, as part of 'highly active antiretroviral therapy' (section 5.3.1) in patients who require treatment for both HIV and chronic hepatitis B. If patients infected with both HIV and chronic hepatitis B only require treatment for chronic hepatitis B, they should receive antivirals that are not active against HIV. Management of these patients should be co-ordinated between HIV and hepatology specialists.

> **NICE guidance**
> **Adefovir dipivoxil and peginterferon alfa-2a for chronic hepatitis B (February 2006)**
> Peginterferon alfa-2a is an option for the initial treatment of chronic hepatitis B.
> Adefovir dipivoxil is recommended as an option for the treatment of chronic hepatitis B if:
> - treatment with interferon alfa or peginterferon alfa-2a has been unsuccessful, or
> - a relapse occurs after successful initial therapy, or
> - treatment with interferon alfa or peginterferon alfa-2a is poorly tolerated or contra-indicated.
>
> Adefovir dipivoxil should not be given before treatment with lamivudine. It may be used either alone or in combination with lamivudine when treatment with lamivudine has resulted in viral resistance, or if lamivudine resistance is likely to occur rapidly and adversely affect the outcome.

Chronic Hepatitis C Before starting treatment, the genotype of the infecting hepatitis C virus should be determined and the viral load measured as this may affect the choice and duration of treatment. A combination of **ribavirin** (see p. 342) and **peginterferon alfa** (section 8.2.4) is used for the treatment of chronic hepatitis C (see NICE guidance, below). The combination of ribavirin and interferon alfa is less effective than the combination of peginterferon alfa and ribavirin. Peginterferon alfa alone should be used if ribavirin is contra-indicated or not tolerated. Ribavirin monotherapy is ineffective.

> **NICE guidance**
> **Peginterferon alfa and ribavirin for mild chronic hepatitis C (August 2006)**
> The combination of peginterferon alfa and ribavirin can be used for treating mild chronic hepatitis C in patients over 18 years. Alternatively, treatment can be delayed until the disease has reached a moderate stage ('watchful waiting'). Peginterferon alfa alone can be used if ribavirin is contra-indicated or not tolerated.

> **NICE guidance**
> **Peginterferon alfa, interferon alfa, and ribavirin for moderate to severe chronic hepatitis C (January 2004)**
> The combination of peginterferon alfa and ribavirin should be used for treating moderate to severe chronic hepatitis C in patients aged over 18 years:
> - not previously treated with interferon alfa or peginterferon alfa;
> - treated previously with interferon alfa alone or in combination with ribavirin;
> - whose condition did not respond to peginterferon alfa alone or responded but subsequently relapsed.
>
> Peginterferon alfa alone should be used if ribavirin is contra-indicated or not tolerated. Interferon alfa for either monotherapy or combined therapy should be used only if neutropenia and thrombocytopenia are a particular risk. Patients receiving interferon alfa may be switched to peginterferon alfa.
> Full guidance available at www.nice.org.uk/TA075.

ADEFOVIR DIPIVOXIL

Indications chronic hepatitis B infection with *either* compensated liver disease with evidence of viral replication, and histologically documented active liver inflammation and fibrosis *or* decompensated liver disease

Cautions monitor liver function tests every 3 months, and viral and serological markers for hepatitis B every 3–6 months; discontinue if deterioration in liver function, hepatic steatosis, progressive hepatomegaly or unexplained lactic acidosis; recurrent hepatitis may occur on discontinuation; monitor renal function every 3 months, more frequently in renal impairment (Appendix 3) or in patients receiving nephrotoxic drugs; pregnancy (Appendix 4); elderly; HIV infection (particularly if uncontrolled—theoretical risk of HIV resistance)

Contra-indications breast-feeding (Appendix 5)

Side-effects nausea, vomiting, dyspepsia, abdominal pain, flatulence, diarrhoea; asthenia, headache; renal failure; hypophosphataemia; rash and pruritus

Dose
- ADULT over 18 years, 10 mg once daily

Hepsera® (Gilead) PoM
Tablets, adefovir dipivoxil 10 mg, net price 30-tab pack = £315.00

ENTECAVIR

Indications chronic hepatitis B infection with compensated liver disease, evidence of viral replication, and histologically documented active liver inflammation or fibrosis

Cautions monitor liver function tests, and viral and serological markers for hepatitis B every 3 months; discontinue if deterioration in liver function, hepatic steatosis, progressive hepatomegaly or unexplained lactic acidosis; recurrent hepatitis may occur on discontinuation; renal impairment (Appendix 3); pregnancy (Appendix 4)

Contra-indications breast-feeding (Appendix 5)

Side-effects nausea, vomiting, dyspepsia, diarrhoea, raised serum amylase and lipase; headache, fatigue, dizziness, sleep disturbances; *less commonly* thrombocytopenia

Dose

- ADULT over 18 years, not previously treated with nucleoside analogues, 500 micrograms once daily
- ADULT over 18 years with lamivudine-resistant chronic hepatitis B, 1 mg once daily

Counselling To be taken at least 2 hours before or 2 hours after food

Baraclude® (Bristol-Myers Squibb) ▼ PoM

Tablets, f/c, entecavir (as monohydrate) 500 micrograms (white), net price 30-tab pack = £378.00; 1 mg (pink), 30-tab pack = £378.00. Counselling, administration

Oral solution, entecavir (as monohydrate) 50 micrograms/mL, net price 210-mL pack (orange-flavoured) = £441.00. Counselling, administration

TELBIVUDINE

Indications chronic hepatitis B infection with compensated liver disease, evidence of viral replication, and histologically documented active liver inflammation or fibrosis

Cautions monitor liver function tests every 3 months and viral and serological markers of hepatitis B every 3–6 months; discontinue if deterioration in liver function, hepatic steatosis, progressive hepatomegaly or unexplained lactic acidosis; recurrent hepatitis may occur on discontinuation; renal impairment (Appendix 3); pregnancy (Appendix 4)

Counselling Patients should be advised to promptly report unexplained muscle pain, tenderness or weakness

Contra-indications breast-feeding (Appendix 5)

Side-effects nausea, diarrhoea, abdominal pain, raised serum amylase and lipase; cough; dizziness, headache, fatigue; rash; *less commonly* arthralgia, myalgia, and myopathy

Dose

- ADULT and CHILD over 16 years, 600 mg once daily

Sebivo® (Novartis) ▼ PoM

Tablets, f/c, telbivudine 600 mg, net price 28-tab pack = £290.33. Counselling, muscle effects

5.3.4 Influenza

For advice on immunisation against influenza, see section 14.4.

Oseltamivir and **zanamivir** reduce replication of influenza A and B viruses by inhibiting viral neuraminidase. They are most effective for the treatment of influenza if started within a few hours of the onset of symptoms; they are licensed for use within 48 hours (within 36 hours for zanamivir in children) of the first symptoms. In otherwise healthy individuals they reduce the duration of symptoms by about 1–1.5 days. Oseltamivir or zanamivir can reduce the risk of complications from influenza in the elderly and in patients with chronic disease (see also NICE guidance, below).

Oseltamivir and zanamivir are licensed for post-exposure prophylaxis of influenza when influenza is circulating in the community. Oseltamivir should be given within 48 hours of exposure to influenza while zanamivir should be given within 36 hours of exposure to influenza (see also NICE guidance, below). Oseltamivir and zanamivir are also licensed for use in exceptional circumstances (e.g. when vaccination does not cover the infecting strain) to prevent influenza in an epidemic.

NICE guidance

Oseltamivir, zanamivir, and amantadine for prophylaxis and treatment of influenza (February and September 2003)

The drugs described here are not a substitute for vaccination, which remains the most effective way of preventing illness from influenza. When influenza A or influenza B is circulating in the community:

- amantadine is **not** recommended for post-exposure prophylaxis, seasonal prophylaxis, or treatment of influenza;
- oseltamivir and zanamivir are **not** recommended for seasonal prophylaxis against influenza;
- oseltamivir or zanamivir are **not** recommended for post-exposure prophylaxis, or treatment of otherwise healthy individuals with influenza;
- oseltamivir is recommended for post-exposure prophylaxis in at-risk adults and adolescents over 13 years [oseltamivir now licensed for children over 1 year[1]] who are not effectively protected by influenza vaccine and who can commence oseltamivir within 48 hours of close contact with someone suffering from influenza-like illness; prophylaxis is also recommended for residents in care establishments (regardless of influenza vaccination) who can commence oseltamivir within 48 hours if influenza-like illness is present in the establishment;
- oseltamivir and zanamivir are recommended (in accordance with UK licensing) to treat at-risk adults who can start treatment within 48 hours of the onset of symptoms; oseltamivir is recommended for at-risk children who can start treatment within 48 hours of the onset of symptoms;

At-risk patients include those aged over 65 years *or* those who have one or more of the following conditions:

- chronic respiratory disease (including chronic obstructive pulmonary disease and asthma) [but see cautions under Zanamivir below];
- significant cardiovascular disease (excluding hypertension);
- chronic renal disease;
- immunosuppression;
- diabetes mellitus.

Community-based virological surveillance schemes including those run by the Health Protection Agency and the Royal College of General Practitioners should be used to indicate when influenza is circulating in the community.

1. The Department of Health in England has advised (February 2006) that it is appropriate to apply these recommendations to children over 1 year.

5 Infections

Amantadine is licensed for prophylaxis and treatment of influenza A but it is no longer recommended (see NICE guidance).

Information on pandemic influenza and avian influenza may be found at www.dh.gov.uk/pandemicflu and at www.hpa.org.uk

AMANTADINE HYDROCHLORIDE

Indications see under Dose; parkinsonism (section 4.9.1)

Cautions see section 4.9.1

Contra-indications see section 4.9.1

Side-effects see section 4.9.1

Dose

- Influenza A (see also notes above), ADULT and CHILD over 10 years, treatment, 100 mg daily for 4–5 days; prophylaxis, 100 mg daily usually for 6 weeks *or* with influenza vaccination for 2–3 weeks after vaccination

Lysovir® (Alliance) PoM

Capsules, red-brown, amantadine hydrochloride 100 mg, net price 5-cap pack = £2.40, 14-cap pack = £4.80. Counselling, driving

Symmetrel® (Alliance) PoM

Section 4.9.1

OSELTAMIVIR

Indications see notes above

Cautions renal impairment (Appendix 3); pregnancy (Appendix 4); breast-feeding (Appendix 5)

Side-effects nausea, vomiting, abdominal pain, dyspepsia, diarrhoea; headache, fatigue, insomnia, dizziness; conjunctivitis, epistaxis; rash; *very rarely* hepatitis, Stevens-Johnson syndrome, and toxic epidermal necrolysis; neuropsychiatric disorders also reported (in children and adolescents)

Dose

- Prevention of influenza, ADULT and ADOLESCENT over 13 years, 75 mg once daily for 10 days for post-exposure prophylaxis; for up to 6 weeks during an epidemic; CHILD 1–13 years, body-weight under 15 kg, 30 mg once daily, body-weight 15–23 kg, 45 mg once daily, body-weight 23–40 kg, 60 mg once daily, body-weight over 40 kg, adult dose
- Treatment of influenza, ADULT and ADOLESCENT over 13 years, 75 mg every 12 hours for 5 days; CHILD 1–13 years, body-weight under 15 kg, 30 mg every 12 hours, body-weight 15–23 kg, 45 mg every 12 hours, body-weight 23–40 kg, 60 mg every 12 hours, body-weight over 40 kg, adult dose

[1]**Tamiflu®** (Roche) ▼ PoM

Capsules, oseltamivir (as phosphate) 30 mg (yellow), net price 10-cap pack = £8.18; 45 mg (grey), 10-cap pack = £16.36; 75 mg (grey-yellow), 10-cap pack = £16.36. Label: 9

Suspension, sugar-free, tutti-frutti-flavoured, oseltamivir (as phosphate) for reconstitution with water, 60 mg/5 mL, net price 75 mL = £16.36. Label: 9
Excipients include sorbitol 1.7 g/5 mL

1. NHS except for the treatment and prophylaxis of influenza as indicated in the notes above and NICE guidance; endorse prescription 'SLS'

ZANAMIVIR

Indications see notes above

Cautions asthma and chronic pulmonary disease (risk of bronchospasm—short-acting bronchodilator should be available; avoid in severe asthma unless close monitoring possible and appropriate facilities available to treat bronchospasm); uncontrolled chronic illness; other inhaled drugs should be administered before zanamivir; pregnancy (Appendix 4)

Contra-indications breast-feeding (Appendix 5)

Side-effects *very rarely*, bronchospasm, respiratory impairment, angioedema, urticaria, and rash

Dose

- By inhalation of powder, post-exposure prophylaxis of influenza, ADULT and CHILD over 5 years, 10 mg once daily for 10 days
  Prevention of influenza during an epidemic, ADULT and CHILD over 12 years, 10 mg once daily for up to 28 days
  Treatment of influenza, ADULT and CHILD over 5 years, 10 mg twice daily for 5 days

[1]**Relenza®** (GSK) PoM

Dry powder for inhalation disks containing 4 blisters of zanamivir 5 mg/blister, net price 5 disks with *Diskhaler®* device = £24.55

1. NHS except for the treatment of influenza as indicated in the notes above and NICE guidance; endorse prescription 'SLS'

5.3.5 Respiratory syncytial virus

Ribavirin (tribavirin) inhibits a wide range of DNA and RNA viruses. It is licensed for administration by inhalation for the treatment of severe bronchiolitis caused by the respiratory syncytial virus (RSV) in infants, especially when they have other serious diseases. However, there is no evidence that ribavirin produces clinically relevant benefit in RSV bronchiolitis. Ribavirin is given by mouth with peginterferon alfa or interferon alfa for the treatment of chronic hepatitis C infection (see Viral Hepatitis, p. 339). Ribavirin is also effective in Lassa fever [unlicensed indication].

Palivizumab is a monoclonal antibody licensed for preventing serious lower respiratory-tract disease caused by respiratory syncytial virus in children at high risk of the disease; it should be prescribed under specialist supervision and on the basis of the likelihood of hospitalisation. Palivizumab should be considered for children under 6 months with haemodynamically significant left-to-right shunt congenital heart disease or who have pulmonary hypertension. It should also be considered for children under 2 years *either* with chronic lung disease requiring oxygen at home (or have been on prolonged oxygen treatment) *or* with severe congenital immunodeficiency. Palivizumab can also be used for the first 6–12 months of life in a child born at under 35 weeks gestation who is considered by the specialist to be at special risk of hospitalisation.

PALIVIZUMAB

Indications see notes above

Cautions moderate to severe acute infection or febrile illness; thrombocytopenia; serum-palivizumab concentration may be reduced after cardiac surgery

Contra-indications hypersensitivity to humanised monoclonal antibodies

Side-effects fever, injection-site reactions, nervousness; *less commonly* diarrhoea, vomiting, constipation, haemorrhage, rhinitis, cough, wheeze, pain, drowsiness, asthenia, hyperkinesia, leucopenia, and rash; *rarely* apnoea, hypersensitivity reactions (including anaphylaxis)

Dose

- By intramuscular injection (preferably in anterolateral thigh), 15 mg/kg once a month during season of RSV risk (child undergoing cardiac bypass surgery, 15 mg/kg as soon as stable after surgery, then once a month during season of risk); injection volume over 1 mL should be divided between more than one site

Synagis® (Abbott) ▼ PoM

Injection, powder for reconstitution, palivizumab, net price 50-mg vial = £360.40; 100-mg vial = £663.11

RIBAVIRIN
(Tribavirin)

Indications severe respiratory syncytial virus bronchiolitis in infants and children; in combination with peginterferon alfa or interferon alfa for chronic hepatitis C in patients without liver decompensation (see also section 5.3.3)

Cautions

Specific cautions for inhaled treatment Maintain standard supportive respiratory and fluid management therapy; monitor electrolytes closely; monitor equipment for precipitation; pregnant women (and those planning pregnancy) should avoid exposure to aerosol

Specific cautions for oral treatment Exclude pregnancy before treatment; effective contraception essential during treatment and for 4 months after treatment in women and for 7 months after treatment in men; routine monthly pregnancy tests recommended; condoms must be used if partner of male patient is pregnant (ribavirin excreted in semen); renal impairment (Appendix 3); cardiac disease (assessment including ECG recommended before and during treatment—discontinue if deterioration); gout; determine full blood count, platelets, electrolytes, serum creatinine, liver function tests and uric acid before starting treatment and then on weeks 2 and 4 of treatment, then as indicated clinically—adjust dose if adverse reactions or laboratory abnormalities develop (consult product literature); test thyroid function before treatment and then every 3 months in children

Interactions: Appendix 1 (Ribavirin)

Contra-indications pregnancy (**important teratogenic risk**: see Cautions and Appendix 4); breast-feeding

Specific contra-indications for oral treatment Severe cardiac disease, including unstable or uncontrolled cardiac disease in previous 6 months; haemoglobinopathies; severe debilitating medical conditions; severe hepatic dysfunction or decompensated cirrhosis (Appendix 2); autoimmune disease (including autoimmune hepatitis); uncontrolled severe psychiatric condition; history of severe psychiatric condition in children

Side-effects

Specific side-effects for inhaled treatment Worsening respiration, bacterial pneumonia, and pneumothorax reported; rarely non-specific anaemia and haemolysis

Specific side-effects for oral treatment Haemolytic anaemia (anaemia may be improved by epoetin); also (in combination with peginterferon alfa or interferon alfa) nausea, vomiting, dyspepsia, abdominal pain, peptic ulcer, flatulence, diarrhoea, constipation, colitis, pancreatitis, appetite changes, weight loss, pulmonary embolism, chest pain, tachycardia, palpitation, syncope, peripheral oedema, changes in blood pressure, flushing, dyspnoea, cough, interstitial pneumonitis, sleep disturbances, abnormal dreams, asthenia, impaired concentration and memory, psychoses, anxiety, depression, suicidal ideation (more frequent in children), dizziness, tremor, hypertonia, ataxia, dysphonia, peripheral neuropathy, influenza-like symptoms, headache, hyperglycaemia, thyroid disorders, menstrual disturbances, reduced libido, impotence, prostatitis, micturition disorders, leucopenia, thrombocytopenia, aplastic anaemia, lymphadenopathy, hypocalcaemia, hyperuricaemia, myalgia, arthralgia, systemic lupus erythematosus, sarcoidosis, eye changes including blurred vision, rhinitis, tinnitus, hearing impairment, dry mouth, stomatitis, glossitis, taste disturbance, pharyngitis, gingivitis, rash (including very rarely Stevens-Johnson syndrome and toxic epidermal necrolysis), pruritus, urticaria, photosensitivity, psoriasis, alopecia, dry skin, increased sweating; in children also growth retardation (including decrease in height and weight), Raynaud's disease, hypertriglyceridaemia, hyperkinesia, testicular pain, virilism, tooth disorders, and skin discoloration

Dose

- See preparations below

Copegus® (Roche) PoM

Tablets, f/c, ribavirin 200 mg (pink), net price 42-tab pack = £115.62, 112-tab pack = £308.31, 168-tab pack = £462.47; 400 mg (red-brown), 56-tab pack = £308.31. Label: 21

Dose chronic hepatitis C (in combination with interferon alfa or peginterferon alfa), ADULT over 18 years, body-weight under 75 kg, 400 mg in the morning and 600 mg in the evening; body-weight 75 kg and over, 600 mg twice daily

Note Chronic hepatitis C genotype 2 or 3, or patients infected with HIV and hepatitis C require a lower dose of *Copegus®* (in combination with peginterferon alfa), usual dose 400 mg twice daily

Rebetol® (Schering-Plough) PoM

Capsules, ribavirin 200 mg, net price 84-cap pack = £275.65, 140-cap pack = £459.42, 168-cap pack = £551.30. Label: 21

Dose chronic hepatitis C, ADULT over 18 years (in combination with interferon alfa or peginterferon alfa), body-weight under 65 kg, 400 mg twice daily; body-weight 65–85 kg, 400 mg in the morning and 600 mg in the evening; body-weight over 85 kg, 600 mg twice daily; CHILD AND ADOLESCENT 3–17 years (in combination with interferon alfa), body-weight under 47 kg, 15 mg/kg daily in 2 divided doses; body-weight 47–49 kg, 200 mg in the morning and 400 mg in the evening; body-weight 50–65 kg, 400 mg twice daily; body-weight over 65kg, as adult

Virazole® (Valeant) PoM

Inhalation, ribavirin 6 g for reconstitution with 300 mL water for injections. Net price 3 × 6-g vials = £349.00

Dose bronchiolitis, by aerosol inhalation *or* nebulisation (via small particle aerosol generator) of solution containing 20 mg/mL for 12–18 hours for at least 3 days; max. 7 days

5.4 Antiprotozoal drugs

5.4.1 Antimalarials
5.4.2 Amoebicides
5.4.3 Trichomonacides
5.4.4 Antigiardial drugs
5.4.5 Leishmaniacides
5.4.6 Trypanocides
5.4.7 Drugs for toxoplasmosis
5.4.8 Drugs for pneumocystis pneumonia

Advice on specific problems available from:

Advice for healthcare professionals

HPA (Health Protection Agency) Malaria Reference Laboratory	(020) 7636 3924 (prophylaxis only)
National Travel Health Network and Centre	0845 602 6712
Travel Medicine Team, Health Protection Scotland (registered users of Travax only) www.travax.nhs.uk (for registered users of the NHS Travax website only)	(0141) 300 1100 (weekdays 2–4 p.m. only)
Birmingham	(0121) 424 0357
Liverpool	(0151) 708 9393
London	0845 155 5000 (treatment)
Oxford	(01865) 225 430

Advice for travellers

Hospital for Tropical Diseases Travel Healthline	020 7950 7799

www.fitfortravel.nhs.uk

WHO advice on international travel and health www.who.int/ith

5.4.1 Antimalarials

Recommendations on the prophylaxis and treatment of malaria reflect guidelines agreed by UK malaria specialists.

The centres listed above should be consulted for advice on special problems.

Treatment of malaria

If the infective species is **not known**, or if the infection is **mixed**, initial treatment should be as for *falciparum malaria* with quinine, *Malarone®* (proguanil with atovaquone), or *Riamet®* (artemether with lumefantrine). Falciparum malaria can progress rapidly in unprotected individuals and antimalarial treatment should be considered in those with features of severe malaria and possible exposure, even if the initial blood tests for the organism are negative.

Falciparum malaria (treatment)

Falciparum malaria (malignant malaria) is caused by *Plasmodium falciparum*. In most parts of the world *P. falciparum* is now resistant to chloroquine which should not therefore be given for treatment.

Quinine, *Malarone®* (proguanil with atovaquone), or *Riamet®* (artemether with lumefantrine) can be given *by mouth* if the patient can swallow and retain tablets and there are no serious manifestations (e.g. impaired consciousness); quinine should be given *by intravenous infusion* (see below) if the patient is seriously ill or unable to take tablets. Mefloquine is now rarely used for treatment because of concerns about resistance.

Oral. The adult dosage regimen for **quinine** *by mouth* is:
600 mg (of quinine salt[1]) every 8 hours for 5–7 days
together with or followed by
either **doxycycline** 200 mg once daily for 7 days
or **clindamycin** 450 mg every 8 hours for 7 days [unlicensed indication].
If the parasite is likely to be sensitive, ***Fansidar®***, 3 tablets as a single dose may be given together with or after a course of quinine.

Alternatively, ***Malarone®*** or ***Riamet®*** may be given instead of quinine. It is not necessary to give doxycycline, clindamycin or *Fansidar®* after *Malarone®* or *Riamet®* treatment.

The adult dose of ***Malarone®*** *by mouth* is:
4 ('standard') tablets once daily for 3 days.

The dose of ***Riamet®*** *by mouth* for adult with body-weight over 35 kg is:
4 tablets initially, followed by 5 further doses of 4 tablets each given at 8, 24, 36, 48, and 60 hours (total 24 tablets over 60 hours).

Parenteral. If the patient is seriously ill or unable to take tablets, **quinine** should be given *by intravenous infusion*. The adult dosage regimen for quinine *by infusion* is:
loading dose[2] of 20 mg/kg[3] (up to maximum 1.4 g) of quinine salt[1] infused over 4 hours *then 8 hours after the start of the loading dose,* maintenance dose of 10 mg/kg[4] (up to maximum 700 mg) of quinine salt[1] infused over 4 hours every 8 hours (until patient can swallow tablets to complete the 7-day course *together with or followed by either* doxycycline or clindamycin as above).
Specialist advice should be sought in difficult cases (e.g. very high parasite count, deterioration on optimal doses of quinine, infection acquired in quinine-resistant areas of south east Asia) because intravenous **artesunate** may be available for 'named-patient' use.

1. Valid for quinine hydrochloride, dihydrochloride, and sulphate; not valid for quinine bisulphate which contains a correspondingly smaller amount of quinine.
2. In intensive care units the loading dose can alternatively be given as quinine salt[1] 7 mg/kg infused over 30 minutes followed immediately by 10 mg/kg over 4 hours then (after 8 hours) maintenance dose as described.
3. **Important:** the loading dose of 20 mg/kg should **not** be used if the patient has received quinine or mefloquine during the previous 12 hours.
4. Maintenance dose should be reduced to 5–7 mg/kg of salt in patients with renal impairment, severe hepatic impairment, or if parenteral treatment is required for more than 48 hours.

Children

Oral. **Quinine** is well tolerated by children although the salts are bitter. The dosage regimen for quinine *by mouth* for children is:

10 mg/kg (of quinine salt[1]) every 8 hours for 7 days
together with or followed by
Fansidar® as a single dose: up to 4 years and body-weight over 5 kg ½ tablet, 5–6 years 1 tablet, 7–9 years 1½ tablets, 10–14 years 2 tablets, 14–18 years 3 tablets
or **clindamycin** 7–13 mg/kg (max. 450 mg) every 8 hours for 7 days [unlicensed indication]
or in children over 12 years, **doxycycline** 200 mg once daily for 7 days

Alternatively, ***Malarone®*** or ***Riamet®*** may be given instead of quinine; it is not necessary to give clindamycin, doxycycline, or *Fansidar®* after *Malarone®* or *Riamet®* treatment. The dose regimen for *Malarone® by mouth* for children over 40 kg is the same as for adults (see above); the dose regimen for *Malarone®* for smaller children is reduced as follows:

body-weight 5–8 kg, 2 'paediatric' tablets once daily for 3 days; body-weight 9–10 kg, 3 'paediatric' tablets once daily for 3 days; body-weight 11–20 kg, 1 'standard' tablet once daily for 3 days; body-weight 21–30 kg, 2 'standard' tablets once daily for 3 days; body-weight 31–40 kg, 3 'standard' tablets once daily for 3 days.

The dose regimen of *Riamet® by mouth* for children over 12 years and body-weight over 35 kg is the same as for adults (see above). The dose regimen for *Riamet®* for children under 12 years is as follows:

body-weight 5–15 kg 1 tablet initially, followed by 5 further doses of 1 tablet each given at 8, 24, 36, 48, and 60 hours (total 6 tablets over 60 hours); body-weight 15–25 kg 2 tablets initially, followed by 5 further doses of 2 tablets each given at 8, 24, 36, 48, and 60 hours (total 12 tablets over 60 hours); body-weight 25–35 kg 3 tablets initially, followed by 5 further doses of 3 tablets each given at 8, 24, 36, 48, and 60 hours (total 18 tablets over 60 hours)

Parenteral. The dose regimen for quinine *by intravenous infusion* for children is calculated on a mg/kg basis as for adults (see above).

Pregnancy Falciparum malaria is particularly dangerous in pregnancy, especially in the last trimester. The adult treatment doses of oral and intravenous quinine given above (including the loading dose) can safely be given to pregnant women. Clindamycin 450 mg every 8 hours for 7 days [unlicensed indication] should be given with or after quinine. Doxycycline should be avoided in pregnancy (affects teeth and skeletal development); *Fansidar®*, *Malarone®*, and *Riamet®* are also best avoided until more information is available.

1. Valid for quinine hydrochloride, dihydrochloride, and sulphate; not valid for quinine bisulphate which contains a correspondingly smaller amount of quinine.
2. For the treatment of chloroquine-resistant benign malaria, *Malarone®* [unlicensed indication], quinine, or *Riamet®* [unlicensed indication] can be used; as with chloroquine, primaquine should be given for radical cure.

Benign malarias (treatment)

Benign malaria is usually caused by *Plasmodium vivax* and less commonly by *P. ovale* and *P. malariae*. **Chloroquine**[2] is the drug of choice for the treatment of benign malarias (but chloroquine-resistant *P. vivax* infection has been reported from Indonesia, New Guinea and some adjacent islands).

The adult dosage regimen for **chloroquine** *by mouth* is:

initial dose of 600 mg of base *then*
a single dose of 300 mg of base after 6 to 8 hours *then*
a single dose of 300 mg of base daily for 2 days
(approximate total cumulative dose of 25 mg/kg of base)

Chloroquine alone is adequate for *P. malariae* infections but in the case of *P. vivax* and *P. ovale*, a *radical cure* (to destroy parasites in the liver and thus prevent relapses) is required. This is achieved with **primaquine**[3] given after chloroquine; in *P. vivax* infection primaquine is given in an adult dosage of 30 mg daily for 14 days and for *P. ovale* infection it is given in an adult dosage of 15 mg daily for 14 days.

Children The dosage regimen of chloroquine for benign malaria in children is:

initial dose of 10 mg/kg of base (max. 600 mg) *then*
a single dose of 5 mg/kg of base (max. 300 mg) after 6–8 hours *then*
a single dose of 5 mg/kg of base (max. 300 mg) daily for 2 days

For a *radical cure*, children are then given primaquine[3]; in *P. vivax* infection primaquine is given in a dose of 500 micrograms/kg daily for 14 days, and for *P. ovale* infection it is given in a dose of 250 micrograms/kg daily for 14 days.

Pregnancy The adult treatment doses of chloroquine can be given for benign malaria. In the case of *P. vivax* or *P. ovale*, however, the radical cure with primaquine should be **postponed** until the pregnancy is over; instead chloroquine should be continued at a dose of 300 mg each week during the pregnancy.

3. Before starting primaquine, blood should be tested for glucose-6-phosphate dehydrogenase (G6PD) activity since the drug can cause haemolysis in G6PD-deficient patients. Specialist advice should be obtained in G6PD deficiency; in mild G6PD deficiency primaquine in a dose for adults of 45 mg once a week (children 750 micrograms/kg once a week; max. 45 mg once a week) for 8 weeks, has been found useful and without undue harmful effects.

Prophylaxis against malaria

The recommendations on prophylaxis reflect guidelines agreed by UK malaria specialists; the advice is aimed at residents of the UK who travel to endemic areas. The choice of drug for a particular individual should take into account:

- risk of exposure to malaria;
- extent of drug resistance;
- efficacy of the recommended drugs;
- side-effects of the drugs;
- patient-related factors (e.g. age, pregnancy, renal or hepatic impairment, compliance with prophylactic regimen).

Protection against bites **Prophylaxis is not absolute**, and breakthrough infection can occur with any of the drugs recommended. Personal protection against being bitten is very important. Mosquito nets impregnated with permethrin provide the most effective barrier protection against insects; mats and vaporised insecticides are also useful. Diethyltoluamide (DEET) 20–50% in lotions, sprays, or roll-on formulations is safe and effective when applied to the skin of adults and children over 2 months of age. It can also be used during pregnancy and breast-feeding. The duration of protection varies according to the concentration of DEET and is longest for DEET 50%. Long sleeves and trousers worn after dusk also provide protection.

Length of prophylaxis In order to determine tolerance and to establish habit, prophylaxis should generally be started one week (preferably 2–3 weeks in the case of mefloquine) before travel into an endemic area (or if not possible at earliest opportunity up to 1 or 2 days before travel); *Malarone*® or doxycycline prophylaxis should be started 1–2 days before travel. Prophylaxis should be continued for **4 weeks after leaving** (except for *Malarone*® prophylaxis which should be stopped 1 week after leaving).

In those requiring long-term prophylaxis, chloroquine and proguanil may be used for periods of over 5 years. Mefloquine is licensed for up to 1 year (although it has been used for up to 3 years without undue problems). Doxycycline can be used for up to 2 years. *Malarone*® is licensed for up to 28 days but can be used for up to 1 year (and possibly longer) with caution. Specialist advice should be sought for long-term prophylaxis.

Return from malarial region It is important to be aware that **any illness** that occurs within 1 year and **especially within 3 months of return might be malaria** even if all recommended precautions against malaria were taken. Travellers should be **warned** of this and told that if they develop any illness **particularly within 3 months** of their return they should go **immediately** to a doctor and specifically mention their exposure to malaria.

Children Prophylactic doses are based on guidelines agreed by UK malaria experts and may differ from advice in product literature. Weight is a better guide than age. If in doubt telephone centres listed on p. 344.

Epilepsy Both chloroquine and mefloquine are unsuitable for malaria prophylaxis in individuals with a history of epilepsy. In areas *without chloroquine resistance* proguanil 200 mg daily alone is recommended; in areas *with chloroquine resistance*, doxycycline or *Malarone*® may be considered; the metabolism of doxycycline may be influenced by antiepileptics (see **interactions:** Appendix 1 (tetracyclines)).

Asplenia Asplenic individuals (or those with severe splenic dysfunction) are at particular risk of severe malaria. If travel to malarious areas is unavoidable, rigorous precautions are required against contracting the disease.

Renal impairment Avoidance (or dosage reduction) of proguanil is recommended since it is excreted by the kidneys. *Malarone*® should not be used for prophylaxis in patients with creatinine clearance less than 30 mL/minute. Chloroquine is only partially excreted by the kidneys and reduction of the dose for prophylaxis is not required except in severe impairment. Mefloquine is considered to be appropriate to use in renal impairment and does not require dosage reduction. Doxycycline is also considered to be appropriate.

Pregnancy Travel to malarious areas should be avoided during pregnancy; if travel is unavoidable, effective prophylaxis must be used. Chloroquine and proguanil can be given in the usual doses during pregnancy, but these drugs are not appropriate for most areas because their effectiveness has declined, particularly in Sub-Saharan Africa; in the case of proguanil, folic acid 5 mg daily should be given. The centres listed on p. 344 should be consulted for advice on prophylaxis in chloroquine-resistant areas. The manufacturer advises that prophylaxis with mefloquine should be avoided as a matter of principle but studies of mefloquine in pregnancy (including use in the first trimester) indicate that it can be considered for travel to chloroquine-resistant areas. Doxycycline is contra-indicated during pregnancy. *Malarone*® should be avoided during pregnancy unless there is no suitable alternative.

Breast-feeding Prophylaxis is required in **breast-fed infants**; although antimalarials are present in milk, the amounts are too variable to give reliable protection.

Anticoagulants Travellers taking warfarin should begin chemoprophylaxis at least 1 week (2–3 weeks for mefloquine) before departure. The INR should be stable before departure. It should be measured before starting chemoprophylaxis, 7 days after starting, and after completing the course. For prolonged stays, the INR should be checked at regular intervals.

Specific recommendations

Where a journey requires two regimens, the regimen for the higher risk area should be used for the whole journey. Those travelling to remote or little-visited areas may require expert advice.

> Risk may vary in different parts of a country—check under all risk levels

> **WARNING** Settled immigrants (or long-term visitors) to the UK may be unaware that they will have **lost some of their immunity** and also that the areas where they previously lived **may now be malarious**

5 Infections

North Africa, the Middle East, and Central Asia

Very low risk Risk *very low* in Algeria, Egypt (but *low risk* in El Faiyum, see below), Georgia (south-east, July–October), Kyrgystan (but *low risk* in south-west, see below), Libya, rural Morocco, most tourist areas of Turkey (but *low risk* in Adana and border with Syria, see below), Uzbekistan (extreme south-east only):

> chemoprophylaxis not recommended but avoid mosquito bites and consider malaria if fever presents

Low risk Risk *low* in Armenia (June–October), Azerbaijan (southern border areas, June–September), Egypt (El Faiyum only, June–October), Iran (northern border with Azerbaijan, May–October; *variable risk* in rural south-east provinces; see below), rural north Iraq (May–November), Kyrgystan (south-west, May–October), north border of Syria (May–October), Turkey (plain around Adana and east of there, border with Syria, March–November), Turkmenistan (south-east only, June–October):

preferably

> chloroquine *or* (if chloroquine not appropriate) proguanil hydrochloride

Variable risk Risk *variable* and *chloroquine resistance present* in Afghanistan (below 2000 m, May–November), Iran (rural south-east provinces, March–November, see also *Low risk* above); Oman (remote rural areas only), Saudi Arabia (south-west and rural areas of western region; no risk in Mecca, Medina, Jeddah, or high-altitude areas of Asir Province), Tajikistan (June–October), Yemen (no risk in Sana'a):

> chloroquine + proguanil hydrochloride *or* (if chloroquine + proguanil not appropriate) doxycycline

---

Sub-Saharan Africa

No chemoprophylaxis recommended for Cape Verde (some risk on São Tiago) and Mauritius (but avoid mosquito bites and consider malaria if fever presents)

Very high risk Risk *very high* (or *locally very high*) and *chloroquine resistance very widespread* in Angola, Benin, Botswana (northern half, November–June), Burkina Faso, Burundi, Cameroon, Central African Republic, Chad, Comoros, Congo, Democratic Republic of the Congo (formely Zaïre), Djibouti, Equatorial Guinea, Eritrea, Ethiopia (below 2000 m; no risk in Addis Ababa), Gabon, Gambia, Ghana, Guinea, Guinea-Bissau, Ivory Coast, Kenya, Liberia, Madagascar, Malawi, Mali, Mauritania (all year in south; July–October in north), Mozambique, Namibia (all year along Kavango and Kunene rivers; November–June in northern third), Niger, Nigeria, Principe, Rwanda, São Tomé, Senegal, Sierra Leone, Somalia, South Africa (north-east, low-altitude areas of Northern Province and Mpumalanga, Kruger National Park, and north-east KwaZulu-Natal as far south as Tugela river), Sudan, Swaziland, Tanzania, Togo, Uganda, Zambia, Zimbabwe (all year in Zambezi valley; November–June in other areas below 1200 m; risk negligible in Harare and Bulawayo):

> mefloquine *or* doxycycline *or Malarone*®

Note In Zimbabwe and neighbouring countries, pyrimethamine with dapsone (also known as *Deltaprim*®) prophylaxis is used by local residents (sometimes with chloroquine)—this regimen is not recommended.

South Asia

Low risk Risk low in Bangladesh (but *high risk* in Chittagong Hill Tracts, see below), India (Kerala [southern states], Tamil Nadu, Karnataka, Southern Andhra Pradesh [including Hyderabad and Mumbai], Rajasthan [including Jaipur], Uttar Pradesh [including Aggra], Haryana, Uttaranchal, Himachal Pradesh, Jammu, Kashmir, Punjab, Delhi; *variable risk* in other areas, see below; *high risk* in Assam), Sri Lanka (but *variable risk* north of Vavuniya, see below):

> chemoprophylaxis not recommended but avoid mosquito bites and consider malaria if fever present

Variable risk Risk *variable* and *chloroquine resistance usually moderate* in southern districts of Bhutan, India (*low risk* in some areas, see above; *high risk* in Assam, see below), Nepal (below 1500 m, especially Terai districts; no risk in Kathmandu), Pakistan (below 2000 m), Sri Lanka (north of Vavuniya; *low risk* in other areas, see above):

> chloroquine + proguanil hydrochloride *or* (if chloroquine + proguanil not appropriate) mefloquine *or* doxycycline *or Malarone*®

High risk Risk *high* and *chloroquine resistance high* in Bangladesh (only in Chittagong Hill Tracts; *low risk* in other areas, see above), India (Assam only; see also *low risk* and *variable risk* above):

> mefloquine *or* doxycycline *or Malarone*® *or* (if mefloquine, doxycycline, or *Malarone*® not appropriate) chloroquine + proguanil hydrochloride

---

South-East Asia

Very low risk Risk *very low* in Bali, Brunei, main tourist areas of China (but *substantial risk* in Yunnan and Hainan, see below; *chloroquine prophylaxis* appropriate for other remote areas), Hong Kong, Korea (both North and South), Malaysia (both East and West including Cameron Highlands, but *substantial risk* in Sabah [except Kota Kinabalu], and *variable risk* in deep forests, see below), Singapore, Thailand (**important**: regional risk exists, see under *Great risk*, below), Vietnam (cities, coast between Ho Chi Minh and Hanoi, and Mekong River until close to Cambodian border; *substantial risk* in other areas, see below):

chemoprophylaxis not recommended but avoid mosquito bites and consider malaria if fever presents

Variable risk Risk *variable* and *some chloroquine resistance* in Indonesia (*very low risk* in Bali, and cities but *substantial risk* in Irian Jaya [West Papua] and Lombok, see below), rural Philippines below 600 m (no risk in cities, Cebu, Bohol, and Catanduanes), deep forests of peninsular Malaysia and Sarawak (but *substantial risk* in Sabah, see below):

chloroquine + proguanil hydrochloride *or* (if chloroquine + proguanil not appropriate) mefloquine *or Malarone®*

Substantial risk Risk *substantial* and *drug resistance common* in Cambodia (no risk in Phnom Penh; for western provinces, see below), China (Yunnan and Hainan; *chloroquine prophylaxis* appropriate for other remote areas; see also *Very low risk* above), East Timor, Irian Jaya [West Papua], Laos (no risk in Vientiane), Lombok, Malaysia (Sabah; see also *Very low risk* and *Variable risk* above), Myanmar (formerly Burma; see also *Great risk* below), Vietnam (*very low risk* in some areas, see above):

mefloquine *or* doxycycline *or Malarone®*

Great risk and drug resistance present Risk *great and widespread chloroquine and mefloquine resistance present* in western provinces of Cambodia, borders of Thailand with Cambodia, Laos and Myanmar (*very low risk* in Chang Ri and Kwai Bridge, see above), Myanmar (eastern Shan State):

doxycycline *or Malarone®*

Oceania

Risk Risk *high* and *chloroquine resistance high* in Papua New Guinea (below 1800 m), Solomon Islands, Vanuatu:

doxycycline *or* mefloquine *or Malarone®*

Central and South America and the Caribbean

Variable to low risk Risk *variable to low* in Argentina (rural areas along northern borders only), rural Belize (except Belize district), rural Costa Rica (below 500 m), Dominican Republic, El Salvador (Santa Ana province in west), Guatemala (below 1500 m), Haiti, Honduras, Mexico (states of Oaxaca and Chiapas), Nicaragua, Panama (west of Panama Canal but *variable to high risk* east of Panama Canal, see below), rural Paraguay:

chloroquine *or* (if chloroquine not appropriate) proguanil hydrochloride

Variable to high risk Risk *variable to high* and *chloroquine resistance present* in rural areas of Bolivia (below 2500 m), Ecuador (below 1500 m; no malaria in Galapagos Islands and Guayaquil; see below for Esmeraldas Province), Panama (east of Panama Canal), Peru (rural areas east of the Andes and west of the Amazon basin area below 1500 m; see below for Amazon basin area), Venezuela (north of Orinoco river; *high risk* south of and including Orinoco river and Amazon basin area, see below; Caracas free of malaria):

chloroquine + proguanil hydrochloride *or* (if chloroquine + proguanil not appropriate) mefloquine *or* doxycycline *or Malarone®*

High risk Risk *high* and *marked chloroquine resistance* in Bolivia (Amazon basin area; see also *variable to high risk* above), Brazil (throughout 'Legal Amazon' area which includes the Amazon basin area, Mato Grosso and Maranhao only; elsewhere *very low risk*—no chemoprophylaxis), Colombia (most areas below 800 m), Ecuador (Esmeraldas Province; *variable to high risk* in other areas, see above), French Guiana, all interior regions of Guyana, Peru (Amazon basin area), Suriname (except Paramaribo and coast), Venezuela (Amazon basin area, areas south of and including Orinoco river):

mefloquine *or* doxycycline *or Malarone®*

Standby treatment

Travellers visiting remote, malarious areas for prolonged periods should carry standby treatment if they are likely to be more than 24 hours away from medical care. Self-medication should be **avoided** if medical help is accessible.

In order to avoid excessive self-medication, the traveller should be provided with **written instructions** that urgent medical attention should be sought if fever (38°C or more) develops 7 days (or more) after arriving in a malarious area and that self-treatment is indicated if medical help is not available within 24 hours of fever onset.

In view of the continuing emergence of resistant strains and of the different regimens required for different areas expert advice should be sought on the best treatment course for an individual traveller.

A drug used for chemoprophylaxis should not be considered for standby treatment for the same traveller.

5 Infections

Artemether with lumefantrine

Artemether with lumefantrine is licensed for the *treatment of acute uncomplicated falciparum malaria.*

ARTEMETHER WITH LUMEFANTRINE

Indications treatment of acute uncomplicated falciparum malaria; treatment of benign malaria [unlicensed indication]

Cautions electrolyte disturbances, concomitant use with other drugs known to cause QT-interval prolongation; hepatic impairment (Appendix 2); renal impairment (Appendix 3); pregnancy (Appendix 4); monitor patients unable to take food (greater risk of recrudescence); **interactions**: Appendix 1 (artemether with lumefantrine)

Driving Dizziness may affect performance of skilled tasks (e.g. driving)

Contra-indications history of arrhythmias, of clinically relevant bradycardia, and of congestive heart failure accompanied by reduced left ventricular ejection fraction; family history of sudden death or of congenital QT interval prolongation; breast-feeding (Appendix 5)

Side-effects abdominal pain, anorexia, diarrhoea, vomiting, nausea; palpitation; cough; headache, dizziness, sleep disturbances, asthenia, paraesthesia; arthralgia, myalgia; pruritus, rash; *less commonly* ataxia, hypoaesthesia

Dose

- Treatment of malaria, see p. 344

Riamet® (Novartis) ▼ PoM

Tablets, yellow, artemether 20 mg, lumefantrine 120 mg, net price 24-tab pack = £22.50. Label: 21, counselling, driving

Note Tablets may be crushed just before administration

Chloroquine

Chloroquine is used for the *prophylaxis of malaria* in areas of the world where the *risk of chloroquine-resistant falciparum malaria is still low.* It is also used with proguanil when chloroquine-resistant falciparum malaria is present but this regimen may not give optimal protection (see specific recommendations by country, p. 346). Chloroquine is **no longer recommended** for the *treatment of falciparum malaria* owing to widespread resistance, nor is it recommended if the infective species is *not known* or if the infection is *mixed*; in these cases treatment should be with quinine, *Malarone®*, or *Riamet®* (for details, see p. 344). It is still recommended for the *treatment of benign malarias* (for details, see p. 345).

CHLOROQUINE

Indications chemoprophylaxis and treatment of malaria; rheumatoid arthritis and lupus erythematosus (section 10.1.3)

Cautions renal impairment (see notes above), pregnancy (but for malaria benefit outweighs risk, see Appendix 4, Antimalarials), may exacerbate psoriasis, neurological disorders (avoid for prophylaxis if history of epilepsy, see notes above), may aggravate myasthenia gravis, severe gastro-intestinal disorders, G6PD deficiency (see section 9.1.5); ophthalmic examination and long-term therapy, see under Chloroquine, section 10.1.3; avoid concurrent therapy with hepatotoxic drugs—other **interactions**: Appendix 1 (chloroquine and hydroxychloroquine)

Side-effects gastro-intestinal disturbances, headache; also hypotension, convulsions, visual disturbances, depigmentation or loss of hair, skin reactions (rashes, pruritus); rarely, bone-marrow suppression, hypersensitivity reactions such as urticaria and angioedema; other side-effects (not usually associated with malaria prophylaxis or treatment), see under Chloroquine, section 10.1.3; very toxic in **overdosage**—immediate advice from poisons centres essential (see also p. 32)

Dose

Note Doses expressed as chloroquine base

- Prophylaxis of malaria, preferably started 1 week before entering endemic area and continued for 4 weeks after leaving (see notes above), 300 mg once weekly; INFANT up to 12 weeks body-weight under 6 kg, 37.5 mg once weekly; 12 weeks–1 year body-weight 6–10 kg, 75 mg once weekly; CHILD 1–4 years body-weight 10–16 kg, 112.5 mg once weekly; 4–8 years body-weight 16–25 kg, 150 mg once weekly; 8–13 years body-weight 25–45 kg, 225 mg once weekly; over 13 years body-weight over 45 kg, adult dose
- Treatment of benign malarias, see p. 345

Counselling Warn travellers about **importance** of avoiding mosquito bites, **importance** of taking prophylaxis regularly, and **importance** of immediate visit to doctor if ill within 1 year and **especially** within 3 months of return. For details, see notes above

Note Chloroquine doses in BNF may differ from those in product literature

Chloroquine sulphate (Beacon) PoM

Injection, chloroquine sulphate 54.5 mg/mL (≡ chloroquine base 40 mg/mL), net price 5-mL amp = 79p

[1]**Avloclor®** (AstraZeneca) PoM

Tablets, scored, chloroquine phosphate 250 mg (≡ chloroquine base 155 mg). Net price 20-tab pack = £1.22. Label: 5, counselling, prophylaxis, see above

[1]**Malarivon®** (Wallace Mfg) PoM

Syrup, chloroquine phosphate 30 mg/5 mL (≡ chloroquine base 50 mg/5 mL), net price 75 mL = £3.35. Label: 5, counselling, prophylaxis, see above

[2]**Nivaquine®** (Beacon)

Syrup, golden, chloroquine sulphate 68 mg/5 mL (≡ chloroquine base 50 mg/5 mL), net price 100 mL = £5.15. Label: 5, counselling, prophylaxis, see above

With proguanil

For cautions and side-effects of proguanil see Proguanil; for dose see Chloroquine and Proguanil

[2]**Paludrine/Avloclor®** (AstraZeneca)

Tablets, travel pack of 14 tablets of chloroquine phosphate 250 mg (≡ chloroquine base 155 mg) and 98 tablets of proguanil hydrochloride 100 mg, net price 112-tab pack = £8.79. Label: 5, 21, counselling, prophylaxis, see above

1. Can be sold to the public provided it is licensed and labelled for the prophylaxis of malaria. Drugs for malaria prophylaxis not prescribable on the NHS; health authorities may investigate circumstances under which antimalarials are prescribed
2. Drugs for malaria prophylaxis not prescribable on the NHS; health authorities may investigate circumstances under which antimalarials prescribed

Mefloquine

Mefloquine is used for the *prophylaxis of malaria* in areas of the world where there is a *high risk of chloroquine-resistant falciparum malaria* (for details, see specific recommendations by country, p. 346).

Mefloquine is now rarely used for the *treatment of falciparum malaria* because of increased resistance. It is rarely used for the treatment of benign malarias because better tolerated alternatives are available. Mefloquine should not be used for treatment if it has been used for prophylaxis.

The CSM has advised that travellers should be informed about adverse reactions of mefloquine and, if they occur, medical advice should be sought on alternative antimalarials before the next dose is due; the patient information leaflet, which describes adverse reactions should always be provided when dispensing mefloquine.

MEFLOQUINE

Indications chemoprophylaxis of malaria, treatment of malaria, see notes above

Cautions pregnancy (see notes under Prophylaxis against malaria; Appendix 4)—manufacturer advises **avoid** pregnancy during and for 3 months after; breast-feeding (Appendix 5); avoid for chemoprophylaxis in severe hepatic impairment; cardiac conduction disorders; epilepsy (avoid for prophylaxis); not recommended in infants under 3 months (5 kg); **interactions:** Appendix 1 (mefloquine)

Driving Dizziness or a disturbed sense of balance may affect performance of skilled tasks (e.g. driving); effects may persist for up to 3 weeks

Contra-indications hypersensitivity to quinine; avoid for prophylaxis if history of psychiatric disorders (including depression) or convulsions

Side-effects nausea, vomiting, diarrhoea, abdominal pain; dizziness, loss of balance, headache, sleep disorders (insomnia, drowsiness, abnormal dreams); also neuropsychiatric reactions (including sensory and motor neuropathies, tremor, ataxia, anxiety, depression, suicidal ideation, panic attacks, agitation, hallucinations, psychosis, convulsions), tinnitus and vestibular disorders, visual disturbances, circulatory disorders (hypotension and hypertension), chest pain, tachycardia, bradycardia, cardiac conduction disorders, dyspnoea, muscle weakness, myalgia, arthralgia, rash, urticaria, pruritus, alopecia, asthenia, malaise, fatigue, fever, loss of appetite, leucopenia or leucocytosis, thrombocytopenia; rarely Stevens-Johnson syndrome, AV block, encephalopathy and anaphylaxis

Dose

- Prophylaxis of malaria, preferably started 2½ weeks before entering endemic area and continued for 4 weeks after leaving (see notes above), ADULT and CHILD body-weight over 45 kg, 250 mg once weekly; body-weight 6–16 kg, 62.5 mg once weekly; body-weight 16–25 kg, 125 mg once weekly; body-weight 25–45 kg, 187.5 mg once weekly
- Treatment of malaria, see notes above

Counselling See CSM advice in notes above. Also warn travellers about **importance** of avoiding mosquito bites, **importance** of taking prophylaxis regularly, and **importance** of immediate visit to doctor if ill within 1 year and **especially** within 3 months of return. For details, see notes above

Note Mefloquine doses in BNF may differ from those in product literature

[1]**Lariam**® (Roche) PoM
Tablets, scored, mefloquine (as hydrochloride) 250 mg. Net price 8-tab pack = £14.53. Label: 21, 25, 27, counselling, driving, prophylaxis, see above
Note Tablet may be crushed and mixed with food such as jam or honey just before administration

1. Drugs for malaria prophylaxis not prescribable on the NHS; health authorities may investigate circumstances under which antimalarials prescribed

Primaquine

Primaquine is used to eliminate the liver stages of *P. vivax or P. ovale following chloroquine treatment* (for details, see p. 345).

PRIMAQUINE

Indications adjunct in the treatment of *Plasmodium vivax* and *P. ovale* malaria (eradication of liver stages)

Cautions G6PD deficiency (test blood, see under Benign Malarias (treatment), p. 345); systemic diseases associated with granulocytopenia (e.g. rheumatoid arthritis, lupus erythematosus); pregnancy (Appendix 4) and breast-feeding; **interactions:** Appendix 1 (primaquine)

Side-effects nausea, vomiting, anorexia, abdominal pain; less commonly methaemoglobinaemia, haemolytic anaemia especially in G6PD deficiency, leucopenia

Dose

- Treatment of benign malarias, see p. 345

Primaquine (Non-proprietary)
Tablets, primaquine (as phosphate) 7.5 mg or 15 mg
Available on a named-patient basis from specialist importing companies, see p. 888

Proguanil

Proguanil is used (usually *with chloroquine*, but occasionally *alone*) for the *prophylaxis of malaria*, (for details, see specific recommendations by country, p. 346).

Proguanil used alone is not suitable for the *treatment of malaria*; however, *Malarone*® (a combination of atovaquone with proguanil) is licensed for the treatment of acute uncomplicated falciparum malaria. *Malarone*® is also used for the *prophylaxis of falciparum malaria* in areas of *widespread mefloquine or chloroquine resistance. Malarone*® is also used as an alternative to mefloquine or doxycycline. *Malarone*® is particularly suitable for short trips to highly chloroquine-resistant areas because it needs to be taken only for 7 days after leaving an endemic area.

PROGUANIL HYDROCHLORIDE

Indications chemoprophylaxis of malaria

Cautions renal impairment (see notes under Prophylaxis against malaria and Appendix 3); pregnancy (Appendix 4); **interactions:** Appendix 1 (proguanil)

Side-effects mild gastric intolerance, diarrhoea, and constipation; occasionally mouth ulcers and stomatitis; *very rarely* cholestasis, vasculitis, skin reactions, and hair loss

Dose

- Prophylaxis of malaria, preferably started 1 week before entering endemic area and continued for 4 weeks after leaving (see notes above), 200 mg once daily; INFANT up to 12 weeks body-weight under 6 kg, 25 mg once daily; 12 weeks–1 year body-weight 6–10 kg, 50 mg once daily; CHILD 1–4 years body-weight 10–16 kg, 75 mg once daily; 4–8 years body-weight 16–25 kg, 100 mg once daily; 8–13 years, body-weight 25–45 kg, 150 mg once daily; over 13 years body-weight over 45 kg, adult dose

Counselling Warn travellers about **importance** of avoiding mosquito bites, **importance** of taking prophylaxis regularly, and **importance** of immediate visit to doctor if ill within 1 year and **especially** within 3 months of return. For details, see notes above

Note Proguanil doses in BNF may differ from those in product literature.

[1]**Paludrine®** (AstraZeneca)
Tablets, scored, proguanil hydrochloride 100 mg. Net price 98-tab pack = £7.43. Label: 21, counselling, prophylaxis, see above
Note Tablet may be crushed and mixed with food such as milk, jam, or honey just before administration

With chloroquine
See under Chloroquine

PROGUANIL HYDROCHLORIDE WITH ATOVAQUONE

Indications treatment of acute uncomplicated falciparum malaria and prophylaxis of falciparum malaria, particularly where resistance to other antimalarial drugs suspected; treatment of benign malaria [unlicensed indication]

Cautions diarrhoea or vomiting (reduced absorption of atovaquone); efficacy not evaluated in cerebral or complicated malaria (including hyperparasitaemia, pulmonary oedema or renal failure); renal impairment (Appendix 3); pregnancy (Appendix 4); breast-feeding (Appendix 5); **interactions**: see Appendix 1 (proguanil, atovaquone)

Side-effects abdominal pain, nausea, vomiting, diarrhoea; cough; headache, dizziness, insomnia, abnormal dreams, anorexia, fever; rash, pruritus; *less frequently* mouth ulcers, stomatitis, blood disorders, hyponatraemia, and hair loss; also reported, hepatitis, cholestasis, and vasculitis

Dose

- See preparations

Counselling Warn travellers about **importance** of avoiding mosquito bites, **importance** of taking prophylaxis regularly, and **importance** of immediate visit to doctor if ill within 1 year and **especially** within 3 months of return. For details, see notes above

[1]**Malarone®** (GSK) PoM
Tablets ('standard'), pink, f/c, proguanil hydrochloride 100 mg, atovaquone 250 mg. Net price 12-tab pack = £22.92. Label: 21, counselling, prophylaxis, see above
Dose prophylaxis of malaria, started 1–2 days before entering endemic area and continued for 1 week after leaving, ADULT and CHILD over 40 kg, 1 tablet daily
Treatment of malaria, ADULT and CHILD body-weight over 40 kg, 4 tablets once daily for 3 days; CHILD body-weight 11–21 kg 1 tablet daily for 3 days; body-weight 21–31 kg 2 tablets once daily for 3 days; body-weight 31–40 kg 3 tablets once daily for 3 days

[1]**Malarone® Paediatric** (GSK) ▼ PoM
Paediatric tablets, pink, f/c proguanil hydrochloride 25 mg, atovaquone 62.5 mg, net price 12-tab pack = £7.64. Label: 21, counselling, prophylaxis, see above
Dose prophylaxis of malaria, started 1–2 days before entering endemic area and continued for 1 week after leaving, CHILD body-weight 11–21 kg, 1 tablet once daily; body-weight 21–31 kg, 2 tablets once daily; body-weight 31–40 kg, 3 tablets once daily; body-weight over 40 kg use *Malarone®* ('standard') tablets
Treatment of malaria, CHILD body-weight 5–9 kg, 2 tablets once daily for 3 days; body-weight 9–11 kg, 3 tablets once daily for 3 days; body-weight 11 kg and over use *Malarone®* ('standard') tablets
Note Tablets may be crushed and mixed with food or milky drink just before administration

Pyrimethamine

Pyrimethamine should not be used alone, but is used with sulfadoxine (in *Fansidar®*).

Fansidar® is not recommended for the *prophylaxis of malaria*, but it is used in the treatment of *falciparum malaria* and can be used *with (or following) quinine.*

PYRIMETHAMINE

Indications malaria (but used only in combined preparations incorporating sulfadoxine); toxoplasmosis—section 5.4.7

Cautions hepatic or renal impairment, pregnancy (Appendix 4); breast-feeding (Appendix 5); blood counts required with prolonged treatment; history of seizures—avoid large loading doses; **interactions:** Appendix 1 (pyrimethamine)

Side-effects depression of haematopoiesis with high doses, rashes, insomnia

Dose

- Malaria, no dose stated because not recommended alone, see Pyrimethamine with Sulfadoxine below
- Toxoplasmosis, section 5.4.7

Daraprim® (GSK) PoM
Tablets, scored, pyrimethamine 25 mg. Net price 30-tab pack = £2.17

PYRIMETHAMINE WITH SULFADOXINE

Indications adjunct to quinine in treatment of *Plasmodium falciparum* malaria; **not** recommended for prophylaxis

Cautions see under Pyrimethamine and under Co-trimoxazole (section 5.1.8); pregnancy (Appendix 4); breast-feeding (Appendix 5); not recommended for prophylaxis (severe side-effects on long-term use); **interactions:** Appendix 1 (pyrimethamine, sulphonamides)

Contra-indications see under Pyrimethamine and under Co-trimoxazole (section 5.1.8); sulphonamide allergy

Side-effects see under Pyrimethamine and under Co-trimoxazole (section 5.1.8); pulmonary infiltrates (e.g. eosinophilic or allergic alveolitis) reported—discontinue if cough or shortness of breath

Dose

- Treatment of falciparum malaria, see p. 344
- Prophylaxis, not recommended by UK malaria experts

1. Drugs for malaria prophylaxis not prescribable on the NHS; health authorities may investigate circumstances under which antimalarials prescribed

Fansidar® (Roche) PoM
Tablets, scored, pyrimethamine 25 mg, sulfadoxine 500 mg, net price 3-tab pack = 74p

Quinine

Quinine is not suitable for the *prophylaxis of malaria.*

Quinine is used for the *treatment of falciparum malaria* or if the infective species is *not known* or if the infection is *mixed* (for details see p. 344).

QUININE

Indications falciparum malaria; nocturnal leg cramps, see section 10.2.2

Cautions cardiac disease (including atrial fibrillation, conduction defects, heart block), elderly—monitor ECG during parenteral treatment; renal impairment (Appendix 3); pregnancy (but appropriate for treatment of malaria; Appendix 4); monitor blood glucose and electrolyte concentration during parenteral treatment; G6PD deficiency (see section 9.1.5); **interactions**: Appendix 1 (quinine)

Contra-indications haemoglobinuria, myasthenia gravis, optic neuritis

Side-effects cinchonism, including tinnitus, headache, hot and flushed skin, nausea, abdominal pain, rashes, visual disturbances (including temporary blindness), confusion; hypersensitivity reactions including angioedema, blood disorders (including thrombocytopenia and intravascular coagulation), and acute renal failure; hypoglycaemia (especially after parenteral administration); cardiovascular effects (see Cautions); very toxic in **overdosage**—immediate advice from poisons centres essential (see also p. 32)

Dose

- Treatment of malaria, see p. 344

Note Quinine (anhydrous base) 100 mg ≡ quinine bisulphate 169 mg ≡ quinine dihydrochloride 122 mg ≡ quinine hydrochloride 122 mg ≡ quinine sulphate 121 mg. Quinine bisulphate 300-mg tablets are available but provide less quinine than 300 mg of the dihydrochloride, hydrochloride, or sulphate

Quinine Sulphate (Non-proprietary) PoM
Tablets, coated, quinine sulphate 200 mg, net price 28-tab pack = £1.94; 300 mg, 28-tab pack = £1.86

Quinine Dihydrochloride (Non-proprietary) PoM
Injection, quinine dihydrochloride 300 mg/mL. For dilution and use as an infusion. 1- and 2-mL amps
'Special order' product; contact Martindale or specialist centres (see p. 344)
Note Intravenous injection of quinine is so hazardous that it has been superseded by infusion

Tetracyclines

Doxycycline (section 5.1.3) is used for the *prophylaxis of malaria* in areas of *widespread mefloquine or chloroquine resistance.* Doxycycline is also used as an alternative to mefloquine or *Malarone®* (for details, see specific recommendations by country, p. 346).

Doxycycline is also used as an *adjunct to quinine in the treatment of falciparum malaria* (for details see p. 344).

DOXYCYCLINE

Indications prophylaxis of malaria; adjunct to quinine in treatment of *Plasmodium falciparum* malaria; see also section 5.1.3

Cautions section 5.1.3

Contra-indications section 5.1.3

Side-effects section 5.1.3

Dose

- Prophylaxis of malaria, started 1–2 days before entering endemic area and continued for 4 weeks after leaving (see notes above), 100 mg once daily
- Treatment of falciparum malaria, see p. 344

Preparations
Section 5.1.3

5.4.2 Amoebicides

Metronidazole is the drug of choice for *acute invasive amoebic dysentery* since it is very effective against vegetative forms of *Entamoeba histolytica* in ulcers; it is given in an adult dose of 800 mg three times daily for 5 days. **Tinidazole** is also effective. Metronidazole and tinidazole are also active against amoebae which may have migrated to the liver. Treatment with metronidazole (or tinidazole) is followed by a 10-day course of diloxanide furoate.

Diloxanide furoate is the drug of choice for asymptomatic patients with *E. histolytica* cysts in the faeces; metronidazole and tinidazole are relatively ineffective. Diloxanide furoate is relatively free from toxic effects and the usual course is of 10 days, given alone for chronic infections or following metronidazole or tinidazole treatment.

For *amoebic abscesses* of the liver **metronidazole** is effective; tinidazole is an alternative. Aspiration of the abscess is indicated where it is suspected that it may rupture or where there is no improvement after 72 hours of metronidazole; the aspiration may need to be repeated. Aspiration aids penetration of metronidazole and, for abscesses with more than 100 mL of pus, if carried out in conjunction with drug therapy, may reduce the period of disability.

Diloxanide furoate is not effective against hepatic amoebiasis, but a 10-day course should be given at the completion of metronidazole or tinidazole treatment to destroy any amoebae in the gut.

DILOXANIDE FUROATE

Indications see notes above; chronic amoebiasis and as adjunct to metronidazole or tinidazole in acute amoebiasis

Contra-indications pregnancy (Appendix 4), breast-feeding (Appendix 5)

Side-effects flatulence, vomiting, urticaria, pruritus

Dose

- 500 mg every 8 hours for 10 days; CHILD over 25 kg, 20 mg/kg daily in 3 divided doses for 10 days
  See also notes above

Diloxanide (Sovereign) PoM
Tablets, diloxanide furoate 500 mg, net price 30-tab pack = £42.95. Label: 9

METRONIDAZOLE

Indications see under Dose below; anaerobic infections, section 5.1.11

Cautions section 5.1.11

Side-effects section 5.1.11

Dose

- By mouth, invasive intestinal amoebiasis, 800 mg every 8 hours for 5 days; CHILD 1–3 years 200 mg every 8 hours; 3–7 years 200 mg every 6 hours; 7–10 years 400 mg every 8 hours

  Extra-intestinal amoebiasis (including liver abscess), 400–800 mg every 8 hours for 5–10 days; CHILD 1–3 years 100–200 mg every 8 hours; 3–7 years 100–200 mg every 6 hours; 7–10 years 200–400 mg every 8 hours

  Urogenital trichomoniasis, 200 mg every 8 hours for 7 days *or* 400–500 mg every 12 hours for 5–7 days, *or* 2 g as a single dose; CHILD 1–3 years 50 mg every 8 hours for 7 days; 3–7 years 100 mg every 12 hours; 7–10 years 100 mg every 8 hours

  Giardiasis, 2 g daily for 3 days *or* 400 mg 3 times daily for 5 days *or* 500 mg twice daily for 7–10 days; CHILD 1–3 years 500 mg daily for 3 days; 3–7 years 600–800 mg daily; 7–10 years 1 g daily

Preparations

Section 5.1.11

TINIDAZOLE

Indications see under Dose below; anaerobic infections, section 5.1.11

Cautions section 5.1.11

Side-effects section 5.1.11

Dose

- Intestinal amoebiasis, 2 g daily for 2–3 days; CHILD 50–60 mg/kg daily for 3 days
- Amoebic involvement of liver, 1.5–2 g daily for 3–6 days; CHILD 50–60 mg/kg daily for 5 days
- Urogenital trichomoniasis and giardiasis, single 2 g dose; CHILD single dose of 50–75 mg/kg (repeated once if necessary)

Preparations

Section 5.1.11

5.4.3 Trichomonacides

Metronidazole (section 5.4.2) is the treatment of choice for *Trichomonas vaginalis* infection. Contact tracing is recommended and sexual contacts should be treated simultaneously. If metronidazole is ineffective, **tinidazole** (section 5.4.2) may be tried.

5.4.4 Antigiardial drugs

Metronidazole (section 5.4.2) is the treatment of choice for *Giardia lamblia* infections. Alternative treatments are **tinidazole** (section 5.4.2) or **mepacrine hydrochloride**.

MEPACRINE HYDROCHLORIDE

Indications giardiasis; discoid lupus erythematosus (Antimalarials, section 10.1.3)

Cautions hepatic impairment, elderly, history of psychosis; avoid in psoriasis; **interactions**: Appendix 1 (mepacrine)

Side-effects gastro-intestinal disturbances; dizziness, headache; with large doses nausea, vomiting and occasionally transient acute toxic psychosis and CNS stimulation; on prolonged treatment yellow discoloration of skin and urine, chronic dermatoses (including severe exfoliative dermatitis), hepatitis, aplastic anaemia; also reported blue/black discoloration of palate and nails and corneal deposits with visual disturbances

Dose

- Giardiasis, 100 mg every 8 hours for 5–7 days

Mepacrine Hydrochloride

Tablets, mepacrine hydrochloride 100 mg. Label: 4, 9, 14, 21

Available from BCM Specials [unlicensed—special order]

5.4.5 Leishmaniacides

Cutaneous leishmaniasis frequently heals spontaneously but if skin lesions are extensive or unsightly, treatment is indicated, as it is in visceral leishmaniasis (kala-azar).

Sodium stibogluconate, an organic pentavalent antimony compound, is the treatment of choice for visceral leishmaniasis. The dose is 20 mg/kg daily (max. 850 mg) for at least 20 days by intramuscular or intravenous injection; the dosage varies with different geographical regions and expert advice should be obtained. Skin lesions can also be treated with sodium stibogluconate.

Amphotericin is used with or after an antimony compound for visceral leishmaniasis unresponsive to the antimonial alone; side-effects may be reduced by using liposomal amphotericin (*AmBisome®*—section 5.2) at a dose of 1–3 mg/kg daily for 10–21 days to a cumulative dose of 21–30 mg/kg *or* at a dose of 3 mg/kg for 5 consecutive days followed by a single dose of 3 mg/kg 6 days later. Other lipid formulations of amphotericin (*Abelcet®* and *Amphocil®*) are also likely to be effective but less information is available.

Pentamidine isetionate (pentamidine isethionate) (section 5.4.8) has been used in antimony-resistant visceral leishmaniasis, but although the initial response is often good, the relapse rate is high; it is associated with serious side-effects. Other treatments include paromomycin (available on named-patient basis from specialist importing companies, see p. 888).

SODIUM STIBOGLUCONATE

Indications leishmaniasis

Cautions intravenous injections must be given slowly over 5 minutes (to reduce risk of local thrombosis) and stopped if coughing or substernal pain; mucocutaneous disease (see below); monitor ECG before and during treatment; heart disease (withdraw if conduction disturbances occur); treat intercurrent infection (e.g. pneumonia); hepatic impairment; pregnancy (Appendix 4); breast-feeding (Appendix 5)

Mucocutaneous disease Successful treatment of mucocutaneous leishmaniasis may induce severe inflammation around the lesions (may be life-threatening if pharyngeal or tracheal involvement)—may require corticosteroid

Contra-indications significant renal impairment

Side-effects anorexia, nausea, vomiting, abdominal pain, diarrhoea; ECG changes; coughing (see Cautions); headache, lethargy; arthralgia, myalgia; *rarely* jaundice, flushing, bleeding from nose or gum, substernal pain (see Cautions), vertigo, fever, sweating, and rash; also reported pancreatitis and anaphylaxis; pain and thrombosis on intravenous administration, intramuscular injection also painful

Dose

- See notes above

Pentostam® (GSK) PoM

Injection, sodium stibogluconate equivalent to pentavalent antimony 100 mg/mL. Net price 100-mL bottle = £66.43

Note Injection should be filtered immediately before administration using a filter of 5 microns or less

5.4.6 Trypanocides

The prophylaxis and treatment of trypanosomiasis is difficult and differs according to the strain of organism. Expert advice should therefore be obtained.

5.4.7 Drugs for toxoplasmosis

Most infections caused by *Toxoplasma gondii* are self-limiting, and treatment is not necessary. Exceptions are patients with eye involvement (toxoplasma chorioidoretinitis), and those who are immunosuppressed. Toxoplasmic encephalitis is a common complication of AIDS. The treatment of choice is a combination of pyrimethamine and sulfadiazine (sulphadiazine), given for several weeks (expert advice **essential**). Pyrimethamine is a folate antagonist, and adverse reactions to this combination are relatively common (folinic acid supplements and weekly blood counts needed). Alternative regimens use combinations of pyrimethamine with clindamycin or clarithromycin or azithromycin. Long-term secondary prophylaxis is required after treatment of toxoplasmosis in immunocompromised patients; prophylaxis should continue until immunity recovers.

If toxoplasmosis is acquired in pregnancy, transplacental infection may lead to severe disease in the fetus. Spiramycin (available on named-patient basis from specialist importing companies, see p. 888) may reduce the risk of transmission of maternal infection to the fetus.

5.4.8 Drugs for pneumocystis pneumonia

Pneumonia caused by *Pneumocystis jiroveci (Pneumocystis carinii)* occurs in immunosuppressed patients; it is a common cause of pneumonia in AIDS. Pneumocystis pneumonia should generally be treated by those experienced in its management. Blood gas measurement is used to assess disease severity.

Treatment

Mild to moderate disease **Co-trimoxazole** (section 5.1.8) in high dosage is the drug of choice for the treatment of mild to moderate pneumocystis pneumonia.

Atovaquone is licensed for the treatment of mild to moderate pneumocystis infection in patients who cannot tolerate co-trimoxazole. A combination of **dapsone** 100 mg daily (section 5.1.10) with **trimethoprim** 5 mg/kg every 6–8 hours (section 5.1.8) is given by mouth for the treatment of mild to moderate disease [unlicensed indication].

A combination of **clindamycin** 600 mg by mouth every 8 hours (section 5.1.6) and **primaquine** 30 mg daily by mouth (section 5.4.1) is used in the treatment of mild to moderate disease [unlicensed indication]; this combination is associated with considerable toxicity.

Inhaled **pentamidine isetionate** is sometimes used for mild disease. It is better tolerated than parenteral pentamidine but systemic absorption may still occur.

Severe disease **Co-trimoxazole** (section 5.1.8) in high dosage, given by mouth or by intravenous infusion, is the drug of choice for the treatment of severe pneumocystis pneumonia. **Pentamidine isetionate** given by intravenous infusion is an alternative for patients who cannot tolerate co-trimoxazole, or who have not responded to it. Pentamidine isetionate is a potentially toxic drug that can cause severe hypotension during or immediately after infusion.

Corticosteroid treatment can be lifesaving in those with severe pneumocystis pneumonia (see Adjunctive Therapy below).

Adjunctive therapy In moderate to severe infections associated with HIV infection, prednisolone 50–80 mg daily is given by mouth for 5 days (alternatively, hydrocortisone may be given parenterally); the dose is then reduced to complete 21 days of treatment. Corticosteroid treatment should ideally be started at the same time as the anti-pneumocystis therapy and certainly no later than 24–72 hours afterwards. The corticosteroid should be withdrawn before anti-pneumocystis treatment is complete.

Prophylaxis

Prophylaxis against pneumocystis pneumonia should be given to all patients with a history of the infection. Prophylaxis against pneumocystis pneumonia should also be considered for severely immunocompromised patients. Prophylaxis should continue until immunity recovers sufficiently. It should not be discontinued if the patient has oral candidiasis, continues to lose weight, or is receiving cytotoxic therapy or long-term immunosuppressant therapy.

Co-trimoxazole by mouth is the drug of choice for prophylaxis against pneumocystis pneumonia. It is given in a dose of 960 mg daily or 960 mg on alternate days (3 times a week); the dose may be reduced to co-trimoxazole 480 mg daily to improve tolerance.

Intermittent inhalation of **pentamidine isetionate** is used for prophylaxis against pneumocystis pneumonia in patients unable to tolerate co-trimoxazole. It is effective but patients may be prone to extrapulmonary infection. Alternatively, **dapsone** 100 mg daily (section 5.1.10) can be used. **Atovaquone** 750 mg twice daily has also been used for prophylaxis [unlicensed indication].

ATOVAQUONE

Indications treatment of mild to moderate *Pneumocystis jiroveci (Pneumocystis carinii)* pneumonia in patients intolerant of co-trimoxazole

Cautions initial diarrhoea and difficulty in taking with food may reduce absorption (and require alternative therapy); other causes of pulmonary disease should be sought and treated; elderly; hepatic impairment (Appendix 2); renal impairment (Appendix 3); pregnancy (Appendix 4); avoid breast-feeding (Appendix 5); **interactions:** Appendix 1 (atovaquone)

Side-effects nausea, diarrhoea, vomiting; headache, insomnia; fever; anaemia, neutropenia, hyponatraemia; rash

Dose

- 750 mg twice daily with food (particularly high fat) for 21 days; CHILD not recommended

Wellvone® (GSK) PoM
Suspension, sugar-free, atovaquone 750 mg/5 mL, net price 210 mL (tutti-frutti-flavoured) = £405.31. Label: 21

With proguanil hydrochloride
See section 5.4.1

PENTAMIDINE ISETIONATE

Indications see under Dose (should only be given by specialists)

Cautions risk of severe hypotension following administration (establish baseline blood pressure and administer with patient lying down; monitor blood pressure closely during administration, and at regular intervals, until treatment concluded); hypokalaemia, hypomagnesaemia, coronary heart disease, bradycardia, history of ventricular arrhythmias, concomitant use with other drugs which prolong QT-interval; hypertension or hypotension; hyperglycaemia or hypoglycaemia; leucopenia, thrombocytopenia, or anaemia; carry out laboratory monitoring according to product literature; care required to protect personnel during handling and administration; hepatic impairment; renal impairment (Appendix 3); pregnancy (Appendix 4); breast-feeding (Appendix 5); **interactions:** Appendix 1 (pentamidine isetionate)

Side-effects severe reactions, sometimes fatal, due to hypotension, hypoglycaemia, pancreatitis, and arrhythmias; also leucopenia, thrombocytopenia, acute renal failure, hypocalcaemia; also reported: azotaemia, abnormal liver-function tests, anaemia, hyperkalaemia, nausea and vomiting, dizziness, syncope, flushing, hyperglycaemia, rash, and taste disturbances; Stevens-Johnson syndrome reported; on inhalation, bronchoconstriction (may be prevented by prior use of bronchodilators), cough, and shortness of breath; discomfort, pain, induration, abscess formation, and muscle necrosis at injection site

Dose

- *Pneumocystis jiroveci (Pneumocystis carinii)* pneumonia, by intravenous infusion, 4 mg/kg once daily for at least 14 days (reduced according to product literature in renal impairment)

  By inhalation of nebulised solution (using suitable equipment—consult product literature) 600 mg pentamidine isetionate once daily for 3 weeks; secondary prevention, 300 mg every 4 weeks *or* 150 mg every 2 weeks
- Visceral leishmaniasis (kala-azar, section 5.4.5), by deep intramuscular injection, 3–4 mg/kg on alternate days to max. total of 10 injections; course may be repeated if necessary
- Cutaneous leishmaniasis, by deep intramuscular injection, 3–4 mg/kg once or twice weekly until condition resolves (but see also section 5.4.5)
- Trypanosomiasis, by deep intramuscular injection *or* intravenous infusion, 4 mg/kg daily or on alternate days to total of 7–10 injections

Note Direct intravenous injection should be avoided whenever possible and **never** given rapidly; intramuscular injections should be deep and preferably given into the buttock

Pentacarinat® (JHC) PoM
Injection, powder for reconstitution, pentamidine isetionate, net price 300-mg vial = £30.45
Nebuliser solution, pentamidine isetionate, net price 300-mg bottle = £32.15

Caution in handling Pentamidine isetionate is toxic and personnel should be adequately protected during handling and administration—consult product literature

5.5 Anthelmintics

5.5.1 Drugs for threadworms
5.5.2 Ascaricides
5.5.3 Drugs for tapeworm infections
5.5.4 Drugs for hookworms
5.5.5 Schistosomicides
5.5.6 Filaricides
5.5.7 Drugs for cutaneous larva migrans
5.5.8 Drugs for strongyloidiasis

Advice on prophylaxis and treatment of helminth infections is available from:

Birmingham	(0121) 424 0357
Scottish Centre for Infection and Environmental Health (registered users of Travax only)	(0141) 300 1100 (weekdays 2–4 p.m. only)
Liverpool	(0151) 708 9393
London	(020) 7387 9300 (treatment)

5.5.1 Drugs for threadworms (pinworms, Enterobius vermicularis)

Anthelmintics are effective in threadworm infections, but their use needs to be combined with hygienic measures to break the cycle of auto-infection. All members of the family require treatment.

Adult threadworms do not live for longer than 6 weeks and for development of fresh worms, ova must be swallowed and exposed to the action of digestive juices in the upper intestinal tract. Direct multiplication of worms does not take place in the large bowel. Adult female worms lay ova on the perianal skin which causes pruritus; scratching the area then leads to ova being transmitted on fingers to the mouth, often via food eaten with unwashed hands. Washing hands and scrubbing nails before each meal and after each visit to the toilet is essential. A bath taken immediately after rising will remove ova laid during the night.

Mebendazole is the drug of choice for treating threadworm infection in patients of all ages over 2 years. It is given as a single dose; as reinfection is very common, a second dose may be given after 2 weeks.

Piperazine is available in combination with sennosides as a single-dose preparation.

MEBENDAZOLE

Indications threadworm, roundworm, whipworm, and hookworm infections

Cautions pregnancy (toxicity in *rats*); breast-feeding (Appendix 5); **interactions:** Appendix 1 (mebendazole)

Note The package insert in the *Vermox®* pack includes the statement that it is not suitable for women known to be pregnant or children under 2 years

Side-effects *very rarely* abdominal pain, diarrhoea, convulsions (in infants) and rash (including Stevens-Johnson syndrome and toxic epidermal necrolysis)

Dose

- Threadworms, ADULT and CHILD over 2 years, 100 mg as a single dose; if reinfection occurs second dose may be needed after 2 weeks; CHILD under 2 years, see *BNF for Children*
- Whipworms, ADULT and CHILD over 2 years, 100 mg twice daily for 3 days; CHILD under 2 years, see *BNF for Children*
- Roundworms—section 5.5.2
- Hookworms—section 5.5.4

[1]**Mebendazole** (Non-proprietary) PoM

Tablets, chewable, mebendazole 100 mg

1. Mebendazole tablets can be sold to the public if supplied for oral use in the treatment of enterobiasis in adults and children over 2 years provided its container or package is labelled to show a max. single dose of 100 mg and it is supplied in a container or package containing not more than 800 mg

Vermox® (Janssen-Cilag) PoM

Tablets, orange, scored, chewable, mebendazole 100 mg. Net price 6-tab pack = £1.42

Suspension, mebendazole 100 mg/5 mL. Net price 30 mL = £1.65

PIPERAZINE

Indications threadworm and roundworm infections

Cautions hepatic impairment (Appendix 2); renal impairment (Appendix 3); epilepsy; pregnancy (Appendix 4); packs on sale to the general public carry a warning to avoid in epilepsy, or in liver or kidney disease, and to seek medical advice in pregnancy; breast-feeding (Appendix 5)

Side-effects nausea, vomiting, colic, diarrhoea, allergic reactions including urticaria, bronchospasm, and rare reports of arthralgia, fever, Stevens-Johnson syndrome and angioedema; rarely dizziness, muscular incoordination ('worm wobble'); drowsiness, nystagmus, vertigo, blurred vision, confusion and clonic contractions in patients with neurological or renal abnormalities

Dose

- See under Preparation, below

Piperazine Citrate (Non-proprietary)

Syrup, piperazine hydrate 750 mg/5 mL (as citrate)
Brands include *Ascalix®*

Dose consult product literature

Syrup, piperazine hydrate 4 g/30 mL (as citrate)
Brands include *Ascalix®*

Dose consult product literature

With sennosides

For cautions, contra-indications, side-effects of senna see section 1.6.2

Pripsen® (Thornton & Ross)

Oral powder, piperazine phosphate 4 g, total sennosides (calculated as sennoside B) 15.3 mg/sachet. Net price two-dose sachet pack = £1.47. Label: 13

Dose threadworms, stirred into milk or water, ADULT and CHILD over 6 years, content of 1 sachet as a single dose (bedtime in adults or morning in children), repeated after 14 days; INFANT 3 months–1 year, 1 level 2.5-mL spoonful in the morning, repeated after 14 days; CHILD 1–6 years, 1 level 5-mL spoonful in the morning, repeated after 14 days

Roundworms, first dose as for threadworms; repeat at monthly intervals for up to 3 months if reinfection risk

5.5.2 Ascaricides (common roundworm infections)

Levamisole (available on named-patient basis from specialist importing companies, see p. 888) is very effective against *Ascaris lumbricoides* and is generally considered to be the drug of choice. It is very well tolerated; mild nausea or vomiting has been reported in about 1% of treated patients; it is given as a single dose of 120–150 mg in adults.

Mebendazole (section 5.5.1) is also active against ascaris; the usual dose is 100 mg twice daily for 3 days. **Piperazine** may be given in a single adult dose, see Piperazine, above.

5.5.3 Drugs for tapeworm infections

Taenicides

Niclosamide (available on named-patient basis from specialist importing companies, see p. 888) is the most widely used drug for tapeworm infections and side-effects are limited to occasional gastro-intestinal upset, lightheadedness, and pruritus; it is not effective against larval worms. Fears of developing cysticercosis in *Taenia solium* infections have proved unfounded. All the same, an antiemetic can be given before treatment and a laxative can be given 2 hours after niclosamide.

Praziquantel (available on named-patient basis from Merck (*Cysticide*®)) is as effective as niclosamide and is given as a single dose of 5–10 mg/kg after a light breakfast (a single dose of 25 mg/kg for *Hymenolepis nana*).

Hydatid disease

Cysts caused by *Echinococcus granulosus* grow slowly and asymptomatic patients do not always require treatment. Surgical treatment remains the method of choice in many situations. **Albendazole** (available on named-patient basis from specialist importing companies, see p. 888) is used in conjunction with surgery to reduce the risk of recurrence or as primary treatment in inoperable cases. Alveolar echinococcosis due to *E. multilocularis* is usually fatal if untreated. Surgical removal with albendazole cover is the treatment of choice, but where effective surgery is impossible, repeated cycles of albendazole (for a year or more) may help. Careful monitoring of liver function is particularly important during drug treatment.

5.5.4 Drugs for hookworms (ancylostomiasis, necatoriasis)

Hookworms live in the upper small intestine and draw blood from the point of their attachment to their host. An iron-deficiency anaemia may occur and, if present, effective treatment of the infection requires not only expulsion of the worms but treatment of the anaemia.

Mebendazole (section 5.5.1) has a useful broad-spectrum activity, and is effective against hookworms; the usual dose is 100 mg twice daily for 3 days. **Albendazole** (available on a named-patient basis from specialist importing companies, see p. 888) given as a single dose of 400 mg, is an alternative.

5.5.5 Schistosomicides (bilharziasis)

Adult *Schistosoma haematobium* worms live in the genito-urinary veins and adult *S. mansoni* in those of the colon and mesentery. *S. japonicum* is more widely distributed in veins of the alimentary tract and portal system.

Praziquantel (available on named-patient basis from Merck (*Cysticide*®)) is effective against all human schistosomes. The dose is 20 mg/kg followed after 4–6 hours by one further dose of 20 mg/kg (60 mg/kg in 3 divided doses on one day for *S. japonicum* infections). No serious adverse effects have been reported. Of all the available schistosomicides, it has the most attractive combination of effectiveness, broad-spectrum activity, and low toxicity.

Hycanthone, lucanthone, niridazole, oxamniquine, and sodium stibocaptate have now been superseded.

5.5.6 Filaricides

Diethylcarbamazine (not on UK market) is effective against microfilariae and adults of *Loa loa*, *Wuchereria bancrofti*, and *Brugia malayi*. To minimise reactions treatment is commenced with a dose of diethylcarbamazine citrate 1 mg/kg on the first day and increased gradually over 3 days to 6 mg/kg daily in divided doses (up to 9 mg/kg daily in divided doses for *Loa loa*); this dosage is maintained for a further period. Close medical supervision is necessary particularly in the early phase of treatment.

In heavy infections there may be a febrile reaction, and in heavy *Loa loa* infection there is a small risk of encephalopathy. In such cases treatment must be given under careful in-patient supervision and stopped at the first sign of cerebral involvement (and specialist advice sought).

Ivermectin (available on named-patient basis from specialist importing companies, see p. 888) is very effective in *onchocerciasis* and it is now the drug of choice. A single dose of 150 micrograms/kg by mouth produces a prolonged reduction in microfilarial levels. Retreatment at intervals of 6 to 12 months depending on symptoms must be given until the adult worms die out. Reactions are usually slight and most commonly take the form of temporary aggravation of itching and rash. Diethylcarbamazine or suramin should no longer be used for onchocerciasis because of their toxicity.

5.5.7 Drugs for cutaneous larva migrans (creeping eruption)

Dog and cat hookworm larvae may enter human skin where they produce slowly extending itching tracks usually on the foot. Single tracks can be treated with topical tiabendazole (no commercial preparation available). Multiple infections respond to **ivermectin**, **albendazole** or **tiabendazole** (thiabendazole) by mouth (all available on a named-patient basis from specialist importing companies, see p. 888).

5.5.8 Drugs for strongyloidiasis

Adult *Strongyloides stercoralis* live in the gut and produce larvae which penetrate the gut wall and invade the tissues, setting up a cycle of auto-infection. **Ivermectin** (available on named-patient basis from specialist importing companies, see p. 888) in a dose of 200 micrograms/kg daily for 2 days is the treatment of choice for chronic *Strongyloides* infection. **Albendazole** (available on named-patient basis from specialist importing companies, see p. 888) is an alternative given in a dose of 400 mg twice daily for 3 days, repeated after 3 weeks if necessary.

6 Endocrine system

6.1 Drugs used in diabetes 358
6.1.1 Insulins 359
6.1.1.1 Short-acting insulins 361
6.1.1.2 Intermediate- and long-acting insulins 362
6.1.1.3 Hypodermic equipment 365
6.1.2 Antidiabetic drugs 366
6.1.2.1 Sulphonylureas 366
6.1.2.2 Biguanides 368
6.1.2.3 Other antidiabetics 369
6.1.3 Diabetic ketoacidosis 372
6.1.4 Treatment of hypoglycaemia 372
6.1.5 Treatment of diabetic nephropathy and neuropathy 373
6.1.6 Diagnostic and monitoring agents for diabetes mellitus 374
6.2 Thyroid and antithyroid drugs 376
6.2.1 Thyroid hormones 376
6.2.2 Antithyroid drugs 377
6.3 Corticosteroids 378
6.3.1 Replacement therapy 378
6.3.2 Glucocorticoid therapy 378
6.4 Sex hormones 384
6.4.1 Female sex hormones 384
6.4.1.1 Oestrogens and HRT 384
6.4.1.2 Progestogens 392
6.4.2 Male sex hormones and antagonists 394
6.4.3 Anabolic steroids 397
6.5 Hypothalamic and pituitary hormones and anti-oestrogens 397
6.5.1 Hypothalamic and anterior pituitary hormones and anti-oestrogens 397
6.5.2 Posterior pituitary hormones and antagonists 402
6.6 Drugs affecting bone metabolism 404
6.6.1 Calcitonin and parathyroid hormone 405
6.6.2 Bisphosphonates and other drugs affecting bone metabolism 406
6.7 Other endocrine drugs 410
6.7.1 Bromocriptine and other dopaminergic drugs 410
6.7.2 Drugs affecting gonadotrophins 412
6.7.3 Metyrapone and trilostane 415
6.7.4 Somatomedins 416

This chapter also includes advice on the drug management of the following:

Adrenal suppression during illness, trauma or surgery, p. 380
Serious infections in patients taking corticosteroids, p. 380
Osteoporosis, p. 404
Breast pain (mastalgia), p. 415

6.1 Drugs used in diabetes

6.1.1 Insulins
6.1.2 Antidiabetic drugs
6.1.3 Diabetic ketoacidosis
6.1.4 Treatment of hypoglycaemia
6.1.5 Treatment of diabetic nephropathy and neuropathy
6.1.6 Diagnostic and monitoring agents for diabetes mellitus

Diabetes mellitus occurs because of a lack of insulin or resistance to its action. It is diagnosed by measuring fasting or random blood-glucose concentration (and occasionally by glucose tolerance test). Although there are many subtypes, the two principal classes of diabetes are type 1 diabetes and type 2 diabetes.

Type 1 diabetes, also referred to as insulin-dependent diabetes mellitus (IDDM), occurs as a result of a deficiency of insulin following autoimmune destruction of pancreatic beta cells. Patients with type 1 diabetes require administration of insulin.

Type 2 diabetes, also referred to as non-insulin-dependent diabetes (NIDDM), is due either to reduced secretion of insulin or to peripheral resistance to the action of insulin. Although patients may be controlled on diet alone, many also require oral antidiabetic drugs or insulin (or both) to maintain satisfactory control. In overweight individuals, type 2 diabetes may be prevented by losing weight and increasing physical activity; use of drugs such as orlistat (section 4.5.1) or sibutramine (section 4.5.2) may be considered in obese patients.

Treatment of all forms of diabetes should be aimed at alleviating symptoms and minimising the risk of long-term complications (see below); tight control of diabetes is essential.

Diabetes is a strong risk factor for cardiovascular disease (section 2.12). Other risk factors for cardiovascular disease such as smoking (section 4.10), hypertension (section 2.5), obesity (section 4.5), and hyperlipidaemia (section 2.12) should be addressed. Cardiovascular risk in patients with diabetes can be further reduced by the use of an ACE inhibitor (section 2.5.5.1), low-dose aspirin (section 2.9) and a lipid-regulating drug (section 2.12).

Prevention of diabetic complications Optimal glycaemic control in both type 1 diabetes and type 2 diabetes reduces, in the long term, the risk of microvascular complications including retinopathy, development of proteinuria and to some extent neuropathy. However, a temporary deterioration in established diabetic retinopathy may occur when normalising blood-glucose concentration. For reference to the use of an ACE inhibitor or an angiotensin-II receptor antagonist in the management of diabetic nephropathy, see section 6.1.5.

A measure of the total glycated (or glycosylated) haemoglobin (HbA_1) or a specific fraction (HbA_{1c}) provides a good indication of glycaemic control over the previous 2–3 months. The ideal HbA_{1c} concentration is between 6.5 and 7.5% but this cannot always be achieved, and those on insulin may have significantly increased risks of severe hypoglycaemia. Tight control of blood pressure in hypertensive patients with type 2 diabetes reduces mortality and protects visual acuity (by reducing considerably the risks of maculopathy and retinal photocoagulation) (see also section 2.5).

Driving Drivers with diabetes are required to notify the Driver and Vehicle Licensing Agency (DVLA) of their condition if they are treated with insulin or if they are treated with oral antidiabetic drugs and also have complications. Detailed guidance on eligibility to drive is available from the DVLA (www.dvla.gov.uk/medical.aspx). Driving is not permitted when hypoglycaemic awareness is impaired or frequent hypoglycaemic episodes occur.

Drivers need to be particularly careful to avoid hypoglycaemia (see also above) and should be warned of the problems. Drivers treated with insulin should normally check their blood-glucose concentration before driving and, on long journeys, at 2-hour intervals; these precautions may also be necessary for drivers taking oral antidiabetic drugs who are at particular risk of hypoglycaemia. Drivers treated with insulin should ensure that a supply of sugar is always available in the vehicle and they should avoid driving if their meal is delayed. If hypoglycaemia occurs, or warning signs develop, the driver should:

- stop the vehicle in a safe place;
- switch off the ignition;
- eat or drink a suitable source of sugar;
- wait until recovery is complete before continuing journey; recovery may take 15 minutes or longer and should preferably be confirmed by checking blood-glucose concentration.

6.1.1 Insulins

6.1.1.1 Short-acting insulins
6.1.1.2 Intermediate- and long-acting insulins
6.1.1.3 Hypodermic equipment

Insulin plays a key role in the regulation of carbohydrate, fat, and protein metabolism. It is a polypeptide hormone of complex structure. There are differences in the amino-acid sequence of animal insulins, human insulins and the human insulin analogues. Insulin may be extracted from pork pancreas and purified by crystallisation; it may also be extracted from beef pancreas, but beef insulins are now rarely used. Human sequence insulin may be produced semisynthetically by enzymatic modification of porcine insulin (emp) or biosynthetically by recombinant DNA technology using bacteria (crb, prb) or yeast (pyr).

All insulin preparations are to a greater or lesser extent immunogenic in man but immunological resistance to insulin action is uncommon. Preparations of human sequence insulin should theoretically be less immunogenic, but no real advantage has been shown in trials.

Insulin is inactivated by gastro-intestinal enzymes, and must therefore be given by injection; the subcutaneous route is ideal in most circumstances. Insulin is usually injected into the upper arms, thighs, buttocks, or abdomen; absorption from a limb site may be increased if the limb is used in strenuous exercise after the injection. Generally subcutaneous insulin injections cause few problems; fat hypertrophy does, however, occur but can be minimised by using different injection sites in rotation. Local allergic reactions are rare.

Insulin is needed by all patients with ketoacidosis, and it is likely to be needed by most patients with:

- rapid onset of symptoms;
- substantial loss of weight;
- weakness;
- ketonuria;
- a first-degree relative who has type 1 diabetes.

Insulin is required by almost all children with diabetes. It is also needed for type 2 diabetes when other methods have failed to achieve good control, and temporarily in the presence of intercurrent illness or peri-operatively. Pregnant women with type 2 diabetes should be treated with insulin when diet alone fails.

Management of diabetes with insulin The aim of treatment is to achieve the best possible control of blood-glucose concentration without making the patient obsessional and to avoid disabling hypoglycaemia; close co-operation is needed between the patient and the medical team because good control reduces the risk of complications.

Mixtures of insulin preparations may be required and appropriate combinations have to be determined for the individual patient. For patients with acute-onset diabetes, treatment should be started with a short-acting insulin (e.g. soluble insulin, insulin aspart) given 3 times daily with intermediate-acting insulin at bedtime. For those less severely ill treatment is usually started with a mixture of premixed short- and intermediate-acting insulins (most commonly in a proportion of 30% soluble insulin and 70% isophane insulin) given twice daily; 8 units twice daily is a suitable initial dose for most ambulant patients. The proportion of the short-acting soluble component can be increased in those with excessive postprandial hyperglycaemia.

The dose of insulin is increased gradually, taking care to avoid troublesome hypoglycaemic reactions.

Insulin preparations can be divided into 3 types:

- those of **short** duration which have a relatively rapid onset of action, namely soluble insulin, insulin lispro and insulin aspart;
- those with an **intermediate** action, e.g. isophane insulin and insulin zinc suspension; and
- those whose action is slower in onset and lasts for **long** periods, e.g. insulin zinc suspension.

The duration of action of a particular type of insulin varies considerably from one patient to another, and needs to be assessed individually.

Examples of recommended insulin regimens

- Short-acting insulin mixed with intermediate-acting insulin: twice daily (before meals)
- Short-acting insulin mixed with intermediate-acting insulin: before breakfast
  Short-acting insulin: before evening meal
  Intermediate-acting insulin: at bedtime
- Short-acting insulin: three times daily (before breakfast, midday, and evening meal)
  Intermediate-acting insulin: at bedtime
- Intermediate-acting insulin with or without short-acting insulin: once daily either before breakfast or at bedtime suffices for some patients with type 2 diabetes who need insulin

Insulin requirements may be increased by infection, stress, accidental or surgical trauma, and during puberty. Requirements may be decreased in patients with renal impairment (Appendix 3) or hepatic impairment and in those with some endocrine disorders (e.g. Addison's disease, hypopituitarism) or coeliac disease.

Pregnancy and breast-feeding During pregnancy and breast-feeding, insulin requirements may alter and doses should be assessed frequently by an experienced diabetes physician. The dose of insulin generally needs to be increased in the second and third trimesters of pregnancy.

Insulin administration Insulin is generally given by *subcutaneous injection*. Injection devices ('pens') (section 6.1.1.3) which hold the insulin in a cartridge and meter the required dose are convenient to use. The conventional syringe and needle is still the preferred method of insulin administration by many and is also required for insulins not available in cartridge form.

For intensive insulin regimens multiple subcutaneous injections (3 to 4 times daily) are usually recommended.

Short-acting injectable insulins (soluble insulin, insulin aspart, insulin glulisine, and insulin lispro) can also be given by *continuous subcutaneous infusion* using a portable infusion pump. This device delivers a continuous basal insulin infusion and patient-activated bolus doses at meal times. This technique is appropriate only for patients who suffer recurrent hypoglycaemia or marked morning rise in blood-glucose concentration despite optimised multiple-injection regimens. NICE (February 2003) has also recommended continuous subcutaneous infusion as an option in those who suffer repeated or unpredictable hypoglycaemia despite optimal multiple-injection regimens (including the use of insulin glargine where appropriate). Patients on subcutaneous insulin infusion must be highly motivated, able to monitor their blood-glucose concentration, and have expert training, advice and supervision from an experienced healthcare team.

Soluble insulin by the *intravenous route* is reserved for urgent treatment, and for fine control in serious illness and in the peri-operative period (see under Diabetes and Surgery, below).

Units The word 'unit' should **not** be abbreviated.

Monitoring Many patients now monitor their own blood-glucose concentrations (section 6.1.6). Since blood-glucose concentrations vary substantially throughout the day, 'normoglycaemia' cannot always be achieved throughout a 24-hour period without causing damaging hypoglycaemia. It is therefore best to recommend that patients should maintain a blood-glucose concentration of between 4 and 9 mmol/litre for most of the time (4–7 mmol/litre before meals and less than 9 mmol/litre after meals), while accepting that on occasions, for brief periods, it will be above these values; strenuous efforts should be made to prevent the blood-glucose concentration from falling below 4 mmol/litre. Patients should be advised to look for 'peaks' and 'troughs' of blood glucose, and to adjust their insulin dosage only once or twice weekly. Overall it is ideal to aim for an HbA_{1c} (glycosylated haemoglobin) concentration of 6.5–7.5% or less (reference range 4–6%) but this is not always possible without causing disabling hypoglycaemia; in those at risk of arterial disease, the aim should be to maintain the HbA_{1c} concentration at 6.5% or less. HbA_{1c} should be measured every 3–6 months. Fructosamine can also be used for assessment of control; this is simpler and cheaper but the measurement of HbA_{1c} is generally a more reliable method.

The intake of energy and of simple and complex carbohydrates should be adequate to allow normal growth and development but obesity must be avoided. The carbohydrate intake needs to be regulated and should be distributed throughout the day. Fine control of plasma glucose can be achieved by moving portions of carbohydrate from one meal to another without altering the total intake.

Hypoglycaemia Hypoglycaemia is a potential problem with insulin therapy. All patients must be carefully instructed on how to avoid it.

Loss of warning of hypoglycaemia is common among insulin-treated patients and can be a serious hazard, especially for drivers and those in dangerous occupations. Very tight control of diabetes lowers the blood-glucose concentration needed to trigger hypoglycaemic symptoms; increase in the frequency of hypoglycaemic episodes reduces the warning symptoms experienced by the patient. Beta-blockers can also blunt hypoglycaemic awareness (and also delay recovery).

To restore the warning signs, episodes of hypoglycaemia must be minimised; this involves appropriate adjustment of insulin type, dose and frequency together with suitable timing and quantity of meals and snacks.

Some patients have reported loss of hypoglycaemia warning after transfer to human insulin. Clinical studies do not confirm that human insulin decreases hypoglycaemia awareness. If a patient believes that human insulin is responsible for the loss of warning it is reasonable to revert to animal insulin and essential to educate the patient about avoiding hypoglycaemia. Great care should be taken to specify whether a human or an animal preparation is required.

Few patients are now treated with beef insulins; when undertaking conversion from beef to human insulin, the total dose should be reduced by about 10% with careful monitoring for the first few days. When changing between pork and human-sequence insulins, a dose change is not usually needed, but careful monitoring is still advised.

Diabetes and surgery The following regimen is suitable when surgery in a patient with type 1 diabetes requires intravenous infusion of insulin for 12 hours or longer.

- Give an injection of the patient's usual insulin on the night before the operation.
- Early on the day of the operation, start an intravenous infusion of glucose 5% or 10% containing potassium chloride 10 mmol/litre (provided that the patient is not hyperkalaemic) and infuse at a constant rate appropriate to the patient's fluid requirements (usually 125 mL per hour); make up a solution of soluble insulin 1 unit/mL in sodium chloride 0.9% and infuse intravenously using a syringe pump piggy-backed to the intravenous infusion.
- The rate of the insulin infusion should normally be:
  Blood glucose < 4 mmol/litre, give 0.5 units/hour
  Blood glucose 4–15 mmol/litre, give 2 units/hour
  Blood glucose 15–20 mmol/litre, give 4 units/hour
  Blood glucose > 20 mmol/litre, review.

In resistant cases (such as patients who are in shock or severely ill or those receiving corticosteroids or sympathomimetics) 2–4 times these rates or even more may be needed.

If a syringe pump is not available soluble insulin 16 units/litre should be added to the intravenous infusion of glucose 5% or 10% containing potassium chloride 10 mmol per litre (provided the patient is not hyperkalaemic) and the infusion run at the rate appropriate to the patient's fluid requirements (usually 125 mL per hour) with the insulin dose adjusted as follows:

Blood glucose < 4 mmol/litre, give 8 units/litre

Blood glucose 4–15 mmol/litre, give 16 units/litre

Blood glucose 15–20 mmol/litre, give 32 units/litre

Blood glucose > 20 mmol/litre, review.

The rate of intravenous infusion depends on the volume depletion, cardiac function, age, and other factors. Blood-glucose concentration should be measured preoperatively and then hourly until stable, thereafter every 2 hours. The duration of action of intravenous insulin is only a few minutes and the infusion must not be stopped unless the patient becomes overtly hypoglycaemic (blood glucose < 3 mmol/litre) in which case it should be stopped for up to 30 minutes. The amount of potassium chloride required in the infusion needs to be assessed by regular measurement of plasma electrolytes. Sodium chloride 0.9% infusion should replace glucose 5% or 10% if the blood glucose is persistently above 15 mmol/litre.

Once the patient starts to eat and drink, give subcutaneous insulin before breakfast and stop intravenous insulin 30 minutes later; the dose may need to be 10–20% more than usual if the patient is still in bed or unwell. If the patient was not previously receiving insulin, an appropriate initial dose is 30–40 units daily in four divided doses using soluble insulin before meals and intermediate-acting insulin at bedtime and the dose adjusted from day to day. Patients with hyperglycaemia often relapse after conversion back to subcutaneous insulin calling for one of the following approaches:

- additional doses of soluble insulin at any of the four injection times (before meals or bedtime) *or*
- temporary addition of intravenous insulin infusion (while continuing the subcutaneous regimen) until blood-glucose concentration is satisfactory *or*
- complete reversion to the intravenous regimen (especially if the patient is unwell).

6.1.1.1 Short-acting insulins

Soluble insulin is a short-acting form of insulin. For maintenance regimens it is usual to inject it 15 to 30 minutes before meals.

Soluble insulin is the most appropriate form of insulin for use in diabetic emergencies e.g. diabetic ketoacidosis (section 6.1.3) and at the time of surgery. It can be given intravenously and intramuscularly, as well as subcutaneously.

When injected subcutaneously, soluble insulin has a rapid onset of action (30 to 60 minutes), a peak action between 2 and 4 hours, and a duration of action of up to 8 hours.

When injected intravenously, soluble insulin has a very short half-life of only about 5 minutes and its effect disappears within 30 minutes.

The human insulin analogues, **insulin aspart**, **insulin glulisine**, and **insulin lispro** have a faster onset and shorter duration of action than soluble insulin; as a result, compared to soluble insulin, fasting and preprandial blood-glucose concentration is a little higher, postprandial blood-glucose concentration is a little lower, and hypoglycaemia occurs slightly less frequently. Subcutaneous injection of insulin analogues may be convenient for those who wish to inject shortly before or, when necessary, shortly after a meal. They can also help those susceptible to hypoglycaemia before lunch and those who eat late in the evening and are prone to nocturnal hypoglycaemia. They can also be administered by subcutaneous infusion (see Insulin Administration, above). Insulin aspart and insulin lispro can be administered intravenously and can be used as alternatives to soluble insulin for diabetic emergencies and at the time of surgery.

INSULIN

(Insulin Injection; Neutral Insulin; Soluble Insulin)

A sterile solution of insulin (i.e. bovine or porcine) or of human insulin; pH 6.6–8.0

Indications diabetes mellitus; diabetic ketoacidosis (section 6.1.3)

Cautions see notes above; pregnancy (Appendix 4); reduce dose in renal impairment (Appendix 3); **interactions**: Appendix 1 (antidiabetics)

Side-effects see notes above, transient oedema; local reactions and fat hypertrophy at injection site; *rarely* hypersensitivity reactions including urticaria, rash; overdose causes hypoglycaemia

Dose

- By subcutaneous, intramuscular *or* intravenous injection *or* intravenous infusion, according to requirements

Highly purified animal

Counselling Show container to patient and confirm that patient is expecting the version dispensed

Hypurin® Bovine Neutral (Wockhardt) PoM
Injection, soluble insulin (bovine, highly purified) 100 units/mL. Net price 10-mL vial = £18.48; cartridges (for *Autopen® Classic*) 5 × 1.5 mL = £13.86, 5 × 3 mL = £27.72

Hypurin® Porcine Neutral (Wockhardt) PoM
Injection, soluble insulin (porcine, highly purified) 100 units/mL. Net price 10-mL vial = £16.80; cartridges (for *Autopen® Classic*) 5 × 1.5 mL = £12.60, 5 × 3 mL = £25.20

Pork Actrapid® (Novo Nordisk) PoM
Injection, soluble insulin (porcine, highly purified) 100 units/mL. Net price 10-mL vial = £4.00
Note Not recommended for use in subcutaneous insulin infusion pumps—may precipitate in catheter or needle

Human sequence

Counselling Show container to patient and confirm that patient is expecting the version dispensed

Actrapid® (Novo Nordisk) PoM
Injection, soluble insulin (human, pyr) 100 units/mL. Net price 10-mL vial = £7.48
Note Not recommended for use in subcutaneous insulin infusion pumps—may precipitate in catheter or needle

Humulin S® (Lilly) PoM
Injection, soluble insulin (human, prb) 100 units/mL. Net price 10-mL vial = £16.50; 5 × 3-mL cartridge (for most *Autopen® Classic* or *HumaPen®*) = £28.12

Insuman® Rapid (Aventis Pharma) ▼ PoM
Injection, soluble insulin (human, crb) 100 units/mL, net price 5 × 3-mL cartridge (for *OptiPen® Pro 1*) = £23.43; 5 × 3-mL *Insuman® Rapid OptiSet®* prefilled disposable injection devices (range 2–40 units, allowing 2-unit dosage adjustment) = £27.90
Note Not recommended for use in subcutaneous insulin infusion pumps

Mixed preparations

See Biphasic Isophane Insulin (section 6.1.1.2)

INSULIN ASPART

(Recombinant human insulin analogue)

Indications diabetes mellitus
Cautions see under Insulin; children (use only if benefit likely compared to soluble insulin)
Side-effects see under Insulin
Dose

- By subcutaneous injection, immediately before meals or when necessary shortly after meals, according to requirements
- By subcutaneous infusion, intravenous injection *or* intravenous infusion, according to requirements

NovoRapid® (Novo Nordisk) PoM
Injection, insulin aspart (recombinant human insulin analogue) 100 units/mL, net price 10-mL vial = £17.27; *Penfill®* cartridge (for *NovoPen®* devices) 5 × 3-mL = £29.43; 5 × 3-mL *FlexPen®* prefilled disposable injection devices (range 1–60 units, allowing 1-unit dosage adjustment) = £32.00
Counselling Show container to patient and confirm that patient is expecting the version dispensed

INSULIN GLULISINE

(Recombinant human insulin analogue)

Indications diabetes mellitus
Cautions see under Insulin
Side-effects see under Insulin
Dose

- By subcutaneous injection, immediately before meals or when necessary shortly after meals, according to requirements
- By subcutaneous infusion, according to requirements
- CHILD and ADOLESCENT under 17 years not recommended

Apidra® (Sanofi-Aventis) ▼ PoM
Injection, insulin glulisine (recombinant human insulin analogue) 100 units/mL, net price 10-mL vial = £17.27; 5× 3-mL cartridge (for *OptiPen® Pro 1* and *Autopen® 24*) = £29.45; 5 × 3-mL *OptiClik®* cartridge (for *OptiClik® Pen* NHS) = £31.50; 5 × 3-mL *Apidra® Optiset®* prefilled disposable injection devices (range 2–40 units, allowing 2-unit dosage adjustment) = £29.45; 5 × 3-mL *Apidra® SoloStar®* prefilled disposable injection devices (range 1–80 units, allowing 1-unit dosage adjustment) = £25.00
Counselling Show container to patient and confirm that patient is expecting the version dispensed

INSULIN LISPRO

(Recombinant human insulin analogue)

Indications diabetes mellitus
Cautions see under Insulin; children (use only if benefit likely compared to soluble insulin)
Side-effects see under Insulin
Dose

- By subcutaneous injection shortly before meals or when necessary shortly after meals, according to requirements
- By subcutaneous infusion, *or* intravenous injection, *or* intravenous infusion, according to requirements

Humalog® (Lilly) PoM
Injection, insulin lispro (recombinant human insulin analogue) 100 units/mL. Net price 10-mL vial = £17.28; 5 × 3-mL cartridge (for *Autopen® Classic* or *HumaPen®*) = £29.46; 5 × 3-mL *Humalog®-Pen* prefilled disposable injection devices (range 1–60 units, allowing 1-unit dosage adjustment) = £29.46
Counselling Show container to patient and confirm that patient is expecting the version dispensed

6.1.1.2 Intermediate- and long-acting insulins

When given by subcutaneous injection, intermediate- and long-acting insulins have an onset of action of approximately 1–2 hours, a maximal effect at 4–12 hours, and a duration of 16–35 hours. Some are given twice daily in conjunction with short-acting (soluble) insulin, and others are given once daily, particularly in elderly patients. Soluble insulin can be mixed with intermediate and long-acting insulins (except insulin detemir and insulin glargine) in the syringe, essentially retaining the properties of the two components, although there may be some blunting of the initial effect of the soluble insulin component (especially on mixing with protamine zinc insulin, see below).

Isophane insulin is a suspension of insulin with protamine which is of particular value for initiation of twice-daily insulin regimens. Patients usually mix isophane with soluble insulin but ready-mixed preparations may be appropriate (**biphasic isophane insulin**, **biphasic insulin aspart**, or **biphasic insulin lispro**).

Insulin zinc suspension (30% amorphous, 70% crystalline) has a more prolonged duration of action.

Protamine zinc insulin is usually given once daily with short-acting (soluble) insulin. It has the drawback of binding with the soluble insulin when mixed in the same syringe and is now rarely used.

Insulin glargine and **insulin detemir** are both human insulin analogues with a prolonged duration of action; insulin glargine is given once daily and insulin detemir is given once or twice daily.

> NICE guidance
> Insulin glargine (December 2002)
> Insulin glargine should be available as an option for patients with type 1 diabetes.
> Insulin glargine is **not** recommended for routine use in patients with type 2 diabetes who require insulin, but it may be considered in type 2 diabetes for those:
> - who require assistance with injecting their insulin; *or*
> - whose lifestyle is significantly restricted by recurrent symptomatic hypoglycaemia; *or*
> - who would otherwise need twice-daily basal insulin injections in combination with oral antidiabetic drugs

INSULIN DETEMIR

(Recombinant human insulin analogue—long acting)

Indications diabetes mellitus
Cautions see under Insulin (section 6.1.1.1); pregnancy (Appendix 4)
Side-effects see under Insulin (section 6.1.1.1)
Dose
- By subcutaneous injection, ADULT and CHILD over 6 years, according to requirements

Levemir® (Novo Nordisk) PoM
Injection, insulin detemir (recombinant human insulin analogue) 100 units/mL, net price 5 × 3-mL cartridge (for *NovoPen®* devices) = £39.00; 5 × 3-mL *FlexPen®* prefilled disposable injection device (range 1–60 units, allowing 1-unit dosage adjustment) = £39.00.
Counselling Show container to patient and confirm that patient is expecting the version dispensed

INSULIN GLARGINE

(Recombinant human insulin analogue—long acting)

Indications diabetes mellitus
Cautions see under Insulin (section 6.1.1.1); pregnancy (Appendix 4)
Side-effects see under Insulin (section 6.1.1.1)
Dose
- By subcutaneous injection, ADULT and CHILD over 6 years, according to requirements

Lantus® (Aventis Pharma) ▼ PoM
Injection, insulin glargine (recombinant human insulin analogue) 100 units/mL, net price 10-mL vial = £26.00; 5 × 3-mL cartridge (for *OptiPen® Pro 1* and *Autopen® 24*) = £39.00; 5 × 3-mL *OptiClik®* cartridge (for *OptiClik® Pen* NHS) = £42.00; 5 × 3-mL *Lantus® OptiSet®* prefilled disposable injection devices (range 2–40 units, allowing 2-unit dosage adjustment) = £39.00; 5 × 3-mL *Lantus® SoloStar®* prefilled disposable injection devices (range 1–80 units, allowing 1-unit dosage adjustment) = £42.00
Counselling Show container to patient and confirm that patient is expecting the version dispensed

INSULIN ZINC SUSPENSION

(Insulin Zinc Suspension (Mixed)—long acting)

A sterile neutral suspension of bovine and/or porcine insulin or of human insulin in the form of a complex obtained by the addition of a suitable zinc salt; consists of rhombohedral crystals (10–40 microns) and of particles of no uniform shape (not exceeding 2 microns)

Indications diabetes mellitus
Cautions see under Insulin (section 6.1.1.1)
Side-effects see under Insulin (section 6.1.1.1)
Dose
- By subcutaneous injection, according to requirements

◢Highly purified animal

Hypurin® Bovine Lente (Wockhardt) PoM
Injection, insulin zinc suspension (bovine, highly purified) 100 units/mL. Net price 10-mL vial = £18.48
Counselling Show container to patient and confirm that patient is expecting the version dispensed

ISOPHANE INSULIN

(Isophane Insulin Injection; Isophane Protamine Insulin Injection; Isophane Insulin (NPH)—intermediate acting)

A sterile suspension of bovine or porcine insulin or of human insulin in the form of a complex obtained by the addition of protamine sulphate or another suitable protamine

Indications diabetes mellitus
Cautions see under Insulin (section 6.1.1.1)
Side-effects see under Insulin (section 6.1.1.1); protamine may cause allergic reactions
Dose
- By subcutaneous injection, according to requirements

◢Highly purified animal
Counselling Show container to patient and confirm that patient is expecting the version dispensed

Hypurin® Bovine Isophane (Wockhardt) PoM
Injection, isophane insulin (bovine, highly purified) 100 units/mL. Net price 10-mL vial = £18.48; cartridges (for *Autopen® Classic*) 5 × 1.5 mL = £13.86, 5 × 3 mL = £27.72

Hypurin® Porcine Isophane (Wockhardt) PoM
Injection, isophane insulin (porcine, highly purified) 100 units/mL. Net price 10-mL vial = £16.80; cartridges (for *Autopen® Classic*) 5 × 1.5 mL = £12.60, 5 × 3 mL = £25.20

Pork Insulatard® (Novo Nordisk) PoM
Injection, isophane insulin (porcine, highly purified) 100 units/mL. Net price 10-mL vial = £4.00

Human sequence

Counselling Show container to patient and confirm that patient is expecting the version dispensed

Insulatard® (Novo Nordisk) PoM
Injection, isophane insulin (human, pyr) 100 units/mL. Net price 10-mL vial = £7.48; *Insulatard Penfill®* cartridge (for *Novopen®* devices) 5 × 3 mL = £20.08; 5 × 3-mL *Insulatard InnoLet®* prefilled disposable injection devices (range 1–50 units, allowing 1-unit dosage adjustment) = £20.40

Humulin I® (Lilly) PoM
Injection, isophane insulin (human, prb) 100 units/mL. Net price 10-mL vial = £16.50; 5 × 3-mL cartridge (for *Autopen® Classic* or *HumaPen®*) = £29.94; 5 × 3-mL *Humulin I-Pen®* prefilled disposable injection devices (range 1–60 units, allowing 1-unit dosage adjustment) = £29.94

Insuman® Basal (Aventis Pharma) ▼ PoM
Injection, isophane insulin (human, crb) 100 units/mL, net price 5-mL vial = £5.84; 5 × 3-mL cartridge (for *OptiPen® Pro 1*) = £23.43; 5 × 3-mL *Insuman® Basal OptiSet®* prefilled disposable injection devices (range 2–40 units, allowing 2-unit dosage adjustment) = £27.90

Mixed preparations

See Biphasic Isophane Insulin (below)

PROTAMINE ZINC INSULIN

(Protamine Zinc Insulin Injection—long acting)

A sterile suspension of insulin in the form of a complex obtained by the addition of a suitable protamine and zinc chloride; this preparation was included in BP 1980 but is not included in BP 1988

Indications diabetes mellitus
Cautions see under Insulin (section 6.1.1.1); see also notes above
Side-effects see under Insulin (section 6.1.1.1); protamine may cause allergic reactions
Dose
- By subcutaneous injection, according to requirements

Hypurin® Bovine Protamine Zinc (Wockhardt) PoM
Injection, protamine zinc insulin (bovine, highly purified) 100 units/mL. Net price 10-mL vial = £18.48
Counselling Show container to patient and confirm that patient is expecting the version dispensed

Biphasic insulins

BIPHASIC INSULIN ASPART

(Intermediate-acting insulin)

Indications diabetes mellitus
Cautions see under Insulin and Insulin Aspart (section 6.1.1.1)
Side-effects see under Insulin (section 6.1.1.1); protamine may cause allergic reactions
Dose
- By subcutaneous injection, up to 10 minutes before or soon after a meal, according to requirements

NovoMix® 30 (Novo Nordisk) PoM
Injection, biphasic insulin aspart (recombinant human insulin analogue), 30% insulin aspart, 70% insulin aspart protamine, 100 units/mL, net price 5 × 3-mL *Penfill®* cartridges (for *NovoPen®* devices) = £29.43; 5 × 3-mL *FlexPen®* prefilled disposable injection devices (range 1–60 units, allowing 1-unit dosage adjustment) = £32.00
Counselling Show container to patient and confirm that patient is expecting the version dispensed; the proportions of the two components should be checked **carefully** (the order in which the proportions are stated may not be the same in other countries)

BIPHASIC INSULIN LISPRO

(Intermediate-acting insulin)

Indications diabetes mellitus
Cautions see under Insulin and Insulin Lispro (section 6.1.1.1)
Side-effects see under Insulin (section 6.1.1.1); protamine may cause allergic reactions
Dose
- By subcutaneous injection, up to 15 minutes before or soon after a meal, according to requirements

Humalog® Mix25 (Lilly) PoM
Injection, biphasic insulin lispro (recombinant human insulin analogue), 25% insulin lispro, 75% insulin lispro protamine, 100 units/mL, net price 5 × 3-mL cartridge (for *Autopen® Classic* or *HumaPen®*) = £29.46; 5 × 3-mL prefilled disposable injection devices (range 1–60 units, allowing 1-unit dosage adjustment) = £30.98
Counselling Show container to patient and confirm that patient is expecting the version dispensed; the proportions of the two components should be checked **carefully** (the order in which the proportions are stated may not be the same in other countries)

Humalog® Mix50 (Lilly) PoM
Injection, biphasic insulin lispro (recombinant human insulin analogue), 50% insulin lispro, 50% insulin lispro protamine, 100 units/mL, net price 5 × 3-mL prefilled disposable injection devices (range 1–60 units, allowing 1-unit dosage adjustment) = £29.46
Counselling Show container to patient and confirm that patient is expecting the version dispensed; the proportions of the two components should be checked **carefully** (the order in which the proportions are stated may not be the same in other countries)

BIPHASIC ISOPHANE INSULIN

(Biphasic Isophane Insulin Injection—intermediate acting)

A sterile buffered suspension of either porcine or human insulin complexed with protamine sulphate (or another suitable protamine) in a solution of insulin of the same species

Indications diabetes mellitus
Cautions see under Insulin (section 6.1.1.1)
Side-effects see under Insulin (section 6.1.1.1); protamine may cause allergic reactions
Dose
- By subcutaneous injection, according to requirements

Highly purified animal

Counselling Show container to patient and confirm that patient is expecting the version dispensed; the proportions of the two components should be checked **carefully** (the order in which the proportions are stated may not be the same in other countries)

Hypurin® Porcine 30/70 Mix (Wockhardt) PoM
Injection, biphasic isophane insulin (porcine, highly purified), 30% soluble, 70% isophane, 100 units/mL. Net price 10-mL vial = £16.80; cartridges (for *Autopen® Classic*) 5 × 1.5 mL = £12.60, 5 × 3 mL = £25.20

Human sequence

Counselling Show container to patient and confirm that patient is expecting the version dispensed; the proportions of the two components should be checked **carefully** (the order in which the proportions are stated may not be the same in other countries)

Mixtard® 30 (Novo Nordisk) PoM
Injection, biphasic isophane insulin (human, pyr), 30% soluble, 70% isophane, 100 units/mL. Net price 10-mL vial = £7.48; *Mixtard 30 Penfill®* cartridge (for *Novopen®* devices) 5 × 3 mL = £20.08; 5 × 3-mL *Mixtard 30 InnoLet®* prefilled disposable injection devices (range 1–50 units allowing 1-unit dosage adjustment) = £19.87

Humulin M3® (Lilly) PoM
Injection, biphasic isophane insulin (human, prb), 30% soluble, 70% isophane, 100 units/mL. Net price 10-mL vial = £16.50; 5 × 3-mL cartridge (for most *Autopen® Classic* or *HumaPen®*) = £28.12

Insuman® Comb 15 (Aventis Pharma) ▼ PoM
Injection, biphasic isophane insulin (human, crb), 15% soluble, 85% isophane, 100 units/mL, net price 5 × 3-mL *Insuman® Comb 15 OptiSet®* prefilled disposable injection devices (range 2–40 units, allowing 2-unit dosage adjustment) = £27.90

Insuman® Comb 25 (Aventis Pharma) ▼ PoM
Injection, biphasic isophane insulin (human, crb), 25% soluble, 75% isophane, 100 units/mL, net price 5-mL vial = £5.84; 5 × 3-mL cartridge (for *OptiPen® Pro 1*) = £23.43; 5 × 3-mL *Insuman® Comb 25 OptiSet®* prefilled disposable injection devices (range 2–40 units, allowing 2-unit dosage adjustment) = £27.90

Insuman® Comb 50 (Aventis Pharma) ▼ PoM
Injection, biphasic isophane insulin (human, crb), 50% soluble, 50% isophane, 100 units/mL, net price 5 × 3-mL cartridge (for *OptiPen® Pro 1*) = £23.43; 5 × 3-mL *Insuman® Comb 50 OptiSet®* prefilled disposable injection devices (range 2–40 units, allowing 2-unit dosage adjustment) = £27.90

6.1.1.3 Hypodermic equipment

Patients should be advised on the safe disposal of lancets, single-use syringes, and needles. Suitable arrangements for the safe disposal of contaminated waste must be made before these products are prescribed for patients who are carriers of infectious diseases.

Injection devices

Autopen® (Owen Mumford)
Injection device, *Autopen® 24* (for use with Sanofi-Aventis 3-mL insulin cartridges), allowing 1-unit dosage adjustment, max. 21 units (single-unit version) *or* 2-unit dosage adjustment, max. 42 units (2-unit version), net price (both) = £15.24; *Autopen® Classic* (for use with Lilly and Wockhardt 3-mL insulin cartridges), allowing 1-unit dosage adjustment, max. 21 units (single-unit version) *or* 2-unit dosage adjustment, max. 42 units (2-unit version), net price (all) = £15.48

HumaPen® Ergo (Lilly)
Injection device, for use with *Humulin®* and *Humalog®* 3-mL cartridges; allowing 1-unit dosage adjustment, max. 60 units, net price = £22.39 (available in burgundy and teal)

HumaPen® Luxura (Lilly)
Injection device, for use with *Humulin®* and *Humalog®* 3-mL cartridges; allowing 1-unit dosage adjustment, max. 60 units, net price = £26.36 (available in burgundy and champagne)

HumaPen® Luxura HD (Lilly)
Injection device, for use with *Humulin®* and *Humalog®* 3-mL cartridges; allowing 0.5-unit dosage adjustment, max. 30 units, net price = £26.36

mhi-500® (Medical House)
Needle-free insulin delivery device NHS for use with any 10-mL vial *or* any 3-mL cartridge of insulin (except the Novo Nordisk 3 mL penfills), allowing 0.5-unit dosage adjustment, max. 50 units, net price *3-month consumables pack* for 10-mL adaptor (13 nozzles, 5 insulin vial adaptors) = £23.43, for 3-mL adaptor (13 nozzles, 5 insulin cartridge adaptors) = £35.81; *vial adaptor pack* (6 insulin vial adaptors) = £7.66, *cartridge adaptor pack* (6 insulin cartridge adaptors) = £7.67; *nozzle pack* (6 nozzles) = £7.81

NovoPen® (Novo Nordisk)
Injection device, for use with *Penfill®* insulin cartridges; *NovoPen® Junior* (for 3-mL cartridges), allowing 0.5-unit dosage adjustment, max. 35 units, net price = £24.12; *NovoPen® 3 Demi* (for 3-mL cartridges), allowing 0.5-unit dosage adjustment, max. 35 units, net price = £24.54; *NovoPen® 3 Classic* or *Fun* (for 3-mL cartridges), allowing 1-unit dosage adjustment, max. 70 units, net price = £24.54

OptiClik® (Sanofi-Aventis)
Injection device, for use with *Lantus OptiClik®* or *Apidra Opticlik®* insulin cartridges, allowing 1-unit dosage adjustment, max. 80 units net price = £20.13 (available in blue and grey)

OptiPen® Pro 1 (Aventis Pharma)
Injection device, for use with *Insuman®* insulin cartridges; allowing 1-unit dosage adjustment, max. 60 units, net price = £22.00

SQ-PEN® (Medical House)
Needle-free insulin delivery device for use with any 10-mL vial *or* any 3-mL cartridge of insulin, allowing 1-unit dosage adjustment, max. 50 units, net price *starter pack* (*SQ-PEN®* device, 1 practice nozzle, 1 nozzle, 1 3-mL adaptor, 1 10-mL adaptor) = £147.83, *3-month consumables pack* for 10-mL adaptor (7 nozzles, 5 × 10-mL insulin vial adaptors) = £18.08, for 3-mL adaptor (7 nozzles, 15 × 3-mL insulin cartridge adaptors) = £30.82; *vial adaptor pack* (6 insulin vial adaptors) = £7.66, *cartridge adaptor pack* (6 insulin cartridge adaptors) = £7.66; nozzle pack (5 nozzles) = £10.03

Lancets

Lancets—sterile, single use (Drug Tariff)

[1]*Ascensia Microlet®* 100 = £3.62, 200 = £6.89; *BD Micro-Fine®*+ 100 = £3.16, 200 = £6.13; *Cleanlet Fine®* 100 = £3.19, 200 = £6.13; [1]*Finepoint®* 100 = £3.48; [1]*FreeStyle®* 200 = £6.76; [1]*GlucoMen®* Fine 100 = £3.42, 200 = £6.61; *Hypoguard Supreme®* 100 = £2.75; [1]*Milward Steri-Let®*, 23 gauge, 100 = £3.00, 200 = £5.70, 28 gauge, 100 = £3.00, 200 = £5.70; [1]*Monolet®* 100 = £3.28, 200 = £6.24; *Monolet Extra®* 100 = £3.28; *MPD Ultra Thin®* 100 = £3.30, 200 = £6.50; *Multiclix®* 204 = £8.84; [1]*One Touch UltraSoft®* 100 = £3.49; [2]*Softclix®* 200 = £7.06; [2]*Softclix XL®* 50 = £1.77; *Thin Lancets* (formerly *MediSense Thin®*), 200 = £6.89; [1]*Unilet ComforTouch®* 100 = £3.53, 200 = £6.69; [1]*Unilet General Purpose®* 100 = £3.59, 200 = £6.83; [1]*Unilet General Purpose Superlite®* 100 = £3.60, 200 = £6.82; [3]*Unilet Superlite®* 100 = £3.60, 200 = £6.82; *Unistik 3 Comfort®*, 28-gauge, 100 = £6.24, 200 = £12.20; *Unistik 3 Extra®*, 21-gauge, 100 = £6.24, 200 = £12.20; *Unistik 3 Normal®*, 23-gauge, 100 = £6.24, 200 = £12.20; *Universal®* (formerly *VitalCare®*), 200 = £6.20; *Vitrex Soft®*, 23-gauge, 100 = £3.00, 200 = £5.70; *Vitrex Gentle®* 28-gauge, 100 = £3.19, 200 = £6.13

Compatible finger-pricking devices (unless indicated otherwise, see footnotes), all NHS: *B-D Lancer®*, *Glucolet®*, *Monojector®*, *Penlet II®*, *Soft Touch®*

1. NHS *Autolet®* and NHS *Autolet Impression®* are also compatible finger-pricking devices
2. Use NHS *Softclix®* finger-pricking device
3. Use NHS *Autolet®* or NHS *Glucolet®* finger-pricking devices

Needles

Hypodermic Needle, Sterile single use (Drug Tariff)

For use with reusable glass syringe, sizes 0.5 mm (25G), 0.45 mm (26G), 0.4 mm (27G). Net price 100-needle pack = £2.62

Brands include *Microlance®*, *Monoject®*

Needles for Prefilled and Reusable Pen Injectors (Drug Tariff)

Screw on, needle length 6.1 mm or less, net price 100-needle pack = £12.53; 6.2–9.9 mm, 100-needle pack = £8.89; 10 mm or more, 100-needle pack = £8.89

Brands include *BD Micro-Fine®* +, *NovoFine®*, *Unifine® Pentips*

Snap on, needle length 6.1 mm or less, net price 100-needle pack = £12.02; 6.2–9.9 mm, 100-needle pack = £8.52; 10 mm or more, 100-needle pack = £8.52

Brands include *Penfine®*

Syringes

Hypodermic Syringe (Drug Tariff)

Calibrated glass with Luer taper conical fitting, for use with U100 insulin. Net price 0.5 mL and 1 mL = £15.18

Brands include *Abcare®*

Pre-Set U100 Insulin Syringe (Drug Tariff)

Calibrated glass with Luer taper conical fitting, supplied with dosage chart and strong box, for blind patients. Net price 1 mL = £21.99

U100 Insulin Syringe with Needle (Drug Tariff)

Disposable with fixed or separate needle for single use or single patient-use, colour coded orange. Needle length 8 mm, diameters 0.33 mm (29G), 0.3 mm (30G), net price 10 (with needle), 0.3 mL = £1.32, 0.5 mL = £1.27, 1 mL = £1.27; needle length 12 mm, diameters 0.45 mm (26G), 0.4 mm (27G), 0.36 mm (28G), 0.33 mm (29G), net price 10 (with needle), 0.3 mL = £1.38; 0.5 mL = £1.37; 1 mL = £1.38

Brands include *BD Micro-Fine®*+, *Clinipak®*, *Insupak®*, *Monoject® Ultra*, *Omnikan®*, *Plastipak®*, *Unifine®*

Accessories

Needle Clipping (Chopping) Device (Drug Tariff)

Consisting of a clipper to remove needle from its hub and container from which cut-off needles cannot be retrieved; designed to hold 1500 needles, not suitable for use with lancets. Net price = £1.29

Brands include *BD Safe-Clip®*

Sharpsbin (Drug Tariff)

Net price 1-litre sharpsbin = 85p

6.1.2 Antidiabetic drugs

6.1.2.1 Sulphonylureas
6.1.2.2 Biguanides
6.1.2.3 Other antidiabetics

Oral antidiabetic drugs are used for the treatment of type 2 (non-insulin-dependent) diabetes mellitus. They should be prescribed only if the patient fails to respond adequately to at least 3 months' restriction of energy and carbohydrate intake and an increase in physical activity. They should be used to augment the effect of diet and exercise, and not to replace them.

For patients not adequately controlled by diet and oral hypoglycaemic drugs, insulin may be added to the treatment regimen or substituted for oral therapy. When insulin is added to oral therapy, it is generally given at bedtime as isophane insulin, and when insulin replaces an oral regimen it is generally given as twice-daily injections of a biphasic insulin (or isophane insulin mixed with soluble insulin). Weight gain and hypoglycaemia may be complications of insulin therapy but weight gain may be reduced if the insulin is given in combination with metformin.

6.1.2.1 Sulphonylureas

The sulphonylureas act mainly by augmenting insulin secretion and consequently are effective only when some residual pancreatic beta-cell activity is present; during long-term administration they also have an extrapancreatic action. All may cause hypoglycaemia but this is uncommon and usually indicates excessive dosage. Sulphonylurea-induced hypoglycaemia may persist for many hours and must always be treated in hospital.

Sulphonylureas are considered for patients who are not overweight, or in whom metformin is contra-indicated or not tolerated. Several sulphonylureas are available and choice is determined by side-effects and the duration of action as well as the patient's age and renal function. The long-acting sulphonylureas **chlorpropamide** and **glibenclamide** are associated with a greater risk of hypoglycaemia; for this reason they should be avoided in the elderly and shorter-acting alternatives, such as **gliclazide** or **tolbutamide**, should be used instead. Chlorpropamide also has more side-effects than the other sulphonylureas (see below) and therefore it is no longer recommended.

When the combination of strict diet and sulphonylurea treatment fails other options include:

- combining with metformin (section 6.1.2.2) (reports of increased hazard with this combination remain unconfirmed);
- combining with acarbose (section 6.1.2.3), which may have a small beneficial effect, but flatulence can be a problem;
- combining with pioglitazone or rosiglitazone, but see section 6.1.2.3;
- combining with bedtime isophane insulin (section 6.1.1) but weight gain and hypoglycaemia can occur.

Insulin therapy should be instituted temporarily during intercurrent illness (such as myocardial infarction, coma, infection, and trauma). Sulphonylureas should be omitted on the morning of surgery; insulin is required because of the ensuing hyperglycaemia in these circumstances.

Cautions Sulphonylureas can encourage weight gain and should be prescribed only if poor control and symptoms persist despite adequate attempts at dieting; metformin (section 6.1.2.2) is considered the drug of choice in obese patients. Caution is needed in the elderly and in those with mild to moderate hepatic impairment (Appendix 2) and mild to moderate renal impairment (Appendix 3) because of the hazard of hypoglycaemia. The short-acting tolbutamide may be used in renal impairment, as may gliclazide which is principally metabolised in the liver, but careful monitoring of blood-glucose concentration is essential; care is required to choose the smallest possible dose that produces adequate control of blood glucose.

Contra-indications Sulphonylureas should be avoided where possible in severe hepatic impairment (Appendix 2) and in severe renal impairment (Appendix 3) impairment and in porphyria (section 9.8.2). They should not be used while breast-feeding (Appendix 5), and insulin therapy should be substituted during pregnancy (see also Appendix 4). Sulphonylureas are contra-indicated in the presence of ketoacidosis.

Side-effects Side-effects of sulphonylureas are generally mild and infrequent and include gastro-intestinal disturbances such as nausea, vomiting, diarrhoea and constipation.

Chlorpropamide has appreciably more side-effects, mainly because of its very prolonged duration of action and the consequent hazard of hypoglycaemia and it should no longer be used. It may also cause facial flushing after drinking alcohol; this effect does not normally occur with other sulphonylureas. Chlorpropamide may also enhance antidiuretic hormone secretion and very rarely cause hyponatraemia (hyponatraemia is also reported with glimepiride and glipizide).

Sulphonylureas can occasionally cause a disturbance in liver function, which may rarely lead to cholestatic jaundice, hepatitis and hepatic failure. Hypersensitivity reactions can occur, usually in the first 6–8 weeks of therapy, they consist mainly of allergic skin reactions which progress rarely to erythema multiforme and exfoliative dermatitis, fever and jaundice; photosensitivity has rarely been reported with chlorpropamide and glipizide. Blood disorders are also rare but may include leucopenia, thrombocytopenia, agranulocytosis, pancytopenia, haemolytic anaemia, and aplastic anaemia.

CHLORPROPAMIDE

Indications type 2 diabetes mellitus (for use in diabetes insipidus, see section 6.5.2)

Cautions see notes above; **interactions:** Appendix 1 (antidiabetics)

Contra-indications see notes above

Side-effects see notes above

Dose

- Initially 250 mg daily with breakfast (ELDERLY 100–125 mg but avoid—see notes above), adjusted according to response; max. 500 mg daily

Chlorpropamide (Non-proprietary) PoM
Tablets, chlorpropamide 100 mg, net price 20 = £1.70; 250 mg, 20 = £2.00. Label: 4

GLIBENCLAMIDE

Indications type 2 diabetes mellitus

Cautions see notes above; **interactions:** Appendix 1 (antidiabetics)

Contra-indications see notes above

Side-effects see notes above

Dose

- Initially 5 mg daily with or immediately after breakfast, dose adjusted according to response (ELDERLY avoid, see notes above); max. 15 mg daily

Glibenclamide (Non-proprietary) PoM
Tablets, glibenclamide 2.5 mg, net price 28-tab pack = 29p; 5 mg, 28-tab pack = 34p

Daonil® (Hoechst Marion Roussel) PoM
Tablets, scored, glibenclamide 5 mg. Net price 28-tab pack = £2.69

Euglucon® (Aventis Pharma) PoM
Tablets, glibenclamide 2.5 mg, net price 28-tab pack = £1.72

GLICLAZIDE

Indications type 2 diabetes mellitus

Cautions see notes above; **interactions:** Appendix 1 (antidiabetics)

Contra-indications see notes above

Side-effects see notes above

Dose

- Initially, 40–80 mg daily, adjusted according to response; up to 160 mg as a single dose, with breakfast; higher doses divided; max. 320 mg daily

Gliclazide (Non-proprietary) PoM
Tablets, scored, gliclazide 80 mg, net price 28-tab pack = 66p, 60-tab pack = £1.46
Brands include *DIAGLYK®*

Diamicron® (Servier) PoM
Tablets, scored, gliclazide 80 mg, net price 60-tab pack = £4.56

Modified release

Diamicron® MR (Servier) PoM
Tablets, m/r, gliclazide 30 mg, net price 28-tab pack = £3.08, 56-tab pack = £6.16. Label: 25
Dose initially 30 mg daily with breakfast, adjusted according to response every 4 weeks (after 2 weeks if no decrease in blood glucose); max. 120 mg daily
Note *Diamicron® MR* 30 mg may be considered to be approximately equivalent in therapeutic effect to standard formulation *Diamicron®* 80 mg

GLIMEPIRIDE

Indications type 2 diabetes mellitus

Cautions see notes above; manufacturer recommends regular hepatic and haematological monitoring but limited evidence of clinical value; **interactions**: Appendix 1 (antidiabetics)

Contra-indications see notes above

Side-effects see notes above

Dose

- Initially 1 mg daily, adjusted according to response in 1-mg steps at 1–2 week intervals; usual max. 4 mg daily (exceptionally, up to 6 mg daily may be used); taken shortly before or with first main meal

Glimepiride (Non-proprietary) PoM
Tablets, glimepiride 1 mg, net price 30-tab pack = £3.14; 2 mg, 30-tab pack = £4.92; 3 mg, 30-tab pack = £7.57; 4 mg, 30-tab pack = £9.75

Amaryl® (Hoechst Marion Roussel) PoM
Tablets, all scored, glimepiride 1 mg (pink), net price 30-tab pack = £4.51; 2 mg (green), 30-tab pack = £7.42; 3 mg (yellow), 30-tab pack = £11.19; 4 mg (blue), 30-tab pack = £14.82

GLIPIZIDE

Indications type 2 diabetes mellitus

Cautions see notes above; **interactions:** Appendix 1 (antidiabetics)

Contra-indications see notes above

Side-effects see notes above; also dizziness, drowsiness

Dose

- Initially 2.5–5 mg daily shortly before breakfast or lunch, adjusted according to response; max. 20 mg daily; up to 15 mg may be given as a single dose; higher doses divided

Glipizide (Non-proprietary) PoM
Tablets, glipizide 5 mg, 56-tab pack = £4.08

Glibenese® (Pfizer) PoM
Tablets, scored, glipizide 5 mg. Net price 56-tab pack = £4.36

Minodiab® (Pharmacia) PoM
Tablets, glipizide 2.5 mg, net price 28-tab pack = £1.48; 5 mg (scored), 28-tab pack = £1.26

TOLBUTAMIDE

Indications type 2 diabetes mellitus

Cautions see notes above; **interactions**: Appendix 1 (antidiabetics)

Contra-indications see notes above

Side-effects see notes above; also headache, tinnitus

Dose

- 0.5–1.5 g (max. 2 g) daily in divided doses with or immediately after meals or as a single dose with or immediately after breakfast

Tolbutamide (Non-proprietary) PoM
Tablets, tolbutamide 500 mg. Net price 28-tab pack = £1.66

6.1.2.2 Biguanides

Metformin, the only available biguanide, has a different mode of action from the sulphonylureas, and is not interchangeable with them. It exerts its effect mainly by decreasing gluconeogenesis and by increasing peripheral utilisation of glucose; since it acts only in the presence of endogenous insulin it is effective only if there are some residual functioning pancreatic islet cells.

Metformin is the drug of first choice in overweight patients in whom strict dieting has failed to control diabetes, if appropriate it may also be considered as an option in patients who are not overweight. It is also used when diabetes is inadequately controlled with sulphonylurea treatment. When the combination of strict diet and metformin treatment fails, other options include:

- combining with acarbose (section 6.1.2.3), which may have a small beneficial effect, but flatulence can be a problem;
- combining with insulin (section 6.1.1) but weight gain and hypoglycaemia can be problems (weight gain minimised if insulin given at night);
- combining with a sulphonylurea (section 6.1.2.1) (reports of increased hazard with this combination remain unconfirmed);
- combining with pioglitazone or rosiglitazone (section 6.1.2.3);
- combining with repaglinide or nateglinide (section 6.1.2.3).

Insulin treatment is almost always required in medical and surgical emergencies; insulin should also be substituted before elective surgery (omit metformin on the morning of surgery and give insulin if required).

Hypoglycaemia does not usually occur with metformin; other advantages are the lower incidence of weight gain and lower plasma-insulin concentration. It does not exert a hypoglycaemic action in non-diabetic subjects unless given in overdose.

Gastro-intestinal side-effects are initially common with metformin, and may persist in some patients, particularly when very high doses such as 3 g daily are given.

Metformin can provoke lactic acidosis which is most likely to occur in patients with renal impairment; it should not be used in patients with even mild renal impairment.

Metformin is used for the symptomatic management of polycystic ovary syndrome [unlicensed indication]; it improves insulin sensitivity, may aid weight reduction, helps to normalise menstrual cycle (increasing the rate of spontaneous ovulation), and may improve hirsutism.

METFORMIN HYDROCHLORIDE

Indications diabetes mellitus (see notes above); polycystic ovary syndrome [unlicensed indication]

Cautions see notes above; determine renal function (using an appropriately sensitive method) before treatment and once or twice annually (more frequently in the elderly or if deterioration suspected); **interactions:** Appendix 1 (antidiabetics)

Contra-indications renal impairment (Appendix 3), ketoacidosis, withdraw if tissue hypoxia likely (e.g. sepsis, respiratory failure, recent myocardial infarction, hepatic impairment (Appendix 2)), use of iodine-containing X-ray contrast media (do not restart metformin until renal function returns to normal) and use of general anaesthesia (suspend metformin on the morning of surgery and restart when renal function returns to normal), pregnancy (Appendix 4) and breast-feeding (Appendix 5)

Side-effects anorexia, nausea, vomiting, diarrhoea (usually transient), abdominal pain, metallic taste; *rarely* lactic acidosis (withdraw treatment), decreased vitamin-B_{12} absorption, erythema, pruritus and urticaria; hepatitis also reported

Dose

- Diabetes mellitus, ADULT and CHILD over 10 years initially 500 mg with breakfast for at least 1 week then 500 mg with breakfast and evening meal for at least 1 week then 500 mg with breakfast, lunch and evening meal; usual max. 2 g daily in divided doses
- Polycystic ovary syndrome [unlicensed], initially 500 mg with breakfast for 1 week, then 500 mg with breakfast and evening meal for 1 week, then 1.5–1.7 g daily in 2–3 divided doses

Note Metformin doses in the BNF may differ from those in the product literature

Metformin (Non-proprietary) PoM

Tablets, coated, metformin hydrochloride 500 mg, net price 28-tab pack = 34p, 84-tab pack = £1.60; 850 mg, 56-tab pack = £1.00. Label: 21

Oral solution, sugar-free, metformin hydrochloride 500 mg/5 mL, net price 100 mL = £59.90. Label: 21
Brands include *Metsol®*

Glucophage® (Merck) PoM

Tablets, f/c, metformin hydrochloride 500 mg, net price 84-tab pack = £2.88; 850 mg, 56-tab pack = £3.20. Label: 21

Modified release

Glucophage® SR (Merck) PoM

Tablets, m/r, metformin hydrochloride 500 mg, net price 28 tab-pack = £3.20, 56 tab-pack = £6.40. Label: 21, 25

Dose initially 500 mg once daily, increased every 10–15 days, max. 2 g once daily with evening meal; if control not achieved use 1 g twice daily with meals and if control still not achieved change to standard-release tablets

Note Patients taking less than 2 g daily of the standard-release metformin may start with the same daily dose of *Glucophage® SR*; not suitable if dose of standard-release tablets more than 2 g daily. The *Scottish Medicines Consortium* has advised (December 2005) that *Glucophage® SR* is not recommended for the treatment of type 2 diabetes

With pioglitazone

See section 6.1.2.3

With rosiglitazone

See section 6.1.2.3

6.1.2.3 Other antidiabetics

Acarbose, an inhibitor of intestinal alpha glucosidases, delays the digestion and absorption of starch and sucrose. It has a small but significant effect in lowering blood glucose and is used either on its own or as an adjunct to metformin or to sulphonylureas when they prove inadequate. Postprandial hyperglycaemia in type 1 (insulin-dependent) diabetes can be reduced by acarbose, but it has been little used for this purpose. Flatulence deters some from using acarbose although this side-effect tends to decrease with time.

Nateglinide and **repaglinide** stimulate insulin release. Both drugs have a rapid onset of action and short duration of activity, and should be administered shortly before each main meal. Repaglinide may be given as monotherapy for patients who are not overweight or for those in whom metformin is contra-indicated or not tolerated, or it may be given in combination with metformin. Nateglinide is licensed only for use with metformin.

The thiazolidinediones, **pioglitazone** and **rosiglitazone**, reduce peripheral insulin resistance, leading to a reduction of blood-glucose concentration. Either drug can be used alone or in combination with metformin or with a sulphonylurea (if metformin inappropriate); the combination of a thiazolidinedione plus metformin is preferred to a thiazolidinedione plus sulphonylurea, particularly for obese patients. Inadequate response to a combination of metformin and sulphonylurea may indicate failing insulin release; the introduction of pioglitazone or rosiglitazone has a limited role in these circumstances and the initiation of insulin is often more appropriate. Blood-glucose control may deteriorate temporarily when a thiazolidinedione is substituted for an oral antidiabetic drug that is being used in combination with another. Long-term benefits of the thiazolidinediones have not yet been demonstrated. The *Scottish Medicines Consortium* accepts use of a thiazolidinedione (rosiglitazone (June 2006) pioglitazone (February 2007)) with metformin and a sulphonylurea, for patients (especially if overweight) whose glycaemic control is inadequate despite the use of 2 oral hypoglycaemic drugs and who are unable or unwilling to take insulin; treatment should be initiated and monitored by an experienced diabetes physician.

MHRA/CHM advice
Rosiglitazone and pioglitazone cardiovascular safety (December 2007 and February 2008)

Rosiglitazone and pioglitazone should not be used in patients with heart failure or history of heart failure; incidence of heart failure is increased when rosiglitazone or pioglitazone is combined with insulin. Rosiglitazone should not be used in patients with acute coronary syndrome. Patients should be closely monitored for signs of heart failure. Rosiglitazone may be associated with a small increased risk of cardiac ischaemia particularly in combination with insulin. Roziglitazone is not recommended for use in patients with ischaemic heart disease or peripheral arterial disease; in patients with history of ischaemic heart disease rosiglitazone should only be used after careful evaluation of the patient's individual risk. The combination of rosiglitazone and insulin should be used only in exceptional cases, and under close supervision.

NICE guidance
Pioglitazone and rosiglitazone for type 2 diabetes mellitus (August 2003)

Use of a thiazolidinedione (pioglitazone or rosiglitazone) as second-line therapy added to either metformin or a sulphonylurea is **not** recommended [see also notes above], except for:

- patients who are unable to tolerate metformin and sulphonylurea in combination therapy, *or*
- patients in whom either metformin or a sulphonylurea is contra-indicated.

In such cases, the thiazolidinedione should replace whichever drug in the combination is poorly tolerated or contra-indicated.

Sitagliptin, an inhibitor of dipeptidylpeptidase-4, increases insulin secretion and lowers glucagon secretion. It is licensed for use in type 2 diabetes in combination with metformin or a thiazolidinedione when treatment with either metformin or a thiazolidinedione fails to achieve adequate glycaemic control.

Exenatide, a synthetic form of exendin-4, is an incretin mimetic which increases insulin secretion, suppresses glucagon secretion, and slows gastric emptying. It is given by subcutaneous injection for the treatment of type 2 diabetes in combination with metformin or a suphonylurea, or both, in patients who have not achieved adequate glycaemic control with these drugs alone or in combination.

ACARBOSE

Indications diabetes mellitus inadequately controlled by diet or by diet with oral antidiabetic drugs

Cautions monitor liver function; may enhance hypoglycaemic effects of insulin and sulphonylureas (hypoglycaemic episodes may be treated with oral glucose but not with sucrose); **interactions:** Appendix 1 (antidiabetics)

Contra-indications inflammatory bowel disease, predisposition to partial intestinal obstruction; hernia, previous abdominal surgery; hepatic impairment; renal impairment (Appendix 3); pregnancy (Appendix 4); breast-feeding (Appendix 5)

Side-effects flatulence, soft stools, diarrhoea (may need to reduce dose or withdraw), abdominal distention and pain; *rarely*, nausea, abnormal liver function tests and skin reactions; *very rarely* ileus, oedema, jaundice, and hepatitis

Note Antacids unlikely to be beneficial for treating side-effects

Dose

- Initially 50 mg daily increased to 50 mg 3 times daily, then increased if necessary after 6–8 weeks to 100 mg 3 times daily; max. 200 mg 3 times daily; CHILD and ADOLESCENT under 18 years not recommended

Counselling Tablets should be chewed with first mouthful of food or swallowed whole with a little liquid immediately before food. To counteract possible hypoglycaemia, patients receiving insulin or a sulphonylurea as well as acarbose need to carry glucose (not sucrose—acarbose interferes with sucrose absorption)

Glucobay® (Bayer) PoM

Tablets, acarbose 50 mg, net price 90-tab pack = £6.60; 100 mg (scored), 90-tab pack = £12.51. Counselling, administration

EXENATIDE

Indications type 2 diabetes mellitus in combination with metformin or sulphonylurea (or with both) when metformin or a sulphonylurea or both inadequate

Cautions elderly; renal impairment (Appendix 3—avoid if creatinine clearance less than 30 mL/minute); **interactions:** Appendix 1 (antidiabetics)

Contra-indications ketoacidosis; severe gastro-intestinal disease; pregnancy (Appendix 4); breast-feeding (Appendix 5)

Side-effects gastro-intestinal disturbances including nausea, vomiting, diarrhoea, dyspepsia, abdominal pain and distension, gastro-oesophageal reflux disease, decreased appetite; headache, dizziness, asthenia; hypoglycaemia; increased sweating, injection-site reactions; antibody formation; *very rarely* anaphylactic reactions; also reported constipation, flatulence, dehydration, taste disturbance, pancreatitis, drowsiness, rash, pruritus, urticaria, and angioedema

Dose

- By subcutaneous injection, ADULT over 18 years, initially 5 micrograms twice daily within 1 hour before 2 main meals (at least 6 hours apart), increased if necessary after at least 1 month to max. 10 micrograms twice daily

Counselling If a dose is missed, continue with the next scheduled dose—do not administer **after** a meal. Some oral medications should be taken at least 1 hour before or 4 hours after exenatide injection—consult product literature for details

Byetta® (Lilly) ▼ PoM

Injection, exenatide 250 micrograms/mL, net price 5 microgram/dose prefilled pen (60 doses) = £68.24, 10 microgram/dose prefilled pen (60 doses) = £68.24. Counselling, administration

NATEGLINIDE

Indications type 2 diabetes mellitus in combination with metformin (section 6.1.2.2) when metformin alone inadequate

Cautions substitute insulin during intercurrent illness (such as myocardial infarction, coma, infection, and trauma) and during surgery (omit nateglinide on morning of surgery and recommence when eating and drinking normally); elderly, debilitated and malnourished patients; moderate hepatic impairment (avoid if severe—Appendix 2); **interactions:** Appendix 1 (antidiabetics)

Contra-indications ketoacidosis; pregnancy (Appendix 4) and breast-feeding (Appendix 5)

Side-effects hypoglycaemia; hypersensitivity reactions including pruritus, rashes and urticaria

Dose

- Initially 60 mg 3 times daily within 30 minutes before main meals, adjusted according to response up to max. 180 mg 3 times daily; CHILD and ADOLESCENT under 18 years not recommended

Starlix® (Novartis) PoM

Tablets, f/c, nateglinide 60 mg (pink), net price 84-tab pack = £22.71; 120 mg (yellow), 84-tab pack = £25.88; 180 mg (red), 84-tab pack = £25.88

PIOGLITAZONE

Indications type 2 diabetes mellitus (alone or combined with metformin or a sulphonylurea, or with both—see also notes above)

Cautions monitor liver function (see below); cardiovascular disease or in combination with insulin (risk of heart failure—see MHRA/CHM advice p. 369); substitute insulin during peri-operative period (omit pioglitazone on morning of surgery and recommence when eating and drinking normally); increased risk of bone fractures in females in feet, lower leg, hands, and lower arms; **interactions:** Appendix 1 (antidiabetics)

Liver toxicity Rare reports of liver dysfunction; monitor liver function before treatment, and periodically thereafter; advise patients to seek immediate medical attention if symptoms such as nausea, vomiting, abdominal pain, fatigue and dark urine develop; discontinue if jaundice occurs

Contra-indications hepatic impairment, history of heart failure, pregnancy (Appendix 4), breast-feeding (Appendix 5)

Side-effects gastro-intestinal disturbances, weight gain, oedema, anaemia, headache, visual disturbances, dizziness, arthralgia, hypoaesthesia, haematuria, impotence; *less commonly* hypoglycaemia, fatigue, insomnia, vertigo, sweating, altered blood lipids, proteinuria; see also Liver Toxicity above

Dose

- Initially 15–30 mg once daily increased to 45 mg once daily according to response

Actos® (Takeda) ▼ PoM
Tablets, pioglitazone (as hydrochloride) 15 mg, net price 28-tab pack = £24.14; 30 mg, 28-tab pack = £33.54; 45 mg, 28-tab pack = £36.96

With metformin

For cautions, contra-indications, and side-effects of metformin, see section 6.1.2.2

Competact® (Takeda) ▼ PoM
Tablets, f/c, pioglitazone (as hydrochloride) 15 mg, metformin hydrochloride 850 mg, net price 56-tab pack = £31.56. Label: 21

Dose type 2 diabetes not controlled by metformin alone, 1 tablet twice daily; CHILD and ADOLESCENT under 18 years not recommended

Note Titration with the individual components (pioglitazone and metformin) desirable before initiating *Competact®*

REPAGLINIDE

Indications type 2 diabetes mellitus (as monotherapy or in combination with metformin when metformin alone inadequate)

Cautions substitute insulin during intercurrent illness (such as myocardial infarction, coma, infection, and trauma) and during surgery (omit repaglinide on morning of surgery and recommence when eating and drinking normally); debilitated and malnourished patients; renal impairment; **interactions**: Appendix 1 (antidiabetics)

Contra-indications ketoacidosis; severe hepatic impairment; pregnancy (Appendix 4) and breast-feeding (Appendix 5)

Side-effects abdominal pain, diarrhoea, constipation, nausea, vomiting; *rarely* hypoglycaemia, hypersensitivity reactions including pruritus, rashes, vasculitis, urticaria, and visual disturbances

Dose

- Initially 500 micrograms within 30 minutes before main meals (1 mg if transferring from another oral hypoglycaemic), adjusted according to response at intervals of 1–2 weeks; up to 4 mg may be given as a single dose, max. 16 mg daily; CHILD and ADOLESCENT under 18 years and ELDERLY over 75 years, not recommended

Prandin® (Daiichi Sankyo) PoM
Tablets, repaglinide 500 micrograms, net price 30-tab pack = £3.92, 90-tab pack = £11.76; 1 mg (yellow), 30-tab pack = £3.92, 90-tab pack = £11.76; 2 mg (peach), 90-tab pack = £11.76
Formerly marketed as *NovoNorm®*

ROSIGLITAZONE

Indications type 2 diabetes mellitus (alone *or* combined with metformin *or* with a sulphonylurea *or* with both—see also notes above)

Cautions monitor liver function (see below); cardiovascular disease or in combination with insulin (risk of heart failure and ischaemic heart disease—see MHRA/CHM advice p. 369); substitute insulin during peri-operative period (omit rosiglitazone on morning of surgery and recommence when eating and drinking normally); increased risk of bone fracture in females in feet, hands, and upper arms; renal impairment (Appendix 3); **interactions**: Appendix 1 (antidiabetics)

Liver toxicity Rare reports of liver dysfunction reported; monitor liver function before treatment and periodically thereafter; advise patients to seek immediate medical attention if symptoms such as nausea, vomiting, abdominal pain, fatigue, anorexia and dark urine develop; discontinue if jaundice occurs or liver enzymes significantly raised

Contra-indications hepatic impairment, history of heart failure or acute coronary syndrome, pregnancy (Appendix 4), breast-feeding (Appendix 5)

Side-effects gastro-intestinal disturbances, cardiac ischaemia, headache, anaemia, altered blood lipids, weight gain, oedema, hypoglycaemia, bone fracture; *less commonly* increased appetite, heart failure, fatigue, paraesthesia, alopecia, dyspnoea; *rarely* pulmonary oedema, onset or worsening of macular oedema; *very rarely* angioedema, urticaria; see also Liver Toxicity above

Dose

- Initially 4 mg daily; may be increased after 8 weeks to 8 mg daily (in 1–2 divided doses) according to response; CHILD and ADOLESCENT under 18 years not recommended

Avandia® (GSK) PoM
Tablets, f/c, rosiglitazone (as maleate) 4 mg (orange), net price 28-tab pack = £24.74, 56-tab pack = £49.48; 8 mg (red/brown), 28-tab pack = £50.78

With metformin

For cautions, contra-indications, and side-effects of metformin, see section 6.1.2.2

Avandamet (GSK) ▼ PoM
Avandamet® 2 mg/500 mg tablets, f/c, pink, rosiglitazone (as maleate) 2 mg, metformin hydrochloride 500 mg, net price 112-tab pack = £52.45.Label: 21
Avandamet® 2 mg/1 g tablets, f/c, yellow, rosiglitazone (as maleate) 2 mg, metformin hydrochloride 1 g, net price 56-tab pack = £27.71. Label: 21
Avandamet® 4 mg/1 g tablets, f/c, pink, rosiglitazone (as maleate) 4 mg, metformin hydrochloride 1 g, net price 56-tab pack = £52.45. Label: 21

Dose type 2 diabetes mellitus not controlled by metformin alone, initially one *Avandamet®* 2 mg/1 g tablet twice daily, increased after 8 weeks according to response up to two *Avandamet®* 2 mg/500 mg tablets twice daily or one *Avandamet®* 4 mg/1 g tablet twice daily; max. 8 mg rosiglitazone and 2 g metformin hydrochloride daily; CHILD and ADOLESCENT under 18 years not recommended

Note Titration with the individual components (rosiglitazone and metformin) desirable before initiating *Avandamet®*

SITAGLIPTIN

Indications type 2 diabetes mellitus (in combination with metformin or a thiazolidinedione, when metformin or thiazolidinedione is inadequate)

Cautions renal impairment (Appendix 3); **interactions**: Appendix 1 (antidiabetics)

Contra-indications ketoacidosis; pregnancy (Appendix 4); breast-feeding (Appendix 5)

Side-effects gastro-intestinal disturbances; peripheral oedema; upper respiratory tract infection, nasopharyngitis; pain; osteoarthritis; *less commonly* anorexia, headache, drowsiness, dizziness, hypoglycaemia, osteoarthritis

Dose

- ADULT over 18 years, 100 mg once daily

Januvia® (MSD) ▼ PoM

Tablets, beige, f/c, sitagliptin (as phosphate) 100 mg, net price 28-tab pack = £33.26

6.1.3 Diabetic ketoacidosis

Soluble insulin, used intravenously, is the most appropriate form of insulin for the management of diabetic ketoacidotic and hyperosmolar non-ketotic coma. It is preferable to use the type of soluble insulin that the patient has been using previously. It is necessary to achieve and to maintain an adequate plasma-insulin concentration until the metabolic disturbance is brought under control.

Insulin is best given by intravenous infusion, using an infusion pump, and diluted to 1 unit/mL (care in mixing, see Appendix 6). Adequate plasma-insulin concentration can usually be maintained with infusion rates of 6 units/hour for adults and 0.1 units/kg/hour for children. Blood glucose is expected to decrease by about 5 mmol/litre/hour; if the response is inadequate the infusion rate can be doubled or quadrupled. When the blood-glucose concentration has fallen to 10 mmol/litre the infusion rate can be reduced to 3 units/hour for adults (about 0.05 units/kg/hour for children) and continued until the patient is ready to take food by mouth. The insulin infusion should not be stopped before subcutaneous insulin has been started.

No matter how large, a bolus intravenous injection of insulin can provide an adequate plasma concentration for a short time only; therefore if facilities for intravenous infusion are not available the insulin is given by *intramuscular injection*. An initial loading dose of 20 units intramuscularly is followed by 6 units intramuscularly every hour until the blood-glucose concentration falls to 10 mmol/litre; intramuscular injections are then given every 2 hours. Although absorption of insulin is usually rapid after intramuscular injection, it may be impaired in the presence of hypotension and poor tissue perfusion; moreover insulin may accumulate during treatment and late hypoglycaemia should be watched for and treated appropriately.

Intravenous replacement of fluid and electrolytes (section 9.2.2) with **sodium chloride** intravenous infusion is an essential part of the management of ketoacidosis; **potassium chloride** is included in the infusion as appropriate to prevent the hypokalaemia induced by the insulin. **Sodium bicarbonate** infusion (1.26% or 2.74%) is used only in cases of extreme acidosis and shock since the acid-base disturbance is normally corrected by the insulin. When the blood glucose has fallen to approximately 10 mmol/litre **glucose** 5% is infused (maximum 2 litres in 24 hours), but insulin infusion must continue.

6.1.4 Treatment of hypoglycaemia

Initially glucose 10–20 g is given by mouth either in liquid form or as granulated sugar or sugar lumps. Approximately 10 g of glucose is available from 2 teaspoons of sugar, 3 sugar lumps, *GlucoGel*® (formerly known as *Hypostop Gel*® glucose 10 g/25 g tube, available from BBI Healthcare), and non-diet versions of *Lucozade*® *Energy Original* 55 mL, *Coca-Cola*® 90 mL, *Ribena*® *Original* 15 mL (to be diluted). If necessary this may be repeated in 10–15 minutes. After initial treatment, a snack providing sustained availability of carbohydrate (e.g. a sandwich, fruit, milk, and biscuits) or the next meal, if it is due, can prevent blood-glucose concentration from falling again.

Hypoglycaemia which causes unconsciousness is an emergency. **Glucagon**, a polypeptide hormone produced by the alpha cells of the islets of Langerhans, increases plasma-glucose concentration by mobilising glycogen stored in the liver. In hypoglycaemia, if sugar cannot be given by mouth, glucagon can be given by injection. Carbohydrates should be given as soon as possible to restore liver glycogen; glucagon is not appropriate for chronic hypoglycaemia. It may be issued to close relatives of insulin-treated patients for emergency use in hypoglycaemic attacks. It is often advisable to prescribe on an 'if necessary' basis to hospitalised insulin-treated patients, so that it may be given rapidly by the nurses during an hypoglycaemic emergency. If not effective in 10 minutes intravenous glucose should be given.

Alternatively, 50 mL of **glucose intravenous infusion 20%** (section 9.2.2) may be given intravenously into a large vein through a large-gauge needle; care is required since this concentration is irritant especially if extravasation occurs. Alternatively, 25 mL of glucose intravenous infusion 50% may be given, but this higher concentration is more irritant and viscous making administration difficult. Glucose intravenous infusion 10% may also be used but larger volumes are needed. Close monitoring is necessary in the case of an overdose with a long-acting insulin because further administration of glucose may be required. Patients whose hypoglycaemia is caused by an oral antidiabetic drug should be transferred to hospital because the hypoglycaemic effects of these drugs may persist for many hours.

For advice on the emergency management of hypoglycaemia in dental practice, see p. 23

GLUCAGON

Indications see notes above and under Dose

Cautions see notes above, insulinoma, glucagonoma; ineffective in chronic hypoglycaemia, starvation, and adrenal insufficiency

Contra-indications phaeochromocytoma

Side-effects nausea, vomiting, abdominal pain, hypokalaemia, hypotension, rarely hypersensitivity reactions

Dose

- Insulin-induced hypoglycaemia, by subcutaneous, intramuscular, *or* intravenous injection, ADULT and CHILD over 8 years (or body-weight over 25 kg), 1 mg; CHILD under 8 years (or body-weight under 25 kg), 500 micrograms; if no response within 10 minutes intravenous glucose must be given
- Diagnostic aid, consult product literature
- Beta-blocker poisoning, see p. 32

Note 1 unit of glucagon = 1 mg of glucagon

[1]**GlucaGen® HypoKit** (Novo Nordisk) PoM
Injection, powder for reconstitution, glucagon (rys) as hydrochloride with lactose, net price 1-mg vial with prefilled syringe containing water for injection = £11.52

1. PoM restriction does not apply where administration is for saving life in emergency

Chronic hypoglycaemia

Diazoxide, administered by mouth, is useful in the management of patients with chronic hypoglycaemia from excess endogenous insulin secretion, either from an islet cell tumour or islet cell hyperplasia. It has no place in the management of acute hypoglycaemia.

DIAZOXIDE

Indications chronic intractable hypoglycaemia (for use in hypertensive crisis see section 2.5.1)

Cautions ischaemic heart disease, pregnancy (Appendix 4), labour, impaired renal function (Appendix 3); haematological examinations and blood pressure monitoring required during prolonged treatment; growth, bone, and developmental checks in children; **interactions:** Appendix 1 (diazoxide)

Side-effects anorexia, nausea, vomiting, hyperuricaemia, hypotension, oedema, tachycardia, arrhythmias, extrapyramidal effects; hypertrichosis on prolonged treatment

Dose

- By mouth, ADULT and CHILD, initially 5 mg/kg daily in 2–3 divided doses

Eudemine® (Celltech) PoM
Tablets, diazoxide 50 mg. Net price 20 = £9.29
Injection, see section 2.5.1

6.1.5 Treatment of diabetic nephropathy and neuropathy

Diabetic nephropathy

Regular review of diabetic patients should include an annual test for urinary protein (using *Albustix®*) and serum creatinine measurement. If the urinary protein test is negative, the urine should be tested for microalbuminuria (the earliest sign of nephropathy). If reagent strip tests (*Micral-Test II®* NHS or *Micro-bumintest®* NHS) are used and prove positive, the result should be confirmed by laboratory analysis of a urine sample. Provided there are no contra-indications, all diabetic patients with nephropathy causing proteinuria or with established microalbuminuria (at least 3 positive tests) should be treated with an ACE inhibitor (section 2.5.5.1) or an angiotensin-II receptor antagonist (section 2.5.5.2) even if the blood pressure is normal; in any case, to minimise the risk of renal deterioration, blood pressure should be carefully controlled (section 2.5).

ACE inhibitors can potentiate the hypoglycaemic effect of insulin and oral antidiabetic drugs; this effect is more likely during the first weeks of combined treatment and in patients with renal impairment.

For the treatment of hypertension in diabetes, see section 2.5.

Diabetic neuropathy

Optimal diabetic control is beneficial for the management of *painful neuropathy* in patients with type 1 diabetes (see also section 4.7.3). **Paracetamol** or a **non-steroidal anti-inflammatory drug** such as ibuprofen (section 10.1.1) may relieve *mild to moderate pain*.

The **tricyclic antidepressants** amitriptyline and nortriptyline (section 4.3.1) are the drugs of choice for painful diabetic neuropathy [unlicensed use]; amitriptyline is given in a dose of 25–75 mg daily (higher doses under specialist supervision). Other classes of antidepressants do not appear to be effective. **Gabapentin** (section 4.8.1) is licensed for the treatment of neuropathic pain and is an effective alternative to a tricyclic antidepressant.

Duloxetine (section 4.3.4) is licensed for the treatment of diabetic neuropathic pain.

Carbamazepine and **phenytoin** [both unlicensed] (section 4.8.1) may be useful for shooting or stabbing pain, but adverse effects are common; carbamazepine 200–800 mg daily in divided doses has been used.

Capsaicin cream 0.075% (section 10.3.2) is licensed for painful diabetic neuropathy and may have some effect, but it produces an intense burning sensation during the initial treatment period.

Neuropathic pain may respond partially to some **opioid analgesics**, such as methadone, oxycodone and tramadol, and they may have a role when other treatments have failed.

In *autonomic neuropathy* diabetic diarrhoea can often be managed by 2 or 3 doses of **tetracycline** 250 mg [unlicensed use] (section 5.1.3). Otherwise **codeine phosphate** (section 1.4.2) is the best drug, but other antidiarrhoeal preparations can be tried. An **antiemetic** which promotes gastric transit, such as metoclopramide or domperidone (section 4.6), is helpful for gastroparesis. In rare cases when an antiemetic does not help, erythromycin (especially when given intravenously) may be beneficial but this needs confirmation.

For the management of erectile dysfunction, see section 7.4.5.

In *neuropathic postural hypotension* increased salt intake and the use of the **mineralocorticoid** fludrocortisone 100–400 micrograms daily [unlicensed use] (section 6.3.1) help by increasing plasma volume, but uncomfortable oedema is a common side-effect. Fludrocortisone can also be combined with **flurbiprofen** (section 10.1.1) and **ephedrine hydrochloride** (section 3.1.1.2) [both unlicensed]. **Midodrine** [unlicensed], an alpha agonist, may also be useful in postural hypotension.

Gustatory sweating can be treated with an **antimuscarinic** such as propantheline bromide (section 1.2); side-effects are common. For the management of hyperhidrosis, see section 13.12.

In some patients with *neuropathic oedema*, **ephedrine hydrochloride** [unlicensed use] 30–60 mg 3 times daily offers effective relief.

6.1.6 Diagnostic and monitoring agents for diabetes mellitus

Blood monitoring

Blood **glucose** monitoring gives a direct measure of the glucose concentration at the time of the test and can detect hypoglycaemia as well as hyperglycaemia. Patients should be properly trained in the use of blood glucose monitoring systems and to take appropriate action on the results obtained. Inadequate understanding of the normal fluctuations in blood glucose may lead to confusion and inappropriate action. It is ideal for patients to observe the 'peaks' and 'troughs' of blood glucose over 24 hours and make adjustments of their insulin no more than once or twice weekly. Daily alterations to the insulin dose are highly undesirable (except during illness).

Blood glucose monitoring is best carried out by means of a meter. Visual colour comparison is sometimes used but is much less satisfactory. Meters give a more precise reading and are useful for patients with poor eyesight or who are colour blind.

Note In the UK blood-glucose concentration is expressed in mmol/litre and Diabetes UK advises that these units should be used for self-monitoring of blood glucose. In other European countries units of mg/100 mL (or mg/dL) are commonly used. It is advisable to check that the meter is pre-set in the correct units.

◢Test strips

Active® (Roche Diagnostics)
Reagent strips, for blood glucose monitoring, range 0.6–33.3 mmol/litre, for use with *Glucotrend®* and *Accu-Chek® Active* NHS meters only. Net price 50-strip pack = £14.47

Advantage Plus® (Roche Diagnostics)
Sensor strips, for blood glucose monitoring, range 0.6–33.3 mmol/litre, for use with *Accu-Chek® Advantage* NHS meter only. Net price 50-strip pack = £14.47

Ascensia® Autodisc (Bayer Diagnostics)
Sensor discs, for blood glucose monitoring, range 0.6–33.3 mmol/litre, for use with *Ascensia Breeze®* NHS and *Ascensia Esprit® 2* NHS meters only. Net price 5 × 10-disc pack = £14.33

Ascensia® Microfill (Bayer Diagnostics)
Sensor strips, for blood glucose monitoring, range 0.6–33.3 mmol/litre, for use with *Contour®* NHS meter only. Net price 50-strip pack = £14.45

Aviva® (Roche Diagnostics)
Sensor strips, for blood glucose monitoring, range 0.6–33.3 mmol/litre, for use with *Accu-Chek® Aviva* NHS meter only. Net price 50-strip pack = £14.20

BM-Accutest® (Roche Diagnostics)
Reagent strips, for blood glucose monitoring, range 1.1–33.3 mmol/litre, for use with *Accutrend®* NHS meters only. Net price 50-strip pack = £14.03

Breeze 2® (Bayer)
Sensor discs, for blood glucose monitoring, range 0.6–33.3 mmol/litre, for use with the Breeze 2® NHS meter only. Net price 5 × 10-disc pack = £14.06

Compact® (Roche Diagnostics)
Reagent strips, for blood glucose monitoring, range 0.6–33.3 mmol/litre, for use with *Accu-Chek® Compact* and *Accu-Chek® Compact Plus* NHS meters only. Net price 3 × 17-strip pack = £14.59

FreeStyle® (Abbott)
Sensor strips, for blood glucose monitoring, range 1.1–27.8 mmol/litre, for use with *FreeStyle®* NHS meters only. Net price 50-strip pack = £14.33

Freestyle Lite® (Abbott)
Sensor strips, for blood glucose monitoring, range 1.1–27.8 micromol/litre, for use with *Freestyle® Lite* NHS meter only. Net price 50-strip pack = £14.33

GlucoMen® (Menarini Diagnostics)
Sensor strips, for blood glucose monitoring, range 1.1–33.3 mmol/litre, for use with *GlucoMen® Glycó* NHS meter only. Net price 50-strip pack = £13.15

GlucoMen® Visio Sensor (Menarini Diagnostics)
Sensor strips, for blood glucose monitoring, range 1.1–33.3 mmol/litre, for use with *GlucoMen® Visio* NHS meter. Net price 50-strip pack = £13.97

Glucotide® (Bayer Diagnostics) NHS
Reagent strips, for blood glucose monitoring, range 0.6–33.3 mmol/litre, for use with *Glucometer® 4* NHS meter only. Net price 50-strip pack = £15.33

Hypoguard® Supreme (Hypoguard)
Reagent strips, for blood glucose monitoring, range 2.2–27.7 mmol/litre, for use with *Hypoguard® Supreme* NHS meters. Net price 50-strip pack = £12.00

MediSense G2® (Abbott)
Sensor strips, for blood glucose monitoring, range 1.1–33.3 mmol/litre, for use with *MediSense® Precision QID* NHS meter only. Net price 50-strip pack = £13.41

MediSense® Soft-Sense Plus (Abbott)
Sensor strips, for blood glucose monitoring, range 1.7–25 mmol/litre, for use with *Optium Xceed®* meter only. Net price 50-strip pack = £14.23

One Touch® (LifeScan)
Reagent strips, for blood glucose monitoring, range 0–33.3 mmol/litre, for use with *One Touch® II*, *Profile* and *Basic* NHS meters only. Net price 50-strip pack = £14.09

One Touch® Ultra (LifeScan)
Sensor strips, for blood glucose monitoring, range 1.1–33.3 mmol/litre, for use with *One Touch® Ultra* meter only. Net price 50-strip pack = £14.24

Optium® β-ketone test strips (Abbott)
Reagent Strips, for blood ketone monitoring, range 0–8.0 mmol/litre, for use with *Optium®* NHS or *Optium Xceed®* NHS meters only. Net price 10-strip pack = £18.80

Optium Plus® (Abbott)
Sensor strips (formerly *Medisense® Optium Plus*), for blood glucose monitoring, range 1.1–33.3 mmol/litre, for use with *Optium Xceed* NHS meter only. Net price 50-strip pack = £14.24

PocketScan® (LifeScan)
Sensor strips, for blood glucose monitoring, range 1.1–33.3 mmol/litre, for use with *PocketScan®* NHS meter only. Net price 50-strip pack = £13.92

Prestige® Smart System (DiagnoSys)
Reagent strips, for blood glucose monitoring, range 1.4–33.3 mmol/litre, for use with *Prestige® Smart System* NHS meter only. Net price 50-strip pack = £14.23

TrueTrack® Smart System (ADL)
Sensor strips, for blood glucose monitoring, range 1.1–33.3 mmol/litre, for use with *TrueTrack® Smart System* NHS meter only. Net price 50-strip pack = £13.97

Meters

Accu-Chek® Aviva (Roche Diagnostics)
Meter, for blood glucose monitoring (for use with *Aviva®* test strips). *Accu-Chek® Aviva* system = £7.79

Accu-Chek® Compact Plus (Roche Diagnostics) NHS
Meter, for blood glucose monitoring (for use with *Compact®* test strips). *Accu-Chek® Compact Plus* system = £7.79

Ascensia Breeze® (Bayer Diagnostics) NHS
Meter, for blood glucose monitoring (for use with *Ascensia® Autodisc* test sensor discs)

Ascensia Esprit® 2 (Bayer Diagnostics) NHS
Meter, for blood glucose monitoring (for use with *Ascensia® Glucodisc* test sensor discs) = £17.49

Contour® (Bayer Diagnostics) NHS
Meter, for blood glucose monitoring (for use with *Ascensia® Microfill* sensor strips) = £19.97

FreeStyle® (Abbott) NHS
Meters for blood glucose monitoring (for use with *FreeStyle®* and *FreeStyle Lite®* test strips). *FreeStyle Lite®* meter = £7.79; *FreeStyle Freedon Lite®* meter = £5.99

GlucoMen® Glycó (Menarini Diagnostics) NHS
Meter, for blood glucose monitoring (for use with *GlucoMen®* sensor strips)

GlucoMen® PC (Menarini Diagnostics) NHS
Meter, for blood glucose monitoring (for use with *GlucoMen®* sensor strips)

GlucoMen® Visio (Menarini Diagnostics) NHS
Meter, for blood glucose monitoring (for use with *GlucoMen® Visio Sensor* strips) = £12.99

Hypoguard® Supreme (Hypoguard) NHS
Meters, for blood glucose monitoring (for use with *Hypoguard® Supreme* test strips). *Hypoguard® Supreme Plus* meter = £35.00; *Hypoguard® Supreme Extra* meter = £45.00

One Touch® (LifeScan) NHS
Meters, for blood glucose monitoring (for use with *One Touch®* test strips). *One Touch® Basic* system pack = £9.38, *One Touch® Profile* system pack = £18.38

One Touch® Ultra (LifeScan) NHS
Meter, for blood glucose monitoring (for use with *One Touch® Ultra* test strips) = £10.00

Optium® Xceed (Abbott) NHS
Meter, for blood glucose monitoring (for use with *Med-iSense® Soft-Sense* and *Optium® Plus* test strips) and for blood ketone monitoring (for use with *Optium®* ß-ketone test strips). Net price starter pack = £14.99

PocketScan® (LifeScan) NHS
Meter, for blood glucose monitoring (for use with *PocketScan®* test strips). *Complete PocketScan® System* = £17.50

Prestige® Smart System (DiagnoSys) NHS
Meter, for blood glucose monitoring (for use with *Prestige® Smart System* test strips) = £5.63

TrueTrack® Smart System (ADL) NHS
Meter, for blood glucose monitoring (for use with *TrueTrack® Smart System* test strips) = £5.63

Urinalysis

Urine testing for glucose is useful in patients who find blood glucose monitoring difficult. Tests for glucose range from reagent strips specific to glucose to reagent tablets which detect all reducing sugars. Few patients still use *Clinitest®*; *Clinistix®* is suitable for screening purposes only. Tests for ketones by patients are rarely required unless they become unwell.

Microalbuminuria can be detected with *Micral-Test II®* NHS or *Microbumintest®* NHS but this should be followed by confirmation in the laboratory, since false positive results are common.

Glucose

Clinistix® (Bayer Diagnostics)
Reagent strips, for detection of glucose in urine. Net price 50-strip pack = £3.18

Clinitest® (Bayer Diagnostics) NHS
Reagent tablets, for detection of glucose and other reducing substances in urine. Pocket set (test tube, dropper and 36 tablets), net price = £4.02, 36-tab pack = £2.00, 6-test tube pack = £3.70, 6-dropper pack = £3.80

Diabur-Test 5000® (Roche Diagnostics)
Reagent strips, for detection of glucose in urine. Net price 50-strip pack = £2.74

Diastix® (Bayer Diagnostics)
Reagent strips, for detection of glucose in urine. Net price 50-strip pack = £2.71

Medi-Test® Glucose (BHR)
Reagent strips, for detection of glucose in urine. Net price 50-strip pack = £2.17

Ketones

Ketostix® (Bayer Diagnostics)
Reagent strips, for detection of ketones in urine. Net price 50-strip pack = £2.87

Ketur Test® (Roche Diagnostics)
Reagent strips, for detection of ketones in urine. Net price 50-strip pack = £2.63

Protein

Albustix® (Bayer Diagnostics)
Reagent strips, for detection of protein in urine. Net price 50-strip pack = £3.94

Medi-Test® Protein 2 (BHR)
Reagent strips, for detection of protein in urine. Net price 50-strip pack = £3.03

Other reagent strips available for urinalysis include:

Combur-3 Test® NHS (glucose and protein—Roche Diagnostics), *Clinitek Microalbumin®* NHS (albumin and creatinine—Bayer Diagnostics), *Ketodiastix®* NHS (glucose and ketones—Bayer Diagnostics), *Medi-Test Combi 2®* NHS (glucose and protein—BHR), *Micral-Test II®* NHS (albumin—Roche Diagnostics), *Microalbustix®* NHS (albumin and creatinine—Bayer Diagnostics), *Microbumintest®* NHS (albumin—Bayer Diagnostics), *Uristix®* NHS (glucose and protein—Bayer Diagnostics)

Glucose tolerance test

The **glucose** tolerance test is now rarely needed for the diagnosis of diabetes when symptoms of hyperglycaemia are present, though it is still required to establish the presence of gestational diabetes. This generally involves giving anhydrous glucose 75 g (equivalent to

6 Endocrine system

Glucose BP 82.5 g) by mouth to the fasting patient, and measuring blood-glucose concentrations at intervals.

The appropriate amount of glucose should be given with 200–300 mL fluid. Anhydrous glucose 75 g may alternatively be given as 113 mL *Polycal®* (Nutricia Clinical) with extra fluid to administer a total volume of 200–300 mL.

6.2 Thyroid and antithyroid drugs

6.2.1 Thyroid hormones
6.2.2 Antithyroid drugs

6.2.1 Thyroid hormones

Thyroid hormones are used in hypothyroidism (myxoedema), and also in diffuse non-toxic goitre, Hashimoto's thyroiditis (lymphadenoid goitre), and thyroid carcinoma. Neonatal hypothyroidism requires prompt treatment for normal development. **Levothyroxine sodium** (thyroxine sodium) is the treatment of choice for *maintenance* therapy.

In infants and children with congenital hypothyroidism and juvenile myxoedema, the dose of levothyroxine should be titrated according to clinical response, growth assessment, and measurements of plasma thyroxine and thyroid-stimulating hormone. See *BNF for Children* (section 6.2.1) for suitable dosage regimens.

Liothyronine sodium has a similar action to levothyroxine but is more rapidly metabolised and has a more rapid effect; 20 micrograms is equivalent to 100 micrograms of levothyroxine. Its effects develop after a few hours and disappear within 24 to 48 hours of discontinuing treatment. It may be used in *severe hypothyroid states* when a rapid response is desired.

Liothyronine by intravenous injection is the treatment of choice in *hypothyroid coma*. Adjunctive therapy includes intravenous fluids, hydrocortisone, and treatment of infection; assisted ventilation is often required.

LEVOTHYROXINE SODIUM
(Thyroxine sodium)

Indications hypothyroidism; see also notes above

Cautions panhypopituitarism or predisposition to adrenal insufficiency (initiate corticosteroid therapy before starting levothyroxine), elderly, cardiovascular disorders (including hypertension, myocardial insufficiency or myocardial infarction, see Initial Dosage below), long-standing hypothyroidism, diabetes insipidus, diabetes mellitus (dose of antidiabetic drugs including insulin may need to be increased); pregnancy (Appendix 4); **interactions:** Appendix 1 (thyroid hormones)

Initial dosage Baseline ECG is valuable because changes induced by hypothyroidism can be confused with ischaemia. If metabolism increases too rapidly (causing diarrhoea, nervousness, rapid pulse, insomnia, tremors and sometimes anginal pain where there is latent myocardial ischaemia), reduce dose or withhold for 1–2 days and start again at a lower dose

Contra-indications thyrotoxicosis

Side-effects usually at excessive dosage (see Initial Dosage above) include diarrhoea, vomiting, anginal pain, arrhythmias, palpitation, tachycardia, tremor, restlessness, excitability, insomnia; headache, flushing, sweating, fever, heat intolerance, weight-loss, muscle cramp, and muscular weakness; transient hair loss in children; hypersensitivity reactions including rash, pruritus and oedema also reported

Dose

- ADULT, initially 50–100 micrograms once daily, preferably before breakfast, adjusted in steps of 25–50 micrograms every 3–4 weeks according to response (usual maintenance dose 100–200 micrograms once daily); in cardiac disease, severe hypothyroidism, and patients over 50 years, initially 25 micrograms once daily, adjusted in steps of 25 micrograms every 4 weeks according to response; usual maintenance dose 50–200 micrograms once daily; CHILD under 12 years see *BNF for Children* (section 6.2.1)
- Congenital hypothyroidism and juvenile myxoedema, see *BNF for Children* (section 6.2.1)

Levothyroxine (Non-proprietary) PoM

Tablets, levothyroxine sodium 25 micrograms, net price 28-tab pack = £1.40; 50 micrograms, 28-tab pack = 66p; 100 micrograms, 28-tab pack = 63p

Brands include *Eltroxin®*

Oral solution, levothyroxine sodium 25 micrograms/5 mL, net price 100 mL = £42.75; 50 micrograms/5 mL, 100 mL = £44.90; 100 micrograms/5 mL, 100 mL = £52.75

Brands include *Evotrox®* (sugar-free)

LIOTHYRONINE SODIUM
(L-Tri-iodothyronine sodium)

Indications see notes above

Cautions see under Levothyroxine Sodium; pregnancy (Appendix 4); breast-feeding (Appendix 5); **interactions:** Appendix 1 (thyroid hormones)

Contra-indications see under Levothyroxine Sodium

Side-effects see under Levothyroxine Sodium

Dose

- By mouth, initially 10–20 micrograms daily gradually increased to 60 micrograms daily in 2–3 divided doses; ELDERLY smaller initial doses; CHILD, adult dose reduced in proportion to body-weight
- By slow intravenous injection, hypothyroid coma, 5–20 micrograms repeated every 12 hours or as often as every 4 hours if necessary; alternatively 50 micrograms initially then 25 micrograms every 8 hours reducing to 25 micrograms twice daily

Liothyronine sodium (Goldshield) PoM

Tablets, scored, liothyronine sodium 20 micrograms, net price 28-tab pack = £9.15

Triiodothyronine (Goldshield) PoM
Injection, powder for reconstitution, liothyronine sodium (with dextran). Net price 20-microgram amp = £37.92

6.2.2 Antithyroid drugs

Antithyroid drugs are used for hyperthyroidism either to prepare patients for thyroidectomy or for long-term management. In the UK carbimazole is the most commonly used drug. Propylthiouracil may be used in patients who suffer sensitivity reactions to carbimazole as sensitivity is not necessarily displayed to both drugs Both drugs act primarily by interfering with the synthesis of thyroid hormones.

> **CSM warning (neutropenia and agranulocytosis)**
> Doctors are reminded of the importance of recognising bone marrow suppression induced by carbimazole and the need to stop treatment promptly.
> 1. Patient should be asked to report symptoms and signs suggestive of infection, especially sore throat.
> 2. A white blood cell count should be performed if there is any clinical evidence of infection.
> 3. Carbimazole should be stopped promptly if there is clinical or laboratory evidence of neutropenia.

Carbimazole is given in a dose of 15 to 40 mg daily; occasionally a larger dose may be required. This dose is continued until the patient becomes euthyroid, usually after 4 to 8 weeks and the dose is then gradually reduced to a maintenance dose of 5 to 15 mg. Therapy is usually given for 12 to 18 months. Children may be given carbimazole in an initial dose of 250 micrograms/kg three times daily, adjusted according to response; treatment in children should be undertaken by a specialist. Rashes and pruritus are common but they can be treated with antihistamines without discontinuing therapy; alternatively propylthiouracil can be substituted. All patients should be advised to report any sore throat immediately because of the rare complication of agranulocytosis (see CSM warning, above).

Propylthiouracil is given in a dose of 200 to 400 mg daily in adults and this dose is maintained until the patient becomes euthyroid; the dose may then be gradually reduced to a maintenance dose of 50 to 150 mg daily.

Antithyroid drugs only need to be given once daily because of their prolonged effect on the thyroid. Overtreatment can result in the rapid development of hypothyroidism and should be avoided particularly during pregnancy because it can cause fetal goitre.

A combination of carbimazole, 40 to 60 mg daily with levothyroxine, 50 to 150 micrograms daily, may be used in a *blocking-replacement regimen*; therapy is usually given for 18 months. The blocking-replacement regimen is **not** suitable during pregnancy.

Iodine has been used as an adjunct to antithyroid drugs for 10 to 14 days before partial thyroidectomy; however, there is little evidence of a beneficial effect. Iodine should not be used for long-term treatment because its antithyroid action tends to diminish.

Radioactive sodium iodide (^{131}I) solution is used increasingly for the treatment of thyrotoxicosis at all ages, particularly where medical therapy or compliance is a problem, in patients with cardiac disease, and in patients who relapse after thyroidectomy.

Propranolol is useful for rapid relief of thyrotoxic symptoms and may be used in conjunction with antithyroid drugs or as an adjunct to radioactive iodine. Beta-blockers are also useful in neonatal thyrotoxicosis and in supraventricular arrhythmias due to hyperthyroidism. Propranolol has been used in conjunction with iodine to prepare mildly thyrotoxic patients for surgery but it is preferable to make the patient euthyroid with carbimazole. Laboratory tests of thyroid function are not altered by beta-blockers. Most experience in treating thyrotoxicosis has been gained with propranolol but **nadolol** is also used. For doses and preparations of beta-blockers see section 2.4.

Thyrotoxic crisis ('thyroid storm') requires emergency treatment with intravenous administration of fluids, propranolol (5 mg) and hydrocortisone (100 mg every 6 hours, as sodium succinate), as well as oral iodine solution and carbimazole or propylthiouracil which may need to be administered by nasogastric tube.

Pregnancy and breast-feeding Radioactive iodine therapy is contra-indicated during pregnancy. Propylthiouracil and carbimazole can be given but the blocking-replacement regimen (see above) is **not** suitable. Both propylthiouracil and carbimazole cross the placenta and in high doses may cause fetal goitre and hypothyroidism—the lowest dose that will control the hyperthyroid state should be used (requirements in Graves' disease tend to fall during pregnancy). Rarely, carbimazole has been associated with aplasia cutis of the neonate.

Carbimazole and propylthiouracil appear in breast milk but this does not preclude breast-feeding as long as neonatal development is closely monitored and the lowest effective dose is used.

CARBIMAZOLE

Indications hyperthyroidism
Cautions liver disorders, pregnancy, breast-feeding (see notes above)
Side-effects nausea, mild gastro-intestinal disturbances, headache, rashes and pruritus, arthralgia; rarely myopathy, alopecia, bone marrow suppression (including pancytopenia and agranulocytosis, see CSM warning above), jaundice
Dose
- See notes above

Counselling Warn patient to tell doctor **immediately** if sore throat, mouth ulcers bruising, fever, malaise, or non-specific illness develops

Neo-Mercazole® (Amdipharm) PoM
Tablets, both pink carbimazole 5 mg, net price 100-tab pack = £5.15; 20 mg, 100-tab pack = £19.12. Counselling, blood disorder symptoms

IODINE AND IODIDE

Indications thyrotoxicosis (pre-operative)
Cautions pregnancy children; not for long-term treatment
Contra-indications breast-feeding

Side-effects hypersensitivity reactions including coryza-like symptoms, headache, lacrimation, conjunctivitis, pain in salivary glands, laryngitis, bronchitis, rashes; on prolonged treatment depression, insomnia, impotence; goitre in infants of mothers taking iodides

Dose

- See under preparation

Aqueous Iodine Oral Solution

(Lugol's Solution), iodine 5%, potassium iodide 10% in purified water, freshly boiled and cooled, total iodine 130 mg/mL. Net price 100 mL = £1.19. Label: 27

Dose 0.1–0.3 mL 3 times daily well diluted with milk or water

PROPYLTHIOURACIL

Indications hyperthyroidism

Cautions see under Carbimazole; hepatic impairment (Appendix 2), renal impairment (Appendix 3)

Side-effects see under Carbimazole; leucopenia; rarely cutaneous vasculitis, thrombocytopenia, aplastic anaemia, hypoprothrombinaemia, hepatitis, encephalopathy, hepatic necrosis, nephritis, lupus erythematous-like syndromes

Dose

- See notes above

Propylthiouracil (Non-proprietary) PoM

Tablets, propylthiouracil 50 mg. Net price 56-tab pack = £32.90

6.3 Corticosteroids

6.3.1 Replacement therapy

6.3.2 Glucocorticoid therapy

6.3.1 Replacement therapy

The adrenal cortex normally secretes hydrocortisone (cortisol) which has glucocorticoid activity and weak mineralocorticoid activity. It also secretes the mineralocorticoid aldosterone.

In deficiency states, physiological replacement is best achieved with a combination of **hydrocortisone** (section 6.3.2) and the mineralocorticoid **fludrocortisone**; hydrocortisone alone does not usually provide sufficient mineralocorticoid activity for complete replacement.

In *Addison's disease* or following adrenalectomy, **hydrocortisone** 20 to 30 mg daily by mouth is usually required. This is given in 2 doses, the larger in the morning and the smaller in the evening, mimicking the normal diurnal rhythm of cortisol secretion. The optimum daily dose is determined on the basis of clinical response. Glucocorticoid therapy is supplemented by fludrocortisone 50 to 300 micrograms daily.

In *acute adrenocortical insufficiency*, **hydrocortisone** is given intravenously (preferably as sodium succinate) in doses of 100 mg every 6 to 8 hours in sodium chloride intravenous infusion 0.9%.

In *hypopituitarism* glucocorticoids should be given as in adrenocortical insufficiency, but since production of aldosterone is also regulated by the renin-angiotensin system a mineralocorticoid is not usually required. Additional replacement therapy with levothyroxine (section 6.2.1) and sex hormones (section 6.4) should be given as indicated by the pattern of hormone deficiency.

FLUDROCORTISONE ACETATE

Indications mineralocorticoid replacement in adrenocortical insufficiency

Cautions section 6.3.2; **interactions**: Appendix 1 (corticosteroids)

Contra-indications section 6.3.2

Side-effects section 6.3.2

Dose

- 50–300 micrograms daily; CHILD 5 micrograms/kg daily

Florinef® (Squibb) PoM

Tablets, scored, fludrocortisone acetate 100 micrograms. Net price 100-tab pack = £5.36. Label: 10, steroid card

6.3.2 Glucocorticoid therapy

In comparing the relative potencies of corticosteroids in terms of their anti-inflammatory (glucocorticoid) effects it should be borne in mind that high glucocorticoid activity in itself is of no advantage unless it is accompanied by relatively low mineralocorticoid activity (see Disadvantages of Corticosteroids below). The mineralocorticoid activity of **fludrocortisone** (section 6.3.1) is so high that its anti-inflammatory activity is of no clinical relevance. The table below shows equivalent anti-inflammatory doses.

Equivalent anti-inflammatory doses of corticosteroids

This table takes no account of mineralocorticoid effects, nor does it take account of variations in duration of action

Prednisolone 5 mg
≡ Betamethasone 750 micrograms
≡ Cortisone acetate 25 mg
≡ Deflazacort 6 mg
≡ Dexamethasone 750 micrograms
≡ Hydrocortisone 20 mg
≡ Methylprednisolone 4 mg
≡ Triamcinolone 4 mg

The relatively high mineralocorticoid activity of **cortisone** and **hydrocortisone**, and the resulting fluid retention, make them unsuitable for disease suppression on a long-term basis. However, they can be used for adrenal replacement therapy (section 6.3.1); hydrocortisone is preferred because cortisone requires conversion in the liver to hydrocortisone. Hydrocortisone is used on a short-term basis by intravenous injection for the emergency management of some conditions. The relatively moderate anti-inflammatory potency of hydrocortisone also makes it a useful topical corticosteroid for the management of inflammatory skin conditions because side-effects (both topical and systemic) are less marked (section 13.4); cortisone is not active topically.

Prednisolone has predominantly glucocorticoid activity and is the corticosteroid most commonly used by mouth for long-term disease suppression.

Betamethasone and **dexamethasone** have very high glucocorticoid activity in conjunction with insignificant mineralocorticoid activity. This makes them particularly suitable for high-dose therapy in conditions where fluid retention would be a disadvantage.

Betamethasone and dexamethasone also have a long duration of action and this, coupled with their lack of mineralocorticoid action makes them particularly suitable for conditions which require suppression of corticotropin (corticotrophin) secretion (e.g. congenital adrenal hyperplasia). Some esters of betamethasone and of **beclometasone** (beclomethasone) exert a considerably more marked topical effect (e.g. on the skin or the lungs) than when given by mouth; use is made of this to obtain topical effects whilst minimising systemic side-effects (e.g. for skin applications and asthma inhalations).

Deflazacort has a high glucocorticoid activity; it is derived from prednisolone.

Use of corticosteroids

Dosages of corticosteroids vary widely in different diseases and in different patients. If the use of a corticosteroid can save or prolong life, as in exfoliative dermatitis, pemphigus, acute leukaemia or acute transplant rejection, high doses may need to be given, because the complications of therapy are likely to be less serious than the effects of the disease itself.

When long-term corticosteroid therapy is used in some chronic diseases, the adverse effects of treatment may become greater than the disabilities caused by the disease. To minimise side-effects the maintenance dose should be kept as low as possible.

When potentially less harmful measures are ineffective corticosteroids are used topically for the treatment of inflammatory conditions of the skin (section 13.4). Corticosteroids should be avoided or used only under specialist supervision in psoriasis (section 13.5).

Corticosteroids are used both topically (by rectum) and systemically (by mouth or intravenously) in the management of ulcerative colitis and Crohn's disease (section 1.5 and section 1.7.2).

Use can be made of the mineralocorticoid activity of fludrocortisone to treat postural hypotension in autonomic neuropathy (section 6.1.5).

High-dose corticosteroids should be avoided for the management of septic shock. However, there is evidence that administration of lower doses of hydrocortisone (50 mg intravenously every 6 hours) and fludrocortisone (50 micrograms daily by mouth) is of benefit in adrenocortical insufficiency resulting from septic shock.

Dexamethasone and betamethasone have little if any mineralocorticoid action and their long duration of action makes them particularly suitable for suppressing corticotropin secretion in congenital adrenal hyperplasia where the dose should be tailored to clinical response and by measurement of adrenal androgens and 17-hydroxyprogesterone. In common with all glucocorticoids their suppressive action on the hypothalamic-pituitary-adrenal axis is greatest and most prolonged when they are given at night. In most individuals a single dose of 1 mg of dexamethasone at night, is sufficient to inhibit corticotropin secretion for 24 hours. This is the basis of the 'overnight dexamethasone suppression test' for diagnosing Cushing's syndrome.

Betamethasone and dexamethasone are also appropriate for conditions where water retention would be a disadvantage.

A corticosteroid may be used in the management of raised intracranial pressure or cerebral oedema that occurs as a result of malignancy (see also p. 16); high doses of betamethasone or dexamethasone are generally used. However, a corticosteroid should **not** be used for the management of head injury or stroke because it is unlikely to be of benefit and may even be harmful.

In acute hypersensitivity reactions such as angioedema of the upper respiratory tract and anaphylactic shock, corticosteroids are indicated as an adjunct to emergency treatment with adrenaline (epinephrine) (section 3.4.3). In such cases hydrocortisone (as sodium succinate) by intravenous injection in a dose of 100 to 300 mg may be required.

Corticosteroids are preferably used by inhalation in the management of asthma (section 3.2) but systemic therapy in association with bronchodilators is required for the emergency treatment of severe acute asthma (section 3.1.1).

Corticosteroids may also be useful in conditions such as autoimmune hepatitis, rheumatoid arthritis and sarcoidosis; they may also lead to remissions of acquired haemolytic anaemia (section 9.1.3), and some cases of the nephrotic syndrome (particularly in children) and thrombocytopenic purpura (section 9.1.4).

Corticosteroids can improve the prognosis of serious conditions such as systemic lupus erythematosus, temporal arteritis, and polyarteritis nodosa; the effects of the disease process may be suppressed and symptoms relieved, but the underlying condition is not cured, although it may ultimately remit It is usual to begin therapy in these conditions at fairly high dose, such as 40 to 60 mg prednisolone daily, and then to reduce the dose to the lowest commensurate with disease control.

For other references to the use of corticosteroids see Prescribing in Palliative Care, section 8.2.2 (immunosuppression), section 10.1.2 (rheumatic diseases), section 11.4 (eye), section 12.1.1 (otitis externa), section 12.2.1 (allergic rhinitis), and section 12.3.1 (aphthous ulcers).

Administration

Whenever possible *local treatment* with creams, intra-articular injections, inhalations, eye-drops, or enemas should be used in preference to *systemic treatment*. The suppressive action of a corticosteroid on cortisol secretion is least when it is given as a single dose in the morning. In an attempt to reduce pituitary-adrenal suppression further, the total dose for two days can sometimes be taken as a single dose on alternate days; alternate-day administration has not been very successful in the management of asthma (section 3.2). Pituitary-adrenal suppression can also be reduced by means of intermittent therapy with short courses. In some conditions it may be possible to reduce the dose of corticosteroid by adding a small dose of an immunosuppressive drug (section 8.2.1).

Cautions and contra-indications of corticosteroids

Adrenal Suppression

During prolonged therapy with corticosteroids, adrenal atrophy develops and can persist for years after stopping. Abrupt withdrawal after a prolonged period can lead to acute adrenal insufficiency, hypotension or death (see Withdrawal of Corticosteroids, below). Withdrawal can also be associated with fever, myalgia, arthralgia, rhinitis, conjunctivitis, painful itchy skin nodules and weight loss.

To compensate for a diminished adrenocortical response caused by prolonged corticosteroid treatment, any significant intercurrent illness, trauma, or surgical procedure requires a temporary increase in corticosteroid dose, or if already stopped, a temporary re-introduction of corticosteroid treatment. Anaesthetists **must** therefore know whether a patient is taking or has been taking a corticosteroid, to avoid a precipitous fall in blood pressure during anaesthesia or in the immediate postoperative period. A suitable regimen for corticosteroid replacement, in patients who have taken more than 10 mg prednisolone daily (or equivalent) within 3 months of surgery, is:

- *Minor surgery under general anaesthesia*—usual oral corticosteroid dose on the morning of surgery or hydrocortisone 25–50 mg (usually the sodium succinate) intravenously at induction; the usual oral corticosteroid dose is recommenced after surgery
- *Moderate or major surgery*—usual oral corticosteroid dose on the morning of surgery and hydrocortisone 25–50 mg intravenously at induction, followed by hydrocortisone 25–50 mg 3 times a day by intravenous injection for 24 hours after moderate surgery or for 48–72 hours after major surgery; the usual pre-operative oral corticosteroid dose is recommenced on stopping hydrocortisone injections

Patients on long-term corticosteroid treatment should carry a Steroid Treatment Card (see p. 382) which gives guidance on minimising risk and provides details of prescriber, drug, dosage and duration of treatment.

Infections

Prolonged courses of corticosteroids increase susceptibility to infections and severity of infections; clinical presentation of infections may also be atypical. Serious infections e.g. *septicaemia* and *tuberculosis* may reach an advanced stage before being recognised, and *amoebiasis* or *strongyloidiasis* may be activated or exacerbated (exclude before initiating a corticosteroid in those at risk or with suggestive symptoms). Fungal or viral *ocular infections* may also be exacerbated (see also section 11.4.1).

Chickenpox Unless they have had chickenpox, patients receiving oral or parenteral corticosteroids for purposes other than replacement should be regarded as being *at risk of severe chickenpox* (see Steroid Treatment Card). Manifestations of fulminant illness include pneumonia, hepatitis and disseminated intravascular coagulation; rash is not necessarily a prominent feature.

Passive immunisation with varicella–zoster immunoglobulin (section 14.5) is needed for exposed non-immune patients receiving systemic corticosteroids or for those who have used them within the previous 3 months. Confirmed chickenpox warrants specialist care and urgent treatment (section 5.3.2.1). Corticosteroids should not be stopped and dosage may need to be increased.

Topical, inhaled or rectal corticosteroids are less likely to be associated with an increased risk of severe chickenpox.

Measles Patients taking corticosteroids should be advised to take particular care to avoid exposure to measles and to seek immediate medical advice if exposure occurs. Prophylaxis with intramuscular normal immunoglobulin (section 14.5) may be needed.

Withdrawal of corticosteroids

The CSM has recommended that *gradual* withdrawal of systemic corticosteroids should be considered in those whose disease is unlikely to relapse and have

- recently received repeated courses (particularly if taken for longer than 3 weeks)
- taken a short course within 1 year of stopping long-term therapy
- other possible causes of adrenal suppression
- received more than 40 mg daily prednisolone (or equivalent)
- been given repeat doses in the evening
- received more than 3 weeks' treatment

Systemic corticosteroids may be stopped abruptly in those whose disease is unlikely to relapse *and* who have received treatment for 3 weeks or less *and* who are not included in the patient groups described above.

During corticosteroid withdrawal the dose may be reduced rapidly down to physiological doses (equivalent to prednisolone 7.5 mg daily) and then reduced more slowly. Assessment of the disease may be needed during withdrawal to ensure that relapse does not occur.

Psychiatric reactions

Systemic corticosteroids, particularly in high doses, are linked to psychiatric reactions including euphoria, nightmares, insomnia, irritability, mood lability, suicidal thoughts, psychotic reactions, and behavioural disturbances. A serious paranoid state or depression with risk of suicide can be induced, particularly in patients with a history of mental disorder. These reactions frequently subside on reducing the dose or discontinuing the corticosteroid but they may also require specific management. Patients should be advised to seek medical advice if psychiatric symptoms (especially depression and suicidal thoughts) occur and they should also be alert to the rare possibility of such reactions during withdrawal of corticosteroid treatment.

Systemic corticosteroids should be prescribed with care in those predisposed to psychiatric reactions, including those who have previously suffered corticosteroid-induced psychosis, or who have a personal or family history of psychiatric disorders.

Advice to patients

A patient information leaflet should be supplied to every patient when a systemic corticosteroid is prescribed. Patients should especially be advised of the following (for details, see Infections, Adrenal Suppression, Psychiatric Reactions, and Withdrawal of Corticosteroids above):

- **Immunosuppression** Prolonged courses of corticosteroids can increase susceptibility to infection and serious infections can go unrecognised. Unless already immune, patients are at risk of severe **chickenpox** and should avoid close contact with people who have chickenpox or shingles. Similarly, precautions should also be taken against contracting **measles**;
- **Adrenal suppression** If the corticosteroid is given for longer than 3 weeks, treatment must not be stopped abruptly. Adrenal suppression can last for a year or more after stopping treatment and the patient must mention the course of corticosteroid when receiving treatment for any illness or injury;
- **Mood and behaviour changes** Corticosteroid treatment, especially with high doses, can alter mood and behaviour early in treatment—the patient can become confused, irritable and suffer from delusion and suicidal thoughts. These effects can also occur when corticosteroid treatment is being withdrawn. Medical advice should be sought if worrying psychological changes occur;
- **Other serious effects** Serious gastro-intestinal, musculoskeletal, and ophthalmic effects which require medical help can also occur; for details see Side-effects of corticosteroids, below.

Steroid treatment cards (see p. 382) should be issued where appropriate. Doctors and pharmacists can obtain supplies of the card from:

England and Wales
NHS Customer Services, Astron
Causeway Distribution Centre, Oldham Broadway Business Park, Chadderton
Oldham, OL9 9XD
Tel: (0161) 683 2376/2382
Fax: (0161) 683 2396

Scotland
Banner Business Supplies
20 South Gyle Crescent
Edinburgh, EH12 9EB
Tel: (01506) 448 440
Fax: (01256) 448 400

Pregnancy and breast-feeding

Following a review of the data on the safety of systemic corticosteroids used in pregnancy and breast-feeding the CSM has concluded:

- corticosteroids vary in their ability to cross the placenta; betamethasone and dexamethasone cross the placenta readily while 88% of prednisolone is inactivated as it crosses the placenta;
- there is no convincing evidence that systemic corticosteroids increase the incidence of congenital abnormalities such as cleft palate or lip;
- when administration is prolonged or repeated during pregnancy, systemic corticosteroids increase the risk of intra-uterine growth restriction; there is no evidence of intra-uterine growth restriction following short-term treatment (e.g. prophylactic treatment for neonatal respiratory distress syndrome);
- any adrenal suppression in the neonate following prenatal exposure usually resolves spontaneously after birth and is rarely clinically important;
- prednisolone appears in small amounts in breast milk but maternal doses of up to 40 mg daily are unlikely to cause systemic effects in the infant; infants should be monitored for adrenal suppression if the mothers are taking a higher dose.

See also Appendix 4 and Appendix 5.

Other cautions and contra-indications

Other cautions include. children and adolescents (growth restriction possibly irreversible), elderly (close supervision required particularly on long-term treatment); frequent monitoring required if history of tuberculosis (or X-ray changes), hypertension, recent myocardial infarction (rupture reported), congestive heart failure, hepatic impairment (Appendix 2), renal impairment, diabetes mellitus including family history, osteoporosis (post-menopausal women at special risk), glaucoma (including family history), ocular herpes simplex—risk of corneal perforation, severe affective disorders (particularly if history of steroid-induced psychosis—see also Psychiatric Reactions, p. 380), epilepsy, peptic ulcer, hypothyroidism, history of steroid myopathy, ulcerative colitis, diverticulitis, recent intestinal anastomoses, thromboembolic disorders; myasthenia gravis; **interactions:** Appendix 1 (corticosteroids)

Other contra-indications include: systemic infection (unless specific therapy given); avoid live virus vaccines in those receiving immunosuppressive doses (serum antibody response diminished)

Side-effects of corticosteroids

Overdosage or prolonged use can exaggerate some of the normal physiological actions of corticosteroids leading to mineralocorticoid and glucocorticoid side-effects.

Mineralocorticoid side-effects include hypertension, sodium and water retention, and potassium and calcium loss. They are most marked with fludrocortisone, but are significant with cortisone, hydrocortisone, corticotropin, and tetracosactide (tetracosactrin). Mineralocorticoid actions are negligible with the high potency glucocorticoids, betamethasone and dexamethasone, and occur only slightly with methylprednisolone, prednisolone, and triamcinolone.

Glucocorticoid side-effects include diabetes and osteoporosis (section 6.6), which is a danger, particularly in the elderly, as it can result in osteoporotic fractures for example of the hip or vertebrae; in addition high doses are associated with avascular necrosis of the femoral head. Muscle wasting (proximal myopathy) can also occur. Corticosteroid therapy is also weakly linked with peptic ulceration and perforation (the potential advantage of soluble or enteric-coated preparations to reduce the risk is speculative only). See also Psychiatric Reactions, p. 380.

High doses of corticosteroids can cause Cushing's syndrome, with moon face, striae, and acne; it is usually reversible on withdrawal of treatment, but this must

STEROID TREATMENT CARD

I am a patient on STEROID treatment which must not be stopped suddenly

- If you have been taking this medicine for more than three weeks, the dose should be reduced gradually when you stop taking steroids unless your doctor says otherwise.
- Read the patient information leaflet given with the medicine.
- Always carry this card with you and show it to anyone who treats you (for example a doctor, nurse, pharmacist or dentist). For one year after you stop the treatment, you must mention that you have taken steroids.
- If you become ill, or if you come into contact with anyone who has an infectious disease, consult your doctor promptly. If you have never had chickenpox, you should avoid close contact with people who have chickenpox or shingles. If you do come into contact with chickenpox, see your doctor urgently.
- Make sure that the information on the card is kept up to date.

always be gradually tapered to avoid symptoms of acute adrenal insufficiency (**important**: see also Adrenal Suppression, p. 380).

In children, administration of corticosteroids may result in suppression of growth. For the effect of corticosteroids given in pregnancy, see Pregnancy and Breast-feeding, p. 381.

Side-effects can be minimised by using lowest effective dose for minimum period possible.

Other side-effects include: *gastro-intestinal effects*: dyspepsia, abdominal distension, acute pancreatitis, oesophageal ulceration and candidiasis; *musculoskeletal effects*: muscle weakness, vertebral and long bone fractures, tendon rupture; *endocrine effects*: menstrual irregularities and amenorrhoea, hirsutism, weight gain, negative nitrogen and calcium balance, increased appetite; increased susceptibility to and severity of infection, reactivation of dormant tuberculosis; *neuropsychiatric effects*: psychological dependence, insomnia, increased intracranial pressure with papilloedema in children (usually after withdrawal), aggravation of schizophrenia, aggravation of epilepsy; *ophthalmic effects*: glaucoma, papilloedema, posterior subcapsular cataracts, corneal or scleral thinning and exacerbation of ophthalmic viral or fungal disease, increased intra-ocular pressure , exophthalmos; *also* impaired healing, petechiae, ecchymoses, facial erythema, suppression of skin test reactions, urticaria, hyperhydrosis, skin atrophy, bruising, telangiectasia, myocardial rupture following recent myocardial infarction, congestive heart failure, leucocytosis, hyperglycaemia, hypersensitivity reactions (including anaphylaxis), thromboembolism, nausea, malaise, hiccups, headache, vertigo.

For other references to the side-effects of corticosteroids see section 3.2 (asthma), section 11.4 (eye) and section 13.4 (skin).

BETAMETHASONE

Indications suppression of inflammatory and allergic disorders; congenital adrenal hyperplasia; see also notes above; ear (section 12.1.1); eye (section 11.4.1); nose (section 12.2.1); oral ulceration (section 12.3.1)

Cautions see notes above; transient effect on fetal movements and heart rate

Contra-indications see notes above

Side-effects see notes above

Dose

- By mouth, usual range 0.5–5 mg daily; see also Administration (above)
- By intramuscular injection *or* slow intravenous injection *or* infusion, 4–20 mg, repeated up to 4 times in 24 hours; CHILD, by slow intravenous injection, up to 1 year 1 mg, 1–5 years 2 mg, 6–12 years 4 mg, repeated up to 4 times in 24 hours according to response

Betnelan® (Celltech) PoM
Tablets, scored, betamethasone 500 micrograms. Net price 100-tab pack = £4.39. Label: 10, steroid card, 21

Betnesol® (Celltech) PoM
Soluble tablets, pink, scored, betamethasone 500 micrograms (as sodium phosphate). Net price 100-tab pack = £5.17. Label: 10, steroid card, 13, 21
Injection, betamethasone 4 mg (as sodium phosphate) /mL. Net price 1-mL amp = £1.22. Label: 10, steroid card

CORTISONE ACETATE

Indications see under Dose but now superseded, see also notes above

Cautions see notes above

Contra-indications see notes above

Side-effects see notes above

Dose

- For replacement therapy, 25–37.5 mg daily in divided doses

Cortisone (Non-proprietary) PoM
Tablets, cortisone acetate 25 mg, net price 56-tab pack = £10.92. Label: 10, steroid card, 21

DEFLAZACORT

Indications suppression of inflammatory and allergic disorders

Cautions see notes above

Contra-indications see notes above

Side-effects see notes above

Dose

- Usual maintenance 3–18 mg daily (acute disorders, initially up to 120 mg daily); see also Administration (above)

  CHILD 0.25–1.5 mg/kg daily (or on alternate days); see also Administration (above)

Calcort® (Shire) PoM

Tablets, deflazacort 6 mg, net price 60-tab pack = £16.46. Label: 5, 10, steroid card

DEXAMETHASONE

Indications suppression of inflammatory and allergic disorders; diagnosis of Cushing's disease, congenital adrenal hyperplasia; cerebral oedema associated with malignancy; croup (section 3.1); nausea and vomiting with chemotherapy (section 8.1); rheumatic disease (section 10.1.2); eye (section 11.4.1); see also notes above

Cautions see notes above

Contra-indications see notes above

Side-effects see notes above; perineal irritation may follow intravenous administration of the phosphate ester

Dose

- By mouth, usual range 0.5–10 mg daily; CHILD 10–100 micrograms/kg daily; see also Administration (above)
- By intramuscular injection *or* slow intravenous injection *or* infusion (as dexamethasone phosphate), initially 0.5–24 mg; CHILD 200–400 micrograms/kg daily

  Cerebral oedema associated with malignancy (as dexamethasone phosphate), by intravenous injection, 10 mg initially, then 4 mg by intramuscular injection every 6 hours as required for 2–4 days then gradually reduced and stopped over 5–7 days

  Adjunctive treatment of bacterial meningitis, (starting before or with first dose of antibacterial treatment, as dexamethasone phosphate) [unlicensed indication], by intravenous injection, 10 mg every 6 hours for 4 days; CHILD 150 micrograms/kg every 6 hours for 4 days

  Note Dexamethasone 1 mg ≡ dexamethasone phosphate 1.2 mg ≡ dexamethasone sodium phosphate 1.3 mg

Dexamethasone (Non-proprietary) PoM

Tablets, dexamethasone 500 micrograms, net price 20 = 70p; 2 mg, 20 = £2.39. Label: 10, steroid card, 21

Available from Organon

Oral solution, sugar-free, dexamethasone (as dexamethasone sodium phosphate) 2 mg/5 mL, net price 150-mL = £42.30. Label: 10, steroid card, 21

Brands include *Dexsol®*

Injection, dexamethasone phosphate (as dexamethasone sodium phosphate) 4 mg/mL, net price 1-mL amp = £1.00, 2-mL vial = £1.98; 24 mg/mL, 5-mL vial = £16.66. Label: 10, steroid card

Available from Mayne

Injection, dexamethasone (as dexamethasone sodium phosphate) 4 mg/mL, net price 1-mL amp = 91p, 2-mL vial = £1.27. Label: 10, steroid card

Available from Organon

HYDROCORTISONE

Indications adrenocortical insufficiency (section 6.3.1); shock; see also notes above; hypersensitivity reactions e.g. anaphylactic shock and angioedema (section 3.4.3); asthma (section 3.1); severe inflammatory bowel disease (section 1.5); haemorrhoids (section 1.7.2); rheumatic disease (section 10.1.2); eye (section 11 4.1); skin (section 13.4)

Cautions see notes above

Contra-indications see notes above

Side-effects see notes above; phosphate ester associated with paraesthesia and pain (particularly in the perineal region)

Dose

- By mouth, replacement therapy, 20–30 mg daily in divided doses—see section 6.3.1; CHILD 10–30 mg
- By intramuscular injection *or* slow intravenous injection *or* infusion, 100–500 mg, 3–4 times in 24 hours or as required; CHILD by slow intravenous injection up to 1 year 25 mg, 1–5 years 50 mg, 6–12 years 100 mg

Efcortesol®[1] (Sovereign) PoM

Injection, hydrocortisone 100 mg (as sodium phosphate)/mL, net price 1-mL amp = 75p, 5-mL amp = £4.48. Label: 10, steroid card

Note Paraesthesia and pain (particularly in the perineal region) may follow intravenous injection of the phosphate ester

1. PoM restriction does not apply where administration is for saving life in emergency

Hydrocortone® (MSD) PoM

Tablets, scored, hydrocortisone 10 mg, net price 30-tab pack = 70p; 20 mg, 30-tab pack = £1.07. Label: 10, steroid card, 21

Solu-Cortef®[1] (Pharmacia) PoM

Injection, powder for reconstitution, hydrocortisone (as sodium succinate). Net price 100-mg vial = 92p, 100-mg vial with 2-mL amp water for injections = £1.16. Label: 10, steroid card

1. PoM restriction does not apply where administration is for saving life in emergency

METHYLPREDNISOLONE

Indications suppression of inflammatory and allergic disorders; severe inflammatory bowel disease (section 1.5); cerebral oedema associated with malignancy; see also notes above; rheumatic disease (section 10.1.2); skin (section 13.4)

Cautions see notes above; rapid intravenous administration of large doses associated with cardiovascular collapse

Contra-indications see notes above

Side-effects see notes above

Dose

- By mouth, usual range 2–40 mg daily; see also Administration (above)
- By intramuscular injection *or* slow intravenous injection *or* infusion, initially 10–500 mg; graft rejection, up to 1 g daily by intravenous infusion for up to 3 days

Medrone® (Pharmacia) PoM

Tablets, scored, methylprednisolone 2 mg (pink), net price 30-tab pack = £3.23; 4 mg, 30-tab pack = £6.19; 16 mg, 30-tab pack = £17.17; 100 mg (blue), 20-tab pack = £48.32. Label: 10, steroid card, 21

Solu-Medrone® (Pharmacia) PoM
Injection, powder for reconstitution, methylprednisolone (as sodium succinate) (all with solvent). Net price 40-mg vial = £1.58; 125-mg vial = £4.75; 500-mg vial = £9.60; 1-g vial = £17.30; 2-g vial = £32.86. Label: 10, steroid card

Intramuscular depot

Depo-Medrone® (Pharmacia) PoM
Injection (aqueous suspension), methylprednisolone acetate 40 mg/mL. Net price 1-mL vial = £2.87; 2-mL vial = £5.15; 3-mL vial = £7.47. Label: 10, steroid card
Dose by deep intramuscular injection into gluteal muscle, 40–120 mg, a second injection may be given after 2–3 weeks if required

PREDNISOLONE

Indications suppression of inflammatory and allergic disorders; see also notes above; inflammatory bowel disease, section 1.5; asthma, section 3.1 and section 3.2; immunosuppression, section 8.2.2; rheumatic disease, section 10.1.2; eye, section 11.4.1; ear, section 12.1.1

Cautions see notes above

Contra-indications see notes above

Side-effects see notes above

Dose

- By mouth, initially, up to 10–20 mg daily (severe disease, up to 60 mg daily), preferably taken in the morning after breakfast; can often be reduced within a few days but may need to be continued for several weeks or months
  Maintenance, usual range, 2.5–15 mg daily, but higher doses may be needed; cushingoid side-effects increasingly likely with doses above 7.5 mg daily
- By intramuscular injection, prednisolone acetate (section 10.1.2.2), 25–100 mg once or twice weekly

Prednisolone (Non-proprietary) PoM
Tablets, prednisolone 1 mg, net price 28-tab pack = 37p; 5 mg, 28-tab pack = 60p; 25 mg, 56-tab pack = £14.51. Label: 10, steroid card, 21

Tablets, both e/c, prednisolone 2.5 mg (brown), net price 30-tab pack = £3.34; 5 mg (red), 30-tab pack = £3.74. Label: 5, 10, steroid card, 25
Brands include *Deltacortril Enteric®*

Soluble tablets, prednisolone 5 mg (as sodium phosphate), net price 30-tab pack = £3.59. Label: 10, steroid card, 13, 21

Injection, see section 10.1.2.2

TRIAMCINOLONE

Indications suppression of inflammatory and allergic disorders; see also notes above; rheumatic disease, section 10.1.2; mouth, section 12.3.1; skin, section 13.4

Cautions see notes above; high dosage may cause proximal myopathy, avoid in chronic therapy

Contra-indications see notes above

Side-effects see notes above

Dose

- By deep intramuscular injection, into gluteal muscle, 40 mg of acetonide for depot effect, repeated at intervals according to the patient's response; max. single dose 100 mg

Kenalog® Intra-articular/Intramuscular (Squibb) PoM
Injection (aqueous suspension), triamcinolone acetonide 40 mg/mL, net price 1-mL vial = £1.70; 1-mL prefilled syringe = £2.11; 2-mL prefilled syringe = £3.66. Label: 10, steroid card
Note Intramuscular needle with prefilled syringe should be replaced for intra-articular injection

6.4 Sex hormones

6.4.1 Female sex hormones
6.4.2 Male sex hormones and antagonists
6.4.3 Anabolic steroids

6.4.1 Female sex hormones

6.4.1.1 Oestrogens and HRT
6.4.1.2 Progestogens

6.4.1.1 Oestrogens and HRT

Oestrogens are necessary for the development of female secondary sexual characteristics; they also stimulate myometrial hypertrophy with endometrial hyperplasia.

In terms of oestrogenic activity *natural oestrogens* (estradiol (oestradiol), estrone (oestrone), and estriol (oestriol)) have a more appropriate profile for hormone replacement therapy (HRT) than *synthetic oestrogens* (ethinylestradiol (ethinyloestradiol) and mestranol). Tibolone has oestrogenic, progestogenic and weak androgenic activity.

Oestrogen therapy is given cyclically or continuously for a number of gynaecological conditions. If long-term therapy is required a progestogen should normally be added to reduce the risk of cystic hyperplasia of the endometrium (or of endometriotic foci in women who have had a hysterectomy) and possible transformation to cancer.

Oestrogens are no longer used to suppress lactation because of their association with thromboembolism.

Hormone replacement therapy

Hormone replacement therapy (HRT) with small doses of an oestrogen (together with a progestogen in women with an intact uterus) is appropriate for alleviating menopausal symptoms such as vaginal atrophy or vasomotor instability. Oestrogen given systemically in the perimenopausal and postmenopausal period or tibolone given in the postmenopausal period also diminish postmenopausal osteoporosis (section 6.6.1) but other drugs (section 6.6) are preferred. Menopausal atrophic vaginitis may respond to a short course of a topical vaginal oestrogen preparation (section 7.2.1) used for a few weeks and repeated if necessary.

Systemic therapy with an oestrogen or drugs with oestrogenic properties alleviates the symptoms of oestrogen deficiency such as vasomotor symptoms. Tibolone combines oestrogenic and progestogenic activity with weak androgenic activity; it is given continuously, without cyclical progestogen.

HRT increases the risk of venous thromboembolism, of stroke and, after some years of use, endometrial cancer (reduced by a progestogen) and of breast cancer (see below). The CSM advises that the minimum effective dose should be used for the shortest duration. Treatment should be reviewed at least annually and for osteoporosis alternative treatments considered (section 6.6). HRT does not prevent coronary heart disease or protect against a decline in cognitive function and it should **not** be prescribed for these purposes. Experience of treating women over 65 years with HRT is limited.

Clonidine (section 2.5.2 and section 4.7.4.2) may be used to reduce vasomotor symptoms in women who cannot take an oestrogen, but clonidine may cause unacceptable side-effects.

HRT may be used in women with early natural or surgical menopause (before age 45 years), since they are at high risk of osteoporosis. For early menopause, HRT can be given until the approximate age of natural menopause (i.e. until age 50 years). Alternatives to HRT should be considered if osteoporosis is the main concern (section 6.6).

In women with an intact uterus, the addition of a progestogen reduces the risk of endometrial cancer but this should be weighed against the increased risk of breast cancer.

For the treatment of menopausal symptoms the benefits of short-term HRT outweigh the risks in the majority of women, especially in those aged under 60 years.

Risk of breast cancer The CSM has estimated that using *all* types of HRT, including tibolone, increases the risk of breast cancer within 1–2 years of initiating treatment. The increased risk is related to the duration of HRT use (but not to the age at which HRT is started) and this excess risk disappears within about 5 years of stopping.

About 10 in every 1000 women aged 50–59 years not using HRT have breast cancer diagnosed over 5 years (about 20 in every 1000 women over 10 years). In those using oestrogen-only HRT for 5 years, breast cancer is diagnosed in about 2 extra cases in 1000 (about 6 extra cases over 10 years). In those using combined HRT for 5 years, breast cancer is diagnosed in about 6 extra cases in 1000 (about 24 extra cases over 10 years). About 15 in every 1000 women aged 60–69 years not using HRT have breast cancer diagnosed over 5 years (about 30 in every 1000 women over 10 years). In those using oestrogen-only HRT for 5 years about 3 extra cases in 1000 are diagnosed (about 9 extra cases over 10 years), and in those using combined HRT for 5 years, breast cancer is diagnosed in about 9 extra cases in 1000 (about 36 extra cases over 10 years).

Tibolone increases the risk of breast cancer but to a lesser extent than with combined HRT.

Radiological detection of breast cancer may be adversely affected by HRT, as mammographic density can increase; tibolone has only a limited effect on mammographic density.

Risk of endometrial cancer The increased risk of endometrial cancer depends on the dose and duration of oestrogen-only HRT.

The MHRA/CHM has estimated that about 2 in every 1000 women aged 50–59 years not using HRT have endometrial cancer diagnosed over 5 years (about 4 in every 1000 women after 10 years); in those using oestrogen-only HRT for 5 years endometrial cancer is diagnosed in about 4 extra cases in 1000 (about 32 extra cases over 10 years).

About 3 in every 1000 women aged 60–69 years not using HRT have endometrial cancer diagnosed over 5 years (about 6 extra cases over 10 years). In those using oestrogen-only HRT for 5 years, endometrial cancer is diagnosed in about 6 extra cases in 1000 (about 48 extra cases over 10 years).

Evidence suggests an increased risk of endometrial cancer with tibolone. After 2.7 years of use (in women of average age 68 years), 1 extra case of endometrial hyperplasia and 4 extra cases of endometrial cancer were diagnosed compared with placebo users.

The risk of endometrial cancer cannot be reliably estimated in those using combined HRT because the addition of progestogen for at least 12 days per month greatly reduces the additional risk. The risk of endometrial cancer in women who have not used HRT increases with body mass index (BMI); the increased risk of endometrial cancer in users of oestrogen-only HRT or tibolone is more apparent in women who are not overweight.

Risk of ovarian cancer The MHRA/CHM has estimated that about 2 in every 1000 women aged 50–59 years not using HRT have ovarian cancer diagnosed over 5 years (about 4 in every 1000 women over 10 years); this figure rises by less than 1 extra case in 1000 in those using oestrogen-only HRT or combined HRT for 5 years (about 1 extra case over 10 years).

About 3 in every 1000 women aged 60–69 years not using HRT have ovarian cancer diagnosed over 5 years (about 6 in every 1000 women over 10 years); this figure rises by less than 1 extra case in 1000 in those using oestrogen-only HRT or combined HRT for 5 years (about 2 extra cases over 10 years).

Long-term use of combined HRT or oestrogen-only HRT is associated with a small increased risk of ovarian cancer.

Risk of venous thromboembolism Women on combined or oestrogen-only HRT are at an increased risk of deep vein thrombosis and of pulmonary embolism especially in the first year.

The MHRA/CHM has estimated that about 5 in every 1000 women aged 50–59 years not using HRT develop venous thromboembolism over 5 years; this figure rises by about 2 extra cases in 1000 in those using oestrogen-only HRT, and by about 7 extra cases in 1000 in those using combined HRT for 5 years. About 8 in every 1000 women aged 60–69 years not using HRT develop venous thromboembolism over 5 years; this figure rises by about 2 extra cases in 1000 in those using oestrogen-only HRT and by about 10 extra cases in 1000 in those using combined HRT for 5 years.

Limited data does not suggest an increased risk of thromboembolism with tibolone compared to combined HRT or women not taking HRT.

Although the level of risk associated with non-oral routes of administration has not been established, it may be lower for the transdermal route.

In *women who have predisposing factors* (such as a personal or family history of deep vein thrombosis or pulmonary embolism, severe varicose veins, obesity, trauma, or prolonged bed-rest) it may be prudent to review the need for HRT as in some cases the risks of HRT may exceed the benefits. See below for advice on surgery.

Travel involving prolonged immobility further increases the risk of deep vein thrombosis, see under Travel in section 7.3.1.

Risk of stroke Combined HRT or oestrogen-only HRT slightly increases the risk of *stroke*. The MHRA/CHM has estimated that about 4 in every 1000 *women aged 50–59 years* not using HRT have a stroke over 5 years; this figure rises by about 1 extra case in 1000 in those using oestrogen-only HRT or combined HRT for 5 years. About 9 in every 1000 women aged 60–69 years not using HRT have a stroke over 5 years; this figure rises by about 3 extra cases in 1000 in those using oestrogen-only HRT or combined HRT for 5 years.

Tibolone use increases the risk of stroke about 2.2 times from the first year of treatment; risk of stroke is age-dependent and therefore the absolute risk of stroke with tibolone increases with age.

Risk of coronary heart disease HRT does not prevent *coronary heart disease* and should not be prescribed for this purpose. There is an increased risk of coronary heart disease in women who start combined HRT more than 10 years after menopause. The MHRA/CHM estimates about 15 extra cases in 1000 aged 70–79 years over 5 years. Although very little information is available on the risk of coronary heart disease in younger women, studies suggest a lower relative risk compared with older women.

There is insufficient data to draw conclusions on the risk of coronary heart disease with tibolone.

Choice The choice of HRT for an individual depends on an overall balance of indication, risk, and convenience. A woman with an intact uterus normally requires oestrogen with cyclical progestogen for the last 12 to 14 days of the cycle *or* a preparation which involves continuous administration of an oestrogen and a progestogen (*or* one which provides both oestrogenic and progestogenic activity in a single preparation). Continuous combined preparations or tibolone are **not suitable** for use in the perimenopause or within 12 months of the last menstrual period; women who use such preparations may bleed irregularly in the early stages of treatment—if bleeding continues endometrial abnormality should be ruled out and consideration given to changing to cyclical HRT.

An oestrogen alone is suitable for continuous use in women without a uterus. However, in endometriosis, endometrial foci may remain despite hysterectomy and the addition of a progestogen should be considered in these circumstances.

An oestrogen may be given by mouth or it may be given by subcutaneous or transdermal administration, which avoids first-pass metabolism. In the case of subcutaneous implants, recurrence of vasomotor symptoms at supraphysiological plasma concentrations may occur; moreover, there is evidence of prolonged endometrial stimulation after discontinuation (calling for continued cyclical progestogen). For the use of topical HRT preparations see section 7.2.1.

Contraception HRT does **not** provide contraception and a woman is considered potentially fertile for 2 years after her last menstrual period if she is under 50 years, and for 1 year if she is over 50 years. A woman who is under 50 years and free of all risk factors for venous and arterial disease can use a low-oestrogen combined oral contraceptive pill (section 7.3.1) to provide both relief of menopausal symptoms and contraception; it is recommended that the oral contraceptive be stopped at 50 years of age since there are more suitable alternatives. If any potentially fertile woman needs HRT, non-hormonal contraceptive measures (such as condoms) are necessary.

Measurement of follicle-stimulating hormone can help to determine fertility, but high measurements alone (particularly in women aged under 50 years) do not necessarily preclude the possibility of becoming pregnant.

Surgery Major surgery under general anaesthesia, including orthopaedic and vascular leg surgery, is a predisposing factor for venous thromboembolism and it may be prudent to stop HRT 4–6 weeks before surgery (see Risk of Venous Thromboembolism, above); it should be restarted only after full mobilisation. If HRT is continued or if discontinuation is not possible (e.g. in non-elective surgery), prophylaxis with heparin and graduated compression hosiery is advised. Oestrogenic activity may persist after removing an estradiol implant (see above).

Reasons to stop HRT For circumstances in which HRT should be stopped, see p. 429.

OESTROGENS FOR HRT

Note Relates only to small amounts of oestrogens given for hormone replacement therapy

Indications see notes above and under preparations

Cautions prolonged exposure to unopposed oestrogens may increase risk of developing endometrial cancer (see notes above); migraine (or migraine-like headaches); diabetes (increased risk of heart disease); history of breast nodules or fibrocystic disease—closely monitor breast status (risk of breast cancer, see notes above); risk factors for oestrogen-dependent tumours (e.g. breast cancer in first-degree relative); uterine fibroids may increase in size, symptoms of endometriosis may be exacerbated; factors predisposing to thromboembolism (see notes above); presence of antiphospholipid antibodies (increased risk of thrombotic events); increased risk of gall-bladder disease reported; hypophyseal tumours; porphyria (see section 9.8.2); **interactions:** Appendix 1 (oestrogens)

Other conditions The product literature advises caution in other conditions including hypertension, renal disease, asthma, epilepsy, sickle-cell disease, melanoma, otosclerosis, multiple sclerosis, and systemic lupus erythematosus (but care required if antiphospholipid antibodies present, see above). Evidence for caution in these conditions is unsatisfactory and many women with these conditions may stand to benefit from HRT.

Contra-indications pregnancy; oestrogen-dependent cancer, history of breast cancer, active thrombophlebitis, active or recent arterial thromboembolic

6 Endocrine system

disease (e.g. angina or myocardial infarction), venous thromboembolism, or history of recurrent venous thromboembolism (unless already on anticoagulant treatment), liver disease (where liver function tests have failed to return to normal), Dubin-Johnson and Rotor syndromes (or monitor closely), untreated endometrial hyperplasia, undiagnosed vaginal bleeding, breast-feeding

Side-effects see notes above for risks of long-term use; nausea and vomiting, abdominal cramps and bloating, weight changes, breast enlargement and tenderness, premenstrual-like syndrome, sodium and fluid retention, cholestatic jaundice, glucose intolerance, altered blood lipids–may lead to pancreatitis, rashes and chloasma, changes in libido, depression, mood changes, headache, migraine, dizziness, leg cramps (rule out venous thrombosis), vaginal candidiasis, contact lenses may irritate; transdermal delivery systems may cause contact sensitisation (possible severe hypersensitivity reaction on continued exposure), and headache has been reported on vigorous exercise

Withdrawal bleeding Cyclical HRT (where a progestogen is taken for 12–14 days of each 28-day oestrogen treatment cycle) usually results in *regular withdrawal bleeding* towards the end of the progestogen. The aim of continuous combined HRT (where a combination of oestrogen and progestogen is taken, usually in a single tablet, throughout each 28-day treatment cycle) is to avoid bleeding, but *irregular bleeding* may occur during the early treatment stages (if it continues endometrial abnormality should be excluded and consideration given to cyclical HRT instead)

Dose

- See under preparations

Counselling on patches Patch should be removed after 3–4 days (or once a week in case of 7-day patch) and replaced with fresh patch on slightly different site; recommended sites: clean, dry, unbroken areas of skin on trunk below waistline; not to be applied on or near breasts or under waistband. If patch falls off in bath allow skin to cool before applying new patch

◢Conjugated oestrogens with progestogen

Premique® (Wyeth) PoM

Premique® Low Dose tablets, s/c, ivory, conjugated oestrogen (equine) 300 micrograms and medroxyprogesterone acetate 1.5 mg, net price 3 × 28-tab pack = £29.85

Dose menopausal symptoms in women with an intact uterus, 1 tablet daily continuously

Premique® tablets, s/c, blue, conjugated oestrogen (equine) 625 micrograms and medroxyprogesterone acetate 5 mg. Net price 3 × 28-tab pack = £27.14

Dose menopausal symptoms and osteoporosis prophylaxis (see section 6.6), in women with intact uterus, 1 tablet daily continuously (starting on day 1 of menstruation if cycles have not ceased)

Premique® Cycle Calendar pack, all s/c, 14 white tablets, conjugated oestrogens (equine) 625 micrograms; 14 green tablets, conjugated oestrogens (equine) 625 micrograms and medroxyprogesterone acetate 10 mg, net price 3 × 28-tab pack = £24.87

Dose menopausal symptoms and osteoporosis prophylaxis (see section 6.6), 1 white tablet daily for 14 days, starting on day 1 of menstruation (or at any time if cycles have ceased or are infrequent) then 1 green tablet daily for 14 days; subsequent courses are repeated without interval

Prempak-C® (Wyeth) PoM

Prempak C® 0.625 Calendar pack, s/c, 28 maroon tablets, conjugated oestrogens (equine) 625 micrograms; 12 light brown tablets, norgestrel 150 micrograms (≡ levonorgestrel 75 micrograms). Net price 3 × 40-tab pack = £17.67

Dose menopausal symptoms and osteoporosis prophylaxis (see section 6.6), in women with intact uterus, 1 maroon tablet daily continuously, starting on day 1 of menstruation (or at any time if cycles have ceased or are infrequent), and 1 brown tablet daily on days 17–28 of each 28-day treatment cycle; subsequent courses are repeated without interval

Prempak C® 1.25 Calendar pack, s/c, 28 yellow tablets, conjugated oestrogens (equine) 1.25 mg; 12 light brown tablets, norgestrel 150 micrograms (≡ levonorgestrel 75 micrograms). Net price 3 × 40-tab pack = £17.37

Dose see under 0.625 Calendar pack, but taking 1 yellow tablet daily continuously (instead of 1 maroon tablet) if symptoms not fully controlled with lower strength

◢Estradiol with progestogen

Angeliq® (Schering Health) PoM

Tablets, f/c, red, estradiol 1mg, drospirenone 2 mg. Net price 3 × 28-tab pack = £25.80

Dose menopausal symptoms and osteoporosis prophylaxis (see section 6.6), in women with intact uterus, 1 tablet daily continuously (if changing from cyclical HRT begin treatment the day after finishing oestrogen plus progestogen phase)

Cautions use with care if an increased concentration of potassium might be hazardous; renal impairment (Appendix 3)

Note Unsuitable for use in perimenopausal women or within 12 months of last menstrual period—see choice above

Climagest® (Novartis) PoM

Climagest® 1-mg tablets, 16 grey-blue, estradiol valerate 1 mg; 12 white, estradiol valerate 1 mg and norethisterone 1 mg. Net price 28-tab pack = £5.74; 3 × 28-tab pack = £16.69

Dose menopausal symptoms, 1 grey-blue tablet daily for 16 days, starting on day 1 of menstruation (or at any time if cycles have ceased or are infrequent) then 1 white tablet for 12 days; subsequent courses are repeated without interval

Climagest® 2-mg tablets, 16 blue, estradiol valerate 2 mg; 12 yellow, estradiol valerate 2 mg and norethisterone 1 mg. Net price 28-tab pack = £5.74; 3 × 28-tab pack = £16.39

Dose see *Climagest® 1-mg*, but starting with 1 blue tablet daily (instead of 1 grey-blue tablet) if symptoms not controlled with lower strength

Climesse® (Novartis) PoM

Tablets, pink, estradiol valerate 2 mg, norethisterone 700 micrograms. Net price 1 × 28-tab pack = £10.34; 3 × 28-tab pack = £31.03

Dose menopausal symptoms and osteoporosis prophylaxis (see section 6.6), in women with intact uterus, 1 tablet daily continuously

Note Unsuitable for use in perimenopausal women or within 12 months of last menstrual period—see Choice above

Clinorette® (ReSource Medical) PoM

Tablets, f/c, 16 white, estradiol 2 mg; 12 pink, estradiol 2 mg and norethisterone 1 mg, net price 3 × 28-tab pack = £9.23

Dose menopausal symptoms, in women with intact uterus, 1 white tablet daily for 16 days starting on day 5 of menstruation (or at any time if cycles have ceased or are infrequent), then 1 pink tablet daily for 12 days; subsequent courses repeated without interval

Cyclo-Progynova® (Viatris) PoM

Cyclo-Progynova® 1-mg tablets, all s/c, 11 beige, estradiol valerate 1 mg; 10 brown, estradiol valerate 1 mg and levonorgestrel 250 micrograms. Net price per pack = £3.11

Dose menopausal symptoms, in women with intact uterus, 1 beige tablet daily for 11 days, starting on day 5 of menstruation (or at any time if cycles have ceased or are infrequent), then 1 brown tablet daily for 10 days, followed by a 7-day interval

Cyclo-Progynova® 2-mg tablets, all s/c, 11 white, estradiol valerate 2 mg; 10 brown, estradiol valerate 2 mg and norgestrel 500 micrograms (≡ levonorgestrel 250 micrograms). Net price per pack = £3.11

Dose menopausal symptoms and osteoporosis prophylaxis (see section 6.6) as *Cyclo-Progynova® 1-mg*, but starting with 1 white tablet daily for 11 days, then 1 brown tablet daily for 10 days, followed by a 7-day interval

Elleste-Duet® (Pharmacia) PoM

Elleste-Duet® 1-mg tablets, 16 white, estradiol 1 mg; 12 green, estradiol 1 mg and norethisterone acetate 1 mg. Net price 3 × 28-tab pack = £9.72

Dose menopausal symptoms, 1 white tablet daily for 16 days starting on day 1 of menstruation (or at any time if cycles have ceased or are infrequent), then 1 green tablet daily for 12 days; subsequent courses are repeated without interval

Elleste-Duet® 2-mg tablets, 16 orange, estradiol 2 mg; 12 grey, estradiol 2 mg, norethisterone acetate 1 mg. Net price 3 × 28-tab pack = £9.72

Dose menopausal symptoms and osteoporosis prophylaxis (see section 6.6), 1 orange tablet daily for 16 days, starting on day 1 of menstruation (or at any time if cycles have ceased or are infrequent) then 1 grey tablet daily for 12 days; subsequent courses are repeated without interval

Elleste-Duet Conti® tablets, f/c, grey, estradiol 2 mg, norethisterone acetate 1 mg. Net price 3 × 28-tab pack = £17.97

Dose menopausal symptoms and osteoporosis prophylaxis (see section 6.6), in women with intact uterus, 1 tablet daily on a continuous basis (if changing from cyclical HRT begin treatment at the end of scheduled bleed)

Note Unsuitable for use in perimenopausal women or within 12 months of last menstrual period—see Choice above

Estracombi® (Novartis) PoM

Combination pack, self-adhesive patches of *Estraderm TTS® 50* (releasing estradiol approx. 50 micrograms/24 hours) and of *Estragest TTS®* (releasing estradiol approx. 50 micrograms/24 hours and norethisterone acetate 250 micrograms/24 hours); net price 1-month pack (4 of each) = £13.37, 3-month pack (12 of each) = £40.11. Counselling, administration

Dose menopausal symptoms and osteoporosis prophylaxis (see section 6.6), in women with intact uterus, starting within 5 days of onset of menstruation (or any time if cycles have ceased or are infrequent), 1 *Estraderm TTS® 50* patch to be applied twice weekly for 2 weeks followed by 1 *Estragest TTS®* patch twice weekly for 2 weeks; subsequent courses are repeated without interval

Evorel® (Janssen-Cilag) PoM

Evorel® Conti patches, self-adhesive, (releasing estradiol approx. 50 micrograms/24 hours and norethisterone acetate approx. 170 micrograms/24 hours), net price 8-patch pack = £12.00, 24-patch pack = £35.99. Counselling, administration

Dose menopausal symptoms and osteoporosis prophylaxis (see section 6.6), in women with intact uterus, 1 patch to be applied twice weekly continuously

Evorel® Sequi combination pack, 4 self-adhesive patches of *Evorel® 50* (releasing estradiol approx. 50 micrograms/24 hours) and 4 self-adhesive patches of *Evorel® Conti* (releasing estradiol approx. 50 micrograms/24 hours and norethisterone acetate approx. 170 micrograms/24 hours), net price 8-patch pack = £10.23. Counselling, administration

Dose menopausal symptoms and osteoporosis prophylaxis (see section 6.6), in women with intact uterus, 1 *Evorel® 50* patch to be applied twice weekly for 2 weeks followed by 1 *Evorel® Conti* patch twice weekly for 2 weeks; subsequent courses are repeated without interval

Femapak® (Solvay) PoM

Femapak® 40 combination pack of 8 self-adhesive patches of *Fematrix® 40* (releasing estradiol approx. 40 micrograms/24 hours) and 14 tablets of *Duphaston®* (dydrogesterone 10 mg). Net price per pack = £7.61. Counselling, administration

Dose see under *Femapak® 80*

Femapak® 80 combination pack of 8 self-adhesive patches of *Fematrix® 80* (releasing estradiol approx. 80 micrograms/24 hours) and 14 tablets of *Duphaston®* (dydrogesterone 10 mg). Net price per pack = £8.06. Counselling, administration

Dose menopausal symptoms (and osteoporosis prophylaxis (see section 6.6) in case of *Femapak® 80* **only**), in women with intact uterus, starting within 5 days of onset of menstruation (or any time if cycles have ceased or are infrequent), apply 1 patch twice weekly continuously and take 1 tablet daily on days 15–28 of each 28-day treatment cycle; therapy should be initiated with *Femapak® 40* in those with menopausal symptoms, prolonged oestrogen deficiency or anticipated intolerance to higher strengths, subsequently adjusted to lowest effective dose

Femoston® (Solvay) PoM

Femoston® 1/10 tablets, both f/c, 14 white, estradiol 1 mg; 14 grey, estradiol 1 mg, dydrogesterone 10 mg. Net price 3 × 28-tab pack = £13.47

Dose menopausal symptoms and osteoporosis prophylaxis (see section 6.6), in women with intact uterus, 1 white tablet daily for 14 days, starting within 5 days of onset of menstruation (or any time if cycles have ceased or are infrequent) then 1 grey tablet for 14 days; subsequent courses repeated without interval

Femoston® 2/10 tablets, both f/c, 14 red, estradiol 2 mg; 14 yellow, estradiol 2 mg, dydrogesterone 10 mg. Net price 3 × 28-tab pack = £13.47

Dose menopausal symptoms and osteoporosis prophylaxis (see section 6.6), in women with intact uterus, 1 red tablet daily for 14 days, starting within 5 days of onset of menstruation (or any time if cycles have ceased or are infrequent) then 1 yellow tablet daily for 14 days; subsequent courses repeated without interval; where therapy required for menopausal symptoms alone, *Femoston® 1/10* given initially and *Femoston® 2/10* substituted if symptoms not controlled

Femoston®-conti tablets, f/c, salmon, estradiol 1 mg, dydrogesterone 5 mg, net price 3 × 28-tab pack = £22.44

Dose menopausal symptoms and osteoporosis prophylaxis (see section 6.6), in women with intact uterus, 1 tablet daily continuously (if changing from cyclical HRT begin treatment the day after finishing oestrogen plus progestogen phase)

Note Unsuitable for use in perimenopausal women or within 12 months of last menstrual period—see Choice above

FemSeven® Conti (Merck) PoM

Patches, self-adhesive (releasing estradiol approx. 50 micrograms/24 hours and levonorgestrel approx. 7 micrograms/24 hours); net price 4-patch pack = £15.48, 12-patch pack = £ 44.12. Counselling, administration

Dose menopausal symptoms in women with intact uterus, 1 patch to be applied once a week continuously

Note Unsuitable for use in perimenopausal women or within 12 months of last menstrual period—see Choice above

FemSeven® Sequi (Merck) PoM

Combination pack, self-adhesive patches of *FemSeven® Sequi Phase 1* (releasing estradiol approx. 50 micrograms/24 hours) and of *FemSeven® Sequi Phase 2* (releasing estradiol approx. 50 micrograms/24 hours and levonorgestrel approx. 10 micrograms/24 hours); net price 1-month pack (2 of each) = £13.18, 3-month pack (6 of each) = £37.54. Counselling, administration

Dose menopausal symptoms in women with intact uterus, 1 *Phase 1* patch applied once a week for 2 weeks followed by 1 *Phase 2* patch once a week for 2 weeks; subsequent courses are repeated without interval

FemTab® Sequi (Merck) PoM
Tablets, both s/c, 16 white, estradiol valerate 2 mg; 12 pink, estradiol valerate 2 mg, levonorgestrel 75 micrograms, net price 3 × 28-tab pack = £15.15
Dose menopausal symptoms and osteoporosis prophylaxis (see section 6.6), in women with intact uterus, 1 white tablet daily for 16 days, starting on day 5 of menstruation (or any time if cycles have ceased or are infrequent) then 1 pink tablet daily for 12 days; subsequent courses are repeated without interval

Indivina® (Orion) PoM
Indivina® 1 mg/2.5 mg tablets, estradiol valerate 1 mg, medroxyprogesterone acetate 2.5 mg, net price 3 × 28-tab pack = £21.49
Indivina® 1 mg/5 mg tablets, estradiol valerate 1 mg, medroxyprogesterone acetate 5 mg, net price 3 × 28-tab pack = £21.49
Indivina® 2 mg/5 mg tablets, estradiol valerate 2 mg, medroxyprogesterone acetate 5 mg, net price 3 × 28-tab pack = £21.49
Dose menopausal symptoms and osteoporosis prophylaxis (see section 6.6), in women with intact uterus, 1 tablet daily continuously; initiate therapy with *Indivina® 1 mg/2.5 mg* tablets and adjust according to response; start at end of scheduled bleed if changing from cyclical HRT
Note Less suitable for use in perimenopausal women or within 3 years of last menstrual period—see Choice above

Kliofem® (Novo Nordisk) PoM
Tablets, f/c yellow, estradiol 2 mg, norethisterone acetate 1 mg. Net price 3 × 28-tab pack = £11.43
Dose menopausal symptoms and osteoporosis prophylaxis (see section 6.6), in women with intact uterus, 1 tablet daily continuously; start at end of scheduled bleed if changing from cyclical HRT
Note Unsuitable for use in perimenopausal women or within 12 months of last menstrual period—see Choice above

Kliovance® (Novo Nordisk) PoM
Tablets, f/c, estradiol 1 mg, norethisterone acetate 500 micrograms, net price 3 × 28-tab pack = £14.67
Dose menopausal symptoms and osteoporosis prophylaxis (see section 6.6), in women with intact uterus, 1 tablet daily continuously; start at end of scheduled bleed if changing from cyclical HRT
Note Unsuitable for use in perimenopausal women or within 12 months of last menstrual period—see Choice above

Novofem (Novo Nordisk) PoM
Tablets, f/c, 16 red, estradiol 1 mg; 12 white, estradiol 1 mg, norethisterone acetate 1 mg, net price 3 × 28-tab pack = £13.50
Dose menopausal symptoms and osteoporosis prophylaxis (see section 6.6), in women with intact uterus, 1 red tablet daily for 16 days then 1 white tablet daily for 12 days; subsequent courses are repeated without interval; start treatment with red tablet at any time or if changing from cyclical HRT, start treatment the day after finishing oestrogen plus progestogen phase

Nuvelle® (Schering Health) PoM
Nuvelle® tablets, all s/c, 16 white, estradiol valerate 2 mg; 12 pink, estradiol valerate 2 mg and levonorgestrel 75 micrograms. Net price 3 × 28-tab pack = £12.87
Dose menopausal symptoms and osteoporosis prophylaxis (see section 6.6), in women with intact uterus, 1 white tablet daily for 16 days, starting on day 5 of menstruation (or any time if cycles have ceased or are infrequent) then 1 pink tablet daily for 12 days; subsequent courses are repeated without interval
Nuvelle® Continuous tablets, f/c, pink, estradiol 2 mg, norethisterone acetate 1 mg, net price 3 × 28-tab pack = £16.85
Dose menopausal symptoms and osteoporosis prophylaxis (see section 6.6), in women with intact uterus, 1 tablet daily continuously; start at end of scheduled bleed if changing from cyclical HRT
Note Unsuitable for use in perimenopausal women or within 12 months of last menstrual period—see Choice above

Tridestra® (Orion) PoM
Tablets, 70 white, estradiol valerate 2 mg; 14 blue, estradiol valerate 2 mg and medroxyprogesterone acetate 20 mg; 7 yellow, inactive. Net price 91-tab pack = £21.40
Dose menopausal symptoms and osteoporosis prophylaxis (see section 6.6), in women with intact uterus, 1 white tablet daily for 70 days, then 1 blue tablet daily for 14 days, then 1 yellow tablet daily for 7 days; subsequent courses are repeated without interval

Trisequens® (Novo Nordisk) PoM
Tablets, 12 blue, estradiol 2 mg; 10 white, estradiol 2 mg, norethisterone acetate 1 mg; 6 red, estradiol 1 mg, net price 3 × 28-tab pack = £11.10
Dose menopausal symptoms and osteoporosis prophylaxis (see section 6.6), in women with intact uterus, 1 blue tablet daily, starting on day 5 of menstruation (or at any time if cycles have ceased or are infrequent), then 1 tablet daily in sequence (without interruption)

Conjugated oestrogens only

Premarin® (Wyeth) PoM
Tablets, all s/c, conjugated oestrogens (equine) 300 micrograms (green) net price 3 × 28-tab pack = £9.72; 625 micrograms (maroon), 3 × 28-tab pack = £9.72; 1.25 mg (yellow), 3 × 28-tab pack = £13.19
Dose menopausal symptoms, 0.3–1.25 mg daily continuously; osteoporosis prophylaxis (see section 6.6), 0.625–1.25 mg daily continuously; with cyclical progestogen for 12–14 days of each cycle in women with intact uterus

Estradiol only

Estradiol Implants (Organon) PoM
Implant, estradiol 25 mg, net price each = £12.95; 50 mg, each = £21.08
Dose *by implantation*, oestrogen replacement, and osteoporosis prophylaxis (see section 6.6) (with cyclical progestogen for 12–14 days of each cycle in women with intact uterus, see notes above), 25–100 mg as required (usually every 4–8 months) according to oestrogen levels—check before each implant
Note On cessation of treatment or if implants are removed from those with intact uterus, cyclical progesterone should be continued until withdrawal bleed stops

Bedol® (ReSource Medical) PoM
Tablets, f/c, estradiol 2 mg, net price 3 × 28-tab pack = £5.07
Dose menopausal symptoms, with cyclical progestogen for 12–14 days of each cycle in women with intact uterus, 2 mg daily starting on day 1–5 of menstruation (or at any time if cycles have ceased or are infrequent)

Climaval® (Novartis) PoM
Tablets, estradiol valerate 1 mg (grey-blue), net price 1 × 28-tab pack = £3.06, 3 × 28-tab pack = £9.19; 2 mg (blue), 1 × 28-tab pack = £3.06, 3 × 28-tab pack = £9.19
Dose menopausal symptoms (if patient has had a hysterectomy), 1–2 mg daily

Elleste-Solo® (Pharmacia) PoM
Elleste-Solo® 1-mg tablets, estradiol 1 mg. Net price 3 × 28-tab pack = £5.34
Dose menopausal symptoms, with cyclical progestogen for 12–14 days of each cycle in women with intact uterus, 1 mg daily starting on day 1 of menstruation (or at any time if cycles have ceased or are infrequent)
Elleste-Solo® 2-mg tablets, orange, estradiol 2 mg. Net price 3 × 28-tab pack = £5.34
Dose menopausal symptoms not controlled with lower strength and osteoporosis prophylaxis (see section 6.6), with cyclical progestogen for 12–14 days of each cycle in women with intact uterus, 2 mg daily starting on day 1 of menstruation (or at any time if cycles have ceased or are infrequent)

Elleste Solo® MX (Pharmacia) PoM

Patches, self-adhesive, estradiol, *MX 40 patch* (releasing approx. 40 micrograms/24 hours), net price 8-patch pack = £5.19; *MX 80 patch* (releasing approx. 80 micrograms/24 hours), 8-patch pack = £5.99. Counselling, administration.

Dose menopausal symptoms (and osteoporosis prophylaxis in case of *Elleste Solo MX 80®* **only**; see section 6.6), 1 patch to be applied twice weekly continuously starting within 5 days of onset of menstruation (or at any time if cycles have ceased or are infrequent); with cyclical progestogen for 12–14 days of each cycle in women with intact uterus; therapy should be initiated with *MX 40* in those with menopausal symptoms, prolonged oestrogen deficiency or anticipated intolerance to higher strength, dosage may be increased if required, subsequently adjusted to lowest effective dose

Estraderm MX® (Novartis) PoM

Patches, self-adhesive, estradiol, *MX 25 patch* (releasing approx. 25 micrograms/24 hours), net price 8-patch pack = £5.72, 24-patch pack = £17.15; *MX 50 patch* (releasing approx. 50 micrograms/24 hours), 8-patch pack = £5.74, 24-patch pack = £17.15, 20-patch pack (hosp. only) = £13.04; *MX 75 patch* (releasing approx. 75 micrograms/24 hours), 8-patch pack = £6.69, 24-patch pack = £20.08; *MX 100 patch* (releasing approx. 100 micrograms/24 hours), 8-patch pack = £6.94, 24-patch pack = £20.83. Counselling, administration

Dose menopausal symptoms (and osteoporosis prophylaxis in case of *Estraderm MX® 50* and *75* **only**; see section 6.6), 1 patch to be applied twice weekly continuously, with cyclical progestogen for 12 days of each cycle in women with intact uterus; therapy should be initiated with *MX 50* for first month, subsequently adjusted to lowest effective dose

Estraderm TTS® (Novartis) PoM

Patches, self-adhesive, estradiol, *TTS 25 patch* (releasing approx. 25 micrograms/24 hours), net price, 8-patch pack = £7.45, 24-patch pack = £22.36; *TTS 50 patch* (releasing approx. 50 micrograms/24 hours), 8-patch pack = £7.48, 24-patch pack = £22.43; *TTS 100 patch* (releasing approx. 100 micrograms/24 hours), 8-patch pack = £9.02, 24-patch pack = £27.16, 20-patch pack (hosp. only) = £16.76. Counselling, administration

Dose menopausal symptoms (and osteoporosis prophylaxis in case of *Estraderm TTS® 50* **only**; see section 6.6), 1 patch to be applied twice weekly continuously, with cyclical progestogen for 12 days of each cycle in women with intact uterus; therapy should be initiated with *TTS 50* for first month, subsequently adjusted to lowest effective dose

Estradot® (Novartis) PoM

Patches, self-adhesive, estradiol, *'25' patch* (releasing approx. 25 micrograms/24 hours), net price 8-patch pack = £5.20; *'37.5' patch* (releasing approx. 37.5 micrograms/24 hours), 8-patch pack = £5.21; *'50' patch* (releasing approx. 50 micrograms/24 hours), 8-patch pack = £5.22; *'75' patch* (releasing approx. 75 micrograms/24 hours), 8-patch pack = £6.08; *'100' patch* (releasing approx. 100 micrograms/24 hours), 8-patch pack = £6.31. Counselling, administration

Dose menopausal symptoms (all strengths) and osteoporosis prophylaxis (*Estradot® '50', '75',* and *'100'* **only**; see section 6.6), 1 patch to be applied twice weekly continuously, with cyclical progestogen for 12 days of each cycle in women with intact uterus; for osteoporosis prophylaxis therapy should be initiated with *'50' patch*

Evorel® (Janssen-Cilag) PoM

Patches, self-adhesive, estradiol, *'25' patch* (releasing approx. 25 micrograms/24 hours), net price 8-patch pack = £2.86; *'50' patch* (releasing approx. 50 micrograms/24 hours), 8-patch pack = £3.24, 24-patch pack = £9.72; *'75' patch* (releasing approx. 75 micrograms/24 hours), 8-patch pack = £3.44; *'100' patch* (releasing approx. 100 micrograms/24 hours), 8-patch pack = £3.57. Counselling, administration

Dose menopausal symptoms and osteoporosis prophylaxis (except *Evorel® 25*; see section 6.6), 1 patch to be applied twice weekly continuously, with cyclical progestogen for at least 12 days of each cycle in women with intact uterus; therapy should be initiated with *'50' patch* for first month, subsequently adjusted to lowest effective dose

Fematrix® (Solvay) PoM

Fematrix® 40 patch, self-adhesive, estradiol, *'40' patch* (releasing approx. 40 micrograms/24 hours). Net price 8-patch pack = £4.95. Counselling, administration

Dose menopausal symptoms, 1 patch to be applied twice weekly continuously starting within 5 days of onset of menstruation (or at any time if cycles have ceased or are infrequent), with cyclical progestogen for 12–14 days of each cycle in women with intact uterus; *'80' patch* may be used if required (subsequently adjusted to lowest effective dose)

Fematrix® 80 patch, self-adhesive, estradiol (releasing approx. 80 micrograms/24 hours). Net price 8-patch pack = £5.40. Counselling, administration

Dose menopausal symptoms and osteoporosis prophylaxis (see section 6.6), as for *Fematrix® 40*; therapy should be initiated with *Fematrix® 40* in those with menopausal symptoms, prolonged oestrogen deficiency or anticipated intolerance to higher strength

FemSeven® (Merck) PoM

Patches, self-adhesive, estradiol, *'50' patch* (releasing approx. 50 micrograms/24 hours), net price 4-patch pack = £6.04, 12-patch pack = £18.02; *'75' patch* (releasing approx. 75 micrograms/24 hours), net price 4-patch pack = £6.98; *'100' patch* (releasing approx. 100 micrograms/24 hours), net price 4-patch pack = £7.28. Counselling, administration

Dose menopausal symptoms and osteoporosis prophylaxis (see section 6.6), 1 patch to be applied once a week continuously, with cyclical progestogen for at least 10 days of each cycle in women with intact uterus; therapy should be initiated with *FemSeven® 50* patches for the first few months, subsequently adjusted according to response

Oestrogel® (Ferring) PoM

Gel, estradiol 0.06%, net price 64-dose pump pack = £7.39. Counselling, administration

Dose menopausal symptoms and osteoporosis prophylaxis (see section 6.6), 2 measures (estradiol 1.5 mg) to be applied over an area twice that of the template provided once daily continuously, starting within 5 days of menstruation (or anytime if cycles have ceased or are infrequent), with cyclical progestogen for 12 days of each cycle in women with intact uterus; for menopausal symptoms may be increased if necessary after 1 month to max. 4 measures daily

Counselling Apply gel to clean, dry, intact skin such as arms, shoulders or inner thighs and allow to dry for 5 minutes before covering with clothing. Not to be applied on or near breasts or on vulval region. Avoid skin contact with another person (particularly male) and avoid other skin products or washing the area for at least 1 hour after application

Progynova® (Schering Health) PoM

Tablets, both s/c, estradiol valerate 1 mg (beige), net price 3 × 28-tab pack = £6.56; 2 mg (blue), 3 × 28-tab pack = £6.56

Dose menopausal symptoms, 1–2 mg daily continuously; osteoporosis prophylaxis (see section 6.6), 2 mg daily continuously; with cyclical progestogen for 12 days of each cycle in women with intact uterus

Progynova® TS (Schering Health) PoM

Patches, self-adhesive, *Progynova® TS 50* (releasing estradiol approx. 50 micrograms/24 hours), net price 12-patch pack = £16.71; *Progynova® TS 100* (releasing estradiol approx. 100 micrograms/24 hours), 12-patch pack = £18.39. Counselling, administration

Dose menopausal symptoms, 1 patch to be applied once a week on a continuous or cyclical basis (1 patch per week for three weeks followed by a 7-day patch-free interval); therapy should be initiated with *Progynova*® *TS 50* and adjusted to lowest effective dose; osteoporosis prophylaxis (see section 6.6), 1 *Progynova*® *TS 50* patch to be applied once a week on a continuous basis (with cyclical progestogen for 10–14 days of each cycle in women with intact uterus)

Note Women receiving *Progynova*® *TS 100* patches for menopausal symptoms may continue with this strength for osteoporosis prophylaxis (see section 6.6)

Sandrena® (Organon) PoM

Gel, estradiol (0.1%), 500 microgram/500 mg sachet, net price 28-sachet pack = £5.28, 1 mg/1 g sachet, 28-sachet pack = £6.08. Counselling, administration

Excipients include propylene glycol (see section 13.1.3)

Dose menopausal symptoms, estradiol 1 mg (1 g gel) to be applied once daily over area 1–2 times size of hand; with cyclical progestogen for 12–14 days of each cycle in women with intact uterus; dose may be adjusted after 2–3 cycles to a usual dose of estradiol 0.5–1.5 mg (0.5–1.5 g gel) daily

Counselling Apply gel to intact areas of skin such as lower trunk or thighs, using right and left sides on alternate days. Wash hands after application. Not to be applied on the breasts or face and avoid contact with eyes. Allow area of application to dry for 5 minutes and do not wash area for at least 1 hour

Zumenon® (Solvay) PoM

Tablets, f/c, estradiol 1 mg, net price 84-tab pack = £6.89; 2 mg (red), 84-tab pack = £6.89

Dose menopausal symptoms, initially 1 mg daily starting on day 5 of menstruation (or any time if cycles have ceased or are infrequent) adjusted to 1–4 mg daily according to response; osteoporosis prophylaxis (see section 6.6), 2 mg daily; with cyclical progestogen for 10–14 days of each cycle in women with intact uterus

Estradiol, estriol and estrone

Hormonin® (Shire) PoM

Tablets, pink, estradiol 600 micrograms, estriol 270 micrograms, estrone 1.4 mg. Net price 84-tab pack = £6.61

Dose menopausal symptoms and osteoporosis prophylaxis (see section 6.6), 1–2 tablets daily, with cyclical progestogen for 12–14 days of each cycle in women with intact uterus

Note *Hormonin*® tablets can be given continuously or cyclically (21 days out of 28)

Estriol only

Ovestin® (Organon) PoM

Tablets, scored, estriol 1 mg. Net price 30-tab pack = £3.91. Label: 25

Dose genito-urinary symptoms associated with oestrogen-deficiency states, 0.5–3 mg daily, as single dose, for up to 1 month, then 0.5–1 mg daily until restoration of epithelial integrity (short-term use); infertility due to poor cervical penetration, 0.25–1 mg daily on days 6–15 of cycle

Estropipate only

Harmogen® (Pharmacia) PoM

Tablets, peach, scored, estropipate 1.5 mg. Net price 28-tab pack = £3.77

Dose menopausal symptoms and osteoporosis prophylaxis (see section 6.6), 1.5 mg daily continuously (with cyclical progestogen for 10–13 days of each cycle in women with intact uterus); up to 3 mg daily (in single or divided doses) for vasomotor symptoms and menopausal vaginitis

TIBOLONE

Indications short-term treatment of symptoms of oestrogen deficiency (including women being treated with gonadotrophin releasing hormone analogues); osteoporosis prophylaxis in women at risk of fractures (second-line)

Cautions see notes above and under Oestrogens for HRT; vaginal bleeding (investigate for endometrial cancer if bleeding continues beyond 6 months or after stopping treatment); renal impairment, history of liver disease (Appendix 2), epilepsy, migraine, diabetes mellitus, hypercholesterolaemia; withdraw if signs of thromboembolic disease, abnormal liver function tests or cholestatic jaundice; see also Note below; **interactions** Appendix 1 (tibolone)

Contra-indications see notes above and under Oestrogens for HRT; hormone-dependent tumours, history of cardiovascular or cerebrovascular disease (e.g. thrombophlebitis, thromboembolism), uninvestigated vaginal bleeding, severe liver disease, pregnancy, breast-feeding

Side-effects see notes above; also abdominal pain, weight changes, vaginal bleeding, leucorrhoea, facial hair, and *rarely* amnesia; gastro-intestinal disturbances, oedema, dizziness, headache, migraine, depression, breast cancer (see notes above and section 6.4.1.1), arthralgia, myalgia, visual disturbances, seborrhoeic dermatitis, rash and pruritus also reported

Dose

- 2.5 mg daily

Note Unsuitable for use in the premenopause (unless being treated with gonadotrophin-releasing hormone analogue) and as (or with) an oral contraceptive; also unsuitable for use within 12 months of last menstrual period (may cause irregular bleeding); induce withdrawal bleed with progestogen if transferring from another form of HRT

Livial® (Organon) PoM

Tablets, tibolone 2.5 mg. Net price 28-tab pack = £10.77; 3 × 28-tab pack = £32.29

Ethinylestradiol

Ethinylestradiol (ethinyloestradiol) is licensed for short-term treatment of symptoms of oestrogen deficiency, for osteoporosis prophylaxis if other drugs (section 6.6) cannot be used and for the treatment of female hypogonadism and menstrual disorders.

Ethinylestradiol is occasionally used under **specialist supervision** for the management of *hereditary haemorrhagic telangiectasia* (but evidence of benefit is limited). Side-effects include nausea, fluid retention, and thrombosis. Impotence and gynaecomastia have been reported in men.

For use in prostate cancer, see section 8.3.1.

ETHINYLESTRADIOL
(Ethinyloestradiol)

Indications see notes above

Cautions cardiovascular disease (sodium retention with oedema, thromboembolism), hepatic impairment (jaundice), see also under Combined Hormonal Contraceptives (section 7.3.1) and under Oestrogen for HRT (above)

Contra-indications see under Combined Hormonal Contraceptives (section 7.3.1) and under Oestrogen for HRT (above)

Side-effects feminising effects in men; see also under Combined Hormonal Contraceptives (section 7.3.1) and under Oestrogen for HRT (above)

Dose

- Menopausal symptoms and osteoporosis prophylaxis, (with progestogen for 12–14 days per cycle in women with intact uterus), 10–50 micrograms daily for 21 days, repeated after 7-day tablet-free period
- Female hypogonadism, 10–50 micrograms daily, usually on cyclical basis; initial oestrogen therapy should be followed by combined oestrogen and progestogen therapy
- Menstrual disorders, 20–50 micrograms daily from day 5 to 25 of each cycle, with progestogen added either throughout the cycle or from day 15 to 25

Ethinylestradiol (Non-proprietary) PoM

Tablets, ethinylestradiol 10 micrograms, net price 21-tab pack = £14.29; 50 micrograms, 21-tab pack = £17.04; 1 mg, 28-tab pack = £31.74

Raloxifene

Raloxifene is licensed for the treatment and prevention of *postmenopausal osteoporosis*; unlike hormone replacement therapy, raloxifene does not reduce menopausal vasomotor symptoms.

Raloxifene may reduce the incidence of oestrogen-receptor-positive breast cancer but its role in established breast cancer is not yet clear. The manufacturer advises avoiding its use during treatment for breast cancer.

RALOXIFENE HYDROCHLORIDE

Indications treatment and prevention of postmenopausal osteoporosis

Cautions risk factors for venous thromboembolism (discontinue if prolonged immobilisation); breast cancer (see notes above); history of oestrogen-induced hypertriglyceridaemia (monitor serum triglycerides); **interactions:** Appendix 1 (raloxifene)

Contra-indications history of venous thromboembolism, undiagnosed uterine bleeding, endometrial cancer, hepatic impairment, cholestasis, severe renal impairment; pregnancy and breast-feeding

Side-effects venous thromboembolism, thrombophlebitis, hot flushes, leg cramps, peripheral oedema, influenza-like symptoms; rarely rashes, gastro-intestinal disturbances, hypertension, headache (including migraine), breast discomfort

Dose

- 60 mg once daily

Evista® (Lilly) PoM

Tablets, f/c, raloxifene hydrochloride 60 mg, net price 28-tab pack = £17.06; 84-tab pack = £59.59

6.4.1.2 Progestogens

There are two main groups of progestogen, progesterone and its analogues (dydrogesterone and medroxyprogesterone) and testosterone analogues (norethisterone and norgestrel). The newer progestogens (desogestrel, norgestimate, and gestodene) are all derivatives of norgestrel; levonorgestrel is the active isomer of norgestrel and has twice its potency. Progesterone and its analogues are less androgenic than the testosterone derivatives and neither progesterone nor dydrogesterone causes virilisation.

Where endometriosis requires drug treatment, it may respond to a progestogen, e.g. norethisterone, administered on a continuous basis. Danazol, gestrinone, and gonadorelin analogues are also available (section 6.7.2).

Although oral progestogens have been used widely for menorrhagia they are relatively ineffective compared with tranexamic acid (section 2.11) or, particularly where dysmenorrhoea is also a factor, mefenamic acid (section 10.1.1); the levonorgestrel-releasing intrauterine system (section 7.3.2.3) may be particularly useful for women also requiring contraception. Oral progestogens have also been used for severe dysmenorrhoea, but where contraception is also required in younger women the best choice is a combined oral contraceptive (section 7.3.1).

Progestogens have also been advocated for the alleviation of premenstrual symptoms, but no convincing physiological basis for such treatment has been shown.

Progestogens have been used for the prevention of spontaneous abortion in women with a history of recurrent miscarriage (habitual abortion) but there is no evidence of benefit and they are **not** recommended for this purpose. In pregnant women with antiphospholipid antibody syndrome who have suffered recurrent miscarriage, administration of low-dose aspirin (section 2.9) and a prophylactic dose of a low molecular weight heparin (section 2.8.1) may decrease the risk of fetal loss (use under specialist supervision only).

Hormone replacement therapy In women with a uterus a progestogen needs to be added to long-term oestrogen therapy for hormone replacement, to prevent cystic hyperplasia of the endometrium and possible transformation to cancer; it can be added on a cyclical or a continuous basis (see section 6.4.1.1). Combined packs incorporating suitable progestogen tablets are available, see p. 387.

Oral contraception Desogestrel, etynodiol (ethynodiol), gestodene, levonorgestrel, norethisterone, and norgestimate are used in combined oral contraceptives and in progestogen-only contraceptives (section 7.3.1 and section 7.3.2).

Cancer Progestogens also have a role in neoplastic disease (section 8.3.2).

Cautions Progestogens should be used with caution in conditions that may worsen with fluid retention e.g. epilepsy, hypertension, migraine, asthma, cardiac or renal dysfunction, and in those susceptible to thromboembolism (particular caution with high dose). Care is also required in liver impairment (avoid if severe), and in those with a history of depression. Progestogens can decrease glucose tolerance and diabetes should be monitored closely. For **interactions** see Appendix 1 (progestogens).

Contra-indications Progestogens should be avoided in patients with a history of liver tumours, and in severe liver impairment. They are also contra-indicated in those with genital or breast cancer (unless progestogens are being used in the management of these conditions), severe arterial disease, undiagnosed vaginal bleeding and porphyria (section 9.8.2). Progestogens should not be used if there is a history during pregnancy of idiopathic jaundice, severe pruritus, or pemphigoid gestationis.

Side-effects Side-effects of progestogens include menstrual disturbances, premenstrual-like syndrome (including bloating, fluid retention, breast tenderness), weight change, nausea, headache, dizziness, insomnia, drowsiness, depression, change in libido; also skin reactions (including urticaria, pruritus, rash, and acne), hirsutism and alopecia. Jaundice and anaphylactoid reactions have also been reported.

DYDROGESTERONE

Indications see under Dose and notes above
Cautions see notes above; breast-feeding (Appendix 5)
Contra-indications see notes above
Side-effects see notes above
Dose
- Endometriosis, 10 mg 2–3 times daily from day 5 to 25 of cycle or continuously
- Infertility, irregular cycles, 10 mg twice daily from day 11 to 25 for at least 6 cycles (but not recommended)
- Recurrent miscarriage, 10 mg twice daily from day 11 to 25 of cycle until conception, then continuously until week 20 of pregnancy and then gradually reduced (but not recommended, see notes above)
- Dysfunctional uterine bleeding, 10 mg twice daily (together with an oestrogen) for 5–7 days to arrest bleeding; 10 mg twice daily (together with an oestrogen) from day 11 to 25 of cycle to prevent bleeding
- Dysmenorrhoea (but see notes above), 10 mg twice daily from day 5 to 25 of cycle
- Amenorrhoea, 10 mg twice daily from day 11 to 25 of cycle with oestrogen therapy from day 1 to 25 of cycle
- Premenstrual syndrome, 10 mg twice daily from day 12 to 26 of cycle increased if necessary (but not recommended, see notes above)
- Hormone replacement therapy, with continuous oestrogen therapy, see under *Duphaston® HRT* below

Duphaston® (Solvay) PoM
Tablets, scored, dydrogesterone 10 mg. Net price 60-tab pack = £4.04

Duphaston® HRT (Solvay) PoM
Tablets, scored, dydrogesterone 10 mg. Net price 42-tab pack = £2.83
Dose 10 mg daily on days 15–28 of each 28-day oestrogen HRT cycle, increased to 10 mg twice daily if withdrawal bleed is early or endometrial biopsy shows inadequate progestational response

MEDROXYPROGESTERONE ACETATE

Indications see under Dose; contraception (section 7.3.2.2); malignant disease (section 8.3.2)
Cautions see notes above; breast-feeding (Appendix 5)
Contra-indications see notes above; pregnancy (Appendix 4)
Side-effects see notes above; indigestion
Dose
- By mouth, 2.5–10 mg daily for 5–10 days beginning on day 16 to 21 of cycle, repeated for 2 cycles in dysfunctional uterine bleeding and 3 cycles in secondary amenorrhoea
- Mild to moderate endometriosis, 10 mg 3 times daily for 90 consecutive days, beginning on day 1 of cycle
- Progestogenic opposition of oestrogen HRT, 10 mg daily for the last 14 days of each 28-day oestrogen HRT cycle

Provera® (Pharmacia) PoM
Tablets, all scored, medroxyprogesterone acetate 2.5 mg (orange), net price 30-tab pack = £1.84; 5 mg (blue), 10-tab pack = £1.23; 10 mg (white), 10-tab pack = £2.47, 90-tab pack = £22.16

Climanor® (ReSource Medical) PoM
Tablets, f/c medroxyprogesterone acetate 5 mg, net price 28-tab pack = £3.27

Combined preparations
Section 6.4.1.1

NORETHISTERONE

Indications see under Dose; HRT (section 6.4.1.1); contraception (section 7.3.1 and section 7.3.2); malignant disease (section 8.3.2)
Cautions see notes above; breast-feeding (Appendix 5)
Contra-indications see notes above; pregnancy (Appendix 4)
Side-effects see notes above
Dose
- Endometriosis by mouth, 10–15 mg daily for 4–6 months or longer, starting on day 5 of cycle (if spotting occurs increase dose to 20–25 mg daily, reduced once bleeding has stopped)
- Dysfunctional uterine bleeding, menorrhagia (but see notes above), by mouth, 5 mg 3 times daily for 10 days to arrest bleeding; to prevent bleeding 5 mg twice daily from day 19 to 26
- Dysmenorrhoea (but see notes above), by mouth, 5 mg 3 times daily from day 5 to 24 for 3–4 cycles
- Premenstrual syndrome (but not recommended, see notes above), by mouth, 5 mg 2–3 times daily from day 19 to 26 for several cycles
- Postponement of menstruation, by mouth, 5 mg 3 times daily starting 3 days before expected onset (menstruation occurs 2–3 days after stopping)

Tablets of 5 mg

Norethisterone (Non-proprietary) PoM
Tablets, norethisterone 5 mg, net price 30-tab pack = £3.60

Primolut N® (Schering Health) PoM
Tablets, norethisterone 5 mg. Net price 30-tab pack = £2.01

Utovlan® (Pharmacia) PoM
Tablets, norethisterone 5 mg, net price 30-tab pack = £1.40, 90-tab pack = £4.21

Combined preparations
Section 6.4.1.1

PROGESTERONE

Indications see under preparations
Cautions see notes above; breast-feeding (Appendix 5)
Contra-indications see notes above; missed or incomplete abortion
Side-effects see notes above; injection-site reactions; pain, diarrhoea and flatulence can occur with rectal administration

Dose
- See under preparations

Crinone® (Serono) PoM
Vaginal gel, progesterone 90 mg/application (8%), 15 = £32.73
Dose by vagina, infertility due to inadequate luteal phase, insert 1 applicatorful daily starting either after documented ovulation or on day 18–21 of cycle. *In vitro* fertilisation, daily application continued for 30 days after laboratory evidence of pregnancy

Cyclogest® (Actavis) PoM
Pessaries, progesterone 200 mg, net price 15 = £7.46; 400 mg, 15 = £10.80
Dose by vagina *or* rectum, premenstrual syndrome and postnatal depression, 200 mg daily to 400 mg twice daily; for premenstrual syndrome start on day 12–14 and continue until onset of menstruation (but not recommended, see notes above); rectally if barrier methods of contraception are used, in patients who have recently given birth or in those who suffer from vaginal infection or recurrent cystitis

Gestone® (Nordic) PoM
Injection, progesterone 50 mg/mL, 1-mL amp = 45p, 2-mL amp = 75p
Dose by deep intramuscular injection into buttock, dysfunctional uterine bleeding, 5–10 mg daily for 5–10 days until 2 days before expected onset of menstruation
Recurrent miscarriage due to inadequate luteal phase (but not recommended, see notes above) or following *in vitro* fertilisation *or* gamete intra-fallopian transfer, 25–100 mg 2–7 times a week from day 15, or day of embryo *or* gamete transfer, until 8–16 weeks of pregnancy; max. 200 mg daily

Utrogestan® (Ferring) PoM
Capsules, progesterone (micronised) 100 mg, net price 30-cap pack = £5.70; 200 mg 15-cap pack = £5.70. Counselling, administration
Excipients include arachis (peanut) oil
Counselling Capsules should be taken at bedtime on an empty stomach
Dose progestogenic opposition of oestrogen HRT 200 mg once daily on days 15–26, *or* 100 mg once daily on days 1–25, of each 28-day oestrogen HRT cycle

6.4.2 Male sex hormones and antagonists

Androgens cause masculinisation; they may be used as replacement therapy in castrated adults and in those who are hypogonadal due to either pituitary or testicular disease. In the normal male they inhibit pituitary gonadotrophin secretion and depress spermatogenesis. Androgens also have an anabolic action which led to the development of anabolic steroids (section 6.4.3).

Androgens are useless as a treatment of impotence and impaired spermatogenesis unless there is associated hypogonadism; they should not be given until the hypogonadism has been properly investigated. Treatment should be under expert supervision.

When given to patients with hypopituitarism they can lead to normal sexual development and potency but not to fertility. If fertility is desired, the usual treatment is with gonadotrophins or pulsatile gonadotrophin-releasing hormone (section 6.5.1) which will stimulate spermatogenesis as well as androgen production.

Caution should be used when androgens or chorionic gonadotrophin are used in treating boys with delayed puberty since the fusion of epiphyses is hastened and may result in short stature; skeletal maturation should be monitored.

Intramuscular depot preparations of **testosterone esters** are preferred for replacement therapy. Testosterone enantate, propionate or undecanoate, or alternatively *Sustanon®*, which consists of a mixture of testosterone esters and has a longer duration of action, may be used. Satisfactory replacement therapy can sometimes be obtained with 1 mL of *Sustanon 250®*, given by intramuscular injection once a month, although more frequent dose intervals are often necessary. Implants of testosterone can be used for hypogonadism; the implants are replaced every 4 to 5 months.

Testosterone implants can be used in postmenopausal women as an adjunct to hormone replacement therapy. A testosterone patch is also licensed to improve libido in *surgically induced* menopausal women (receiving concomitant oestrogen therapy).

TESTOSTERONE AND ESTERS

Indications see under preparations

Cautions cardiac, renal, or hepatic impairment (Appendix 2), elderly, ischaemic heart disease, hypertension, epilepsy, migraine, diabetes mellitus, skeletal metastases (risk of hypercalcaemia), undertake regular examination of the prostate and breast during treatment; monitor full blood count, lipid profile and liver function; pre-pubertal boys (see notes above and under Side-effects); **interactions**: Appendix 1 (testosterone)
Women Regularly assess for androgenic side-effects; women should be advised to report any signs of virilisation e.g. deepening of the voice or hirsutism

Contra-indications breast cancer in men, prostate cancer, history of primary liver tumours, hypercalcaemia, pregnancy (Appendix 4), breast-feeding (Appendix 5), nephrotic syndrome

Side-effects prostate abnormalities and prostate cancer, headache, depression, gastro-intestinal bleeding, nausea, vomiting, cholestatic jaundice, changes in libido, gynaecomastia, polycythaemia, anxiety, irritability, nervousness, asthenia, paraesthesia, hypertension, electrolyte disturbances including sodium retention with oedema and hypercalcaemia, weight gain; increased bone growth, muscle cramps, arthralgia; androgenic effects such as hirsutism, male-pattern baldness, seborrhoea, acne, pruritus, excessive frequency and duration of penile erection, precocious sexual development and premature closure of epiphyses in pre-pubertal males, suppression of spermatogenesis in men and virilism in women; *rarely* liver tumours; sleep apnoea also reported; *with patches, buccal tablets, and gel*, local irritation and allergic reactions (including burn-like lesions with *patches*), and taste disturbances

Dose
- See under preparations

Oral

Restandol® Testocaps (Organon) PoM
Capsules, orange, testosterone undecanoate 40 mg in oily solution. Net price 30-cap pack = £8.89; 60-cap pack = £17.79. Label: 21, 25
Dose androgen deficiency, 120–160 mg daily for 2–3 weeks; maintenance 40–120 mg daily

Buccal

Striant® SR (Ardana) PoM

Mucoadhesive buccal tablets, m/r, testosterone 30 mg, net price 60-tab pack = £45.84. Counselling, see under Dose below

Dose hypogonadism, 30 mg every 12 hours; CHILD and ADOLESCENT under 18 years not recommended

Counselling Place rounded side of tablet on gum above front teeth and hold lip firmly over the gum for 30 seconds. If tablet detaches within 4 hours of next dose, replace with new tablet which is considered the second dose for the day.

Intramuscular

Testosterone Enantate (Cambridge) PoM

Injection (oily), testosterone enantate 250 mg/mL. Net price 1-mL amp = £9.33

Dose by slow intramuscular injection, hypogonadism, initially 250 mg every 2–3 weeks; maintenance 250 mg every 3–6 weeks

Breast cancer, 250 mg every 2–3 weeks

Nebido® (Schering Health) ▼ PoM

Injection (oily), testosterone undecanoate 250 mg/mL. Net price 4-mL amp = £76.70

Dose by deep intramuscular injection, hypogonadism in men over 18 years, 1 g every 10–14 weeks; if necessary, second dose may be given after 6 weeks to achieve rapid steady state plasma testosterone levels and then every 10–14 weeks

Sustanon 100® (Organon) PoM

Injection (oily), testosterone propionate 20 mg, testosterone phenylpropionate 40 mg, and testosterone isocaproate 40 mg/mL. Net price 1-mL amp = £1.09

Excipients include arachis (peanut) oil, benzyl alcohol (see Excipients p. 2)

Dose by deep intramuscular injection, androgen deficiency, 1 mL every 2 weeks

Sustanon 250® (Organon) PoM

Injection (oily), testosterone propionate 30 mg, testosterone phenylpropionate 60 mg, testosterone isocaproate 60 mg, and testosterone decanoate 100 mg/mL. Net price 1-mL amp = £2.55

Excipients include arachis (peanut) oil, benzyl alcohol (see Excipients p. 2)

Dose by deep intramuscular injection, androgen deficiency, 1 mL usually every 3 weeks

Virormone® (Nordic) PoM

Injection, testosterone propionate 50 mg/mL. Net price 2-mL amp = 45p

Dose by intramuscular injection, androgen deficiency, 50 mg 2–3 times weekly

Delayed puberty, 50 mg weekly

Breast cancer in women, 100 mg 2–3 times weekly

Implant

Testosterone (Organon) PoM

Implant, testosterone 100 mg, net price = £7.40; 200 mg = £13.79

Dose by implantation, male hypogonadism, 100–600 mg; 600 mg usually maintains plasma-testosterone concentration within the normal range for 4–5 months

Postmenopausal women, 50–100 mg every 4–8 months, as an adjunct to oestrogen replacement therapy

Transdermal preparations

Andropatch® (GSK) PoM

Patches, self-adhesive, releasing testosterone approx. 2.5 mg/24 hours, net price 60-patch pack = £49.10; releasing testosterone approx. 5 mg/24 hours, net price 30-patch pack = £49.10. Counselling, administration

Dose androgen deficiency in men (over 15 years) associated with primary or secondary hypogonadism, apply to clean, dry, unbroken skin on back, abdomen, upper arms or thighs, removing after 24 hours and siting replacement patch on a different area (with an interval of 7 days before using the same site); initially apply patches equivalent to testosterone 5 mg/24 hours (2.5 mg/24 hours in non-virilised patients) at night (approx. 10 p.m.), then adjust to 2.5 mg to 7.5 mg every 24 hours according to plasma-testosterone concentration (those with a body-weight over 130 kg may require 7.5 mg every 24 hours)

Intrinsa® (Procter & Gamble) ▼ PoM

Patches, self-adhesive, releasing testosterone approx. 300 micrograms/24 hours, net price 8-patch pack = £28.00. Counselling, administration

Dose hypoactive sexual desire disorder associated with surgically induced menopause (in women receiving concomitant oestrogen therapy (section 6.4.1.1)), apply 1 patch twice weekly continuously to clean, dry, unbroken skin on lower abdomen below waistline; site replacement patch on a different area (avoid using same area for 7 days); assess treatment after 3–6 months, discontinue if no benefit

Note Not recommended for women naturally menopausal or those taking conjugated oestrogens. Safety and efficacy of use beyond 1 year not established

Testim® (Ipsen) ▼ PoM

Gel, testosterone 50 mg/5 g tube, net price 30-tube pack = £33.00. Counselling, administration

Excipients include propylene glycol (see section 13.1.3)

Dose hypogonadism due to testosterone deficiency in men (over 18 years), 50 mg testosterone (5 g gel) applied once daily; subsequent application adjusted according to response; max. 100 mg (10 g gel) daily

Counselling Squeeze entire content of tube on to one palm and apply as a thin layer on clean, dry, healthy skin of shoulder or upper arm, preferably in the morning after washing or bathing (if 2 tubes required use 1 per shoulder or upper arm); rub in and allow to dry before putting on clothing to cover site; wash hands with soap after application; avoid washing application site for at least 6 hours

Avoid skin contact with application sites to prevent testosterone transfer to other people, especially pregnant women and children—consult product literature

Testogel® (Schering Health) PoM

Gel, testosterone 50 mg/5 g sachet, net price 30-sachet pack = £33.00. Counselling, administration

Dose hypogonadism due to androgen deficiency in men (over 18 years), 50 mg testosterone (5 g gel) to be applied once daily; subsequent application adjusted according to response in 25-mg (2.5 g gel) increments to max. 100 mg (10 g gel) daily

Counselling Apply thin layer of gel on clean, dry, healthy skin such as shoulders, arms or abdomen, immediately after sachet is opened. Not to be applied on genital area as high alcohol content may cause local irritation. Allow to dry for 3–5 minutes before dressing. Wash hands with soap and water after applying gel, avoid shower or bath for at least 6 hours

Avoid skin contact with gel application sites to prevent testosterone transfer to other people, especially pregnant women and children—consult product literature

Tostran® (ProStrakan) PoM

Gel, testosterone 2% (10 mg/metered application), net price 60 g multidose dispenser = £26.67. Counselling, administration

Excipients include butylhydroxytoluene, propylene glycol (see section 13.1.3)

Dose hypogonadism due to testosterone deficiency in men (over 18 years), initially 60 mg testosterone (3 g gel) applied once daily; subsequent applications adjusted according to response; max. 80 mg (4 g gel) daily

Counselling Apply gel on clean, dry, intact skin of abdomen or both inner thighs, preferably in the morning. Gently rub in with a finger until dry before dressing. Wash hands with soap and water after applying gel; avoid washing application site for at least 2 hours. Not to be applied on genital area.

Avoid skin contact with gel application sites to prevent testosterone transfer to other people, especially pregnant women and children—consult product literature

MESTEROLONE

Indications see under Dose
Cautions see under Testosterone and Esters
Contra-indications see under Testosterone and Esters
Side-effects see under Testosterone and Esters but spermatogenesis unimpaired
Dose
- Androgen deficiency and male infertility associated with hypogonadism, 25 mg 3–4 times daily for several months, reduced to 50–75 mg daily in divided doses for maintenance; CHILD not recommended

Pro-Viron® (Schering Health) PoM
Tablets, scored, mesterolone 25 mg. Net price 30-tab pack = £4.44

Anti-androgens

Cyproterone acetate

Cyproterone acetate is an anti-androgen used in the treatment of severe hypersexuality and sexual deviation in the male. It inhibits spermatogenesis and produces reversible infertility (but is not a male contraceptive); abnormal sperm forms are produced. Fully informed consent is recommended and an initial spermatogram. As hepatic tumours have been produced in *animal* studies, careful consideration should be given to the risk/benefit ratio before treatment. Cyproterone acetate is also used as an adjunct in prostatic cancer (section 8.3.4.2) and in the treatment of acne and hirsutism in women (section 13.6.2).

6 Endocrine system

CYPROTERONE ACETATE

Indications see notes above; prostate cancer (section 8.3.4.2)
Cautions ineffective for male hypersexuality in chronic alcoholism (relevance to prostate cancer not known); blood counts initially and throughout treatment; monitor hepatic function regularly (liver function tests should be performed before treatment, see also under Side-effects below); monitor adrenocortical function regularly; diabetes mellitus (see also Contra-indications)
Driving Fatigue and lassitude may impair performance of skilled tasks (e.g. driving)
Contra-indications (do not apply in prostate cancer) hepatic disease (Appendix 2), severe diabetes (with vascular changes); sickle-cell anaemia, malignant or wasting disease, severe depression, history of thrombo-embolic disorders; youths under 18 years (may arrest bone maturation and testicular development)
Side-effects fatigue and lassitude, breathlessness, weight changes, reduced sebum production (may clear acne), changes in hair pattern, gynaecomastia (rarely leading to galactorrhoea and benign breast nodules); rarely hypersensitivity reactions, rash and osteoporosis; inhibition of spermatogenesis (see notes above); hepatotoxicity reported (including jaundice, hepatitis and hepatic failure usually in men given 200–300 mg daily for prostatic cancer, see section 8.3.4.2 for details and warnings)
Dose
- Male hypersexuality, 50 mg twice daily after food

Cyproterone Acetate (Non-proprietary) PoM
Tablets, cyproterone acetate 50 mg, net price 56-tab pack = £31.54. Label: 21 counselling, driving

Androcur® (Schering Health) PoM
Tablets, scored, cyproterone acetate 50 mg. Net price 56-tab pack = £25.89. Label: 21 counselling, driving

Dutasteride and finasteride

Dutasteride and **finasteride** are specific inhibitors of the enzyme 5α-reductase, which metabolises testosterone into the more potent androgen, dihydrotestosterone. This inhibition of testosterone metabolism leads to reduction in prostate size, with improvement in urinary flow rate and in obstructive symptoms. Dutasteride and finasteride are alternatives to alpha-blockers (section 7.4.1) particularly in men with a significantly enlarged prostate. Finasteride is also licensed for use with doxazosin in the management of benign prostatic hyperplasia.

A low strength of finasteride is licensed for treating male-pattern baldness in men (section 13.9).

Cautions Dutasteride and finasteride decrease serum concentration of prostate cancer markers such as prostate-specific antigen; reference values may need adjustment. Both dutasteride and finasteride are excreted in semen and use of a condom is recommended if sexual partner is pregnant or likely to become pregnant. Women of childbearing potential should avoid handling crushed or broken tablets of finasteride and leaking capsules of dutasteride.

Contra-indications Dutasteride and finasteride are contra-indicated in women, children, and adolescents.

Side-effects The side-effects of dutasteride and finasteride include impotence, decreased libido, ejaculation disorders, and breast tenderness and enlargement.

DUTASTERIDE

Indications benign prostatic hyperplasia
Cautions see notes above; **interactions:** Appendix 1 (dutasteride)
Contra-indications see notes above; also severe hepatic impairment
Side-effects see notes above
Dose
- 500 micrograms daily (may require 6 months' treatment before benefit is obtained)

Avodart® (GSK) PoM
Capsules, yellow, dutasteride 500 micrograms, net price 30-cap pack = £24.81. Label: 25

FINASTERIDE

Indications benign prostatic hyperplasia; male-pattern baldness in men (section 13.9)
Cautions see notes above; also obstructive uropathy
Side-effects see notes above; also testicular pain, hypersensitivity reactions (including lip and face swelling, pruritus and rash)
Dose
- 5 mg daily, review treatment after 6 months (may require several months' treatment before benefit is obtained)

Proscar® (MSD) PoM
Tablets, blue, f/c, finasteride 5 mg. Net price 28-tab pack = £13.94

6.4.3 Anabolic steroids

Anabolic steroids have some androgenic activity but they cause less virilisation than androgens in women. They are used in the treatment of some *aplastic anaemias* (section 9.1.3). Anabolic steroids have been given for osteoporosis in women but they are no longer advocated for this purpose.

The protein-building properties of anabolic steroids have not proved beneficial in the clinical setting. Their use as body builders or tonics is quite unjustified; some athletes abuse them.

NANDROLONE

Indications osteoporosis in postmenopausal women (but not recommended, see notes above); aplastic anaemia (section 9.1.3)

Cautions cardiac and renal impairment, hepatic impairment (Appendix 2), hypertension, diabetes mellitus, epilepsy, migraine; monitor skeletal maturation in young patients; skeletal metastases (risk of hypercalcaemia); **interactions:** Appendix 1 (anabolic steroids)

Contra-indications severe hepatic impairment, prostate cancer, male breast cancer, pregnancy (Appendix 4) and breast-feeding, porphyria (section 9.8.2)

Side-effects acne, sodium retention with oedema, virilisation with high doses including voice changes (sometimes irreversible), amenorrhoea, inhibition of spermatogenesis, premature epiphyseal closure; abnormal liver-function tests reported with high doses; liver tumours reported occasionally on prolonged treatment with anabolic steroids

Dose
- See below

Deca-Durabolin® (Organon) PoM
Injection (oily), nandrolone decanoate 50 mg/mL, net price 1-mL amp = £3.29
Excipients include arachis (peanut) oil, benzyl alcohol (see Excipients, p. 2)
Dose by deep intramuscular injection, 50 mg every 3 weeks

6.5 Hypothalamic and pituitary hormones and anti-oestrogens

6.5.1 Hypothalamic and anterior pituitary hormones and anti-oestrogens

6.5.2 Posterior pituitary hormones and antagonists

Use of preparations in these sections requires detailed prior investigation of the patient and *should be reserved for specialist centres.*

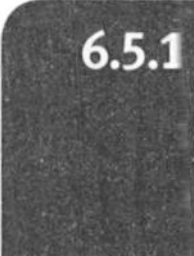

6.5.1 Hypothalamic and anterior pituitary hormones and anti-oestrogens

Anti-oestrogens

The anti-oestrogens **clomifene** (clomiphene) and **tamoxifen** (section 8.3.4.1) are used in the treatment of female infertility due to oligomenorrhoea or secondary amenorrhoea (e.g. associated with polycystic ovarian disease). They induce gonadotrophin release by occupying oestrogen receptors in the hypothalamus, thereby interfering with feedback mechanisms; chorionic gonadotrophin is sometimes used as an adjunct. Patients should be warned that there is a risk of multiple pregnancy (*rarely* more than twins).

CLOMIFENE CITRATE
(Clomiphene Citrate)

Indications anovulatory infertility—see notes above

Cautions see notes above; polycystic ovary syndrome (cysts may enlarge during treatment), ovarian hyperstimulation syndrome, uterine fibroids, ectopic pregnancy, incidence of multiple births increased (consider ultrasound monitoring), visual symptoms (discontinue and initiate ophthalmological examination); breast-feeding (Appendix 5)
CSM Advice. The CSM has recommended that clomifene should not normally be used for longer than 6 cycles (possibly increased risk of ovarian cancer)

Contra-indications hepatic disease (Appendix 2), ovarian cysts, hormone-dependent tumours or abnormal uterine bleeding of undetermined cause, pregnancy (exclude before treatment; Appendix 4)

Side-effects visual disturbances (withdraw), ovarian hyperstimulation (withdraw), hot flushes, abdominal discomfort, occasionally nausea, vomiting, depression, insomnia, breast tenderness, headache, intermenstrual spotting, menorrhagia, endometriosis, convulsions, weight gain, rashes, dizziness, hair loss

Dose
- 50 mg daily for 5 days, starting within about 5 days of onset of menstruation (preferably on 2nd day) or at any time (normally preceded by a progestogen-induced withdrawal bleed) if cycles have ceased; second course of 100 mg daily for 5 days may be given in absence of ovulation; most patients who are going to respond will do so to first course; 3 courses should constitute adequate therapeutic trial; long-term cyclical therapy not recommended—see CSM advice, above

Clomifene (Non-proprietary) PoM
Tablets, clomifene citrate 50 mg, net price 30-tab pack = £11.11

Clomid® (Aventis Pharma) PoM
Tablets, yellow, scored, clomifene citrate 50 mg. Net price 30-tab pack = £8.80

Anterior pituitary hormones

Corticotrophins

Tetracosactide (tetracosactrin), an analogue of corticotropin (ACTH), is used to test adrenocortical function; failure of the plasma cortisol concentration to rise after administration of tetracosactide indicates adrenocortical insufficiency.

Both corticotropin and tetracosactide were formerly used as alternatives to corticosteroids in conditions such as Crohn's disease or rheumatoid arthritis; their value was limited by the variable and unpredictable therapeutic response and by the waning of their effect with time.

TETRACOSACTIDE
(Tetracosactrin)

Indications see notes above
Cautions as for corticosteroids, section 6.3.2; **important**: risk of anaphylaxis (medical supervision; consult product literature); **interactions**: Appendix 1 (corticosteroids)
Contra-indications as for corticosteroids, section 6.3.2; avoid injections containing benzyl alcohol in neonates (see under preparations)
Side-effects as for corticosteroids, section 6.3.2
Dose
- See under preparations below

Synacthen® (Alliance) PoM
Injection, tetracosactide 250 micrograms (as acetate)/mL. Net price 1-mL amp = £2.93
Dose diagnostic (30-minute test), by intramuscular *or* intravenous injection, 250 micrograms as a single dose

Synacthen Depot® (Alliance) PoM
Injection (aqueous suspension), tetracosactide acetate 1 mg/mL, with zinc phosphate complex. Net price 1-mL amp = £4.18
Excipients include benzyl alcohol (avoid in neonates, see Excipients p. 2)
Dose diagnostic (5-hour test), by intramuscular injection, 1 mg as a single dose
Note Formerly used therapeutically by intramuscular injection, in an initial dose of 1 mg daily (or every 12 hours in acute cases); reduced to 1 mg every 2–3 days, then 1 mg weekly (or 500 micrograms every 2–3 days) but value was limited (see notes above)

Gonadotrophins

Follicle-stimulating hormone (FSH) and luteinising hormone (LH) together (as in **human menopausal gonadotrophin**), follicle-stimulating hormone alone (as in **follitropin**), or chorionic gonadotrophin, are used in the treatment of infertility in women with proven hypopituitarism or who have not responded to clomifene, or in superovulation treatment for assisted conception (such as *in vitro* fertilisation).

The gonadotrophins are also occasionally used in the treatment of hypogonadotrophic hypogonadism and associated oligospermia. There is no justification for their use in primary gonadal failure.

Chorionic gonadotrophin has also been used in delayed puberty in the male to stimulate endogenous testosterone production, but has little advantage over testosterone (section 6.4.2).

CHORIONIC GONADOTROPHIN
(Human Chorionic Gonadotrophin; HCG)

A preparation of a glycoprotein fraction secreted by the placenta and obtained from the urine of pregnant women having the action of the pituitary luteinising hormone

Indications see notes above
Cautions cardiac or renal impairment, asthma, epilepsy, migraine; prepubertal boys (risk of premature epiphyseal closure or precocious puberty)
Contra-indications androgen-dependent tumours
Side-effects oedema (particularly in males—reduce dose), headache, tiredness, mood changes, gynaecomastia, local reactions; may aggravate ovarian hyperstimulation, multiple pregnancy
Dose
- By subcutaneous *or* intramuscular injection, according to patient's response

Choragon® (Ferring) PoM
Injection, powder for reconstitution, chorionic gonadotrophin. Net price 5000-unit amp (with solvent) = £3.26. For intramuscular injection

Pregnyl® (Organon) PoM
Injection, powder for reconstitution, chorionic gonadotrophin. Net price 1500-unit amp = £2.20; 5000-unit amp = £3.27 (both with solvent). For subcutaneous or intramuscular injection

CHORIOGONADOTROPIN ALFA
(Human chorionic gonadotropin)

Indications see notes above
Cautions rule out infertility caused by hypothyroidism, adrenocortical deficiency, hyperprolactinaemia, tumours of the pituitary or hypothalamus
Contra-indications ovarian enlargement or cyst (unless caused by polycystic ovarian disease); ectopic pregnancy in previous 3 months; active thromboembolic disorders; hypothalamus, pituitary, ovarian, uterine or mammary malignancy
Side-effects nausea, vomiting, abdominal pain; headache, tiredness; injection-site reactions; ovarian hyperstimulation syndrome; rarely diarrhoea, depression, irritability, breast pain; ectopic pregnancy and ovarian torsion reported
Dose
- By subcutaneous injection, according to patient's response

Ovitrelle® (Serono) ▼ PoM
Injection, choriogonadotropin alfa, net price 6500-unit/0.5 mL (250-micrograms/0.5 mL) prefilled syringe = £33.31

FOLLITROPIN ALFA and BETA
(Recombinant human follicle stimulating hormone)

Indications see notes above
Cautions see under Human Menopausal Gonadotrophins; porphyria
Contra-indications see under Human Menopausal Gonadotrophins

6 Endocrine system

Side-effects see under Human Menopausal Gonadotrophins

Dose

- By subcutaneous *or* intramuscular injection, according to patient's response

Follitropin alfa

Gonal-F® (Serono) PoM

Injection, powder for reconstitution, follitropin alfa. Net price 75-unit amp = £22.31; 450 units/0.75 mL, multidose vial = £133.86; 1050 units/1.75 mL, multidose vial = £312.34 (all with solvent). For subcutaneous injection

Injection, prefilled pen, follitropin alfa 600 units/mL, net price 0.5 mL (300 units) = £97.08, 0.75 mL (450 units) = £145.62, 1.5 mL (900 units) = £291.24. For subcutaneous injection

Follitropin alfa with lutropin alfa

Pergoveris® (Serono) PoM

Injection, powder for reconstitution, follitropin alfa 150 units (11 micrograms), lutropin alfa 75 units (3 micrograms), net price per vial (with solvent) = £60.29. For subcutaneous injection

Electrolytes Na^{+} <1 mmol/vial

Follitropin beta

Puregon® (Organon) PoM

Injection, follitropin beta 100 units/mL, net price 0.5-mL (50-unit) vial = £18.74; 200 units/mL, 0.5-mL (100-unit) vial = £37.48; 300 units/mL, 0.5-mL (150-unit) vial = £50.62; 400 units/mL, 0.5-mL (200-unit) vial = £67.49; 0.36-mL (300-unit) cartridge = £101.23, 0.72-mL (600-unit) cartridge = £202.47, 1.08-mL (900-unit) cartridge = £303.66, (cartridges for use with *Puregon®* pen). For subcutaneous (cartridges and vials) or intramuscular injection (vials)

Excipients may include neomycin and streptomycin

HUMAN MENOPAUSAL GONADOTROPHINS

Indications see notes above

Cautions rule out infertility caused by adrenal or thyroid disorders, hyperprolactinaemia

Contra-indications ovarian cysts (not caused by polycystic ovarian syndrome); tumours of pituitary, hypothalamus, breast, uterus, ovaries, testes or prostate; vaginal bleeding of unknown cause; pregnancy and breast-feeding

Side-effects ovarian hyperstimulation, increased risk of multiple pregnancy and miscarriage, hypersensitivity reactions, gastro-intestinal disturbances, headache, joint pain, fever, injection site reactions, *very rarely* thromboembolism; gynaecomastia, acne, and weight gain reported in men

Dose

- By deep intramuscular *or* subcutaneous injection, according to patient's response

Menotrophin

Purified extract of human post-menopausal urine containing follicle-stimulating hormone (FSH) and luteinising hormone (LH) in a ratio of 1:1

Merional® (Pharmasure) PoM

Injection, powder for reconstitution, menotrophin as follicle-stimulating hormone 75 units and luteinising hormone 75 units, net price per vial (with solvent) = £13.95; follicle-stimulating hormone 150 units, luteinising hormone 150 units, net price per vial (with solvent) = £27.90. For intramuscular injection

Menopur® (Ferring) PoM

Injection, powder for reconstitution, menotrophin as follicle-stimulating hormone 75 units and luteinising hormone 75 units, net price per vial (with solvent) = £13.65. For intramuscular or subcutaneous injection

Urofollitropin

Purified extract of human post-menopausal urine containing follicle-stimulating hormone (FSH)

Fostimon® (Pharmasure) PoM

Injection, powder for reconstitution, urofollitropin as follicle-stimulating hormone 75 units, net price per vial (with solvent) = £13.95; follicle-stimulating hormone 150 units, net price per vial (with solvent) = £27.90. For intramuscular or subcutaneous injection

LUTROPIN ALFA

(Recombinant human luteinising hormone)

Indications see notes above

Cautions rule out infertility caused by hypothyroidism, adrenocortical deficiency, hyperprolactinaemia, tumours of the pituitary or hypothalamus

Contra-indications ovarian enlargement or cyst (unless caused by polycystic ovarian disease); undiagnosed vaginal bleeding; tumours of hypothalamus and pituitary; ovarian, uterine or mammary carcinoma

Side-effects nausea, vomiting, abdominal and pelvic pain; headache, somnolence; injection-site reactions; ovarian hyperstimulation syndrome, ovarian cyst, breast pain, ectopic pregnancy; thromboembolism, adnexal torsion, and haemoperitoneum

Dose

- By subcutaneous injection, in conjunction with follicle-stimulating hormone, according to response

Luveris® (Serono) PoM

Injection, powder for reconstitution, lutropin alfa, net price 75-unit vial = £33.31 (with solvent)

Growth hormone

Growth hormone is used to treat deficiency of the hormone in children and in adults (see NICE guidance below). In children it is used in Prader-Willi syndrome, Turner's syndrome and in chronic renal insufficiency; growth hormone has also recently been licensed for use in short children considered small for gestational age at birth.

Growth hormone of human origin (HGH; somatotrophin) has been replaced by a growth hormone of human sequence, **somatropin**, produced using recombinant DNA technology.

> **NICE guidance**
> Somatropin in children with growth failure (May 2002)
> Treatment with somatropin is recommended for children with:
> - proven growth-hormone deficiency;
> - Turner's syndrome;
> - Prader-Willi syndrome;
> - chronic renal insufficiency before puberty.
>
> Treatment should be initiated and monitored by a paediatrician with expertise in managing growth-hormone disorders; treatment can be continued under a shared-care protocol by a general practitioner.
> Treatment should be discontinued if the response is poor (i.e. an increase in growth velocity of less than 50% from baseline) in the first year of therapy.
> In children with chronic renal insufficiency, treatment should be stopped after renal transplantation and not restarted for at least a year

> **NICE guidance**
> Somatropin for adults with growth hormone deficiency (August 2003)
> Somatropin is recommended in adults **only** if the following 3 criteria are fulfilled:
> - Severe growth hormone deficiency, established by an appropriate method,
> - Impaired quality of life, measured by means of a specific questionnaire,
> - Already receiving treatment for another pituitary hormone deficiency.
>
> Somatropin treatment should be discontinued if the quality of life has not improved sufficiently by 9 months.
> Severe growth hormone deficiency developing after linear growth is complete but before the age of 25 years should be treated with growth hormone; treatment should continue until adult peak bone mass has been achieved. Treatment for adult-onset growth hormone deficiency should be stopped only when the patient and the patient's physician consider it appropriate.
> Treatment with somatropin should be initiated and managed by a physician with expertise in growth hormone disorders; maintenance treatment can be prescribed in the community under a shared-care protocol.

Mecasermin, a human insulin-like growth factor-I (rhIGF-I), is licensed to treat growth failure in children and adolescents with severe primary insulin-like growth factor-I deficiency (section 6.7.4).

SOMATROPIN
(Synthetic Human Growth Hormone)

Indications see under Dose

Cautions diabetes mellitus (adjustment of antidiabetic therapy may be necessary), papilloedema (see under Side-effects), relative deficiencies of other pituitary hormones (notably hypothyroidism—manufacturers recommend periodic thyroid function tests but limited evidence of clinical value), history of malignant disease, disorders of the epiphysis of the hip (monitor for limping), resolved intracranial hypertension (monitor closely), initiation of treatment close to puberty not recommended in child born small for gestational age; Silver-Russell syndrome; rotate subcutaneous injection sites to prevent lipoatrophy; breast-feeding (Appendix 5); **interactions:** Appendix 1 (somatropin)

Contra-indications evidence of tumour activity (complete antitumour therapy and ensure intracranial lesions inactive before starting); not to be used after renal transplantation or for growth promotion in children with closed epiphyses (or near closure in Prader-Willi syndrome); severe obesity or severe respiratory impairment in Prader-Willi syndrome; pregnancy (interrupt treatment if pregnancy occurs, Appendix 4)

Side-effects headache, funduscopy for papilloedema recommended if severe or recurrent headache, visual problems, nausea and vomiting occur—if papilloedema confirmed consider benign intracranial hypertension (rare cases reported); fluid retention (peripheral oedema), arthralgia, myalgia, carpal tunnel syndrome, paraesthesia, antibody formation, hypothyroidism, insulin resistance, hyperglycaemia, hypoglycaemia, reactions at injection site; leukaemia in children with growth hormone deficiency also reported

Dose
- Gonadal dysgenesis (Turner's syndrome), by subcutaneous injection, 45–50 micrograms/kg daily *or* 1.4 mg/m² daily
- Deficiency of growth hormone in children, by subcutaneous *or* intramuscular injection, 23–39 micrograms/kg daily *or* 0.7–1 mg/m² daily
- Growth disturbance in short children born small for gestational age whose growth has not caught up by 4 years or later, by subcutaneous injection, 35 micrograms/kg daily or 1 mg/m² daily
- Prader-Willi syndrome, by subcutaneous injection in children with growth velocity greater than 1 cm/year, in combination with energy-restricted diet, 35 micrograms/kg daily *or* 1 mg/m² daily; max. 2.7 mg daily
- Chronic renal insufficiency in children (renal function decreased to less than 50%), by subcutaneous injection, 45–50 micrograms/kg daily *or* 1.4 mg/m² daily (higher doses may be needed) adjusted if necessary after 6 months
- Adult growth hormone deficiency, by subcutaneous injection, initially 150–300 micrograms daily, gradually increased if required to max. 1 mg daily; use minimum effective dose (requirements may decrease with age)

Note Dose formerly expressed in units; somatropin 1 mg ≡ 3 units

Genotropin® (Pharmacia) PoM
Injection, two-compartment cartridge containing powder for reconstitution, somatropin (rbe) and diluent, net price 5.3-mg (16-unit) cartridge = £122.87, 12-mg (36-unit) cartridge = £278.20. For use with *Genotropin® Pen* NHS device (available free of charge from clinics). For subcutaneous injection
MiniQuick injection, two-compartment single-dose syringe containing powder for reconstitution, somatropin (rbe) and diluent, net price 0.2-mg (0.6-unit) syringe = £4.64; 0.4-mg (1.2-unit) syringe = £9.27; 0.6-mg (1.8-unit) syringe = £13.91; 0.8-mg (2.4-unit) syringe = £18.55; 1-mg (3-unit) syringe = £23.18; 1.2-mg (3.6-unit) syringe = £27.82; 1.4-mg (4.2-unit)

syringe = £32.46; 1.6-mg (4.8-unit) syringe = £37.09; 1.8-mg (5.4-unit) syringe = £41.73; 2-mg (6-unit) syringe = £46.37. For subcutaneous injection

Humatrope® (Lilly) PoM
Injection, powder for reconstitution, somatropin (rbe), net price 6-mg (18-unit) cartridge = £137.25; 12-mg (36-unit) cartridge = £274.50; 24-mg (72-unit) cartridge = £549.00; all supplied with diluent. For subcutaneous or intramuscular injection; cartridges for subcutaneous injection

Norditropin® (Novo Nordisk) PoM
SimpleXx injection, somatropin (epr) 3.3 mg (10 units)/mL, net price 1.5-mL (5-mg, 15-unit) cartridge = £115.90; 6.7 mg (20 units)/mL, 1.5-mL (10-mg, 30-unit) cartridge = £231.80; 10 mg (30 units)/mL, 1.5-mL (15-mg, 45-unit) cartridge = £347.70. For use with appropriate *NordiPen®* NHS device (available free of charge from clinics). For subcutaneous injection

NutropinAq® (Ipsen) PoM
Injection, somatropin (rbe), net price 10 mg (30 units) 2-ml cartridge = £230.00. For use with *NutropinAq® Pen* NHS device (available free of charge from clinics). For subcutaneous injection

Omnitrope® (Sandoz) ▼ PoM
Injection, powder for reconstitution, somatropin (rbe), net price 5-mg (15-unit) vial (with diluent) = £91.33. For use with *Omnitrope Pen L®* NHS device (available free of charge from clinics). For subcutaneous injection
Excipients include benzyl alcohol (avoid in neonates, see Excipients, p. 2)

Saizen® (Serono) PoM
Injection, powder for reconstitution, somatropin (rmc), net price 1.33-mg (4-unit) vial (with diluent) = £29.28; 3.33-mg (10-unit) vial (with diluent) = £73.20. For subcutaneous or intramuscular injection
Click.easy®, powder for reconstitution, somatropin (rmc), net price 8-mg (24-unit) vial (in *Click.easy®* device with diluent) = £175.68. For use with *One.click®* NHS autoinjector device *or Cool.Click®* NHS needle-free device (both available free of charge from clinics). For subcutaneous injection

Zomacton® (Ferring) PoM
Injection, powder for reconstitution, somatropin (rbe), net price 4-mg (12-unit) vial (with diluent) = £81.32. For use with *ZomaJet® 2* NHS needle-free device or with *Auto-Jector®* NHS (both available free of charge from clinics) or with needles and syringes. For subcutaneous injection
Excipients include benzyl alcohol (avoid in neonates, see Excipients p. 2)

Growth hormone receptor antagonists

Pegvisomant is a genetically modified analogue of human growth hormone and is a highly selective growth hormone receptor antagonist. Pegvisomant is licensed for the treatment of acromegaly in patients with inadequate response to surgery, radiation, or both, and to treatment with somatostatin analogues. Pegvisomant should be initiated only by physicians experienced in the treatment of acromegaly.

PEGVISOMANT

Indications see notes above
Cautions liver disease (monitor liver enzymes every 4–6 weeks for 6 months or if symptoms of hepatitis develop); diabetes mellitus (adjustment of antidiabetic therapy may be necessary); possible increase in female fertility
Contra-indications pregnancy and breast-feeding
Side-effects diarrhoea, constipation, nausea, vomiting, abdominal distension, dyspepsia, flatulence, elevated liver enzymes; hypertension; headache, asthenia, dizziness, drowsiness, tremor, sleep disturbances; influenza-like syndrome, weight gain, hyperglycaemia, hypoglycaemia; arthralgia, myalgia; injection-site reactions, sweating, pruritus, rash; fatigue; hypercholesterolaemia; less commonly thrombocytopenia, leucopenia, leucocytosis, bleeding tendency
Dose
- By subcutaneous injection, initially 80 mg, then 10 mg daily, increased in steps of 5 mg daily according to response; max. 30 mg daily; CHILD not recommended

Somavert® (Pfizer) ▼ PoM
Injection, powder for reconstitution, pegvisomant, net price 10-mg vial = £50.00; 15-mg vial = £75.00; 20-mg vial = £100.00 (all with solvent)

Thyrotrophin

Thyrotropin alfa is a recombinant form of thyrotrophin (thyroid stimulating hormone). It is licensed for use with or without radioiodine imaging, together with serum thyroglobulin testing, for the detection of thyroid remnants and thyroid cancer in post-thyroidectomy patients.

THYROTROPIN ALFA
(Recombinant human thyroid stimulating hormone, rhTSH)

Indications see notes above and product literature
Cautions presence of thyroglobulin autoantibodies may give false negative results
Contra-indications hypersensitivity to bovine or human thyrotrophin; pregnancy; breast-feeding
Side-effects nausea, vomiting; headache, dizziness, fatigue; *less commonly* asthenia, paraesthesia, back pain, influenza-like symptoms, rash, urticaria; *rarely* diarrhoea; *very rarely* palpitation, flushing, dyspnoea, pain at site of metastases, tremor, arthralgia, myalgia, hyperhydrosis, and injection-site reactions including pain, pruritus, and rash
Dose
- By intramuscular injection into the gluteal muscle, 900 micrograms every 24 hours for 2 doses, consult product literature

Thyrogen® (Genzyme) PoM
Injection, powder for reconstitution, thyrotropin alfa 900 micrograms/vial, net price = £232.50

Hypothalamic hormones

Gonadorelin when injected intravenously in normal subjects leads to a rapid rise in plasma concentrations of both luteinising hormone (LH) and follicle-stimulating hormone (FSH). It has not proved to be very helpful, however, in distinguishing hypothalamic from pituitary lesions. **Gonadorelin analogues** are indicated in endometriosis and infertility (section 6.7.2) and in breast and prostate cancer (section 8.3.4).

Protirelin is a hypothalamic releasing hormone which stimulates the release of thyrotrophin from the pituitary. It is licensed for the diagnosis of mild hyperthyroidism or hypothyroidism, but its use has been superseded by immunoassays for thyroid-stimulating hormone.

GONADORELIN
(Gonadotrophin-releasing hormone; GnRH; LH–RH)

Indications see preparations below

Cautions pituitary adenoma

Side-effects rarely, nausea, headache, abdominal pain, increased menstrual bleeding; rarely, hypersensitivity reaction on repeated administration of large doses; irritation at injection site

Dose

- See under preparations

HRF® (Intrapharm) PoM

Injection, powder for reconstitution, gonadorelin. Net price 100-microgram vial (with diluent) = £13.72 (hosp. only)

Excipients include benzyl alcohol (avoid in neonates, see Excipients p. 2)

Dose for assessment of pituitary function (adults), by subcutaneous *or* intravenous injection, 100 micrograms

PROTIRELIN
(Thyrotrophin-releasing hormone; TRH)

Indications assessment of thyroid function and thyroid stimulating hormone reserve

Cautions severe hypopituitarism, myocardial ischaemia, bronchial asthma and obstructive airways disease, pregnancy, breast-feeding (Appendix 5)

Side-effects after rapid intravenous administration desire to micturate, flushing, dizziness, nausea, strange taste; transient increase in pulse rate and blood pressure; rarely bronchospasm

Dose

- By intravenous injection, 200 micrograms; CHILD under 12 years 1 microgram/kg

Protirelin (Cambridge) PoM

Injection, protirelin 100 micrograms/mL. Net price 2-mL amp = £12.03

6.5.2 Posterior pituitary hormones and antagonists

Posterior pituitary hormones

Diabetes insipidus **Vasopressin** (antidiuretic hormone, ADH) is used in the treatment of *pituitary* ('cranial') *diabetes insipidus* as is its analogue **desmopressin**. Dosage is tailored to produce a slight diuresis every 24 hours to avoid water intoxication. Treatment may be required for a limited period only in diabetes insipidus following trauma or pituitary surgery.

Desmopressin is more potent and has a longer duration of action than vasopressin; unlike vasopressin it has no vasoconstrictor effect. It is given by mouth or intranasally for maintenance therapy, and by injection in the postoperative period or in unconscious patients. Desmopressin is also used in the differential diagnosis of diabetes insipidus. Following a dose of 2 micrograms intramuscularly or 20 micrograms intranasally, restoration of the ability to concentrate urine after water deprivation confirms a diagnosis of cranial diabetes insipidus. Failure to respond occurs in nephrogenic diabetes insipidus.

In *nephrogenic* and *partial pituitary diabetes insipidus* benefit may be gained from the paradoxical antidiuretic effect of thiazides (section 2.2.1) e.g. chlortalidone 100 mg twice daily reduced to maintenance dose of 50 mg daily.

Chlorpropamide (section 6.1.2.1) is also useful in partial pituitary diabetes insipidus, and probably acts by sensitising the renal tubules to the action of remaining endogenous vasopressin; it is given in doses of up to 350 mg daily in adults and 200 mg daily in children, care being taken to avoid hypoglycaemia. Carbamazepine (section 4.8.1) is also sometimes useful (in a dose of 200 mg once or twice daily) [unlicensed]; its mode of action may be similar to that of chlorpropamide.

Other uses Desmopressin is also used to boost factor VIII concentration in mild to moderate haemophilia and in von Willebrand's disease; it is also used to test fibrinolytic response. For a comment on use of desmopressin in nocturnal enuresis see section 7.4.2.

Vasopressin infusion is used to control variceal bleeding in portal hypertension, prior to more definitive treatment and with variable results. Terlipressin, a derivative of vasopressin, is used similarly.

Oxytocin, another posterior pituitary hormone, is indicated in obstetrics (section 7.1.1).

VASOPRESSIN

Indications pituitary diabetes insipidus; bleeding from oesophageal varices

Cautions heart failure, hypertension, asthma, epilepsy, migraine or other conditions which might be aggravated by water retention; renal impairment (see also Contra-indications); pregnancy (Appendix 4); avoid fluid overload

Contra-indications vascular disease (especially disease of coronary arteries) unless extreme caution, chronic nephritis (until reasonable blood nitrogen concentrations attained)

Side-effects fluid retention, pallor, tremor, sweating, vertigo, headache, nausea, vomiting, belching, abdominal cramps, desire to defaecate, hypersensitivity reactions (including anaphylaxis), constriction of coronary arteries (may cause anginal attacks and myocardial ischaemia), peripheral ischaemia and rarely gangrene

Dose

- By subcutaneous *or* intramuscular injection, diabetes insipidus, 5–20 units every four hours
- By intravenous infusion, initial control of variceal bleeding, 20 units over 15 minutes

▲Synthetic vasopressin

Pitressin® (Goldshield) PoM
Injection, argipressin (synthetic vasopressin) 20 units/mL. Net price 1-mL amp = £17.14 (hosp. only)

DESMOPRESSIN

Indications see under Dose

Cautions see under Vasopressin; less pressor activity, but still considerable caution in renal impairment (Appendix 3), in cardiovascular disease and in hypertension (not indicated for nocturnal enuresis or nocturia in these circumstances); elderly (avoid for nocturnal enuresis and nocturia in those over 65 years); also considerable caution in cystic fibrosis; in nocturia and nocturnal enuresis limit fluid intake to minimum from 1 hour before dose until 8 hours afterwards; in nocturia periodic blood pressure and weight checks needed to monitor for fluid overload; pregnancy (Appendix 4) **interactions:** Appendix 1 (desmopressin)

Hyponatraemic convulsions The CSM has advised that patients being treated for primary nocturnal enuresis should be warned to avoid fluid overload (including during swimming) and to stop taking desmopressin during an episode of vomiting or diarrhoea (until fluid balance normal). The risk of hyponatraemic convulsions can also be minimised by keeping to the recommended starting doses and by avoiding concomitant use of drugs which increase secretion of vasopressin (e.g. tricyclic antidepressants)

Contra-indications cardiac insufficiency and other conditions treated with diuretics; psychogenic polydipsia and polydipsia in alcohol dependence

Side-effects fluid retention, and hyponatraemia (in more serious cases with convulsions) on administration without restricting fluid intake; stomach pain, headache, nausea, vomiting, allergic reactions, and emotional disturbance in children also reported; epistaxis, nasal congestion, rhinitis with nasal spray

Dose

- By mouth (as desmopressin acetate)

  Diabetes insipidus, treatment, ADULT and CHILD initially 300 micrograms daily (in 3 divided doses); maintenance, 300–600 micrograms daily in 3 divided doses; range 0.2–1.2 mg daily

  Primary nocturnal enuresis (if urine concentrating ability normal), ADULT (under 65 years) and CHILD over 5 years (preferably over 7 years) 200 micrograms at bedtime, only increased to 400 micrograms if lower dose not effective (**important:** see also Cautions); withdraw for at least 1 week for reassessment after 3 months

  Postoperative polyuria or polydipsia, adjust dose according to urine osmolality
- Sublingually (as desmopressin base)

  Diabetes insipidus, treatment, ADULT and CHILD initially 180 micrograms daily in 3 divided doses; range 120–720 micrograms daily

  Polyuria or polydipsia after hypophysectomy, adjust dose according to urine osmolality
- Intranasally (as desmopressin acetate)

  Diabetes insipidus, diagnosis, ADULT and CHILD 20 micrograms (limit fluid intake to 500 mL from 1 hour before to 8 hours after administration)

  Diabetes insipidus, treatment, ADULT 10–40 micrograms daily (in 1–2 divided doses); CHILD 5–20 micrograms daily; infants may require lower doses

  Nocturia associated with multiple sclerosis (when other treatments have failed), ADULT (under 65 years) 10–20 micrograms at bedtime (**important:** see also Cautions), dose not to be repeated within 24 hours

  Renal function testing (empty bladder at time of administration and limit fluid intake to 500 mL from 1 hour before until 8 hours after administration), ADULT 40 micrograms; INFANT under 1 year 10 micrograms (restrict fluid intake to 50% at next 2 feeds to avoid fluid overload), CHILD 1–15 years 20 micrograms

  Mild to moderate haemophilia and von Willebrand's disease, ADULT 300 micrograms (one 150-microgram spray into each nostril) 30 minutes before surgery or when bleeding; may be repeated at intervals of 12 hours (or at intervals of at least 3 days if self-administered)

  Fibrinolytic response testing, ADULT 300 micrograms (one 150-microgram spray into each nostril); blood sampled after 1 hour for fibrinolytic activity
- By injection (as desmopressin acetate)

  Diabetes insipidus, diagnosis (subcutaneous *or* intramuscular), ADULT and CHILD 2 micrograms (limit fluid intake to 500 mL from 1 hour before to 8 hours after administration)

  Diabetes insipidus, treatment (subcutaneous, intramuscular *or* intravenous), ADULT 1–4 micrograms daily; INFANT and CHILD 400 nanograms

  Renal function testing (empty bladder at time of administration and limit fluid intake to 500 mL from 1 hour before until 8 hours after administration) (subcutaneous *or* intramuscular), ADULT and CHILD 2 micrograms INFANT 400 nanograms (restrict fluid intake to 50% at next 2 feeds)

  Mild to moderate haemophilia and Von Willebrand's disease, (subcutaneous *or* intravenous), ADULT and CHILD over 1 month 300 nanograms/kg as a single dose immediately before surgery or after trauma; may be repeated at intervals of 12 hours

  Fibrinolytic response testing, (subcutaneous *or* intravenous), ADULT and CHILD 300 nanograms/kg; blood sampled after 20 minutes for fibrinolytic activity

  Lumbar-puncture-associated headache, consult product literature

Desmopressin acetate (Non-proprietary) PoM
Nasal spray, desmopressin acetate 10 micrograms/metered spray, net price 6-mL unit (60 metered sprays) = £22.73. Counselling, fluid intake, see above
Brands include *Presinex®*
Note Children requiring dose of less than 10 micrograms should be given *DDAVP®* intranasal solution

DDAVP® (Ferring) PoM
Tablets, both scored, desmopressin acetate 100 micrograms, net price 90-tab pack = £45.48; 200 micrograms, 90-tab pack = £90.96. Counselling, fluid intake, see above
Sublingual tablets (DDAVP® Melt), desmopressin (as acetate) 60 micrograms, net price 100-tab pack =

6 Endocrine system

£50.53; 120 micrograms, 100-tab pack = £101.07; 240 micrograms, 100-tab pack = £202.14. Label: 26, counselling, fluid intake, see above

Intranasal solution, desmopressin acetate 100 micrograms/mL. Net price 2.5-mL dropper bottle and catheter = £9.72. Counselling, fluid intake, see above

Injection, desmopressin acetate 4 micrograms/mL. Net price 1-mL amp = £1.10

Desmotabs® (Ferring) PoM
Tablets, scored, desmopressin acetate 200 micrograms, net price 30-tab pack = £30.34. Counselling, fluid intake, see above

DesmoMelt® (Ferring) PoM
Sublingual tablets, desmopressin (as acetate) 120 micrograms, net price 30-tab pack = £30.34; 240 micrograms, 30-tab pack = £60.68. Label: 26, counselling, fluid intake, see above

Desmospray® (Ferring) PoM
Nasal spray, desmopressin acetate 10 micrograms/metered spray. Net price 6-mL unit (60 metered sprays) = £26.04. Counselling, fluid intake, see above
Note Children requiring dose of less than 10 micrograms should be given *DDAVP® intranasal solution*

Octim® (Ferring) PoM
Nasal spray, desmopressin acetate 150 micrograms/metered spray, net price 2.5-mL unit (25 metered sprays) = £600.00. Counselling, fluid intake, see above

Injection, desmopressin acetate 15 micrograms/mL, net price 1-mL amp = £20.00

TERLIPRESSIN

Indications bleeding from oesophageal varices
Cautions see under Vasopressin
Contra-indications see under Vasopressin
Side-effects see under Vasopressin, but effects milder
Dose
- By intravenous injection, 2 mg followed by 1 or 2 mg every 4 to 6 hours until bleeding is controlled, for up to 72 hours

Glypressin® (Ferring) PoM
Injection, terlipressin, powder for reconstitution. Net price 1-mg vial with 5 mL diluent = £19.44 (hosp. only)

Antidiuretic hormone antagonists

Demeclocycline (section 5.1.3) can be used in the treatment of hyponatraemia resulting from inappropriate secretion of antidiuretic hormone, if fluid restriction alone does not restore sodium concentration or is not tolerable. Demeclocycline is thought to act by directly blocking the renal tubular effect of antidiuretic hormone. Initially 0.9–1.2 g is given daily in divided doses, reduced to 600–900 mg daily for maintenance.

6.6 Drugs affecting bone metabolism

6.6.1 Calcitonin and parathyroid hormone
6.6.2 Bisphosphonates and other drugs affecting bone metabolism

See also calcium (section 9.5.1.1), phosphorus (section 9.5.2), vitamin D (section 9.6.4), and oestrogens in postmenopausal osteoporosis (section 6.4.1.1).

Osteoporosis

Osteoporosis occurs most commonly in postmenopausal women and in those taking long-term oral corticosteroids (glucocorticosteroids). Other risk factors for osteoporosis include low body weight, cigarette smoking, excess alcohol intake, lack of physical activity, family history of osteoporosis, and early menopause.

> Those at risk of osteoporosis should maintain an adequate intake of **calcium and vitamin D** and any deficiency should be corrected by increasing dietary intake or taking supplements.

Elderly patients, especially those who are housebound or live in residential or nursing homes, are at increased risk of calcium and vitamin D deficiency and may benefit from supplements (section 9.5.1.1 and section 9.6.4). Reversible secondary causes of osteoporosis such as hyperthyroidism, hyperparathyroidism, osteomalacia or hypogonadism should be excluded, in both men and women, before treatment for osteoporosis is initiated.

Postmenopausal osteoporosis The **bisphosphonates** (alendronic acid, disodium etidronate, and risedronate, section 6.6.2) are effective for preventing postmenopausal osteoporosis. **Hormone replacement therapy** (HRT section 6.4.1.1) is an option where other therapies are contra-indicated, cannot be tolerated, or if there is a lack of response. The CSM has advised that HRT should **not** be considered first-line therapy for long-term prevention of osteoporosis in women over 50 years of age. HRT is of most benefit for the prophylaxis of postmenopausal osteoporosis if started early in menopause and continued for up to 5 years, but bone loss resumes (possibly at an accelerated rate) on stopping HRT. **Calcitonin** (section 6.6.1) may be considered for those at high risk of osteoporosis for whom a bisphosphonate is unsuitable. Women of Afro-Caribbean origin appear to be less susceptible to osteoporosis than those who are white or of Asian origin.

Postmenopausal osteoporosis may be *treated* with a **bisphosphonate** (section 6.6.2). The bisphosphonates (such as alendronate, etidronate, and risedronate) decrease the risk of vertebral fracture; alendronate and risedronate have also been shown to reduce non-vertebral fractures. If bisphosphonates are unsuitable **calcitriol** (section 9.6.4), **calcitonin** or **strontium ranelate** (section 6.6.2) may be considered. Calcitonin [unlicensed indication] may also be useful for pain relief for up to 3 months after a vertebral fracture if other analgesics are ineffective. **Parathyroid hormone**, and **teriparatide** (section 6.6.1) have been introduced for the treatment of postmenopausal oestoporosis.

Raloxifene (section 6.4.1.1) is licensed for the *prophylaxis* and *treatment* of vertebral fractures in postmenopausal women.

> NICE guidance
>
> Bisphosphonates, selective oestrogen receptor modulators and parathyroid hormone for secondary prevention of osteoporotic fragility fractures in postmenopausal women (January 2005)
>
> **Bisphosphonates** are recommended as treatment options for the secondary prevention of osteoporotic fractures in susceptible postmenopausal women. In women who cannot take a bisphosphonate or who have suffered a fragility fracture despite treatment for a year and whose bone mineral density declines below the pretreatment level, the selective oestrogen receptor modulator **raloxifene** is an alternative. The parathyroid hormone fragment **teriparatide** is recommended for women over 65 years who cannot take a bisphosphonate (or in whom bisphosphonate has failed to prevent a fracture) and have:
>
> - either an extremely low bone mineral density
> - or a very low bone mineral density, suffered more than 2 fractures, and have other risk factors for fractures (e.g. body mass index under 19 kg/m^2, premature menopause, prolonged immobility, history of maternal hip fracture under the age of 75 years).

Corticosteroid-induced osteoporosis To reduce the risk of osteoporosis doses of oral corticosteroids should be as low as possible and courses of treatment as short as possible. The risk of osteoporosis may be related to cumulative dose of corticosteroids; even intermittent courses can therefore increase the risk. The greatest rate of bone loss occurs during the first 6–12 months of corticosteroid use and so early steps to prevent the development of osteoporosis are important. Long-term use of high-dose inhaled corticosteroids may also contribute to corticosteroid-induced osteoporosis(-section 3.2).

Patients taking (or who are likely to take) the equivalent of prednisolone 7.5 mg or more each day for 3 months or longer should be assessed and where necessary given prophylactic treatment; those aged over 65 years are at greater risk. Patients taking oral corticosteroids who have sustained a low-trauma fracture should receive treatment for osteoporosis. The therapeutic options for *prophylaxis* and *treatment* of corticosteroid-induced osteoporosis are the same:

- a bisphosphonate such as alendronate, etidronate or risedronate;
- calcitriol.
- hormone replacement (HRT in women, (section 6.4.1) testosterone in men (section 6.4.2))

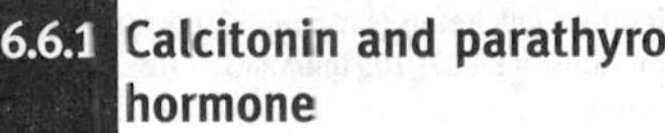

6.6.1 Calcitonin and parathyroid hormone

Calcitonin is involved with parathyroid hormone in the regulation of bone turnover and hence in the maintenance of calcium balance and homoeostasis. **Calcitonin (salmon)** (**salcatonin**, synthetic or recombinant salmon calcitonin) is used to lower the plasma-calcium concentration in some patients with hypercalcaemia (notably when associated with malignant disease). Calcitonin is licensed for treatment of Paget's disease of bone. It can also be used in the prevention and treatment of postmenopausal osteoporosis (see section 6.6).

Recombinant **parathyroid hormone**, and **teriparatide** (a recombinant fragment of parathyroid hormone), have been introduced for the treatment of postmenopausal osteoporosis. *The Scottish Medicines Consortium* has advised that teriparatide (December 2003) and parathyroid hormone (February 2007) should be initiated by specialists experienced in the treatment of osteoporosis.

Cinacalcet (section 9.5.1.2) is licensed for the treatment of hypercalcaemia in parathyroid carcinoma.

CALCITONIN (SALMON)/ SALCATONIN

Indications see under Dose

Cautions history of allergy (skin test advised); renal impairment; heart failure; pregnancy (Appendix 4), breast-feeding (Appendix 5)

Contra-indications hypocalcaemia

Side-effects nausea, vomiting, diarrhoea, abdominal pain; flushing; dizziness, headache, taste disturbances; musculoskeletal pain; with nasal spray nose and throat irritation, rhinitis, sinusitis and epistaxis; *less commonly* diuresis, oedema, cough, visual disturbances, injection-site reactions, rash, hypersensitivity reactions including pruritus

Dose

- Hypercalcaemia of malignancy (see also section 9.5.1.2), ADULT over 18 years, by subcutaneous *or* intramuscular injection, 100 units every 6–8 hours adjusted according to response; max. 400 units every 6–8 hours; in severe or emergency cases, by intravenous infusion, up to 10 units/kg over at least 6 hours
- Paget's disease of bone, ADULT over 18 years, by subcutaneous *or* intramuscular injection, 50 units 3 times weekly to 100 units daily adjusted according to response
- Postmenopausal osteoporosis to reduce risk of vertebral fractures, intranasally, 200 units (1 spray) into one nostril daily, with dietary calcium and vitamin D supplements (section 9.5.1.1 and section 9.6.4)
- Prevention of acute bone loss due to sudden immobility, ADULT over 18 years, by subcutaneous *or* intramuscular injection, 100 units daily in 1–2 divided doses for 2–4 weeks, reduced to 50 units daily at start of mobilisation and continued until fully mobile

Miacalcic® (Novartis) PoM

Nasal spray▼, calcitonin (salmon) 200 units/ metered spray, net price 2-mL unit (approx. 14 metered sprays) = £20.99

Injection, calcitonin (salmon) 50 units/mL, net price 1-mL amp = £4.27; 100 units/mL, 1-mL amp = £8.55; 200 units/mL, 2-mL vial = £30.75
For subcutaneous or intramuscular injection and for dilution and use as an intravenous infusion

PARATHYROID HORMONE
(Human recombinant parathyroid hormone)

Indications treatment of osteoporosis in postmenopausal women at high risk of fractures (to reduce the risk of vertebral fractures) (see also notes above)

Cautions monitor serum or urinary calcium concentration at 1, 3 and 6 months after initiation of treatment (consult product literature for guidance if serum calcium concentration raised); active or previous urolithiasis; concomitant cardiac glycosides; renal impairment (Appendix 3)

Contra-indications previous radiation therapy to skeleton, pre-existing hypercalcaemia, metabolic bone disease (including hyperparathyroidism and Paget's disease), unexplained raised levels of alkaline phosphatase; avoid in severe hepatic impairment; pregnancy; breast-feeding

Side-effects nausea, vomiting, dyspepsia, constipation, diarrhoea; palpitation; headache, dizziness, fatigue, asthenia; transient hypercalcaemia, hypercalciuria; muscle cramp, pain in extremities, back pain; injection-site reactions; *less commonly* abdominal pain, altered sense of smell, taste disturbance, anorexia, influenza, hyperuricaemia

Dose
- By subcutaneous injection, 100 micrograms daily, max. duration of treatment 24 months

Preotact® (Nycomed) ▼ PoM
Injection, dual-chamber cartridge containing powder for reconstitution, parathyroid hormone (rdna) and diluent, net price 1.61-mg (14-dose) cartridge = £130.20. For use with *Preotact®* pen device.

TERIPARATIDE

Indications treatment of osteoporosis in postmenopausal women and in men at increased risk of fractures (see also notes above)

Cautions moderate renal impairment (avoid if severe)

Contra-indications pre-existing hypercalcaemia, skeletal malignancies or bone metastases, metabolic bone diseases, including Paget's disease and hyperparathyroidism, unexplained raised alkaline phosphatase, previous radiation therapy to the skeleton; pregnancy; breast-feeding

Side-effects gastro-intestinal disorders (including nausea, reflux and haemorrhoids); palpitation; dyspnoea; headache, fatigue, asthenia, depression, dizziness, vertigo; anaemia, increased sweating, muscle cramps, sciatica, myalgia, arthralgia; *less commonly* urinary disorders, hypercalaemia; injection-site reactions; *rarely* hypersensitivity reactions

Dose
- By subcutaneous injection, 20 micrograms daily; max. duration of treatment 18 months

Forsteo® (Lilly) ▼ PoM
Injection, teriparatide 250 micrograms/mL, net price 3-mL prefilled pen = £271.88
Note 3-ml prefilled pen intended for 28 doses

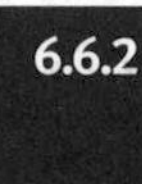

6.6.2 Bisphosphonates and other drugs affecting bone metabolism

Bisphosphonates

Bisphosphonates are adsorbed onto hydroxyapatite crystals in bone, slowing both their rate of growth and dissolution, and therefore reducing the rate of bone turnover. Bisphosphonates have an important role in the prophylaxis and treatment of osteoporosis and corticosteroid-induced osteoporosis; **alendronic acid** or **risedronate sodium** are considered the drugs of choice for these conditions, but **disodium etidronate** may be considered if these drugs are unsuitable or not tolerated (see also section 6.6).

Bisphosphonates are also used in the treatment of *Paget's disease*, hypercalcaemia of malignancy (section 9.5.1.2). and in bone metastases in breast cancer (section 8.3.4.1). Disodium etidronate can impair bone mineralisation when used continuously or in high doses (such as in the treatment of *Paget's disease*).

Osteonecrosis of the jaw Osteonecrosis of the jaw has been reported in patients receiving intravenous bisphosphonates and, rarely, in those taking oral bisphosphonates. Adequate oral hygiene should be maintained during and after treatment with bisphosphonates. Ideally in patients with concomitant risk factors, such as cancer, chemotherapy treatment, corticosteroid treatment, or poor oral hygiene, remedial dental work should be carried out before starting bisphosphonate treatment.

ALENDRONIC ACID

Indications see under Dose

Cautions upper gastro-intestinal disorders (dysphagia, symptomatic oesophageal disease, gastritis, duodenitis, or ulcers—see also under Contra-indications and Side-effects); history (within 1 year) of ulcers, active gastro-intestinal bleeding, or surgery of the upper gastro-intestinal tract; renal impairment (Appendix 3); correct disturbances of calcium and mineral metabolism (e.g. vitamin-D deficiency, hypocalcaemia) before starting and monitor serum calcium during treatment; consider preventive dental treatment before initiating bisphosphonate (risk of osteonecrosis of the jaw, see notes above); exclude other causes of osteoporosis; **interactions**: Appendix 1 (bisphosphonates)

Contra-indications abnormalities of oesophagus and other factors which delay emptying (e.g. stricture or achalasia), hypocalcaemia, pregnancy (Appendix 4) and breast-feeding (Appendix 5)

Side-effects oesophageal reactions (see below), abdominal pain and distension, dyspepsia, regurgitation, melaena, diarrhoea or constipation, flatulence, musculoskeletal pain, headache; *rarely* rash, pruritus, erythema, photosensitivity, uveitis, scleritis, transient decrease in serum calcium and phosphate; nausea, vomiting, gastritis, peptic ulceration, and hypersensitivity reactions (including urticaria and angioedema) also reported; myalgia, malaise and fever at initiation of treatment; *very rarely* severe skin reactions (including Stevens-Johnson syndrome), osteonecrosis (see notes above)

Oesophageal reactions Severe oesophageal reactions (oesophagitis, oesophageal ulcers, oesophageal stricture and oesophageal erosions) have been reported; patients should be advised to stop taking the tablets and to seek medical attention if they develop symptoms of oesophageal irritation such as dysphagia, new or worsening heartburn, pain on swallowing or retrosternal pain

Dose

- Treatment of postmenopausal osteoporosis and osteoporosis in men, 10 mg daily *or* (in postmenopausal osteoporosis) 70 mg once weekly
- Prevention of postmenopausal osteoporosis, 5 mg daily
- Prevention and treatment of corticosteroid-induced osteoporosis, 5 mg daily (postmenopausal women not receiving hormone replacement therapy, 10 mg daily)

Counselling Tablets should be swallowed whole with plenty of water while sitting or standing; to be taken on an empty stomach at least 30 minutes before breakfast (or another oral medicine); patient should stand or sit upright for at least 30 minutes after taking tablet

Alendronic acid (Non-proprietary) PoM
Tablets, alendronic acid (as sodium alendronate) 10 mg, net price 28-tab pack = £8.45.Counselling, administration

Fosamax® (MSD) PoM
Tablets, alendronic acid (as sodium alendronate) 10 mg, 28-tab pack = £23.12. Counselling, administration

Alendronic Acid Once-Weekly (Non-proprietary) PoM
Tablets, alendronic acid (as sodium alendronate) 70 mg, net price 4-tab pack = £3.91.Counselling, administration

Fosamax® Once Weekly (MSD) PoM
Tablets, alendronic acid (as sodium alendronate) 70 mg, net price 4-tab pack = £22.80. Counselling, administration

With colecalciferol

For cautions, contra-indications, and side-effects of colecalciferol, see section 9.6.4

Fosavance® (MSD) ▼ PoM
Tablets, alendronic acid (as sodium alendronate) 70 mg, colecalciferol 70 micrograms (2 800 units), net price 4-tab pack = £22.80. Counselling, administration

Dose treatment of postmenopausal osteoporosis in women at risk of vitamin D deficiency, 1 tablet once weekly

Counselling Tablets should be swallowed whole with plenty of water while sitting or standing; to be taken on an empty stomach at least 30 minutes before breakfast (or another oral medicine); patient should stand or sit upright for at least 30 minutes after taking tablet

DISODIUM ETIDRONATE

Indications see under Dose

Cautions consider preventive dental treatment before initiating bisphosphonate (risk of osteonecrosis of the jaw, see notes above); renal impairment (Appendix 3); **interactions:** Appendix 1 (bisphosphonates)

Contra-indications moderate to severe renal impairment; pregnancy (Appendix 4) and breast-feeding (Appendix 5); not indicated for osteoporosis in presence of hypercalcaemia or hypercalciuria or for osteomalacia

Side-effects nausea, diarrhoea or constipation, abdominal pain; increased bone pain in Paget's disease, also increased risk of fractures with high doses in Paget's disease (discontinue if fractures occur); rarely exacerbation of asthma, skin reactions (including angioedema, rash, urticaria and pruritus), transient hyperphosphataemia, headache, paraesthesia, peripheral neuropathy reported; blood disorders (including leucopenia, agranulocytosis and pancytopenia) also reported; *very rarely* osteonecrosis (see notes above)

Dose

- Paget's disease of bone, by mouth, 5 mg/kg as a single daily dose for up to 6 months; doses above 10 mg/kg daily for up to 3 months may be used with caution but doses above 20 mg/kg daily are not recommended; after interval of not less than 3 months may be repeated where evidence of reactivation—including biochemical indices (avoid premature retreatment)

  Monitoring Serum phosphate, serum alkaline phosphatase and (if possible) urinary hydroxyproline should be measured before starting and at intervals of 3 months—consult product literature for further details

- Osteoporosis, see under *Didronel PMO®*

Counselling Avoid food for at least 2 hours before and after oral treatment, particularly calcium-containing products e.g.milk; also avoid iron and mineral supplements and antacids

Didronel® (Procter & Gamble Pharm.) PoM
Tablets, disodium etidronate 200 mg. Net price 60-tab pack = £20.68. Counselling, food and calcium (see above)

With calcium carbonate

For cautions and side-effects of calcium carbonate see section 9.5.1.1

Didronel PMO® (Procter & Gamble Pharm.) PoM
Tablets, 14 white, disodium etidronate 400 mg; 76 pink, effervescent, calcium carbonate 1.25 g (*Cacit®*). Net price per pack = £21.12. Label: 10, patient information leaflet, counselling, food and calcium (see above)

Dose treatment of osteoporosis, prevention of bone loss in postmenopausal women (particularly if hormone replacement therapy inappropriate), and prevention and treatment of corticosteroid-induced osteoporosis, given in 90-day cycles, 1 *Didronel®* tablet daily for 14 days, then 1 *Cacit®* tablet daily for 76 days

DISODIUM PAMIDRONATE

Disodium pamidronate was formerly called aminohydroxypropylidenediphosphonate disodium (APD)

Indications see under Dose

Cautions renal impairment (Appendix 3); assess renal function before each dose; hepatic impairment (Appendix 2); cardiac disease (especially in elderly); previous thyroid surgery (risk of hypocalcaemia); monitor serum electrolytes, calcium and phosphate—possibility of convulsions due to electrolyte changes; avoid concurrent use with other bisphosphonates; consider preventive dental treatment before initiating bisphosphonate (risk of osteonecrosis of the jaw, see notes above); **interactions:** Appendix 1 (bisphosphonates)

Driving Patients should be warned against driving or operating machinery immediately after treatment (somnolence or dizziness can occur)

Contra-indications pregnancy (Appendix 4); breast-feeding (Appendix 5)

6 Endocrine system

Side-effects hypophosphataemia, fever and influenza-like symptoms (sometimes accompanied by malaise, rigors, fatigue and flushes); nausea, vomiting, anorexia, abdominal pain, diarrhoea, constipation; symptomatic hypocalcaemia (paraesthesia, tetany), hypomagnesaemia, headache, insomnia, drowsiness; hypertension; anaemia, thrombocytopenia, lymphocytopenia; rash; arthralgia, myalgia; rarely muscle cramps, dyspepsia, agitation, confusion, dizziness, lethargy; leucopenia, hypotension, pruritus, hyperkalaemia or hypokalaemia, and hypernatraemia; osteonecrosis (see also notes above), isolated cases of seizures, hallucinations, haematuria, acute renal failure, deterioration of renal disease, conjunctivitis and other ocular symptoms; reactivation of herpes simplex and zoster also reported; also injection-site reactions

Dose

- By slow intravenous infusion (via cannula in a relatively large vein), see also Appendix 6

  Hypercalcaemia of malignancy, according to serum calcium concentration 15–60 mg in single infusion or in divided doses over 2–4 days; max. 90 mg per treatment course

  Osteolytic lesions and bone pain in bone metastases associated with breast cancer or multiple myeloma, 90 mg every 4 weeks (or every 3 weeks to coincide with chemotherapy in breast cancer)

  Paget's disease of bone, 30 mg once a week for 6 weeks (total dose 180 mg) *or* 30 mg in first week then 60 mg every other week (total dose 210 mg); max. total 360 mg (in divided doses of 60 mg) per treatment course; may be repeated every 6 months
- CHILD not recommended

Calcium and vitamin D supplements Oral supplements are advised for those with Paget's disease at risk of calcium or vitamin D deficiency (e.g. through malabsorption or lack of exposure to sunlight) to minimise potential risk of hypocalcaemia

Disodium pamidronate (Non-proprietary) PoM

Concentrate for intravenous infusion, disodium pamidronate 3 mg/mL, net price 5-mL vial = £27.50, 10-mL vial = £55.00; 6 mg/mL, 10-mL vial = £110.00; 9 mg/mL, 10-mL vial = £165.00

Aredia Dry Powder® (Novartis) PoM

Injection, powder for reconstitution, disodium pamidronate, for use as an infusion. Net price 15-mg vial = £29.83; 30-mg vial = £59.66; 90-mg vial = £170.45 (all with diluent)

IBANDRONIC ACID

Indications see under Dose

Cautions consider preventive dental treatment before initiating bisphosphonate (risk of osteonecrosis of the jaw, see notes above); renal impairment (Appendix 3); monitor renal function and serum calcium, phosphate and magnesium; cardiac disease (avoid fluid overload); **interactions:** Appendix 1 (bisphosphonates)

Contra-indications pregnancy (Appendix 4); breast-feeding (Appendix 5)

Side-effects hypocalcaemia, hypophosphataemia, influenza-like symptoms (including fever, chills, and muscle pain), bone pain; oesophageal reactions (see below), diarrhoea, nausea, vomiting, gastritis, abdominal pain, dyspepsia, pharyngitis; headache, asthenia, rash; *rarely* anaemia, hypersensitivity reactions (pruritus, bronchospasm and angioedema reported); urticaria; injection-site reactions; *very rarely* osteonecrosis (see notes above)

Oesophageal reactions Severe oesophageal reactions reported with all **oral** bisphosphonates; patients should be advised to stop tablets and seek medical attention for symptoms of oesophageal irritation such as dysphagia, pain on swallowing, retrosternal pain, or heartburn

Dose

- Reduction of bone damage in bone metastases in breast cancer, by mouth, 50 mg daily, *or* by intravenous infusion, 6 mg every 3–4 weeks
- Hypercalcaemia of malignancy by intravenous infusion, according to serum calcium concentration, 2–4 mg in single infusion
- Treatment of postmenopausal osteoporosis, by mouth, 150 mg once a month *or* by intravenous injection over 15–30 seconds, 3 mg every 3 months
- CHILD not recommended

Counselling Tablets should be swallowed whole with plenty of water while sitting or standing; to be taken on an empty stomach at least 30 minutes (*Bondronat®* tablets, 50 mg) or 1 hour (*Bonviva®* tablets, 150 mg) before breakfast or another oral medicine; patient should continue to fast, and stand or sit upright for at least 30 minutes (50-mg tablet) or 1 hour (150-mg tablet) after taking tablet

Bondronat® (Roche) ▼ PoM

Tablets, f/c, ibandronic acid 50 mg, net price 28-tab pack = £195.00. Counselling, administration

Concentrate for intravenous infusion, ibandronic acid 1 mg/mL, net price 2-mL amp = £94.86, 6-mL vial = £195.00

Bonviva® (Roche) ▼ PoM

Tablets, f/c, ibandronic acid 150 mg, net price 1-tab pack = £21.45, 3-tab pack = £64.35. Counselling, administration

Injection, ibandronic acid 1 mg/mL, net price 3-mL prefilled syringe = £80.00

RISEDRONATE SODIUM

Indications see under Dose

Cautions oesophageal abnormalities and other factors which delay transit or emptying (e.g. stricture or achalasia—see also under Side-effects); renal impairment (Appendix 3); correct hypocalcaemia before starting, correct other disturbances of bone and mineral metabolism (e.g. vitamin-D deficiency) at onset of treatment; consider preventive dental treatment before initiating bisphosphonate (risk of osteonecrosis of the jaw, see notes above); **interactions:** Appendix 1 (bisphosphonates)

Contra-indications hypocalcaemia (see Cautions above), pregnancy (Appendix 4) and breast-feeding (Appendix 5)

Side-effects gastro-intestinal disturbances (including abdominal pain, dyspepsia, nausea, diarrhoea, constipation); dizziness, headache; influenza-like symptoms, musculoskeletal pain; *rarely* oesophageal stricture, oesophagitis, oesophageal ulcer, dysphagia, gastritis, duodenitis, glossitis, peripheral oedema, weight loss, myasthenia, arthralgia, apnoea, bronchitis, sinusitis, rash, nocturia, ambylopia, corneal lesion, dry eye, tinnitus, iritis; *very rarely* hypersensitivity reactions including angioedema, osteonecrosis (see notes above)

Dose

- Paget's disease of bone, 30 mg daily for 2 months; may be repeated if necessary after at least 2 months

- Treatment of postmenopausal osteoporosis to reduce risk of vertebral or hip fractures, 5 mg daily *or* 35 mg once weekly
- Prevention of osteoporosis (including corticosteroid-induced osteoporosis) in postmenopausal women, 5 mg daily
- CHILD not recommended

Counselling Swallow tablets whole with full glass of water; on rising, take on an empty stomach at least 30 minutes before first food or drink of the day or, if taking at any other time of the day, avoid food and drink for at least 2 hours before or after risedronate (particularly avoid calcium-containing products e.g. milk, also avoid iron and mineral supplements and antacids); stand or sit upright for at least 30 minutes; do not take tablets at bedtime or before rising

Actonel® (Procter & Gamble Pharm.) PoM
Tablets, f/c, risedronate sodium 5 mg (yellow), net price 28-tab pack = £19.10; 30 mg (white), 28-tab pack = £152.81. Counselling, administration, food and calcium (see above)

Actonel Once a Week® (Procter & Gamble Pharm.) PoM
Tablets, f/c, risedronate sodium 35 mg (orange), net price 4-tab pack = £20.30. Counselling, administration, food and calcium (see above)

SODIUM CLODRONATE

Indications see under Dose

Cautions monitor renal and hepatic function and white cell count; also monitor serum calcium and phosphate periodically; renal dysfunction reported in patients receiving concomitant NSAIDs; maintain adequate fluid intake during treatment; consider preventive dental treatment before initiating bisphosphonate (risk of osteonecrosis of the jaw, see notes above); renal impairment—avoid if severe (Appendix 3); **interactions:** Appendix 1 (bisphosphonates)

Contra-indications acute gastro-intestinal inflammatory conditions; pregnancy (Appendix 4); breast-feeding (Appendix 5)

Side-effects nausea, diarrhoea; skin reactions; bronchospasm; *very rarely* osteonecrosis (see notes above)

Dose

- Osteolytic lesions, hypercalcaemia and bone pain associated with skeletal metastases in patients with breast cancer or multiple myeloma, by mouth, 1.6 g daily in single or 2 divided doses increased if necessary to a max. of 3.2 g daily

  Counselling Avoid food for 1 hour before and after treatment, particularly calcium-containing products e.g. milk; also avoid iron and mineral supplements and antacids; maintain adequate fluid intake
- Hypercalcaemia of malignancy, by slow intravenous infusion, 300 mg daily for max. 7–10 days *or* by single-dose infusion of 1.5 g

Bonefos® (Schering Health) PoM
Capsules, yellow, sodium clodronate 400 mg, net price 120-cap pack = £161.97. Counselling, food and calcium

Tablets, f/c, scored, sodium clodronate 800 mg, net price 60-tab pack = £169.62. Counselling, food and calcium

Concentrate (= intravenous solution), sodium clodronate 60 mg/mL, for dilution and use as infusion. Net price 5-mL amp = £12.82

Loron® (Roche) PoM
Loron 520® tablets, f/c, scored, sodium clodronate 520 mg. Net price 60-tab pack = £161.99. Label: 10, patient information leaflet, counselling, food and calcium

Dose 2 tablets daily in single or two divided doses; may be increased to max. 4 tablets daily

TILUDRONIC ACID

Indications Paget's disease of bone

Cautions renal impairment (monitor renal function regularly, see under Contra-indications); correct disturbances of calcium metabolism (e.g. vitamin D deficiency, hypocalcaemia) before starting; avoid concomitant use of indometacin; consider preventive dental treatment before initiating bisphosphonate (risk of osteonecrosis of the jaw, see notes above); **interactions:** Appendix 1 (bisphosphonates)

Contra-indications renal impairment (avoid if creatinine clearance less than 30 mL/minute; Appendix 3), juvenile Paget's disease, pregnancy (Appendix 4) and breast-feeding (Appendix 5)

Side-effects stomach pain, nausea, diarrhoea; rarely asthenia, dizziness, headache and skin reactions; *very rarely* osteonecrosis (see notes above)

Dose

- 400 mg daily as a single dose for 12 weeks; may be repeated if necessary after 6 months

  Counselling Avoid food for 2 hours before and after treatment, particularly calcium-containing products e.g. milk; also avoid antacids

Skelid® (Sanofi-Synthelabo) PoM
Tablets, tiludronic acid (as tiludronate disodium) 200 mg. Net price 28-tab pack = £99.00. Counselling, food and calcium

ZOLEDRONIC ACID

Indications see under Preparations

Cautions monitor serum electrolytes, calcium, phosphate and magnesium; assess renal function before each dose; ensure adequate hydration; renal impairment (Appendix 3); severe hepatic impairment (Appendix 2); cardiac disease (avoid fluid overload); consider preventive dental treatment before initiating bisphosphonate (risk of osteonecrosis of the jaw, see notes above); **interactions:** Appendix 1 (bisphosphonates)

Contra-indications pregnancy (Appendix 4), breast-feeding (Appendix 5)

Side-effects hypophosphataemia, anaemia, influenza-like symptoms including bone pain, myalgia, arthralgia, fever and rigors; gastro-intestinal disturbances; headache, conjunctivitis, renal impairment (rarely acute renal failure); *less commonly* taste disturbance, dry mouth, stomatitis, chest pain, hypertension, hypotension, dyspnoea, cough, dizziness, paraesthesia, tremor, anxiety, sleep disturbance, blurred vision, weight gain, pruritus, rash, sweating, muscle cramps, haematuria, proteinuria, hypersensitivity reactions (including angioedema), asthenia, peripheral oedema, thrombocytopenia, leucopenia, hypomagnesaemia, hypokalaemia, also injection-site reactions; *rarely* bradycardia, confusion, hyperkalaemia, hypernatraemia, pancytopenia, osteonecrosis of the jaw (see also notes above); *very rarely* uveitis and episcleritis

Dose

- See under Preparations

Aclasta® (Novartis) ▼ PoM

Intravenous infusion, zoledronic acid 50 micrograms/mL, net price 100-mL bottle = £283.74

Dose Treatment of Paget's disease of bone, by intravenous infusion, 5 mg as a single dose over at least 15 minutes

Note Correct any hypocalcaemia before treatment; following infusion, at least 500 mg elemental calcium twice daily (with vitamin D) for at least 10 days is recommended

Treatment of postmenopausal osteoporosis, by intravenous infusion, 5 mg over at least 15 minutes once a year

Zometa® (Novartis) PoM

Concentrate for intravenous infusion, zoledronic acid, 800 micrograms/mL, net price 5-mL (4-mg) vial = £195.00

Dose Reduction of bone damage in advanced malignancies involving bone, by intravenous infusion, 4 mg every 3–4 weeks

Note Calcium 500 mg daily and vitamin D 400 units daily should also be taken

Hypercalcaemia of malignancy, by intravenous infusion, 4 mg as a single dose

CHILD not recommended

Strontium ranelate

Strontium ranelate stimulates bone formation and reduces bone resorption. It is licensed for the treatment of postmenopausal osteoporosis. The *Scottish Medicines Consortium* has advised (July 2005) that strontium ranelate should be restricted to use when bisphosphonates are contra-indicated or not tolerated and then only in women aged over 75 years with a previous fracture and low bone mineral density or in other women at equivalent risk.

STRONTIUM RANELATE

Indications treatment of postmenopausal osteoporosis to reduce risk of vertebral and hip fractures

Cautions predisposition to thromboembolism; interferes with colorimetric measurements of calcium in blood and urine; renal impairment (Appendix 3); **interactions**: Appendix 1 (strontium ranelate)

Contra-indications pregnancy, breast-feeding

Side-effects nausea, diarrhoea; venous thromboembolism; headache; dermatitis, eczema; *very rarely* vomiting, abdominal pain, stomatitis, and hypersensitivity reactions, including rash, pruritus, urticaria and angioedema—see Severe Allergic Reactions, below

> **Severe allergic reactions**
>
> Severe allergic reactions, including drug rash with eosinophilia and systemic symptoms (DRESS), have been reported in patients taking strontium ranelate. DRESS starts with rash, fever, swollen glands, and increased white cell count, and it can affect the liver, kidneys and lungs; DRESS can also be fatal.
>
> Patients should be advised to stop taking strontium ranelate and consult their doctor immediately if skin rash develops. Treatment with strontium ranelate should not be restarted.

Dose

- 2 g once daily in water, preferably at bedtime

Counselling Avoid food for 2 hours before and after taking granules, particularly calcium-containing products e.g. milk; also preferably avoid concomitant antacids containing aluminium and magnesium hydroxides for 2 hours after taking granules

Protelos® (Servier) ▼ PoM

Granules, yellow, strontium ranelate, 2 g/sachet, net price 28-sachets = £25.60. Label: 5, 13, counselling, food and calcium

Excipients include aspartame (section 9.4.1)

6.7 Other endocrine drugs

6.7.1 Bromocriptine and other dopaminergic drugs

6.7.2 Drugs affecting gonadotrophins

6.7.3 Metyrapone and trilostane

6.7.4 Somatomedins

6.7.1 Bromocriptine and other dopaminergic drugs

Bromocriptine is a stimulant of dopamine receptors in the brain; it also inhibits release of prolactin by the pituitary. Bromocriptine is used for the treatment of galactorrhoea, and for the treatment of prolactinomas (when it reduces both plasma prolactin concentration and tumour size). Bromocriptine also inhibits the release of growth hormone and is sometimes used in the treatment of acromegaly, but somatostatin analogues (such as octreotide, section 8.3.4.3) are more effective.

Cabergoline has actions and uses similar to those of bromocriptine, but its duration of action is longer. It has similar side-effects to bromocriptine, however patients intolerant of bromocriptine may be able to tolerate cabergoline (and *vice versa*).

Quinagolide is a non-ergot dopamine D_2 agonist; it has actions and uses similar to those of ergot-derived dopamine agonists, but its side-effects differ slightly.

Cautions see notes below; also bromocriptine and cabergoline should be used with caution in patients with a history of peptic ulcer, particularly in acromegalic patients. Treatment should be withdrawn if gastro-intestinal bleeding occurs. In hyperprolactinaemic patients, the source of the hyperprolactinaemia should be established (i.e. exclude pituitary tumour before treatment). Gynaecological assessment is recommended annually in premenopausal women (postmenopausal, 6 monthly), preferably including cervical and endometrial cytology. Bromocriptine and cabergoline should be used with caution in patients with Raynaud's syndrome and cardiovascular disease (see also Contra-indications under Bromocriptine, below). Monitor for fibrotic disease (see Fibrotic Reactions, below). Caution is also advised in patients with a history of serious mental disorders (especially psychotic disorders) and in those with porphyria (see section 9.8.2)

Contra-indications Bromocriptine and cabergoline should not be used in patients with a hypersensitivity to ergot alkaloids. They should also be avoided in pre-eclampsia (see also Contra-indications under Bromocriptine, below).

Side-effects Nausea, constipation, and headache are common side-effects of bromocriptine and cabergoline. Paraesthesia has been reported rarely. Other reported side-effects include hypotension (see also Hypotensive Reactions, below), dyskinesia, pathological gambling, increased libido, hypersexuality, leg cramps, allergic skin reactions, alopecia and peripheral oedema. Bromocriptine and cabergoline have been associated with pleuritis, pleural effusion, pericardial effusion, constrictive pericarditis, and retroperitoneal, pleural, and pulmonary fibrosis (see Fibrotic Reactions).

Hypotensive reactions Hypotensive reactions may be disturbing in some patients during the first few days of treatment with bromocriptine, cabergoline, or quinagolide—monitor blood pressure for a few days after starting treatment and following dosage increases; particular care should be exercised when driving or operating machinery; tolerance may be reduced by alcohol

> **Fibrotic reactions**
> The CSM has advised that ergot-derived dopamine-receptor agonists, bromocriptine, cabergoline, lisuride [discontinued], and pergolide have been associated with pulmonary, retroperitoneal, and pericardial fibrotic reactions.
> Before starting treatment with these ergot derivatives it may be appropriate to measure the erythrocyte sedimentation rate and serum creatinine and to obtain a chest X-ray. Patients should be monitored for dyspnoea, persistent cough, chest pain, cardiac failure, and abdominal pain or tenderness. If long-term treatment is expected, then lung-function tests may also be helpful.

> **Sudden onset of sleep**
> Excessive daytime sleepiness and sudden onset of sleep can occur with dopaminergic drugs.
> Patients starting treatment with these drugs should be warned of the possibility of these effects and of the need to exercise caution when driving or operating machinery.
> Patients who have suffered excessive sedation or sudden onset of sleep, should refrain from driving or operating machines, until those effects have stopped recurring.

Suppression of lactation Although bromocriptine and cabergoline are licensed to suppress lactation, they are **not** recommended for routine suppression (or for the relief of symptoms of postpartum pain and engorgement) that can be adequately treated with simple analgesics and breast support. If a dopamine-receptor agonist is required, cabergoline is preferred. Quinagolide is not licensed for the suppression of lactation.

BROMOCRIPTINE

Indications see notes above and under Dose; parkinsonism (section 4.9.1)

Cautions see notes above; also specialist evaluation—monitor for pituitary enlargement, particularly during pregnancy; monitor visual field to detect secondary field loss in macroprolactinoma; contraceptive advice if appropriate (oral contraceptives may increase prolactin concentration); avoid breast-feeding for about 5 days if lactation prevention fails; hepatic impairment (Appendix 2); **interactions**: Appendix 1 (bromocriptine)

Contra-indications see notes above; also hypertension in postpartum women or in puerperium (see also below)

Postpartum or puerperium Should not be used postpartum or in puerperium in women with high blood pressure, coronary artery disease or symptoms (or history) of serious mental disorder; monitor blood pressure carefully (especially during first few days) in postpartum women. Very rarely hypertension, myocardial infarction, seizures or stroke (both sometimes preceded by severe headache or visual disturbances) and mental disorders have been reported in postpartum women given bromocriptine for lactation suppression—caution with antihypertensive therapy and avoid other ergot alkaloids. Discontinue immediately if hypertension, unremitting headache or signs of CNS toxicity develop

Side-effects see notes above; also drowsiness (see also Sudden Onset of Sleep, above), nasal congestion; *less commonly* vomiting, postural hypotension, fatigue, dizziness, dry mouth; also, particularly with *high doses*, confusion, psychomotor excitation, hallucinations; *rarely* diarrhoea, gastro-intestinal bleeding, gastric ulcer, abdominal pain, tachycardia, bradycardia, arrhythmia, insomnia, psychosis, visual disturbances, tinnitus; *very rarely* vasospasm of fingers and toes particularly in patients with Raynaud's syndrome, and effects like neuroleptic malignant syndrome on withdrawal; urinary incontinence, leucopenia, thrombocytopenia, hyponatraemia, reversible hearing loss, pathological gambling, increased libido, and hypersexuality also reported

Dose

- Prevention or suppression of lactation (but see notes above and under Cautions), 2.5 mg on day 1 (prevention) or daily for 2–3 days (suppression); then 2.5 mg twice daily for 14 days
- Hypogonadism, galactorrhoea, infertility, initially 1–1.25 mg at bedtime, increased gradually; usual dose 7.5 mg daily in divided doses, increased if necessary to max. 30 mg daily, usual dose in infertility without hyperprolactinaemia, 2.5 mg twice daily
- Acromegaly initially 1–1.25 mg at bedtime, increase gradually to 5 mg every 6 hours
- Prolactinoma, initially 1–1.25 mg at bedtime; increased gradually to 5 mg every 6 hours (occasional patients may require up to 30 mg daily)
- CHILD under 15 years, not recommended

Bromocriptine (Non-proprietary) PoM
Tablets, bromocriptine (as mesilate) 2.5 mg, net price 30-tab pack = £10.57. Label: 21, counselling, hypotensive reactions, driving, see notes above

Parlodel® (Meda) PoM
Tablets, both scored, bromocriptine (as mesilate) 1 mg, net price 100-tab pack = £9.90; 2.5 mg, 30-tab pack = £5.78. Label: 21, counselling, hypotensive reactions, driving, see notes above
Capsules, bromocriptine (as mesilate) 5 mg (blue/white), net price 100-cap pack = £37.57; 10 mg (white), 100-cap pack = £69.50. Label: 21, counselling, hypotensive reactions, driving, see notes above

CABERGOLINE

Indications see notes above and under Dose

Cautions see notes above; also severe hepatic impairment (Appendix 2); monthly pregnancy tests during the amenorrhoeic period; advise non-hormonal contraception if pregnancy not desired (see also

6 Endocrine system

Contra-indications, below); **interactions**: Appendix 1 (cabergoline)

Contra-indications see notes above; history of puerperal psychosis; exclude pregnancy before starting and discontinue 1 month before intended conception (ovulatory cycles persist for 6 months)—discontinue if pregnancy occurs during treatment (specialist advice needed; Appendix 4); avoid breast-feeding if lactation prevention fails (Appendix 5); history of pulmonary, pericardial, or retroperitoneal fibrotic disorders (see Fibrotic Reactions in notes above); cardiac valvulopathy

Side-effects see notes above; also drowsiness (see also Sudden Onset of Sleep, above), dyspepsia, gastritis, epigastric and abdominal pain, angina, syncope, depression, confusion, hallucinations, breast pain; *rarely* vomiting, palpitation, epistaxis, digital vasospasm, hot flushes, transient hemianopia, muscle weakness; *also reported* cardiac valvulopathy, erythromelalgia

Dose

- Prevention of lactation (but see notes above and under Contra-indications), during first day postpartum, 1 mg as a single dose; suppression of established lactation (but see notes above) 250 micrograms every 12 hours for 2 days
- Hyperprolactinaemic disorders, 500 micrograms weekly (as a single dose *or* as 2 divided doses on separate days) increased at monthly intervals in steps of 500 micrograms until optimal therapeutic response (usually 1 mg weekly, range 0.25–2 mg weekly) with monthly monitoring of serum prolactin levels; reduce initial dose and increase more gradually if patient intolerant; over 1 mg weekly give as divided doses; up to 4.5 mg weekly has been used in hyperprolactinaemic patients
- Parkinsonism, section 4.9.1
- CHILD under 16 years, not recommended

Cabergoline (Non-proprietary) PoM

Tablet, scored, cabergoline 500 micrograms, net price 8-tab pack = £28.88. Label: 21, counselling, hypotensive reactions, driving, see notes above

Note Dispense in original container (contains dessicant)

Dostinex® (Pharmacia) PoM

Tablets, scored, cabergoline 500 micrograms. Net price 8-tab pack = £30.04. Label: 21, counselling, hypotensive reactions, driving, see notes above

Note Dispense in original container (contains dessicant)

QUINAGOLIDE

Indications see notes above and under Dose

Cautions see notes above; history of psychotic illness; advise non-hormonal contraception if pregnancy not desired; discontinue if pregnancy occurs during treatment (specialist advice needed; Appendix 4); **interactions**: Appendix 1 (quinagolide)

Contra-indications hypersensitivity to quinagolide (but not ergot alkaloids); hepatic impairment (Appendix 2); renal impairment (Appendix 3); breast-feeding (Appendix 5)

Side-effects nausea, vomiting, anorexia, abdominal pain, constipation or diarrhoea; syncope, hypotension (see also notes above), oedema, flushing; nasal congestion; headache, dizziness, fatigue, insomnia; *rarely* sudden onset of sleep (see notes above); *very rarely* psychosis

Dose

- Hyperprolactinaemia, 25 micrograms at bedtime for 3 days; increased at intervals of 3 days in steps of 25 micrograms to usual maintenance dose of 75–150 micrograms daily; for doses higher than 300 micrograms daily increase in steps of 75–150 micrograms at intervals of not less than 4 weeks; CHILD not recommended

Norprolac® (Ferring) PoM

Tablets, quinagolide (as hydrochloride) 75 micrograms (white), net price 30-tab pack = £30.00; starter pack of 3 × 25-microgram tabs (pink) with 3 × 50-microgram tabs (blue) = £5.00. Label: 21, counselling, hypotensive reactions

6.7.2 Drugs affecting gonadotrophins

Danazol inhibits pituitary gonadotrophins; it combines androgenic activity with antioestrogenic and antiprogestogenic activity. It is licensed for the treatment of *endometriosis* and for the relief of severe pain and tenderness in *benign fibrocystic breast disease* where other measures have proved unsatisfactory. It may also be effective in the long-term management of *hereditary angioedema* [unlicensed indication].

Gestrinone has general actions similar to those of danazol and is indicated for the treatment of endometriosis.

Cetrorelix and **ganirelix** are luteinising hormone releasing hormone antagonists, which inhibit the release of gonadotrophins (luteinising hormone and follicle-stimulating hormone). They are used in the treatment of infertility by assisted reproductive techniques.

CETRORELIX

Indications adjunct in the treatment of female infertility (under specialist supervision)

Contra-indications pregnancy, breast-feeding (Appendix 5), moderate renal impairment (Appendix 3), moderate hepatic impairment (Appendix 2)

Side-effects nausea, headache, injection site reactions; rarely hypersensitivity reactions

Dose

- By subcutaneous injection into the lower abdominal wall,

  either 250 micrograms in the morning, starting on day 5 or 6 of ovarian stimulation with gonadotrophins (*or* each evening starting on day 5 of ovarian stimulation); continue throughout administration of gonadotrophin including day of ovulation induction (*or* evening before ovulation induction)

  or 3 mg on day 7 of ovarian stimulation with gonadotrophins; if ovulation induction not possible on day 5 after 3-mg dose, additional 250 micrograms once daily until day of ovulation induction

Cetrotide® (Serono) PoM

Injection, powder for reconstitution, cetrorelix (as acetate), net price 250-micrograms vial = £24.00; 3-mg vial = £168.00 (both with solvent)

DANAZOL

Indications see notes above and under Dose

Cautions cardiac, hepatic, or renal impairment (avoid if severe), elderly, polycythaemia, epilepsy, diabetes mellitus, hypertension, migraine, lipoprotein disorder, history of thrombosis or thromboembolic disease; withdraw if virilisation (may be irreversible on continued use); non-hormonal contraceptive methods should be used, if appropriate; **interactions:** Appendix 1 (danazol)

Contra-indications pregnancy (Appendix 4), ensure that patients with amenorrhoea are not pregnant; breast-feeding (Appendix 5); severe hepatic, renal or cardiac impairment; thromboembolic disease; undiagnosed genital bleeding; androgen-dependent tumours; porphyria (section 9.8.2)

Side-effects nausea, dizziness, skin reactions including rashes, photosensitivity and exfoliative dermatitis, fever, backache, nervousness, mood changes, anxiety, changes in libido, vertigo, fatigue, epigastric and pleuritic pain, headache, weight gain; menstrual disturbances, vaginal dryness and irritation, flushing and reduction in breast size; musculo-skeletal spasm, joint pain and swelling, hair loss; androgenic effects including acne, oily skin, oedema, hirsutism, voice changes and rarely clitoral hypertrophy (see also Cautions); temporary alteration in lipoproteins and other metabolic changes, insulin resistance; thrombotic events; leucopenia, thrombocytopenia, eosinophilia, reversible erythrocytosis or polycythaemia reported; headache and visual disturbances may indicate benign intracranial hypertension; rarely cholestatic jaundice, pancreatitis, peliosis hepatis and benign hepatic adenomata

Dose

Note In women of child-bearing potential, treatment should start during menstruation, preferably on day 1

- Endometriosis, 200–800 mg daily in up to 4 divided doses, adjusted to achieve amenorrhoea, usually for 3–6 months
- Severe pain and tenderness in benign fibrocystic breast disease not responding to other treatment, 300 mg daily in divided doses usually for 3–6 months
- Hereditary angioedema [unlicensed indication], initially 200 mg 2–3 times daily, then reduced according to response

Danazol (Non-proprietary) PoM
Capsules, danazol 100 mg, net price 28-cap pack = £19.02, 60-cap pack = £17.04; 200 mg, 56-cap pack = £64.18

Danol® (Sanofi-Synthelabo) PoM
Capsules, danazol 100 mg (grey/white), net price 60-cap pack = £17.04; 200 mg (pink/white), 60-cap pack = £33.75

GANIRELIX

Indications adjunct in the treatment of female infertility (under specialist supervision)

Contra-indications pregnancy (Appendix 4), breast-feeding (Appendix 5); renal impairment (avoid if creatinine clearance less than 20 mL/minute; Appendix 3); moderate hepatic impairment (Appendix 2)

Side-effects nausea, headache, malaise, injection site reactions; *very rarely* hypersensitivity reactions including rash, facial oedema, and dyspnoea also reported

Dose

- By subcutaneous injection preferably into the upper leg (rotate injection sites to prevent lipoatrophy), 250 micrograms in the morning (or each afternoon) starting on day 6 of ovarian stimulation with gonadotrophins; continue throughout administration of gonadotrophins including day of ovulation induction (if administering in afternoon, give last dose in afternoon *before* ovulation induction)

Orgalutran® (Organon) PoM
Injection, ganirelix, 500 micrograms/mL, net price 0.5-mL prefilled syringe = £22.32

GESTRINONE

Indications endometriosis

Cautions cardiac dysfunction; renal impairment (avoid if creatinine clearance less than 20 mL/minute); **interactions:** Appendix 1 (gestrinone)

Contra-indications pregnancy (use non-hormonal method of contraception); breast-feeding (Appendix 5); severe cardiac or hepatic impairment; metabolic or vascular disorders associated with previous sex hormone treatment

Side-effects spotting; acne, oily skin, fluid retention, weight gain, hirsutism, voice change; liver enzyme disturbances; headache; gastro-intestinal disturbances; change in libido, flushing, decrease in breast size; nervousness, depression, change in appetite; muscle cramp

Dose

- 2.5 mg twice weekly starting on first day of cycle with second dose 3 days later, repeated on same two days preferably at same time each week; duration of treatment usually 6 months

Missed doses One missed dose—2.5 mg as soon as possible and maintain original sequence; two or more missed doses—discontinue, re-start on first day of new cycle (following negative pregnancy test)

Dimetriose® (Sanofi-Aventis) PoM
Capsules, gestrinone 2.5 mg, net price 8-cap pack = £103.91

Gonadorelin analogues

Administration of **gonadorelin analogues** produces an initial phase of stimulation; continued administration is followed by down-regulation of gonadotrophin-releasing hormone receptors, thereby reducing the release of gonadotrophins (follicle stimulating hormone and luteinising hormone) which in turn leads to inhibition of androgen and oestrogen production.

Gonadorelin analogues are used in the treatment of endometriosis, precocious puberty, infertility, anaemia due to uterine fibroids (together with iron supplementation), breast cancer (section 8.3.4.1), prostate cancer (section 8.3.4.2) and before intra-uterine surgery. Use of leuprorelin and triptorelin for 3 to 4 months before surgery reduces the uterine volume, fibroid size and associated bleeding. For women undergoing hysterectomy or myomectomy, a vaginal procedure is made more feasible following the use of a gonadorelin analogue.

Cautions Non-hormonal, barrier methods of contraception should be used during entire treatment period with gonadorelin analogues; also use with caution in patients with metabolic bone disease because decrease in bone mineral density can occur.

Contra-indications Gonadorelin analogues are contra-indicated for use longer than 6 months (do not repeat), where there is undiagnosed vaginal bleeding, in pregnancy (Appendix 4; exclude pregnancy—also give first injection during menstruation or shortly afterwards *or* use barrier contraception for 1 month beforehand) and in breast-feeding.

Side-effects Side-effects of the gonadorelin analogues related to the inhibition of oestrogen production include menopausal-like symptoms (e.g. hot flushes, increased sweating, vaginal dryness, dyspareunia and loss of libido) and a decrease in trabecular bone density; these effects can be reduced by hormone replacement (e.g. with an oestrogen and a progestogen or with tibolone). Side-effects of gonadorelin analogues also include headache (rarely migraine) and hypersensitivity reactions including urticaria, pruritus, rash, asthma and anaphylaxis; when treating uterine fibroids, bleeding associated with fibroid degeneration can occur; spray formulations can cause irritation of the nasal mucosa including nose bleeds; local reactions at injection site can occur; other side-effects also reported with some gonadorelin analogues include palpitation, hypertension, ovarian cysts (may require withdrawal), changes in breast size, musculoskeletal pain or weakness, visual disturbances, paraesthesia, changes in scalp and body hair, oedema of the face and extremities, weight changes, and mood changes including depression.

BUSERELIN

Indications see under Dose; prostate cancer (section 8.3.4.2)

Cautions see notes above; polycystic ovarian disease, depression, hypertension, diabetes

Contra-indications see notes above; hormone-dependent tumours

Side-effects see notes above; initially withdrawal bleeding and subsequently breakthrough bleeding, leucorrhoea; nausea, vomiting, constipation, diarrhoea; anxiety, memory and concentration disturbances, sleep disturbances, nervousness, dizziness, drowsiness; breast tenderness, lactation; abdominal pain; fatigue; increased thirst, changes in appetite; acne, dry skin, splitting nails, dry eyes; altered blood lipids, leucopenia, thrombocytopenia; hearing disturbances; reduced glucose tolerance

Dose

- Endometriosis, intranasally, 300 micrograms (one 150-microgram spray in each nostril) 3 times daily (starting on days 1 or 2 of menstruation); max. duration of treatment 6 months (do not repeat)
- Pituitary desensitisation before induction of ovulation by gonadotrophins for *in vitro* fertilisation (under specialist supervision), by subcutaneous injection, 200–500 micrograms daily given as a single injection (occasionally up to 500 micrograms twice daily may be needed) starting in early follicular phase (day 1) *or*, after exclusion of pregnancy, in midluteal phase (day 21) and continued until down-regulation achieved (usually about 1–3 weeks) then maintained during gonadotrophin administration (stopping gonadotrophin and buserelin on administration of chorionic gonadotrophin at appropriate stage of follicular development)

  Intranasally, 150 micrograms (one spray in one nostril) 4 times daily during waking hours (occasionally up to 300 micrograms 4 times daily may be needed) starting in early follicular phase (day 1) *or*, after exclusion of pregnancy, in midluteal phase (day 21) and continued until down-regulation achieved (usually about 2–3 weeks) then maintained during gonadotrophin administration (stopping gonadotrophin and buserelin on administration of chorionic gonadotrophin at appropriate stage of follicular development)

Counselling Avoid use of nasal decongestants before and for at least 30 minutes after treatment

Suprecur® (Aventis Pharma) PoM

Nasal spray, buserelin (as acetate) 150 micrograms/metered spray. Net price 2 × 100-dose pack (with metered dose pumps) = £91.19. Counselling, nasal decongestants

Injection, buserelin (as acetate) 1mg/mL. Net price 5.5-mL vial = £28.64

GOSERELIN

Indications see under Dose; prostate cancer (section 8.3.4.2); early and advanced breast cancer (section 8.3.4.1)

Cautions see notes above; polycystic ovarian disease

Contra-indications see notes above

Side-effects see notes above; withdrawal bleeding

Dose

- By subcutaneous injection into anterior abdominal wall

  Endometriosis, 3.6 mg every 28 days; max. duration of treatment 6 months (do not repeat)

  Endometrial thinning before intra-uterine surgery, 3.6 mg (may be repeated after 28 days if uterus is large or to allow flexible surgical timing)

  Before surgery in women who have anaemia due to uterine fibroids, 3.6 mg every 28 days (with supplementary iron); max. duration of treatment 3 months

  Pituitary desensitisation before induction of ovulation by gonadotrophins for *in vitro* fertilisation (under specialist supervision), after exclusion of pregnancy, 3.6 mg to achieve pituitary down-regulation (usually 1–3 weeks) then gonadotrophin is administered (stopping gonadotrophin on administration of chorionic gonadotrophin at appropriate stage of follicular development)

Preparation

Section 8.3.4.2

LEUPRORELIN ACETATE

Indications see under Dose; prostate cancer (section 8.3.4.2)

Cautions see notes above; family history of osteoporosis; chronic use of other drugs which reduce bone density including alcohol and tobacco; diabetes

Contra-indications see notes above

Side-effects see notes above; breast tenderness; nausea, vomiting, diarrhoea, anorexia; fever, chills; sleep disturbances, dizziness, fatigue, leucopenia, thrombocytopenia, altered blood lipids, pulmonary embolism; spinal fracture, paralysis, hypotension and worsening of depression also reported

Dose

- By subcutaneous *or* intramuscular injection (as *Prostap® SR*)
  Endometriosis, 3.75 mg as a single dose in first 5 days of menstrual cycle then every month for max. 6 months (course not to be repeated)
  Endometrial thinning before intra-uterine surgery, 3.75 mg as a single dose (given between days 3 and 5 of menstrual cycle) 5–6 weeks before surgery
  Reduction of size of uterine fibroids and of associated bleeding before surgery, 3.75 mg as a single dose every month usually for 3–4 months (max. 6 months)
- By intramuscular injection (as *Prostap® 3*)
  Endometriosis, 11.25 mg as a single dose in first 5 days of menstrual cycle then every 3 months for max. 6 months (course not to be repeated)

Preparations
Section 8.3.4.2

NAFARELIN

Indications see under Dose
Cautions see notes above
Contra-indications see notes above
Side-effects see notes above; acne
Dose

- Endometriosis, women over 18 years, 200 micrograms twice daily as one spray in one nostril in the morning and one spray in the other nostril in the evening (starting on days 2–4 of menstruation), max. duration of treatment 6 months (do not repeat)
- Pituitary desensitisation before induction of ovulation by gonadotrophins for *in vitro* fertilisation (under specialist supervision), 400 micrograms (one spray in each nostril) twice daily starting in early follicular phase (day 2) or, after exclusion of pregnancy, in midluteal phase (day 21) and continued until down-regulation achieved (usually within 4 weeks) then maintained (usually for 8–12 days) during gonadotrophin administration (stopping gonadotrophin and nafarelin on administration of chorionic gonadotrophin at follicular maturity); discontinue if down-regulation not achieved within 12 weeks

Counselling Avoid use of nasal decongestants before and for at least 30 minutes after treatment; repeat dose if sneezing occurs during or immediately after administration

Synarel® (Pharmacia) PoM
Nasal spray, nafarelin (as acetate) 200 micrograms/metered spray. Net price 30-dose unit = £32.28; 60-dose unit = £55.66. Label: 10, patient information leaflet, counselling, see above

TRIPTORELIN

Indications endometriosis, precocious puberty, reduction in size of uterine fibroids; advanced prostate cancer (section 8.3.4.2)
Cautions see notes above
Contra-indications see notes above
Side-effects see notes above; asthenia
Dose

- See under preparations below

Decapeptyl® SR (Ipsen) PoM
Injection, (powder for suspension), m/r, triptorelin (as acetate), net price 4.2-mg vial (with diluent) = £69.00

Dose by intramuscular injection, endometriosis and reduction in size of uterine fibroids, 3 mg every 4 weeks starting during first 5 days of menstrual cycle; for uterine fibroids continue treatment for at least 3 months; max. duration of treatment 6 months (not to be repeated)

Note Each 4.2-mg vial includes an overage to allow administration of 3-mg dose

Injection, (powder for suspension), m/r, triptorelin (as acetate), net price 15-mg vial (with diluent) = £207.00

Dose by intramuscular injection, endometriosis, 11.25 mg every 3 months starting during first 5 days of menstrual cycle; max. duration of treatment 6 months (not to be repeated)
Precocious puberty (girls under 8 years, boys under 9 years), 11.25 mg every 3 months; discontinue when bone maturation consistent with age over 12 years in girls or over 13–14 years in boys

Note Each 15-mg vial includes an overage to allow administration of 11.25-mg dose

Gonapeptyl Depot® (Ferring) PoM
Injection, (powder for suspension), triptorelin (as acetate), net price 3.75-mg prefilled syringe (with prefilled syringe of vehicle) = £85.00

Dose by subcutaneous *or* deep intramuscular injection, endometriosis and reduction in size of uterine fibroids, 3.75 mg every 4 weeks starting during first 5 days of menstrual cycle; for uterine fibroids continue treatment for 3–4 months; max. duration of treatment 6 months (not to be repeated)
Precocious puberty (girls under 9 years, boys under 10 years), body-weight over 30 kg, initially 3.75 mg every 2 weeks for 3 doses, then every 3–4 weeks; body-weight 20–30 kg, initially 2.5 mg every 2 weeks for 3 doses, then every 3–4 weeks; body-weight under 20 kg, initially 1.875 mg every 2 weeks for 3 doses, then every 3–4 weeks; discontinue when bone maturation consistent with age over 12 years in girls or over 13 years in boys

Breast pain (mastalgia)

Once any serious underlying cause for breast pain has been ruled out, most women will respond to reassurance and reduction in dietary fat; withdrawal of an oral contraceptive or of hormone replacement therapy may help to resolve the pain.

Mild, non-cyclical breast pain is treated with simple analgesics (section 4.7.1); moderate to severe pain, cyclical pain or symptoms that persist for longer than 6 months may require specific drug treatment.

Danazol (section 6.7.2) is licensed for the relief of severe pain and tenderness in benign fibrocystic breast disease which has not responded to other treatment.

Tamoxifen (section 8.3.4.1) may be a useful adjunct in the treatment of mastalgia [unlicensed indication] especially when symptoms can definitely be related to cyclic oestrogen production; it may be given on the days of the cycle when symptoms are predicted.

Treatment for breast pain should be reviewed after 6 months and continued if necessary. Symptoms recur in about 50% of women within 2 years of withdrawal of therapy but may be less severe.

6.7.3 Metyrapone and trilostane

Metyrapone is a competitive inhibitor of 11β-hydroxylation in the adrenal cortex; the resulting inhibition of cortisol (and to a lesser extent aldosterone) production leads to an increase in ACTH production which, in turn, leads to increased synthesis and release of cortisol precursors. It may be used as a test of anterior pituitary function.

Although most types of *Cushing's syndrome* are treated surgically, that which occasionally accompanies carcinoma of the bronchus is not usually amenable to surgery. Metyrapone has been found helpful in controlling the symptoms of the disease; it is also used in other forms of Cushing's syndrome to prepare the patient for surgery. The dosages used are either low, and tailored to cortisol production, or high, in which case corticosteroid replacement therapy is also needed.

Trilostane reversibly inhibits 3β-hydroxysteroid dehydrogenase / delta 5-4 isomerase in the adrenal cortex; the resulting inhibition of the synthesis of mineralocorticoids and glucocorticoids may be useful in *Cushing's syndrome* and *primary hyperaldosteronism*. Trilostane appears to be less effective than metyrapone for Cushing's syndrome (where it is tailored to corticosteroid production). It also has a minor role in postmenopausal breast cancer that has relapsed following initial oestrogen antagonist therapy (corticosteroid replacement therapy is also required). **Ketoconazole** (section 5.2) is also used by specialists for the management of *Cushing's syndrome* [unlicensed indication].

METYRAPONE

Indications see notes above and under Dose (specialist supervision in hospital)

Cautions gross hypopituitarism (risk of precipitating acute adrenal failure); hypertension on long-term administration; hypothyroidism or hepatic impairment (delayed response); many drugs interfere with diagnostic estimation of steroids; avoid in porphyria (section 9.8.2)

Driving Drowsiness may affect the performance of skilled tasks (e.g. driving)

Contra-indications adrenocortical insufficiency (see Cautions); pregnancy (Appendix 4), breast-feeding (Appendix 5)

Side-effects occasional nausea, vomiting, dizziness, headache, hypotension, sedation; rarely abdominal pain, allergic skin reactions, hypoadrenalism, hirsutism

Dose

- Differential diagnosis of ACTH-dependent Cushing's syndrome, 750 mg every 4 hours for 6 doses; CHILD 15 mg/kg (minimum 250 mg) every 4 hours for 6 doses
- Management of Cushing's syndrome, range 0.25–6 g daily, tailored to cortisol production; see notes above
- Resistant oedema due to increased aldosterone secretion in cirrhosis, nephrotic syndrome, and congestive heart failure (with glucocorticoid replacement therapy) 3 g daily in divided doses

Metopirone® (Alliance) PoM

Capsules, ivory, metyrapone 250 mg. Net price 100-tab pack = £41.44. Label: 21, counselling, driving

TRILOSTANE

Indications see notes above and under Dose (specialist supervision)

Cautions breast cancer (concurrent corticosteroid replacement therapy needed, see under Dose), adrenal cortical hyperfunction (tailored to cortisol and electrolytes, concurrent corticosteroid therapy may be needed, see under Dose); hepatic and renal impairment; **interactions:** Appendix 1 (trilostane)

Contra-indications pregnancy (use non-hormonal method of contraception; Appendix 4); breast-feeding; children

Side-effects flushing, tingling and swelling of mouth, rhinorrhoea, nausea, vomiting, diarrhoea, and rashes reported; rarely granulocytopenia

Dose

- Adrenal cortical hyperfunction, 240 mg daily in divided doses for at least 3 days then tailored according to response with regular monitoring of plasma electrolytes and circulating corticosteroids (both mineralocorticoid and glucocorticoid replacement therapy may be needed); usual dose: 120–480 mg daily (may be increased to 960 mg)
- Postmenopausal breast cancer (with glucocorticoid replacement therapy) following relapse to initial oestrogen receptor antagonist therapy, initially 240 mg daily increased every 3 days in steps of 240 mg to a maintenance dose of 960 mg daily (720 mg daily if not tolerated)

Modrenal® (Bioenvision) PoM

Capsules, trilostane 60 mg (pink/black), net price 100-cap pack = £49.50; 120 mg (pink/yellow), 100-cap pack = £98.50. Label: 21

6.7.4 Somatomedins

Somatomedins are a group of polypeptide hormones structurally related to insulin and commonly known as insulin-like growth factors (IGFs). **Mecasermin**, a human insulin-like growth factor-I (rhIGF-I), is the principal mediator of the somatotropic effects of human growth hormone and is used to treat growth failure in children and adolescents with severe primary insulin-like growth factor-I deficiency.

MECASERMIN

(Recombinant human insulin-like growth factor-I; rhIGF-I)

Indications see notes above

Cautions correct hypothyroidism before initiating treatment; diabetes mellitus (adjustment of antidiabetic therapy may be necessary), monitor ECG before and on termination of treatment (and during treatment if ECG abnormal), papilloedema (see under Side-effects), monitor for disorders of the epiphysis of the hip (monitor for limping), monitor for signs of tonsillar hypertrophy (snoring, sleep apnoea, and chronic middle ear effusions); pregnancy (Appendix 4)

Contra-indications evidence of tumour activity (discontinue treatment), breast-feeding

Side-effects headache, funduscopy for papilloedema recommended if severe or recurrent headache, visual problems, nausea and vomiting occur—if papilloedema confirmed consider benign intracranial hypertension (rare cases reported); cardiomegaly, ventricular hypertrophy, tachycardia; convulsions, sleep apnoea, night terrors, dizziness, nervousness; tonsillar hypertrophy (see Cautions above); hypoglycaemia (especially in first month, and in younger children),

6 Endocrine system

hyperglycaemia, gynaecomastia; arthralgia, myalgia; visual disturbance, impaired hearing; antibody formation; injection-site reactions (rotate site)

Dose

- By subcutaneous injection, ADOLESCENT and CHILD over 2 years, initially 40 micrograms/kg twice daily for 1 week, if tolerated increase dose in steps of 40 micrograms/kg to max. 120 micrograms/kg twice daily; discontinue if no response within 1 year

Counselling Dose should be administered just before or after food; do not increase dose if a dose is missed

Note Reduce dose if hypoglycaemia occurs despite adequate food intake; withhold injection if patient unable to eat

Increlex® (Ipsen) ▼ PoM

Injection, mecasermin 10 mg/mL, net price 4-mL vial = £384.00. Counselling, administration

Excipients include benzyl alcohol (avoid in neonates, see Excipients, p. 2)

7 Obstetrics, gynaecology, and urinary-tract disorders

7.1 Drugs used in obstetrics **418**
7.1.1 Prostaglandins and oxytocics 418
7.1.1.1 Ductus arteriosus 421
7.1.2 Mifepristone 422
7.1.3 Myometrial relaxants 423
7.2 Treatment of vaginal and vulval conditions **424**
7.2.1 Preparations for vaginal atrophy 424
7.2.2 Vaginal and vulval infections 425
7.3 Contraceptives **427**
7.3.1 Combined hormonal contraceptives 427
7.3.2 Progestogen-only contraceptives 432
7.3.2.1 Oral progestogen-only contraceptives 432
7.3.2.2 Parenteral progestogen-only contraceptives 433
7.3.2.3 Intra-uterine progestogen-only device 434
7.3.3 Spermicidal contraceptives 435
7.3.4 Contraceptive devices 435
7.3.5 Emergency contraception 437
7.4 Drugs for genito-urinary disorders **438**
7.4.1 Drugs for urinary retention 438
7.4.2 Drugs for urinary frequency, enuresis, and incontinence 440
7.4.3 Drugs used in urological pain 443
7.4.4 Bladder instillations and urological surgery 443
7.4.5 Drugs for erectile dysfunction 444

This chapter also includes advice on the drug management of the following:
- emergency contraception, p. 437
- induction of abortion, below
- induction and augmentation of labour, below
- nocturnal enuresis, p. 442
- premature labour, p. 423
- prevention and treatment of post-partum haemorrhage, p. 419
- priapism, p. 445

For hormonal therapy of gynaecological disorders see section 6.4.1, section 6.5.1 and section 6.7.2.

7.1 Drugs used in obstetrics

7.1.1 Prostaglandins and oxytocics
7.1.2 Mifepristone
7.1.3 Myometrial relaxants

Because of the complexity of dosage regimens in obstetrics, in all cases **detailed specialist literature** should be consulted.

7.1.1 Prostaglandins and oxytocics

Prostaglandins and oxytocics are used to induce abortion or induce or augment labour and to minimise blood loss from the placental site. They include oxytocin, carbetocin, ergometrine, and the prostaglandins. All induce uterine contractions with varying degrees of pain according to the strength of contractions induced.

Induction of abortion **Gemeprost**, administered vaginally as pessaries is the preferred prostaglandin for the medical induction of late therapeutic abortion. Gemeprost ripens the cervix before surgical abortion, particularly in primigravidas. The prostaglandin **misoprostol** is given by mouth or by vaginal administration to induce medical abortion [unlicensed indication]; intravaginal use ripens the cervix before surgical abortion [unlicensed indication]. Extra-amniotic **dinoprostone** is rarely used nowadays.

Pre-treatment with **mifepristone** (section 7.1.2) can facilitate the process of medical abortion. It sensitises the uterus to subsequent administration of a prostaglandin and, therefore, abortion occurs in a shorter time and with a lower dose of prostaglandin.

Induction and augmentation of labour **Dinoprostone** is available as vaginal tablets, pessaries and vaginal gels for the induction of labour. The intravenous solution is rarely used; it is associated with more side-effects.

Oxytocin (*Syntocinon®*) is administered by slow intravenous infusion, using an infusion pump, to induce or augment labour, usually in conjunction with amniotomy. Uterine activity must be monitored carefully and hyperstimulation avoided. Large doses of oxytocin may result in excessive fluid retention.

Misoprostol is given orally or vaginally for the induction of labour [unlicensed indication].

> **NICE guidance**
> **Induction of labour (June 2001)**
> NICE has recommended that:
> - dinoprostone is preferable to oxytocin for induction of labour in women with intact membranes, regardless of parity or cervical favourability;
> - dinoprostone or oxytocin are equally effective for the induction of labour in women with ruptured membranes, regardless of parity or cervical favourability;
> - oxytocin should not be started for 6 hours following administration of vaginal prostaglandins;
> - when used to induce labour, the recommended dose of oxytocin by intravenous infusion[1] is initially 0.001–0.002 units/minute increased at intervals of at least 30 minutes until a maximum of 3–4 contractions occur every 10 minutes (0.012 units/minute is often adequate); the maximum recommended rate is 0.032 units/minute (licensed max. 0.02 units/minute)
>
> 1. Oxytocin should be used in standard dilutions of 10 units/500 mL (infusing 3 mL/hour delivers 0.001 unit/minute) or, for higher doses, 30 units/500 mL (infusing 1 mL/hour delivers 0.001 unit/minute).

Prevention and treatment of haemorrhage Bleeding due to incomplete abortion can be controlled with **ergometrine** and **oxytocin** (*Syntometrine*®) given intramuscularly, the dose is adjusted according to the patient's condition and blood loss. This is commonly used before surgical evacuation of the uterus, particularly when surgery is delayed. Oxytocin and ergometrine combined are more effective in early pregnancy than either drug alone.

Active management of the third stage of labour reduces the risk of postpartum haemorrhage; ergometrine 500 micrograms with oxytocin 5 units (*Syntometrine*® 1 mL) is given by intramuscular injection on delivery of the anterior shoulder or, at the latest, immediately after the baby is delivered. Alternatively, oxytocin may be given alone by intramuscular injection [unlicensed], particularly if ergometrine is inappropriate (e.g. in pre-eclampsia); oxytocin alone causes less nausea, vomiting, and hypertension than when given with ergometrine.

In excessive uterine bleeding, any placental products remaining in the uterus should be removed. Oxytocic drugs are used to treat postpartum haemorrhage caused by uterine atony as follows:

- oxytocin 5–10 units by intravenous injection, followed in severe cases by intravenous infusion of oxytocin 5–30 units in 500 mL infusion fluid at a rate that controls uterine atony
- ergometrine by intramuscular injection
- ergometrine 250–500 micrograms by intravenous injection (use with caution—risk of hypertension)
- ergometrine 500 micrograms with oxytocin 5 units (*Syntometrine*® 1 mL) by intramuscular injection

Carboprost has an important role in severe postpartum haemorrhage unresponsive to ergometrine and oxytocin.

Misoprostol [unlicensed] may be an alternative in postpartum haemorrhage unresponsive to ergometrine, oxytocin, and carboprost.

CARBETOCIN

Indications prevention of uterine atony and postpartum haemorrhage after caesarean section

Cautions hyponatraemia; monitor blood pressure for up to 8 hours in pre-eclampsia or eclampsia; cardiovascular disease, epilepsy, migraine, asthma

Contra-indications hepatic impairment, renal impairment

Side-effects nausea, vomiting, abdominal pain; flushing, hypotension; headache, tremor; pruritus; *rarely* metallic taste, tachycardia, chest pain, dyspnoea, dizziness, back pain, anaemia, sweating, and chills

Dose

- By intravenous injection, a single dose of 100 micrograms, as soon as possible after delivery, preferably before removal of placenta

Pabal® (Ferring) ▼ PoM
Injection, carbetocin 100 micrograms/mL, net price 1-mL amp = £18.00

CARBOPROST

Indications postpartum haemorrhage due to uterine atony in patients unresponsive to ergometrine and oxytocin

Cautions history of glaucoma or raised intra-ocular pressure, asthma, hypertension, hypotension, anaemia, jaundice, diabetes, epilepsy; uterine scars; excessive dosage may cause uterine rupture; **interactions**: Appendix 1 (prostaglandins)

Contra-indications untreated pelvic infection; cardiac, renal, pulmonary, or hepatic disease

Side-effects nausea, vomiting and diarrhoea, hyperthermia and flushing, bronchospasm; less frequent effects include raised blood pressure, dyspnoea, and pulmonary oedema; chills, headache, diaphoresis, dizziness; cardiovascular collapse also reported; erythema and pain at injection site reported

Dose

- By deep intramuscular injection, 250 micrograms repeated if necessary at intervals of 1½ hours (in severe cases the interval may be reduced but should not be less than 15 minutes); total dose should not exceed 2 mg (8 doses)

Hemabate® (Pharmacia) PoM
Injection, carboprost as trometamol salt (tromethamine salt) 250 micrograms/mL, net price 1-mL amp = £18.20 (hosp. only)

DINOPROSTONE

Indications see notes above and under preparations below

Cautions history of asthma, glaucoma and raised intra-ocular pressure; cardiac, hepatic or renal impairment; hypertension; history of epilepsy; uterine scarring; monitor uterine activity and fetal status (particular care if history of uterine hypertony); uterine rupture; see also notes above; monitor for disseminated intravascular coagulation after parturition; risk factors for disseminated intravascular coagulation; effect of oxytocin enhanced (care needed in monitoring uterine activity when used in sequence); **interactions**: Appendix 1 (prostaglandins)

Contra-indications active cardiac, pulmonary, renal or hepatic disease; placenta praevia or unexplained vaginal bleeding during pregnancy, ruptured membranes, major cephalopelvic disproportion or fetal malpresentation, history of caesarean section or major uterine surgery, untreated pelvic infection, fetal distress, grand multiparas and multiple pregnancy, history of difficult or traumatic delivery; avoid extra-amniotic route in cervicitis or vaginitis

Side-effects nausea, vomiting, diarrhoea; other side-effects include uterine hypertonus, severe uterine contractions, pulmonary or amniotic fluid embolism, abruptio placenta, fetal distress, maternal hypertension, bronchospasm, rapid cervical dilation, fever, backache; uterine hypercontractility with or without fetal bradycardia, low Apgar scores; cardiac arrest, uterine rupture, stillbirth or neonatal death also reported; vaginal symptoms (warmth, irritation, pain); after intravenous administration—flushing, shivering, headache, dizziness, temporary pyrexia and raised white blood cell count; disseminated intravascular coagulation reported; also local tissue reaction and erythema after intravenous administration and possibility of infection after extra-amniotic administration

Dose

- See under preparations, below

Important Do not confuse dose of *Prostin E2®* vaginal **gel** with that of *Prostin E2®* vaginal **tablets**—not bioequivalent.

Propess® (Ferring) PoM

Pessaries (within retrieval device), releasing dinoprostone approx. 10 mg over 24 hours; net price 1-pessary pack = £30.00

Dose by vagina, cervical ripening and induction of labour at term, 1 pessary (in retrieval device) inserted high into posterior fornix and removed when cervical ripening adequate; if oxytocin necessary, remove 30 minutes before oxytocin infusion; remove if cervical ripening inadequate after 24 hours (dose not to be repeated)

Prostin E2® (Pharmacia) PoM

Intravenous solution, for dilution and use as an infusion, dinoprostone 1 mg/mL, net price 0.75-mL amp = £8.52; 10 mg/mL, 0.5-mL amp = £18.40 (both hosp. only; rarely used, consult product literature for dose and indications)

Extra-amniotic solution, dinoprostone 10 mg/mL. Net price 0.5-mL amp (with diluent) = £18.40 (hosp. only; less commonly used nowadays, consult product literature for dose and indications)

Vaginal gel, dinoprostone 400 micrograms/mL, net price 2.5 mL (1 mg) = £13.28; 800 micrograms/mL, 2.5 mL (2 mg) = £13.28

Dose by vagina, induction of labour, inserted high into posterior fornix (avoid administration into cervical canal), 1 mg (unfavourable primigravida 2 mg), followed after 6 hours by 1–2 mg if required; max. [gel] 3 mg (unfavourable primigravida 4 mg)

Vaginal tablets, dinoprostone 3 mg. Net price 8-vaginal tab pack = £106.23

Dose by vagina, induction of labour, inserted high into posterior fornix, 3 mg, followed after 6–8 hours by 3 mg if labour is not established; max. 6 mg [vaginal tablets]

Note *Prostin E2 Vaginal Gel* and *Vaginal Tablets* are **not** bioequivalent

ERGOMETRINE MALEATE

Indications see notes above

Cautions cardiac disease, hypertension, multiple pregnancy; porphyria (section 9.8.2); hepatic impairment (avoid if severe; Appendix 2); renal impairment (avoid if severe; Appendix 3); **interactions:** Appendix 1 (ergot alkaloids)

Contra-indications induction of labour, first and second stages of labour, vascular disease, severe cardiac disease, sepsis, severe hypertension, eclampsia

Side-effects nausea, vomiting, headache, dizziness, tinnitus, abdominal pain, chest pain, palpitation, dyspnoea, bradycardia, transient hypertension, vasoconstriction; stroke, myocardial infarction and pulmonary oedema also reported

Dose

- See notes above

Ergometrine (Non-proprietary) PoM

Injection, ergometrine maleate 500 micrograms/mL. Net price 1-mL amp = 60p

With oxytocin

Syntometrine® (Alliance) PoM

Injection, ergometrine maleate 500 micrograms, oxytocin 5 units/mL. Net price 1-mL amp = £1.31

Dose by intramuscular injection, 1 mL; by intravenous injection, no longer recommended

GEMEPROST

Indications see under Dose

Cautions obstructive airways disease, cardiovascular insufficiency, raised intra-ocular pressure, cervicitis or vaginitis; **interactions:** Appendix 1 (prostaglandins)

Important For warnings relating to use of gemeprost in a patient undergoing induction of abortion with mifepristone, see under Mifepristone and Note below

Contra-indications unexplained vaginal bleeding, uterine scarring, placenta praevia

Side-effects vaginal bleeding and uterine pain; nausea, vomiting, or diarrhoea; headache, muscle weakness, dizziness, flushing, chills, backache, dyspnoea, chest pain, palpitation and mild pyrexia; uterine rupture reported (most commonly in multiparas or if history of uterine surgery or if given with intravenous oxytocics); also reported severe hypotension, coronary artery spasm and myocardial infarction

Dose

- By vagina, cervical ripening prior to first trimester surgical abortion, 1 mg inserted into posterior fornix 3 hours before surgery
- Second trimester abortion, 1 mg inserted into posterior fornix every 3 hours for max. of 5 administrations; second course may begin 24 hours after start of treatment (if treatment fails pregnancy should be terminated by another method)
- Second trimester intra-uterine death, 1 mg inserted into posterior fornix every 3 hours for max. of 5 administrations only; monitor for coagulopathy

Note If used in combination with mifepristone, carefully monitor blood pressure and pulse for 3 hours

Gemeprost (Beacon) PoM

Pessaries, gemeprost 1 mg. Net price 5-pessary pack = £215.00

OXYTOCIN

Indications see under Dose and notes above

Cautions induction or enhancement of labour—presence of borderline cephalopelvic disproportion (avoid if significant), secondary uterine inertia, mild or moderate pregnancy-induced hypertension or cardiac disease, women over 35 years or with history of lower-uterine segment caesarean section (see also under Contra-indications below); risk factors for disseminated intravascular coagulation; monitor for disseminated intravascular coagulation after parturition; avoid large infusion volumes and restrict fluid intake by mouth (risk of hyponatraemia and water-intoxication—see also Appendix 6); effects enhanced by concomitant prostaglandins (very careful monitoring of uterine activity); caudal block anaesthesia (may enhance hypertensive effects of sympathomimetic vasopressors); see also **interactions**: Appendix 1 (oxytocin)

Contra-indications hypertonic uterine contractions, fetal distress; any condition where spontaneous labour or vaginal delivery inadvisable; avoid prolonged administration in oxytocin-resistant uterine inertia, severe pre-eclamptic toxaemia, or severe cardiovascular disease

Side-effects nausea, vomiting; arrhythmia; headache; *rarely* disseminated intravascular coagulation, rash and anaphylactoid reactions (with dyspnoea, hypotension, or shock); uterine spasm (may occur at low doses), uterine hyperstimulation (usually with excessive doses—may cause fetal distress, asphyxia, and death, or may lead to hypertonicity, tetanic contractions, soft-tissue damage or uterine rupture); water intoxication and hyponatraemia associated with high doses with large infusion volumes of electrolyte-free fluid (see also under Dose below); placental abruption and amniotic fluid embolism also reported on overdose

Dose

- Induction of labour for medical reasons or stimulation of labour in hypotonic uterine inertia, by intravenous infusion, see NICE guidance above; max. 5 units in 1 day (may be repeated next day starting again at 0.001–0.002 units/minute)

  Important Careful monitoring of fetal heart rate and uterine motility essential for dose titration (**avoid** intravenous injection during labour); discontinue immediately in uterine hyperactivity or fetal distress
- Caesarean section, by slow intravenous injection immediately after delivery, 5 units
- Prevention of postpartum haemorrhage, after delivery of placenta, by slow intravenous injection, 5 units (if infusion used for induction or enhancement of labour, increase rate during third stage and for next few hours).

  Important Avoid rapid intravenous injection (may transiently reduce blood pressure)

  Note Can be given in a dose of 10 units by intramuscular injection [unlicensed route] instead of oxytocin with ergometrine (*Syntometrine*®), see notes above
- Treatment of postpartum haemorrhage, by slow intravenous injection, 5–10 units, followed in severe cases by intravenous infusion of 5–30 units in 500 mL infusion fluid at a rate sufficient to control uterine atony

  Important Avoid rapid intravenous injection (may transiently reduce blood pressure); prolonged administration, see warning below
- Incomplete, inevitable, or missed abortion, by slow intravenous injection, 5 units followed if necessary by intravenous infusion, 0.02–0.04 units/minute or faster

Important Prolonged intravenous administration at high doses with large volume of fluid (as possible in inevitable or missed abortion or postpartum haemorrhage) may cause water intoxication with hyponatraemia. To avoid: use electrolyte-containing diluent (i.e. not glucose), increase oxytocin concentration to reduce fluid, restrict fluid intake by mouth; monitor fluid and electrolytes.

Note Oxytocin doses in the BNF may differ from those in the product literature

Syntocinon® (Alliance) PoM

Injection, oxytocin, net price 5 units/mL, 1-mL amp = 89p; 10 units/mL, 1-mL amp = £1.01

With ergometrine

See *Syntometrine*®, p. 420

7.1.1.1 Ductus arteriosus

Maintenance of patency

Alprostadil (prostaglandin E_1) is used to maintain patency of the ductus arteriosus in neonates with congenital heart defects, prior to corrective surgery in centres where intensive care is immediately available. See *BNF for Children* (section 2.14) for further advice on maintaining the patency of the ductus arteriosus.

ALPROSTADIL

Indications congenital heart defects in neonates prior to corrective surgery; erectile dysfunction (section 7.4.5)

Cautions see notes above; history of haemorrhage, avoid in hyaline membrane disease, monitor arterial pressure; **interactions**: Appendix 1 (prostaglandins)

Side-effects apnoea (particularly in neonates under 2 kg), flushing, bradycardia, hypotension, tachycardia, cardiac arrest, oedema, diarrhoea, fever, convulsions, disseminated intravascular coagulation, hypokalaemia; cortical proliferation of long bones and weakening of the wall of the ductus arteriosus and of pulmonary artery may follow prolonged use; gastric-outlet obstruction reported

Dose

- By intravenous infusion, initially 10 nanograms/kg/minute, adjusted according to response in steps of 5–10 nanograms/kg/minute; max. 100 nanograms/kg/minute (but associated with increased side-effects)

  Note Alprostadil doses in BNF may differ from those in product literature

Prostin VR® (Pharmacia) PoM

Intravenous solution, alprostadil 500 micrograms/mL in alcohol. For dilution and use as an infusion. Net price 1-mL amp = £75.19 (hosp. only)

Closure of ductus arteriosus

Indometacin (indomethacin) is used to close a patent ductus arteriosus in premature babies, probably by inhibiting prostaglandin synthesis. See *BNF for Children* (section 2.14) for further advice on closure of the ductus arteriosus.

INDOMETACIN
(Indomethacin)

Indications patent ductus arteriosus in premature babies (under specialist supervision in neonatal intensive care unit); uncomplicated premature labour [unlicensed indication] (section 7.1.3); rheumatoid disease (section 10.1.1)

Cautions may mask symptoms of infection; may reduce urine output by 50% or more (monitor carefully—see also under Anuria or Oliguria, below) and precipitate renal impairment especially if extracellular volume depleted, heart failure, sepsis, or hepatic impairment, or if receiving nephrotoxic drugs; may induce hyponatraemia; monitor renal function and electrolytes; inhibition of platelet aggregation (monitor for bleeding); **interactions**: Appendix 1 (NSAIDs)

Anuria or oliguria If anuria or marked oliguria (urinary output less than 0.6 mL/kg/hour) at time of scheduled second or third dose, delay until renal function returns to normal

Contra-indications untreated infection, bleeding (especially with active intracranial haemorrhage or gastro-intestinal bleeding); thrombocytopenia, coagulation defects, necrotising enterocolitis, renal impairment

Side-effects haemorrhagic, renal, gastro-intestinal (including necrotising enterocolitis), metabolic, and coagulation disorders; pulmonary hypertension, intracranial bleeding, fluid retention, and exacerbation of infection

Dose

- By intravenous injection, over 20–30 minutes (using a suitable syringe driver), 3 doses at intervals of 12–24 hours (provided urine output remains adequate), NEONATE under 48 hours, 200 micrograms/kg then 100 micrograms/kg then 100 micrograms/kg; NEONATE 2–7 days, 200 micrograms/kg then 200 micrograms/kg then 200 micrograms/kg; NEONATE over 7 days, 200 micrograms/kg then 250 micrograms/kg then 250 micrograms/kg; solution prepared with 1–2 mL sodium chloride 0.9% or water for injections (not glucose and no preservatives)

  If ductus arteriosus reopens a second course of 3 injections may be given 48 hours after first course

Indocid PDA® (IDIS) PoM

Injection, powder for reconstitution, indometacin (as sodium trihydrate). Net price 3 × 1-mg vials = £43.50 (hosp. only)

7.1.2 Mifepristone

Mifepristone, an antiprogestogenic steroid, sensitises the myometrium to prostaglandin-induced contractions and ripens the cervix. For termination of pregnancy, a single dose of mifepristone is followed by vaginal administration of the prostaglandin gemeprost. Although mifepristone is licensed for use in a dose of 600 mg, for medical abortion, a dose of 200 mg is effective for gestation of up to 24 weeks. Guidelines of the Royal College of Obstetricians and Gynaecologists (September 2004) include the following [unlicensed] regimens for inducing medical abortion:

- For gestation up to 9 weeks, mifepristone 200 mg by mouth followed 1–3 days later by misoprostol 800 micrograms vaginally; in women at more than 7 weeks gestation (49–63 days), if the abortion has not occurred 4 hours after misoprostol, a further dose of misoprostol 400 micrograms may be given vaginally or by mouth
- For gestation between 9 and 13 weeks, mifepristone 200 mg by mouth followed 36–48 hours later by misoprostol 800 micrograms vaginally followed if necessary by a maximum of 4 further doses at 3-hourly intervals of misoprostol 400 micrograms vaginally or by mouth
- For gestation between 13 and 24 weeks, mifepristone 200 mg by mouth followed 36–48 hours later by misoprostol 800 micrograms vaginally then a maximum of 4 further doses at 3-hourly intervals of misoprostol 400 micrograms by mouth

MIFEPRISTONE

Indications see under dose

Cautions asthma (avoid if severe and uncontrolled); haemorrhagic disorders and anticoagulant therapy; prosthetic heart valve or history of endocarditis (see section 5.1 table 2); smokers aged over 35 years (increased risk of cardiovascular events); adrenal suppression (may require corticosteroid); not recommended in hepatic or renal impairment; breast-feeding (Appendix 5); avoid aspirin and NSAIDs for analgesia; **interactions**: Appendix 1 (mifepristone)

Important For warnings relating to use of gemeprost in a patient undergoing induction of abortion with mifepristone, see under Gemeprost

Contra-indications uncontrolled severe asthma; suspected ectopic pregnancy (use other specific means of termination); chronic adrenal failure, porphyria (section 9.8.2)

Side-effects nausea, vomiting, gastro-intestinal cramps; uterine contractions, vaginal bleeding (sometimes severe) may occur between administration of mifepristone and surgery (and rarely abortion may occur before surgery); *less commonly* hypersensitivity reactions including rash, urticaria, and facial oedema; *rarely* malaise, headache, fever, hot flushes, dizziness, chills

Dose

- Medical termination of intra-uterine pregnancy of up to 63 days gestation, by mouth, mifepristone 600 mg (200 mg may be effective) as a single dose under medical supervision, followed 36–48 hours later (unless abortion already complete) by gemeprost 1 mg by vagina and observed for at least 3 hours (or until bleeding or pain at acceptable level); follow-up visit 10–14 days later to verify complete expulsion (if treatment fails essential that pregnancy be terminated by another method)
- Cervical ripening before mechanical cervical dilatation for termination of pregnancy, 36–48 hours before procedure, by mouth, mifepristone 600 mg as a single dose under medical supervision
- Termination of pregnancy of 13–24 weeks gestation (in combination with gemeprost), by mouth, mifepristone 600 mg (200 mg may be effective) as a single dose under medical supervision followed 36–48 hours later by gemeprost 1 mg by vagina every 3 hours up to max. 5 mg; if abortion does not occur, 24 hours after start of treatment repeat course of gemeprost 1 mg by vagina up to max. 5 mg (if treatment fails pregnancy should be terminated by another method); follow-up visit after appropriate interval to assess vaginal bleeding recommended

  Note Careful monitoring of blood pressure and pulse essential for 3 hours after administration of gemeprost pessary (risk of profound hypotension)
- Labour induction in fetal death *in utero*, by mouth, mifepristone 600 mg daily as a single dose for 2 days under medical supervision; if labour not started within 72 hours of first dose, another method should be used

Mifegyne® (Exelgyn) PoM

Tablets, yellow, mifepristone 200 mg. Net price 3-tab pack = £41.83 (supplied to NHS hospitals and premises approved under Abortion Act 1967). Label: 10, patient information leaflet

7.1.3 Myometrial relaxants

Tocolytic drugs postpone *premature labour* and they are used with the aim of reducing harm to the child. However, there is no satisfactory evidence that the use of these drugs reduces mortality. The greatest benefit is gained by using the delay to administer corticosteroid therapy or to implement other measures which improve perinatal health (including transfer to a unit with neonatal intensive care facility).

The oxytocin receptor antagonist, **atosiban**, is licensed for the inhibition of uncomplicated premature labour *between 24 and 33 weeks* of gestation. Atosiban may be preferable to a beta$_2$ agonist because it has fewer side-effects.

The dihydropyridine calcium-channel blocker **nifedipine** (section 2.6.2) also has fewer side-effects than a beta$_2$ agonist. Nifedipine [unlicensed indication] can be given initially in a dose of 20 mg followed by 10–20 mg 3–4 times daily adjusted according to uterine activity.

A beta$_2$ agonist (**ritodrine**, **salbutamol** or **terbutaline**) is used for inhibiting uncomplicated premature labour between 24 and 33 weeks of gestation and it may permit a delay in delivery of at least 48 hours. Prolonged therapy should be avoided since risk to the mother increases after 48 hours and there is a lack of evidence of benefit from further treatment; maintenance treatment is therefore **not recommended**.

Indometacin (indomethacin) (section 10.1.1), a cyclo-oxygenase inhibitor, also inhibits labour [unlicensed indication] and it can be useful in situations where a beta$_2$ agonist is not appropriate; however, there are concerns about neonatal complications such as transient impairment of renal function and premature closure of ductus arteriosus.

Atosiban

ATOSIBAN

Indications uncomplicated premature labour (see notes above)

Cautions monitor blood loss after delivery; intra-uterine growth restriction; abnormal placental site; hepatic impairment (Appendix 2); renal impairment (Appendix 3)

Contra-indications eclampsia and severe pre-eclampsia, intra-uterine infection, intra-uterine fetal death, antepartum haemorrhage (requiring immediate delivery), placenta praevia, abruptio placenta, intra-uterine growth restriction with abnormal fetal heart rate, premature rupture of membranes after 30 weeks' gestation

Side-effects nausea, vomiting, tachycardia, hypotension, headache, dizziness, hot flushes, hyperglycaemia, injection-site reaction; *less commonly* pruritus, rash, fever, insomnia

Dose

- By intravenous injection, initially 6.75 mg over 1 minute, then by intravenous infusion 18 mg/hour for 3 hours, then 6 mg/hour for up to 45 hours; max. duration of treatment 48 hours

Tractocile® (Ferring) PoM

Injection, atosiban (as acetate) 7.5 mg/mL, net price 0.9-mL (6.75-mg) vial = £18.60

Concentrate for intravenous infusion, atosiban (as acetate) 7.5 mg/mL, net price 5-mL vial = £53.35

Beta$_2$ agonists

Cautions Beta$_2$ agonists should be used with caution in patients with suspected cardiovascular disease (such patients should be assessed by a cardiologist before initiating therapy—see also Contra-indications, below), hypertension, mild to moderate pre-eclampsia, hyperthyroidism, and hypokalaemia (particular risk with potassium-depleting diuretics—see also CSM advice, p. 150). It is important to monitor pulse rate (should not exceed 140 beats per minute), ECG (discontinue treatment if signs of myocardial ischaemia), and the patient's fluid and electrolyte status (avoid over-hydration—discontinue drug immediately and initiate diuretic therapy if pulmonary oedema occurs). Beta$_2$ agonists should also be used with caution in diabetes—monitor blood glucose (risk of hyperglycaemia and ketoacidosis, especially with intravenous beta$_2$ agonist).

Contra-indications Beta$_2$ agonists are contra-indicated in cardiac disease and in patients with significant risk factors for myocardial ischaemia; they should also be avoided in antepartum haemorrhage, intra-uterine infection, intra-uterine fetal death, placenta praevia, abruptio placenta, threatened miscarriage, cord compression, and eclampsia or severe pre-eclampsia.

Side-effects Side-effects of the beta$_2$ agonists include nausea, vomiting, pulmonary oedema (see Cautions above and under Ritodrine dose), palpitation, tachycardia, arrhythmias, myocardial ischaemia, peripheral vasodilation, headache, tremor, hyperglycaemia, hypokalaemia (see Cautions), muscle cramps and tension, and hypersensitivity reactions (including angioedema, urticaria, rash, bronchospasm, hypotension, and collapse).

RITODRINE HYDROCHLORIDE

Indications uncomplicated premature labour (see notes above)

Cautions see notes above; **interactions:** Appendix 1 (sympathomimetics *and* sympathomimetics, beta$_2$)

Contra-indications see notes above

Side-effects see notes above; also reported flushing, sweating; salivary gland enlargement; leucopenia and agranulocytosis on prolonged administration (several weeks); liver function abnormalities (including increased transaminases and hepatitis)

Dose

- By intravenous infusion (**important:** minimum fluid volume, see below), initially 50 micrograms/minute, increased gradually according to response by 50 micrograms/minute every 10 minutes until contractions stop or maternal heart rate reaches 140 beats per minute; continue for 12–48 hours after contractions cease (usual rate 150–350 micrograms/minute); max. rate 350 micrograms/minute; or by intramuscular injection, 10 mg every 3–8 hours continued for 12–48 hours after contractions have ceased; then by mouth (but see notes above), 10 mg 30 minutes before termination of intravenous infusion, repeated every 2 hours for 24 hours, followed by 10–20 mg every 4–6 hours, max. oral dose 120 mg daily

Important Manufacturer states that although *fatal pulmonary oedema* associated with ritodrine infusion is almost certainly multifactorial in origin, evidence suggests that **fluid overload** may be the most important single factor. The volume of infusion should therefore be kept to a minimum; for further guidance see Appendix 6. For specific guidance on infusion rates, consult product literature

Yutopar® (Durbin) PoM
Tablets, yellow, scored, ritodrine hydrochloride 10 mg, net price 90-tab pack = £30.40

Injection, ritodrine hydrochloride 10 mg/mL, net price 5-mL amp = £3.55

SALBUTAMOL
(Albuterol)

Indications uncomplicated premature labour (see notes above); asthma (section 3.1.1)

Cautions see notes above; **interactions:** Appendix 1 (sympathomimetics, beta$_2$)

Contra-indications see notes above

Side-effects see notes above

Dose

- By intravenous infusion, initially 10 micrograms/minute, rate increased gradually according to response at 10-minute intervals until contractions diminish then increase rate slowly until contractions cease (max. rate 45 micrograms/minute); maintain rate for 1 hour after contractions have stopped, then gradually reduce by 50% every 6 hours; then by mouth (but see notes above), 4 mg every 6–8 hours

Preparations
Section 3.1.1.1

TERBUTALINE SULPHATE

Indications uncomplicated premature labour (see notes above); asthma (section 3.1.1)

Cautions see notes above; **interactions:** Appendix 1 (sympathomimetics, beta$_2$)

Contra-indications see notes above

Side-effects see notes above; also reported sleep disturbances and behavioural disturbances

Dose

- By intravenous infusion, 5 micrograms/minute for 20 minutes, increased every 20 minutes in steps of 2.5 micrograms/minute until contractions have ceased (more than 10 micrograms/minute should **seldom** be given—20 micrograms/minute should **not** be exceeded), continue for 1 hour then decrease every 20 minutes in steps of 2.5 micrograms/minute to lowest dose that maintains suppression, continue at this level for 12 hours then by mouth (but see notes above), 5 mg every 8 hours for as long as is desirable to prolong pregnancy (or alternatively follow the intravenous infusion by subcutaneous injection 250 micrograms every 6 hours for a few days then by mouth as above)

Preparations
Section 3.1.1.1

7.2 Treatment of vaginal and vulval conditions

7.2.1 Preparations for vaginal atrophy
7.2.2 Vaginal and vulval infections

Symptoms are often restricted to the vulva, but infections almost invariably involve the vagina which should also be treated. Applications to the vulva alone are likely to give only symptomatic relief without cure.

Aqueous medicated douches may disturb normal vaginal acidity and bacterial flora.

Topical anaesthetic agents give only symptomatic relief and may cause sensitivity reactions. They are indicated only in cases of pruritus where specific local causes have been excluded.

Systemic drugs are required in the treatment of infections such as gonorrhoea and syphilis (section 5.1).

7.2.1 Preparations for vaginal atrophy

Topical HRT

A cream containing an oestrogen may be applied on a short-term basis to improve the vaginal epithelium in *menopausal atrophic vaginitis.* It is **important** to bear in mind that topical oestrogens should be used in the **smallest effective** amount to minimise systemic effects. Modified-release vaginal tablets and an impregnated vaginal ring are now also available.

The risk of endometrial hyperplasia and carcinoma is increased when *systemic* oestrogens are administered alone for prolonged periods (section 6.4.1.1). The endometrial safety of long-term or repeated use of *topical* vaginal oestrogens is uncertain; treatment should be reviewed at least annually, with special consideration given to any symptoms of endometrial hyperplasia or carcinoma.

Topical oestrogens are also used in postmenopausal women before vaginal surgery for prolapse when there is epithelial atrophy.

For a general comment on hormone replacement therapy, including the role of topical oestrogens, see section 6.4.1.1.

OESTROGENS, TOPICAL

Indications see notes above

Cautions see notes above; see also Oestrogens for HRT (section 6.4.1.1); interrupt treatment periodically to assess need for continued treatment

Contra-indications see notes above; see also Oestrogens for HRT (section 6.4.1.1); pregnancy and breast-feeding

Side-effects see notes above; see also Oestrogens for HRT (section 6.4.1.1); local irritation

Ortho-Gynest® (Janssen-Cilag) PoM

Intravaginal cream, estriol 0.01%. Net price 80 g with applicator = £2.53

Excipients include arachis (peanut) oil

Condoms damages latex condoms and diaphragms

Dose insert 1 applicatorful daily, preferably in evening; reduced to 1 applicatorful twice a week; attempts to reduce or discontinue should be made at 3–6 month intervals with re-examination

Pessaries, estriol 500 micrograms. Net price 15 pessaries = £4.92

Excipients include butylated hydroxytoluene

Condoms damages latex condoms and diaphragms

Dose insert 1 pessary daily, preferably in the evening, until improvement occurs; maintenance 1 pessary twice a week; attempts to reduce or discontinue should be made at 3–6 month intervals with re-examination

Ovestin® (Organon) PoM

Intravaginal cream, estriol 0.1%. Net price 15 g with applicator = £4.63

Excipients include cetyl alcohol, polysorbates, stearyl alcohol

Condoms effect on latex condoms and diaphragms not yet known

Dose insert 1 applicator-dose daily for 2–3 weeks, then reduce to twice a week (discontinue every 2–3 months for 4 weeks to assess need for further treatment); vaginal surgery, 1 applicator-dose daily for 2 weeks before surgery, resuming 2 weeks after surgery

Premarin® (Wyeth) PoM

Vaginal cream, conjugated oestrogens (equine) 625 micrograms/g. Net price 42.5 g with calibrated applicator = £2.19

Excipients include cetyl alcohol, propylene glycol

Condoms effect on latex condoms and diaphragms not yet known

Dose insert 1–2 g daily starting on day 5 of cycle (or at any time if cycles have ceased) for 3 weeks, repeated after a 1-week interval

Vagifem® (Novo Nordisk) PoM

Vaginal tablets, f/c, m/r, estradiol 25 micrograms in disposable applicators. Net price 15-applicator pack = £8.80

Excipients none as listed in section 13.1.3

Condoms no evidence of damage to latex condoms and diaphragms

Dose insert 1 tablet daily for 2 weeks then reduce to 1 tablet twice weekly; discontinue after 3 months to assess need for further treatment

◢Vaginal ring

Estring® (Pharmacia) PoM

Vaginal ring, releasing estradiol approx. 7.5 micrograms/24 hours. Net price 1-ring pack = £31.42. Label: 10, patient information leaflet

Dose for postmenopausal urogenital conditions (not suitable for vasomotor symptoms or osteoporosis prophylaxis), to be inserted into upper third of vagina and worn continuously; replace after 3 months; max. duration of continuous treatment 2 years

Non-hormonal preparations

Replens MD® and *Sylk®* are acidic, non-hormonal vaginal moisturisers; *Replens MD®* provides a high moisture content for up to 3 days.

7.2.2 Vaginal and vulval infections

Effective specific treatments are available for the common vaginal infections.

Fungal infections

Candidal vulvitis can be treated locally with cream but is almost invariably associated with vaginal infection which should also be treated. *Vaginal candidiasis* is treated primarily with antifungal pessaries or cream inserted high into the vagina (including during menstruation). Single-dose preparations offer an advantage when compliance is a problem. Local irritation may occur on application of vaginal antifungal products.

Imidazole drugs (clotrimazole, econazole, and miconazole) are effective against candida in short courses of 3 to 14 days according to the preparation used. Vaginal applications may be supplemented with antifungal cream for vulvitis and to treat other superficial sites of infection.

Nystatin cream is used in cases of vulvitis and infection of other superficial sites. Nystatin stains clothing yellow.

Oral treatment of vaginal infection with **fluconazole** or **itraconazole** (section 5.2) is also effective; oral ketoconazole has been associated with fatal hepatotoxicity (see section 5.2 for CSM warning).

Recurrent vulvovaginal candidiasis Recurrence of vulvovaginal candidiasis is particularly likely if there are predisposing factors such as antibacterial therapy, pregnancy, diabetes mellitus and possibly oral contraceptive use. Reservoirs of infection may also lead to recontamination and should be treated; these include other skin sites such as the digits, nail beds, and umbilicus as well as the gastro-intestinal tract and the bladder. The partner may also be the source of re-infection and, if symptomatic, should be treated with cream at the same time.

Treatment against candida may need to be extended for 6 months in recurrent vulvovaginal candidiasis. Some recommended regimens [all unlicensed] include:

- fluconazole (section 5.2) by mouth 100 mg (as a single dose) every week for 6 months
- clotrimazole vaginally 500-mg pessary (as a single dose) every week for 6 months
- itraconazole (section 5.2) by mouth 400 mg (as 2 divided doses on one day) every month for 6 months.

PREPARATIONS FOR VAGINAL AND VULVAL CANDIDIASIS

Side-effects occasional local irritation

Clotrimazole (Non-proprietary)

Cream (topical), clotrimazole 1%, net price 20 g = £2.83, 50 g = £3.80

Condoms check with manufacturer of cream for effect on latex condoms and diaphragms

Dose apply to anogenital area 2–3 times daily

Pessary, clotrimazole 500 mg, net price 1 pessary with applicator = £3.40

Dose insert 1 pessary at night as a single dose; can be repeated once if necessary

Canesten® (Bayer Consumer Care)

Cream (topical), clotrimazole 1%. Net price 20 g = £2.14; 50 g = £3.80

Excipients include benzyl alcohol, cetostearyl alcohol, polysorbates

Condoms damages latex condoms and diaphragms

Dose apply to anogenital area 2–3 times daily

Thrush Cream (topical), clotrimazole 2%, net price 20 g = £3.99
Excipients include benzyl alcohol, cetostearyl alcohol, polysorbates
Condoms damages latex condoms and diaphragms
Dose apply to anogenital area 2–3 times daily

Vaginal cream (*10% VC®*) PoM, clotrimazole 10%. Net price 5-g applicator pack = £5.62
Excipients include benzyl alcohol, cetostearyl alcohol, polysorbates
Condoms damages latex condoms and diaphragms
Dose insert 5 g at night as a single dose; can be repeated once if necessary
Note Brands for sale to the public include *Canesten® Internal Cream*

Cream Combi, clotrimazole 10% vaginal cream and 2% topical cream, net price 5-g vaginal cream (with applicator) and 10-g topical cream = £5.76
Excipients include benzyl alcohol, cetostearyl alcohol, polysorbates
Condoms damages latex condoms and diaphragms
Dose see under individual components

Pessaries, clotrimazole 100 mg, net price 6 pessaries with applicator = £3.63; 200 mg, 3 pessaries with applicator = £3.63
Condoms damages latex condoms and diaphragms
Dose insert 200 mg for 3 nights *or* 100 mg for 6 nights; course can be repeated once if necessary

Pessary, clotrimazole 500 mg. Net price 1 with applicator = £3.25
Excipients none as listed in section 13.1.3
Condoms damages latex condoms and diaphragms
Dose insert 1 pessary at night as a single dose; can be repeated once if necessary

Combi, clotrimazole 500-mg pessary and cream (topical) 2%. Net price 1 pessary and 10 g cream = £5.21
Condoms damages latex condoms and diaphragms
Dose see under individual components

Ecostatin® (Squibb)
Cream (topical), econazole nitrate 1%. Net price 15 g = £1.49; 30 g = £2.75
Excipients include butylated hydroxyanisole, fragrance
Condoms damages latex condoms and diaphragms
Dose apply to anogenital area twice daily

Pessaries PoM, econazole nitrate 150 mg. Net price 3 with applicator = £3.35
Excipients none as listed in section 13.1.3
Condoms damages latex condoms and diaphragms
Dose insert 1 pessary for 3 nights; course can be repeated once if necessary

Pessary (*Ecostatin-1®*) PoM, econazole nitrate 150 mg, formulated for single-dose therapy. Net price 1 pessary with applicator = £3.35
Excipients none as listed in section 13.1.3
Condoms damages latex condoms and diaphragms
Dose insert 1 pessary at night as a single dose; can be repeated once if necessary

Twinpack PoM, econazole nitrate 150-mg pessaries and cream 1%. Net price 3 pessaries and 15 g cream = £4.35
Condoms damages latex condoms and diaphragms
Dose see under individual components

Gyno-Daktarin® (Janssen-Cilag) PoM
Intravaginal cream, miconazole nitrate 2%. Net price 78 g with applicators = £4.60
Excipients include butylated hydroxyanisole
Condoms damages latex condoms and diaphragms
Dose insert 5-g applicatorful once daily for 10–14 days *or* twice daily for 7 days; course can be repeated once if necessary; *topical*, apply to anogenital area twice daily

Pessaries, miconazole nitrate 100 mg. Net price 14 = £3.12
Excipients none as listed in section 13.1.3
Condoms damages latex condoms and diaphragms
Dose insert 1 pessary daily for 14 days or 1 pessary twice daily for 7 days; course can be repeated once if necessary

Ovule (= vaginal capsule) (*Gyno-Daktarin 1®*), miconazole nitrate 1.2 g in a fatty basis. Net price 1 ovule = £3.12
Excipients include hydroxybenzoates (parabens)
Condoms damages latex condoms and diaphragms
Dose insert 1 ovule at night as a single dose; can be repeated once if necessary

Gyno-Pevaryl® (Janssen-Cilag) PoM
Cream, econazole nitrate 1%. Net price 15 g = £1.40; 30 g = £3.21
Excipients none as listed in section 13.1.3
Condoms damages latex condoms and diaphragms
Dose insert 5-g applicatorful intravaginally and apply to vulva at night for at least 14 nights; course can be repeated once if necessary

Pessaries, econazole nitrate 150 mg. Net price 3 pessaries = £2.95
Excipients none as listed in section 13.1.3
Condoms damages latex condoms and diaphragms
Dose ADULT and ADOLESCENT over 16 years, insert 1 pessary for 3 nights; course can be repeated once if necessary

Pessary (*Gyno-Pevaryl 1®*), econazole nitrate 150 mg, formulated for single-dose therapy. Net price 1 pessary with applicator = £3.13
Excipients none as listed in section 13.1.3
Condoms damages latex condoms and diaphragms
Dose ADULT and ADOLESCENT over 16 years, insert 1 pessary at night as a single dose; can be repeated once if necessary

Nizoral® (Janssen-Cilag) PoM
Cream (topical), ketoconazole 2%. Net price 30 g = £3.54
Excipients include polysorbates, propylene glycol, stearyl alcohol
Condoms effect on latex condoms and diaphragms not yet known
Dose apply to anogenital area once or twice daily

Nystan® (Squibb) PoM
Cream and *Ointment*, see section 13.10.2

Vaginal cream, nystatin 100 000 units/4-g application. Net price 60 g with applicator = £2.58
Excipients include benzyl alcohol, propylene glycol
Condoms damages latex condoms and diaphragms
Dose insert 1–2 applicatorfuls at night for at least 14 nights; course can be repeated once if necessary

Other infections

Vaginal preparations intended to restore normal acidity may prevent recurrence of vaginal infections and permit the re-establishment of the normal vaginal flora.

Trichomonal infections commonly involve the lower urinary tract as well as the genital system and need systemic treatment with metronidazole or tinidazole (section 5.1.11).

Bacterial infections with Gram-negative organisms are particularly common in association with gynaecological operations and trauma. Metronidazole is effective against certain Gram-negative organisms, especially *Bacteroides* spp. and can be used prophylactically in gynaecological surgery.

Topical vaginal products containing povidone–iodine can be used to treat vaginitis due to candidal, trichomonal, non-specific, or mixed infections; they are also used for the pre-operative preparation of the vagina. Clindamycin cream and metronidazole gel are also indicated for bacterial vaginosis.

The antiviral drugs aciclovir, famciclovir, and valaciclovir can be used in the treatment of genital infection due to *herpes simplex virus,* the HSV type 2 being a major cause of genital ulceration. They have a beneficial effect on virus shedding and healing, generally giving relief from pain and other symptoms. See section 5.3.2.1 for systemic preparations, and section 13.10.3 for topical preparations.

PREPARATIONS FOR OTHER VAGINAL INFECTIONS

Dalacin® (Pharmacia) PoM

Cream, clindamycin 2% (as phosphate). Net price 40-g pack with 7 applicators = £10.86

Excipients include benzyl alcohol, cetostearyl alcohol, polysorbates, propylene glycol

Condoms damages latex condoms and diaphragms

Side-effects irritation, cervicitis and vaginitis; poorly absorbed into the blood—very low likelihood of systemic effects (section 5.1.6)

Dose bacterial vaginosis, insert 5-g applicatorful at night for 3–7 nights

Zidoval® (3M) PoM

Vaginal gel, metronidazole 0.75%. Net price 40-g pack with 5 applicators = £4.31

Excipients include disodium edetate, hydroxybenzoates (parabens), propylene glycol

Cautions not recommended during menstruation; some absorption may occur, see section 5.1.11 for systemic effects

Side-effects local effects including irritation, candidiasis, abnormal discharge, pelvic discomfort

Dose bacterial vaginosis, insert 5-g applicatorful at night for 5 nights

7.3 Contraceptives

7.3.1 Combined hormonal contraceptives
7.3.2 Progestogen-only contraceptives
7.3.3 Spermicidal contraceptives
7.3.4 Contraceptive devices
7.3.5 Emergency contraception

Hormonal contraception is the most effective method of fertility control, but has major and minor side-effects, especially for certain groups of women.

Intra-uterine devices are a highly effective method of contraception but may produce undesirable local side-effects. They are most suitable for older parous women, but less appropriate for younger nulliparous women and for those with an increased risk of pelvic inflammatory disease.

Barrier methods alone (condoms, diaphragms, and caps) are less effective but can be very reliable for well-motivated couples if used in conjunction with a **spermicide**. Occasionally sensitivity reactions occur. A female condom (*Femidom®*) is also available; it is prelubricated but does not contain a spermicide.

7.3.1 Combined hormonal contraceptives

Oral contraceptives containing an oestrogen and a progestogen ('combined oral contraceptives') are the most effective preparations for general use. Advantages of combined oral contraceptives include:

- reliable and reversible;
- reduced dysmenorrhoea and menorrhagia;
- reduced incidence of premenstrual tension;
- less symptomatic fibroids and functional ovarian cysts;
- less benign breast disease;
- reduced risk of ovarian and endometrial cancer;
- reduced risk of pelvic inflammatory disease, which may be a risk with intra-uterine devices.

Combined oral contraceptives containing a fixed amount of an oestrogen and a progestogen in each active tablet are termed 'monophasic'; those with varying amounts of the two hormones according to the stage of the cycle are termed 'biphasic' and 'triphasic'. A transdermal patch containing an oestrogen with a progestogen is also available.

Choice The oestrogen content of combined oral contraceptives ranges from 20 to 40 micrograms. Generally a preparation with the lowest oestrogen and progestogen content which gives good cycle control and minimal side-effects in the individual woman is chosen.

- *Low strength preparations* (containing ethinylestradiol 20 micrograms) are particularly appropriate for women with risk factors for circulatory disease, provided a combined oral contraceptive is otherwise suitable. It is recommended that the combined oral contraceptive is not continued beyond 50 years of age since more suitable alternatives exist.
- *Standard strength preparations* (containing ethinylestradiol 30 or 35 micrograms or in 30–40 microgram *phased* preparations) are appropriate for standard use—but see Risk of Venous Thromboembolism below. Phased preparations are generally reserved for women who *either* do not have withdrawal bleeding *or* who have breakthrough bleeding with monophasic products.

The progestogens desogestrel, drospirenone, and gestodene (in combination with ethinylestradiol) may be considered for women who have side-effects (such as acne, headache, depression, weight gain, breast symptoms, and breakthrough bleeding) with other progestogens. However, women should be advised that desogestrel and gestodene have also been associated with an increased risk of *venous thromboembolism.* Drospirenone, a derivative of spironolactone, has anti-androgenic and anti-mineralocorticoid activity; it should be used with care if an increased concentration of potassium might be hazardous. The progestogen norelgestromin is combined with ethinylestradiol in a transdermal patch.

Risk of venous thromboembolism There is an increased risk of venous thromboembolic disease (particularly during the first year) in users of oral contraceptives but this risk is considerably smaller than that associated with pregnancy (about 60 cases of venous thromboembolic disease per 100 000 pregnancies). In all cases the risk of venous thromboembolism increases with age and in the presence of other risk factors for venous thromboembolism (e.g. obesity). The risk of venous thromboembolism with transdermal patches is not yet known.

The incidence of venous thromboembolism in healthy, non-pregnant women who are not taking an oral contraceptive is about 5 cases per 100 000 women per year. For those using combined oral contraceptives containing second-generation progestogens e.g. levonorgestrel, this incidence is about 15 per 100 000 women per year of use. Some studies have reported a greater risk of venous thromboembolism in women using preparations containing the third-generation progestogens desogestrel and gestodene; the incidence in these women is about 25 per 100 000 women per year of use.

The absolute risk of venous thromboembolism in women using combined oral contraceptives containing these third-generation progestogens remains very small and well below the risk associated with pregnancy. Provided that women are informed of the relative risks of venous thromboembolism and accept them, the choice of oral contraceptive is for the woman together with the prescriber jointly to make in light of her individual medical history and any contra-indications.

Travel Women taking oral contraceptives, or using the patch are at an increased risk of deep-vein thrombosis during travel involving long periods of immobility (over 5 hours). The risk may be reduced by appropriate exercise during the journey and possibly by wearing graduated compression hosiery.

Missed pill The critical time for loss of contraceptive protection is when a pill is omitted at the *beginning* or *end* of a cycle (which lengthens the pill-free interval).

If a woman forgets to take a pill, it should be taken as soon as she remembers, and the next one taken at the normal time (even if this means taking 2 pills together). A missed pill is one that is 24 or more hours late. If a woman misses only one pill, she should take an active pill as soon as she remembers and then resume normal pill-taking. No additional precautions are necessary.

If a woman misses 2 or more pills (especially from the first 7 in a packet), she may not be protected. She should take an active pill as soon as she remembers and then resume normal pill-taking. In addition, she must either abstain from sex or use an additional method of contraception such as a condom for the next 7 days. If these 7 days run beyond the end of the packet, the next packet should be started at once, omitting the pill-free interval (or, in the case of *everyday* (ED) pills, omitting the 7 inactive tablets).

Emergency contraception (section 7.3.5) is recommended if 2 or more combined oral contraceptive tablets are missed from the first 7 tablets in a packet and unprotected intercourse has occurred since finishing the last packet.

Delayed application or detached patch If a patch is partly detached for less than 24 hours, reapply to the same site or replace with a new patch immediately; no additional contraception is needed and the next patch should be applied on the usual change day. If a patch remains detached for more than 24 hours or if the user is not aware when the patch became detached then stop the current contraceptive cycle and start a new cycle by applying a new patch, giving a new 'Day 1'; an additional non-hormonal contraceptive must be used concurrently for the first 7 days of the new cycle.

If application of a new patch at the start of a new cycle is delayed, contraceptive protection is lost. A new patch should be applied as soon as remembered giving a new 'Day 1'; additional non-hormonal methods of contraception should be used for the first 7 days of the new cycle. If intercourse has occurred during this extended patch-free interval, a possibility of fertilisation should be considered. If application of a patch in the middle of the cycle is delayed (i.e. the patch is not changed on day 8 or day 15):

- for up to 48 hours, apply a new patch immediately; next patch change day remains the same and no additional contraception is required.
- for more than 48 hours, contraceptive protection may have been lost. Stop the current cycle and start a new 4-week cycle immediately by applying a new patch giving a new 'Day 1'; additional non-hormonal contraception should be used for the first 7 days of the new cycle.

If the patch is not removed at the end of the cycle (day 22), remove it as soon as possible and start the next cycle on the usual 'change day', after day 28; no additional contraception is required.

Diarrhoea and vomiting Vomiting and persistent, severe diarrhoea can interfere with the absorption of combined oral contraceptives. If vomiting occurs within 2 hours of taking a combined oral contraceptive another pill should be taken as soon as possible. In cases of persistent vomiting or severe diarrhoea lasting more than 24 hours, additional precautions should be used during and for 7 days after recovery (see also under Missed pill, above). If the vomiting and diarrhoea occurs during the last 7 tablets, the next pill-free interval should be omitted (in the case of ED tablets the inactive ones should be omitted).

Interactions The effectiveness of both *combined* and *progestogen-only* oral contraceptives can be considerably reduced by interaction with drugs that induce hepatic enzyme activity (e.g. **carbamazepine**, **griseofulvin**, **modafinil**, **nelfinavir**, **nevirapine**, **oxcarbazepine**, **phenytoin**, **phenobarbital**, **primidone**, **ritonavir**, **St John's Wort**, **topiramate**, and, above all, **rifabutin** and **rifampicin**). A condom together with a long-acting method, such as an injectable contraceptive, may be more suitable for patients with HIV infection or at risk of HIV infection; advice on the possibility of interaction with antiretroviral drugs should be sought from HIV specialists.

For a *short course of an enzyme-inducing drug*, the dose of combined oral contraceptives should be adjusted to provide ethinylestradiol 50 micrograms or more daily [unlicensed use]; furthermore, additional contraceptive precautions should be taken whilst taking the enzyme-inducing drug and for 4 weeks after stopping it.

Women requiring a *long-term course of an enzyme-inducing drug* should be encouraged to consider a contraceptive method that is unaffected by the interacting drug. In women unable to use an alternative method of contraception (for rifampicin and rifabutin see also below), a regimen of combined oral contraceptives should be taken which provides a daily intake of ethinylestradiol 50 micrograms or more [unlicensed use]; 'tricycling' (i.e. taking 3 or 4 packets of monophasic tablets without a break followed by a short tablet-free interval of 4 days) is recommended (but women should be warned of uncertainty about the effectiveness of this regimen). **Rifampicin** and **rifabutin** are such potent enzyme-inducing drugs that an alternative method of contraception (such as an IUD) is **always** recommended. Since enzyme activity does not return to normal for several weeks after stopping an enzyme-inducing drug, appropriate contraceptive measures are required for 4 to 8 weeks after stopping.

The effectiveness of contraceptive patches can also be reduced by drugs that induce hepatic enzyme activity. Additional contraceptive precautions are required whilst taking the enzyme-inducing drug and for 4 weeks after stopping. If concomitant administration runs beyond the 3 weeks of patch treatment, a new treatment cycle should be started immediately without a patch-free break. For women taking enzyme-inducing drugs over a long period, another method of contraception should be considered.

Some antibacterials that do not induce liver enzymes (e.g. ampicillin, doxycycline) may reduce the efficacy of *combined* oral contraceptives by impairing the bacterial flora responsible for recycling ethinylestradiol from the large bowel. Additional contraceptive precautions should be taken whilst taking a short course of an antibacterial drug that is not enzyme-inducing and for 7 days after stopping. If these 7 days run beyond the end of a packet the next packet should be started immediately without a break (in the case of ED tablets the inactive ones should be omitted). If the antibacterial course *exceeds 3 weeks*, the bacterial flora develop antibacterial resistance and additional precautions become unnecessary unless a new antibacterial is prescribed; additional precautions are also unnecessary if a woman starting a *combined* oral contraceptive has been on a course of antibacterial therapy for 3 weeks or more.

It is possible that some antibacterials affect the efficacy of contraceptive patches. Additional contraceptive precautions are recommended during concomitant use and for 7 days after discontinuation of an antibacterial that is not enzyme-inducing (except tetracycline). If concomitant administration runs beyond the 3 weeks of patch treatment, a new treatment cycle should be started immediately without a patch-free break. If the antibacterial course exceeds 3 weeks, additional precautions become unnecessary unless a new antibacterial is prescribed; additional precautions are also unnecessary if a woman starting a contraceptive patch has been on a course of antibacterial therapy for 3 weeks or more.

Surgery Oestrogen-containing contraceptives should preferably be discontinued (and adequate alternative contraceptive arrangements made) 4 weeks before major elective surgery and all surgery to the legs or surgery which involves prolonged immobilisation of a lower limb; they should normally be recommenced at the first menses occurring at least 2 weeks after full mobilisation. A depot injection of a progestogen-only contraceptive may be offered and the oestrogen-containing contraceptive restarted later—if preferred before the next injection would be due. When discontinuation of an oestrogen-containing contraceptive is not possible, e.g. after trauma or if a patient admitted for an elective procedure is still on an oestrogen-containing contraceptive, thromboprophylaxis (with heparin and graduated compression hosiery) is advised. These recommendations do not apply to minor surgery with short duration of anaesthesia, e.g. laparoscopic sterilisation or tooth extraction, or to women using oestrogen-free hormonal contraceptives (whether by mouth or by injection).

Reason to stop immediately Combined hormonal contraceptives or hormone replacement therapy (HRT) should be stopped (pending investigation and treatment), if any of the following occur:

- sudden severe chest pain (even if not radiating to left arm);
- sudden breathlessness (or cough with blood-stained sputum);
- unexplained swelling or severe pain in calf of one leg;
- severe stomach pain;
- serious neurological effects including unusual severe, prolonged headache especially if first time or getting progressively worse *or* sudden partial or complete loss of vision *or* sudden disturbance of hearing or other perceptual disorders *or* dysphasia *or* bad fainting attack or collapse *or* first unexplained epileptic seizure *or* weakness, motor disturbances, very marked numbness suddenly affecting one side or one part of body;
- hepatitis, jaundice, liver enlargement;
- blood pressure above systolic 160 mmHg and diastolic 100 mmHg;
- prolonged immobility after surgery or leg injury;
- detection of a risk factor which contra-indicates treatment (see Cautions and Contra-indications under Combined Hormonal Contraceptives below or under Oestrogens for HRT (section 6.4.1.1)).

COMBINED HORMONAL CONTRACEPTIVES

Indications contraception; menstrual symptoms (section 6.4.1.2)

Cautions risk factors for venous thromboembolism (see below and also notes above), arterial disease and migraine, see below; personal or family history of hypertriglyceridaemia (increased risk of pancreatitis); hyperprolactinaemia (seek specialist advice); history of severe depression especially if induced by hormonal contraceptive; undiagnosed breast mass; gene mutations associated with breast cancer (e.g. BRCA 1); sickle-cell disease; inflammatory bowel disease including Crohn's disease; reduced efficacy of contraceptive patch in women with body-weight $\geq$ 90 kg; **interactions**: see above and Appendix 1 (oestrogens, progestogens)

Risk factors for venous thromboembolism See also notes above. Use **with caution** if any of following factors present but **avoid** if two or more factors present:

- *family history of venous thromboembolism* in first-degree relative aged under 45 years (avoid contraceptive containing desogestrel or gestodene, *or* if known prothrombotic coagulation abnormality e.g. factor V Leiden or antiphospholipid antibodies (including lupus anticoagulant));
- *obesity*—body mass index above 30 kg/m² (avoid if body mass index above 39 kg/m²);
- *long-term immobilisation* e.g. in a wheelchair (avoid if confined to bed or leg in plaster cast);
- history of superficial thrombophlebitis.

7 Obstetrics, gynaecology, and urinary-tract disorders

Risk factors for arterial disease Use with **caution** if any one of following factors present but **avoid** if two or more factors present:

- *family history of arterial disease* in first degree relative aged under 45 years (avoid if atherogenic lipid profile);
- *diabetes mellitus* (avoid if diabetes complications present);
- *hypertension*—blood pressure above *systolic 140 mmHg* and *diastolic 90 mmHg* (avoid if blood pressure above *systolic 160 mmHg* and *diastolic 95 mmHg*);
- *smoking* (avoid if smoking 40 or more cigarettes daily);
- *age* over 35 years (avoid if over 50 years);
- *obesity* (avoid if body mass index above 39 kg/m^2);
- *migraine*—see below.

Migraine Women should report any increase in headache frequency or onset of focal symptoms (discontinue immediately and refer urgently to neurology expert if focal neurological symptoms not typical of aura persist for more than 1 hour—see also Reason to stop immediately in notes above); **contra-indicated** in

- migraine with typical focal aura,
- severe migraine regularly lasting over 72 hours despite treatment,
- migraine treated with ergot derivatives;

use with **caution** in

- migraine without focal aura,
- migraine controlled with 5HT$_1$ agonist (section 4.7.4.1).

Contra-indications pregnancy (Appendix 4); personal history of venous or arterial thrombosis, severe or multiple risk factors for arterial disease or for venous thromboembolism (see above), heart disease associated with pulmonary hypertension or risk of embolus; sclerosing treatment for varicose veins; migraine (see above); transient cerebral ischaemic attacks without headaches; liver disease including disorders of hepatic excretion (e.g. Dubin-Johnson or Rotor syndromes), infective hepatitis (until liver function returns to normal); systemic lupus erythematosus; porphyria (section 9.8.2); liver tumour; gallstones; active trophoblastic disease (until return to normal of urine and plasma gonadotrophin concentration); history of haemolytic uraemic syndrome or history during pregnancy of pruritus, cholestatic jaundice, chorea, pemphigoid gestationis; history of breast cancer but can be used after 5 years if no evidence of disease and non-hormonal methods unacceptable; undiagnosed vaginal bleeding; breast-feeding (until weaning or for 6 months after birth—Appendix 5)

Side-effects nausea, vomiting, abdominal cramps, changes in body-weight, liver impairment, hepatic tumours; fluid retention, thrombosis (more common when factor V Leiden present or in blood groups A, B, and AB; see also notes above), hypertension, changes in lipid metabolism; headache, depression, chorea, nervousness, irritability; changes in libido, breast tenderness, enlargement, and secretion; reduced menstrual loss, 'spotting' in early cycles, absence of withdrawal bleeding, amenorrhoea after discontinuation, changes in vaginal discharge, cervical erosion; contact lenses may irritate, visual disturbances; leg cramps; skin reactions, chloasma, photosensitivity; rarely gallstones and systemic lupus erythematosus

Breast cancer There is a small increase in the risk of having breast cancer diagnosed in women taking the combined oral contraceptive pill; this relative risk may be due to an earlier diagnosis. In users of combined oral contraceptive pills the cancers are more likely to be localised to the breast. The most important factor for diagnosing breast cancer appears to be the age at which the contraceptive is stopped rather than the duration of use; any increase in the rate of diagnosis diminishes gradually during the 10 years after stopping and disappears by 10 years. The CSM has advised that a possible small increase in the risk of breast cancer should be weighed against the benefits and evidence of the protective effect against cancers of the ovary and endometrium

Dose

- By mouth, each tablet should be taken at approximately same time each day; if delayed by longer than 24 hours contraceptive protection may be lost

  21-day combined (monophasic) preparations, 1 tablet daily for 21 days; subsequent courses repeated after a 7-day interval (during which withdrawal bleeding occurs); first course usually started on day 1 of cycle—if starting on day 4 of cycle or later additional precautions (barrier methods) necessary during first 7 days

  Every day (ED) combined (monophasic) preparations, 1 *active* tablet starting on day 1 of cycle (see also under preparations below)—if starting on day 4 of cycle or later additional precautions (barrier methods) necessary during first 7 days; withdrawal bleeding occurs when *inactive* tablets being taken; subsequent courses repeated without interval

  Biphasic and triphasic preparations, see under individual preparations below

  Changing to combined preparation containing different progesterone *21-day combined preparations:* continue current pack until last tablet and start first tablet of new brand the next day. If a 7-day break is taken before starting new brand, additional precautions (barrier methods) should be used during first 7 days of taking the new brand.

  Every Day (ED) combined preparations: start the new brand (first tablet of a *21-day preparation* or the first *active* tablet of an *ED preparation*) the day after taking the last *active* tablet of previous brand (omitting the *inactive* tablets).

  Changing from progesterone-only tablet Start on day 1 of menstruation or any day if amenorrhoea present and pregnancy has been excluded.

  Secondary amenorrhoea (exclude pregnancy) Start any day, additional precautions (barrier methods) necessary during first 7 days.

  After childbirth (not breast-feeding) Start 3 weeks after birth (increased risk of thrombosis if started earlier); later than 3 weeks postpartum additional precautions (barrier methods) necessary for first 7 days.

  Not recommended if woman breast-feeding—oral progestogen-only contraceptive preferred.

  After abortion or miscarriage Start same day.

- By transdermal application, apply first patch on day 1 of cycle, change patch on days 8 and 15; remove third patch on day 22 and apply new patch after 7-day patch-free interval to start subsequent contraceptive cycle

  Note If first patch applied later than day 1, additional precaution (abstinence or barrier methods) should be used for the next 7 days

  Changing from combined oral contraception Apply patch on the first day of withdrawal bleeding; if no withdrawal bleeding within 5 days of taking last *active* tablet, rule out pregnancy before applying first patch. Unless patch is applied on first day of withdrawal bleeding, additional precautions (barrier methods) should be used concurrently for first 7 days

  Changing from progesterone-only method From an implant, apply first patch on the day implant removed; from an injection, apply first patch when next injection due; from oral progestogen, first patch may be started on any day after stopping pill. For all methods additional precautions (barrier methods) should be used concurrently for first 7 days

  After childbirth (not breast-feeding) Start 4 weeks after birth; if started later than 4 weeks after birth additional precautions (barrier methods) should be used for first 7 days

  After abortion or miscarriage Before 20 weeks' gestation start immediately; no additional contraception required if started immediately. After 20 weeks' gestation start on day 21 after abortion or on the first day of first spontaneous menstruation; additional precautions (barrier methods) should be used for first 7 days after applying the patch

Low strength (oral)

Ethinylestradiol with Norethisterone

Loestrin 20® (Galen) PoM

Tablets, blue, norethisterone acetate 1 mg, ethinylestradiol 20 micrograms. Net price 3 × 21-tab pack = £2.70

Dose 1 tablet daily for 21 days; subsequent courses repeated after 7-day tablet-free interval (during which withdrawal bleeding occurs); for starting routines see under Dose above

Ethinylestradiol with Desogestrel

See Risk of Venous Thromboembolism in notes above before prescribing

Mercilon® (Organon) PoM

Tablets, desogestrel 150 micrograms, ethinylestradiol 20 micrograms. Net price 3 × 21-tab pack = £7.97

Dose 1 tablet daily for 21 days; subsequent courses repeated after 7-day tablet-free interval (during which withdrawal bleeding occurs); for starting routines see under Dose above

Ethinylestradiol with Gestodene

See Risk of Venous Thromboembolism in notes above before prescribing

Femodette® (Schering Health) PoM

Tablets, s/c, gestodene 75 micrograms, ethinylestradiol 20 micrograms, net price 3 × 21-tab pack = £9.45

Dose 1 tablet daily for 21 days; subsequent courses repeated after 7-day tablet-free interval (during which withdrawal bleeding occurs); for starting routines see under Dose above

Sunya 20/75® (Stragen) PoM

Tablets, s/c, gestodene 75 micrograms, ethinylestradiol 20 micrograms, net price 3 × 21-tab pack = £6.62

Dose 1 tablet daily for 21 days; subsequent courses repeated after 7-day tablet-free interval (during which withdrawal bleeding occurs); for starting routines see under Dose above

Low strength (transdermal)

Ethinylestradiol with Norelgestromin

Evra® (Janssen-Cilag) ▼ PoM

Patches, self-adhesive (releasing ethinylestradiol approx. 20 micrograms/24 hours and norelgestromin approx. 150 micrograms/24 hours); net price 9-patch pack = £16.26. Counselling, administration

Dose 1 patch to be applied once weekly for three weeks, followed by a 7-day patch-free interval; subsequent courses repeated after 7-day patch-free interval (during which withdrawal bleeding occurs); for starting routines see under Dose above

Note Adhesives or bandages should not be used to hold patch in place. If patch no longer sticky do not reapply but use a new patch.

The *Scottish Medicines Consortium* has advised (September 2003) that *Evra®* patches should be restricted for use in women who are likely to comply poorly with combined oral contraceptives

Standard strength

Ethinylestradiol with Levonorgestrel

Logynon® (Schering Health) PoM

6 light brown tablets, ethinylestradiol 30 micrograms, levonorgestrel 50 micrograms;

5 white tablets, ethinylestradiol 40 micrograms, levonorgestrel 75 micrograms;

10 ochre tablets, ethinylestradiol 30 micrograms, levonorgestrel 125 micrograms.

Net price 3 × 21-tab pack = £4.12

Dose 1 tablet daily for 21 days, starting with light brown tablet marked 1 on day 1 of cycle; repeat after 7-day tablet-free interval

Logynon ED® (Schering Health) PoM

6 light brown tablets, ethinylestradiol 30 micrograms, levonorgestrel 50 micrograms;

5 white tablets, ethinylestradiol 40 micrograms, levonorgestrel 75 micrograms;

10 ochre tablets, ethinylestradiol 30 micrograms, levonorgestrel 125 micrograms;

7 white, inactive tablets.

Net price 3 × 28-tab pack = £4.12

Dose 1 tablet daily for 28 days, starting on day 1 of cycle with active tablet (withdrawal bleeding occurs when inactive tablets being taken); subsequent courses repeated without interval; for starting routines see under Dose above

Microgynon 30® (Schering Health) PoM

Tablets, s/c, levonorgestrel 150 micrograms, ethinylestradiol 30 micrograms. Net price 3 × 21-tab pack = £2.99

Dose 1 tablet daily for 21 days; subsequent courses repeated after 7-day tablet-free interval (during which withdrawal bleeding occurs); for starting routines see under Dose above

Microgynon 30 ED® (Schering Health) PoM

Tablets, beige, levonorgestrel 150 micrograms, ethinylestradiol 30 micrograms, white inactive tablets. Net price 3 × 28-tab (7 are inactive) pack = £2.69

Dose 1 tablet daily for 28 days starting on day 1 of cycle with active tablet (withdrawal bleeding occurs when inactive tablets being taken); subsequent courses repeated without interval; for starting routines see also under Dose above

Ovranette® (Wyeth) PoM

Tablets, levonorgestrel 150 micrograms, ethinylestradiol 30 micrograms. Net price 3 × 21-tab pack = £2.29

Dose 1 tablet daily for 21 days; subsequent courses repeated after 7-day tablet-free interval (during which withdrawal bleeding occurs); for starting routines see under Dose above

Trinordiol® (Wyeth) PoM

6 light brown tablets, ethinylestradiol 30 micrograms, levonorgestrel 50 micrograms;

5 white tablets, ethinylestradiol 40 micrograms, levonorgestrel 75 micrograms;

10 ochre tablets, ethinylestradiol 30 micrograms, levonorgestrel 125 micrograms.

Net price 3 × 21-tab pack = £4.04

Dose 1 tablet daily for 21 days, starting with light brown tablet marked 1 on day 1 of cycle; repeat after 7-day tablet-free interval

Ethinylestradiol with Norethisterone

BiNovum® (Janssen-Cilag) PoM

7 white tablets ethinylestradiol 35 micrograms, norethisterone 500 micrograms

14 peach tablets, ethinylestradiol 35 micrograms, norethisterone 1mg.

Net price 3 × 21-tab pack = £2.08

Dose 1 tablet daily for 21 days, starting with white tablet on day 1 of cycle; repeat after 7-day tablet-free interval

Brevinor® (Pharmacia) PoM

Tablets, blue, norethisterone 500 micrograms, ethinylestradiol 35 micrograms. Net price 3 × 21-tab pack = £1.99

Dose 1 tablet daily for 21 days; subsequent courses repeated after 7-day tablet-free interval (during which withdrawal bleeding occurs); for starting routines see under Dose above

Loestrin 30® (Galen) PoM

Tablets, pale green, norethisterone acetate 1.5 mg, ethinylestradiol 30 micrograms. Net price 3 × 21-tab pack = £3.90

Dose 1 tablet daily for 21 days; subsequent courses repeated after 7-day tablet-free interval (during which withdrawal bleeding occurs); for starting routines see under Dose above

Norimin® (Pharmacia) PoM

Tablets, norethisterone 1 mg, ethinylestradiol 35 micrograms. Net price 3 × 21-tab pack = £2.28

Dose 1 tablet daily for 21 days; subsequent courses repeated after 7-day tablet-free interval (during which withdrawal bleeding occurs); for starting routines see under Dose above

Ovysmen® (Janssen-Cilag) PoM

Tablets, norethisterone 500 micrograms, ethinylestradiol 35 micrograms. Net price 3 × 21-tab pack = £1.58

Dose 1 tablet daily for 21 days; subsequent courses repeated after 7-day tablet-free interval (during which withdrawal bleeding occurs); for starting routines see under Dose above

Synphase® (Pharmacia) PoM

7 blue tablets, ethinylestradiol 35 micrograms, norethisterone 500 micrograms;

9 white tablets, ethinylestradiol 35 micrograms, norethisterone 1 mg;

5 blue tablets, ethinylestradiol 35 micrograms, norethisterone 500 micrograms.

Net price 21-tab pack = £1.20

Dose 1 tablet daily for 21 days, starting with blue tablet marked 1 on day 1 of cycle; repeat after 7-day tablet-free interval

TriNovum® (Janssen-Cilag) PoM

7 white tablets, ethinylestradiol 35 micrograms, norethisterone 500 micrograms;

7 light peach tablets, ethinylestradiol 35 micrograms, norethisterone 750 micrograms;

7 peach tablets, ethinylestradiol 35 micrograms, norethisterone 1 mg.

Net price 3 × 21-tab pack = £2.89

Dose 1 tablet daily for 21 days, starting with white tablet on day 1 of cycle; repeat after 7-day tablet-free interval

◢Ethinylestradiol with Norgestimate

Cilest® (Janssen-Cilag) PoM

Tablets, blue, norgestimate 250 micrograms, ethinylestradiol 35 micrograms. Net price 3 × 21-tab pack = £5.97, 6 × 21-tab pack = £11.94

Dose 1 tablet daily for 21 days; subsequent courses repeated after 7-day tablet-free interval (during which withdrawal bleeding occurs); for starting routines see under Dose above

◢Ethinylestradiol with Desogestrel

See Risk of Venous Thromboembolism in notes above before prescribing

Marvelon® (Organon) PoM

Tablets, desogestrel 150 micrograms, ethinylestradiol 30 micrograms. Net price 3 × 21-tab pack = £6.70

Dose 1 tablet daily for 21 days; subsequent courses repeated after 7-day tablet-free interval (during which withdrawal bleeding occurs); for starting routines see under Dose above

◢Ethinylestradiol with Drospirenone

Yasmin® (Schering Health) PoM

Tablets, f/c, yellow, drospirenone 3 mg, ethinylestradiol 30 micrograms. Net price 3 × 21-tab pack = £14.70

Cautions use with care if increased concentration of potassium might be hazardous; renal impairment (Appendix 3)

Dose 1 tablet daily for 21 days; subsequent courses repeated after 7-day tablet-free interval (during which withdrawal bleeding occurs); for starting routines see under Dose above

Note The *Scottish Medicines Consortium* has advised (March 2003) that *Yasmin®* is not recommended

◢Ethinylestradiol with Gestodene

See Risk of Venous Thromboembolism in notes above before prescribing

Femodene® (Schering Health) PoM

Tablets, s/c, gestodene 75 micrograms, ethinylestradiol 30 micrograms. Net price 3 × 21-tab pack = £7.18

Dose 1 tablet daily for 21 days; subsequent courses repeated after 7-day tablet-free interval (during which withdrawal bleeding occurs); for starting routines see under Dose above

Femodene® ED (Schering Health) PoM

Tablets, s/c, gestodene 75 micrograms, ethinylestradiol 30 micrograms. Net price 3 × 28-tab (7 are inactive) pack = £7.18

Dose 1 tablet daily for 28 days, starting on day 1 of cycle with active tablet (withdrawal bleeding occurs when inactive tablets being taken); subsequent courses repeated without interval; for starting routines see under Dose above

Katya 30/75® (Stragen) PoM

Tablets, s/c, gestodene 75 micrograms, ethinylestradiol 30 micrograms. Net price 3 × 21-tab pack = £5.03

Dose 1 tablet daily for 21 days; subsequent courses repeated after 7-day tablet-free interval (during which withdrawal bleeding occurs); for starting routines see under Dose above

Triadene® (Schering Health) PoM

6 beige tablets, ethinylestradiol 30 micrograms, gestodene 50 micrograms;

5 dark brown tablets, ethinylestradiol 40 micrograms, gestodene 70 micrograms;

10 white tablets, ethinylestradiol 30 micrograms, gestodene 100 micrograms.

Net price 3 × 21-tab pack = £9.54

Dose 1 tablet daily for 21 days, starting with beige tablet marked 'start' on day 1 of cycle; repeat after 7-day tablet-free interval

◢Mestranol with Norethisterone

Norinyl-1® (Pharmacia) PoM

Tablets, norethisterone 1 mg, mestranol 50 micrograms. Net price 3 × 21-tab pack = £2.19

Dose 1 tablet daily for 21 days; subsequent courses repeated after 7-day tablet-free interval (during which withdrawal bleeding occurs); for starting routines see under Dose above

◢Ethinylestradiol with cyproterone acetate

See Co-cyprindiol (section 13.6.2)

7.3.2 Progestogen-only contraceptives

7.3.2.1 Oral progestogen-only contraceptives
7.3.2.2 Parenteral progestogen-only contraceptives
7.3.2.3 Intra-uterine progestogen-only device

7.3.2.1 Oral progestogen-only contraceptives

Oral progestogen-only preparations may offer a suitable alternative when oestrogens are contra-indicated (including those patients with venous thrombosis or a past history or predisposition to venous thrombosis), but have a higher failure rate than combined preparations. They are suitable for older women, for heavy smokers, and for those with hypertension, valvular heart disease, diabetes mellitus, and migraine. Menstrual irregularities (oligomenorrhoea, menorrhagia) are more common but tend to resolve on long-term treatment.

Interactions Effectiveness of oral progestogen-only preparations is not affected by antibacterials that do not induce liver enzymes. The efficacy of oral progestogen-only preparations is, however, reduced by enzyme-inducing drugs and an additional or alternative contraceptive method is recommended during treatment with an enzyme-inducing drug and for at least 4 weeks afterwards—see p. 428 and Appendix 1 (progestogens).

Surgery All progestogen-only contraceptives (including those given by injection) are suitable for use as an alternative to combined oral contraceptives before major elective surgery, before all surgery to the legs, or before surgery which involves prolonged immobilisation of a lower limb.

Starting routine One tablet daily, on a continuous basis, starting on day 1 of cycle and taken at the same time each day (if delayed by longer than 3 hours contraceptive protection may be lost). Additional contraceptive precautions are not necessary when initiating treatment.

Changing from a combined oral contraceptive Start on the day following completion of the combined oral contraceptive course without a break (or in the case of ED tablets omitting the inactive ones).

After childbirth Start any time after 3 weeks postpartum (increased risk of breakthrough bleeding if started earlier)—lactation is not affected.

Missed pill The following advice is now recommended by family planning organisations:

> 'If you forget a pill, take it as soon as you remember and carry on with the next pill at the right time. If the pill was more than 3 hours (12 hours for *Cerazette*®) overdue you are not protected. Continue normal pill-taking but you must also use another method, such as the condom, for the next 2 days.'

The Faculty of Family Planning and Reproductive Health Care recommends emergency contraception (see p. 437) if one or more progestogen-only contraceptive tablets are missed or taken more than 3 hours (12 hours for *Cerazette*®) late and unprotected intercourse has occurred before 2 further tablets have been correctly taken.

Diarrhoea and vomiting Vomiting and persistent, severe diarrhoea can interfere with the absorption of oral progestogen-only contraceptives. If vomiting occurs within 2 hours of taking an oral progestogen-only contraceptive, another pill should be taken as soon as possible. If a replacement pill is not taken within 3 hours (12 hours for *Cerazette*®) of the normal time for taking the progestogen-only pill, or in cases of persistent vomiting or very severe diarrhoea, additional precautions should be used during illness and for 2 days after recovery (see also under Missed pill above).

ORAL PROGESTOGEN-ONLY CONTRACEPTIVES
(Progestogen-only pill, 'POP')

Indications contraception

Cautions arterial disease; sex-steroid dependent cancer; past ectopic pregnancy; malabsorption syndromes; active trophoblastic disease (until return to normal of urine and plasma gonadotrophin concentration); functional ovarian cysts; active liver disease; recurrent cholestatic jaundice; history of jaundice in pregnancy; **interactions**: p. 428 and Appendix 1 (progestogens)

Other conditions The product literature advises caution in patients with history of thromboembolism, hypertension, diabetes mellitus and migraine; evidence for caution in these conditions is unsatisfactory

Contra-indications pregnancy; undiagnosed vaginal bleeding; severe arterial disease; liver tumour; porphyria (section 9.8.2); history of breast cancer but can be used after 5 years if no evidence of disease and non-hormonal contraceptive methods unacceptable

Side-effects menstrual irregularities (see also notes above); nausea, vomiting, headache, dizziness, breast discomfort, depression, skin disorders, disturbance of appetite, weight changes, changes in libido

Breast cancer There is a small increase in the risk of having breast cancer diagnosed in women using, or who have recently used, a progestogen-only contraceptive pill; this relative risk may be due to an earlier diagnosis. The most important risk factor appears to be the age at which the contraceptive is stopped rather than the duration of use; the risk disappears gradually during the 10 years after stopping and there is no excess risk by 10 years. The CSM has advised that a possible small increase in the risk of breast cancer should be weighed against the benefits

Dose

- 1 tablet daily at same time each day, starting on day 1 of cycle then continuously; if administration delayed for 3 hours (12 hours for *Cerazette*®) or more it should be regarded as a 'missed pill', see notes above

Cerazette® (Organon) PoM
Tablets, f/c, desogestrel 75 micrograms. Net price 3 × 28-tab pack = £8.85

The *Scottish Medicines Consortium* has advised (September 2003) that *Cerazette*® should be restricted for use in women who cannot tolerate oestrogen-containing contraceptives or in whom these preparations are contra-indicated

Femulen® (Pharmacia) PoM
Tablets, etynodiol diacetate 500 micrograms. Net price 3 × 28-tab pack = £3.31

Micronor® (Janssen-Cilag) PoM
Tablets, norethisterone 350 micrograms. Net price 3 × 28-tab pack = £1.76

Norgeston® (Schering Health) PoM
Tablets, s/c, levonorgestrel 30 micrograms. Net price 35-tab pack = 98p

Noriday® (Pharmacia) PoM
Tablets, norethisterone 350 micrograms. Net price 3 × 28-tab pack = £2.10

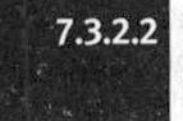

7.3.2.2 Parenteral progestogen-only contraceptives

Medroxyprogesterone acetate (*Depo-Provera*®) is a long-acting progestogen given by intramuscular injection; it is as effective as the combined oral preparations but because of its prolonged action it should never be given without *full counselling backed by the patient information leaflet*. It may be used as a short-term or long-term contraceptive for women who have been counselled about the likelihood of menstrual disturbance and the potential for a delay in return to full fertility. Delayed return of fertility and irregular cycles may occur after discontinuation of treatment but there is no evidence of permanent infertility. Heavy bleeding has been reported in patients given medroxyprogesterone acetate in the immediate puerperium (the first dose is best delayed until 6 weeks after birth). If the woman is not breast-feeding, the first injection may be given within 5 days postpartum (she should be warned that the risk of heavy or prolonged bleeding may be increased).

Reduction in bone mineral density and, rarely, osteoporosis and osteoporotic fractures have also been reported with medroxyprogesterone acetate. The reduction in bone mineral density occurs in the first 2–3 years of use and then stabilises. See also CSM advice below.

CSM advice

The CSM has advised that:

- in adolescents, medroxyprogesterone acetate (*Depo-Provera*®) be used only when other methods of contraception are inappropriate;
- in all women, benefits of using medroxyprogesterone acetate beyond 2 years should be evaluated against risks;
- in women with risk factors for osteoporosis a method of contraception other than medroxyprogesterone acetate should be considered.

Norethisterone enantate (*Noristerat*®) is a long-acting progestogen given as an oily injection which provides contraception for 8 weeks; it is used as short-term interim contraception e.g. before vasectomy becomes effective.

An **etonogestrel-releasing implant** (*Implanon*®), consisting of a single flexible rod, is also available; the rod is inserted subdermally into the lower surface of the upper arm and it provides effective contraception for up to 3 years. In women with a body mass index greater than 35 kg/m^2, blood etonogestrel concentrations are lower and therefore the implant may not provide effective contraception during the third year; earlier replacement should be considered in such patients. Local reactions such as bruising and itching may occur at the insertion site. The contraceptive effect of *Implanon*® is rapidly reversed on removal of the implant. *The doctor or nurse administering (or removing) the system should be fully trained in the technique and should provide full counselling backed by the patient information leaflet.*

The cautions, contra-indications, and side-effects of oral progestogen-only contraceptives apply to parenteral progestogen-only contraceptives, except that parenteral preparations reliably inhibit ovulation and therefore protect against ectopic pregnancy and functional ovarian cysts.

Interactions Effectiveness of parenteral progestogen-only contraceptives is not affected by antibacterials that do not induce liver enzymes. However, effectiveness of norethisterone and etonogestrel (but not medroxyprogesterone acetate) may be reduced by enzyme-inducing drugs; additional contraceptive precautions should be taken whilst taking the enzyme-inducing drug and for 4 weeks after stopping it *or* an alternative contraceptive method should be considered if *long-term* use of the enzyme-inducing drug is contemplated.

PARENTERAL PROGESTOGEN-ONLY CONTRACEPTIVES

Indications contraception, see also notes above and under preparations (roles vary according to preparation)

Cautions see notes above and under preparations; possible risk of breast cancer, see oral progestogen-only contraceptives (section 7.3.2.1); history during pregnancy of pruritus or of deterioration of otosclerosis, disturbances of lipid metabolism; **interactions**: see notes above and Appendix 1 (progestogens)

Counselling Full counselling backed by *patient information leaflet* required before administration

Contra-indications see notes above; history of breast cancer but can be used after 5 years if no evidence of disease and non-hormonal contraceptive methods unacceptable

Side-effects see notes above; injection-site reactions

Dose

- See under preparations

Injectable preparations

Depo-Provera® (Pharmacia) PoM

Injection (aqueous suspension), medroxyprogesterone acetate 150 mg/mL, net price 1-mL prefilled syringe = £6.01, 1-mL vial = £5.01. Counselling, see patient information leaflet

Dose by deep intramuscular injection, 150 mg within first 5 days of cycle or within first 5 days after parturition (delay until 6 weeks after parturition if breast-feeding); for long-term contraception, repeated every 12 weeks (if interval greater than 12 weeks and 5 days, rule out pregnancy before next injection and advise patient to use additional contraceptive measures (e.g. barrier) for 14 days after the injection)

Noristerat® (Schering Health) PoM

Injection (oily), norethisterone enantate 200 mg/mL, net price 1-mL amp = £3.59. Counselling, see patient information leaflet

Dose by deep intramuscular injection given very slowly *into gluteal muscle*, short-term contraception, 200 mg within first 5 days of cycle or immediately after parturition (duration 8 weeks); may be repeated once after 8 weeks (withhold breast-feeding for neonates with severe or persistent jaundice requiring medical treatment)

Implants

Implanon® (Organon) PoM

Implant, containing etonogestrel 68 mg in each flexible rod, net price = £81.00. Counselling, see patient information leaflet

Dose by subdermal implantation, no previous hormonal contraceptive, 1 implant inserted during first 5 days of cycle; parturition or abortion in second trimester, 1 implant inserted between days 21–28 after delivery or abortion (if inserted after 28 days additional precautions necessary for next 7 days); abortion in first trimester, 1 implant inserted immediately; changing from an oral contraceptive, consult product literature; remove within 3 years of insertion

7.3.2.3 Intra-uterine progestogen-only device

The progestogen-only intra-uterine system, *Mirena*®, releases **levonorgestrel** directly into the uterine cavity. It is licensed for use as a contraceptive, for the treatment of primary menorrhagia and for the prevention of endometrial hyperplasia during oestrogen replacement therapy. This may therefore be a contraceptive method of choice for women who have excessively heavy menses.

The effects of the progestogen-only intra-uterine system are mainly local and hormonal including prevention of endometrial proliferation, thickening of cervical mucus, and suppression of ovulation in some women (in some cycles). In addition to the progestogenic activity, the intra-uterine system itself may contribute slightly to the contraceptive effect. Return of fertility after removal is rapid and appears to be complete.

Advantages of the progestogen-only intra-uterine system over copper intra-uterine devices are that there may be an improvement in any dysmenorrhoea and a reduction in blood loss; there is also evidence that the frequency of pelvic inflammatory disease may be reduced (particularly in the youngest age groups who are most at risk).

In primary menorrhagia, menstrual bleeding is reduced significantly within 3–6 months of inserting the progestogen-only intra-uterine system, probably because it prevents endometrial proliferation. Another treatment should be considered if menorrhagia does not improve within this period (section 6.4.1.2).

Cautions and contra-indications Generally the cautions and contra-indications for the progestogen-only intra-uterine system are as for standard intra-uterine devices (section 7.3.4), but the risk of ectopic pregnancy is considerably smaller. Although the progestogen-only intra-uterine system produces little systemic progestogenic activity, it is usually avoided for 5 years after any evidence of breast cancer. However, the system can be considered for a woman in long-term remission from breast cancer who has menorrhagia and requires effective contraception. Since levonorgestrel is released close to the site of the main contraceptive action (on cervical mucus and endometrium) progestogenic side-effects and interactions are less likely; in particular, enzyme-inducing drugs are unlikely to significantly reduce the contraceptive effect of the progestogen-only intra-uterine system and additional contraceptive precautions are not required.

Side-effects Initially, changes in the pattern and duration of menstrual bleeding (spotting or prolonged bleeding) are common; endometrial disorders should be ruled out before insertion and the patient should be fully counselled (and provided with a patient information leaflet). Improvement in progestogenic side-effects, such as mastalgia and mood changes, and in the bleeding pattern usually occurs a few months after insertion and bleeding may often become very light or absent. Functional ovarian cysts (usually asymptomatic) can occur and usually resolve spontaneously (ultrasound monitoring recommended).

INTRA-UTERINE PROGESTOGEN-ONLY SYSTEM

Indications see under Dose

Cautions see notes above; active liver disease; liver tumour; in case of pregnancy—remove system (teratogenicity cannot be excluded); advanced uterine atrophy; not suitable for emergency contraception; interactions: see notes above and Appendix 1 (progestogens)

Contra-indications see notes above

Side-effects see notes above; also abdominal pain; peripheral oedema; nervousness; salpingitis and pelvic inflammatory disease; pelvic pain, back pain; *rarely* hirsutism, hair loss, pruritus, migraine, rash

Mirena® (Schering Health) PoM

Intra-uterine system, T-shaped plastic frame (impregnated with barium sulphate and with threads attached to base) with polydimethylsiloxane reservoir releasing levonorgestrel 20 micrograms/24 hours. Net price = £83.16. Counselling, see patient information leaflet

Dose Contraception and menorrhagia, insert into uterine cavity within 7 days of onset of menstruation (anytime if replacement) or immediately after first-trimester termination by curettage; postpartum insertions should be delayed until 6 weeks after delivery; effective for 5 years.

Prevention of endometrial hyperplasia during oestrogen replacement therapy, insert during last days of menstruation or withdrawal bleeding or anytime if amenorrhoeic; effective for 4 years

7.3.3 Spermicidal contraceptives

Spermicidal contraceptives are useful additional safeguards but do not give adequate protection if used alone except where fertility is already significantly diminished (section 6.4.1.1); they are suitable for use with barrier methods. They have two components: a spermicide and a vehicle which itself may have some inhibiting effect on sperm activity.

Spermicidal contraceptives are not suitable for use in those with or at high risk of sexually transmitted diseases (including HIV); high frequency use of the spermicide nonoxinol '9' has been associated with genital lesions, which may increase the risk of acquiring these infections.

> **CSM advice**
> Products such as petroleum jelly (*Vaseline®*), baby oil and oil-based vaginal and rectal preparations are likely to damage condoms and contraceptive diaphragms made from latex rubber, and may render them less effective as a barrier method of contraception and as a protection from sexually transmitted diseases (including HIV).

Gygel® (Marlborough)

Gel, nonoxinol '9' 2%, net price 30 g = £4.25

Excipients include hydroxybenzoates (parabens), propylene glycol, sorbic acid

Condoms No evidence of harm to latex condoms and diaphragms

7.3.4 Contraceptive devices

Intra-uterine devices

The intra-uterine device (IUD) is suitable for older parous women and as a second-line contraceptive in young nulliparous women who should be carefully screened because they have an increased background risk of pelvic inflammatory disease.

Smaller devices have been introduced to minimise side-effects; these consist of a plastic carrier wound with copper wire or fitted with copper bands; some also have a central core of silver to prevent fragmentation of the copper. Fertility declines with age and therefore a copper intra-uterine device which is fitted in a woman over the age of 40, may remain in the uterus until menopause. The intra-uterine device *Gyne-T 380®* (Janssen-Cilag) is no longer available, but some women may have the device in place until 2009. The intra-uterine devices *Multiload® Cu250* and *Multiload® Cu250 Short* (Organon) have been discontinued, but some women may have the devices in place until 2011.

A frameless, copper-bearing intra-uterine device (*GyneFix®*) is also available. It consists of a knotted, polypropylene thread with 6 copper sleeves; the device is anchored in the uterus by inserting the knot into the uterine fundus. *The healthcare professional inserting (or removing) the device should be fully trained in the technique and should provide full counselling backed by the patient information leaflet.*

The timing and technique of fitting an intra-uterine device are critical for its subsequent performance and call for proper training and experience. Devices should not be fitted during the heavy days of the period; they are best fitted after the end of menstruation and before the calculated time of implantation. The main excess risk of infection occurs in the first 20 days after insertion and is believed to be related to existing carriage of a sexually transmitted disease, therefore pre-screening (at least for chlamydia) should ideally be performed. The woman should be advised to attend *as an emergency* if she experiences sustained pain during the next 20 days.

An intra-uterine device should not be removed in mid-cycle unless an additional contraceptive was used for the previous 7 days. If removal is essential post-coital contraception should be considered.

If an intra-uterine device fails and the woman wishes to continue to full-term the device should be removed in the first trimester if possible.

INTRA-UTERINE CONTRACEPTIVE DEVICES

Indications see notes above

Cautions see notes above; also anaemia, menorrhagia (progestogen intra-uterine system might be preferable, section 7.3.2.3), endometriosis, severe primary dysmenorrhoea, history of pelvic inflammatory disease, diabetes, fertility problems, nulliparity and young age, severely scarred uterus (including after endometrial resection) or severe cervical stenosis; valvular heart disease or history of endocarditis (Table 2, section 5.1); drug- or disease-induced immunosuppression (risk of infection—avoid if marked immunosuppression); epilepsy (risk of seizure at time of insertion); increased risk of expulsion if inserted before uterine involution; gynaecological examination before insertion, 6–8 weeks after then annually but counsel women to see doctor promptly in case of significant symptoms, especially pain; anticoagulant therapy (avoid if possible); remove if pregnancy occurs; if pregnancy occurs, increased likelihood that it may be ectopic

Contra-indications pregnancy, severe anaemia, recent sexually transmitted infection (if not fully investigated and treated), unexplained uterine bleeding, distorted or small uterine cavity, genital malignancy, active trophoblastic disease (until return to normal of urine and plasma gonadotrophin concentration), pelvic inflammatory disease, established or marked immunosuppression; *copper devices:* copper allergy, Wilson's disease, medical diathermy

Side-effects uterine or cervical perforation, displacement, expulsion; pelvic infection may be exacerbated, menorrhagia, dysmenorrhoea, allergy; *on insertion:* pain (alleviated by NSAID such as ibuprofen 30 minutes before insertion) and bleeding, occasionally epileptic seizure and vasovagal attack

Flexi-T® 300 (FP)
Intra-uterine device, copper wire, surface area approx. 300 mm² wound on vertical stem of T-shaped plastic carrier, impregnated with barium sulphate for radio-opacity, monofilament thread attached to base of vertical stem; preloaded in inserter, net price = £9.29
For uterine length over 5 cm; replacement every 5 years (see also notes above)

Flexi-T® + 380 (FP)
Intra-uterine device, copper wire, surface area approx. 380 mm² wound on vertical stem of T-shaped plastic carrier with copper sleeve on each arm, impregnated with barium sulphate for radio-opacity, monofilament thread attached to base of vertical stem; preloaded in inserter, net price = £10.06
For uterine length over 6 cm; replacement every 5 years (see also notes above)

GyneFix® (FP)
Intra-uterine device, 6 copper sleeves with surface area of 330 mm² on polypropylene thread, net price = £26.12
Suitable for all uterine sizes; replacement every 5 years

Load® 375 (Durbin)
Intra-uterine device, copper wire, surface area approx. 375 mm², wound on vertical stem of U-shaped plastic carrier, impregnated with barium sulphate for radio-opacity, monofilament thread attached to base of vertical stem; preloaded in inserter, net price = £8.00
For uterine length over 7 cm; replacement every 5 years (see also notes above)

Mini TT 380® Slimline (Durbin)
Intra-uterine device, copper wire, wound on vertical stem of T-shaped plastic carrier with copper sleeves fitted flush on to distal portion of each horizontal arm, total surface area approx. 380 mm², impregnated with barium sulphate for radio-opacity, thread attached to base of vertical stem; easy-loading system, no capsule, net price = £11.70
For minimum uterine length 5 cm; replacement every 5 years (see also notes above)

Multiload® Cu375 (Organon)
Intra-uterine device, as *Load® 375*, with copper surface area approx. 375 mm² and vertical stem length 3.5 cm, net price = £9.24
For uterine length 6–9 cm; replacement every 5 years (see notes above)

Nova-T® 380 (Schering Health)
Intra-uterine device, copper wire with silver core, surface area approx. 380 mm² wound on vertical stem of T-shaped plastic carrier, impregnated with barium sulphate for radio-opacity, threads attached to base of vertical stem, net price = £13.50
For uterine length 6.5–9 cm; replacement every 5 years (see notes above)

T-Safe® CU 380 A (FP)
Intra-uterine device, copper wire, wound on vertical stem of T-shaped plastic carrier with copper collar on the distal portion of each arm, total surface area approx. 380 mm², impregnated with barium sulphate for radio-opacity, threads attached to base of vertical stem, net price = £10.09
For uterine length 6.5–9 cm; replacement every 10 years (see notes above)

TT 380® Slimline (Durbin)
Intra-uterine device, copper wire wound on vertical stem of T-shaped plastic carrier, with copper sleeves fitted flush on to distal portion of each horizontal arm, total surface area approx. 380 mm², impregnated with barium sulphate for radio-opacity, thread attached to base of vertical stem; easy-loading system, no capsule, net price = £11.70
For uterine length 6.5–9 cm; replacement every 10 years (see also notes above)

UT 380 Short® (Durbin)
Intra-uterine device, copper wire wound on vertical stem of T-shaped plastic carrier, total surface area approx. 380 mm², impregnated with barium sulphate for radio-opacity, thread attached to base of vertical stem; net price = £10.53
For uterine length 5–7 cm; replacement every 5 years (see also notes above)

UT 380 Standard® (Durbin)
Intra-uterine device, copper wire, surface area approx. 380 mm², wound on vertical stem of T-shaped plastic carrier, impregnated with barium sulphate for radio-opacity, thread attached to base of vertical stem; net price = £10.53
For uterine length 6.5–9 cm; replacement every 5 years (see also notes above)

Other contraceptive devices

Contraceptive caps

Type A contraceptive pessary
Opaque rubber, sizes 1 (50 mm), 2 (55 mm), 3 (60 mm), 4 (65 mm), 5 (75 mm), net price = £6.85

Type B contraceptive pessary
Opaque rubber, sizes 22 to 31 mm (rising in steps of 3 mm), net price = £8.46

Type C contraceptive pessary
Opaque rubber, sizes 1 to 3 (42, 48, and 54 mm), net price = £7.26

Silicone contraceptive pessary
Silicone, sizes 22, 26, and 30 mm, net price = £15.00
Brands include *FemCap®*

Contraceptive diaphragms

Type A Diaphragm with flat metal spring
Transparent rubber with flat metal spring, sizes 55–95 mm (rising in steps of 5 mm), net price = £5.78
Brands include *Reflexions®*

Type B Diaphragm with coiled metal spring
Opaque rubber with coiled metal spring, sizes 60–100 mm (rising in steps of 5 mm), net price = £6.59
Brands include *Ortho®*
Silicone with coiled metal spring, sizes 60–90 mm (rising in steps of 5 mm), net price = £8.35
Brands include *Milex Omniflex®*

Type C Arcing Spring Diaphragm
Opaque rubber with arcing spring, sizes 60–95 mm (rising in steps of 5 mm), net price = £7.49
Brands include *All-Flex®*
Silicone with arcing spring, sizes 60–90 mm (rising in steps of 5 mm), net price = £8.35
Brands include *Milex Arcing Style®*

Fertility thermometer

Fertility (Ovulation) Thermometer (Zeal)
Mercury in glass thermometer, range 35 to 39°C (graduated in 0.1°C), net price = £1.89
For monitoring ovulation for the fertility awareness method of contraception

7.3.5 Emergency contraception

Hormonal methods

Hormonal emergency contraception involves the use of **levonorgestrel**. It is effective if taken within 72 hours (3 days) of unprotected intercourse; taking the dose as soon as possible increases efficacy. Levonorgestrel may also be used between 72 and 120 hours after unprotected intercourse [unlicensed use] but efficacy decreases with time. Hormonal emergency contraception is less effective than insertion of an intra-uterine device (see below).

If vomiting occurs within 2 hours of taking levonorgestrel, a replacement dose should be given. If an anti-emetic is required domperidone is preferred.

When prescribing hormonal emergency contraception the doctor should explain:

- that the next period may be early or late;
- that a barrier method of contraception needs to be used until the next period;
- the need to return promptly if any lower abdominal pain occurs because this could signify an ectopic pregnancy and also in 3 to 4 weeks if the subsequent menstrual bleed is abnormally light, heavy or brief, or is absent, or if she is otherwise concerned).

Intra-uterine pregnancy despite treatment: see Appendix 4 (levonorgestrel).

Interactions The effectiveness of hormonal emergency contraception is reduced by enzyme-inducing drugs; a copper intra-uterine device can be offered instead or the dose of levonorgestrel should be increased to a total of 3 mg taken as a single dose [unlicensed dose—advise women accordingly]. There is no need to increase the dose for emergency contraception if the patient is taking antibacterials that are not enzyme inducers.

LEVONORGESTREL

Indications emergency contraception

Cautions see notes above; past ectopic pregnancy; severe malabsorption syndromes; active trophoblastic disease (until return to normal of urine and plasma gonadotrophin concentration); pregnancy (see notes above and Appendix 4); breast-feeding (Appendix 5); **interactions**: see notes above and Appendix 1 (progestogens)

Contra-indications porphyria (section 9.8.2)

Side-effects menstrual irregularities (see also notes above), nausea, low abdominal pain, fatigue, headache, dizziness, breast tenderness, vomiting

Dose

- 1.5 mg as a single dose as soon as possible after coitus (preferably within 12 hours but no later than after 72 hours)

[1]Levonelle® One Step (Schering Health)
Tablets, levonorgestrel 1.5 mg, net price 1-tab pack = £13.83

1. Can be sold to women over 16 years; when supplying emergency contraception to the public, pharmacists should refer to guidance issued by the Royal Pharmaceutical Society of Great Britain

Levonelle® 1500 (Schering Health) PoM
Tablets, levonorgestrel 1.5 mg, net price 1-tab pack = £5.11

Intra-uterine device

Insertion of an intra-uterine device is more effective than the hormonal methods of emergency contraception. A copper intra-uterine contraceptive device (section 7.3.4) can be inserted up to 120 hours (5 days) after unprotected intercourse; sexually transmitted diseases should be tested for and insertion of the device should usually be covered by antibacterial prophylaxis (e.g. azithromycin 1 g as a single dose). If intercourse has occurred more than 5 days previously, the device can still be inserted up to 5 days after the earliest likely calculated ovulation (i.e. within the minimum period before implantation).

7.4 Drugs for genito-urinary disorders

7.4.1 Drugs for urinary retention
7.4.2 Drugs for urinary frequency, enuresis, and incontinence
7.4.3 Drugs used in urological pain
7.4.4 Bladder instillations and urological surgery
7.4.5 Drugs for erectile dysfunction

For drugs used in the treatment of urinary-tract infections see section 5.1.13.

7.4.1 Drugs for urinary retention

Acute retention is painful and is treated by catheterisation.

Chronic retention is painless and often long-standing. Catheterisation is unnecessary unless there is deterioration of renal function. After the cause has initially been established and treated, drugs may be required to increase detrusor muscle tone.

Benign prostatic hyperplasia is treated either surgically or medically with alpha-blockers (see below). Dutasteride and finasteride (section 6.4.2) are alternatives to alpha-blockers, particularly in men with a significantly enlarged prostate.

Alpha-blockers

The selective alpha-blockers, **alfuzosin**, **doxazosin**, **indoramin**, **prazosin**, **tamsulosin** and **terazosin** relax smooth muscle in benign prostatic hyperplasia producing an increase in urinary flow-rate and an improvement in obstructive symptoms.

Cautions Since selective alpha-blockers reduce blood pressure, patients receiving antihypertensive treatment may require reduced dosage and specialist supervision. Caution may be required in the elderly and in patients with hepatic impairment (Appendix 2) and renal impairment (Appendix 3). For **interactions** see Appendix 1 (alpha-blockers).

Contra-indications Alpha-blockers should be avoided in patients with a history of postural hypotension and micturition syncope.

Side-effects Side-effects of selective alpha-blockers include drowsiness, hypotension (notably postural hypotension), syncope, asthenia, depression, headache, dry mouth, gastro-intestinal disturbances (including nausea, vomiting, diarrhoea, constipation), oedema, blurred vision, rhinitis, erectile disorders (including priapism), tachycardia, and palpitations. Hypersensitivity reactions including rash, pruritus and angioedema have also been reported.

ALFUZOSIN HYDROCHLORIDE

Indications see notes above
Cautions see notes above
Contra-indications see notes above; severe hepatic impairment
Side-effects see notes above; also flushes and chest pain
Dose
- 2.5 mg 3 times daily, max. 10 mg daily; ELDERLY initially 2.5 mg twice daily

First dose effect First dose may cause collapse due to hypotensive effect (therefore should be taken on retiring to bed). Patient should be warned to lie down if symptoms such as dizziness, fatigue or sweating develop, and to remain lying down until they abate completely

Xatral® (Sanofi-Synthelabo) PoM
Tablets, f/c, alfuzosin hydrochloride 2.5 mg, net price 60-tab pack = £21.20. Label: 3, counselling, see dose above

Modified release
Besavar® XL (Winthrop) PoM
Tablets, m/r, yellow/white, alfuzosin hydrochloride 10 mg, net price 30-tab pack = £13.28. Label: 3, 21, 25, counselling, see above
Dose benign prostatic hyperplasia 10 mg once daily
Acute urinary retention associated with benign prostatic hyperplasia in men over 65 years, 10 mg once daily for 2–3 days during catheterisation and for one day after removal; max. 4 days

Xatral® XL (Sanofi-Synthelabo) PoM
Tablets, m/r, yellow/white, alfuzosin hydrochloride 10 mg, net price 10-tab pack = £4.42, 30-tab pack = £13.28. Label: 3, 21, 25, counselling, see above
Dose benign prostatic hyperplasia 10 mg once daily
Acute urinary retention associated with benign prostatic hyperplasia in men over 65 years, 10 mg once daily for 2–3 days during catheterisation and for one day after removal; max. 4 days

DOXAZOSIN

Indications see notes above and section 2.5.4
Cautions see notes above and section 2.5.4
Contra-indications see notes above
Side-effects see notes above and section 2.5.4

Dose

- Initially 1 mg daily; dose may be doubled at intervals of 1–2 weeks according to response, up to max. 8 mg daily; usual maintenance 2–4 mg daily

Preparations
Section 2.5.4

INDORAMIN

Indications see notes above and section 2.5.4
Cautions see notes above and section 2.5.4
Contra-indications see notes above and section 2.5.4
Side-effects see notes above and section 2.5.4
Dose

- 20 mg twice daily; increased if necessary by 20 mg every 2 weeks to max. 100 mg daily in divided doses; ELDERLY, 20 mg at night may be adequate

Doralese® (Chemidex) PoM
Tablets, yellow, f/c, indoramin 20 mg, net price 60-tab pack = £25.85. Label: 2

PRAZOSIN

Indications see notes above and section 2.5.4
Cautions see notes above and section 2.5.4
Contra-indications see notes above and section 2.5.4
Side-effects see notes above and section 2.5.4; also paraesthesia, arthralgia, epistaxis, nervousness, dyspnoea, hallucinations, and alopecia
Dose

- Initially 500 micrograms twice daily for 3–7 days, subsequently adjusted according to response; usual maintenance (and max.) 2 mg twice daily; ELDERLY initiate with lowest possible dose

First dose effect First dose may cause collapse due to hypotensive effect (therefore should be taken on retiring to bed). Patient should be warned to lie down if symptoms such as dizziness, fatigue or sweating develop, and to remain lying down until they abate completely

Preparations
Section 2.5.4

TAMSULOSIN HYDROCHLORIDE

Indications see notes above
Cautions see notes above; also cataract surgery (risk of intraoperative floppy iris syndrome)
Contra-indications see notes above; severe hepatic impairment
Side-effects see notes above
Dose

- 400 micrograms daily as a single dose

Tamsulosin hydrochloride (Non-proprietary) PoM
Capsules, m/r, tamsulosin hydrochloride 400 micrograms, net price 30-cap pack = £6.85. Label: 25
Brands include *Bazetham® MR, Contiflo® XL, Diffundox® XL, Omnic® MR, Stronazon® MR, Tabphyn® MR*

Flomaxtra® XL (Astellas) PoM
Tablets, m/r, tamsulosin hydrochloride 400 micrograms. Net price 30-tab pack = £17.55. Label: 25

TERAZOSIN

Indications see notes above and section 2.5.4
Cautions see notes above and section 2.5.4
Contra-indications see notes above
Side-effects see notes above and section 2.5.4; also weight gain, paraesthesia, dyspnoea, thrombocytopenia, nervousness, decreased libido, back pain and pain in extremities
Dose

- Initially 1 mg at bedtime; if necessary dose may be doubled at intervals of 1–2 weeks according to response, up to max. 10 mg once daily; usual maintenance 5–10 mg daily

First dose effect First dose may cause collapse due to hypotensive effect (therefore should be taken on retiring to bed). Patient should be warned to lie down if symptoms such as dizziness, fatigue or sweating develop, and to remain lying down until they abate completely

Terazosin (Non-proprietary) PoM
Tablets, terazosin (as hydrochloride) 2 mg, net price 28-tab pack = £3.06; 5 mg, 28-tab pack = £4.51; 10 mg, 28-tab pack = £11.77. Label: 3, counselling, see dose above

Hytrin® (Amdipharm) PoM
Tablets, terazosin (as hydrochloride) 2 mg (yellow) net price, 28-tab pack = £4.57; 5 mg (tan), 28-tab pack = £8.57; 10 mg (blue), 28-tab pack = £17.14; starter pack (for benign prostatic hyperplasia) of 7 × 1-mg tab with 14 × 2-mg tab and 7 × 5-mg tab = £10.97. Label: 3, counselling, see dose above

Parasympathomimetics

The parasympathomimetic **bethanechol** increases detrusor muscle contraction. However, it has only a limited role in the relief of urinary retention; its use has been superseded by catheterisation.

Distigmine inhibits the breakdown of acetylcholine. It may help patients with an upper motor neurone neurogenic bladder.

BETHANECHOL CHLORIDE 

Indications urinary retention, but see notes above
Cautions autonomic neuropathy (use lower initial dose); **interactions**: Appendix 1 (parasympathomimetics)
Contra-indications peptic ulcer; intestinal or urinary obstruction; conditions where increased motility of the urinary or gastro-intestinal tract could be harmful; cardiovascular disorders (including recent myocardial infarction, bradycardia, and heart block); hypotension; obstructive airways disease; epilepsy; parkinsonism; hyperthyroidism; pregnancy (Appendix 4); breast-feeding
Side-effects nausea, vomiting, diarrhoea, abdominal pain, increased salivation, eructation; flushing, hypotension, bradycardia; bronchoconstriction, rhinorrhoea; headache; increased lacrimation; increased sweating
Dose

- 10–25 mg 3–4 times daily half an hour before food

Myotonine® (Glenwood) PoM
Tablets, scored, bethanechol chloride 10 mg, net price 20 = £1.01; 25 mg, 20 = £1.30. Label: 22

DISTIGMINE BROMIDE

Indications postoperative urinary retention (see notes above), neurogenic bladder; myasthenia gravis (section 10.2.1)

Cautions peptic ulcer; conditions where increased motility of the urinary or gastro-intestinal tract could be harmful; oesophagitis; cardiovascular disease; bronchospasm; epilepsy; parkinsonism; pregnancy (Appendix 4); breast-feeding; **interactions**: Appendix 1 (parasympathomimetics)

Contra-indications intestinal or urinary obstruction; severe circulatory insufficiency; asthma

Side-effects abdominal pain, diarrhoea, increased salivation; bradycardia, AV block, hypotension; dyspnoea; muscle twitching; increased lacrimation, miosis; increased sweating

Dose

- Urinary retention, 5 mg daily, half an hour before breakfast
- Neurogenic bladder, 5 mg daily or on alternate days, half an hour before breakfast

Ubretid® (Rhône-Poulenc Rorer) PoM

Tablets, scored, distigmine bromide 5 mg, net price 30-tab pack = £41.22. Label: 22

7.4.2 Drugs for urinary frequency, enuresis, and incontinence

Urinary incontinence

Incontinence in adults which arises from detrusor instability is managed by combining drug therapy with conservative methods for managing urge incontinence such as pelvic floor exercises and bladder training; stress incontinence is generally managed by non-drug methods. **Duloxetine**, an inhibitor of serotonin and noradrenaline re-uptake can be added and is licensed for the treatment of moderate to severe stress incontinence in women; it may be more effective when used as an adjunct to pelvic floor exercises.

Involuntary detrusor contractions cause urgency and urge incontinence, usually with frequency and nocturia. Antimuscarinic drugs reduce these contractions and increase bladder capacity. **Oxybutynin** also has a direct relaxant effect on urinary smooth muscle. Side-effects limit the use of oxybutynin but they may be reduced by starting at a lower dose. A modified-release preparation of oxybutynin is effective and has fewer side-effects; a transdermal patch is also available. The efficacy and side-effects of **tolterodine** are comparable to those of modified-release oxybutynin. **Flavoxate** has less marked side-effects but it is also less effective. **Darifenacin**, **propiverine**, **solifenacin**, and **trospium** are newer antimuscarinic drugs licensed for urinary frequency, urgency, and incontinence. The need for continuing antimuscarinic drug therapy should be reviewed after 3–6 months.

Propantheline and tricyclic antidepressants were used for urge incontinence but they are little used now because of their side-effects. The use of imipramine is limited by its potential to cause cardiac side-effects.

Purified bovine collagen implant (*Contigen®*, Bard) is indicated for *urinary incontinence* caused by intrinsic sphincter deficiency (poor or non-functioning bladder outlet mechanism). The implant should be inserted only by surgeons or physicians trained in the technique for injection of the implant.

Cautions Antimuscarinic drugs should be used with caution in the elderly (especially if frail), in those with autonomic neuropathy, and in those susceptible to angle-closure glaucoma. They should also be used with caution in hiatus hernia with reflux oesophagitis, hepatic impairment (Appendix 2), and renal impairment (Appendix 3). Antimuscarinics can worsen hyperthyroidism, coronary artery disease, congestive heart failure, hypertension, prostatic hyperplasia, arrhythmias, and tachycardia. For **interactions** see Appendix 1 (antimuscarinics).

Contra-indications Antimuscarinic drugs should be avoided in patients with myasthenia gravis, significant bladder outflow obstruction or urinary retention, severe ulcerative colitis, toxic megacolon, and in gastro-intestinal obstruction or intestinal atony.

Side-effects Side-effects of antimuscarinic drugs include dry mouth, gastro-intestinal disturbances including constipation, blurred vision, dry eyes, drowsiness, difficulty in micturition (less commonly urinary retention), palpitation, and skin reactions (including dry skin, rash, and photosensitivity); also headache, diarrhoea, angioedema, arrhythmias, and tachycardia. Central nervous system stimulation, such as restlessness, disorientation, hallucination, and convulsion may occur; children are at higher risk of these effects. Antimuscarinic drugs can reduce sweating, leading to heat sensations and fainting in hot environments or in patients with fever, and *very rarely* may precipitate angle-closure glaucoma.

DARIFENACIN

Indications urinary frequency, urgency, and incontinence

Cautions see notes above; breast-feeding (Appendix 5)

Contra-indications see notes above; pregnancy (Appendix 4)

Side-effects see notes above; also *less commonly* ulcerative stomatitis, flatulence, taste disturbance, oedema, hypertension, dyspnoea, cough, rhinitis, weakness, dizziness, insomnia, impotence, and vaginitis

Dose

- ADULT over 18 years, 7.5 mg once daily, increased if necessary after 2 weeks to 15 mg once daily

Emselex® (Novartis) ▼ PoM

Tablets, m/r, darifenacin (as hydrobromide) 7.5 mg (white), net price 28-tab pack = £26.13; 15 mg (peach), 28-tab pack = £26.13. Label: 3, 25

Note The *Scottish Medicines Consortium* has advised (May 2007) that darifenacin (*Emselex®*) is accepted for restricted use as a second-line drug for the symptomatic treatment of urge incontinence, urinary frequency, and urgency in patients with overactive bladder syndrome

DULOXETINE

Indications moderate to severe stress urinary incontinence in women; major depressive disorder (section 4.3.4); diabetic neuropathy (section 4.3.4)

Cautions elderly; cardiac disease; hypertension (avoid if uncontrolled); history of mania; history of seizures; raised intra-ocular pressure, susceptibility to angle-closure glaucoma; bleeding disorders or concomitant use of drugs that increase risk of bleeding; **interactions**: Appendix 1 (duloxetine)

Withdrawal Nausea, vomiting, headache, anxiety, dizziness, paraesthesia, sleep disturbances, and tremor are the most common features of abrupt withdrawal or marked reduction of the dose; dose should be reduced over at least 1–2 weeks

Contra-indications hepatic impairment; renal impairment (avoid if creatinine clearance less than 30 mL/minute); pregnancy (Appendix 4); breast-feeding (Appendix 5)

Side-effects nausea, vomiting, dyspepsia, constipation, diarrhoea, abdominal pain, weight changes, decreased appetite, flatulence, dry mouth; palpitation, hot flush; insomnia, abnormal dreams, paraesthesia, drowsiness, anxiety, headache, dizziness, fatigue, weakness, tremor, nervousness, anorexia; sexual dysfunction; visual disturbances; sweating, pruritus; *less commonly* gastritis, halitosis, hepatitis, bruxism, tachycardia, hypertension, postural hypotension, syncope, raised cholesterol, vertigo, taste disturbance, cold extremities, impaired temperature regulation, impaired attention, movement disorders, muscle twitching, musculoskeletal pain, thirst, stomatitis, hypothyroidism, urinary disorders, and photosensitivity; *rarely* mania and angle-closure glaucoma; *also reported* supraventricular arrhythmia, chest pain, hallucinations, suicidal behaviour (see Suicidal Behaviour and Antidepressant Therapy, p. 202), seizures, hypersensitivity reactions including urticaria, angioedema, rash (including Stevens-Johnson syndrome) and anaphylaxis, hyponatraemia (see Hyponatraemia and Antidepressant Therapy, p. 202)

Dose

- ADULT over 18 years, 40 mg twice daily, assess for benefit and tolerability after 2–4 weeks

  Note Initial dose of 20 mg twice daily for 2 weeks can minimise side-effects

Yentreve® (Lilly) ▼ PoM

Capsules, duloxetine (as hydrochloride) 20 mg (blue), net price 28-cap pack = £15.40, 56-cap pack = £30.80; 40 mg (orange/blue), 56-cap pack = £30.80. Label: 2

Cymbalta® (Lilly) ▼ PoM

Section 4.3.4 (major depressive episode and diabetic neuropathy)

FLAVOXATE HYDROCHLORIDE

Indications urinary frequency and incontinence, dysuria, urgency; bladder spasms due to catheterisation, cytoscopy, or surgery

Cautions see notes above; pregnancy (Appendix 4), breast-feeding (Appendix 5)

Contra-indications see notes above; gastro-intestinal haemorrhage

Side-effects see notes above; also dizziness, vertigo, fatigue, eosinophilia, leucopenia, urticaria, erythema, and pruritus

Dose

- ADULT and ADOLESCENT over 12 years, 200 mg 3 times daily

Urispas 200® (Recordati) PoM

Tablets, f/c, flavoxate hydrochloride 200 mg, net price 90-tab pack = £11.87

OXYBUTYNIN HYDROCHLORIDE

Indications urinary frequency, urgency and incontinence, neurogenic bladder instability, and nocturnal enuresis associated with overactive bladder

Cautions see notes above; pregnancy (Appendix 4), porphyria (section 9.8.2)

Contra-indications see notes above; breast-feeding (Appendix 5)

Side-effects see notes above; also dizziness; *less commonly* anorexia, facial flushing; *rarely* night terrors; application site reactions with *patches*

Dose

- Initially 2.5–5 mg 2–3 times daily increased if necessary to max. 5 mg 4 times daily; ELDERLY initially 2.5–3 mg twice daily, increased to 5 mg twice daily according to response and tolerance; CHILD over 5 years, neurogenic bladder instability, 2.5–3 mg twice daily increased to 5 mg twice daily (max. 5 mg 3 times daily); CHILD over 7 years, nocturnal enuresis associated with overactive bladder, 2.5–3 mg twice daily increased to 5 mg 2–3 times daily (last dose before bedtime)

Oxybutynin Hydrochloride (Non-proprietary) PoM

Tablets, oxybutynin hydrochloride 2.5 mg, net price 56-tab pack = £3.28; 3 mg, 56-tab pack = £9.15; 5 mg, 56-tab pack = £9.68, 84-tab pack = £2.86. Label: 3

Cystrin® (Sanofi-Synthelabo) PoM

Tablets, oxybutynin hydrochloride 3 mg, net price 56-tab pack = £9.15; 5 mg (scored), 84-tab pack = £22.88. Label: 3

Ditropan® (Sanofi-Synthelabo) PoM

Tablets, both blue, scored, oxybutynin hydrochloride 2.5 mg, net price 84-tab pack = £6.86; 5 mg, 84-tab pack = £13.34. Label: 3

Elixir, oxybutynin hydrochloride 2.5 mg/5 mL. Net price 150-mL pack = £5.74. Label: 3

Modified release

Lyrinel® XL (Janssen-Cilag) PoM

Tablets, m/r, oxybutynin hydrochloride 5 mg (yellow), net price 30-tab pack = £10.49; 10 mg (pink), 30-tab pack = £20.98. Label: 3, 25

Dose Initially 5 mg once daily, adjusted according to response in steps of 5 mg at weekly intervals; max. 20 mg once daily; CHILD over 6 years, neurogenic bladder instability, initially 5 mg once daily, adjusted according to response in steps of 5 mg at weekly intervals; max. 15 mg once daily

Note Patients taking immediate-release oxybutynin may be transferred to the nearest equivalent daily dose of *Lyrinel® XL*

Transdermal preparations

Kentera® (UCB Pharma) PoM

Patches, self-adhesive, oxybutynin 36 mg (releasing oxybutynin approx. 3.9 mg/24 hours), net price 8-patch pack = £27.20. Label: 3, counselling, administration

Dose ADULT over 18 years, urinary frequency, urgency and incontinence, apply 1 patch twice weekly to clean, dry, unbroken skin on abdomen, hip or buttock, remove after every 3–4 days and site replacement patch on a different area (avoid using same area for 7 days)

Note The *Scottish Medicines Consortium* has advised (July 2005) that *Kentera®* should be restricted for use in patients who benefit from oral oxybutynin but cannot tolerate its side-effects

PROPANTHELINE BROMIDE

Indications adult enuresis

Cautions see notes above; ulcerative colitis, pregnancy (Appendix 4) and breast-feeding (Appendix 5)

Contra-indications see notes above

Side-effects see notes above; also facial flushing

Dose

- Initially 15 mg 3 times daily at least one hour before food and 30 mg at bedtime, subsequently adjusted according to response (max. 120 mg daily)

Preparations

Section 1.2

PROPIVERINE HYDROCHLORIDE

Indications urinary frequency, urgency and incontinence; neurogenic bladder instability

Cautions see notes above

Contra-indications see notes above; moderate to severe hepatic impairment; pregnancy (Appendix 4) and breast-feeding (Appendix 5)

Side-effects see notes above

Dose

- 15 mg 1–3 times daily, increased if necessary to max. 15 mg 4 times daily; CHILD not recommended

Detrunorm® (Amdipharm) PoM

Tablets, pink, s/c, propiverine hydrochloride 15 mg, net price 56-tab pack = £24.45. Label: 3

Modified release

Detrunorm® XL (Amdipharm) PoM

Capsules, orange/white, m/r, propiverine hydrochloride 30 mg, net price 28-cap pack = £24.45. Label: 3, 25

Dose urinary frequency, urgency, and incontinence, 30 mg once daily; CHILD not recommended

SOLIFENACIN SUCCINATE

Indications urinary frequency, urgency and urge incontinence

Cautions see notes above; neurogenic bladder disorder; pregnancy (Appendix 4)

Contra-indications see notes above; severe hepatic impairment (Appendix 2); haemodialysis; breast-feeding (Appendix 5)

Side-effects see notes above; gastro-oesophageal reflux, altered taste; fatigue; oedema

Dose

- 5 mg daily, increased if necessary to 10 mg once daily; CHILD not recommended

Note Max. 5 mg daily with concomitant itraconazole, ketoconazole, nelfinavir or ritonavir

Vesicare® (Astellas) PoM

Tablets, f/c, solifenacin succinate 5 mg (yellow), net price 30-tab pack = £27.62; 10 mg (pink), 30-tab pack = £35.91. Label: 3

TOLTERODINE TARTRATE

Indications urinary frequency, urgency and incontinence

Cautions see notes above

Contra-indications see notes above; pregnancy (Appendix 4) and breast-feeding (Appendix 5)

Side-effects see notes above; also dyspepsia, fatigue, flatulence, chest pain, dry eyes, peripheral oedema, paraesthesia

Dose

- ADULT over 18 years, 2 mg twice daily; reduce to 1 mg twice daily if necessary to minimise side-effects

Detrusitol® (Pharmacia) PoM

Tablets, f/c, tolterodine tartrate 1 mg, net price 56-tab pack = £29.03; 2 mg, 56-tab pack = £30.56. Label: 3

Modified release

Detrusitol® XL (Pharmacia) PoM

Capsules, blue, m/r, tolterodine tartrate 4 mg, net price 28-cap pack = £29.03. Label: 3, 25

Dose ADULT over 18 years, 4 mg once daily (dose form not appropriate for hepatic and renal impairment)

TROSPIUM CHLORIDE

Indications urinary frequency, urgency and incontinence

Cautions see notes above; pregnancy (Appendix 4); breast-feeding (Appendix 5)

Contra-indications see notes above

Side-effects see notes above; also flatulence, chest pain, dyspnoea, rash and asthenia

Dose

- 20 mg twice daily before food; CHILD not recommended

Regurin® (Galen) PoM

Tablets, brown, f/c, trospium chloride 20 mg, net price 60-tab pack = £26.00. Label: 23

Nocturnal enuresis

Nocturnal enuresis is a common occurrence in young children but persists in as many as 5% by 10 years of age. Treatment is not appropriate in children under 5 years and it is usually not needed in those aged under 7 years and in cases where the child and parents are not anxious about the bedwetting; however, children over 10 years usually require prompt treatment. An **enuresis alarm** should be first-line treatment for well-motivated children aged over 7 years because it may achieve a more sustained reduction of enuresis than use of drugs. Use of an alarm may be combined with drug therapy if either method alone is unsuccessful.

Drug therapy is not usually appropriate for children under 7 years of age; it can be used when alternative measures have failed, preferably on a short-term basis, to cover periods away from home for example. The possible side-effects of the various drugs should be borne in mind when they are prescribed.

Desmopressin (section 6.5.2), an analogue of vasopressin, is used for nocturnal enuresis; it is given by oral or by sublingual administration. Particular care is needed to avoid fluid overload. Treatment should not be continued for longer than 3 months without stopping for 1 week for full re-assessment. Desmopressin should not be given intranasally for nocturnal enuresis due to an increased incidence of side-effects.

Tricyclics (section 4.3.1) such as **amitriptyline**, **imipramine**, and less often **nortriptyline** are also used, but behavioural disturbances can occur and relapse is common after withdrawal. Treatment should not normally exceed 3 months unless a full physical examination is made and the child is fully re-assessed; toxicity following overdosage with tricyclics is of particular concern.

7.4.3 Drugs used in urological pain

The acute pain of *ureteric colic* may be relieved with **pethidine** (section 4.7.2). **Diclofenac** by injection or as suppositories (section10.1.1) is also effective and compares favourably with pethidine; other non-steroidal anti-inflammatory drugs are occasionally given by injection.

Lidocaine (lignocaine) gel is a useful topical application in *urethral pain* or to relieve the discomfort of catheterisation (section 15.2).

Alkalinisation of urine

Alkalinisation of urine can be undertaken with **potassium citrate**. The alkalinising action may relieve the discomfort of *cystitis* caused by lower urinary tract infections. **Sodium bicarbonate** is used as a urinary alkalinising agent in some metabolic and renal disorders (section 9.2.1.3).

POTASSIUM CITRATE

Indications relief of discomfort in mild urinary-tract infections; alkalinisation of urine

Cautions renal impairment (avoid if creatinine clearance less than 10 mL/minute; Appendix 3), cardiac disease; elderly; **interactions**: Appendix 1 (potassium salts)

Side-effects hyperkalaemia on prolonged high dosage, mild diuresis

Potassium Citrate Mixture BP (Potassium Citrate Oral Solution)
Oral solution, potassium citrate 30%, citric acid monohydrate 5% in a suitable vehicle with a lemon flavour. Extemporaneous preparations should be recently prepared according to the following formula: potassium citrate 3 g, citric acid monohydrate 500 mg, syrup 2.5 mL, quillaia tincture 0.1 mL, lemon spirit 0.05 mL, double-strength chloroform water 3 mL, water to 10 mL. Contains about 28 mmol K^{+}/10 mL. Label: 27

Dose 10 mL 3 times daily well diluted with water

Proprietary brands of potassium citrate are on sale to the public for the relief of discomfort in mild urinary-tract infections

SODIUM BICARBONATE

Indications relief of discomfort in mild urinary-tract infections; alkalinisation of urine

Cautions hepatic impairment (Appendix 2); renal impairment (Appendix 3), cardiac disease, pregnancy; patients on sodium-restricted diet; elderly; avoid prolonged use; **interactions**: Appendix 1 (antacids)

Side-effects belching, alkalosis on prolonged use

Dose

- 3 g in water every 2 hours until urinary pH exceeds 7; maintenance of alkaline urine 5–10 g daily

Preparations
Section 9.2.1 3

SODIUM CITRATE

Indications relief of discomfort in mild urinary-tract infections

Cautions renal impairment, cardiac disease, hypertension, pregnancy, patients on a sodium-restricted diet; elderly

Side-effects mild diuresis

Note Proprietary brands of sodium citrate are on sale to the public for the relief of discomfort in mild urinary-tract infections

Acidification of urine

Urine acidification is difficult; it is very occasionally used in the management of recurrent urinary-tract infections and to prevent renal stone formation, especially in patients with paraplegia or with a neurogenic bladder. Methenamine (section 5.1.13) requires acid urine for its antimicrobial activity.

Ammonium chloride may be used for urinary acidification but tolerance can develop rapidly. Vomiting and, with large doses, hypokalaemia and acidosis can also occur. Ammonium chloride oral solution needs to be prepared extemporaneously and may not be readily available. **Ascorbic acid** is less suitable for urine acidification because it is not always reliable and high doses, which can lead to renal stones in those with hyperoxaluria, are required.

For pH-modifying solutions for the maintenance of indwelling urinary catheters, see section 7.4.4.

Other preparations for urinary disorders

A terpene mixture (*Rowatinex*®) is claimed to be of benefit in *urolithiasis* for the expulsion of calculi.

Rowatinex® (Rowa) PoM
Capsules, yellow, e/c, anethol 4 mg, borneol 10 mg, camphene 15 mg, cineole 3 mg, fenchone 4 mg, pinene 31 mg. Net price 50 = £7.35. Label: 25

Dose 1–2 capsules 3–4 times daily before food; CHILD not recommended

7.4.4 Bladder instillations and urological surgery

Bladder infection Various solutions are available as irrigations or washouts.

Aqueous **chlorhexidine** (section 13.11.2) can be used in the management of common infections of the bladder but it is ineffective against most *Pseudomonas* spp. Solutions containing chlorhexidine 1 in 5000 (0.02%) are used but they may irritate the mucosa and cause burning and haematuria (in which case they should be discontinued); sterile **sodium chloride solution 0.9%** (physiological saline) is usually adequate and is preferred as a mechanical irrigant.

Continuous bladder irrigation with **amphotericin** 50 micrograms/mL (section 5.2) may be of value in mycotic infections.

Dissolution of blood clots Clot retention is usually treated by irrigation with sterile **sodium chloride solution 0.9%** but sterile **sodium citrate solution for bladder irrigation 3%** may also be helpful.

Bladder cancer Bladder instillations of **doxorubicin** (section 8.1.2), **mitomycin** (section 8.1.2), and **thiotepa** (section 8.1.1) are used for recurrent superficial bladder tumours. Such instillations reduce systemic side-effects; adverse effects on the bladder (e.g. micturition disorders and reduction in bladder capacity) may occur.

Instillation of **epirubicin** (section 8.1.2) is used for treatment and prophylaxis of certain forms of superficial bladder cancer; instillation of **doxorubicin** (section 8.1.2) is also used for some papillary tumours.

Instillation of **BCG** (Bacillus Calmette-Guérin), a live attenuated strain derived from *Mycobacterium bovis* (section 8.2.4), is licensed for the treatment of primary or recurrent bladder carcinoma *in-situ* and for the prevention of recurrence following transurethral resection.

Interstitial cystitis **Dimethyl sulfoxide** (dimethyl sulphoxide) may be used for symptomatic relief in patients with interstitial cystitis (Hunner's ulcer). 50 mL of a 50% solution (*Rimso-50*®—available on named-patient basis from Britannia) is instilled into the bladder, retained for 15 minutes, and voided by the patient. Treatment is repeated at intervals of 2 weeks. Bladder spasm and hypersensitivity reactions may occur and long-term use requires ophthalmic, renal, and hepatic assessment at intervals of 6 months.

SODIUM CITRATE

Indications bladder washouts, see notes above

Sterile Sodium Citrate Solution for Bladder Irrigation
sodium citrate 3%, dilute hydrochloric acid 0.2%, in purified water, freshly boiled and cooled, and sterilised

Urological surgery

There is a high risk of fluid absorption from the irrigant used in endoscopic surgery within the urinary tract; if this occurs in excess, hypervolaemia, haemolysis, and renal failure may result. **Glycine irrigation solution 1.5%** is the irrigant of choice for transurethral resection of the prostate gland and bladder tumours; **sterile sodium chloride solution 0.9%** (physiological saline) is used for percutaneous renal surgery.

GLYCINE

Indications bladder irrigation during urological surgery; see notes above
Cautions see notes above
Side-effects see notes above

Glycine Irrigation Solution (Non-proprietary)
Irrigation solution, glycine 1.5% in water for injections

Maintenance of indwelling urinary catheters

The deposition which occurs in catheterised patients is usually chiefly composed of phosphate and to minimise this the catheter (if latex) should be changed at least as often as every 6 weeks. If the catheter is to be left for longer periods a silicone catheter should be used together with the appropriate use of catheter maintenance solutions. Repeated blockage usually indicates that the catheter needs to be changed.

CATHETER PATENCY SOLUTIONS

Chlorhexidine 0.02%
Brands include *Uriflex C*®, 100-mL sachet = £2.40; *Uro-Tainer Chlorhexidine*®, 100-mL sachet = £2.60

Sodium chloride 0.9%
Brands include *OptiFlo S*®, 50- and 100-mL sachets = £3.20; *Uriflex S*®, 100-mL sachet = £2.40; *Uriflex SP*®, with integral drug additive port, 100-mL sachet = £2.40; *Uro-Tainer Sodium Chloride*®, 50- and 100-mL sachets = £2.99; *Uro-Tainer M*®, with integral drug additive port, 50- and 100-mL sachets = £2.90

Solution G
Citric acid 3.23%, magnesium oxide 0.38%, sodium bicarbonate 0.7%, disodium edetate 0.01%. Brands include *OptiFlo G*®, 50- and 100-mL sachets = £3.40; *Uriflex G*®, 100-mL sachet = £2.40; *Uro-Tainer*® *Twin Suby G*, 2 × 30-mL = £4.10

Solution R
Citric acid 6%, gluconolactone 0.6%, magnesium carbonate 2.8%, disodium edetate 0.01%. Brands include *OptiFlo R*®, 50- and 100-mL sachets = £3.40; *Uriflex R*®, 100-mL sachet = £2.40; *Uro-Tainer*® *Twin Solutio R*, 2 × 30-mL = £4.10

7.4.5 Drugs for erectile dysfunction

Reasons for failure to produce a satisfactory erection include *psychogenic, vascular, neurogenic,* and *endocrine abnormalities*; impotence can also be drug-induced. Intracavernosal injection or urethral application of vasoactive drugs under careful medical supervision is used for both diagnostic and therapeutic purposes.

Erectile disorders may also be treated with drugs given by mouth which increase the blood flow to the penis. Drugs should be used with caution if the penis is deformed (e.g. in angulation, cavernosal fibrosis, and Peyronie's disease).

Priapism If priapism occurs with alprostadil, treatment should not be delayed more than 6 hours and is as follows:

Initial therapy by penile aspiration—using aseptic technique a 19–21 gauge butterfly needle inserted into the corpus cavernosum and 20–50 mL of blood aspirated; if necessary the procedure may be repeated on the opposite side.

If initial aspiration is unsuccessful a second 19-21 gauge butterfly needle can be inserted into the opposite corpus cavernosum and sterile physiological saline introduced through the first needle and drained through the second.

If aspiration and lavage of corpora are unsuccessful, *cautious* intracavernosal injection of a sympathomimetic (section 2.7.2) with action on alpha-adrenergic receptors, continuously monitoring blood pressure and pulse (*extreme caution:* coronary heart disease, hypertension, cerebral ischaemia or if taking antidepressant) as follows:

- intracavernosal injections of phenylephrine 100–200 micrograms (0.5–1 mL of a 200 microgram/mL solution) every 5–10 minutes; max. total dose 1 mg [unlicensed indication] [*important:* if suitable strength of phenylephrine injection not available may be specially prepared by diluting 0.1 mL of the phenylephrine 1% (10 mg/mL) injection (section 2.7.2) to 5 mL with sodium chloride 0.9%];
  alternatively
- intracavernosal injections of adrenaline 10–20 micrograms (0.5–1 mL of a 20 microgram/mL solution) every 5–10 minutes; max. total dose 100 micrograms [unlicensed indication] [*important:* if suitable strength of adrenaline not available may be specially prepared by diluting 0.1 mL of the adrenaline 1 in 1000 (1 mg/mL, section 3.4.3) injection to 5 mL with sodium chloride 0.9%];
  alternatively
- intracavernosal injection of metaraminol (*caution: has been associated with fatal hypertensive crises*); metaraminol 1 mg (0.1 mL of 10 mg/mL metaraminol injection, section 2.7.2) is diluted to 50 mL with sodium chloride injection 0.9% and given carefully by slow injection into the corpora in 5-mL injections every 15 minutes [unlicensed indication].

If necessary the sympathomimetic injections can be followed by further aspiration of blood through the same butterfly needle.

If sympathomimetics unsuccessful, urgent surgical referral for management (possibly including shunt procedure).

Prescribing on the NHS Drug treatments for erectile dysfunction may only be prescribed on the NHS under certain circumstances (see individual preparations). The Department of Health (England) has recommended that treatment should also be available from specialist services (commissioned by Health Authorities and Primary Care Groups, and operating under local agreement) when the condition is causing severe distress; specialist centres should use form FP10(HP) or form HBP in Scotland or form WP10HP in Wales and endorse them 'SLS' if the treatment is to be dispensed in the community. The following criteria should be considered when assessing distress:

- significant disruption to normal social and occupational activities;
- a marked effect on mood, behaviour, social and environmental awareness;
- a marked effect on interpersonal relationships.

Alprostadil

Alprostadil (prostaglandin E_1) is given by intracavernosal injection or intraurethral application for the management of erectile dysfunction (after exclusion of treatable medical causes); it is also used as a diagnostic test.

ALPROSTADIL

Indications erectile dysfunction (including aid to diagnosis); neonatal congenital heart defects (section 7.1.1.1)

Cautions priapism—patients should be instructed to report any erection lasting 4 hours or longer—for management, see section 7.4.5; anatomical deformations of penis (painful erection more likely)—follow up regularly to detect signs of penile fibrosis (consider discontinuation if angulation, cavernosal fibrosis or Peyronie's disease develop); **interactions:** Appendix 1 (prostaglandins)

Contra-indications predisposition to prolonged erection (as in sickle cell anaemia, multiple myeloma or leukaemia); not for use with other agents for erectile dysfunction, in patients with penile implants or when sexual activity medically inadvisable; urethral application also contra-indicated in urethral stricture, severe hypospadia, severe curvature, balanitis, urethritis

Side-effects hypotension, hypertension; dizziness, headache; penile pain, other localised pain (buttocks, leg, testicular, abdominal); influenza-like syndrome; urethral burning, urethral bleeding; injection site reactions including penile fibrosis, penile oedema, penile rash, haematoma, haemosiderin deposits; *less commonly* nausea, dry mouth, vasodilatation, syncope, supraventricular extrasystole, rapid pulse, asthenia, leg cramps, pelvic pain, scrotal or testicular oedema, scrotal erythema, testicular thickening, micturation difficulties, haematuria, mydriasis, and sweating; local reactions including penile warmth, pruritus, irritation, penile numbness or sensitivity, balantitis, phimosis, priapism (see section 7.4.5 and under Cautions), abnormal ejaculation; *rarely* vertigo, urinary-tract infection, and hypersensitivity reactions (including rash, erythema, urticaria, and anaphylaxis)

Dose

- See under preparations below

Intracavernosal injection

[1]**Caverject®** (Pharmacia) PoM NHS

Injection, powder for reconstitution, alprostadil, net price 5-microgram vial = £7.73; 10-microgram vial = £9.24; 20-microgram vial = £11.94; 40-microgram vial = £21.58 (all with diluent-filled syringe, needles and swabs)

Caverject® Dual Chamber, double-chamber cartridges (containing alprostadil and diluent), net price 10-microgram cartridge (for doses 2.5–10 micrograms) = £7.35; 20-microgram cartridge (for doses 5–20 micrograms) = £9.50 (both with needles)

Dose by direct intracavernosal injection, ADULT over 18 years, erectile dysfunction, first dose 2.5 micrograms, second dose 5 micrograms (if some response to first dose) *or* 7.5 micrograms (if no response to first dose), increasing in steps of 5–10 micrograms to obtain dose suitable for producing erection lasting not more than 1 hour (neurological dysfunction, first dose 1.25 micrograms, second dose 2.5 micrograms, third dose 5 micrograms, increasing in steps of 5–10 micrograms to obtain suitable dose); if no response to dose then next higher dose can be given within 1 hour, if there is a response the next dose should not be given for at least 24 hours; usual dose 5–20 micrograms; max. 60 micrograms; max. frequency of injection not more than 3 times per week with at least 24 hour interval between injections

Note The first dose must be given by medically trained personnel; self-administration may only be undertaken after proper training

Aid to diagnosis, 10–20 micrograms as a single dose (where evidence of neurological dysfunction, initially 5 micrograms and max. 10 micrograms)—consult product literature for details

[1]**Viridal® Duo** (Schwarz) PoM NHS

Starter Pack (hosp. only), contents as for *Continuation Pack* below plus *Duoject* applicator, 10-microgram starter pack = £20.13, 20-microgram starter pack = £24.54, 40-microgram starter pack = £29.83; *Continuation Pack*, 2 double-chamber cartridges (containing alprostadil and diluent), 2 needles, swabs, 10-microgram continuation pack = £16.55, 20-microgram continuation pack = £21.39, 40-microgram continuation pack = £27.22; *Duoject®* applicator available free of charge from Schwarz

Dose by direct intracavernosal injection, ADULT over 18 years, erectile dysfunction, initially 5 micrograms (2.5 micrograms in neurogenic erectile dysfunction) increasing in steps of 2.5–5 micrograms to obtain dose suitable for producing erection not lasting more than 1 hour; usual range 10–20 micrograms; max. 40 micrograms; max. frequency of injection not more than 2–3 times per week with at least 24 hour interval between injections; reduce dose if erection lasts longer than 2 hours

Note The first dose must be given by medically trained personnel; self-administration may only be undertaken after proper training

1. NHS except to treat erectile dysfunction in men who:

- have diabetes, multiple sclerosis, Parkinson's disease, poliomyelitis, prostate cancer, severe pelvic injury, single gene neurological disease, spina bifida, or spinal cord injury;
- are receiving dialysis for renal failure;
- have had radical pelvic surgery, prostatectomy (including transurethral resection of the prostate), or kidney transplant;
- were receiving *Caverject®*, *Erecnos®*, *MUSE®*, *Viagra®*, or *Viridal®* for erectile dysfunction, at the expense of the NHS, on 14 September 1998;
- are suffering severe distress as a result of impotence (prescribed in specialist centres only, see notes above).

The prescription must be endorsed 'SLS'.

Urethral application

Counselling If partner pregnant barrier contraception should be used

[1]**MUSE®** (Meda) PoM NHS

Urethral application, alprostadil, net price 125-microgram single-use applicator = £9.89, 250-microgram single-use applicator = £10.76, 500-microgram single-use applicator = £10.76, 1-mg single-use applicator = £11.01 (all strengths also available in packs of 6 applicators)

Condoms no evidence of harm to latex condoms and diaphragms

Dose by direct urethral application, ADULT over 18 years, erectile dysfunction, initially 250 micrograms adjusted according to response (usual range 0.125–1 mg); max. 2 doses in 24 hours and 7 doses in 7 days)

Note The first dose must be given by medically trained personnel; self-administration may only be undertaken after proper training

Aid to diagnosis, 500 micrograms as a single dose

Phosphodiesterase type-5 inhibitors

Sildenafil, **tadalafil** and **vardenafil** are phosphodiesterase type-5 inhibitors licensed for the treatment of erectile dysfunction; they are not recommended for use with other treatments for erectile dysfunction. The patient should be assessed appropriately before prescribing sildenafil, tadalafil or vardenafil. Since these drugs are given by mouth there is a potential for drug interactions.

Cautions Sildenafil, tadalafil, and vardenafil should be used with caution in cardiovascular disease, left ventricular outflow obstruction, anatomical deformation of the penis (e.g. angulation, cavernosal fibrosis, Peyronie's disease), and in those with a predisposition to priapism (e.g. in sickle-cell disease, multiple myeloma, or leukaemia).

Contra-indications Sildenafil, tadalafil, and vardenafil are contra-indicated in patients receiving nitrates, in patients in whom vasodilation or sexual activity are inadvisable, or in patients with a previous history of non-arteritic anterior ischaemic optic neuropathy. In the absence of information, manufacturers contra-indicate these drugs in hypotension (avoid if systolic blood pressure below 90 mmHg), recent stroke, unstable angina, and myocardial infarction.

Side-effects The side-effects of sildenafil, tadalafil, and vardenafil include dyspepsia, nausea, vomiting, headache (including migraine), flushing, dizziness, myalgia, back pain, visual disturbances (non-arteritic anterior ischaemic optic neuropathy has been reported—stop drug if sudden visual impairment occurs), and nasal congestion. *Less common* side-effects include painful red eyes, palpitation, hypotension, hypertension, epistaxis. Other side-effects reported rarely include syncope, hypersensitivity reactions (including rash, facial oedema, and Stevens-Johnson syndrome), and priapism. Serious cardiovascular events (including arrhythmia, unstable angina, and myocardial infarction), sudden hearing loss (discontinue drug and seek medical advice), and retinal vascular occlusion have also been reported.

SILDENAFIL

Indications erectile dysfunction; pulmonary hypertension (section 2.5.1)

Cautions see notes above; also hepatic impairment (Appendix 2—avoid if severe); renal impairment (Appendix 3); bleeding disorders or active peptic ulceration; **interactions**: Appendix 1 (sildenafil)

Contra-indications see notes above; also hereditary degenerative retinal disorders

Side-effects see notes above

Dose

- ADULT over 18 years initially 50 mg approx. 1 hour before sexual activity, subsequent doses adjusted according to response to 25–100 mg as a single dose as needed; max. 1 dose in 24 hours (max. single dose 100 mg)
  Note Onset of effect may be delayed if taken with food

[1]**Viagra®** (Pfizer) PoM NHS
Tablets, all blue, f/c, sildenafil (as citrate), 25 mg, net price 4-tab pack = £16.59, 8-tab pack = £33.19; 50 mg, 4-tab pack = £19.34, 8-tab pack = £38.67; 100 mg, 4-tab pack = £23.50, 8-tab pack = £46.99

Revatio® (Pfizer) ▼ PoM
Section 2.5.1 (pulmonary hypertension)

TADALAFIL

Indications erectile dysfunction

Cautions see notes above; also hepatic impairment (Appendix 2); renal impairment (Appendix 3); **interactions**: Appendix 1 (tadalafil)

Contra-indications see notes above; also moderate heart failure, uncontrolled arrhythmias, uncontrolled hypertension

Side-effects see notes above; also increased sweating and abdominal pain reported

Dose

- ADULT over 18 years, initially 10 mg at least 30 minutes before sexual activity, subsequent doses adjusted according to response to 20 mg as a single dose; max. 1 dose in 24 hours (but daily use not recommended)
  Note Effect may persist for longer than 24 hours

[1]**Cialis®** (Lilly) PoM NHS
Tablets, f/c, tadalafil 10 mg (light yellow), net price 4-tab pack = £24.99; 20 mg (yellow), 4-tab pack = £24.99; 8-tab pack = £49.97

1. NHS except to treat erectile dysfunction in men who:

- have diabetes, multiple sclerosis, Parkinson's disease, poliomyelitis, prostate cancer, severe pelvic injury, single gene neurological disease, spina bifida, or spinal cord injury;
- are receiving dialysis for renal failure;
- have had radical pelvic surgery, prostatectomy (including transurethral resection of the prostate), or kidney transplant;
- were receiving *Caverject®*, *Erecnos®*, *MUSE®*, *Viagra®*, or *Viridal®* for erectile dysfunction, at the expense of the NHS, on 14 September 1998;
- are suffering severe distress as a result of impotence (prescribed in specialist centres only, see notes above).

The prescription must be endorsed 'SLS'.

VARDENAFIL

Indications erectile dysfunction

Cautions see notes above; also hepatic impairment (Appendix 2—avoid if severe); renal impairment (Appendix 3); bleeding disorders or active peptic ulceration; susceptibility to prolongation of QT interval (including concomitant use of drugs which prolong QT interval); **interactions**: Appendix 1 (vardenafil)

Contra-indications see notes above; also hereditary degenerative retinal disorders

Side-effects see notes above; also *less commonly* drowsiness, dyspnoea, increased lacrimation, photosensitivity; *rarely* anxiety, seizures, transient amnesia, hypertonia, and raised intra-ocular pressure

Dose

- ADULT over 18 years, initially 10 mg (ELDERLY and patients on alpha-blocker therapy 5 mg) approx. 25–60 minutes before sexual activity, subsequent doses adjusted according to response up to max. 20 mg as a single dose; max. 1 dose in 24 hours
  Note Onset of effect may be delayed if taken with high-fat meal

[1]**Levitra®** (Bayer) PoM NHS
Tablets, all orange, f/c, vardenafil (as hydrochloride trihydrate) 5 mg, net price 4-tab pack = £16.58, 8-tab pack = £33.19; 10 mg, 4-tab pack = £22.24, 8-tab pack = £44.47; 20 mg, 4-tab pack = £23.50, 8-tab pack = £46.99

Papaverine and phentolamine

Although not licensed the smooth muscle relaxant **papaverine** has also been given by intracavernosal injection for erectile dysfunction. Patients with neurological or psychogenic impotence are more sensitive to the effect of papaverine than those with vascular abnormalities. **Phentolamine** is added if the response is inadequate [unlicensed indication].

Persistence of the erection for longer than 4 hours is an emergency, see advice in section 7.4.5.

8 Malignant disease and immunosuppression

8.1 Cytotoxic drugs 448
8.1.1 Alkylating drugs 452
8.1.2 Anthracyclines and other cytotoxic antibiotics 454
8.1.3 Antimetabolites 456
8.1.4 Vinca alkaloids and etoposide 461
8.1.5 Other antineoplastic drugs 462
8.2 Drugs affecting the immune response 473
8.2.1 Antiproliferative immunosuppressants 473
8.2.2 Corticosteroids and other immunosuppressants 474
8.2.3 Rituximab and alemtuzumab 477
8.2.4 Other immunomodulating drugs 478
8.3 Sex hormones and hormone antagonists in malignant disease 482
8.3.1 Oestrogens 482
8.3.2 Progestogens 483
8.3.3 Androgens 483
8.3.4 Hormone antagonists 483
8.3.4.1 Breast cancer 483
8.3.4.2 Prostate cancer and gonadorelin analogues 486
8.3.4.3 Somatostatin analogues 488

8.1 Cytotoxic drugs

8.1.1 Alkylating drugs
8.1.2 Anthracyclines and other cytotoxic antibiotics
8.1.3 Antimetabolites
8.1.4 Vinca alkaloids and etoposide
8.1.5 Other antineoplastic drugs

The chemotherapy of cancer is complex and should be confined to specialists in oncology. Cytotoxic drugs have both anti-cancer activity and the potential to damage normal tissue. Chemotherapy may be given with a curative intent or it may aim to prolong life or to palliate symptoms. In an increasing number of cases chemotherapy may be combined with radiotherapy or surgery or both as either neoadjuvant treatment (initial chemotherapy aimed at shrinking the primary tumour, thereby rendering local therapy less destructive or more effective) or as adjuvant treatment (which follows definitive treatment of the primary disease, when the risk of sub-clinical metastatic disease is known to be high). All chemotherapy drugs cause side-effects and a balance has to be struck between likely benefit and acceptable toxicity.

CRM guidelines on handling cytotoxic drugs:

1. Trained personnel should reconstitute cytotoxics;
2. Reconstitution should be carried out in designated areas;
3. Protective clothing (including gloves) should be worn;
4. The eyes should be protected and means of first aid should be specified;
5. Pregnant staff should not handle cytotoxics;
6. Adequate care should be taken in the disposal of waste material, including syringes, containers, and absorbent material.

Intrathecal chemotherapy

A Health Service Circular (HSC 2003/010) provides guidance on the introduction of safe practice in NHS Trusts where intrathecal chemotherapy is administered. Support for training programmes is also available.

Copies, and further information may be obtained from:

Department of Health
PO Box 777
London SE1 6XH
Fax: 01623 724524

It is also available from the Department of Health website (www.dh.gov.uk)

Combinations of cytotoxic drugs are frequently more toxic than single drugs but have the advantage in certain tumours of enhanced response, reduced development of drug resistance and increased survival. However for some tumours, single-agent chemotherapy remains the treatment of choice.

> Most cytotoxic drugs are teratogenic and all may cause life-threatening toxicity; administration should be confined to those experienced in their use.
> Because of the complexity of dosage regimens in the treatment of malignant disease, dose statements have been omitted from some of the drug entries in this chapter. *In all cases detailed specialist literature should be consulted.*
> Prescriptions should **not** be repeated except on the instructions of a specialist.

Cytotoxic drugs fall into a number of classes, each with characteristic antitumour activity, sites of action, and toxicity. A knowledge of sites of metabolism and excretion is important because impaired drug handling as a result of disease is not uncommon and may result in enhanced toxicity.

Side-effects of cytotoxic drugs

Side-effects common to most cytotoxic drugs are discussed below whilst side-effects characteristic of a particular drug or class of drugs (e.g. neurotoxicity with vinca alkaloids) are mentioned in the appropriate sections. Manufacturers' product literature should be consulted for full details of side-effects associated with individual drugs.

Extravasation of intravenous drugs A number of cytotoxic drugs will cause severe local tissue necrosis if leakage into the extravascular compartment occurs. To reduce the risk of extravasation injury it is recommended that cytotoxic drugs are administered by appropriately trained staff. For information on the prevention and management of extravasation injury see section 10.3.

Oral mucositis A sore mouth is a common complication of cancer chemotherapy; it is most often associated with fluorouracil, methotrexate, and the anthracyclines. It is best to prevent the complication. Good mouth care (rinsing the mouth frequently and effective brushing of the teeth with a soft brush 2–3 times daily) is probably beneficial. For fluorouracil, sucking ice chips during short infusions of the drug is also helpful.

Once a sore mouth has developed, treatment is much less effective. Saline mouthwashes should be used but there is no good evidence to support the use of antiseptic or anti-inflammatory mouthwashes. In general, mucositis is self-limiting but with poor oral hygiene it can be a focus for blood-borne infection.

Tumour lysis syndrome Tumour lysis syndrome can occur as a result of massive cell breakdown following treatment of cancer sensitive to the chemotherapy. Features include hyperkalaemia, hyperuricaemia (see below), and hyperphosphataemia with hypocalcaemia; renal damage and arrhythmias can follow.

Hyperuricaemia Hyperuricaemia, which may be present in high-grade lymphoma and leukaemia, can be markedly worsened by chemotherapy and is associated with acute renal failure. Allopurinol (section 10.1.4) should be started 24 hours before treating such tumours and patients should be adequately hydrated. The dose of mercaptopurine or azathioprine should be reduced if allopurinol needs to be given concomitantly (see Appendix 1).

Rasburicase (section 10.1.4), a recombinant urate oxidase, is licensed for hyperuricaemia in patients with haematological malignancy, for details, see p. 557. It rapidly reduces plasma uric acid and may be of particular value in reducing complications following treatment of leukaemias or bulky lymphomas.

Nausea and vomiting Nausea and vomiting cause considerable distress to many patients who receive chemotherapy and, to a lesser extent, abdominal radiotherapy; it may lead to refusal of further treatment. Symptoms may be acute (occurring within 24 hours of treatment), delayed (first occurring more than 24 hours after treatment, or anticipatory (occurring prior to subsequent doses). Delayed and anticipatory symptoms are more difficult to control than acute symptoms and require different management.

Patients vary in their susceptibility to drug-induced nausea and vomiting; those affected more often include women, patients under 50 years of age, anxious patients, and those who experience motion sickness. Susceptibility also increases with repeated exposure to the cytotoxic drug.

Drugs may be divided according to their emetogenic potential and some examples are given below, but the symptoms vary according to the dose, to other drugs administered and to individual susceptibility.

Mildly emetogenic treatment—fluorouracil, etoposide, methotrexate (less than 100 mg/m^2), the vinca alkaloids, and abdominal radiotherapy.

Moderately emetogenic treatment—the taxanes, doxorubicin, intermediate and low doses of cyclophosphamide, mitoxantrone (mitozantrone), and high doses of methotrexate (0.1–1.2 g/m^2).

Highly emetogenic treatment—cisplatin, dacarbazine, and high doses of cyclophosphamide.

Prevention of acute symptoms. For patients at *low risk of emesis*, pretreatment with domperidone or, in adults over 20 years, with metoclopramide, continued for up to 24 hours after chemotherapy, is often effective (section 4.6). If metoclopramide or domperidone are not sufficiently effective, additional drugs such as dexamethasone (6–10 mg by mouth) or lorazepam (1–2 mg by mouth) may be used.

For patients at *high risk of emesis* or when other treatment is inadequate, a specific ($5HT_3$) serotonin antagonist (section 4.6), usually given by mouth, is often highly effective, particularly when used with dexamethasone; adding the neurokinin receptor antagonist, aprepitant (section 4.6) can improve control of cisplatin-related nausea and vomiting.

Prevention of delayed symptoms. Dexamethasone, given by mouth, is the drug of choice for preventing delayed symptoms; it is used alone or with metoclopramide or prochlorperazine. The $5HT_3$ antagonists may be less effective for delayed symptoms.

Prevention of anticipatory symptoms. Good symptom control is the best way to prevent anticipatory symptoms. Lorazepam can be helpful for its amnesic, sedative, and anxiolytic effects.

Bone-marrow suppression All cytotoxic drugs except vincristine and bleomycin cause bone-marrow depression. This commonly occurs 7 to 10 days after administration, but is delayed for certain drugs, such as carmustine, lomustine, and melphalan. Peripheral blood counts must be checked before each treatment, and doses should be reduced or therapy delayed if bone-marrow has not recovered.

Fever in a neutropenic patient (neutrophil count less than 1.0×10^9/litre) requires immediate broad-spectrum antibacterial therapy. Patients at low risk (those receiving chemotherapy for solid tumours, lymphoma or chronic leukaemia) can be treated with oral ciprofloxacin with or without co-amoxiclav (initially in hospital). All other patients should receive parenteral broad-spectrum antibacterial therapy. Appropriate bacteriological investigations should be conducted as soon as possible.

In selected patients, the duration and the severity of neutropenia can be reduced by the use of recombinant human granulocyte-colony stimulating factors, section 9.1.6.

Symptomatic anaemia is usually treated with red blood cell transfusions. Epoetin administered subcutaneously is also effective but not widely used.

Alopecia Reversible hair loss is a common complication, although it varies in degree between drugs and individual patients. No pharmacological methods of preventing this are available.

Reproductive function Most cytotoxic drugs are teratogenic and should not be administered during pregnancy, especially during the first trimester.

Contraceptive advice should be offered where appropriate before cytotoxic therapy begins (and should cover the duration of contraception required after therapy has ended). Regimens that do not contain an alkylating drug may have less effect on fertility, but those with an alkylating drug carry the risk of causing permanent male sterility (there is no effect on potency). Pre-treatment counselling and consideration of sperm storage may be appropriate. Women are less severely affected, though the span of reproductive life may be shortened by the onset of a premature menopause. No increase in fetal abnormalities or abortion-rate has been recorded in patients who remain fertile after cytotoxic chemotherapy.

Thromboembolism Venous thromboembolism can be a complication of cancer itself, but chemotherapy can also increase the risk.

Drugs for cytotoxic-induced side-effects

Anthracycline side-effects

Anthracycline-induced cardiotoxicity The anthracycline cytotoxic drugs are associated with dose-related, cumulative, and potentially life-threatening cardiotoxic side-effects.

Dexrazoxane, an iron chelator, is licensed for the prevention of chronic cumulative cardiotoxicity caused by doxorubicin or epirubicin treatment in advanced or metastatic cancer patients who have previously received anthracycline therapy. Patients receiving dexrazoxane should still be monitored for cardiac toxicity. The myelosuppressive effects of dexrazoxane may be additive to those of chemotherapy.

Anthracycline extravasation Dexrazoxane is licensed for the treatment of anthracycline extravasation. The first dose should be given as soon as possible and within six hours after the injury. For further information on the prevention and management of extravasation injury, see section 10.3.

> Local guidelines for the management of extravasation should be followed or specialist advice sought.

DEXRAZOXANE

Indications see notes above and under preparations

Cautions monitor full blood count; hepatic impairment (Appendix 2); renal impairment (Appendix 3)

Contra-indications pregnancy (Appendix 4); breast-feeding

Side-effects nausea, vomiting, dyspepsia, abdominal pain, diarrhoea, stomatitis, dry mouth, anorexia; dyspnoea; dizziness, syncope, asthenia, paraesthesia, tremor, fatigue, drowsiness; pyrexia; vaginal haemorrhage; myalgia; bone-marrow suppression; conjunctivitis; alopecia, pruritus; peripheral oedema, injection-site reactions including phlebitis

Dose

- See under preparations

Cardioxane® (Novartis) ▼ PoM

Intravenous infusion, powder for reconstitution, dexrazoxane (as hydrochloride), net price 500-mg vial = £156.57

Dose prevention of anthracycline-induced cardiotoxicity, ADULT over 18 years, by intravenous infusion (30 minutes prior to anthracycline administration), 20 times the doxorubicin-equivalent dose or 10 times the epirubicin-equivalent dose

Savene® (TopoTarget) ▼ PoM

Intravenous infusion, powder for reconstitution, dexrazoxane (as hydrochloride), net price 10 x 500-mg vials (with diluent) = £6750.00

Dose anthracycline extravasation, ADULT over 18 years, by intravenous infusion, 1 g/m² (max. 2 g) daily for 2 days, then 500 mg/m² for 1 day

Note Local coolants such as ice packs should be removed at least 15 minutes before administration

Chemotherapy-induced mucositis and myelosuppression

Folinic acid (given as calcium folinate) is used to counteract the folate-antagonist action of methotrexate and thus speed recovery from methotrexate-induced mucositis or myelosuppression ('folinic acid rescue').

Folinic acid is also used in the management of methotrexate overdose, together with other measures to maintain fluid and electrolyte balance, and to manage possible renal failure.

Folinic acid does not counteract the antibacterial activity of folate antagonists such as trimethoprim.

When folinic acid and fluorouracil are used together in metastatic colorectal cancer the response-rate improves compared to that with fluorouracil alone.

The calcium salt of **levofolinic acid**, a single isomer of folinic acid, is also used for rescue therapy following methotrexate administration, for cases of methotrexate overdose, and for use with fluorouracil for colorectal cancer. The dose of calcium levofolinate is generally half that of calcium folinate.

The disodium salt of folinic acid is also licensed for rescue therapy following methotrexate therapy and for use with fluorouracil for colorectal cancer.

Palifermin, a human keratinocyte growth factor, is licensed for the management of oral mucositis in patients with haematological malignancies receiving myeloablative therapy with autologous haematopoietic stem-cell support.

CALCIUM FOLINATE
(Calcium leucovorin)

Indications see notes above

Cautions avoid simultaneous administration of methotrexate; **not** indicated for pernicious anaemia or other megaloblastic anaemias due to vitamin B_{12} deficiency; pregnancy (Appendix 4) and breast-feeding (Appendix 5); **interactions:** Appendix 1 (folates)

Important Intrathecal injection **contra-indicated**

Side-effects hypersensitivity reactions; *rarely* pyrexia after parenteral use

Dose

Note Doses expressed as folinic acid

- Prevention of methotrexate-induced adverse effects, usually started 24 hours after start of methotrexate infusion, by intramuscular injection, *or* by intravenous injection, *or* by intravenous infusion, 15 mg, repeated every 6 hours for 24 hours (may be continued by mouth); consult local treatment protocol for further information
- Suspected methotrexate overdosage, by intravenous injection or by intravenous infusion (at a max. rate of 160 mg/minute), initial dose equal to or exceeding dose of methotrexate; consult poisons information service (p. 27) for advice on continuing management
- Adjunct to fluorouracil in colorectal cancer, consult product literature

Calcium Folinate (Non-proprietary) PoM

Tablets, scored, folinic acid (as calcium salt) 15 mg, net price 10-tab pack = £37.85, 30-tab pack = £85.74

Brands include *Refolinon®*

Note Not all strengths and pack sizes are available from all manufacturers

Injection, folinic acid (as calcium salt) 3 mg/mL, net price 1-mL amp = £2.28, 10-mL amp = £4.62; 7.5 mg/mL, net price 2-mL amp = £7.80; 10 mg/mL, net price 5-mL vial = £19.41, 10-mL vial = £35.09, 30-mL vial = £94.69, 35-mL vial = £90.98

Brands include *Lederfolin®*

Note Not all strengths and pack sizes are available from all manufacturers

Injection, powder for reconstitution, folinic acid (as calcium salt), net price 15-mg vial = £4.46; 30-mg vial = £8.36

CALCIUM LEVOFOLINATE
(Calcium levoleucovorin)

Indications see notes above

Cautions see Calcium Folinate

Side-effects see Calcium Folinate

Dose

Note Doses expressed as levofolinic acid

- Prevention of methotrexate-induced adverse effects, (usually started 24 hours after beginning of methotrexate infusion), by intramuscular injection, *or* by intravenous injection *or* by intravenous infusion, usually 7.5 mg every 6 hours for 10 doses
- Suspected methotrexate overdosage, by intravenous injection *or* by intravenous infusion (at a max. rate of 160 mg/minute), initial dose at least 50% of the dose of methotrexate; consult poisons information service (p. 27) for advice on continuing management
- Adjunct to fluorouracil in colorectal cancer, consult product literature

Isovorin® (Wyeth) ▼ PoM

Injection, levofolinic acid (as calcium salt) 10 mg/mL, net price 2.5-mL vial = £12.09, 5-mL vial = £26.00, 17.5-mL vial = £84.63

DISODIUM FOLINATE

Indications see notes above

Cautions see Calcium Folinate

Side-effects see Calcium Folinate

Dose

- As an antidote to methotrexate, see Calcium Folinate
- Adjunct to fluorouracil in colorectal cancer, consult product literature

Sodiofolin® (Medac) PoM

Injection, folinic acid (as disodium salt) 50 mg/mL, net price 2-mL vial = £35.09, 8-mL vial = £126.25, 18-mL vial = £284.07

PALIFERMIN

Indications see notes above

Cautions pregnancy (Appendix 4)

Contra-indications breast-feeding

Side-effects taste disturbance, thickening and discoloration of tongue; fever; oedema; arthralgia; rash, pruritus, erythema

Dose

- By intravenous injection, 60 micrograms/kg once daily for 3 doses (third dose given 24–48 hours before myeloablative therapy) then 3 further doses at least 24 hours after myeloablative therapy, starting on same day as (but after) stem-cell infusion; CHILD not recommended

Kepivance® (Amgen) ▼ PoM

Injection, powder for reconstitution, palifermin, net price 6.25-mg vial = £544.24

Urothelial toxicity

Haemorrhagic cystitis is a common manifestation of urothelial toxicity which occurs with the oxazaphosphorines, cyclophosphamide and ifosfamide; it is caused by the metabolite acrolein. **Mesna** reacts specifically with this metabolite in the urinary tract, preventing toxicity. Mesna is used routinely (preferably by mouth) in patients receiving ifosfamide, and in patients receiving cyclophosphamide by the intravenous route at a high dose (e.g. more than 2 g) or in those who experienced urothelial toxicity when given cyclophosphamide previously.

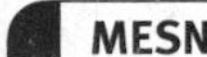

MESNA

Indications see notes above

Contra-indications hypersensitivity to thiol-containing compounds

Side-effects nausea, vomiting, colic, diarrhoea, fatigue, headache, limb and joint pains, depression, irritability, rash, hypotension and tachycardia; rarely hypersensitivity reactions (more common in patients with auto-immune disorders)

Dose

Note Doses calculated according to oxazaphosphorine (cyclophosphamide or ifosfamide) treatment—for details consult product literature

- By mouth, dose is given 2 hours *before* oxazaphosphorine treatment and repeated 2 and 6 hours *after* treatment
- By intravenous injection, dose is given *with* oxazaphosphorine treatment and repeated 4 and 8 hours *after* treatment

Uromitexan® (Baxter) PoM

Tablets, f/c, mesna 400 mg, net price 10-tab pack = £21.10; 600 mg, 10-tab pack = £27.40

Injection, mesna 100 mg/mL. Net price 4-mL amp = £1.95; 10-mL amp = £4.38

Note For oral administration contents of ampoule are taken in a flavoured drink such as orange juice or cola which may be stored in a refrigerator for up to 24 hours in a sealed container

8.1.1 Alkylating drugs

Extensive experience is available with these drugs, which are among the most widely used in cancer chemotherapy. They act by damaging DNA, thus interfering with cell replication. In addition to the side-effects common to many cytotoxic drugs (section 8.1), there are two problems associated with prolonged usage. Firstly, gametogenesis is often severely affected (section 8.1). Secondly, prolonged use of these drugs, particularly when combined with extensive irradiation, is associated with a marked increase in the incidence of acute non-lymphocytic leukaemia.

Cyclophosphamide is used for the treatment of chronic lymphocytic leukaemia, the lymphomas, soft-tissue and osteogenic sarcoma, and solid tumours. It is given by mouth or intravenously; it is inactive until metabolised by the liver. A urinary metabolite of cyclophosphamide, acrolein, can cause haemorrhagic cystitis; this is a rare but serious complication; increased fluid intake for 24–48 hours after intravenous injection, can prevent this complication. When high-dose therapy (e.g. more than 2 g intravenously) is used or when the patient is considered to be at high risk of cystitis (e.g. because of pelvic irradiation) mesna (given initially intravenously then by mouth) can also help prevent cystitis—see under Urothelial Toxicity (section 8.1).

Ifosfamide is related to cyclophosphamide and is given intravenously; mesna (section 8.1) is routinely given with it to reduce urothelial toxicity.

Chlorambucil is used to treat chronic lymphocytic leukaemia, non-Hodgkin's lymphoma, Hodgkin's disease, and Waldenstrom's macroglobulinaemia. It is given by mouth. Side-effects, apart from bone-marrow suppression, are uncommon. However, patients occasionally develop severe widespread rashes which can progress to Stevens-Johnson syndrome or to toxic epidermal necrolysis. If a rash occurs further chlorambucil is contra-indicated and cyclophosphamide is substituted.

Melphalan is licensed for the treatment of multiple myeloma, advanced ovarian adenocarcinoma, advanced breast cancer, childhood neuroblastoma, and polycythaemia vera. Melphalan is also licensed for regional arterial perfusion in localised malignant melanoma of the extremities and localised soft-tissue sarcoma of the extremities. Interstitial pneumonitis and life-threatening pulmonary fibrosis are associated with melphalan.

Busulfan (busulphan) is given by mouth to treat chronic myeloid leukaemia. Busulfan given by mouth or intravenously, followed by cyclophosphamide, is also licensed as conditioning treatment before haematopoietic stem-cell transplantation in adults and children. Frequent blood tests are necessary because excessive myelosuppression may result in irreversible bone-marrow aplasia. Rarely, progressive pulmonary fibrosis is associated with busulfan. Skin hyperpigmentation is a common side-effect of oral therapy.

Lomustine is a lipid-soluble nitrosourea and is given by mouth. It is used mainly to treat Hodgkin's disease resistant to conventional therapy, malignant melanoma and certain solid tumours. Bone-marrow toxicity is delayed, and the drug is therefore given at intervals of 4 to 6 weeks. Permanent bone-marrow damage can occur with prolonged use. Nausea and vomiting are common and moderately severe.

Carmustine given intravenously has similar activity to lomustine; it is given to patients with multiple myeloma, non-Hodgkin's lymphomas, and brain tumours. Cumulative renal damage and delayed pulmonary fibrosis may occur with intravenous use. Carmustine implants are licensed for intralesional use in adults for the treatment of recurrent glioblastoma multiforme as an adjunct to surgery. Carmustine implants are also licensed for high-grade malignant glioma as adjunctive treatment to surgery and radiotherapy.

NICE guidance (carmustine implants and temozolomide for the treatment of newly diagnosed high-grade glioma)
See p. 465

Estramustine is a combination of an oestrogen and chlormethine used predominantly in prostate cancer. It is given by mouth and has both an antimitotic effect and (by reducing testosterone concentration) a hormonal effect.

Treosulfan is given by mouth or by intravenous or intraperitoneal administration and is used to treat ovarian cancer. Skin pigmentation is a common side-effect and allergic alveolitis, pulmonary fibrosis and haemorrhagic cystitis occur rarely.

Thiotepa is usually used as an intracavitary drug for the treatment of malignant effusions or bladder cancer (section 7.4.4). It is also occasionally used to treat breast cancer, but requires parenteral administration.

Mitobronitol is occasionally used to treat chronic myeloid leukaemia; it is available on a named-patient basis from specialist importing companies, see p. 888.

BUSULFAN
(Busulphan)

Indications see notes above

Cautions see section 8.1 and notes above; monitor cardiac function; previous radiation therapy; avoid in porphyria (section 9.8.2); hepatic impairment (Appendix 2); **interactions:** Appendix 1 (busulfan)

Contra-indications pregnancy (Appendix 4); breast-feeding

Side-effects see section 8.1 and notes above; also hepatotoxicity (including hepatic veno-occlusive disease, hyperbilirubinaemia, jaundice and fibrosis); cardiac tamponade at high doses in thalassaemic patients; pneumonia; skin hyperpigmentation

Dose

- Chronic myeloid leukaemia, induction of remission, by mouth, 60 micrograms/kg daily (max. 4 mg); maintenance, usually 0.5–2 mg daily
- Conditioning treatment before haematopoietic stem-cell transplantation, by mouth *or* by intravenous infusion, consult product literature

Busilvex® (Fabre) ▼ PoM
Concentrate for intravenous infusion, busulfan 6 mg/mL, net price 10-mL vial = £201.25

Myleran® (GSK) PoM
Tablets, f/c, busulfan 2 mg, net price 25-tab pack = £5.20

CARMUSTINE

Indications see notes above

Cautions see section 8.1 and notes above

Contra-indications pregnancy (Appendix 4), breast-feeding

Side-effects see section 8.1 and notes above; irritant to tissues

BiCNU® (Bristol-Myers Squibb) PoM
Injection, powder for reconstitution, carmustine. Net price 100-mg vial (with diluent) = £12.50

Gliadel® (Link) PoM
Implant, carmustine 7.7 mg, net price = £650.38

CHLORAMBUCIL

Indications see notes above

Cautions see section 8.1 and notes above; history of epilepsy and children with nephrotic syndrome (increased risk of seizures); hepatic impairment (Appendix 2); avoid in porphyria (section 9.8.2)

Contra-indications pregnancy (Appendix 4), breast-feeding

Side-effects see section 8.1 and notes above

Dose

- Hodgkin's disease, used alone, 200 micrograms/kg daily for 4–8 weeks
- Non-Hodgkin's lymphoma, used alone, initially 100–200 micrograms/kg daily for 4–8 weeks then dose reduced or given intermittently
- Chronic lymphocytic leukaemia, initially 150 micrograms/kg daily until leucocyte count sufficiently reduced; maintenance (started 4 weeks after end of first course) 100 micrograms/kg daily
- Waldenstrom's macroglobulinaemia, 6–12 mg daily until leucopenia occurs, then reduce to 2–8 mg daily

Leukeran® (GSK) PoM
Tablets, f/c, brown, chlorambucil 2 mg, net price 25-tab pack = £8.36

CYCLOPHOSPHAMIDE

Indications see notes above; rheumatoid arthritis (section 10.1 3)

Cautions see section 8.1 and notes above; hepatic impairment (Appendix 2); renal impairment (Appendix 3); avoid in porphyria (section 9.8.2); **interactions:** Appendix 1 (cyclophosphamide)

Contra-indications haemorrhagic cystitis; pregnancy (Appendix 4), breast-feeding (Appendix 5)

Side-effects see section 8.1 and notes above; also anorexia; cardiotoxicity at high doses; interstitial pulmonary fibrosis; inappropriate secretion of antidiuretic hormone, disturbances of carbohydrate metabolism; urothelial toxicity; pigmentation of palms, nails, and soles

Cyclophosphamide (Non-proprietary) PoM
Tablets, s/c, cyclophosphamide (anhydrous) 50 mg, net price 20 = £2.12. Label: 27
Injection, powder for reconstitution, cyclophosphamide, net price 500-mg vial = £2.88; 1-g vial = £5.04

Endoxana® (Baxter) PoM
Tablets, s/c, cyclophosphamide 50 mg, net price 100-tab pack = £12.00. Label: 23, 25, 27
Injection, powder for reconstitution, cyclophosphamide. Net price 200-mg vial = £1.86; 500-mg vial = £3.54; 1-g vial = £6.18

ESTRAMUSTINE PHOSPHATE

Indications prostate cancer

Cautions see section 8.1; hepatic impairment (Appendix 2); renal impairment (Appendix 3)

Contra-indications peptic ulceration, cardiac disease

Side-effects see section 8.1; also gynaecomastia, altered liver function, cardiovascular disorders (angina and rare reports of myocardial infarction)

Dose

- 0.14–1.4 g daily in divided doses (usual initial dose 560 mg daily)

Counselling Each dose should be taken not less than 1 hour before or 2 hours after meals and should not be taken with dairy products

Estracyt® (Pharmacia) PoM
Capsules, estramustine phosphate 140 mg (as disodium salt). Net price 100-cap pack = £171.28. Label: 23, counselling, see above

IFOSFAMIDE

Indications see notes above

Cautions see section 8.1 and notes above; ensure satisfactory electrolyte balance and renal function before each course (risk of tubular dysfunction, Fanconi's syndrome or diabetes insipidus if renal toxicity not treated promptly); renal impairment (avoid if serum creatinine concentration greater than 120 micromol/litre; Appendix 3); **interactions:** Appendix 1 (ifosfamide)

Contra-indications myelosuppression; urinary-tract obstruction; acute infection (including urinary-tract infection); urothelial damage; hepatic impairment; pregnancy (Appendix 4), breast-feeding

Side-effects see section 8.1 and notes above; also drowsiness, confusion, disorientation, restlessness, psychosis; urothelial toxicity, renal toxicity (see Cautions, above)

Mitoxana® (Baxter) PoM
Injection, powder for reconstitution, ifosfamide. Net price 1-g vial = £27.03; 2-g vial = £45.49 (hosp. only)

LOMUSTINE

Indications see notes above
Cautions see section 8.1 and notes above
Contra-indications severe renal impairment; coeliac disease; pregnancy (Appendix 4); breast-feeding
Side-effects see section 8.1 and notes above
Dose

- Used alone, 120–130 mg/m² body-surface every 6–8 weeks

Lomustine (Medac) PoM
Capsules, blue/clear, lomustine 40 mg. Net price 20-cap pack = £396.19

Note The brand name *CCNU®* has been used for lomustine capsules

MELPHALAN

Indications see notes above
Cautions see section 8.1 and notes above; renal impairment (Appendix 3); **interactions:** Appendix 1 (melphalan)
Contra-indications pregnancy (Appendix 4); breast-feeding
Side-effects see section 8.1 and notes above
Dose

- By mouth, multiple myeloma, dose may vary according to regimen; typical dose 150 micrograms/kg daily for 4 days, repeated every 6 weeks
  Ovarian adenocarcinoma, 200 micrograms/kg daily for 5 days, repeated every 4–8 weeks
  Advanced breast cancer, 150 micrograms/kg daily for 5 days, repeated every 6 weeks
  Polycythaemia vera, initially, 6–10 mg daily reduced after 5–7 days to 2–4 mg daily until satisfactory response then further reduce to 2–6 mg **per week**
- By intravenous injection *or* infusion and regional arterial perfusion, consult product literature

Alkeran® (GSK) PoM
Tablets, melphalan 2 mg, net price 25 = £11.46
Injection, powder for reconstitution, melphalan 50 mg (as hydrochloride). Net price 50-mg vial (with solvent-diluent) = £27.61

THIOTEPA

Indications see notes above and section 7.4.4
Cautions see section 8.1; **interactions:** Appendix 1 (thiotepa)
Contra-indications pregnancy (Appendix 4); breast-feeding
Side-effects see section 8.1

Thiotepa (Goldshield) PoM
Injection, powder for reconstitution, thiotepa, net price 15-mg vial = £5.20

TREOSULFAN

Indications see notes above
Cautions see section 8.1
Contra-indications pregnancy; breast-feeding
Side-effects see section 8.1 and notes above
Dose

- Consult product literature

Treosulfan (Medac) PoM
Capsules, treosulfan 250 mg. Net price 20 = £67.25
Label: 25
Injection, powder for reconstitution, treosulfan. Net price 1 g = £39.44; 5 g = £152.41 (both in infusion bottle with transfer needle)

8.1.2 Anthracyclines and other cytotoxic antibiotics

Drugs in this group are widely used. Many cytotoxic antibiotics act as radiomimetics and simultaneous use of radiotherapy should be **avoided** as it may result in markedly enhanced toxicity.

Daunorubicin, doxorubicin, epirubicin and idarubicin are anthracycline antibiotics. Mitoxantrone (mitozantrone) is an anthracycline derivative.

Doxorubicin is used to treat the acute leukaemias, Hodgkin's and non-Hodgkin's lymphomas, paediatric malignancies and some solid tumours. It is given by injection into a fast-running infusion, commonly at 21-day intervals. Extravasation can cause severe tissue necrosis. Doxorubicin is largely excreted in the bile and an elevated bilirubin concentration is an indication for reducing the dose. Supraventricular tachycardia related to drug administration is an uncommon complication. Higher cumulative doses are associated with cardiomyopathy and it is usual to limit total cumulative doses to 450 mg/m² because symptomatic and potentially fatal heart failure is common above this dose. Patients with cardiac disease, hypertension, the elderly, and those who have received myocardial irradiation should be treated cautiously. Cardiac monitoring may assist in determining safe dosage. Some evidence suggests that weekly low-dose administration may be less cardiotoxic. Doxorubicin is also given by bladder instillation for the treatment of transitional cell carcinoma, papillary bladder tumours and carcinoma *in-situ*.

Liposomal formulations of doxorubicin for intravenous use are also available. They may reduce the incidence of cardiotoxicity and lower the potential for local necrosis, but infusion reactions, sometimes severe, may occur. Hand-foot syndrome (painful, macular reddening skin eruptions) occurs commonly with liposomal doxorubicin and may be dose limiting. It can occur after 2–3 treatment cycles and may be prevented by cooling hands and feet and avoiding socks, gloves, or tight-fitting footwear for 4–7 days after treatment.

The *Scottish Medicines Consortium* has advised (December 2003) that pegylated liposomal doxorubicin is **not** recommended for metastatic breast cancer.

NICE guidance (paclitaxel, pegylated liposomal doxorubicin and topotecan for second-line or subsequent treatment of advanced ovarian cancer)
See p. 466

Epirubicin is structurally related to doxorubicin and clinical trials suggest that it is as effective in the treatment of breast cancer. A maximum cumulative dose of 0.9–1 g/m² is recommended to help avoid cardiotoxicity. Like doxorubicin it is given intravenously and by bladder instillation.

Idarubicin has general properties similar to those of doxorubicin; it is mostly used in the treatment of haematological malignancies. Idarubicin is given intravenously and it may also be given by mouth.

Daunorubicin also has general properties similar to those of doxorubicin. It should be given by intravenous infusion and is indicated for acute leukaemias. A liposomal formulation for intravenous use is licensed for AIDS-related Kaposi's sarcoma.

Use with trastuzumab
Concomitant use of anthracyclines with trastuzumab (section 8.1.5) is associated with cardiotoxicity; for details, see p. 472.

Mitoxantrone (mitozantrone) is structurally related to doxorubicin; it is used for metastatic breast cancer. Mitoxantrone is also licensed for use in the treatment of non-Hodgkin's lymphoma and adult non-lymphocytic leukaemia. It is given intravenously and is well tolerated but myelosuppression and dose-related cardiotoxicity occur; cardiac examinations are recommended after a cumulative dose of 160 mg/m².

Bleomycin is given intravenously or intramuscularly to treat metastatic germ cell cancer and, in some regimens, non-Hodgkin's lymphoma. It causes little bone-marrow suppression but dermatological toxicity is common and increased pigmentation particularly affecting the flexures and subcutaneous sclerotic plaques may occur. Mucositis is also relatively common and an association with Raynaud's phenomenon is reported. Hypersensitivity reactions manifest by chills and fevers commonly occur a few hours after drug administration and may be prevented by simultaneous administration of a corticosteroid, for example hydrocortisone intravenously. The principal problem associated with the use of bleomycin is progressive pulmonary fibrosis. This is dose-related, occurring more commonly at cumulative doses greater than 300 000 units (see Bleomycin, below) and in the elderly. Basal lung crepitations or suspicious chest X-ray changes are an indication to stop therapy with this drug. Patients who have received extensive treatment with bleomycin (e.g. cumulative dose more than 100 000 units—see Bleomycin below) may be at risk of developing respiratory failure if a general anaesthetic is given with high inspired oxygen concentrations. Anaesthetists should be warned of this.

Dactinomycin is principally used to treat paediatric cancers; it is given intravenously. Its side-effects are similar to those of doxorubicin, except that cardiac toxicity is not a problem.

Mitomycin is given intravenously to treat upper gastro-intestinal and breast cancers and by bladder instillation for superficial bladder tumours. It causes delayed bone-marrow toxicity and therefore it is usually administered at 6-weekly intervals. Prolonged use may result in permanent bone-marrow damage. It may also cause lung fibrosis and renal damage.

BLEOMYCIN

Indications squamous cell carcinoma; see also notes above

Cautions see section 8.1 and notes above; renal impairment (Appendix 3); caution in handling—irritant to tissues

Contra-indications pregnancy (Appendix 4); breast-feeding

Side-effects see section 8.1 and notes above

Bleomycin (Non-proprietary) PoM
Injection, powder for reconstitution, bleomycin (as sulphate). Net price 15 000-unit vial = £15.56
Note To conform to the European Pharmacopoeia vials previously labelled as containing '15 units' of bleomycin are now labelled as containing 15 000 units. The amount of bleomycin in the vial has not changed.
Brands include *Bleo-Kyowc*®

DACTINOMYCIN
(Actinomycin D)

Indications see notes above

Cautions see section 8.1 and notes above; caution in handling—irritant to tissues

Contra-indications pregnancy (Appendix 4); breast-feeding

Side-effects see section 8.1 and notes above

Cosmegen Lyovac® (Ovation) PoM
Injection, powder for reconstitution, dactinomycin, net price 500-microgram vial = £6.75

DAUNORUBICIN

Indications see notes above

Cautions see section 8.1 and notes above; hepatic impairment (Appendix 2), renal impairment (Appendix 3); caution in handling—irritant to tissues

Contra-indications pregnancy (Appendix 4); breast-feeding

Side-effects see section 8.1 and notes above

Daunorubicin (Non-proprietary) PoM
Injection, powder for reconstitution, daunorubicin (as hydrochloride), net price 20-mg vial = £44.76
Note The brand name *Cerubidin*® was formerly used.

Lipid formulation

DaunoXome® (Gilead) PoM
Concentrate for intravenous infusion, daunorubicin encapsulated in liposomes. For dilution before use. Net price 50-mg vial = £137.67
For advanced AIDS-related Kaposi's sarcoma

DOXORUBICIN HYDROCHLORIDE

Indications see notes above and section 7.4.4

Cautions see section 8.1 and notes above; hepatic impairment (Appendix 2); caution in handling—irritant to tissues; **interactions**: Appendix 1 (doxorubicin)

Contra-indications see notes above; severe hepatic impairment; severe myocardial insufficiency, recent myocardial infarction, severe arrhythmias; previous treatment with maximum cumulative doses of doxorubicin or other anthracyclines; intravesical use in urinary infections, bladder inflammation, and in urethral stenosis with catheterisation difficulties; pregnancy (Appendix 4); breast-feeding

Side-effects see section 8.1 and notes above

Doxorubicin (Non-proprietary) PoM

Injection, powder for reconstitution, doxorubicin hydrochloride, net price 10-mg vial = £18.72; 50-mg vial = £96.86

Note The brand name *Adriamycin*® was formerly used

Injection, doxorubicin hydrochloride 2 mg/mL, net price 5-mL vial = £20.60, 25-mL vial = £103.00, 100-mL vial = £412.00

Lipid formulation

Caelyx® (Schering-Plough) PoM

Concentrate for intravenous infusion, pegylated doxorubicin hydrochloride 2 mg/mL encapsulated in liposomes. For dilution before use. Net price 10-mL vial = £382.51, 25-mL vial = £813.49

For AIDS-related Kaposi's sarcoma in patients with low CD4 count and extensive mucocutaneous or visceral disease, for advanced ovarian cancer when platinum-based chemotherapy has failed, and as monotherapy for metastatic breast cancer with increased cardiac risk

Myocet® (Zeneus) ▼ PoM

Injection, powder for reconstitution, doxorubicin hydrochloride (as doxorubicin–citrate complex) encapsulated in liposomes, net price 50-mg vial (with vials of liposomes and buffer) = £464.50

For use with cyclophosphamide for metastatic breast cancer

EPIRUBICIN HYDROCHLORIDE

Indications see notes above and section 7.4.4

Cautions see section 8.1 and notes above; hepatic impairment (Appendix 2); caution in handling—irritant to tissues; **interactions:** Appendix 1 (epirubicin)

Contra-indications pregnancy (Appendix 4); breast-feeding

Side-effects see section 8.1 and notes above

Pharmorubicin® Rapid Dissolution (Pharmacia) PoM

Injection, powder for reconstitution, epirubicin hydrochloride. Net price 10-mg vial = £19.31; 20-mg vial = £38.62; 50-mg vial = £96.54

Pharmorubicin® Solution for Injection (Pharmacia) PoM

Injection, epirubicin hydrochloride 2 mg/mL, net price 5-mL vial = £19.31, 25-mL vial = £96.54, 100-mL vial = £386.16

IDARUBICIN HYDROCHLORIDE

Indications advanced breast cancer after failure of first-line chemotherapy (not including anthracyclines); acute leukaemias—see notes above

Cautions see section 8.1 and notes above; hepatic impairment (Appendix 2); renal impairment (avoid if creatinine clearance less than 10 mL/minute; Appendix 3); caution in handling—irritant to tissues

Contra-indications pregnancy (Appendix 4); breast-feeding

Side-effects see section 8.1 and notes above

Dose

- By mouth, acute non-lymphocytic leukaemia, monotherapy, 30 mg/m² daily for 3 days *or* in combination therapy, 15–30 mg/m² daily for 3 days

  Advanced breast cancer, monotherapy, 45 mg/m² as a single dose *or* 15 mg/m² daily for 3 consecutive days; repeat every 3–4 weeks

Note Max. cumulative dose by mouth (for all indications) 400 mg/m²

- By intravenous administration, consult product literature

Zavedos® (Pharmacia) PoM

Capsules, idarubicin hydrochloride, 5 mg (red), net price 1-cap pack = £34.56; 10 mg (red/white), 1-cap pack = £69.12; 25 mg (white), 1-cap pack = £172.80. Label: 25

Injection, powder for reconstitution, idarubicin hydrochloride, net price 5-mg vial = £87.36; 10-mg vial = £174.72

MITOMYCIN

Indications see notes above and section 7.4.4

Cautions see section 8.1 and notes above; caution in handling—irritant to tissues

Contra-indications pregnancy (Appendix 4); breast-feeding

Side-effects see section 8.1 and notes above

Mitomycin C Kyowa® (Kyowa Hakko) PoM

Injection, powder for reconstitution, mitomycin. Net price 2-mg vial = £5.88; 10-mg vial = £19.37; 20-mg vial = £36.94; 40-mg vial = £73.88 (hosp. only)

MITOXANTRONE
(Mitozantrone)

Indications see notes above

Cautions see section 8.1 and notes above; intrathecal administration not recommended

Contra-indications pregnancy (Appendix 4); breast-feeding

Side-effects see section 8.1 and notes above

Mitoxantrone (Non-proprietary) PoM

Concentrate for intravenous infusion, mitoxantrone (as hydrochloride) 2 mg/mL, net price 10-mL vial = £100.00

Onkotrone® (Baxter) PoM

Concentrate for intravenous infusion, mitoxantrone (as hydrochloride) 2 mg/mL, net price 10-mL vial = £121.85, 12.5-mL vial = £152.33, 15-mL vial = £203.04

8.1.3 Antimetabolites

Antimetabolites are incorporated into new nuclear material or combine irreversibly with vital cellular enzymes, preventing normal cellular division.

Methotrexate inhibits the enzyme dihydrofolate reductase, essential for the synthesis of purines and pyrimidines. It is given by mouth, intravenously, intramuscularly, or intrathecally.

Methotrexate is used as maintenance therapy for childhood acute lymphoblastic leukaemia. Other uses include choriocarcinoma, non-Hodgkin's lymphoma, and a number of solid tumours. Intrathecal methotrexate is used in the CNS prophylaxis of childhood acute lymphoblastic leukaemia, and as a therapy for established meningeal cancer or lymphoma.

Methotrexate causes myelosuppression, mucositis, and rarely pneumonitis. It is **contra-indicated** in significant renal impairment because it is excreted primarily by the kidney. It is also contra-indicated in patients with severe hepatic impairment. It should also be **avoided** in the presence of significant pleural effusion or ascites because it can accumulate in these fluids, and its subsequent return to the circulation may cause myelosuppression. Systemic toxicity may follow intrathecal administration and blood counts should be carefully monitored.

Folinic acid (section 8.1) following methotrexate administration helps to prevent methotrexate-induced mucositis or myelosuppression.

Capecitabine, which is metabolised to fluorouracil, is given by mouth. It is used as monotherapy for metastatic colorectal cancer; it has been shown to be of similar efficacy as a combination of fluorouracil and folinic acid. Capecitabine is also licensed for adjuvant treatment of advanced colon cancer following surgery. It is also licensed for second-line treatment of locally advanced or metastatic breast cancer either in combination with docetaxel (where previous therapy included an anthracycline) or alone (after failure of a taxane and anthracycline regimen or where further anthracycline treatment is not indicated). Capecitabine is also licensed for the first-line treatment of advanced gastric cancer in combination with a platinum-based regimen.

> NICE guidance
> **Capecitabine and oxaliplatin in the adjuvant treatment of stage III (Dukes' C) colon cancer (April 2006)**
> Capecitabine alone *or* oxaliplatin combined with fluorouracil and folinic acid are options for adjuvant treatment following surgery for stage III (Dukes' C) colon cancer.

> NICE guidance
> **Capecitabine and tegafur with uracil for metastatic colorectal cancer (May 2003)**
> Capecitabine or tegafur with uracil (in combination with folinic acid) is an option for the first-line treatment of metastatic colorectal cancer.

> NICE guidance
> **Capecitabine for locally advanced or metastatic breast cancer (May 2003)**
> Capecitabine in combination with docetaxel should be used in preference to docetaxel monotherapy for locally advanced or metastatic breast cancer in people for whom anthracycline-containing regimens are unsuitable or have failed.
> Capecitabine monotherapy is recommended as an option for people with locally advanced or metastatic breast cancer who have not previously received capecitabine in combination therapy and for whom anthracycline and taxane-containing regimens have failed or further anthracycline therapy is contra-indicated.

Cytarabine acts by interfering with pyrimidine synthesis. It is given subcutaneously, intravenously, or intrathecally. Its predominant use is in the induction of remission of acute myeloblastic leukaemia. It is a potent myelosuppressant and requires careful haematological monitoring. A liposomal formulation of cytarabine for intrathecal use is licensed for lymphomatous meningitis.

Fludarabine is licensed for the initial treatment of advanced B-cell chronic lymphocytic leukaemia (CLL) or after first-line treatment in patients with sufficient bone-marrow reserves; it is given by mouth or by intravenous injection or by intravenous infusion. Fludarabine is generally well tolerated but it does cause myelosuppression, which may be cumulative. Immunosuppression is also common (see panel on cladribine and fludarabine below) and co-trimoxazole is often used to prevent pneumocystis infection. Immune-mediated haemolytic anaemia, thrombocytopenia, and neutropenia are less common side-effects.

The *Scottish Medicines Consortium* has advised (October 2006) that fludarabine is accepted for restricted use for the treatment of B-cell chronic lymphocytic leukaemia (CLL) in patients with sufficient bone marrow reserves. First-line treatment should only be initiated in patients with advanced disease, Rai stages III/IV (Binet stage C), or Rai stages I/II (Binet stage A/B) where the patient has disease-related symptoms or evidence of progressive disease.

> NICE guidance
> **Fludarabine monotherapy for the first-line treatment of chronic lymphocytic leukaemia (February 2007)**
> Fludarabine monotherapy, is **not** recommended for the first-line treatment of chronic lymphocytic leukaemia.

Cladribine is given by intravenous infusion for the treatment of hairy cell leukaemia. It is also given for chronic lymphocytic leukaemia in patients who have failed to respond to standard regimens containing an alkylating agent. Cladribine produces severe myelosuppression, with neutropenia, anaemia, and thrombocytopenia; haemolytic anamia has also been reported. High doses of cladribine have been associated with acute renal failure and severe neurotoxicity.

> **Cladribine** and **fludarabine** have a potent and prolonged immunosuppressive effect and only irradiated blood products should be administered to prevent potentially fatal graft-versus-host reaction. Prescribers should consult specialist literature when using highly immunosuppressive drugs.

Clofarabine is licensed for the treatment of acute lymphoblastic leukaemia in patients aged 1 to 21 years who have relapsed or are refractory after receiving at least two previous regimens. It is given by intravenous infusion.

Nelarabine is licensed for the treatment of T-cell acute lymphoblastic leukaemia and T-cell lymphoblastic lymphoma in patients who have relapsed or who are refractory after receiving at least two previous regimens. It is given by intravenous infusion. Neurotoxicity is common with nelarabine and close monitoring for neurological adverse events is strongly recommended—discontinue if neurotoxicity occurs.

Gemcitabine is used intravenously; it is given alone for palliative treatment or with cisplatin as first-line treatment for locally advanced or metastatic non-small cell lung cancer. It is also used in the treatment of locally advanced or metastatic pancreatic cancer (see NICE guidance below). Combined with cisplatin, gemcitabine is also licensed for the treatment of advanced bladder cancer. Combined with paclitaxel, gemcitabine is also licensed for the treatment of metastatic breast cancer which has relapsed after previous chemotherapy including an anthracycline (see NICE guidance below). Gemcitabine is generally well tolerated but it can cause mild gastro-intestinal side-effects and rashes; renal impairment, pulmonary toxicity and influenza-like symptoms have also been reported. Haemolytic uraemic syndrome has been reported rarely and gemcitabine should be discontinued if signs of microangiopathic haemolytic anaemia occur.

The *Scottish Medicines Consortium* has advised (November 2006) that gemcitabine is accepted for restricted use for the treatment of metastatic breast cancer, which has relapsed following previous chemotherapy including an anthracycline (unless contra-indicated).

NICE guidance

Gemcitabine for the treatment of metastatic breast cancer (January 2007)

Gemcitabine, in combination with paclitaxel, is an option for the treatment of metastatic breast cancer **only** when docetaxel monotherapy or docetaxel plus capecitabine are also considered appropriate.

NICE guidance

Gemcitabine for the treatment of pancreatic cancer (May 2001)

Gemcitabine is an option for first-line chemotherapy for patients with advanced or metastatic adenocarcinoma of the pancreas and a Karnofsky score of at least 50 [Karnofsky score is a measure of the ability to perform ordinary tasks].

Gemcitabine is not recommended for patients who can have potentially curative surgery. There is insufficient evidence about its use for second-line treatment of pancreatic adenocarcinoma.

Fluorouracil is usually given intravenously because absorption following oral administration is unpredictable. It is used to treat a number of solid tumours, including gastro-intestinal tract cancers and breast cancer. It is commonly used with folinic acid in advanced colorectal cancer. It may also be used topically for certain malignant and pre-malignant skin lesions. Toxicity is unusual, but may include myelosuppression, mucositis, and rarely a cerebellar syndrome. On prolonged infusion, a desquamative hand–foot syndrome may occur.

Pemetrexed inhibits thymidylate transferase and other folate-dependent enzymes. It is licensed for use with cisplatin for the treatment of unresectable malignant pleural mesothelioma which has not previously been treated with chemotherapy; it is given by intravenous infusion. Pemetrexed used alone is also licensed for the treatment of locally advanced or metastatic non-small cell lung cancer which has previously been treated with chemotherapy. Common adverse effects include myelosuppression, gastro-intestinal toxicity, and skin disorders.

The *Scottish Medicines Consortium* has advised (July 2005) that pemetrexed in combination with cisplatin is accepted for restricted use for the treatment of chemotherapy-naive patients with stage III/IV unresectable malignant pleural mesothelioma.

NICE guidance

Pemetrexed for the treatment of non-small cell lung cancer (August 2007)

Pemetrexed is **not** recommended for the treatment of locally advanced or metastatic non-small cell lung cancer.

Patients currently receiving pemetrexed should have the option to continue therapy until they and their clinicians consider it appropriate to stop.

Raltitrexed, a thymidylate synthase inhibitor, is given intravenously for palliation of advanced colorectal cancer when fluorouracil and folinic acid cannot be used. It is probably of similar efficacy to fluorouracil. Raltitrexed is generally well tolerated, but can cause marked myelosuppression and gastro-intestinal side-effects.

NICE guidance (irinotecan, oxaliplatin and raltitrexed for advanced colorectal cancer)

See p. 466

Mercaptopurine is used as maintenance therapy for the acute leukaemias and in the management of ulcerative colitis and Crohn's disease (section 1.5). Azathioprine, which is metabolised to mercaptopurine, is generally used as an immunosuppressant (section 8.2.1 and section 10.1.3). The dose of both drugs should be reduced if the patient is receiving allopurinol since it interferes with their metabolism.

Tegafur (in combination with uracil) is given by mouth, together with calcium folinate, in the management of metastatic colorectal cancer. Tegafur is a prodrug of fluorouracil; uracil inhibits the degradation of fluorouracil. Tegafur (with uracil) has been shown to be of similar efficacy as a combination of fluorouracil and folinic acid for metastatic colorectal cancer. For NICE guidance on capecitabine and tegafur with uracil for metastatic colorectal cancer, see above.

Tioguanine (thioguanine) is given by mouth for the treatment of acute leukaemias and chronic myeloid leukaemia. It can be given at various stages of treatment in short-term cycles. Long-term therapy is no longer recommended because of the high risk of liver toxicity; treatment with tioguanine should be discontinued if liver toxicity develops.

CAPECITABINE

Indications see notes above

Cautions see section 8.1; history of significant cardiovascular disease, arrhythmias; monitor plasma-calcium concentration; diabetes mellitus; renal impairment (avoid if creatinine clearance less than 30 mL/minute; Appendix 3); **interactions:** Appendix 1 (fluorouracil)

Contra-indications hepatic impairment (Appendix 2); pregnancy (Appendix 4); breast-feeding

Side-effects see section 8.1 and notes above; hand–foot (desquamative) syndrome; diarrhoea

Dose

- Stage III colon cancer, ADULT over 18 years 1.25 g/m² twice daily for 14 days, followed by a 7-day interval, given as 3-week cycles for a total of 8 cycles
- Metastatic colorectal cancer, ADULT over 18 years 1.25 g/m² twice daily for 14 days; subsequent courses repeated after a 7-day interval
- Advanced gastric cancer, ADULT over 18 years 1 g/m² twice daily for 14 days; subsequent courses repeated after a 7-day interval

  Note The first dose should be taken on the evening of day 1 and last dose on the morning of day 15; dose differs in combination with epirubicin—consult product literature
- Breast cancer, ADULT over 18 years 1.25g/m² twice daily for 14 days; subsequent courses repeated after a 7-day interval

Xeloda® (Roche) ▼ PoM
Tablets, f/c, peach, capecitabine 150 mg, net price 60-tab pack = £44.47; 500 mg, 120-tab pack = £295.06. Label: 21

CLADRIBINE

Indications see notes above
Cautions see section 8.1 and notes above; use irradiated blood only; hepatic impairment (Appendix 2); renal impairment (Appendix 3)
Contra-indications pregnancy (Appendix 4); breast-feeding
Side-effects see section 8.1 and notes above; also constipation, diarrhoea, abdominal pain, flatulence; oedema, tachycardia; cough, dyspnoea; dizziness, insomnia, anxiety, headache; chills, asthenia, malaise; myalgia, arthralgia; sweating, rash, pruritus, and purpura

Leustat® (Janssen-Cilag) PoM
Concentrate for intravenous infusion, cladribine 1 mg/mL. For dilution and use as an infusion, net price 10-mL vial = £169.53
For hairy cell leukaemia and for B-cell chronic lymphocytic leukaemia in patients who have failed to respond to standard regimens containing an alkylating agent

Litak® (Lipomed) ▼ PoM
Injection (for subcutaneous use only—no dilution required), cladribine 2 mg/mL, net price 5-mL vial = £165.00
For hairy cell leukaemia

CLOFARABINE

Indications see notes above
Cautions see section 8.1 and notes above; hepatic impairment (Appendix 2); renal impairment (avoid in severe renal impairment; Appendix 3)
Contra-indications pregnancy (Appendix 4); breast-feeding
Side-effects see section 8.1; also jaundice; tachycardia, flushing, hypotension, pericardial effusion, haematoma; dyspnoea, cough; anxiety, agitation, dizziness, drowsiness, headache, paraesthesia, peripheral neuropathy, restlessness; rash, pruritus, sweating

Evoltra® (Bioenvision) ▼ PoM
Concentrate for intravenous infusion, clofarabine 1 mg/mL, net price 20-mL vial = £1200.00
Electrolytes Na^+ 3.08 mmol/vial

CYTARABINE

Indications see notes above
Cautions see section 8.1 and notes above; hepatic impairment (Appendix 2); **interactions:** Appendix 1 (cytarabine)
Contra-indications pregnancy (Appendix 4); breast-feeding
Side-effects see section 8.1 and notes above

Cytarabine (Non-proprietary) PoM
Injection (for intravenous, subcutaneous, or intrathecal use), cytarabine 20 mg/mL, net price 5-mL vial = £4.00
Injection (for intravenous or subcutaneous use), cytarabine 20 mg/mL, net price 5-mL vial = £3.90, 25-mL vial = £19.50; 100 mg/mL, 1-mL vial = £4.00, 5-mL vial = £20.00, 10-mL vial = £39.00, 20-mL vial = £77.50

◢Lipid formulation for intrathecal use

DepoCyte® (Napp) ▼ PoM
Intrathecal injection, cytarabine encapsulated in liposomes, net price 50-mg vial = £1223.75
For lymphomatous meningitis
Note The *Scottish Medicines Consortium* does not recommend (April 2005) *Depocyte®* for the intrathecal treatment of lymphomatous meningitis

FLUDARABINE PHOSPHATE

Indications see notes above
Cautions see section 8.1 and notes above; use irradiated blood only; monitor for neurological toxicity; renal impairment (avoid if creatinine clearance less than 30 mL/minute; Appendix 3) **interactions:** Appendix 1 (fludarabine)
Contra-indications haemolytic anaemia, pregnancy (Appendix 4); breast-feeding
Side-effects see section 8.1 and notes above; also diarrhoea, anorexia; oedema; pneumonia; peripheral neuropathy, visual disturbances; chills, fever, malaise, weakness; rash

Dose

- By mouth, ADULT 40 mg/m² for 5 days every 28 days usually for 6 cycles
- By intravenous injection *or* infusion, consult product literature

Fludara® (Schering Health) PoM
Tablets, f/c, pink, fludarabine phosphate 10 mg, net price 15-tab pack = £279.00, 20-tab pack = £372.00
Injection, powder for reconstitution, fludarabine phosphate. Net price 50-mg vial = £156.00

FLUOROURACIL

Indications see notes above; pre-malignant and malignant skin lesions (section 13.8.1)
Cautions see section 8.1 and notes above; caution in handling—irritant to tissues; hepatic impairment (Appendix 2); **interactions**: Appendix 1 (fluorouracil)
Contra-indications pregnancy (Appendix 4); breast-feeding
Side-effects see section 8.1 and notes above; also local irritation with topical preparation

Dose

- By mouth, maintenance 15 mg/kg weekly; max. in one day 1 g
- By intravenous injection *or* infusion *or* by intra-arterial infusion, consult product literature

Fluorouracil (Non-proprietary) PoM
Capsules, fluorouracil 250 mg.
Available from Cambridge on a named-patient basis
Injection, fluorouracil (as sodium salt) 25 mg/mL, net price 10-mL vial = £3.20, 20-mL vial = £6.40, 100-mL vial = £32.00; 50 mg/mL, 10-mL vial = £6.40, 20-mL vial = £12.80, 50-mL vial = £32.00, 100-mL vial = £64.00

GEMCITABINE

Indications see notes above
Cautions see section 8.1 and notes above; hepatic impairment (Appendix 2); renal impairment (Appendix 3)
Contra-indications pregnancy (Appendix 4); breast-feeding
Side-effects see section 8.1 and notes above

Gemzar® (Lilly) PoM
Injection, powder for reconstitution, gemcitabine (as hydrochloride), net price 200-mg vial = £32.55; 1-g vial = £162.76 (both hosp. only)

MERCAPTOPURINE

Indications acute leukaemias and chronic myeloid leukaemia; inflammatory bowel disease [unlicensed indication] (section 1.5)
Cautions see section 8.1 and notes above; monitor liver function—hepatic impairment (Appendix 2); renal impairment (Appendix 3); **interactions:** Appendix 1 (mercaptopurine)
Contra-indications pregnancy (Appendix 4); breast-feeding
Side-effects see section 8.1 and notes above; also hepatotoxicity; *rarely* intestinal ulceration, pancreatitis
Dose

- Initially 2.5 mg/kg daily

Puri-Nethol® (GSK) PoM
Tablets, yellow, scored, mercaptopurine 50 mg, net price 25-tab pack = £18.78

METHOTREXATE

Indications see notes above and under Dose; rheumatoid arthritis (section 10.1.3); psoriasis (section 13.5.3)
Cautions see section 8.1, notes above and section 10.1.3; hepatic impairment (Appendix 2); renal impairment (avoid if creatinine clearance less than 20 mL/minute; Appendix 3); **interactions:** Appendix 1 (methotrexate)
Contra-indications pregnancy (Appendix 4); breast-feeding
Side-effects see section 8.1, notes above and section 10.1.3
Dose

- By mouth, leukaemia in children (maintenance), 15 mg/m² weekly in combination with other drugs

> **Important**
> Note that the above dose is a **weekly** dose. To avoid error with low-dose methotrexate, it is recommended that:
>
> - the patient is carefully advised of the **dose** and **frequency** and the reason for taking methotrexate and any other prescribed medicine (e.g. folic acid);
> - only one strength of methotrexate tablet (usually 2.5 mg) is prescribed and dispensed;
> - the prescription and the dispensing label clearly show the dose and frequency of methotrexate administration;
> - the patient is warned to report immediately the onset of any feature of blood disorders (e.g. sore throat, bruising, and mouth ulcers), liver toxicity (e.g. nausea, vomiting, abdominal discomfort, and dark urine), and respiratory effects (e.g. shortness of breath).

- By intravenous injection *or* infusion, *or* by intra-arterial infusion, *or* by intramuscular injection, *or* intrathecal administration, consult product literature

Methotrexate (Non-proprietary) PoM
Injection, methotrexate (as sodium salt) 2.5 mg/mL, net price 2-mL vial = £1.68; 25 mg/mL, 2-mL vial = £2.62, 20-mL vial = £25.07
Injection, methotrexate 100 mg/mL (not for intrathecal use), net price 10-mL vial = £78.33, 50-mL vial = £380.07

Oral preparations
Section 10.1.3

NELARABINE

Indications see notes above
Cautions see section 8.1 and notes above; previous or concurrent intrathecal chemotherapy or craniospinal irradiation (increased risk of neurotoxicity)
Driving May affect performance of skilled tasks (e.g. driving)
Contra-indications pregnancy (Appendix 4); breast-feeding
Side-effects see section 8.1; also abdominal pain, constipation, taste disturbance, anorexia, diarrhoea; hypotension, oedema; pleural effusion, wheezing, dyspnoea, cough; confusion, seizures, amnesia, drowsiness, peripheral neurological disorders, hypoesthesia, paraesthesia, ataxia, demyelination, tremor, dizziness, headache, asthenia, fatigue; pyrexia; electrolyte disturbances; blurred vision; muscle weakness, myalgia, arthralgia; benign and malignant tumours also reported

Atriance® (GSK) ▼ PoM
Intravenous Infusion, nelarabine 5 mg/mL, net price 50-mL vial = £222.00
Electrolytes Na^+ 3.75 mmol/vial

PEMETREXED

Indications see notes above
Cautions see section 8.1 and notes above; prophylactic folic acid and vitamin-B_{12} supplementation required (consult product literature)
Contra-indications pregnancy (Appendix 4); breast-feeding (Appendix 5)
Side-effects see section 8.1 and notes above

Alimta® (Lilly) ▼ PoM
Injection, powder for reconstitution, pemetrexed 500 mg (as disodium), net price 500-mg vial = £800.00

RALTITREXED

Indications see notes above

Cautions see section 8.1 and notes above; hepatic impairment (Appendix 2); renal impairment (avoid if creatinine clearance less than 25 mL/minute; Appendix 3)

Contra-indications pregnancy (Appendix 4); breast-feeding

Side-effects see section 8.1 and notes above

Tomudex® (AstraZeneca) PoM
Injection, powder for reconstitution, raltitrexed. Net price 2-mg vial = £121.86

TEGAFUR WITH URACIL

Indications see notes above

Cautions see section 8.1; cardiac disease; renal impairment; hepatic impairment (avoid if severe—Appendix 2); **interactions:** Appendix 1 (fluorouracil)

Contra-indications pregnancy (Appendix 4); breast-feeding

Side-effects see section 8.1 and notes above

Dose

- ADULT, tegafur 300 mg/m² (with uracil 672 mg/m²) daily in 3 divided doses for 28 days; subsequent courses repeated after 7-day interval; for dose adjustment due to toxicity, consult product literature

Uftoral® (Merck Serono) ▼ PoM
Capsules, tegafur 100 mg, uracil 224 mg, net price 36-cap pack = £96.12, 120-cap pack = £320.40. Label: 23

TIOGUANINE
(Thioguanine)

Indications see notes above

Cautions see section 8.1 and notes above; monitor liver function weekly; hepatic impairment (Appendix 2); renal impairment (Appendix 3); **interactions:** Appendix 1 (tioguanine)

Contra-indications pregnancy (Appendix 4); breast-feeding

Side-effects see section 8.1 and notes above

Dose

- 100–200 mg/m² daily

Lanvis® (GSK) PoM
Tablets, yellow, scored, tioguanine 40 mg. Net price 25-tab pack = £45.41

8.1.4 Vinca alkaloids and etoposide

The vinca alkaloids, **vinblastine**, **vincristine**, and **vindesine**, are used to treat a variety of cancers including leukaemias, lymphomas, and some solid tumours (e.g. breast and lung cancer). **Vinorelbine** is a semi-synthetic vinca alkaloid, it is given intravenously for the treatment of advanced breast cancer (see also NICE guidance below) and for advanced non-small cell lung cancer. An oral preparation of vinorelbine is also licensed to treat advanced non-small cell lung cancer.

Neurotoxicity, usually as peripheral or autonomic neuropathy, occurs with all vinca alkaloids and is a limiting side-effect of vincristine; it occurs less often with vindesine, vinblastine, and vinorelbine. Patients with neurotoxicity commonly have peripheral paraesthesia, loss of deep tendon reflexes, abdominal pain, and constipation; ototoxicity has been reported. If symptoms of neurotoxicity are severe, doses should be reduced. Motor weakness can also occur, and increasing motor weakness calls for discontinuation of these drugs. Recovery from neurotoxic effects is usually slow but complete.

Myelosuppression is the dose-limiting side-effect of vinblastine, vindesine, and vinorelbine; vincristine causes negligible myelosuppression. The vinca alkaloids may cause reversible alopecia. They cause severe local irritation and care must be taken to avoid extravasation.

> Vinblastine, vincristine, vindesine, and vinorelbine injections are **for intravenous administration only**. Inadvertent intrathecal administration can cause severe neurotoxicity, which is usually fatal.

> **NICE guidance**
> **Vinorelbine for advanced breast cancer (December 2002)**
> Vinorelbine monotherapy is an option for the second-line (or subsequent) treatment of advanced breast cancer where anthracycline-based regimens have failed or are unsuitable.
> Vinorelbine monotherapy is not recommended as first-line treatment for advanced breast cancer.
> Insufficient information is available to recommend the routine use of vinorelbine in combination with other therapies for advanced breast cancer.

Etoposide may be given orally or by slow intravenous infusion, the oral dose being double the intravenous dose. A preparation containing etoposide phosphate can be given by intravenous injection or infusion. Etoposide is usually given daily for 3–5 days and courses should not be repeated more frequently than at intervals of 21 days. It has particularly useful activity in small cell carcinoma of the bronchus, the lymphomas, and testicular cancer. Toxic effects include alopecia, myelosuppression, nausea, and vomiting.

ETOPOSIDE

Indications see notes above

Cautions see section 8.1 and notes above; renal impairment (Appendix 3); **interactions:** Appendix 1 (etoposide)

Contra-indications see section 8.1 and notes above; severe hepatic impairment; pregnancy (Appendix 4); breast-feeding

Side-effects see section 8.1 and notes above; irritant to tissues

Dose

- By mouth, 120–240 mg/m² daily for 5 days
- By intravenous infusion, consult product literature

Etoposide (Non-proprietary) PoM
Concentrate for intravenous infusion, etoposide 20 mg/mL, net price 5-mL vial = £12.15, 10-mL vial = £29.00, 25-mL vial = £60.75
Brands include *Eposin®*

Etopophos® (Bristol-Myers Squibb) PoM
Injection, powder for reconstitution, etoposide (as phosphate), net price 100-mg vial = £27.78 (hosp. only)

Vepesid® (Bristol-Myers Squibb) PoM
Capsules, both pink, etoposide 50 mg, net price 20 = £105.97; 100 mg, 10-cap pack = £92.60 (hosp. only). Label: 23

VINBLASTINE SULPHATE

Indications see notes above
Cautions see section 8.1 and notes above; hepatic impairment (Appendix 2); caution in handling; **interactions:** Appendix 1 (vinblastine)
Contra-indications see section 8.1 and notes above; pregnancy (Appendix 4); breast-feeding
Important Intrathecal injection **contra-indicated**
Side-effects see section 8.1 and notes above; irritant to tissues

Vinblastine (Non-proprietary) PoM
Injection, vinblastine sulphate 1 mg/mL. Net price 10-mL vial = £13.09

Velbe® (Genus) PoM
Injection, powder for reconstitution, vinblastine sulphate. Net price 10-mg amp = £14.15

VINCRISTINE SULPHATE

Indications see notes above
Cautions see section 8.1 and notes above; hepatic impairment (Appendix 2); neuromuscular disease; caution in handling; **interactions:** Appendix 1 (vincristine)
Contra-indications see section 8.1 and notes above; pregnancy (Appendix 4); breast-feeding
Important Intrathecal injection **contra-indicated**
Side-effects see section 8.1 and notes above; irritant to tissues

Vincristine (Non-proprietary) PoM
Injection, vincristine sulphate 1 mg/mL. Net price 1-mL vial = £10.92; 2-mL vial = £21.17; 5-mL vial = £44.16

Oncovin® (Genus) PoM
Injection, vincristine sulphate 1 mg/mL, net price 1-mL vial = £14.18; 2-mL vial = £28.05

VINDESINE SULPHATE

Indications see notes above
Cautions see section 8.1 and notes above; hepatic impairment (Appendix 2); neuromuscular disease; caution in handling
Contra-indications see section 8.1 and notes above; pregnancy (Appendix 4); breast-feeding
Important Intrathecal injection **contra-indicated**
Side-effects see section 8.1 and notes above; irritant to tissues

Eldisine® (Genus) PoM
Injection, powder for reconstitution, vindesine sulphate, net price 5-mg vial = £78.30 (hosp. only)

VINORELBINE

Indications see notes above
Cautions see section 8.1 and notes above; hepatic impairment (Appendix 2); caution in handling
Contra-indications see section 8.1 and notes above; pregnancy (Appendix 4); breast-feeding
Important Intrathecal injection **contra-indicated**
Side-effects see section 8.1 and notes above; irritant to tissues
Dose
- By mouth, 60 mg/m² once weekly for 3 weeks, increased if tolerated to 80 mg/m² once weekly; max. 160 mg once weekly
- By intravenous injection *or* infusion, consult product literature

Vinorelbine (Non-proprietary) PoM
Concentrate for intravenous infusion, vinorelbine (as tartrate) 10 mg/mL, net price 1-mL vial = £32.95, 5-mL vial = £153.98

Navelbine® (Fabre) PoM
Concentrate for intravenous infusion, vinorelbine (as tartrate) 10 mg/mL. Net price 1-mL vial = £29.75; 5-mL vial = £139.98

Capsules▼, vinorelbine (as tartrate) 20 mg (brown), net price 1-cap pack = £43.98; 30 mg (pink), 1-cap pack = £65.98. Label: 21, 25

8.1.5 Other antineoplastic drugs

Amsacrine

Amsacrine has an action and toxic effects similar to those of doxorubicin (section 8.1.2) and is given *intravenously*. It is occasionally used in acute myeloid leukaemia. Side-effects include myelosuppression and mucositis; electrolytes should be monitored as fatal arrhythmias have occurred in association with hypokalaemia.

AMSACRINE

Indications see notes above
Cautions see section 8.1 and notes above; reduce dose in renal or hepatic impairment; also caution in handling—irritant to skin and tissues
Contra-indications pregnancy (Appendix 4); breast-feeding
Side-effects see section 8.1 and notes above

Amsidine® (Goldshield) PoM
Concentrate for intravenous infusion, amsacrine 5 mg (as lactate)/mL, when reconstituted by mixing two solutions. Net price 1.5-mL (75-mg) amp with 13.5-mL diluent vial = £54.08 (hosp. only)
Note Use glass apparatus for reconstitution

Arsenic trioxide

Arsenic trioxide is licensed for acute promyelocytic leukaemia in patients who have relapsed or failed to respond to previous treatment with a retinoid and chemotherapy.

ARSENIC TRIOXIDE

Indications see notes above

Cautions see section 8.1; correct electrolyte abnormalities before treatment; ECG required before and during treatment—consult product literature; avoid concomitant administration with drugs causing QT interval prolongation, hypokalaemia, and hypomagnesaemia; previous treatment with anthracyclines (increased risk of QT interval prolongation); renal impairment (Appendix 3)

Contra-indications pregnancy (Appendix 4); breast-feeding

Side-effects see section 8.1; leucocyte activation syndrome (requires immediate treatment—consult product literature); hyperglycaemia, hypokalaemia, leucocytosis, QT interval prolongation, atrial fibrillation, atrial flutter, haemorrhage, dyspnoea, pleuritic pain, musculoskeletal pain, paraesthesia, fatigue

Trisenox® (Cephalon) ▼ PoM
Concentrate for intravenous infusion, arsenic trioxide 1 mg/mL, net price 10-mL amp = £250.90

Bevacizumab

Bevacizumab is an inhibitor of vascular endothelial growth factor. It is licensed for first-line treatment of metastatic colorectal cancer in combination with *either* fluorouracil and folinic acid *or* fluorouracil, folinic acid, and irinotecan (but see NICE guidance below). It is also licensed for first-line treatment of metastatic breast cancer in combination with paclitaxel. Bevacizumab, in combination with platinum-based chemotherapy, is licensed for first-line treatment of unresectable advanced, metastatic or recurrent non-small cell lung cancer other than predominantly squamous cell histology. Bevacizumab is given by intravenous infusion.

NICE guidance

Bevacizumab and cetuximab for the treatment of metastatic colorectal cancer (January 2007)

- Bevacizumab in combination with fluorouracil plus folinic acid, with or without irinotecan, is **not** recommended for the first-line treatment of metastatic colorectal cancer;
- Cetuximab in combination with irinotecan is **not** recommended for the second-line or subsequent treatment of metastatic colorectal cancer after the failure of an irinotecan-containing chemotherapy regimen;
- Patients currently receiving bevacizumab or cetuximab should have the option to continue therapy until they and their consultants consider it appropriate to stop.

BEVACIZUMAB

Indications see notes above

Cautions see section 8.1; intra-abdominal inflammation (risk of gastro-intestinal perforation); withhold treatment for elective surgery and avoid for at least 28 days after major surgery or until wound fully healed; history of hypertension (increased risk of proteinuria—discontinue if nephrotic syndrome); uncontrolled hypertension; monitor blood pressure; history of arterial thromboembolism; history of cardiovascular disease (increased risk of cardiovascular events especially in the elderly); monitor for congestive heart failure; increased risk of haemorrhage (especially tumour-associated haemorrhage); monitor for reversible posterior leuccencephalopathy syndrome (presenting as seizures, headache, altered mental status, visual disturbance or cortical blindness, with or without hypertension)

Contra-indications pregnancy (Appendix 4); breast-feeding (Appendix 5); untreated CNS metastases

Side-effects see section 8.1; gastro-intestinal perforation, intestinal obstruction, abdominal pain, diarrhoea, constipation, taste disturbances; mucocutaneous bleeding, haemorrhage, hypoxia, arterial thromboembolism, congestive heart failure, syncope, supraventricular tachycardia, hypertension (see also Cautions); dyspnoea, rhinitis; anorexia, somnolence, headache, peripheral neuropathy, asthenia, lethargy; pyrexia; proteinuria; dehydration; eye disorders; impaired wound healing, hand-foot syndrome, exfoliative dermatitis, dry skin, skin discoloration and tracheoesophageal fistula formation also reported

Avastin® (Roche) ▼ PoM
Concentrate for intravenous infusion, bevacizumab 25 mg/mL, net price 4-ml (100-mg) vial = £242.66, 16-ml (400-mg) vial = £924.40

Bexarotene

Bexarotene is an agonist at the retinoid X receptor, which is involved in the regulation of cell differentiation and proliferation. It is associated with little myelosuppression or immunosuppression. Bexarotene can cause regression of cutaneous T-cell lymphoma. The main adverse effects are hyperlipidaemia, hypothyroidism, leucopenia, headache, rash, and pruritus.

The *Scottish Medicines Consortium* has advised (November 2002) that bexarotene is recommended for restricted use as a second-line treatment for patients with advanced cutaneous T-cell lymphoma.

BEXAROTENE

Indications skin manifestations of cutaneous T-cell lymphoma refractory to previous systemic treatment

Cautions see section 8.1 and notes above; hyperlipidaemia (avoid if uncontrolled), hypothyroidism (avoid if uncontrolled); hypersensitivity to retinoids; **interactions:** Appendix 1 (bexarotene)

Contra-indications see section 8.1 and notes above; history of pancreatitis, hypervitaminosis A, hepatic impairment; pregnancy (Appendix 4); breast-feeding

Side-effects see section 8.1 and notes above

Dose

- Initially 300 mg/m² daily as a single dose with a meal; adjust dose according to response

Targretin® (Zeneus) PoM
Capsules, bexarotene 75 mg in a liquid suspension, net price 100-cap pack = £937.50

Bortezomib

Bortezomib, a proteasome inhibitor, is licensed for multiple myeloma which has progressed despite the use of at least one therapy, and where the patient has already had bone-marrow transplantation or cannot have it. It is given by intravenous injection. Peripheral neuropathy, thrombocytopenia, gastro-intestinal disturbances, pyrexia, postural hypotension, and fatigue are among the most common side-effects.

> NICE guidance
> Bortezomib monotherapy for relapsed multiple myeloma (October 2007)
> Bortezomib monotherapy is an option for the treatment of progressive multiple myeloma in patients who are at first relapse having received one prior therapy and who have undergone, or are unsuitable for, bone-marrow transplantation, under the following circumstances:
> - the response to bortezomib is measured using serum M protein after a maximum of four cycles of treatment, and treatment is continued only in patients who have a reduction in serum M protein of 50% or more (where serum M protein is not measurable, an appropriate alternative biochemical measure of response should be used) **and**
> - the manufacturer rebates the full cost of bortezomib if there is an inadequate response (as defined above) after four cycles of treatment.
>
> Patients currently receiving bortezomib monotherapy who do not meet the above criteria should have the option to continue therapy until they and their clinicians consider it appropriate to stop.

BORTEZOMIB

Indications see notes above
Cautions see section 8.1 and notes above; hepatic impairment (avoid if severe; Appendix 2); renal impairment (Appendix 3); pregnancy (Appendix 4); monitor blood-glucose concentration in patients on oral antidiabetics
Contra-indications breast-feeding
Side-effects see section 8.1 and notes above

Velcade® (Ortho Biotech) ▼ PoM
Injection, powder for reconstitution, bortezomib (as mannitol boronic ester), net price 3.5-mg vial = £762.38

Cetuximab

Cetuximab is licensed, in combination with irinotecan, for the treatment of metastatic colorectal cancer in patients with tumours expressing epidermal growth factor receptor in whom previous chemotherapy, that has included irinotecan, has failed (but see NICE guidance under Bevacizumab on p. 463). Cetuximab is also licensed, in combination with radiotherapy, for the treatment of locally advanced squamous cell cancer of the head and neck.

Cetuximab is given by intravenous infusion. Patients must receive an antihistamine before the first infusion; an antihistamine is also recommended before subsequent infusions of cetuximab. Resuscitation facilities should be available and treatment should be initiated by a specialist.

CETUXIMAB

Indications see notes above and product literature
Cautions cardiopulmonary disease, pulmonary disease—discontinue if interstitial lung disease; pregnancy (Appendix 4)
Contra-indications breast-feeding (Appendix 5)
Side-effects infusion-related side-effects including nausea, vomiting, headache, dizziness, chills, fever, hypersensitivity reactions such as rash, urticaria, airway obstruction, dyspnoea (possibly delayed onset), hypotension; skin reactions including acne, pruritus, dry skin, desquamation, hypertrichosis, and nail disorders; conjunctivitis; hypomagnesaemia also reported

Erbitux® (Merck) ▼ PoM
Intravenous infusion, cetuximab 2 mg/mL, net price 50-mL vial = £136.50; 5 mg/mL, 20-mL vial = £136.50, 100-mL vial = £682.50

Crisantaspase

Crisantaspase is the enzyme asparaginase produced by *Erwinia chrysanthemi.* It is given *intramuscularly, intravenously*, or *subcutaneously* almost exclusively in acute lymphoblastic leukaemia. Facilities for the management of anaphylaxis should be available. Side-effects also include nausea, vomiting, fever, pancreatitis, CNS depression, neurotoxicity, liver function changes, coagulation disorders, and blood lipid changes; careful monitoring is therefore necessary and the urine is tested for glucose because of a risk of hyperglycaemia.

CRISANTASPASE

Indications see notes above
Cautions see notes above
Contra-indications pregnancy (Appendix 4); breast-feeding
Side-effects see notes above

Erwinase® (OPi) PoM
Injection, powder for reconstitution, crisantaspase. Net price 10 000-unit vial = £194.77

Dacarbazine and temozolomide

Dacarbazine is used to treat metastatic melanoma and, in combination therapy, soft tissue sarcomas. It is also a component of a commonly used combination for Hodgkin's disease (ABVD—doxorubicin [previously *Adriamycin®*], bleomycin, vinblastine, and dacarbazine). It is given *intravenously*. The predominant side-effects are myelosuppression and severe nausea and vomiting.

Temozolomide is structurally related to dacarbazine. It is given by mouth and is licensed for the initial treatment of glioblastoma multiforme (in combination with radiotherapy) and for second-line treatment of malignant glioma.

> **NICE guidance**
> **Temozolomide for the treatment of recurrent malignant glioma (brain cancer) (April 2001)**
> Temozolomide may be considered for the treatment of recurrent malignant glioma, which has not responded to first-line chemotherapy.

> **NICE guidance**
> **Carmustine implants and temozolomide for the treatment of newly diagnosed high-grade glioma (June 2007)**
> Temozolomide is an option for the treatment of newly diagnosed glioblastoma multiforme in patients with a WHO performance status of 0 or 1.
> Carmustine implants are an option for the treatment of newly diagnosed high-grade (Grade 3 or 4) glioma **only** for patients in whom at least 90% of the tumour has been resected.
> Treatment with carmustine implants should be provided only within specialist centres.

DACARBAZINE

Indications see notes above
Cautions see section 8.1; hepatic impairment (Appendix 2); renal impairment (avoid if creatinine clearance less than 10 mL/minute; Appendix 3); caution in handling
Contra-indications pregnancy (Appendix 4); breast-feeding
Side-effects see section 8.1 and notes above; *rarely* liver necrosis due to hepatic vein thrombosis; irritant to skin and tissues

Dacarbazine (Non-proprietary) PoM
Injection, powder for reconstitution, dacarbazine (as citrate), net price 100-mg vial = £5.05; 200-mg vial = £7.16; 500-mg vial = £16.50; 600-mg vial = £22.50; 1-g vial = £31.80

TEMOZOLOMIDE

Indications see notes above
Cautions see section 8.1; severe hepatic impairment and renal impairment; **interactions**: Appendix 1 (temozolomide)
Contra-indications pregnancy (Appendix 4); breast-feeding
Side-effects see section 8.1
Dose

- Consult product literature; CHILD under 3 years not recommended

Temodal® (Schering-Plough) PoM
Capsules, temozolomide 5 mg (green/white), net price 5-cap pack = £17.30; 20 mg (yellow/white), 5-cap pack = £69.20; 100 mg (pink/white), 5-cap pack = £346.00; 250 mg (white), 5-cap pack = £865.00.
Label: 23, 25

Hydroxycarbamide

Hydroxycarbamide (hydroxyurea) is an orally active drug used mainly in the treatment of chronic myeloid leukaemia. It is also licensed for the treatment of cancer of the cervix in conjunction with radiotherapy. It is occasionally used for polycythaemia (the usual treatment is venesection). Myelosuppression, nausea, and skin reactions are the most common toxic effects.

HYDROXYCARBAMIDE
(Hydroxyurea)

Indications see notes above
Cautions see section 8.1 and notes above; renal impairment; **interactions**: Appendix 1 (hydroxycarbamide)
Contra-indications pregnancy (Appendix 4); breast-feeding
Side-effects see section 8.1 and notes above
Dose

- 20–30 mg/kg daily *or* 80 mg/kg every third day

Hydroxycarbamide (Non-proprietary) PoM
Capsules, hydroxycarbamide 500 mg, net price 20 = £2.22

Hydrea® (Squibb) PoM
Capsules, pink/green, hydroxycarbamide 500 mg. Net price 20 = £2.39

Mitotane

Mitotane is licensed for the symptomatic treatment of advanced or inoperable adrenocortical carcinoma. It selectively inhibits the activity of the adrenal cortex, necessitating corticosteroid replacement therapy (section 6.3.1); the dose of glucocorticoid should be increased in case of shock, trauma, or infection.

Gastro-intestinal side-effects such as anorexia, nausea, and vomiting, and endocrine side-effects, such as hypogonadism and thyroid disorders, are very common with mitotane; neurotoxicity occurs in many patients.

MITOTANE

Indications see notes above
Cautions see section 8.1 and notes above; risk of accumulation in overweight patients; monitor plasma-mitotane concentration—consult product literature; hepatic impairment (Appendix 2); renal impairment (avoid if creatinine clearance less than 30 mL/minute; Appendix 3); **interactions**: Appendix 1 (mitotane)
Driving CNS effects may affect performance of skilled tasks (e.g. driving)
Counselling Warn patient to contact doctor immediately if injury, infection or illness occurs (because of risk of acute adrenal insufficiency)
Contra-indications pregnancy (Appendix 4); breast-feeding
Side-effects see section 8.1 and notes above; also gastro-intestinal disturbances (including nausea, vomiting, diarrhoea, epigastric discomfort), anorexia, liver disorders; hypercholesterolaemia, hypertriglyceridaemia; ataxia, confusion, asthenia, myasthenia, paraesthesia, drowsiness, neuropathy, cognitive impairment, movement disorder, dizziness, headache; gynaecomastia; prolonged bleeding time, leucopenia, thrombocytopenia, anaemia; rash; *rarely* hypersalivation, hypertension, postural hypotension, flushing, pyrexia, haematuria, proteinuria, haemorrhagic cystitis, hypouricaemia, visual disturbances and ocular disorders

Dose

- ADULT over 18 years, initially 2–3 g daily, (up to 6 g daily in severe illness) in 2–3 divided doses, adjusted according to plasma-mitotane concentration; reduce dose or interrupt treatment if signs of toxicity; discontinue if inadequate response after 3 months
  Note Plasma-mitotane concentration for optimum response 14–20 mg/litre

Lysodren® (HRA Pharma) ▼ PoM
Tablets, scored, mitotane 500 mg, net price 100-tab pack = £460.40. Label: 2, 10, 21, counselling, driving, adrenal suppression

Pentostatin

Pentostatin is highly active in hairy cell leukaemia. It is given *intravenously* on alternate weeks and is capable of inducing prolonged complete remission. It is potentially toxic, causing myelosuppression, immunosuppression and a number of other side-effects which may be severe. Its use is probably best confined to specialist centres.

PENTOSTATIN

Indications see notes above
Cautions see section 8.1 and notes above; **interactions**: Appendix 1 (pentostatin)
Contra-indications pregnancy (Appendix 4); breast-feeding
Side-effects see section 8.1 and notes above

Nipent® (EuroGen) PoM
Injection, powder for reconstitution, pentostatin. Net price 10-mg vial = £863.78

Platinum compounds

Carboplatin is widely used in the treatment of advanced ovarian cancer and lung cancer (particularly the small cell type). It is given *intravenously*. The dose of carboplatin is determined according to renal function rather than body surface area. Carboplatin can be given on an outpatient basis and is better tolerated than cisplatin; nausea and vomiting are reduced in severity and nephrotoxicity, neurotoxicity, and ototoxicity are much less of a problem than with cisplatin. It is, however, more myelosuppressive than cisplatin.

Cisplatin is used alone or in combination for the treatment of testicular, lung, cervical, bladder, head and neck, and ovarian cancer (but carboplatin is preferred for ovarian cancer). It is given *intravenously*. Cisplatin requires intensive intravenous hydration and treatment may be complicated by severe nausea and vomiting. Cisplatin is toxic, causing nephrotoxicity (monitoring of renal function is essential), ototoxicity, peripheral neuropathy, hypomagnesaemia and myelosuppression. It is, however, increasingly given in a day-care setting.

Oxaliplatin is licensed in combination with fluorouracil and folinic acid, for the treatment of metastatic colorectal cancer and as adjuvant treatment of colon cancer after resection of the primary tumour; it is given by intravenous infusion. Neurotoxic side-effects (including sensory peripheral neuropathy) are dose limiting. Other side-effects include gastro-intestinal disturbances, ototoxicity, and myelosuppression. Manufacturers advise renal function monitoring in moderate impairment.

NICE guidance
Irinotecan, oxaliplatin, and raltitrexed for advanced colorectal cancer (August 2005)
A combination of fluorouracil and folinic acid with either irinotecan or oxaliplatin are options for first-line treatment for advanced colorectal cancer.
Irinotecan alone or fluorouracil and folinic acid with oxaliplatin are options for patients who require further treatment subsequently.
Raltitrexed is **not** recommended for the treatment of advanced colorectal cancer. Its use should be confined to clinical studies.

NICE guidance (capecitabine and oxaliplatin in the adjuvant treatment of stage III (Dukes' C) colon cancer)
See p. 457

NICE guidance
Paclitaxel for ovarian cancer (January 2003)
Either paclitaxel in combination with a platinum compound (cisplatin or carboplatin) *or* a platinum compound alone are alternatives for the first-line treatment of ovarian cancer (usually following surgery).

NICE guidance
Paclitaxel, pegylated liposomal doxorubicin, and topotecan for second-line or subsequent treatment of advanced ovarian cancer (May 2005)
Paclitaxel, combined with a platinum compound (carboplatin or cisplatin), is an option for advanced cancer that relapses 6 months or more after completing initial platinum-based chemotherapy. Paclitaxel alone is an option for advanced ovarian cancer that does not respond to, or relapses within 6 months of completing initial platinum-based chemotherapy.
Pegylated liposomal doxorubicin is an option for advanced ovarian cancer that does not respond to, or relapses within 12 months of completing initial platinum-based chemotherapy.
Paclitaxel alone or pegylated liposomal doxorubicin are options for advanced ovarian cancer in patients who are allergic to platinum compounds. Topotecan alone is an option only for advanced ovarian cancer that does not respond to, or relapses within 6 months of completing initial platinum-based chemotherapy or in those allergic to platinum compounds *and* for whom paclitaxel alone or pegylated liposomal doxorubicin are inappropriate.

CARBOPLATIN

Indications see notes above
Cautions see section 8.1 and notes above; renal impairment (avoid if creatinine clearance less than 20 mL/minute; Appendix 3); **interactions**: Appendix 1 (platinum compounds)
Contra-indications pregnancy (Appendix 4); breast-feeding
Side-effects see section 8.1 and notes above

Carboplatin (Non-proprietary) PoM
Injection, carboplatin 10 mg/mL, net price 5-mL vial = £22.04, 15-mL vial = £56.29, 45-mL vial = £168.85, 60-mL vial = £260.00

Paraplatin® (Bristol-Myers Squibb) PoM
Concentrate for intravenous infusion, carboplatin 10 mg/mL, net price 5-mL vial = £21.26, 15-mL vial = £61.22, 45-mL vial = £183.66, 60-mL vial = £244.88

CISPLATIN

Indications see notes above
Cautions see section 8.1 and notes above; **interactions:** Appendix 1 (platinum compounds)
Contra-indications renal impairment (Appendix 3); pregnancy (Appendix 4); breast-feeding
Side-effects see section 8.1 and notes above

Cisplatin (Non-proprietary) PoM
Injection, cisplatin 1 mg/mL, net price 10-mL vial = £5.85, 50-mL vial = £25.37, 100-mL vial = £50.22
Injection, powder for reconstitution, cisplatin, net price 50-mg vial = £17.00

OXALIPLATIN

Indications metastatic colorectal cancer in combination with fluorouracil and folinic acid; colon cancer—see notes above
Cautions see section 8.1 and notes above; **interactions:** Appendix 1 (platinum compounds)
Contra-indications see section 8.1; peripheral neuropathy with functional impairment; renal impairment (avoid if creatinine clearance less than 30 mL/minute; Appendix 3); pregnancy (Appendix 4); breast-feeding
Side-effects see section 8.1 and notes above

Oxaliplatin (Non-proprietary) PoM
Injection, powder for reconstitution, oxaliplatin, net price 50-mg vial = £156.75, 100-mg vial= £313.50

Eloxatin® (Sanofi-Aventis) PoM
Concentrate for intravenous infusion, oxaliplatin 5 mg/mL, net price 10-mL vial = £165.00, 20-mL vial = £330.00

Porfimer sodium and temoporfin

Porfimer sodium and **temoporfin** are used in the photodynamic treatment of various tumours. The drugs accumulate in malignant tissue and are activated by laser light to produce a cytotoxic effect.

Porfimer sodium is licensed for photodynamic therapy of non-small cell lung cancer and obstructing oesophageal cancer. Temoporfin is licensed for photodynamic therapy of advanced head and neck cancer.

The *Scottish Medicines Consortium* has advised (May 2004) that temoporfin is **not** recommended for the palliative treatment of advanced head and neck cancer.

PORFIMER SODIUM

Indications non-small cell lung cancer; oesophageal cancer; see notes above
Cautions see section 8.1; avoid exposure of skin and eyes to direct sunlight or bright indoor light for at least 30 days
Contra-indications see section 8.1; severe hepatic impairment; tracheo-oesophageal or broncho-oesophageal fistula; porphyria (section 9.8.2); pregnancy (Appendix 4); breast-feeding (Appendix 5)
Side-effects see section 8.1; photosensitivity (see Cautions above—sunscreens offer no protection), constipation

Photofrin (Sinclair) ▼ PoM
Injection, powder for reconstitution, porfimer sodium, net price 15-mg vial = £154.00; 75-mg vial = £770.00

TEMOPORFIN

Indications advanced head and neck squamous cell carcinoma refractory to, or unsuitable for, other treatments
Cautions see section 8.1; avoid exposure of skin and eyes to direct sunlight or bright indoor light for at least 15 days after administration; avoid prolonged exposure of injection site arm to direct sunlight for 6 months after administration, if extravasation occurs protect area from light for at least 3 months; **interactions:** Appendix 1 (temoporfin)
Contra-indications see section 8.1; porphyria (section 9.8.2) or other diseases exacerbated by light; elective surgery or ophthalmic slit-lamp examination for 30 days after administration; concomitant photosensitising treatment; pregnancy (Appendix 4); breast-feeding (Appendix 5)
Side-effects see section 8.1; also constipation, dysphagia; haemorrhage, oedema; giddiness, trismus, facial pain; injection site pain blistering, scarring, erythema, skin necrosis, hyperpigmentation, photosensitivity (see Cautions above; sunscreens ineffective)

Foscan® (Biolitec) ▼ PoM
Injection, temoporfin 4 mg/mL, net price 5-mL vial = £4400.00

Procarbazine

Procarbazine is most often used in Hodgkin's disease. It is given *by mouth*. Toxic effects include nausea, myelosuppression, and a hypersensitivity rash preventing further use of this drug. It is a mild monoamine-oxidase inhibitor and dietary restriction is rarely considered necessary. Alcohol ingestion may cause a disulfiram-like reaction.

PROCARBAZINE

Indications see notes above
Cautions see section 8.1 and notes above; hepatic impairment—avoid if severe; renal impairment (avoid if creatinine clearance less than 10 mL/minute; Appendix 3); **interactions:** Appendix 1 (procarbazine)
Contra-indications pregnancy (Appendix 4); breast-feeding
Side-effects see section 8.1 and notes above
Dose

- Used alone, initially 50 mg daily, increased by 50 mg daily to 250–300 mg daily in divided doses; maintenance (on remission) 50–150 mg daily to cumulative total of at least 6 g

Procarbazine (Cambridge) PoM
Capsules, ivory, procarbazine (as hydrochloride) 50 mg, net price 50-cap pack = £181.04. Label: 4

Protein kinase inhibitors

Dasatinib, erlotinib, imatinib, sorafenib, and sunitinib are protein kinase inhibitors.

Dasatinib, a tyrosine kinase inhibitor, is licensed for the treatment of chronic myeloid leukaemia in those who have resistance to or intolerance of previous therapy, including imatinib. It is also licensed for acute lymphoblastic leukaemia in those who have resistance to or intolerance of previous therapy.

Erlotinib, a tyrosine kinase inhibitor, is licensed in combination with gemcitabine for the treatment of metastatic pancreatic cancer. It is also licensed for the treatment of locally advanced or metastatic non-small cell lung cancer after failure of previous chemotherapy.

The *Scottish Medicines Consortium* has advised (June 2006) that erlotinib is accepted for restricted use for the treatment of locally advanced or metastatic non-small cell lung cancer, after failure of at least one chemotherapy regimen. Erlotinib is restricted to use in patients who would otherwise be eligible for treatment with docetaxel monotherapy.

Imatinib, a tyrosine kinase inhibitor, is licensed for the treatment of newly diagnosed chronic myeloid leukaemia where bone marrow transplantation is not considered first-line treatment, and for chronic myeloid leukaemia in chronic phase after failure of interferon alfa, or in accelerated phase, or in blast crisis (see NICE guidance below). It is also licensed for c-kit (CD117)-positive unresectable or metastatic malignant gastro-intestinal stromal tumours (GIST). Imatinib is licensed for the treatment of newly diagnosed acute lymphoblastic leukaemia in combination with other chemotherapy, and as monotherapy for relapsed or refractory acute lymphoblastic leukaemia. Imatinib is also licensed for the treatment of unresectable dermatofibrosarcoma protuberans and for patients with recurrent or metastatic dermatofibrosarcoma protuberans who cannot have surgery.

Recently imatinib has also been licensed for the treatment of myelodysplastic/myeloproliferative diseases associated with platelet-derived growth factor receptor gene rearrangement and for the treatment of advanced hypereosinophilic syndrome and chronic eosinophilic leukaemia.

The *Scottish Medicines Consortium* has advised (March 2002) that imatinib should be used for chronic myeloid leukaemia only under specialist supervision in accordance with British Society of Haematology guidelines (November 2001).

> **NICE guidance**
> **Imatinib for chronic myeloid leukaemia (October 2003)**
> Imatinib is recommended as first-line treatment for Philadelphia-chromosome-positive chronic myeloid leukaemia in the chronic phase and as an option for patients presenting in the accelerated phase or with blast crisis, provided that imatinib has not been used previously.
> Where imatinib has failed to stop disease progression from chronic phase to accelerated phase or to blast crisis, continued use is recommended only as part of further clinical study.

Sorafenib, an inhibitor of multiple kinases, is licensed for the treatment of advanced renal cell carcinoma when treatment with interferon alfa or interleukin-2 has failed or is contra-indicated. It is also licensed for the treatment of hepatocellular carcinoma.

Sunitinib, a tyrosine kinase inhibitor, is licensed for the treatment of advanced or metastatic renal cell carcinoma. It is also licensed for the treatment of unresectable or metastatic malignant gastro-intestinal stromal tumours (GIST) after failure of imatinib.

DASATINIB

Indications see notes above

Cautions see section 8.1; susceptibility to QT-interval prolongation; hypokalaemia; hypomagnesaemia; hepatic impairment (Appendix 2); pregnancy (Appendix 4 and section 8.1); **interactions**: Appendix 1 (dasatinib)

Contra-indications breast-feeding

Side-effects see section 8.1; also diarrhoea, anorexia, weight gain, abdominal pain, taste disturbance, constipation, dyspepsia, colitis, gastritis; arrhythmias, congestive cardiac failure, chest pain, flushing, haemorrhage (including gastro-intestinal and CNS haemorrhage), palpitation; dyspnoea, cough, oedema (including pleural effusion); depression, dizziness, headache, insomnia, neuropathy; influenza-like symptoms; musculoskeletal pain; visual disturbances; acne, dry skin, sweating, pruritus, urticaria; *less commonly* pancreatitis, hepatitis, cholestasis, hypertension, hypotension, transient ischaemic attack, thrombophlebitis, syncope, pulmonary hypertension, asthma, convulsions, amnesia, tremor, drowsiness, vertigo, gynaecomastia, irregular menstruation, urinary frequency, proteinuria, hypocalcaemia, rhabdomyolysis, tinnitus, hypersensitivity reactions (including dermatitis, photosensitivity), pigmentation and nail disorders

Dose

- Chronic phase chronic myeloid leukaemia, ADULT over 18 years 100 mg once daily, increased if necessary to max. 140 mg once daily
- Accelerated and blast phase chronic myeloid leukaemia, ADULT over 18 years 70 mg twice daily, increased if necessary to max. 100 mg twice daily
- Acute lymphoblastic leukaemia, ADULT over 18 years 70 mg twice daily increased if necessary to max. 100 mg twice daily

Sprycel® (Bristol-Myers Squibb) ▼ PoM
Tablets, f/c, dasatinib (as monohydrate) 20 mg, net price 56-tab pack = £1216.43; 50 mg, 56-tab pack = £2432.85; 70 mg, 56-tab pack = £2432.85. Label: 25

ERLOTINIB

Indications see notes above

Cautions see section 8.1; pre-existing liver disease or concomitant use with hepatotoxic drugs—monitor liver function; hepatic impairment (Appendix 2); **interactions:** Appendix 1 (erlotinib)

Contra-indications renal impairment (avoid if creatinine clearance less than 15 mL/minute; Appendix 3); pregnancy (Appendix 4); breast-feeding (Appendix 5)

Side-effects see section 8.1; diarrhoea, abdominal pain, dyspepsia, flatulence; anorexia, depression, headache; fatigue, rigor; conjunctivitis; rash, pruritus, dry skin; *less commonly* interstitial lung disease—discontinue if unexplained symptoms such as dyspnoea, cough or fever occur; *rarely* hepatic failure

8 Malignant disease and immunosuppression

Dose

- Non-small cell lung cancer, 150 mg once daily
- Pancreatic cancer, 100 mg once daily in combination with gemcitabine

Tarceva® (Roche) ▼ PoM
Tablets, f/c, white-yellow, erlotinib (as hydrochloride) 25 mg, net price 30-tab pack = £378.30; 100 mg, 30-tab pack = £1324.14; 150 mg, 30-tab pack = £1631.53. Label: 23

IMATINIB

Indications see notes above

Cautions see section 8.1; cardiac disease; monitor liver function and for symptoms of fluid retention; hepatic impairment (Appendix 2); renal impairment (Appendix 3); **interactions:** Appendix 1 (imatinib)

Contra-indications pregnancy (Appendix 4 and section 8.1); breast-feeding

Side-effects see section 8.1; also abdominal pain, anorexia, constipation, diarrhoea, flatulence, gastro-oesophageal reflux, taste disturbance; oedema (including pulmonary oedema, pleural effusion, and ascites); dyspnoea; dizziness, headache, insomnia, paraesthesia; influenza-like symptoms; cramps, arthralgia, swelling of joint muscles; visual disturbances; epistaxis; dry skin, sweating, rash, pruritus; *less commonly* dry mouth, gastric ulceration, pancreatitis, jaundice, hepatitis, heart failure, tachycardia, haemorrhage, syncope, hypertension, hypotension, flushing, cold extremities, cough, acute respiratory failure, depression, drowsiness, anxiety, peripheral neuropathy, migraine, impaired memory, vertigo, decreased libido, gynaecomastia, menorrhagia, electrolyte disturbances, renal failure, urinary frequency, gout, tinnitus; *rarely* intestinal obstruction, gastro-intestinal perforation, colitis, diverticulitis, hepatic necrosis, thromboembolism, pulmonary fibrosis, interstitial pneumonitis, increased intracranial pressure, convulsions, confusion, aseptic necrosis of bone, angioedema, photosensitivity, skin pigmentation, exfoliative dermatitis, Stevens-Johnson syndrome

Dose

- Chronic phase chronic myeloid leukaemia, ADULT 400 mg once daily, increased if necessary to max. 800 mg daily (in 2 divided doses); CHILD (chronic and advanced phase) 2–18 years 340 mg/m² (max. 800 mg) daily (in 1–2 divided doses), increased to 570 mg/m² (max. 800 mg) daily if necessary (consult product literature)
- Accelerated phase and blast crisis chronic myeloid leukaemia, ADULT 600 mg once daily, increased if necessary to max. 800 mg daily (in 2 divided doses)
- Acute lymphoblastic leukaemia, ADULT 600 mg once daily
- Gastro-intestinal stromal tumours, ADULT 400 mg once daily
- Dermatofibrosarcoma protuberans, ADULT 800 mg daily in 2 divided doses
- Myelodysplastic/myeloproliferative diseases, ADULT 400 mg once daily
- Advanced hypereosinophilic syndrome and chronic eosinophilic leukaemia, ADULT 100–400 mg once daily

Glivec® (Novartis) ▼ PoM
Tablets, f/c, imatinib (as mesilate) 100 mg (yellow-brown, scored), net price 60-tab pack = £802.04; 400 mg (yellow), 30-tab pack = £1604.08. Label: 21, 27
Counselling Tablets may be dispersed in water or apple juice

SORAFENIB

Indications see notes above

Cautions major surgical procedures; cardiac ischaemia; hepatic impairment (Appendix 2); pregnancy (Appendix 4); **interactions:** Appendix 1 (sorafenib)

Contra-indications breast-feeding

Side-effects see section 8.1; also diarrhoea, constipation, dyspepsia, dysphagia, anorexia, hypertension, haemorrhage, flushing, hoarseness, fatigue, asthenia, depression, peripheral neuropathy, fever, erectile dysfunction, hypophosphataemia, arthralgia, myalgia, tinnitus, rash, pruritus, erythema, dry skin, desquamation, acne, hand-foot skin reaction; *less commonly* reversible posterior leucoencephalopathy, myocardial infarction, congestive heart failure, hypertensive crisis, and gastro-intestinal perforations

Dose

- ADULT over 18 years, 400 mg twice daily

Nexavar® (Bayer) ▼ PoM
Tablets, f/c, red, sorafenib (as tosylate) 200 mg, net price 112-tab pack = £2504.60. Label: 23

SUNITINIB

Indications see notes above

Cautions see section 8.1; monitor for signs and symptoms of congestive cardiac failure (consider interrupting or stopping treatment); susceptibility to QT-interval prolongation; hypertension; pregnancy (Appendix 4 and section 8.1); **interactions:** Appendix 1 (sunitinib)

Contra-indications breast-feeding

Side-effects see section 8.1; also abdominal pain, anorexia, taste disturbance; hypertension, oedema; fatigue, dizziness, headache, paraesthesia; hypothyroidism; arthralgia, myalgia; lacrimation; epistaxis; skin and hair discoloration, hand-foot syndrome, and rash; gastro-intestinal perforation, pancreatitis, hepatic failure, and seizures reported

Dose

- 50 mg daily for 4 weeks, followed by a 2-week treatment-free period to complete 6-week cycle; adjust dose in steps of 12.5 mg according to tolerability; dose range 37.5–87.5 mg daily

Sutent® (Pfizer) ▼ PoM
Capsules, sunitinib (as malate) 12.5 mg (orange), net price 30-cap pack = £840.75; 25 mg (caramel), 30-cap pack = £1681.50; 50 mg (caramel/orange), 30-cap pack = £3363.00

Taxanes

Paclitaxel is a member of the taxane group of drugs. It is given by *intravenous infusion*. Paclitaxel given with carboplatin or cisplatin is used for the treatment of ovarian cancer (see NICE guidance p. 466); the combination is also considered appropriate for women whose ovarian cancer is initially considered inoperable. Paclitaxel is also used in the secondary treatment of metastatic breast cancer (see NICE guidance, below). There is limited evidence to support its use in non-small cell lung cancer. Routine premedication with a corticosteroid, an antihistamine and a histamine H_2-receptor antagonist is recommended to prevent severe hypersensitivity reactions; hypersensitivity reactions may occur rarely despite premedication, although more commonly only bradycardia or asymptomatic hypotension occur.

Other side-effects of paclitaxel include myelosuppression, peripheral neuropathy, and cardiac conduction defects with arrhythmias (which are nearly always asymptomatic). It also causes alopecia and muscle pain; nausea and vomiting is mild to moderate.

Docetaxel is licensed for use in locally advanced or metastatic breast cancer and non-small cell lung cancer resistant to other cytotoxic drugs (see NICE guidance on breast cancer, below) or for initial chemotherapy in combination with other cytotoxic drugs. It is also licensed for hormone-resistant prostate cancer, for use with other cytotoxic drugs for gastric adenocarcinoma and head and neck cancer, and for adjuvant treatment of operable node-positive breast cancer. Its side-effects are similar to those of paclitaxel but persistent fluid retention (commonly as leg oedema that worsens during treatment) can be resistant to treatment; hypersensitivity reactions also occur. Dexamethasone by mouth is recommended for reducing fluid retention and hypersensitivity reactions.

NICE guidance

Docetaxel for the adjuvant treatment of early node-positive breast cancer (September 2006)

Docetaxel, in combination with doxorubicin and cyclophosphamide, is an option for the adjuvant treatment of women with early node-positive breast cancer.

NICE guidance

Paclitaxel for the adjuvant treatment of early node-positive breast cancer (September 2006)

Paclitaxel is **not** recommended for the adjuvant treatment of early node-positive breast cancer.

NICE guidance

Taxanes for the treatment of breast cancer (September 2001)

Both docetaxel and paclitaxel are options for the treatment of *advanced* breast cancer where initial cytotoxic chemotherapy (including an anthracycline) has failed or is inappropriate.

NICE guidance (paclitaxel, pegylated liposomal doxorubicin and topotecan for second-line or subsequent treatment of advanced ovarian cancer)

See p. 466

NICE guidance

Docetaxel for the treatment of hormone-refractory metastatic prostate cancer (June 2006)

Docetaxel is an option for hormone-refractory metastatic prostate cancer and a Karnofsky score of at least 60% [Karnofsky score is a measure of the ability to perform ordinary tasks].

DOCETAXEL

Indications adjuvant treatment of operable node-positive breast cancer, in combination with doxorubicin and cyclophosphamide; with doxorubicin for initial chemotherapy of advanced or metastatic breast cancer; alone or with capecitabine for advanced or metastatic breast cancer where cytotoxic chemotherapy with anthracycline or alkylating drug has failed; with trastuzumab for initial chemotherapy of metastatic breast cancer; advanced or metastatic non-small cell lung cancer where first-line chemotherapy has failed; with cisplatin for unresectable, advanced or metastatic non-small cell lung cancer; with prednisolone for hormone-refractory metastatic prostate cancer; with cisplatin and 5-fluorouracil for initial treatment of metastatic gastric adenocarcinoma, including adenocarcinoma of the gastroesophageal junction, and as induction treatment for inoperable locally advanced squamous cell carcinoma of the head and neck

Cautions see section 8.1 and notes above; hepatic impairment (Appendix 2); **interactions:** Appendix 1 (docetaxel)

Contra-indications pregnancy (Appendix 4); breast-feeding

Side-effects see section 8.1 and notes above

Taxotere® (Sanofi-Aventis) PoM

Concentrate for intravenous infusion, docetaxel 40 mg/mL. Net price 0.5-mL vial = £162.75, 2-mL vial = £534.75 (both with diluent) (hosp. only)

PACLITAXEL

Indications ovarian cancer (advanced or residual disease following laparotomy) in combination with cisplatin; metastatic ovarian cancer where platinum-containing therapy has failed; locally advanced or metastatic breast cancer (in combination with other cytotoxics or alone if other cytotoxics have failed or are inappropriate); adjuvant treatment of node-positive breast cancer following treatment with anthracycline and cyclophosphamide; non-small cell lung cancer (in combination with cisplatin) when surgery or radiotherapy not appropriate; advanced AIDS-related Kaposi's sarcoma where liposomal anthracycline therapy has failed

Cautions see section 8.1 and notes above; **interactions:** Appendix 1 (paclitaxel)

Contra-indications see section 8.1 and notes above; severe hepatic impairment; pregnancy (Appendix 4); breast-feeding

Side-effects see section 8.1 and notes above

Paclitaxel (Non-proprietary) PoM

Concentrate for intravenous infusion, paclitaxel 6 mg/mL, net price 5-mL vial = £111.41, 16.7-mL vial

= £333.91, 25-mL vial = £500.86, 50-mL vial = £1001.72

Excipients include polyoxyl castor oil (risk of anaphylaxis, see Excipients, p. 2)

Taxol® (Bristol-Myers Squibb) PoM

Concentrate for intravenous infusion, paclitaxel 6 mg/mL, net price 5-mL vial = £116.05, 16.7-mL vial = £347.82, 25-mL vial = £521.73, 50-mL vial = £1043.46 (hosp. only)

Excipients include polyoxyl castor oil (risk of anaphylaxis, see Excipients, p. 2)

Topoisomerase I inhibitors

Irinotecan and topotecan inhibit topoisomerase I, an enzyme involved in DNA replication.

Irinotecan is licensed for metastatic colorectal cancer in combination with fluorouracil and folinic acid or as monotherapy when treatment containing fluorouracil has failed. It is also licensed in combination with cetuximab for the treatment of epidermal growth factor receptor-expressing metastatic colorectal cancer after failure of chemotherapy that has included irinotecan. Irinotecan is also licensed in combination with 5-fluorouracil, folinic acid and bevacizumab for the first-line treatment of metastatic carcinoma of the colon or rectum. Irinotecan is given by intravenous infusion.

NICE guidance (irinotecan, oxaliplatin and raltitrexed for advanced colorectal cancer)
See p. 466

Topotecan is given by intravenous infusion in metastatic ovarian cancer when first-line or subsequent therapy has failed.

In addition to dose-limiting myelosuppression, side-effects of irinotecan and topotecan include gastro-intestinal effects (delayed diarrhoea requiring prompt treatment may follow irinotecan treatment), asthenia, alopecia, and anorexia.

The *Scottish Medicines Consortium* has advised (November 2007) that topotecan is accepted for restricted use in combination with cisplatin for treatment of recurrent carcinoma of the cervix after radiotherapy and for stage IVB disease; it is restricted to patients who are cisplatin-naive.

NICE guidance (paclitaxel, pegylated liposomal doxorubicin and topotecan for second-line or subsequent treatment of advanced ovarian cancer)
See p. 466

IRINOTECAN HYDROCHLORIDE

Indications see notes above

Cautions see section 8.1 and notes above; raised plasma-bilirubin concentration (see under Contra-indications and Appendix 2)

Contra-indications see section 8.1 and notes above, also chronic inflammatory bowel disease, bowel obstruction; plasma bilirubin concentration more than 3 times the upper limit of reference range; renal impairment (Appendix 3); pregnancy (Appendix 4); breast-feeding

Side-effects see section 8.1 and notes above; also acute cholinergic syndrome (with early diarrhoea) and delayed diarrhoea (consult product literature), interstitial pulmonary disease

Campto® (Pfizer) PoM

Concentrate for intravenous infusion, irinotecan hydrochloride 20 mg/mL, net price 2-mL vial = £53.00; 5-mL vial = £130.00

TOPOTECAN

Indications metastatic ovarian cancer where first-line or subsequent therapy has failed

Cautions see section 8.1 and notes above; renal impairment (avoid if creatinine clearance less than 20 mL/minute; Appendix 3)

Contra-indications see section 8.1 and notes above; severe hepatic impairment; pregnancy (Appendix 4); breast-feeding

Side-effects see section 8.1 and notes above

Hycamtin® (Merck) PoM

Intravenous infusion, powder for reconstitution, topotecan (as hydrochloride), net price 1-mg vial = £97.65; 4-mg vial = £290.62

Trabectedin

Trabectedin is licensed for the treatment of advanced soft tissue sarcoma when treatment with anthracyclines and ifosfamide has failed or is contra-indicated.

Trabectedin is given by intravenous infusion. Dexamethasone by intravenous infusion should be given concomitantly for its antiemetic and hepatoprotective effects.

TRABECTEDIN

Indications see notes above

Cautions see section 8.1 and notes above; measure creatine phosphokinase, renal function and hepatic function before starting (consult product literature); monitor haematological and hepatic parameters weekly during first 2 cycles and at least once between treatments in subsequent cycles; concomitant use with hepatotoxic drugs (avoid alcohol); hepatic impairment (Appendix 2)

Contra-indications raised bilirubin; renal impairment (avoid if creatinine clearance less than 30 mL/minute; Appendix 3); pregnancy (Appendix 4); breast-feeding (Appendix 5)

Side-effects see section 8.1; also abdominal pain, constipation, diarrhoea, dyspepsia, taste disturbance, hepatobiliary disorders; hypotension, oedema, flushing; dyspnoea, cough; headache, insomnia, peripheral neuropathy, paraesthesia, dizziness, anorexia, asthenia, fatigue; pyrexia; hypokalaemia, dehydration, increased blood creatine phosphokinase; myalgia, arthralgia, back pain

Yondelis® (Pharma Mar) ▼ PoM
Injection, powder for reconstitution, trabectedin, net price 250-microgram vial = £363.00; 1-mg vial = £1366.00

Trastuzumab

Trastuzumab is licensed for the treatment of early breast cancer which overexpresses human epidermal growth factor receptor-2 (HER2) (see NICE guidance, below).

Trastuzumab is also licensed, in combination with paclitaxel or docetaxel, for metastatic breast cancer in patients with HER2-positive tumours who have not received chemotherapy for metastatic breast cancer and in whom anthracycline treatment is inappropriate.

Trastuzumab is also licensed, in combination with an aromatase inhibitor, for metastatic breast cancer in postmenopausal patients with hormone-receptor positive HER2-positive tumours not previously treated with trastuzumab.

Trastuzumab is also licensed as monotherapy for metastatic breast cancer in patients with tumours that overexpress HER2 who have received at least 2 chemotherapy regimens including, where appropriate, an anthracycline and a taxane; women with oestrogen-receptor-positive breast cancer should also have received hormonal therapy.

Trastuzumab is given by intravenous infusion. Resuscitation facilities should be available and treatment should be initiated by a specialist.

> NICE guidance
> Trastuzumab for the adjuvant treatment of early-stage HER2-positive breast cancer (August 2006)
> Trastuzumab is an option for women with early-stage HER2-positive breast cancer following surgery, chemotherapy (neoadjuvant or adjuvant), and radiotherapy (if appropriate).

Use with anthracyclines Concomitant use of trastuzumab with anthracyclines (section 8.1.2) is associated with cardiotoxicity. The use of anthracyclines even after stopping trastuzumab can increase the risk of cardiotoxicity and if possible should be avoided for up to 24 weeks. If an anthracycline needs to be used, cardiac function should be monitored closely.

TRASTUZUMAB

Indications see notes above and product literature

Cautions see section 8.1 and notes above; symptomatic heart failure, history of hypertension, coronary artery disease, uncontrolled arrhythmias; pregnancy (Appendix 4)

Cardiotoxicity Monitor cardiac function before and during treatment—for details of monitoring and managing cardiotoxicity, consult product literature

Contra-indications see section 8.1 and notes above; severe dyspnoea at rest; breast-feeding (Appendix 5)

Side-effects infusion-related side-effects including chills, fever, hypersensitivity reactions such as anaphylaxis, urticaria, and angioedema; gastro-intestinal symptoms; cardiotoxicity (see also above), chest pain, hypotension; pulmonary events (possibly delayed onset); headache, taste disturbance, anxiety, malaise, depression, insomnia, drowsiness, dizziness, paraesthesia, tremor, asthenia, peripheral neuropathy, hypertonia; mastitis, urinary-tract infection; leucopenia, ecchymosis, oedema, weight loss; arthralgia, myalgia, arthritis, bone pain, leg cramps; rash, pruritus, sweating, dry skin, alopecia, acne, nail disorders

Herceptin® (Roche) ▼ PoM
Intravenous infusion, powder for reconstitution, trastuzumab, net price 150-mg vial = £407.40

Tretinoin

Tretinoin is licensed for the induction of remission in acute promyelocytic leukaemia. It is used in previously untreated patients as well as in those who have relapsed after standard chemotherapy or who are refractory to it.

TRETINOIN

Note Tretinoin is the acid form of vitamin A

Indications see notes above; acne (section 13.6.1); photodamage (section 13.8.1)

Cautions exclude pregnancy before starting treatment and ensure effective contraception is used during and for at least 1 month after treatment; monitor haematological and coagulation profile, liver function, serum calcium and plasma lipids before and during treatment; increased risk of thromboembolism during first month of treatment; hepatic impairment (Appendix 2); renal impairment (Appendix 3); **interactions**: Appendix 1 (retinoids)

Contra-indications pregnancy (**important teratogenic risk**: see Cautions and Appendix 4) and breast-feeding

Side-effects retinoic acid syndrome (fever, dyspnoea, acute respiratory distress, pulmonary infiltrates, pleural effusion, hyperleukocytosis, hypotension, oedema, weight gain, hepatic, renal and multi-organ failure) requires immediate treatment—consult product literature; gastro-intestinal disturbances, pancreatitis; arrhythmias, flushing, oedema; headache, benign intracranial hypertension (mainly in children—consider dose reduction if intractable headache in children), shivering, dizziness, confusion, anxiety, depression, insomnia, paraesthesia, visual and hearing disturbances; raised liver enzymes, serum creatinine and lipids; bone and chest pain, alopecia, erythema, rash, pruritus, sweating, dry skin and mucous membranes, cheilitis; thromboembolism, hypercalcaemia, and genital ulceration reported

Dose

- ADULT and CHILD 45 mg/m^2 daily in 2 divided doses, max. duration of treatment 90 days (consult product literature for details of concomitant chemotherapy)

Vesanoid® (Roche) PoM
Capsules, yellow/brown, tretinoin 10 mg. Net price 100-cap pack = £170.52. Label: 21, 25

8.2 Drugs affecting the immune response

8.2.1 Antiproliferative immunosuppressants
8.2.2 Corticosteroids and other immunosuppressants
8.2.3 Rituximab and alemtuzumab
8.2.4 Other immunomodulating drugs

Immunosuppressant therapy

Immunosuppressants are used to suppress rejection in organ transplant recipients and to treat a variety of chronic inflammatory and autoimmune diseases. Solid organ transplant patients are usually maintained on a corticosteroid combined with a calcineurin inhibitor (ciclosporin or tacrolimus), *or* with an antiproliferative drug (azathioprine or mycophenolate mofetil), *or* with both. Specialist management is required and other immunomodulators may be used to initiate treatment or to treat rejection.

Impaired immune responsiveness Modification of tissue reactions caused by corticosteroids and other immunosuppressants may result in the rapid *spread of infection*. Corticosteroids may suppress clinical signs of infection and allow diseases such as septicaemia or tuberculosis to reach an advanced stage before being recognised—**important:** for advice on measles and chickenpox (varicella) exposure, see Immunoglobulins (section 14.5). For advice on the use of live vaccines in individuals with impaired immune response, see section 14.1. For general comments and warnings relating to corticosteroids and immunosuppressants see section 6.3.2 (under Prednisolone).

Pregnancy Transplant patients immunosuppressed with azathioprine should not discontinue it on becoming pregnant; there is no evidence that azathioprine is teratogenic. However, there have been reports of premature birth and low birth-weight following exposure to azathioprine, particularly in combination with corticosteroids. Spontaneous abortion has been reported following maternal or paternal exposure.

There is less experience of ciclosporin in pregnancy but it does not appear to be any more harmful than azathioprine. The use of these drugs during pregnancy needs to be supervised in specialist units.

Manufacturers contra-indicate the use of tacrolimus and mycophenolate in pregnancy (Appendix 4).

8.2.1 Antiproliferative immunosuppressants

Azathioprine is widely used for transplant recipients and it is also used to treat a number of auto-immune conditions, usually when corticosteroid therapy alone provides inadequate control. It is metabolised to mercaptopurine, and doses should be reduced when allopurinol is given concurrently.

Blood tests and monitoring for signs of myelosuppression are essential in long-term treatment with azathioprine. The enzyme thiopurine methyltransferase (TPMT) metabolises azathioprine; the risk of myelosuppression is increased in those with a low activity of the enzyme, particularly in the very few individuals who are homozygous for low TPMT activity.

Mycophenolate mofetil is metabolised to mycophenolic acid which has a more selective mode of action than azathioprine. It is licensed for the prophylaxis of acute rejection in renal, hepatic or cardiac transplantation when used in combination with ciclosporin and corticosteroids. There is evidence that compared with similar regimens incorporating azathioprine, mycophenolate mofetil reduces the risk of acute rejection episodes; the risk of opportunistic infections (particularly due to tissue-invasive cytomegalovirus) and the occurrence of blood disorders such as leucopenia may be higher.

Cyclophosphamide (section 8.1.1) is less commonly prescribed as an immunosuppressant.

AZATHIOPRINE

Indications see notes above; also rheumatoid arthritis (section 10.1.3)

Cautions monitor for toxicity throughout treatment; monitor full blood count weekly (more frequently with higher doses or if hepatic or renal impairment) for first 4 weeks (manufacturer advises weekly monitoring for 8 weeks but evidence of practical value unsatisfactory), thereafter reduce frequency of monitoring to at least every 3 months; hepatic impairment (Appendix 2); renal impairment (Appendix 3); reduce dose in elderly; pregnancy (see section 8.2)—treatment should not generally be initiated during pregnancy; **interactions:** Appendix 1 (azathioprine)

Bone marrow suppression Patients should be warned to report immediately any signs or symptoms of bone marrow suppression e.g. inexplicable bruising or bleeding, infection

Contra-indications hypersensitivity to azathioprine or mercaptopurine; breast-feeding

Side-effects hypersensitivity reactions (including malaise, dizziness, vomiting, diarrhoea, fever, rigors, myalgia, arthralgia, rash, hypotension and interstitial nephritis—calling for immediate withdrawal); dose-related bone marrow suppression (see also Cautions); liver impairment, cholestatic jaundice, hair loss and increased susceptibility to infections and colitis in patients also receiving corticosteroids; nausea; rarely pancreatitis, pneumonitis, hepatic veno-occlusive disease

Dose

- By mouth, *or* (if oral administration not possible—intravenous solution very irritant, see below) by intravenous injection over at least 1 minute (followed by 50 mL sodium chloride intravenous infusion), *or* by intravenous infusion

  Autoimmune conditions, 1–3 mg/kg daily, adjusted according to response (consider withdrawal if no improvement in 3 months)

  Suppression of transplant rejection, initially up to 5 mg/kg then 1–4 mg/kg daily according to response

  Note Intravenous injection is alkaline and very irritant, intravenous route should therefore be used **only** if oral route not feasible, see also Appendix 6

8 Malignant disease and immunosuppression

Azathioprine (Non-proprietary) PoM
Tablets, azathioprine 25 mg, net price 28-tab pack = £8.05; 50 mg, 56-tab pack = £9.48. Label: 21
Brands include *Azamune®*, *Immunoprin®*

Imuran® (GSK) PoM
Tablets, both f/c, azathioprine 25 mg (orange), net price 100-tab pack = £10.99; 50 mg (yellow), 100-tab pack = £7.99. Label: 21

Injection, powder for reconstitution, azathioprine (as sodium salt). Net price 50-mg vial = £15.38

MYCOPHENOLATE MOFETIL

Indications prophylaxis of acute renal, cardiac, or hepatic transplant rejection (in combination with ciclosporin and corticosteroids) under specialist supervision

Cautions full blood counts every week for 4 weeks then twice a month for 2 months then every month in the first year (possibly interrupt treatment if neutropenia develops); elderly (increased risk of infection, gastro-intestinal haemorrhage and pulmonary oedema); children (higher incidence of side-effects may call for temporary reduction of dose or interruption); active serious gastro-intestinal disease (risk of haemorrhage, ulceration and perforation); delayed graft function; increased susceptibility to skin cancer (avoid exposure to strong sunlight); **interactions**: Appendix 1 (mycophenolate)

Bone marrow suppression Patients should be warned to report immediately any signs or symptoms of bone marrow suppression e.g. infection and inexplicable bruising or bleeding

Contra-indications pregnancy (exclude before starting and avoid for 6 weeks after discontinuation) (Appendix 4); breast-feeding (Appendix 5)

Side-effects gastro-intestinal disturbances (including diarrhoea, vomiting, and abdominal pain), gastro-intestinal ulceration and bleeding, abnormal liver function tests, hepatitis, jaundice, pancreatitis; oedema, tachycardia, hypertension, hypotension, vasodilatation; cough, dyspnoea; insomnia, agitation, tremor, dizziness, headache; influenza-like syndrome, infections (viral, bacterial, and fungal); hyperglycaemia; renal impairment; increased risk of malignancies, particularly of the skin; blood disorders (including leucopenia, anaemia, thrombocytopenia, pancytopenia), disturbances of electrolytes and blood lipids; arthralgia; alopecia, acne, and rash

Dose

- Renal transplantation, by mouth, 1 g twice daily starting within 72 hours of transplantation *or* by intravenous infusion, 1 g twice daily starting within 24 hours of transplantation for max. 14 days (then transfer to oral therapy); CHILD and ADOLESCENT 2–18 years, by mouth 600 mg/m² twice daily (max. 2 g daily)

  Note Tablets and capsules not appropriate for dose titration in children with body surface area less than 1.25 m²

- Cardiac transplantation, by mouth, 1.5 g twice daily starting within 5 days of transplantation
- Hepatic transplantation, by intravenous infusion, 1 g twice daily starting within 24 hours of transplantation for 4 days (up to max. 14 days), then by mouth, 1.5 g twice daily as soon as is tolerated

CellCept® (Roche) PoM
Capsules, blue/brown, mycophenolate mofetil 250 mg, net price 100-cap pack = £87.33

Tablets, lavender, mycophenolate mofetil 500 mg, net price 50-tab pack = £87.33

Oral suspension, mycophenolate mofetil 1 g/5 mL when reconstituted with water, net price 175 mL = £122.25

Intravenous infusion, powder for reconstitution, mycophenolate mofetil (as hydrochloride), net price 500-mg vial = £9.69

Mycophenolic acid

Myfortic® (Novartis) PoM
Tablets, e/c, mycophenolic acid (as mycophenolate sodium) 180 mg (green), net price 120-tab pack = £99.71; 360 mg (orange), 120-tab pack = £199.41. Label: 25

Dose renal transplantation, 720 mg twice daily starting within 72 hours of transplantation

Equivalence to mycophenolate mofetil Mycophenolic acid 720 mg is approximately equivalent to mycophenolate mofetil 1 g but avoid unnecessary switching because of pharmacokinetic differences

8.2.2 Corticosteroids and other immunosuppressants

Prednisolone (section 6.3.2) is widely used in oncology. It has a marked antitumour effect in acute lymphoblastic leukaemia, Hodgkin's disease, and the non-Hodgkin lymphomas. It has a role in the palliation of symptomatic end-stage malignant disease when it may enhance appetite and produce a sense of well-being (see also Prescribing in Palliative Care, p. 17).

The corticosteroids are also powerful immunosuppressants. They are used to prevent organ transplant rejection, and in high dose to treat rejection episodes.

Ciclosporin (cyclosporin), a calcineurin inhibitor, is a potent immunosuppressant which is virtually non-myelotoxic but markedly nephrotoxic. It has an important role in organ and tissue transplantation, for prevention of graft rejection following bone marrow, kidney, liver, pancreas, heart, lung, and heart-lung transplantation, and for prophylaxis and treatment of graft-versus-host disease.

Tacrolimus is also a calcineurin inhibitor. Although not chemically related to ciclosporin it has a similar mode of action and side-effects, but the incidence of neurotoxicity appears to be greater; cardiomyopathy has also been reported. Disturbance of glucose metabolism also appears to be significant; hypertrichosis appears to be less of a problem than with ciclosporin.

Sirolimus is a potent non-calcineurin inhibiting immunosuppressant introduced recently for renal transplantation. It can cause hyperlipidaemia.

Basiliximab and **daclizumab** are monoclonal antibodies that prevent T-lymphocyte proliferation; they are used for prophylaxis of acute rejection in allogenic renal transplantation. They are given with ciclosporin and corticosteroid immunosuppression regimens; their use should be confined to specialist centres.

NICE guidance
Immunosuppressive therapy for renal transplantation in adults (September 2004)
Immunosuppressive therapy for renal transplantation in children and adolescents (April 2006)

For induction therapy in the prophylaxis of organ rejection, either basiliximab or daclizumab are options for combining with a calcineurin inhibitor. For each individual, ciclosporin or tacrolimus is chosen as the calcineurin inhibitor on the basis of side-effects.

Mycophenolate mofetil [mycophenolic acid also available but not licensed for use in children, see p. 474] is recommended as part of an immunosuppressive regimen only if:

- the calcineurin inhibitor is not tolerated, particularly if nephrotoxicity endangers the transplanted kidney; *or*
- there is very high risk of nephrotoxicity from the calcineurin inhibitor, requiring a reduction in the dose of the calcineurin inhibitor or its avoidance.

Sirolimus is recommended as a component of immunosuppressive regimen **only if** intolerance necessitates the withdrawal of a calcineurin inhibitor.

These recommendations may not be consistent with the marketing authorisation of some of the products.

BASILIXIMAB

Indications see notes above

Contra-indications pregnancy (Appendix 4) and breast-feeding

Side-effects *rarely* severe hypersensitivity reactions; cytokine release syndrome also reported; for side-effects of regimen see under Ciclosporin (below) and Prednisolone (section 6.3.2)

Dose

- By intravenous injection *or* by intravenous infusion, 20 mg within 2 hours before transplant surgery and 20 mg 4 days after surgery; withhold second dose if severe hypersensitivity or graft loss occurs; CHILD and ADOLESCENT 1–17 years, body-weight under 35 kg, 10 mg within 2 hours before transplant surgery and 10 mg 4 days after surgery; body-weight over 35 kg, adult dose

Simulect® (Novartis) PoM
Injection, powder for reconstitution, basiliximab, net price 10-mg vial = £758.69, 20-mg vial = £842.38 (both with water for injections) . For intravenous infusion

CICLOSPORIN
(Cyclosporin)

Indications see notes above, and under Dose; atopic dermatitis and psoriasis (section 13.5.3); rheumatoid arthritis (section 10.1.3)

Cautions monitor kidney function—dose dependent increase in serum creatinine and urea during first few weeks may necessitate dose reduction in transplant patients (exclude rejection if kidney transplant) or discontinuation in non-transplant patients; monitor liver function (dosage adjustment based on bilirubin and liver enzymes may be needed); monitor blood pressure—discontinue if hypertension develops that cannot be controlled by antihypertensives; hyperuricaemia; monitor serum potassium especially in renal dysfunction (risk of hyperkalaemia); monitor serum magnesium; measure blood lipids before treatment and thereafter as appropriate; pregnancy (see p. 473) and breast-feeding (Appendix 5); porphyria (section 9.8.2); use with tacrolimus specifically contra-indicated and apart from specialist use in transplant patients preferably avoid other immunosuppressants with the exception of corticosteroids (increased risk of infection and lymphoma); **interactions:** Appendix 1 (ciclosporin)

Additional cautions in nephrotic syndrome *Contra-indicated* in uncontrolled hypertension, uncontrolled infections, and malignancy; reduce dose by 25–50% if serum creatinine more than 30% above baseline on more than one measurement; in renal impairment initially 2.5 mg/kg daily; in long-term management, perform renal biopsies at yearly intervals

Additional cautions Atopic Dermatitis and Psoriasis, section 13.5.3; Rheumatoid Arthritis, section 10.1.3

Side-effects dose-dependent increase in serum creatinine and urea during first few weeks (see also under Cautions); less commonly renal structural changes on long-term administration; also hypertrichosis, headache, tremor, hypertension (especially in heart transplant patients), hepatic dysfunction, fatigue, gingival hypertrophy, gastro-intestinal disturbances, burning sensation in hands and feet (usually during first week); *occasionally* rash (possibly allergic), mild anaemia, hyperkalaemia, hyperuricaemia, gout, hypomagnesaemia, hypercholesterolaemia, hyperglycaemia, weight increase, oedema, pancreatitis, neuropathy, confusion, paraesthesia, convulsions, benign intracranial hypertension (discontinue), dysmenorrhoea or amenorrhoea; myalgia, muscle weakness, cramps, myopathy, gynaecomastia (in patients receiving concomitant spironolactone), colitis and cortical blindness also reported; thrombocytopenia (sometimes with haemolytic uraemic syndrome) also reported; incidence of malignancies and lymphoproliferative disorders similar to that with other immunosuppressive therapy

Dose

- Organ transplantation, used alone, ADULT and CHILD over 3 months 10–15 mg/kg by mouth 4–12 hours before transplantation followed by 10–15 mg/kg daily for 1–2 weeks postoperatively then reduced gradually to 2–6 mg/kg daily for maintenance (dose should be adjusted according to blood-ciclosporin concentration and renal function); dose lower if given concomitantly with other immunosuppressant therapy (e.g. corticosteroids); if necessary one-third corresponding oral dose can be given by intravenous infusion over 2–6 hours
- Bone-marrow transplantation, prevention and treatment of graft-versus-host disease, ADULT and CHILD over 3 months 3–5 mg/kg daily by intravenous infusion over 2–6 hours from day before transplantation to 2 weeks postoperatively (or 12.5–15 mg/kg daily by mouth) then 12.5 mg/kg daily by mouth for 3–6 months then tailed off (may take up to a year after transplantation)
- Nephrotic syndrome, by mouth, 5 mg/kg daily in 2 divided doses; CHILD 6 mg/kg daily in 2 divided doses; maintenance treatment reduce to lowest effective dose according to proteinuria and serum

creatinine measurements; discontinue after 3 months if no improvement in glomerulonephritis or glomerulosclerosis (after 6 months in membranous glomerulonephritis)

Conversion Any conversion between brands should be undertaken very carefully and the manufacturer contacted for further information. Currently only *Neoral®* remains available for oral use; *Sandimmun®* capsules and oral solution and *SangCya®* oral solution are available on named-patient basis only for patients who cannot be transferred to another brand of oral ciclosporin

> Because of differences in bioavailability, the brand of oral ciclosporin to be dispensed should be specified by the prescriber

Neoral® (Novartis) PoM

Capsules, ciclosporin 10 mg (yellow/white), net price 60-cap pack = £18.98; 25 mg (blue/grey), 30-cap pack = £13.86; 50 mg (yellow/white), 30-cap pack = £30.68; 100 mg (blue/grey), 30-cap pack = £57.89. Counselling, administration

Oral solution, yellow, sugar-free, ciclosporin 100 mg/mL, net price 50 mL = £94.71. Counselling, administration

Counselling Total daily dose should be taken in 2 divided doses. Avoid grapefruit or grapefruit juice for 1 hour before dose

Mix solution with orange juice (or squash) or apple juice (to improve taste) or with water immediately before taking (and rinse with more to ensure total dose). Do not mix with grapefruit juice. Keep medicine measure away from other liquids (including water)

Sandimmun® (Novartis) PoM

Concentrate for intravenous infusion (oily), ciclosporin 50 mg/mL. To be diluted before use. Net price 1-mL amp = £1.94; 5-mL amp = £9.17

Excipients include polyoxyl castor oil (risk of anaphylaxis, see Excipients, p. 2)

Note Observe for at least 30 minutes after starting infusion and at frequent intervals thereafter

DACLIZUMAB

Indications see notes above

Contra-indications pregnancy and breast-feeding

Side-effects severe hypersensitivity reactions reported rarely; for side-effects of regimen see under Ciclosporin (above) and Prednisolone (section 6.3.2)

Dose

- By intravenous infusion, ADULT and CHILD, 1 mg/kg within the 24-hour period before transplantation, then 1 mg/kg every 14 days for a total of 5 doses

Zenapax® (Roche) ▼ PoM

Concentrate for intravenous infusion, daclizumab 5 mg/mL, net price 5-mL = £223.68

SIROLIMUS

Indications prophylaxis of organ rejection in kidney allograft recipients (initially in combination with ciclosporin and corticosteroid, then with corticosteroid only); see also under Dose

Cautions monitor kidney function when given with ciclosporin; Afro-Caribbean patients may require higher doses; hepatic impairment (Appendix 2); renal impairment (Appendix 3); food may affect absorption (administer at the same time with respect to food); **interactions:** Appendix 1 (sirolimus)

Contra-indications pregnancy (Appendix 4); breast-feeding (Appendix 5)

Side-effects abdominal pain, diarrhoea, stomatitis, abnormal liver-function tests (elevated transaminases); oedema, tachycardia, hyperlipidaemias (including hypercholesterolaemia, hypertriglyceridaemia), venous thromboembolism; pneumonitis; pyrexia, increased susceptibility to infection (especially urinary-tract infection); proteinuria, haemolytic uraemic syndrome, increase in serum creatinine in patients also receiving ciclosporin; anaemia, thrombocytopenia, thrombotic thrombocytopenic purpura, leucopenia, neutropenia, hypokalaemia, hypophosphataemia, hyperglycaemia, lymphocele; arthralgia, osteonecrosis; epistaxis; acne, rash, impaired healing; *less commonly* pancreatitis, pulmonary embolism, pulmonary haemorrhage, pericardial effusion, nephrotic syndrome, susceptibility to lymphoma and other malignancies particularly of the skin, pancytopenia; *rarely* interstitial lung disease, hepatic necrosis, lymphoedema, and hypersensitivity reactions including anaphylactic reactions, angioedema, exfoliative dermatitis, and hypersensitivity vasculitis

Dose

- Initially 6 mg, after surgery, then 2 mg once daily (dose adjusted according to blood-sirolimus concentration) in combination with ciclosporin and corticosteroid for 2–3 months (sirolimus given 4 hours after ciclosporin); ciclosporin should then be withdrawn over 4–8 weeks (if not possible, sirolimus should be discontinued and an alternate immunosuppressive regimen used)

Note Pre-dose ('trough') blood-sirolimus concentration (using chromatographic assay) when used with ciclosporin should be 4–12 micrograms/litre; after withdrawal of ciclosporin pre-dose blood-sirolimus concentration should be 12–20 micrograms/litre; close monitoring of blood-sirolimus concentration required in hepatic impairment, during treatment with potent inducers or inhibitors of metabolism and after discontinuing them

When changing between oral solution and tablets, measurement of serum 'trough' blood-sirolimus concentration after 1–2 weeks is recommended

Rapamune® (Wyeth) ▼ PoM

Tablets, coated, sirolimus 1 mg, net price 30-tab pack = £90.00; 2 mg, 30-tab pack = £180.00

Oral solution, sirolimus 1 mg/mL, net price 60 mL = £169.00. Counselling, administration

Counselling Mix solution with at least 60 mL water or orange juice in a glass or plastic container immediately before taking; refill container with at least 120 mL and drink immediately (to ensure total dose). Do not mix with any other liquids

TACROLIMUS

Indications prophylaxis of organ rejection in liver, kidney, and heart allograft recipients and allograft rejection resistant to conventional immunosuppressive regimens, see also notes above; moderate to severe atopic eczema (section 13.5.3)

Cautions see under Ciclosporin; also monitor ECG (**important**: also echocardiography, see CSM warning below), visual status, blood glucose, haematological and neurological parameters and whole blood 'trough' concentrations of tacrolimus (especially during episodes of diarrhoea); hepatic impairment (Appendix 2); **interactions:** Appendix 1 (tacrolimus)

Driving May affect performance of skilled tasks (e.g. driving)

Contra-indications hypersensitivity to macrolides; pregnancy (exclude before starting—if contraception needed non-hormonal methods should be used, Appendix 4); breast-feeding (Appendix 5); avoid concurrent administration with ciclosporin (care if patient has previously received ciclosporin)

Side-effects gastro-intestinal disturbances including dyspepsia, and inflammatory and ulcerative disorders; hepatic dysfunction, jaundice, bile-duct and gallbladder abnormalities; hypertension (*less frequently* hypotension), tachycardia, angina, arrhythmias, thromboembolic and ischaemic events, *rarely* myocardial hypertrophy, cardiomyopathy (**important**: see CSM warning below); dyspnoea, pleural effusion; tremor, headache, insomnia, paraesthesia, confusion, depression, dizziness, anxiety, convulsions, incoordination, encephalopathy, psychosis; visual and hearing abnormalities; haematological effects including anaemia, leucocytosis, leucopenia, thrombocytopenia, coagulation disorders; altered acid-base balance and glucose metabolism, electrolyte disturbances including hyperkalaemia (*less frequently* hypokalaemia); altered renal function including increased serum creatinine; hypophosphataemia, hypercalcaemia, hyperuricaemia; muscle cramps, arthralgia; pruritus, alopecia, rash, sweating, acne, photosensitivity; susceptibility to lymphoma and other malignancies particularly of the skin; *less commonly* ascites, pancreatitis, atelectasis, kidney damage and renal failure, myasthenia, hirsutism; *rarely* Stevens-Johnson syndrome

CSM Warning Cardiomyopathy has been reported in children given tacrolimus after transplantation. Patients should be monitored carefully by echocardiography for hypertrophic changes; dose reduction or discontinuation should be considered if these occur

Dose

- Liver transplantation, starting 12 hours after transplantation, by mouth, 100–200 micrograms/kg daily in 2 divided doses *or* by intravenous infusion over 24 hours, 10–50 micrograms/kg daily for up to max. 7 days (then transfer to oral therapy); CHILD by mouth, 300 micrograms/kg daily in 2 divided doses *or* by intravenous infusion over 24 hours, 50 micrograms/kg daily for up to max. 7 days (then transfer to oral therapy)
- Renal transplantation, starting within 24 hours of transplantation, by mouth, 200–300 micrograms/kg daily in 2 divided doses *or* by intravenous infusion over 24 hours, 50–100 micrograms/kg daily for up to max. 7 days (then transfer to oral therapy); CHILD by mouth, 300 micrograms/kg daily in 2 divided doses *or* by intravenous infusion over 24 hours, 75–100 micrograms/kg daily for up to max. 7 days (then transfer to oral therapy)
- Heart transplantation (with or without antibody induction) starting within 5 days of transplantation, by mouth, 75 micrograms/kg daily in 2 divided doses *or* by intravenous infusion over 24 hours, 10–20 micrograms/kg daily for up to max. 7 days (then transfer to oral therapy); CHILD, without antibody induction, initially by intravenous infusion over 24 hours, 30–50 micrograms/kg daily, then by mouth, 300 micrograms/kg daily in 2 divided doses as soon as clinically possible (give 8–12 hours after discontinuing intravenous infusion); following antibody induction, by mouth, 100–300 micrograms/kg daily in 2 divided doses
- Maintenance treatment, dose adjusted according to response
- Rejection therapy, seek specialist advice

Prograf® (Astellas) PoM

Capsules, tacrolimus 500 micrograms (yellow), net price 50-cap pack = £65.69; 1 mg (white), 50-cap pack = £85.22, 100-cap pack = £170.43; 5 mg (greyish-red), 50-cap pack = £314.84. Label: 23, counselling, driving

Concentrate for intravenous infusion, tacrolimus 5 mg/mL. To be diluted before use. Net price 1-mL amp = £62.05

Excipients include polyoxyl castor oil (risk of anaphylaxis, see Excipients, p. 2)

Modified release

Advagraf® (Astellas) PoM

Capsules, m/r, tacrolimus 500 micrograms (yellow/orange), net price 50-cap pack = £42.22; 1 mg (white/orange), 50-cap pack = £84.43, 100-cap pack = £168.87; 5 mg (red/orange), 50-cap pack = £422.17. Label: 23, 25 counselling, driving

Dose Liver transplantation, starting 12–18 hours after transplantation, by mouth, 100–200 micrograms/kg once daily in the morning

Renal transplantation, starting within 24 hours of transplantation, by mouth, 200–300 micrograms/kg once daily in the morning

Rejection therapy, seek specialist advice

CHILD not recommended

Equivalence to *Prograf®* Manufacturer advises that conversion from oral *Prograf®* to *Advagraf®* should be on a 1:1 (mg:mg) total daily dose basis; tacrolimus trough levels should be measured prior to conversion and within 2 weeks of conversion to *Advagraf®*, and if necessary dose adjustment made to maintain similar systemic exposure

8.2.3 Rituximab and alemtuzumab

Rituximab is a monoclonal antibody which causes lysis of B lymphocytes. It is licensed for the treatment of chemotherapy-resistant or relapsed stage III–IV follicular lymphoma and in combination with other chemotherapy, for previously untreated stage III-IV follicular lymphoma (see NICE guidance below). Rituximab is also licensed for maintenance therapy in patients with relapsed or refractory follicular lymphoma that has responded to induction therapy with chemotherapy (with or without rituximab). It is also licensed for use in combination with other chemotherapy for the treatment of diffuse large B-cell non-Hodgkin's lymphoma (see NICE guidance below). Full resuscitation facilities should be at hand and as with other cytotoxics, treatment should be undertaken under the close supervision of a specialist. See section 10.1.3 for the role of rituximab in rheumatoid arthritis.

Rituximab should be used with caution in patients receiving cardiotoxic chemotherapy or with a history of cardiovascular disease because exacerbation of angina, arrhythmia, and heart failure have been reported. Transient hypotension occurs frequently during infusion and antihypertensives may need to be withheld for 12 hours before infusion.

Infusion-related side-effects (including cytokine release syndrome) are reported commonly with rituximab and occur predominantly during the first infusion; they include fever and chills, nausea and vomiting, allergic reactions (such as rash, pruritus, angioedema, bronchospasm and dyspnoea), flushing and tumour pain. Patients should be given an analgesic and an antihistamine before each dose of rituximab to reduce these effects. Premedication with a corticosteroid should also be considered. The infusion may have to be stopped temporarily and the infusion-related effects treated—consult product literature for appropriate management. Evidence of pulmonary infiltration and features of tumour lysis syndrome should be sought if infusion-related effects occur.

Fatalities following **severe** cytokine release syndrome (characterised by severe dyspnoea) and associated with features of tumour lysis syndrome have occurred 1–2 hours after infusion of rituximab. Patients with a high tumour burden as well as those with pulmonary insufficiency or infiltration are at increased risk and should be monitored **very closely** (and a slower rate of infusion considered).

> **NICE guidance**
> **Rituximab for the treatment of follicular lymphoma (September 2006)**
> Rituximab, in combination with cyclophosphamide, vincristine, and prednisolone is an option for the treatment of symptomatic stage III and IV follicular lymphoma in previously untreated patients.

> **NICE guidance**
> **Rituximab for recurrent or refractory stage III or IV follicular non-Hodgkin's lymphoma (March 2002)**
> For stage III or IV follicular lymphoma, rituximab is recommended only if the disease is resistant to other chemotherapy or if the patient cannot tolerate such treatment. In these circumstances rituximab should be used as part of a prospective study.

> **NICE guidance**
> **Rituximab for aggressive non-Hodgkin's lymphoma (September 2003)**
> Rituximab, in combination with cyclophosphamide, doxorubicin, vincristine, and prednisolone, is recommended for first-line treatment of CD20-positive diffuse large-B-cell lymphoma at clinical stage II, III or IV.
> The use of rituximab for localised (stage I) disease should be limited to clinical trials.

Alemtuzumab, another monoclonal antibody that causes lysis of B lymphocytes, is licensed for use in patients with chronic lymphocytic leukaemia which has failed to respond to treatment with an alkylating drug, or which has remitted for only a short period (less than 6 months) following fludarabine treatment. In common with rituximab, it causes infusion-related side-effects including cytokine release syndrome (see above) and premedication with an analgesic, an antihistamine, and a corticosteroid is recommended.

ALEMTUZUMAB

Indications see notes above
Cautions see notes above—for full details consult product literature
Contra-indications pregnancy (Appendix 4); breast-feeding (Appendix 5); for full details consult product literature
Side-effects see notes above—for full details (including monitoring and management of side-effects) consult product literature
Dose
- Consult product literature

MabCampath® (Schering Health) ▼ PoM
Concentrate for intravenous infusion, alemtuzumab 30 mg/mL, net price 1-mL vial = £274.83

RITUXIMAB

Indications see notes above; severe active rheumatoid arthritis (section 10.1.3)
Cautions see notes above—for full details consult product literature; pregnancy (Appendix 4)
Contra-indications breast-feeding (Appendix 5)
Side-effects see notes above—but for full details (including monitoring and management of side-effects) consult product literature

MabThera® (Roche) PoM
Concentrate for intravenous infusion, rituximab 10 mg/mL, net price 10-mL vial = £174.63, 50-mL vial = £873.15

8.2.4 Other immunomodulating drugs

Interferon alfa

Interferon alfa has shown some antitumour effect in certain lymphomas and solid tumours. Interferon alfa preparations are also used in the treatment of chronic hepatitis B, and chronic hepatitis C ideally in combination with ribavirin (section 5.3.3). Side-effects are dose-related, but commonly include anorexia, nausea, influenza-like symptoms, and lethargy. Ocular side-effects and depression (including suicidal behaviour) have also been reported. Myelosuppression may occur, particularly affecting granulocyte counts. Cardiovascular problems (hypotension, hypertension, and arrhythmias), nephrotoxicity and hepatotoxicity have been reported. Hypertriglyceridaemia, sometimes severe, has been observed; monitoring of lipid concentration is recommended. Other side-effects include hypersensitivity reactions, thyroid abnormalities, hyperglycaemia, alopecia, psoriasiform rash, confusion, coma and seizures (usually with high doses in the elderly).

Polyethylene glycol-conjugated ('pegylated') derivatives of interferon alfa (**peginterferon alfa-2a** and **peginterferon alfa-2b**) are available; pegylation increases the persistence of the interferon in the blood. The peginterferons are licensed for the treatment of chronic hepatitis C, ideally in combination with ribavirin (see section 5.3.3). Peginterferon alfa-2a is also licensed for the treatment of chronic hepatitis B.

> **NICE guidance (adefovir dipivoxil and peginterferon alfa-2a for chronic hepatitis B)**
> See p. 340

> **NICE guidance (peginterferon alfa, interferon alfa, and ribavirin for chronic hepatitis C)**
> See p. 340

INTERFERON ALFA

Indications see under preparations

Cautions consult product literature; **interactions:** Appendix 1 (interferons)

Contra-indications consult product literature; avoid injections containing benzyl alcohol in neonates (see under preparations below); pregnancy (Appendix 4); breast-feeding (Appendix 5)

Side-effects see notes above and consult product literature

Dose

- Consult product literature

IntronA® (Schering-Plough) PoM

Injection, interferon alfa-2b (rbe) 10 million units/mL, net price 1-mL vial = £43.17, 2.5-mL vial = £108.00. For subcutaneous injection or intravenous infusion

Injection pen, interferon alfa-2b (rbe), net price 15 million units/mL, 1.5-mL cartridge = £77.76; 25 million units/mL, 1.5-mL cartridge = £129.60; 50 million units/mL, 1.5-mL cartridge = £259.20. For subcutaneous injection

Note Each 1.5-mL multidose cartridge delivers 6 doses of 0.2 mL i.e. a total of 1.2 mL

For chronic myelogenous leukaemia (as monotherapy or in combination with cytarabine), hairy cell leukaemia, follicular lymphoma, lymph or liver metastases of carcinoid tumour, chronic hepatitis B, chronic hepatitis C, adjunct to surgery in malignant melanoma and maintenance of remission in multiple myeloma

Roferon-A® (Roche) PoM

Injection, interferon alfa-2a (rbe). Net price 6 million units/mL, 0.5-mL (3 million-unit) prefilled syringe = £15.07; 9 million units/mL, 0.5-mL (4.5 million-unit) prefilled syringe = £22.60; 12 million units/mL, 0.5-mL (6 million-unit) prefilled syringe = £30.12; 18 million units/mL, 0.5-mL (9 million-unit) prefilled syringe = £45.19; 36 million units/mL, 0.5-mL (18 million-unit) prefilled syringe = £90.39; 30 million units/mL, 0.6-mL (18 million-unit) cartridge = £90.39, for use with *Roferon* pen device. For subcutaneous injection (cartridges, vials, and prefilled syringes) and intramuscular injection (cartridges and vials)

Excipients include benzyl alcohol (avoid in neonates, see Excipients, p. 2)

For AIDS-related Kaposi's sarcoma, hairy cell leukaemia, chronic myelogenous leukaemia, recurrent or metastatic renal cell carcinoma, progressive cutaneous T-cell lymphoma, chronic hepatitis B and chronic hepatitis C, follicular non-Hodgkin's lymphoma, adjunct to surgery in malignant melanoma

Viraferon® (Schering-Plough) PoM

Injection, interferon alfa-2b (rbe) 6 million units/mL, net price 3-mL vial = £90.40. For subcutaneous injection

Injection pen, interferon alfa-2b (rbe), net price 15 million units/mL, 1.5-mL cartridge = £90.40. For subcutaneous injection

Note 1.5-mL multidose cartridge delivers 6 doses of 0.2 mL each

For chronic hepatitis B and chronic hepatitis C

PEGINTERFERON ALFA

Indications see under preparations

Cautions consult product literature; **interactions:** Appendix 1 (interferons)

Contra-indications consult product literature

Side-effects see notes above and consult product literature

Dose

- Consult product literature

Pegasys® (Roche) PoM

Injection, peginterferon alfa-2a, net price 135-microgram prefilled syringe = £114.39, 180-microgram prefilled syringe = £132.06. For subcutaneous injection

Combined with ribavirin for chronic hepatitis C; as monotherapy for chronic hepatitis C if ribavirin not tolerated or contra-indicated (see section 5.3.3); as monotherapy for chronic hepatitis B

PegIntron® (Schering-Plough) PoM

Injection, powder for reconstitution, peginterferon alfa-2b (rbe), net price 50-microgram vial = £62.78, 80-microgram vial = £108.00, 100-microgram vial = £125.55, 120-microgram vial = £162.00, 150-microgram vial = £202.50 (all with injection equipment and water for injections). For subcutaneous injection

Combined with ribavirin for chronic hepatitis C; as monotherapy for chronic hepatitis C if ribavirin not tolerated or contra-indicated (see section 5.3.3)

ViraferonPeg® (Schering-Plough) PoM

Injection, powder for reconstitution, peginterferon alfa-2b (rbe), net price 50-microgram vial = £62.78, 80-microgram vial = £100.44, 100-microgram vial = £125.55, 120-microgram vial = £150.66, 150-microgram vial = £188.33 (all with injection equipment and water for injections). For subcutaneous injection

Injection, prefilled pen, powder for reconstitution, peginterferon alfa-2b (rbe), net price 50-microgram pen = £69.05, 80-microgram pen = £118.80, 100-microgram pen = £138.11, 120-microgram pen = £165.73, 150-microgram pen = £207.16 (all with needles and swabs). For subcutaneous injection

Combined with ribavirin for chronic hepatitis C; as monotherapy for chronic hepatitis C if ribavirin not tolerated or contra-indicated (see section 5.3.3)

Interferon beta

Interferon beta is licensed for use in patients with *relapsing, remitting multiple sclerosis* (characterised by at least two attacks of neurological dysfunction over the previous 2 or 3 years, followed by complete or incomplete recovery) who are able to walk unaided. Not all patients respond and a deterioration in the bouts has been observed in some. It is also licensed for use in patients with a single demyelinating event with an active inflammatory process, if it is severe enough to require treatment with an intravenous corticosteroid, and they are at high risk of developing multiple sclerosis. Interferon beta-1b is also licensed for use in patients with *secondary progressive multiple sclerosis* but its role in this condition has not been confirmed.

Interferon beta should not be used in those with severe depressive illness (or suicidal ideation), or in decompensated liver disease. Caution is advised in those with severe hepatic or renal impairment or a history of cardiac disorders, depressive disorders (avoid in severe depression or in those with suicidal ideation), seizures, or severe myelosuppression. Patients should be monitored for signs of hepatic injury. Side-effects reported most frequently include irritation at injection site (including inflammation, hypersensitivity, necrosis) and influenza-like symptoms (fever, chills, myalgia, or malaise) but these decrease over time; nausea and vomiting occur occasionally. Other side-effects include hypersensitivity reactions (including anaphylaxis and urticaria), blood disorders, menstrual disorders, mood and personality changes, suicide attempts, confusion and convulsions; alopecia, hepatitis, and thyroid dysfunction have been reported rarely with interferon beta-1b.

NICE guidance

Interferon beta and glatiramer for multiple sclerosis (January 2002)

Interferon beta and glatiramer acetate are **not** recommended for the treatment of multiple sclerosis in the NHS in England and Wales.

Patients who are currently receiving interferon beta or glatiramer acetate for multiple sclerosis, whether as routine therapy or as part of a clinical trial, should have the option to continue treatment until they and their consultant consider it appropriate to stop, having regard to the established criteria for withdrawal from treatment.

Provision of disease-modifying therapies for multiple sclerosis

The Department of Health, the National Assembly for Wales, the Scottish Executive, the Northern Ireland Department of Health, Social Services & Public Safety, and the manufacturers have reached agreement on a risk-sharing scheme for the NHS supply of interferon beta and glatiramer acetate for multiple sclerosis. Health Service Circular (HSC 2002/004) explains how patients can participate in the scheme. It is available on the Department of Health website (www.dh.gov.uk)

INTERFERON BETA

Indications see notes above and under preparations

Cautions see notes above and consult product literature

Contra-indications see notes above and consult product literature; pregnancy (Appendix 4—advise contraceptive measures if appropriate), breast-feeding (Appendix 5)

Side-effects see notes above and consult product literature

Dose

- Consult product literature

◢Interferon beta-1a

Avonex® (Biogen) PoM

Injection, interferon beta-1a 60 micrograms (12 million units)/mL, net price 0.5-mL (30-microgram, 6 million-unit) prefilled syringe = £174.25. For intramuscular injection

Injection, powder for reconstitution, interferon beta-1a, net price 30-microgram (6 million-unit) vial with diluent = £174.25. For intramuscular injection

For relapsing, remitting multiple sclerosis or for a single demyelinating event with an active inflammatory process (if it is severe enough to require intravenous corticosteroid and patient at high risk of developing multiple sclerosis)

Rebif® (Serono) PoM

Injection, interferon beta-1a, net price 22-microgram (6 million-unit) prefilled syringe = £48.16; 44-microgram (12 million-unit) prefilled syringe = £57.32; starter pack of 6 × 8.8–microgram (2.4 million-unit) prefilled syringes with 6 × 22–microgram (6 million-unit) prefilled syringes = £586.19. For subcutaneous injection

For relapsing, remitting multiple sclerosis

◢Interferon beta-1b

Betaferon® (Schering Health) PoM

Injection, powder for reconstitution, interferon beta-1b. Net price 300-microgram (9.6 million-unit) vial with diluent = £39.78. For subcutaneous injection

Note An autoinjector device (*Betaject® Light*) is available from Schering Health

For relapsing, remitting multiple sclerosis, for secondary progressive multiple sclerosis with active disease, or for a single demyelinating event with an active inflammatory process (if severe enough to require intravenous corticosteroid and patient at high risk of developing multiple sclerosis)

Aldesleukin

Aldesleukin (recombinant interleukin-2) is licensed for metastatic renal cell carcinoma; it is usually given by subcutaneous injection. It is now rarely given by intravenous infusion because of an association with a capillary leak syndrome, which can cause pulmonary oedema and hypotension. Aldesleukin produces tumour shrinkage in a small proportion of patients, but it has not been shown to increase survival. Bone-marrow, hepatic, renal, thyroid, and CNS toxicity is common. It is for use in **specialist units only**. **Interactions:** Appendix 1 (aldesleukin)

Proleukin® (Novartis) PoM

Injection, powder for reconstitution, aldesleukin. Net price 18-million unit vial = £112.00. For subcutaneous injection

Injection, powder for reconstitution, aldesleukin. Net price 18-million unit vial = £112.00. For intravenous infusion but see notes above

For metastatic renal cell carcinoma, **excluding** patients in whom all three of the following prognostic factors are present: performance status of Eastern Co-operative Oncology Group of 1 or greater, more than one organ with metastatic disease sites, and a period of less than 24 months between initial diagnosis of primary tumour and date of evaluation of treatment.

BCG bladder instillation

BCG (**Bacillus Calmette-Guérin**) is a live attenuated strain derived from *Mycobacterium bovis*. It is licensed as a bladder instillation for the treatment of primary or recurrent bladder carcinoma and for the prevention of recurrence following transurethral resection.

BACILLUS CALMETTE-GUÉRIN

Indications see notes above; BCG immunisation (section 14.4)

Cautions screen for active tuberculosis (contra-indicated if tuberculosis confirmed); traumatic catheterisation or urethral or bladder injury (delay administration until mucosal damage healed)

Contra-indications impaired immune response, HIV infection, urinary-tract infection, severe haematuria, tuberculosis, fever of unknown origin; pregnancy and breast-feeding

Side-effects cystitis, dysuria, urinary frequency, haematuria, malaise, fever, influenza-like syndrome; also systemic BCG infection (with fatalities)—consult product literature; rarely hypersensitivity reactions (such as arthralgia and rash), orchitis, transient urethral obstruction, bladder contracture, renal abscess; ocular symptoms reported

Dose

- Consult product literature

ImmuCyst® (Cambridge) PoM
Bladder instillation, freeze-dried powder containing attenuated *Mycobacterium bovis* prepared from the Connaught strain of bacillus of Calmette and Guérin, net price 81-mg vial = £89.00

OncoTICE® (Organon) PoM
Bladder instillation, freeze-dried powder containing attenuated *Mycobacterium bovis* prepared from the TICE strain of bacillus of Calmette and Guérin, net price 12.5-mg vial = £80.00

Glatiramer acetate

Glatiramer is an immunomodulating drug comprising synthetic polypeptides. It is licensed for reducing the frequency of relapses in ambulatory patients with relapsing-remitting multiple sclerosis who have had at least 2 clinical relapses in the past 2 years. Initiation of treatment with glatiramer should be supervised by a specialist.

NICE guidance (interferon beta and glatiramer for multiple sclerosis)
See p. 480

Provision of disease-modifying therapies for multiple sclerosis
See p. 480

GLATIRAMER ACETATE

Indications see notes above

Cautions cardiac disorders; renal impairment (Appendix 3); breast-feeding (Appendix 5)

Contra-indications pregnancy (Appendix 4)

Side-effects flushing, chest pain, palpitation, tachycardia, and dyspnoea may occur within minutes of injection; nausea, constipation, diarrhoea; syncope, anxiety, asthenia, depression, dizziness, headache, tremor, sweating; oedema, lymphadenopathy; hypertonia, back pain, arthralgia, influenza-like symptoms; injection-site reactions, rash; *rarely* convulsions, hypersensitivity reactions

Dose

- By subcutaneous injection, ADULT over 18 years, 20 mg daily

Copaxone® (Teva) PoM
Injection, glatiramer acetate 20 mg/mL, net price 1-mL prefilled syringe = £16.00

Lenalidomide and thalidomide

Lenalidomide is an immunomodulating drug with anti-neoplastic, anti-angiogenic, and pro-erythropoietic properties. It is licensed, in combination with dexamethasone, for the treatment of multiple myeloma in patients who have received at least one previous therapy.

The most serious side-effects of lenalidomide are venous thromboembolism and severe neutropenia. Lenalidomide is structurally related to thalidomide and there is a risk of teratogenesis. Pregnancy must be excluded before starting treatment and women of child-bearing age must use effective contraception (oral combined hormonal contraceptives and copper-releasing intrauterine devices not recommended). Women must be registered with a pregnancy prevention programme (see under Cautions below).

Thalidomide [unlicensed drug] should **always** be given under specialist supervision because of its teratogenic potential. It has immunomodulatory and anti-inflammatory activity; it is used in the treatment of refractory myeloma and can delay progression of early disease. It is used alone or in combination with a corticosteroid and an alkylating drug. Thalidomide can cause drowsiness, constipation, and on prolonged use, peripheral neuropathy. It should **never** be given to women of child-bearing potential.

LENALIDOMIDE

Indications see notes above

Cautions see notes above; exclude pregnancy before starting (perform pregnancy test on initiation or in the 3 days prior to initiation—women must practice effective contraception at least 1 month before, during, and for at least 1 month after treatment); monitor full blood count (including differential white cell count and platelet count) before treatment and every week for the first 8 weeks then every 4 weeks (reduce dose or interrupt treatment if neutropenia or thrombocytopenia develop—consult product literature); concomitant drugs that increase the risk of thromboembolism; monitor thyroid function; renal impairment (Appendix 3); **interactions:** Appendix 1 (lenalidomide)

Thromboembolism Patients and their carers should be made aware of the symptoms of thromboembolism and advised to report sudden breathlessness, chest pain, or swelling of a limb

Neutropenia and thrombocytopenia Patients and their carers should be made aware of the symptoms of neutropenia and advised to seek medical advice if symptoms suggestive of neutropenia (such as fever, sore throat) or of thrombocytopenia (such as bleeding) develop

Contra-indications pregnancy (**important teratogenic risk:** see Cautions above and Appendix 4); breast-feeding

Side-effects hypotension, deep vein thrombosis; dyspnoea; tremor, hypoaesthesia, fatigue, asthenia; neutropenia, thrombocytopenia, anaemia, lymphopenia, leucopenia; muscle cramp; pruritus, rash

Dose

- ADULT over 18 years, 25 mg once daily for 21 consecutive days of a 28-day cycle; for doses of dexamethasone, consult product literature

Revlimid® (Celgene) ▼ PoM
Capsules, lenalidomide, 5 mg (white), net price 21-cap pack = £3570.00; 10 mg (blue/yellow), 21-cap pack = £3780.00; 15 mg (blue/white), 21-cap pack = £3969.00; 25 mg (white), 21-cap pack = £4368.00. Label: 25, counselling, symptoms of thromboembolism, neutropenia or thrombocytopenia, patient information leaflet

Note Patient, prescriber, and supplying pharmacy must be registered with Celgene Ltd and comply with a pregnancy prevention programme

Natalizumab

Natalizumab is a monoclonal antibody that inhibits the migration of leucocytes into the central nervous system, hence reducing inflammation and demyelination. It is licensed for use in patients with highly active *relapsing-remitting multiple sclerosis* despite treatment with interferon beta or those with rapidly evolving severe relapsing-remitting multiple sclerosis.

Natalizumab is associated with an increased risk of opportunistic infection and progressive multifocal leucoencephalopathy (PML). Patients should be monitored for new or worsening neurological symptoms or signs of PML—treatment should be suspended until PML has been excluded. If a patient develops an opportunistic infection or PML, natalizumab should be permanently discontinued.

Infusion-related side-effects include nausea, vomiting, flushing, headache, dizziness, fatigue, rigors, pyrexia, arthralgia, urticaria, and pruritus. Patients should be observed for hypersensitivity reactions during the infusion and for 1 hour after completion of the infusion. Natalizumab should be discontinued permanently if hypersensitivity reaction occurs.

The *Scottish Medicines Consortium* has advised (August 2007) that natalizumab is accepted for restricted use as single disease-modifying therapy in highly active relapsing-remitting multiple sclerosis only in patients with rapidly evolving severe relapsing-remitting multiple sclerosis defined by 2 or more disabling relapses in 1 year and with 1 or more gadolinium-enhancing lesions on brain magnetic resonance imaging (MRI) or a significant increase in T2 lesion load compared with a previous MRI.

> **NICE guidance**
> **Natalizumab for the treatment of adults with highly active relapsing-remitting multiple sclerosis (August 2007)**
> Natalizumab is an option for the treatment only of rapidly evolving severe relapsing-remitting multiple sclerosis (RES). RES is defined by 2 or more disabling relapses in 1 year, and 1 or more gadolinium-enhancing lesions on brain magnetic resonance imaging (MRI) or a significant increase in T2 lesion load compared with a previous MRI. Patients currently receiving natalizumab who do not meet the above criteria, should have the option to continue therapy until they and their consultants consider it appropriate to stop.

NATALIZUMAB

Indications see notes above

Cautions prior treatment with immunosuppressants; see also notes above and consult product literature

Contra-indications progressive multifocal leucoencephalopathy; active infection (see notes above); concurrent use of interferon beta or glatiramer acetate; immunosuppression; active malignancies; pregnancy (Appendix 4); breast-feeding (Appendix 5)

Side-effects see notes above

Dose

- By intravenous infusion, ADULT over 18 years, 300 mg once every 4 weeks

Tysabri® (Biogen) ▼ PoM
Concentrate for intravenous infusion, natalizumab 20 mg/mL, net price 15-mL vial = £1130.00

8.3 Sex hormones and hormone antagonists in malignant disease

8.3.1 Oestrogens
8.3.2 Progestogens
8.3.3 Androgens
8.3.4 Hormone antagonists

Hormonal manipulation has an important role in the treatment of breast, prostate, and endometrial cancer, and a more marginal role in the treatment of hypernephroma. These treatments are not curative, but may provide excellent palliation of symptoms in selected patients, sometimes for a period of years. Tumour response, and treatment toxicity should be carefully monitored and treatment changed if progression occurs or side-effects exceed benefit.

8.3.1 Oestrogens

Diethylstilbestrol (stilboestrol) is sometimes used to treat prostate cancer, but it is not usually used first-line because of its side-effects. It is occasionally used in postmenopausal women with breast cancer. Toxicity is common and dose-related side-effects include nausea, fluid retention, and venous and arterial thrombosis. Impotence and gynaecomastia always occur in men, and withdrawal bleeding may be a problem in women. Hypercalcaemia and bone pain may also occur in breast cancer.

Ethinylestradiol (ethinyloestradiol) is the most potent oestrogen available; unlike other oestrogens it is only slowly metabolised in the liver. Ethinylestradiol is licensed for the palliative treatment of prostate cancer.

DIETHYLSTILBESTROL
(Stilboestrol)

Indications see notes above

Cautions cardiovascular disease

Contra-indications hepatic impairment (Appendix 2)

Side-effects sodium retention with oedema, thromboembolism, jaundice, feminising effects in men; see also notes above

Dose

- Breast cancer, 10–20 mg daily
- Prostate cancer, 1–3 mg daily

Diethylstilbestrol (Non-proprietary) PoM
Tablets, diethylstilbestrol 1 mg, net price 28 = £37.24; 5 mg, 28 = £210.21

ETHINYLESTRADIOL
(Ethinyloestradiol)

Indications see notes above; other indications (section 6.4.1.1)

Cautions see section 6.4.1.1; **interactions:** Appendix 1 (oestrogens)
Contra-indications see section 6.4.1.1
Side-effects see section 6.4.1.1
Dose
- Prostate cancer (palliative), 0.15–1.5 mg daily

Preparations
Section 6.4.1.1

8.3.2 Progestogens

Progestogens have a role in the treatment of endometrial cancer; their use in breast cancer and renal cell cancer has declined. Progestogens are now rarely used to treat prostate cancer. **Medroxyprogesterone** or **megestrol** are usually chosen and can be given orally; high-dose or parenteral treatment cannot be recommended. Side-effects are mild but may include nausea, fluid retention, and weight gain.

MEDROXYPROGESTERONE ACETATE

Indications see notes above; contraception (section 7.3.2.2); other indications (section 6.4.1.2)
Cautions see section 6.4.1.2 and notes above; **interactions:** Appendix 1 (progestogens)
Contra-indications see section 6.4.1.2 and notes above
Side-effects see section 6.4.1.2 and notes above; glucocorticoid effects at high dose may lead to a cushingoid syndrome
Dose
- See preparations below

Provera® (Pharmacia) PoM
Tablets, medroxyprogesterone acetate 100 mg (scored), net price 60-tab pack = £29.98, 100-tab pack = £49.94; 200 mg (scored), 30-tab pack = £29.65, 400 mg, 30-tab pack = £58.67
Dose endometrial and renal cell cancer, 200–400 mg daily; breast cancer, 400–800 mg daily
Tablets, medroxyprogesterone acetate 2.5 mg, 5 mg and 10 mg, see section 6.4.1.2

MEGESTROL ACETATE

Indications see notes above
Cautions see under Medroxyprogesterone acetate (section 6.4.1.2) and notes above; **interactions:** Appendix 1 (progestogens)
Contra-indications see under Medroxyprogesterone acetate (section 6.4.1.2) and notes above
Side-effects see under Medroxyprogesterone acetate (section 6.4.1.2) and notes above
Dose
- Breast cancer, 160 mg daily in single or divided doses
- Endometrial cancer, 40–320 mg daily in divided doses

Megace® (Bristol-Myers Squibb) PoM
Tablets, scored, megestrol acetate 160 mg (off-white), 30-tab pack = £20.72

NORETHISTERONE

Indications see notes above, other indications (section 6.4.1.2)
Cautions see section 6.4.1.2 and notes above; **interactions:** Appendix 1 (progestogens)
Contra-indications see section 6.4.1.2 and notes above
Side-effects see section 6.4.1.2 and notes above
Dose
- Breast cancer, 40 mg daily, increased to 60 mg daily if required

Preparations
Section 6.4.1.2

8.3.3 Androgens

Testosterone esters (section 6.4.2) have largely been superseded by other drugs for breast cancer.

8.3.4 Hormone antagonists

8.3.4.1 Breast cancer

The management of patients with breast cancer involves surgery, radiotherapy, drug therapy, or a combination of these.

For operable breast cancer, treatment before surgery (neoadjuvant therapy) reduces the size of the tumour and facilitates breast-conserving surgery; hormone antagonist therapy (e.g. letrozole) is chosen for steroid hormone-receptor-positive breast cancer and chemotherapy for steroid hormone-receptor-negative tumours or for younger women.

Early breast cancer All women should be considered for adjuvant therapy following surgical removal of the tumour. Adjuvant therapy is used to eradicate the micro-metastases that cause relapses. Choice of adjuvant treatment is determined by the risk of recurrence, steroid hormone-receptor status of the primary tumour, and menopausal status.

Adjuvant therapy comprises either cytotoxic chemotherapy or hormone-antagonist therapy. Women with steroid hormone-receptor-positive breast cancer are considered for hormone-antagonist therapy (preceded by cytotoxic chemotherapy if necessary) whilst women with steroid hormone-receptor-negative breast cancer should be considered for cytotoxic chemotherapy.

The oestrogen-receptor antagonist **tamoxifen** is effective in premenopausal, perimenopausal, and postmenopausal women. The aromatase inhibitors **anastrozole**, **exemestane**, and **letrozole** are effective in postmenopausal women **only**. Adjuvant hormone antagonist therapy reduces the risk of cancer in the other breast and should generally be continued for 5 years following removal of the tumour. In those considered for extended adjuvant therapy, 5 years of tamoxifen is followed by an aromatase inhibitor such as letrozole for a further 3 years.

Trastuzumab is licensed for use in early breast cancer which overexpresses human epidermal growth factor-2 (HER2) in women who have received surgery, chemotherapy and radiotherapy (as appropriate).

Premenopausal women may also benefit from treatment with a gonadorelin analogue or ovarian ablation.

Advanced breast cancer Tamoxifen is used in postmenopausal women with oestrogen-receptor-positive tumours, long disease-free interval following treatment for early breast cancer, and disease limited to bone or soft tissues. However, aromatase inhibitors, such as anastrozole or letrozole, may be more effective and are regarded as preferred treatment in postmenopausal women. Ovarian ablation or a gonadorelin analogue (section 8.3.4.2) should be considered in premenopausal women.

Progestogens such as medroxyprogesterone acetate continue to have a role in postmenopausal women with advanced breast cancer. They are as effective as tamoxifen, but they are not as well tolerated; they are less effective than the aromatase inhibitors.

Cytotoxic chemotherapy is preferred for advanced steroid hormone-receptor-negative tumours and for aggressive disease, particularly where metastases involve visceral sites (e.g. the liver) or where the disease-free interval following treatment for early breast cancer is short.

Chemoprevention Recent evidence suggests that tamoxifen prophylaxis can reduce breast cancer in women at high risk of the disease. However, the adverse effects of tamoxifen preclude its routine use in most women.

Cytotoxic drugs used in breast cancer An anthracycline combined with fluorouracil (section 8.1.3) and cyclophosphamide (section 8.1.1), and sometimes also with methotrexate (section 8.1.3) is effective. Cyclophosphamide, methotrexate, and fluorouracil can be useful if an anthracycline is inappropriate (e.g. in cardiac disease).

Metastatic disease The choice of chemotherapy regimen will be influenced by whether the patient has previously received adjuvant treatment and the presence of any co-morbidity.

For women who have not previously received chemotherapy, an anthracycline such as doxorubicin or epirubicin combined with cyclophosphamide is the standard initial therapy for metastatic breast disease.

Patients with anthracycline-refractory or resistant disease should be considered for treatment with a taxane (section 8.1.5) either alone or in combination with trastuzumab if they have tumours that overexpress HER2. Other cytotoxic drugs with activity against breast cancer include capecitabine (section 8.1.3), mitoxantrone, mitomycin (both section 8.1.2), and vinorelbine (section 8.1.4). Trastuzumab alone (section 8.1.5) is an option for chemotherapy-resistant cancers that overexpress HER2.

Oestrogen-receptor antagonists **Tamoxifen** is an oestrogen-receptor antagonist that is licensed for breast cancer and anovulatory infertility (section 6.5.1).

Fulvestrant is licensed for the treatment of oestrogen-receptor-positive metastatic or locally advanced breast cancer in postmenopausal women in whom disease progresses or relapses while on, or after, other anti-oestrogen therapy.

Toremifene is licensed for steroid hormone-receptor-positive metastatic breast cancer in postmenopausal women, but it is not often used.

Aromatase inhibitors Aromatase inhibitors act predominantly by blocking the conversion of androgens to oestrogens in the peripheral tissues. They do not inhibit ovarian oestrogen synthesis and should not be used in premenopausal women.

Anastrozole and **letrozole** are non-steroidal aromatase inhibitors; **exemestane** is a steroidal aromatase inhibitor. Anastrozole and letrozole are at least as effective as tamoxifen for first-line treatment of metastatic breast cancer in postmenopausal women. However, it is not yet known whether the benefits of aromatase inhibitors persist over the long term.

The *Scottish Medicines Consortium* has advised (August 2005) that anastrazole is accepted for restricted use in the adjuvant treatment of postmenopausal women with hormone-receptor-positive early invasive breast cancer.

The *Scottish Medicines Consortium* has advised (October 2005) that exemestane is accepted for restricted use as an adjuvant treatment in postmenopausal women with oestrogen-receptor-positive invasive early breast cancer, following 2–3 years of initial adjuvant tamoxifen therapy.

> NICE guidance
> **Hormonal therapies for the adjuvant treatment of early oestrogen-receptor-positive breast cancer (November 2006)**
> The aromatase inhibitors anastrozole, exemestane, and letrozole, within their licensed indications, are options for the adjuvant treatment of early oestrogen-receptor-positive invasive breast cancer in postmenopausal women.

Gonadorelin analogues Goserelin (section 8.3.4.2), a gonadorelin analogue is licensed for the management of advanced breast cancer in premenopausal women.

Other drugs used in breast cancer Trilostane (section 6.7.3) is licensed for postmenopausal breast cancer. It is quite well tolerated but diarrhoea and abdominal discomfort may be a problem. Trilostane causes adrenal hypofunction and corticosteroid replacement therapy is needed.

The use of **bisphosphonates** (section 6.6.2) in patients with metastatic breast cancer may prevent skeletal complications of bone metastases.

ANASTROZOLE

Indications adjuvant treatment of oestrogen-receptor-positive early breast cancer in postmenopausal women, either as sole therapy or following 2–3 years of tamoxifen therapy; advanced breast cancer in postmenopausal women which is oestrogen-receptor positive or responsive to tamoxifen

Cautions laboratory test for menopause if doubt; susceptibility to osteoporosis (assess bone mineral density before treatment and at regular intervals)

8 Malignant disease and immunosuppression

Contra-indications pregnancy and breast-feeding; moderate or severe hepatic disease; moderate or severe renal impairment; not for premenopausal women

Side-effects hot flushes, vaginal dryness, vaginal bleeding, hair thinning, anorexia, nausea, vomiting, diarrhoea, headache, arthralgia, bone fractures, rash (including Stevens-Johnson syndrome); asthenia and drowsiness—may initially affect ability to drive or operate machinery; slight increases in total cholesterol levels reported; very rarely allergic reactions including angioedema and anaphylaxis

Dose

- 1 mg daily

Arimidex® (AstraZeneca) PoM
Tablets, f/c, anastrozole 1 mg. Net price 28-tab pack = £68.56

EXEMESTANE

Indications adjuvant treatment of oestrogen-receptor-positive early breast cancer in postmenopausal women following 2–3 years of tamoxifen therapy; advanced breast cancer in postmenopausal women in whom anti-oestrogen therapy has failed

Cautions hepatic impairment (Appendix 2); renal impairment (Appendix 3); **interactions:** Appendix 1 (exemestane)

Contra-indications pregnancy and breast-feeding; not indicated for premenopausal women

Side-effects nausea, vomiting, abdominal pain, dyspepsia, constipation, anorexia; dizziness, fatigue, headache, depression, insomnia; hot flushes, sweating; alopecia, rash; *less commonly* drowsiness, asthenia, and peripheral oedema; *rarely* thrombocytopenia, leucopenia

Dose

- 25 mg daily

Aromasin® (Pharmacia) PoM
Tablets, s/c, exemestane 25 mg, net price 30-tab pack = £88.80, 90-tab pack = £266.40. Label: 21

FULVESTRANT

Indications treatment of oestrogen-receptor-positive metastatic or locally advanced breast cancer in postmenopausal women in whom disease progresses or relapses while on, or after, other anti-oestrogen therapy

Cautions hepatic impairment (avoid if severe; Appendix 2)

Contra-indications pregnancy (Appendix 4); breast-feeding (Appendix 5)

Side-effects hot flushes, nausea, vomiting, diarrhoea, anorexia, headache, back pain, rash, asthenia, venous thromboembolism, injection-site reactions, urinary-tract infections; less commonly vaginal haemorrhage, vaginal candidiasis, leucorrhoea, hypersensitivity reactions including angioedema, urticaria

Dose

- By deep intramuscular injection, 250 mg into gluteal muscle every 4 weeks

Faslodex® (AstraZeneca) PoM
Injection (oily), fulvestrant 50 mg/mL, net price 5-mL (250-mg) prefilled syringe = £348.27

LETROZOLE

Indications adjuvant treatment of oestrogen-receptor-positive early breast cancer in postmenopausal women; advanced breast cancer in postmenopausal women (including those in whom other anti-oestrogen therapy has failed); early invasive breast cancer in postmenopausal women after standard adjuvant tamoxifen therapy; pre-operative treatment in postmenopausal women with localised hormone-receptor-positive breast cancer to allow subsequent breast conserving surgery

Cautions renal impairment (Appendix 3); susceptibility to osteoporosis (assess bone mineral density before treatment and at regular intervals)

Contra-indications severe hepatic impairment; not indicated for premenopausal women; pregnancy (Appendix 4) and breast-feeding

Side-effects hot flushes, nausea, vomiting, fatigue, dizziness, headache, dyspepsia, constipation, diarrhoea, depression, anorexia, appetite increase, hypercholesterolaemia, alopecia, increased sweating, rash, peripheral oedema, musculoskeletal pain, osteoporosis, bone fracture; *less commonly* hypertension, palpitation, tachycardia, dyspnoea, cough, drowsiness, insomnia, anxiety, memory impairment, dysaesthesia, taste disturbance, pruritus, dry skin, urticaria, thrombophlebitis, abdominal pain, urinary frequency, urinary-tract infection, vaginal bleeding, vaginal discharge, breast pain, pyrexia, mucosal dryness, stomatitis, cataract, eye irritation, blurred vision, tumour pain, arthritis, leucopenia, general oedema; *rarely* pulmonary embolism, arterial thrombosis, cerebrovascular infarction

Dose

- 2.5 mg daily

Femara® (Novartis) PoM
Tablets, f/c, letrozole 2.5 mg. Net price 14-tab pack = £41.58, 28-tab pack = £83.16

TAMOXIFEN

Indications see under Dose and notes above; mastalgia [unlicensed indication] (section 6.7.2)

Cautions occasional cystic ovarian swellings in premenopausal women; increased risk of thromboembolic events when used with cytotoxics (see also below); breast-feeding (Appendix 5); endometrial changes (**important**: see below); porphyria (section 9.8.2); **interactions:** Appendix 1 (tamoxifen)

Endometrial changes Increased endometrial changes, including hyperplasia, polyps, cancer, and uterine sarcoma reported; prompt investigation required if abnormal vaginal bleeding including menstrual irregularities, vaginal discharge, and pelvic pain or pressure in those receiving (or who have received) tamoxifen.

Contra-indications pregnancy (exclude before commencing and advise non-hormonal contraception if appropriate—Appendix 4)

Side-effects hot flushes, vaginal bleeding and vaginal discharge (**important**: see also Endometrial Changes under Cautions), suppression of menstruation in some premenopausal women, pruritus vulvae, gastro-intestinal disturbances, headache, light-headedness, tumour flare, decreased platelet counts; occasionally oedema, hypercalcaemia if bony metastases, alopecia, rashes, uterine fibroids; also visual disturbances (including corneal changes, cataracts, retinopathy);

leucopenia (sometimes with anaemia and thrombocytopenia), rarely neutropenia; hypertriglyceridaemia reported (sometimes with pancreatitis); thromboembolic events reported (see below); liver enzyme changes (rarely fatty liver, cholestasis, hepatitis); rarely interstitial pneumonitis, hypersensitivity reactions including angioedema, Stevens-Johnson syndrome, bullous pemphigoid; see also notes above

Risk of thromboembolism Tamoxifen can increase the risk of thromboembolism particularly during and immediately after major surgery or periods of immobility. Patients should be made aware of the symptoms of thromboembolism and advised to report sudden breathlessness and any pain in the calf of one leg

Dose

- Breast cancer, 20 mg daily

  CSM advice The CSM has advised that tamoxifen in a dose of 20 mg daily substantially increases survival in early breast cancer, and that no further benefit has been demonstrated with higher doses. Patients should be told of the small risk of endometrial cancer (see under Cautions above) and encouraged to report relevant symptoms early. They can, however, be reassured that the benefits of treatment far outweigh the risks
- Anovulatory infertility, 20 mg daily on days 2, 3, 4 and 5 of cycle; if necessary the daily dose may be increased to 40 mg then 80 mg for subsequent courses; if cycles irregular, start initial course on any day, with subsequent course starting 45 days later *or* on day 2 of cycle if menstruation occurs

Tamoxifen (Non-proprietary) PoM

Tablets, tamoxifen (as citrate) 10 mg, net price 30-tab pack = £1.43; 20 mg, 30-tab pack = £1.57; 40 mg, 30-tab pack = £7.25

Oral solution, tamoxifen (as citrate) 10 mg/5 mL, net price 150 mL = £29.61

Brands include *Soltamox*®

Nolvadex-D® (AstraZeneca) PoM

Tablets, tamoxifen (as citrate) 20 mg, net-price 30-tab pack = £8.71

TOREMIFENE

Indications hormone-dependent metastatic breast cancer in postmenopausal women

Cautions hypercalcaemia may occur (especially if bone metastases and usually at beginning of treatment); **interactions:** Appendix 1 (toremifene)

Endometrial changes There is a risk of increased endometrial changes including hyperplasia, polyps and cancer. Abnormal vaginal bleeding including menstrual irregularities, vaginal discharge and symptoms such as pelvic pain or pressure should be promptly investigated

Contra-indications endometrial hyperplasia, severe hepatic impairment (Appendix 2), history of severe thromboembolic disease; pregnancy and breast-feeding

Side-effects hot flushes, vaginal bleeding or discharge (**important:** see also Cautions), dizziness, oedema, sweating, nausea, vomiting, chest or back pain, fatigue, headache, skin discoloration, weight increase, insomnia, constipation, dyspnoea, paresis, tremor, vertigo, pruritus, anorexia, corneal opacity (reversible), asthenia; thromboembolic events reported; rarely dermatitis, alopecia, emotional lability, depression, jaundice, stiffness

Dose

- 60 mg daily

Fareston® (Orion) PoM

Tablets, toremifene (as citrate) 60 mg. Net price 30-tab pack = £30.37

8.3.4.2 Prostate cancer and gonadorelin analogues

Metastatic cancer of the prostate usually responds to hormonal treatment aimed at androgen depletion. Standard treatments include bilateral subcapsular orchidectomy or use of a gonadorelin analogue (**buserelin, goserelin, leuprorelin**, or **triptorelin**). Response in most patients lasts for 12 to 18 months. No entirely satisfactory therapy exists for disease progression despite this treatment (hormone-refractory prostate cancer), but occasional patients respond to other hormone manipulation e.g. with an anti-androgen. Bone disease can often be palliated with irradiation or, if widespread, with strontium or prednisolone (section 6.3.2).

Gonadorelin analogues

Gonadorelin analogues are as effective as orchidectomy or **diethylstilbestrol** (section 8.3.1) but are expensive and require parenteral administration, at least initially. They cause initial stimulation then depression of luteinising hormone release by the pituitary. During the initial stage (1–2 weeks) increased production of testosterone may be associated with progression of prostate cancer. In susceptible patients this tumour 'flare' may cause spinal cord compression, ureteric obstruction or increased bone pain. When such problems are anticipated, alternative treatments (e.g. orchidectomy) or concomitant use of an anti-androgen such as cyproterone acetate or flutamide (see below) are recommended; anti-androgen treatment should be started 3 days before the gonadorelin analogue and continued for 3 weeks. Gonadorelin analogues are also used in women for breast cancer (section 8.3.4.1) and other indications (section 6.7.2).

Cautions Men at risk of tumour 'flare' (see above) should be monitored closely during the first month of therapy. Caution is required in patients with metabolic bone disease because reduced bone mineral density can occur. The injection site should be rotated.

Side-effects The gonadorelin analogues cause side-effects similar to the menopause in women and orchidectomy in men and include hot flushes and sweating, sexual dysfunction, vaginal dryness or bleeding, and gynaecomastia or changes in breast size. Signs and symptoms of prostate or breast cancer may worsen initially (managed in prostate cancer with anti-androgens, see above). Other side-effects include hypersensitivity reactions (rashes, pruritus, asthma, and rarely anaphylaxis), injection site reactions (see Cautions), headache (rarely migraine), visual disturbances, dizziness, arthralgia and possibly myalgia, hair loss, peripheral oedema, gastro-intestinal disturbances, weight changes, sleep disorders, and mood changes.

Anti-androgens

Cyproterone acetate, **flutamide** and **bicalutamide** are anti-androgens that inhibit the tumour 'flare' which may occur after commencing gonadorelin analogue administration. Cyproterone acetate and flutamide are also licensed for use alone in patients with metastatic prostate cancer refractory to gonadorelin analogue therapy. Bicalutamide is used for prostate cancer either alone or as an adjunct to other therapy, according to the clinical circumstances.

BICALUTAMIDE

Indications locally advanced prostate cancer at high risk of disease progression, either alone or as adjuvant treatment; locally advanced, non-metastatic prostate cancer when surgical castration or other medical intervention inappropriate

Cautions hepatic impairment (Appendix 2), also consider periodic liver function tests; **interactions:** Appendix 1 (bicalutamide)

Side-effects nausea, vomiting, diarrhoea, asthenia, gynaecomastia, breast tenderness, hot flushes, pruritus, dry skin, alopecia, hirsutism, decreased libido, impotence, weight gain; less commonly hypersensitivity reactions including angioneurotic oedema and urticaria, interstitial lung disease; rarely abdominal pain, cardiovascular disorders (including angina, heart failure and arrhythmias), depression, dyspepsia, haematuria, cholestasis, jaundice, thrombocytopenia

Dose

- 150 mg once daily

Note The CSM has advised (October 2003) that bicalutamide should no longer be used for the treatment of localised prostate cancer

Casodex® (AstraZeneca) PoM
Tablets, f/c, bicalutamide 50 mg, net price 28-tab pack = £128.00; 150 mg, 28-tab pack = £240.00

BUSERELIN

Indications advanced prostate cancer; other indications (section 6.7.2)

Cautions depression, see also notes above

Side-effects see notes above; worsening hypertension, palpitation, glucose intolerance, altered blood lipids, thrombocytopenia, leucopenia, nervousness, fatigue, memory and concentration disturbances, anxiety, increased thirst, hearing disorders, musculoskeletal pain; nasal irritation, nose bleeds and altered sense of taste and smell (spray formulation only)

Dose

- By subcutaneous injection, 500 micrograms every 8 hours for 7 days, then intranasally, 1 spray into each nostril 6 times daily (see also notes above)

Counselling Avoid use of nasal decongestants before and for at least 30 minutes after treatment.

Suprefact® (Aventis Pharma) PoM
Injection, buserelin (as acetate) 1 mg/mL. Net price 2 × 5.5-mL vial = £23.69

Nasal spray, buserelin (as acetate) 100 micrograms/metered spray. Net price treatment pack of 4 × 10-g bottle with spray pump = £87.68. Counselling, see above

CYPROTERONE ACETATE

Indications prostate cancer, see under Dose and also notes above; other indications, see section 6.4.2

Cautions in prostate cancer, blood counts initially and throughout treatment; hepatic impairment (Appendix 2; see also under side-effects below); monitor hepatic function (liver function tests should be performed before treatment, see also under Side-effects below); monitor adrenocortical function regularly; risk of recurrence of thromboembolic disease; diabetes mellitus, sickle-cell anaemia, severe depression (in other indications some of these are contra-indicated, see section 6.4.2)

Driving Fatigue and lassitude may impair performance of skilled tasks (e.g. driving)

Contra-indications none in prostate cancer; for contra-indications relating to other indications see section 6.4.2

Side-effects see section 6.4.2

Hepatotoxicity Direct hepatic toxicity including jaundice, hepatitis and hepatic failure have been reported (usually after several months) in patients treated with cyproterone acetate 200–300 mg daily. Liver function tests should be performed before and regularly during treatment and whenever symptoms suggestive of hepatotoxicity occur—if confirmed cyproterone should normally be withdrawn unless the hepatotoxicity can be explained by another cause such as metastatic disease (in which case cyproterone should be continued only if the perceived benefit exceeds the risk)

Dose

- Flare with initial gonadorelin therapy, 300 mg daily in 2–3 divided doses, reduced to 200 mg daily in 2–3 divided doses if necessary
- Long-term palliative therapy where gonadorelin analogues or orchidectomy contra-indicated, not tolerated, or where oral therapy preferred, 200–300 mg daily in 2–3 divided doses
- Hot flushes with gonadorelin therapy or after orchidectomy, initially 50 mg daily, adjusted according to response to 50–150 mg daily in 1–3 divided doses

Cyproterone Acetate (Non-proprietary) PoM
Tablets, cyproterone acetate 50 mg, net price 56-tab pack = £31.54; 100 mg, 84-tab pack = £77.55. Label: 21, counselling, driving

Cyprostat® (Schering Health) PoM
Tablets, scored, cyproterone acetate 50 mg, net price 168-tab pack = £77.68; 100 mg, 84-tab pack = £77.68. Label: 21, counselling, driving

FLUTAMIDE

Indications advanced prostate cancer, see also notes above

Cautions cardiac disease (oedema reported); hepatic impairment, also liver function tests, monthly for first 4 months, periodically thereafter and at the first sign or symptom of liver disorder (e.g. pruritus, dark urine, persistent anorexia, jaundice, abdominal pain, unexplained influenza-like symptoms); avoid excessive alcohol consumption; **interactions:** Appendix 1 (flutamide)

Side-effects gynaecomastia (sometimes with galactorrhoea); nausea, vomiting, diarrhoea, increased appetite, insomnia, tiredness; other side-effects reported include decreased libido, reduced sperm count, gastric and chest pain, hypertension, headache, dizziness, oedema, blurred vision, thirst, rash, pruritus, haemolytic anaemia, systemic lupus erythematosus-like syndrome, and lymphoedema; hepatic injury (with transaminase abnormalities, cholestatic jaundice, hepatic necrosis, hepatic encephalopathy and occasional fatality) reported

Dose

- 250 mg 3 times daily (see also notes above)

Flutamide (Non-proprietary) PoM
Tablets, flutamide 250 mg. Net price 84-tab pack = £21.94

Drogenil® (Schering-Plough) PoM
Tablets, yellow, scored, flutamide 250 mg, net price 84-tab pack = £65.10

GOSERELIN

Indications prostate cancer; advanced breast cancer; oestrogen-receptor positive early breast cancer (section 8.3.4.1); other indications (section 6.7.2)

Cautions see notes above; breast-feeding (Appendix 5)

Contra-indications pregnancy (Appendix 4); undiagnosed vaginal bleeding

Side-effects see notes above; also transient changes in blood pressure, paraesthesia, rarely hypercalcaemia (in patients with metastatic breast cancer)

Dose

- See under preparations below

Zoladex® (AstraZeneca) PoM
Implant, goserelin 3.6 mg (as acetate) in *SafeSystem®* syringe applicator. Net price each = £84.14
Dose breast cancer and prostate cancer by subcutaneous injection into anterior abdominal wall, 3.6 mg every 28 days (see also notes above)

Zoladex® LA (AstraZeneca) PoM
Implant, goserelin 10.8 mg (as acetate) in *SafeSystem®* syringe applicator. Net price each = £267.48
Dose prostate cancer, by subcutaneous injection into anterior abdominal wall, 10.8 mg every 12 weeks (see also notes above)

LEUPRORELIN ACETATE

Indications advanced prostate cancer; other indications (section 6.7.2)

Cautions see notes above and section 6.7.2

Side-effects see notes above and section 6.7.2; also fatigue, muscle weakness, paraesthesia, hypertension, palpitation, alteration of glucose tolerance and of blood lipids; hypotension, jaundice, thrombocytopenia and leucopenia reported

Dose

- See under preparations below

Prostap® SR (Wyeth) PoM
Injection (microsphere powder for reconstitution), leuprorelin acetate, net price 3.75-mg vial with 1-mL vehicle-filled syringe = £125.40
Dose advanced prostate cancer, by subcutaneous *or* by intramuscular injection, 3.75 mg every 4 weeks (see also notes above)

Prostap® 3 (Wyeth) PoM
Injection (microsphere powder for reconstitution), leuprorelin acetate, net price 11.25-mg vial with 2-mL vehicle-filled syringe = £376.20
Dose advanced prostate cancer, by subcutaneous injection, 11.25 mg every three months (see also notes above)

TRIPTORELIN

Indications advanced prostate cancer; endometriosis, precocious puberty, reduction in size of uterine fibroids (section 6.7.2)

Cautions see notes above

Side-effects see notes above; also dry mouth, transient hypertension, paraesthesia, and increased dysuria

Dose

- See under preparations below

Decapeptyl® SR (Ipsen) PoM
Injection (powder for suspension), m/r, triptorelin (as acetate), net price 4.2-mg vial (with diluent) = £69.00
Dose by intramuscular injection, advanced prostate cancer, 3 mg every 4 weeks
Note Each 4.2-mg vial includes an overage to allow administration of a 3-mg dose
Injection (powder for suspension), m/r, triptorelin (as acetate), net price 15-mg vial (with diluent) = £207.00
Dose by intramuscular injection, advanced prostate cancer, 11.25 mg every 3 months (see also notes above)
Note Each 15-mg vial includes an overage to allow administration of an 11.25-mg dose

Gonapeptyl Depot® (Ferring) PoM
Injection (powder for suspension), triptorelin (as acetate), net price 3.75-mg prefilled syringe (with prefilled syringe of vehicle) = £85.00
Dose by subcutaneous *or* deep intramuscular injection, advanced prostate cancer, 3.75 mg every 4 weeks (see also notes above)

8.3.4.3 Somatostatin analogues

Lanreotide and **octreotide** are analogues of the hypothalamic release-inhibiting hormone somatostatin. They are indicated for the relief of symptoms associated with neuroendocrine (particularly carcinoid) tumours and acromegaly. Additionally, lanreotide is licensed for the treatment of thyroid tumours and octreotide is also licensed for the prevention of complications following pancreatic surgery; octreotide may also be valuable in reducing vomiting in palliative care (see p. 18) and in stopping variceal bleeding [unlicensed indication]—see also vasopressin and terlipressin (section 6.5.2).

Cautions Growth hormone-secreting pituitary tumours can expand causing serious complications; during treatment with somatostatin analogues patients should be monitored for signs of tumour expansion (e.g. visual field defects). Ultrasound examination of the gallbladder is recommended before treatment and at intervals of 6–12 months during treatment (avoid abrupt withdrawal of short-acting octreotide—see Side-effects below). In insulinoma an increase in the depth and duration of hypoglycaemia may occur (observe patients when initiating treatment and changing doses); in diabetes mellitus, insulin or oral antidiabetic requirements may be reduced.

Side-effects Gastro-intestinal disturbances including anorexia, nausea, vomiting, abdominal pain and bloating, flatulence, diarrhoea, and steatorrhoea may occur. Postprandial glucose tolerance may be impaired and rarely persistent hyperglycaemia occurs with chronic administration; hypoglycaemia has also been reported. Gallstones have been reported after long-term treatment (abrupt withdrawal of subcutaneous octreotide is associated with biliary colic and pancreatitis). Pain and irritation may occur at the injection site and sites should be rotated. Rarely, pancreatitis has been reported shortly after administration.

LANREOTIDE

Indications see notes above

Cautions see notes above; pregnancy (Appendix 4); breast-feeding (Appendix 5); **interactions**: Appendix 1 (lanreotide)

Side-effects see notes above; also reported asthenia, fatigue, raised bilirubin; *less commonly* skin nodule, hot flushes, leg pain, malaise, headache, tenesmus, decreased libido, drowsiness, pruritus, increased sweating; *rarely* hypothyroidism (monitor as necessary)

Dose

- See under preparations

Somatuline® LA (Ipsen) PoM

Injection (copolymer microparticles for aqueous suspension), lanreotide (as acetate) 30-mg vial (with vehicle) = £340.00

Dose by intramuscular injection, acromegaly and neuroendocrine (particularly carcinoid) tumours, initially 30 mg every 14 days, frequency increased to every 7–10 days according to response

Thyroid tumours, 30 mg every 14 days, frequency increased to every 10 days according to response

Somatuline Autogel® (Ipsen)

Injection, prefilled syringe, lanreotide (as acetate) 60 mg = £573.00; 90 mg = £765.00; 120 mg = £989.00

Dose by deep subcutaneous injection into the gluteal region, acromegaly (if somatostatin analogue not given previously), initially 60 mg every 28 days, adjusted according to response; for patients treated previously with somatostatin analogue, consult product literature for initial dose

Neuroendocrine (particularly carcinoid) tumours, initially 60–120 mg every 28 days, adjusted according to response

OCTREOTIDE

Indications see under Dose

Cautions see notes above; hepatic impairment; pregnancy (Appendix 4); breast-feeding (Appendix 5); monitor thyroid function on long-term therapy; **interactions**: Appendix 1 (octreotide)

Side-effects see notes above; *rarely* altered liver function tests, hepatitis and transient alopecia

Dose

- Symptoms associated with carcinoid tumours with features of carcinoid syndrome, VIPomas, glucagonomas, by subcutaneous injection, initially 50 micrograms once or twice daily, gradually increased according to response to 200 micrograms 3 times daily (higher doses required exceptionally); maintenance doses variable; in carcinoid tumours discontinue after 1 week if no effect; if rapid response required, initial dose by intravenous injection (with ECG monitoring and after dilution to a concentration of 10–50% with sodium chloride 0.9% injection)
- Acromegaly, short-term treatment before pituitary surgery *or* long-term treatment in those inadequately controlled by other treatment *or* until radiotherapy becomes fully effective by subcutaneous injection, 100–200 micrograms 3 times daily; discontinue if no improvement within 3 months
- Prevention of complications following pancreatic surgery, consult product literature

Sandostatin® (Novartis) PoM

Injection, octreotide (as acetate) 50 micrograms/mL, net price 1-mL amp = £3.72; 100 micrograms/mL, 1-mL amp = £6.53; 200 micrograms/mL 5-mL vial = £69.66; 500 micrograms/mL, 1-mL amp = £33.87

Depot preparation

Sandostatin Lar® (Novartis) PoM

Injection (microsphere powder for aqueous suspension), octreotide (as acetate) 10-mg vial = £637.50; 20-mg vial = £850.00; 30-mg vial = £1062.50 (all supplied with 2.5-mL diluent-filled syringe)

Dose acromegaly (test dose by subcutaneous injection 50–100 micrograms if subcutaneous octreotide not previously given), neuroendocrine (particularly carcinoid) tumour adequately controlled by subcutaneous octreotide, by deep intramuscular injection into gluteal muscle, initially 20 mg every 4 weeks for 3 months then adjusted according to response; max. 30 mg every 4 weeks

For acromegaly, start depot octreotide 1 day after the last dose of subcutaneous octreotide (for pituitary surgery give last dose of depot octreotide at least 3 weeks before surgery); for neuroendocrine tumours, continue subcutaneous octreotide for 2 weeks after first dose of depot octreotide

9 Nutrition and blood

9.1 **Anaemias and some other blood disorders** 490
9.1.1 Iron-deficiency anaemias 490
9.1.1.1 Oral iron 490
9.1.1.2 Parenteral iron 492
9.1.2 Drugs used in megaloblastic anaemias 493
9.1.3 Drugs used in hypoplastic, haemolytic, and renal anaemias 495
9.1.4 Drugs used in platelet disorders 500
9.1.5 G6PD deficiency 500
9.1.6 Drugs used in neutropenia 501
9.2 **Fluids and electrolytes** 503
9.2.1 Oral preparations for fluid and electrolyte imbalance 503
9.2.1.1 Oral potassium 503
9.2.1.2 Oral sodium and water 504
9.2.1.3 Oral bicarbonate 505
9.2.2 Parenteral preparations for fluid and electrolyte imbalance 506
9.2.2.1 Electrolytes and water 506
9.2.2.2 Plasma and plasma substitutes 508
9.3 **Intravenous nutrition** 511
9.4 **Oral nutrition** 516
9.4.1 Foods for special diets 516
9.4.2 Enteral nutrition 516
9.5 **Minerals** 517
9.5.1 Calcium and magnesium 517
9.5.1.1 Calcium supplements 517
9.5.1.2 Hypercalcaemia and hypercalciuria 518
9.5.1.3 Magnesium 519
9.5.2 Phosphorus 519
9.5.2.1 Phosphate supplements 519
9.5.2.2 Phosphate-binding agents 520
9.5.3 Fluoride 521
9.5.4 Zinc 522
9.5.5 Selenium 522
9.6 **Vitamins** 522
9.6.1 Vitamin A 523
9.6.2 Vitamin B group 523
9.6.3 Vitamin C 524
9.6.4 Vitamin D 525
9.6.5 Vitamin E 527
9.6.6 Vitamin K 527
9.6.7 Multivitamin preparations 528
9.7 **Bitters and tonics** 528
9.8 **Metabolic disorders** 528
9.8.1 Drugs used in metabolic disorders 528
9.8.2 Acute porphyrias 532

9.1 Anaemias and some other blood disorders

9.1.1 Iron-deficiency anaemias
9.1.2 Drugs used in megaloblastic anaemias
9.1.3 Drugs used in hypoplastic, haemolytic, and renal anaemias
9.1.4 Drugs used in platelet disorders
9.1.5 G6PD deficiency
9.1.6 Drugs used in neutropenia

Before initiating treatment for anaemia it is essential to determine which type is present. Iron salts may be harmful and result in iron overload if given alone to patients with anaemias other than those due to iron deficiency.

9.1.1 Iron-deficiency anaemias

9.1.1.1 Oral iron
9.1.1.2 Parenteral iron

Treatment with an iron preparation is justified only in the presence of a demonstrable iron-deficiency state. Before starting treatment, it is important to exclude any serious underlying cause of the anaemia (e.g. gastric erosion, gastro-intestinal cancer).

Prophylaxis with an iron preparation is justifiable in individuals who have additional risk factors for iron deficiency (e.g. poor diet). Prophylaxis may also be appropriate in malabsorption, menorrhagia, pregnancy, after subtotal or total gastrectomy, in haemodialysis patients, and in the management of low birth-weight infants such as preterm neonates.

9.1.1.1 Oral iron

Iron salts should be given by mouth unless there are good reasons for using another route.

Ferrous salts show only marginal differences between one another in efficiency of absorption of iron, but ferric salts are much less well absorbed. Haemoglobin regeneration rate is little affected by the type of salt used provided sufficient iron is given, and in most patients the speed of response is not critical. Choice of preparation is thus usually decided by the incidence of side-effects and cost.

The oral dose of elemental iron for deficiency should be 100 to 200 mg daily. It is customary to give this as dried **ferrous sulphate**, 200 mg (≡ 65 mg elemental iron) three times daily; a dose of ferrous sulphate 200 mg once or twice daily may be effective for prophylaxis or for mild iron deficiency.

Iron content of different iron salts

Iron salt	Amount	Content of ferrous iron
Ferrous fumarate	200 mg	65 mg
Ferrous gluconate	300 mg	35 mg
Ferrous sulphate	300 mg	60 mg
Ferrous sulphate, dried	200 mg	65 mg

Therapeutic response The haemoglobin concentration should rise by about 100–200 mg/100 mL (1–2 g/litre) per day *or* 2 g/100 mL (20 g/litre) over 3–4 weeks. When the haemoglobin is in the reference range, treatment should be continued for a further 3 months to replenish the iron stores. Epithelial tissue changes such as atrophic glossitis and koilonychia are usually improved, but the response is often slow.

Side-effects Gastro-intestinal irritation can occur with iron salts. Nausea and epigastric pain are dose-related but the relationship between dose and altered bowel habit (constipation or diarrhoea) is less clear. Oral iron, particularly modified-release preparations, can exacerbate diarrhoea in patients with inflammatory bowel disease; care is also needed in patients with intestinal strictures and diverticular disease.

Iron preparations taken orally can be constipating, particularly in older patients, occasionally leading to faecal impaction.

If side-effects occur, the dose may be reduced; alternatively, another iron salt may be used but an improvement in tolerance may simply be a result of a lower content of elemental iron. The incidence of side-effects due to ferrous sulphate is no greater than with other iron salts when compared on the basis of equivalent amounts of elemental iron.

Iron preparations are a common cause of accidental overdose in children. For the treatment of **iron overdose**, see Emergency Treatment of Poisoning, p. 32.

Compound preparations Some oral preparations contain ascorbic acid to aid absorption of the iron but the therapeutic advantage of such preparations is minimal and cost may be increased.

There is no justification for the inclusion of other ingredients, such as the B group of vitamins (except folic acid for pregnant women, see Iron and Folic Acid, p. 492 and on p. 494).

Modified-release preparations Modified-release preparations of iron are licensed for once-daily dosage, but have no therapeutic advantage and should not be used. These preparations are formulated to release iron gradually; the low incidence of side-effects may reflect the small amounts of iron available for absorption as the iron is carried past the first part of the duodenum into an area of the gut where absorption may be poor.

FERROUS SULPHATE

Indications iron-deficiency anaemia
Cautions interactions: Appendix 1 (iron)
Side-effects see notes above
Dose

- See under preparations below and notes above

Counselling Although iron preparations are best absorbed on an empty stomach they may be taken after food to reduce gastro-intestinal side-effects; they may discolour stools

Ferrous Sulphate (Non-proprietary)
Tablets, coated, dried ferrous sulphate 200 mg (65 mg iron), net price 28-tab pack = £2.40
Dose prophylactic, 1 tablet daily; therapeutic, 1 tablet 2–3 times daily

Ironorm® Drops (Wallace Mfg)
Oral drops, ferrous sulphate 125 mg (25 mg iron)/mL. Net price 15-mL = £3.35
Dose ADULT and CHILD over 6 years, 0.6 mL daily; INFANT and CHILD up to 6 years, 0.3 mL daily

Modified-release preparations

Feospan® (Intrapharm) NHS
Spansule® (= capsules m/r), clear/red, enclosing green and brown pellets, dried ferrous sulphate 150 mg (47 mg iron). Net price 30-cap pack = £1.43. Label: 25
Dose 1–2 capsules daily; CHILD over 1 year, 1 capsule daily; can be opened and sprinkled on food

Ferrograd® (Teofarma)
Tablets, f/c, m/r, red, dried ferrous sulphate 325 mg (105 mg iron). Net price 30-tab pack = £1.18. Label: 25
Dose ADULT and CHILD over 12 years, 1 tablet daily before food

FERROUS FUMARATE

Indications iron-deficiency anaemia
Cautions interactions: Appendix 1 (iron)
Side-effects see notes above
Dose

- See under preparations below and notes above

Fersaday® (Goldshield)
Tablets, brown, f/c, ferrous fumarate 322 mg (100 mg iron). Net price 28-tab pack = 79p
Dose prophylactic, 1 tablet daily; therapeutic, 1 tablet twice daily

Fersamal® (Goldshield)
Tablets, brown, ferrous fumarate 210 mg (68 mg iron). Net price 20 = 29p
Dose 1–2 tablets 3 times daily

Syrup, brown, ferrous fumarate approx. 140 mg (45 mg iron)/5 mL. Net price 200 mL = £3.11
Dose 10–20 mL twice daily; PRETERM NEONATE 0.6–2.4 mL/kg daily; CHILD up to 6 years 2.5–5 mL twice daily

Galfer® (Thornton & Ross)
Capsules, red/green, ferrous fumarate 305 mg (100 mg iron). Net price 20 = 36p
Dose 1 capsule 1–2 times daily before food

Syrup, brown, sugar-free ferrous fumarate 140 mg (45 mg iron)/5 mL. Net price 300 mL = £4.86
Dose 10 mL 1–2 times daily before food; CHILD (full-term infant and young child) 2.5–5 mL 1–2 times daily

FERROUS GLUCONATE

Indications iron-deficiency anaemia
Cautions interactions: Appendix 1 (iron)
Side-effects see notes above
Dose
- See under preparation below and notes above

Ferrous Gluconate (Non-proprietary)
Tablets, red, coated, ferrous gluconate 300 mg (35 mg iron). Net price 20 = 73p
Dose prophylactic, 2 tablets daily before food; therapeutic, 4–6 tablets daily in divided doses before food; CHILD 6–12 years, prophylactic and therapeutic, 1–3 tablets daily

POLYSACCHARIDE–IRON COMPLEX

Indications iron-deficiency anaemia
Cautions interactions: Appendix 1 (iron)
Side-effects see notes above
Dose
- See under preparation below and notes above

Niferex® (Tillomed)
Elixir, brown, sugar-free, polysaccharide–iron complex equivalent to 100 mg of iron/5 mL. Net price 240-mL pack = £6.06; NHS[1] 30-mL dropper bottle for paediatric use = £2.16. Counselling, use of dropper
Dose prophylactic, 2.5 mL daily; therapeutic, 5 mL 1–2 times daily (once daily if required during second and third trimester of pregnancy); PRETERM NEONATE, NEONATE, and INFANT (from dropper bottle) 1 drop (approx. 500 micrograms iron) per 450 g body-weight 3 times daily; CHILD 2–6 years 2.5 mL daily, 6–12 years 5 mL daily

1. except 30 mL paediatric dropper bottle for prophylaxis and treatment of iron deficiency in infants born prematurely; endorse prescription 'SLS'

SODIUM FEREDETATE
(Sodium ironedetate)

Indications iron-deficiency anaemia
Cautions interactions: Appendix 1 (iron)
Side-effects see notes above
Dose
- See under preparation below and notes above

Sytron® (Link)
Elixir, sugar-free, sodium feredetate 190 mg equivalent to 27.5 mg of iron/5 mL. Net price 100 mL = 89p
Dose 5 mL increasing gradually to 10 mL 3 times daily; PRETERM NEONATE, NEONATE, and INFANT under 1 year 2.5 mL twice daily (smaller doses should be used initially); CHILD 1–5 years 2.5 mL 3 times daily, 6–12 years 5 mL 3 times daily

Iron and folic acid

These preparations are used during pregnancy in women who are at high risk of developing iron and folic acid deficiency; they should be distinguished from those used for the prevention of neural tube defects in women planning a pregnancy (see p. 494).

It is important to note that the small doses of folic acid contained in these preparations are inadequate for the treatment of megaloblastic anaemias.

Fefol® (Intrapharm) NHS
Spansule® (= capsules m/r), clear/green, enclosing brown, yellow, and white pellets, dried ferrous sulphate 150 mg (47 mg iron), folic acid 500 micrograms. Net price 30-cap pack = £1.69. Label: 25
Dose 1 capsule daily

Ferrograd Folic® (Teofarma)
Tablets, f/c, red/yellow, dried ferrous sulphate 325 mg (105 mg iron) for sustained release, folic acid 350 micrograms. Net price 30-tab pack = £1.32. Label: 25
Dose ADULT and CHILD over 12 years, 1 tablet daily before food

Galfer FA® (Thornton & Ross)
Capsules, red/yellow, ferrous fumarate 305 mg (100 mg iron), folic acid 350 micrograms. Net price 30-cap pack = £1.10
Dose 1 capsule daily before food

Pregaday® (Celltech)
Tablets, brown, f/c, ferrous fumarate equivalent to 100 mg iron, folic acid 350 micrograms. Net price 28-tab pack =£1.25
Dose 1 tablet daily

Compound iron preparations

There is no justification for prescribing compound iron preparations, except for preparations of iron and folic acid for prophylactic use in pregnancy (see above).

Ferrograd C® (Teofarma) NHS
Tablets, f/c, red, dried ferrous sulphate 325 mg (105 mg iron) for sustained release, ascorbic acid 500 mg (as sodium salt). Net price 30-tab pack = £1.71. Label: 25
Dose ADULT and CHILD over 12 years, 1 tablet daily before food

Givitol® (Galen) NHS
Capsules, red/maroon, ferrous fumarate 305 mg (100 mg iron) with vitamins B group and C. Net price 20 = 88p
Dose 1 capsule daily before food

9.1.1.2 Parenteral iron

Iron can be administered parenterally as iron dextran or iron sucrose. Parenteral iron is generally reserved for use when oral therapy is unsuccessful because the patient cannot tolerate oral iron, or does not take it reliably, or if there is continuing blood loss, or in malabsorption.

Also, many patients with chronic renal failure who are receiving haemodialysis (and some who are receiving peritoneal dialysis) require iron by the intravenous route on a regular basis (see also Erythropoietin, section 9.1.3).

With the exception of patients with severe renal failure receiving haemodialysis, parenteral iron does not produce a faster haemoglobin response than oral iron provided that the oral iron preparation is taken reliably and is absorbed adequately.

Iron dextran, a complex of ferric hydroxide with dextrans, and **iron sucrose**, a complex of ferric hydroxide with sucrose, are used for the parenteral administration of iron. Anaphylactoid reactions can occur with parenteral administration of iron complexes and patients should be given a small test dose initially.

IRON DEXTRAN

A complex of ferric hydroxide with dextran containing 5% (50 mg/mL) of iron

Indications iron-deficiency anaemia, see notes above

Cautions oral iron not to be given until 5 days after last injection; hepatic impairment (Appendix 2); renal impairment (Appendix 3); pregnancy (Appendix 4)

Anaphylaxis Anaphylactic reactions can occur with parenteral iron and a test dose is recommended before *each* dose; the patient should be carefully observed for 60 minutes after the first test dose and for 15 minutes after subsequent test doses (subsequent test doses not necessary for intramuscular administration). Facilities for cardiopulmonary resuscitation must be at hand; risk of allergic reactions increased in immune or inflammatory conditions

Contra-indications history of allergic disorders including asthma and eczema; infection; active rheumatoid arthritis

Side-effects *less commonly* nausea, vomiting, abdominal pain, flushing, dyspnoea, anaphylactic reactions (see Anaphylaxis above), numbness, cramps, blurred vision, pruritus, and rash; *rarely* diarrhoea, chest pain, hypotension, angioedema, arrhythmias, tachycardia, dizziness, restlessness, fatigue, seizures, tremor, impaired consciousness, myalgia, arthralgia, sweating, and injection-site reactions; *very rarely* hypertension, palpitation, headache, paraesthesia, haemolysis, and transient deafness

Dose

- By deep intramuscular injection into the gluteal muscle *or* by slow intravenous injection *or* by intravenous infusion, calculated according to body-weight and iron deficit, consult product literature CHILD under 14 years, not recommended

CosmoFer® (Vitaline) PoM
Injection, iron (as iron dextran) 50 mg/mL, net price 2-mL amp = £7.97

IRON SUCROSE

A complex of ferric hydroxide with sucrose containing 2% (20 mg/mL) of iron

Indications iron-deficiency anaemia, see notes above

Cautions oral iron therapy should not be given until 5 days after last injection; pregnancy (Appendix 4)

Anaphylaxis Anaphylactic reactions can occur with parenteral iron and a test dose is recommended before the first dose; the patient should be carefully observed for 15 minutes. Facilities for cardiopulmonary resuscitation must be at hand

Contra-indications history of allergic disorders including asthma, eczema and anaphylaxis; liver disease; infection

Side-effects taste disturbances; *less commonly* nausea, vomiting, abdominal pain, diarrhoea, hypotension, tachycardia, flushing, palpitation, chest pain, bronchospasm, dyspnoea, headache, dizziness, fever, myalgia, pruritus, rash, and injection-site reactions; rarely peripheral oedema, anaphylactic reactions (see Anaphylaxis above), fatigue, asthenia, and paraesthesia; confusion, arthralgia, and increased sweating also reported

Dose

- By slow intravenous injection *or* by intravenous infusion, calculated according to body-weight and iron deficit, consult product literature; CHILD not recommended

Venofer® (Syner-Med) PoM
Injection, iron (as iron sucrose) 20 mg/mL, net price 5-mL amp = £8.50

9.1.2 Drugs used in megaloblastic anaemias

Most megaloblastic anaemias result from a lack of either vitamin B_{12} or folate, and it is essential to establish in every case which deficiency is present and the underlying cause. In emergencies, when delay might be dangerous, it is sometimes necessary to administer both substances after the bone marrow test while plasma assay results are awaited. Normally, however, appropriate treatment should be instituted only when the results of tests are available.

One cause of megaloblastic anaemia in the UK is *pernicious anaemia* in which lack of gastric intrinsic factor resulting from an autoimmune gastritis causes malabsorption of vitamin B_{12}.

Vitamin B_{12} is also needed in the treatment of megaloblastosis caused by *prolonged nitrous oxide anaesthesia*, which inactivates the vitamin, and in the rare syndrome of *congenital transcobalamin II deficiency*.

Vitamin B_{12} should be given prophylactically after *total gastrectomy* or *total ileal resection* (or after *partial gastrectomy* if a vitamin B_{12} absorption test shows vitamin B_{12} malabsorption).

Apart from dietary deficiency, all other causes of vitamin B_{12} deficiency are attributable to malabsorption. There is little place for the use of low-dose vitamin B_{12} orally and none for vitamin B_{12} intrinsic factor complexes given by mouth. Vitamin B_{12} in larger oral doses of 1–2 mg daily [unlicensed] may be effective.

Hydroxocobalamin has completely replaced cyanocobalamin as the form of vitamin B_{12} of choice for therapy; it is retained in the body longer than cyanocobalamin and thus for maintenance therapy can be given at intervals of up to 3 months. Treatment is generally initiated with frequent administration of intramuscular injections to replenish the depleted body stores. Thereafter, maintenance treatment, which is usually for life, can be instituted. There is no evidence that doses larger than those recommended provide any additional benefit in vitamin B_{12} neuropathy.

Folic acid has few indications for long-term therapy since most causes of folate deficiency are self-limiting or will yield to a short course of treatment. It should not be used in undiagnosed megaloblastic anaemia unless vitamin B_{12} is administered concurrently otherwise neuropathy may be precipitated (see above).

In *folate-deficient megaloblastic anaemia* (e.g. because of poor nutrition, pregnancy, or antiepileptic drugs), daily folic acid supplementation for 4 months brings about haematological remission and replenishes body stores.

For *prophylaxis in chronic haemolytic states* or *in renal dialysis*, folic acid is given daily or sometimes weekly, depending on the diet and the rate of haemolysis.

For *prophylaxis in pregnancy*, see Prevention of Neural Tube Defects below.

Folinic acid is also effective in the treatment of folate-deficient megaloblastic anaemia but it is generally used in association with cytotoxic drugs (see section 8.1); it is given as calcium folinate.

Prevention of neural tube defects Folic acid supplements taken before and during pregnancy can reduce the occurrence of neural tube defects. The risk of a neural tube defect occurring in a child should be assessed and folic acid given as follows:

> Women at a low risk of neural tube defects should be advised to take folic acid as a medicinal or food supplement at a dose of 400 micrograms daily before conception and until week 12 of pregnancy. Women who have not been taking folic acid and who suspect they are pregnant should start at once and continue until week 12 of pregnancy.
>
> Couples are at a high risk of conceiving a child with a neural tube defect if either partner has a neural tube defect (or either partner has a family history of neural tube defects), if they have had a previous pregnancy affected by a neural tube defect, or if the woman has coeliac disease (or other malabsorption state), diabetes mellitus, sickle-cell anaemia, or is taking antiepileptic medicines (see also section 4.8.1).
>
> Women in the high risk group who wish to become pregnant (or who are at risk of becoming pregnant) should be advised to take folic acid 5 mg daily and continue until week 12 of pregnancy (women with sickle-cell disease should continue taking their normal dose of folic acid 5 mg daily throughout pregnancy).

There is **no** justification for prescribing multiple-ingredient vitamin preparations containing vitamin B_{12} or folic acid.

HYDROXOCOBALAMIN

Indications see under dose below

Cautions should not be given before diagnosis fully established but see also notes above; **interactions:** Appendix 1 (hydroxocobalamin)

Side-effects nausea, headache, dizziness; fever, hypersensitivity reactions including rash and pruritus; injection-site pain; hypokalaemia during initial treatment

Dose

- By intramuscular injection, pernicious anaemia and other macrocytic anaemias without neurological involvement, initially 1 mg 3 times a week for 2 weeks then 1 mg every 3 months

  Pernicious anaemia and other macrocytic anaemias with neurological involvement, initially 1 mg on alternate days until no further improvement, then 1 mg every 2 months

  Prophylaxis of macrocytic anaemias associated with vitamin-B_{12} deficiency, 1 mg every 2–3 months

  Tobacco amblyopia and Leber's optic atrophy, initially 1 mg daily for 2 weeks, then 1 mg twice weekly until no further improvement, thereafter 1 mg every 1–3 months

  CHILD see *BNF for Children*
- Cyanide poisoning [not licensed], see p. 33

Hydroxocobalamin (Non-proprietary) PoM

Injection, hydroxocobalamin 1 mg/mL. Net price 1-mL amp = £2.46

Note The BP directs that when vitamin B_{12} injection is prescribed or demanded hydroxocobalamin injection shall be dispensed or supplied

Brands include *Cobalin-H®* NHS, *Neo-Cytamen®* NHS

CYANOCOBALAMIN

Indications see notes above

Dose

- By mouth, vitamin-B_{12} deficiency of dietary origin, 50–150 micrograms or more daily taken between meals; CHILD 50–105 micrograms daily in 1–3 divided doses
- By intramuscular injection, initially 1 mg repeated 10 times at intervals of 2–3 days, maintenance 1 mg every month, but see notes above

Cyanocobalamin (Non-proprietary)

[1]Tablets NHS, cyanocobalamin 50 micrograms. Net price 50-tab pack = £4.07

Brands include *Cytacon®* NHS

Liquid NHS, cyanocobalamin 35 micrograms/5 mL. Net price 200 mL = £2.77

Brands include *Cytacon®* NHS

Injection PoM, cyanocobalamin 1 mg/mL. Net price 1-mL amp = £1.67

Brands include *Cytamen®* NHS

Note The BP directs that when vitamin B_{12} injection is prescribed or demanded hydroxocobalamin injection shall be dispensed or supplied

1. NHS except to treat or prevent vitamin-B_{12} deficiency in a patient who is a vegan or who has a proven vitamin-B_{12} deficiency of dietary origin; endorse prescription 'SLS'; currently available brands may not be suitable for vegans—cyanocobalamin injection may be a suitable alternative

FOLIC ACID

Indications see notes above and under dose

Cautions should never be given alone for pernicious anaemia and other vitamin-B_{12} deficiency states (may precipitate subacute combined degeneration of the spinal cord); **interactions:** Appendix 1 (folates)

Dose

- Folate-deficient megaloblastic anaemia, by mouth, ADULT and CHILD over 1 year, 5 mg daily for 4 months (until term in pregnant women); up to 15 mg daily may be required in malabsorption states; maintenance, 5 mg every 1–7 days; CHILD under 1 year, 500 micrograms/kg daily for up to 4 months; maintenance 500 micrograms/kg every 1–7 days
- Prevention of neural tube defects, by mouth, see notes above
- Prevention of methotrexate-induced side-effects in rheumatic disease [unlicensed], by mouth, ADULT over 18 years 5 mg once weekly; CHILD 2–18 years see *BNF for Children*

9 Nutrition and blood

- Prophylaxis in chronic haemolytic states, by mouth, ADULT 5 mg every 1–7 days depending on underlying disease
- Prophylaxis of folate deficiency in dialysis, by mouth, ADULT 5 mg every 1–7 days; CHILD 1–12 years 250 micrograms/kg (max. 10 mg) once daily, CHILD 12–18 years 5–10 mg once daily

[1] **Folic Acid** (Non-proprietary) (PoM)
Tablets, folic acid 400 micrograms, net price 90-tab pack = £2.24; 5 mg, 28-tab pack = 40p

Syrup, folic acid 2.5 mg/5 mL, net price 150 mL = £9.16; 400 micrograms/5 mL, 150 mL = £1.40
Brands include *Folicare®*, *Lexpec®* (sugar-free)

Injection, folic acid 15 mg, net price 1-mL amp = £1.34
'Special order' [unlicensed] product; contact BCM Specials

1. Can be sold to the public provided daily doses do not exceed 500 micrograms

9.1.3 Drugs used in hypoplastic, haemolytic, and renal anaemias

Anabolic steroids (section 6.4.3), pyridoxine, antilymphocyte immunoglobulin, and various corticosteroids are used in hypoplastic and haemolytic anaemias.

Antilymphocyte globulin given intravenously through a central line over 12–18 hours each day for 5 days produces a response in about 50% of cases of acquired *aplastic anaemia*; the response rate may be increased when ciclosporin is given as well. Severe reactions are common in the first 2 days and profound immunosuppression can occur; antilymphocyte globulin should be given under specialist supervision with appropriate resuscitation facilities. Alternatively, oxymetholone tablets (available on a named-patient basis from Cambridge) can be used in aplastic anaemia at a dose of 1–5 mg/kg daily for 3 to 6 months.

It is unlikely that dietary deprivation of **pyridoxine** (section 9.6.2) produces clinically relevant haematological effects. However, certain forms of *sideroblastic anaemia* respond to pharmacological doses, possibly reflecting its role as a co-enzyme during haemoglobin synthesis. Pyridoxine is indicated in both *idiopathic acquired* and *hereditary sideroblastic anaemias*. Although complete cures have not been reported, some increase in haemoglobin can occur; the dose required is usually high, up to 400 mg daily. *Reversible sideroblastic anaemias* respond to treatment of the underlying cause but in pregnancy, haemolytic anaemias, and alcohol dependence, or during isoniazid treatment, pyridoxine is also indicated.

Hydroxycarbamide (hydroxyurea, section 8.1.5) can reduce the frequency of crises in *sickle-cell disease* and reduce the need for blood transfusions [unlicensed indication].

Corticosteroids (see section 6.3) have an important place in the management of a wide variety of haematological disorders. They include conditions with an immune basis such as *autoimmune haemolytic anaemia*, *immune thrombocytopenias* and *neutropenias*, and *major transfusion reactions*. They are also used in chemotherapy schedules for many types of *lymphoma*, *lymphoid leukaemias*, and *paraproteinaemias*, including *multiple myeloma*.

Eculizumab is licensed for the treatment of paroxysmal nocturnal haemoglobinuria.

Erythropoietins

Epoetins (recombinant human erythropoietins) are used to treat the symptomatic anaemia associated with erythropoietin deficiency in chronic renal failure, to increase the yield of autologous blood in normal individuals and to shorten the period of symptomatic anaemia in patients receiving cytotoxic chemotherapy. Epoetin beta is also used for the prevention of anaemia in preterm neonates of low birth-weight; only unpreserved formulations should be used in neonates because other preparations may contain benzyl alcohol (see Excipients, p. 2). Epoetin delta is licensed for the treatment of symptomatic anaemia associated with chronic renal failure.

Darbepoetin, is a hyperglycosylated derivative of epoetin; it has a longer half-life and can be administered less frequently than epoetin.

Methoxy polyethylene glycol-epoetin beta (pegzerepoetin alfa) is a continuous erythropoietin receptor activator that is licensed for the treatment of symptomatic anaemia associated with chronic kidney disease. It has a longer duration of action than epoetin.

Other factors which contribute to the anaemia of chronic renal failure such as iron or folate deficiency should be corrected before treatment and monitored during therapy. Supplemental iron may improve the response in resistant patients. Aluminium toxicity, concurrent infection or other inflammatory disease can impair the response to erythropoietin.

MHRA/CHM advice (Erythropoietins—target haemoglobin concentration)

Overcorrection of haemoglobin concentration in patients with chronic kidney disease may increase the risk of death and serious cardiovascular events, and in patients with cancer may increase the risk of thrombosis and related complications:

- patients may be treated with erythropoietins for the licensed indications in chronic kidney disease or cancer in patients receiving chemotherapy *only* if symptoms of anaemia are present;
- the target haemoglobin concentration range is 10–12 g/100 mL;
- haemoglobin concentrations higher than 12 g/100 mL should be avoided;
- the aim of treatment is to relieve symptoms of anaemia and to avoid the need for blood transfusion; the haemoglobin concentration should not be increased beyond that which provides adequate control of symptoms of anaemia (in some patients, this may be achieved at concentrations lower than the normal range).

See also MHRA/CHM advice below.

> **MHRA/CHM advice (Erythropoietins—tumour progression and survival in patients with cancer)**
> Clinical trial data show a consistent, unexplained excess mortality and increased risk of tumour progression in patients with anaemia associated with cancer who have been treated with erythropoietins *outside* of the licensed indications (i.e. overcorrected haemoglobin concentration or patients who have *not* received chemotherapy):
> - erythropoietins licensed for the treatment of *symptomatic* anaemia associated with cancer, are licensed only for patients who are receiving chemotherapy;
> - currently erythropoietins have not been shown to influence survival in patients treated within the licensed cancer indications.
>
> See also MHRA/CHM advice above.

> **CSM advice (pure red cell aplasia)**
> There have been very rare reports of pure red cell aplasia in patients treated with epoetin alfa. The CSM has advised that in patients developing epoetin alfa failure with a diagnosis of pure red cell aplasia, treatment with epoetin alfa must be discontinued and testing for erythropoietin antibodies considered. Patients who develop pure red cell aplasia should **not** be switched to another form of erythropoietin.

DARBEPOETIN ALFA

Indications see under Dose below

Cautions see Epoetin; hepatic disease; pregnancy (Appendix 4); **interactions:** Appendix 1 (epoetin)

Contra-indications see Epoetin; breast-feeding (Appendix 5)

Side-effects see Epoetin; also, peripheral oedema, injection-site pain; isolated reports of pure red cell aplasia (discontinue therapy)—see also CSM advice above

Dose

- Symptomatic anaemia associated with chronic renal failure in patients on dialysis (see also MHRA/CHM advice, p. 495), ADULT and CHILD over 11 years, by subcutaneous *or* intravenous injection, initially 450 nanograms/kg once weekly, adjusted according to response by approx. 25% of initial dose at intervals of at least 4 weeks; maintenance dose, given once weekly *or* once every 2 weeks
- Symptomatic anaemia associated with chronic renal failure in patients not on dialysis (see also MHRA/CHM advice, p. 495), ADULT and CHILD over 11 years, by subcutaneous *or* intravenous injection, initially 450 nanograms/kg once weekly *or* by subcutaneous injection, initially 750 nanograms/kg once every 2 weeks; adjusted according to response by approx. 25% of initial dose at intervals of at least 4 weeks; maintenance dose, given once weekly *or* once every 2 weeks *or* once every month

Note Reduce maintenance dose by 25% if haemoglobin rise exceeds 2 g/100 mL per month (see also MHRA/CHM advice, p. 495). When changing route give same dose then adjust according to weekly or fortnightly haemoglobin measurements. Adjust doses at 2-week intervals during maintenance treatment

- Symptomatic anaemia in adults with non-myeloid malignancies receiving chemotherapy (see also MHRA/CHM advice, p. 495), by subcutaneous injection, initially 6.75 micrograms/kg once every 3 weeks (if response inadequate after 9 weeks further treatment may not be effective) *or* 2.25 micrograms/kg once weekly; if adequate response obtained or if rise in haemoglobin greater than 2 g/100 mL in 4 weeks, reduce dose by 25–50%

Note Darbepoetin alfa doses in the BNF may differ from those in the product literature

Aranesp® (Amgen) PoM

Injection, prefilled syringe, darbepoetin alfa, 25 micrograms/mL, net price 0.4 mL (10 micrograms) = £15.59; 40 micrograms/mL, 0.375 mL (15 micrograms) = £23.38, 0.5 mL (20 micrograms) = £31.17; 100 micrograms/mL, 0.3 mL (30 micrograms) = £46.76, 0.4 mL (40 micrograms) = £62.34, 0.5 mL (50 micrograms) = £77.93; 200 micrograms/mL, 0.3 mL (60 micrograms) = £93.51, 0.4 mL (80 micrograms) = £124.68, 0.5 mL (100 micrograms) = £155.85, 0.65 mL (130 micrograms) = £202.61; 500 micrograms/mL, 0.3 mL (150 micrograms) = £233.78, 0.6 mL (300 micrograms) = £467.55, 1 mL (500 micrograms) = £779.25

Injection (*Aranesp® SureClick*), prefilled disposable injection device, darbepoetin alfa, 40 micrograms/mL, net price 0.5 mL (20 micrograms) = £31.17; 100 micrograms/mL, 0.4 mL (40 micrograms) = £62.34; 200 micrograms/mL, 0.3 mL (60 micrograms) = £93.51, 0.4 mL (80 micrograms) = £124.68, 0.5 mL (100 micrograms) = £155.85, 0.65 mL (130 micrograms) = £202.61; 500 micrograms/mL, 0.3 mL (150 micrograms) = £233.78, 0.6 mL (300 micrograms) = £467.55, 1 mL (500 micrograms) = £779.25

EPOETIN ALFA, BETA, and DELTA

(Recombinant human erythropoietins)

Note The prescriber must specify which epoetin is required

Indications see under preparations, below

Cautions inadequately treated or poorly controlled blood pressure (monitor closely blood pressure, reticulocyte counts, haemoglobin, and electrolytes), interrupt treatment if blood pressure uncontrolled; sudden stabbing migraine-like pain is warning of hypertensive crisis; sickle-cell disease (lower target haemoglobin concentration may be appropriate), exclude other causes of anaemia (e.g. folic acid or vitamin B_{12} deficiency) and give iron supplements if necessary (see also notes above); ischaemic vascular disease; thrombocytosis (monitor platelet count for first 8 weeks); epilepsy; malignant disease; chronic liver failure (Appendix 2); increase in heparin dose may be needed; risk of thrombosis may be increased when used for anaemia in adults receiving cancer chemotherapy; risk of thrombosis may be increased when used for anaemia before orthopaedic surgery—avoid in cardiovascular disease including recent myocardial infarction or cerebrovascular accident; pregnancy (Appendix 4) and breast-feeding (Appendix 5); **interactions:** Appendix 1 (epoetin)

Contra-indications pure red cell aplasia following erythropoietin (see also CSM advice above); uncontrolled hypertension; patients unable to receive thromboprophylaxis; avoid injections containing benzyl alcohol in neonates (see under preparations, below)

Side-effects diarrhoea, nausea; dose-dependent increase in blood pressure or aggravation of hypertension; in isolated patients with normal or low blood pressure, hypertensive crisis with encephalopathy-like symptoms and generalised tonic-clonic seizures requiring immediate medical attention; headache; dose-dependent increase in platelet count (but thrombocytosis rare) regressing during treatment; influenza-like symptoms (may be reduced if intravenous injection given over 5 minutes); thromboembolic events; shunt thrombosis especially if tendency to hypotension or arteriovenous shunt complications; very rarely sudden loss of response because of pure red cell aplasia, particularly following subcutaneous administration in patients with chronic renal failure (discontinue erythropoietin therapy)—see also CSM advice above, hyperkalaemia, hypersensitivity reactions (including anaphylaxis), and skin reactions

Dose

- See under preparations, below

◢Epoetin alfa

Eprex® (Janssen-Cilag) PoM

Injection, prefilled syringe, epoetin alfa, net price 1000 units = £7.54; 2000 units = £15.08; 3000 units = £22.63; 4000 units = £30.17; 5000 units = £37.71; 6000 units = £45.25; 8000 units = £60.34; 10 000 units = £75.42; 20 000 units = £150.84; 30 000 units = £226.26; 40 000 units = £301.68. An auto-injector device is available for use with prefilled syringes

Dose symptomatic anaemia associated with chronic renal failure in patients on haemodialysis (see also MHRA/CHM advice, p. 495), by intravenous injection over 1–5 minutes *or* by subcutaneous injection (max. 1 mL per injection site), initially 50 units/kg 3 times weekly adjusted according to response in steps of 25 units/kg 3 times weekly at intervals of at least 4 weeks; maintenance dose, usually a total of 75–300 units/kg weekly (as a single dose or in divided doses); CHILD by intravenous injection initially as for adults; maintenance dose (when haemoglobin concentration of 9.5–11 g/100 mL achieved), body-weight under 10 kg usually 75–150 units/kg 3 times weekly, body-weight 10–30 kg usually 60–150 units/kg 3 times weekly, body-weight over 30 kg usually 30–100 units/kg 3 times weekly

Note Intravenous route preferred; epoetin alfa doses in the BNF may differ from those in the product literature

Symptomatic anaemia associated with chronic renal failure in adults on peritoneal dialysis (see also MHRA/CHM advice, p. 495), by intravenous injection over 1–5 minutes *or* by subcutaneous injection (max. 1 mL per injection site), initially 50 units/kg twice weekly; maintenance dose 25–50 units/kg twice weekly

Note Intravenous route preferred; epoetin alfa doses in the BNF may differ from those in the product literature

Severe symptomatic anaemia of renal origin in adults with renal insufficiency not yet on dialysis (see also MHRA/CHM advice, p. 495), by intravenous injection over 1–5 minutes *or* by subcutaneous injection (max. 1 mL per injection site), initially 50 units/kg 3 times weekly increased according to response in steps of 25 units/kg 3 times weekly at intervals of at least 4 weeks; maintenance dose 17–33 units/kg 3 times weekly; max. 200 units/kg 3 times weekly

Note Intravenous route preferred; epoetin alfa doses in the BNF may differ from those in the product literature

Symptomatic anaemia in adults receiving cancer chemotherapy (see also MHRA/CHM advice, p. 495), by subcutaneous injection (max. 1 mL per injection site), 150 units/kg 3 times weekly (*or* 450 units/kg once weekly), increased if appropriate rise in haemoglobin (or reticulocyte count) not achieved after 4 weeks to 300 units/kg 3 times weekly; discontinue if inadequate response after 4 weeks at higher dose; reduce dose by 25–50% if haemoglobin rise exceeds 2 g/100 mL per month

Note Epoetin alfa doses in the BNF may differ from those in the product literature

To increase yield of autologous blood (to avoid homologous blood) in predonation programme in moderate anaemia *either* when large volume of blood required *or* when sufficient blood cannot be saved for elective major surgery, by intravenous injection over 1–5 minutes, 600 units/kg twice weekly for 3 weeks before surgery; consult product literature for details and advice on ensuring high iron stores

Moderate anaemia (haemoglobin concentration 10–13 g/100 mL) before elective orthopaedic surgery in adults with expected moderate blood loss to reduce exposure to allogeneic transfusion or if autologous transfusion unavailable, by subcutaneous injection (max. 1 mL per injection site), 600 units/kg every week for 3 weeks before surgery and on day of surgery *or* 300 units/kg daily for 15 days starting 10 days before surgery; consult product literature for details

◢Epoetin beta

NeoRecormon® (Roche) PoM

Injection, prefilled syringe, epoetin beta, net price 500 units = £3.90; 1000 units = £7.79; 2000 units = £15.59; 3000 units = £23.38; 4000 units = £31.17; 5000 units = £38.97; 6000 units = £46.76; 10 000 units = £77.93; 20 000 units = £155.87; 30 000 units = £233.81

Excipients include phenylalanine up to 300 micrograms/syringe (section 9.4.1)

Multidose injection, powder for reconstitution, epoetin beta, net price 50 000-unit vial = £419.01; 100 000-unit vial = £838.01 (both with solvent)

Excipients include phenylalanine up to 5 mg/vial (section 9.4.1), benzyl alcohol (avoid in neonates, see Excipients p. 2)

Note Avoid contact of reconstituted injection with glass; use only plastic materials

Reco-Pen, (for subcutaneous use), double-chamber cartridges (containing epoetin beta and solvent), net price 10 000-unit cartridge = £77.93; 20 000-unit cartridge = £155.87; for use with *Reco-Pen* injection device and needles (both available free from Roche)

Excipients include phenylalanine up to 300 micrograms/cartridge (section 9.4.1), benzyl alcohol (avoid in neonates, see Excipients, p. 2)

Dose symptomatic anaemia associated with chronic renal failure in dialysis patients, symptomatic anaemia of renal origin in patients not yet on dialysis (see also MHRA/CHM advice, p. 495), ADULT and CHILD

By subcutaneous injection, initially 20 units/kg 3 times weekly for 4 weeks, increased according to response at intervals of 4 weeks in steps of 20 units/kg 3 times weekly; maintenance dose, initially reduce dose by half then adjust according to response at intervals of 1–2 weeks; weekly maintenance dose given as a single dose or in divided doses; max. 720 units/kg weekly (see also MHRA/CHM advice, p. 495)

Note Epoetin beta doses in the BNF may differ from those in the product literature

By intravenous injection over 2 minutes, initially 40 units/kg 3 times weekly for 4 weeks, increased according to response to 80 units/kg 3 times weekly with further increases if needed at intervals of 4 weeks in steps of 20 units/kg 3 times weekly; maintenance dose, initially reduce dose by half then adjust according to response at intervals of 1–2 weeks; max. 720 units/kg weekly (see also MHRA/CHM advice, p. 495)

Note Epoetin beta doses in the BNF may differ from those in the product literature

Prevention of anaemia of prematurity in neonates with birth-weight of 0.75–1.5 kg and gestational age of less than 34 weeks, by subcutaneous injection (of single-dose, unpreserved injection), 250 units/kg 3 times weekly preferably starting within 3 days of birth and continued for 6 weeks

Symptomatic anaemia in adults with non-myeloid malignancies receiving chemotherapy (see also MHRA/CHM advice, p. 495), by subcutaneous injection, initially 450 units/kg weekly (as a single dose or in 3–7 divided doses), increased if necessary after 4 weeks (if a rise in haemoglobin of at least 1 g/100 mL not achieved) to 900 units/kg weekly (as a single dose or in 3–7 divided doses); reduce dose by 25–50% if haemoglobin rise exceeds 2 g/100 mL per month; adjust dose to ensure haemoglobin concentration does not exceed 12 g/100 mL; max 900 units/kg weekly (see also MHRA/CHM advice, p. 495)

Note Discontinue treatment if haemoglobin concentration does not increase by at least 1 g/100 mL after 8 weeks of therapy (response unlikely); epoetin beta doses in the BNF may differ from those in the product literature

To increase yield of autologous blood (to avoid homologous blood) in predonation programme in moderate anaemia when blood-conserving procedures are insufficient or unavailable, consult product literature

▲Epoetin delta

Dynepo® (Shire) ▼ PoM

Injection, prefilled syringe, epoetin delta, net price 1000 units = £5.66; 2000 units = £11.31; 3000 units = £16.97; 4000 units = £22.63; 5000 units = £28.28; 6000 units = £33.94; 8000 units = £45.25; 10 000 units = £56.57

Dose symptomatic anaemia associated with chronic renal failure

By intravenous injection, ADULT over 18 years, initially 50 units/kg 3 times weekly, adjusted according to response at intervals of at least 4 weeks

By subcutaneous injection, ADULT over 18 years, initially 50 units/kg twice weekly, adjusted according to response at intervals of at least 4 weeks

Note See also MHRA/CHM advice, p. 495

Reduce dose by 25% if haemoglobin rise exceeds 2.5 g/100 mL per month, or if haemoglobin reaches 12 g/100 mL; increase dose by 50% if haemoglobin rise is below 0.7 g/100 mL per month, or if haemoglobin falls below 10 g/100 mL (unless symptoms of anaemia controlled— see also MHRA/CHM advice, p. 495); anaemia failing to respond to doses of 20 000 units/week should be investigated further. Subcutaneous route preferred in patients not on dialysis

Epoetin delta doses in the BNF may differ from those in the product literature

METHOXY POLYETHYLENE GLYCOL-EPOETIN BETA

(Pegzerepoetin alfa)

Indications see under Dose below

Cautions see Epoetin; severe liver disease (Appendix 2); pregnancy (Appendix 4); breast-feeding (Appendix 5)

Contra-indications see Epoetin

Side-effects see Epoetin; also hot flushes reported

Dose

- Symptomatic anaemia associated with chronic kidney disease in patients *not* currently treated with erythropoietin, ADULT over 18 years, by subcutaneous *or* intravenous injection, initially 600 nanograms/kg once every 2 weeks, adjusted according to response at intervals of at least 4 weeks; maintenance dose of double the previous fortnightly dose may be given every 4 weeks (see also MHRA/CHM advice, p. 495)

  Note Reduce dose by 25% if haemoglobin rise exceeds 2 g/100 mL per month, or if haemoglobin concentration approaches 12 g/100 mL; increase dose by 25% if rise in haemoglobin concentration is less than 1 g/100 mL per month

- Symptomatic anaemia associated with chronic kidney disease in patients currently treated with erythropoietin; ADULT over 18 years, by subcutaneous *or* intravenous injection, consult product literature (see also MHRA/CHM advice, p. 495)

Note Methoxy polyethylene glycol-epoetin beta doses in the BNF may differ from those in the product literature

Mircera® (Roche) ▼ PoM

Injection, prefilled syringe, methoxy polyethylene glycol-epoetin beta, net price 50 micrograms/0.3 mL = £77.93; 75 micrograms/0.3 mL = £116.89; 100 micrograms/0.3 mL = £155.85; 150 micrograms/0.3 mL = £233.78; 200 micrograms/0.3 mL = £311.70; 250 micrograms/0.3 mL = £389.63

Iron overload

Severe tissue iron overload can occur in aplastic and other refractory anaemias, mainly as the result of repeated blood transfusions. It is a particular problem in refractory anaemias with hyperplastic bone marrow, especially *thalassaemia major*, where excessive iron absorption from the gut and inappropriate iron therapy can add to the tissue siderosis.

Iron overload associated with haemochromatosis can be treated with repeated venesection. Venesection may also be used for patients who have received multiple transfusions and whose bone marrow has recovered. Where venesection is contra-indicated, the long-term administration of the iron chelating compound **desferrioxamine mesilate** is useful. Subcutaneous infusions of desferrioxamine are given over 8–12 hours, 3–7 times a week. The dose should reflect the degree of iron overload. For children starting therapy (and who have low iron overload) the dose should not exceed 30 mg/kg. For established overload the dose is usually between 20 and 50 mg/kg daily. Desferrioxamine (up to 2 g per unit of blood) may also be given at the time of blood transfusion, provided that the desferrioxamine is **not** added to the blood and is **not** given through the same line as the blood (but the two may be given through the same cannula).

Iron excretion induced by desferrioxamine is enhanced by administration of ascorbic acid (vitamin C, section 9.6.3) in a dose of 200 mg daily (100 mg in infants); it should be given separately from food since it also enhances iron absorption. Ascorbic acid should not be given to patients with cardiac dysfunction; in patients with normal cardiac function ascorbic acid should be introduced 1 month after starting desferrioxamine.

Desferrioxamine infusion can be used to treat *aluminium overload* in dialysis patients; theoretically 100 mg of desferrioxamine binds with 4.1 mg of aluminium.

Deferasirox, an oral iron chelator, is licensed for the treatment of chronic iron overload in adults and children over 6 years with thalassaemia major who receive frequent blood transfusions (more than 7 mL/kg/month packed red blood cells). It is also licensed for chronic iron overload when desferrioxamine is contra-indicated or inadequate in patients with thalassaemia major who receive infrequent blood transfusions (less than 7 mL/kg/month packed red blood cells), in patients with other anaemias, and in children aged 2 to 5 years.

The *Scottish Medicines Consortium* has advised (January 2007) that deferasirox is accepted for restricted use for the treatment of chronic iron overload associated with the treatment of rare acquired or inherited anaemias requiring recurrent blood transfusions. It is not recommended for patients with myelodysplastic syndromes.

Deferiprone, an oral iron chelator, is licensed for the treatment of iron overload in patients with thalassaemia major in whom desferrioxamine is contra-indicated or is not tolerated. Blood dyscrasias, particularly agranulocytosis, have been reported with deferiprone.

DEFERASIROX

Indications see notes above

Cautions eye and ear examinations required before treatment and annually during treatment; monitor body-weight, height, and sexual development in children annually; test liver function monthly; see also hepatic impairment (Appendix 2); measure baseline serum creatinine and monitor renal function weekly during the first month of treatment and monthly thereafter; test for proteinuria monthly; see also renal impairment (Appendix 3); pregnancy (Appendix 4); breast-feeding (Appendix 5); **interactions**: Appendix 1 (deferasirox)

Side-effects gastro-intestinal disturbances; headache; proteinuria; pruritus, rash; *less commonly* hepatitis, cholelithiasis, oedema, fatigue, anxiety, sleep disorder, dizziness, pyrexia, pharyngitis, glucosuria, disturbances of hearing and vision (including lens opacity and maculopathy), and skin pigmentation; acute renal failure, blood disorders (including agranulocytosis, neutropenia, and thrombocytopenia), hypersensitivity reactions (including anaphylaxis and angioedema) also reported

Dose

- ADULT and CHILD over 2 years initially 10–30 mg/kg once daily according to serum-ferritin concentration and amount of transfused blood (consult product literature); maintenance, adjust dose every 3–6 months in steps of 5–10 mg/kg according to serum-ferritin concentration; max. 30 mg/kg daily

Exjade® (Novartis) ▼ PoM
Dispersible tablets, deferasirox 125 mg, net price 28-tab pack = £117.60; 250 mg, 28-tab pack = £235.20; 500 mg, 28-tab pack = £470.40. Label: 13, 22, counselling, administration
Counselling Tablets may be dispersed in water, orange juice, or apple juice; if necessary resuspend residue

DEFERIPRONE

Indications see notes above

Cautions monitor neutrophil count weekly and discontinue treatment if neutropenia develops; monitor plasma-zinc concentration; hepatic impairment (Appendix 2); renal impairment (Appendix 3)
Blood disorders Patients or their carers should be told how to recognise signs of neutropenia and advised to seek immediate medical attention if symptoms such as fever or sore throat develop

Contra-indications pregnancy (contraception advised in women of child-bearing potential; **important teratogenic risk**: see Appendix 4); breast-feeding (Appendix 5)

Side-effects gastro-intestinal disturbances (reducing dose and increasing gradually may improve tolerance); red-brown urine discoloration; neutropenia, agranulocytosis; zinc deficiency; arthropathy

Dose

- ADULT and CHILD over 6 years 25 mg/kg 3 times daily (max. 100 mg/kg daily)

Ferriprox® (Swedish Orphan) PoM
Tablets, f/c, scored, deferiprone 500 mg, net price 100-tab pack = £152.39. Label: 14, counselling, blood disorders

DESFERRIOXAMINE MESILATE
(Deferoxamine Mesilate)

Indications see notes above; iron poisoning, see Emergency Treatment of Poisoning, p. 32

Cautions renal impairment; eye and ear examinations before treatment and at 3-month intervals during treatment; monitor body-weight and height in children at 3-month intervals—risk of growth retardation with excessive doses; aluminium-related encephalopathy (may exacerbate neurological dysfunction); pregnancy (Appendix 4); breast-feeding (Appendix 5); **interactions**: Appendix 1 (desferrioxamine)

Side-effects hypotension (especially when given too rapidly by intravenous injection), disturbances of hearing and vision (including lens opacity and retinopathy); injection-site reactions, gastro-intestinal disturbances, asthma, fever, headache, arthralgia and myalgia; *very rarely* anaphylaxis, acute respiratory distress syndrome, neurological disturbances (including dizziness, neuropathy and paraesthesia), Yersinia and mucormycosis infections, rash, renal impairment, and blood dyscrasias

Dose

- See notes above; iron poisoning, see Emergency Treatment of Poisoning, p. 32

Note For full details and warnings relating to administration, consult product literature

Desferrioxamine mesilate (Non-proprietary) PoM
Injection, powder for reconstitution, desferrioxamine mesilate, net price 500-mg vial = £4.26; 2-g vial = £17.05

Desferal® (Novartis) PoM
Injection, powder for reconstitution, desferrioxamine mesilate, net price 500-mg vial = £4.44, 2-g vial = £17.77

Paroxysmal nocturnal haemoglobinuria

Eculizumab, a recombinant monoclonal antibody, inhibits terminal complement activation at the C5 protein and thereby reduces haemolysis. It is licensed for the treatment of paroxysmal nocturnal haemoglobinuria, a severe and disabling form of haemolytic anaemia.

ECULIZUMAB

Indications paroxysmal nocturnal haemoglobinuria (specialist use only)

Cautions active systemic infection; intravascular haemolysis—monitor serum lactate dehydrogenase during treatment and for at least 8 weeks after discontinuation
Meningococcal infection Vaccinate against *Neisseria meningitidis* at least 2 weeks prior to treatment (tetravalent vaccine against serotypes A, C, W135 and Y recommended); revaccinate according to current medical guidelines. Advise patient to report promptly any signs of meningococcal infection. Other immunisations should also be up to date (section 14.1)

Contra-indications unresolved *Neisseria meningitidis* infection; patients unvaccinated against *Neisseria meningitidis* (see Cautions above); known or suspected hereditary complement deficiencies; pregnancy (Appendix 4); breast-feeding (Appendix 5)

Side-effects gastro-intestinal disturbances; nasopharyngitis, sinusitis, cough, pharyngolaryngeal pain, epistaxis; headache, fatigue, dizziness, insomnia; infection (including meningococcal infection), pyrexia, influenza-like symptoms; muscle cramp, pain in extremities; rash, pruritus

Dose

- By intravenous infusion, ADULT over 18 years, initially 600 mg once a week for 4 weeks, then 900 mg on week 5; maintenance, 900 mg once every 12–16 days

Soliris® (Alexion) ▼ PoM

Concentrate for intravenous infusion, eculizumab 10 mg/mL, net price 30-mL vial = £3150.00. Counselling, meningococcal infection, patient information card

Electrolytes Na^+ 5 mmol/vial

9.1.4 Drugs used in platelet disorders

Acute idiopathic thrombocytopenic purpura is usually self-limiting in children. In adults, idiopathic thrombocytopenic purpura can be treated with a **corticosteroid**, e.g. prednisolone 1 mg/kg daily, gradually reducing the dose over several weeks. Splenectomy is considered if a satisfactory platelet count is not achieved or if there is a relapse on reducing the dose of corticosteroid or withdrawing it.

Immunoglobulin preparations (section 14.5), are also used in idiopathic thrombocytopenic purpura or where a temporary rapid rise in platelets is needed, as in pregnancy or pre-operatively; they are also used for children often in preference to a corticosteroid. **Anti-D (Rh_0) immunoglobulin** (section 14.5) is effective in raising the platelet count in about 80% of unsplenectomised rhesus-positive individuals; its effects may last longer than normal immunoglobulin for intravenous use, but further doses are usually required.

Other therapy that has been tried in refractory idiopathic thrombocytopenic purpura includes azathioprine (section 8.2.1), cyclophosphamide (section 8.1.1), vincristine (section 8.1.4), ciclosporin (section 8.2.2), and danazol (section 6.7.2). Rituximab (section 8.2.3) may also be effective and in some cases induces prolonged remission. For patients with chronic severe thrombocytopenia refractory to other therapy, tranexamic acid (section 2.11) may be given to reduce the severity of haemorrhage.

Anagrelide inhibits platelet formation. It is licensed for essential thrombocythaemia in patients at risk of thrombo-haemorrhagic events who have not responded adequately to other drugs or who cannot tolerate other drugs.

ANAGRELIDE

Indications essential thrombocythaemia in at-risk patients who have not responded adequately to other therapy or who are intolerant of it (initiated under specialist supervision)

Cautions cardiac disease; assess cardiac function before and during treatment; concomitant aspirin in patients with a history of haemorrhage or severely raised platelet count; monitor full blood count (monitor platelet count every 2 days for 1 week, then weekly until maintenance dose established), liver function, serum creatinine and urea; hepatic impairment (Appendix 2); renal impairment (Appendix 3); **interactions:** Appendix 1 (anagrelide)

Driving Dizziness may affect performance of skilled tasks (e.g. driving)

Contra-indications pregnancy (Appendix 4); breast-feeding (Appendix 5)

Side-effects gastro-intestinal disturbances; palpitation, tachycardia, fluid retention; headache, dizziness, fatigue; anaemia; rash; *less commonly* pancreatitis, gastro-intestinal haemorrhage, congestive heart failure, hypertension, arrhythmias, syncope, chest pain, dyspnoea, sleep disturbances, paraesthesia, hypoaesthesia, depression, confusion, amnesia, fever, weight changes, impotence, blood disorders, myalgia, arthralgia, epistaxis, dry mouth, alopecia, skin discoloration, and pruritus; *rarely* gastritis, colitis, postural hypotension, myocardial infarction, vasodilatation, pulmonary hypotension, pulmonary infiltrates, impaired co-ordination, dysarthria, asthenia, tinnitus, renal failure, nocturia, visual disturbances, and gingival bleeding; allergic alveolitis also reported

Dose

- Initially 500 micrograms twice daily adjusted according to response in steps of 500 micrograms daily at weekly intervals to max. 10 mg daily (max. single dose 2.5 mg); usual dose range 1–3 mg daily in divided doses

Xagrid® (Shire) ▼ PoM

Capsules, anagrelide (as hydrochloride), 500 micrograms, net price 100-cap pack = £337.14. Counselling, driving, see above

9.1.5 G6PD deficiency

Glucose 6-phosphate dehydrogenase (G6PD) deficiency is highly prevalent in individuals originating from most parts of Africa, from most parts of Asia, from Oceania, and from Southern Europe; it can also occur, rarely, in any other individuals. G6PD deficiency is more common in males than it is in females.

Individuals with G6PD deficiency are susceptible to developing acute haemolytic anaemia on taking a number of common drugs. They are also susceptible to developing acute haemolytic anaemia upon ingestion of fava beans (broad beans, *Vicia faba*); this is termed *favism* and can be more severe in children or when the fresh fava beans are eaten raw.

When prescribing drugs for patients with G6PD deficiency, the following three points should be kept in mind:

- G6PD deficiency is genetically heterogeneous; susceptibility to the haemolytic risk from drugs varies; thus, a drug found to be safe in some G6PD-deficient individuals may not be equally safe in others;
- manufacturers do not routinely test drugs for their effects in G6PD-deficient individuals;
- the risk and severity of haemolysis is almost always dose-related.

The lists below should be read with these points in mind. Ideally, information about G6PD deficiency should be available before prescribing a drug listed below. However, in the absence of this information, the possibility of haemolysis should be considered, especially if the patient belongs to a group in which G6PD deficiency is common.

A very few G6PD-deficient individuals with chronic non-spherocytic haemolytic anaemia have haemolysis even in the absence of an exogenous trigger. These patients must be regarded as being at high risk of severe exacerbation of haemolysis following administration of any of the drugs listed below.

Drugs with definite risk of haemolysis in most G6PD-deficient individuals

Dapsone and other sulphones (higher doses for dermatitis herpetiformis more likely to cause problems)
Methylthioninium chloride (methylene blue)
Niridazole [not on UK market]
Nitrofurantoin
Pamaquin [not on UK market]
Primaquine (30 mg weekly for 8 weeks has been found to be without undue harmful effects in African and Asian people, see section 5.4.1)
Quinolones (including ciprofloxacin, moxifloxacin, nalidixic acid, norfloxacin, and ofloxacin)
Sulphonamides (including co-trimoxazole; some sulphonamides, e.g. sulfadiazine, have been tested and found not to be haemolytic in many G6PD-deficient individuals)

Drugs with possible risk of haemolysis in some G6PD-deficient individuals

Aspirin (acceptable up to a dose of at least 1 g daily in most G6PD-deficient individuals)
Chloroquine (acceptable in acute malaria)
Menadione, water-soluble derivatives (e.g. menadiol sodium phosphate)
Probenecid [not on UK market]
Quinidine (acceptable in acute malaria) [not on UK market]
Quinine (acceptable in acute malaria)
Rasburicase

Note Naphthalene in mothballs also causes haemolysis in individuals with G6PD deficiency

9.1.6 Drugs used in neutropenia

Recombinant human granulocyte-colony stimulating factor (rhG-CSF) stimulates the production of neutrophils and may reduce the duration of chemotherapy-induced neutropenia and thereby reduce the incidence of associated sepsis; there is as yet no evidence that it improves overall survival. **Filgrastim** (unglycosylated rhG-CSF) and **lenograstim** (glycosylated rhG-CSF) have similar effects; both have been used in a variety of clinical settings but they do not have any clear-cut routine indications. In congenital neutropenia filgrastim usually elevates the neutrophil count with appropriate clinical response. Prolonged use may be associated with an increased risk of myeloid malignancy. **Pegfilgrastim** is a polyethylene glycol-conjugated ('pegylated') derivative of filgrastim; pegylation increases the duration of filgrastim activity.

Treatment with recombinant human growth factors should only be prescribed by those experienced in their use.

Cautions Recombinant human growth factors should be used with caution in patients with pre-malignant or malignant myeloid conditions. Full blood counts including differential white cell and platelet counts should be monitored. Treatment should be withdrawn in patients who develop signs of pulmonary infiltration. There have been reports of pulmonary infiltrates leading to acute respiratory distress syndrome—patients with a history of pulmonary infiltrates or pneumonia may be at higher risk. Splenic rupture following administration of granulocyte-colony stimulating factors has been reported—monitor spleen size. Recombinant human growth factors should be used with caution in patients with sickle-cell disease. Recombinant human growth factors are not recommended in pregnancy (Appendix 4) or breast-feeding (Appendix 5).

Side-effects Side-effects of granulocyte-colony stimulating factors include gastro-intestinal disturbances (including nausea, vomiting, and diarrhoea), anorexia, headache, asthenia, fever, musculoskeletal pain, bone pain, rash, alopecia, injection-site reactions, and leucocytosis. *Less commonly* chest pain, hypersensitivity reactions (including anaphylaxis and bronchospasm) and arthralgia. *Rarely* pulmonary side-effects, particularly interstitial pneumonia, can occur (see Cautions above).

FILGRASTIM

(Recombinant human granulocyte-colony stimulating factor, G-CSF)

Indications (specialist use only) reduction in duration of neutropenia and incidence of febrile neutropenia in cytotoxic chemotherapy for malignancy (except chronic myeloid leukaemia and myelodysplastic syndromes); reduction in duration of neutropenia (and associated sequelae) in myeloablative therapy followed by bone-marrow transplantation; mobilisation of peripheral blood progenitor cells for harvesting and subsequent autologous or allogeneic infusion; severe congenital neutropenia, cyclic neutropenia, or idiopathic neutropenia and history of severe or recurrent infections (distinguish carefully from other haematological disorders, consult product literature); persistent neutropenia in advanced HIV infection

Cautions see notes above; also reduced myeloid precursors; regular morphological and cytogenetic bone-marrow examinations recommended in severe congenital neutropenia (possible risk of myelodysplastic syndromes or leukaemia); secondary acute myeloid leukaemia, sickle-cell disease; monitor spleen size (risk of rupture); osteoporotic bone disease (monitor bone density if given for more than 6 months); **interactions**: Appendix 1 (filgrastim)

Contra-indications severe congenital neutropenia (Kostmann's syndrome) with abnormal cytogenetics

Side-effects see notes above; also splenic enlargement, hepatomegaly, transient hypotension, epistaxis, urinary abnormalities (including dysuria, proteinuria, and haematuria), osteoporosis, exacerbation of rheumatoid arthritis, cutaneous vasculitis, thrombocytopenia, anaemia, transient decrease in blood glucose, raised uric acid

Dose

- Cytotoxic-induced neutropenia, preferably by subcutaneous injection *or* by intravenous infusion (over 30 minutes), ADULT and CHILD, 500 000 units/kg daily started at least 24 hours after cytotoxic chemotherapy, continued until neutrophil count in normal range, usually for up to 14 days (up to 38 days in acute myeloid leukaemia)
- Myeloablative therapy followed by bone-marrow transplantation, by intravenous infusion over 30 minutes or over 24 hours *or* by subcutaneous infusion over 24 hours, 1 million units/kg daily, started at least 24 hours following cytotoxic chemotherapy (and within 24 hours of bone-marrow infusion), then adjusted according to neutrophil count (consult product literature)
- Mobilisation of peripheral blood progenitor cells for autologous infusion, used alone, by subcutaneous injection *or* by subcutaneous infusion over 24 hours, 1 million units/kg daily for 5–7 days; used following adjunctive myelosuppressive chemotherapy (to improve yield), by subcutaneous injection, 500 000 units/kg daily, started the day after completing chemotherapy and continued until neutrophil count in normal range; for timing of leucopheresis consult product literature
- Mobilisation of peripheral blood progenitor cells in normal donors for allogeneic infusion, by subcutaneous injection, ADULT under 60 years and ADOLESCENT over 16 years, 1 million units/kg daily for 4–5 days; for timing of leucopheresis consult product literature
- Severe chronic neutropenia, by subcutaneous injection, ADULT and CHILD, in severe congenital neutropenia, initially 1.2 million units/kg daily in single or divided doses (initially 500 000 units/kg daily in idiopathic or cyclic neutropenia), adjusted according to response (consult product literature)
- Persistent neutropenia in HIV infection, by subcutaneous injection, initially 100 000 units/kg daily, increased as necessary until neutrophil count in normal range (usual max. 400 000 units/kg daily), then adjusted to maintain neutrophil count in normal range (consult product literature)

Neupogen® (Amgen) PoM

Injection, filgrastim 30 million-units (300 micrograms)/mL, net price 1-mL vial = £68.41

Injection (Singleject®), filgrastim 60 million-units (600 micrograms)/mL, net price 0.5-mL prefilled syringe = £68.41; 96 million-units (960 micrograms)/mL, 0.5-mL prefilled syringe = £109.11

LENOGRASTIM

(Recombinant human granulocyte-colony stimulating factor, rHuG-CSF)

Indications (specialist use only) reduction in the duration of neutropenia and associated complications following bone-marrow transplantation for non-myeloid malignancy or following treatment with cytotoxic chemotherapy associated with a significant incidence of febrile neutropenia; mobilisation of peripheral blood progenitor cells for harvesting and subsequent infusion

Cautions see notes above; also pre-malignant myeloid conditions; reduced myeloid precursors; sickle cell disease; monitor spleen size (risk of rupture)

Side-effects see notes above; also splenic rupture, cutaneous vasculitis, acute febrile neutrophilic dermatosis, toxic epidermal necrolysis

Dose

- Following bone-marrow transplantation, by intravenous infusion, ADULT and CHILD over 2 years 19.2 million units/m² daily started the day after transplantation, continued until neutrophil count stable in acceptable range (max. 28 days)
- Cytotoxic-induced neutropenia, by subcutaneous injection, ADULT 19.2 million units/m² daily started the day after completion of chemotherapy, continued until neutrophil count stable in acceptable range (max. 28 days)
- Mobilisation of peripheral blood progenitor cells, used alone, by subcutaneous injection, ADULT 1.28 million units/kg daily for 4–6 days (5–6 days in healthy donors); used following adjunctive myelosuppressive chemotherapy (to improve yield), by subcutaneous injection, 19.2 million units/m² daily, started the day after completion of chemotherapy and continued until neutrophil count in acceptable range; for timing of leucopheresis consult product literature

Granocyte® (Chugai) PoM

Injection, powder for reconstitution, lenograstim, net price 13.4 million-unit (105-microgram) vial = £42.00; 33.6 million-unit (263-microgram) vial = £67.09 (both with 1-mL prefilled syringe water for injections)

PEGFILGRASTIM

(Pegylated recombinant methionyl human granulocyte-colony stimulating factor)

Indications (specialist use only) reduction in duration of neutropenia and incidence of febrile neutropenia in cytotoxic chemotherapy for malignancy (except chronic myeloid leukaemia and myelodysplastic syndromes)

Cautions see notes above; also acute leukaemia and myelosuppressive chemotherapy; sickle-cell disease; monitor spleen size (risk of rupture); **interactions:** Appendix 1 (filgrastim)

Side-effects see notes above; also *rarely* thrombocytopenia; *very rarely* acute febrile neutrophilic dermatosis, cutaneous vasculitis, and splenic rupture

Dose

Note Dose expressed as filgrastim

- By subcutaneous injection, ADULT over 18 years, 6 mg (0.6 mL) for each chemotherapy cycle, starting 24 hours after chemotherapy

Neulasta® (Amgen) PoM

Injection, pegfilgrastim (expressed as filgrastim) 10 mg/mL, net price 0.6-mL (6-mg) prefilled syringe = £714.24; *SureClick®* prefilled disposable injection device 0.6 mL (6 mg) = £714.24

9.2 Fluids and electrolytes

9.2.1 Oral preparations for fluid and electrolyte imbalance
9.2.2 Parenteral preparations for fluid and electrolyte imbalance

The following tables give a selection of useful electrolyte values:

Electrolyte concentrations—intravenous fluids

Intravenous infusion	Millimoles per litre Na$^+$	K$^+$	HCO_3^-	Cl$^-$	Ca^{2+}
Normal plasma values	142	4.5	26	103	2.5
Sodium Chloride 0.9%	150	—	—	150	—
Compound Sodium Lactate (Hartmann's)	131	5	29	111	2
Sodium Chloride 0.18% and Glucose 4%	30	—	—	30	—
Potassium Chloride 0.3% and Glucose 5%	—	40	—	40	—
Potassium Chloride 0.3% and Sodium Chloride 0.9%	150	40	—	190	—
To correct metabolic acidosis					
Sodium Bicarbonate 1.26%	150	—	150	—	—
Sodium Bicarbonate 8.4% for cardiac arrest	1000	—	1000	—	—
Sodium Lactate (m/6)	167	—	167	—	—

Electrolyte content—gastro-intestinal secretions

Type of fluid	Millimoles per litre H$^+$	Na$^+$	K$^+$	HCO_3^-	Cl$^-$
Gastric	40–60	20–80	5–20	—	100–150
Biliary	—	120–140	5–15	30–50	80–120
Pancreatic	—	120–140	5–15	70–110	40–80
Small bowel	—	120–140	5–15	20–40	90–130

Faeces, vomit, or aspiration should be saved and analysed where possible if abnormal losses are suspected; where this is impracticable the approximations above may be helpful in planning replacement therapy

9.2.1 Oral preparations for fluid and electrolyte imbalance

9.2.1.1 Oral potassium
9.2.1.2 Oral sodium and water
9.2.1.3 Oral bicarbonate

Sodium and potassium salts, which may be given by mouth to prevent deficiencies or to treat established deficiencies of mild or moderate degree, are discussed in this section. Oral preparations for removing excess potassium and preparations for oral rehydration therapy are also included here. Oral bicarbonate, for metabolic acidosis, is also described in this section.

For reference to calcium, magnesium, and phosphate, see section 9.5.

9.2.1.1 Oral potassium

Compensation for potassium loss is especially necessary:

- in those taking digoxin or anti-arrhythmic drugs, where potassium depletion may induce arrhythmias;
- in patients in whom secondary hyperaldosteronism occurs, e.g. renal artery stenosis, cirrhosis of the liver, the nephrotic syndrome, and severe heart failure;
- in patients with excessive losses of potassium in the faeces, e.g. chronic diarrhoea associated with intestinal malabsorption or laxative abuse.

Measures to compensate for potassium loss may also be required in the elderly since they frequently take inadequate amounts of potassium in the diet (but see below for **warning** on **renal insufficiency**). Measures may also be required during long-term administration of drugs known to induce potassium loss (e.g. corticosteroids). Potassium supplements are **seldom required** with the small doses of diuretics given to treat hypertension; **potassium-sparing diuretics** (rather than potassium supplements) are recommended for prevention of hypokalaemia due to diuretics such as furosemide (frusemide) or the thiazides when these are given to eliminate oedema.

Dosage If potassium salts are used for the *prevention of hypokalaemia*, then doses of potassium chloride 2 to 4 g (approx. 25 to 50 mmol) daily (in divided doses) by mouth are suitable in patients taking a normal diet. *Smaller doses* must be used if there is *renal insufficiency (common in the elderly)* otherwise there is **danger of hyperkalaemia**. Potassium salts cause nausea and vomiting therefore poor compliance is a major limitation to their effectiveness; where appropriate, potassium-sparing diuretics are preferable (see also above). Regular monitoring of plasma-potassium concentration is essential in those receiving potassium supplements. When there is *established potassium depletion* larger doses may be necessary, the quantity depending on the severity of any continuing potassium loss (monitoring of plasma-potassium concentration and specialist advice would be required). Potassium depletion is frequently associated with chloride depletion and with metabolic alkalosis, and these disorders require correction.

Administration Potassium salts are preferably given as a liquid (or effervescent) preparation, rather than modified-release tablets; they should be given as the chloride (the use of effervescent potassium tablets BPC 1968 should be restricted to *hyperchloraemic states*, section 9.2.1.3).

Salt substitutes A number of salt substitutes which contain significant amounts of potassium chloride are readily available as health food products (e.g. *LoSalt*® and *Ruthmol*®). These should not be used by patients with renal failure as potassium intoxication may result.

9 Nutrition and blood

POTASSIUM CHLORIDE

Indications potassium depletion (see notes above)

Cautions elderly, renal impairment (avoid if creatinine clearance less than 10 mL/minute; Appendix 3); intestinal stricture, history of peptic ulcer, hiatus hernia (for sustained-release preparations); **important:** special hazard if given with drugs liable to raise plasma-potassium concentration such as potassium-sparing diuretics, ACE inhibitors, or ciclosporin, for other **interactions**: Appendix 1 (potassium salts)

Contra-indications plasma-potassium concentration above 5 mmol/litre

Side-effects nausea and vomiting (severe symptoms may indicate obstruction), oesophageal or small bowel ulceration

Dose

- See notes above

Note Do not confuse Effervescent Potassium Tablets BPC 1968 (section 9.2.1.3) with effervescent potassium chloride tablets. Effervescent Potassium Tablets BPC 1968 do not contain chloride ions and their use should be restricted to hyperchloraemic states (section 9.2.1.3). Effervescent Potassium Chloride Tablets BP are usually available in two strengths, one containing 6.7 mmol each of K^+ and Cl^- (corresponding to *Kloref®*), the other containing 12 mmol K^+ and 8 mmol Cl^- (corresponding to *Sando-K®*). Generic prescriptions must specify the strength required.

Kay-Cee-L® (Geistlich)
Syrup, red, sugar-free, potassium chloride 7.5% (1 mmol/mL each of K^+ and Cl^-). Net price 500 mL = £3.74. Label: 21

Kloref® (Alpharma)
Tablets, effervescent, betaine hydrochloride, potassium benzoate, bicarbonate, and chloride, equivalent to potassium chloride 500 mg (6.7 mmol each of K^+ and Cl^-). Net price 50 = £2.71. Label: 13, 21
Note May be difficult to obtain

Sando-K® (HK Pharma)
Tablets, effervescent, potassium bicarbonate and chloride equivalent to potassium 470 mg (12 mmol of K^+) and chloride 285 mg (8 mmol of Cl^-). Net price 20 = £1.53. Label: 13, 21

Modified-release preparations

Avoid unless effervescent tablets or liquid preparations inappropriate

Slow-K® (Alliance)
Tablets, m/r, orange, s/c, potassium chloride 600 mg (8 mmol each of K^+ and Cl^-). Net price 20 = 54p. Label: 25, 27, counselling, swallow whole with fluid during meals while sitting or standing

Potassium removal

Ion-exchange resins may be used to remove excess potassium in *mild hyperkalaemia* or in *moderate hyperkalaemia* when there are no ECG changes.

Severe hyperkalaemia Severe hyperkalaemia calls for urgent treatment with 10–30 mL of calcium gluconate 10% by intravenous injection to temporarily protect against myocardial excitability. An intravenous injection of soluble insulin (5–10 units) with 50 mL glucose 50% given over 5–15 minutes, reduces serum-potassium concentration; this is repeated if necessary or a continuous infusion instituted; occasionally haemodialysis is needed.

POLYSTYRENE SULPHONATE RESINS

Indications hyperkalaemia associated with anuria or severe oliguria, and in dialysis patients

Cautions children (impaction of resin with excessive dosage or inadequate dilution); monitor for electrolyte disturbances (stop if plasma-potassium concentration below 5 mmol/litre); pregnancy and breast-feeding; sodium-containing resin in congestive heart failure, hypertension, renal impairment, and oedema; **interactions**: Appendix 1 (sodium polystyrene sulphonate)

Contra-indications obstructive bowel disease; oral administration or reduced gut motility in neonates; avoid calcium-containing resin in hyperparathyroidism, multiple myeloma, sarcoidosis, or metastatic carcinoma

Side-effects rectal ulceration following rectal administration; colonic necrosis reported following enemas containing sorbitol; sodium retention, hypercalcaemia, gastric irritation, anorexia, nausea and vomiting, constipation (discontinue treatment—avoid magnesium-containing laxatives), diarrhoea; calcium-containing resin may cause hypercalcaemia (in dialysed patients and occasionally in those with renal impairment), hypomagnesaemia

Dose

- By mouth, 15 g 3–4 times daily in water (not fruit squash which has a high potassium content) or as a paste; CHILD 0.5–1 g/kg daily in divided doses
- By rectum, as an enema, 30 g in methylcellulose solution, retained for 9 hours followed by irrigation to remove resin from colon; NEONATE and CHILD, 0.5–1 g/kg daily

Calcium Resonium® (Sanofi-Synthelabo)
Powder, buff, calcium polystyrene sulphonate. Net price 300 g = £47.55. Label: 13

Resonium A® (Sanofi-Synthelabo)
Powder, buff, sodium polystyrene sulphonate. Net price 454 g = £70.24. Label: 13

9.2.1.2 Oral sodium and water

Sodium chloride is indicated in states of sodium depletion and usually needs to be given intravenously (section 9.2.2). In chronic conditions associated with mild or moderate degrees of sodium depletion, e.g. in salt-losing bowel or renal disease, oral supplements of sodium chloride or sodium bicarbonate (section 9.2.1.3), according to the acid-base status of the patient, may be sufficient.

SODIUM CHLORIDE

Indications sodium depletion—see also 9.2.2.1; nebuliser diluent (section 3.1.5); eye (section 11.8.1); oral hygiene (section 12.3.4); wound irrigation (section 13.11.1)

Slow Sodium® (HK Pharma)
Tablets, m/r, sodium chloride 600 mg (approx. 10 mmol each of Na^+ and Cl^-). Net price 100-tab pack = £6.05. Label: 25
Dose prophylaxis of sodium chloride deficiency 4–8 tablets daily with water (in severe depletion up to max. 20 tablets daily)
Chronic renal salt wasting, up to 20 tablets daily with appropriate fluid intake
CHILD see *BNF for Children*

Oral rehydration therapy (ORT)

As a worldwide problem *diarrhoea* is by far the most important indication for fluid and electrolyte replacement. Intestinal absorption of sodium and water is enhanced by glucose (and other carbohydrates). Replacement of fluid and electrolytes lost through diarrhoea can therefore be achieved by giving solutions containing sodium, potassium, and glucose or another carbohydrate such as rice starch.

Oral rehydration solutions should:

- enhance the absorption of water and electrolytes;
- replace the electrolyte deficit adequately and safely;
- contain an alkalinising agent to counter acidosis;
- be slightly hypo-osmolar (about 250 mmol/litre) to prevent the possible induction of osmotic diarrhoea;
- be simple to use in hospital and at home;
- be palatable and acceptable, especially to children;
- be readily available.

It is the policy of the World Health Organization (WHO) to promote a single oral rehydration solution but to use it flexibly (e.g. by giving extra water between drinks of oral rehydration solution to moderately dehydrated infants).

Oral rehydration solutions used in the UK are lower in sodium (50–60 mmol/litre) than the WHO formulation since, in general, patients suffer less severe sodium loss.

Rehydration should be rapid over 3 to 4 hours (except in hypernatraemic dehydration in which case rehydration should occur more slowly over 12 hours). The patient should be reassessed after initial rehydration and if still dehydrated rapid fluid replacement should continue.

Once rehydration is complete further dehydration is prevented by encouraging the patient to drink normal volumes of an appropriate fluid and by replacing continuing losses with an oral rehydration solution; in infants, breast-feeding or formula feeds should be offered between oral rehydration drinks.

For intravenous rehydration see section 9.2.2.

ORAL REHYDRATION SALTS (ORS)

Indications fluid and electrolyte loss in diarrhoea, see notes above

Dose

- According to fluid loss, usually 200–400 mL solution after every loose motion; INFANT 1–1½ times usual feed volume; CHILD 200 mL after every loose motion

UK formulations

Note After reconstitution any unused solution should be discarded no later than 1 hour after preparation unless stored in a refrigerator when it may be kept for up to 24 hours

Dioralyte® (Sanofi-Aventis)

Oral powder, sodium chloride 470 mg, potassium chloride 300 mg, disodium hydrogen citrate 530 mg, glucose 3.56 g/sachet, net price 6-sachet pack = £2.11, 20-sachet pack (black currant- or citrus-flavoured or natural) = £6.99

Note Reconstitute 1 sachet with 200 mL of water (freshly boiled and cooled for infants); 5 sachets reconstituted with 1 litre of water provide Na^+ 60 mmol, K^+ 20 mmol, Cl^- 60 mmol, citrate 10 mmol, and glucose 90 mmol

Dioralyte® Relief (Sanofi-Aventis)

Oral powder, sodium chloride 350 mg, potassium chloride 300 mg, sodium citrate 580 mg, cooked rice powder 6 g/sachet, net price 6-sachet pack (apricot-, black currant- or raspberry-flavoured) = £2.35, 20-sachet pack (apricot-flavoured) = £7.42

Note Reconstitute 1 sachet with 200 mL of water (freshly boiled and cooled for infants); 5 sachets when reconstituted with 1 litre of water provide Na^+ 60 mmol, K^+ 20 mmol, Cl^- 50 mmol and citrate 10 mmol; contains aspartame (section 9.4.1)

Electrolade® (Thornton & Ross)

Oral powder, sodium chloride 236 mg, potassium chloride 300 mg, sodium bicarbonate 500 mg, anhydrous glucose 4 g/sachet (banana-, black currant-, lemon and lime-, or orange-flavoured). Net price 6-sachet (plain or multiflavoured) pack = £1.33, 20-sachet (single- or multiflavoured) pack = £4.99

Note Reconstitute 1 sachet with 200 mL of water (freshly boiled and cooled for infants); 5 sachets when reconstituted with 1 litre of water provide Na^+ 50 mmol, K^+ 20 mmol, Cl^- 40 mmol, HCO_3^- 30 mmol, and glucose 111 mmol

Rapolyte® (KoGEN)

Oral powder, sodium chloride 350 mg, potassium chloride 300 mg, sodium citrate 600 mg, anhydrous glucose 4 g, net price 20-sachet pack (black currant- or raspberry-flavoured) = £4.28

Note Reconstitute 1 sachet with 200 mL of water (freshly boiled and cooled for infants); 5 sachets when reconstituted with 1 litre of water provide Na^+ 60 mmol, K^+ 20 mmol, Cl^- 50 mmol, citrate 10 mmol, and glucose 110 mmol

WHO formulation

Oral Rehydration Salts (Non-proprietary)

Oral powder, sodium chloride 2.6 g, potassium chloride 1.5 g, sodium citrate 2.9 g, anhydrous glucose 13.5 g. To be dissolved in sufficient water to produce 1 litre (providing Na^+ 75 mmol, K^+ 20 mmol, Cl^- 65 mmol, citrate 10 mmol, glucose 75 mmol/litre)

Note Recommended by the WHO and the United Nations Children's Fund but not commonly used in the UK.

9.2.1.3 Oral bicarbonate

Sodium bicarbonate is given by mouth for *chronic acidotic states* such as uraemic acidosis or renal tubular acidosis. The dose for correction of metabolic acidosis is not predictable and the response must be assessed; sodium bicarbonate 4.8 g daily (57 mmol each of Na^+ and HCO_3^-) or more may be required. For severe metabolic acidosis, sodium bicarbonate can be given intravenously (section 9.2.2).

Sodium bicarbonate may also be used to increase the pH of the urine (see section 7.4.3); for use in dyspepsia see section 1.1.1.

Sodium supplements may increase blood pressure or cause fluid retention and pulmonary oedema in those at risk; hypokalaemia may be exacerbated.

Where *hyperchloraemic acidosis* is associated with potassium deficiency, as in some renal tubular and gastro-intestinal disorders it may be appropriate to give oral **potassium bicarbonate**, although acute or severe deficiency should be managed by intravenous therapy.

SODIUM BICARBONATE

Indications see notes above

Cautions see notes above; avoid in respiratory acidosis; **interactions**: Appendix 1 (antacids)

Dose

- See notes above

Sodium Bicarbonate (Non-proprietary)

Capsules, sodium bicarbonate 500 mg (approx. 6 mmol each of Na^+ and HCO_3^-). Net price 56-cap pack = £16.97

Tablets, sodium bicarbonate 600 mg, net price 100 = £2.48

Important Oral solutions of sodium bicarbonate are required occasionally; these need to be obtained on special order and the strength of sodium bicarbonate should be stated on the prescription

POTASSIUM BICARBONATE

Indications see notes above

Cautions cardiac disease, renal impairment (avoid if creatinine clearance less than 10 mL/minute; Appendix 3); **interactions:** Appendix 1 (potassium salts)

Contra-indications hypochloraemia; plasma-potassium concentration above 5 mmol/litre

Side-effects nausea and vomiting

Dose

- See notes above

Potassium Tablets, Effervescent (Non-proprietary)

Effervescent tablets, potassium bicarbonate 500 mg, potassium acid tartrate 300 mg, each tablet providing 6.5 mmol of K^+. To be dissolved in water before administration. Net price 56 = £33.05. Label: 13, 21

Note These tablets do not contain chloride; for effervescent tablets containing potassium and chloride, see under Potassium Chloride, section 9.2.1.1

9.2.2 Parenteral preparations for fluid and electrolyte imbalance

9.2.2.1 Electrolytes and water

9.2.2.2 Plasma and plasma substitutes

9.2.2.1 Electrolytes and water

Solutions of electrolytes are given intravenously, to meet normal fluid and electrolyte requirements or to replenish substantial deficits or continuing losses, when the patient is nauseated or vomiting and is unable to take adequate amounts by mouth. When intravenous administration is not possible, fluid (as sodium chloride 0.9% or glucose 5%) can also be given by subcutaneous infusion (hypodermoclysis).

The nature and severity of the electrolyte imbalance must be assessed from the history and clinical and biochemical investigations. Sodium, potassium, chloride, magnesium, phosphate, and water depletion can occur singly and in combination with or without disturbances of acid-base balance; for reference to the use of magnesium and phosphates, see section 9.5.

Isotonic solutions may be infused safely into a peripheral vein. Solutions more concentrated than plasma, e.g. 20% glucose, are best given through an indwelling catheter positioned in a large vein.

Intravenous sodium

Sodium chloride in isotonic solution provides the most important extracellular ions in near physiological concentration and is indicated in *sodium depletion* which may arise from such conditions as gastro-enteritis, diabetic ketoacidosis, ileus, and ascites. In a severe deficit of from 4 to 8 litres, 2 to 3 litres of isotonic sodium chloride may be given over 2 to 3 hours; thereafter the infusion can usually be at a slower rate. Excessive administration should be avoided; the jugular venous pressure should be assessed, the bases of the lungs should be examined for crepitations, and in elderly or seriously ill patients it is often helpful to monitor the right atrial (central) venous pressure.

Chronic hyponatraemia arising from inappropriate secretion of antidiuretic hormone should ideally be corrected by fluid restriction. However, if sodium chloride is required for acute or chronic hyponatraemia, regardless of the cause, the deficit should be corrected slowly to avoid the risk of osmotic demyelination syndrome and the rise in plasma-sodium concentration should not exceed 10 mmol/litre in 24 hours. In severe hyponatraemia, sodium chloride 1.8% may be used cautiously.

Compound sodium lactate (Hartmann's solution) can be used instead of isotonic sodium chloride solution during surgery or in the initial management of the injured or wounded.

Sodium chloride and glucose solutions are indicated when there is combined *water and sodium depletion.* A 1:1 mixture of isotonic sodium chloride and 5% glucose allows some of the water (free of sodium) to enter body cells which suffer most from dehydration while the sodium salt with a volume of water determined by the normal plasma Na^+ remains extracellular. Maintenance fluid should accurately reflect daily requirements and close monitoring is required to avoid fluid and electrolyte imbalance. Illness or injury increase the secretion of anti-diuretic hormone and therefore the ability to excrete excess water may be impaired. Injudicious use of solutions such as sodium chloride 0.18% and glucose 4% may also cause dilutional hyponatraemia especially in children and the elderly; if necessary, guidance should be sought from a clinician experienced in the management of fluid and electrolytes.

Combined sodium, potassium, chloride, and water depletion may occur, for example, with severe diarrhoea or persistent vomiting; replacement is carried out with sodium chloride intravenous infusion 0.9% and glucose intravenous infusion 5% with potassium as appropriate.

SODIUM CHLORIDE

Indications electrolyte imbalance—see also section 9.2.1.2; nebuliser diluent (section 3.1.5); eye (section 11.8.1); oral hygiene (section 12.3.4); wound irrigation (section 13.11.1)

Cautions restrict intake in impaired renal function, cardiac failure, hypertension, peripheral and pulmonary oedema, toxaemia of pregnancy

Side-effects administration of large doses may give rise to sodium accumulation, oedema, and hyperchloraemic acidosis

Dose

- See notes above

Sodium Chloride Intravenous Infusion (Non-proprietary) PoM

Intravenous infusion, usual strength sodium chloride 0.9% (9 g, 150 mmol each of Na^+ and Cl^-/litre), this strength being supplied when normal saline for injection is requested. Net price 2-mL amp = 24p; 5-mL amp = 33p; 10-mL amp = 46p; 20-mL amp = £1.04; 50-mL amp = £2.01

In hospitals, 500- and 1000-mL packs, and sometimes other sizes, are available

Note The term 'normal saline' should **not** be used to describe sodium chloride intravenous infusion 0.9%; the term 'physiological saline' is acceptable but it is preferable to give the composition (i.e. sodium chloride intravenous infusion 0.9%).

With other ingredients

Sodium Chloride and Glucose Intravenous Infusion (Non-proprietary) PoM

Intravenous infusion, sodium chloride 0.18% (Na^+ and Cl^- each 30 mmol/litre), glucose 4%

In hospitals, usually 500-mL packs and sometimes other sizes are available

Intravenous infusion, sodium chloride 0.45% (Na^+ and Cl^- each 75 mmol/litre), glucose 2.5%

In hospitals, usually 500-mL packs and sometimes other sizes are available

Intravenous infusion, sodium chloride 0.45% (Na^+ and Cl^- each 75 mmol/litre), glucose 5%

In hospitals, usually 500-mL packs and sometimes other sizes are available

Intravenous infusion, sodium chloride 0.9% (Na^+ and Cl^- each 150 mmol/litre), glucose 5%

In hospitals, usually 500-mL packs and sometimes other sizes are available

Note See above for warning on hyponatraemia especially in children and elderly

Ringer's Solution for Injection PoM

Calcium chloride (dihydrate) 322 micrograms, potassium chloride 300 micrograms, sodium chloride 8.6 mg/mL, providing the following ions (in mmol/litre), Ca^{2+} 2.2, K^+ 4, Na^+ 147, Cl^- 156

In hospitals, 500- and 1000-mL packs, and sometimes other sizes, are available

Sodium Lactate Intravenous Infusion, Compound (Non-proprietary) PoM

(Hartmann's Solution for Injection; Ringer-Lactate Solution for Injection)

Intravenous infusion, sodium chloride 0.6%, sodium lactate 0.25%, potassium chloride 0.04%, calcium chloride 0.027% (containing Na^+ 131 mmol, K^+ 5 mmol, Ca^{2+} 2 mmol, HCO_3^- (as lactate) 29 mmol, Cl^- 111 mmol/litre)

In hospitals, 500- and 1000-mL packs, and sometimes other sizes, are available

Intravenous glucose

Glucose solutions (5%) are used mainly to replace water deficit and should be given alone only when there is no significant loss of electrolytes; prolonged administration of glucose solutions without electrolytes can lead to hyponatraemia and other electrolyte disturbances. Average water requirements in a healthy adult are 1.5 to 2.5 litres daily and this is needed to balance unavoidable losses of water through the skin and lungs and to provide sufficient for urinary excretion. Water depletion (dehydration) tends to occur when these losses are not matched by a comparable intake, as may occur in coma or dysphagia or in the elderly or apathetic who may not drink enough water on their own initiative.

Excessive loss of water without loss of electrolytes is uncommon, occurring in fevers, hyperthyroidism, and in uncommon water-losing renal states such as diabetes insipidus or hypercalcaemia. The volume of glucose solution needed to replace deficits varies with the severity of the disorder, but usually lies within the range of 2 to 6 litres.

Glucose solutions are also used to correct and prevent hypoglycaemia and to provide a source of energy in those too ill to be fed adequately by mouth; glucose solutions are a key component of parenteral nutrition (section 9.3).

Glucose solutions are given in regimens with calcium and insulin for the emergency management of *hyperkalaemia* (see p. 504). They are also given, after correction of hyperglycaemia, during treatment of diabetic ketoacidosis, when they must be accompanied by continuing insulin infusion.

GLUCOSE
(Dextrose Monohydrate)

Note Glucose BP is the monohydrate but Glucose Intravenous Infusion BP is a sterile solution of anhydrous glucose or glucose monohydrate, potency being expressed in terms of anhydrous glucose

Indications fluid replacement (see notes above), provision of energy (section 9.3); hypoglycaemia (section 6.1.4)

Side-effects glucose injections especially if hypertonic may have a low pH and may cause venous irritation and thrombophlebitis

Dose

- Water replacement, see notes above; energy source, 1–3 litres daily of 20–50% solution

Glucose Intravenous Infusion (Non-proprietary) PoM

Intravenous infusion, glucose or anhydrous glucose (potency expressed in terms of anhydrous glucose), usual strength 5% (50 mg/mL) and 10% (100 mg/mL); 25% solution, net price 25-mL amp = £2.21; 50% solution,[1] 25-mL amp = £3.80, 50-mL amp = £1.63

In hospitals, 500- and 1000-mL packs, and sometimes other sizes and strengths, are available; also available as *Min-I-Jet® Glucose*, 50% in 50-mL disposable syringe[1]

1. PoM restriction does not apply where administration is for saving life in emergency

Intravenous potassium

Potassium chloride and sodium chloride intravenous infusion is the initial treatment for the correction of *severe hypokalaemia* and when sufficient potassium cannot be taken by mouth. Ready-mixed infusion solutions should be used when possible; alternatively, potassium chloride concentrate, as ampoules containing 1.5 g (K^+ 20 mmol) in 10 mL, is **thoroughly mixed** with 500 mL of sodium chloride 0.9% intravenous infusion and given slowly over 2 to 3 hours, with specialist advice and ECG monitoring in difficult cases. Higher concentrations of potassium chloride may be given in very severe depletion, but require specialist advice.

Repeated measurement of plasma-potassium concentration is necessary to determine whether further infusions are required and to avoid the development of hyperkalaemia, which is especially likely in renal impairment.

Initial potassium replacement therapy should **not** involve glucose infusions, because glucose may cause a further decrease in the plasma-potassium concentration.

POTASSIUM CHLORIDE

Indications electrolyte imbalance; see also oral potassium supplements, section 9.2.1.1

Cautions for intravenous infusion the concentration of solution should not usually exceed 3 g (40 mmol)/litre; specialist advice and ECG monitoring (see notes above); renal impairment (avoid if creatinine clearance less than 10 mL/minute; Appendix 3); **interactions:** Appendix 1 (potassium salts)

Side-effects rapid infusion toxic to heart

Dose

- By slow intravenous infusion, depending on the deficit or the daily maintenance requirements, see also notes above

Potassium Chloride and Glucose Intravenous Infusion (Non-proprietary) PoM

Intravenous infusion, usual strength potassium chloride 0.3% (3 g, 40 mmol each of K^+ and Cl^-/litre) or 0.15% (1.5 g, 20 mmol each of K^+ and Cl^-/litre) with 5% of anhydrous glucose

In hospitals, 500- and 1000-mL packs, and sometimes other sizes, are available

Potassium Chloride and Sodium Chloride Intravenous Infusion (Non-proprietary) PoM

Intravenous infusion, usual strength potassium chloride 0.15% (1.5 g/litre) with sodium chloride 0.9% (9 g/litre), containing K^+ 20 mmol, Na^+ 150 mmol, and Cl^- 170 mmol/litre *or* potassium chloride 0.3% (3 g/litre) with sodium chloride 0.9% (9 g/litre), containing K^+ 40 mmol, Na^+ 150 mmol, and Cl^- 190 mmol/litre

In hospitals, 500- and 1000-mL packs, and sometimes other sizes, are available

Potassium Chloride, Sodium Chloride, and Glucose Intravenous Infusion (Non-proprietary) PoM

Intravenous infusion, sodium chloride 0.45% (4.5 g, Na^+ 75 mmol/litre) with 5% of anhydrous glucose and usually sufficient potassium chloride to provide K^+ 10–40 mmol/litre (to be specified by the prescriber)

In hospitals, 500- and 1000-mL packs, and sometimes other sizes, are available

Intravenous infusion, sodium chloride 0.18% (1.8 g, Na^+ 30 mmol/litre) with 4% of anhydrous glucose and usually sufficient potassium chloride to provide K^+ 10–40 mmol/litre (to be specified by the prescriber)

In hospitals, 500- and 1000-mL packs, and sometimes other sizes, are available

Potassium Chloride Concentrate, Sterile (Non-proprietary) PoM

Sterile concentrate, potassium chloride 15% (150 mg, approximately 2 mmol each of K^+ and Cl^-/mL). Net price 10-mL amp = 48p

Important Must be diluted with **not less** than 50 times its volume of sodium chloride intravenous infusion 0.9% or other suitable diluent and **mixed well**

Solutions containing 10 and 20% of potassium chloride are also available in both 5- and 10-mL ampoules

Bicarbonate and lactate

Sodium bicarbonate is used to control severe *metabolic acidosis* (pH < 7.1) particularly that caused by loss of bicarbonate (as in renal tubular acidosis or from excessive gastro-intestinal losses). Mild metabolic acidosis associated with volume depletion should first be managed by appropriate fluid replacement, because acidosis usually resolves as tissue and renal perfusion are restored. In more severe metabolic acidosis or when the acidosis remains unresponsive to correction of anoxia or hypovolaemia, sodium bicarbonate (1.26%) can be infused over 3–4 hours with plasma-pH and electrolyte monitoring. In severe shock, for example in cardiac arrest (section 2.7.1), metabolic acidosis can develop without sodium or volume depletion; in these circumstances sodium bicarbonate is best given as a small volume of hypertonic solution, such as 50 mL of 8.4% solution intravenously; plasma-pH and electrolytes should be monitored.

Sodium lactate intravenous infusion is no longer used in metabolic acidosis because of the risk of producing lactic acidosis, particularly in seriously ill patients with poor tissue perfusion or impaired hepatic function.

SODIUM BICARBONATE

Indications metabolic acidosis

Dose

- By slow intravenous injection, a strong solution (up to 8.4%), or by continuous intravenous infusion, a weaker solution (usually 1.26%), an amount appropriate to the body base deficit (see notes above)

Sodium Bicarbonate Intravenous Infusion PoM

Usual strength sodium bicarbonate 1.26% (12.6 g, 150 mmol each of Na^+ and HCO_3^-/litre); various other strengths available

In hospitals, 500- and 1000-mL packs, and sometimes other sizes, are available

Min-I-Jet® Sodium Bicarbonate (Celltech) PoM

Intravenous injection, sodium bicarbonate in disposable syringe, net price 4.2%, 10 mL = £5.82; 8.4%, 10 mL = £6.00, 50 mL = £8.14

SODIUM LACTATE

Indications see notes above

Sodium Lactate (Non-proprietary) PoM

Intravenous infusion, sodium lactate M/6, contains the following ions (in mmol/litre), Na^+ 167, HCO_3^- (as lactate) 167

Water

Water for Injections PoM

Net price 1-mL amp = 18p; 2-mL amp = 17p; 5-mL amp = 28p; 10-mL amp = 31p; 20-mL amp = 92p; 50-mL amp = £1.91; 100-mL vial = 23p

9.2.2.2 Plasma and plasma substitutes

Plasma and plasma substitutes ('colloids') contain large molecules that do not readily leave the intravascular space where they exert osmotic pressure to maintain circulatory volume. Compared to fluids containing electrolytes such as sodium chloride and glucose ('crystalloids'), a smaller volume of colloid is required to produce the same expansion of blood volume, thereby shifting salt and water from the extravascular space. If resuscitation requires a volume of fluid that exceeds the maximum dose of the colloid then crystalloids can be given; packed red cells may also be required.

Albumin solutions, prepared from whole blood, contain soluble proteins and electrolytes but no clotting factors, blood group antibodies, or plasma cholinesterases; they may be given without regard to the recipient's blood group.

Albumin should usually be used after the acute phase of illness, to correct a plasma-volume deficit in patients with salt and water retention and oedema; hypoalbuminaemia itself is not an appropriate indication. The use of albumin solutions in acute plasma or blood loss may be wasteful; plasma substitutes are more appropriate. Concentrated albumin solutions may also be used to obtain a diuresis in hypoalbuminaemic patients (e.g. in hepatic cirrhosis).

Recent evidence does not support the previous view that the use of albumin increases mortality.

> Plasma and plasma substitutes are often used in very ill patients whose condition is unstable. Therefore, close monitoring is required and fluid and electrolyte therapy should be adjusted according to the patient's condition at all times.

ALBUMIN SOLUTION

(Human Albumin Solution)

A solution containing protein derived from plasma, serum, or normal placentas; at least 95% of the protein is albumin. The solution may be isotonic (containing 4–5% protein) or concentrated (containing 15–25% protein).

Indications see under preparations, and also notes above

Cautions history of cardiac or circulatory disease (administer slowly to avoid rapid rise in blood pressure and cardiac failure, and monitor cardiovascular and respiratory function); increased capillary permeability; correct dehydration when administering concentrated solution

Contra-indications cardiac failure; severe anaemia

Side-effects hypersensitivity reactions (including anaphylaxis) with nausea, vomiting, increased salivation, fever, tachycardia, hypotension and chills reported

Isotonic solutions

Indications: acute or sub-acute loss of plasma volume e.g. in burns, pancreatitis, trauma, and complications of surgery; plasma exchange

Available as: *Human Albumin Solution 4.5%* (50-, 100-, 250- and 400-mL bottles—Baxter Bioscience); *Human Albumin Solution 5%* (100-, 250- and 500-mL bottles—Grifols); *Albutein® 5%* (250- and 500-mL bottles—Grifols); *Octalbin® 5%* (100- and 200-mL bottles—Octapharm); *Zenalb® 4.5%* (50-, 100-, 250-, and 500-mL bottles—BPL)

Concentrated solutions (20–25%)

Indications: severe hypoalbuminaemia associated with low plasma volume and generalised oedema where salt and water restriction with plasma volume expansion are required; adjunct in the treatment of hyperbilirubinaemia by exchange transfusion in the newborn; paracentesis of large volume ascites associated with portal hypertension

Available as: *Human Albumin Solution 20%* (50- and 100-mL vials—Baxter Bioscience); *Human Albumin Solution 20%* (50- and 100-mL bottles—Grifols); *Albutein® 20%* (50- and 100-mL bottles—Grifols); *Albutein® 25%* (20-, 50-, and 100-mL vials—Grifols); *Octalbin® 20%* (50- and 100-mL bottles—Octapharm); *Zenalb® 20%* (50- and 100-mL bottles—BPL)

Plasma substitutes

Dextrans, **gelatin** and the **etherified starches** (hetastarch, pentastarch, and tetrastarch) are macromolecular substances which are metabolised slowly; they may be used at the outset to expand and maintain blood volume in shock arising from conditions such as burns or septicaemia. Plasma substitutes may be used as an immediate short-term measure to treat haemorrhage until blood is available. They are rarely needed when shock is due to sodium and water depletion because, in these circumstances, the shock responds to water and electrolyte repletion. See also section 2.7.1 for the management of shock.

Plasma substitutes should **not** be used to maintain plasma volume in conditions such as burns or peritonitis where there is loss of plasma protein, water and electrolytes over periods of several days or weeks. In these situations, plasma or plasma protein fractions containing large amounts of albumin should be given.

Large volumes of *some* plasma substitutes can increase the risk of bleeding through depletion of coagulation factors.

Dextran 70 by intravenous infusion is used predominantly for volume expansion. Dextran 40 intravenous infusion is used in an attempt to improve peripheral blood flow in ischaemic disease of the limbs. Dextrans 40 and 70 have also been used in the prophylaxis of thromboembolism but are now rarely used for this purpose.

Dextrans may interfere with blood group cross-matching or biochemical measurements and these should be carried out before infusion is begun.

> Plasma and plasma substitutes are often used in very ill patients whose condition is unstable. Therefore, close monitoring is required and fluid and electrolyte therapy should be adjusted according to the patient's condition at all times.

Cautions Plasma substitutes should be used with caution in patients with cardiac disease, liver disease, or renal impairment; urine output should be monitored. Care should be taken to avoid haematocrit concentration from falling below 25–30% and the patient should be monitored for hypersensitivity reactions.

Side-effects Hypersensitivity reactions may occur including, rarely, severe anaphylactoid reactions. Transient increase in bleeding time may occur.

DEXTRAN 40

Dextrans of weight average molecular weight about '40 000'

Indications conditions associated with peripheral local slowing of the blood flow; prophylaxis of post-surgical thromboembolic disease (but see notes above)

Cautions see notes above; can interfere with some laboratory tests (see also above); correct dehydration beforehand, give adequate fluids during therapy and, where possible, monitor central venous pressure; pregnancy (Appendix 4)

Side-effects see notes above

Dose

- By intravenous infusion, initially 500–1000 mL; further doses are given according to the patient's condition (see notes above)

Dextran 40® (Baxter) PoM
Intravenous infusion, dextran 40 intravenous infusion in glucose intravenous infusion 5% or in sodium chloride intravenous infusion 0.9%. Net price 500-mL bag (both) = £4.56

DEXTRAN 70

Dextrans of weight average molecular weight about '70 000'

Indications short-term blood volume expansion; prophylaxis of post-surgical thromboembolic disease (but see notes above)

Cautions see notes above; can interfere with some laboratory tests (see also above); where possible, monitor central venous pressure; pregnancy (Appendix 4)

Side-effects see notes above

Dose

- By intravenous infusion, after moderate to severe haemorrhage or in the shock phase of burn injury (initial 48 hours), 500–1000 mL rapidly initially followed by 500 mL later if necessary (see also notes above); total dosage should not exceed 20 mL/kg during initial 24 hours; CHILD total dosage should not exceed 20 mL/kg

9 Nutrition and blood

Dextran 70® (Baxter) PoM
Intravenous infusion, dextran 70 intravenous infusion in glucose intravenous infusion 5% or in sodium chloride intravenous infusion 0.9%. Net price 500-mL bag (both) = £4.56

Hypertonic solution

RescueFlow® (Vitaline) PoM
Intravenous infusion, dextran 70 intravenous infusion 6% in sodium chloride intravenous infusion 7.5%. Net price 250-mL bag = £28.50
Cautions see notes above; severe hyperglycaemia and hyperosmolality
Dose initial treatment of hypovolaemia with hypotension induced by traumatic injury, by intravenous infusion over 2–5 minutes, 250 mL, followed immediately by administration of isotonic fluids

GELATIN

Note The gelatin is partially degraded

Indications low blood volume

Cautions see notes above

Side-effects see notes above

Dose

- By intravenous infusion, initially 500–1000 mL of a 3.5–4% solution (see notes above)

Gelofusine® (Braun) PoM
Intravenous infusion, succinylated gelatin (modified fluid gelatin, average molecular weight 30 000) 40 g (4%), Na^+ 154 mmol, Cl^- 120 mmol/litre, net price 500-mL *Ecobag®* = £4.70, 1-litre *Ecobag®* = £9.45

Haemaccel® (KoRa) PoM
Intravenous infusion, polygeline (gelatin derivative, average molecular weight 30 000) 35 g (3.5%), Na^+ 145 mmol, K^+ 5.1 mmol, Ca^{2+} 6.25 mmol, Cl^- 145 mmol/litre net price 500–mL bottle = £5.00

Volplex® (Maelor) PoM
Intravenous infusion, succinylated gelatin (modified fluid gelatin, average molecular weight 30 000) 40 g (4%), Na^+ 154 mmol, Cl^- 125 mmol/litre, net price 500-mL bag = £4.70, 1-litre bag = £9.09

ETHERIFIED STARCH

A starch composed of more than 90% of amylopectin that has been etherified with hydroxyethyl groups; hetastarch has a higher degree of etherification than pentastarch

Indications low blood volume

Cautions see notes above; children

Side-effects see notes above; also pruritus, raised serum amylase

Dose

- See under preparations below

Hetastarch

Hetastarch (Non-proprietary) PoM
Intravenous infusion, hetastarch (weight average molecular weight 450 000) 6% in sodium chloride intravenous infusion 0.9%, net price 500-mL bag = £8.00
Dose by intravenous infusion, 500–1000 mL; usual daily max. 1500 mL (see notes above)

Pentastarch

Pentastarch (Non-proprietary) PoM
Intravenous infusion, pentastarch (weight average molecular weight 200 000), net price (both in sodium chloride intravenous infusion 0.9%) 6%, 500-mL bag = £7.85; 10%, 500-mL bag = £9.24
Dose by intravenous infusion, pentastarch 6%, 500–1000 mL; max. 2500 mL daily; pentastarch 10%, 500–1000 mL; max. 1500 mL daily (see notes above)

HAES-steril® (Fresenius Kabi) PoM
Intravenous infusion, pentastarch (weight average molecular weight 200 000) 10% in sodium chloride intravenous infusion 0.9%, net price 500 mL = £16.50
Dose by intravenous infusion, up to 1500 mL daily (see notes above)

Hemohes® (Braun) PoM
Intravenous infusion, pentastarch (weight average molecular weight 200 000), net price (both in sodium chloride intravenous infusion 0.9%) 6%, 500 mL = £12.50; 10%, 500 mL = £16.50
Cautions see notes above
Dose by intravenous infusion, pentastarch 6%, up to 2500 mL daily; pentastarch 10%, up to 1500 mL daily (see notes above)

Infukoll® (Beacon) PoM
Intravenous infusion, pentastarch (weight average molecular weight 200 000) 6% in sodium chloride intravenous infusion 0.9%, net price 500-mL bag = £10.00
Dose by intravenous infusion, up to 2 500 mL daily (see notes above)

Tetrastarch

Venofundin® (Braun) PoM

Intravenous infusion, hydroxyethyl starch (weight average molecular weight 130 000) 6% in sodium chloride intravenous infusion 0.9%, net price 500-mL bag = £12.90

Dose by intravenous infusion, up to 50 mL/kg daily (see notes above)

Voluven® (Fresenius Kabi) PoM

Intravenous infusion, hydroxyethyl starch (weight average molecular weight 130 000) 6% in sodium chloride intravenous infusion 0.9%, net price 500-mL bag = £12.50

Dose by intravenous infusion, up to 50 mL/kg daily (see notes above)

Hypertonic solution

HyperHAES® (Fresenius Kabi) PoM

Intravenous infusion, hydroxyethyl starch (weight average molecular weight 200 000) 6% in sodium chloride intravenous infusion 7.2%, net price 250-mL bag = £28.00

Cautions see notes above; also diabetes

Dose by intravenous injection over 2–5 minutes, 4 mL/kg as a single dose, followed immediately by administration of appropriate replacement fluids

9.3 Intravenous nutrition

When adequate feeding through the alimentary tract is not possible, nutrients may be given by intravenous infusion. This may be in addition to ordinary oral or tube feeding—**supplemental parenteral nutrition**, or may be the sole source of nutrition—**total parenteral nutrition** (TPN). Indications for this method include preparation of undernourished patients for surgery, chemotherapy, or radiation therapy; severe or prolonged disorders of the gastro-intestinal tract; major surgery, trauma, or burns; prolonged coma or refusal to eat; and some patients with renal or hepatic failure. The composition of proprietary preparations available is given in the table Proprietary Infusion Fluids for Parenteral Feeding, p. 512.

Parenteral nutrition requires the use of a solution containing amino acids, glucose, fat, electrolytes, trace elements, and vitamins. This is now commonly provided by the pharmacy in the form of a 3-litre bag. A single dose of vitamin B_{12}, as hydroxocobalamin, is given by intramuscular injection; regular vitamin B_{12} injections are not usually required unless total parenteral nutrition continues for many months. Folic acid is given in a dose of 15 mg once or twice each week, usually in the nutrition solution. Other vitamins are usually given daily; they are generally introduced in the parenteral nutrition solution. Alternatively, if the patient is able to take small amounts by mouth, vitamins may be given orally.

The nutrition solution is infused through a central venous catheter inserted under full surgical precautions. Alternatively infusion through a peripheral vein may be used for supplementary as well as total parenteral nutrition for periods of up to a month, depending on the availability of peripheral veins; factors prolonging cannula life and preventing thrombophlebitis include the use of soft polyurethane paediatric cannulas and use of feeds of low osmolality and neutral pH. Only nutritional fluids should be given by the dedicated intravenous line.

Before starting, the patient should be well oxygenated with a near normal circulating blood volume and attention should be given to renal function and acid-base status. Appropriate biochemical tests should have been carried out beforehand and serious deficits corrected. Nutritional and electrolyte status must be monitored throughout treatment.

Complications of long-term parenteral nutrition include gall bladder sludging, gall stones, cholestasis and abnormal liver function tests. For details of the prevention and management of parenteral nutrition complications, specialist literature should be consulted.

Protein is given as mixtures of essential and non-essential synthetic L-amino acids. Ideally, all essential amino acids should be included with a wide variety of non-essential ones to provide sufficient nitrogen together with electrolytes (see also section 9.2.2). Solutions vary in their composition of amino acids; they often contain an energy source (usually glucose) and electrolytes.

Energy is provided in a ratio of 0.6 to 1.1 megajoules (150–250 kcals) per gram of protein nitrogen. Energy requirements must be met if amino acids are to be utilised for tissue maintenance. A mixture of carbohydrate and fat energy sources (usually 30–50% as fat) gives better utilisation of amino acids than glucose alone.

Glucose is the preferred source of carbohydrate, but if more than 180 g is given per day frequent monitoring of blood glucose is required, and insulin may be necessary. Glucose in various strengths from 10 to 50% must be infused through a central venous catheter to avoid thrombosis.

In total parenteral nutrition regimens, it is necessary to provide adequate phosphate in order to allow phosphorylation of the glucose and to prevent hypophosphataemia; between 20 and 30 mmol of phosphate is required daily.

Fructose and sorbitol have been used in an attempt to avoid the problem of hyperosmolar hyperglycaemic non-ketotic acidosis but other metabolic problems may occur, as with xylitol and ethanol which are now rarely used.

Fat emulsions have the advantages of a high energy to fluid volume ratio, neutral pH, and iso-osmolarity with plasma, and provide essential fatty acids. Several days of adaptation may be required to attain maximal utilisation. Reactions include occasional febrile episodes (usually only with 20% emulsions) and rare anaphylactic responses. Interference with biochemical measurements such as those for blood gases and calcium may occur if samples are taken before fat has been cleared. Daily checks are necessary to ensure complete clearance from the plasma in conditions where fat metabolism may be disturbed. **Additives may only be mixed with fat emulsions where compatibility is known.**

Administration. Because of the complex requirements relating to parenteral nutrition full details relating to administration have been omitted. In all cases *product literature and other specialist literature should be consulted.*

Proprietary Infusion Fluids for Parenteral Feeding

Preparation	Nitrogen g/litre	[1,2]Energy kJ/litre	Electrolytes mmol/litre					Other components/litre
			K^+	Mg^{2+}	Na^+	$Acet^-$	Cl^-	
Aminoplasmal 5% E (Braun) Net price 500 mL = £9.02	8		25	2.6	43	59	29	dihydrogen phosphate 9 mmol, malic acid 1.01 g
Aminoplasmal 10% (Braun) Net price 500 mL = £17.06	16						57	
Aminoven 25 (Fresenius Kabi) Net price 500 mL = £22.00	25.7							
Clinimix N9G20E (Baxter) Net price (dual compartment bag of amino acids with electrolytes 1000 mL and glucose 20% with calcium 1000 mL) = £29.00	4.55	1680	30	2.5	35	50	40	Ca^{2+} 2.25 mmol, phosphate 15 mmol, anhydrous glucose 100 g
Clinimix N14G30E (Baxter) Net price (dual compartment bag of amino acids with electrolytes 1000 mL and glucose 30% with calcium 1000 mL) = £33.00	7	2520	30	2.5	35	70	40	Ca^{2+} 2.25 mmol, phosphate 15 mmol, anhydrous glucose 150 g
ClinOleic 20% (Baxter) Net price 100 mL = £6.28; 250 mL = £10.08; 500 mL = £13.88		8360						purified olive and soya oil 200 g, glycerol 22.5 g, egg phosphatides 12 g
Glamin (Fresenius Kabi) Net price 250 mL = £14.16; 500 mL = £26.38	22.4					62		
Hyperamine 30 (Braun) Net price 500 mL = £23.67	30				5			
Intrafusin 22 (Fresenius Kabi) Net price 500 mL = £17.80	22.8							
Intralipid 10% (Fresenius Kabi) Net price 100 mL = £4.70; 500 mL = £10.30		4600						soya oil 100 g, glycerol 22 g, purified egg phospholipids 12 g, phosphate 15 mmol
Intralipid 20% (Fresenius Kabi) Net price 100 mL = £7.05; 250 mL = £11.60; 500 mL = £15.45		8400						soya oil 200 g, glycerol 22 g, purified egg phospholipids 12 g, phosphate 15 mmol
Intralipid 30% (Fresenius Kabi) Net price 333 mL = £17.30		12600						soya oil 300 g, glycerol 16.7 g, purified egg phospholipids 12 g, phosphate 15 mmol
Ivelip 10% (Baxter) Net price 500 mL = £9.08		4600						soya oil 100 g, glycerol 25 g
Ivelip 20% (Baxter) Net price 100 mL = £6.28; 500 mL = £13.88		8400						soya oil 200 g, glycerol 25 g
Kabiven (Fresenius Kabi) Net price (triple compartment bag of amino acids and electrolytes 300 mL, 450 mL, 600 mL, or 750 mL; glucose 526 mL, 790 mL, 1053 mL, or 1316 mL; lipid emulsion 200 mL, 300 mL, 400 mL, or 500 mL) 1026 mL = £35.00, 1540 mL = £50.00, 2053 mL = £67.00, 2566 mL = £70.00	5.3	3275	23	4	31	38	45	Ca^{2+} 2 mmol, phosphate 9.7 mmol, anhydrous glucose 97 g, soya oil 39 g
Kabiven Peripheral (Fresenius Kabi) Net price (triple compartment bag of amino acids and electrolytes 300 mL, 400 mL, or 500 mL; glucose 885 mL, 1180 mL, or 1475 mL; lipid emulsion 255 mL, 340 mL, or 425 mL) 1440 mL = £35.00, 1920 mL = £50.00, 2400 mL = £64.00	3.75	2625	17	2.8	22	27	33	Ca^{2+} 1.4 mmol, phosphate 7.5 mmol, anhydrous glucose 67.5 g, soya oil 35.4 g

1. *Note.* 1000 kcal = 4200 kJ; 1000 kJ = 238.8 kcal. All entries are PoM
2. Excludes protein- or amino acid-derived energy

Preparation	Nitrogen g/litre	[1,2]Energy kJ/litre	Electrolytes mmol/litre					Other components/litre
			K^+	Mg^{2+}	Na^+	Acet⁻	Cl^-	
Lipidem (Braun) Net price 100 mL = £18.00; 250 mL = £30.00; 500 mL = £38.00		7900						omega-3-acid triglycerides 20 g, soya oil 80 g, medium-chain triglycerides 100 g
Lipofundin MCT/LCT 10% (Braun) Net price 100 mL = £7.70; 500 mL = £12.90		4430						soya oil 50 g, medium-chain triglycerides 50 g
Lipofundin MCT/LCT 20% (Braun) Net price 100 mL = £12.51; 250 mL = £11.30; 500 mL = £19.18		8000						soya oil 100 g, medium-chain triglycerides 100 g
Nutracel 400 (Baxter) Net price 500 mL = £2.43		3400		18		0.16	66	Ca^{2+} 15 mmol, Mn^{2+} 10 micromol, Zn^{2+} 80 micromol, anhydrous glucose 200 g
Nutracel 800 (Baxter) Net price 1000 mL = £4.19		3400		9		0.08	33	Ca^{2+} 7.5 mmol, Mn^{2+} 5 micromol, Zn^{2+} 40 micromol, anhydrous glucose 200 g
NuTRIflex Lipid peri (Braun) Net price (triple compartment bag of amino acids 500 mL or 1000 mL; glucose 500 mL or 1000 mL; lipid emulsion 20% 250 mL or 500 mL) 1250 mL = £43.38, 2500 mL = £65.05	4.56	2664	24	2.4	40	32	38.4	Ca^{2+} 2.4 mmol, Zn^{2+} 24 micromol, phosphate 6 mmol, anhydrous glucose 64 g, soya oil 20 g, medium-chain triglycerides 20 g
NuTRIflex Lipid plus (Braun) Net price (triple compartment bag of amino acids 500 mL, 750 mL or 1000 mL; glucose 500 mL, 750 mL or 1000 mL; lipid emulsion 20% 250 mL, 375 mL or 500 mL) 1250 mL = £47.17, 1875 mL = £60.23, 2500 mL = £69.27	5.44	3600	28	3.2	40	36	36	Ca^{2+} 3.2 mmol, Zn^{2+} 24 micromol, phosphate 12 mmol, anhydrous glucose 120 g, soya oil 20 g, medium-chain triglycerides 20 g
NuTRIflex Lipid plus without Electrolytes (Braun) Net price (triple compartment bag of amino acids 500 mL, 750 mL or 1000 mL; glucose 500 mL, 750 mL or 1000 mL; lipid emulsion 20% 250 mL, 375 mL or 500 mL) 1250 mL = £47.17, 1875 mL = £60.23, 2500 mL = £69.27	5.44	3600						anhydrous glucose 120 g, soya oil 20 g, medium-chain triglycerides 20 g
NuTRIflex Lipid special (Braun) Net price (triple compartment bag of amino acids 500 mL, 750 mL or 1000 mL; glucose 500 mL, 750 mL or 1000 mL; lipid emulsion 20% 250 mL, 375 mL or 500 mL) 1250 mL = £57.69, 1875 mL = £75.58, 2500 mL = £89.21	8	4004	37.6	4.24	53.6	48	48	Ca^{2+} 4.24 mmol, Zn^{2+} 32 micromol, phosphate 16 mmol, anhydrous glucose 144 g, soya oil 20 g, medium-chain triglycerides 20 g
NuTRIflex Lipid special without Electrolytes (Braun) Net price (triple compartment bag of amino acids 500 mL, 750 mL or 1000 mL; glucose 500 mL, 750 mL or 1000 mL; lipid emulsion 20% 250 mL, 375 mL or 500 mL) 1250 mL = £57.69, 1875 mL = £75.58, 2500 mL = £89.21	8	4004						anhydrous glucose 144 g, soya oil 20 g, medium-chain triglycerides 20 g
OliClinomel N4-550E (Baxter) Net price (triple compartment bag of amino acids with electrolytes 1000 mL; glucose 20% 1000 mL; lipid emulsion 10% 500 mL) 2500 mL = £69.30	3.6	2184	16	2.2	21	30	33	Ca^{2+} 2 mmol, phosphate 8.5 mmol, refined olive and soya oil 20 g, anhydrous glucose 80 g

1. *Note.* 1000 kcal = 4200 kJ; 1000 kJ = 238.8 kcal. All entries are PoM
2. Excludes protein- or amino acid-derived energy

Preparation	Nitrogen g/litre	[1,2]Energy kJ/litre	Electrolytes mmol/litre K$^+$	Mg^{2+}	Na$^+$	Acet$^-$	Cl$^-$	Other components/litre
OliClinomel N4-720E (Baxter) Net price (triple compartment bag of amino acids with electrolytes 1000 mL; glucose 20% 1000 mL; lipid emulsion 20% 500 mL) 2500 mL = £69.30	3.64	3024	24	2	28	40	40	Ca^{2+} 1.8 mmol, phosphate 8 mmol, refined olive and soya oil 40 g, anhydrous glucose 80 g
OliClinomel N5-800E (Baxter) Net price (triple compartment bag of amino acids with electrolytes 800 mL or 1000 mL; glucose 25% 800 mL or 1000 mL; lipid emulsion 20% 400 mL or 500 mL) 2000 mL = £60.39, 2500 mL = £65.34	4.6	3360	24	2.2	32	49	44	Ca^{2+} 2 mmol, phosphate 10 mmol, refined olive and soya oil 40 g, anhydrous glucose 100 g
OliClinomel N6-900E (Baxter) Net price (triple compartment bag of amino acids with electrolytes 800 mL or 1000 mL; glucose 30% 800 mL or 1000 mL; lipid emulsion 20% 400 mL or 500 mL) 2000 mL = £70.40, 2500 mL = £75.90	5.6	3696	24	2.2	32	53	46	Ca^{2+} 2 mmol, phosphate 10 mmol, refined olive and soya oil 40 g, anhydrous glucose 120 g
OliClinomel N7-1000 (Baxter) Net price (triple compartment bag of amino acids 600 mL; glucose 40% 600 mL; lipid emulsion 20% 300 mL) 1500 mL = £43.70	6.6	4368				37	16	phosphate 3 mmol, refined olive and soya oil 40 g, anhydrous glucose 160 g
OliClinomel N7-1000E (Baxter) Net price (triple compartment bag of amino acids with electrolytes 800 mL; glucose 40% 800 mL; lipid emulsion 20% 400 mL) 2000 mL = £66.33	6.6	4368	24	2.2	32	57	48	Ca^{2+} 2 mmol, phosphate 10 mmol, refined olive and soya oil 40 g, anhydrous glucose 160 g
OliClinomel N8-800 (Baxter) Net price (triple compartment bag of amino acids 800 mL; glucose 31.25% 800 mL; lipid emulsion 15% 400 mL) 2000 mL = £77.10	8.25	3360				42.5	20	phosphate 2.25 mmol, refined olive and soya oil 30 g, anhydrous glucose 125 g
Omegaven (Fresenius Kabi) Net price 100 mL = £22.50		4700						highly refined fish oil 100 g, glycerol 25 g, egg phosphatide 12 g
Plasma-Lyte 148 (water) (Baxter) Net price 1000 mL = £1.59			5	1.5	140	27	98	gluconate 23 mmol
Plasma-Lyte 148 (dextrose 5%) (Baxter) Net price 1000 mL = £1.59		840	5	1.5	140	27	98	gluconate 23 mmol, anhydrous glucose 50 g
Plasma-Lyte M (dextrose 5%) (Baxter) Net price 1000 mL = £1.33		840	16	1.5	40	12	40	Ca^{2+} 2.5 mmol, lactate 12 mmol, anhydrous glucose 50 g
[3]Primene 10% (Baxter) Net price 100 mL = £5.78, 250 mL = £7.92	15						19	
SMOFlipid (Fresenius Kabi) Net price 500 mL = £20.50		8400						fish oil 30 g, olive oil 50 g, soya oil 60 g, medium-chain triglycerides 60 g
StructoKabiven Electrolyte Free (Fresenius Kabi) Net price (triple compartment bag of amino acids 500 mL, 750 mL or 1000 mL; glucose 42% 298 mL, 446 mL or 595 mL; lipid emulsion 188 mL, 281 mL or 375 mL) 986 mL = £66.50, 1477 mL = £69.00, 1970 mL = £74.00	8	3685				74.5		phosphate 2.8 mmol, anhydrous glucose 127 g, glycerol 4.23 g, egg phospholipids 4.56 g, purified structured triglyceride 38.5 g (contains coconut oil, palm kernel oil and soya oil trigylcerides)
Structolipid 20% (Fresenius Kabi) Net price 500 mL = £16.09		8200						purified structured triglyceride 200 g (contains coconut oil, palm kernel oil, and soya oil triglycerides)

1. *Note.* 1000 kcal = 4200 kJ; 1000 kJ = 238.8 kcal. All entries are PoM
2. Excludes protein- or amino acid-derived energy
3. For use in neonates and children only

Preparation	Nitrogen g/litre	[1,2]Energy kJ/litre	Electrolytes mmol/litre					Other components/litre
			K^+	Mg^{2+}	Na^+	$Acet^-$	Cl^-	
Synthamin 9 (Baxter) Net price 500 mL = £6.66; 1000 mL = £12.34	9.1		60	5	70	100	70	acid phosphate 30 mmol
Synthamin 9 EF (electrolyte-free) (Baxter) Net price 500 mL = £6.66; 1000 mL = £12.34	9.1					44	22	
Synthamin 14 (Baxter) Net price 500 mL = £9.64; 1000 mL = £17.13; 3000 mL = £48.98	14		60	5	70	140	70	acid phosphate 30 mmol
Synthamin 14 EF (electrolyte-free) (Baxter) Net price 500 mL = £9.87; 1000 mL = £17.51	14					68	34	
Synthamin 17 (Baxter) Net price 500 mL = £12.66; 1000 mL = £23.00	16.5		60	5	70	150	70	acid phosphate 30 mmol
Synthamin 17 EF (electrolyte-free) (Baxter) Net price 500 mL = £12.66; 1000 mL = £23.00	16.5					82	40	
Vamin 9 Glucose (Fresenius Kabi) Net price 100 mL = £3.80; 500 mL = £7.70; 1000 mL = £13.40	9.4	1700	20	1.5	50		50	Ca^{2+} 2.5 mmol, anhydrous glucose 100 g
Vamin 14 (Fresenius Kabi) Net price 500 mL = £10.80; 1000 mL = £14.67	13.5		50	8	100	135	100	Ca^{2+} 5 mmol, SO_4^{2-} 8 mmol
Vamin 14 (Electrolyte-Free) (Fresenius Kabi) Net price 500 mL = £10.80; 1000 mL = £18.30	13.5					90		
Vamin 18 (Electrolyte-Free) (Fresenius Kabi) Net price 500 mL = £13.70; 1000 mL = £26.70	18					110		
Vaminolact (Fresenius Kabi) Net price 100 mL = £4.20; 500 mL = £9.70	9.3							

Supplementary preparations

Compatibility with the infusion solution must be ascertained before adding supplementary preparations.

Addiphos® (Fresenius Kabi) PoM
Solution, sterile, phosphate 40 mmol, K^+ 30 mmol, Na^+ 30 mmol/20 mL. For addition to *Vamin®* solutions and glucose intravenous infusions. Net price 20-mL vial = £1.53

Additrace® (Fresenius Kabi) PoM
Solution, trace elements for addition to *Vamin®* solutions and glucose intravenous infusions, traces of Fe^{3+}, Zn^{2+}, Mn^{2+}, Cu^{2+}, Cr^{3+}, Se^{4+}, Mo^{6+}, F^-, I^-. For adults and children over 40 kg. Net price 10-mL amp = £2.31

Cernevit® (Baxter) PoM
Solution, *dl*-alpha tocopherol 11.2 units, ascorbic acid 125 mg, biotin 69 micrograms, colecalciferol 220 units, cyanocobalamin 6 micrograms, folic acid 414 micrograms, glycine 250 mg, nicotinamide 46 mg, pantothenic acid (as dexpanthenol) 17.25 mg, pyridoxine hydrochloride 5.5 mg, retinol (as palmitate) 3500 units, riboflavin (as dihydrated sodium phosphate) 4.14 mg, thiamine (as cocarboxylase tetrahydrate) 3.51 mg. Dissolve in 5 mL water for injections. Net price per vial = £2.90

Decan® (Baxter) PoM
Solution, trace elements for addition to infusion solutions, Fe^{2+}, Zn^{2+}, Cu^{2+}, Mn^{2+}, F^-, Co^{2+}, I^-, Se^{4+}, Mo^{6+}, Cr^{3+}. For adults and children over 40 kg. Net price 40-mL vial = £2.00

Dipeptiven® (Fresenius Kabi) PoM
Solution, *N*(2)-L-alanyl-L-glutamine 200 mg/mL (providing L-alanine 82 mg, L-glutamine 134.6 mg). For addition to infusion solutions containing amino acids. Net price 50 mL = £15.90, 100 mL = £29.60

Dose amino acid supplement for hypercatabolic or hypermetabolic states, 300–400 mg/kg daily; max. 400 mg/kg daily, dose not to exceed 20% of total amino acid intake

1. *Note.* 1000 kcal = 4200 kJ; 1000 kJ = 238.8 kcal. All entries are PoM
2. Excludes protein- or amino acid-derived energy

Glycophos® Sterile Concentrate (Fresenius Kabi) PoM
Solution, sterile, phosphate 20 mmol, Na^+ 40 mmol/ 20 mL. For addition to *Vamin®* and *Vaminolact®* solutions, and glucose intravenous infusions. Net price 20-mL vial = £4.25

Peditrace® (Fresenius Kabi) PoM
Solution, trace elements for addition to *Vaminolact®*, *Vamin® 14 Electrolyte-Free* solutions and glucose intravenous infusions, traces of Zn^{2+}, Cu^{2+}, Mn^{2+}, Se^{4+}, F^-, I^-. For use in neonates (when kidney function established, usually second day of life), infants, and children. Net price 10-mL vial = £3.88
Cautions reduced biliary excretion especially in cholestatic liver disease or in markedly reduced urinary excretion (careful biochemical monitoring required); total parenteral nutrition exceeding 1 month (measure serum manganese concentration and check liver function before commencing treatment and regularly during treatment)—discontinue if manganese concentration raised or if cholestasis develops

Solivito N® (Fresenius Kabi) PoM
Solution, powder for reconstitution, biotin 60 micrograms, cyanocobalamin 5 micrograms, folic acid 400 micrograms, glycine 300 mg, nicotinamide 40 mg, pyridoxine hydrochloride 4.9 mg, riboflavin sodium phosphate 4.9 mg, sodium ascorbate 113 mg, sodium pantothenate 16.5 mg, thiamine mononitrate 3.1 mg. Dissolve in water for injections or glucose intravenous infusion for adding to glucose intravenous infusion or *Intralipid®*; dissolve in *Vitlipid N®* or *Intralipid®* for adding to *Intralipid®* only. Net price per vial = £2.32

Vitlipid N® (Fresenius Kabi) PoM
Emulsion, adult, vitamin A 330 units, ergocalciferol 20 units, *dl*-alpha tocopherol 1 unit, phytomenadione 15 micrograms/mL. For addition to *Intralipid®*. For adults and children over 11 years. Net price 10-mL amp = £2.32
Emulsion, infant, vitamin A 230 units, ergocalciferol 40 units, *dl*-alpha tocopherol 0.7 unit, phytomenadione 20 micrograms/mL. For addition to *Intralipid®*. Net price 10-mL amp = £2.32

9.4 Oral nutrition

9.4.1 Foods for special diets
9.4.2 Enteral nutrition

9.4.1 Foods for special diets

These are preparations that have been modified to eliminate a particular constituent from a food or are nutrient mixtures formulated as substitutes for the food. They are for patients who either cannot tolerate or cannot metabolise certain common constituents of food.

Phenylketonuria Phenylketonuria (phenylalaninaemia), which results from the inability to metabolise phenylalanine, is managed by restricting its dietary intake to a small amount sufficient for tissue building and repair. **Aspartame** (as a sweetener in some foods and medicines) contributes to the phenylalanine intake and may affect control of phenylketonuria. Where the presence of aspartame is specified in the product literature this is indicated in the BNF against the preparation.

Coeliac disease Coeliac disease, which results from an intolerance to gluten, is managed by completely eliminating gluten from the diet.

ACBS
In certain clinical conditions some foods may have the characteristics of drugs and the Advisory Committee on Borderline Substances advises as to the circumstances in which such foods may be regarded as drugs and so can be prescribed in the NHS. Prescriptions for these foods issued in accordance with the advice of this committee and endorsed 'ACBS' will normally not be investigated. See Appendix 7 for details of these foods and a listing by clinical condition (consult Drug Tariff for late amendments).

Preparations
For preparations on the ACBS list see Appendix 7

9.4.2 Enteral nutrition

The body's reserves of protein rapidly become exhausted in severely ill patients, especially during chronic illness or in those with severe burns, extensive trauma, pancreatitis, or intestinal fistula. Much can be achieved by frequent meals and by persuading the patient to take supplementary snacks of ordinary food between the meals.

However, extra calories, protein, other nutrients, and vitamins are often best given by supplementing ordinary meals with sip or tube feeds of one of the nutritionally complete foods.

When patients cannot feed normally at all, for example, patients with severe facial injury, oesophageal obstruction, or coma, a diet composed solely of nutritionally complete foods must be given. This is planned by a dietitian who will take into account the protein and total energy requirement of the patient and decide on the form and relative contribution of carbohydrate and fat to the energy requirements.

There are a number of nutritionally complete foods available and their use reduces an otherwise heavy workload in hospital or in the home. Most contain protein derived from milk or soya. Some contain protein hydrolysates or free amino acids and are only appropriate for patients who have diminished ability to break down protein, as may be the case in inflammatory bowel disease or pancreatic insufficiency.

Even when nutritionally complete feeds are being given it may be important to monitor water and electrolyte balance. Extra minerals (e.g. magnesium and zinc) may be needed in patients where gastro-intestinal secretions are being lost. Additional vitamins may also be needed.

Regular haematological and biochemical tests may be needed particularly in the unstable patient.

Some feeds are supplemented with vitamin K; for drug interactions of vitamin K see Appendix 1 (vitamins).

Children Infants and young children have special requirements and in most situations liquid feeds prepared for adults are totally unsuitable and should not be given. Expert advice should be sought.

Preparations
See Appendix 7

9.5 Minerals

9.5.1 Calcium and magnesium
9.5.2 Phosphorus
9.5.3 Fluoride
9.5.4 Zinc
9.5.5 Selenium

See section 9.1.1 for iron salts.

9.5.1 Calcium and magnesium

9.5.1.1 Calcium supplements
9.5.1.2 Hypercalcaemia and hypercalciuria
9.5.1.3 Magnesium

9.5.1.1 Calcium supplements

Calcium supplements are usually only required where dietary calcium intake is deficient. This dietary requirement varies with age and is relatively greater in childhood, pregnancy, and lactation, due to an increased demand, and in old age, due to impaired absorption. In osteoporosis, a calcium intake which is double the recommended amount reduces the rate of bone loss. If the actual dietary intake is less than the recommended amount, a supplement of as much as 40 mmol is appropriate, see also Osteoporosis, p. 404 and Vitamin D, p. 525.

In hypocalcaemic tetany an initial intravenous injection of 10 mL of calcium gluconate injection 10% (providing approximately 2.25 mmol of calcium) should be followed by the continuous infusion of about 40 mL daily (providing approximately 9 mmol of calcium), but plasma calcium should be monitored. This regimen can also be used immediately to temporarily reduce the toxic effects of hyperkalaemia.

CALCIUM SALTS

Indications see notes above; calcium deficiency

Cautions renal impairment; sarcoidosis; history of nephrolithiasis; avoid calcium chloride in respiratory acidosis or respiratory failure; **interactions:** Appendix 1 (antacids, calcium salts)

Contra-indications conditions associated with hypercalcaemia and hypercalciuria (e.g. some forms of malignant disease)

Side-effects gastro-intestinal disturbances; bradycardia, arrhythmias; *with injection*, peripheral vasodilatation, fall in blood pressure, injection-site reactions

Dose

- By mouth, daily in divided doses, see notes above
- By slow intravenous injection, acute hypocalcaemia, calcium gluconate 1–2 g (Ca^{2+} 2.25–4.5 mmol); CHILD obtain paediatric advice

Oral preparations

Calcium Gluconate (Non-proprietary)
Tablets, calcium gluconate 600 mg (calcium 53.4 mg or Ca^{2+} 1.35 mmol), net price 20 = £1.43. Label: 24
Effervescent tablets, calcium gluconate 1 g (calcium 89 mg or Ca^{2+} 2.23 mmol), net price 28-tab pack = £4.62. Label: 13
Note Each tablet usually contains 4.46 mmol Na^+

Calcium Lactate (Non-proprietary)
Tablets, calcium lactate 300 mg (calcium 39 mg or Ca^{2+} 1 mmol), net price 84 = £3.11

Adcal® (ProStrakan)
Chewable tablets, fruit flavour, calcium carbonate 1.5 g (calcium 600 mg or Ca^{2+} 15 mmol), net price 100-tab pack = £7.25. Label: 24

Cacit® (Procter & Gamble Pharm.)
Tablets, effervescent, pink, calcium carbonate 1.25 g, providing calcium citrate when dispersed in water (calcium 500 mg or Ca^{2+} 12.6 mmol), net price 76-tab pack = £12.54. Label: 13

Calcichew® (Shire)
Tablets (chewable), orange flavour, calcium carbonate 1.25 g (calcium 500 mg or Ca^{2+} 12.6 mmol), net price 100-tab pack = £9.33. Label: 24
Forte tablets (chewable), orange flavour, scored, calcium carbonate 2.5 g (calcium 1 g or Ca^{2+} 25 mmol), net price 60-tab pack = £13.16. Label: 24
Excipients include aspartame (section 9.4.1)

Calcium-500 (Martindale)
Tablets, pink, f/c, calcium carbonate 1.25 g (calcium 500 mg or Ca^{2+} 12.5 mmol). Net price 100-tab pack = £9.46. Label: 25

Calcium-Sandoz® (Alliance)
Syrup, orange flavour, calcium glubionate 1.09 g, calcium lactobionate 727 mg (calcium 108.3 mg or Ca^{2+} 2.7 mmol)/5 mL. Net price 300 mL = £3.39

Sandocal® (Novartis Consumer Health)
Sandocal-400 tablets, effervescent, orange flavour, calcium lactate gluconate 930 mg, calcium carbonate 700 mg, anhydrous citric acid 1.189 g, providing calcium 400 mg (Ca^{2+} 10 mmol). Net price 5 × 20-tab pack = £6.87. Label: 13
Excipients include aspartame (section 9.4.1)
Sandocal-1000 tablets, effervescent, orange flavour, calcium lactate gluconate 2.263 g, calcium carbonate 1.75 g, anhydrous citric acid 2.973 g providing 1 g

calcium (Ca^{2+} 25 mmol). Net price 3 × 10-tab pack = £6.17. Label: 13
Excipients include aspartame (section 9.4.1)

Parenteral preparations

Calcium Gluconate (Non-proprietary) PoM
Injection, calcium gluconate 10% (calcium 8.4 mg or Ca^{2+} 226 micromol/mL). Net price 10-mL amp = 60p

Calcium Chloride (Non-proprietary) PoM
Injection, calcium chloride dihydrate 10% (calcium 27.3 mg or Ca^{2+} 680 micromol/mL). Net price 10-mL disposable syringe = £4.64
Brands include *Minijet® Calcium Chloride 10%*

Injection, calcium chloride dihydrate 13.4% (calcium 36 mg or Ca^{2+} 910 micromol/mL). Net price 10-mL amp = £14.94

With vitamin D

Section 9.6.4

With disodium etidronate

Section 6.6.2

9.5.1.2 Hypercalcaemia and hypercalciuria

Severe hypercalcaemia Severe hypercalcaemia calls for urgent treatment before detailed investigation of the cause. Dehydration should be corrected first with intravenous infusion of **sodium chloride 0.9%**. Drugs (such as thiazides and vitamin D compounds) which promote hypercalcaemia, should be discontinued and dietary calcium should be restricted.

If *severe hypercalcaemia persists* drugs which inhibit mobilisation of calcium from the skeleton may be required. The **bisphosphonates** are useful and disodium pamidronate (section 6.6.2) is probably the most effective.

Corticosteroids (section 6.3) are widely given, but may only be useful where hypercalcaemia is due to sarcoidosis or vitamin D intoxication; they often take several days to achieve the desired effect.

Calcitonin (section 6.6.1) is relatively non-toxic but is expensive and its effect can wear off after a few days despite continued use; it is rarely effective where bisphosphonates have failed to reduce serum calcium adequately.

After treatment of severe hypercalcaemia the underlying cause must be established. *Further treatment* is governed by the same principles as for initial therapy. Salt and water depletion and drugs promoting hypercalcaemia should be avoided; oral administration of a bisphosphonate may be useful.

Hyperparathyroidism **Cinacalcet** is licensed for the treatment of secondary hyperparathyroidism in dialysis patients with end-stage renal disease and for the treatment of hypercalcaemia in parathyroid carcinoma. Cinacalcet reduces parathyroid hormone which leads to a decrease in serum calcium concentrations.

Parathyroidectomy may be indicated for hyperparathyroidism.

> **NICE guidance**
> **Cinacalcet for the treatment of secondary hyperparathyroidism in patients with end-stage renal disease on maintenance dialysis therapy (January 2007)**
> Cinacalcet is not recommended for the routine treatment of secondary hyperparathyroidism in patients with end-stage renal disease on maintenance dialysis therapy.
> Cinacalcet is recommended for the treatment of refractory secondary hyperparathyroidism in patients with end-stage renal disease (including those with calciphylaxis) **only** in those:
> - who have 'very uncontrolled' plasma concentration of intact parathyroid hormone (defined as greater than 85 picomol/litre) refractory to standard therapy, and a normal or high adjusted serum calcium concentration,
> **and**
> - in whom surgical parathyroidectomy is contra-indicated, in that the risks of surgery outweigh the benefits.
>
> Response to treatment should be monitored regularly and treatment should be continued only if a reduction in the plasma concentration of intact parathyroid hormone of 30% or greater is seen within 4 months of treatment.

Hypercalciuria Hypercalciuria should be investigated for an underlying cause, which should be treated. Where a cause is not identified (idiopathic hypercalciuria), the condition is managed by increasing fluid intake and giving bendroflumethiazide in a dose of 2.5 mg daily (a higher dose is not usually necessary). Reducing dietary calcium intake may be beneficial but severe restriction of calcium intake has not proved beneficial and may even be harmful.

CINACALCET

Indications see under Dose

Cautions measure serum-calcium concentration before initiation of treatment and within 1 week after starting treatment or adjusting dose, then monthly for secondary hyperparathyroidism and every 2–3 months for parathyroid carcinoma; treatment should not be initiated in patients with hypocalcaemia; in secondary hyperparathyroidism measure parathyroid hormone concentration 1–4 weeks after starting treatment or adjusting dose, then every 1–3 months; dose adjustment may be necessary if smoking started or stopped during treatment; hepatic impairment (Appendix 2); pregnancy (Appendix 4); **interactions**: Appendix 1 (cinacalcet)

Contra-indications breast-feeding (Appendix 5)

Side-effects nausea, vomiting; anorexia, dizziness, paraesthesia, asthenia; reduced testosterone concentrations; myalgia; rash; *less commonly* dyspepsia, seizures

Dose
- Secondary hyperparathyroidism in patients with end-stage renal disease on dialysis, ADULT over 18 years, 30 mg once daily, adjusted every 2–4 weeks to max. 180 mg daily
- Hypercalcaemia of parathyroid carcinoma, ADULT over 18 years, initially 30 mg twice daily, adjusted every 2–4 weeks according to response up to max. 90 mg 4 times daily

Mimpara® (Amgen) PoM

Tablets, green, f/c, cinacalcet (as hydrochloride) 30 mg, net price 28-tab pack = £126.28; 60 mg, 28-tab pack = £232.96; 90 mg, 28-tab pack = £349.44. Label: 21

9.5.1.3 Magnesium

Magnesium is an essential constituent of many enzyme systems, particularly those involved in energy generation; the largest stores are in the skeleton.

Magnesium salts are not well absorbed from the gastro-intestinal tract, which explains the use of magnesium sulphate (section 1.6.4) as an osmotic laxative.

Magnesium is excreted mainly by the kidneys and is therefore retained in renal failure, but significant *hypermagnesaemia* (causing muscle weakness and arrhythmias) is rare.

Hypomagnesaemia Since magnesium is secreted in large amounts in the gastro-intestinal fluid, excessive losses in diarrhoea, stoma or fistula are the most common causes of *hypomagnesaemia*; deficiency may also occur in alcoholism or as a result of treatment with certain drugs. Hypomagnesaemia often causes secondary hypocalcaemia, and also hypokalaemia and hyponatraemia.

Symptomatic *hypomagnesaemia* is associated with a deficit of 0.5–1 mmol/kg; up to 160 mmol Mg^{2+} over up to 5 days may be required to replace the deficit (allowing for urinary losses). Magnesium is given initially by intravenous infusion or by intramuscular injection of **magnesium sulphate**; the intramuscular injection is painful. Plasma magnesium concentration should be measured to determine the rate and duration of infusion and the dose should be reduced in renal impairment. To prevent *recurrence of the deficit*, magnesium may be given by mouth in a dose of 24 mmol Mg^{2+} daily in divided doses; a suitable preparation is magnesium glycerophosphate tablets [not licensed, available from a specialist importing company]. For maintenance (e.g. in intravenous nutrition), parenteral doses of magnesium are of the order of 10–20 mmol Mg^{2+} daily (often about 12 mmol Mg^{2+} daily).

Arrhythmias Magnesium sulphate has also been recommended for the emergency treatment of *serious arrhythmias*, especially in the presence of hypokalaemia (when hypomagnesaemia may also be present) and when salvos of rapid ventricular tachycardia show the characteristic twisting wave front known as *torsade de pointes* (see also section 2.3.1). The usual dose of magnesium sulphate by intravenous injection is 8 mmol Mg^{2+} over 10–15 minutes (repeated once if necessary).

Myocardial infarction Limited evidence that magnesium sulphate prevents arrhythmias and reperfusion injury in patients with suspected myocardial infarction has not been confirmed by large studies. Routine use of magnesium sulphate for this purpose is not recommended. For the management of myocardial infarction, see section 2.10.1.

Eclampsia and pre-eclampsia Magnesium sulphate is the drug of choice for the prevention of recurrent seizures in *eclampsia*; see also Appendix 4. Regimens may vary between hospitals. Calcium gluconate injection is used for the management of magnesium toxicity.

Magnesium sulphate is also of benefit in women with *pre-eclampsia* in whom there is concern about developing eclampsia. The patient should be monitored carefully (see under Magnesium Sulphate).

MAGNESIUM SULPHATE

Indications see notes above; constipation (section 1.6.4); severe acute asthma (section 3.1); paste for boils (section 13.10.5)

Cautions see notes above; hepatic impairment (Appendix 2); renal impairment (Appendix 3); in severe hypomagnesaemia administer initially via controlled infusion device (preferably syringe pump); monitor blood pressure, respiratory rate, urinary output and for signs of overdosage (loss of patellar reflexes, weakness, nausea, sensation of warmth, flushing, drowsiness, double vision, and slurred speech); pregnancy (Appendix 4); **interactions:** Appendix 1 (magnesium, parenteral)

Side-effects generally associated with hypermagnesaemia, nausea, vomiting, thirst, flushing of skin, hypotension, arrhythmias, coma, respiratory depression, drowsiness, confusion, loss of tendon reflexes, muscle weakness, colic and diarrhoea following oral administration

Dose

- Hypomagnesaemia, see notes above
- Prevention of seizure recurrence in eclampsia, initially by intravenous injection over 5–15 minutes, 4 g, followed by intravenous infusion, 1 g/hour for at least 24 hours after last seizure; if seizure recurs, additional dose by intravenous injection, 2 g (4 g if body-weight over 70 kg)
- Prevention of seizures in pre-eclampsia [unlicensed indication], initially by intravenous infusion over 5–15 minutes, 4 g followed by intravenous infusion, 1 g/hour for 24 hours; if seizure occurs, additional dose by intravenous injection, 2 g

Intravenous administration For intravenous injection concentration of magnesium sulphate should not exceed 20% (dilute 1 part of magnesium sulphate injection 50% with at least 1.5 parts of water for injections)

Note Magnesium sulphate 1 g equivalent to Mg^{2+} approx. 4 mmol

Magnesium Sulphate (Non-proprietary) PoM

Injection, magnesium sulphate 20% (Mg^{2+} approx. 0.8 mmol/mL), net price 20-mL (4-g) amp = £2.75; 50% (Mg^{2+} approx. 2 mmol/mL), 2-mL (1-g) amp = £3.47, 4-mL (2-g) prefilled syringe = £6.40, 5-mL (2.5-g) amp = £2.50, 10-mL (5-g) amp = £3.35; 10-mL (5-g) prefilled syringe = £4.95

Brands include *Minijet® Magnesium Sulphate 50%*

9.5.2 Phosphorus

9.5.2.1 Phosphate supplements
9.5.2.2 Phosphate-binding agents

9.5.2.1 Phosphate supplements

Oral phosphate supplements may be required in addition to vitamin D in a small minority of patients with hypophosphataemic vitamin D-resistant rickets. Diarrhoea is a common side-effect and should prompt a reduction in dosage.

Phosphate infusion is occasionally needed in alcohol dependence or in phosphate deficiency arising from use of parenteral nutrition deficient in phosphate supplements; phosphate depletion also occurs in severe diabetic ketoacidosis. For *established hypophosphataemia*, monobasic potassium phosphate may be infused at a rate of 9 mmol every 12 hours. In critically ill patients, the dose of phosphate can be increased up to 500 micromol/kg (approx. 30 mmol in adults), infused over 6–12 hours, according to severity. Excessive doses of phosphates may cause hypocalcaemia and metastatic calcification; it is **essential** to monitor closely plasma concentrations of calcium, phosphate, potassium, and other electrolytes.

For phosphate requirements in *total parenteral nutrition* regimens, see section 9.3.

Phosphates (Fresenius Kabi) PoM
Intravenous infusion, phosphates (providing PO_4^{3-} 100 mmol/litre), net price 500 mL (*Polyfusor®*) = £3.75.
For the treatment of moderate to severe hypophosphatemia

Phosphate-Sandoz® (HK Pharma)
Tablets, effervescent, anhydrous sodium acid phosphate 1.936 g, sodium bicarbonate 350 mg, potassium bicarbonate 315 mg, equivalent to phosphorus 500 mg (phosphate 16.1 mmol), sodium 468.8 mg (Na^+ 20.4 mmol), potassium 123 mg (K^+ 3.1 mmol). Net price 20 = £3.29. Label: 13
Dose vitamin D-resistant hypophosphataemic osteomalacia, 4–6 tablets daily; CHILD under 5 years 2–3 tablets daily

9 Nutrition and blood

9.5.2.2 Phosphate-binding agents

Aluminium-containing and calcium-containing preparations are used as phosphate-binding agents in the management of hyperphosphataemia complicating renal failure. Calcium-containing phosphate-binding agents are contra-indicated in hypercalcaemia or hypercalciuria. Phosphate-binding agents which contain aluminium may increase plasma aluminium in dialysis patients.

Sevelamer is licensed for the treatment of hyperphosphataemia in patients on haemodialysis or peritoneal dialysis.

Lanthanum is licensed for the control of hyperphosphataemia in chronic renal failure patients on haemodialysis or continuous ambulatory peritoneal dialysis (CAPD).

ALUMINIUM HYDROXIDE

Indications hyperphosphataemia; dyspepsia (section 1.1)
Cautions hyperaluminaemia; see also notes above; **interactions:** Appendix 1 (antacids)
Side-effects see section 1.1.1

Alu-Cap® (3M)
Capsules, green/red, dried aluminium hydroxide 475 mg (low Na^+). Net price 120-cap pack = £3.75
Dose phosphate-binding agent in renal failure, 4–20 capsules daily in divided doses with meals

CALCIUM SALTS

Indications hyperphosphataemia
Cautions see notes above; **interactions:** Appendix 1 (antacids, calcium salts)
Side-effects hypercalcaemia

Adcal® section 9.5.1.1

Calcichew® section 9.5.1.1

Calcium-500 section 9.5.1.1

Phosex® (Vitaline)
Tablets, yellow, calcium acetate 1 g (calcium 250 mg or Ca^{2+} 6.2 mmol), net price 180-tab pack = £19.79. Label: 25
Dose phosphate-binding agent (with meals) in renal failure, according to the requirements of the patient

LANTHANUM

Indications hyperphosphataemia in patients on haemodialysis or continuous ambulatory peritoneal dialysis (CAPD)
Cautions acute peptic ulcer; ulcerative colitis; Crohn's disease; bowel obstruction; hepatic impairment; breast-feeding (Appendix 5); **interactions**: Appendix 1 (lanthanum)
Contra-indications pregnancy (Appendix 4)
Side-effects gastro-intestinal disturbances; hypocalcaemia; *less commonly* anorexia, increased appetite, taste disturbances, dry mouth, thirst, stomatitis, chest pain, peripheral oedema, headache, dizziness, vertigo, asthenia, fatigue, malaise, hyperglycaemia, hyperparathyroidism, hypercalcaemia, hyperphosphataemia, hypophosphataemia, eosinophilia, arthralgia, myalgia, osteoporosis, sweating, alopecia, pruritus, and erythematous rash; accumulation of lanthanum in bone, and transient changes in QT interval also reported
Dose
- ADULT over 18 years, initially 750 mg daily in divided doses with or immediately after meals adjusted according to plasma-phosphate concentration every 2–3 weeks (usual dose range 1.5–3 g daily in divided doses)

Fosrenol® (Shire) ▼ PoM
Tablets (chewable), lanthanum (as carbonate hydrate) 500 mg, net price 90-tab pack = £114.13; 750 mg, 90-tab pack = £152.17; 1 g, 90-tab pack = £161.33. Label: 21, 24

SEVELAMER

Indications hyperphosphataemia in patients on haemodialysis or peritoneal dialysis
Cautions pregnancy (Appendix 4); breast-feeding (Appendix 5); gastro-intestinal disorders; **interactions**: Appendix 1 (sevelamer)
Contra-indications bowel obstruction
Side-effects gastro-intestinal disturbances; hypotension, hypertension; headache; pruritus and rash; *very rarely* intestinal obstruction
Dose
- ADULT over 18 years, initially 2.4–4.8 g daily in 3 divided doses with meals, then adjusted according to plasma-phosphate concentration (usual dose range 2.4–12 g daily in 3 divided doses)

Renagel® (Genzyme) PoM
Tablets, f/c, sevelamer 800 mg, net price 180-tab pack = £122.76. Label: 25, Counselling, with meals

9.5.3 Fluoride

Availability of adequate fluoride confers significant resistance to dental caries. It is now considered that the topical action of fluoride on enamel and plaque is more important than the systemic effect.

Where the fluoride content of the drinking water is less than 700 micrograms per litre (0.7 parts per million), daily administration of fluoride tablets or drops is a suitable means of supplementation. Systemic fluoride supplements should not be prescribed without reference to the fluoride content of the local water supply. Infants need not receive fluoride supplements until the age of 6 months.

Dentifrices which incorporate sodium fluoride or monofluorophosphate are also a convenient source of fluoride.

Individuals who are either particularly caries prone or medically compromised may be given additional protection by use of fluoride rinses or by application of fluoride gels. Rinses may be used daily or weekly; daily use of a less concentrated rinse is more effective than weekly use of a more concentrated one. High-strength gels must be applied on a regular basis under professional supervision; extreme caution is necessary to prevent children from swallowing any excess. Less concentrated gels are available for home use. Varnishes are also available and are particularly valuable for young or disabled children since they adhere to the teeth and set in the presence of moisture.

> Fluoride mouthwash, oral drops, tablets and toothpaste are prescribable on form FP10D (GP14 in Scotland, WP10D in Wales; for details see preparations, below).
> There are also arrangements for health authorities to supply fluoride tablets in the course of pre-school dental schemes, and they may also be supplied in school dental schemes.
> Fluoride gels are not prescribable on form FP10D (GP14 in Scotland, WP10D in Wales).

FLUORIDES

Note Sodium fluoride 2.2 mg provides approx. 1 mg fluoride ion

Indications prophylaxis of dental caries—see notes above

Contra-indications not for areas where drinking water is fluoridated

Side-effects occasional white flecks on teeth with recommended doses; rarely yellowish-brown discoloration if recommended doses are exceeded

Dose

Note Dose expressed as fluoride ion (F^-)

- Water content less than F^- 300 micrograms/litre (0.3 parts per million), CHILD up to 6 months none; 6 months–3 years F^- 250 micrograms daily, 3–6 years F^- 500 micrograms daily, over 6 years F^- 1 mg daily
- Water content between F^- 300 and 700 micrograms/litre (0.3–0.7 parts per million), CHILD up to 3 years none, 3–6 years F^- 250 micrograms daily, over 6 years F^- 500 micrograms daily
- Water content above F^- 700 micrograms/litre (0.7 parts per million), supplements not advised

Note These doses reflect the recommendations of the British Dental Association, the British Society of Paediatric Dentistry and the British Association for the Study of Community Dentistry (*Br Dent J* 1997; **182**: 6–7)

Tablets

Counselling Tablets should be sucked or dissolved in the mouth and taken preferably in the evening

En-De-Kay® (Manx)

Fluotabs 3–6 years, orange-flavoured, scored, sodium fluoride 1.1 mg (F^- 500 micrograms). Net price 200-tab pack = £2.38

Fluotabs 6+ years, orange-flavoured, scored, sodium fluoride 2.2 mg (F^- 1 mg). Net price 200-tab pack = £2.38

Dental prescribing on NHS May be prescribed as Sodium Fluoride Tablets

Fluor-a-day® (Dental Health)

Tablets, buff, sodium fluoride 1.1 mg (F^- 500 micrograms), net price 200-tab pack = £1.91; 2.2 mg (F^- 1 mg), 200-tab pack = £1.91

Dental prescribing on NHS May be prescribed as Sodium Fluoride Tablets

FluoriGard® (Colgate-Palmolive)

Tablets 0.5, purple, grape-flavoured, scored, sodium fluoride 1.1 mg (F^- 500 micrograms). Net price 200-tab pack = £1.91

Tablets 1.0, orange, orange-flavoured, scored, sodium fluoride 2.2 mg (F^- 1 mg). Net price 200-tab pack = £1.91

Dental prescribing on NHS May be prescribed as Sodium Fluoride Tablets

Oral drops

Note Fluoride supplements not considered necessary below 6 months of age (see notes above)

En-De-Kay® (Manx)

Fluodrops® (= paediatric drops), sugar-free, sodium fluoride 550 micrograms (F^- 250 micrograms)/0.15 mL. Net price 60 mL = £2.38

Dental prescribing on NHS Corresponds to Sodium Fluoride Oral Drops DPF 0.37% equivalent to sodium fluoride 80 micrograms (F^- 36 micrograms)/drop

Mouthwashes

Rinse mouth for 1 minute and spit out

Counselling Avoid eating, drinking, or rinsing mouth for 15 minutes after use

Duraphat® (Colgate-Palmolive)

Weekly dental rinse (= mouthwash), blue, sodium fluoride 0.2%. Net price 150 mL = £2.25. Counselling, see above

Dose CHILD 6 years and over, for *weekly* use, rinse with 10 mL

Dental prescribing on NHS May be prescribed as Sodium Fluoride Mouthwash 0.2%

En-De-Kay® (Manx)

Daily fluoride mouthrinse (= mouthwash), blue, sodium fluoride 0.05%. Net price 250 mL = £1.51

Dose CHILD 6 years and over, for *daily* use, rinse with 10 mL

Dental prescribing on NHS May be prescribed as Sodium Fluoride Mouthwash 0.05%

Fluorinse (= mouthwash), red, sodium fluoride 2%. Net price 100 mL = £4.97. Counselling, see above

Dose CHILD 8 years and over, for *daily* use, dilute 5 drops to 10 mL of water; for *weekly* use, dilute 20 drops to 10 mL

Dental prescribing on NHS May be prescribed as Sodium Fluoride Mouthwash 2%

FluoriGard® (Colgate-Palmolive)
Daily dental rinse (= mouthwash), blue, sodium fluoride 0.05%. Net price 500 mL = £3.05. Counselling, see above

Dose CHILD 6 years and over, for *daily* use, rinse with 10 mL

Dental prescribing on NHS May be prescribed as Sodium Fluoride Mouthwash 0.05%

Gels

FluoriGard® (Colgate-Palmolive)
Gel-Kam (= gel), stannous fluoride 0.4% in glycerol basis. Net price 100 mL = £2.97. Counselling, see below

Dose ADULT and CHILD 3 years and over, for *daily* use, using a toothbrush, apply onto all tooth surfaces

Counselling Swish between teeth for 1 minute before spitting out. Avoid eating, drinking, or rinsing mouth for at least 30 minutes after use

Toothpastes

Duraphat® (Colgate-Palmolive) PoM
Duraphat® '2800 ppm' toothpaste, sodium fluoride 0.619%. Net price 75 mL = £3.26, dual pack (2×75 mL) = £5.54. Counselling, see below

Dose ADULT and CHILD over 10 years, apply 1 cm twice daily using a toothbrush

Counselling Brush teeth for 1 minute before spitting out. Avoid drinking or rinsing mouth for 30 minutes after use

Dental prescribing on NHS May be prescribed as Sodium Fluoride Toothpaste 0.619%

Duraphat® '5000 ppm' toothpaste, sodium fluoride 1.1%. Net price 51 g = £4.45. Counselling, see below

Dose ADULT and ADOLESCENT over 16 years, apply 2 cm 3 times daily after meals using a toothbrush

Counselling Brush teeth for 3 minutes before spitting out

Dental prescribing on NHS May be prescribed as Sodium Fluoride Toothpaste 1.1%

9.5.4 Zinc

Zinc supplements should be given only when there is good evidence of deficiency (hypoproteinaemia spuriously lowers plasma-zinc concentration) or in zinc-losing conditions. Zinc deficiency can occur as a result of inadequate diet or malabsorption; excessive loss of zinc can occur in trauma, burns, and protein-losing conditions. A zinc supplement is given until clinical improvement occurs, but it may need to be continued in severe malabsorption, metabolic disease (section 9.8.1), or in zinc-losing states.

Parenteral nutrition regimens usually include trace amounts of zinc (section 9.3). If necessary, further zinc can be added to intravenous feeding regimens. A suggested dose for intravenous nutrition is elemental zinc 6.5 mg (Zn^{2+} 100 micromol) daily.

ZINC SULPHATE

Indications zinc deficiency or supplementation in zinc-losing conditions

Cautions acute renal failure (may accumulate); **interactions:** Appendix 1 (zinc)

Side-effects abdominal pain, dyspepsia, nausea, vomiting, diarrhoea, gastric irritation, gastritis; irritability, headache, lethargy

Dose

- See preparation below and notes above

Zinc Sulphate (Non-proprietary) PoM
Injection, zinc sulphate 14.6 mg/mL (zinc 50 micromol/mL), net price 10 mL vial = £2.50

Solvazinc® (KoGEN)
Effervescent tablets, yellow-white, zinc sulphate monohydrate 125 mg (45 mg zinc). Net price 30 = £4.32. Label: 13, 21

Dose ADULT and CHILD over 30 kg, 1 tablet in water 1–3 times daily after food; CHILD under 10 kg, ½ tablet daily; 10–30 kg, ½ tablet 1–3 times daily

9.5.5 Selenium

Selenium deficiency can occur as a result of inadequate diet or prolonged parenteral nutrition. A selenium supplement should be given only when there is good evidence of deficiency.

SELENIUM

Indications selenium deficiency

Cautions interactions: Appendix 1 (selenium)

Dose

- By mouth *or* by intramuscular injection *or* by intravenous injection, 100–500 micrograms daily

Selenase® (Oxford Nutrition) PoM
Oral solution, selenium (as sodium selenite pentahydrate) 50 micrograms/mL, net price 2-mL amp = 53p, 10-mL bottle = £3.08

Injection, selenium (as sodium selenite pentahydrate) 50 micrograms/mL, net price 2-mL amp = 93p, 10-mL vial = £3.75

9.6 Vitamins

9.6.1 Vitamin A
9.6.2 Vitamin B group
9.6.3 Vitamin C
9.6.4 Vitamin D
9.6.5 Vitamin E
9.6.6 Vitamin K
9.6.7 Multivitamin preparations

Vitamins are used for the prevention and treatment of specific deficiency states or where the diet is known to be inadequate; they may be prescribed in the NHS to prevent or treat deficiency but not as dietary supplements.

Their use as general 'pick-me-ups' is of unproven value and, in the case of preparations containing vitamin A or D, may actually be harmful if patients take more than the prescribed dose. The 'fad' for mega-vitamin therapy with water-soluble vitamins, such as ascorbic acid and pyridoxine, is unscientific and can be harmful.

Dietary reference values for vitamins are available in the Department of Health publication:

Dietary Reference Values for Food Energy and Nutrients for the United Kingdom: Report of the Panel on Dietary Reference Values of the Committee on Medical Aspects of Food Policy. *Report on Health and Social Subjects 41*. London: HMSO, 1991

Dental patients Most patients who develop a nutritional deficiency despite an adequate intake of vitamins have malabsorption and if this is suspected the patient should be referred to a medical practitioner.

It is unjustifiable to treat stomatitis or glossitis with mixtures of vitamin preparations; this delays diagnosis and correct treatment.

9.6.1 Vitamin A

Deficiency of vitamin A (retinol) is associated with ocular defects (particularly xerophthalmia) and an increased susceptibility to infections, but deficiency is rare in the UK (even in disorders of fat absorption).

Massive overdose can cause rough skin, dry hair, an enlarged liver, and a raised erythrocyte sedimentation rate and raised serum calcium and serum alkaline phosphatase concentrations.

In view of evidence suggesting that high levels of vitamin A may cause birth defects, women who are (or may become) pregnant are advised not to take vitamin A supplements (including tablets and fish-liver oil drops), except on the advice of a doctor or an antenatal clinic; nor should they eat liver or products such as liver paté or liver sausage.

VITAMIN A
(Retinol)

Indications see notes above
Cautions see notes above; **interactions:** Appendix 1 (vitamins)
Side-effects see notes above
Dose
- See notes above and under preparations

Vitamins A and D

Halibut-liver Oil (Non-proprietary)
Capsules, vitamin A 4000 units [also contains vitamin D]. Net price 100-cap pack = 93p

Vitamins A and D (Non-proprietary)
Capsules, vitamin A 4000 units, vitamin D 400 units. Net price 84-cap pack = £2.61

Halycitrol® (LAB) NHS
Emulsion, vitamin A 4600 units, vitamin D 380 units/5 mL. Net price 114 mL = £1.77
Dose 5 mL daily but see notes above

Vitamins A, C and D

Healthy Start Children's Vitamin Drops (Non-proprietary)
Oral drops, vitamin A 5000 units, vitamin D 2000 units, ascorbic acid 150 mg/mL
Available free of charge to children under 4 years through the Healthy Start Scheme; otherwise available direct to the public from maternity and child health clinics
Dose prevention of vitamin deficiency, CHILD 1 month–5 years, 5 drops daily (5 drops contain vitamin A approx. 700 units, vitamin D approx. 300 units, ascorbic acid approx. 20 mg)
Note *Healthy Start Vitamins for women* (containing ascorbic acid, vitamin D, and folic acid) are also available to women during pregnancy and until their baby is one year old, through the Healthy Start Scheme

9.6.2 Vitamin B group

Deficiency of the B vitamins, other than deficiency of vitamin B_{12} (section 9.1.2), is rare in the UK and is usually treated by preparations containing thiamine (B_1), riboflavin (B_2), and nicotinamide, which is used in preference to nicotinic acid, as it does not cause vasodilatation. Other members (or substances traditionally classified as members) of the vitamin B complex such as aminobenzoic acid, biotin, choline, inositol, and pantothenic acid or panthenol may be included in vitamin B preparations but there is no evidence of their value.

The severe deficiency states Wernicke's encephalopathy and Korsakoff's psychosis, especially as seen in chronic alcoholism, are best treated initially by the parenteral administration of B vitamins (*Pabrinex®*), followed by oral administration of thiamine in the longer term. Anaphylaxis has been reported with parenteral B vitamins (see CSM advice, below).

As with other vitamins of the B group, pyridoxine (B_6) deficiency is rare, but it may occur during isoniazid therapy (section 5.1.9) or penicillamine treatment in Wilson's disease (section 9.8.1) and is characterised by peripheral neuritis. High doses of pyridoxine are given in some metabolic disorders, such as hyperoxaluria, and it is also used in sideroblastic anaemia (section 9.1.3). There is evidence to suggest that pyridoxine in a dose not exceeding 100 mg daily may provide some benefit in premenstrual syndrome. It has been tried for a wide variety of other disorders, but there is little sound evidence to support the claims of efficacy, and overdosage induces toxic effects.

Nicotinic acid inhibits the synthesis of cholesterol and triglyceride (see section 2.12). Folic acid and vitamin B_{12} are used in the treatment of megaloblastic anaemia (section 9.1.2). Folinic acid (available as calcium folinate) is used in association with cytotoxic therapy (section 8.1).

RIBOFLAVIN
(Riboflavine, vitamin B_2)

Indications see notes above

Preparations
Injections of vitamins B and C, see under Thiamine

Oral vitamin B complex preparations
See p. 524

THIAMINE
(Vitamin B_1)

MHRA/CHM advice
Although potentially serious allergic adverse reactions may rarely occur during, or shortly after, parenteral administration, the CHM has recommended that:
1. This should not preclude the use of parenteral thiamine in patients where this route of administration is required, particularly in patients at risk of Wernicke-Korsakoff syndrome where treatment with thiamine is essential;
2. Intravenous administration should be by infusion over 30 minutes;
3. Facilities for treating anaphylaxis (including resuscitation facilities) should be available when parenteral thiamine is administered.

Indications see notes above
Cautions anaphylactic shock may occasionally follow injection (see MHRA/CHM advice above); breast-feeding (Appendix 5)

Dose

- Mild chronic deficiency, 10–25 mg daily; severe deficiency, 200–300 mg daily

Thiamine (Non-proprietary)
Tablets, thiamine hydrochloride 50 mg, net price 20 = 79p; 100 mg, 20 = £1.23
Brands include *Benerva®* (NHS)

Pabrinex® (Link) (PoM)
I/M High potency injection, for intramuscular use only, ascorbic acid 500 mg, nicotinamide 160 mg, pyridoxine hydrochloride 50 mg, riboflavin 4 mg, thiamine hydrochloride 250 mg/7 mL. Net price 7 mL (in 2 amps) = £1.96
I/V High potency injection, for intravenous use only, ascorbic acid 500 mg, anhydrous glucose 1 g, nicotinamide 160 mg, pyridoxine hydrochloride 50 mg, riboflavin 4 mg, thiamine hydrochloride 250 mg/10 mL. Net price 10 mL (in 2 amps) = £1.96
Parenteral vitamins B and C for rapid correction of severe depletion or malabsorption (e.g. in alcoholism, after acute infections, postoperatively, or in psychiatric states), maintenance of vitamins B and C in chronic intermittent haemodialysis
Dose see MHRA/CHM advice above
Coma or delirium from alcohol, from opioids, or from barbiturates, collapse following narcosis, by intravenous infusion of *I/V High potency*, 2–3 pairs every 8 hours
Psychosis following narcosis or electroconvulsive therapy, toxicity from acute infections, by intravenous infusion of *I/V High potency* or by deep intramuscular injection into the gluteal muscle of *I/M High potency*, 1 pair twice daily for up to 7 days
Haemodialysis, by intravenous infusion of *I/V High potency* (in sodium chloride intravenous infusion 0.9%) 1 pair every 2 weeks

Oral vitamin B complex preparations
See below

PYRIDOXINE HYDROCHLORIDE
(Vitamin B_6)

Indications see under Dose
Cautions interactions: Appendix 1 (vitamins)
Side-effects sensory neuropathy reported with high doses given for extended periods
Dose

- Deficiency states, 20–50 mg up to 3 times daily
- Isoniazid neuropathy, prophylaxis 10 mg daily [or 20 mg daily if suitable product not available]; therapeutic, 50 mg three times daily
- Idiopathic sideroblastic anaemia, 100–400 mg daily in divided doses
- Premenstrual syndrome, 50–100 mg daily (see notes above)

Prolonged use of pyridoxine in a dose of 10 mg daily is considered safe but the long-term use of pyridoxine in a dose of 200 mg or more daily has been associated with neuropathy. The safety of long-term pyridoxine supplementation with doses above 10 mg daily has not been established.

Pyridoxine (Non-proprietary)
Tablets, pyridoxine hydrochloride 10 mg, net price 20 = 34p; 20 mg, 20 = 34p; 50 mg, 28 = 60p

Injections of vitamins B and C
See under Thiamine

NICOTINAMIDE

Indications see notes above; acne vulgaris, see section 13.6.1

Nicotinamide (Non-proprietary)
Tablets, nicotinamide 50 mg. Net price 20 = £1.37

Injections of vitamins B and C
See under Thiamine

Oral vitamin B complex preparations

Note Other multivitamin preparations are in section 9.6.7.

Vitamin B Tablets, Compound
Tablets, nicotinamide 15 mg, riboflavin 1 mg, thiamine hydrochloride 1 mg. Net price 20 = 7p
Dose prophylactic, 1–2 tablets daily

Vitamin B Tablets, Compound, Strong
Tablets, brown, f/c or s/c, nicotinamide 20 mg, pyridoxine hydrochloride 2 mg, riboflavin 2 mg, thiamine hydrochloride 5 mg. Net price 28-tab pack = £1.43
Dose treatment of vitamin-B deficiency, 1–2 tablets 3 times daily
Dental prescribing on NHS Vitamin B Tablets, Compound Strong may be prescribed

Vigranon B® (Wallace Mfg) (NHS)
Syrup, thiamine hydrochloride 5 mg, riboflavin 2 mg, nicotinamide 20 mg, pyridoxine hydrochloride 2 mg, panthenol 3 mg/5 mL. Net price 150 mL = £2.41

Other compounds

Potassium aminobenzoate has been used in the treatment of various disorders associated with excessive fibrosis such as scleroderma but its therapeutic value is **doubtful**.

Potaba® (Glenwood)
Capsules, potassium aminobenzoate 500 mg. Net price 20 = £1.59. Label: 21
Tablets, potassium aminobenzoate 500 mg. Net price 20 = £1.12. Label: 21
Envules® (= powder in sachets), potassium aminobenzoate 3 g. Net price 40 sachets = £17.21. Label: 13, 21
Dose Peyronie's disease, scleroderma, 12 g daily in divided doses after food

9.6.3 Vitamin C
(Ascorbic acid)

Vitamin C therapy is essential in scurvy, but less florid manifestations of vitamin C deficiency are commonly found, especially in the elderly. It is rarely necessary to prescribe more than 100 mg daily except early in the treatment of scurvy.

Severe scurvy causes gingival swelling and bleeding margins as well as petechiae on the skin. This is, however, exceedingly rare and a patient with these signs is more likely to have leukaemia. Investigation should not be delayed by a trial period of vitamin treatment.

Claims that vitamin C ameliorates colds or promotes wound healing have not been proved.

ASCORBIC ACID

Indications prevention and treatment of scurvy

Cautions interactions: Appendix 1 (vitamins)

Dose

- Prophylactic, 25–75 mg daily; therapeutic, not less than 250 mg daily in divided doses

Ascorbic Acid (Non-proprietary)

Tablets, ascorbic acid 50 mg, net price 28 = £1.21; 100 mg, 28 = £1.26; 200 mg, 28 = £1.28; 500 mg (label: 24), 28 = £2.60

Brands include *Redoxon®* NHS

Dental prescribing on NHS Ascorbic Acid Tablets may be prescribed

Injection, ascorbic acid 100 mg/mL. Net price 5-mL amp = £2.51

Available from UCB Pharma

9.6.4 Vitamin D

Note The term Vitamin D is used for a range of compounds which possess the property of preventing or curing rickets. They include ergocalciferol (calciferol, vitamin D_2), colecalciferol (vitamin D_3), dihydrotachysterol, alfacalcidol (1α-hydroxycholecalciferol), and calcitriol (1,25-dihydroxycholecalciferol).

Simple vitamin D deficiency can be prevented by taking an oral supplement of only 10 micrograms (400 units) of ergocalciferol (calciferol, vitamin D_2) or colecalciferol (vitamin D_3) daily. Vitamin D deficiency can occur in people whose exposure to sunlight is limited and in those whose diet is deficient in vitamin D. In these individuals, ergocalciferol or colecalciferol in a dose of 20 micrograms (800 units) daily by mouth can prevent vitamin D deficiency. Since there is no plain tablet of this strength available, **calcium and ergocalciferol tablets** can be given (although the calcium is unnecessary).

Preparations containing calcium and colecalciferol are available for the management of calcium and vitamin D deficiency, or for those at high risk of deficiency (see also Osteoporosis, p. 404 and Calcium Supplements, p. 517).

Vitamin D deficiency caused by *intestinal malabsorption* or *chronic liver disease* usually requires vitamin D in pharmacological doses, such as **ergocalciferol tablets** up to 1 mg (40 000 units) daily; the hypocalcaemia of *hypoparathyroidism* often requires doses of up to 2.5 mg (100 000 units) daily in order to achieve normocalcaemia.

Vitamin D requires hydroxylation by the kidney to its active form therefore the hydroxylated derivatives **alfacalcidol** or **calcitriol** should be prescribed if patients with *severe renal impairment* require vitamin D therapy. Calcitriol is also licensed for the management of postmenopausal osteoporosis.

Paricalcitol, a synthetic vitamin D analogue, is licensed for the prevention and treatment of secondary hyperparathyroidism associated with chronic renal failure (section 9.5.1.2).

Important. All patients receiving pharmacological doses of vitamin D should have the plasma-calcium concentration checked at intervals (initially weekly) and whenever nausea or vomiting are present. Breast milk from women taking pharmacological doses of vitamin D may cause hypercalcaemia if given to an infant.

ERGOCALCIFEROL

(Calciferol, Vitamin D_2)

Indications see notes above

Cautions take care to ensure correct dose in infants; monitor plasma calcium in patients receiving high doses and in renal impairment; **interactions**: Appendix 1 (vitamins)

Contra-indications hypercalcaemia; metastatic calcification

Side-effects symptoms of overdosage include anorexia, lassitude, nausea and vomiting, diarrhoea, constipation, weight loss, polyuria, sweating, headache, thirst, vertigo, and raised concentrations of calcium and phosphate in plasma and urine

Dose

- See notes above

Daily supplements

Note There is no plain vitamin D tablet available for treating simple deficiency (see notes above). Alternatives include vitamins capsules (section 9.6.7), preparations of vitamins A and D (section 9.6.1), and calcium and ergocalciferol tablets (see below).

Calcium and Ergocalciferol (Non-proprietary) **(Calcium and Vitamin D)**

Tablets, calcium lactate 300 mg, calcium phosphate 150 mg (calcium 97 mg or Ca^{2+} 2.4 mmol), ergocalciferol 10 micrograms (400 units). Net price 28-tab pack = £1.54. Counselling, crush before administration or may be chewed

Pharmacological strengths (see notes above)

Note The BP directs that when calciferol is prescribed or demanded, colecalciferol or ergocalciferol should be dispensed or supplied

Ergocalciferol (Non-proprietary)

Tablets, ergocalciferol 250 micrograms (10 000 units), net price 20 = £4.40; 1.25 mg (50 000 units) may also be available

Important When the strength of the tablets ordered or prescribed is not clear, the intention of the prescriber with respect to the strength (expressed in micrograms or milligrams per tablet) should be ascertained.

Injection, ergocalciferol, 7.5 mg (300 000 units)/mL in oil, net price 1-mL amp = £7.07, 2-mL amp = £8.01

ALFACALCIDOL

(1α-Hydroxycholecalciferol)

Indications see notes above

Cautions see under Ergocalciferol; also nephrolithiasis

Contra-indications see under Ergocalciferol

Side-effects see under Ergocalciferol; also *rarely* nephrocalcinosis, pruritus, rash, urticaria

Dose

- By mouth *or* by intravenous injection over 30 seconds, ADULT and CHILD over 20 kg, initially 1 microgram daily (elderly 500 nanograms), adjusted to avoid hypercalcaemia; maintenance usually 0.25–1 microgram daily; NEONATE and PRETERM NEONATE initially 50–100 nanograms/kg daily, CHILD under 20 kg initially 50 nanograms/kg daily

Alfacalcidol (Non-proprietary) PoM

Capsules, alfacalcidol 250 nanograms net price 30-cap pack = £6.31; 500 nanograms 30-cap pack = £12.57; 1 microgram 30-cap pack = £18.94

One-Alpha® (LEO) PoM
Capsules, alfacalcidol 250 nanograms (white), net price 30-cap pack = £3.37; 500 nanograms (red), 30-cap pack = £6.27; 1 microgram (brown), 30-cap pack = £8.75
Excipients include sesame oil

Oral drops, sugar-free, alfacalcidol 2 micrograms/mL (1 drop contains approx. 100 nanograms), net price 10 mL = £22.49
Excipients include alcohol
Note The concentration of alfacalcidol in *One-Alpha® drops* is **10 times greater** than that of the former presentation *One-Alpha® solution*.

Injection, alfacalcidol 2 micrograms/mL, net price 0.5-mL amp = £2.16, 1-mL amp = £4.11
Note Contains propylene glycol and should be used with caution in small preterm neonates

CALCITRIOL
(1,25-Dihydroxycholecalciferol)

Indications see notes above
Cautions see under Ergocalciferol; monitor plasma calcium, phosphate, and creatinine during dosage titration
Contra-indications see under Ergocalciferol
Side-effects see under Ergocalciferol
Dose
- By mouth, renal osteodystrophy, initially 250 nanograms daily, or on alternate days (in patients with normal or only slightly reduced plasma-calcium concentration), increased if necessary in steps of 250 nanograms at intervals of 2–4 weeks; usual dose 0.5–1 microgram daily; CHILD not established
Established postmenopausal osteoporosis, 250 nanograms twice daily (monitor plasma-calcium concentration and creatinine, consult product literature)
- By intravenous injection (or injection through catheter after haemodialysis), hypocalcaemia in dialysis patients with chronic renal failure, initially 500 nanograms (approx. 10 nanograms/kg) 3 times a week, increased if necessary in steps of 250–500 nanograms at intervals of 2–4 weeks; usual dose 0.5–3 micrograms 3 times a week; CHILD not established
Moderate to severe secondary hyperparathyroidism in dialysis patients, initially 0.5–4 micrograms 3 times a week, increased if necessary in steps of 250–500 nanograms at intervals of 2–4 weeks; max. 8 micrograms 3 times a week

Rocaltrol® (Roche) PoM
Capsules, calcitriol 250 nanograms (red/white), net price 20 = £3.83; 500 nanograms (red), 20 = £6.85

Calcijex® (Abbott) PoM
Injection, calcitriol 1 microgram/mL, net price 1-mL amp = £5.14; 2 micrograms/mL, 1-mL amp = £10.28

COLECALCIFEROL
(Cholecalciferol, vitamin D_3)

Indications see notes above
Cautions see under Ergocalciferol
Contra-indications see under Ergocalciferol
Side-effects see under Ergocalciferol

Adcal-D_3® (ProStrakan)
Tablets (chewable) (lemon or tutti-frutti flavour), calcium carbonate 1.5 g (calcium 600 mg or Ca^{2+} 15 mmol), colecalciferol 10 micrograms (400 units), net price 56-tab pack = £4.06, 112-tab pack = £7.99. Label: 24

Dissolve® (effervescent tablets), lemon flavour, calcium carbonate 1.5 g (calcium 600 mg or Ca^{2+} 15 mmol), colecalciferol 10 micrograms (400 units), net price 56-tab pack = £4.99. Label: 13

Cacit® D3 (Procter & Gamble Pharm.)
Granules, effervescent, lemon flavour, calcium carbonate 1.25 g (calcium 500 mg or Ca^{2+} 12.6 mmol), colecalciferol 11 micrograms (440 units)/sachet. Net price 30-sachet pack = £4.31. Label: 13

Calceos® (KoGEN)
Tablets (chewable), lemon flavour, calcium carbonate 1.25 g (calcium 500 mg or Ca^{2+} 12.6 mmol), colecalciferol 10 micrograms (400 units). Net price 60-tab pack = £3.90. Label: 24

Calcichew-D_3® (Shire)
Tablets (chewable), orange flavour, calcium carbonate 1.25 g (calcium 500 mg or Ca^{2+} 12.6 mmol), colecalciferol 5 micrograms (200 units). Net price 100-tab pack = £15.02. Label: 24
Excipients include aspartame (section 9.4.1)

Calcichew-D_3® Forte (Shire)
Tablets (chewable), lemon flavour, calcium carbonate 1.25 g (calcium 500 mg or Ca^{2+} 12.6 mmol), colecalciferol 10 micrograms (400 units). Net price 60-tab pack = £4.50, 100-tab pack = £7.50. Label: 24
Excipients include aspartame (section 9.4.1)

Calfovit D3® (Menarini)
Powder, lemon flavour, calcium phosphate 3.1 g (calcium 1.2 g or Ca^{2+} 30 mmol), colecalciferol 20 micrograms (800 units), net price 30-sachet pack = £4.32. Label: 13, 21

With alendronic acid
Section 6.6.2

DIHYDROTACHYSTEROL

Indications see notes above
Cautions see under Ergocalciferol
Contra-indications see under Ergocalciferol
Side-effects see under Ergocalciferol

AT 10® (Intrapharm)
Oral solution, dihydrotachysterol 250 micrograms/mL. Net price 15-mL dropper bottle = £22.87
Excipients include arachis (peanut) oil
Dose acute, chronic, and latent forms of hypocalcaemic tetany due to hypoparathyroidism, consult product literature

PARICALCITOL

Indications see notes above
Cautions monitor plasma calcium and phosphate during dose titration and at least monthly when stabilised; monitor parathyroid hormone concentration; pregnancy (Appendix 4); breast-feeding (Appendix 5); **interactions**: Appendix 1 (vitamins)
Contra-indications see under Ergocalciferol
Side-effects see under Ergocalciferol; also hypercalcaemia, hyperphosphataemia; pruritus, rash; taste disturbance

Dose

- By slow intravenous injection—consult product literature; max. initial dose 40 micrograms

Zemplar® (Abbott) ▼ PoM
Injection, paricalcitol 5 micrograms/mL, net price 5 × 1-mL amp = £62.00, 5 × 2-mL amp = £124.00
Excipients include propylene glycol, see Excipients, p. 2

9.6.5 Vitamin E (Tocopherols)

The daily requirement of vitamin E has not been well defined but is probably about 3 to 15 mg daily. There is little evidence that oral supplements of vitamin E are essential in adults, even where there is fat malabsorption secondary to cholestasis. In young children with congenital cholestasis, abnormally low vitamin E concentrations may be found in association with neuromuscular abnormalities, which usually respond only to the parenteral administration of vitamin E.

Vitamin E has been tried for various other conditions but there is little scientific evidence of its value.

ALPHA TOCOPHERYL ACETATE

Indications see notes above

Cautions predisposition to thrombosis; increased risk of necrotising enterocolitis in neonate weighing less than 1.5 kg

Side-effects diarrhoea and abdominal pain with doses more than 1 g daily

Vitamin E Suspension (Cambridge)
Suspension, alpha tocopheryl acetate 500 mg/5 mL. Net price 100 mL = £21.25
Dose malabsorption in cystic fibrosis, 100–200 mg daily; CHILD 1 month–1 year 50 mg daily; 1–12 years, 100 mg daily
Malabsorption in abetalipoproteinaemia, ADULT and CHILD 50–100 mg/kg daily
Malabsorption in chronic cholestasis and severe liver disease, CHILD see *BNF for Children*

Note Tablets containing tocopheryl acetate 100 mg are available on a named-patient basis from Bell and Croyden (*Ephynal®*)

9.6.6 Vitamin K

Vitamin K is necessary for the production of blood clotting factors and proteins necessary for the normal calcification of bone.

Because vitamin K is fat soluble, patients with fat malabsorption, especially in biliary obstruction or hepatic disease, may become deficient. For oral administration to prevent vitamin K deficiency in malabsorption syndromes, a water-soluble preparation, **menadiol sodium phosphate** must be used; the usual dose is about 10 mg daily.

Oral coumarin anticoagulants act by interfering with vitamin K metabolism in the hepatic cells and their effects can be antagonised by giving vitamin K; for British Society for Haematology Guidelines, see section 2.8.2.

Vitamin K deficiency bleeding Neonates are relatively deficient in vitamin K and those who do not receive supplements of vitamin K are at risk of serious bleeding including intracranial bleeding. The Chief Medical Officer and the Chief Nursing Officer have recommended that all newborn babies should receive vitamin K to prevent vitamin K deficiency bleeding (haemorrhagic disease of the newborn). An appropriate regimen should be selected after discussion with parents in the antenatal period.

Vitamin K (as **phytomenadione**) 1 mg may be given by a single intramuscular injection at birth; this prevents vitamin K deficiency bleeding in virtually all babies.

Alternatively, vitamin K may be given by mouth, and arrangements must be in place to ensure the appropriate regimen is followed. Two doses of a colloidal (mixed micelle) preparation of phytomenadione 2 mg should be given in the first week. For exclusively breast-fed babies, a third dose of phytomenadione 2 mg is given at 1 month of age; the third dose is omitted in formula-fed babies because formula feeds contain vitamin K.

MENADIOL SODIUM PHOSPHATE

Indications see notes above

Cautions G6PD deficiency (section 9.1.5) and vitamin E deficiency (risk of haemolysis); **interactions:** Appendix 1 (vitamins)

Contra-indications neonates and infants, late pregnancy

Dose

- See notes above

Menadiol Phosphate (Cambridge)
Tablets, menadiol sodium phosphate equivalent to 10 mg of menadiol phosphate. Net price 100-tab pack = £48.25

PHYTOMENADIONE (Vitamin K_1)

Indications see notes above

Cautions intravenous injections should be given very slowly (see also below); pregnancy (Appendix 4); **interactions:** Appendix 1 (vitamins)

Dose

- See notes above and section 2.8.2

Konakion® (Roche) PoM
Tablets, s/c, phytomenadione 10 mg, net price 10-tab pack = £1.65. To be chewed or allowed to dissolve slowly in the mouth (Label: 24)

Colloidal formulation

Konakion® MM (Roche) PoM
Injection, phytomenadione 10 mg/mL in a mixed micelles vehicle. Net price 1-mL amp = 40p
Excipients include glycocholic acid 54.6 mg/amp, lecithin
Cautions reduce dose in elderly; liver impairment (glycocholic acid may displace bilirubin); reports of anaphylactoid reactions
Note *Konakion® MM* may be administered by slow intravenous injection or by intravenous infusion in glucose 5% (see Appendix 6); not for intramuscular injection

Konakion® MM Paediatric (Roche) ▼ PoM
Injection, phytomenadione 10 mg/mL in a mixed micelles vehicle. Net price 0.2-mL amp = £1.00
Excipients include glycocholic acid 10.9 mg/amp, lecithin
Cautions parenteral administration in neonate of less than 2.5 kg (increased risk of kernicterus)
Note *Konakion® MM Paediatric* may be administered *by mouth* or *by intramuscular injection* or *by intravenous injection*

9.6.7 Multivitamin preparations

Vitamins

Capsules, ascorbic acid 15 mg, nicotinamide 7.5 mg, riboflavin 500 micrograms, thiamine hydrochloride 1 mg, vitamin A 2500 units, vitamin D 300 units. Net price 20 = 22p

Abidec® (Chefaro UK)

Drops, vitamins A, B group, C, and D. Net price 25 mL (with dropper) = £2.08

Excipients include arachis (peanut) oil

Note Contains 1333 units of vitamin A (as palmitate) per 0.6-mL dose

Dalivit® (LPC)

Oral drops, vitamins A, B group, C, and D, net price 25 mL = £2.98, 50 mL = £4.85

Note Contains 5000 units of vitamin A (as palmitate) per 0.6-mL dose

Vitamin and mineral supplements and adjuncts to synthetic diets

Forceval® (Alliance)

Capsules, brown/red, vitamins (ascorbic acid 60 mg, biotin 100 micrograms, cyanocobalamin 3 micrograms, folic acid 400 micrograms, nicotinamide 18 mg, pantothenic acid 4 mg, pyridoxine 2 mg, riboflavin 1.6 mg, thiamine 1.2 mg, vitamin A 2500 units, vitamin D_2 400 units, vitamin E 10 mg, minerals and trace elements (calcium 100 mg, chromium 200 micrograms, copper 2 mg, iodine 140 micrograms, iron 12 mg, magnesium 30 mg, manganese 3 mg, molybdenum 250 micrograms, phosphorus 77 mg, potassium 4 mg, selenium 50 micrograms, zinc 15 mg). Net price 30-cap pack = £4.94, 45-cap pack = £6.47; 90-cap pack = £11.93. Label: 25

Dose vitamin and mineral deficiency and as adjunct in synthetic diets, ADULT 1 capsule daily one hour after a meal

Junior capsules, brown, vitamins (ascorbic acid 25 mg, biotin 50 micrograms, cyanocobalamin 2 micrograms, folic acid 100 micrograms, nicotinamide 7.5 mg, pantothenic acid 2 mg, pyridoxine 1 mg, riboflavin 1 mg, thiamine 1.5 mg, vitamin A 1250 units, vitamin D_2 200 units, vitamin E 5 mg, vitamin K_1 25 micrograms), minerals and trace elements (chromium 50 micrograms, copper 1 mg, iodine 75 micrograms, iron 5 mg, magnesium 1 mg, manganese 1.25 mg, molybdenum 50 micrograms, selenium 25 micrograms, zinc 5 mg). Net price 30-cap pack = £3.52, 60-cap pack = £6.69

Dose vitamin and mineral deficiency and as adjunct in synthetic diets, CHILD over 5 years, 2 capsules daily

Ketovite® (Paines & Byrne)

Tablets [PoM], yellow, ascorbic acid 16.6 mg, riboflavin 1 mg, thiamine hydrochloride 1 mg, pyridoxine hydrochloride 330 micrograms, nicotinamide 3.3 mg, calcium pantothenate 1.16 mg, alpha tocopheryl acetate 5 mg, inositol 50 mg, biotin 170 micrograms, folic acid 250 micrograms, acetomenaphthone 500 micrograms. Net price 100-tab pack = £4.17

Dose prevention of vitamin deficiency in disorders of carbohydrate or amino-acid metabolism and adjunct in restricted, specialised, or synthetic diets, 1 tablet 3 times daily; use with *Ketovite® Liquid* for complete vitamin supplementation

Liquid, pink, sugar-free, vitamin A 2500 units, ergocalciferol 400 units, choline chloride 150 mg, cyanocobalamin 12.5 micrograms/5 mL. Net price 150-mL pack = £2.70

Dose prevention of vitamin deficiency in disorders of carbohydrate or amino-acid metabolism and adjunct in restricted, specialised, or synthetic diets, 5 mL daily; use with *Ketovite® Tablets* for complete vitamin supplementation

9.7 Bitters and tonics

Mixtures containing simple and aromatic bitters, such as alkaline gentian mixture, are traditional remedies for loss of appetite. All depend on suggestion.

Gentian Mixture, Alkaline, BP (Alkaline Gentian Oral Solution)

Mixture, concentrated compound gentian infusion 10%, sodium bicarbonate 5% in a suitable vehicle. Extemporaneous preparations should be recently prepared according to the following formula: concentrated compound gentian infusion 1 mL, sodium bicarbonate 500 mg, double-strength chloroform water 5 mL, water to 10 mL

Dose 10 mL 3 times daily in water before meals

Effico® (Forest) [NHS]

Tonic, orange-red, thiamine hydrochloride 180 micrograms, nicotinamide 2.1 mg, caffeine 20.2 mg, compound gentian infusion 0.31 mL/5 mL. Net price 300-mL pack = £2.46, 500-mL pack = £3.13

Labiton® (LAB) [NHS]

Tonic, brown, thiamine hydrochloride 375 micrograms, caffeine 3.5 mg, kola nut dried extract 3.025 mg, alcohol 1.4 mL/5 mL. Net price 200 mL = £2.62

Metatone® (Chefaro UK) [NHS]

Tonic, thiamine hydrochloride 500 micrograms, calcium glycerophosphate 45.6 mg, manganese glycerophosphate 5.7 mg, potassium glycerophosphate 45.6 mg, sodium glycerophosphate 22.8 mg/5 mL. Net price 300 mL = £2.79

9.8 Metabolic disorders

9.8.1 Drugs used in metabolic disorders
9.8.2 Acute porphyrias

This section covers drugs used in metabolic disorders and not readily classified elsewhere.

9.8.1 Drugs used in metabolic disorders

Wilson's disease

Penicillamine (see also section 10.1.3) is used in Wilson's disease (hepatolenticular degeneration) to aid the elimination of copper ions. See below for other indications.

Trientine is used for the treatment of Wilson's disease only in patients intolerant of penicillamine; it is **not** an alternative to penicillamine for rheumatoid arthritis or cystinuria. Penicillamine-induced systemic lupus erythematosus may not resolve on transfer to trientine.

Zinc prevents the absorption of copper in Wilson's disease. Symptomatic patients should be treated initially with a chelating agent because zinc has a slow onset of action. When transferring from chelating treatment to zinc maintenance therapy, chelating treatment should be co-administered for 2–3 weeks until zinc produces its maximal effect.

PENICILLAMINE

Indications see under Dose below
Cautions see section 10.1.3
Contra-indications see section 10.1.3
Side-effects see section 10.1.3
Dose

- Wilson's disease, 1.5–2 g daily in divided doses before food; max. 2 g daily for 1 year; maintenance 0.75–1 g daily; ELDERLY 20 mg/kg daily in divided doses, adjusted according to response; CHILD up to 20 mg/kg daily in divided doses, minimum 500 mg daily
- Autoimmune hepatitis (used rarely; after disease controlled with corticosteroids), initially 500 mg daily in divided doses increased slowly over 3 months; usual maintenance dose 1.25 g daily; ELDERLY not recommended
- Cystinuria, therapeutic, 1–3 g daily in divided doses before food, adjusted to maintain urinary cystine below 200 mg/litre; prophylactic (maintain urinary cystine below 300 mg/litre) 0.5–1 g at bedtime; maintain adequate fluid intake (at least 3 litres daily); CHILD and ELDERLY minimum dose to maintain urinary cystine below 200 mg/litre
- Severe active rheumatoid arthritis, section 10.1.3
- Copper and lead poisoning, see Emergency Treatment of Poisoning

Preparations
Section 10.1.3

TRIENTINE DIHYDROCHLORIDE

Indications Wilson's disease in patients intolerant of penicillamine
Cautions see notes above; pregnancy (Appendix 4); interactions: Appendix 1 (trientine)
Side-effects nausea, rash; rarely anaemia
Dose

- 1.2–2.4 g daily in 2–4 divided doses before food; CHILD initially 0.6–1.5 g daily in 2–4 divided doses before food, adjusted according to response

Trientine Dihydrochloride (Univar) PoM
Capsules, trientine dihydrochloride 300 mg. Label: 6, 22

ZINC ACETATE

Indications Wilson's disease (initiated under specialist supervision)
Cautions portal hypertension (risk of hepatic decompensation when switching from chelating agent); monitor full blood count and serum cholesterol; pregnancy (Appendix 4); **interactions**: Appendix 1 (zinc)
Contra-indications breast-feeding
Side-effects gastric irritation (usually transient; may be reduced if first dose taken mid-morning or with a little protein); *less commonly* sideroblastic anaemia and leucopenia
Dose
Note Dose expressed as elemental zinc

- Wilson's disease, 50 mg 3 times daily (max. 50 mg 5 times daily), adjusted according to response; CHILD 1–6 years, 25 mg twice daily; 6–16 years, body-weight under 57 kg, 25 mg 3 times daily, body-weight over 57 kg, 50 mg 3 times daily; ADOLESCENT 16–18 years, 50 mg 3 times daily

Wilzin® (Orphan Europe) ▼ PoM
Capsules, zinc (as acetate) 25 mg (blue), net price 250-cap pack = £123.00; 50 mg (orange), 250-cap pack = £233.00. Label: 23

Carnitine deficiency

Carnitine is available for the management of primary carnitine deficiency due to inborn errors of metabolism or of secondary deficiency in haemodialysis patients.

CARNITINE

Indications primary and secondary carnitine deficiency
Cautions diabetes mellitus; renal impairment; monitoring of free and acyl carnitine in blood and urine recommended; pregnancy (Appendix 4) and breast-feeding
Side-effects nausea, vomiting, abdominal pain, diarrhoea, body odour; side-effects may be dose-related—monitor tolerance during first week and after any dose increase
Dose

- Primary deficiency, by mouth, up to 200 mg/kg daily in 2–4 divided doses; higher doses of up to 400 mg/kg daily occasionally required; by intravenous injection over 2–3 minutes, up to 100 mg/kg daily in 3–4 divided doses
- Secondary deficiency, by intravenous injection over 2–3 minutes, 20 mg/kg after each dialysis session (dosage adjusted according to carnitine concentration); maintenance, by mouth, 1 g daily

Carnitor® (Sigma-Tau) PoM
Oral liquid, L-carnitine 100 mg/mL (10%), net price 10 × 10-mL (1-g) single-dose bottle = £35.00
Paediatric solution, L-carnitine 300 mg/mL (30%), net price 20 mL = £21.00
Excipients include sorbitol
Injection, L-carnitine 200 mg/mL. Net price 5-mL amp = £11.90

Fabry's disease

Agalsidase alfa and **agalsidase beta**, enzymes produced by recombinant DNA technology, are licensed for long-term enzyme replacement therapy in Fabry's disease (a lysosomal storage disorder caused by deficiency of alpha-galactosidase A).

AGALSIDASE ALFA and BETA

Indications (specialist use only) Fabry's disease

Cautions pregnancy (Appendix 4); breast-feeding (Appendix 5); **interactions:** Appendix 1 (agalsidase beta)

Infusion-related reactions Infusion-related reactions very common, calling for use of antihistamine, antipyretic and corticosteroid; consult product literature for details

Side-effects nausea, vomiting, oedema, hypertension, hypersensitivity reactions, fever, headache, tremor, myalgia, injection-site pain; *commonly* abdominal pain, bradycardia, tachycardia, palpitation, fatigue, drowsiness, paraesthesia, neuropathic pain, dizziness, anaemia, proteinuria, visual disturbances, abnormal tear secretion, tinnitus, acne, pruritus and rash

Fabrazyme® (Genzyme) PoM
Intravenous infusion, powder for reconstitution, agalsidase beta, net price 5-mg vial = £325.50; 35-mg vial = £2269.20
Dose By intravenous infusion, ADULT and CHILD over 8 years 1 mg/kg every 2 weeks

Replagal® (Shire) PoM
Concentrate for intravenous infusion, agalsidase alfa 1 mg/mL, net price 1-mL vial = £356.85; 3.5-mL vial = £1161.57
Dose By intravenous infusion, ADULT over 18 years 200 micrograms/kg every 2 weeks

Gaucher's disease

Imiglucerase, an enzyme produced by recombinant DNA technology, is administered as enzyme replacement therapy for non-neurological manifestations of type I or type III Gaucher's disease, a familial disorder affecting principally the liver, spleen, bone marrow, and lymph nodes.

Miglustat, an inhibitor of glucosylceramide synthase, is licensed for the treatment of mild to moderate type I Gaucher's disease in patients for whom imiglucerase is unsuitable; it is given by mouth.

IMIGLUCERASE

Indications (specialist use only) non-neurological manifestations of type I or type III Gaucher's disease

Cautions pregnancy (Appendix 4); breast-feeding (Appendix 5); monitor for imiglucerase antibodies; when stabilised, monitor all parameters and response to treatment at intervals of 6–12 months

Side-effects hypersensitivity reactions (including urticaria, angioedema, hypotension, flushing, tachycardia); less commonly nausea, vomiting, diarrhoea, abdominal cramps, headache, dizziness, paraesthesia, fatigue, fever, arthralgia, injection-site reactions

Dose

- By intravenous infusion, initially 60 units/kg once every 2 weeks (2.5 units/kg 3 times a week or 15 units/kg once every 2 weeks may improve haematological parameters and organomegaly, but not bone parameters); maintenance, adjust dose according to response

Cerezyme® (Genzyme) PoM
Intravenous infusion, powder for reconstitution, imiglucerase, net price 200-unit vial = £553.35; 400-unit vial = £1106.70
Electrolytes Na^+ 0.62 mmol/200-unit vial, 1.24 mmol/400-unit vial

MIGLUSTAT

Indications mild to moderate type I Gaucher's disease (specialist supervision only)

Cautions hepatic impairment (Appendix 2); renal impairment (Appendix 3); monitor cognitive and neurological function

Contra-indications pregnancy (Appendix 4); men should not father a child during or within 3 months of treatment; breast-feeding (Appendix 5)

Side-effects diarrhoea, flatulence, abdominal pain, constipation, nausea, vomiting, weight changes; tremor, dizziness, headache; leg cramps; visual disturbances; commonly dyspepsia, decreased appetite, peripheral neuropathy, cognitive dysfunction

Dose

- ADULT over 18 years, 100 mg 3 times daily; reduced if not tolerated to 100 mg 1–2 times daily

Zavesca® (Actelion) ▼ PoM
Capsules, miglustat 100 mg, net price 84-cap pack = £4015.00 (hospital only)

Mucopolysaccharidosis

Laronidase, an enzyme produced by recombinant DNA technology, is licensed for long-term replacement therapy in the treatment of non-neurological manifestations of mucopolysaccharidosis I, a lysosomal storage disorder caused by deficiency of alpha-L- iduronidase.

Idursulfase, an enzyme produced by recombinant DNA technology, is licensed for long-term replacement therapy in mucopolysaccharidosis II (Hunter syndrome), a lysosomal storage disorder caused by deficiency of iduronate-2-sulfatase.

Galsulfase, a recombinant form of human N-acetylgalactosamine-4-sulfatase, is licensed for long-term replacement therapy in mucopolysaccharidosis VI (Maroteaux-Lamy syndrome).

Infusion-related reactions often occur with administration of laronidase, idursulfase, and galsulfase; they can be managed by slowing the infusion rate or interrupting the infusion, and can be minimized by pre-treatment with an antihistamine and an antipyretic; recurrent reactions may require a corticosteroid—consult product literature for details.

LARONIDASE

Indications (specialist use only) non-neurological manifestations of mucopolysaccharidosis I

Cautions monitor immunoglobulin G (IgG) antibody concentration; pregnancy (Appendix 4); breast-feeding (Appendix 5); **interactions:** Appendix 1 (laronidase)

Infusion-related reactions Infusion-related reactions very common—see notes above

Side-effects nausea, vomiting, diarrhoea, abdominal pain; cold extremities, pallor, flushing, tachycardia, angioedema, blood pressure changes; dyspnoea, cough; headache, paraesthesia, dizziness, fatigue, restlessness; influenza-like symptoms; musculoskeletal pain, pain in extremities; rash pruritus, urticaria, alopecia, infusion-site reactions, anaphylaxis; also reported bronchospasm and respiratory arrest

Dose

- By intravenous infusion, 100 units/kg once weekly; CHILD see *BNF for Children*

Aldurazyme® (Genzyme) ▼ PoM
Concentrate for intravenous infusion, laronidase 100 units/mL, net price 5-mL vial = £460.35

IDURSULFASE

Indications (specialist use only) mucopolysaccharidosis II

Cautions severe respiratory disease; acute febrile respiratory illness (consider delaying treatment); breast-feeding (Appendix 5)

Infusion-related reactions Infusion-related reactions very common—see notes above

Contra-indications women of child-bearing potential (see Pregnancy—Appendix 4)

Side-effects gastro-intestinal disturbances, swollen tongue; arrhythmia, chest pain, cyanosis, peripheral oedema, hypertension, hypotension, flushing, pulmonary embolism; bronchospasm, cough, wheezing, tachypnoea, dyspnoea; headache, dizziness, tremor; pyrexia; arthralgia; increased lacrimation; facial oedema, urticaria, pruritus, rash, infusion-site swelling, erythema, and eczema; anaphylaxis also reported

Dose

- By intravenous infusion, ADULT and CHILD over 5 years, 500 micrograms/kg once weekly

Elaprase® (Shire) ▼ PoM
Concentrate for intravenous infusion, idursulfase 2 mg/mL, net price 3-mL vial = £1985.00

GALSULFASE

Indications (specialist use only) mucopolysaccharidosis VI

Cautions respiratory disease; acute febrile or respiratory illness (consider delaying treatment); pregnancy (Appendix 4)

Infusion-related reactions Infusion-related reactions very common—see notes above

Contra-indications breast-feeding (Appendix 5)

Side-effects abdominal pain, umbilical hernia, gastroenteritis; chest pain, hypertension; dyspnoea, apnoea, nasal congestion; rigors, malaise, areflexia; pharyngitis; conjunctivitis, corneal opacity; ear pain; facial oedema

Dose

- By intravenous infusion, ADULT and CHILD over 5 years, 1 mg/kg once weekly

Naglazyme® (BioMarin) ▼ PoM
Concentrate for intravenous infusion, galsulfase 1 mg/mL, net price 5-mL vial = £982.00

Nephropathic cystinosis

Mercaptamine (cysteamine) is available for the treatment of nephropathic cystinosis.

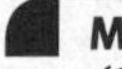

MERCAPTAMINE
(Cysteamine)

Indications (specialist use only) nephropathic cystinosis

Cautions leucocyte-cystine concentration and haematological monitoring required—consult product literature; dose of phosphate supplement may need to be adjusted

Contra-indications pregnancy and breast-feeding; hypersensitivity to mercaptamine or penicillamine

Side-effects breath and body odour, nausea, vomiting, diarrhoea, anorexia, lethargy, fever, rash; also reported dehydration, hypertension, abdominal discomfort, gastroenteritis, drowsiness, encephalopathy, headache, nervousness, depression; anaemia, leucopenia; *rarely* gastro-intestinal ulceration and bleeding, seizures, hallucinations, urticaria, interstitial nephritis

Dose

- Initial doses should be one-sixth to one-quarter of the expected maintenance dose, increased gradually over 4–6 weeks
- Maintenance, ADULT and CHILD over 50 kg body-weight, 2 g daily in 4 divided doses
  CHILD up to 12 years, 1.3 g/m² (approx. 50 mg/kg) daily in 4 divided doses

Cystagon® (Orphan Europe) PoM
Capsules, mercaptamine (as bitartrate) 50 mg, net price 100-cap pack = £44.00; 150 mg, 100-cap pack = £125.00

Note CHILD under 6 years at risk of aspiration, capsules can be opened and contents sprinkled on food (at a temperature suitable for eating); avoid adding to acidic drinks (e.g. orange juice)

Pompe disease

Alglucosidase alfa, an enzyme produced by recombinant DNA technology, is licensed for long-term replacement therapy in Pompe disease, a lysosomal storage disorder caused by deficiency of acid alpha-glucosidase.

ALGLUCOSIDASE ALFA

Indications (specialist use only) Pompe disease

Cautions cardiac and respiratory dysfunction—monitor closely; pregnancy (Appendix 4)

Infusion-related reactions Infusion-related reactions very common, calling for use of antihistamine, antipyretic or corticosteroid; consult product literature for details

Contra-indications breast-feeding (Appendix 5)

Side-effects nausea, vomiting; flushing, tachycardia, blood pressure changes, cold extremities, cyanosis, facial oedema; cough, tachypnoea, bronchospasm; headache, agitation, tremor, irritability, restlessness, paraesthesia, dizziness; pyrexia, rigors; antibody formation; sweating, rash, pruritus, and urticaria; anaphylaxis

Dose

- By intravenous infusion, 20 mg/kg every 2 weeks

Myozyme® (Genzyme) ▼ PoM
Intravenous infusion, powder for reconstitution, alglucosidase alfa, net price 50-mg vial = £368.59

Tyrosinaemia type I

Nitisinone is licensed for the treatment of hereditary tyrosinaemia type I in combination with dietary restriction of tyrosine and phenylalanine.

NITISINONE
(NTBC)

Indications hereditary tyrosinaemia type I (specialist use only)

Cautions slit-lamp examination of eyes recommended before treatment; monitor liver function regularly; monitor platelet and white blood cell count every 6 months

Contra-indications pregnancy (Appendix 4); breast-feeding (Appendix 5)

Side-effects thrombocytopenia, leucopenia, granulocytopenia; conjunctivitis, photophobia, corneal opacity, keratitis, eye pain; *less commonly* leucocytosis, blepharitis, pruritus, exfoliative dermatitis, and erythematous rash

Dose

- ADULT, NEONATE and CHILD initially 500 micrograms/kg twice daily, adjusted according to response; max. 2 mg/kg daily

  Note Capsules can be opened and the contents suspended in a small amount of water or formula diet and taken immediately

Orfadin® (Swedish Orphan) PoM
Capsules, nitisinone 2 mg, net price 60-cap pack = £564.00; 5 mg, 60-cap pack = £1127.00; 10 mg, 60-cap pack = £2062.00

Urea cycle disorders

Sodium phenylbutyrate is used in the management of urea cycle disorders. It is indicated as adjunctive therapy in all patients with neonatal-onset disease and in those with late-onset disease who have a history of hyperammonaemic encephalopathy.

Carglumic acid is licensed for the treatment of hyperammonaemia due to *N*-acetylglutamate synthase deficiency.

CARGLUMIC ACID

Indications hyperammonaemia due to *N*-acetylglutamate synthase deficiency (initiated under specialist supervision)

Cautions pregnancy (Appendix 4) and breast-feeding (Appendix 5)

Side-effects raised serum transaminases, sweating

Dose

- ADULT and CHILD initially 100 mg/kg daily in 2–4 divided doses immediately before food (max. 250 mg/kg daily), adjusted according to plasma–ammonia concentration; maintenance 10–100 mg/kg daily in 2–4 divided doses

Carbaglu® (Orphan Europe) ▼ PoM
Dispersible tablets, carglumic acid 200 mg, net price 5-tab pack = £226.00, 60-tab pack = £2685.00. Label: 13

SODIUM PHENYLBUTYRATE

Indications adjunct in long-term treatment of urea cycle disorders (under specialist supervision)

Cautions congestive heart failure, hepatic and renal impairment

Contra-indications pregnancy (Appendix 4); breast-feeding (Appendix 5)

Side-effects amenorrhoea and irregular menstrual cycles, decreased appetite, body odour, taste disturbances; less commonly nausea, vomiting, abdominal pain, peptic ulcer, pancreatitis, rectal bleeding, arrhythmia, oedema, syncope, depression, headache, rash, weight gain, renal tubular acidosis, aplastic anaemia, ecchymoses

Dose

- ADULT and CHILD over 20 kg, 9.9–13 g/m² daily in divided doses with meals (max. 20 g daily); CHILD less than 20 kg, 450–600 mg/kg daily in divided doses with meals

Ammonaps® (Swedish Orphan) PoM
Tablets, sodium phenylbutyrate 500 mg. Contains Na^+ 2.7 mmol/tablet. Net price 250-tab pack = £493.00

Granules, sodium phenylbutyrate 940 mg/g. Contains Na^+ 5.4 mmol/g. Net price 266-g pack = £860.00

Note Granules should be mixed with food before taking

9.8.2 Acute porphyrias

The acute porphyrias (acute intermittent porphyria, variegate porphyria, hereditary coproporphyria, and 5-aminolaevulinic acid dehydratase deficiency porphyria) are hereditary disorders of haem biosynthesis; they have a prevalence of about 1 in 10 000 of the population.

Great care must be taken when prescribing for patients with acute porphyria, since certain drugs can induce acute porphyric crises. Since acute porphyrias are hereditary, relatives of affected individuals should be screened and advised about the potential danger of certain drugs.

Treatment of serious or life-threatening conditions should not be withheld from patients with acute porphyria. When there is no safe alternative, urinary porphobilinogen excretion should be measured regularly; if it increases or symptoms occur, the drug can be withdrawn and the acute attack treated.

Haem arginate is administered by short intravenous infusion as haem replacement in moderate, severe, or unremitting acute porphyria crises.

Supplies of haem arginate may be obtained outside office hours from the on-call pharmacist at:

St Thomas' Hospital, London (020) 7188 7188

HAEM ARGINATE
(Human hemin)

Indications acute porphyrias (acute intermittent porphyria, porphyria variegata, hereditary coproporphyria)

Cautions pregnancy (Appendix 4); breast feeding (Appendix 5)

Side-effects rarely hypersensitivity reactions and fever; pain and thrombophlebitis at injection site

Dose

- By intravenous infusion, ADULT and CHILD 3 mg/kg once daily (max. 250 mg daily) for 4 days; if response inadequate, repeat 4-day course with close biochemical monitoring

Normosang® (Orphan Europe) ▼ PoM
Concentrate for intravenous infusion, haem arginate 25 mg/mL, net price 10-mL amp = £281.25

Drugs unsafe for use in acute porphyrias

The following list contains drugs on the UK market that have been classified as 'unsafe' in porphyria because they have been shown to be porphyrinogenic in animals or *in vitro*, or have been associated with acute attacks in patients. Absence of a drug from the following lists does not necessarily imply that the drug is safe. For many drugs no information about porphyria is available.

An up-to-date list of drugs considered **safe** in acute porphyrias is available at www.wmic.wales.nhs.uk/porphyria_info.php

Further information may be obtained from:
www.porphyria-europe.org

and also from:

Welsh Medicines Information Centre
University Hospital of Wales
Cardiff, CF14 4XW
Tel: (029) 2074 2979/3877

Note Quite modest changes in chemical structure can lead to changes in porphyrinogenicity but where possible general statements have been made about groups of drugs; these should be checked first.

Unsafe Drug Groups (check *first*)

Amphetamines
Anabolic Steroids
Antidepressants[1]
Antihistamines[2]
Barbiturates[3]
Calcium channel blockers[4]
Contraceptives, hormonal[5]
Ergot Derivatives[6]
Gold Salts
Hormone Replacement Therapy[5]
Imidazole antifungals
Non-nucleoside reverse transcriptase inhibitors[7]
Progestogens[5]
Protease inhibitors[7]
Statins[8]
Sulphonamides[9]
Sulphonylureas[10]
Tetracyclines
Triazole antifungals

Unsafe Drugs (check groups above *first*)

Aceclofenac
Alcohol
Amiodarone
Azapropazone
Bosentan
Bromocriptine
Buspirone
Busulfan
Cabergoline
Carbamazepine
Carisoprodol
Chloral Hydrate[11]
Chlorambucil[12]
Chloramphenicol
Chloroform[13]
Clindamycin
Clonidine
Cocaine
Colistin
Cyclophosphamide[12]
Cycloserine
Danazol
Dapsone
Dexfenfluramine
Diazepam[14]
Diclofenac
Erythromycin
Etamsylate
Ethosuximide
Etomidate
Fenfluramine
Flupentixol
Griseofulvin
Halothane
Hydralazine
Indapamide
Isometheptene Mucate
Isoniazid
Ketamine
Ketorolac
Lidocaine (lignocaine)[15]
Mebeverine
Mefenamic Acid[12]
Meprobamate
Methyldopa
Metoclopramide[12]
Metolazone
Metronidazole[12]
Metyrapone
Mifepristone
Minoxidil[12]
Nalidixic Acid
Nitrofurantoin
Orphenadrine
Oxcarbazepine
Oxybutynin
Oxycodone[16]
Pentazocine[16]
Pentoxifylline (oxpentifylline)
Phenoxybenzamine
Phenytoin
Pivmecillinam
Porfimer
Probenecid
Pyrazinamide
Rifabutin[17]
Rifampicin[17]
Spironolactone
Sulfinpyrazone
Sulpiride
Tamoxifen
Temoporfin
Theophylline[18]
Tiagabine
Tinidazole
Topiramate
Tramadol[16]
Triclofos[11]
Trimethoprim
Valproate[14]
Xipamide
Zidovudine[7]
Zuclopenthixol

1. Includes tricyclic (and related) antidepressants and MAOIs; fluoxetine and mianserin thought to be safe.
2. Alimemazine (trimeprazine), chlorphenamine, desloratadine, ketotifen, loratadine, and promethazine thought to be safe.
3. Includes primidone and thiopental.
4. Diltiazem may be used with caution if safer alternative not available
5. Progestogens are more porphyrinogenic than oestrogens; oestrogens may be safe at least in replacement doses. Progestogens should be avoided whenever possible by all women susceptible to acute porphyria; however, when non-hormonal contraception is inappropriate, progestogens may be used with extreme caution if the potential benefit outweighs risk. The risk of an acute attack is greatest in women who have had a previous attack or are aged under 30 years. Long-acting progestogen preparations should **never** be used in those at risk of acute porphyria.
6. Includes ergometrine (oxytocin probably safe) and pergolide.
7. Contact Welsh Medicines Information Centre for further advice.
8. Rosuvastatin is thought to be safe.
9. Includes co-trimoxazole and sulfasalazine.
10. Glipizide is thought to be safe.
11. Although evidence of hazard is uncertain, manufacturer advises avoid.
12. May be used with caution if safer alternative not available.
13. Small amounts in medicines probably safe.
14. Status epilepticus has been treated successfully with intravenous diazepam.
15. When used for local anaesthesia, bupivacaine, lidocaine (lignocaine), prilocaine, and tetracaine are thought to be safe.
16. Buprenorphine, codeine, diamorphine, dihydrocodeine, fentanyl, methadone, morphine, and pethidine are thought to be safe.
17. Rifamycins have been used in a few patients without evidence of harm—use with caution if safer alternative not available.
18. Includes aminophylline.

10 Musculoskeletal and joint diseases

10.1 Drugs used in rheumatic diseases and gout 534
10.1.1 Non-steroidal anti-inflammatory drugs 535
10.1.2 Corticosteroids 544
10.1.2.1 Systemic corticosteroids 544
10.1.2.2 Local corticosteroid injections 545
10.1.3 Drugs that suppress the rheumatic disease process 546
10.1.4 Gout and cytotoxic-induced hyperuricaemia 555
10.1.5 Other drugs for rheumatic diseases 557
10.2 Drugs used in neuromuscular disorders 557
10.2.1 Drugs that enhance neuromuscular transmission 557
10.2.2 Skeletal muscle relaxants 559
10.3 Drugs for the relief of soft-tissue inflammation 562
10.3.1 Enzymes 562
10.3.2 Rubefacients and other topical antirheumatics 563

This chapter also includes advice on the drug management of the following:

- dental and orofacial pain, p. 536
- extravasation, p. 562
- myasthenia gravis, p. 557
- osteoarthritis and soft-tissue disorders, below
- rheumatoid arthritis and other inflammatory disorders, below

For treatment of septic arthritis see Table 1, section 5.1.

10.1 Drugs used in rheumatic diseases and gout

10.1.1 Non-steroidal anti-inflammatory drugs
10.1.2 Corticosteroids
10.1.3 Drugs that suppress the rheumatic disease process
10.1.4 Gout and cytotoxic-induced hyperuricaemia
10.1.5 Other drugs for rheumatic diseases

Rheumatoid arthritis and other inflammatory disorders

A non-steroidal anti-inflammatory drug (NSAID) is indicated for pain and stiffness resulting from inflammatory rheumatic disease. Drugs are also used to influence the disease process itself (section 10.1.3). For rheumatoid arthritis these disease-modifying antirheumatic drugs (DMARDs) include penicillamine, gold salts, antimalarials (chloroquine and hydroxychloroquine), drugs that affect the immune response, and sulfasalazine; corticosteroids may also be of value (section 10.1.2.1). Drugs which may affect the disease process in psoriatic arthritis include sulfasalazine, gold salts, azathioprine, methotrexate (section 10.1.3), and etanercept. For long-term control of gout uricosuric drugs and allopurinol (section 10.1.4) can be used.

Osteoarthritis and soft-tissue disorders

In osteoarthritis (sometimes called degenerative joint disease or osteoarthrosis) non-drug measures such as weight reduction and exercise should be encouraged. For pain relief in osteoarthritis and soft-tissue disorders, paracetamol (section 4.7.1) is often adequate and should be used first. Alternatively, a low dose of a NSAID (e.g. ibuprofen up to 1.2 g daily) can be used. If pain relief with either drug is inadequate, both paracetamol (in a full dose of 4 g daily) and a low dose of a NSAID can be used; if necessary the dose of the NSAID can be increased or a low dose of an opioid analgesic given with paracetamol (as co-codamol 8/500 or co-dydramol 10/500).

Topical treatment, including application of a NSAID or capsaicin 0.025% (section 10.3.2), may provide some pain relief in osteoarthritis.

Intra-articular corticosteroid injections (section 10.1.2.2) may produce temporary benefit in osteoarthritis, especially if associated with soft-tissue inflammation.

Hyaluronic acid and its derivatives are available for osteoarthritis of the knee. Sodium hyaluronate (*Durolane*®, *Fermathron*®, *Orthovisc*®, *Ostenil*®, *Suplasyn*®, *Synocrom*®) or hylan G-F 20 (*Synvisc*®) is injected intra-articularly to supplement natural hyaluronic acid in the synovial fluid. These injections may reduce pain over 1–6 months but they are associated with short-term increase in knee inflammation.

Glucosamine (section 10.1.5) is licensed for symptomatic relief of mild to moderate osteoarthritis of the knee.

10.1.1 Non-steroidal anti-inflammatory drugs

In *single doses* non-steroidal anti-inflammatory drugs (NSAIDs) have analgesic activity comparable to that of paracetamol (section 4.7.1), but paracetamol is preferred, particularly in the elderly (see also Prescribing for the Elderly, p. 20).

In regular *full dosage* NSAIDs have both a lasting analgesic and an anti-inflammatory effect which makes them particularly useful for the treatment of continuous or regular pain associated with inflammation. Therefore, although paracetamol often gives adequate pain control in osteoarthritis, NSAIDs are more appropriate than paracetamol or the opioid analgesics in the *inflammatory arthritides* (e.g. rheumatoid arthritis) and in some cases of *advanced osteoarthritis*. NSAIDs can also be of benefit in the less well defined conditions of *back pain* and *soft-tissue disorders*.

Choice Differences in anti-inflammatory activity between NSAIDs are small, but there is considerable variation in individuals' tolerance to these drugs and their response to them. About 60% of patients will respond to any NSAID; of the others, those who do not respond to one may well respond to another. Pain relief starts soon after taking the first dose and a full analgesic effect should normally be obtained within a week, whereas an anti-inflammatory effect may not be achieved (or may not be clinically assessable) for up to 3 weeks. If appropriate responses are not obtained within these times, another NSAID should be tried.

NSAIDs reduce the production of prostaglandins by inhibiting the enzyme cyclo-oxygenase. They vary in their selectivity for inhibiting different types of cyclo-oxygenase; selective inhibition of cyclo-oxygenase-2 improves gastro-intestinal tolerance. A number of other factors also determine susceptibility to gastro-intestinal effects and a NSAID should be chosen on the basis of the incidence of gastro-intestinal and other side-effects.

Ibuprofen is a propionic acid derivative with anti-inflammatory, analgesic, and antipyretic properties. It has fewer side-effects than other non-selective NSAIDs but its anti-inflammatory properties are weaker. Doses of 1.6 to 2.4 g daily are needed for rheumatoid arthritis and it is unsuitable for conditions where inflammation is prominent, such as acute gout. **Dexibuprofen** is the active enantiomer of ibuprofen. It has similar properties to ibuprofen and is licensed for the relief of mild to moderate pain and inflammation.

Other propionic acid derivatives:

Naproxen is one of the first choices because it combines good efficacy with a low incidence of side-effects (but more than ibuprofen, see CSM comment below).

Fenbufen is claimed to be associated with less gastro-intestinal bleeding, but there is a high risk of rashes (see p. 540).

Fenoprofen is as effective as naproxen, and **flurbiprofen** may be slightly more effective. Both are associated with slightly more gastro-intestinal side-effects than ibuprofen.

Ketoprofen has anti-inflammatory properties similar to ibuprofen and has more side-effects (see also CSM comment below). **Dexketoprofen**, an isomer of ketoprofen, has been introduced for the short-term relief of mild to moderate pain.

Tiaprofenic acid is as effective as naproxen; it has more side-effects than ibuprofen (**important:** reports of severe cystitis, see CSM advice on p. 544).

Drugs with properties similar to those of propionic acid derivatives:

Azapropazone is similar in effect to naproxen; it has a tendency to cause rashes and is associated with an increased risk of severe gastro-intestinal toxicity (**important:** see CSM restrictions on p. 537).

Diclofenac and **aceclofenac** have actions and side-effects similar to those of naproxen.

Etodolac has efficacy comparable to naproxen; it is licensed for symptomatic relief of osteoarthritis and rheumatoid arthritis.

Indometacin (indomethacin) has an action equal to or superior to that of naproxen, but with a high incidence of side-effects including headache, dizziness, and gastro-intestinal disturbances (see also CSM comment below).

Mefenamic acid has minor anti-inflammatory properties. It has occasionally been associated with diarrhoea and haemolytic anaemia which require discontinuation of treatment.

Meloxicam is licensed for the short-term relief of pain in osteoarthritis and for long-term treatment of rheumatoid arthritis and ankylosing spondylitis.

Nabumetone is comparable in effect to naproxen.

Piroxicam is as effective as naproxen and has a long duration of action which permits once-daily administration. However, it has more gastro-intestinal side-effects than most other NSAIDs, and is associated with more frequent serious skin reactions (**important:** see CHMP advice, p. 543).

Sulindac is similar in tolerance to naproxen.

Tenoxicam is similar in activity and tolerance to naproxen. Its long duration of action allows once-daily administration.

Tolfenamic acid is licensed for the treatment of migraine (section 4.7.4.1)

Ketorolac and the selective inhibitor of cyclo-oxygenase-2, **parecoxib**, are licensed for the short-term management of postoperative pain (section 15.1.4.2).

The selective inhibitors of cyclo-oxygenase-2, **etoricoxib** and **celecoxib**, are as effective as non-selective NSAIDs such as diclofenac and naproxen. Short-term data indicate that the risk of serious upper gastro-intestinal events is lower with selective inhibitors compared to non-selective NSAIDs; this advantage may be lost in patients who require concomitant low-dose aspirin. There are concerns about the cardiovascular safety of cyclo-oxygenase-2 selective inhibitors (see below).

Celecoxib and **etoricoxib** are licensed for the relief of pain in osteoarthritis and for rheumatoid arthritis; celecoxib is also licensed for symptomatic relief of ankylosing spondylitis, and etoricoxib is also licensed for the relief of pain from acute gout.

NSAIDs and cardiovascular events

Cyclo-oxygenase-2 selective inhibitors are associated with an increased risk of thrombotic events (e.g. myocardial infarction and stroke) and should not be used in preference to non-selective NSAIDs except when specifically indicated (i.e. for patients at a particularly high risk of developing gastroduodenal ulceration or bleeding) *and* after assessing their cardiovascular risk.

Non-selective NSAIDs may also be associated with a small increased risk of thrombotic events particularly when used at high doses and for long-term treatment. **Diclofenac** (150 mg daily) and **ibuprofen** (2.4 g daily) are associated with an increased risk of thrombotic events. The increased risk for diclofenac is similar to that of licensed doses of **etoricoxib**. **Naproxen** is associated with a lower thrombotic risk, and low doses of ibuprofen (1.2 g daily or less) have not been associated with an increased risk of myocardial infarction. A small increased thrombotic risk cannot be excluded for other NSAIDs.

The CHM has advised (October 2006) that the lowest effective dose of NSAID or cyclo-oxygenase-2 selective inhibitor should be prescribed for the shortest period to control symptoms and that the need for long-term treatment should be reviewed periodically.

Dental and orofacial pain Most mild to moderate dental pain and inflammation is effectively relieved by NSAIDs. Those used for dental pain include **ibuprofen**, **diclofenac**, and **aspirin**.

In an appraisal of the relative safety of 7 non-selective NSAIDs, the CSM assessed ibuprofen to have the lowest risk of serious gastro-intestinal side-effects (see p. 537).

For further information on the management of dental and orofacial pain, see p. 224.

Cautions and contra-indications NSAIDs should be used with caution in the elderly (risk of serious side-effects and fatalities, see also Prescribing for the Elderly p. 20), in allergic disorders (they are **contra-indicated** in patients with a history of hypersensitivity to aspirin or any other NSAID—which includes those in whom attacks of asthma, angioedema, urticaria or rhinitis have been precipitated by aspirin or any other NSAID), during pregnancy and breast-feeding (see Appendix 4 and Appendix 5), and in coagulation defects. Long-term use of some NSAIDs is associated with reduced female fertility, which is reversible on stopping treatment.

In patients with renal, cardiac, or hepatic impairment caution is required since NSAIDs may impair renal function (see also under Side-effects, below and Appendix 2 and Appendix 3); the dose should be kept as **low as possible** and renal function should be **monitored**.

All NSAIDs are contra-indicated in severe heart failure. The selective inhibitors of cyclo-oxygenase-2 (celecoxib, etoricoxib, and parecoxib) are **contra-indicated** in ischaemic heart disease, cerebrovascular disease, peripheral arterial disease, and moderate or severe heart failure. The selective inhibitors of cyclo-oxygenase-2 should be used with caution in patients with a history of cardiac failure, left ventricular dysfunction, hypertension, in patients with oedema for any other reason, and in patients with risk factors for heart disease.

The CSM has advised that non-selective NSAIDs are contra-indicated in patients with previous or active peptic ulceration and that selective inhibitors of cyclo-oxygenase-2 are contra-indicated in active peptic ulceration (see also **CSM advice** below). While it is preferable to avoid NSAIDs in patients with active or previous gastro-intestinal ulceration or bleeding, and to withdraw them if gastro-intestinal lesions develop, nevertheless patients with serious rheumatic diseases (e.g. rheumatoid arthritis) are usually dependent on NSAIDs for effective relief of pain and stiffness. For advice on the prophylaxis and treatment of NSAID-associated peptic ulcers, see section 1.3.

For **interactions** of NSAIDs, see Appendix 1 (NSAIDs).

Side-effects Gastro-intestinal discomfort, nausea, diarrhoea, and occasionally bleeding and ulceration occur (see also CSM advice below). Systemic as well as local effects of NSAIDs contribute to gastro-intestinal damage; taking oral formulations with milk or food, or using enteric-coated formulations, or changing the route of administration may only partially reduce symptoms such as dyspepsia. Those at risk of duodenal or gastric ulceration (including the elderly) who need to continue NSAID treatment should receive either a selective inhibitor of cyclo-oxygenase-2 alone, or a non-selective NSAID with gastroprotective treatment (section 1.3).

Other side-effects include hypersensitivity reactions (particularly rashes, angioedema, and bronchospasm—see CSM advice below), headache, dizziness, nervousness, depression, drowsiness, insomnia, vertigo, hearing disturbances such as tinnitus, photosensitivity, and haematuria. Blood disorders have also occurred. Fluid retention may occur (rarely precipitating congestive heart failure); blood pressure may be raised.

Renal failure may be provoked by NSAIDs, especially in patients with renal impairment (**important**, see also under Cautions above). Rarely, papillary necrosis or interstitial fibrosis associated with NSAIDs may lead to renal failure.

Hepatic damage, alveolitis, pulmonary eosinophilia, pancreatitis, eye changes, Stevens-Johnson syndrome and toxic epidermal necrolysis are other rare side-effects. Induction of or exacerbation of colitis has been reported. Aseptic meningitis has been reported rarely with NSAIDs; patients with connective-tissue disorders such as systemic lupus erythematosus may be especially susceptible.

Overdosage: see Emergency Treatment of Poisoning, p. 29.

CSM advice (gastro-intestinal side-effects)

All NSAIDs are associated with serious gastro-intestinal toxicity; the risk is higher in the elderly. Evidence on the relative safety of 7 **non-selective** NSAIDs indicates differences in the risks of serious upper gastro-intestinal side-effects. **Azapropazone** is associated with the *highest risk* (**important:** see also CSM restrictions below) and **ibuprofen** with the *lowest*; **piroxicam**, **ketoprofen**, **indometacin**, **naproxen** and **diclofenac** are associated with *intermediate risks* (possibly higher in the case of piroxicam, see also CHMP advice, p. 543). **Selective inhibitors of cyclo-oxygenase-2** are associated with a *lower risk* of serious upper gastro-intestinal side-effects than non-selective NSAIDs.

Recommendations are that NSAIDs associated with a low risk e.g. ibuprofen are *generally preferred*, to start at the *lowest recommended dose*, not to use more than one oral NSAID at a time, and to remember that all NSAIDs (including selective inhibitors of cyclo-oxygenase-2) are *contra-indicated* in patients with active peptic ulceration. The CSM also contra-indicates non-selective NSAIDs in patients with a history of peptic ulceration.

The combination of a NSAID and low-dose aspirin can increase the risk of gastro-intestinal side-effects; this combination should be used only if absolutely necessary and the patient should be monitored closely.

CSM warning (asthma)

Any degree of worsening of asthma may be related to the ingestion of NSAIDs, either prescribed or (in the case of ibuprofen and others) purchased over the counter.

ACECLOFENAC

Indications pain and inflammation in rheumatoid arthritis, osteoarthritis and ankylosing spondylitis

Cautions see notes above; avoid in porphyria (section 9.8.2); breast-feeding (Appendix 5); **interactions:** Appendix 1 (NSAIDs)

Contra-indications see notes above

Side-effects see notes above

Dose

- 100 mg twice daily; CHILD not recommended

Preservex® (UCB Pharma) PoM

Tablets, f/c, aceclofenac 100 mg, net price 60-tab pack = £9.45. Label: 21

ACEMETACIN

(Glycolic acid ester of indometacin)

Indications pain and inflammation in rheumatic disease and other musculoskeletal disorders; post-operative analgesia

Cautions see under Indometacin and notes above; breast-feeding (Appendix 5); **interactions:** Appendix 1 (NSAIDs)

Driving Dizziness may affect performance of skilled tasks (e.g. driving)

Contra-indications see notes above

Side-effects see under Indometacin and notes above

Dose

- 120 mg daily in divided doses with food, increased if necessary to 180 mg daily; CHILD not recommended

Emflex® (Merck) PoM

Capsules, yellow/orange, acemetacin 60 mg, net price 90-cap pack = £28.20. Label: 21, counselling, driving

AZAPROPAZONE

Indications see under CSM restrictions

CSM restrictions CSM *has restricted* azapropazone to use in rheumatoid arthritis, ankylosing spondylitis and acute gout only when other NSAIDs have been tried and failed, *has* **contra-indicated** it in patients with a history of peptic ulceration, and *has reduced* the maximum daily dose to 600 mg for rheumatoid arthritis and ankylosing spondylitis in patients over 60 years, and those with impaired renal function

Cautions see notes above; **interactions**: Appendix 1 (NSAIDs)

Contra-indications see notes above; also porphyria (section 9.8.2); history of inflammatory bowel disease or blood disorder

Side-effects see notes above; also photosensitivity, see CSM advice below

Photosensitivity CSM has reminded of the need to advise patients taking azapropazone to avoid direct exposure to sunlight (or to use sunscreen preparations)

Dose

- Rheumatoid arthritis and ankylosing spondylitis, 1.2 g daily in 2 or 4 divided doses; ELDERLY over 60 years, 300 mg twice daily; CHILD not recommended
- Acute gout, 1.8 g daily in divided doses until acute symptoms subside (usually by day 4) *then* 1.2 g daily in divided doses until symptoms resolve—consider alternative therapy if symptoms persist; ELDERLY over 60 years, 1.8 g daily in divided doses for the first 24 hours *then* 1.2 g daily in divided doses, reduced to 600 mg daily in divided doses as soon as possible (preferably by day 4) until acute symptoms resolve—consider alternative therapy if symptoms persist; CHILD not recommended

Rheumox® (Goldshield) PoM

Capsules, orange, azapropazone 300 mg, net price 100-cap pack = £15.50. Label: 11, 21, counselling, photosensitivity (see above)

CELECOXIB

Indications pain and inflammation in osteoarthritis, rheumatoid arthritis, and ankylosing spondylitis

Cautions see notes above; **interactions**: Appendix 1 (NSAIDs)

Contra-indications see notes above; sulphonamide sensitivity; inflammatory bowel disease

Side-effects see notes above; flatulence, insomnia, pharyngitis, sinusitis; *less commonly* stomatitis, constipation, palpitation, fatigue, paraesthesia, muscle cramps; *rarely* taste disturbance, alopecia; *very rarely* aggravation of epilepsy

Dose

- Osteoarthritis, 200 mg daily in 1–2 divided doses, increased if necessary to max. 200 mg twice daily; CHILD not recommended
- Rheumatoid arthritis, 100 mg twice daily, increased if necessary to 200 mg twice daily; CHILD not recommended
- Ankylosing spondylitis, 200 mg daily in 1–2 divided doses, increased if necessary to max. 400 mg daily in 1–2 divided doses; CHILD not recommended

Note Discontinue if no improvement after 2 weeks on max. dose

Celebrex® (Pharmacia) PoM
Capsules, celecoxib 100 mg (white/blue), net price 60-cap pack = £21.55; 200 mg (white/gold), 30-cap pack = £21.55

DEXIBUPROFEN

Indications pain and inflammation associated with osteoarthritis and other musculoskeletal disorders; mild to moderate pain and inflammation including dysmenorrhoea and dental pain

Cautions see notes above; systemic lupus erythematosus and other connective tissue disorders; breast-feeding (Appendix 5); **interactions**: Appendix 1 (NSAIDs)

Contra-indications see notes above

Side-effects see notes above

Dose

- 600–900 mg daily in up to 3 divided doses; increased if necessary to max. 1.2 g daily (900 mg daily for dysmenorrhoea); max. single dose 400 mg (300 mg for dysmenorrhoea); CHILD not recommended

Seractil® (Genus) ▼ PoM
Tablets, f/c, dexibuprofen 300 mg, net price 60-tab pack = £9.47; 400 mg (scored) 60-tab pack = £9.47. Label: 21

DEXKETOPROFEN

Indications short-term treatment of mild to moderate pain including dysmenorrhoea

Cautions see notes above; breast-feeding (Appendix 5); **interactions**: Appendix 1 (NSAIDs)

Contra-indications see notes above

Side-effects see notes above

Dose

- 12.5 mg every 4–6 hours *or* 25 mg every 8 hours; max. 75 mg daily; ELDERLY initially max. 50 mg daily; CHILD not recommended

Keral® (Menarini) PoM
Tablets, f/c, scored, dexketoprofen (as trometamol) 25 mg, net price 20-tab pack = £3.67, 50-tab pack = £9.18. Label: 22

DICLOFENAC SODIUM

Indications pain and inflammation in rheumatic disease (including juvenile idiopathic arthritis) and other musculoskeletal disorders; acute gout; postoperative pain

Cautions see notes above; **interactions**: Appendix 1 (NSAIDs)

Contra-indications see notes above; porphyria (section 9.8.2); avoid injections containing benzyl alcohol in neonates (see preparations below)

Intravenous use Additional contra-indications include concomitant NSAID or anticoagulant use (including low-dose heparin), history of haemorrhagic diathesis, history of confirmed or suspected cerebrovascular bleeding, operations with high risk of haemorrhage, history of asthma, moderate or severe renal impairment, hypovolaemia, dehydration

Side-effects see notes above; suppositories may cause rectal irritation; injection site reactions

Dose

- By mouth, 75–150 mg daily in 2–3 divided doses
- By deep intramuscular injection into the gluteal muscle, acute exacerbations of pain and postoperative pain, 75 mg once daily (twice daily in severe cases) for max. of 2 days
  Ureteric colic, 75 mg then a further 75 mg after 30 minutes if necessary
- By intravenous infusion (in hospital setting), 75 mg repeated if necessary after 4–6 hours for max. 2 days
  Prevention of postoperative pain, initially after surgery 25–50 mg over 15–60 minutes then 5 mg/hour for max. 2 days
- By rectum in suppositories, 75–150 mg daily in divided doses
- Max. total daily dose by any route 150 mg
- CHILD 1–12 years, juvenile arthritis, by mouth *or* by rectum, 1–3 mg/kg daily in divided doses (25 mg e/c tablets, 12.5 mg and 25 mg suppositories only)
- CHILD 6–12 years, postoperative pain, by rectum, 1–2 mg/kg daily in divided doses (12.5 mg and 25 mg suppositories only) for max. 4 days

Diclofenac Sodium (Non-proprietary) PoM
Tablets, e/c, diclofenac sodium 25 mg, net price 84-tab pack = £1.20; 50 mg, 84-tab pack = £2.03. Label: 5, 25

Note Other brands include *Defenac®*, *Dicloflex®*, *Diclozip®*, *Fenactol®*, *Flamrase®*

Dental prescribing on NHS Diclofenac Sodium Tablets may be prescribed

Suppositories, diclofenac sodium 100 mg, net price 10 = £3.04

Brands include *Econac®*

Injection, diclofenac sodium 25 mg/mL. Net price 3-mL amp = 83p

Note Licensed for intramuscular use

Voltarol® (Novartis) PoM
Tablets, e/c, diclofenac sodium 25 mg (yellow), net price 84-tab pack = £3.67; 50 mg (brown), 84-tab pack = £5.71. Label: 5, 25

Dispersible tablets, sugar-free, pink, diclofenac, equivalent to diclofenac sodium 50 mg, net price 21-tab pack = £6.19. Label: 13, 21

Note Voltarol Dispersible tablets are more suitable for **short-term** use in acute conditions for which treatment required for no more than 3 months (no information on use beyond 3 months)

Injection, diclofenac sodium 25 mg/mL, net price 3-mL amp = 83p

Excipients include benzyl alcohol (avoid in neonates, see Excipients, p. 2), propylene glycol

Suppositories, diclofenac sodium 12.5 mg, net price 10 = 71p; 25 mg, 10 = £1.26; 50 mg, 10 = £2.07; 100 mg, 10 = £3.70

▲Diclofenac potassium

Voltarol® Rapid (Novartis) PoM

Tablets, s/c, diclofenac potassium 25 mg (red), net price 28-tab pack = £4.04; 50 mg (brown), 28-tab pack = £7.73

Dose rheumatic disease, musculoskeletal disorders, acute gout, postoperative pain, 75–150 mg daily in 2–3 divided doses; CHILD over 14 years, 75–100 mg daily in 2–3 divided doses

Migraine, 50 mg at onset, repeated after 2 hours if necessary then after 4–6 hours; max. 200 mg in 24 hours; CHILD not recommended

▲Modified release

Diclomax SR® (Provalis) PoM

Capsules, m/r, yellow, diclofenac sodium 75 mg, net price 56-cap pack = £12.10. Label: 21, 25

Dose 1 capsule 1–2 times daily *or* 2 capsules once daily, preferably with food; CHILD not recommended

Diclomax Retard® (Provalis) PoM

Capsules, m/r, diclofenac sodium 100 mg, net price 28-tab pack = £8.27. Label: 21, 25

Dose 1 capsule daily preferably with food; CHILD not recommended

Motifene® 75 mg (Daiichi Sankyo) PoM

Capsules, e/c, m/r, diclofenac sodium 75 mg (enclosing e/c pellets containing diclofenac sodium 25 mg and m/r pellets containing diclofenac sodium 50 mg), net price 56-cap pack = £8.00. Label: 25

Dose 1 capsule 1-2 times daily; CHILD not recommended

Voltarol® 75 mg SR (Novartis) PoM

Tablets, m/r, f/c, pink, diclofenac sodium 75 mg, net price 28-tab pack = £8.08; 56-tab pack = £16.15. Label: 21, 25

Dose 75 mg 1–2 times daily preferably with food; CHILD not recommended

Note Other brands of modified-release tablets containing diclofenac sodium 75 mg include *Defenac® SR, Dexomon® 75 SR, Dicloflex® 75 SR, Fenactol® 75 mg SR, Flamatak® 75 MR, Flamrase® SR, Flexotard® MR 75, Rheumatac® Retard 75, Rhumalgan® CR, Slofenac® SR, Volsaid® Retard 75*

Voltarol® Retard (Novartis) PoM

Tablets, m/r, f/c, red, diclofenac sodium 100 mg. Net price 28-tab pack = £11.84. Label: 21, 25

Dose 1 tablet daily preferably with food; CHILD not recommended

Note Other brands of modified-release tablets containing diclofenac sodium 100 mg include *Defenac® Retard, Dexomon® Retard 100, Dicloflex® Retard, Fenactol® Retard 100 mg, Flamatak® 100 MR, Flamrase® SR, Rhumalgan® CR, Slofenac® SR, Volsaid® Retard 100*

▲With misoprostol

For **cautions, contra-indications**, and **side-effects** of misoprostol, see section 1.3.4

Arthrotec® (Pharmacia) PoM

Arthrotec® 50 tablets, diclofenac sodium (in e/c core) 50 mg, misoprostol 200 micrograms, net price 60-tab pack = £13.31; Label: 21, 25

Dose prophylaxis against NSAID-induced gastroduodenal ulceration in patients requiring diclofenac for rheumatoid arthritis or osteoarthritis, 1 tablet 2–3 times daily with food; CHILD not recommended

Arthrotec® 75 tablets, diclofenac sodium (in e/c core) 75 mg, misoprostol 200 micrograms, net price 60-tab pack = £17.59. Label: 21, 25

Dose prophylaxis against NSAID-induced gastroduodenal ulceration in patients requiring diclofenac for rheumatoid arthritis or osteoarthritis, 1 tablet twice daily with food; CHILD not recommended

▲Topical preparations

Section 10.3.2

ETODOLAC

Indications pain and inflammation in rheumatoid arthritis and osteoarthritis

Cautions see notes above; breast-feeding (Appendix 5); **interactions**: Appendix 1 (NSAIDs)

Contra-indications see notes above

Side-effects see notes above; also flatulence, constipation, vomiting, ulcerative stomatitis, gastritis, vasculitis, palpitation, dyspnoea, confusion, fatigue, paraesthesia, tremor, urinary frequency, dysuria, pyrexia, and pruritus

Dose

- ADULT over 18 years, 600 mg daily in 1–2 divided doses

Etodolac (Non-proprietary) PoM

Capsules, etodolac 300 mg, net price 60-cap pack = £8.14

Brands include *Eccoxolac®*

▲Modified release

Etopan XL® (Taro) PoM

Tablets, m/r, f/c, grey, etodolac 600 mg, net price 30-tab pack = £15.50. Label: 25

Dose 1 tablet daily; CHILD not recommended

Lodine SR® (Shire) PoM

Tablets, m/r, f/c, light-grey, etodolac 600 mg, net price 30-tab pack = £15.50. Label: 25

Dose 1 tablet daily; CHILD not recommended

ETORICOXIB

Indications pain and inflammation in osteoarthritis and in rheumatoid arthritis; acute gout

Cautions see notes above; also dehydration; monitor blood pressure; hepatic impairment (avoid if severe; Appendix 2); renal impairment (avoid if creatinine clearance less than 30 mL/minute; Appendix 3); **interactions**: Appendix 1 (NSAIDs)

Contra-indications see notes above; inflammatory bowel disease; uncontrolled hypertension; breast-feeding (Appendix 5)

Side-effects see notes above; also flatulence, palpitation, fatigue, influenza-like symptoms, ecchymosis; *less commonly* dry mouth, taste disturbance, mouth ulcer, constipation, appetite and weight change, atrial fibrillation, chest pain, flushing, cough, dyspnoea, epistaxis, anxiety, mental acuity impaired, paraesthesia, infection, electrolyte disturbance, myalgia and arthralgia; *very rarely* confusion and hallucinations

Dose

- Osteoarthritis, ADULT and CHILD over 16 years, 30 mg once daily, increased if necessary to 60 mg once daily
- Rheumatoid arthritis, ADULT and CHILD over 16 years, 90 mg once daily
- Acute gout, ADULT and CHILD over 16 years, 120 mg once daily for max. 8 days

Arcoxia® (MSD) ▼ PoM

Tablets, f/c, etoricoxib 30 mg (blue-green), net price 28-tab pack = £13.99; 60 mg (dark green), 28-tab pack

= £20.11; 90 mg (white), 28-tab pack = £22.96; 120 mg (pale green), 7-tab pack = £5.74

FENBUFEN

Indications pain and inflammation in rheumatic disease and other musculoskeletal disorders

Cautions see notes above; breast-feeding (Appendix 5); **interactions:** Appendix 1 (NSAIDs)

Contra-indications see notes above

Side-effects see notes above, but also high risk of rashes especially in seronegative rheumatoid arthritis, psoriatic arthritis and in women (discontinue immediately); erythema multiforme and Stevens-Johnson syndrome reported; also allergic interstitial lung disorders (may follow rashes)

Dose

- 300 mg in the morning and 600 mg at bed-time *or* 450 mg twice daily; CHILD under 14 years not recommended

Fenbufen (Non-proprietary) PoM

Capsules, fenbufen 300 mg, net price 84-cap pack = £20.71. Label: 21

Tablets, fenbufen 300 mg, net price 84-tab pack = £6.60; 450 mg, 56-tab pack = £18.80. Label: 21

Lederfen® (Goldshield) PoM

Capsules, dark blue, fenbufen 300 mg. Net price 84-cap pack = £20.71. Label: 21

Tablets, both light blue, f/c, fenbufen 300 mg, net price 84-tab pack = £6.00; 450 mg, 56-tab pack = £6.49. Label: 21

FENOPROFEN

Indications pain and inflammation in rheumatic disease and other musculoskeletal disorders; mild to moderate pain

Cautions see notes above; breast-feeding (Appendix 5); **interactions:** Appendix 1 (NSAIDs)

Contra-indications see notes above

Side-effects see notes above; upper respiratory-tract infection, nasopharyngitis, and cystitis also reported

Dose

- 300–600 mg 3–4 times daily with food; max. 3 g daily; CHILD not recommended

Fenopron® (Typharm) PoM

Tablets, both orange, fenoprofen (as calcium salt) 300 mg (*Fenopron®* 300), net price 100-tab pack = £9.45; 600 mg (*Fenopron®* 600, scored), 100-tab pack = £18.29. Label: 21

FLURBIPROFEN

Indications pain and inflammation in rheumatic disease and other musculoskeletal disorders; mild to moderate pain including dysmenorrhoea; migraine; postoperative analgesia; sore throat (section 12.3.1)

Cautions see notes above; breast-feeding (Appendix 5); **interactions:** Appendix 1 (NSAIDs)

Contra-indications see notes above

Side-effects see notes above; also vomiting, ulcerative stomatitis; *less commonly* gastritis, paraesthesia, confusion, hallucinations, and fatigue

Dose

- ADULT and CHILD over 12 years, 150–200 mg daily in 2–4 divided doses, increased in acute conditions to 300 mg daily
- Dysmenorrhoea, ADULT and CHILD over 12 years, initially 100 mg, then 50–100 mg every 4–6 hours; max. 300 mg daily

Flurbiprofen (Non-proprietary) PoM

Tablets, flurbiprofen 50 mg, net price 20 = £4.64; 100 mg, 20 = £9.49. Label: 21

Froben® (Abbott) PoM

Tablets, yellow, s/c, flurbiprofen 50 mg, net price 20 = £2.18; 100 mg, 20 = £4.13. Label: 21

Modified release

Froben SR® (Abbott) PoM

Capsules, m/r, yellow, flurbiprofen 200 mg, net price 30-cap pack = £7.84. Label: 21, 25

Dose ADULT and CHILD over 12 years, 1 capsule daily, preferably in the evening

IBUPROFEN

Indications pain and inflammation in rheumatic disease (including juvenile idiopathic arthritis) and other musculoskeletal disorders; mild to moderate pain including dysmenorrhoea; postoperative analgesia; migraine; dental pain; fever and pain in children; post-immunisation pyrexia (section 14.1)

Cautions see notes above; breast-feeding (Appendix 5); **interactions:** Appendix 1 (NSAIDs)

Contra-indications see notes above

Side-effects see notes above; **overdosage:** see Emergency Treatment of Poisoning, p. 29

Dose

- ADULT and CHILD over 12 years, initially 300–400 mg 3–4 times daily; increased if necessary to max. 2.4 g daily; maintenance dose of 0.6–1.2 g daily may be adequate
- Pain and fever in children, CHILD 1–3 months, see *BNF for Children*; CHILD 3–6 months (body-weight over 5 kg), 50 mg 3 times daily (max. 30 mg/kg daily in 3–4 divided doses); CHILD 6 months–1 year, 50 mg 3–4 times daily (max. 30 mg/kg daily in 3–4 divided doses); CHILD 1–4 years, 100 mg 3 times daily (max. 30 mg/kg daily in 3–4 divided doses); CHILD 4–7 years, 150 mg 3 times daily (max. 30 mg/kg daily in 3–4 divided doses); CHILD 7–10 years, 200 mg 3 times daily (up to 30 mg/kg daily (max. 2.4 g) in 3–4 divided doses); CHILD 10–12 years, 300 mg 3 times daily (up to 30 mg/kg daily (max. 2.4 g) in 3–4 divided doses)
- Rheumatic disease in children (including juvenile idiopathic arthritis), CHILD 3 months–18 years (body-weight over 5 kg), 30–40 mg/kg (max. 2.4 g) daily in 3–4 divided doses; in systemic juvenile idiopathic arthritis up to 60 mg/kg (max. 2.4 g) daily [unlicensed] in 4–6 divided doses

[1]Ibuprofen (Non-proprietary) PoM

Tablets, coated, ibuprofen 200 mg, net price 84-tab pack = £2.03; 400 mg, 84-tab pack = £2.40; 600 mg, 84-tab pack = £3.74. Label: 21

Brands include *Arthrofen®*, *Ebufac®*, *Rimafen®*

1. Can be sold to the public in certain circumstances; for exemptions see *Medicines, Ethics and Practice*, No. 31, London, Pharmaceutical Press, 2007 (and subsequent editions as available)

Oral suspension, ibuprofen 100 mg/5 mL, net price 100 mL = £2.69, 150 mL = £2.71, 500 mL = £8.88. Label: 21

Note Sugar-free versions are available and can be ordered by specifying 'sugar-free' on the prescription

Brands include *Calprofen®*, *Fenpaed®*, *Feverfen®*, *Nurofen® for Children*, *Orbifen® for Children*

Dental prescribing on NHS Ibuprofen Tablets and Ibuprofen Oral Suspension Sugar-free may be prescribed

Brufen® (Abbott) PoM

Tablets, f/c, ibuprofen 200 mg, net price 100-tab pack = £4.08; 400 mg, 100-tab pack = £8.16; 600 mg, 100-tab pack = £12.24. Label: 21

Syrup, orange, ibuprofen 100 mg/5 mL, net price 500 mL (orange-flavoured) = £8.88. Label: 21

Granules, effervescent, ibuprofen 600 mg/sachet, net price 20-sachet pack = £6.80. Label: 13, 21

Electrolytes Na^+ approx. 9 mmol/sachet

Modified release

Brufen Retard® (Abbott) PoM

Tablets, m/r, ibuprofen 800 mg, net price 56-tab pack = £6.74. Label: 25, 27

Dose ADULT and CHILD over 12 years, 2 tablets daily as a single dose, preferably in the early evening, increased in severe cases to 3 tablets daily in 2 divided doses

Fenbid® (Goldshield) PoM

Spansule® (= capsule m/r), maroon/pink, enclosing off-white pellets, ibuprofen 300 mg, net price 120-cap pack = £9.64. Label: 25

Dose ADULT and CHILD over 12 years, initially 2 capsules twice daily, increased in severe cases to 3 capsules twice daily; then 1–2 capsules twice daily

Topical preparations

Section 10.3.2

INDOMETACIN
(Indomethacin)

Indications pain and moderate to severe inflammation in rheumatic disease and other acute musculoskeletal disorders; acute gout; dysmenorrhoea; closure of ductus arteriosus (section 7.1.1.1); premature labour (section 7.1.3)

Cautions see notes above; also epilepsy, parkinsonism, psychiatric disturbances; during prolonged therapy ophthalmic and blood examinations particularly advisable; avoid rectal administration in proctitis and haemorrhoids; breast-feeding (Appendix 5); **interactions:** Appendix 1 (NSAIDs)

Driving Dizziness may affect performance of skilled tasks (e.g. driving)

Contra-indications see notes above

Side-effects see notes above; frequently gastro-intestinal disturbances (including diarrhoea), headache, dizziness, and light-headedness; also gastro-intestinal ulceration and bleeding; rarely, drowsiness, confusion, insomnia, convulsions, psychiatric disturbances, depression, syncope, blood disorders (particularly thrombocytopenia), hypertension, hyperglycaemia, blurred vision, corneal deposits, peripheral neuropathy, and intestinal strictures; suppositories may cause rectal irritation and occasional bleeding

Dose

- By mouth, rheumatic disease, 50–200 mg daily in divided doses, with food; CHILD not recommended
  Acute gout, 150–200 mg daily in divided doses
  Dysmenorrhoea, up to 75 mg daily
- By rectum in suppositories, 100 mg at night and in the morning if required; CHILD not recommended
  Combined oral and rectal treatment, max. total daily dose 150–200 mg

Indometacin (Non-proprietary) PoM

Capsules, indometacin 25 mg, net price 28-cap pack = £1.23; 50 mg, 28-cap pack = £2.40. Label: 21, counselling, driving, see above

Brands include *Flexacid®*

Suppositories, indometacin 100 mg. Net price 10 = £11.43. Counselling, driving, see above

Modified release

Indometacin m/r preparations PoM

Capsules, m/r, indometacin 75 mg. Label: 21, 25, counselling, driving see above

Brands include *Indolar SR®*, *Pardelprin®*, *Slo-Indo®*

Dose 1 capsule 1–2 times daily; CHILD not recommended

KETOPROFEN

Indications pain and mild inflammation in rheumatic disease and other musculoskeletal disorders, and after orthopaedic surgery; acute gout; dysmenorrhoea

Cautions see notes above; breast-feeding (Appendix 5); **interactions:** Appendix 1 (NSAIDs)

Contra-indications see notes above

Side-effects see notes above; pain may occur at injection site (occasionally tissue damage); suppositories may cause rectal irritation

Dose

- By mouth, rheumatic disease, 100–200 mg daily in 2–4 divided doses; CHILD not recommended
  Pain and dysmenorrhoea, 50 mg up to 3 times daily; CHILD not recommended
- By rectum in suppositories, rheumatic disease, 100 mg at bedtime; CHILD not recommended
  Combined oral and rectal treatment, max. total daily dose 200 mg
- By deep intramuscular injection into the gluteal muscle, 50–100 mg every 4 hours (max. 200 mg in 24 hours) for up to 3 days; CHILD not recommended

Ketoprofen (Non-proprietary) PoM

Capsules, ketoprofen 50 mg, net price 28-cap pack = £9.17; 100 mg, 56-cap pack = £15.14. Label: 21

Orudis® (Sanofi-Aventis) PoM

Capsules, ketoprofen 50 mg (green/purple), net price 112-cap pack = £16.07; 100 mg (pink), 56-cap pack = £16.12. Label: 21

Suppositories, ketoprofen 100 mg. Net price 10 = £6.92

Oruvail® (Sanofi-Aventis) PoM

Injection, ketoprofen 50 mg/mL. Net price 2-mL amp = £1.11

Modified release

Oruvail® (Sanofi-Aventis) PoM

Capsules, all m/r, enclosing white pellets, ketoprofen 100 mg (pink/purple), net price 56-cap pack = £24.90;

150 mg (pink), 28-cap pack = £14.21; 200 mg (pink/white), 28-cap pack = £24.82. Label: 21, 25

Dose 100–200 mg once daily with food; CHILD not recommended

Note Other brands of modified-release capsules containing ketoprofen 100 mg and 200 mg include *Ketocid®* 200 mg, *Ketovail®*, *Larafen CR®* 200 mg, *Tiloket® CR*

Topical preparations

Section 10.3.2

MEFENAMIC ACID

Indications pain and inflammation in rheumatoid arthritis and osteoarthritis; postoperative pain; mild to moderate pain; dysmenorrhoea and menorrhagia

Cautions see notes above; epilepsy; breast-feeding (Appendix 5); porphyria (section 9.8.2); **interactions:** Appendix 1 (NSAIDs)

Contra-indications see notes above; inflammatory bowel disease

Side-effects see notes above; also diarrhoea or rashes (withdraw treatment), vomiting, flatulence, constipation, ulcerative stomatitis; *less commonly* paraesthesia and fatigue; *rarely* hypotension, palpitation, glucose intolerance, thrombocytopenia, haemolytic anaemia (positive Coombs' test), and aplastic anaemia reported

Dose

- ADULT over 18 years, 500 mg 3 times daily
- CHILD 12–18 years, acute pain including dysmenorrhoea, menorrhagia, 500 mg 3 times daily
- CHILD under 12 years not recommended

Mefenamic Acid (Non-proprietary) PoM

Capsules, mefenamic acid 250 mg. Net price 100-cap pack = £5.94. Label: 21

Tablets, mefenamic acid 500 mg, net price 28-tab pack = £2.17. Label: 21

Suspension, mefenamic acid 50 mg/5 mL. Net price 125 mL = £79.98. Label: 21

Excipients include ethanol

Ponstan® (Chemidex) PoM

Capsules, blue/ivory, mefenamic acid 250 mg, net price 100-cap pack = £8.17. Label: 21

Forte tablets, yellow, mefenamic acid 500 mg, net price 100-tab pack = £15.72. Label: 21

MELOXICAM

Indications pain and inflammation in rheumatic disease; exacerbation of osteoarthritis (short-term); ankylosing spondylitis

Cautions see notes above; avoid rectal administration in proctitis or haemorrhoids; breast-feeding (Appendix 5); **interactions:** Appendix 1 (NSAIDs)

Contra-indications see notes above; renal failure (unless receiving dialysis); severe heart failure

Side-effects see notes above

Dose

- By mouth, osteoarthritis, 7.5 mg daily, increased if necessary to max. 15 mg once daily

  Rheumatoid arthritis, ankylosing spondylitis, 15 mg once daily, may be reduced to 7.5 mg daily; ELDERLY 7.5 mg daily
- By rectum, in suppositories, osteoarthritis, 7.5 mg daily, increased if necessary to max. 15 mg once daily

  Rheumatoid arthritis, ankylosing spondylitis, 15 mg once daily, may be reduced to 7.5 mg daily; ELDERLY 7.5 mg daily
- CHILD under 15 years not recommended

Meloxicam (Non-proprietary) PoM

Tablets, meloxicam 7.5 mg, net price 30-tab pack = £4.22; 15 mg, 30-tab pack = £5.67. Label: 21

Mobic® (Boehringer Ingelheim) PoM

Tablets, yellow, scored, meloxicam 7.5 mg, net price 30-tab pack = £9.30; 15 mg, 30-tab pack = £12.93. Label: 21

Suppositories, meloxicam 7.5 mg, net price 12 = £3.72; 15 mg, 12 = £5.58

NABUMETONE

Indications pain and inflammation in osteoarthritis and rheumatoid arthritis

Cautions see notes above; breast-feeding (Appendix 5); **interactions:** Appendix 1 (NSAIDs)

Contra-indications see notes above

Side-effects see notes above

Dose

- 1 g at night; severe or persistent symptoms 0.5–1 g in morning and 1 g at night; ELDERLY 0.5–1 g daily; CHILD not recommended

Nabumetone (Non-proprietary) PoM

Tablets, nabumetone 500 mg, net price 56-tab pack = £11.20. Label: 21

Relifex® (Meda) PoM

Tablets, red, f/c, nabumetone 500 mg. Net price 56-tab pack = £6.18. Label: 21

Suspension, sugar-free, nabumetone 500 mg/5 mL. Net price 300-mL pack = £24.08. Label: 21

NAPROXEN

Indications pain and inflammation in rheumatic disease (including juvenile idiopathic arthritis) and other musculoskeletal disorders; dysmenorrhoea; acute gout

Cautions see notes above; breast-feeding (Appendix 5); **interactions:** Appendix 1 (NSAIDs)

Contra-indications see notes above

Side-effects see notes above

Dose

- Rheumatic disease, 0.5–1 g daily in 1–2 divided doses; CHILD (over 5 years), juvenile idiopathic arthritis, 10 mg/kg daily in 2 divided doses
- Acute musculoskeletal disorders and dysmenorrhoea, 500 mg initially, then 250 mg every 6–8 hours as required; max. dose after first day 1.25 g daily; CHILD under 16 years not recommended
- Acute gout, 750 mg initially, then 250 mg every 8 hours until attack has passed; CHILD under 16 years not recommended

Naproxen (Non-proprietary) PoM

Tablets, naproxen 250 mg, net price 28-tab pack = 89p; 500 mg, 28-tab pack = £1.57. Label: 21

Brands include *Arthroxen®*

Tablets, e/c, naproxen 250 mg, net price 56-tab pack = £5.23; 375 mg, 56-tab pack = £6.96; 500 mg, 56-tab pack = £9.11. Label: 5, 25

Naprosyn® (Roche) PoM
Tablets, all scored, naproxen 250 mg (buff), net price 56-tab pack = £4.55; 500 mg (buff), 56-tab pack = £9.09. Label: 21
Tablets, e/c, (*Naprosyn EC®*), naproxen 250 mg, net price 56-tab pack = £4.55; 375 mg, 56-tab pack = £6.82; 500 mg, 56-tab pack = £9.09. Label: 5, 25

Synflex® (Roche) PoM
Tablets, blue, naproxen sodium 275 mg. Net price 60-tab pack = £7.54. Label: 21
Note 275 mg naproxen sodium ≡ 250 mg naproxen
Dose musculoskeletal disorders, postoperative analgesia, 550 mg twice daily when necessary, preferably after food; max. 1.1 g daily; CHILD under 16 years not recommended
Dysmenorrhoea and acute gout, initially 550 mg then 275 mg every 6–8 hours as required; max. of 1.375 g on first day and 1.1 g daily thereafter; CHILD under 16 years not recommended
Migraine, 825 mg at onset, then 275–550 mg at least 30 minutes after initial dose; max. 1.375 g in 24 hours; CHILD under 16 years not recommended

With misoprostol

For **cautions, contra-indications**, and **side-effects** of misoprostol, see section 1.3.4

Napratec® (Pharmacia) PoM
Combination pack, 56 yellow scored tablets, naproxen 500 mg; 56 white scored tablets, misoprostol 200 micrograms. Net price = £23.76. Label: 21
Dose patients requiring naproxen for rheumatoid arthritis, osteoarthritis, or ankylosing spondylitis, with prophylaxis against NSAID-induced gastroduodenal ulceration, 1 naproxen 500-mg tablet and 1 misoprostol 200-microgram tablet taken together twice daily with food; CHILD not recommended

PIROXICAM

Indications pain and inflammation in rheumatic disease (including juvenile idiopathic arthritis) and other musculoskeletal disorders; acute gout
Cautions see notes above and CHMP advice below; breast-feeding (Appendix 5); **interactions**: Appendix 1 (NSAIDs)
Contra-indications see notes above
Side-effects see notes above; pain at injection site (occasionally tissue damage)
Dose

- By mouth, rheumatic disease, initially 20 mg daily, increased if necessary to 30 mg daily in single or divided doses; CHILD (over 6 years), juvenile idiopathic arthritis, under 15 kg, 5 mg daily; 16–25 kg, 10 mg; 26–45 kg, 15 mg; over 46 kg, 20 mg (but see CHMP advice below)
  Acute musculoskeletal disorders, 40 mg daily in single or divided doses for 2 days, then 20 mg daily for 7–14 days (but see CHMP advice below); CHILD not recommended
  Acute gout, 40 mg initially, then 40 mg daily in single or divided doses for 4–6 days (but see CHMP advice below); CHILD not recommended
- By deep intramuscular injection into gluteal muscle, for initial treatment of acute conditions (but see CHMP advice below), as dose by mouth (on short-term basis); CHILD not recommended

CHMP advice
Piroxicam (June 2007)
The CHMP has recommended restrictions on the use of piroxicam because of the increased risk of gastro-intestinal side effects and serious skin reactions. The CHMP has advised that:

- piroxicam should be initiated only by physicians experienced in treating inflammatory or degenerative rheumatic diseases
- piroxicam should not be used as first-line treatment
- in adults, use of piroxicam should be limited to the symptomatic relief of osteoarthritis, rheumatoid arthritis, and ankylosing spondylitis
- piroxicam dose should not exceed 20 mg daily
- piroxicam should no longer be used for the treatment of acute painful and inflammatory conditions
- treatment should be reviewed 2 weeks after initiating piroxicam, and periodically thereafter
- concomitant administration of a gastro-protective agent (section 1.3) should be considered

Note Topical preparations containing piroxicam are not affected by these restrictions

Piroxicam (Non-proprietary) PoM
Capsules, piroxicam 10 mg, net price 56-cap pack = £3.00; 20 mg, 28-cap pack = £2.86. Label: 21
Dispersible tablets, piroxicam 10 mg, net price 56-tab pack = £9.96; 20 mg, 28-tab pack = £25.62. Label: 13, 21

Brexidol® (Trinity) PoM
Tablets, yellow scored, piroxicam (as betadex) 20 mg, net price 30-tab pack = £14.66. Label: 21
Dose osteoarthritis, rheumatic disease and acute musculoskeletal disorders, 1 tablet daily (may be halved in elderly); CHILD not recommended

Feldene® (Pfizer) PoM
Capsules, piroxicam 10 mg (red/blue), net price 56-cap pack = £7.20; 20 mg (white), 28-cap pack = £7.20. Label: 21
Tablets, (*Feldene Melt®*), piroxicam 20 mg, net price 28-tab pack = £9.83. Label: 10, patient information leaflet, 21
Excipients include aspartame equivalent to phenylalanine 140 micrograms/tablet (section 9.4.1)
Note *Feldene Melt®* tablets can be taken by placing on tongue or by swallowing
Injection, piroxicam 20 mg/mL, net price 1-mL amp = 84p

Topical preparations

Section 10.3.2

SULINDAC

Indications pain and inflammation in rheumatic disease and other musculoskeletal disorders; acute gout
Cautions see notes above; also history of renal stones and ensure adequate hydration; breast-feeding (Appendix 5); **interactions**: Appendix 1 (NSAIDs)
Contra-indications see notes above
Side-effects see notes above; jaundice with fever, cholestasis, hepatitis, hepatic failure; also urine discoloration occasionally reported
Dose

- 200 mg twice daily with food (may be reduced according to response); max. 400 mg daily; acute gout should respond within 7 days limit treatment of periarticular disorders to 7–10 days; CHILD not recommended

Sulindac (Non-proprietary) PoM
Tablets, sulindac 100 mg, net price 56-tab pack = £16.91; 200 mg, 56-tab pack = £34.33. Label: 21

Clinoril® (MSD) PoM
Tablets, both yellow, scored, sulindac 100 mg, net price 60-tab pack = £6.73; 200 mg, 60-tab pack = £12.96. Label: 21

TENOXICAM

Indications pain and inflammation in rheumatic disease and other musculoskeletal disorders
Cautions see notes above; breast-feeding (Appendix 5); **interactions**: Appendix 1 (NSAIDs)
Contra-indications see notes above
Side-effects see notes above
Dose
- Rheumatic disease, 20 mg daily; CHILD not recommended
- Acute musculoskeletal disorders, 20 mg daily for 7 days (max. 14 days); CHILD not recommended

Mobiflex® (Roche) PoM
Tablets, yellow, f/c, tenoxicam 20 mg. Net price 30-tab pack = £12.92. Label: 21

TIAPROFENIC ACID

Indications pain and inflammation in rheumatic disease and other musculoskeletal disorders
Cautions see notes above; breast-feeding (Appendix 5); **interactions**: Appendix 1 (NSAIDs)
Contra-indications see notes above; also active bladder or prostate disease (or symptoms) and history of recurrent urinary-tract disorders—if urinary symptoms develop discontinue immediately and perform urine tests and culture; see also CSM advice below

> **CSM advice**
> Following reports of **severe cystitis** the CSM has recommended that tiaprofenic acid should not be given to patients with urinary-tract disorders and should be stopped if urinary symptoms develop. Patients should be advised to stop taking tiaprofenic acid and to report to their doctor promptly if they develop urinary-tract symptoms (such as increased frequency, nocturia, urgency, pain on urinating, or blood in urine)

Side-effects see notes above
Dose
- 300 mg twice daily; CHILD not recommended

Surgam® (Sanofi-Aventis) PoM
Tablets, tiaprofenic acid 300 mg, net price 56-tab pack = £15.56. Label: 21

Aspirin

Aspirin (section 4.7.1) was the traditional first choice anti-inflammatory analgesic but most physicians now prefer to start treatment with another NSAID.

10.1.2 Corticosteroids

10.1.2.1 Systemic corticosteroids

The general actions, uses, and cautions of corticosteroids are described in section 6.3. Treatment with corticosteroids in rheumatic diseases should be reserved for specific indications, e.g. when other anti-inflammatory drugs are unsuccessful. Corticosteroids can induce osteoporosis, and prophylaxis should be considered on long-term treatment (section 6.6).

In severe, possibly life-threatening, situations a high initial dose of corticosteroid is given to induce remission and the dose is then reduced gradually and discontinued altogether. Relapse may occur as the dose of corticosteroid is reduced, particularly if the reduction is too rapid. The tendency is therefore to increase the maintenance dose and consequently the patient becomes dependent on corticosteroids. For this reason pulse doses of corticosteroids (e.g. methylprednisolone up to 1 g intravenously on 3 consecutive days) are used to suppress highly active inflammatory disease while longer-term treatment with a disease-modifying drug is commenced.

Prednisolone 7.5 mg daily may reduce the rate of joint destruction in moderate to severe *rheumatoid arthritis* of less than 2 years' duration. The reduction in joint destruction must be distinguished from mere symptomatic improvement (which lasts only 6 to 12 months at this dose) and care should be taken to avoid increasing the dose above 7.5 mg daily. Evidence supports maintenance of this anti-erosive dose for 2–4 years only after which treatment should be tapered off to reduce long-term adverse effects.

Polymyalgia rheumatica and *giant cell (temporal) arteritis* are always treated with corticosteroids. The usual initial dose of prednisolone in polymyalgia rheumatica is 10–15 mg daily and in giant cell arteritis 40–60 mg daily (the higher dose being used if visual symptoms occur). Treatment should be continued until remission of disease activity and doses are then reduced gradually to about 7.5–10 mg daily for maintenance. Relapse is common if therapy is stopped prematurely. Many patients require treatment for at least 2 years and in some patients it may be necessary to continue long-term low-dose corticosteroid treatment.

Polyarteritis nodosa and *polymyositis* are usually treated with corticosteroids. An initial dose of 60 mg of prednisolone daily is often used and reduced to a maintenance dose of 10–15 mg daily.

Systemic lupus erythematosus is treated with corticosteroids when necessary using a similar dosage regimen to that for polyarteritis nodosa and polymyositis (above). Patients with pleurisy, pericarditis, or other systemic manifestations will respond to corticosteroids. It may then be possible to reduce the dosage; alternate-day treatment is sometimes adequate, and the drug may be gradually withdrawn. In some mild cases corticosteroid treatment may be stopped after a few months. Many mild cases of systemic lupus erythematosus do not require corticosteroid treatment. Alternative treatment with anti-inflammatory analgesics, and possibly chloroquine or hydroxychloroquine, should be considered.

Ankylosing spondylitis should not be treated with long-term corticosteroids; rarely, pulse doses may be needed and may be useful in extremely active disease that does not respond to conventional treatment.

10.1.2.2 Local corticosteroid injections

Corticosteroids are injected locally for an anti-inflammatory effect. In inflammatory conditions of the joints, particularly in rheumatoid arthritis, they are given by *intra-articular injection* to relieve pain, increase mobility, and reduce deformity in one or a few joints. Full aseptic precautions are essential; infected areas should be avoided. Occasionally an acute inflammatory reaction develops after an intra-articular or soft-tissue injection of a corticosteroid. This may be a reaction to the microcrystalline suspension of the corticosteroid used, but must be distinguished from sepsis introduced into the injection site.

Smaller amounts of corticosteroids may also be injected directly into soft tissues for the relief of inflammation in conditions such as *tennis* or *golfer's elbow* or *compression neuropathies.* In *tendinitis,* injections should be made into the tendon sheath and not directly into the tendon (due to the absence of a true tendon sheath, the Achilles tendon should not be injected). A soluble preparation (e.g. containing betamethasone or dexamethasone sodium phosphate) is preferred for injection into the carpal tunnel.

Hydrocortisone acetate or one of the synthetic analogues is generally used for local injection. Intra-articular corticosteroid injections can cause flushing and may affect the hyaline cartilage. Each joint should usually be treated **no more** than 3 times in one year.

Corticosteroid injections are also injected into soft tissues for the treatment of skin lesions (see section 13.4).

LOCAL CORTICOSTEROID INJECTIONS

Indications local inflammation of joints and soft tissues (for details, consult product literature)

Cautions see notes above and consult product literature; see also section 6.3.2

Contra-indications see notes above and consult product literature; avoid injections containing benzyl alcohol in neonates (see preparations below)

Side-effects see notes above and consult product literature

Dose

- See under preparations

▲Betamethasone

Betnesol® (UCB Pharma) PoM

Injection, betamethasone (as sodium phosphate) 4 mg/mL, net price 1-mL amp = £1.22.

▲Dose calculated as dexamethasone

Dexamethasone (Organon) PoM

Injection, dexamethasone 4 mg/mL (as sodium phosphate) (≡ dexamethasone sodium phosphate 5.2 mg/mL ≡ dexamethasone phosphate 4.8 mg/mL). Net price 1-mL amp = 83p; 2-mL vial = £1.27

Dose by intra-articular *or* intrasynovial injection (for details consult product literature), 0.6–3 mg (calculated as dexamethasone) according to size; where appropriate may be repeated at intervals of 3–21 days according to response

▲Dose calculated as dexamethasone phosphate

Dexamethasone (Mayne) PoM

Injection, dexamethasone phosphate 4 mg/mL (as sodium phosphate) (≡ dexamethasone 3.3 mg/mL ≡ dexamethasone sodium phosphate 4.4 mg/mL), net price 1-mL amp = £1.00; 2-mL vial = £1.98

Dose by intra-articular *or* intrasynovial injection (for details consult product literature), 0.4–4 mg (calculated as dexamethasone phosphate) according to size (by soft-tissue infiltration 2–6 mg); where appropriate may be repeated at intervals of 3–21 days

▲Hydrocortisone acetate

Hydrocortistab® (Sovereign) PoM

Injection, (aqueous suspension), hydrocortisone acetate 25 mg/mL. Net price 1-mL amp = £5.72

Dose by intra-articular *or* intrasynovial injection (for details consult product literature), 5–50 mg according to size; where appropriate may be repeated at intervals of 21 days; not more than 3 joints should be treated on any one day; CHILD 5–30 mg (divided)

▲Methylprednisolone acetate

Depo-Medrone® (Pharmacia) PoM

Injection (aqueous suspension), methylprednisolone acetate 40 mg/mL. Net price 1-mL vial = £2.87; 2-mL vial = £5.15; 3-mL vial = £7.47

Dose by intra-articular *or* intrasynovial injection (for details consult product literature), 4–80 mg, according to size; where appropriate may be repeated at intervals of 7–35 days; also for intralesional injection

Depo-Medrone® with Lidocaine (Pharmacia) PoM

Injection (aqueous suspension), methylprednisolone acetate 40 mg, lidocaine hydrochloride 10 mg/mL. Net price 1-mL vial = £3.28; 2-mL vial = £5.88

Dose by intra-articular *or* intrasynovial injection (for details consult product literature), 4–80 mg, according to size; where appropriate may be repeated at intervals of 7–35 days

▲Prednisolone acetate

Deltastab® (Sovereign) PoM

Injection (aqueous suspension), prednisolone acetate 25 mg/mL. Net price 1-mL amp = £5.73

Dose by intra-articular *or* intrasynovial injection (for details consult product literature), 5–25 mg according to size; not more than 3 joints should be treated on any one day; where appropriate may be repeated when relapse occurs

For intramuscular injection, see section 6.3.2

▲Triamcinolone acetonide

Adcortyl® Intra-articular/Intradermal (Squibb) PoM

Injection (aqueous suspension), triamcinolone acetonide 10 mg/mL. Net price 1-mL amp = £1.02; 5-mL vial = £4.14

Excipients include benzyl alcohol (avoid in neonates, see Excipients, p. 2)

Dose by intra-articular injection *or* intrasynovial injection (for details consult product literature), 2.5–15 mg according to size (for larger doses use *Kenalog®*); where appropriate may be repeated when relapse occurs

By intradermal injection, (for details consult product literature): 2–3 mg; max. 5 mg at any one site (total max. 30 mg); where appropriate may be repeated at intervals of 1–2 weeks

CHILD under 6 years not recommended

Kenalog® Intra-articular/Intramuscular (Squibb) PoM

Injection (aqueous suspension), triamcinolone acetonide 40 mg/mL, net price 1-mL vial = £1.70;

1-mL prefilled syringe = £2.11; 2-mL prefilled syringe = £3.66

Note Intramuscular needle with prefilled syringe should be replaced for intra-articular injection

Dose by intra-articular *or* intrasynovial injection (for details consult product literature), 5–40 mg according to size; total max. 80 mg (for doses below 5 mg use *Adcortyl® Intra-articular/Intradermal*); where appropriate may be repeated when relapse occurs; CHILD under 6 years not recommended

For intramuscular injection, see section 6.3.2

10.1.3 Drugs that suppress the rheumatic disease process

Certain drugs such as those affecting the immune response can suppress the disease process in *rheumatoid arthritis* and *psoriatic arthritis*; gold, penicillamine, hydroxychloroquine, chloroquine, and sulfasalazine can also suppress the disease process in *rheumatoid arthritis* while sulfasalazine and possibly gold can suppress the disease process in *psoriatic arthritis*. Unlike NSAIDs, disease-modifying anti-rheumatic drugs (DMARDs) can affect the progression of disease but may require 2–6 months of treatment for a full therapeutic response. Since in the first few months of treatment, the course of rheumatoid arthritis is unpredictable and the diagnosis uncertain, it is usual to start treatment with an NSAID alone. However, disease-modifying anti-rheumatic drugs should be initiated by specialists as soon as diagnosis, progression, and severity of the disease have been confirmed. Response to a disease-modifying anti-rheumatic drug may allow the dose of the NSAID to be reduced.

Disease-modifying antirheumatic drugs can improve not only the symptoms of inflammatory joint disease but also extra-articular manifestations such as vasculitis. They reduce the erythrocyte sedimentation rate, C-reactive protein, and sometimes the titre of rheumatoid factor; some also retard erosive damage as judged radiologically.

Choice The choice of a disease-modifying anti-rheumatic drug should take into account co-morbidity and patient preference. Sulfasalazine, methotrexate, intramuscular gold and penicillamine are similar in efficacy. However, **sulfasalazine** or **methotrexate** are often used first because they may be better tolerated.

Penicillamine and drugs that affect the immune response ('immunomodulators') are also sometimes used in rheumatoid arthritis where there are troublesome extra-articular features such as vasculitis, and in patients who are taking high doses of corticosteroids. Response to the drugs often produces a striking reduction in requirements of both corticosteroids and other drugs. **Gold** and **penicillamine** are effective in *palindromic rheumatism*. *Systemic* and *discoid lupus erythematosus* are sometimes treated with **chloroquine** or **hydroxychloroquine**.

If a disease-modifying anti-rheumatic drug does not lead to an objective benefit within 6 months (or within 3 months for inhibitors of tumour necrosis factor), it should be replaced by a different one.

In some circumstances, and under specialist supervision, combining two or more disease-modifying anti-rheumatic drugs can be considered.

Juvenile idiopathic arthritis Many children with *juvenile idiopathic arthritis* (juvenile chronic arthritis) do not require disease-modifying antirheumatic drugs. Methotrexate is effective [unlicensed indication]; sulfasalazine is an alternative [unlicensed indication] but it should be avoided in *systemic-onset juvenile idiopathic arthritis*. Gold and penicillamine are no longer used. For the role of etanercept in *polyarticular-course juvenile idiopathic arthritis*, see p. 552

Gold

Gold can be given by intramuscular injection as sodium aurothiomalate or by mouth as auranofin.

Sodium aurothiomalate must be given by deep intramuscular injection and the area gently massaged. A test dose of 10 mg must be given followed by doses of 50 mg at weekly intervals until there is definite evidence of remission. Benefit is not to be expected until about 300–500 mg has been given; it should be discontinued if there is no remission after 1 g has been given. In patients who do respond, the interval between injections is then gradually increased to 4 weeks and treatment is continued for up to 5 years after complete remission. If relapse occurs the dosage frequency may be immediately increased to 50 mg weekly and only once control has been obtained again should the dosage frequency be decreased; if no response is seen within 2 months, alternative treatment should be sought. It is important to avoid complete relapse since second courses of gold are not usually effective. Children can be given 1 mg/kg weekly to a maximum of 50 mg weekly, the intervals being gradually increased to 4 weeks according to response; an initial test dose is given corresponding to one-tenth to one-fifth of the calculated dose.

Auranofin is given by mouth. If there is no response after 6 months treatment should be discontinued. Auranofin is less effective than parenteral gold.

Gold therapy should be discontinued in the presence of blood disorders, gastro-intestinal bleeding (associated with ulcerative enterocolitis), or unexplained proteinuria (associated with immune complex nephritis) which is repeatedly above 300 mg/litre. Urine tests and full blood counts (including total and differential white cell and platelet counts) must therefore be performed before starting treatment with gold and before each intramuscular injection; in the case of oral treatment the urine and blood tests should be carried out monthly. Rashes with pruritus often occur after 2 to 6 months of intramuscular treatment and may necessitate discontinuation of treatment; the most common side-effect of oral therapy, diarrhoea with or without nausea or abdominal pain, may respond to bulking agents (such as bran) or temporary reduction in dosage.

SODIUM AUROTHIOMALATE

Indications active progressive rheumatoid arthritis, juvenile idiopathic arthritis

Cautions see notes above; hepatic impairment (Appendix 2), renal impairment (Appendix 3), pregnancy (Appendix 4), breast-feeding (Appendix 5); elderly, history of urticaria, eczema, colitis, drugs which cause blood disorders; annual chest X-ray

Contra-indications severe renal and hepatic disease (see notes above); history of blood disorders or bone marrow aplasia, exfoliative dermatitis, systemic lupus erythematosus, necrotising enterocolitis, pulmonary fibrosis; porphyria (section 9.8.2)

Side-effects severe reactions (occasionally fatal) in up to 5% of patients; mouth ulcers, skin reactions (including, on prolonged parenteral treatment, irreversible pigmentation in sun-exposed areas), proteinuria, blood disorders (sometimes sudden and fatal); rarely colitis, peripheral neuritis, pulmonary fibrosis, hepatotoxicity with cholestatic jaundice, nephrotic syndrome, alopecia

Dose

- By deep intramuscular injection, administered on expert advice, see notes above

  Counselling Warn patient to tell doctor immediately if sore throat, fever, infection, non-specific illness, unexplained bleeding and bruising, purpura, mouth ulcers, metallic taste, or rashes develop; also ask patients to report immediately any breathlessness or cough

Myocrisin® (Sanofi-Aventis) PoM

Injection, sodium aurothiomalate 20 mg/mL, net price 0.5-mL (10-mg) amp = £3.80; 100 mg/mL, 0.5-mL (50-mg) amp = £11.23. Counselling, blood disorder symptoms

AURANOFIN

Indications active progressive rheumatoid arthritis

Cautions see under Sodium Aurothiomalate; hepatic impairment (Appendix 2); pregnancy (Appendix 4); breast-feeding (Appendix 5); also inflammatory bowel disease

Blood counts Withdraw if platelet count falls below 100 000/mm³ or if signs and symptoms suggestive of thrombocytopenia occur, see also notes above

Contra-indications see under Sodium Aurothiomalate

Side-effects diarrhoea most common (reduced by bulking agents such as bran); see also under Sodium Aurothiomalate

Dose

- Administered on expert advice, 6 mg daily (initially in 2 divided doses then if tolerated as single dose), if response inadequate after 6 months, increase to 9 mg daily (in 3 divided doses), discontinue if no response after a further 3 months; CHILD not recommended

  Counselling Warn patient to tell doctor immediately if sore throat, fever, infection, non-specific illness, unexplained bleeding and bruising, purpura, mouth ulcers, metallic taste, or rashes develop; also ask patients to report immediately any breathlessness or cough

  Note The package insert for *Ridaura®* also advises that patients must also report immediately if conjunctivitis or hair loss develops

Ridaura® (Astellas) PoM

Tablets, yellow, f/c, auranofin 3 mg. Net price 60-tab pack = £25.20. Label: 21, counselling, blood disorder symptoms (see above)

Penicillamine

Penicillamine has a similar action to gold. More patients are able to continue treatment than with gold but side-effects are common.

Patients should be warned not to expect improvement for at least 6 to 12 weeks after treatment is initiated. Penicillamine should be discontinued if there is no improvement within 1 year.

Blood counts, including platelets, and urine examinations should be carried out before starting treatment and then every 1 or 2 weeks for the first 2 months then every 4 weeks to detect blood disorders and proteinuria (they should also be carried out in the week after any dose increase). A reduction in platelet count calls for discontinuation with subsequent re-introduction at a lower dosage and then, if possible, gradual increase. Proteinuria, associated with immune complex nephritis, occurs in up to 30% of patients, but may resolve despite continuation of treatment; treatment may be continued provided that renal function tests remain normal, oedema is absent, and the 24-hour urinary excretion of protein does not exceed 2 g.

Nausea may occur but is not usually a problem provided that penicillamine is taken before food or on retiring and that low initial doses are used and only gradually increased. Loss of taste can occur about 6 weeks after treatment is started but usually returns 6 weeks later irrespective of whether treatment is discontinued; mineral supplements are not recommended. Rashes are a common side-effect. Those that occur in the first few months of treatment disappear when the drug is stopped and treatment may then be re-introduced at a lower dose level and gradually increased. Late rashes are more resistant and often necessitate discontinuation of treatment.

Patients who are hypersensitive to penicillin may react rarely to penicillamine.

PENICILLAMINE

Indications see notes above and under Dose

Cautions see notes above; renal impairment (Appendix 3); pregnancy (Appendix 4); concomitant nephrotoxic drugs (increased risk of toxicity); gold treatment (avoid concomitant use if adverse reactions to gold); **interactions**: Appendix 1 (penicillamine)

Blood counts and urine tests See notes above. Longer intervals may be adequate in cystinuria and Wilson's disease. Consider withdrawal if platelet count falls below 120 000/mm³ or white blood cells below 2500/mm³ or if 3 successive falls within reference range (can restart at reduced dose when counts return to within reference range but permanent withdrawal necessary if recurrence of leucopenia or thrombocytopenia)

Counselling Warn patient to tell doctor immediately if sore throat, fever, infection, non-specific illness, unexplained bleeding and bruising, purpura, mouth ulcers, or rashes develop

Contra-indications lupus erythematosus

Side-effects (see also notes above) initially nausea, anorexia, fever, and skin reactions; taste loss (mineral supplements not recommended); blood disorders including thrombocytopenia, leucopenia, agranulocytosis and aplastic anaemia; proteinuria, rarely haematuria (withdraw immediately); haemolytic anaemia, nephrotic syndrome, lupus erythematosus-like syndrome, myasthenia gravis-like syndrome, polymyositis (rarely with cardiac involvement), dermatomyositis, mouth ulcers, stomatitis, alopecia, bronchiolitis and pneumonitis, pemphigus, Goodpasture's syndrome, and Stevens-Johnson syndrome also reported; male and female breast enlargement reported; in non-rheumatoid conditions rheumatoid arthritis-like syndrome also reported; late rashes (consider withdrawing treatment)

Dose

- Severe active rheumatoid arthritis, administered on expert advice, ADULT initially 125–250 mg daily before food for 1 month increased by similar amounts at intervals of not less than 4 weeks to usual maintenance of 500–750 mg daily in divided doses; max. 1.5 g daily; if remission sustained for 6 months, reduction of daily dose by 125–250 mg every 12 weeks may be attempted; ELDERLY initially up to 125 mg daily before food for 1 month increased by similar amounts at intervals of not less than 4 weeks; max. 1 g daily; CHILD maintenance of 15–20 mg/kg daily (initial dose lower and increased at intervals of 4 weeks over a period of 3-6 months)

- Wilson's disease, autoimmune hepatitis, and cystinuria, section 9.8.1
- Lead poisoning, see Emergency Treatment of Poisoning, p. 34

Penicillamine (Non-proprietary) PoM
Tablets, penicillamine 125 mg, net price 56-tab pack = £13.22; 250 mg, 56-tab pack = £21.28. Label: 6, 22, counselling, blood disorder symptoms (see above)

Distamine® (Alliance) PoM
Tablets, all f/c, penicillamine 125 mg, net price 20 = £1.96; 250 mg, 20 = £3.41. Label: 6, 22, counselling, blood disorder symptoms (see above)

Antimalarials

The antimalarial **hydroxychloroquine** is used to treat rheumatoid arthritis of moderate inflammatory activity; **chloroquine** is also licensed for treating inflammatory disorders but is used much less frequently and is generally reserved for use if other drugs have failed. These drugs are effective for mild systemic lupus erythematosus, particularly involving the skin and joints. Chloroquine and hydroxychloroquine should not be used for psoriatic arthritis.

Chloroquine and hydroxychloroquine are better tolerated than gold or penicillamine. Retinopathy (see below) rarely occurs provided that the recommended doses are not exceeded; in the elderly it is difficult to distinguish drug-induced retinopathy from ageing changes.

Mepacrine (section 5.4.4) is sometimes used in discoid lupus erythematosus [unlicensed].

Cautions Chloroquine and hydroxychloroquine should be used with caution in hepatic impairment (Appendix 2) and in renal impairment (Appendix 3). Manufacturers recommend regular ophthalmological examination but the evidence of practical value is unsatisfactory (see advice of the Royal College of Ophthalmologists, below). It is not necessary to withdraw an antimalarial drug during pregnancy (Appendix 4) if the rheumatic disease is well controlled. Chloroquine and hydroxychloroquine are present in breast milk and breast-feeding (Appendix 5) should be avoided when they are used to treat rheumatic disease; chloroquine can, however, be used for malaria during pregnancy and breast-feeding (section 5.4.1). Both should be used with caution in neurological disorders (especially in those with a history of epilepsy), in severe gastro-intestinal disorders, in G6PD deficiency (section 9.1.5), in porphyria, and in the elderly (see also above). Chloroquine and hydroxychloroquine may exacerbate psoriasis and aggravate myasthenia gravis. Concurrent use of hepatotoxic drugs should be avoided; other **interactions**: Appendix 1 (chloroquine and hydroxychloroquine).

Screening for ocular toxicity
A review group convened by the Royal College of Ophthalmologists has updated guidelines for screening to prevent ocular toxicity on long-term treatment with chloroquine, hydroxychloroquine, and mepacrine (*Ocular toxicity with hydroxychloroquine: guidelines for screening 2004*). Chloroquine should be considered (for treating chronic inflammatory conditions) **only** if other drugs have failed. All patients taking chloroquine should receive ocular examination according to a protocol arranged locally between the prescriber and the ophthalmologist. Mepacrine has negligible ocular toxicity. The following recommendations relate to hydroxychloroquine, which is only rarely associated with toxicity.

Before treatment:

- Assess renal and liver function (adjust dose if impaired)
- Ask patient about visual impairment (not corrected by glasses). If impairment or eye disease present, assessment by an optometrist is advised and any abnormality should be referred to an ophthalmologist
- Record near visual acuity of each eye (with glasses where appropriate) using a standard reading chart
- Initiate hydroxychloroquine treatment if no abnormality detected (at a dose not exceeding hydroxychloroquine sulphate 6.5 mg/kg daily)

During treatment:

- Ask patient about visual symptoms and monitor visual acuity annually using the standard reading chart
- Refer to ophthalmologist if visual acuity changes or if vision blurred and warn patient to stop treatment and seek prescribing doctor's advice
- A child treated for juvenile idiopathic arthritis should receive slit-lamp examination routinely to check for uveitis
- If long-term treatment is required (more than 5 years), individual arrangement should be agreed with the local ophthalmologist

Note To avoid excessive dosage in obese patients, the dose of hydroxychloroquine and chloroquine should be calculated on the basis of lean body weight. Ocular toxicity is unlikely if the dose of chloroquine phosphate does not exceed 4 mg/kg daily (equivalent to chloroquine base approx. 2.5 mg/kg daily)

Side-effects The side-effects of chloroquine and hydroxychloroquine include gastro-intestinal disturbances, headache and skin reactions (rashes, pruritus); those occurring less frequently include ECG changes, convulsions, visual changes, retinal damage (see above), keratopathy, ototoxicity, hair depigmentation, hair loss, and discoloration of skin, nails, and mucous membranes. Side-effects that occur rarely include blood disorders (including thrombocytopenia, agranulocytosis, and aplastic anaemia), mental changes (including emotional disturbances and psychosis), myopathy (including cardiomyopathy and neuromyopathy), acute generalised exanthematous pustulosis, exfoliative dermatitis, Stevens-Johnson syndrome, photosensitivity, and hepatic damage. **Important**: very toxic in overdosage—immediate advice from poisons centres essential (see also p. 32).

CHLOROQUINE

Indications active rheumatoid arthritis (including juvenile idiopathic arthritis), systemic and discoid lupus erythematosus; malaria (section 5.4.1)

Cautions see notes above

Side-effects see notes above

Dose

- Administered on expert advice, by mouth, chloroquine (base) 150 mg daily; max. 2.5 mg/kg daily, see recommendations above; CHILD up to 3 mg/kg daily

Note Chloroquine base 150 mg ≡ chloroquine sulphate 200 mg ≡ chloroquine phosphate 250 mg (approx.).

Preparations

Section 5.4.1

HYDROXYCHLOROQUINE SULPHATE

Indications active rheumatoid arthritis (including juvenile idiopathic arthritis), systemic and discoid lupus erythematosus; dermatological conditions caused or aggravated by sunlight

Cautions see notes above

Side-effects see notes above

Dose

- Administered on expert advice, initially 400 mg daily in divided doses; maintenance 200–400 mg daily; max. 6.5 mg/kg daily (but not exceeding 400 mg daily), see recommendations above; CHILD, up to 6.5 mg/kg daily (max. 400 mg daily)

Plaquenil® (Sanofi-Synthelabo) PoM

Tablets, f/c, hydroxychloroquine sulphate 200 mg. Net price 60-tab pack = £5.46. Label: 5, 21

Drugs affecting the immune response

Methotrexate is a disease-modifying antirheumatic drug suitable for moderate to severe rheumatoid arthritis. **Azathioprine**, **ciclosporin**, **cyclophosphamide**, **leflunomide**, and the **cytokine modulators** (adalimumab, anakinra, etanercept, and infliximab) are considered more toxic and they are used in cases that have not responded to other disease-modifying drugs.

Methotrexate is usually given in an initial dose of 7.5 mg by mouth once a week, adjusted according to response to a maximum of 15 mg once a week (occasionally 20 mg once a week). Regular full blood counts (including differential white cell count and platelet count), renal and liver-function tests are required. In patients who experience mucosal or gastro-intestinal side-effects with methotrexate, folic acid 5 mg every week may help to reduce the frequency of such side-effects.

Azathioprine is usually given in a dose of 1.5 to 2.5 mg/kg daily in divided doses. Blood counts are needed to detect possible neutropenia or thrombocytopenia (usually resolved by reducing the dose). Nausea, vomiting, and diarrhoea may occur, usually starting early during the course of treatment, and may necessitate withdrawal of the drug; herpes zoster infection may also occur.

Leflunomide acts on the immune system as a disease-modifying antirheumatic drug. Its therapeutic effect starts after 4–6 weeks and improvement may continue for a further 4–6 months. Leflunomide, which is similar in efficacy to sulfasalazine and methotrexate, may be chosen when these drugs cannot be used. The active metabolite of leflunomide persists for a long period; active procedures to wash the drug out are required in case of serious adverse effects, or before starting treatment with another disease-modifying antirheumatic drug, or, in men or women, before conception. Side-effects of leflunomide include bone-marrow toxicity; its immunosuppressive effects increase the risk of infection and malignancy.

Ciclosporin (cyclosporin) is licensed for severe active rheumatoid arthritis when conventional second-line therapy is inappropriate or ineffective. There is some evidence that ciclosporin may retard the rate of erosive progression and improve symptom control in those who respond only partially to methotrexate.

Cyclophosphamide (section 8.1.1) may be used at a dose of 1 to 1.5 mg/kg daily by mouth for rheumatoid arthritis with severe systemic manifestations [unlicensed indication]; it is toxic and regular blood counts (including platelet counts) should be carried out. Cyclophosphamide can also be given intravenously in a dose of 0.5 to 1 g (with prophylactic mesna) for *severe systemic rheumatoid arthritis* and for other connective tissue diseases (especially with active vasculitis), repeated initially at fortnightly then at monthly intervals (according to clinical response and haematological monitoring).

Drugs that affect the immune response are also used in the management of severe cases of *systemic lupus erythematosus* and other connective tissue disorders. They are often given in conjunction with corticosteroids for patients with severe or progressive renal disease. They may be used in cases of *polymyositis* that are resistant to corticosteroids. They are used for their corticosteroid-sparing effect in patients whose corticosteroid requirements are excessive. **Azathioprine** is usually used.

Azathioprine and methotrexate are used in the treatment of *psoriatic arthropathy* [unlicensed indication] for severe or progressive cases that are not controlled with anti-inflammatory drugs.

AZATHIOPRINE

Indications see notes above; transplantation rejection, see section 8.2.1

Cautions see section 8.2.1

Contra-indications see section 8.2.1

Side-effects see section 8.2.1

Dose

- By mouth, initially, rarely more than 3 mg/kg daily, reduced according to response; maintenance 1–3 mg/kg daily; consider withdrawal if no improvement within 3 months

Preparations

Section 8.2.1

CICLOSPORIN
(Cyclosporin)

Indications severe active rheumatoid arthritis when conventional second-line therapy inappropriate or ineffective; graft-versus-host disease (section 8.2.2); atopic dermatitis and psoriasis (section 13.5.3).

Cautions see section 8.2.2

Additional cautions in rheumatoid arthritis *Contra-indicated* in abnormal renal function, uncontrolled hypertension (see also below), uncontrolled infections, and malignancy. Measure serum creatinine at least twice before treatment and monitor every 2 weeks for first 3 months, then every 4 weeks (or more frequently if dose increased or concomitant NSAIDs introduced or increased (see also *interactions:* Appendix 1 (ciclosporin)), reduce dose if serum creatinine increases more than 30% above baseline in more than 1 measurement; if above 50%, reduce dose by 50% (even if within normal range) and discontinue if reduction not successful within 1 month; monitor blood pressure (discontinue if hypertension develops that cannot be controlled by antihypertensive therapy); monitor hepatic function if concomitant NSAIDs given.

Side-effects see section 8.2.2

Dose

- By mouth, administered in accordance with expert advice, initially 2.5 mg/kg daily in 2 divided doses, if necessary increased gradually after 6 weeks; max. 4 mg/kg daily (discontinue if response insufficient after 3 months); dose adjusted according to response for maintenance and treatment reviewed after 6 months (continue only if benefits outweigh risks); CHILD and under 18 years, not recommended

Important For preparations and counselling and for advice on conversion between the preparations, see section 8.2.2

Preparations

Section 8.2.2

LEFLUNOMIDE

Indications moderate to severe active rheumatoid arthritis; active psoriatic arthritis

Cautions renal impairment (Appendix 3); impaired bone-marrow function including anaemia, leucopenia or thrombocytopenia (avoid if significant and due to causes other than rheumatoid arthritis); recent treatment with other hepatotoxic or myelotoxic disease-modifying antirheumatic drugs (avoid concomitant use); history of tuberculosis; exclude pregnancy before treatment; effective contraception **essential** during treatment and for at least 2 years after treatment in women and at least 3 months after treatment in men (plasma concentration monitoring required; waiting time before conception may be reduced with washout procedures—consult product literature and see Washout Procedure below); monitor full blood count (including differential white cell count and platelet count) before treatment and every 2 weeks for 6 months then every 8 weeks; monitor liver function—(see Hepatotoxicity below); monitor blood pressure; washout procedures recommended for serious adverse effects and before switching to other disease-modifying antirheumatic drugs (consult product literature and see below); **interactions:** Appendix 1 (leflunomide)

Hepatotoxicity Potentially life-threatening hepatotoxicity reported usually in the first 6 months; monitor liver function before treatment and every 2 weeks for first 6 months then every 8 weeks. Discontinue treatment (and institute washout procedure—consult product literature and see Washout Procedure below) or reduce dose according to liver-function abnormality; if liver-function abnormality persists after dose reduction, discontinue treatment and institute washout procedure

Washout procedure To aid drug elimination in case of serious adverse effect, or before starting another disease-modifying antirheumatic drug, or before conception (see also Appendix 4), stop treatment and give *either* colestyramine 8 g 3 times daily for 11 days *or* activated charcoal 50 g 4 times daily for 11 days; the concentration of the active metabolite after washout should be less than 20 micrograms/litre (measured on 2 occasions 14 days apart) in men or women before conception—consult product literature

Contra-indications severe immunodeficiency; serious infection; hepatic impairment (Appendix 2); severe hypoproteinaemia; pregnancy (**important teratogenic risk:** see Cautions and Appendix 4); breast-feeding (Appendix 5)

Side-effects diarrhoea, nausea, vomiting, anorexia, oral mucosal disorders, abdominal pain, weight loss; increase in blood pressure; headache, dizziness, asthenia, paraesthesia; tenosynovitis; alopecia, eczema, dry skin, rash, pruritus; leucopenia; rarely taste disturbances, anxiety, tendon rupture, urticaria, anaemia, thrombocytopenia, eosinophilia, hyperlipidaemia, hypokalaemia, hypophosphataemia, hepatic dysfunction (see Hepatotoxicity above); also reported, pancreatitis, anaphylaxis, interstitial lung disease, severe infection, pancytopenia, vasculitis, Stevens-Johnson syndrome, toxic epidermal necrolysis (discontinue and initiate washout procedure—consult product literature)

Dose

- Rheumatoid arthritis, ADULT over 18 years, initially 100 mg once daily for 3 days then maintenance, 10–20 mg once daily
- Psoriatic arthritis, ADULT over 18 years, initially 100 mg once daily for 3 days then maintenance, 20 mg once daily

Arava® (Aventis Pharma) PoM

Tablets, f/c, leflunomide 10 mg, net price 30-tab pack = £51.13; 20 mg (ochre), 30-tab pack = £51.13; 100 mg, 3-tab pack = £25.56. Label: 4

METHOTREXATE

Indications moderate to severe active rheumatoid arthritis; Crohn's disease; malignant disease (section 8.1.3); psoriasis (section 13.5.3)

Cautions section 8.1; see CSM advice below (blood count, liver and pulmonary toxicity); extreme caution in blood disorders (avoid if severe); peptic ulceration, ulcerative colitis, diarrhoea and ulcerative stomatitis (withdraw if stomatitis develops—may be first sign of gastro-intestinal toxicity); risk of accumulation in pleural effusion or ascites—drain before treatment; porphyria (section 9.8.2); renal impairment (avoid if creatinine clearance less than 20 mL/minute; Appendix 3); **interactions:** see below and Appendix 1 (methotrexate)

> **CSM advice**
>
> In view of reports of blood dyscrasias (including fatalities) and liver cirrhosis with low-dose methotrexate, the CSM has advised:
>
> - full blood count and renal and liver function tests before starting treatment and repeated weekly until therapy stabilised, thereafter patients should be monitored every 2–3 months
> - that patients should be advised to report all symptoms and signs suggestive of infection, especially sore throat
>
> Treatment with folinic acid (as calcium folinate, section 8.1) may be required in acute toxicity

Blood count Haematopoietic suppression can occur abruptly; factors likely to increase toxicity include advanced age, renal impairment, and concomitant administration of another anti-folate drug. A profound drop in white-cell or platelet count calls for immediate withdrawal of methotrexate and introduction of supportive therapy

Liver toxicity Liver cirrhosis reported. Treatment should not be started or should be discontinued if any abnormality of liver function tests or liver biopsy is present or develops during therapy. Abnormalities may return to normal within 2 weeks after which treatment may be recommenced if judged appropriate

Pulmonary toxicity Pulmonary toxicity may be a special problem in rheumatoid arthritis (patient to seek medical attention if dyspnoea, cough or fever); monitor for symptoms at each visit—discontinue if pneumonitis suspected.

Aspirin and other NSAIDs If aspirin or other NSAIDs are given concurrently the dose of methotrexate should be carefully monitored. Patients should be advised to avoid self-medication with over-the-counter aspirin or ibuprofen

Contra-indications see Cautions above, hepatic impairment (Appendix 2), pregnancy (following administration to a woman or a man, avoid conception for **at least 3 months** after stopping—Appendix 4), breast-feeding (Appendix 5), active infection and immunodeficiency syndromes

Side-effects section 8.1; also anorexia, abdominal discomfort, dyspepsia, gastro-intestinal ulceration and bleeding, diarrhoea, toxic megacolon, hepatotoxicity (see Cautions above); hypotension, pericarditis, pericardial tamponade; pulmonary oedema, pleuritic pain, pulmonary fibrosis, interstitial pneumonitis (see also Pulmonary Toxicity above); anaphylactic reactions, urticaria; dizziness, fatigue, chills, fever, drowsiness, malaise, headache, mood changes, abnormal cranial sensations, neurotoxicity, confusion, paraesthesia; precipitation of diabetes; menstrual disturbances, vaginitis, cystitis, reduced libido, impotence; blood disorders; haematuria, dysuria, renal failure; osteoporosis, arthralgia, myalgia, vasculitis; conjunctivitis, visual disturbance; rash, pruritus, Stevens-Johnson syndrome, toxic epidermal necrolysis, photosensitivity, changes in nail and skin pigmentation, telangiectasia, acne, furuncolosis, ecchymosis; injection-site reactions

Dose

- Moderate to severe active rheumatoid arthritis, by mouth, 7.5 mg once weekly, adjusted according to response; max. weekly dose 20 mg
- Severe active rheumatoid arthritis, by subcutaneous *or* by intramuscular *or* by intravenous injection, 7.5 mg once weekly, increased according to response by 2.5 mg weekly; max. weekly dose 25 mg
- Refractory Crohn's disease [unlicensed indication], by intramuscular injection, induction of remission, 25 mg once weekly; maintenance, 15 mg once weekly

> **Important**
>
> Note that the above dose is a **weekly** dose. To avoid error with low-dose methotrexate, it is recommended that:
>
> - the patient is carefully advised of the **dose** and **frequency** and the reason for taking methotrexate and any other prescribed medicine (e.g. folic acid);
> - only one strength of methotrexate tablet (usually 2.5 mg) is prescribed and dispensed;
> - the prescription and the dispensing label clearly show the dose and frequency of methotrexate administration;
> - the patient is warned to report immediately the onset of any feature of blood disorders (e.g. sore throat, bruising, and mouth ulcers), liver toxicity (e.g. nausea, vomiting, abdominal discomfort, and dark urine), and respiratory effects (e.g. shortness of breath).

Methotrexate (Non-proprietary) PoM

Tablets, yellow, methotrexate 2.5 mg, net price 28-tab pack = £3.27. Counselling, dose, NSAIDs

Brands include *Maxtrex®*

Tablets, yellow, methotrexate 10 mg, net price 20 (Mayne) = £11.01; (Pharmacia, *Maxtrex®*) = £9.03. Counselling, dose, NSAIDs

Parenteral preparations

See also section 8.1.3

Metoject® (Medac) PoM

Injection, prefilled syringe, methotrexate (as disodium salt) 10 mg/mL, net price 0.75 mL (7.5 mg) = £14.85, 1 mL (10 mg) = £15.29, 1.5 mL (15 mg) = £16.57, 2 mL (20 mg) = £17.84, 2.5 mL (25 mg) = £18.48

Cytokine modulators

Cytokine modulators should be used under specialist supervision.

Adalimumab, etanercept, and infliximab inhibit the activity of tumour necrosis factor alpha (TNF-α).

> **NICE guidance**
>
> **Adalimumab for the treatment of psoriatic arthritis (August 2007)**
>
> Adalimumab is an option for the treatment of active and progressive psoriatic arthritis in adults with at least 3 tender joints and at least 3 swollen joints, who have not responded adequately to at least 2 standard disease-modifying antirheumatic drugs (used alone or in combination). Adalimumab should be used under specialist supervision and should be discontinued if there is an inadequate response after 12 weeks.

> **NICE guidance**
>
> **Adalimumab, etanercept and infliximab for the treatment of rheumatoid arthritis (October 2007)**
>
> The tumour necrosis factor alpha (TNF-α) inhibitors adalimumab, etanercept, and infliximab are options for the treatment of adults with active rheumatoid arthritis who have failed to respond to at least 2 disease-modifying antirheumatic drugs (DMARDs), including methotrexate (unless contra-indicated). TNF-α inhibitors should be given in combination with methotrexate; however, where methotrexate cannot be used because of intolerance or contra-indications, adalimumab or etanercept may be given as monotherapy.
>
> Adalimumab, etanercept and infliximab should be withdrawn if response is not adequate within 6 months. Response to treatment should be monitored at least every 6 months in patients who respond initially; treatment should be withdrawn if response is not maintained. An alternative TNF-α inhibitor may be considered for patients in whom treatment is withdrawn due to intolerance before the initial 6-month assessment of efficacy.
>
> Use of TNF-α inhibitors for the treatment of severe, active and progressive rheumatoid arthritis in adults not previously treated with methotrexate or other DMARDs is not recommended.

NICE guidance
Etanercept and infliximab for the treatment of adults with psoriatic arthritis (July 2006)
Etanercept is recommended for severe active psoriatic arthritis in adults with at least 3 tender joints and at least 3 swollen joints, and who have not responded adequately to 2 other disease-modifying antirheumatic drugs (used alone or in combination); infliximab [in combination with methotrexate, unless contra-indicated or not tolerated] is recommended for those intolerant to etanercept.
Etanercept or infliximab should be used under specialist supervision and should be withdrawn if inadequate response after 12 weeks.

NICE guidance
Etanercept for the treatment of juvenile idiopathic arthritis (March 2002)
Etanercept is recommended in children aged 4–17 years with active polyarticular-course juvenile idiopathic arthritis who have not responded adequately to methotrexate or who are intolerant of it. Etanercept should be used under specialist supervision according to the guidelines of the British Society for Paediatric and Adolescent Rheumatology [previously the British Paediatric Rheumatology Group].

Etanercept should be withdrawn if severe side-effects develop or if there is no response after 6 months or if the initial response is not maintained. There is no evidence to support treatment for longer than 2 years; a decision to continue therapy should be based on disease activity and clinical effectiveness in individual cases.

Prescribers of etanercept should register consenting patients with the Biologics Registry of the British Society for Paediatric and Adolescent Rheumatology.

Adalimumab is licensed for moderate to severe active *rheumatoid arthritis* when response to other disease-modifying antirheumatic drugs (including methotrexate) has been inadequate (see also NICE guidance, above); it may also be used for severe, active, and progressive disease in adults not previously treated with methotrexate. In the treatment of rheumatoid arthritis, adalimumab should be used in combination with methotrexate, but it may be given alone if methotrexate is inappropriate. Adalimumab is also licensed for the treatment of active and progressive *psoriatic arthritis* (see also NICE guidance, above) and severe active *ankylosing spondylitis* that have not responded adequately to other disease-modifying antirheumatic drugs. For the role of adalimumab in Crohn's disease, see section 1.5.

Etanercept is licensed for the treatment of moderate to severe active *rheumatoid arthritis* either alone or in combination with methotrexate when the response to other disease-modifying antirheumatic drugs is inadequate (see also NICE guidance). It is also licensed for the treatment of active and progressive *psoriatic arthritis* inadequately responsive to other disease-modifying antirheumatic drugs, and for severe *ankylosing spondylitis* inadequately responsive to conventional therapy. For the role of etanercept in psoriasis see section 13.5.3.

Infliximab is licensed for the treatment of active *rheumatoid arthritis* in combination with methotrexate when the response to other disease-modifying antirheumatic drugs is inadequate (see also NICE guidance). It is also licensed for the treatment of *ankylosing spondylitis*, in patients with severe axial symptoms who have not responded adequately to conventional therapy, and in combination with methotrexate (or alone if methotrexate is not tolerated or is contra-indicated) for the treatment of active and progressive *psoriatic arthritis* which has not responded adequately to disease-modifying antirheumatic drugs. For the role of infliximab in psoriasis, see section 13.5.3.

Rituximab is licensed in combination with methotrexate for the treatment of severe active *rheumatoid arthritis* in patients whose condition has not responded adequately to other disease-modifying antirheumatic drugs (including one or more tumour necrosis factor inhibitors) or who are intolerant of them (see also NICE guidance, below). For the role of rituximab in malignant disease, see section 8.2.3.

NICE guidance
Rituximab for the treatment of rheumatoid arthritis (August 2007)
Rituximab, in combination with methotrexate, is an option for the treatment of severe active rheumatoid arthritis in adults who have not had an adequate response to, or are intolerant of, other disease-modifying antirheumatic drugs (DMARDs), including treatment with at least 1 tumour necrosis factor alpha (TNF-α) inhibitor.
Treatment with rituximab plus methotrexate should be continued only if there is an adequate response to therapy; repeat courses should be given no more frequently than every 6 months.

Side-effects Adalimumab, etanercept, infliximab, and rituximab have been associated with infections, sometimes severe, including tuberculosis, septicaemia, and hepatitis B reactivation. Other side-effects include nausea, abdominal pain, worsening heart failure, hypersensitivity reactions, fever, headache, depression, antibody formation (including lupus erythematosus-like syndrome), pruritus, injection-site reactions, and blood disorders (including anaemia, leucopenia, thrombocytopenia, pancytopenia, and aplastic anaemia).

Anakinra inhibits the activity of interleukin-1. Anakinra (in combination with methotrexate) is licensed for the treatment of *rheumatoid arthritis* which has not responded to methotrexate alone; it is not, however, recommended for routine management of *rheumatoid arthritis*, see NICE guidance below.

The *Scottish Medicines Consortium* has advised (October 2003) that anakinra is **not** recommended for rheumatoid arthritis.

NICE guidance
Anakinra for rheumatoid arthritis (November 2003)
Anakinra is not recommended for the treatment of rheumatoid arthritis except when used in a controlled long-term clinical study. Patients receiving anakinra for rheumatoid arthritis should continue treatment until they and their consultant consider it appropriate to stop.

Abatacept prevents the full activation of T-lymphocytes. It is licensed for moderate to severe active *rheumatoid arthritis* in combination with methotrexate, in patients unresponsive or intolerant to other disease-modifying antirheumatic drugs (including at least one tumour necrosis factor (TNF) inhibitor). Abatacept is not recommended for use in combination with TNF inhibitors.

The *Scottish Medicines Consortium* has advised (August 2007) that abatacept is **not** recommended for the treatment of moderate to severe active rheumatoid arthritis.

ABATACEPT

Indications see under Cytokine Modulators, above

Cautions predisposition to infections (screen for latent tuberculosis and viral hepatitis); not to be initiated until active infections are controlled; elderly (increased risk of side-effects); **interactions:** Appendix 1 (abatacept)

Contra-indications severe infection (see also Cautions); pregnancy (Appendix 4); breast-feeding (Appendix 5)

Side-effects abdominal pain, diarrhoea, dyspepsia, nausea; flushing, hypertension; cough; dizziness, fatigue, headache; infection, rhinitis; rash; *less commonly* gastritis, stomatitis, tachycardia, bradycardia, palpitation, hypotension, dyspnoea, paraesthesia, weight gain, depression, anxiety, amenorrhoea, basal cell carcinoma, thrombocytopenia, leucopenia, arthralgia, pain in extremities, conjunctivitis, visual disturbance, vertigo, bruising, alopecia, and dry skin

Dose

- By intravenous infusion, ADULT over 18 years, body-weight less than 60 kg, 500 mg, repeated 2 weeks and 4 weeks after initial infusion, then every 4 weeks; body-weight 60–100 kg, 750 mg repeated 2 weeks and 4 weeks after initial infusion, then every 4 weeks; body-weight over 100 kg, 1 g repeated 2 weeks and 4 weeks after initial infusion, then every 4 weeks

Note Discontinue if no response within 6 months

Orencia® (Bristol-Myers Squibb) ▼ PoM

Intravenous infusion, powder for reconstitution, abatacept, net price 250-mg vial = £252.00

Electrolytes Na^+ <0.5 mmol/vial

ADALIMUMAB

Indications see under Cytokine Modulators above; Crohn's disease (section 1.5)

Cautions predisposition to infection; monitor for infections before, during, and for 5 months after treatment (see also Tuberculosis below); do not initiate until active infections are controlled; hepatitis B virus—monitor for active infection; heart failure (discontinue if symptoms develop or worsen; avoid in moderate or severe heart failure); demyelinating CNS disorders (risk of exacerbation); **interactions:** Appendix 1 (adalimumab)

Tuberculosis Patients should be evaluated for tuberculosis before treatment. Active tuberculosis should be treated with standard treatment (section 5.1.9) for at least 2 months before starting adalimumab. Patients who have previously received adequate treatment for tuberculosis can start adalimumab but should be monitored every 3 months for possible recurrence. In patients without active tuberculosis but who were previously not treated adequately, chemoprophylaxis should ideally be completed before starting adalimumab. Patients should be advised to seek medical attention if symptoms suggestive of tuberculosis (e.g. persistent cough, weight loss, and fever) develop

Contra-indications pregnancy (Appendix 4); breast-feeding (Appendix 5); severe infection (see also Cautions)

Side-effects see under Cytokine Modulators and Cautions above; also diarrhoea, constipation, vomiting, oesophagitis, dyspepsia, gastritis, hepatitis, rectal bleeding, enteritis, mouth ulcer, hypertension, chest pain, arrhythmia, syncope, palpitation, myocardial infarction, tachycardia, angina, flushing, vascular occlusion, haematoma, aneurysm, dysphonia, oedema, cough, sore throat, asthma, dyspnoea, nasal congestion, sleep disturbance, fatigue, dizziness, mood disorders, appetite disorders, anxiety, tremor, paraesthesia, neuralgia, demyelinating disorders, migraine, goitre, menstrual disorders, haematuria, proteinuria, malignancy, electrolyte disturbances, hyperlipidaemia, musculoskeletal pain, rhabdomyolysis, eye disorders, tinnitus, hearing loss, rash, ecchymosis, and alopecia

Dose

- By subcutaneous injection, rheumatoid arthritis, ADULT over 18 years, 40 mg on alternate weeks; if necessary increased to 40 mg weekly in patients receiving adalimumab alone

  Psoriatic arthritis, ankylosing spondylitis, ADULT over 18 years, 40 mg on alternate weeks

Note Discontinue treatment if no response after 12 weeks

Humira® (Abbott) ▼ PoM

Injection, adalimumab, net price 40-mg prefilled pen or prefilled syringe = £357.50. Counselling, tuberculosis

ANAKINRA

Indications see under Cytokine Modulators above

Cautions predisposition to infections; history of asthma (risk of serious infection); renal impairment (avoid if creatinine clearance less than 30 mL/minute; Appendix 3); **interactions:** Appendix 1 (anakinra)

Blood disorders Neutropenia reported commonly. Monitor neutrophil count before treatment, then every month for 6 months, then every 3 months—discontinue if neutropenia develops. Patients should be instructed to seek medical advice if symptoms suggestive of neutropenia (such as fever, sore throat, infection) develop

Contra-indications pregnancy (Appendix 4); breast-feeding (Appendix 5); neutropenia

Side-effects injection-site reactions, headache; infections, neutropenia (see also Cautions), and antibody formation

Dose

- By subcutaneous injection, ADULT over 18 years, 100 mg once daily

Kineret® (Amgen) PoM

Injection, anakinra, net price 100-mg prefilled syringe = £19.03. Counselling, blood disorder symptoms

ETANERCEPT

Indications see under Cytokine Modulators above; severe, active and progressive rheumatoid arthritis in patients not previously treated with methotrexate; psoriasis (section 13.5.3)

Cautions predisposition to infection (avoid if predisposition to septicaemia); significant exposure to herpes zoster virus—interrupt treatment and consider varicella–zoster immunoglobulin; hepatitis B virus—monitor for active infection; heart failure (risk of exacerbation); demyelinating CNS disorders (risk of exacerbation); history of blood disorders; **interactions:** Appendix 1 (etanercept)

Tuberculosis Patients should be evaluated for tuberculosis before treatment. Active tuberculosis should be treated with standard treatment (section 5.1.9) for at least 2 months before starting etanercept. Patients who have previously received adequate treatment for tuberculosis can start etanercept but should be monitored every 3 months for possible recurrence. In patients without active tuberculosis but who were previously not treated adequately, chemoprophylaxis should ideally be completed before starting etanercept. Patients should be advised to seek medical attention if symptoms suggestive of tuberculosis (e.g. persistent cough, weight loss, and fever) develop

Blood disorders Patients should be advised to seek medical attention if symptoms suggestive of blood disorders (such as fever, sore throat, bruising, or bleeding) develop

Contra-indications active infection; avoid injections containing benzyl alcohol in neonates (see preparations below); pregnancy (Appendix 4); breast-feeding (Appendix 5)

Side-effects see under Cytokine Modulators above; also rash; *rarely* demyelinating disorders, seizures, and cutaneous vasculitis; *also reported* appendicitis, cholecystitis, gastritis, gastro-intestinal haemorrhage, intestinal obstruction, liver damage, oesophagitis, pancreatitis, ulcerative colitis, vomiting, cerebral ischaemia, hypertension, hypotension, myocardial infarction, thrombophlebitis, thromboembolism, asthma, dyspnoea, aseptic meningitis, confusion, paresis, paraesthesia, vertigo, lymphadenopathy, diabetes mellitus, haematuria, malignancy, renal calculi, renal impairment, bone fracture, bursitis, polymyositis, scleritis, and cutaneous ulcer

Dose

- By subcutaneous injection, rheumatoid arthritis, psoriatic arthritis, ankylosing spondylitis, ADULT over 18 years, 25 mg twice weekly *or* 50 mg once weekly

  Polyarticular-course juvenile idiopathic arthritis, CHILD and ADOLESCENT 4–17 years, 400 micrograms/kg (max. 25 mg) twice weekly, with an interval of 3–4 days between doses

  Plaque psoriasis, ADULT over 18 years, 25 mg twice weekly; max. treatment duration 24 weeks; discontinue if no response after 12 weeks

Enbrel® (Wyeth) ▼ PoM

Injection, powder for reconstitution, etanercept, net price 25-mg vial (with solvent) = £89.38. Label: 10, alert card, counselling, tuberculosis and blood disorders

Paediatric injection, powder for reconstitution, etanercept, net price 25-mg vial (with solvent) = £89.38. Label: 10, alert card, counselling, tuberculosis and blood disorders

Excipients include benzyl alcohol (avoid in neonates, see Excipients, p. 2)

Injection, etanercept, net price 25-mg prefilled syringe = £89.38; 50-mg prefilled syringe = £178.75. Label: 10, alert card, counselling, tuberculosis and blood disorders

INFLIXIMAB

Indications see under Cytokine Modulators above; severe, active and progressive rheumatoid arthritis in patients not previously treated with methotrexate; psoriasis; inflammatory bowel disease (section 1.5)

Cautions predisposition to infection; monitor for infections before, during, and for 6 months after treatment (see also Tuberculosis below); hepatitis B virus—monitor for active infection; heart failure (discontinue if symptoms develop or worsen; avoid in moderate or severe heart failure); demyelinating CNS disorders (risk of exacerbation); history of malignancy (consider discontinuing treatment if malignancy develops); history of prolonged immunosuppressant or PUVA treatment in patients with psoriasis; **interactions:** Appendix 1 (infliximab)

Tuberculosis Patients should be evaluated for tuberculosis before treatment. Active tuberculosis should be treated with standard treatment (section 5.1.9) for at least 2 months before starting infliximab. Patients who have previously received adequate treatment for tuberculosis can start infliximab but should be monitored every 3 months for possible recurrence. In patients without active tuberculosis but who were previously not treated adequately, chemoprophylaxis should ideally be completed before starting infliximab. Patients should be advised to seek medical attention if symptoms suggestive of tuberculosis (e.g. persistent cough, weight loss, and fever) develop

Hypersensitivity reactions Hypersensitivity reactions (including fever, chest pain, hypotension, hypertension, dyspnoea, pruritus, urticaria, serum sickness-like reactions, angioedema, anaphylaxis) reported during or within 1–2 hours after infusion (risk greatest during first or second infusion or in patients who discontinue other immunosuppressants. All patients should be observed carefully for 1–2 hours after infusion and resuscitation equipment should be available for immediate use. Prophylactic antipyretics, antihistamines, or hydrocortisone may be administered. Monitor for symptoms of delayed hypersensitivity if readministered after a prolonged period. Patients should be advised to keep Alert card with them at all times and seek medical advice if symptoms of delayed hypersensitivity develop

Contra-indications severe infections (see also under Cautions); pregnancy (Appendix 4); breast-feeding (Appendix 5)

Side-effects see under Cytokine Modulators and Cautions above; also diarrhoea, dyspepsia; flushing, chest pain; dyspnoea; dizziness, fatigue; sinusitis; rash, sweating, dry skin; *less commonly* constipation, gastro-oesophageal reflux, diverticulitis, cholecystitis, palpitation, arrhythmia, hypertension, hypotension, vasospasm, cyanosis, bradycardia, syncope, oedema, thrombophlebitis, epistaxis, bronchospasm, pleurisy, confusion, agitation, nervousness, amnesia, drowsiness, insomnia, vaginitis, demyelinating disorders, antibody formation, myalgia, arthralgia, endophthalmitis, abnormal skin pigmentation, ecchymosis, cheilitis, and alopecia; *rarely* hepatitis, intestinal stenosis, intestinal perforation, gastro-intestinal haemorrhage, pancreatitis, circulatory failure, meningitis, seizure, neuropathy, paraesthesia, lymphoma, and transverse myelitis; *very rarely* pericardial effusion

Dose

- By intravenous infusion, rheumatoid arthritis (in combination with methotrexate), ADULT over 18 years, 3 mg/kg, repeated 2 weeks and 6 weeks after initial infusion, then every 8 weeks; if response inadequate after 12 weeks, dose may be increased in steps of 1.5 mg/kg every 8 weeks, up to max. 7.5 mg/kg every 8 weeks; alternatively, 3 mg/kg may be given every 4 weeks; discontinue if no response by 12 weeks of initial infusion or after dose adjustment

  Ankylosing spondylitis, ADULT over 18 years, 5 mg/kg, repeated 2 weeks and 6 weeks after initial infusion, then every 6–8 weeks; discontinue if no response by 6 weeks of initial infusion

  Psoriatic arthritis (in combination with methotrexate), ADULT over 18 years, 5 mg/kg, repeated 2 weeks and 6 weeks after initial infusion, then every 8 weeks

Psoriasis, ADULT over 18 years, 5 mg/kg, repeated 2 weeks and 6 weeks after initial infusion, then every 8 weeks; discontinue if no response by 14 weeks of initial infusion

Remicade® (Schering-Plough) ▼ PoM
Intravenous infusion, powder for reconstitution, infliximab, net price 100-mg vial = £419.62. Label: 10, alert card, counselling, tuberculosis and hypersensitivity reactions

RITUXIMAB

Indications see under Cytokine Modulators above; malignant disease (section 8.2.3)
Cautions section 8.2.3; predisposition to infection; hepatitis B virus—monitor for active infection
Contra-indications section 8.2.3; severe infection
Side-effects section 8.2.3 and under Cytokine Modulators above; *also* dyspepsia; hypertension, hypotension; rhinitis, sore throat; asthenia, paraesthesia, migraine; arthralgia, muscle spasm; urticaria
Dose
- By intravenous infusion, rheumatoid arthritis (in combination with methotrexate), 1 g, repeated 2 weeks after initial infusion; CHILD not recommended

Preparations
Section 8.2.3

Sulfasalazine

Sulfasalazine (sulphasalazine) has a beneficial effect in suppressing the inflammatory activity of rheumatoid arthritis. Side-effects include rashes, gastro-intestinal intolerance and, especially in patients with rheumatoid arthritis, occasional leucopenia, neutropenia, and thrombocytopenia. These haematological abnormalities occur usually in the first 3 to 6 months of treatment and are reversible on cessation of treatment. Close monitoring of full blood counts (including differential white cell count and platelet count) is necessary initially, and at monthly intervals during the first 3 months (liver function tests also being performed at monthly intervals for the first 3 months). Although the manufacturer recommends renal function tests, evidence of practical value is unsatisfactory.

SULFASALAZINE
(Sulphasalazine)

Indications active rheumatoid arthritis; ulcerative colitis, see section 1.5 and notes above
Cautions see section 1.5 and notes above
The CSM has recommended that patients should be advised to report any unexplained bleeding, bruising, purpura, sore throat, fever or malaise. A blood count should be performed and the drug stopped immediately if there is suspicion of a blood dyscrasia.
Contra-indications see section 1.5 and notes above
Side-effects see section 1.5 and notes above
Dose
- By mouth, administered on expert advice, as enteric-coated tablets, initially 500 mg daily, increased by 500 mg at intervals of 1 week to a max. of 2–3 g daily in divided doses

Sulfasalazine (Non-proprietary) PoM
Tablets, e/c, sulfasalazine 500 mg. Net price 112-tab pack = £18.33. Label: 5, 14, 25, counselling, blood disorder symptoms (see CSM recommendation above), contact lenses may be stained
Brands include *Sulazine EC®*

Salazopyrin EN-Tabs® (Pharmacia) PoM
Tablets, e/c, yellow, f/c, sulfasalazine 500 mg. Net price 112-tab pack = £8.43. Label: 5, 14, 25, counselling, blood disorder symptoms (see CSM recommendation above), contact lenses may be stained

10.1.4 Gout and cytotoxic-induced hyperuricaemia

It is important to distinguish drugs used for the treatment of acute attacks of gout from those used in the long-term control of the disease. The latter exacerbate and prolong the acute manifestations if started during an attack.

Acute attacks of gout

Acute attacks of gout are usually treated with high doses of **NSAIDs** such as diclofenac, etoricoxib, indometacin, ketoprofen, naproxen, or sulindac (section 10.1.1). Colchicine is an alternative. Aspirin is *not* indicated in gout. Allopurinol and uricosurics are not effective in treating an acute attack and may prolong it indefinitely if started during the acute episode.

Colchicine is probably as effective as NSAIDs. Its use is limited by the development of toxicity at higher doses, but it is of value in patients with heart failure since, unlike NSAIDs, it does not induce fluid retention; moreover, it can be given to patients receiving anticoagulants.

Oral or parenteral **corticosteroids** are an effective alternative in those who cannot tolerate NSAIDs or who are resistant to other treatments. Intra-articular injection of a corticosteroid can be used in acute monoarticular gout [unlicensed indication]. A corticosteroid by intramuscular injection can be effective in podagra.

COLCHICINE

Indications acute gout, short-term prophylaxis during initial therapy with allopurinol and uricosuric drugs; prophylaxis of familial Mediterranean fever (recurrent polyserositis) [unlicensed]
Cautions elderly, gastro-intestinal disease, cardiac, hepatic impairment, renal impairment (avoid if creatinine clearance less than 10 mL/minute; Appendix 3); breast-feeding (Appendix 5); **interactions**: Appendix 1 (colchicine)
Contra-indications pregnancy (Appendix 4)
Side-effects most common are nausea, vomiting, and abdominal pain; excessive doses may also cause profuse diarrhoea, gastro-intestinal haemorrhage, rashes, renal and hepatic damage. Rarely peripheral neuritis, myopathy, alopecia, inhibition of spermatogenesis, and with prolonged treatment blood disorders

Dose

- Treatment of gout, initially 1 mg, then 500 micrograms no more frequently than every 4 hours until pain relieved or vomiting or diarrhoea occur, max. 6 mg per course; course not to be repeated within 3 days
- Prevention of gout attacks during initial treatment with allopurinol or uricosuric drugs, 500 micrograms 2–3 times daily
- Prophylaxis of familial Mediterranean fever [unlicensed], 0.5–2 mg daily

Colchicine (Non-proprietary) PoM

Tablets, colchicine 500 micrograms, net price 20 = £4.80

Long-term control of gout

Frequent recurrence of acute attacks of gout, the presence of tophi, or signs of chronic gouty arthritis may call for the initiation of long-term ('interval') treatment. For long-term control of gout the formation of uric acid from purines may be reduced with the xanthine-oxidase inhibitor allopurinol, or the uricosuric drug sulfinpyrazone may be used to increase the excretion of uric acid in the urine. Treatment should be continued indefinitely to prevent further attacks of gout by correcting the hyperuricaemia. These drugs should never be started during an acute attack; they are usually started 1–2 weeks after the attack has settled. The initiation of treatment may precipitate an acute attack therefore colchicine or an anti-inflammatory analgesic should be used as a prophylactic and continued for at least one month after the hyperuricaemia has been corrected (usually about 3 months of prophylaxis). However, if an acute attack develops during treatment, then the treatment should continue at the same dosage and the acute attack treated in its own right.

Allopurinol is a well-tolerated drug which is widely used. It is especially useful in patients with renal impairment or urate stones where uricosuric drugs cannot be used; it is *not* indicated for the treatment of asymptomatic hyperuricaemia. It may cause rashes.

Sulfinpyrazone (sulphinpyrazone) can be used instead of allopurinol, or in conjunction with it in cases that are resistant to treatment.

Probenecid (available on a named-patient basis) is a uricosuric drug used to prevent nephrotoxicity associated with cidofovir (section 5.3.2.2).

Benzbromarone (available on a named-patient basis) is a uricosuric drug that may be used in patients with mild renal impairment.

Crystallisation of urate in the urine may occur with the uricosuric drugs and it is important to ensure an adequate urine output especially in the first few weeks of treatment. As an additional precaution the urine may be rendered alkaline.

Aspirin and salicylates antagonise the uricosuric drugs; they do not antagonise allopurinol but are nevertheless *not* indicated in gout.

ALLOPURINOL

Indications prophylaxis of gout and of uric acid and calcium oxalate renal stones; prophylaxis of hyperuricaemia associated with cancer chemotherapy

Cautions administer prophylactic colchicine or NSAID (*not* aspirin or salicylates) until at least 1 month after hyperuricaemia corrected; ensure adequate fluid intake (2–3 litres/day); for hyperuricaemia associated with cancer therapy, allopurinol treatment should be started before cancer therapy; hepatic impairment (Appendix 2); renal impairment (Appendix 3); pregnancy (Appendix 4); breast-feeding (Appendix 5); **interactions**: Appendix 1 (allopurinol)

Contra-indications not a treatment for acute gout but continue if attack develops when already receiving allopurinol, and treat attack separately (see notes above)

Side-effects rashes (**withdraw** therapy; if rash mild re-introduce cautiously but **discontinue** immediately if recurrence—hypersensitivity reactions occur rarely and include exfoliation, fever, lymphadenopathy, arthralgia, and eosinophilia resembling Stevens-Johnson or Lyell's syndrome, vasculitis, hepatitis, renal impairment, and very rarely seizures); gastro-intestinal disorders; rarely malaise, headache, vertigo, drowsiness, visual and taste disturbances, hypertension, alopecia, hepatotoxicity, paraesthesia and neuropathy, gynaecomastia, blood disorders (including leucopenia, thrombocytopenia, haemolytic anaemia and aplastic anaemia)

Dose

- Initially 100 mg daily, preferably after food, then adjusted according to plasma or urinary uric acid concentration; usual maintenance dose in mild conditions 100–200 mg daily, in moderately severe conditions 300–600 mg daily, in severe conditions 700–900 mg daily; doses over 300 mg daily given in divided doses; CHILD under 15 years, (in neoplastic conditions, enzyme disorders) 10–20 mg/kg daily (max. 400 mg daily)

Allopurinol (Non-proprietary) PoM

Tablets, allopurinol 100 mg, net price 28-tab pack = 43p; 300 mg, 28-tab pack = 83p. Label: 8, 21, 27
Brands include *Caplenal®*, *Cosuric®*, *Rimapurinol®*

Zyloric® (GSK) PoM

Tablets, allopurinol 100 mg, net price 100-tab pack = £10.19; 300 mg, 28-tab pack = £7.31. Label: 8, 21, 27

PROBENECID

Indications prevention of nephrotoxicity associated with cidofovir (section 5.3.2.2)

Cautions ensure adequate fluid intake (about 2–3 litres daily) and render urine alkaline if uric acid overload is high; peptic ulceration; transient false-positive Benedict's test; G6PD-deficiency (section 9.1.5); **interactions:** Appendix 1 (probenecid)

Contra-indications history of blood disorders, nephrolithiasis, porphyria (section 9.8.2), acute gout attack; avoid aspirin and salicylates; renal impairment (avoid if creatinine clearance less than 30 mL/minute; Appendix 3)

Side-effects gastro-intestinal disturbances, urinary frequency, headache, flushing, dizziness, alopecia, anaemia, haemolytic anaemia, sore gums; hypersensitivity reactions including anaphylaxis, dermatitis, pruritus, urticaria, fever and Stevens-Johnson syndrome; rarely nephrotic syndrome, hepatic necrosis, leucopenia, aplastic anaemia; toxic epidermal necrolysis reported with concurrent colchicine

Dose

- Used with cidofovir, see section 5.3.2.2

Probenecid (Non-proprietary) PoM
Tablets, probenecid 500 mg. Label: 12, 21, 27
Available on named-patient basis from specialist importing companies, see p. 888

SULFINPYRAZONE
(Sulphinpyrazone)

Indications gout prophylaxis, hyperuricaemia
Cautions see under Probenecid; regular blood counts advisable; cardiac disease (may cause salt and water retention); renal impairment (avoid if creatinine clearance less than 10 mL/minute; Appendix 3); **interactions**: Appendix 1 (sulfinpyrazone)
Contra-indications see under Probenecid; avoid in hypersensitivity to NSAIDs
Side-effects gastro-intestinal disturbances, occasionally allergic skin reactions, salt and water retention; rarely blood disorders, gastro-intestinal ulceration and bleeding, acute renal failure, raised liver enzymes, jaundice and hepatitis
Dose

- Initially 100–200 mg daily with food (or milk) increasing over 2–3 weeks to 600 mg daily (rarely 800 mg daily), continued until serum uric acid concentration normal then reduced for maintenance (maintenance dose may be as low as 200 mg daily)

Anturan® (Amdipharm) PoM
Tablets, both yellow, s/c, sulfinpyrazone 100 mg, net price 84-tab pack = £5.66; 200 mg, 84-tab pack = £11.25. Label: 12, 21

Hyperuricaemia associated with cytotoxic drugs

Allopurinol is used to prevent hyperuricaemia associated with cytotoxic drugs—see section 8.1 (Hyperuricaemia) and Allopurinol above.

Rasburicase is licensed for the prophylaxis and treatment of acute hyperuricaemia, before and during initiation of chemotherapy, in patients with haematological malignancy and a high tumour burden at risk of rapid lysis.

RASBURICASE

Indications prophylaxis and treatment of acute hyperuricaemia with initial chemotherapy for haematological malignancy
Cautions monitor closely for hypersensitivity; atopic allergies; may interfere with test for uric acid—consult product literature
Contra-indications G6PD deficiency (section 9.1.5); pregnancy (Appendix 4); breast-feeding (Appendix 5)
Side-effects fever; *less commonly* nausea, vomiting, diarrhoea, headache, hypersensitivity reactions (including rash, bronchospasm and anaphylaxis); haemolytic anaemia, methaemoglobinaemia
Dose

- By intravenous infusion, 200 micrograms/kg once daily for up to 7 days according to plasma-uric acid concentration

Fasturtec® (Sanofi-Synthelabo) PoM
Intravenous infusion, powder for reconstitution, rasburicase, net price 1.5-mg vial (with solvent) = £57.88; 7.5-mg vial (with solvent) = £241.20

10.1.5 Other drugs for rheumatic diseases

Glucosamine

Glucosamine is a natural substance found in mucopolysaccharides, mucoproteins, and chitin. It is licensed for symptomatic relief of mild to moderate osteoarthritis of the knee, however the mechanism of action is not understood.

GLUCOSAMINE

Indications symptomatic relief of mild to moderate osteoarthritis of the knee
Cautions impaired glucose tolerance (monitor blood-glucose concentration before treatment and periodically thereafter); predisposition to cardiovascular disease (monitor cholesterol); asthma; **interactions**: Appendix 1 (glucosamine)
Contra-indications shellfish allergy; pregnancy (Appendix 4); breast-feeding (Appendix 5)
Side-effects nausea, abdominal pain, indigestion, diarrhoea, constipation; headache, fatigue; *less commonly* flushing, rash, pruritus; hypercholesterolaemia also reported
Dose

- ADULT over 18 years, 1.25 g once daily; review treatment if no benefit after 2–3 months

Alateris® (Ransom) ▼ PoM
Tablets, glucosamine (as hydrochloride) 625 mg, net price 60-tab pack = £18.40

10.2 Drugs used in neuromuscular disorders

10.2.1 Drugs that enhance neuromuscular transmission
10.2.2 Skeletal muscle relaxants

10.2.1 Drugs that enhance neuromuscular transmission

Anticholinesterases are used as first-line treatment in *ocular myasthenia gravis* and as an adjunct to immunosuppressant therapy for *generalised myasthenia gravis*.

Corticosteroids are used when anticholinesterases do not control symptoms completely. A second-line immunosuppressant such as azathioprine is frequently used to reduce the dose of corticosteroid.

Plasmapheresis or infusion of intravenous immunoglobulin [unlicensed indication] may induce temporary remission in severe relapses, particularly where bulbar or respiratory function is compromised or before thymectomy.

Anticholinesterases

Anticholinesterase drugs enhance neuromuscular transmission in voluntary and involuntary muscle in myasthenia gravis. They prolong the action of acetylcholine by inhibiting the action of the enzyme acetylcholinesterase. Excessive dosage of these drugs can impair neuromuscular transmission and precipitate cholinergic crises by causing a depolarising block. This may be difficult to distinguish from a worsening myasthenic state.

Muscarinic side-effects of anticholinesterases include increased sweating, increased salivary and gastric secretions, increased gastro-intestinal and uterine motility, and bradycardia. These parasympathomimetic effects are antagonised by atropine.

Edrophonium has a very brief action and it is therefore used mainly for the diagnosis of myasthenia gravis. However, such testing should be performed only by those experienced in its use; other means of establishing the diagnosis are available. A single test-dose usually causes substantial improvement in muscle power (lasting about 5 minutes) in patients with the disease (if respiration already impaired, *only* in conjunction with someone skilled at intubation).

Edrophonium can also be used to determine whether a patient with myasthenia is receiving inadequate or excessive treatment with cholinergic drugs. If treatment is excessive an injection of edrophonium will either have no effect or will intensify symptoms (if respiration already impaired, *only* in conjunction with someone skilled at intubation). Conversely, transient improvement may be seen if the patient is being inadequately treated. The test is best performed just before the next dose of anticholinesterase.

Neostigmine produces a therapeutic effect for up to 4 hours. Its pronounced muscarinic action is a disadvantage, and simultaneous administration of an antimuscarinic drug such as atropine or propantheline may be required to prevent colic, excessive salivation, or diarrhoea. In severe disease neostigmine can be given every 2 hours. The maximum that most patients can tolerate is 180 mg daily.

Pyridostigmine is less powerful and slower in action than neostigmine but it has a longer duration of action. It is preferable to neostigmine because of its smoother action and the need for less frequent dosage. It is particularly preferred in patients whose muscles are weak on waking. It has a comparatively mild gastro-intestinal effect but an antimuscarinic drug may still be required. It is inadvisable to exceed a total daily dose of 450 mg in order to avoid acetylcholine receptor down-regulation. Immunosuppressant therapy is usually considered if the dose of pyridostigmine exceeds 360 mg daily.

Distigmine has the longest action but the danger of a cholinergic crisis caused by accumulation of the drug is greater than with shorter-acting drugs; it is rarely used in the management of myasthenia gravis.

Neostigmine and edrophonium are also used to reverse the actions of the non-depolarising neuromuscular blocking drugs (see section 15.1.6).

NEOSTIGMINE

Indications myasthenia gravis; other indications (section 15.1.6)

Cautions asthma (*extreme* caution), bradycardia, arrhythmias, recent myocardial infarction, epilepsy, hypotension, parkinsonism, vagotonia, peptic ulceration, hyperthyroidism, renal impairment (Appendix 3), pregnancy (Appendix 4), breast-feeding (Appendix 5); atropine or other antidote to muscarinic effects may be necessary (particularly when neostigmine is given by injection), but not given routinely because it may mask signs of overdosage; **interactions:** Appendix 1 (parasympathomimetics)

Contra-indications intestinal or urinary obstruction

Side-effects nausea, vomiting, increased salivation, diarrhoea, abdominal cramps (more marked with higher doses); signs of overdosage include bronchoconstriction, increased bronchial secretions, lacrimation, excessive sweating, involuntary defaecation and micturition, miosis, nystagmus, bradycardia, heart block, arrhythmias, hypotension, agitation, excessive dreaming, and weakness eventually leading to fasciculation and paralysis

Dose

- By mouth, neostigmine bromide 15–30 mg at suitable intervals throughout day, total daily dose 75–300 mg (but see also notes above); NEONATE 1–5 mg every 4 hours, half an hour before feeds; CHILD up to 6 years initially 7.5 mg, 6–12 years initially 15 mg, usual total daily dose 15–90 mg
- By subcutaneous *or* intramuscular injection, neostigmine metilsulfate 1–2.5 mg at suitable intervals throughout day (usual total daily dose 5–20 mg); NEONATE 50–250 micrograms every 4 hours half an hour before feeds; CHILD 200–500 micrograms as required

Neostigmine (Non-proprietary) PoM

Tablets, scored, neostigmine bromide 15 mg. Net price 20 = £6.07

Injection, neostigmine metilsulfate 2.5 mg/mL. Net price 1-mL amp = 57p

DISTIGMINE BROMIDE

Indications myasthenia gravis (but rarely used); urinary retention and other indications (section 7.4.1)

Cautions see section 7.4.1

Contra-indications see section 7.4.1

Side-effects see section 7.4.1

Dose

- Initially 5 mg daily half an hour before breakfast, increased at intervals of 3–4 days if necessary to a max. of 20 mg daily; CHILD up to 10 mg daily according to age

Preparations

Section 7.4.1

EDROPHONIUM CHLORIDE

Indications see under Dose and notes above; reversal of non-depolarising neuromuscular blockade and diagnosis of dual block (section 15.1.6)

Cautions see under Neostigmine; have resuscitation facilities; *extreme* caution in respiratory distress (see notes above) and in asthma

Note Severe cholinergic reactions can be counteracted by injection of atropine sulphate (which should always be available)

Contra-indications see under Neostigmine

Side-effects see under Neostigmine

Dose

- Diagnosis of myasthenia gravis, by intravenous injection, 2 mg followed after 30 seconds (if no adverse reaction has occurred) by 8 mg; in adults without suitable veins, by intramuscular injection, 10 mg
- Detection of overdosage or underdosage of cholinergic drugs, by intravenous injection, 2 mg (preferably just before next dose of anticholinesterase, see notes above)
- CHILD by intravenous injection, 20 micrograms/kg followed after 30 seconds (if no adverse reaction has occurred) by 80 micrograms/kg

Edrophonium (Cambridge) PoM
Injection, edrophonium chloride 10 mg/mL. Net price 1-mL amp = £6.55

PYRIDOSTIGMINE BROMIDE

Indications myasthenia gravis

Cautions see under Neostigmine; weaker muscarinic action

Contra-indications see under Neostigmine

Side-effects see under Neostigmine

Dose

- By mouth, 30–120 mg at suitable intervals throughout day, total daily dose 0.3–1.2 g (but see also notes above); NEONATE 5–10 mg every 4 hours, 30–60 minutes before feeds; CHILD up to 6 years initially 30 mg, 6–12 years initially 60 mg, usual total daily dose 30–360 mg

Mestinon® (Valeant) PoM
Tablets, scored, pyridostigmine (as bromide) 60 mg. Net price 20 = £4.21

Immunosuppressant therapy

Corticosteroids (section 6.3) are established as treatment for myasthenia gravis; although they are commonly given on alternate days there is little evidence of benefit over daily administration. Corticosteroid treatment is usually initiated under in-patient supervision and all patients should receive osteoporosis prophylaxis (section 6.6).

In *generalised myasthenia gravis* small initial doses of prednisolone (10 mg on alternate days) are increased in steps of 10 mg on alternate days to 1–1.5 mg/kg (max. 100 mg) on alternate days. When given daily, prednisolone is started at 5 mg daily and then increased in steps of 5 mg daily to 60 mg daily or occasionally up to 80 mg daily (0.75–1 mg/kg daily). About 10% of patients experience a transient but very serious worsening of symptoms in the first 2–3 weeks, especially if the corticosteroid is started at a high dose. However, ventilated patients may be started on 1.5 mg/kg (max. 100 mg) on alternate days. Smaller doses of corticosteroid are usually required in *ocular myasthenia*. Once clinical remission has occurred (usually after 2–6 months), the dose of prednisolone should be reduced slowly to the minimum effective dose (usually 10–40 mg on alternate days).

In generalised myasthenia gravis **azathioprine** (section 8.2.1) is usually started at the same time as the corticosteroid and it allows a lower maintenance dose of the corticosteroid to be used; azathioprine is initiated at a low dose, which is increased over 3–4 weeks to 2–2.5 mg/kg daily. **Ciclosporin** (section 8.2.2), **methotrexate** (section 8.1.3), or **mycophenolate mofetil** (section 8.2.1) can be used in patients unresponsive or intolerant to other treatments [unlicensed indications].

10.2.2 Skeletal muscle relaxants

The drugs described below are used for the relief of chronic muscle spasm or spasticity associated with multiple sclerosis or other neurological damage; they are not indicated for spasm associated with minor injuries. They act principally on the central nervous system with the exception of dantrolene, which has a peripheral site of action. They differ in action from the muscle relaxants used in anaesthesia (section 15.1.5), which block transmission at the neuromuscular junction.

The underlying cause of spasticity should be treated and any aggravating factors (e.g. pressure sores, infection) remedied. Skeletal muscle relaxants are effective in most forms of spasticity except the rare alpha variety. The major disadvantage of treatment with these drugs is that reduction in muscle tone can cause a loss of splinting action of the spastic leg and trunk muscles and sometimes lead to an increase in disability.

Dantrolene acts directly on skeletal muscle and produces fewer central adverse effects making it a drug of choice. The dose should be increased slowly.

Baclofen inhibits transmission at spinal level and also depresses the central nervous system. The dose should be increased slowly to avoid the major side-effects of sedation and muscular hypotonia (other adverse events are uncommon).

Diazepam can also be used. Sedation and occasionally extensor hypotonus are disadvantages. Other benzodiazepines also have muscle-relaxant properties. Muscle-relaxant doses of benzodiazepines are similar to anxiolytic doses (section 4.1.2).

Tizanidine is an alpha$_2$-adrenoceptor agonist indicated for spasticity associated with multiple sclerosis or spinal cord injury.

BACLOFEN

Indications chronic severe spasticity resulting from disorders such as multiple sclerosis or traumatic partial section of spinal cord

Cautions renal impairment (Appendix 3); psychiatric illness, Parkinson's disease, cerebrovascular disease, elderly; respiratory impairment, epilepsy; history of peptic ulcer; diabetes; hypertonic bladder sphincter; pregnancy (Appendix 4); avoid abrupt withdrawal (risk of hyperactive state, may exacerbate spasticity, and precipitate autonomic dysfunction including hyperthermia, psychiatric reactions and convulsions, see also under Withdrawal below); **interactions:** Appendix 1 (muscle relaxants)

Withdrawal CSM has advised that serious side-effects can occur on abrupt withdrawal; to minimise risk, discontinue by gradual dose reduction over at least 1–2 weeks (longer if symptoms occur)

Driving Drowsiness may affect performance of skilled tasks (e.g. driving); effects of alcohol enhanced

Contra-indications peptic ulceration

Side-effects frequently sedation, drowsiness, muscular hypotonia, nausea, urinary disturbances; occasionally lassitude, confusion, speech disturbance, dizziness, ataxia, hallucinations, nightmares, headache, euphoria, insomnia, depression, anxiety, agitation, tremor, nystagmus, paraesthesias, seizures, myalgia, fever, respiratory or cardiovascular depression, hypotension, dry mouth, gastro-intestinal disturbances, sexual dysfunction, visual disorders, rash, pruritus, urticaria, hyperhidrosis, angioedema; rarely taste alterations, blood sugar changes, and paradoxical increase in spasticity

Dose

- By mouth, 5 mg 3 times daily, preferably with or after food, gradually increased; max. 100 mg daily (discontinue if no benefit within 6 weeks); CHILD 0.75–2 mg/kg daily (over 10 years, max. 2.5 mg/kg daily) *or* 2.5 mg 4 times daily increased gradually according to age to maintenance: 1–2 years 10–20 mg daily, 2–6 years 20–30 mg daily, 6–10 years 30–60 mg daily
- By intrathecal injection, see preparation below

Baclofen (Non-proprietary) PoM

Tablets, baclofen 10 mg, net price 84-tab pack = £1.77. Label: 2, 8

Oral solution, baclofen 5 mg/5 mL, net price 300 mL = £8.95. Label: 2, 8

Brands include *Lyflex*® (sugar-free)

Lioresal® (Novartis) PoM

Tablets, scored, baclofen 10 mg. Net price 84-tab pack = £10.84. Label: 2, 8

Excipients include gluten

Liquid, sugar-free, raspberry-flavoured, baclofen 5 mg/5 mL. Net price 300 mL = £8.95. Label: 2, 8

By intrathecal injection

Lioresal® (Novartis) PoM

Intrathecal injection, baclofen, 50 micrograms/mL, net price 1-mL amp (for test dose) = £2.74; 500 micrograms/mL, 20-mL amp (for use with implantable pump) = £60.77; 2 mg/mL, 5-mL amp (for use with implantable pump) = £60.77

Important: consult product literature for details on dose testing and titration—important to monitor patients closely in appropriately equipped and staffed environment during screening and immediately after pump implantation. Resuscitation equipment must be available for immediate use

Dose by intrathecal injection, specialist use only, severe chronic spasticity unresponsive to oral antispastic drugs (or where side-effects of oral therapy unacceptable) *or* as alternative to ablative neurosurgical procedures, initial *test dose* 25–50 micrograms over at least 1 minute via catheter or lumbar puncture, increased in 25-microgram steps (not more often than every 24 hours) to max. 100 micrograms to determine appropriate dose *then dose-titration phase*, most often using infusion pump (implanted into chest wall or abdominal wall tissues) to establish *maintenance dose* (ranging from 12 micrograms to 2 mg daily for spasticity of spinal origin *or* 22 micrograms to 1.4 mg daily for spasticity of cerebral origin) retaining some spasticity to avoid sensation of paralysis; CHILD 4–18 years (spasticity of cerebral origin only), initial *test dose* 25 micrograms then titrated as for ADULT to *maintenance dose* (ranging from 24 micrograms to 1.2 mg daily in children under 12 years)

DANTROLENE SODIUM

Indications chronic severe spasticity of voluntary muscle; malignant hyperthermia (section 15.1.8)

Cautions impaired cardiac and pulmonary function; test liver function before and at intervals during therapy; therapeutic effect may take a few weeks to develop but if treatment is ineffective it should be discontinued after 4–6 weeks; avoid when spasticity is useful, for example, locomotion; **interactions:** Appendix 1 (muscle relaxants).

Driving Drowsiness may affect performance of skilled tasks (e.g. driving); effects of alcohol enhanced

Contra-indications hepatic impairment (may cause severe liver damage); acute muscle spasm; pregnancy (Appendix 4); breast-feeding (Appendix 5)

Side-effects transient drowsiness, dizziness, weakness, malaise, fatigue, diarrhoea (withdraw if severe, discontinue treatment if recurs on re-introduction), anorexia, nausea, headache, rash; less frequently constipation, dysphagia, speech and visual disturbances, confusion, nervousness, insomnia, depression, seizures, chills, fever, increased urinary frequency; rarely, tachycardia, erratic blood pressure, dyspnoea, haematuria, possible crystalluria, urinary incontinence or retention, pleural effusion, pericarditis, dose-related hepatotoxicity (occasionally fatal) may be more common in women over 30 especially those taking oestrogens

Dose

- Initially 25 mg daily, may be increased at weekly intervals to max. of 100 mg 4 times daily; usual dose 75 mg 3 times daily; CHILD not recommended

Dantrium® (Procter & Gamble Pharm.) PoM

Capsules, both orange/brown, dantrolene sodium 25 mg, net price 20 = £2.46; 100 mg, 20 = £8.61. Label: 2

DIAZEPAM

Indications muscle spasm of varied aetiology, including tetanus; other indications (section 4.1.2, section 4.8, section 15.1.4.1)

Cautions see section 4.1.2; special precautions for intravenous injection (section 4.8.2)

Contra-indications see section 4.1.2

Side-effects see section 4.1.2; also hypotonia

Dose

- Muscle spasm, by mouth, 2–15 mg daily in divided doses, increased if necessary in spastic conditions to 60 mg daily according to response

Cerebral spasticity in selected cases, CHILD 2–40 mg daily in divided doses

By intramuscular *or* by slow intravenous injection (into a large vein at a rate of not more than

5 mg/minute), in acute muscle spasm, 10 mg repeated if necessary after 4 hours

Note Only use intramuscular route when oral and intravenous routes not possible; special precautions for intravenous injection see section 4.8.2

- Tetanus, ADULT and CHILD, by intravenous injection, 100–300 micrograms/kg repeated every 1–4 hours; by intravenous infusion (*or* by nasoduodenal tube), 3–10 mg/kg over 24 hours, adjusted according to response

◢Preparations
Section 4.1.2

TIZANIDINE

Indications spasticity associated with multiple sclerosis or spinal cord injury or disease

Cautions elderly, renal impairment (Appendix 3), pregnancy (Appendix 4), breast-feeding (Appendix 5), monitor liver function monthly for first 4 months and in those who develop unexplained nausea, anorexia or fatigue; concomitant administration of drugs that prolong QT interval; **interactions:** Appendix 1 (muscle relaxants)

Driving Drowsiness may affect performance of skilled tasks (e.g. driving); effects of alcohol enhanced

Contra-indications severe hepatic impairment

Side-effects drowsiness, fatigue, dizziness, dry mouth, nausea, gastro-intestinal disturbances, hypotension; also reported, bradycardia, insomnia, hallucinations and altered liver enzymes (discontinue if persistently raised—consult product literature); rarely acute hepatitis

Dose

- ADULT over 18 years, initially 2 mg daily as a single dose increased according to response at intervals of at least 3–4 days in steps of 2 mg daily (and given in divided doses) usually up to 24 mg daily in 3–4 divided doses; max. 36 mg daily

Tizanidine (Non-proprietary) PoM
Tablets, tizanidine (as hydrochloride) 2 mg net price 120-tab pack = £31.96; 4 mg, 120-tab pack = £43.58. Label: 2

Zanaflex® (Cephalon) PoM
Tablets, scored, tizanidine (as hydrochloride) 2 mg, net price 120-tab pack = £63.00; 4 mg, 120-tab pack = £80.00. Label: 2

Other muscle relaxants

The clinical efficacy of carisoprodol, meprobamate (section 4.1.2), and methocarbamol as muscle relaxants is **not** well established, although they have been included in compound analgesic preparations.

CARISOPRODOL ◢

Indications short-term symptomatic relief of muscle spasm (but see notes above)

Cautions see under Meprobamate (section 4.1.2); breast-feeding (Appendix 5); **interactions:** Appendix 1 (muscle relaxants)

Contra-indications see under Meprobamate (section 4.1.2); porphyria (section 9.8.2)

Side-effects see under Meprobamate (section 4.1.2); drowsiness is common

Dose

- 350 mg 3 times daily; ELDERLY half adult dose or less

Carisoma® (Forest) PoM ◢
Tablets, carisoprodol 125 mg, net price 100 = £6.65; 350 mg, 100 = £7.45. Label: 2

METHOCARBAMOL ◢

Indications short-term symptomatic relief of muscle spasm (but see notes above)

Cautions hepatic impairment (Appendix 2); renal impairment (Appendix 3); pregnancy (Appendix 4); breast-feeding (Appendix 5); **interactions:** Appendix 1 (muscle relaxants)

Driving Drowsiness may affect performance of skilled tasks (e.g. driving); effects of alcohol enhanced

Contra-indications coma or pre-coma, brain damage, epilepsy, myasthenia gravis

Side-effects nausea, vomiting, dyspepsia; hypersensitivity reactions (including urticaria, angioedema, anaphylaxis); fever, headache, drowsiness, dizziness, confusion, amnesia, restlessness, anxiety, tremor, seizures; blurred vision, nasal congestion; rash, pruritus; leucopenia, cholestatic jaundice

Dose

- 1.5 g 4 times daily; may be reduced to 750 mg 3 times daily; ELDERLY up to 750 mg 4 times daily may be sufficient; CHILD not recommended

Robaxin® (Shire) PoM ◢
750 Tablets, f/c, scored, methocarbamol 750 mg, net price 20 = £2.53. Label: 2

Nocturnal leg cramps

Quinine salts (section 5.4.1) 200–300 mg at bedtime are effective in reducing the frequency of nocturnal leg cramps by about 25% in ambulatory patients. It may take up to 4 weeks for improvement to become apparent; if there is benefit, quinine treatment is continued. Patients should be monitored closely during the early stages for adverse effects as well as for benefit. Treatment should be interrupted at intervals of approximately 3 months to assess the need for further quinine treatment. Quinine is very toxic in overdosage and accidental fatalities have occurred in children (see also below).

QUININE

Indications see notes above; malaria (section 5.4.1)

Cautions see section 5.4.1 and notes above

Contra-indications see section 5.4.1

Side-effects see section 5.4.1; **important:** very toxic in **overdosage**—immediate advice from poison centres essential (see also p. 32)

Dose

- See notes above

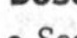

◢Preparations
Section 5.4.1

10.3 Drugs for the relief of soft-tissue inflammation

10.3.1 Enzymes
10.3.2 Rubefacients and other topical antirheumatics

Extravasation

Local guidelines for the management of extravasation should be followed where they exist or specialist advice sought.

Extravasation injury follows leakage of drugs or intravenous fluids from the veins or inadvertent administration into the subcutaneous or subdermal tissue. It must be dealt with **promptly** to prevent tissue necrosis.

Acidic or alkaline preparations and those with an osmolarity greater than that of plasma can cause extravasation injury; excipients including alcohol and polyethylene glycol have also been implicated. Cytotoxic drugs commonly cause extravasation injury. In addition, certain patients such as the very young and the elderly are at increased risk. Those receiving anticoagulants are more likely to lose blood into surrounding tissues if extravasation occurs, while those receiving sedatives or analgesics may not notice the early signs or symptoms of extravasation.

Prevention of extravasation Precautions should be taken to avoid extravasation; ideally, drugs likely to cause extravasation injury should be given through a central line and patients receiving repeated doses of hazardous drugs peripherally should have the cannula resited at regular intervals. Attention should be paid to the manufacturers' recommendations for administration. Placing a glyceryl trinitrate patch (section 2.6.1) distal to the cannula may improve the patency of the vessel in patients with small veins or in those whose veins are prone to collapse.

Patients should be asked to report any pain or burning at the site of injection immediately.

Management of extravasation If extravasation is suspected the infusion should be stopped immediately but the cannula should not be removed until after an attempt has been made to aspirate the area (through the cannula) in order to remove as much of the drug as possible. Aspiration is sometimes possible if the extravasation presents with a raised bleb or blister at the injection site and is surrounded by hardened tissue, but it is often unsuccessful if the tissue is soft or soggy. **Corticosteroids** are usually given to treat inflammation, although there is little evidence to support their use in extravasation. Hydrocortisone or dexamethasone (section 6.3.2) can be given either locally by subcutaneous injection or intravenously at a site distant from the injury. **Antihistamines** (section 3.4.1) and **analgesics** (section 4.7) may be required for symptom relief.

The management of extravasation beyond these measures is not well standardised and calls for specialist advice. Treatment depends on the nature of the offending substance; one approach is to localise and neutralise the substance whereas another is to spread and dilute it.

The first method may be appropriate following extravasation of vesicant drugs and involves administration of an antidote (if available) and the application of cold compresses 3–4 times a day (consult specialist literature for details of specific antidotes). Spreading and diluting the offending substance involves infiltrating the area with physiological saline, applying warm compresses, elevating the affected limb, and administering **hyaluronidase** (section 10.3.1). A saline flush-out technique (involving flushing the subcutaneous tissue with physiological saline) may be effective but requires specialist advice. Hyaluronidase should **not** be administered following extravasation of vesicant drugs (unless it is either specifically indicated or used in the saline flush-out technique). **Dexrazoxane** (section 8.1) is licensed for the treatment of anthracycline-induced extravasation.

10.3.1 Enzymes

Hyaluronidase is used to render the tissues more readily permeable to injected fluids, e.g. for introduction of fluids by subcutaneous infusion (termed hypodermoclysis).

HYALURONIDASE

Indications enhance permeation of subcutaneous or intramuscular injections, local anaesthetics and subcutaneous infusions; promote resorption of excess fluids and blood

Cautions infants or elderly (control speed and total volume and avoid overhydration especially in renal impairment)

Contra-indications do not apply direct to cornea; avoid sites where infection or malignancy; not for anaesthesia in unexplained premature labour; not to be used to reduce swelling of bites or stings; not for intravenous administration

Side-effects oedema; *rarely* local irritation, infection, bleeding, bruising; occasional severe allergy (including anaphylaxis)

Dose

- With subcutaneous or intramuscular injection, 1500 units dissolved directly in solution to be injected (ensure compatibility)
- With local anaesthetics, 1500 units mixed with local anaesthetic solution (ophthalmology, 15 units/mL)
- Hypodermoclysis, 1500 units dissolved in 1 mL water for injections or 0.9% sodium chloride injection, administered before start of 500–1000 mL infusion fluid
- Extravasation (see notes above) or haematoma, 1500 units dissolved in 1 mL water for injections or 0.9% sodium chloride injection, infiltrated into affected area (as soon as possible after extravasation)

Hyalase® (CP) PoM
Injection, powder for reconstitution, hyaluronidase (ovine). Net price 1500-unit amp = £7.60

10 Musculoskeletal and joint diseases

10.3.2 Rubefacients and other topical antirheumatics

Rulefacients act by counter-irritation. Pain, whether sup:rficial or deep-seated, is relieved by any method whih itself produces irritation of the skin. Counter-irrittion is comforting in painful lesions of the muscles, tenons, and joints, and in non-articular rheumatism. Rubfacients probably all act through the same essential mecanism and differ mainly in intensity and duration of acion.

Theise of a NSAID by mouth is effective for relieving musuloskeletal pain. **Topical NSAIDs** (e.g. felbinac, ibupfen, ketoprofen, and piroxicam) may provide somslight relief of pain in musculoskeletal conditions.

A pnaration containing **capsaicin** 0.025% is licensed for t symptomatic relief of osteoarthritis. It may need to bused for 1–2 weeks before pain is relieved. A high strength of capsaicin 0.075% cream is licensed for symptomatic relief of postherpetic neuralgia (sectn 4.7.3) after lesions have healed, and relief of pain diabetic neuropathy (section 6.1.5).

Topal NSAIDs and counter-irritants

Cauts Apply with gentle massage only. Avoid contact h eyes, mucous membranes, and inflamed or brokekin; discontinue if rash develops. Hands should be wed immediately after use. Not for use with occlue dressings. Topical application of large amou can result in systemic effects, including hypersensity and asthma (renal disease has also been repon. Not generally suitable for children. Patient packsrry a **warning** to avoid during **pregnancy** or **breaseding**.

Hypensitivity For NSAID hypersensitivity and asthmarning, see p. 536 and p. 537

Photosensitivity Patients should be advised against excesexposure to sunlight of area treated in order to avossibility of photosensitivity

Ketopn (Non-proprietary) PoM
Gel,profen 2.5%, net price 30 g = £2.43, 50 g = £3.00 g = £3.28
Dosey 2–4 times daily for up to 7 days (usual max. 15 g daily)

Piroxi (Non-proprietary) PoM
Gel, icam 0.5%, net price 60 g = £2.71; 112 g = £2.2(
Dose 3–4 times daily

▲Propry preparations

Feldenfizer) PoM
Gel, cam 0.5%. Net price 60 g = £6.00; 112 g = £9.41 7.5 g starter pack, hosp. only)
Excipiude benzyl alcohol, propylene glycol
Dose 3–4 times daily; therapy should be reviewed after 4 weeks

Fenbidte Gel (Goldshield) PoM
Gel, fen 10%, net price 100 g = £6.50
Excipiude benzyl alcohol
Dose p to 4 times daily; therapy should be reviewed after 14 day

Ibugel® Forte (Dermal) PoM
Forte gel, ibuprofen 10%, net price 100 g = £6.05
Excipients none as listed in section 13.1.3
Dose apply up to 3 times daily

Oruvail® (Rhône-Poulenc Rorer) PoM
Gel, ketoprofen 2.5%. Net price 100 g = £5.87
Excipients include fragrance
Dose apply 2–4 times daily for up to 7 days (usual recommended dose 15 g daily)

Pennsaid® (Dimethaid) PoM
Cutaneous solution, diclofenac sodium 16 mg/mL in dimethyl sulfoxide, net price 60 mL = £16.00
Excipients include propylene glycol
Dose pain in osteoarthritis of superficial joints, apply 0.5–1 mL 4 times daily

Powergel® (Menarini) PoM
Gel, ketoprofen 2.5%. Net price 50 g = £3.06; 100 g = £5.89
Excipients include hydroxybenzoates (parabens), fragrance
Dose apply 2–3 times daily for up to max. 10 days

Traxam® (Goldshield) PoM
Foam, felbinac 3.17%. Net price 100 g = £7.30. Label: 15
Excipients include cetostearyl alcohol

Gel, felbinac 3%. Net price 100 g = £7.00
Excipients none as listed in section 13.1.3
Dose apply 2–4 times daily; max. 25 g daily; therapy should be reviewed after 14 days
Note Felbinac is an active metabolite of the NSAID fenbufen

Voltarol Emulgel® (Novartis) PoM
Gel, diclofenac diethylammonium salt 1.16% (equivalent to diclofenac sodium 1%). Net price 20 g (hosp. only) = £1.55; 100 g = £7.00
Excipients include propylene glycol, fragrance
Dose apply 3–4 times daily; therapy should be reviewed after 14 days (or after 28 days for osteoarthritis)

Voltarol Gel Patch® (Novartis) PoM
Gel patch, diclofenac epolamine (equivalent to 140 mg diclofenac sodium per patch), net price 10-patch pack = £14.09
Excipients include hydroxybenzoates (parabens), propylene glycol
Dose ADULT and CHILD over 15 years, ankle sprain, apply 1 patch daily for up to 3 days; epicondylitis, apply 1 patch twice daily for up to 14 days
Note The *Scottish Medicines Consortium* has advised (September 2005) that *Voltarol Gel Patch®* is not recommended for the treatment of pain in epicondylitis and ankle sprain

Capsaicin

Cautions Avoid contact with eyes, and inflamed or broken skin. Hands should be washed immediately after use. Not for use under tight bandages. Avoid taking a hot shower or bath just before or after applying capsaicin—burning sensation enhanced.

Side-effects Transient burning sensation can occur during initial treatment, particularly if too much cream is used, or if the frequency of administration is less than 3–4 times daily.

Zacin® (Zeneus) PoM
Cream, capsaicin 0.025%. net price 45 g = £15.04.
Excipients include benzyl alcohol, cetyl alcohol
Dose symptomatic relief in osteoarthritis, apply a small amount 4 times daily

Axsain® (Zeneus) PoM
Cream, capsaicin 0.075%. net price 45 g = £12.15.
Excipients include benzyl alcohol, cetyl alcohol
Dose post-herpetic neuralgia (**important: after** lesions have healed), apply a small amount up to 3–4 times daily; for painful diabetic neuropathy, under supervision of hospital consultant, apply 3–4 times daily for 8 weeks then review

Poultices

Kaolin Poultice
Poultice, heavy kaolin 52.7%, thymol 0.05%, boric acid 4.5%, peppermint oil 0.05%, methyl salicylate 0.2%, glycerol 42.5%. Net price 200 g = £2.29
Dose warm and apply directly or between layers of muslin; avoid application of overheated poultice

Kaolin Poultice K/L Pack® (K/L)
Kaolin poultice Net price 4 × 100-g pouches = £6.40

11 Eye

11.1 **Administration of drugs to the eye** 565
11.2 **Control of microbial contamination** 566
11.3 **Anti-infective eye preparations** 566
11.3.1 Antibacterials 566
11.3.2 Antifungals 568
11.3.3 Antivirals 568
11.4 **Corticosteroids and other anti-inflammatory preparations** 568
11.4.1 Corticosteroids 568
11.4.2 Other anti-inflammatory preparations 570
11.5 **Mydriatics and cycloplegics** 571
11.6 **Treatment of glaucoma** 572
11.7 **Local anaesthetics** 577
11.8 **Miscellaneous ophthalmic preparations** 577
11.8.1 Tear deficiency, ocular lubricants, and astringents 577
11.8.2 Ocular diagnostic and peri-operative preparations and photodynamic treatment 579
11.9 **Contact lenses** 581

11.1 Administration of drugs to the eye

Drugs are most commonly administered to the eye by topical application as eye drops or eye ointments. Where a higher drug concentration is required within the eye, a local injection may be necessary.

Eye-drop dispenser devices are available to aid the instillation of eye drops from plastic bottles especially amongst the elderly, visually impaired, arthritic, or otherwise physically limited patients.

Eye drops and eye ointments Eye drops are generally instilled into the pocket formed by gently pulling down the lower eyelid and keeping the eye closed for as long as possible after application; one drop is all that is needed. A small amount of eye ointment is applied similarly; the ointment melts rapidly and blinking helps to spread it.

When two different eye-drop preparations are used at the same time of day, dilution and overflow may occur when one immediately follows the other. The patient should therefore leave an interval of at least 5 minutes between the two.

Systemic effects may arise from absorption of drugs into the general circulation from conjunctival vessels or from the nasal mucosa after the excess preparation has drained down through the tear ducts. The extent of systemic absorption following ocular administration is highly variable; nasal drainage of drugs is associated with eye drops much more often than with eye ointments. Pressure on the lacrimal punctum for at least a minute after applying eye drops reduces nasolacrimal drainage and therefore decreases systemic absorption from the nasal mucosa.

For warnings relating to eye drops and contact lenses, see section 11.9.

Eye lotions These are solutions for the irrigation of the conjunctival sac. They act mechanically to flush out irritants or foreign bodies as a first-aid treatment. Sterile sodium chloride 0.9% solution (section 11.8.1) is usually used. Clean water will suffice in an emergency.

Other preparations Subconjunctival injection may be used to administer anti-infective drugs, mydriatics, or corticosteroids for conditions not responding to topical therapy. The drug diffuses through the cornea and sclera to the anterior and posterior chambers and vitreous humour. However, because the dose-volume is limited (usually not more than 1 mL), this route is suitable only for drugs which are readily soluble.

Drugs such as antimicrobials and corticosteroids may be administered systemically to treat susceptible eye conditions.

Preservatives and sensitisers Information on preservatives and on substances identified as skin sensitisers (see section 13.1.3) is provided under preparation entries.

11.2 Control of microbial contamination

Preparations for the eye should be sterile when issued. Eye drops in multiple-application containers include a preservative but care should nevertheless be taken to avoid contamination of the contents during use.

Eye drops in multiple-application containers for *domiciliary use* should not be used for more than 4 weeks after first opening (unless otherwise stated).

Eye drops for use in *hospital wards* are normally discarded 1 week after first opening. Individual containers should be provided for each patient. A separate bottle should be supplied for each eye only if there are special concerns about contamination. Containers used before an operation should be discarded at the time of the operation and fresh containers supplied. A fresh supply should also be provided upon discharge from hospital; in specialist ophthalmology units, it may be acceptable to issue eye-drop bottles that have been dispensed to the patient on the day of discharge.

In *out-patient departments* single-application packs should preferably be used; if multiple-application packs are used, they should be discarded at the end of each day. In clinics for eye diseases and in accident and emergency departments, where the dangers of infection are high, single-application packs should be used; if a multiple-application pack is used, it should be discarded after single use.

Diagnostic dyes (e.g. fluorescein) should be used only from single-application packs.

In *eye surgery* single-application containers should be used if possible; if a multiple-application pack is used, it should be discarded after single use. Preparations used during intra-ocular procedures and others that may penetrate into the anterior chamber must be isotonic and without preservatives and buffered if necessary to a neutral pH. Specially formulated fluids should be used for intra-ocular surgery; intravenous infusion preparations are not suitable for this purpose. For all surgical procedures, a previously unopened container is used for each patient.

11.3 Anti-infective eye preparations

11.3.1 Antibacterials
11.3.2 Antifungals
11.3.3 Antivirals

Eye infections Most acute superficial eye infections can be treated topically. Blepharitis and conjunctivitis are often caused by staphylococci; keratitis and endophthalmitis may be bacterial, viral, or fungal.

Bacterial *blepharitis* is treated by application of an antibacterial eye ointment to the conjunctival sac or to the lid margins. Systemic treatment may occasionally be required and is usually undertaken after culturing organisms from the lid margin and determining their antimicrobial sensitivity; antibiotics such as the tetracyclines given for 3 months or longer may be appropriate.

Most cases of acute bacterial conjunctivitis are self-limiting; where treatment is appropriate, antibacterial eye drops or an eye ointment are used. A poor response might indicate viral or allergic conjunctivitis. *Gonococcal conjunctivitis* is treated with systemic and topical antibacterials.

Corneal ulcer and *keratitis* require specialist treatment and may call for hospital admission for intensive therapy.

Endophthalmitis is a medical emergency which also calls for specialist management and often requires parenteral, subconjunctival, or intra-ocular administration of antimicrobials.

11.3.1 Antibacterials

Bacterial infections are generally treated topically with eye drops and eye ointments. Systemic administration is sometimes appropriate in blepharitis.

Chloramphenicol has a broad spectrum of activity and is the drug of choice for *superficial eye infections*. Chloramphenicol eye drops are well tolerated and the recommendation that chloramphenicol eye drops should be avoided because of an increased risk of aplastic anaemia is not well founded.

Other antibacterials with a broad spectrum of activity include the quinolones, **ciprofloxacin**, **levofloxacin**, and **ofloxacin**; **gentamicin** and **neomycin** are also active against a wide variety of bacteria. Gentamicin, ciprofloxacin, levofloxacin, ofloxacin, and **polymyxin B** are effective for infections caused by *Pseudomonas aeruginosa*.

Ciprofloxacin eye drops are licensed for *corneal ulcers*; intensive application (especially in the first 2 days) is required throughout the day and night.

Trachoma which results from chronic infection with *Chlamydia trachomatis* can be treated with **azithromycin** by mouth [unlicensed indication].

Fusidic acid is useful for staphylococcal infections.

Propamidine isetionate is of little value in bacterial infections but is specific for the rare but potentially devastating condition of *acanthamoeba keratitis* (see also section 11.9).

With corticosteroids Many antibacterial preparations also incorporate a corticosteroid but such mixtures should **not** be used unless a patient is under close specialist supervision. In particular they should not be prescribed for undiagnosed 'red eye' which is sometimes caused by the herpes simplex virus and may be difficult to diagnose (section 11.4).

Administration Frequency of application depends on the severity of the infection and the potential for irreversible ocular damage; antibacterial eye preparations are usually administered as follows.

Eye drops Apply 1 drop at least every 2 hours then reduce frequency as infection is controlled and continue for 48 hours after healing.

Eye ointment Apply *either* at night (if eye drops used during the day) *or* 3–4 times daily (if eye ointment used alone).

CHLORAMPHENICOL

Indications see notes above

Side-effects transient stinging; see also notes above

Dose

- See Administration in notes above

[1]**Chloramphenicol** (Non-proprietary) PoM

Eye drops, chloramphenicol 0.5%. Net price 10 mL = £1.20

Eye ointment, chloramphenicol 1%. Net price 4 g = £1.57

1. Chloramphenicol 0.5% eye drops (in max. pack size 10 mL) and 1% eye ointment (in max. pack size 4 g) can be sold to the public for treatment of acute bacterial conjunctivitis in adults and children over 2 years; max. duration of treatment 5 days

Chloromycetin® (Goldshield) PoM

Redidrops (= eye drops), chloramphenicol 0.5%. Net price 5 mL = £1.65; 10 mL = £1.85

Excipients include phenylmercuric acetate

Ophthalmic ointment (= eye ointment), chloramphenicol 1%. Net price 4 g = £1.85

Single use

Minims® Chloramphenicol (Chauvin) PoM

Eye drops, chloramphenicol 0.5%. Net price 20 × 0.5 mL = £4.92

CIPROFLOXACIN

Indications superficial bacterial infections, see notes above; corneal ulcers

Cautions not recommended for children under 1 year; pregnancy (Appendix 4); breast-feeding (Appendix 5)

Side-effects local burning and itching; lid margin crusting; hyperaemia; taste disturbances; corneal staining, keratitis, lid oedema, lacrimation, photophobia, corneal infiltrates; nausea and visual disturbances reported

Dose

- Superficial bacterial infection, see Administration in notes above
- Corneal ulcer, apply *eye drops* throughout day and night, day 1 apply every 15 minutes for 6 hours then every 30 minutes, day 2 apply every hour, days 3–14 apply every 4 hours (max. duration of treatment 21 days)

  Apply *eye ointment* throughout day and night; apply 1.25 cm ointment every 1-2 hours for 2 days then every 4 hours for next 12 days

Ciloxan® (Alcon) PoM

Ophthalmic solution (= eye drops), ciprofloxacin (as hydrochloride) 0.3%. Net price 5 mL = £4.94

Excipients include benzalkonium chloride

Eye ointment▼, ciprofloxacin (as hydrochloride) 0.3%. Net price 3.5 g = £5.49

FUSIDIC ACID

Indications see notes above

Dose

- See under preparation below

Fucithalmic® (LEO) PoM

Eye drops, m/r, fusidic acid 1% in gel basis (liquifies on contact with eye). Net price 5 g = £2.09

Excipients include benzalkonium chloride, disodium edetate

Dose apply twice daily

GENTAMICIN

Indications see notes above

Dose

- See Administration in notes above

Genticin® (Roche) PoM

Drops (for ear or eye), gentamicin 0.3% (as sulphate). Net price 10 mL = £1.78

Excipients include benzalkonium chloride

Single use

Minims® Gentamicin Sulphate (Chauvin) PoM

Eye drops, gentamicin 0.3% (as sulphate). Net price 20 × 0.5 mL = £5.75

LEVOFLOXACIN

Indications see notes above

Cautions not recommended for children under 1 year; pregnancy (Appendix 4); breast-feeding (Appendix 5)

Side-effects transient ocular irritation, visual disturbances, lid margin crusting, lid or conjunctival oedema, hyperaemia, conjunctival follicles, photophobia, headache, rhinitis

Dose

- See Administration in notes above

Oftaquix® (Kestrel Ophthalmics) ▼ PoM

Eye drops, levofloxacin 0.5%, net price 5 mL = £6.95

Excipients include benzalkonium chloride

NEOMYCIN SULPHATE

Indications see notes above

Dose

- See Administration in notes above

Neomycin (Non-proprietary) PoM

Eye drops, neomycin sulphate 0.5% (3500 units/mL). Net price 10 mL = £3.11

Eye ointment, neomycin sulphate 0.5% (3500 units/g). Net price 3 g = £2.44

With other antibacterials

Neosporin® (PLIVA) PoM

Eye drops, gramicidin 25 units, neomycin sulphate 1700 units, polymyxin B sulphate 5000 units/mL. Net price 5 mL = £4.86

Excipients include thiomersal

Dose apply 2–4 times daily or more frequently if required

With hydrocortisone

Section 12.1.1

OFLOXACIN

Indications see notes above
Cautions pregnancy (Appendix 4); breast-feeding (Appendix 5); not to be used for more than 10 days
Side-effects local irritation including photophobia; dizziness, numbness, nausea and headache reported
Dose
- See Administration in notes above

Exocin® (Allergan) PoM
Ophthalmic solution (= eye drops), ofloxacin 0.3%. Net price 5 mL = £2.17
Excipients include benzalkonium chloride

POLYMYXIN B SULPHATE

Indications see notes above
Side-effects local irritation and dermatitis
Dose
- See Administration in notes above

With other antibacterials
Polyfax® (PLIVA) PoM
Eye ointment, polymyxin B sulphate 10 000 units, bacitracin zinc 500 units/g. Net price 4 g = £3.26

PROPAMIDINE ISETIONATE

Indications local treatment of infections (but see notes above)
Dose
- See preparations

Brolene® (Aventis Pharma)
Eye drops, propamidine isetionate 0.1%. Net price 10 mL = £2.80
Excipients include benzalkonium chloride
Dose apply 4 times daily
Note Eye drops containing propamidine isetionate 0.1% also available from Typharm (*Golden Eye Drops*)

Eye ointment, dibromopropamidine isetionate 0.15%. Net price 5 g = £2.92
Dose apply 1–2 times daily
Note Eye ointment containing dibromopropamidine isetionate 0.15% also available from Typharm (*Golden Eye Ointment*)

11.3.2 Antifungals

Fungal infections of the cornea are rare but can occur after agricultural injuries, especially in hot and humid climates. Orbital mycosis is rarer, and when it occurs it is usually because of a direct spread of infection from the paranasal sinuses. Increasing age, debility, or immunosuppression may encourage fungal proliferation. The spread of infection through blood occasionally produces a metastatic endophthalmitis.

Many different fungi are capable of producing ocular infection; they may be identified by appropriate laboratory procedures.

Antifungal preparations for the eye are not generally available. Treatment will normally be carried out at specialist centres, but requests for information about supplies of preparations not available commercially should be addressed to the Strategic Health Authority (or equivalent), or to the nearest hospital ophthalmology unit, or to Moorfields Eye Hospital, City Road, London EC1V 2PD (tel. (020) 7253 3411).

11.3.3 Antivirals

Herpes simplex infections producing, for example, dendritic corneal ulcer can be treated with **aciclovir**.

Slow-release ocular implants containing **ganciclovir** (available on a named-patient basis from specialist importing companies, see p. 888) may be inserted surgically to treat immediate sight-threatening CMV retinitis. Local treatments do not protect against systemic infection or infection in the other eye. For systemic treatment of CMV retinitis, see section 5.3.2.2.

ACICLOVIR
(Acyclovir)

Indications local treatment of herpes simplex infections
Side-effects local irritation and inflammation, superficial punctate keratopathy; *rarely* blepharitis; *very rarely* hypersensitivity reactions including angioedema
Dose
- Apply 5 times daily (continue for at least 3 days after complete healing)

Zovirax® (GSK) PoM
Eye ointment, aciclovir 3%. Net price 4.5 g = £9.92
Tablets, section 5.3.2.1
Injection, section 5.3.2.1
Cream, section 13.10.3

11.4 Corticosteroids and other anti-inflammatory preparations

11.4.1 Corticosteroids
11.4.2 Other anti-inflammatory preparations

11.4.1 Corticosteroids

Corticosteroids administered locally to the eye or given by mouth are effective for treating anterior segment inflammation, including that which results from surgery.

Topical corticosteroids should normally only be used under expert supervision; three main dangers are associated with their use:

- a 'red eye', where the diagnosis is unconfirmed, may be due to herpes simplex virus, and a corticosteroid may aggravate the condition, leading to corneal ulceration, with possible damage to vision and even loss of the eye. Bacterial, fungal and amoebic infections pose a similar hazard;
- 'steroid glaucoma' may follow the use of corticosteroid eye preparations in susceptible individuals;
- a 'steroid cataract' may follow prolonged use.

Other side-effects of ocular corticosteroids include thinning of the cornea and sclera.

Combination products containing a corticosteroid with an anti-infective drug are sometimes used after ocular surgery to reduce inflammation and prevent infection; use of combination products is otherwise rarely justified.

Systemic corticosteroids (section 6.3.2) may be useful for ocular conditions. The risk of producing a 'steroid cataract' increases with the dose and duration of corticosteroid use.

BETAMETHASONE

Indications local treatment of inflammation (short-term)

Cautions see notes above

Side-effects see notes above

Dose

- Apply eye drops every 1–2 hours until controlled then reduce frequency; apply eye ointment 2–4 times daily *or* at night when used with eye drops

Betnesol® (Celltech) PoM

Drops (for ear, eye, or nose), betamethasone sodium phosphate 0.1%. Net price 10 mL = £2.32

Excipients include benzalkonium chloride, disodium edetate

Eye ointment, betamethasone sodium phosphate 0.1%. Net price 3 g = £1.41

Vista-Methasone® (Martindale) PoM

Drops (for ear, eye, or nose), betamethasone sodium phosphate 0.1%. Net price 5 mL = £1.02; 10 mL = £1.16

Excipients include benzalkonium chloride

With neomycin

Betnesol-N® (Celltech) PoM

Drops (for ear, eye, or nose), see section 12.1.1

Eye ointment, betamethasone sodium phosphate 0.1%, neomycin sulphate 0.5%. Net price 3 g = £1.28

Note May be difficult to obtain

Vista-Methasone N® (Martindale) PoM

Drops (for ear, eye, or nose), see section 12.1.1

DEXAMETHASONE

Indications local treatment of inflammation (short-term)

Cautions see notes above

Side-effects see notes above

Dose

- Apply eye drops 4–6 times daily; severe conditions every 30–60 minutes until controlled then reduce frequency

  Apply eye ointment 3–4 times daily *or* at night when used with eye drops

Maxidex® (Alcon) PoM

Eye drops, dexamethasone 0.1%, hypromellose 0.5%. Net price 5 mL = £1.49; 10 mL = £2.95

Excipients include benzalkonium chloride, disodium edetate, polysorbate 80

Single use

Minims® Dexamethasone (Chauvin) PoM

Eye drops, dexamethasone sodium phosphate 0.1%. Net price 20 × 0.5 mL = £6.95

Excipients include disodium edetate

With antibacterials

Maxitrol® (Alcon) PoM

Eye drops, dexamethasone 0.1%, neomycin 0.35% (as sulphate), polymyxin B sulphate 6000 units/mL. Net price 5 mL = £1.77

Excipients include benzalkonium chloride, polysorbate 20

Eye ointment, dexamethasone 0.1%, neomycin 0.35% (as sulphate), polymyxin B sulphate 6000 units/g. Net price 3.5 g = £1.52

Excipients include hydroxybenzoates (parabens), wool fat

Sofradex® (Sanofi-Aventis) PoM

Drops (for ear or eye), see section 12.1.1

Tobradex® (Alcon) PoM

Eye drops, dexamethasone 0.1%, tobramycin 0.3%. Net price 5 mL = £5.65

Excipients include benzalkonium chloride, disodium edetate

FLUOROMETHOLONE

Indications local treatment of inflammation (short-term)

Cautions see notes above

Side-effects see notes above

Dose

- Apply 2–4 times daily (initially every hour for 24–48 hours then reduce frequency)

FML® (Allergan) PoM

Ophthalmic suspension (= eye drops), fluorometholone 0.1%, polyvinyl alcohol (*Liquifilm®*) 1.4%. Net price 5 mL = £1.71; 10 mL = £2.95

Excipients include benzalkonium chloride, disodium edetate, polysorbate 80

HYDROCORTISONE ACETATE

Indications local treatment of inflammation (short-term)

Cautions see notes above

Side-effects see notes above

Hydrocortisone (Non-proprietary) PoM

Eye drops, hydrocortisone acetate 1%. Net price 10 mL = £3.21

Eye ointment, hydrocortisone acetate 0.5%, net price 3 g = £2.40; 1%, 3 g = £2.42; 2.5%, 3 g = £2.44

With neomycin

Neo-Cortef® (PLIVA) PoM

Ointment (for ear or eye), see section 12.1.1

Note May be difficult to obtain

PREDNISOLONE

Indications local treatment of inflammation (short-term)

Cautions see notes above

Side-effects see notes above

Dose

- Apply every 1–2 hours until controlled then reduce frequency

Predsol® (Celltech) PoM

Drops (for ear or eye), prednisolone sodium phosphate 0.5%. Net price 10 mL = £2.00

Excipients include benzalkonium chloride, disodium edetate

Pred Forte® (Allergan) PoM

Eye drops, prednisolone acetate 1%. Net price 5 mL = £1.52; 10 mL = £3.05

Excipients include benzalkonium chloride, disodium edetate, polysorbate 80

Dose apply 2–4 times daily

Single use

Minims® Prednisolone Sodium Phosphate (Chauvin) PoM
Eye drops, prednisolone sodium phosphate 0.5%. Net price 20 × 0.5 mL = £5.75
Excipients include disodium edetate

With neomycin

Predsol-N® (Celltech) PoM
Drops (for ear or eye), see section 12.1.1

RIMEXOLONE

Indications local treatment of inflammation (short-term)
Cautions see notes above
Side-effects see notes above
Dose
- Postoperative inflammation, apply 4 times daily for 2 weeks, beginning 24 hours after surgery
- Steroid-responsive inflammation, apply at least 4 times daily for up to 4 weeks
- Uveitis, apply every hour during daytime in week 1, then every 2 hours in week 2, then 4 times daily in week 3, then twice daily for first 4 days of week 4, then once daily for remaining 3 days of week 4

Vexol® (Alcon) ▼ PoM
Eye drops, rimexolone 1%, net price 5 mL = £5.95
Excipients include benzalkonium chloride, disodium edetate, polysorbate 80

11.4.2 Other anti-inflammatory preparations

Other preparations used for the topical treatment of inflammation and allergic conjunctivitis include antihistamines, lodoxamide, and sodium cromoglicate.

Eye drops of **antihistamines** such **antazoline** (with xylometazoline as *Otrivine-Antistin®*), **azelastine**, **epinastine**, **ketotifen** and **olopatadine** may be used for allergic conjunctivitis.

Sodium cromoglicate (sodium cromoglycate) and **nedocromil sodium** eye drops can be useful for vernal keratoconjunctivitis and other allergic forms of conjunctivitis.

Lodoxamide eye drops are used for allergic conjunctival conditions including seasonal allergic conjunctivitis.

Diclofenac eye drops (section 11.8.2) and **emedastine** eye drops are also licensed for seasonal allergic conjunctivitis.

ANTAZOLINE SULPHATE

Indications allergic conjunctivitis

Otrivine-Antistin® (Novartis Consumer Health)
Eye drops, antazoline sulphate 0.5%, xylometazoline hydrochloride 0.05%. Net price 10 mL = £2.35
Excipients include benzalkonium chloride, disodium edetate
Dose ADULT and CHILD over 5 years apply 2–3 times daily
Note Xylometazoline is a sympathomimetic; it should be used with caution in patients susceptible to angle-closure glaucoma; absorption of antazoline and xylometazoline may result in systemic side-effects and the possibility of interaction with other drugs

AZELASTINE HYDROCHLORIDE

Indications allergic conjunctivitis
Side-effects mild transient irritation; bitter taste reported
Dose
- Seasonal allergic conjunctivitis, ADULT and CHILD over 4 years, apply twice daily, increased if necessary to 4 times daily
- Perennial conjunctivitis, ADULT and ADOLESCENT over 12 years, apply twice daily, increased if necessary to 4 times daily; max. duration of treatment 6 weeks

Optilast® (Viatris) PoM
Eye drops, azelastine hydrochloride 0.05%. Net price 8 mL = £6.40
Excipients include benzalkonium chloride, disodium edetate
Note Azelastine 0.05% eye drops can be sold to the public (in max. pack size of 6 mL) for treatment of seasonal and perennial allergic conjunctivitis in adults and children over 12 years

EMEDASTINE

Indications seasonal allergic conjunctivitis
Side-effects transient burning or stinging; blurred vision, local oedema, keratitis, irritation, dry eye, lacrimation, corneal infiltrates (discontinue) and staining; photophobia; headache, and rhinitis occasionally reported
Dose
- ADULT and CHILD over 3 years, apply twice daily

Emadine® (Alcon) PoM
Eye drops, emedastine 0.05% (as difumarate), net price 5 mL = £7.69
Excipients include benzalkonium chloride

EPINASTINE HYDROCHLORIDE

Indications seasonal allergic conjunctivitis
Side-effects burning; *less commonly* dry mouth, taste disturbance; nasal irritation, rhinitis; headache, blepharoptosis, conjunctival oedema and hyperaemia, dry eye, local irritation, photophobia, visual disturbance; pruritus
Dose
- ADULT and ADOLESCENT over 12 years, apply twice daily; max. duration of treatment 8 weeks

Relestat® (Allergan) PoM
Eye drops, epinastine hydrochloride 500 micrograms/mL, net price 5 mL = £9.90
Excipients include benzalkonium chloride, disodium edetate

KETOTIFEN

Indications seasonal allergic conjunctivitis
Side-effects burning or stinging, punctate corneal epithelial erosion; *less commonly* dry eye, subconjunctival haemorrhage, photophobia; headache, drowsiness, skin reactions, and dry mouth also reported
Dose
- ADULT and CHILD over 3 years, apply twice daily

Zaditen® (Novartis) PoM
Eye drops, ketotifen (as fumarate) 250 micrograms/mL, net price 5 mL = £9.75
Excipients include benzalkonium chloride

LODOXAMIDE

Indications allergic conjunctivitis

Side-effects burning, stinging, itching, and lacrimation; flushing and dizziness reported

Dose

- ADULT and CHILD over 4 years, apply 4 times daily

Alomide® (Alcon) PoM

Ophthalmic solution (= eye drops), lodoxamide 0.1% (as trometamol). Net price 10 mL = £5.48

Excipients include benzalkonium chloride, disodium edetate

Note Lodoxamide 0.1% eye drops can be sold to the public for treatment of allergic conjunctivitis in adults and children over 4 years

NEDOCROMIL SODIUM

Indications allergic conjunctivitis; seasonal keratoconjunctivitis

Side-effects burning and stinging; distinctive taste reported

Dose

- Seasonal and perennial conjunctivitis, ADULT and CHILD over 6 years, apply twice daily increased if necessary to 4 times daily; max. 12 weeks treatment for seasonal allergic conjunctivitis
- Seasonal keratoconjunctivitis, ADULT and CHILD over 6 years, apply 4 times daily

Rapitil® (Aventis Pharma) PoM

Eye drops, nedocromil sodium 2%. Net price 5 mL = £5.12

Excipients include benzalkonium chloride, disodium edetate

OLOPATADINE

Indications seasonal allergic conjunctivitis

Side-effects local irritation; less commonly keratitis, dry eye, local oedema, photophobia; headache, asthenia, dizziness; dry nose also reported

Dose

- ADULT and CHILD over 3 years, apply twice daily; max. duration of treatment 4 months

Opatanol® (Alcon) PoM

Eye drops, olopatadine (as hydrochloride) 1 mg/mL, net price 5 mL = £4.11

Excipients include benzalkonium chloride

SODIUM CROMOGLICATE
(Sodium cromoglycate)

Indications allergic conjunctivitis; seasonal keratoconjunctivitis

Side-effects burning and stinging

Dose

- ADULT and CHILD apply eye drops 4 times daily

[1]**Sodium Cromoglicate** (Non-proprietary) PoM

Eye drops, sodium cromoglicate 2%. Net price 13.5 mL = £1.97

Brands include *Hay-Crom® Aqueous, Opticrom® Aqueous, Vividrin®*)

1. Sodium cromoglicate 2% eye drops can be sold to the public (in max. pack size of 10 mL) for treatment of acute seasonal and perennial allergic conjunctivitis

11.5 Mydriatics and cycloplegics

Antimuscarinics dilate the pupil and paralyse the ciliary muscle; they vary in potency and duration of action.

Short-acting, relatively weak mydriatics, such as **tropicamide** 0.5%, facilitate the examination of the fundus of the eye. **Cyclopentolate** 1% or **atropine** are preferable for producing cycloplegia for refraction in young children. Atropine ointment 1% is sometimes preferred for children aged under 5 years because the ointment formulation reduces systemic absorption. Atropine, which has a longer duration of action, is also used for the treatment of anterior uveitis mainly to prevent posterior synechiae, often with **phenylephrine** 10% eye drops (2.5% in children, the elderly, and those with cardiac disease). **Homatropine** 1% is also used in the treatment of anterior segment inflammation, and may be preferred for its shorter duration of action.

Cautions Darkly pigmented iris is more resistant to pupillary dilatation and caution should be exercised to avoid overdosage. Mydriasis can precipitate acute angle-closure glaucoma in a few patients, usually aged over 60 years and hypermetropic (long-sighted), who are predisposed to the condition because of a shallow anterior chamber. Phenylephrine may interact with systemically administered monoamine-oxidase inhibitors; other **interactions**: Appendix 1 (sympathomimetics).

Driving Patients should be warned not to drive for 1–2 hours after mydriasis.

Side-effects Ocular side-effects of mydriatics and cycloplegics include transient stinging and raised intra-ocular pressure; on prolonged administration, local irritation, hyperaemia, oedema and conjunctivitis can occur. Contact dermatitis can occur with the antimuscarinic mydriatic drugs, especially atropine.

Systemic side-effects of atropine and cyclopentolate can occur in children and the elderly; see under Atropine Sulphate (section 1.2) for systemic side-effects of antimuscarinic drugs.

Antimuscarinics

ATROPINE SULPHATE

Indications refraction procedures in young children; anterior uveitis—see also notes above

Cautions risk of systemic effects with eye drops in infants under 3 months—eye ointment preferred; see also notes above

Side-effects see notes above

Atropine (Non-proprietary) PoM

Eye drops, atropine sulphate 0.5%, net price 10 mL = £2.32; 1%, 10 mL = 91p

Eye ointment, atropine sulphate 1%. Net price 3 g = £2.97

Single use

Minims® Atropine Sulphate (Chauvin) PoM

Eye drops, atropine sulphate 1%. Net price 20 × 0.5 mL = £4.92

CYCLOPENTOLATE HYDROCHLORIDE

Indications see notes above
Cautions see notes above
Side-effects see notes above

Mydrilate® (Intrapharm) PoM
Eye drops, cyclopentolate hydrochloride 0.5%, net price 5 mL = 97p; 1%, 5 mL = £1.19
Excipients include benzalkonium chloride

Single use
Minims® Cyclopentolate Hydrochloride (Chauvin) PoM
Eye drops, cyclopentolate hydrochloride 0.5% and 1%. Net price 20 × 0.5 mL (both) = £4.92

HOMATROPINE HYDROBROMIDE

Indications see notes above
Cautions see notes above
Side-effects see notes above

Homatropine (Non-proprietary) PoM
Eye drops, homatropine hydrobromide 1%, net price 10 mL = £2.14; 2%, 10 mL = £2.26

TROPICAMIDE

Indications see notes above
Cautions see notes above
Side-effects see notes above

Mydriacyl® (Alcon) PoM
Eye drops, tropicamide 0.5%, net price 5 mL = £1.36; 1%, 5 mL = £1.68
Excipients include benzalkonium chloride, disodium edetate

Single use
Minims® Tropicamide (Chauvin) PoM
Eye drops, tropicamide 0.5% and 1%. Net price 20 × 0.5 mL (both) = £5.75

Sympathomimetics

PHENYLEPHRINE HYDROCHLORIDE

Indications mydriasis; see also notes above
Cautions children and elderly (avoid 10% strength); cardiovascular disease (avoid or use 2.5% strength only); tachycardia; hyperthyroidism; diabetes; see also notes above
Side-effects eye pain and stinging; blurred vision, photophobia; systemic effects include arrhythmias, hypertension, coronary artery spasm; *very rarely* angle-closure glaucoma

Phenylephrine (Non-proprietary)
Eye drops, phenylephrine hydrochloride 10%. Net price 10 mL = £3.38

Single use
Minims® Phenylephrine Hydrochloride (Chauvin)
Eye drops, phenylephrine hydrochloride 2.5%, net price 20 × 0.5 mL = £5.75; 10%, 20 × 0.5 mL = £5.75
Excipients include disodium edetate, sodium metabisulphite

11.6 Treatment of glaucoma

Glaucoma describes a group of disorders characterised by a loss of visual field associated with cupping of the optic disc and optic nerve damage. While glaucoma is generally associated with raised intra-ocular pressure, it can occur when the intra-ocular pressure is within the normal range.

The commonest form of glaucoma is *primary open-angle glaucoma* (chronic simple glaucoma; wide-angle glaucoma), where the obstruction is in the trabecular meshwork. The condition is often asymptomatic and the patient may present with significant loss of visual-field. *Primary angle closure glaucoma* (acute closed-angle glaucoma, narrow-angle glaucoma) results from blockage of aqueous humour flow into the anterior chamber and is a medical emergency.

Only drugs that reduce intra-ocular pressure are available for managing glaucoma; they act by a variety of mechanisms. A topical beta-blocker or a prostaglandin analogue is commonly the drug of first choice. It may be necessary to combine these drugs or add others, such as miotics, sympathomimetics, and carbonic anhydrase inhibitors, to control intra-ocular pressure.

For urgent reduction of intra-ocular pressure and before surgery, mannitol 20% (up to 500 mL) is given by slow intravenous infusion until the intra-ocular pressure has been satisfactorily reduced. Acetazolamide by intravenous injection can also be used for the emergency management of raised intra-ocular pressure.

Standard antiglaucoma therapy is used if supplementary treatment is required after iridotomy, iridectomy, or a drainage operation in either primary open-angle or acute closed-angle glaucoma.

Beta-blockers

Topical application of a beta-blocker to the eye reduces intra-ocular pressure effectively in *primary open-angle glaucoma*, probably by reducing the rate of production of aqueous humour. Administration by mouth also reduces intra-ocular pressure but this route is not used since side-effects may be troublesome.

Beta-blockers used as eye drops include **betaxolol**, **carteolol**, **levobunolol**, **metipranolol**, and **timolol**.

Cautions, contra-indications and side-effects Systemic absorption may follow topical application to the eyes, therefore eye drops containing a beta-blocker are contra-indicated in patients with bradycardia, heart block, or uncontrolled heart failure. **Important**: for a warning to avoid in asthma see CSM advice below. Consider also other cautions, contra-indications and side-effects of beta-blockers (p. 84). Local side-effects of eye drops include ocular stinging, burning, pain, itching, erythema, dry eyes and allergic reactions including anaphylaxis and blepharoconjunctivitis; occasionally corneal disorders have been reported.

CSM advice The CSM has advised that beta-blockers, even those with apparent cardioselectivity, should not be used in patients with asthma or a history of obstructive airways disease, unless no alternative treatment is available. In such cases the risk of inducing bronchospasm should be appreciated and appropriate precautions taken.

Interactions Since systemic absorption may follow topical application the possibility of interactions, in particular, with drugs such as verapamil should be borne in mind. See also Appendix 1 (beta-blockers).

BETAXOLOL HYDROCHLORIDE

Indications see notes above
Cautions see notes above
Contra-indications see notes above
Side-effects see notes above
Dose
- Apply twice daily

Betoptic® (Alcon) PoM
Ophthalmic solution (= eye drops), betaxolol (as hydrochloride) 0.5%, net price 5 mL = £2.00
Excipients include benzalkonium chloride, disodium edetate

Ophthalmic suspension (= eye drops), m/r, betaxolol (as hydrochloride) 0.25%, net price 5 mL = £2.80
Excipients include benzalkonium chloride, disodium edetate

Unit dose eye drop suspension, m/r, betaxolol (as hydrochloride) 0.25%, net price 50 × 0.25 mL = £14.49

CARTEOLOL HYDROCHLORIDE

Indications see notes above
Cautions see notes above
Contra-indications see notes above
Side-effects see notes above
Dose
- Apply twice daily

Teoptic® (Novartis) PoM
Eye drops, carteolol hydrochloride 1%, net price 5 mL = £4.60; 2%, 5 mL = £5.40
Excipients include benzalkonium chloride

LEVOBUNOLOL HYDROCHLORIDE

Indications see notes above
Cautions see notes above
Contra-indications see notes above
Side-effects see notes above; anterior uveitis occasionally reported
Dose
- Apply once or twice daily

Levobunolol (Non-proprietary) PoM
Eye drops, levobunolol hydrochloride 0.5%. Net price 5 mL = £2.40

Betagan® (Allergan) PoM
Eye drops, levobunolol hydrochloride 0.5%, polyvinyl alcohol (*Liquifilm®*) 1.4%. Net price 5-mL = £1.85
Excipients include benzalkonium chloride, disodium edetate, sodium metabisulphite

Unit dose eye drops, levobunolol hydrochloride 0.5%, polyvinyl alcohol (*Liquifilm®*) 1.4%. Net price 30 × 0.4 mL = £9.98
Excipients include disodium edetate

METIPRANOLOL

Indications see notes above but in chronic open-angle glaucoma **restricted** to patients allergic to preservatives or to those wearing soft contact lenses (in whom benzalkonium chloride should be avoided)
Cautions see notes above
Contra-indications see notes above
Side-effects see notes above; granulomatous anterior uveitis reported (discontinue treatment)
Dose
- Apply twice daily

Minims® Metipranolol (Chauvin) PoM
Eye drops, metipranolol 0.1%, net price 20 × 0.5 mL = £10.19; 0.3%, 20 × 0.5 mL = £11.09

TIMOLOL MALEATE

Indications see notes above
Cautions see notes above
Contra-indications see notes above
Side-effects see notes above
Dose
- Apply twice daily; long-acting preparations, see under preparations below

Timolol (Non-proprietary) PoM
Eye drops, timolol (as maleate) 0.25%, net price 5 mL = £2.51; 0.5%, 5 mL = £2.00

Timoptol® (MSD) PoM
Eye drops, in *Ocumeter®* metered-dose unit, timolol (as maleate) 0.25%, net price 5 mL = £3.12; 0.5%, 5 mL = £3.12
Excipients include benzalkonium chloride

Unit dose eye drops, timolol (as maleate) 0.25%, net price 30 × 0.2 mL = £8.45; 0.5%, 30 × 0.2 mL = £9.65

Once-daily preparations

Nyogel® (Novartis) PoM
Eye gel (= eye drops), timolol (as maleate) 0.1%, net price 5 g = £2.85
Excipients include benzalkonium chloride
Dose apply once daily

Timoptol®-LA (MSD) PoM
Ophthalmic gel-forming solution (= eye drops), timolol (as maleate) 0.25%, net price 2.5 mL = £3.12; 0.5%, 2.5 mL = £3.12
Excipients include benzododecinium bromide
Dose apply once daily

With bimatoprost
See under Bimatoprost

With brimonidine
See under Brimonidine

With dorzolamide
See under Dorzolamide

With latanoprost
See under Latanoprost

With travoprost
See under Travoprost

Prostaglandin analogues

Latanoprost and **travoprost** are prostaglandin analogues which increase uveoscleral outflow; **bimatoprost** is a related drug. They are used to reduce intra-ocular pressure in ocular hypertension or in open-angle glaucoma. Patients receiving prostaglandin analogues should be monitored for any changes to eye coloration since an increase in the brown pigment in the iris may occur; particular care is required in those with mixed coloured irides and those receiving treatment to one eye only.

BIMATOPROST

Indications raised intra-ocular pressure in open-angle glaucoma; ocular hypertension

Cautions see under Latanoprost and notes above

Side-effects see under Latanoprost; also ocular pruritus, allergic conjunctivitis, cataract, conjunctival oedema, eye discharge, photophobia, superficial punctate keratitis, headache; hypertension

Dose

- Apply once daily, preferably in the evening; CHILD and ADOLESCENT under 18 years, not recommended

Lumigan® (Allergan) PoM
Eye drops, bimatoprost 300 micrograms/mL, net price 3 mL = £11.46, triple pack (3 × 3 mL) = £32.66
Excipients include benzalkonium chloride

With timolol

For cautions, contra-indications, and side-effects of timolol, see section 11.6, Beta-blockers

Ganfort® (Allergan) ▼ PoM
Eye drops, bimatoprost 300 micrograms/mL, timolol (as maleate) 5 mg/mL, net price 3-mL = £14.58
Excipients include benzalkonium chloride
Dose for raised intra-ocular pressure in patients with open-angle glaucoma or ocular hypertension when beta-blocker or prostaglandin analogue alone not adequate; apply once daily, preferably in the morning

LATANOPROST

Indications raised intra-ocular pressure in open-angle glaucoma; ocular hypertension

Cautions before initiating treatment, advise patients of possible change in eye colour; monitor for eye colour change (see also notes above); aphakia, or pseudophakia with torn posterior lens capsule or anterior chamber lenses; risk factors for iritis, uveitis, and cystoid macular oedema; brittle or severe asthma; not to be used within 5 minutes of use of thiomersal-containing preparations; pregnancy (Appendix 4); breast-feeding (Appendix 5)

Side-effects brown pigmentation particularly in those with mixed-colour irides; blepharitis, ocular irritation and pain; darkening, thickening and lengthening of eye lashes; conjunctival hyperaemia; transient punctate epithelial erosion; skin rash; *less commonly* eyelid oedema and rash; *rarely* dyspnoea, exacerbation of asthma, iritis, uveitis, local oedema, darkening of palpebral skin; *very rarely* chest pain, exacerbation of angina

Dose

- Apply once daily, preferably in the evening; CHILD not recommended

Xalatan® (Pharmacia) PoM
Eye drops, latanoprost 50 micrograms/mL, net price 2.5 mL = £13.14
Excipients include benzalkonium chloride

With timolol

For cautions, contra-indications, and side-effects of timolol, see section 11.6, Beta-blockers

Xalacom® (Pharmacia) PoM
Eye drops, latanoprost 50 micrograms, timolol (as maleate) 5 mg/mL, net price 2.5 mL = £15.07
Excipients include benzalkonium chloride
Dose for raised intra-ocular pressure in patients with open-angle glaucoma and ocular hypertension when beta-blocker alone not adequate; apply once daily

TRAVOPROST

Indications raised intra-ocular pressure in open-angle glaucoma; ocular hypertension

Cautions see under Latanoprost and notes above

Side-effects see under Latanoprost; also headache, ocular pruritus, photophobia, and keratitis reported; rarely, hypotension, bradycardia, conjunctivitis, browache

Dose

- Apply once daily, preferably in the evening; CHILD and ADOLESCENT under 18 years, not recommended

Travatan® (Alcon) PoM
Eye drops, travoprost 40 micrograms/mL, net price 2.5 mL = £10.50
Excipients include benzalkonium chloride

With timolol

For cautions, contra-indications, and side-effects of timolol, see section 11.6, Beta-blockers

DuoTrav® (Alcon) ▼ PoM
Eye drops, travoprost 40 micrograms, timolol (as maleate) 5 mg/mL, net price 2.5mL = £12.52
Excipients include benzalkonium chloride, disodium edetate
Dose for raised intraocular pressure in patients with open-angle glaucoma or ocular hypertension when beta-blocker or prostaglandin analogue alone not adequate; apply once daily; CHILD and ADOLESCENT under 18 years, not recommended

Sympathomimetics

Dipivefrine is a pro-drug of adrenaline (epinephrine). It is claimed to pass more rapidly than adrenaline through the cornea and is then converted to the active form.

Adrenaline probably acts both by reducing the rate of production of aqueous humour and by increasing the outflow through the trabecular meshwork. Because it is a mydriatic, adrenaline should be used with caution in patients susceptible to angle-closure glaucoma, unless an iridectomy has been carried out. Side-effects include severe smarting and redness of the eye; adrenaline should be used with caution in patients with hypertension and heart disease.

Brimonidine, a selective $alpha_2$-adrenoceptor agonist, is licensed for the reduction of intra-ocular pressure in open-angle glaucoma or ocular hypertension in patients for whom beta-blockers are inappropriate; it may also be used as adjunctive therapy when intra-ocular pressure is inadequately controlled by other antiglaucoma therapy.

Apraclonidine (section 11.8.2) is another $alpha_2$-adrenoceptor agonist. Eye drops containing apraclonidine 0.5% are used for a short term to delay laser treatment or surgery for glaucoma in patients not adequately controlled by another drug; eye drops containing 1% are used for control of intra-ocular pressure after anterior segment laser surgery.

BRIMONIDINE TARTRATE

Indications raised intra-ocular pressure, see notes above

Cautions severe cardiovascular disease; cerebral or coronary insufficiency, Raynaud's syndrome, postural hypotension, depression, hepatic or renal impairment;

pregnancy, breast-feeding; **interactions:** Appendix 1 (alpha$_2$-adrenoceptor stimulants)

Driving Drowsiness may affect performance of skilled tasks (e.g. driving)

Side-effects ocular reactions including conjunctival hyperaemia, stinging, pruritus, allergy, and conjunctival folliculosis, visual disturbances, blepharitis, epiphora, corneal erosion, superficial punctuate keratitis, eye pain, discharge, dryness, and irritation, eyelid inflammation, oedema, pruritus conjunctivitis, photophobia; also, hypertension, headache, depression, dry mouth, fatigue, drowsiness; *less commonly*, taste disturbances, palpitation, dizziness, syncope, rhinitis, nasal dryness

Dose

- Apply twice daily

Alphagan® (Allergan) PoM

Eye drops, brimonidine tartrate 0.2%, net price 5 mL = £6.85

Excipients include benzalkonium chloride

With timolol

For cautions, contra-indications, and side-effects of timolol, see section 11.6, Beta-blockers

Combigan® (Allergan) ▼ PoM

Eye drops, brimonidine tartrate 0.2%, timolol (as maleate) 0.5%, net price 5-mL = £10.00

Excipients include benzalkonium chloride

Dose for raised intra-ocular pressure in open-angle glaucoma and for ocular hypertension when beta-blocker alone not adequate, apply twice daily

DIPIVEFRINE HYDROCHLORIDE

Indications see notes above

Contra-indications see notes above

Side-effects see notes above

Dose

- Apply twice daily

Propine® (Allergan) PoM

Eye drops, dipivefrine hydrochloride 0.1%, net price 5 mL = £3.81, 10 mL = £4.77

Excipients include benzalkonium chloride, disodium edetate

Carbonic anhydrase inhibitors and systemic drugs

The **carbonic anhydrase inhibitors**, acetazolamide, brinzolamide, and dorzolamide, reduce intra-ocular pressure by reducing aqueous humour production. Systemic use also produces weak diuresis.

Acetazolamide is given by mouth or by intravenous injection (intramuscular injections are painful because of the alkaline pH of the solution). It is used as an adjunct to other treatment for reducing intra-ocular pressure. Acetazolamide is a sulphonamide; blood disorders, rashes, and other sulphonamide-related side-effects occur occasionally. It is not generally recommended for long-term use; electrolyte disturbances and metabolic acidosis that occur may be corrected by administering potassium bicarbonate (as effervescent potassium tablets, section 9.2.1.3).

Dorzolamide and **brinzolamide** are topical carbonic anhydrase inhibitors. They are licensed for use in patients resistant to beta-blockers or those in whom beta-blockers are contra-indicated. They are used alone or as an adjunct to a topical beta-blocker. Systemic absorption may rarely give rise to sulphonamide-like side-effects and may require discontinuation if severe.

The **osmotic diuretics**, intravenous hypertonic **mannitol** (section 2.2.5) or **glycerol** by mouth, are useful short-term ocular hypotensive drugs.

ACETAZOLAMIDE

Indications reduction of intra-ocular pressure in open-angle glaucoma, secondary glaucoma, and peri-operatively in angle-closure glaucoma; diuresis (section 2.2.7); epilepsy

Cautions not generally recommended for prolonged use but if given monitor blood count and plasma electrolyte concentration; pulmonary obstruction (risk of acidosis); elderly; pregnancy (Appendix 4); avoid extravasation at injection site (risk of necrosis); **interactions:** Appendix 1 (diuretics)

Contra-indications hypokalaemia, hyponatraemia, hyperchloraemic acidosis; severe hepatic impairment; renal impairment (Appendix 3); sulphonamide hypersensitivity

Side-effects nausea, vomiting, diarrhoea, taste disturbance; loss of appetite, paraesthesia, flushing, headache, dizziness, fatigue, irritability, depression; thirst, polyuria; reduced libido; metabolic acidosis and electrolyte disturbances on long-term therapy; occasionally, drowsiness, confusion, hearing disturbances, urticaria, melaena, glycosuria, haematuria, abnormal liver function, renal calculi, blood disorders including agranulocytosis and thrombocytopenia, rashes including Stevens-Johnson syndrome and toxic epidermal necrolysis; rarely, photosensitivity, liver damage, flaccid paralysis, convulsions; transient myopia reported

Dose

- Glaucoma, by mouth *or* by intravenous injection, 0.25–1 g daily in divided doses
- Epilepsy, by mouth *or* by intravenous injection, 0.25–1 g daily in divided doses; CHILD 8–30 mg/kg daily, max. 750 mg daily

Note Dose by intramuscular injection, as for intravenous injection but preferably avoided because of alkalinity

Diamox® (Goldshield) PoM

Tablets, acetazolamide 250 mg. Net price 112-tab pack = £12.68. Label: 3

Sodium Parenteral (= injection), powder for reconstitution, acetazolamide (as sodium salt). Net price 500-mg vial = £14.76

Modified release

Diamox® SR (Goldshield) PoM

Capsules, m/r, two-tone orange, enclosing orange f/c pellets, acetazolamide 250 mg. Net price 30-cap pack = £13.88. Label: 3, 25

Dose glaucoma, 1–2 capsules daily

BRINZOLAMIDE

Indications adjunct to beta-blockers or used alone in raised intra-ocular pressure in ocular hypertension and in open-angle glaucoma if beta-blocker alone inadequate or inappropriate

Cautions hepatic impairment; pregnancy (Appendix 4); **interactions:** Appendix 1 (brinzolamide)

Contra-indications renal impairment (creatinine clearance less than 30 mL/minute), hyperchloraemic acidosis; breast-feeding

Side-effects local irritation, taste disturbance; less commonly nausea, dyspepsia, dry mouth, chest pain, epistaxis, haemoptysis, dyspnoea, rhinitis, pharyngitis, bronchitis, paraesthesia, depression, dizziness, headache, dermatitis, alopecia, corneal erosion

Dose

- Apply twice daily increased to 3 times daily if necessary

Azopt® (Alcon) PoM
Eye drops, brinzolamide 10 mg/mL, net price 5 mL = £6.90
Excipients include benzalkonium chloride, disodium edetate

DORZOLAMIDE

Indications raised intra-ocular pressure in ocular hypertension, open-angle glaucoma, pseudo-exfoliative glaucoma *either* as adjunct to beta-blocker *or* used alone in patients unresponsive to beta-blockers or if beta-blockers contra-indicated

Cautions hepatic impairment; systemic absorption follows topical application; history of renal calculi; chronic corneal defects, history of intra-ocular surgery; **interactions:** Appendix 1 (dorzolamide)

Contra-indications renal impairment (Appendix 3); hyperchloraemic acidosis; pregnancy and breast-feeding

Side-effects nausea, bitter taste, dry mouth; headache, asthenia; ocular irritation, blurred vision, lacrimation, conjunctivitis, superficial punctuate keratitis, eyelid inflammation; *less commonly* iridocyclitis; *rarely* hypersensitivity reactions (including urticaria, angioedema, bronchospasm), dizziness, paraesthesia, urolithiasis, eyelid crusting, transient myopia, corneal oedema, epistaxis, throat irritation

Dose

- Used alone, apply 3 times daily
- With topical beta-blocker, apply twice daily

Trusopt® (MSD) PoM
Ophthalmic solution (= eye drops), in *Ocumeter® Plus* metered-dose unit, dorzolamide (as hydrochloride) 2%, net price 5 mL = £6.33
Excipients include benzalkonium chloride

Unit dose eye drops, dorzolamide (as hydrochloride) 2%, net price 60 × 0.2 mL = £24.18

With timolol

For cautions, contra-indications, and side-effects of timolol, see section 11.6, Beta-blockers

Cosopt® (MSD) PoM
Ophthalmic solution (= eye drops), dorzolamide (as hydrochloride) 2%, timolol (as maleate) 0.5%, net price 5 mL = £10.05
Excipients include benzalkonium chloride

Unit dose eye drops, dorzolamide (as hydrochloride) 2%, timolol (as maleate) 0.5%, net price 60 × 0.2 mL = £28.59

Miotics

The small pupil is an unfortunate side-effect of these drugs (except when pilocarpine is used temporarily before an operation for *angle-closure glaucoma*). They act by opening up the inefficient drainage channels in the trabecular meshwork resulting from contraction or spasm of the ciliary muscle.

Miotics used in the management of raised intra-ocular pressure include pilocarpine.

Cautions A darkly pigmented iris may require higher concentration of the miotic or more frequent administration and care should be taken to avoid overdosage. Retinal detachment has occurred in susceptible individuals and those with retinal disease; therefore fundus examination is advised before starting treatment with a miotic. Care is also required in conjunctival or corneal damage. Intra-ocular pressure and visual fields should be monitored in those with chronic simple glaucoma and those receiving long-term treatment with a miotic. Miotics should be used with caution in cardiac disease, hypertension, asthma, peptic ulceration, urinary-tract obstruction, and Parkinson's disease.
Counselling Blurred vision may affect performance of skilled tasks (e.g. driving) particularly at night or in reduced lighting

Contra-indications Miotics are contra-indicated in conditions where pupillary constriction is undesirable such as acute iritis, anterior uveitis and some forms of secondary glaucoma. They should be avoided in acute inflammatory disease of the anterior segment.

Side-effects Ciliary spasm leads to headache and browache which may be more severe in the initial 2–4 weeks of treatment (a particular disadvantage in patients under 40 years of age). Ocular side-effects include burning, itching, smarting, blurred vision, conjunctival vascular congestion, myopia, lens changes with chronic use, vitreous haemorrhage, and pupillary block. Systemic side-effects (see under Parasympathomimetics, section 7.4.1) are rare following application to the eye.

PILOCARPINE

Indications see notes above; dry mouth (section 12.3.5)

Cautions see notes above

Contra-indications see notes above

Side-effects see notes above

Dose

- Apply up to 4 times daily; long-acting preparations, see under preparations below

Pilocarpine Hydrochloride (Non-proprietary) PoM
Eye drops, pilocarpine hydrochloride 0.5%, net price 10 mL = £1.39; 1%, 10 mL = £2.62; 2%, 10 mL = £2.50; 3%, 10 mL = £1.64; 4%, 10 mL = £3.34

Single use

Minims® Pilocarpine Nitrate (Chauvin) PoM
Eye drops, pilocarpine nitrate 2% and 4%, net price 20 × 0.5 mL (both) = £4.92

Long acting

Pilogel® (Alcon) PoM
Ophthalmic gel, pilocarpine hydrochloride 4%, net price 5 g = £6.86
Excipients include benzalkonium chloride, disodium edetate
Dose apply 1–1.5 cm gel once daily at bedtime

11.7 Local anaesthetics

Oxybuprocaine and tetracaine (amethocaine) are probably the most widely used topical local anaesthetics. Proxymetacaine causes less initial stinging and is useful for children. Oxybuprocaine or a combined preparation of lidocaine (lignocaine) and fluorescein is used for tonometry. Tetracaine produces a more profound anaesthesia and is suitable for use before minor surgical procedures, such as the removal of corneal sutures. It has a temporary disruptive effect on the corneal epithelium. Lidocaine, with or without adrenaline (epinephrine), is injected into the eyelids for minor surgery, while retrobulbar or peribulbar injections are used for surgery of the globe itself. Local anaesthetics should never be used for the management of ocular symptoms.

Local anaesthetic eye drops should be avoided in preterm neonates because of the immaturity of the metabolising enzyme system.

LIDOCAINE HYDROCHLORIDE
(Lignocaine hydrochloride)

Indications local anaesthetic

Minims® Lignocaine and Fluorescein (Chauvin) PoM
Eye drops, lidocaine hydrochloride 4%, fluorescein sodium 0.25%. Net price 20 × 0.5 mL = £6.93

OXYBUPROCAINE HYDROCHLORIDE
(Benoxinate hydrochloride)

Indications local anaesthetic

Minims® Oxybuprocaine Hydrochloride (Chauvin) PoM
Eye drops, oxybuprocaine hydrochloride 0.4%. Net price 20 × 0.5 mL = £4.92

PROXYMETACAINE HYDROCHLORIDE

Indications local anaesthetic

Minims® Proxymetacaine (Chauvin) PoM
Eye drops, proxymetacaine hydrochloride 0.5%. Net price 20 × 0.5 mL = £6.95

With fluorescein

Minims® Proxymetacaine and Fluorescein (Chauvin) PoM
Eye drops, proxymetacaine hydrochloride 0.5%, fluorescein sodium 0.25%. Net price 20 × 0.5 mL = £7.95

TETRACAINE HYDROCHLORIDE
(Amethocaine hydrochloride)

Indications local anaesthetic

Minims® Amethocaine Hydrochloride (Chauvin) PoM
Eye drops, tetracaine hydrochloride 0.5% and 1%. Net price 20 × 0.5 mL (both) = £5.75

11.8 Miscellaneous ophthalmic preparations

11.8.1 Tear deficiency, ocular lubricants, and astringents
11.8.2 Ocular diagnostic and peri-operative preparations and photodynamic treatment

Certain eye drops, e.g. amphotericin, ceftazidime, cefuroxime, colistin, desferrioxamine, dexamethasone, gentamicin and vancomycin may be prepared aseptically from material supplied for injection.

11.8.1 Tear deficiency, ocular lubricants, and astringents

Chronic soreness of the eyes associated with reduced or abnormal tear secretion (e.g. in Sjögren's syndrome) often responds to tear replacement therapy or pilocarpine given by mouth (section 12.3.5). The severity of the condition and patient preference will often guide the choice of preparation.

Hypromellose is the traditional choice of treatment for tear deficiency. It may need to be instilled frequently (e.g. hourly) for adequate relief. Ocular surface mucin is often abnormal in tear deficiency and the combination of hypromellose with a mucolytic such as **acetylcysteine** can be helpful.

The ability of **carbomers** to cling to the eye surface may help reduce frequency of application to 4 times daily.

Polyvinyl alcohol increases the persistence of the tear film and is useful when the ocular surface mucin is reduced.

Povidone eye drops are also used in the management of tear deficiency.

Sodium chloride 0.9% drops are sometimes useful in tear deficiency, and can be used as 'comfort drops' by contact lens wearers, and to facilitate lens removal. Special presentations of sodium chloride 0.9% and other irrigation solutions are used routinely for intraocular surgery.

Eye ointments containing a **paraffin** may be used to lubricate the eye surface, especially in cases of recurrent corneal epithelial erosion. They may cause temporary visual disturbance and are best suited for application before sleep. Ointments should not be used during contact lens wear.

Zinc sulphate is a traditional astringent that is now little used.

ACETYLCYSTEINE

Indications tear deficiency, impaired or abnormal mucus production

Dose

- Apply 3–4 times daily

Ilube® (Alcon) PoM
Eye drops, acetylcysteine 5%, hypromellose 0.35%. Net price 10 mL = £4.63
Excipients include benzalkonium chloride, disodium edetate

11 Eye

CARBOMERS
(Polyacrylic acid)

Note Synthetic high molecular weight polymers of acrylic acid cross-linked with either allyl ethers of sucrose or allyl ethers of pentaerithrityl

Indications dry eyes including keratoconjunctivitis sicca, unstable tear film

Dose

- Apply 3–4 times daily or as required

GelTears® (Chauvin)
Gel (= eye drops), carbomer 980 (polyacrylic acid) 0.2%, net price 10 g = £2.80
Excipients include benzalkonium chloride

Liposic® (Chauvin)
Gel (= eye drops), carbomer 980 (polyacrylic acid) 0.2%, net price 10 g = £2.96
Excipients include cetrimide

Liquivisc® (Allergan)
Gel (= eye drops), carbomer 974P (polyacrylic acid) 0.25%, net price 10 g = £1.99
Excipients include benzalkonium chloride
Note May be difficult to obtain

Viscotears® (Novartis)
Liquid gel (= eye drops), carbomer 980 (polyacrylic acid) 0.2%, net price 10 g = £3.12
Excipients include cetrimide, disodium edetate

Liquid gel (= eye drops), carbomer 980 (polyacrylic acid) 0.2%, net price 30 × 0.6-mL single-dose units = £5.75

CARMELLOSE SODIUM

Indications dry eye conditions

Dose

- Apply as required

Celluvisc® (Allergan)
Eye drops, carmellose sodium 0.5%, net price 30 × 0.4 mL = £5.75, 90 × 0.4 mL = £15.53; 1%, 30 × 0.4 mL = £5.75, 60 × 0.4 mL = £10.99

HYDROXYETHYLCELLULOSE

Indications tear deficiency

Minims® Artificial Tears (Chauvin)
Eye drops, hydroxyethylcellulose 0.44%, sodium chloride 0.35%. Net price 20 × 0.5 mL = £5.75

HYPROMELLOSE

Indications tear deficiency

Note The Royal Pharmaceutical Society of Great Britain has stated that where it is not possible to ascertain the strength of hypromellose prescribed, the prescriber should be contacted to clarify the strength intended.

Hypromellose (Non-proprietary)
Eye drops, hypromellose 0.3%, net price 10 mL = 89p
Brands include *Artelac®*

Isopto Alkaline® (Alcon)
Eye drops, hypromellose 1%, net price 10 mL = 99p
Excipients include benzalkonium chloride

Isopto Plain® (Alcon)
Eye drops, hypromellose 0.5%, net price 10 mL = 85p
Excipients include benzalkonium chloride

Tears Naturale® (Alcon)
Eye drops, dextran '70' 0.1%, hypromellose 0.3%, net price 15 mL = £1.68
Excipients include benzalkonium chloride, disodium edetate

Single use

Artelac® SDU (Pharma-Global)
Eye drops, hypromellose 0.32%, net price 30 × 0.5 mL = £13.60

LIQUID PARAFFIN

Indications dry eye conditions

Lacri-Lube® (Allergan)
Eye ointment, white soft paraffin 57.3%, liquid paraffin 42.5%, wool alcohols 0.2%. Net price 3.5 g = £2.28, 5 g = £2.96

Lubri-Tears® (Alcon)
Eye ointment, white soft paraffin 60%, liquid paraffin 30%, wool fat 10%. Net price 5 g = £2.29

PARAFFIN, YELLOW, SOFT

Indications see notes above

Simple Eye Ointment
Ointment, liquid paraffin 10%, wool fat 10%, in yellow soft paraffin. Net price 4 g = £2.68

POLYVINYL ALCOHOL

Indications tear deficiency

Liquifilm Tears® (Allergan)
Ophthalmic solution (= eye drops), polyvinyl alcohol 1.4%. Net price 15 mL = £1.93
Excipients include benzalkonium chloride, disodium edetate

Ophthalmic solution (= eye drops), polyvinyl alcohol 1.4%, povidone 0.6%. Net price 30 × 0.4 mL = £5.35

Sno Tears® (Chauvin)
Eye drops, polyvinyl alcohol 1.4%. Net price 10 mL = £1.06
Excipients include benzalkonium chloride, disodium edetate

POVIDONE

Indications dry eye conditions

Dose

- Apply 4 times daily or as required

Oculotect® (Novartis)
Eye drops, povidone 5%. Net price 20 × 0.4 mL = £3.40

SODIUM CHLORIDE

Indications irrigation, including first-aid removal of harmful substances

Sodium Chloride 0.9% Solutions
See section 13.11.1

Balanced Salt Solution
Solution (sterile), sodium chloride 0.64%, sodium acetate 0.39%, sodium citrate 0.17%, calcium chloride 0.048%, magnesium chloride 0.03%, potassium chloride 0.075%
For intra-ocular or topical irrigation during surgical procedures
Brands include *Iocare®*

■Single use

Minims® Saline (Chauvin)

Eye drops, sodium chloride 0.9%. Net price 20 × 0.5 mL = £4.92

ZINC SULPHATE

Indications see notes above

Cautions see notes above

Zinc Sulphate (Non-proprietary)

Eye drops, zinc sulphate 0.25%. Net price 10 mL = £3.15

11.8.2 Ocular diagnostic and peri-operative preparations and photodynamic treatment

Ocular diagnostic preparations

Fluorescein sodium is used in diagnostic procedures and for locating damaged areas of the cornea due to injury or disease.

FLUORESCEIN SODIUM

Indications detection of lesions and foreign bodies

Minims® Fluorescein Sodium (Chauvin)

Eye drops, fluorescein sodium 1% or 2%. Net price 20 × 0.5 mL (both) = £4.92

■With local anaesthetic

Section 11.7

Ocular peri-operative drugs

Drugs used to prepare the eye for surgery, drugs that are injected into the anterior chamber at the time of surgery, and those used after eye surgery, are included here.

Non-steroidal anti-inflammatory eye drops such as **diclofenac**, **flurbiprofen**, and **ketorolac**, are used for the prophylaxis and treatment of inflammation, pain, and other symptoms associated with ocular surgery or laser treatment of the eye. Diclofenac and flurbiprofen are also used to prevent miosis during ocular surgery.

Apraclonidine, an alpha$_2$-adrenoreceptor agonist, reduces intra-ocular pressure possibly by reducing the production of aqueous humour. It is used to control increases in intra-ocular pressure associated with ocular surgery and as short-term treatment to reduce intra-ocular pressure prior to surgery.

Intra-ocular **sodium hyaluronate** is used during surgical procedures on the eye.

Acetylcholine, instilled into the anterior chamber of the eye during surgery, rapidly produces miosis which lasts approximately 20 minutes. If prolonged miosis is required, it can be applied again.

Balanced salt solution is used routinely during intra-ocular surgery (section 11.8.1).

ACETYLCHOLINE CHLORIDE

Indications cataract surgery, penetrating keratoplasty, iridectomy, and other anterior segment surgery requiring rapid complete miosis

Contra-indications pregnancy; breast-feeding

Side-effects *rarely* bradycardia, hypotension, breathing difficulty, sweating, flushing

Miochol-E® (Novartis) PoM

Intra-ocular irrigation, powder for reconstitution, acetylcholine chloride 10 mg/mL (1%) when reconstituted, net price 20-mg vial (with solvent) = £9.10

APRACLONIDINE

Note Apraclonidine is a derivative of clonidine

Indications control of intra-ocular pressure

Cautions history of angina, severe coronary insufficiency, recent myocardial infarction, heart failure, cerebrovascular disease, vasovagal attack, chronic renal failure; depression; pregnancy and breast-feeding; monitor intra-ocular pressure and visual fields; loss of effect may occur over time; suspend treatment if reduction in vision occurs in end-stage glaucoma; monitor for excessive reduction in intra-ocular pressure following peri-operative use; **interactions:** Appendix 1 (alpha$_2$-adrenoceptor stimulants)

Driving Drowsiness may affect performance of skilled tasks (e.g. driving)

Contra-indications history of severe or unstable and uncontrolled cardiovascular disease

Side-effects dry mouth, taste disturbance; hyperaemia, ocular pruritus, discomfort and lacrimation (withdraw if ocular intolerance including oedema of lids and conjunctiva); headache, asthenia, dry nose; lid retraction, conjunctival blanching and mydriasis reported after peri-operative use; since absorption may follow topical application systemic effects (see Clonidine Hydrochloride, section 2.5.2) may occur

Dose

- See under preparations below

Iopidine® (Alcon) PoM

Ophthalmic solution (= eye drops), apraclonidine 1% (as hydrochloride). Net price 12 × 2 single use 0.25-mL units = £81.90

Dose control or prevention of postoperative elevation of intra-ocular pressure after anterior segment laser surgery, apply 1 drop 1 hour before laser procedure then 1 drop immediately after completion of procedure; CHILD not recommended

Iopidine 0.5% ophthalmic solution (= eye drops), apraclonidine 0.5% (as hydrochloride). Net price 5 mL = £11.45

Excipients include benzalkonium chloride

Dose short-term adjunctive treatment of chronic glaucoma in patients not adequately controlled by another drug (see note below), apply 1 drop 3 times daily usually for max. 1 month; CHILD not recommended

Note May not provide additional benefit if patient already using two drugs that suppress the production of aqueous humour

DICLOFENAC SODIUM

Indications inhibition of intra-operative miosis during cataract surgery (but does not possess intrinsic mydriatic properties); postoperative inflammation in cataract surgery, strabismus surgery or argon laser trabeculoplasty; pain in corneal epithelial defects after photorefractive keratectomy, radial keratotomy or accidental trauma; seasonal allergic conjunctivitis (section 11.4.2)

Voltarol® Ophtha Multidose (Novartis) PoM
Eye drops, diclofenac sodium 0.1%, net price 5 mL = £6.68
Excipients include benzalkonium chloride, disodium edetate, propylene glycol

Single use

Voltarol® Ophtha (Novartis) PoM
Eye drops, diclofenac sodium 0.1%. Net price pack of 5 single-dose units = £4.00, 40 single-dose units = £32.00

FLURBIPROFEN SODIUM

Indications inhibition of intra-operative miosis (but does not possess intrinsic mydriatic properties); anterior segment inflammation following postoperative and post-laser trabeculoplasty when corticosteroids contra-indicated

Ocufen® (Allergan) PoM
Ophthalmic solution (= eye drops), flurbiprofen sodium 0.03%, polyvinyl alcohol (*Liquifilm®*) 1.4%. Net price 40 × 0.4 mL = £37.15

KETOROLAC TROMETAMOL

Indications prophylaxis and reduction of inflammation and associated symptoms following ocular surgery

Acular® (Allergan) PoM
Eye drops, ketorolac trometamol 0.5%. Net price 5 mL = £5.00
Excipients include benzalkonium chloride, disodium edetate

Subfoveal choroidal neovascularisation

Pegaptanib and **ranibizumab** are vascular endothelial growth factor inhibitors licensed for the treatment of neovascular (wet) age-related macular degeneration; they are given by intravitreal injection by specialists experienced in the management of this condition.

Verteporfin is licensed for use in the photodynamic treatment of age-related macular degeneration associated with predominantly classic subfoveal choroidal neovascularisation *or* with pathological myopia (see NICE guidance below). Following intravenous infusion, verteporfin is activated by local irradiation using non-thermal red light to produce cytotoxic derivatives. Only specialists experienced in the management of these conditions should use it.

> NICE guidance
> **Photodynamic therapy for wet age-related macular degeneration (September 2003)**
> Photodynamic therapy is recommended for wet age-related macular degeneration with a confirmed diagnosis of classic (no occult) subfoveal choroidal neovascularisation and best-corrected visual acuity of 6/60 or better.
> Photodynamic therapy is **not** recommended for wet age-related macular degeneration with predominantly classic but partly occult subfoveal choroidal neovascularisation *except* in clinical studies.

PEGAPTANIB SODIUM

Indications see notes above—specialist use only

Cautions monitor intra-ocular pressure following injection; pregnancy (Appendix 4); breast-feeding (Appendix 5)

Contra-indications ocular or periocular infection

Side-effects rhinorrhoea; headache; eye pain, anterior chamber inflammation, raised intra-ocular pressure, punctate keratitis, vitreous floaters, cataract, conjunctival and retinal haemorrhage, local oedema, conjunctivitis, corneal dystrophy, dry eye, endophthalmitis, eye discharge, eye irritation, macular degeneration, mydriasis, periorbital haematoma, photophobia, flashing lights, vitreous disorders; *less commonly* vomiting, dyspepsia, palpitation, chest pain, hypertension, aortic aneurysm, influenza-like symptoms, nightmares, depression, back pain, asthenopia, blepharitis, corneal deposits, vitreous haemorrhage, chalazion, retinal exudates, eyelid ptosis, decreased intra-ocular pressure, injection-site reactions, retinal detachment, occlusion of retinal blood vessels, ectropion, eye movement disorder, pupillary disorder, iritis, optic nerve cupping, nasopharyngitis, deafness, vertigo, eczema, changes in hair colour, rash, pruritus, night sweats

Dose

- By intravitreal injection, 300 micrograms once every 6 weeks into the affected eye

Note For further information on administration, consult product literature

Macugen® (Pfizer) ▼ PoM
Solution for intravitreal injection, pegaptanib (as sodium salt), net price 300-microgram vial = £514.00

RANIBIZUMAB

Indications see notes above—specialist use only

Cautions monitor intra-ocular pressure and for signs of ocular infection following injection; pregnancy (Appendix 4); breast-feeding (Appendix 5)

Contra-indications ocular or periocular infection; severe intra-ocular inflammation

Side-effects nausea; hypertension; headache; bronchitis; anaemia; arthalgia, back pain; conjunctival and retinal haemorrhage, eye pain, vitreous floaters, raised intra-ocular pressure, vitreous detachment, intra-ocular inflammation, eye irritation, cataract, visual disturbance, blepharitis, subretinal fibrosis, ocular hyperaemia, dry eye, posterior capsule opacification, injection-site reactions, increased lacrimation, eye pruritus, conjunctivitis, maculopathy, retinal disorders; *less commonly* atrial fibrillation, cough, wheezing, increased upper airway secretions, iritis, iridocyclitis, keratitis, corneal disorders, vitreous disorders, photophobia, anterior chamber inflammation, angle-closure glaucoma, endophthalmitis, uveitis, eyelid oedema and irritation, blindness, hypopyon, and lichenoid keratosis

Dose

- By intravitreal injection, initially 500 micrograms once a month for 3 months into the affected eye, thereafter monitor visual acuity once a month; if necessary subsequent doses may be given at least 1 month apart

Note For further information on administration, consult product literature

Antimicrobial eye drops should be administered into the affected eye for 3 days before and 3 days after each injection

Lucentis® (Novartis) ▼ PoM

Solution for intravitreal injection, ranibizumab 10 mg/mL, net price 0.3-mL vial = £761.20

VERTEPORFIN

Indications see notes above—specialist use only

Cautions photosensitivity—avoid exposure of unprotected skin and eyes to bright light during infusion and for 48 hours afterwards; hepatic impairment (avoid if severe), biliary obstruction; avoid extravasation; pregnancy (Appendix 4)

Contra-indications porphyria; breast-feeding (Appendix 5)

Side-effects visual disturbances (including blurred vision, flashing lights, visual-field defects), nausea, back pain, asthenia, pruritus, hypercholesterolaemia, fever; *rarely* lacrimation disorder, subretinal or vitreous haemorrhage, hypersensitivity reactions (including chest pain, syncope, headache, dizziness, dyspnoea, urticaria, sweating, changes in blood pressure and in heart rate); injection-site reactions including pain, oedema, inflammation, haemorrhage, discoloration and blistering

Dose

- By intravenous infusion over 10 minutes, 6 mg/m²

Note For information on administration and light activation, consult product literature

Visudyne® (Novartis) PoM

Injection, powder for reconstitution, verteporfin, net price 15-mg vial = £850.00

11.9 Contact lenses

Note Some recommendations in this section involve non-licensed indications.

For cosmetic reasons many people prefer to wear contact lenses rather than spectacles; contact lenses are also sometimes required for medical indications. Visual defects are corrected by either rigid ('hard' or gas permeable) lenses or soft (hydrogel or silicone hydrogel) lenses; soft lenses are the most popular type, because they are the most comfortable, although they may not give the best vision. Lenses should usually be worn for a specified number of hours each day. Continuous (extended) wear involves much greater risks to eye health and is not recommended except where medically indicated.

Contact lenses require meticulous care. Poor compliance with directions for use, and with daily cleaning and disinfection, can result in complications including ulcerative keratitis and conjunctival problems (such as purulent or papillary conjunctivitis). One-day disposable lenses, which are worn only once and therefore require no maintenance or storage, are becoming increasingly popular.

Acanthamoeba keratitis, a sight-threatening condition, is associated with ineffective lens cleaning and disinfection or the use of contaminated lens cases. The condition is especially associated with the use of soft lenses (including frequently replaced lenses). *Acanthamoeba keratitis* is treated, by specialists, with intensive use of polihexanide (polyhexamethylene biguanide), propamidine isetionate (section 11.3.1), chlorhexidine, and neomycin (section 11.3.1) drops sometimes used in combination.

Contact lenses and drug treatment Special care is required in prescribing eye preparations for contact lens users. Some drugs and preservatives in eye preparations can accumulate in hydrogel lenses and may induce toxic reactions. Therefore, unless medically indicated, the lenses should be removed before instillation and not worn during the period of treatment. Alternatively, unpreserved drops can be used. Eye drops may, however, be instilled over rigid corneal contact lenses. Ointment preparations should never be used in conjunction with contact lens wear; oily eye drops should also be avoided.

Many drugs given systemically can also have adverse effects on contact lens wear. These include oral contraceptives (particularly those with a higher oestrogen content), drugs which reduce blink rate (e.g. anxiolytics, hypnotics, antihistamines, and muscle relaxants), drugs which reduce lacrimation (e.g. antihistamines, antimuscarinics, phenothiazines and related drugs, some beta-blockers, diuretics, and tricyclic antidepressants), and drugs which increase lacrimation (including ephedrine and hydralazine). Other drugs that may affect contact lens wear are isotretinoin (can cause conjunctival inflammation) aspirin (salicylic acid appears in tears and can be absorbed by contact lenses—leading to irritation), and rifampicin and sulfasalazine (can discolour lenses).

12 Ear, nose, and oropharynx

12.1 Drugs acting on the ear **582**
12.1.1 Otitis externa 582
12.1.2 Otitis media 585
12.1.3 Removal of ear wax 585
12.2 Drugs acting on the nose **586**
12.2.1 Drugs used in nasal allergy 586
12.2.2 Topical nasal decongestants 588
12.2.3 Nasal preparations for infection 589
12.3 Drugs acting on the oropharynx **590**
12.3.1 Drugs for oral ulceration and inflammation 590
12.3.2 Oropharyngeal anti-infective drugs 592
12.3.3 Lozenges and sprays 594
12.3.4 Mouthwashes, gargles, and dentifrices 594
12.3.5 Treatment of dry mouth 595

This chapter also includes advice on the drug management of the following:

allergic rhinitis, p. 586
nasal polyps, p. 586
oropharyngeal infections, p. 592
periodontitis, p. 590

12.1 Drugs acting on the ear

12.1.1 Otitis externa
12.1.2 Otitis media
12.1.3 Removal of ear wax

12.1.1 Otitis externa

Otitis externa is an inflammatory reaction of the meatal skin. It is important to exclude an underlying chronic otitis media before treatment is commenced. Many cases recover after thorough cleansing of the external ear canal by suction or dry mopping. A frequent problem in resistant cases is the difficulty in applying lotions and ointments satisfactorily to the relatively inaccessible affected skin. The most effective method is to introduce a ribbon gauze dressing or sponge wick soaked with **corticosteroid** ear drops or with an astringent such as **aluminium acetate** solution. When this is not practical, the ear should be gently cleansed with a probe covered in cotton wool and the patient encouraged to lie with the affected ear uppermost for ten minutes after the canal has been filled with a liberal quantity of the appropriate solution.

If infection is present, a topical anti-infective which is not used systemically (such as **neomycin** or **clioquinol**) may be used, but for only about a week as excessive use may result in fungal infections; these may be difficult to treat and require expert advice. Sensitivity to the anti-infective or solvent may occur and resistance to antibacterials is a possibility with prolonged use. Aluminium acetate ear drops are also effective against bacterial infection and inflammation of the ear. **Chloramphenicol** may be used but the ear drops contain propylene glycol and cause hypersensitivity reactions in about 10% of patients. Solutions containing an anti-infective and a corticosteroid (such as *Locorten-Vioform®*) are used for treating cases where infection is present with inflammation and eczema. In view of reports of ototoxicity in patients with a perforated tympanic membrane (eardrum), the CSM has stated that treatment with a topical aminoglycoside antibiotic is contraindicated in those with a tympanic perforation. However, many specialists do use these drops cautiously in the presence of a perforation in patients with otitis media (section 12.1.2) and where other measures have failed for otitis externa.

A solution of **acetic acid** 2% acts as an antifungal and antibacterial in the external ear canal. It may be used to treat mild otitis externa but in severe cases an anti-inflammatory preparation with or without an anti-infective drug is required. A proprietary preparation containing acetic acid 2% (*EarCalm®* spray) is on sale to the public.

For severe pain associated with otitis externa, a simple analgesic, such as **paracetamol** (section 4.7.1) or **ibu-**

profen (section 10.1.1), can be used. A systemic antibacterial (Table 1, section 5.1) can be used if there is spreading cellulitis or if the patient is systemically unwell. When a resistant staphylococcal infection (a boil) is present in the external auditory meatus, **flucloxacillin** is the drug of choice; **ciprofloxacin** (or an aminoglycoside) may be needed in pseudomonal infections which may occur if the patient has diabetes or is immunocompromised.

The skin of the pinna adjacent to the ear canal is often affected by eczema. Topical corticosteroid creams and ointments (section 13.4) are then required, but prolonged use should be avoided.

Astringent preparations

ALUMINIUM ACETATE

Indications inflammation in otitis externa (see notes above)

Dose

- Insert into meatus or apply on a ribbon gauze dressing or sponge wick which should be kept saturated with the ear drops

Aluminium Acetate (Non-proprietary)
Ear drops 13%, aluminium sulphate 2.25 g, calcium carbonate 1 g, tartaric acid 450 mg, acetic acid (33%) 2.5 mL, purified water 7.5 mL
Available from manufacturers of 'special order' products

Ear drops 8%, dilute 8 parts aluminium acetate ear drops (13%) with 5 parts purified water. Must be freshly prepared

Anti-inflammatory preparations

Corticosteroids

Topical corticosteroids are used to treat inflammation and eczema in otitis externa.

Cautions Prolonged use of topical corticosteroid ear preparations should be avoided.

Contra-indications Corticosteroid ear preparations should be avoided in the presence of an untreated ear infection. If infection is present, the corticosteroid should be used in combination with a suitable anti-infective (see notes above).

Side-effects Local sensitivity reactions may occur.

BETAMETHASONE SODIUM PHOSPHATE

Indications eczematous inflammation in otitis externa (see notes above)
Cautions see notes above
Contra-indications see notes above
Side-effects see notes above

Betnesol® (Celltech) PoM
Drops (for ear, eye, or nose), betamethasone sodium phosphate 0.1%. Net price 10 mL = £2.32
Excipients include benzalkonium chloride, disodium edetate
Dose ear, apply 2–3 drops every 2–3 hours; reduce frequency when relief obtained; eye, section 11.4.1; nose, section 12.2.1

Vista-Methasone® (Martindale) PoM
Drops (for ear, eye, or nose), betamethasone sodium phosphate 0.1%. Net price 5 mL = £1.10; 10 mL = £1.25
Excipients include benzalkonium chloride, disodium edetate
Dose ear, apply 2–3 drops every 3–4 hours; reduce frequency when relief obtained; eye, section 11.4.1; nose, section 12.2.1

With antibacterial

Betnesol-N® (Celltech) PoM
Drops (for ear, eye, or nose), betamethasone sodium phosphate 0.1%, neomycin sulphate 0.5%. Net price 10 mL = £2.39
Excipients include benzalkonium chloride, disodium edetate
Dose ear, apply 2–3 drops 3–4 times daily; eye, section 11.4.1; nose, section 12.2.3

Vista-Methasone N® (Martindale) PoM
Drops (for ear, eye, or nose), betamethasone sodium phosphate 0.1%, neomycin sulphate 0.5%. Net price 5 mL = £1.09; 10 mL = £1.20
Excipients include thiomersal
Dose ear, apply 2–3 drops every 3–4 hours; reduce frequency when relief obtained; eye, section 11.4.1; nose, section 12.2.3

DEXAMETHASONE

Indications eczematous inflammation in otitis externa (see notes above)
Cautions see notes above
Contra-indications see notes above
Side-effects see notes above

With antibacterial

Otomize® (GSK Consumer Healthcare) PoM
Ear spray, dexamethasone 0.1%, neomycin sulphate 3250 units/mL, glacial acetic acid 2%. Net price 5-mL pump-action aerosol unit = £4.24
Excipients include hydroxybenzoates (parabens)
Dose ear, apply 1 metered spray 3 times daily

Sofradex® (Sanofi-Aventis) PoM
Drops (for ear or eye), dexamethasone (as sodium metasulphobenzoate) 0.05%, framycetin sulphate 0.5%, gramicidin 0.005%. Net price 10 mL = £5.21
Excipients include polysorbate 80
Dose ear, apply 2–3 drops 3–4 times daily; eye, section 11.4.1

FLUMETASONE PIVALATE
(Flumethasone Pivalate)

Indications eczematous inflammation in otitis externa (see notes above)
Cautions see notes above
Contra-indications see notes above
Side-effects see notes above

With antibacterial

Locorten-Vioform® (Amdipharm) PoM
Ear drops, flumetasone pivalate 0.02%, clioquinol 1%. Net price 7.5 mL = £1.47
Contra-indications iodine sensitivity
Dose ADULT and CHILD over 2 years apply 2–3 drops into the ear twice daily for 7–10 days
Note Clioquinol stains skin and clothing

HYDROCORTISONE

Indications eczematous inflammation in otitis externa (see notes above)
Cautions see notes above
Contra-indications see notes above
Side-effects see notes above

With antibacterial

Gentisone® HC (Roche) PoM
Ear drops, hydrocortisone acetate 1%, gentamicin 0.3% (as sulphate). Net price 10 mL = £3.69
Excipients include benzalkonium chloride, disodium edetate
Dose ear, apply 2–4 drops 3–4 times daily and at night

Neo-Cortef® (PLIVA) PoM
Ointment (for ear or eye), hydrocortisone acetate 1.5%, neomycin sulphate 0.5%. Net price 3.9 g = £1.53
Excipients include wool fat
Dose ear, apply 1–2 times daily; eye, see section 11.4.1
Note May be difficult to obtain

Otosporin® (GSK) PoM
Ear drops, hydrocortisone 1%, neomycin sulphate 3400 units, polymyxin B sulphate 10 000 units/mL. Net price 5 mL = £2.00; 10 mL = £4.00
Excipients include cetostearyl alcohol, hydroxybenzoates (parabens), polysorbate 20
Dose ADULT and CHILD over 3 years, ear, apply 3 drops 3–4 times daily

PREDNISOLONE SODIUM PHOSPHATE

Indications eczematous inflammation in otitis externa (see notes above)
Cautions see notes above
Contra-indications see notes above
Side-effects see notes above

Predsol® (Celltech) PoM
Drops (for ear or eye), prednisolone sodium phosphate 0.5%. Net price 10 mL = £2.00
Excipients include benzalkonium chloride, disodium edetate
Dose ear, apply 2–3 drops every 2–3 hours; reduce frequency when relief obtained; eye, section 11.4.1

With antibacterial

Predsol-N® (Celltech) PoM
Drops (for ear or eye), prednisolone sodium phosphate 0.5%, neomycin sulphate 0.5%. Net price 10 mL = £2.36
Excipients include benzalkonium chloride, disodium edetate
Dose ear, apply 2–3 drops 3–4 times daily; eye, section 11.4.1

TRIAMCINOLONE ACETONIDE

Indications eczematous inflammation in otitis externa (see notes above)
Cautions see notes above
Contra-indications see notes above
Side-effects see notes above

With antibacterial

Tri-Adcortyl Otic® (Squibb) PoM
Ear ointment, triamcinolone acetonide 0.1%, gramicidin 0.025%, neomycin 0.25% (as sulphate), nystatin 100 000 units/g in *Plastibase®*. Net price 10 g = £1.58
Dose ear, ADULT and CHILD over 1 year, apply 2–3 times daily

Anti-infective preparations

CHLORAMPHENICOL

Indications bacterial infection in otitis externa (but see notes above)
Cautions avoid prolonged use (see notes above)
Side-effects high incidence of sensitivity reactions to vehicle

Chloramphenicol (Non-proprietary) PoM
Ear drops, chloramphenicol in propylene glycol, net price 5%, 10 mL = £1.41; 10%, 10 mL = £1.40
Dose ear, apply 2–3 drops 2–3 times daily

CLIOQUINOL

Indications mild bacterial or fungal infections in otitis externa (see notes above)
Cautions avoid prolonged use (see notes above); manufacturer advises avoid in perforated tympanic membrane (but used by specialists for short periods)
Side-effects local sensitivity; stains skin and clothing

With corticosteroid

Locorten-Vioform® see Flumetasone, p. 583

CLOTRIMAZOLE

Indications fungal infection in otitis externa (see notes above)
Side-effects occasional local irritation or sensitivity

Canesten® (Bayer Consumer Care)
Solution, clotrimazole 1% in polyethylene glycol 400 (macrogol 400). Net price 20 mL = £2.43
Dose ear, apply 2–3 times daily continuing for at least 14 days after disappearance of infection; skin, section 13.10.2

FRAMYCETIN SULPHATE

Indications bacterial infection in otitis externa (see notes above)
Cautions avoid prolonged use (see notes above)
Contra-indications perforated tympanic membrane (see notes above)
Side-effects local sensitivity

With corticosteroid

Sofradex® see Dexamethasone, p. 583

GENTAMICIN

Indications bacterial infection in otitis externa (see notes above)
Cautions avoid prolonged use (see notes above)
Contra-indications perforated tympanic membrane (but see also notes above and section 12.1.2)
Side-effects local sensitivity

Genticin® (Roche) PoM
Drops (for ear or eye), gentamicin 0.3% (as sulphate). Net price 10 mL = £1.91
Excipients include benzalkonium chloride
Dose ear, apply 2–3 drops 3–4 times daily and at night; eye, section 11.3.1

With corticosteroid

Gentisone® HC see Hydrocortisone, above

NEOMYCIN SULPHATE

Indications bacterial infection in otitis externa (see notes above)
Cautions avoid prolonged use (see notes above)
Contra-indications perforated tympanic membrane (see notes above)
Side-effects local sensitivity

With corticosteroid
Betnesol-N® see Betamethasone, p. 583

Neo-Cortef® see Hydrocortisone, p. 584

Otomize® see Dexamethasone, p. 583

Otosporin® see Hydrocortisone, p. 584

Predsol-N® see Prednisolone, p. 584

Tri-Adcortyl Otic® see Triamcinolone, p. 584

Vista-Methasone N® see Betamethasone, p. 583

12.1.2 Otitis media

Acute otitis media Acute otitis media is the commonest cause of severe pain in small children. Many infections, especially those accompanying coryza, are caused by viruses. Most uncomplicated cases resolve without antibacterial treatment and a **simple analgesic**, such as paracetamol, may be sufficient. In children without systemic features, a **systemic antibacterial** may be started after 72 hours if there is no improvement, or earlier in immunocompromised patients, in children under 2 years, or if there is deterioration (Table 1, section 5.1). Topical treatment of acute otitis media is ineffective and there is no place for drops containing a local anaesthetic. Perforation of the tympanic membrane in patients with *acute otitis media* usually heals spontaneously without treatment; if there is no improvement, e.g. pain or discharge persists, a systemic antibacterial (Table 1, section 5.1) can be given.

Otitis media with effusion Otitis media with effusion ('glue ear') occurs in about 10% of children and in 90% of children with cleft palates. Systemic antibacterials are not usually required. If 'glue ear' persists for more than a month or two, the child should be referred for assessment and follow up because of the risk of long-term hearing impairment which can delay language development. Untreated or resistant glue ear may be responsible for some types of *chronic otitis media*.

Chronic otitis media Opportunistic organisms are often present in the debris, keratin, and necrotic bone of the middle ear and mastoid in patients with chronic otitis media. The mainstay of treatment is thorough cleansing with aural microsuction which may completely resolve long-standing infection. Local cleansing of the meatal and middle ear may be followed by treatment with a sponge wick or ribbon gauze dressing soaked with corticosteroid ear drops or with an astringent such as aluminium acetate solution; this is particularly beneficial for discharging ears or infections of the mastoid cavity. An antibacterial ear ointment may also be used. Acute exacerbations of chronic infection may also require systemic treatment with amoxicillin (or erythromycin if penicillin-allergic); treatment is adjusted according to the results of sensitivity testing. Parenteral antibacterials are required if *Pseudomonas aeruginosa* and *Proteus* spp. are present.

The CSM has stated that topical treatment with ototoxic antibacterials is contra-indicated in the presence of a perforation (section 12.1.1). However, many specialists use ear drops containing **aminoglycosides** (e.g. neomycin) or **polymyxins** if the otitis media has failed to settle with systemic antibacterials; it is considered that the pus in the middle ear associated with otitis media carries a higher risk of ototoxicity than the drops themselves. Ciprofloxacin or ofloxacin ear drops [both unlicensed; available on named-patient basis from a specialist importing company] or eye drops used in the ear [unlicensed indication] are an effective alternative to aminoglycoside ear drops for chronic otitis media in patients with perforation of the tympanic membrane.

12.1.3 Removal of ear wax

Wax is a normal bodily secretion which provides a protective film on the meatal skin and need only be removed if it causes deafness or interferes with a proper view of the ear drum. Syringing is generally best avoided in young children, in patients with a history of recurrent otitis externa, a history of ear-drum perforation, or previous ear surgery. A person who has hearing in one ear only should not have that ear syringed because even a very slight risk of damage is unacceptable in this situation.

Wax may be removed by syringing with water (warmed to body temperature). If necessary, wax can be softened using simple remedies such as **olive oil** ear drops or **almond oil** ear drops; **sodium bicarbonate** ear drops are also effective but may cause dryness of the ear canal. If the wax is hard and impacted the drops may be used twice daily for a few days before syringing; otherwise the wax may be softened on the day of syringing. The patient should lie with the affected ear uppermost for 5 to 10 minutes after a generous amount of the softening remedy has been introduced into the ear. Some proprietary preparations containing organic solvents can irritate the meatal skin, and in most cases the simple remedies indicated above are just as effective and less likely to cause irritation. Docusate sodium or urea–hydrogen peroxide are ingredients in a number of proprietary preparations for softening ear wax.

Almond Oil (Non-proprietary)
Ear drops, almond oil in a suitable container
Allow to warm to room temperature before use

Olive Oil (Non-proprietary)
Ear drops, olive oil in a suitable container
Allow to warm to room temperature before use

Sodium Bicarbonate (Non-proprietary)
Ear drops, sodium bicarbonate 5%, net price 10 mL = £1.25

Cerumol® (LAB)
Ear drops, chlorobutanol 5%, paradichlorobenzene 2%, arachis (peanut) oil 57.3%. Net price 11 mL = £1.76

Exterol® (Dermal)
Ear drops, urea–hydrogen peroxide complex 5% in glycerol. Net price 8 mL = £1.83

Molcer® (Wallace Mfg)
Ear drops, docusate sodium 5%. Net price 15 mL = £1.90
Excipients include propylene glycol

Otex® (DDD)
Ear drops, urea–hydrogen peroxide 5%. Net price 8 mL = £2.64

Waxsol® (Norgine)
Ear drops, docusate sodium 0.5%. Net price 10 mL = £1.26

12.2 Drugs acting on the nose

12.2.1 Drugs used in nasal allergy
12.2.2 Topical nasal decongestants
12.2.3 Nasal preparations for infection

Rhinitis is often self-limiting but bacterial sinusitis may require treatment with antibacterials (Table 1, section 5.1). There are few indications for nasal sprays and drops except in allergic rhinitis and perennial rhinitis (section 12.2.1). Many nasal preparations contain sympathomimetic drugs which may damage the nasal cilia (section 12.2.2). **Sodium chloride 0.9%** solution may be used as a douche or 'sniff' following endonasal surgery.

Nasal polyps Short-term use of corticosteroid nasal drops helps to shrink nasal polyps; to be effective, the drops must be administered with the patient in the 'head down' position. A short course of a systemic corticosteroid (section 6.3.2) may be required initially to shrink large polyps. A corticosteroid nasal spray can be used to maintain the reduction in swelling and also for the initial treatment of small polyps.

12.2.1 Drugs used in nasal allergy

Mild allergic rhinitis is controlled by **antihistamines** (see also section 3.4.1) or topical **nasal corticosteroids**; systemic nasal decongestants are of doubtful value (section 3.10). Topical nasal decongestants can be used for a short period to relieve congestion and allow penetration of a topical nasal corticosteroid.

More persistent symptoms and nasal congestion can be relieved by topical nasal **corticosteroids** or **cromoglicate** (cromoglycate); although it may be less effective, cromoglicate is often the first choice in children. The topical antihistamine **azelastine** is useful for controlling breakthrough symptoms in allergic rhinitis. Topical antihistamines are considered less effective than topical corticosteroids but probably more effective than cromoglicate. In seasonal allergic rhinitis (e.g. hay fever), treatment should begin 2 to 3 weeks before the season commences and may have to be continued for several months; continuous treatment may be required for years in perennial rhinitis.

Montelukast (section 3.3.2) can be used in patients with seasonal allergic rhinitis and concomitant asthma; montelukast is less effective than topical nasal corticosteroids.

Sometimes allergic rhinitis is accompanied by vasomotor rhinitis. In this situation, the addition of topical nasal ipratropium bromide (section 12.2.2) can reduce watery rhinorrhoea.

Very disabling symptoms occasionally justify the use of **systemic corticosteroids** for short periods (section 6.3), for example, in students taking important examinations. They may also be used at the beginning of a course of treatment with a corticosteroid spray to relieve severe mucosal oedema and allow the spray to penetrate the nasal cavity.

Pregnancy If a pregnant woman cannot tolerate the symptoms of allergic rhinitis, treatment with nasal beclometasone or sodium cromoglicate may be considered.

Antihistamines

AZELASTINE HYDROCHLORIDE

Indications allergic rhinitis

Side-effects irritation of nasal mucosa; bitter taste (if applied incorrectly)

Rhinolast® (Viatris) PoM
Nasal spray, azelastine hydrochloride 140 micrograms (0.14 mL)/metered spray. Net price 22 mL (with metered pump) = £11.09
Excipients include sodium edetate

Dose ADULT and CHILD over 5 years, 140 micrograms (1 spray) into each nostril twice daily

Note Preparations of azelastine hydrochloride can be sold to the public for nasal administration in aqueous form (other than by aerosol) if supplied for the treatment of seasonal allergic rhinitis or perennial allergic rhinitis in adults and children over 5 years, subject to max. single dose of 140 micrograms per nostril, max. daily dose of 280 micrograms per nostril, and a pack size limit of 36 doses

Corticosteroids

Nasal preparations containing corticosteroids (beclometasone, betamethasone, budesonide, flunisolide, fluticasone, mometasone, and triamcinolone) have a useful role in the prophylaxis and treatment of allergic rhinitis (see notes above).

Cautions Corticosteroid nasal preparations should be avoided in the presence of untreated nasal infections, and also after nasal surgery (until healing has occurred); they should also be avoided in pulmonary tuberculosis. Patients transferred from systemic corticosteroids may experience exacerbation of some symptoms. Systemic absorption may follow nasal administration particularly if high doses are used or if treatment is prolonged; for cautions and side-effects of systemic corticosteroids, see section 6.3.2. The risk of systemic effects may be greater with nasal drops than with nasal sprays; drops are administered incorrectly more often than sprays. The CSM recommends that the height of children receiving prolonged treatment with nasal corticosteroids is monitored; if growth is slowed, referral to a paediatrician should be considered.

Side-effects Local side-effects include dryness, irritation of nose and throat, epistaxis and rarely ulceration; nasal septal perforation (usually following nasal surgery)

and raised intra-ocular pressure or glaucoma may also occur rarely. Headache, smell and taste disturbances may also occur. Hypersensitivity reactions, including bronchospasm, have been reported.

BECLOMETASONE DIPROPIONATE
(Beclomethasone Dipropionate)

Indications prophylaxis and treatment of allergic and vasomotor rhinitis

Cautions see notes above

Side-effects see notes above

Dose

- ADULT and CHILD over 6 years, 100 micrograms (2 sprays) into each nostril twice daily; max. total 400 micrograms (8 sprays) daily; when symptoms controlled, dose reduced to 50 micrograms (1 spray) into each nostril twice daily

[1]**Beclometasone** (Non-proprietary) PoM

Nasal spray, beclometasone dipropionate 50 micrograms/metered spray. Net price 200-spray unit = £3.97

Brands include *Nasobec Aqueous*®

1. Can be sold to the public for nasal administration (other than by aerosol) if supplied for the prevention and treatment of allergic rhinitis in adults over 18 years subject to max. single dose of 100 micrograms per nostril, max. daily dose of 200 micrograms per nostril for max. 3 months, and a pack size of 20 mg

Beconase® (A&H) PoM

Nasal spray (aqueous suspension), beclometasone dipropionate 50 micrograms/metered spray. Net price 200-spray unit with applicator = £2.19

Excipients include benzalkonium chloride, polysorbate 80

BETAMETHASONE SODIUM PHOSPHATE

Indications non-infected inflammatory conditions of nose

Cautions see notes above

Side-effects see notes above

Betnesol® (Celltech) PoM

Drops (for ear, eye, or nose), betamethasone sodium phosphate 0.1%, net price 10 mL = £2.32

Excipients include benzalkonium chloride, disodium edetate

Dose nose, 2–3 drops into each nostril 2–3 times daily; ear, section 12.1.1; eye, section 11.4.1

Vista-Methasone® (Martindale) PoM

Drops (for ear, eye, or nose), betamethasone sodium phosphate 0.1%. Net price 5 mL = £1.02, 10 mL = £1.16

Excipients include benzalkonium chloride, disodium edetate

Dose nose, 2–3 drops into each nostril twice daily; ear, section 12.1.1; eye, section 11.4.1

BUDESONIDE

Indications prophylaxis and treatment of allergic and vasomotor rhinitis; nasal polyps

Cautions see notes above; **interactions**: Appendix 1 (corticosteroids)

Side-effects see notes above

Dose

- See preparations

[1]**Budesonide** (Non-proprietary) PoM

Nasal spray, budesonide 100 micrograms/metered spray, net price 100-spray unit = £4.49

Dose rhinitis, ADULT and CHILD over 12 years, 200 micrograms (2 sprays) into each nostril once daily in the morning *or* 100 micrograms (1 spray) into each nostril twice daily; when control achieved reduce to 100 micrograms (1 spray) into each nostril once daily

Nasal polyps, ADULT and CHILD over 12 years, 100 micrograms (1 spray) into each nostril twice daily for up to 3 months

1. Can be sold to the public for nasal administration (other than by aerosol) if supplied for the prevention and treatment of seasonal allergic rhinitis in adults over 18 years subject to max. single dose of 200 micrograms per nostril, max. daily dose of 200 micrograms per nostril for max. period of 3 months, and a pack size of 10 mg

Rhinocort Aqua® (AstraZeneca) PoM

Nasal spray, budesonide 64 micrograms/metered spray. Net price 120-spray unit = £4.49

Excipients include disodium edetate, polysorbate 80, potassium sorbate

Dose rhinitis, ADULT and CHILD over 12 years, 128 micrograms (2 sprays) into each nostril once daily in the morning *or* 64 micrograms (1 spray) into each nostril twice daily; when control achieved reduce to 64 micrograms (1 spray) into each nostril once daily; max. duration of treatment 3 months

Nasal polyps, ADULT and CHILD over 12 years, 64 micrograms (1 spray) into each nostril twice daily for up to 3 months

FLUNISOLIDE

Indications prophylaxis and treatment of allergic rhinitis

Cautions see notes above

Side-effects see notes above

Syntaris® (IVAX) PoM

Aqueous nasal spray, flunisolide 25 micrograms/metered spray. Net price 240-spray unit with pump and applicator = £5.05

Excipients include benzalkonium chloride, butylated hydroxytoluene, disodium edetate, polysorbate 20, propylene glycol

Dose ADULT, 50 micrograms (2 sprays) into each nostril twice daily, increased if necessary to max. 3 times daily then reduced for maintenance; CHILD 5–14 years initially 25 micrograms (1 spray) into each nostril up to 3 times daily

FLUTICASONE PROPIONATE

Indications prophylaxis and treatment of allergic rhinitis and perennial rhinitis; nasal polyps

Cautions see notes above; **interactions**: Appendix 1 (corticosteroids)

Side-effects see notes above

Dose

- Rhinitis, 100 micrograms (2 sprays) into each nostril once daily, preferably in the morning, increased to max. twice daily if required; when control achieved reduce to 50 micrograms (1 spray) into each nostril once daily; CHILD 4–11 years, 50 micrograms (1 spray) into each nostril once daily, preferably in the morning, increased to max. twice daily if required
- Nasal polyps, see *Flixonase Nasule®* below

Flixonase® (A&H) PoM

Aqueous nasal spray, fluticasone propionate 50 micrograms/metered spray. Net price 150-spray unit with applicator = £11.69

Excipients include benzalkonium chloride, polysorbate 80

Note Preparations of fluticasone propionate can be sold to the public for nasal administration (other than by pressurised nasal spray) if supplied for the prevention and treatment of allergic rhinitis in adults over 18 years, subject to max. single dose of 100 micrograms per nostril, max. daily dose of

200 micrograms per nostril for max. 3 months, and a pack size of 3 mg

Flixonase Nasule® (A&H) PoM
Nasal drops, fluticasone propionate 400 micrograms/unit dose, net price 28 × 0.4-mL units = £13.76
Excipients include polysorbate 20
Dose nasal polyps, ADULT and ADOLESCENT over 16 years, 200 micrograms (approx. 6 drops) into each nostril once or twice daily; consider alternative treatment if no improvement after 4–6 weeks

Nasofan® (IVAX) PoM
Aqueous nasal spray fluticasone propionate 50 micrograms/metered spray. Net price 150-spray unit = £10.52
Excipients include benzalkonium chloride, polysorbate 80

MOMETASONE FUROATE

Indications see preparations
Cautions see notes above
Side-effects see notes above

Nasonex® (Schering-Plough) PoM
Nasal spray, mometasone furoate 50 micrograms/metered spray. Net price 140-spray unit = £7.83
Excipients include benzalkonium chloride, polysorbate 80
Dose prophylaxis and treatment of allergic rhinitis, ADULT and CHILD over 12 years, 100 micrograms (2 sprays) into each nostril once daily, increased if necessary to max. 200 micrograms (4 sprays) into each nostril once daily; when control achieved reduce to 50 micrograms (1 spray) into each nostril once daily; CHILD 6–11 years, 50 micrograms (1 spray) into each nostril once daily
Nasal polyps, ADULT over 18 years, 100 micrograms (2 sprays) into each nostril once daily, increased if necessary after 5–6 weeks to 100 micrograms (2 sprays) into each nostril twice daily (consider alternative treatment if no improvement after further 5–6 weeks); reduce dose when control achieved

TRIAMCINOLONE ACETONIDE

Indications prophylaxis and treatment of allergic rhinitis
Cautions see notes above
Side-effects see notes above

Nasacort® (Aventis Pharma) PoM
Aqueous nasal spray, triamcinolone acetonide 55 micrograms/metered spray. Net price 120-spray unit = £7.39
Excipients include benzalkonium chloride, disodium edetate, polysorbate 80
Dose ADULT and CHILD over 12 years 110 micrograms (2 sprays) into each nostril once daily; when control achieved, reduce to 55 micrograms (1 spray) into each nostril once daily; CHILD 6–12 years, 55 micrograms (1 spray) into each nostril once daily
Note Preparations of triamcinolone acetonide can be sold to the public for nasal administration as a non-pressurised nasal spray if supplied for the symptomatic treatment of seasonal allergic rhinitis in adults over 18 years, subject to max. daily dose of 110 micrograms per nostril for max. 3 months, and a pack size of 3.575 mg

Cromoglicate

SODIUM CROMOGLICATE
(Sodium Cromoglycate)

Indications prophylaxis of allergic rhinitis
Side-effects local irritation; rarely transient bronchospasm

Rynacrom® (Sanofi-Aventis)
4% aqueous nasal spray, sodium cromoglicate 4% (5.2 mg/spray). Net price 22 mL with pump = £17.76
Excipients include benzalkonium chloride, disodium edetate
Dose ADULT and CHILD, 1 spray into each nostril 2–4 times daily

Vividrin® (Pharma-Global)
Nasal spray, sodium cromoglicate 2%. Net price 15 mL = £9.85
Excipients include benzalkonium chloride, edetic acid, polysorbate 80
Dose ADULT and CHILD, 1 spray into each nostril 4–6 times daily

12.2.2 Topical nasal decongestants

The nasal mucosa is sensitive to changes in atmospheric temperature and humidity and these alone may cause slight nasal congestion. The nose and nasal sinuses produce a litre of mucus in 24 hours and much of this finds its way silently into the stomach via the nasopharynx. Slight changes in the nasal airway, accompanied by an awareness of mucus passing along the nasopharynx causes some patients to be inaccurately diagnosed as suffering from chronic sinusitis. These symptoms are particularly noticeable in the later stages of the common cold. **Sodium chloride** 0.9% given as nasal drops may relieve nasal congestion by helping to liquefy mucous secretions.

Symptoms of nasal congestion associated with vasomotor rhinitis and the common cold can be relieved by the short-term use (usually not longer than 7 days) of decongestant nasal drops and sprays. These all contain sympathomimetic drugs which exert their effect by vasoconstriction of the mucosal blood vessels which in turn reduces oedema of the nasal mucosa. They are of limited value because they can give rise to a rebound congestion (rhinitis medicamentosa) on withdrawal, due to a secondary vasodilation with a subsequent temporary increase in nasal congestion. This in turn tempts the further use of the decongestant, leading to a vicious cycle of events. **Ephedrine nasal drops** is the safest sympathomimetic preparation and can give relief for several hours. The more potent sympathomimetic drugs oxymetazoline, and xylometazoline are more likely to cause a rebound effect. All of these preparations may cause a hypertensive crisis if used during treatment with a monoamine-oxidase inhibitor including moclobemide.

Non-allergic watery rhinorrhoea often responds well to treatment with the antimuscarinic **ipratropium bromide**.

Inhalation of **warm moist air** is useful in the treatment of symptoms of acute infective conditions. The addition of volatile substances such as menthol and eucalyptus may encourage the use of warm moist air (section 3.8).

Systemic nasal decongestants—see section 3.10.

Sinusitis and oral pain Sinusitis affecting the maxillary antrum can cause pain in the upper jaw. Where this is associated with blockage of the opening from the sinus into the nasal cavity, it may be helpful to relieve the congestion with inhalation of warm moist air (section 3.8) or with **ephedrine nasal drops** (see above). For antibacterial treatment of sinusitis, see Table 1, section 5.1.

Sympathomimetics

EPHEDRINE HYDROCHLORIDE

Indications nasal congestion

Cautions see notes above; also avoid excessive or prolonged use; caution in infants under 3 months (no good evidence of value—if irritation occurs might narrow nasal passage); **interactions**: Appendix 1 (sympathomimetics)

Side-effects local irritation, nausea, headache; after excessive use tolerance with diminished effect, rebound congestion; cardiovascular effects also reported

Dose

- See below

Ephedrine (Non-proprietary)

Nasal drops, ephedrine hydrochloride 0.5%, net price 10 mL = £1.25; 1%, 10 mL = £1.31

Note The BP directs that if no strength is specified 0.5% drops should be supplied

Dose 1–2 drops into each nostril up to 3 or 4 times daily when required; CHILD over 3 months, 1–2 drops of 0.5% solution into each nostril 3–4 times daily; max. duration 7 days

Dental prescribing on NHS Ephedrine nasal drops may be prescribed

XYLOMETAZOLINE HYDROCHLORIDE

Indications nasal congestion

Cautions see under Ephedrine Hydrochloride and notes above

Side-effects see under Ephedrine Hydrochloride and notes above

Dose

- See below

Xylometazoline (Non-proprietary)

Nasal drops, xylometazoline hydrochloride 0.1%, net price 10 mL = £1.91

Dose 2–3 drops into each nostril 2–3 times daily when required; max. duration 7 days; not recommended for children under 12 years

Brands include *Otradrops*®, *Otrivine*® NHS

Paediatric nasal drops, xylometazoline hydrochloride 0.05%, net price 10 mL = £1.59

Dose CHILD over 3 months 1–2 drops into each nostril 1–2 times daily when required (not recommended for infants under 3 months of age, doctor's advice only under 2 years); max. duration 7 days

Brands include *Otradrops*®, *Otrivine*® NHS, *Tixycolds*®

Nasal spray, xylometazoline hydrochloride 0.1%, net price 10 mL = £1.91

Dose 1 spray into each nostril 2–3 times daily when required; max. duration 7 days; not recommended for children under 12 years

Brands include *Otraspray*®, *Otrivine*® NHS

Antimuscarinic

IPRATROPIUM BROMIDE

Indications rhinorrhoea associated with allergic and non-allergic rhinitis

Cautions see section 3.1.2; avoid spraying near eyes

Side-effects epistaxis, nasal dryness, and irritation; less frequently nausea, headache, and pharyngitis; *very rarely* antimuscarinic effects such as gastro-intestinal motility disturbances, palpitations, and urinary retention

Dose

- ADULT and CHILD over 12 years, 42 micrograms (2 sprays) into each nostril 2–3 times daily

Rinatec® (Boehringer Ingelheim) PoM

Nasal spray 0.03%, ipratropium bromide 21 micrograms/metered spray. Net price 180-dose unit = £4.55

Excipients include benzalkonium chloride, disodium edetate

12.2.3 Nasal preparations for infection

There is **no** evidence that topical anti-infective nasal preparations have any therapeutic value in rhinitis or sinusitis; for elimination of nasal staphylococci, see below.

Systemic treatment of sinusitis—see Table 1 section 5.1

Betnesol-N® (Celltech) PoM

Drops (for ear, eye, or nose), betamethasone sodium phosphate 0.1%, neomycin sulphate 0.5%. Net price 10 mL = £2.39

Excipients include benzalkonium chloride, disodium edetate

Dose nose, 2–3 drops into each nostril 2–3 times daily; eye, section 11.4.1; ear, section 12.1.1

Vista-Methasone N® (Martindale) PoM

Drops (for ear, eye, or nose), betamethasone sodium phosphate 0.1%, neomycin sulphate 0.5%. Net price 5 mL = £1.09, 10 mL = £1.20

Excipients include thiomersal

Dose nose, 2–3 drops into each nostril twice daily; eye, section 11.4.1; ear, section 12.1.1

Nasal staphylococci

Elimination of organisms such as staphylococci from the nasal vestibule can be achieved by the use of a cream containing **chlorhexidine and neomycin** (*Naseptin*®), but re-colonisation frequently occurs. Coagulase-positive staphylococci are present in the noses of 40% of the population.

A nasal ointment containing **mupirocin** is also available; it should probably be held in reserve for resistant cases. In hospital or in care establishments, mupirocin nasal ointment should be reserved for the eradication (in both patients and staff) of nasal carriage of meticillin-resistant *Staphylococcus aureus* (MRSA). The ointment should be applied 3 times daily for 5 days and a sample taken 2 days after treatment to confirm eradication. The course may be repeated if the sample is positive (and the throat is not colonised). To avoid the development of resistance, the treatment course should not exceed 7 days and the course should not be repeated on more than one occasion. If the MRSA strain is mupirocin-resistant or does not respond after 2 courses, consider alternative products such as chlorhexidine and neomycin cream.

Bactroban Nasal® (GSK) PoM
Nasal ointment, mupirocin 2% (as calcium salt) in white soft paraffin basis. Net price 3 g = £5.80
Dose for eradication of nasal carriage of staphylococci, including meticillin-resistant *Staphylococcus aureus* (MRSA), apply 2–3 times daily to the inner surface of each nostril

Naseptin® (Alliance) PoM
Cream, chlorhexidine hydrochloride 0.1%, neomycin sulphate 0.5%, net price 15 g = £1.58
Excipients include arachis (peanut) oil, cetostearyl alcohol
Dose for eradication of nasal carriage of staphylococci, apply to nostrils 4 times daily for 10 days; for preventing nasal carriage of staphylococci apply to nostrils twice daily

12.3 Drugs acting on the oropharynx

12.3.1 Drugs for oral ulceration and inflammation
12.3.2 Oropharyngeal anti-infective drugs
12.3.3 Lozenges and sprays
12.3.4 Mouthwashes, gargles, and dentifrices
12.3.5 Treatment of dry mouth

12.3.1 Drugs for oral ulceration and inflammation

Ulceration of the oral mucosa may be caused by trauma (physical or chemical), recurrent aphthae, infections, carcinoma, dermatological disorders, nutritional deficiencies, gastro-intestinal disease, haematopoietic disorders, and drug therapy (see also Chemotherapy-induced mucositis and myelosuppression, section 8.1). It is important to establish the diagnosis in each case as the majority of these lesions require specific management in addition to local treatment. Local treatment aims to protect the ulcerated area, to relieve pain, to reduce inflammation, or to control secondary infection. Patients with an unexplained mouth ulcer of more than 3 weeks' duration require urgent referral to hospital to exclude oral cancer.

Simple mouthwashes A **saline** mouthwash (section 12.3.4) may relieve the pain of traumatic ulceration. The mouthwash is made up with warm water and used at frequent intervals until the discomfort and swelling subsides.

Antiseptic mouthwashes Secondary bacterial infection may be a feature of any mucosal ulceration; it can increase discomfort and delay healing. Use of **chlorhexidine** mouthwash (section 12.3.4) is often beneficial and may accelerate healing of recurrent aphthae.

Mechanical protection **Carmellose gelatin paste** may relieve some discomfort arising from ulceration by protecting the ulcer site. The paste adheres to dry mucosa, but is difficult to apply effectively to some parts of the mouth.

Corticosteroids Topical corticosteroid therapy may be used for some forms of oral ulceration. In the case of aphthous ulcers it is most effective if applied in the 'prodromal' phase.
Thrush or other types of candidiasis are recognised complications of corticosteroid treatment.

Hydrocortisone oromucosal tablets are allowed to dissolve next to an ulcer and are useful in recurrent aphthae and erosive lichenoid lesions.

Triamcinolone dental paste is designed to keep the corticosteroid in contact with the mucosa for long enough to permit penetration of the lesion, but is difficult for patients to apply properly.

Beclometasone dipropionate inhaler 50–100 micrograms sprayed twice daily on the oral mucosa is used to manage oral ulceration [unlicensed indication]. Alternatively, **betamethasone** soluble tablets dissolved in water can be used as a mouthwash to treat oral ulceration [unlicensed indication].

Systemic corticosteroid therapy (section 6.3.2) is reserved for severe conditions such as pemphigus vulgaris.

Local analgesics Local analgesics have a limited role in the management of oral ulceration. When applied topically their action is of a relatively short duration so that analgesia cannot be maintained continuously throughout the day. The main indication for a topical local analgesic is to relieve the pain of otherwise intractable oral ulceration particularly when it is due to major aphthae. For this purpose lidocaine (lignocaine) 5% ointment or lozenges containing a local anaesthetic are applied to the ulcer. Lidocaine 10% solution as spray (section 15.2) can be applied thinly to the ulcer [unlicensed indication] using a cotton bud. When local anaesthetics are used in the mouth care must be taken not to produce anaesthesia of the pharynx before meals as this might lead to choking.

Benzydamine mouthwash or spray may be useful in reducing the discomfort associated with a variety of ulcerative conditions. It has also been found to be effective in reducing the discomfort of post-irradiation mucositis. Some patients find the full-strength mouthwash causes some stinging and, for them, it should be diluted with an equal volume of water. **Flurbiprofen** lozenges are licensed for the relief of sore throat.

Choline salicylate dental gel has some analgesic action and may provide relief for recurrent aphthae, but excessive application or confinement under a denture irritates the mucosa and can itself cause ulceration. Benefit in teething may merely be due to pressure of application (comparable with biting a teething ring); excessive use can lead to salicylate poisoning.

Other preparations **Doxycycline** rinsed in the mouth may be of value for recurrent aphthous ulceration.

Periodontitis Low-dose doxycycline (*Periostat®*) is licensed as an adjunct to scaling and root planing for the treatment of periodontitis; a low dose of doxycycline reduces collagenase activity without inhibiting bacteria associated with periodontitis. For anti-infectives used in the treatment of destructive (refractory) forms of periodontal disease, see section 12.3.2 and Table 1, section 5.1. For mouthwashes used for oral hygiene and plaque inhibition, see section 12.3.4.

BENZYDAMINE HYDROCHLORIDE

Indications painful inflammatory conditions of oropharynx

Side-effects occasional numbness or stinging; rarely hypersensitivity reactions

Difflam® (3M)

Oral rinse, green, benzydamine hydrochloride 0.15%, net price 200 mL (*Difflam® Sore Throat Rinse*) = £2.63; 300 mL = £4.01

Dose ADULT and ADOLESCENT over 12 years, rinse or gargle, using 15 mL (dilute with an equal volume of water if stinging occurs) every 1½–3 hours as required, usually for not more than 7 days

Dental prescribing on NHS May be prescribed as Benzydamine Mouthwash 0.15%

Spray, benzydamine hydrochloride 0.15%. Net price 30-mL unit = £3.17

Dose ADULT, 4–8 sprays onto affected area every 1½–3 hours; CHILD under 6 years 1 spray per 4 kg body-weight to max. 4 sprays every 1½–3 hours; 6–12 years 4 sprays every 1½–3 hours

Dental prescribing on NHS May be prescribed as Benzydamine Oromucosal Spray 0.15%

CARMELLOSE SODIUM

Indications mechanical protection of oral and perioral lesions

Orabase® (ConvaTec)

Protective paste (= oral paste), carmellose sodium 16.7%, pectin 16.7%, gelatin 16.7%, in *Plastibase®*. Net price 30 g = £2.02; 100 g = £4.48

Dose apply a thin layer when necessary after meals

Dental prescribing on NHS May be prescribed as Carmellose Gelatin Paste

Orahesive® (ConvaTec)

Powder, carmellose sodium, pectin, gelatin, equal parts. Net price 25 g = £2.33

Dose sprinkle on the affected area

CORTICOSTEROIDS

Indications oral and perioral lesions

Contra-indications untreated oral infection; manufacturer of triamcinolone contra-indicates use on tuberculous and viral lesions

Side-effects occasional exacerbation of local infection; thrush or other candidal infections

[1]**Adcortyl in Orabase®** (Squibb) PoM

Oral paste, triamcinolone acetonide 0.1% in adhesive basis. Net price 10 g = £1.18

Dose ADULT and CHILD, apply a thin layer 2–4 times daily; do not rub in; use limited to 5 days for children and short-term use also advised for elderly

Dental prescribing on NHS May be prescribed as Triamcinolone Dental Paste

1. A 5-g tube is on sale to the public for the treatment of common mouth ulcers for max. 5 days

Betnesol® (Celltech) PoM

Soluble tablets, pink, scored, betamethasone 500 micrograms (as sodium phosphate). net price 100-tab pack = £5.17 Label: 10, steroid card, 13, 21

Dose oral ulceration, [unlicensed indication] ADULT and CHILD over 12 years, 500 micrograms dissolved in 20 ml water and rinsed around the mouth 4 times daily; not to be swallowed

Dental prescribing on the NHS May be prescribed as Betamethasone Soluble Tablets 500 micrograms

Corlan® (UCB Pharma)

Pellets (= oromucosal tablets), hydrocortisone 2.5 mg (as sodium succinate). Net price 20 = £2.54

Dose ADULT and CHILD over 12 years, 1 lozenge 4 times daily, allowed to dissolve slowly in the mouth in contact with the ulcer; CHILD under 12 years, only on medical advice

Dental prescribing on NHS May be prescribed as Hydrocortisone Oromucosal Tablets

DOXYCYCLINE

Indications see preparations; oral herpes (section 12.3.2); other indications (section 5.1.3)

Cautions section 5.1.3; monitor for superficial fungal infection, particularly, if predisposition to oral candidiasis

Contra-indications section 5.1.3

Side-effects section 5.1.3; fungal superinfection

Dose

- See preparations

Note Doxycycline stains teeth; avoid in children under 12 years of age

Periostat® (Alliance) PoM

Tablets, f/c, doxycycline (as hyclate) 20 mg, net price 56-tab pack = £16.50. Label: 6, 11, 27, counselling, posture

Dose periodontitis (as an adjunct to gingival scaling and root planing), 20 mg twice daily for 3 months; CHILD under 12 years not recommended

Counselling Tablets should be swallowed whole with plenty of fluid (at least 100 mL), while sitting or standing

Dental prescribing on NHS May be prescribed as Doxycycline Tablets 20 mg

Local application

For recurrent aphthous ulceration, the contents of a 100 mg doxycycline capsule can be stirred into a small amount of water then rinsed around the mouth for 2–3 minutes 4 times daily usually for 3 days; it should preferably not be swallowed [unlicensed indication].

FLURBIPROFEN

Indications relief of sore throat

Cautions see section 10.1.1

Contra-indications see section 10.1.1

Side-effects taste disturbance, mouth ulcers (move lozenge around mouth); see also section 10.1.1

Strefen® (Crookes)

Lozenges, flurbiprofen 8.75 mg, net price 16 = £2.08

Dose ADULT and CHILD over 12 years, allow 1 lozenge to dissolve slowly in the mouth every 3–6 hours, max. 5 lozenges in 24 hours, for max. 3 days

LOCAL ANAESTHETICS

Indications relief of pain in oral lesions

Cautions avoid prolonged use; hypersensitivity; pregnancy (Appendix 4); avoid anaesthesia of the pharynx before meals—risk of choking

Lidocaine (Non-proprietary)

Ointment, lidocaine 5% in a water-miscible basis, net price 15 g = 80p

Dose rub sparingly and gently on affected areas

Dental prescribing on NHS Lidocaine 5% Ointment may be prescribed

Xylocaine® (AstraZeneca)

Spray (= pump spray), lidocaine 10% (100 mg/g) supplying 10 mg lidocaine/spray; 500 spray doses per container. Net price 50-mL bottle = £3.13

Dose apply thinly to the ulcer [unlicensed indication] using a cotton bud

Dental prescribing on NHS May be prescribed as Lidocaine Spray 10%

Preparations on sale to the public

Many mouth ulcer preparations, throat lozenges, and throat sprays on sale to the public contain a **local anaesthetic**. To identify the active ingredients in such preparations, consult the product literature of the manufacturer.

Note The correct proprietary name should be ascertained—many products have very similar names but different active ingredients

SALICYLATES

Indications mild oral and perioral lesions

Cautions not to be applied to dentures—leave at least 30 minutes before re-insertion of dentures; frequent application, especially in children, may give rise to salicylate poisoning

Note CSM warning on aspirin and Reye's syndrome does not apply to salicylates in topical preparations such as teething gels and oral paints

Choline salicylate

Choline Salicylate Dental Gel, BP

Oral gel, choline salicylate 8.7% in a flavoured gel basis, net price 15 g = £1.79

Brands include *Bonjela®* (sugar-free)

Dose apply ½-inch of gel with gentle massage not more often than every 3 hours; CHILD over 4 months ¼-inch of gel not more often than every 3 hours; max. 6 applications daily

Dental prescribing on NHS Choline Salicylate Dental Gel may be prescribed

Salicylic acid

Pyralvex® (Norgine)

Oral paint, brown, rhubarb extract (anthraquinone glycosides 0.5%), salicylic acid 1%. Net price 10 mL with brush = £3.38

Dose ADULT and CHILD over 12 years, apply 3–4 times daily

12.3.2 Oropharyngeal anti-infective drugs

The most common cause of a sore throat is a viral infection which does not benefit from anti-infective treatment. Streptococcal sore throats require systemic **penicillin** therapy (Table 1, section 5.1). Acute ulcerative gingivitis (Vincent's infection) responds to systemic **metronidazole** (section 5.1.11).

Preparations administered in the dental surgery for the local treatment of periodontal disease include gels of metronidazole (*Elyzol®*, Colgate-Palmolive) and of minocycline (*Dentomycin®*, Blackwell).

Oropharyngeal fungal infections

Fungal infections of the mouth are usually caused by *Candida* spp. (candidiasis or candidosis). Different types of oropharyngeal candidiasis are managed as follows:

Thrush Acute pseudomembranous candidiasis (thrush), is usually an acute infection but it may persist for months in patients receiving inhaled corticosteroids, cytotoxics or broad-spectrum antibacterials. Thrush also occurs in patients with serious systemic disease associated with reduced immunity such as leukaemia, other malignancies, and HIV infection. Any predisposing condition should be managed appropriately. When thrush is associated with corticosteroid inhalers, rinsing the mouth with water (or cleaning a child's teeth) immediately after using the inhaler may avoid the problem. Treatment with **nystatin**, **amphotericin**, or **miconazole** may be needed. **Fluconazole** (section 5.2) is effective for unresponsive infections or if a topical antifungal drug cannot be used or if the patient has dry mouth. Topical therapy may not be adequate in immunocompromised patients and an oral triazole antifungal is preferred (section 5.2).

Acute erythematous candidiasis Acute erythematous (atrophic) candidiasis is a relatively uncommon condition associated with corticosteroid and broad-spectrum antibacterial use and with HIV disease. It is usually treated with **fluconazole** (section 5.2).

Denture stomatitis Patients with denture stomatitis (chronic atrophic candidiasis), should cleanse their dentures thoroughly and leave them out as often as possible during the treatment period. To prevent recurrence of the problem, dentures should not normally be worn at night. New dentures may be required if these measures fail despite good compliance.

Miconazole oral gel can be applied to the fitting surface of the denture before insertion (for short periods only). Alternatively, **amphotericin** lozenges can be allowed to dissolve slowly in the mouth but they are less effective at resolving the stomatitis. Denture stomatitis is not always associated with candidiasis and other factors such as mechanical or chemical irritation, bacterial infection, or rarely allergy to the dental base material, may be the cause.

Chronic hyperplastic candidiasis Chronic hyperplastic candidiasis (candidal leucoplakia) carries an increased risk of malignancy; biopsy is essential—this type of candidiasis may be associated with varying degrees of dysplasia, with oral cancer present in a high proportion of cases. Chronic hyperplastic candidiasis is treated with a systemic antifungal such as **fluconazole** (section 5.2) to eliminate candidal overlay. Patients should avoid the use of tobacco.

Angular cheilitis Angular cheilitis (angular stomatitis) is characterised by soreness, erythema and fissuring at the angles of the mouth. It is commonly associated with denture stomatitis but may represent a nutritional deficiency or it may be related to orofacial granulomatosis or HIV infection. Both yeasts (*Candida* spp.) and bacteria (*Staphylococcus aureus* and beta-haemolytic streptococci) are commonly involved as interacting, infective factors. A reduction in facial height related to ageing and tooth loss with maceration in the deep occlusive folds that may subsequently arise, predisposes to such infection. While the underlying cause is being identified and treated, it is often helpful to apply **miconazole** and **hydrocortisone** cream or ointment (see p. 604), **miconazole** cream (see p. 630), **nystatin** ointment (see p. 630), or **sodium fusidate** ointment (see p. 629).

Immunocompromised patients For advice on prevention of fungal infections in immunocompromised patients see p. 321.

Drugs used in oropharyngeal candidiasis
Amphotericin and **nystatin** are not absorbed from the gastro-intestinal tract and are applied locally (as lozenges or suspension) to the mouth for treating local fungal infections. Nystatin ointment is available for perioral lesions (see p. 630). **Miconazole** is applied locally (as an oral gel) in the mouth but it is absorbed to the extent that potential interactions need to be considered. Miconazole may be more effective than amphotericin or nystatin for some types of candidiasis, particularly chronic hyperplastic candidiasis or chronic mucocutaneous candidiasis (chronic thrush). Miconazole also has some activity against Gram-positive bacteria including streptococci and staphylococci. **Fluconazole** (section 5.2) is given by mouth for infections that do not respond to topical therapy. It is reliably absorbed and effective. **Itraconazole** (section 5.2) can be used for fluconazole-resistant infections.

If candidal infection fails to respond to 1 to 2 weeks of treatment with antifungal drugs the patient should be sent for investigation to eliminate the possibility of underlying disease. Persistent infection may also be caused by reinfection from the genito-urinary or gastro-intestinal tract. Infection can be eliminated from these sources by appropriate anticandidal therapy; the patient's partner may also require treatment to prevent reinfection.

For the role of antiseptic mouthwashes in the prevention of oral candidiasis in immunocompromised patients and treatment of denture stomatitis, see section 12.3.4.

AMPHOTERICIN

Indications oral and perioral fungal infections

Side-effects mild gastro-intestinal disturbances reported

Fungilin® (Squibb) PoM
Lozenges, yellow, amphotericin 10 mg. Net price 60-lozenge pack = £3.67. Label: 9, 24, counselling, after food
Dose allow 1 lozenge to dissolve slowly in the mouth 4 times daily for 10–15 days (continued for 48 hours after lesions have resolved); increase to 8 daily if infection severe
Dental prescribing on NHS May be prescribed as Amphotericin Lozenges

MICONAZOLE

Indications see under Dose

Cautions pregnancy (Appendix 4); breast-feeding; avoid in porphyria (section 9.8.2); **interactions:** Appendix 1 (antifungals, imidazole)

Contra-indications hepatic impairment

Side-effects nausea and vomiting, diarrhoea (with long-term treatment); rarely allergic reactions; isolated reports of hepatitis

Dose
- Prevention and treatment of oral and intestinal fungal infections, 5–10 mL in the mouth after food 4 times daily; retain near oral lesions before swallowing; NEONATE see *BNF for Children*; CHILD 1 month–2 years 2.5 mL twice daily, 2–6 years 5 mL twice daily, over 6 years 5 mL 4 times daily; treatment continued for 48 hours after lesions have healed
- Localised lesions, smear small amount on affected area with clean finger 4 times daily for 5–7 days (dental prostheses should be removed at night and brushed with gel); treatment continued for 48 hours after lesions have healed

[1]**Daktarin®** (Janssen-Cilag) PoM
Oral gel, sugar-free, orange-flavoured, miconazole 24 mg/mL (20 mg/g). Net price 15-g tube = £2.45, 80-g tube = £4.65. Label: 9, counselling, hold in mouth, after food
Dental prescribing on NHS May be prescribed as Miconazole Oromucosal Gel

1. 15-g tube can be sold to the public

NYSTATIN

Indications oral and perioral fungal infections

Side-effects oral irritation and sensitisation, nausea reported; see also p. 326

Dose
- Treatment, ADULT and CHILD, 100 000 units 4 times daily after food usually for 7 days (continued for 48 hours after lesions have resolved)

Note Unlicensed for treating candidiasis in NEONATE

Nystan® (Squibb) PoM
Oral suspension, yellow, nystatin 100 000 units/mL. Net price 30 mL with pipette = £1.91. Label: 9, counselling, use of pipette, hold in mouth, after food
Dental prescribing on NHS Nystatin Oral Suspension may be prescribed

Oropharyngeal viral infections

The management of primary herpetic gingivostomatitis is a soft diet, adequate fluid intake, and analgesics as required, including local use of **benzydamine** (section 12.3.1). The use of chlorhexidine mouthwash (section 12.3.4) will control plaque accumulation if toothbrushing is painful and will also help to control secondary infection in general.

In the case of severe herpetic stomatitis, a systemic antiviral such as aciclovir is required (section 5.3.2.1). Valaciclovir and famciclovir are suitable alternatives for oral lesions associated with herpes zoster. Aciclovir and valaciclovir are also used for the prevention of frequently recurring herpes simplex lesions of the mouth, particularly when implicated in the initiation of erythema multiforme. See section 13.10.3 for the treatment of labial herpes simplex infections.

Herpes infections of the mouth may also respond to rinsing the mouth with **doxycycline**, (see p. 591).

12.3.3 Lozenges and sprays

There is no convincing evidence that antiseptic lozenges and sprays have a beneficial action and they sometimes irritate and cause sore tongue and sore lips. Some of these preparations also contain local anaesthetics which relieve pain but may cause sensitisation.

12.3.4 Mouthwashes, gargles, and dentifrices

Superficial infections of the mouth are often helped by warm mouthwashes which have a mechanical cleansing effect and cause some local hyperaemia. However, to be effective, they must be used frequently and vigorously. A warm saline mouthwash is ideal and can be prepared either by dissolving half a teaspoonful of salt in a glassful of warm water or by diluting **compound sodium chloride mouthwash** with an equal volume of warm water. **Mouthwash solution-tablets** are used to remove unpleasant tastes.

Mouthwashes containing an oxidising agent, such as **hydrogen peroxide**, may be useful in the treatment of acute ulcerative gingivitis (Vincent's infection) since the organisms involved are anaerobes. It also has a mechanical cleansing effect arising from frothing when in contact with oral debris.

Chlorhexidine is an effective antiseptic which has the advantage of inhibiting plaque formation on the teeth. It does not, however, completely control plaque deposition and is not a substitute for effective toothbrushing. Moreover, chlorhexidine preparations do not penetrate significantly into stagnation areas and are therefore of little value in the control of dental caries or of periodontal disease once pocketing has developed. Chlorhexidine mouthwash is used in the treatment of denture stomatitis. It is also used in the prevention of oral candidiasis in immunocompromised patients. Chlorhexidine mouthwash reduces the incidence of alveolar osteitis following tooth extraction. Chlorhexidine mouthwash should not be used for the prevention of endocarditis in patients undergoing dental procedures.

Chlorhexidine can be used as a mouthwash, spray or gel for secondary infection in mucosal ulceration and for controlling gingivitis, as an adjunct to other oral hygiene measures. These preparations may also be used instead of toothbrushing where there is a painful periodontal condition (e.g. primary herpetic stomatitis) or if the patient has a haemorrhagic disorder, or is disabled. Chlorhexidine preparations are of little value in the control of acute necrotising ulcerative gingivitis.

There is no convincing evidence that gargles are effective.

CHLORHEXIDINE GLUCONATE

Indications see under preparations below

Side-effects mucosal irritation (if desquamation occurs, discontinue treatment or dilute mouthwash with an equal volume of water); taste disturbance; reversible brown staining of teeth, and of silicate or composite restorations; tongue discoloration; parotid gland swelling reported

Note Chlorhexidine gluconate may be incompatible with some ingredients in toothpaste; leave an interval of at least 30 minutes between using mouthwash and toothpaste

Chlorhexidine (Non-proprietary)

Mouthwash, chlorhexidine gluconate 0.2%, net price 300 mL = £2.02

Dose oral hygiene and plaque inhibition, oral candidiasis, gingivitis, and management of aphthous ulcers, rinse mouth with 10 mL for about 1 minute twice daily

Denture stomatitis, cleanse and soak dentures in mouthwash solution for 15 minutes twice daily

Dental prescribing on NHS Chlorhexidine Mouthwash may be prescribed

Chlorohex® (Colgate-Palmolive)

Chlorohex 1200® mouthwash, chlorhexidine gluconate 0.12% (mint-flavoured). Net price 300 mL = £2.00

Dose oral hygiene and plaque inhibition, rinse mouth with 15 mL for about 30 seconds twice daily

Corsodyl® (GSK Consumer Healthcare)

Dental gel, chlorhexidine gluconate 1%. Net price 50 g = £1.21

Dose oral hygiene and plaque inhibition and gingivitis, brush on the teeth once or twice daily

Oral candidiasis and management of aphthous ulcers, apply to affected areas once or twice daily

Dental prescribing on NHS May be prescribed as Chlorhexidine Gluconate Gel 1%

Mouthwash, chlorhexidine gluconate 0.2%. Net price 300 mL (original or mint) = £1.93, 600 mL (mint) = £3.85

Dose oral hygiene and plaque inhibition, oral candidiasis, gingivitis, and management of aphthous ulcers, rinse mouth with 10 mL for about 1 minute twice daily

Denture stomatitis, cleanse and soak dentures in mouthwash solution for 15 minutes twice daily

Oral spray, chlorhexidine gluconate 0.2% (mint-flavoured). Net price 60 mL = £4.10

Dose oral hygiene and plaque inhibition, oral candidiasis, gingivitis, and management of aphthous ulcers, apply as required to tooth, gingival, or ulcer surfaces using up to 12 actuations (approx. 0.14 mL/actuation) twice daily

Dental prescribing on NHS May be prescribed as Chlorhexidine Oral Spray

With chlorobutanol

Eludril® (Fabre)

Mouthwash or *gargle*, chlorhexidine gluconate 0.1%, chlorobutanol 0.5% (mint-flavoured), net price 90 mL = £1.36, 250 mL = £2.83, 500 mL = £5.06

Dose oral hygiene and plaque inhibition, use 10–15 mL (diluted with warm water in measuring cup provided) 2–3 times daily

Denture disinfection, soak previously cleansed dentures in mouthwash (diluted with 2 volumes of water) for 60 minutes

HEXETIDINE

Indications oral hygiene

Side-effects local irritation; *very rarely* taste disturbance and transient anaesthesia

Oraldene® (Pfizer Consumer)
Mouthwash or *gargle*, red or blue-green (mint-flavoured), hexetidine 0.1%. Net price 100 mL = £1.31; 200 mL = £2.02
Dose ADULT and CHILD over 6 years, use 15 mL undiluted 2–3 times daily

HYDROGEN PEROXIDE

Indications oral hygiene, see notes above
Side-effects hypertrophy of papillae of tongue on prolonged used

Hydrogen Peroxide Mouthwash, BP
Mouthwash, consists of Hydrogen Peroxide Solution 6% (= approx. 20 volume) BP
Dose rinse the mouth for 2–3 minutes with 15 mL diluted in half a tumblerful of warm water 2–3 times daily
Dental prescribing on NHS Hydrogen Peroxide Mouthwash may be prescribed

Peroxyl® (Colgate-Palmolive)
Mouthwash, hydrogen peroxide 1.5%, net price 300 mL = £2.81
Dose rinse the mouth with 10 mL for about 1 minute up to 4 times daily (after meals and at bedtime)

SODIUM CHLORIDE

Indications oral hygiene, see notes above

Sodium Chloride Mouthwash, Compound, BP
Mouthwash, sodium bicarbonate 1%, sodium chloride 1.5% in a suitable vehicle with a peppermint flavour.
Dose extemporaneous preparations should be prepared according to the following formula: sodium chloride 1.5 g, sodium bicarbonate 1 g, concentrated peppermint emulsion 2.5 mL, double-strength chloroform water 50 mL, water to 100 mL
To be diluted with an equal volume of warm water
Dental prescribing on NHS Compound Sodium Chloride Mouthwash may be prescribed

THYMOL

Indications oral hygiene, see notes above

Mouthwash Solution-tablets
Consist of tablets which may contain antimicrobial, colouring, and flavouring agents in a suitable soluble effervescent basis to make a mouthwash suitable for dental purposes.
Dose dissolve 1 tablet in a tumblerful of warm water
Note Mouthwash solution tablets may contain ingredients such as thymol
Dental prescribing on NHS Mouthwash Solution-tablets may be prescribed

12.3.5 Treatment of dry mouth

Dry mouth (xerostomia) may be caused by drugs with antimuscarinic (anticholinergic) side-effects (e.g. antispasmodics, tricyclic antidepressants, and some antipsychotics), by diuretics, by irradiation of the head and neck region or by damage to or disease of the salivary glands. Patients with a persistently dry mouth may develop a burning or scalded sensation and have poor oral hygiene; they may develop increased dental caries, periodontal disease, intolerance of dentures, and oral infections (particularly candidiasis). Dry mouth may be relieved in many patients by simple measures such as frequent sips of cool drinks or sucking pieces of ice or sugar-free fruit pastilles. Sugar-free chewing gum stimulates salivation in patients with residual salivary function.

Artificial saliva can provide useful relief of dry mouth. A properly balanced artificial saliva should be of a neutral pH and contain electrolytes (including fluoride) to correspond approximately to the composition of saliva. The acidic pH of some artificial saliva products may be inappropriate. Of the proprietary preparations, *Luborant®* is licensed for any condition giving rise to a dry mouth; *Biotène Oralbalance®*, *BioXtra®*, *Glandosane®*, *Saliva Orthana®*, and *Saliveze®*, have ACBS approval for dry mouth associated only with radiotherapy or sicca syndrome. *Salivix®* pastilles, which act locally as salivary stimulants, are also available and have similar ACBS approval. *SST* tablets may be prescribed for dry mouth in patients with salivary gland impairment (and patent salivary ducts). *Salinum®* may also be prescribed for relief of symptoms of dry mouth.

Pilocarpine tablets are licensed for the treatment of xerostomia following irradiation for head and neck cancer and for dry mouth and dry eyes (xerophthalmia) in Sjögren's syndrome. They are effective only in patients who have some residual salivary gland function, and therefore should be withdrawn if there is no response.

Local treatment

AS Saliva Orthana® (AS Pharma)
Oral spray, gastric mucin (porcine) 3.5%, xylitol 2%, sodium fluoride 4.2 mg/litre, with preservatives and flavouring agents, pH neutral. Net price 50-mL bottle = £4.25; 450-mL refill = £29.69
Dose ACBS: patients suffering from dry mouth as a result of having (or having undergone) radiotherapy, or sicca syndrome, spray 2–3 times onto oral and pharyngeal mucosa, when required
Lozenges, mucin 65 mg, xylitol 59 mg, in a sorbitol basis, pH neutral. Net price 30-lozenge pack = £3.02
Dose ACBS: patients suffering from dry mouth as a result of having (or having undergone) radiotherapy, or sicca syndrome
Note *AS Saliva Orthana®* lozenges do not contain fluoride
Dental prescribing on NHS *AS Saliva Orthana®* Oral Spray and Lozenges may be prescribed

Biotène Oralbalance® (Angliar)
Saliva replacement gel, lactoperoxidase, lactoferrin, lysozyme, glucose oxidase, xylitol in a gel basis, net price 50-g tube = £4.10, 24 × 12.4-mL tube = £30.40 (for hospital use)
Dose ACBS: patients suffering from dry mouth as a result of having (or having undergone) radiotherapy, or sicca syndrome, apply to gums and tongue as required
Note Avoid use with toothpastes containing detergents (including foaming agents)
Dental prescribing on NHS *Biotène Oralbalance®* Saliva Replacement Gel may be prescribed

BioXtra® (Molar)
Gel, lactoperoxidase, lactoferrin, lysozyme, whey colostrum, xylitol and other ingredients, net price 40-mL tube = £2.95, 50-mL spray = £2.95
Dose ACBS: patients suffering from dry mouth as a result of having (or having undergone) radiotherapy, or sicca syndrome, apply to oral mucosa as required
Dental prescribing on NHS *BioXtra®* Gel may be prescribed

Glandosane® (Fresenius Kabi)
Aerosol spray, carmellose sodium 500 mg, sorbitol 1.5 g, potassium chloride 60 mg, sodium chloride 42.2 mg, magnesium chloride 2.6 mg, calcium chloride 7.3 mg, and dipotassium hydrogen phosphate 17.1 mg/50 g, pH 5.75. Net price 50-mL unit (neutral, lemon or peppermint flavoured) = £4.48

Dose ACBS: patients suffering from dry mouth as a result of having (or having undergone) radiotherapy, or sicca syndrome, spray onto oral and pharyngeal mucosa as required

Dental prescribing on NHS *Glandosane®* Aerosol Spray may be prescribed

Luborant® (Goldshield)
Oral spray, pink, sorbitol 1.8 g, carmellose sodium (sodium carboxymethylcellulose) 390 mg, dibasic potassium phosphate 48.23 mg, potassium chloride 37.5 mg, monobasic potassium phosphate 21.97 mg, calcium chloride 9.972 mg, magnesium chloride 3.528 mg, sodium fluoride 258 micrograms/60 mL, with preservatives and colouring agents. Net price 60-mL unit = £3.96

Dose saliva deficiency, 2–3 sprays onto oral mucosa up to 4 times daily, or as directed

Note May be difficult to obtain

Dental prescribing on NHS *Luborant®* Oral Spray may be prescribed as Artificial Saliva

Salinum® (Crawford)
Liquid, sugar-free, linseed extract (containing polysaccharides) with dipotassium phosphate buffer and preservatives, pH 6–7, net price 300-mL bottle = £13.50

Dose symptomatic treatment of dry mouth, approx. 2 mL rinsed around the mouth and then swallowed, when required

Saliveze® (Wyvern)
Oral spray, carmellose sodium (sodium carboxymethylcellulose), calcium chloride, magnesium chloride, potassium chloride, sodium chloride, and dibasic sodium phosphate, pH neutral. Net price 50-mL bottle (mint-flavoured) = £3.50

Dose ACBS: patients suffering from dry mouth as a result of having (or having undergone) radiotherapy, or sicca syndrome, 1 spray onto oral mucosa as required

Dental prescribing on NHS *Saliveze®* Oral Spray may be prescribed

Salivix® (KoGEN)
Pastilles, sugar-free, reddish-amber, acacia, malic acid and other ingredients. Net price 50-pastille pack = £2.86

Dose ACBS: patients suffering from dry mouth as a result of having (or having undergone) radiotherapy, or sicca syndrome, suck 1 pastille when required

Dental prescribing on NHS *Salivix®* Pastilles may be prescribed

SST (Medac)
Tablets, sugar-free, citric acid, malic acid and other ingredients in a sorbitol base, net price 100-tab pack = £4.86

Dose symptomatic treatment of dry mouth in patients with impaired salivary gland function and patent salivary ducts, allow 1 tablet to dissolve slowly in the mouth when required

Systemic treatment

PILOCARPINE HYDROCHLORIDE

Indications xerostomia following irradiation for head and neck cancer (see also notes above); dry mouth and dry eyes in Sjögren's syndrome

Cautions asthma and chronic obstructive pulmonary disease (avoid if uncontrolled, see Contra-indications), cardiovascular disease (avoid if uncontrolled); cholelithiasis or biliary-tract disease, peptic ulcer, hepatic impairment (Appendix 2), renal impairment; risk of increased urethral smooth muscle tone and renal colic; maintain adequate fluid intake to avoid dehydration associated with excessive sweating; cognitive or psychiatric disturbances; susceptibility to angle-closure glaucoma; **interactions**: Appendix 1 (parasympathomimetics)

Counselling Blurred vision or dizziness may affect performance of skilled tasks (e.g. driving) particularly at night or in reduced lighting

Contra-indications uncontrolled asthma and chronic obstructive pulmonary disease (increased bronchial secretions and increased airways resistance); uncontrolled cardiorenal disease; acute iritis; pregnancy (Appendix 4); breast-feeding

Side-effects dyspepsia, diarrhoea, abdominal pain, nausea, vomiting, constipation; flushing, hypertension, palpitation, headache, dizziness, asthenia, influenza-like symptoms, sweating; increased urinary frequency; visual disturbances, lacrimation, ocular pain, conjunctivitis; rhinitis; rash, pruritus; *less commonly* flatulence, urinary urgency

Dose

- Xerostomia following irradiation for head and neck cancer, 5 mg 3 times daily with or immediately after meals (last dose always with evening meal); if tolerated but response insufficient after 4 weeks, may be increased to max. 30 mg daily in divided doses; max. therapeutic effect normally within 4–8 weeks; discontinue if no improvement after 2–3 months; CHILD not recommended
- Dry mouth and dry eyes in Sjögren's syndrome, 5 mg 4 times daily (with meals and at bedtime); if tolerated but response insufficient, may be increased to max. 30 mg daily in divided doses; discontinue if no improvement after 2–3 months; CHILD not recommended

Salagen® (Novartis) PoM
Tablets, f/c, pilocarpine hydrochloride 5 mg. Net price 84-tab pack = £51.43. Label: 21, 27, counselling, driving

13 Skin

13.1	**Management of skin conditions**	**597**
13.1.1	Vehicles	597
13.1.2	Suitable quantities for prescribing	598
13.1.3	Excipients and sensitisation	598
13.2	**Emollient and barrier preparations**	**598**
13.2.1	Emollients	598
13.2.1.1	Emollient bath additives	601
13.2.2	Barrier preparations	602
13.3	**Topical local anaesthetics and antipruritics**	**603**
13.4	**Topical corticosteroids**	**604**
13.5	**Preparations for eczema and psoriasis**	**610**
13.5.1	Preparations for eczema	610
13.5.2	Preparations for psoriasis	611
13.5.3	Drugs affecting the immune response	616
13.6	**Acne and rosacea**	**618**
13.6.1	Topical preparations for acne	618
13.6.2	Oral preparations for acne	621
13.7	**Preparations for warts and calluses**	**622**
13.8	**Sunscreens and camouflagers**	**624**
13.8.1	Sunscreen preparations	624
13.8.2	Camouflagers	626
13.9	**Shampoos and other preparations for scalp and hair conditions**	**626**
13.10	**Anti-infective skin preparations**	**628**
13.10.1	Antibacterial preparations	628
13.10.1.1	Antibacterial preparations only used topically	628
13.10.1.2	Antibacterial preparations also used systemically	629
13.10.2	Antifungal preparations	630
13.10.3	Antiviral preparations	633
13.10.4	Parasiticidal preparations	633
13.10.5	Preparations for minor cuts and abrasions	636
13.11	**Skin cleansers and antiseptics**	**637**
13.11.1	Alcohols and saline	637
13.11.2	Chlorhexidine salts	637
13.11.3	Cationic surfactants and soaps	638
13.11.4	Iodine	638
13.11.5	Phenolics	639
13.11.6	Oxidisers and dyes	639
13.11.7	Preparations for promotion of wound healing	639
13.12	**Antiperspirants**	**640**
13.13	**Topical circulatory preparations**	**640**

This chapter also includes advice on the drug management of the following:

candidiasis, p. 630
crab lice, p. 634
dermatophytoses, p. 630
head lice, p. 634
hirsutism, p. 627
nappy rash, p. 602
photodamage, p. 625
pityriasis versicolor, p. 630
scabies, p. 634

For further information on wound management products and elastic hosiery see Appendix 8, p. 850

13.1 Management of skin conditions

13.1.1 Vehicles

Both vehicle and active ingredients are important in the treatment of skin conditions; the vehicle alone may have more than a mere placebo effect. The vehicle affects the degree of hydration of the skin, has a mild anti-inflammatory effect, and aids the penetration of active drug.

Applications are usually viscous solutions, emulsions, or suspensions for application to the skin (including the scalp) or nails.

Collodions are painted on the skin and allowed to dry to leave a flexible film over the site of application.

Creams are emulsions of oil and water and are generally well absorbed into the skin. They may contain an antimicrobial preservative unless the active ingredient or basis is intrinsically bactericidal and fungicidal. Generally, creams are cosmetically more acceptable than ointments because they are less greasy and easier to apply.

Gels consist of active ingredients in suitable hydrophilic or hydrophobic bases; they generally have a high water content. Gels are particularly suitable for application to the face and scalp.

Lotions have a cooling effect and may be preferred to ointments or creams for application over a hairy area. Lotions in alcoholic basis can sting if used on broken skin. *Shake lotions* (such as calamine lotion) contain insoluble powders which leave a deposit on the skin surface.

Ointments are greasy preparations which are normally anhydrous and insoluble in water, and are more occlusive than creams. They are particularly suitable for chronic, dry lesions. The most commonly used ointment bases consist of soft paraffin or a combination of soft, liquid and hard paraffin. Some ointment bases have both *hydrophilic and lipophilic* properties; they may have occlusive properties on the skin surface, encourage hydration, and also be miscible with water; they often have a mild anti-inflammatory effect. *Water-soluble ointments* contain macrogols which are freely soluble in water and are therefore readily washed off; they have a limited but useful role where ready removal is desirable.

Pastes are stiff preparations containing a high proportion of finely powdered solids such as zinc oxide and starch suspended in an ointment. They are used for circumscribed lesions such as those which occur in lichen simplex, chronic eczema, or psoriasis. They are less occlusive than ointments and can be used to protect inflamed, lichenified, or excoriated skin.

Dusting powders are used only rarely. They reduce friction between opposing skin surfaces. Dusting powders should not be applied to moist areas because they can cake and abrade the skin. Talc is a lubricant but it does not absorb moisture whereas starch is less lubricant but absorbs water.

Dilution The BP directs that creams and ointments should **not** normally be diluted but that should dilution be necessary care should be taken, in particular, to prevent microbial contamination. The appropriate diluent should be used and heating should be avoided during mixing; excessive dilution may affect the stability of some creams. Diluted creams should normally be used within 2 weeks of their preparation.

13.1.2 Suitable quantities for prescribing

Suitable quantities of dermatological preparations to be prescribed for specific areas of the body

	Creams and Ointments	Lotions
Face	15–30 g	100 mL
Both hands	25–50 g	200 mL
Scalp	50–100 g	200 mL
Both arms or both legs	100–200 g	200 mL
Trunk	400 g	500 mL
Groins and genitalia	15–25 g	100 mL

These amounts are usually suitable for an adult for twice daily application for 1 week. The recommendations do not apply to corticosteroid preparations—for suitable quantities of corticosteroid preparations see section 13.4.

13.1.3 Excipients and sensitisation

Excipients in topical products rarely cause problems. If a patch test indicates allergy to an excipient, then products containing the substance should be avoided. The following excipients in topical preparations may rarely be associated with sensitisation; the presence of these excipients is indicated in the entries for topical products. See also Excipients under General Guidance, p. 2.

- Beeswax
- Benzyl alcohol
- Butylated hydroxyanisole
- Butylated hydroxytoluene
- Cetostearyl alcohol (including cetyl and stearyl alcohol)
- Chlorocresol
- Edetic acid (EDTA)
- Ethylenediamine
- Fragrances
- Hydroxybenzoates (parabens)
- Imidurea
- Isopropyl palmitate
- *N*-(3-Chloroallyl)hexaminium chloride (quaternium 15)
- Polysorbates
- Propylene glycol
- Sodium metabisulphite
- Sorbic acid
- Wool fat and related substances including lanolin[1]

13.2 Emollient and barrier preparations

13.2.1 **Emollients**
13.2.2 **Barrier preparations**

Borderline substances The preparations marked 'ACBS' are regarded as drugs when prescribed in accordance with the advice of the Advisory Committee on Borderline Substances for the clinical conditions listed. Prescriptions issued in accordance with this advice and endorsed 'ACBS' will normally not be investigated. See Appendix 7 for listing by clinical condition.

13.2.1 Emollients

Emollients soothe, smooth and hydrate the skin and are indicated for all dry or scaling disorders. Their effects are short-lived and they should be applied frequently even after improvement occurs. They are useful in dry and eczematous disorders, and to a lesser extent in psoriasis (section 13.5.2). Light emollients such as **aqueous cream** are suitable for many patients with dry skin but a wide range of more greasy preparations including **white soft paraffin**, **emulsifying ointment**, and **liquid and white soft paraffin ointment** are available; the severity of the condition, patient preference and site of application will often guide the choice of

1. Purified versions of wool fat have reduced the problem

emollient; emollients should be applied in the direction of hair growth. Ointments may exacerbate acne and folliculitis. Some ingredients may rarely cause sensitisation (section 13.1.3) and this should be suspected if an eczematous reaction occurs.

Fire hazard with paraffin-based emollients
Emulsifying ointment *or* 50% Liquid Paraffin and 50% White Soft Paraffin Ointment in contact with dressings and clothing is easily ignited by a naked flame. The risk will be greater when these preparations are applied to large areas of the body, and clothing or dressings become soaked with the ointment. Patients should be told to keep away from fire or flames, and not to smoke when using these preparations. The risk of fire should be considered when using large quantities of any paraffin-based emollient.

Preparations such as **aqueous cream** and **emulsifying ointment** can be used as soap substitutes for hand washing and in the bath; the preparation is rubbed on the skin before rinsing off completely. The addition of a bath oil (section 13.2.1.1) may also be helpful.

Preparations containing an antibacterial (section 13.10) should be avoided unless infection is present or is a frequent complication.

Urea is a hydrating agent used in the treatment of dry, scaling conditions (including ichthyosis) and may be useful in elderly patients. It is occasionally used with other topical agents such as corticosteroids to enhance penetration of the skin.

Non-proprietary emollient preparations

Aqueous Cream, BP
Cream, emulsifying ointment 30%, [1]phenoxyethanol 1% in freshly boiled and cooled purified water, net price 500 g = £1.49
Excipients include cetostearyl alcohol
1. The BP permits use of alternative antimicrobials provided their identity and concentration are stated on the label

Emulsifying Ointment, BP
Ointment, emulsifying wax 30%, white soft paraffin 50%, liquid paraffin 20%, net price 500 g = £2.37
Excipients include cetostearyl alcohol

Hydrous Ointment, BP
Ointment, (oily cream), dried magnesium sulphate 0.5%, phenoxyethanol 1%, wool alcohols ointment 50%, in freshly boiled and cooled purified water, net price 500 g = £2.00

Liquid and White Soft Paraffin Ointment, NPF
Ointment, liquid paraffin 50%, white soft paraffin 50%, net price 500 g = £3.94

Paraffin, White Soft, BP
White petroleum jelly, net price 100 g = 61p

Paraffin, Yellow Soft, BP
Yellow petroleum jelly, net price 100 g = 33p

Proprietary emollient preparations

Aveeno® (J&J)
Cream, colloidal oatmeal in emollient basis, net price 100 mL = £3.78
Excipients include benzyl alcohol, cetyl alcohol, isopropyl palmitate
ACBS: For endogenous and exogenous eczema, xeroderma, ichthyosis, and senile pruritus (pruritus of the elderly) associated with dry skin

Lotion, colloidal oatmeal in emollient basis, net price 400-mL pump pack = £6.42
Excipients include benzyl alcohol, cetyl alcohol, isopropyl palmitate
ACBS: as for *Aveeno® Cream*

Cetraben® (Genus)
Emollient cream, white soft paraffin 13.2%, light liquid paraffin 10.5%, net price 50-g pump pack = £1.17, 150-g pump pack = £2.88, 500-g pump pack = £5.61
Excipients include cetostearyl alcohol, hydroxybenzoates (parabens)
For inflamed, damaged, dry or chapped skin including eczema

Decubal® Clinic (Alpharma)
Cream, isopropyl myristate 17%, glycerol 8.5%, wool fat 6%, dimeticone 5%, net price 50 g = £1.02, 100 g = £1.98
Excipients include cetyl alcohol, polysorbates, sorbic acid, wool fat
For dry skin conditions including ichthyosis, psoriasis, dermatitis and hyperkeratosis

Dermamist® (Alliance)
Spray application, white soft paraffin 10% in a basis containing liquid paraffin, fractionated coconut oil, net price 250-mL pressurised aerosol unit = £9.22
Excipients none as listed in section 13.1.3
For dry skin conditions including eczema, ichthyosis, pruritus of the elderly
Note Flammable

Diprobase® (Schering-Plough)
Cream, cetomacrogol 2.25%, cetostearyl alcohol 7.2%, liquid paraffin 6%, white soft paraffin 15%, water-miscible basis used for *Diprosone®* cream, net price 50 g = £1.34; 500-g pump pack = £6.76
Excipients include cetostearyl alcohol, chlorocresol
For dry skin conditions

Ointment, liquid paraffin 5%, white soft paraffin 95%, basis used for *Diprosone®* ointment, net price 50 g = £1.34
Excipients none as listed in section 13.1.3
For dry skin conditions

Doublebase® (Dermal)
Gel, isopropyl myristate 15%, liquid paraffin 15%, net price 100 g = £2.77, 500 g = £6.09
Excipients none as listed in section 13.1.3
For dry chapped or itchy skin conditions

Emollient shower gel, isopropyl myristate 15%, liquid paraffin 15%, net price 200 g = £5.45
Excipients none as listed in section 13.1.3
For dry and chapped skin conditions

Drapolene®
Section 13.2.2

E45® (Crookes)
Cream, light liquid paraffin 12.6%, white soft paraffin 14.5%, hypoallergenic anhydrous wool fat (hypoallergenic lanolin) 1% in self-emulsifying monostearin, net price 50 g = £1.40, 125 g = £2.55, 350 g = £4.46, 500-g pump pack = £6.20
Excipients include cetyl alcohol, hydroxybenzoates (parabens)
For dry skin conditions

Emollient Wash Cream, soap substitute, zinc oxide 5% in an emollient basis, net price 250-mL pump pack = £3.19
Excipients none as listed in section 13.1.3
ACBS: for endogenous and exogenous eczema, xeroderma, ichthyosis and senile pruritus (pruritus of the elderly) associated with dry skin

Lotion, light liquid paraffin 4%, cetomacrogol, white soft paraffin 10%, hypoallergenic anhydrous wool fat

(hypoallergenic lanolin) 1% in glyceryl monostearate, net price 200 mL = £2.40, 500-mL pump pack = £4.50
Excipients include isopropyl palmitate, hydroxybenzoates (parabens), benzyl alcohol
ACBS: for symptomatic relief of dry skin conditions, such as those associated with atopic eczema and contact dermatitis

Emollin® (C D Medical)
Spray, liquid paraffin 50%, white soft paraffin 50% in aerosol basis, net price 240 mL = £5.98
Excipients none as listed in section 13.1.3
For dry skin conditions

Epaderm® (Medlock)
Ointment, emulsifying wax 30%, yellow soft paraffin 30%, liquid paraffin 40%, net price 125 g = £3.55, 500 g = £6.02
Excipients include cetostearyl alcohol
For use as an emollient or soap substitute

Hewletts® (Kestrel)
Cream, hydrous wool fat 4%, zinc oxide 8%, arachis (peanut) oil, oleic acid, white soft paraffin, net price 35 g = £1.43, 400 g = £6.69
Excipients include fragrance
For nursing hygiene and care of skin, and chapped hands

Hydromol® (Alliance)
Cream, sodium pidolate 2.5%, liquid paraffin 13.8%, net price 50 g = £2.04, 100 g = £3.80, 500 g = £12.60
Excipients include cetyl alcohol, hydroxybenzoates (parabens)
For dry skin conditions
Ointment, yellow soft paraffin 30%, emulsifying wax 30%, liquid paraffin 40%, net price 125 g = £2.79, 500 g = £4.74
Excipients include cetostearyl alcohol
For use as an emollient, bath additive, or soap substitute

Kamillosan® (Goldshield)
Ointment, chamomile extracts 10.5% in a basis containing wool fat, net price 50 g = £2.50
Excipients include beeswax, cetostearyl alcohol, hydroxybenzoates (parabens)
For nappy rash, sore nipples, and chapped hands

Keri® (Novartis Consumer Health)
Lotion, mineral oil 16%, with lanolin oil, net price 190-mL pump pack = £3.56, 380-mL pump pack = £5.81
Excipients include fragrance, hydroxybenzoates (parabens), *N*-(3-chloroallyl) hexaminium chloride (quaternium 15), propylene glycol
For dry skin conditions and nappy rash

Linola® Gamma (Linderma)
Cream, evening primrose oil 20%, net price 50 g = £2.83, 250 g = £8.20
Excipients include beeswax, hydroxybenzoates (parabens), propylene glycol
Cautions epilepsy (but hazard unlikely with topical preparations)
For dry skin conditions

Lipobase® (Astellas)
Cream, fatty cream basis used for *Locoid Lipocream®*, net price 50 g = £2.08
Excipients include cetostearyl alcohol, hydroxybenzoates (parabens)
For dry skin conditions, also for use during treatment with topical corticosteroid and as diluent for *Locoid Lipocream®*

Neutrogena® Dermatological Cream (J&J)
Cream, glycerol 40% in an emollient basis, net price 100 g = £3.77
Excipients include cetostearyl alcohol, hydroxybenzoates (parabens)
For dry skin conditions

Oilatum® (Stiefel)
Cream, light liquid paraffin 6%, white soft paraffin 15%, net price 40 g = £1.79, 150 g = £3.38, 500-mL pump pack = £6.35, 1.05-litre pump pack = £14.67; *Oilatum® Junior* 150 g = £3.38, 350 mL = £4.65, 500 mL = £6.35, 1.05-litre pump pack = £14.67
Excipients include benzyl alcohol, cetostearyl alcohol
For dry skin conditions
Shower emollient (gel), light liquid paraffin 70%, net price 150 g = £5.15
Excipients include fragrance
For dry skin conditions including dermatitis

QV® (Crawford)
Cream, glycerol 10%, light liquid paraffin 10%, white soft paraffin 5%, net price 100 g = £1.95, 500 g = £5.60
Excipients include cetostearyl alcohol, hydroxybenzoates (parabens)
For dry skin conditions including eczema, psoriasis, ichthyosis, pruritus
Lotion, white soft paraffin 5%, net price 250 mL = £3.00
Excipients include cetostearyl alcohol, hydroxybenzoates (parabens)
For dry skin conditions including eczema, psoriasis, ichthyosis, pruritus
Wash, glycerol 10%, net price 200 mL = £2.50
Excipients include hydroxybenzoates (parabens)
For dry skin conditions including eczema, psoriasis, ichthyosis, and pruritus, use as soap substitute

Ultrabase® (Valeant)
Cream, water-miscible, containing liquid paraffin and white soft paraffin, net price 50 g = 89p, 500-g pump pack = £6.44
Excipients include fragrance, hydroxybenzoates (parabens), disodium edetate, stearyl alcohol
For dry skin conditions

Unguentum M® (Crookes)
Cream, containing saturated neutral oil, liquid paraffin, white soft paraffin, net price 50 g = £1.41, 100 g = £2.78, 200-mL pump pack = £5.50, 500 g = £8.48
Excipients include cetostearyl alcohol, polysorbate 40, propylene glycol, sorbic acid
For dry skin conditions and nappy rash

Vaseline Dermacare® (Elida Fabergé)
Cream, dimeticone 1%, white soft paraffin 15%, net price 150 mL = £2.11
Excipients include hydroxybenzoates (parabens)
ACBS: for endogenous and exogenous eczema, xeroderma, ichthyosis and senile pruritus (pruritus of the elderly) associated with dry skin
Lotion, dimeticone 1%, liquid paraffin 4%, white soft paraffin 5% in an emollient basis, net price 75 mL = 78p, 200 mL = £1.49
Excipients include disodium edetate, hydroxybenzoates (parabens), wool fat
ACBS: as for *Vaseline Dermacare® Cream*

Zerobase® (Zeroderma)
Cream, liquid paraffin 11%, net price 500-g pump pack = £5.99
Excipients include cetostearyl alcohol, chlorocresol
For dry skin conditions

Preparations containing urea

Aquadrate® (Alliance)
Cream, urea 10%, net price 30 g = £1.37, 100 g = £3.64
Excipients none as listed in section 13.1.3
Dose for dry, scaling and itching skin, apply thinly and rub into area when required

Balneum® Plus (Crookes)
Cream, urea 5%, lauromacrogols 3%, net price 100 g = £3.29, 175-g pump pack = £8.33, 500-g pump pack = £17.09
Excipients include benzyl alcohol, polysorbates
Dose for dry, scaling and itching skin, apply twice daily

Calmurid® (Galderma)
Cream, urea 10%, lactic acid 5%, net price 100 g = £7.36, 500-g pump pack = £28.37
Excipients none as listed in section 13.1.3
Dose for dry, scaling and itching skin, apply a thick layer for 3–5 minutes, massage into area, and remove excess, usually twice daily. Use half-strength cream for 1 week if stinging occurs
Note Can be diluted with aqueous cream (life of diluted cream 14 days)

E45® Itch Relief Cream (Crookes)
Cream, urea 5%, macrogol lauryl ether 3%, net price 50 g = £2.55, 100 g = £3.47, 500-g pump pack = £17.36
Excipients include benzyl alcohol, polysorbates
Dose for dry, scaling, and itching skin, apply twice a day

Eucerin® Intensive (Beiersdorf)
Cream, urea 10%, net price 100 mL = £7.15
Excipients include benzyl alcohol, isopropyl palmitate, wool fat
Dose for dry skin conditions including eczema, ichthyosis, xeroderma, hyperkeratosis, apply thinly and rub into area twice daily
Lotion, urea 10%, net price 250 mL = £7.69
Excipients include benzyl alcohol, isopropyl palmitate
Dose for dry skin conditions including eczema, ichthyosis, xeroderma, hyperkeratosis, apply sparingly and rub into area twice daily

Nutraplus® (Galderma)
Cream, urea 10%, net price 100 g = £4.37
Excipients include hydroxybenzoates (parabens), propylene glycol
Dose for dry, scaling and itching skin, apply 2–3 times daily

◢With antimicrobials

Dermol® (Dermal)
Cream, benzalkonium chloride 0.1%, chlorhexidine hydrochloride 0.1%, isopropyl myristate 10%, liquid paraffin 10%, net price 100-g tube = £3.22, 500-g bottle = £7.45
Excipients include cetostearyl alcohol
Dose for dry and pruritic skin conditions including eczema and dermatitis, apply to skin or use as soap substitute
Dermol® 500 Lotion, benzalkonium chloride 0.1%, chlorhexidine hydrochloride 0.1%, liquid paraffin 2.5%, isopropyl myristate 2.5%, net price 500-mL pump pack = £6.31
Excipients include cetostearyl alcohol
Dose for dry and pruritic skin conditions including eczema and dermatitis, apply to skin or use as soap substitute
Dermol® 200 Shower Emollient, benzalkonium chloride 0.1%, chlorhexidine hydrochloride 0.1%, liquid paraffin 2.5%, isopropyl myristate 2.5%, net price 200 mL = £3.71
Excipients include cetostearyl alcohol
Dose for dry and pruritic skin conditions including eczema and dermatitis, apply to skin or use as soap substitute

13.2.1.1 Emollient bath additives

Emollient bath additives should be added to bath water; hydration can be improved by soaking in the bath for 10–20 minutes. Some bath emollients can be applied to wet skin undiluted and rinsed off. In dry skin conditions soap should be avoided (see section 13.2.1 for soap substitutes). The quantities of bath additives recommended for adults are suitable for an adult-size bath. Proportionately less should be used for a child-size bath or a washbasin; recommended bath additive quantities for children reflect this.
Note These preparations make skin and surfaces slippery—particular care is needed when bathing

Alpha Keri Bath® (Novartis Consumer Health)
Bath oil, liquid paraffin 91.7%, oil-soluble fraction of wool fat 3%, net price 240 mL = £3.45, 480 mL = £6.43
Excipients include fragrance
Dose for dry skin conditions including ichthyosis and pruritus of the elderly, add 10–20 mL/bath (INFANT 5 mL) or apply to wet skin and rinse

Aveeno® (J&J)
Aveeno® Bath oil, colloidal oatmeal, white oat fraction in emollient basis, net price 250 mL = £4.28
Excipients include beeswax, fragrance
Dose ACBS: for endogenous and exogenous eczema, xeroderma, ichthyosis, and senile pruritus (pruritus of the elderly) associated with dry skin, add 30 mL/bath or apply to wet skin and rinse
Aveeno Colloidal® Bath additive, oatmeal, white oat fraction in emollient basis, net price 10 × 50-g sachets = £7.33
Excipients none as listed in section 13.1.3
Dose ACBS: as for Aveeno® Bath oil; add 1 sachet/bath (INFANT half sachet)

Balneum® (Crookes)
Balneum® bath oil, soya oil 84.75%, net price 200 mL = £2.48, 500 mL = £5.38, 1 litre = £10.39
Excipients include butylated hydroxytoluene, propylene glycol, fragrance
Dose for dry skin conditions including those associated with dermatitis and eczema; add 20–60 mL/bath (INFANT 5–15 mL); do not use undiluted
Balneum Plus® bath oil, soya oil 82.95%, mixed lauromacrogols 15%, net price 500 mL = £6.66
Excipients include butylated hydroxytoluene, propylene glycol, fragrance
Dose for dry skin conditions including those associated with dermatitis and eczema where pruritus also experienced; add 20 mL/bath (INFANT 5 mL) or apply to wet skin and rinse

Cetraben® (Genus)
Emollient bath additive, light liquid paraffin 82.8%, net price 500 mL = £5.25
Dose for dry skin conditions, including eczema, add 1–2 capfuls/bath (CHILD ½–1 capful) or apply to wet skin and rinse

Dermalo® (Dermal)
Bath emollient, acetylated wool alcohols 5%, liquid paraffin 65%, net price 500 mL = £3.60
Excipients none as listed in section 13.1.3
Dose for dermatitis, dry skin conditions including ichthyosis and pruritus of the elderly; add 15–20 mL/bath (INFANT and CHILD 5–10 mL) or apply to wet skin and rinse

Diprobath® (Schering-Plough)
Bath additive, isopropyl myristate 39%, light liquid paraffin 46%, net price 500 mL = £6.97
Excipients none as listed in section 13.1.3
Dose for dry skin conditions including dermatitis and eczema; add 25–50 mL/bath (INFANT 10 mL); do not use undiluted

E45® (Crookes)
Emollient bath oil, cetyl dimeticone 5%, liquid paraffin 91%, net price 250 mL = £3.19, 500 mL = £5.11
Excipients none as listed in section 13.1.3
Dose ACBS: for endogenous and exogenous eczema, xeroderma, ichthyosis, and senile pruritus (pruritus of the elderly) associated with dry skin; add 15 mL/bath (CHILD 5–10 mL) or apply to wet skin and rinse

Hydromol Emollient® (Alliance)
Bath additive, isopropyl myristate 13%, light liquid paraffin 37.8%, net price 350 mL = £3.80, 500 mL = £5.14, 1 litre = £9.00
Excipients none as listed in section 13.1.3
Dose for dry skin conditions including eczema, ichthyosis and pruritus of the elderly; add 1–3 capfuls/bath (INFANT ½–2 capfuls) or apply to wet skin and rinse

Imuderm® (Goldshield)

Bath oil, almond oil 30%, light liquid paraffin 69.6%, net price 250 mL = £3.75

Excipients include butylated hydroxyanisole

Dose for dry skin conditions including dermatitis, eczema, pruritus of the elderly, and ichthyosis, add 15–30 mL/bath (INFANT and CHILD 7.5–15 mL) or rub into dry skin until absorbed

Oilatum® (Stiefel)

Emollient bath additive (emulsion), acetylated wool alcohols 5%, liquid paraffin 63.4%, net price 250 mL = £2.75, 500 mL = £4.57

Excipients include isopropyl palmitate, fragrance

Dose for dry skin conditions including dermatitis, pruritus of the elderly and ichthyosis; add 1–3 capfuls/bath (INFANT 0.5–2 capfuls) or apply to wet skin and rinse

Junior Emollient bath additive, light liquid paraffin 63.4%, net price 150 mL = £2.82, 250 mL = £3.25, 300 mL = £5.10, 500 mL = £5.75

Excipients include wool fat, isopropyl palmitate

Dose for dry skin conditions including dermatitis, pruritus of the elderly and ichthyosis; add 1–3 capfuls/bath (INFANT 0.5–2 capfuls) or apply to wet skin and rinse

QV® (Crawford)

Bath oil, light liquid paraffin 85.09%, net price 200 mL = £2.20, 500 mL = £4.50

Excipients include hydroxybenzoates (parabens)

Dose for dry skin conditions including eczema, ichthyosis, and pruritus of the elderly, add 10 mL/bath (CHILD 7 mL, INFANT 4 mL) or apply to wet skin and rinse

With antimicrobials

Dermol® 600 (Dermal)

Bath Emollient, benzalkonium chloride 0.5%, liquid paraffin 25%, isopropyl myristate 25%, net price 600 mL = £7.90

Excipients include polysorbate 60

Dose for dry and pruritic skin conditions including eczema and dermatitis, add up to 30 mL/bath (INFANT up to 15 mL); do not use undiluted

Emulsiderm® (Dermal)

Liquid emulsion, liquid paraffin 25%, isopropyl myristate 25%, benzalkonium chloride 0.5%, net price 300 mL (with 15-mL measure) = £4.03, 1 litre (with 30-mL measure) = £12.55

Excipients include polysorbate 60

Dose for dry skin conditions including eczema and ichthyosis; add 7–30 mL/bath or rub into dry skin until absorbed

Oilatum® Plus (Stiefel)

Bath additive, benzalkonium chloride 6%, triclosan 2%, light liquid paraffin 52.5%, net price 500 mL = £6.98

Excipients include wool fat, isopropyl palmitate

Dose for topical treatment of eczema including eczema at risk from infection; add 1–2 capfuls/bath (CHILD over 6 months 1 mL); do not use undiluted

With tar

Section 13.5.2

13.2.2 Barrier preparations

Barrier preparations often contain water-repellent substances such as **dimeticone** (dimethicone) or other silicones. They are used on the skin around stomas, bedsores, and pressure areas in the elderly where the skin is intact. Where the skin has broken down, barrier preparations have a limited role in protecting adjacent skin. They are no substitute for adequate nursing care and it is doubtful if they are any more effective than **zinc ointments.**

Nappy rash Barrier creams and ointments are used for protection against nappy rash which is usually a local dermatitis. The first line of treatment is to ensure that nappies are changed frequently and that tightly fitting water-proof pants are avoided. The rash may clear when left exposed to the air and a barrier preparation can be helpful. If the rash is associated with a fungal infection, an antifungal cream such as clotrimazole cream (section 13.10.2) is useful. A mild corticosteroid such as hydrocortisone 1% is useful in moderate to severe inflammation, but it should be avoided in neonates. The barrier preparation is applied after the corticosteroid preparation to prevent further damage. Hydrocortisone can be used in combination with antifungal and antibacterial drugs (section 13.4) if there is considerable inflammation, erosion, and infection. Preparations containing hydrocortisone should be applied for no more than a week; the occlusive effect of nappies and water-proof pants may increase absorption (for cautions, see p. 605).

Non-proprietary barrier preparations

Zinc Cream, BP

Cream, zinc oxide 32%, arachis (peanut) oil 32%, calcium hydroxide 0.045%, oleic acid 0.5%, wool fat 8%, in freshly boiled and cooled purified water, net price 50 g = 50p

For nappy and urinary rash and eczematous conditions

Zinc Ointment, BP

Ointment, zinc oxide 15%, in Simple Ointment BP 1988 (which contains wool fat 5%, hard paraffin 5%, cetostearyl alcohol 5%, white soft paraffin 85%), net price 25 g = 22p

For nappy and urinary rash and eczematous conditions

Zinc and Castor Oil Ointment, BP

Ointment, zinc oxide 7.5%, castor oil 50%, arachis (peanut) oil 30.5%, white beeswax 10%, cetostearyl alcohol 2%, net price 100 g = 70p

For nappy and urinary rash

Proprietary barrier preparations

Conotrane® (Astellas)

Cream, benzalkonium chloride 0.1%, dimeticone '350' 22%, net price 100 g = 74p, 500 g = £3.51

Excipients include cetostearyl alcohol, fragrance

For nappy and urinary rash and pressure sores

Drapolene® (Chefaro UK)

Cream, benzalkonium chloride 0.01%, cetrimide 0.2% in a basis containing white soft paraffin, cetyl alcohol and wool fat, net price 100 g = £1.54, 200 g = £2.50, 350 g = £3.75

Excipients include cetyl alcohol, chlorocresol, wool fat

For nappy and urinary rash; minor wounds

Medicaid® (LPC)

Cream, cetrimide 0.5% in a basis containing light liquid paraffin, white soft paraffin, cetostearyl alcohol, glyceryl monostearate, net price 50 g = £1.69

Excipients include cetostearyl alcohol, fragrance, hydroxybenzoates (parabens), wool fat

For nappy rash, minor burns and abrasions

Metanium® (Ransom)

Ointment, titanium dioxide 20%, titanium peroxide 5%, titanium salicylate 3% in a basis containing

dimeticone, light liquid paraffin, white soft paraffin, and benzoin tincture, net price 30 g = £2.01
Excipients none as listed in section 13.1.3
For nappy rash and related disorders

Morhulin® (Thornton & Ross)
Ointment, cod-liver oil 11.4%, zinc oxide 38%, in a basis containing liquid paraffin and yellow soft paraffin, net price 50 g = £1.72
Excipients include wool fat derivative
For minor wounds, varicose ulcers, pressure sores, eczema and nappy rash

Siopel® (Centrapharm)
Barrier cream, dimeticone '1000' 10%, cetrimide 0.3%, arachis (peanut) oil, net price 50 g = £2.15
Excipients include butylated hydroxytoluene, cetostearyl alcohol, hydroxybenzoates (parabens)
For protection against water-soluble irritants

Sprilon® (Ayrton Saunders)
Spray application, dimeticone 1.04%, zinc oxide 12.5%, in a basis containing wool alcohols, cetostearyl alcohol, dextran, white soft paraffin, liquid paraffin, propellants, net price 115-g pressurised aerosol unit = £3.54
Excipients include cetostearyl alcohol, hydroxybenzoates (parabens), wool fat
For urinary rash, pressure sores, leg ulcers, moist eczema, fissures, fistulae and ileostomy care
Note Flammable

Sudocrem® (Forest)
Cream, benzyl alcohol 0.39%, benzyl benzoate 1.01%, benzyl cinnamate 0.15%, hydrous wool fat (hypoallergenic lanolin) 4%, zinc oxide 15.25%, net price 30 g = £1.01, 60 g = £1.13, 125 g = £1.70, 250 g = £2.89, 400 g = £4.08
Excipients include beeswax (synthetic), propylene glycol, fragrance
For nappy rash and pressure sores

Vasogen® (Forest)
Barrier cream, dimeticone 20%, calamine 1.5%, zinc oxide 7.5%, net price 50 g = 80p, 100 g = £1.36
Excipients include hydroxybenzoates (parabens), wool fat
For nappy rash, pressure sores, ileostomy and colostomy care

13.3 Topical local anaesthetics and antipruritics

Pruritus may be caused by systemic disease (such as drug hypersensitivity, obstructive jaundice, endocrine disease, and certain malignant diseases), skin disease (e.g. psoriasis, eczema, urticaria, and scabies) or as a side-effect of opioid analgesics. Where possible the underlying causes should be treated. An **emollient** (section 13.2.1) may be of value where the pruritus is associated with dry skin. Pruritus that occurs in otherwise healthy elderly people can also be treated with an emollient. For advice on the treatment of pruritus in palliative care, see p. 17.

Preparations containing **crotamiton** are sometimes used but are of uncertain value. Preparations containing **calamine** are often ineffective.

A topical preparation containing **doxepin** 5% is licensed for the relief of pruritus in eczema; it can cause drowsiness and there may be a risk of sensitisation.

Pruritus is common in biliary obstruction, especially in primary biliary cirrhosis and drug-induced cholestasis. Oral administration of **colestyramine** (cholestyramine) is the treatment of choice (section 1.9.2).

Topical antihistamines and local anaesthetics are only marginally effective and may occasionally cause sensitisation. For *insect stings* and *insect bites*, a short course of a topical corticosteroid is appropriate. Short treatment with a **sedating antihistamine** (section 3.4.1) may help in insect stings and in intractable pruritus where sedation is desirable. Calamine preparations are of little value for the treatment of insect stings or bites.

For preparations used in *pruritus ani*, see section 1.7.1.

CALAMINE

Indications pruritus

Calamine (Non-proprietary)
Aqueous cream, calamine 4%, zinc oxide 3%, liquid paraffin 20%, self-emulsifying glyceryl monostearate 5%, cetomacrogol emulsifying wax 5%, phenoxyethanol 0.5%, freshly boiled and cooled purified water 62.5%, net price 100 mL = 59p
Lotion (= cutaneous suspension), calamine 15%, zinc oxide 5%, glycerol 5%, bentonite 3%, sodium citrate 0.5%, liquefied phenol 0.5%, in freshly boiled and cooled purified water, net price 200 mL = 63p
Oily lotion (BP 1980), calamine 5%, arachis (peanut) oil 50%, oleic acid 0.5%, wool fat 1%, in calcium hydroxide solution, net price 200 mL = £1.57

CROTAMITON

Indications pruritus (including pruritus after scabies—section 13.10.4); see notes above
Cautions avoid use near eyes and broken skin; use on doctor's advice for children under 3 years
Contra-indications acute exudative dermatoses
Dose
- Pruritus, apply 2–3 times daily; CHILD below 3 years, apply once daily

Eurax® (Novartis Consumer Health)
Cream, crotamiton 10%, net price 30 g = £2.27, 100 g = £3.95
Excipients include beeswax, fragrance, hydroxybenzoates (parabens), stearyl alcohol
Lotion, crotamiton 10%, net price 100 mL = £2.99
Excipients include cetyl alcohol, fragrance, propylene glycol, sorbic acid, stearyl alcohol

DOXEPIN HYDROCHLORIDE

Indications pruritus in eczema; depressive illness (section 4.3.1)
Cautions susceptibility to angle-closure glaucoma, urinary retention, severe liver impairment, mania; avoid application to large areas; pregnancy and breast-feeding; **interactions**: Appendix 1 (antidepressants, tricyclic)
Driving Drowsiness may affect performance of skilled tasks (e.g. driving); effects of alcohol enhanced
Side-effects drowsiness; local burning, stinging, irritation, tingling and rash; systemic side-effects such as

antimuscarinic effects, headache, fever, dizziness, gastro-intestinal disturbances also reported

Dose

- ADULT and CHILD over 12 years, apply thinly 3–4 times daily; usual max. 3 g per application; usual total max. 12 g daily; coverage should be less than 10% of body surface area

Xepin® (CHS) PoM

Cream, doxepin hydrochloride 5%, net price 30 g = £11.70. Label: 2, 10, patient information leaflet

Excipients include benzyl alcohol

TOPICAL LOCAL ANAESTHETICS

Indications relief of local pain, see notes above. See section 15.2 for use in surface anaesthesia

Cautions occasionally cause hypersensitivity

Note Topical local anaesthetic preparations may be absorbed, especially through mucosal surfaces, therefore excessive application should be avoided and they should preferably not be used for more than about 3 days; not generally suitable for young children

TOPICAL ANTIHISTAMINES

Indications see notes above

Cautions may cause hypersensitivity; avoid in eczema; photosensitivity (diphenhydramine); not recommended for longer than 3 days

13.4 Topical corticosteroids

Topical corticosteroids are used for the treatment of inflammatory conditions of the skin (other than those arising from an infection) in particular eczema (section 13.5.1), contact dermatitis, insect stings (p. 36), and eczema of scabies (section 13.10.4). Corticosteroids suppress the inflammatory reaction during use; they are not curative and on discontinuation a rebound exacerbation of the condition may occur. They are generally used to relieve symptoms and suppress signs of the disorder when other measures such as emollients are ineffective.

Topical corticosteroids are of no value in the treatment of urticaria and they are **contra-indicated** in rosacea; they may worsen ulcerated or secondarily infected lesions. They should not be used indiscriminately in pruritus (where they will only benefit if inflammation is causing the itch) and are **not** recommended for acne vulgaris.

Systemic or potent topical corticosteroids should be avoided or given only under specialist supervision in *psoriasis* because, although they may suppress the psoriasis in the short term, relapse or vigorous rebound occurs on withdrawal (sometimes precipitating severe pustular psoriasis). Topical use of potent corticosteroids on widespread psoriasis can lead to systemic as well as to local side-effects. It is reasonable, however, to prescribe a mild to moderate topical corticosteroid for a short period (2–4 weeks) for *flexural* and *facial psoriasis*. It is reasonable to use a more potent corticosteroid such as betamethasone or fluocinonide for psoriasis of the scalp, palms or soles (see below for cautions in psoriasis).

In general, the most potent topical corticosteroids should be reserved for recalcitrant dermatoses such as *chronic discoid lupus erythematosus, lichen simplex chronicus, hypertrophic lichen planus,* and *palmoplantar pustulosis.* Potent corticosteroids should generally be avoided on the face and skin flexures, but specialists occasionally prescribe them for these areas in certain circumstances.

When topical treatment has failed, intralesional corticosteroid injections (section 10.1.2.2) may be used. These are more effective than the very potent topical corticosteroid preparations and should be reserved for severe cases where there are localised lesions such as *keloid scars, hypertrophic lichen planus,* or *localised alopecia areata.*

Perioral lesions **Hydrocortisone** cream 1% can be used for up to 7 days to treat uninfected inflammatory lesions on the lips and on the skin surrounding the mouth. **Hydrocortisone and miconazole** cream or ointment is useful where infection by susceptible organisms and inflammation co-exist, particularly for initial treatment (up to 7 days) e.g. in angular cheilitis (see also p. 593). Organisms susceptible to miconazole include *Candida* spp. and many Gram-positive bacteria including streptococci and staphylococci.

Children Children, especially infants, are particularly susceptible to side-effects. However, concern about the safety of topical corticosteroids in children should not result in the child being undertreated. The aim is to control the condition as well as possible; inadequate treatment will perpetuate the condition. A mild corticosteroid such as hydrocortisone 1% ointment or cream is useful for treating nappy rash (section 13.2.2) and for atopic eczema in childhood (section 13.5.1). A moderately potent or potent corticosteroid may be appropriate for severe atopic eczema on the limbs, for 1–2 weeks only, switching to a less potent preparation as the condition improves. In an acute flare-up of atopic eczema, it may be appropriate to use more potent formulations of topical corticosteroids for a short period to regain control of the condition. A very potent corticosteroid should generally be prescribed under the supervision of a consultant dermatologist. Continuous daily application of a mild corticosteroid such as hydrocortisone 1% is equivalent to a potent corticosteroid such as betamethasone 0.1% applied intermittently. Carers of young children should be advised that treatment should **not** necessarily be reserved to 'treat only the worst areas' and they may need to be advised that patient information leaflets may contain inappropriate advice for the patient's condition.

Choice of formulation Water-miscible corticosteroid *creams* are suitable for moist or weeping lesions whereas *ointments* are generally chosen for dry, lichenified or scaly lesions or where a more occlusive effect is required. *Lotions* may be useful when minimal application to a large or hair-bearing area is required or for the treatment of exudative lesions. *Occlusive polythene or hydrocolloid dressings* increase absorption, but also increase the risk of side-effects; they are therefore used only under supervision on a short-term basis for areas of very thick skin (such as the palms and soles).

The inclusion of urea or salicylic acid also increases the penetration of the corticosteroid.

In the BNF topical corticosteroids for the skin are categorised as 'mild', 'moderately potent', 'potent' or 'very potent' (see below); the **least potent** preparation which is effective should be chosen but dilution should be avoided whenever possible.

Cautions Avoid prolonged use of a topical corticosteroid on the face (and keep away from eyes). In children avoid prolonged use and use potent or very potent corticosteroids under specialist supervision; extreme caution is required in dermatoses of infancy including nappy rash—treatment should be limited to 5–7 days.

Psoriasis The use of potent or very potent corticosteroids in psoriasis can result in rebound relapse, development of generalised pustular psoriasis, and local and systemic toxicity.

Contra-indications Topical corticosteroids are contra-indicated in untreated bacterial, fungal, or viral skin lesions, in acne rosacea, and in perioral dermatitis; potent corticosteroids are contra-indicated in widespread plaque psoriasis (see notes above).

Side-effects *Mild* and *moderately potent* topical corticosteroids are associated with few side-effects but care is required in the use of *potent* and *very potent* corticosteroids. Absorption through the skin can rarely cause adrenal suppression and even Cushing's syndrome (section 6.3.2), depending on the area of the body being treated and the duration of treatment. Absorption is greatest where the skin is thin or raw, and from intertriginous areas; it is increased by occlusion. Local side-effects include:

- spread and worsening of untreated infection;
- thinning of the skin which may be restored over a period after stopping treatment but the original structure may never return;
- irreversible striae atrophicae and telangiectasia;
- contact dermatitis;
- perioral dermatitis;
- acne, or worsening of acne or acne rosacea;
- mild depigmentation which may be reversible;
- hypertrichosis also reported

In order to minimise the side-effects of a topical corticosteroid, it is important to apply it **thinly** to affected areas **only**, no more frequently than **twice daily**, and to use the least potent formulation which is fully effective.

Application Topical corticosteroid preparations should be applied no more frequently than twice daily; once daily is often sufficient.

Topical corticosteroids are spread thinly on the skin; the length of cream or ointment expelled from a tube may be used to specify the quantity to be applied to a given area of skin. This length can be measured in terms of a *fingertip unit* (the distance from the tip of the adult index finger to the first crease). One fingertip unit (approximately 500 mg) is sufficient to cover an area that is twice that of the flat adult palm.

Suitable quantities of corticosteroid preparations to be prescribed for specific areas of the body

	Creams and Ointments
Face and neck	15 to 30 g
Both hands	15 to 30 g
Scalp	15 to 30 g
Both arms	30 to 60 g
Both legs	100 g
Trunk	100 g
Groins and genitalia	15 to 30 g

These amounts are usually suitable for an adult for a single daily application for 2 weeks

Mixing topical preparations on the skin should be avoided where possible; at least 30 minutes should elapse between application of different preparations. The practice of using an emollient immediately before a topical corticosteroid is inappropriate.

Compound preparations The advantages of including other substances (such as antibacterials or antifungals) with corticosteroids in topical preparations are uncertain, but such combinations may have a place where inflammatory skin conditions are associated with bacterial or fungal infection, such as infected eczema. In these cases the antimicrobial drug should be chosen according to the sensitivity of the infecting organism and used regularly for a short period (typically twice daily for 1 week). Longer use increases the likelihood of resistance and of sensitisation.

Topical corticosteroid preparation potencies

Potency of a topical corticosteroid preparation is a result of the formulation as well as the corticosteroid. Therefore, proprietary names are shown below.

Mild

Hydrocortisone 0.1–2.5%, *Dioderm, Efcortelan, Mildison*

- Mild with antimicrobials: *Canesten HC, Daktacort, Econacort, Fucidin H, Nystaform-HC, Synalar 1 in 10 Dilution, Timodine, Vioform-Hydrocortisone*
- Mild with crotamiton: *Eurax-Hydrocortisone*

Moderate

Betnovate-RD, Eumovate, Haelan, Modrasone, Synalar 1 in 4 Dilution, Ultralanum Plain

- Moderate with antimicrobials: *Trimovate*
- Moderate with urea: *Alphaderm, Calmurid HC*

Potent

Betamethasone valerate 0.1%, *Betacap, Bettamousse, Betnovate, Cutivate, Diprosone Elocon,* Hydrocortisone butyrate, *Locoid, Locoid Crelo, Metosyn, Nerisone, Synalar*

- Potent with antimicrobials: *Aureocort, Betnovate-C, Betnovate-N, FuciBET, Locoid C, Lotriderm, Synalar C, Synalar N, Tri-Adcortyl*
- Potent with salicylic acid: *Diprosalic*

Very potent

Clarelux, Dermovate, Nerisone Forte

HYDROCORTISONE

Indications mild inflammatory skin disorders such as eczemas (but for over-the-counter preparations, see below); nappy rash, see notes above and section 13.2.2

Cautions see notes above

Contra-indications see notes above

Side-effects see notes above

Dose

- Apply thinly 1–2 times daily

Hydrocortisone (Non-proprietary) PoM

Cream, hydrocortisone 0.5%, net price, 15 g = £3.54, 30 g = £5.19; 1%, 15 g = £2.48, 30 g = £4.86 Label: 28. Potency: mild

Dental prescribing on NHS Hydrocortisone Cream 1% 15 g may be prescribed

Ointment, hydrocortisone 0.5%, net price 15 g = £4.86 , 30 g = £5.23; 1%, 15 g = £3.11, 30 g = £5.26.Label: 28. Potency: mild

When hydrocortisone cream or ointment is prescribed and no strength is stated, the 1% strength should be supplied

Over-the-counter hydrocortisone preparations

Skin creams and ointments containing hydrocortisone (alone or with other ingredients) can be sold to the public for the treatment of allergic contact dermatitis, irritant dermatitis, insect bite reactions and mild to moderate eczema, to be applied sparingly over the affected area 1–2 times daily for max. 1 week. Over-the-counter hydrocortisone preparations should not be sold without medical advice for children under 10 years or for pregnant women; they should **not** be sold for application to the face, anogenital region, broken or infected skin (including cold sores, acne, and athlete's foot).

Proprietary hydrocortisone preparations

Dioderm® (Dermal) PoM

Cream, hydrocortisone 0.1%, net price 30 g = £2.50. Label: 28. Potency: mild

Excipients include cetostearyl alcohol, propylene glycol

Note Although this contains only 0.1% hydrocortisone, the formulation is designed to provide a clinical activity comparable to that of Hydrocortisone Cream 1% BP

Efcortelan® (GSK) PoM

Cream, hydrocortisone 0.5%, net price, 30 g = 61p; 1%, 30 g = 75p. Label: 28. Potency: mild

Excipients include cetostearyl alcohol, chlorocresol

Ointment, hydrocortisone 0.5%, net price, 30 g = 61p; 1%, 30 g = 75p; 2.5%, 30 g = £1.70. Label: 28. Potency: mild

Excipients none as listed in section 13.1.3

Mildison® (Astellas) PoM

Lipocream, hydrocortisone 1%, net price 30 g = £2.45. Label: 28. Potency: mild

Excipients include cetostearyl alcohol, hydroxybenzoates (parabens)

Compound preparations

Compound preparations with coal tar see section 13.5.2

Alphaderm® (Alliance) PoM

Cream, hydrocortisone 1%, urea 10%, net price 30 g = £1.98; 100 g = £5.86. Label: 28. Potency: moderate

Excipients none as listed in section 13.1.3

Calmurid HC® (Galderma) PoM

Cream, hydrocortisone 1%, urea 10%, lactic acid 5%, net price 30 g = £2.80, 50 g = £4.67. Label: 28. Potency: moderate

Excipients none as listed in section 13.1.3

Note Manufacturer advises dilute to half-strength with aqueous cream for 1 week if stinging occurs then transfer to undiluted preparation (but see section 13.1.1 for advice to avoid dilution where possible)

[1]**Eurax-Hydrocortisone®** (Novartis Consumer Health) PoM

Cream, hydrocortisone 0.25%, crotamiton 10%, net price 30 g = 87p. Label: 28. Potency: mild

Excipients include fragrance, hydroxybenzoates (parabens), propylene glycol, stearyl alcohol

1. A 15-g tube is on sale to the public for treatment of contact dermatitis and insect bites

With antimicrobials

See notes above for comment on compound preparations

[1]**Canesten HC®** (Bayer Consumer Care) PoM

Cream, hydrocortisone 1%, clotrimazole 1%, net price 30 g = £2.42. Label: 28. Potency: mild

Excipients include benzyl alcohol, cetostearyl alcohol

1. A 15-g tube is on sale to the public for the treatment of athlete's foot and fungal infection of skin folds with associated inflammation

Daktacort® (Janssen-Cilag) PoM

Cream, hydrocortisone 1%, miconazole nitrate 2%, net price 30 g = £1.90. Label: 28. Potency: mild

Excipients include butylated hydroxyanisole, disodium edetate

Note A 15-g tube is on sale to the public for the treatment of athlete's foot and candidal intertrigo

Ointment, hydrocortisone 1%, miconazole nitrate 2%, net price 30 g = £2.09. Label: 28. Potency: mild

Excipients none as listed in section 13.1.3

Dental prescribing on NHS May be prescribed as Hydrocortisone and Miconazole Cream or Ointment for max. 7 days

Econacort® (Squibb) PoM

Cream, hydrocortisone 1%, econazole nitrate 1%, net price 30 g = £2.25. Label: 28. Potency: mild

Excipients include butylated hydroxyanisole

Fucidin H® (LEO) PoM

Cream, hydrocortisone acetate 1%, fusidic acid 2%, net price 30 g = £5.30, 60 g = £10.60. Label: 28. Potency: mild

Excipients include butylated hydroxyanisole, cetyl alcohol, potassium sorbate, polysorbate 60

Ointment, hydrocortisone acetate 1%, sodium fusidate 2%, net price 30 g = £3.26, 60 g = £6.53. Label: 28. Potency: mild

Excipients include cetyl alcohol, wool fat

Nystaform-HC® (Typharm) PoM

Cream, hydrocortisone 0.5%, nystatin 100 000 units/g, chlorhexidine hydrochloride 1%, net price 30 g = £2.66. Label: 28. Potency: mild

Excipients include benzyl alcohol, cetostearyl alcohol, polysorbate '60'

Ointment, hydrocortisone 1%, nystatin 100 000 units/g, chlorhexidine acetate 1%, net price 30 g = £2.66. Label: 28. Potency: mild

Excipients none as listed in section 13.1.3

Timodine® (R&C) PoM

Cream, hydrocortisone 0.5%, nystatin 100 000 units/g, benzalkonium chloride solution 0.2%, dimeticone '350' 10%, net price 30 g = £2.38. Label: 28. Potency: mild

Excipients include butylated hydroxyanisole, cetostearyl alcohol, hydroxybenzoates (parabens), sodium metabisulphite, sorbic acid

Vioform-Hydrocortisone® (Novartis Consumer Health) PoM

Cream, hydrocortisone 1%, clioquinol 3%, net price 30 g = £1.46. Label: 28. Potency: mild

Excipients include cetostearyl alcohol

Ointment, hydrocortisone 1%, clioquinol 3%, net price 30 g = £1.46. Label: 28. Potency: mild

Excipients none as listed in section 13.1.3

Note Stains clothing

HYDROCORTISONE BUTYRATE

Indications severe inflammatory skin disorders such as eczemas unresponsive to less potent corticosteroids; psoriasis, see notes above

Cautions see notes above

Contra-indications see notes above

Side-effects see notes above

Dose

- Apply thinly 1–2 times daily

Locoid® (Astellas) PoM

Cream, hydrocortisone butyrate 0.1%, net price 30 g = £2.29, 100 g = £7.05. Label: 28. Potency: potent

Excipients include cetostearyl alcohol, hydroxybenzoates (parabens)

Lipocream, hydrocortisone butyrate 0.1%, net price 30 g = £2.41, 100 g = £7.38. Label: 28. Potency: potent

Excipients include benzyl alcohol, cetostearyl alcohol, hydroxybenzoates (parabens)

Note For bland cream basis see *Lipobase®*, section 13.2.1

Ointment, hydrocortisone butyrate 0.1%, net price 30 g = £2.29, 100 g = £7.05. Label: 28. Potency: potent

Excipients none as listed in section 13.1.3

Scalp lotion, hydrocortisone butyrate 0.1%, in an aqueous isopropyl alcohol basis, net price 100 mL = £9.76. Label: 15, 28. Potency: potent

Excipients none as listed in section 13.1.3

Locoid Crelo® (Astellas) PoM

Lotion (topical emulsion), hydrocortisone butyrate 0.1% in a water-miscible basis, net price 100 g (with applicator nozzle) = £8.44. Label: 28. Potency: potent

Excipients include butylated hydroxytoluene, cetostearyl alcohol, hydroxybenzoates (parabens), propylene glycol

With antimicrobials

See notes above for comment on compound preparations

Locoid C® (Astellas) PoM

Cream, hydrocortisone butyrate 0.1%, chlorquinaldol 3%, net price 30 g = £3.00. Label: 28. Potency: potent

Excipients include cetostearyl alcohol

Note Stains clothing and can darken skin and hair

Ointment, hydrocortisone butyrate 0.1%, chlorquinaldol 3%, in a greasy basis, net price 30 g = £3.00. Label: 28. Potency: potent

Excipients none as listed in section 13.1.3

Note Stains clothing and can darken skin and hair

ALCLOMETASONE DIPROPIONATE

Indications inflammatory skin disorders such as eczemas

Cautions see notes above

Contra-indications see notes above

Side-effects see notes above

Dose

- Apply thinly 1–2 times daily

Modrasone® (PLIVA) PoM

Cream, alclometasone dipropionate 0.05%, net price 50 g = £2.68. Label: 28. Potency: moderate

Excipients include cetostearyl alcohol, chlorocresol, propylene glycol

Ointment, alclometasone dipropionate 0.05%, net price 50 g = £2.68. Label: 28. Potency: moderate

Excipients include beeswax, propylene glycol

BETAMETHASONE ESTERS

Indications severe inflammatory skin disorders such as eczemas unresponsive to less potent corticosteroids; psoriasis, see notes above

Cautions see notes above; use of more than 100 g per week of 0.1% preparation likely to cause adrenal suppression

Contra-indications see notes above

Side-effects see notes above

Dose

- Apply thinly 1–2 times daily

Betamethasone Valerate (Non-proprietary) PoM

Cream, betamethasone (as valerate) 0.1%, net price 30 g = £1.42, 100 g = £4.05. Label: 28. Potency: potent

Ointment, betamethasone (as valerate) 0.1%, net price 30 g = £1.38, 100 g = £4.05. Label: 28. Potency: potent

Betacap® (Dermal) PoM

Scalp application, betamethasone (as valerate) 0.1% in a water-miscible basis containing coconut oil derivative, net price 100 mL = £3.92. Label: 15, 28. Potency: potent

Excipients none as listed in section 13.1.3

Betnovate® (GSK) PoM

Cream, betamethasone (as valerate) 0.1% in a water-miscible basis, net price 30 g = £1.43, 100 g = £4.05. Label: 28. Potency: potent

Excipients include cetostearyl alcohol, chlorocresol

Ointment, betamethasone (as valerate) 0.1% in an anhydrous paraffin basis, net price 30 g = £1.43, 100 g = £4.05. Label 28. Potency: potent

Excipients none as listed in section 13.1.3

Lotion, betamethasone (as valerate) 0.1%, net price 100 mL = £4.86. Label: 28. Potency: potent

Excipients include cetostearyl alcohol, hydroxybenzoates (parabens)

Scalp application, betamethasone (as valerate) 0.1% in a water-miscible basis, net price 100 mL = £5.30. Label: 15, 28. Potency: potent

Excipients none as listed in section 13.1.3

Betnovate-RD® (GSK) PoM

Cream, betamethasone (as valerate) 0.025% in a water-miscible basis (1 in 4 dilution of *Betnovate®* cream), net price 100 g = £3.34. Label: 28. Potency: moderate

Excipients include cetostearyl alcohol, chlorocresol

Ointment, betamethasone (as valerate) 0.025% in an anhydrous paraffin basis (1 in 4 dilution of *Betnovate®* ointment), net price 100 g = £3.34. Label: 28. Potency: moderate

Excipients none as listed in section 13.1.3

Bettamousse® (UCB Pharma) PoM

Foam (= scalp application), betamethasone valerate 0.12% (≡ betamethasone 0.1%), net price 100 g = £9.75. Label: 28. Potency: potent

Excipients include cetyl alcohol, polysorbate 60, propylene glycol, stearyl alcohol

Note Flammable

Diprosone® (Schering-Plough) PoM
Cream, betamethasone (as dipropionate) 0.05%, net price 30 g = £2.24, 100 g = £6.36. Label: 28. Potency: potent
Excipients include cetostearyl alcohol, chlorocresol

Ointment, betamethasone (as dipropionate) 0.05%, net price 30 g = £2.24, 100 g = £6.36. Label: 28. Potency: potent
Excipients none as listed in section 13.1.3

Lotion, betamethasone (as dipropionate) 0.05%, net price 30 mL = £2.83, 100 mL = £8.10. Label: 28. Potency: potent
Excipients none as listed in section 13.1.3

With salicylic acid

See notes above for comment on compound preparations

Diprosalic® (Schering-Plough) PoM
Ointment, betamethasone (as dipropionate) 0.05%, salicylic acid 3%, net price 30 g = £3.30, 100 g = £9.50. Label: 28. Potency: potent
Excipients none as listed in section 13.1.3
Dose apply thinly 1–2 times daily; max. 60 g per week

Scalp application, betamethasone (as dipropionate) 0.05%, salicylic acid 2%, in an alcoholic basis, net price 100 mL = £10.50. Label: 28. Potency: potent
Excipients include disodium edetate
Dose apply a few drops 1–2 times daily

With antimicrobials

See notes above for comment on compound preparations

Betnovate-C® (GSK) PoM
Cream, betamethasone (as valerate) 0.1%, clioquinol 3%, net price 30 g = £1.76. Label: 28. Potency: potent
Excipients include cetostearyl alcohol, chlorocresol
Note Stains clothing

Ointment, betamethasone (as valerate) 0.1%, clioquinol 3%, net price 30 g = £1.76. Label: 28. Potency: potent
Excipients none as listed in section 13.1.3
Note Stains clothing

Betnovate-N® (GSK) PoM
Cream, betamethasone (as valerate) 0.1%, neomycin sulphate 0.5%, net price 30 g = £1.76, 100 g = £4.88. Label: 28. Potency: potent
Excipients include cetostearyl alcohol, chlorocresol

Ointment, betamethasone (as valerate) 0.1%, neomycin sulphate 0.5%, net price 30 g = £1.76, 100 g = £4.88. Label: 28. Potency: potent
Excipients none as listed in section 13.1.3

FuciBET® (LEO) PoM
Cream, betamethasone (as valerate) 0.1%, fusidic acid 2%, net price 30 g = £5.62, 60 g = £11.23. Label: 28. Potency: potent
Excipients include cetostearyl alcohol, chlorocresol

Lotriderm® (PLIVA) PoM
Cream, betamethasone dipropionate 0.064% (≡ betamethasone 0.05%), clotrimazole 1%, net price 30 g = £6.34. Label: 28. Potency: potent
Excipients include benzyl alcohol, cetostearyl alcohol, propylene glycol

CLOBETASOL PROPIONATE

Indications short-term treatment only of severe resistant inflammatory skin disorders such as recalcitrant eczemas unresponsive to less potent corticosteroids; psoriasis, see notes above
Cautions see notes above
Contra-indications see notes above
Side-effects see notes above
Dose
- Apply thinly 1–2 times daily for up to 4 weeks; max. 50 g of 0.05% preparation per week

Clarelux® (Fabre) PoM
Foam(= scalp application), clobetasol propionate 0.05%, net price 100 g = £11.06. Label: 15, 28. Potency: very potent
Excipients include cetyl alcohol, polysorbate 60, propylene glycol, stearyl alcohol
Caution flammable
Note Apply directly to scalp lesions (foam begins to subside immediately on contact with skin)

Dermovate® (GSK) PoM
Cream, clobetasol propionate 0.05%, net price 30 g = £2.86, 100 g = £8.39. Label: 28. Potency: very potent
Excipients include beeswax (or beeswax substitute), cetostearyl alcohol, chlorocresol, propylene glycol

Ointment, clobetasol propionate 0.05%, net price 30 g = £2.86, 100 g = £8.39. Label: 28. Potency: very potent
Excipients include propylene glycol

Scalp application, clobetasol propionate 0.05%, in a thickened alcoholic basis, net price 30 mL = £3.26, 100 mL = £11.06. Label: 15, 28. Potency: very potent
Excipients none as listed in section 13.1.3

Etrivex® (Galderma) PoM
Shampoo, clobetasol propionate 0.05%, net price 125 mL = £11.94. Label: 28. Potency: very potent
Excipients none as listed in section 13.1.3
Dose moderate scalp psoriasis, ADULT over 18 years, apply thinly once daily, rinse off after 15 minutes; reduce frequency of application after clinical improvement; max. duration of treatment 4 weeks

CLOBETASONE BUTYRATE

Indications eczemas and dermatitis of all types; maintenance between courses of more potent corticosteroids
Cautions see notes above
Contra-indications see notes above
Side-effects see notes above
Dose
- Apply thinly 1–2 times daily

[1]**Eumovate®** (GSK) PoM
Cream, clobetasone butyrate 0.05%, net price 30 g = £1.97, 100 g = £5.77. Label: 28. Potency: moderate
Excipients include beeswax substitute, cetostearyl alcohol, chlorocresol

Ointment, clobetasone butyrate 0.05%, net price 30 g = £1.97, 100 g = £5.77. Label: 28. Potency: moderate
Excipients none as listed in section 13.1.3

1. Cream can be sold to the public for short-term symptomatic treatment and control of patches of eczema and dermatitis (but not seborrhoeic dermatitis) in adults and children over 12 years provided pack does not contain more than 15 g

With antimicrobials

See notes above for comment on compound preparations

Trimovate® (GSK) PoM
Cream, clobetasone butyrate 0.05%, oxytetracycline 3% (as calcium salt), nystatin 100 000 units/g, net price 30 g = £3.49. Label: 28. Potency: moderate
Excipients include cetostearyl alcohol, chlorocresol, sodium metabisulphite
Note Stains clothing

DIFLUCORTOLONE VALERATE

Indications severe inflammatory skin disorders such as eczemas unresponsive to less potent corticosteroids; high strength (0.3%), short-term treatment of severe exacerbations; psoriasis, see notes above

Cautions see notes above

Contra-indications see notes above

Side-effects see notes above

Dose

- Apply thinly 1–2 times daily for up to 4 weeks (0.1% preparations) or 2 weeks (0.3% preparations), reducing strength as condition responds; max. 60 g of 0.3% per week

Nerisone® (Meadow) PoM

Cream, diflucortolone valerate 0.1%, net price 30 g = £1.59. Label: 28. Potency: potent
Excipients include disodium edetate, hydroxybenzoates (parabens), stearyl alcohol

Oily cream, diflucortolone valerate 0.1%, net price 30 g = £2.56. Label: 28. Potency: potent
Excipients include beeswax

Ointment, diflucortolone valerate 0.1%, net price 30 g = £1.59. Label: 28. Potency: potent
Excipients none as listed in section 13.1.3

Nerisone Forte® (Meadow) PoM

Oily cream, diflucortolone valerate 0.3%, net price 15 g = £2.09. Label: 28. Potency: very potent
Excipients include beeswax

Ointment, diflucortolone valerate 0.3%, net price 15 g = £2.09. Label: 28. Potency: very potent
Excipients none as listed in section 13.1.3

FLUDROXYCORTIDE
(Flurandrenolone)

Indications inflammatory skin disorders such as eczemas

Cautions see notes above

Contra-indications see notes above

Side-effects see notes above

Dose

- Apply thinly 1–2 times daily

Haelan® (Typharm) PoM

Cream, fludroxycortide 0.0125%, net price 60 g = £3.26. Label: 28. Potency: moderate
Excipients include cetyl alcohol, propylene glycol

Ointment, fludroxycortide 0.0125%, net price 60 g = £3.26. Label: 28. Potency: moderate
Excipients include beeswax, cetyl alcohol, polysorbate

Tape, polythene adhesive film impregnated with fludroxycortide 4 micrograms /cm^2, net price 7.5 cm × 50 cm = £9.27, 7.5 cm × 200 cm = £24.95
Dose for chronic localised recalcitrant dermatoses (but not acute or weeping), cut tape to fit lesion, apply to clean, dry skin shorn of hair, usually for 12 hours daily

FLUOCINOLONE ACETONIDE

Indications inflammatory skin disorders such as eczemas; psoriasis, see notes above

Cautions see notes above

Contra-indications see notes above

Side-effects see notes above

Dose

- Apply thinly 1–2 times daily, reducing strength as condition responds

Synalar® (GP Pharma) PoM

Cream, fluocinolone acetonide 0.025%, net price 30 g = £2.93, 100 g = £8.34. Label: 28. Potency: potent
Excipients include benzyl alcohol, cetostearyl alcohol, polysorbates, propylene glycol

Gel, fluocinolone acetonide 0.025%, net price 30 g = £4.34, 60 g = £7.82. For use on scalp and other hairy areas. Label: 28. Potency: potent
Excipients include hydroxybenzoates (parabens), propylene glycol

Ointment, fluocinolone acetonide 0.025%, net price 30 g = £2.93, 100 g = £8.34. Label 28. Potency: potent
Excipients include propylene glycol, wool fat

Synalar 1 in 4 Dilution® (GP Pharma) PoM

Cream, fluocinolone acetonide 0.00625%, net price 50 g = £3.43. Label: 28. Potency: moderate
Excipients include benzyl alcohol, cetostearyl alcohol, polysorbates, propylene glycol

Ointment, fluocinolone acetonide 0.00625%, net price 50 g = £3.43. Label: 28. Potency: moderate
Excipients include propylene glycol, wool fat

Synalar 1 in 10 Dilution® (GP Pharma) PoM

Cream, fluocinolone acetonide 0.0025%, net price 50 g = £3.25. Label: 28. Potency: mild
Excipients include benzyl alcohol, cetostearyl alcohol, polysorbates, propylene glycol

With antibacterials

See notes above for comment on compound preparations

Synalar C® (GP Pharma) PoM

Cream, fluocinolone acetonide 0.025%, clioquinol 3%, net price 15 g = £1.89. Label: 28. Potency: potent
Excipients include cetostearyl alcohol, disodium edetate, hydroxybenzoates (parabens), polysorbates, propylene glycol

Ointment, fluocinolone acetonide 0.025%, clioquinol 3%, net price 15 g = £1.89. Label: 28. Potency: potent.
Note stains clothing
Excipients include propylene glycol, wool fat

Synalar N® (GP Pharma) PoM

Cream, fluocinolone acetonide 0.025%, neomycin sulphate 0.5%, net price 30 g = £3.09. Label: 28. Potency: potent
Excipients include cetostearyl alcohol, hydroxybenzoates (parabens), polysorbates, propylene glycol

Ointment, fluocinolone acetonide 0.025%, neomycin sulphate 0.5%, in a greasy basis, net price 30 g = £3.09. Label: 28. Potency: potent
Excipients include propylene glycol, wool fat

FLUOCINONIDE

Indications severe inflammatory skin disorders such as eczemas unresponsive to less potent corticosteroids; psoriasis, see notes above

Cautions see notes above

Contra-indications see notes above

Side-effects see notes above

Dose

- Apply thinly 1–2 times daily

Metosyn® (GP Pharma) PoM

FAPG cream, fluocinonide 0.05%, net price 25 g = £2.57, 100 g = £8.68. Label: 28. Potency: potent
Excipients include propylene glycol

Ointment, fluocinonide 0.05%, net price 25 g = £2.28, 100 g = £8.56 Label: 28. Potency: potent
Excipients include propylene glycol, wool fat

FLUOCORTOLONE

Indications severe inflammatory skin disorders such as eczemas unresponsive to less potent corticosteroids; psoriasis, see notes above

Cautions see notes above

Contra-indications see notes above

Side-effects see notes above
Dose

- Apply thinly 1–2 times daily, reducing strength as condition responds

Ultralanum Plain® (Meadow) PoM
Cream, fluocortolone caproate 0.25%, fluocortolone pivalate 0.25%, net price 50 g = £2.95. Label: 28. Potency: moderate
Excipients include disodium edetate, fragrance, hydroxybenzoates (parabens), stearyl alcohol

Ointment, fluocortolone 0.25%, fluocortolone caproate 0.25%, net price 50 g = £2.95. Label: 28. Potency: moderate
Excipients include wool fat, fragrance

FLUTICASONE PROPIONATE

Indications inflammatory skin disorders such as dermatitis and eczemas unresponsive to less potent corticosteroids
Cautions see notes above
Contra-indications see notes above
Side-effects see notes above
Dose

- Apply thinly 1–2 times daily

Cutivate® (GSK) PoM
Cream, fluticasone propionate 0.05%, net price 15 g = £2.41, 50 g = £7.11. Label: 28. Potency: potent
Excipients include cetostearyl alcohol, imidurea, propylene glycol

Ointment, fluticasone propionate 0.005%, net price 15 g = £2.41, 50 g = £7.11. Label: 28. Potency: potent
Excipients include propylene glycol

MOMETASONE FUROATE

Indications severe inflammatory skin disorders such as eczemas unresponsive to less potent corticosteroids; psoriasis, see notes above
Cautions see notes above
Contra-indications see notes above
Side-effects see notes above
Dose

- Apply thinly once daily (to scalp in case of lotion)

Elocon® (Schering-Plough) PoM
Cream, mometasone furoate 0.1%, net price 30 g = £4.54, 100 g = £13.07. Label: 28. Potency: potent
Excipients include stearyl alcohol

Ointment, mometasone furoate 0.1%, net price 30 g = £4.54, 100 g = £13.07. Label: 28. Potency: potent
Excipients none as listed in section 13.1.3

Scalp lotion, mometasone furoate 0.1% in an aqueous isopropyl alcohol basis, net price 30 mL = £4.54. Label: 28. Potency: potent
Excipients include propylene glycol

TRIAMCINOLONE ACETONIDE

Indications severe inflammatory skin disorders such as eczemas unresponsive to less potent corticosteroids; psoriasis, see notes above
Cautions see notes above
Contra-indications see notes above
Side-effects see notes above
Dose

- Apply thinly 1–2 times daily

◢With antimicrobials

See notes above for comment on compound preparations

Aureocort® (Lederle) PoM
Ointment, triamcinolone acetonide 0.1%, chlortetracycline hydrochloride 3%, in an anhydrous greasy basis containing wool fat and white soft paraffin, net price 15 g = £2.70. Label: 28. Potency: potent
Excipients include wool fat
Note Stains clothing

Tri-Adcortyl® (Squibb) PoM
Cream, triamcinolone acetonide 0.1%, gramicidin 0.025%, neomycin (as sulphate) 0.25%, nystatin 100 000 units/g, net price 30 g = £3.15. Label: 28. Potency: potent
Excipients include benzyl alcohol, ethylenediamine, propylene glycol, fragrance

Ointment, triamcinolone acetonide 0.1%, gramicidin 0.025%, neomycin (as sulphate) 0.25%, nystatin 100 000 units/g, net price 30 g = £3.15. Label: 28. Potency: potent
Excipients none as listed in section 13.1.3
Note Not recommended owing to presence of ethylenediamine in the cream and also because combination of antibacterial with antifungal not considered useful in either the cream or ointment

13.5 Preparations for eczema and psoriasis

13.5.1 Preparations for eczema
13.5.2 Preparations for psoriasis
13.5.3 Drugs affecting the immune response

13.5.1 Preparations for eczema

Eczema (dermatitis) has several causes, which may influence treatment. The main types of eczema are irritant, allergic contact, atopic, venous and discoid; different types may co-exist. Lichenification, due to scratching and rubbing, may complicate any chronic eczema. *Atopic eczema* is the most common type and it usually involves dry skin as well as infection and lichenification.

Management of eczema involves the removal or treatment of contributory factors including occupational and domestic irritants. Known or suspected contact allergens should be avoided. Rarely, ingredients in topical medicinal products may sensitise the skin; the BNF lists active ingredients together with excipients that have been associated with skin sensitisation.

Skin dryness and the consequent irritant eczema requires **emollients** (section 13.2.1) applied regularly and liberally to the affected area; this may be supplemented with bath or shower emollients. The use of emollients should continue even if the eczema improves or if other treatment is being used.

Topical corticosteroids (section 13.4) are also required in the management of eczema; the potency of the corticosteroid should be appropriate to the severity and site of the condition. Mild corticosteroids are generally used on the face and on flexures; potent corticosteroids are generally required for use on adults with discoid or lichenified eczema or with eczema on the scalp, limbs, and trunk. Treatment should be reviewed regularly, especially if a potent corticosteroid is required. Bandages (including those containing **zinc** and **ichthammol**) are sometimes applied over topical corticosteroids to treat eczema of the limbs.

For the role of topical **pimecrolimus** and **tacrolimus** in atopic eczema see section 13.5.3.

Infection Bacterial infection (commonly with *Staphylococcus aureus* and occasionally with *Streptococcus pyogenes*) can exacerbate eczema and requires treatment with topical or systemic **antibacterial drugs** (section 13.10.1 and section 5.1). Antibacterial drugs, particularly fusidic acid, should be used in short courses (typically 1 week) to reduce the risk of drug resistance or skin sensitisation. Associated eczema is treated simultaneously with a topical corticosteroid usually of moderate or high potency.

Eczema involving widespread or recurrent infection requires the use of a systemic antibacterial that is active against the infecting organism. Products that combine an antiseptic with an emollient application (section 13.2.1) and with a bath emollient (section 13.2.1.1) may also be used; antiseptic shampoos (section 13.9) may be used on the scalp.

Intertriginous eczema commonly involves candida and bacteria; it is best treated with a mild or moderately potent topical corticosteroid and a suitable antimicrobial drug.

Widespread herpes simplex infection may complicate atopic eczema and treatment with a systemic antiviral drug (section 5.3.2.1) is indicated.

The management of *seborrhoeic dermatitis* is described below.

Management of other features of eczema *Lichenification*, which results from repeated scratching is treated initially with a potent corticosteroid. Bandages containing **ichthammol paste** (to reduce pruritus) and other substances such as **zinc oxide** may be applied over the corticosteroid. **Coal tar** (section 13.5.2) and **ichthammol** can be useful in some cases of *chronic eczema*.

Antihistamines (section 3.4.1) may be of some value in relieving the itch of eczema, usually because of their sedating effect.

Exudative ('*weeping*') *eczema* requires a potent corticosteroid initially; infection may also be present and require specific treatment (see above). **Potassium permanganate** solution (1 in 10 000) can be used in exudating eczema for its antiseptic and astringent effect; treatment should be stopped when exudation stops.

Severe refractory eczema is best managed under specialist supervision; it may require phototherapy or drugs that act on the immune system (section 13.5.3).

Seborrhoeic dermatitis *Seborrhoeic dermatitis* (*seborrhoeic eczema*) is associated with species of the yeast *Malassezia* and affects the scalp, paranasal areas, and eyebrows. Shampoos active against the yeast (including those containing ketoconazole and coal tar, section 13.9) and combinations of mild corticosteroids with suitable antimicrobials (section 13.4) are used.

ICHTHAMMOL

Indications chronic lichenified eczema
Side-effects skin irritation
Dose

- Apply 1–3 times daily

Ichthammol Ointment, BP 1980
Ointment, ichthammol 10%, yellow soft paraffin 45%, wool fat 45%

Zinc and Ichthammol Cream, BP
Cream, ichthammol 5%, cetostearyl alcohol 3%, wool fat 10%, in zinc cream

Zinc Paste and Ichthammol Bandage, BP 1993
See Appendix 8 (section A8.2.9)

13.5.2 Preparations for psoriasis

Psoriasis is characterised by epidermal thickening and scaling. It commonly affects extensor surfaces and the scalp. For mild psoriasis, reassurance and treatment with an emollient may be all that is necessary.

Occasionally psoriasis is provoked or exacerbated by drugs such as lithium, chloroquine and hydroxychloroquine, beta-blockers, non-steroidal anti-inflammatory drugs, and ACE inhibitors. Psoriasis may not be seen until the drug has been taken for weeks or months.

Emollients (section 13.2.1), in addition to their effects on dryness, scaling and cracking, may have an antiproliferative effect in psoriasis. They are particularly useful in *inflammatory psoriasis* and in *plaque psoriasis of palms and soles*, in which irritant factors can perpetuate the condition. Emollients are useful adjuncts to other more specific treatment.

More specific treatment for *chronic stable plaque psoriasis* on extensor surfaces of trunk and limbs involves the use of **vitamin D analogues**, **coal tar**, **dithranol**, and the retinoid **tazarotene**. However, they can irritate the skin and they are not suitable for the more inflammatory forms of psoriasis; their use should be suspended during an inflammatory phase of psoriasis. The efficacy and the irritancy of each substance varies between patients. If a substance irritates significantly, it should be stopped or the concentration reduced; if it is tolerated, its effects should be assessed after 4 to 6 weeks and treatment continued if it is effective.

Widespread *unstable psoriasis* of erythrodermic or generalised pustular type requires urgent specialist assessment. Initial topical treatment should be limited to using emollients frequently and generously; emollients should be prescribed in quantities of 1 kg or more. More localised acute or subacute *inflammatory psoriasis* with hot, spreading or itchy lesions, should be treated topically with emollients or with a corticosteroid of moderate potency.

Calcipotriol and **tacalcitol** are analogues of vitamin D that affect cell division and differentiation. **Calcitriol** is an active form of vitamin D. Vitamin D and its analogues are used as first-line treatment for plaque psoriasis; they do not smell or stain and they may be more acceptable than tar or dithranol products. Of the vitamin D analogues, tacalcitol and calcitriol are less likely to irritate.

Coal tar has anti-inflammatory properties that are useful in chronic plaque psoriasis; it also has antiscaling properties. Crude coal tar (coal tar, BP) is the most effective form, typically in a concentration of 1 to 10% in a soft paraffin base, but few outpatients tolerate the smell and mess. Cleaner extracts of coal tar included in proprietary preparations, are more practicable for home use but they are less effective and improvement takes longer. Contact of coal tar products with normal skin is not normally harmful and they can be used for widespread small lesions; however, irritation, contact allergy, and sterile folliculitis can occur. The milder tar extracts can be used on the face and flexures. Tar baths and tar shampoos are also helpful.

Dithranol is effective for chronic plaque psoriasis. Its major disadvantages are irritation (for which individual susceptibility varies) and staining of skin and of clothing. It should be applied to chronic extensor plaques only, carefully avoiding normal skin. Dithranol is not generally suitable for widespread small lesions nor should it be used in the flexures or on the face. Treatment should be started with a low concentration such as dithranol 0.1%, and the strength increased gradually every few days up to 3%, according to tolerance. Proprietary preparations are more suitable for home use; they are usually washed off after 5 to 60 minutes ('short contact'). Specialist nurses may apply intensive treatment with dithranol paste which is covered by stockinette dressings and usually retained overnight. Dithranol should be discontinued if even a low concentration causes acute inflammation; continued use can result in the psoriasis becoming unstable. When applying dithranol, hands should be protected by gloves or they should be washed thoroughly afterwards.

Tazarotene, a retinoid, seems to be less effective than calcipotriol with a greater incidence of irritation. Although irritation is common, it is minimised by applying tazarotene sparingly to the plaques and avoiding normal skin. Tazarotene is clean and odourless.

A topical **corticosteroid** (section 13.4) is not generally suitable as the sole treatment of extensive chronic plaque psoriasis; any early improvement is not usually maintained and there is a risk of the condition deteriorating or of precipitating an unstable form of psoriasis (e.g. erythrodermic psoriasis or generalised pustular psoriasis). However, it may be appropriate to treat psoriasis in specific sites, such as the face and flexures, usually with a mild corticosteroid, and psoriasis of the scalp, palms, and soles with a potent corticosteroid.

Combining the use of a corticosteroid with another specific topical treatment may be beneficial in chronic plaque psoriasis; the drugs may be used separately at different times of the day or used together in a single formulation. *Eczema* co-existing with psoriasis may be treated with a corticosteroid, or coal tar, or both.

Scalp psoriasis is usually scaly, and the scale may be thick and adherent. This requires softening with an emollient ointment, cream, or oil and usually combined with **salicylic acid** as a keratolytic.

Some preparations prescribed for psoriasis affecting the scalp combine salicylic acid with coal tar or **sulphur**. Preparations containing salicylic acid, sulphur, and coal tar are available as proprietary products. The product should be applied generously and an adequate quantity should be prescribed. It should be left on for at least an hour, often more conveniently overnight, before washing it off. If a corticosteroid lotion or gel is required (e.g. for itch), it can be used in the morning.

Phototherapy **Phototherapy** is available in specialist centres under the supervision of a dermatologist. **Ultraviolet B** (UVB) radiation is usually effective for *chronic stable psoriasis* and for *guttate psoriasis*. It may be considered for patients with moderately severe psoriasis in whom topical treatment has failed, but it may irritate inflammatory psoriasis.

Photochemotherapy combining long-wave ultraviolet A radiation with a psoralen (PUVA) is available in specialist centres under the supervision of a dermatologist. The psoralen, which enhances the effect of irradiation, is administered either by mouth or topically. PUVA is effective in most forms of psoriasis, including *localised palmoplantar pustular psoriasis*. Early adverse effects include phototoxicity and pruritus. Higher cumulative doses exaggerate skin ageing, increase the risk of dysplastic and neoplastic skin lesions, especially squamous cancer, and pose a theoretical risk of cataracts.

Phototherapy combined with coal tar, dithranol, tazarotene, topical vitamin D or vitamin D analogues, or oral acitretin allows reduction of the cumulative dose of phototherapy required to treat psoriasis.

Systemic treatment **Systemic treatment** is required for severe, resistant, unstable or complicated forms of psoriasis, and it should be initiated only under specialist supervision. Systemic drugs for psoriasis include acitretin (see below) and drugs that affect the immune response (such as ciclosporin, hydroxycarbamide, and methotrexate, section 13.5.3).

Systemic corticosteroids should be used only rarely in psoriasis because rebound deterioration may occur on reducing the dose.

Acitretin, a metabolite of etretinate, is a retinoid (vitamin A derivative); it is prescribed by specialists. The main indication for acitretin is *psoriasis*, but it is also used in disorders of keratinisation such as severe *Darier's disease* (keratosis follicularis), and some forms of *ichthyosis*. Although a minority of cases of psoriasis respond well to acitretin alone, it is only moderately effective in many cases and it is combined with other treatments. A therapeutic effect occurs after 2 to 4 weeks and the maximum benefit after 4 to 6 weeks or longer. The manufacturers of acitretin do not recommend continuous treatment for longer than 6 months. However, some patients may benefit from longer treatment, provided that the lowest effective dose is used, patients are monitored carefully for adverse effects, and the need for treatment is reviewed regularly.

Apart from teratogenicity, which remains a risk for 2 years after stopping, acitretin is the least toxic systemic treatment for psoriasis; in women with a potential for child-bearing, the possibility of pregnancy must be excluded before treatment and effective contraception must be used during treatment and for 2 years afterwards (oral progestogen-only contraceptives not considered effective). Common side-effects derive from its widespread but reversible effects on epithelia, such as dry and cracking lips, dry skin and mucosal surfaces, hair thinning, paronychia, and soft and sticky palms and soles. Liver function and blood lipid concentration should be monitored.

Topical preparations for psoriasis

Vitamin D and analogues

Calcipotriol, **calcitriol**, and **tacalcitol** are used for the management of *plaque psoriasis*. They should be avoided by those with calcium metabolism disorders, and used with caution in *generalised pustular* or *erythrodermic exfoliative psoriasis* (enhanced risk of hypercalcaemia). Local skin reactions (itching, erythema, burning, paraesthesia, dermatitis) are common. Hands should be washed thoroughly after application to avoid inadvertent transfer to other body areas. Aggravation of psoriasis has also been reported.

CALCIPOTRIOL

Indications plaque psoriasis

Cautions see notes above; pregnancy (Appendix 4); avoid use on face; avoid excessive exposure to sunlight and sunlamps—if used with UV treatment apply at least 2 hours before UV exposure

Contra-indications see notes above

Side-effects see notes above; also photosensitivity; rarely facial or perioral dermatitis, skin atrophy

Dose

- *cream* or *ointment* apply once or twice daily; max. 100 g weekly (less with *scalp solution*, see below); CHILD over 6 years, apply twice daily; 6–12 years max. 50 g weekly; over 12 years max. 75 g weekly

Note Patient information leaflets for *Dovonex®* cream and ointment advise liberal application (but note max. recommended weekly dose, above)

Calcipotriol (Non-proprietary) PoM

Ointment, calcipotriol 50 micrograms/g, net price 120 g = £24.79

Note Not licensed for use in children under 18 years

Dovonex® (LEO) PoM

Cream, calcipotriol 50 micrograms/g, net price 60 g = £12.02, 120 g = £24.04

Excipients include cetostearyl alcohol, disodium edetate

Scalp solution, calcipotriol 50 micrograms/mL, net price 60 mL = £13.04, 120 mL = £26.07

Excipients include propylene glycol

Dose scalp psoriasis, apply to scalp twice daily; max. 60 mL weekly (less with cream or ointment, see below); CHILD under 18 years, see *BNF for Children*

Note When preparations used together max. total calcipotriol 5 mg in any one week (e.g. scalp solution 60 mL with cream or ointment 30 g *or* cream or ointment 60 g with scalp solution 30 mL)

With betamethasone

For cautions, contra-indications, side-effects, and for comment on the limited role of corticosteroids in psoriasis, see section 13.4.

Dovobet® (LEO) PoM

Ointment, betamethasone 0.05% (as dipropionate), calcipotriol 50 micrograms/g, net price 60 g = £35.00, 120 g = £65.00. Label: 28

Excipients none as listed in section 13.1.3

Dose initial treatment of stable plaque psoriasis, apply once daily to max. 30% of body surface (max. 15 g daily, max. 100 g weekly) for 4 weeks; if necessary, subsequent courses repeated after an interval of at least 4 weeks; CHILD under 18 years see *BNF for Children*

CALCITRIOL
(1,25-Dihydroxycholecalciferol)

Indications mild to moderate plaque psoriasis

Cautions see notes above; liver impairment (Appendix 2); pregnancy (Appendix 4)

Contra-indications see notes above; do not apply under occlusion; renal impairment (Appendix 3)

Side-effects see notes above

Dose

- ADULT and CHILD over 12 years, apply twice daily; not more than 35% of body surface to be treated daily, max. 30 g daily

Silkis® (Galderma) PoM

Ointment, calcitriol 3 micrograms/g, net price 100 g = £16.34

Excipients none as listed in section 13.1.3

TACALCITOL

Indications plaque psoriasis

Cautions see notes above; pregnancy (Appendix 4), breast-feeding (Appendix 5); avoid eyes; monitor plasma calcium if risk of hypercalcaemia or in renal impairment; if used in conjunction with UV treatment, UV radiation should be given in the morning and tacalcitol applied at bedtime

Contra-indications see notes above

Side-effects see notes above

Dose

- ADULT and CHILD over 12 years, apply daily preferably at bedtime; max. 10 g daily

Curatoderm® (Crookes) PoM

Ointment, tacalcitol (as monohydrate) 4 micrograms/g, net price 30 g = £13.40, 60 g = £23.14, 100 g = £30.86

Excipients none as listed in section 13.1.3

Tazarotene

TAZAROTENE

Indications mild to moderate plaque psoriasis affecting up to 10% of skin area

Cautions wash hands immediately after use, avoid contact with eyes, face, intertriginous areas, hair-covered scalp, eczematous or inflamed skin; avoid excessive exposure to UV light (including sunlight, solariums, PUVA or UVB treatment); do not apply emollients or cosmetics within 1 hour of application

Contra-indications pregnancy—women of child-bearing potential must use effective contraception (Appendix 4); breast-feeding (Appendix 5)

Side-effects local irritation (more common with higher concentration and may require discontinuation), pruritus, burning, erythema, desquamation, non-specific rash, contact dermatitis, and worsening of psoriasis; rarely stinging and inflamed, dry or painful skin

Dose

- Apply once daily in the evening usually for up to 12 weeks; CHILD under 18 years not recommended

Zorac® (Allergan) PoM

Gel, tazarotene 0.05%, net price 30 g = £14.09; 0.1%, 30 g = £14.80

Excipients include benzyl alcohol, butylated hydroxyanisole, butylated hydroxytoluene, disodium edetate, polysorbate 40

Tars

TARS

Indications psoriasis and occasionally chronic atopic eczema

Cautions avoid eyes, mucosa, genital or rectal areas, and broken or inflamed skin; use suitable chemical protection gloves for extemporaneous preparation

Contra-indications not for use in sore, acute, or pustular psoriasis or in presence of infection

Side-effects skin irritation and acne-like eruptions, photosensitivity; stains skin, hair, and fabric

Dose

- Apply 1–3 times daily starting with low-strength preparations

Note For shampoo preparations see section 13.9; impregnated dressings see Appendix 8 (section A8.2.9)

Non-proprietary preparations

May be difficult to obtain—some patients may find newer proprietary preparations more acceptable

Calamine and Coal Tar Ointment, BP
Ointment, calamine 12.5 g, strong coal tar solution 2.5 g, zinc oxide 12.5 g, hydrous wool fat 25 g, white soft paraffin 47.5 g
Excipients include wool fat
Dose apply 1–2 times daily

Coal Tar and Salicylic Acid Ointment, BP
Ointment, coal tar 2 g, salicylic acid 2 g, emulsifying wax 11.4 g, white soft paraffin 19 g, coconut oil 54 g, polysorbate '80' 4 g, liquid paraffin 7.6 g
Excipients include cetostearyl alcohol
Dose apply 1–2 times daily

Coal Tar Paste, BP
Paste, strong coal tar solution 7.5%, in compound zinc paste
Dose apply 1–2 times daily

Zinc and Coal Tar Paste, BP
Paste, zinc oxide 6%, coal tar 6%, emulsifying wax 5%, starch 38%, yellow soft paraffin 45%
Excipients include cetostearyl alcohol
Dose apply 1–2 times daily

Proprietary preparations

Carbo-Dome® (Sandoz)
Cream, coal tar solution 10%, in a water-miscible basis, net price 30 g = £4.77, 100 g = £16.38
Excipients include beeswax, hydroxybenzoates (parabens)
Dose psoriasis, apply to skin 2–3 times daily

Clinitar® (CHS)
Cream, coal tar extract 1%, net price 100 g = £10.99
Excipients include cetostearyl alcohol, isopropyl palmitate, propylene glycol
Dose psoriasis and eczema, apply to skin 1–2 times daily

Cocois® (UCB Pharma)
Scalp ointment, coal tar solution 12%, salicylic acid 2%, precipitated sulphur 4%, in a coconut oil emollient basis, net price 40 g (with applicator nozzle) = £6.22, 100 g = £11.69
Excipients include cetostearyl alcohol
Dose scaly scalp disorders including psoriasis, eczema, seborrhoeic dermatitis and dandruff, apply to scalp once weekly as necessary (if severe use daily for first 3–7 days), shampoo off after 1 hour; CHILD 6–12 years, medical supervision required (not recommended under 6 years)

Exorex® (Forest)
Lotion, prepared coal tar 1% in an emollient basis, net price 100 mL = £8.11, 250 mL = £16.24
Excipients include hydroxybenzoates (parabens), polysorbate 80
Dose psoriasis, apply to skin or scalp 2–3 times daily; CHILD under 12 years and ELDERLY, lotion can be diluted with a few drops of water before applying

Psoriderm® (Dermal)
Cream, coal tar 6%, lecithin 0.4%, net price 225 mL = £9.85
Excipients include isopropyl palmitate, propylene glycol
Dose psoriasis, apply to skin or scalp 1–2 times daily
Scalp lotion—section 13.9

Sebco® (Centrapharm)
Scalp ointment, coal tar solution 12%, salicylic acid 2%, precipitated sulphur 4%, in a coconut oil emollient basis, net price 40 g = £4.54, 100 g = £8.52
Excipients include cetostearyl alcohol
Dose scaly scalp disorders including psoriasis, eczema, seborrhoeic dermatitis and dandruff, apply to scalp as necessary (if severe use daily for first 3–7 days), shampoo off after 1 hour; CHILD 6–12 years, medical supervision required (not recommended under 6 years)

Bath preparations

Coal Tar Solution, BP
Solution, coal tar 20%, polysorbate '80' 5%, in alcohol (96%), net price 500 mL = £6.74
Excipients include polysorbates
Dose use 100 mL in a bath
Note Strong Coal Tar Solution BP contains coal tar 40%

Pinetarsol® (Crawford)
Bath oil, tar 2.3% in a light liquid paraffin basis, net price 200 mL = £4.75, 500 mL = £7.95
Excipients include fragrance
Dose eczema and psoriasis, use 15–30 mL in a bath or apply directly to wet skin and rinse after a few minutes; can be used as soap substitute
Gel, tar 1.6%, net price 100 g = £4.95
Dose eczema and psoriasis, apply directly to wet skin and rinse after a few minutes; can be used as soap substitute
Solution, tar 2.3%, net price 200 mL = £4.45, 500 mL = £7.45
Dose eczema and psoriasis, use 15–30 mL in a bath *or* dilute 15 mL with 3 litres of water and apply to affected areas *or* apply solution directly to wet skin and rinse after a few minutes; can be used as soap substitute

Polytar Emollient® (Stiefel)
Bath additive, coal tar solution 2.5%, arachis (peanut) oil extract of coal tar 7.5%, tar 7.5%, cade oil 7.5%, liquid paraffin 35%, net price 500 mL = £5.78
Excipients include isopropyl palmitate
Dose psoriasis, eczema, atopic and pruritic dermatoses, use 2–4 capfuls (15–30 mL) in bath and soak for 20 minutes

Psoriderm® (Dermal)
Bath emulsion, coal tar 40%, net price 200 mL = £2.87
Excipients include polysorbate 20
Dose psoriasis, use 30 mL in a bath and soak for 5 minutes

With corticosteroids

Alphosyl HC® (GSK Consumer Healthcare) PoM
Cream, coal tar extract 5%, hydrocortisone 0.5%, allantoin 2%, net price 100 g = £3.54. Label: 28. Potency: mild
Excipients include beeswax, cetyl alcohol, hydroxybenzoates (parabens), isopropyl palmitate, wool fat
Dose ADULT and CHILD over 5 years, psoriasis, apply thinly twice daily

Dithranol

DITHRANOL
(Anthralin)

Indications subacute and chronic psoriasis, see notes above

Cautions avoid use near eyes and sensitive areas of skin; see also notes above

Contra-indications hypersensitivity; acute and pustular psoriasis

Side-effects local burning sensation and irritation; stains skin, hair, and fabrics

Dose
- See notes above and under preparations

Note Some of these dithranol preparations also contain coal tar or salicylic acid—for cautions, contra-indications, and side-effects see under Tars (above) or under Salicylic Acid

Non-proprietary preparations

[1]**Dithranol Ointment, BP** (PoM)
Ointment, dithranol, in yellow soft paraffin; usual strengths 0.1–2%. Part of basis may be replaced by hard paraffin if a stiffer preparation is required. Label: 28

1. (PoM) if dithranol content more than 1%, otherwise may be sold to the public

Dithranol Paste, BP
Paste, dithranol in zinc and salicylic acid (Lassar's) paste. Usual strengths 0.1–1% of dithranol. Label: 28

Proprietary preparations

Dithrocream® (Dermal)
Cream, dithranol 0.1%, net price 50 g = £3.94; 0.25%, 50 g = £4.23; 0.5%, 50 g = £4.87; 1%, 50 g = £5.67; (PoM) 2%, 50 g = £7.10. Label: 28
Excipients include cetostearyl alcohol, chlorocresol
Dose for application to skin or scalp; 0.1–0.5% suitable for overnight treatment, 1–2% for max. 1 hour

Micanol® (GP Pharma)
Cream, dithranol 1% in a lipid-stabilised basis, net price 50 g = £13.48; (PoM) 3%, 50 g = £16.79. Label: 28
Excipients none as listed in section 13.1.3
Dose for application to skin or scalp, apply 1% cream for up to 30 minutes once daily, if necessary 3% cream can be used under medical supervision
Note At the end of contact time, use plenty of lukewarm (not hot) water to rinse off cream; soap should not be used

Psorin® (LPC)
Ointment, dithranol 0.11%, coal tar 1%, salicylic acid 1.6%, net price 50 g = £9.22, 100 g = £18.44. Label: 28
Excipients include beeswax, wool fat
Dose for application to skin up to twice daily

Scalp gel, dithranol 0.25%, salicylic acid 1.6% in gel basis containing methyl salicylate, net price 50 g = £7.03. Label: 28
Excipients none as listed in section 13.1.3
Dose for application to scalp, initially apply on alternate days for 10–20 minutes; may be increased to daily application for max. 1 hour and then wash off
Note May be difficult to obtain

Salicylic acid

SALICYLIC ACID

For coal tar preparations containing salicylic acid, see under Tars, p. 614; for dithranol preparations containing salicylic acid see under Dithranol, below

Indications hyperkeratotic skin disorders; acne (section 13.6.1); warts and calluses (section 13.7); scalp conditions (section 13.9); fungal nail infections (section 13.10.2)

Cautions see notes above; avoid broken or inflamed skin
Salicylate toxicity If large areas of skin are treated, salicylate toxicity may occur

Side-effects sensitivity, excessive drying, irritation, systemic effects after widespread use (see under Cautions)

Zinc and Salicylic Acid Paste, BP
Paste, (Lassar's Paste), zinc oxide 24%, salicylic acid 2%, starch 24%, white soft paraffin 50%, net price 25 g = 17p
Dose apply twice daily

Oral retinoids for psoriasis

ACITRETIN

Note Acitretin is a metabolite of etretinate

Indications severe extensive psoriasis resistant to other forms of therapy; palmoplantar pustular psoriasis; severe congenital ichthyosis; severe Darier's disease (keratosis follicularis)

Cautions exclude pregnancy before starting (test for pregnancy within 2 weeks before treatment and monthly thereafter; start treatment on day 2 or 3 of menstrual cycle)—women (including those with history of infertility) should avoid pregnancy for at least 1 month before, during, and for at least 2 years after treatment; patients should avoid concomitant tetracycline or methotrexate, high doses of vitamin A (more than 4000–5000 units daily) and use of keratolytics, and should not donate blood during or for at least 1 year after stopping therapy (teratogenic risk); check liver function at start, then every 1–2 weeks for 2 months, then every 3 months; monitor plasma lipids; diabetes (can alter glucose tolerance—initial frequent blood glucose checks); radiographic assessment on long-term treatment; investigate atypical musculoskeletal symptoms; in children use only in exceptional circumstances (premature epiphyseal closure reported); avoid excessive exposure to sunlight and unsupervised use of sunlamps; **interactions:** Appendix 1 (retinoids)

Contra-indications hepatic impairment (Appendix 2); renal impairment (Appendix 3); hyperlipidaemia, pregnancy (**important teratogenic risk:** see Cautions and Appendix 4); breast-feeding

Side-effects dryness of mucous membranes (sometimes erosion), of skin (sometimes scaling, thinning, erythema especially of face, and pruritus), and of conjunctiva (sometimes conjunctivitis and decreased tolerance of contact lenses); sticky skin, dermatitis;

other side-effects reported include palmoplantar exfoliation, epistaxis, epidermal and nail fragility, oedema, paronychia, granulomatous lesions, bullous eruptions, reversible hair thinning and alopecia, myalgia and arthralgia, occasional nausea, headache, malaise, drowsiness, rhinitis, sweating, taste disturbance, and gingivitis; benign intracranial hypertension (discontinue if severe headache, vomiting, diarrhoea, abdominal pain, and visual disturbance occur; **avoid** concomitant tetracyclines); photosensitivity, corneal ulceration, raised liver enzymes, rarely jaundice and hepatitis (**avoid** concomitant methotrexate); raised serum triglycerides or cholesterol; decreased night vision reported; skeletal hyperostosis and extra-osseous calcification reported following long-term administration of etretinate (and premature epiphyseal closure in children, see Cautions)

Dose

- Under expert supervision, initially 25–30 mg daily (Darier's disease 10 mg daily) for 2–4 weeks, then adjusted according to response, usual range 25–50 mg daily; up to 75 mg daily for short periods in psoriasis and ichthyosis; CHILD (**important**: exceptional circumstances only, see Cautions), 500 micrograms/kg daily (occasionally up to 1 mg/kg daily to max. 35 mg daily for limited periods) with careful monitoring of musculoskeletal development

Neotigason® (Roche) PoM

Capsules, acitretin 10 mg (brown/white), net price 60-cap pack = £25.25; 25 mg (brown/yellow), 60-cap pack = £58.59. Label: 10, patient information leaflet, 21

13.5.3 Drugs affecting the immune response

Drugs affecting the immune response are used for eczema or psoriasis. Systemic drugs acting on the immune system are generally used by **specialists** in a hospital setting.

Ciclosporin (cyclosporin) by mouth can be used for *severe psoriasis* and for *severe eczema*. **Azathioprine** (section 8.2.1) or **mycophenolate mofetil** (section 8.2.1) are used for severe refractory eczema [unlicensed indication]. **Hydroxycarbamide** (hydroxyurea) (section 8.1.5) is used by mouth for severe psoriasis [unlicensed indication].

Methotrexate can be used for *severe psoriasis*, the dose being adjusted according to severity of the condition and haematological and biochemical measurements; the usual dose is methotrexate 10 to 25 mg **once weekly**, by mouth. Folic acid may be given to reduce the possibility of methotrexate toxicity.

Etanercept, a cytokine modulator (see p. 553), is used for *severe psoriasis* either refractory to at least 2 systemic treatments and photochemotherapy or in patients intolerant of these treatments. **Efalizumab** (which inhibits T-cell activation) or **infliximab** (a cytokine modulator, see p. 554) are alternatives. Etanercept and infliximab are also licensed for psoriatic arthritis (see p. 552).

> **NICE guidance**
> **Etanercept and efalizumab for plaque psoriasis in adults (July 2006)**
> Etanercept is recommended for severe plaque psoriasis which has failed to respond to standard systemic treatments (including ciclosporin and methotrexate) and to photochemotherapy, or when standard treatments cannot be used because of intolerance or contra-indications. Etanercept should be withdrawn if the response is not adequate after 12 weeks.
> Efalizumab is recommended for severe plaque psoriasis which has failed to respond to etanercept or when etanercept cannot be used because of intolerance or contra-indications. Efalizumab should be withdrawn if the response is not adequate after 12 weeks.

Pimecrolimus by topical application is licensed for *mild to moderate atopic eczema*. **Tacrolimus** is licensed for topical use in *moderate to severe atopic eczema*. Both are drugs whose long-term safety and place in therapy is still being evaluated and they should not usually be considered first-line treatments unless there is a specific reason to avoid or reduce the use of topical corticosteroids. Short-term treatment with topical pimecrolimus or topical tacrolimus should be initiated only by prescribers experienced in treating atopic eczema; continuous long-term treatment should be avoided.

> **NICE guidance**
> **Tacrolimus and pimecrolimus for atopic eczema (August 2004)**
> Topical pimecrolimus and tacrolimus are options for atopic eczema not controlled by maximal topical corticosteroid treatment or if there is a risk of important corticosteroid side-effects (particularly skin atrophy).
> Topical pimecrolimus is recommended for moderate atopic eczema on the face and neck of children aged 2–16 years and topical tacrolimus is recommended for moderate to severe atopic eczema in adults and children over 2 years. Pimecrolimus and tacrolimus should be used within their licensed indications.

For the role of topical corticosteroids in eczema see section 13.5.1 and for comment on their limited role in psoriasis see section 13.4. Short courses of systemic corticosteroids (section 6.3.2) can be given for eczema flares that have not improved despite appropriate topical treatment.

CICLOSPORIN
(Cyclosporin)

Indications see under Dose; transplantation and graft-versus-host disease (section 8.2.2)

Cautions see section 8.2.2

Additional cautions in atopic dermatitis and psoriasis *Contra-indicated* in abnormal renal function, hypertension not under control (see also below), infections not under control, and malignancy (see also below). Dermatological and physical examination, including blood pressure and renal function measurements required at least twice before starting; discontinue if hypertension develops that cannot be controlled by dose reduction or antihypertensive therapy; avoid excessive exposure to sunlight and use of UVB or PUVA; *in atopic dermatitis*, also allow herpes simplex infections to clear before starting (if they occur during treatment withdraw if severe); *Staphylococcus aureus* skin infections not absolute contra-indication providing controlled (but avoid erythromycin unless no other alternative—see also **interactions**: Appendix 1 (ciclosporin)); monitor serum creatinine every 2 weeks during treatment; *in psoriasis*, also exclude malignancies (including those of skin and cervix) before starting (biopsy any lesions not typical of psoriasis) and treat patients with malignant or pre-malignant conditions of skin only after appropriate treatment (and if no other option); monitor serum creatinine every 2 weeks for first 3 months then every 2 months (monthly if dose more than 2.5 mg/kg daily), reducing dose by 25–50% if increases more than 30% above baseline (even if within normal range) and discontinuing if reduction not successful within 1 month; also discontinue if lymphoproliferative disorder develops

Side-effects see section 8.2.2

Dose

- Short-term treatment (usually for max. 8 weeks but can be longer under specialists) of severe atopic dermatitis where conventional therapy ineffective or inappropriate, administered in accordance with expert advice, by mouth, ADULT and CHILD over 16 years, initially 2.5 mg/kg daily in 2 divided doses, if good initial response not achieved within 2 weeks, increase rapidly to max. 5 mg/kg daily; initial dose of 5 mg/kg daily in 2 divided doses if very severe; CHILD under 16 years, see *BNF for Children*
- Severe psoriasis where conventional therapy ineffective or inappropriate, administered in accordance with expert advice, by mouth, ADULT and CHILD over 16 years, initially 2.5 mg/kg daily in 2 divided doses, increased gradually to max. 5 mg/kg daily if no improvement within 1 month (discontinue if response still insufficient after 6 weeks); initial dose of 5 mg/kg daily justified if rapid control required; CHILD under 16 years, see *BNF for Children*

Important For preparations and counselling and for advice on conversion between the preparations, see section 8.2.2

Preparations
Section 8.2.2

EFALIZUMAB

Indications moderate to severe chronic plaque psoriasis for those whose disease is unresponsive to, or who are intolerant of other systemic therapy or photochemotherapy

Cautions low platelet count (monitor platelet count before treatment, monthly during initial therapy then every 3 months), hepatic impairment, renal impairment; **interactions**: Appendix 1 (efalizumab)

Contra-indications immunodeficiency, severe infection, active tuberculosis; history of malignancy; pregnancy and breast-feeding (Appendix 5)

Side-effects hypersensitivity reactions, asthenia, influenza-like symptoms, leucocytosis, arthralgia, exacerbation of psoriasis or development of variant forms including psoriatic arthritis (discontinue treatment); *less commonly* thrombocytopenia and injection-site reactions; also reported inflammatory polyradiculoneuropathy

Dose

- By subcutaneous injection, initially 700 micrograms/kg then 1 mg/kg *weekly*; discontinue if inadequate response after 12 weeks; CHILD and ADOLESCENT not recommended

Raptiva® (Serono) ▼ PoM
Injection, powder for reconstitution, efalizumab, net price 125-mg vial = £169.20 (with 1.3 mL water for injections in prefilled syringe)

METHOTREXATE

Indications severe psoriasis unresponsive to conventional therapy (specialist use only); Crohn's disease (section 1.5); malignant disease (section 8.1.3); rheumatoid arthritis (section 10.1.3)

Cautions section 10.1.3; also photosensitivity—psoriasis lesions aggravated by UV radiation (skin ulceration reported)

Contra-indications section 10.1.3

Side-effects section 10.1.3

Dose

- By mouth *or* by intramuscular *or* intravenous injection, 10–25 mg once weekly, adjusted according to response; ELDERLY consider dose reduction (extreme caution); CHILD 12–18 years see *BNF for Children*

Important
Note that the above dose is a **weekly** dose. To avoid error with low dose methotrexate, it is recommended that:

- the patient is carefully advised of the **dose** and **frequency** and the reason for taking methotrexate and any other prescribed medicine (e.g. folic acid);
- only one **strength** of methotrexate tablet (usually 2.5 mg) is prescribed and dispensed;
- the prescription and the dispensing label clearly show the dose and frequency of methotrexate administration;
- the patient is warned to report immediately the onset of any feature of blood disorders (e.g. sore throat, bruising, and mouth ulcers), liver toxicity (e.g. nausea, vomiting, abdominal discomfort and dark urine), and respiratory effects e.g. shortness of breath).

Preparations
Section 8.1.3 (parenteral) and section 10.1.3 (oral)

PIMECROLIMUS

Indications short-term treatment of mild to moderate atopic eczema (including flares) when topical corticosteroids cannot be used; see also notes above

Cautions UV light (avoid excessive exposure to sunlight and sunlamps), avoid other topical treatments except emollients at treatment site; alcohol consumption (risk of facial flushing and skin irritation)

Contra-indications contact with eyes and mucous membranes, application under occlusion, infection at treatment site; congenital epidermal barrier defects; generalised erythroderma; immunodeficiency; concomitant use with drugs that cause immunosuppression (may be prescribed in exceptional circumstances by specialists); application to malignant or potentially malignant skin lesions

Side-effects burning sensation, pruritus, erythema, skin infections (including folliculitis and *less commonly* impetigo, herpes simplex and zoster, molluscum contagiosum); *rarely* papilloma, skin discoloration, local reactions including pain, paraesthesia, peeling, dryness, oedema, and worsening of eczema; skin malignancy reported

Dose

- Apply twice daily until symptoms resolve (stop treatment if eczema worsens or no response after 6 weeks); CHILD under 2 years not recommended

Elidel® (Novartis) ▼ PoM
Cream, pimecrolimus 1%, net price 30 g = £19.69, 60 g = £37.41, 100 g = £59.07. Label: 4, 28
Excipients include benzyl alcohol, cetyl alcohol, propylene glycol, stearyl alcohol

TACROLIMUS

Indications short-term treatment of moderate to severe atopic eczema (including flares) either unresponsive to, or in patients intolerant of conventional therapy; see also notes above; other indications section 8.2.2

Cautions infection at treatment site, UV light (avoid excessive exposure to sunlight and sunlamps); alcohol consumption (risk of facial flushing and skin irritation); pregnancy

Contra-indications hypersensitivity to macrolides; avoid contact with eyes and mucous membranes, application under occlusion; congenital epidermal barrier defects; generalised erythroderma; immunodeficiency; concomitant use with drugs that cause immunosuppression (may be prescribed in exceptional circumstances by specialists); application to malignant or potentially malignant skin lesions; breast-feeding

Side-effects application-site reactions including rash, irritation, pain and paraesthesia; herpes simplex infection, Kaposi's varicelliform eruption; *less commonly* acne; acne rosacea and skin malignancy also reported

Dose

- ADULT and CHILD over 16 years initially apply 0.1% ointment thinly twice daily until lesion clears (consider other treatment if eczema worsens or no improvement after 2 weeks); reduce to once daily or switch to 0.03% ointment if condition allows; CHILD 2–16 years, initially apply 0.03% ointment twice daily for up to 3 weeks (consider other treatment if eczema worsens or if no improvement after 2 weeks) then reduce to once daily until lesion clears

Protopic® (Astellas) ▼ PoM
Ointment, tacrolimus (as monohydrate) 0.03%, net price 30 g = £19.44, 60 g = £36.94; 0.1%, 30 g = £21.60, 60 g = £41.04. Label: 4, 11, 28
Excipients include beeswax

13.6 Acne and rosacea

13.6.1 Topical preparations for acne
13.6.2 Oral preparations for acne

Acne Treatment of acne should be commenced early to prevent scarring. Patients should be counselled that an improvement may not be seen for at least a couple of months. The choice of treatment depends on whether the acne is predominantly inflammatory or comedonal and its severity.

Mild to moderate acne is generally treated with topical preparations (section 13.6.1). Systemic treatment (section 13.6.2) with oral antibacterials is generally used for *moderate to severe acne* or where topical preparations are not tolerated or are ineffective or where application to the site is difficult. Another oral preparation used for acne is the hormone treatment co-cyprindiol (cyproterone acetate with ethinylestradiol); it is for women only.

Severe acne, acne unresponsive to prolonged courses of oral antibacterials, scarring, or acne associated with psychological problems calls for early referral to a consultant dermatologist who may prescribe isotretinoin for administration by mouth.

Rosacea Rosacea is not comedonal (but may exist with acne which may be comedonal). The pustules and papules of rosacea respond to topical metronidazole (section 13.10.1.2) or to topical azelaic acid (section 13.6.1). Alternatively, oral administration of oxytetracycline or tetracycline 500 mg twice daily (section 5.1.3) or of erythromycin 500 mg twice daily (section 5.1.5) can be used; courses usually last 6–12 weeks and are repeated intermittently. Doxycycline (section 5.1.3) in a dose of 100 mg once daily can be used [unlicensed indication] if oxytetracycline or tetracycline is inappropriate (e.g. in renal impairment). Isotretinoin is occasionally given in refractory cases [unlicensed indication]. Camouflagers (section 13.8.2) may be required for the redness.

13.6.1 Topical preparations for acne

In mild to moderate acne, comedones and inflamed lesions respond well to benzoyl peroxide (see below) or to a topical retinoid (see p. 619). Alternatively, topical application of an antibacterial such as erythromycin or clindamycin may be effective for inflammatory acne. If topical preparations prove inadequate, oral preparations may be needed (section 13.6.2).

Benzoyl peroxide and azelaic acid

Benzoyl peroxide is effective in mild to moderate acne. Both comedones and inflamed lesions respond well to benzoyl peroxide. The lower concentrations seem to be as effective as higher concentrations in reducing inflammation. It is usual to start with a lower strength and to increase the concentration of benzoyl peroxide gradually. Adverse effects include local skin irritation, particularly when therapy is initiated, but the scaling and redness often subside with treatment continued at a reduced frequency of application. If the acne does not respond after 2 months then use of a topical antibacterial should be considered.

Azelaic acid has antimicrobial and anticomedonal properties. It may be an alternative to benzoyl peroxide or to a topical retinoid for treating mild to moderate comedonal acne, particularly of the face. Some patients prefer it because it is less likely to cause local irritation than benzoyl peroxide.

BENZOYL PEROXIDE

Indications acne vulgaris

Cautions avoid contact with eyes, mouth, and mucous membranes; may bleach fabrics and hair; avoid excessive exposure to sunlight

Side-effects skin irritation (reduce frequency or suspend use until irritation subsides and re-introduce at reduced frequency)

Dose

- Apply 1–2 times daily preferably after washing with soap and water, start treatment with lower-strength preparations

Note May bleach clothing

Acnecide® (Galderma)

Gel, benzoyl peroxide 5% in an aqueous gel basis, net price 60 g = £5.10

Excipients include propylene glycol

Brevoxyl® (Stiefel)

Cream, benzoyl peroxide 4% in an aqueous basis, net price 40 g = £3.30

Excipients include cetyl alcohol, fragrance, stearyl alcohol

PanOxyl® (Stiefel)

Aquagel (= aqueous gel), benzoyl peroxide 2.5%, net price 40 g = £1.76; 5%, 40 g = £1.92; 10%, 40 g = £2.13

Excipients include propylene glycol

Cream, benzoyl peroxide 5% in a non-greasy basis, net price 40 g = £1.89

Excipients include isopropyl palmitate, propylene glycol

Gel, benzoyl peroxide 5% in an aqueous alcoholic basis, net price 40 g = £1.51; 10%, 40 g = £1.69

Excipients include fragrance

Wash, benzoyl peroxide 10% in a detergent basis, net price 150 mL = £4.00

Excipients include imidurea

With antimicrobials

Duac® Once Daily (Stiefel) PoM

Gel, benzoyl peroxide 5%, clindamycin 1% (as phosphate) in an aqueous basis, net price 25 g = £9.95, 50 g = £19.90

Excipients include disodium edetate

Dose apply once daily in the evening

Quinoderm® (Ferndale)

Cream, benzoyl peroxide 5%, potassium hydroxyquinoline sulphate 0.5%, in an astringent vanishing-cream basis, net price 50 g = £2.21

Excipients include cetostearyl alcohol, edetic acid (EDTA)

Cream, benzoyl peroxide 10%, potassium hydroxyquinoline sulphate 0.5%, in an astringent vanishing-cream basis, net price 25 g = £1.30, 50 g = £2.49

Excipients include cetostearyl alcohol, edetic acid (EDTA)

AZELAIC ACID

Indications see preparations

Cautions avoid contact with eyes, mouth, and mucous membranes

Side-effects local irritation (reduce frequency or discontinue temporarily); *less commonly* skin discoloration; *very rarely* photosensitisation

Finacea® (Valeant) PoM

Gel, azelaic acid 15%, net price 30 g = £7.48

Excipients include disodium edetate, polysorbate 80, propylene glycol

Dose facial acne vulgaris, ADULT and CHILD over 14 years, apply twice daily; discontinue if no improvement after 1 month

Papulopustular rosacea, ADULT over 18 years, apply twice daily

Skinoren® (Valeant) PoM

Cream, azelaic acid 20%, net price 30 g = £3.74

Excipients include propylene glycol

Dose acne vulgaris, apply twice daily (sensitive skin, once daily for first week). Extended treatment may be required but manufacturer advises period of treatment should not exceed 6 months

Topical antibacterials for acne

For many patients with mild to moderate inflammatory acne, topical antibacterials may be no more effective than topical benzoyl peroxide or tretinoin. Topical antibacterials are probably best reserved for patients who wish to avoid oral antibacterials or who cannot tolerate them. Topical preparations of **erythromycin** and **clindamycin** are effective for inflammatory acne. Topical antibacterials can produce mild irritation of the skin, and on rare occasions cause sensitisation.

Antibacterial resistance of *Propionibacterium acnes* is increasing; there is cross-resistance between erythromycin and clindamycin. To avoid development of resistance:

- when possible use non-antibiotic antimicrobials (such as benzoyl peroxide or azelaic acid);
- avoid concomitant treatment with different oral and topical antibacterials;
- if a particular antibacterial is effective, use it for repeat courses if needed (short intervening courses of benzoyl peroxide or azelaic acid may eliminate any resistant propionibacteria);
- do not continue treatment for longer than necessary (however, treatment with a topical preparation should be continued for at least 6 months).

ANTIBACTERIALS

Indications acne vulgaris

Cautions some manufacturers advise preparations containing alcohol are not suitable for use with benzoyl peroxide

Dalacin T® (Pharmacia) PoM

Topical solution, clindamycin 1% (as phosphate), in an aqueous alcoholic basis, net price (both with applicator) 30 mL = £4.34, 50 mL = £7.23

Excipients include propylene glycol

Dose apply twice daily

Lotion, clindamycin 1% (as phosphate) in an aqueous basis, net price 30 mL = £5.08, 60 mL = £8.47

Excipients include cetostearyl alcohol, hydroxybenzoates (parabens)

Dose apply twice daily

Stiemycin® (Stiefel) PoM

Solution, erythromycin 2% in an alcoholic basis, net price 50 mL = £8.00

Excipients include propylene glycol

Dose apply twice daily

Zindaclin® (Crawford) PoM

Gel, clindamycin 1% (as phosphate), net price 30 g = £8.66

Excipients include propylene glycol

Dose apply once daily

Zineryt® (Astellas) PoM

Topical solution, powder for reconstitution, erythromycin 40 mg, zinc acetate 12 mg/mL when reconstituted with solvent containing ethanol, net price per pack of powder and solvent to provide 30 mL = £7.71, 90 mL = £22.24

Excipients none as listed in section 13.1.3

Dose apply twice daily

Topical retinoids and related preparations for acne

Topical **tretinoin** and its isomer **isotretinoin** are useful for treating comedones and inflammatory lesions in mild to moderate acne. Patients should be warned that some redness and skin peeling may occur initially but settles with time. Several months of treatment may be needed to achieve an optimal response and the treatment should be continued until no new lesions develop.

Isotretinoin is given by mouth in severe acne; see section 13.6.2 for **warnings** relating to use by mouth.

Adapalene, a retinoid-like drug, is licensed for mild to moderate acne. It is less irritant than topical retinoids.

Cautions Topical retinoids should be avoided in severe acne involving large areas. Contact with eyes, nostrils, mouth and mucous membranes, eczematous, broken or sunburned skin should be avoided. These drugs should be used with caution in sensitive areas such as the neck, and accumulation in angles of the nose should be avoided. Exposure to UV light (including sunlight, solariums) should be avoided; if sun exposure is unavoidable, an appropriate sunscreen or protective clothing should be used. Use of retinoids with abrasive cleaners, comedogenic or astringent cosmetics should be avoided. Allow peeling (e.g. resulting from use of benzoyl peroxide) to subside before using a topical retinoid; alternating a preparation that causes peeling with a topical retinoid may give rise to contact dermatitis (reduce frequency of retinoid application).

Contra-indications Topical retinoids are contra-indicated in pregnancy (Appendix 4); women of child-bearing age must use effective contraception (oral progestogen-only contraceptives not considered effective). Tretinoin is contra-indicated in personal or familial history of cutaneous epithelioma.

Side-effects Local reactions include burning, erythema, stinging, pruritus, dry or peeling skin (discontinue if severe). Increased sensitivity to UVB light or sunlight occurs. Temporary changes of skin pigmentation have been reported. Eye irritation and oedema, and blistering or crusting of skin have been reported rarely.

ADAPALENE

Indications mild to moderate acne
Cautions see notes above
Contra-indications see notes above
Side-effects see notes above
Dose
- Apply thinly once daily before retiring

Differin® (Galderma) PoM
Cream, adapalene 0.1%, net price 45 g = £11.40
Excipients include disodium edetate, hydroxybenzoates (parabens)

Gel, adapalene 0.1%, net price 45 g = £11.40
Excipients include disodium edetate, hydroxybenzoates (parabens), propylene glycol

TRETINOIN

Note Tretinoin is the acid form of vitamin A

Indications see preparations; malignant disease (section 8.1.5)
Cautions see notes above
Contra-indications see notes above
Side-effects see notes above
Dose
- See preparations

Retin-A® (Janssen-Cilag) PoM
Cream, tretinoin 0.025%, net price 60 g = £5.61
Excipients include butylated hydroxytoluene, sorbic acid, stearyl alcohol
Dose acne vulgaris, for dry or fair skin, apply thinly 1–2 times daily

Gel, tretinoin 0.01%, net price 60 g = £5.61; 0.025%, 60 g = £5.61
Excipients include butylated hydroxytoluene
Dose acne vulgaris, apply thinly 1–2 times daily

With antibacterial

Aknemycin® Plus (Crookes) PoM
Solution, tretinoin 0.025%, erythromycin 4% in an alcoholic basis, net price 25 mL = £7.05
Excipients none as listed in section 13.1.3
Dose acne, apply thinly 1–2 times daily

ISOTRETINOIN

Note Isotretinoin is an isomer of tretinoin
Important For **indications, cautions, contra-indications** and **side-effects** of isotretinoin **when given by mouth**, see p. 622

Indications see notes above; oral treatment (see section 13.6.2)
Cautions (*topical application* **only**) see notes above
Contra-indications (*topical application* **only**) see notes above
Dose
- Apply thinly 1–2 times daily

Isotrex® (Stiefel) PoM
Gel, isotretinoin 0.05%, net price 30 g = £6.18
Excipients include butylated hydroxytoluene

With antibacterial

Isotrexin® (Stiefel) PoM
Gel, isotretinoin 0.05%, erythromycin 2% in ethanolic basis, net price 30 g = £7.78
Excipients include butylated hydroxytoluene

Other topical preparations for acne

Salicylic acid is available in various preparations for sale direct to the public for the treatment of mild acne. Other products are more suitable for acne; salicylic acid is used mainly for its keratolytic effect.

Preparations containing **sulphur** and **abrasive agents** are not considered beneficial in acne.

Topical **corticosteroids** should **not** be used in acne.

A topical preparation of **nicotinamide** is available for inflammatory acne.

ABRASIVE AGENTS

Indications acne vulgaris (but see notes above)
Cautions avoid contact with eyes; discontinue use temporarily if skin becomes irritated
Contra-indications superficial venules, telangiectasia

Brasivol® (Stiefel)
Paste No. 1, aluminium oxide 38.09% in fine particles, in a soap-detergent basis, net price 75 g = £2.21
Excipients include fragrance, *N*-(3-Chloroallyl)hexaminium chloride (quaternium 15)
Dose use instead of soap 1–3 times daily

CORTICOSTEROIDS

Indications use in acne not recommended (see notes above)
Cautions see section 13.4 and notes above
Contra-indications see section 13.4 and notes above
Side-effects see section 13.4 and notes above

Actinac® (Peckforton) PoM
Lotion (powder for reconstitution with solvent), chloramphenicol 40 mg, hydrocortisone acetate 40 mg, allantoin 24 mg, butoxyethyl nicotinate 24 mg, precipitated sulphur 320 mg/g. Discard 21 days after reconstitution, net price 2 × 6.25-g bottles powder with 2 × 20-mL bottles solvent = £16.28. Label: 28. Potency: mild
Excipients none as listed in section 13.1.3

NICOTINAMIDE

Indications see under preparation
Cautions avoid contact with eyes and mucous membranes (including nose and mouth); reduce frequency of application if excessive dryness, irritation or peeling
Side-effects dryness of skin; also pruritus, erythema, burning and irritation

Nicam® (Dermal)
Gel, nicotinamide 4%, net price 60 g = £7.42
Excipients none as listed in section 13.1.3
Dose inflammatory acne vulgaris, apply twice daily; reduce to once daily or on alternate days if irritation occurs

SALICYLIC ACID

Indications acne; psoriasis (section 13.5.2); warts and calluses (section 13.7); fungal nail infections (section 13.10.2)
Cautions avoid contact with mouth, eyes, mucous membranes; systemic effects after excessive use (see section 4.7.1)
Side-effects local irritation

Acnisal® (Alliance)
Topical solution, salicylic acid 2% in a detergent and emollient basis, net price 177 mL = £4.03.
Excipients include benzyl alcohol
Dose use up to 3 times daily

13.6.2 Oral preparations for acne

Oral antibacterials for acne

Systemic antibacterial treatment is useful for inflammatory acne if topical treatment is not adequately effective or if it is inappropriate. Anticomedonal treatment (e.g. with topical benzoyl peroxide) may also be required.

Either **oxytetracycline** or **tetracycline** (section 5.1.3) is usually given for acne in a dose of 500 mg twice daily. If there is no improvement after the first 3 months another oral antibacterial should be used. Maximum improvement usually occurs after 4 to 6 months but in more severe cases treatment may need to be continued for 2 years or longer.

Doxycycline and **lymecycline** (section 5.1.3) are alternatives to tetracycline. Doxycycline can be used in a dose of 100 mg daily. Lymecycline is given in a dose of 408 mg daily.

Although **minocycline** is as effective as other tetracyclines for acne, it is associated with a greater risk of lupus erythematosus-like syndrome. Minocycline sometimes causes irreversible pigmentation; it is given in a dose of 100 mg once daily *or* 50 mg twice daily.

Erythromycin (section 5.1.5) in a dose of 500 mg twice daily is an alternative for the management of acne but propionibacteria strains resistant to erythromycin are becoming widespread and this may explain poor response.

Trimethoprim (section 5.1.8) in a dose of 300 mg twice daily may be used for acne resistant to other antibacterials [unlicensed indication]. Prolonged treatment with trimethoprim may depress haematopoiesis; it should generally be initiated by specialists.

Concomitant use of different topical and systemic antibacterials is undesirable owing to the increased likelihood of the development of bacterial resistance.

Hormone treatment for acne

Co-cyprindiol (cyproterone acetate with ethinylestradiol) contains an anti-androgen. It is no more effective than an oral broad-spectrum antibacterial but is useful in women who also wish to receive oral contraception. Improvement of acne with co-cyprindiol probably occurs because of decreased sebum secretion which is under androgen control. Some women with moderately severe hirsutism may also benefit because hair growth is also androgen-dependent. Contra-indications of co-cyprindiol include pregnancy and a predisposition to thrombosis.

CSM advice

Venous thromboembolism occurs more frequently in women taking co-cyprindiol than those taking a low-dose combined oral contraceptive. The CSM has reminded prescribers that co-cyprindiol is licensed for use in women with severe acne which has not responded to oral antibacterials and for moderately severe hirsutism; it should not be used solely for contraception. It is contra-indicated in those with a personal or close family history of venous thromboembolism. Women with severe acne or hirsutism may have an inherently increased risk of cardiovascular disease.

CO-CYPRINDIOL

A mixture of cyproterone acetate and ethinylestradiol in the mass proportions 2000 parts to 35 parts, respectively

Indications severe acne in women refractory to prolonged oral antibacterial therapy (but see notes above); moderately severe hirsutism
Cautions see under Combined Hormonal Contraceptives, section 7.3.1
Contra-indications see under Combined Hormonal Contraceptives, section 7.3.1
Side-effects see under Combined Hormonal Contraceptives, section 7.3.1
Dose
- 1 tablet daily for 21 days starting on day 1 of menstrual cycle and repeated after a 7-day interval, usually for several months; withdraw when acne or Hirsutism completely resolved (repeat courses may be given if recurrence)

Co-cyprindiol (Non-proprietary) PoM
Tablets, co-cyprindiol 2000/35 (cyproterone acetate 2 mg, ethinylestradiol 35 micrograms), net price 21-tab pack = £2.62
Brands include *Acnecide®*, *Cicafem®*, *Clairette®*, *Diva®*

13 Skin

Dianette® (Schering Health) PoM
Tablets, beige, s/c, co-cyprindiol 2000/35 (cyproterone acetate 2 mg, ethinylestradiol 35 micrograms), net price 21-tab pack = £3.11

Oral retinoid for acne

The retinoid **isotretinoin** (*Roaccutane®*) reduces sebum secretion. It is used for the systemic treatment of nodulo-cystic and conglobate acne, severe acne, scarring, acne which has not responded to an adequate course of a systemic antibacterial, or acne which is associated with psychological problems. It is also useful in women who develop acne in the third or fourth decades of life, since late onset acne is frequently unresponsive to antibacterials.

Isotretinoin is a toxic drug that should be prescribed **only** by, or under the supervision of, a consultant dermatologist. It is given for at least 16 weeks; repeat courses are not normally required.

Side-effects of isotretinoin include severe dryness of the skin and mucous membranes, nose bleeds, and joint pains. The drug is **teratogenic** and must **not** be given to women of child-bearing age unless they practise effective contraception (oral progestogen-only contraceptives not considered effective) and then only after detailed assessment and explanation by the physician. Women must also be registered with a pregnancy prevention programme (see under Cautions below).

Although a causal link between isotretinoin use and psychiatric changes (including suicidal ideation) has not been established, the possibility should be considered before initiating treatment; if psychiatric changes occur during treatment, isotretinoin should be stopped, the prescriber informed, and specialist psychiatric advice should be sought.

ISOTRETINOIN

Note Isotretinoin is an isomer of tretinoin

Indications see notes above

Cautions exclude pregnancy before starting (perform pregnancy test 2–3 days before expected menstruation, start treatment on day 2 or 3 of menstrual cycle)—women must practice effective contraception at least 1 month before, during, and for at least 1 month after treatment (see also notes above); avoid blood donation during treatment and for at least 1 month after treatment; history of depression; measure hepatic function and serum lipids before treatment, 1 month after starting and then every 3 months (reduce dose or discontinue if transaminase or serum lipids persistently raised); discontinue if uncontrolled hypertriglyceridaemia or pancreatitis; diabetes; dry eye syndrome (associated with risk of keratitis); avoid keratolytics; renal impairment (Appendix 3) **interactions:** Appendix 1 (retinoids)

Counselling Warn patient to avoid wax epilation (risk of epidermal stripping), dermabrasion, and laser skin treatments (risk of scarring) during treatment and for at least 6 months after stopping; patient should avoid exposure to UV light (including sunlight) and use sunscreen and emollient (including lip balm) preparations from the start of treatment.

Contra-indications pregnancy (**important teratogenic risk:** see Cautions above and Appendix 4); breast-feeding; hepatic impairment (Appendix 2); hypervitaminosis A, hyperlipidaemia

Side-effects dryness of skin (with dermatitis, scaling, thinning, erythema, pruritus), epidermal fragility (trauma may cause blistering), dryness of lips (sometimes cheilitis), dryness of eyes (with blepharitis and conjunctivitis), dryness of pharyngeal mucosa (with hoarseness), dryness of nasal mucosa (with epistaxis), headache, myalgia and arthralgia, raised plasma concentration of triglycerides, of glucose, of serum transaminases, and of cholesterol (risk of pancreatitis if triglycerides above 8 g/litre), haematuria and proteinuria, thrombocytopenia, thrombocytosis, neutropenia and anaemia; *rarely* mood changes (depression, suicidal ideation, aggressive behaviour, anxiety)—expert referral required, exacerbation of acne, acne fulminans, allergic skin reactions, and hypersensitivity, alopecia; *very rarely* nausea, inflammatory bowel disease, diarrhoea (discontinue if severe), benign intracranial hypertension (avoid concomitant tetracyclines), convulsions, malaise, drowsiness, lymphadenopathy, increased sweating, hyperuricaemia, raised serum creatinine concentration and glomerulonephritis, hepatitis, tendinitis, bone changes (including reduced bone density, early epiphyseal closure, and skeletal hyperostosis following long-term administration), visual disturbances (papilloedema, corneal opacities, cataracts, decreased night vision, photophobia, blurred vision, colour blindness)—expert referral required and consider withdrawal, decreased tolerance to contact lenses and keratitis, impaired hearing, Gram-positive infections of skin and mucous membranes, allergic vasculitis and granulomatous lesions, paronychia, hirsutism, nail dystrophy, skin hyperpigmentation, photosensitivity

Dose

- 500 micrograms/kg daily increased if necessary to 1 mg/kg (in 1–2 divided doses) for 16–24 weeks (8 weeks if failure or relapse after first course); max. cumulative dose 150 mg/kg per course; CHILD not recommended

Isotretinoin (Non-proprietary) PoM
Capsules, isotretinoin 5 mg, net price 56-cap pack = £15.00; 20 mg, 56-cap pack = £40.00. Label: 10, patient information leaflet, 11, 21

Roaccutane® (Roche) PoM
Capsules, isotretinoin 5 mg (red-violet/white), net price 30-cap pack = £9.08; 20 mg (red-violet/white), 30-cap pack = £25.02. Label: 10, patient information card, 11, 21
Excipients include arachis (peanut) oil

13.7 Preparations for warts and calluses

Warts (verrucas) are caused by a human papillomavirus, which most frequently affects the hands, feet (plantar warts), and the anogenital region (see below); treatment usually relies on local tissue destruction. Warts may regress on their own and treatment is required only if the warts are painful, unsightly, persistent, or cause distress.

Preparations of **salicylic acid, formaldehyde, gluteraldehyde** or **silver nitrate** are available for purchase by the public; they are suitable for the removal of warts on hands and feet. **Salicylic acid** is a useful keratolytic which may be considered first; it is also suitable for the removal of *corns and calluses*. Preparations of salicylic acid in a collodion basis are available but some patients may develop an allergy to colophony in the formulation. An ointment combining **salicylic acid** with **podophyllum resin** (*Posalfilin®*) is available for treating plantar warts. Cryotherapy causes pain, swelling, and blistering and may be no more effective than topical salicylic acid in the treatment of warts.

SALICYLIC ACID

Indications see under preparations; psoriasis (section 13.5.2); acne (section 13.6.1); fungal nail infections (section 13.10.2)

Cautions significant peripheral neuropathy, patients with diabetes at risk of neuropathic ulcers; protect surrounding skin and avoid broken skin; not suitable for application to face, anogenital region, or large areas

Side-effects skin irritation, see notes above

Dose

- See under preparations; advise patient to apply carefully to wart and to protect surrounding skin (e.g. with soft paraffin or specially designed plaster); rub wart surface gently with file or pumice stone once weekly; treatment may need to be continued for up to 3 months

Cuplex® (Crawford)
Gel, salicylic acid 11%, lactic acid 4%, in a collodion basis, net price 5 g = £2.23. Label: 15
Dose for plantar and mosaic warts, corns, and calluses, apply twice daily
Note Contains colophony (see notes above)

Duofilm® (Stiefel)
Paint, salicylic acid 16.7%, lactic acid 16.7%, in flexible collodion, net price 15 mL (with applicator) = £2.25. Label: 15
Dose for plantar and mosaic warts, apply daily

Occlusal® (Alliance)
Cutaneous solution, salicylic acid 26% in polyacrylic solution, net price 10 mL (with applicator) = £3.39. Label: 15
Dose for common and plantar warts, apply daily

Salactol® (Dermal)
Paint, salicylic acid 16.7%, lactic acid 16.7%, in flexible collodion, net price 10 mL (with applicator) = £1.79. Label: 15
Dose for warts, particularly plantar warts, verrucas, corns, and calluses, apply daily
Note Contains colophony (see notes above)

Salatac® (Dermal)
Gel, salicylic acid 12%, lactic acid 4% in a collodion basis, net price 8 g (with applicator) = £3.12. Label: 15
Dose for warts, verrucas, corns, and calluses, apply daily

Verrugon® (Ransom)
Ointment, salicylic acid 50% in a paraffin basis, net price 6 g = £2.83
Dose for plantar warts, apply daily

With podophyllum

Posalfilin® (Norgine)
Ointment, podophyllum resin 20%, salicylic acid 25%, net price 10 g = £3.51
Dose for plantar warts apply daily
Note Owing to the salicylic acid content, not suitable for anogenital warts; owing to the podophyllum content also contra-indicated in pregnancy and breast-feeding

FORMALDEHYDE

Indications see under preparations

Cautions see under Salicylic Acid

Side-effects see under Salicylic Acid

Veracur® (Typharm)
Gel, formaldehyde 0.75% in a water-miscible gel basis, net price 15 g = £2.41.
Dose for warts, particularly plantar warts, apply twice daily

GLUTARALDEHYDE

Indications warts, particularly plantar warts

Cautions protect surrounding skin; not for application to face, mucosa, or anogenital areas

Side-effects rashes, skin irritation (discontinue if severe); stains skin brown

Dose

- Apply twice daily (see also under Salicylic acid)

Glutarol® (Dermal)
Solution (= application), glutaraldehyde 10%, net price 10 mL (with applicator) = £2.17

SILVER NITRATE

Indications warts, verrucas, umbilical granulomas, over-granulating tissue, cauterisation

Cautions protect surrounding skin and avoid broken skin; not suitable for application to face, ano-genital region, or large areas

Side-effects chemical burns on surrounding skin; stains skin and fabric

Dose

- Common warts and verrucas, apply moistened caustic pencil tip for 1–2 minutes; repeat after 24 hours up to max. 3 applications for warts or max. 6 applications for verrucas
Note Instructions in proprietary packs generally incorporate advice to remove dead skin before use by gentle filing and to cover with adhesive dressing after application
- Umbilical granulomas, apply moistened caustic pencil tip (usually containing silver nitrate 40%) for 1–2 minutes while protecting surrounding skin with soft paraffin

Silver nitrate (Non-proprietary)
Caustic pencil, tip containing silver nitrate 40%, potassium nitrate 60%, net price = 93p

AVOCA® (Bray)
Caustic pencil, tip containing silver nitrate 95%, potassium nitrate 5%, net price, treatment pack (including emery file, 6 adhesive dressings and protector pads) = £1.94.

Anogenital warts

The treatment of anogenital warts (condylomata acuminata) should be accompanied by screening for other sexually transmitted diseases. **Podophyllum** and **podophyllotoxin** (the major active ingredient of podophyllum) may be used for *soft, non-keratinised* external anogenital warts; these preparations can cause considerable irritation of the treated area. They can also cause severe systemic toxicity on excessive application including gastro-intestinal, renal, haematological, and CNS effects. Patients with a limited number of external warts or *keratinised* lesions may be better treated with cryotherapy or other forms of physical ablation.

Imiquimod cream is licensed for the treatment of external anogenital warts; it may be used for both keratinised and non-keratinised lesions. It is also licensed for the treatment of superficial basal cell carcinoma and actinic keratosis (section 13.8.1).

Inosine pranobex (section 5.3.2.1) is licensed for adjunctive treatment of genital warts but it has been superseded by more effective drugs.

IMIQUIMOD

Indications see under Dose

Cautions avoid normal or broken skin, and open wounds; not suitable for internal genital warts; uncircumcised males (risk of phimosis or stricture of foreskin); autoimmune disease; immunosuppressed patients; pregnancy

Side-effects local reactions (including itching, burning sensation, erythema, erosion, oedema, excoriation, and scabbing); headache; influenza-like symptoms; myalgia; *less commonly* local ulceration and alopecia; *rarely* Stevens-Johnson syndrome and cutaneous lupus erythematosus-like effect; permanent hypopigmentation or hyperpigmentation reported

Dose

- Warts (external genital and perianal), apply thinly 3 times a week at night until lesions resolve (max. 16 weeks)
- Superficial basal cell carcinoma, apply to lesion (and 1 cm beyond it) on 5 days each week for 6 weeks; assess response 12 weeks after completing treatment
- Actinic keratosis, apply to lesion 3 times a week for 4 weeks; assess response after a 4 week treatment-free interval; repeat 4-week course if lesions persist; max. 2 courses
- CHILD under 18 years, see *BNF for Children*

Important Should be rubbed in and allowed to stay on the treated area for 6–10 hours for warts or for 8 hours for basal cell carcinoma and actinic keratosis, then washed off with mild soap and water (uncircumcised males treating warts under foreskin should wash the area daily). The cream should be washed off before sexual contact

Aldara® (3M) PoM

Cream, imiquimod 5%, net price 12-sachet pack = £51.32. Label: 10, patient information leaflet

Excipients include benzyl alcohol, cetyl alcohol, hydroxybenzoates (parabens), polysorbate 60, stearyl alcohol

Condoms may damage latex condoms and diaphragms

PODOPHYLLUM

Indications see under preparations

Cautions avoid normal skin and open wounds; keep away from face; very irritant to eyes; **important**: see also warnings below

Contra-indications pregnancy and breast-feeding; children

Side-effects see notes above

Podophyllin Paint, Compound, BP PoM

(podophyllum resin 15% in compound benzoin tincture), podophyllum resin 1.5 g, compound benzoin tincture to 10 mL; 5 mL to be dispensed unless otherwise directed. Label: 15

Dose external genital warts, applied weekly in genitourinary clinic (or at a general practitioner's surgery by trained nurses after screening for other sexually transmitted diseases)

Important Should be allowed to stay on the treated area for not longer than 6 hours and then washed off. Care should be taken to avoid splashing the surrounding skin during application (which must be covered with soft paraffin as a protection). Where there are a large number of warts only a few should be treated at any one time as **severe toxicity** caused by absorption of podophyllin has been reported

Podophyllotoxin

Condyline® (Ardern) PoM

Solution, podophyllotoxin 0.5% in alcoholic basis, net price 3.5 mL (with applicators) = £14.49. Label: 15

Dose condylomata acuminata affecting the penis or the female external genitalia, apply twice daily for 3 consecutive days; treatment may be repeated at weekly intervals if necessary for a total of five 3-day treatment courses; direct medical supervision for lesions in the female and for lesions greater than 4 cm^2 in the male; max. 50 single applications ('loops') per session (consult product literature)

Warticon® (Stiefel) PoM

Cream, podophyllotoxin 0.15%, net price 5 g (with mirror) = £15.46

Excipients include butylated hydroxyanisole, cetyl alcohol, hydroxybenzoates (parabens), sorbic acid, stearyl alcohol

Dose condylomata acuminata affecting the penis or the female external genitalia, apply twice daily for 3 consecutive days; treatment may be repeated at weekly intervals if necessary for a total of four 3-day treatment courses; direct medical supervision for lesions greater than 4 cm^2

Solution, blue, podophyllotoxin 0.5% in alcoholic basis, net price 3 mL (with applicators— *Warticon®* [for men]; with applicators and mirror—*Warticon Fem®* [for women]) = £12.88. Label: 15

Dose condylomata acuminata affecting the penis or the female external genitalia, apply twice daily for 3 consecutive days; treatment may be repeated at weekly intervals if necessary for a total of four 3-day treatment courses; direct medical supervision for lesions greater than 4 cm^2; max. 50 single applications ('loops') per session (consult product literature)

13.8 Sunscreens and camouflagers

13.8.1 Sunscreen preparations
13.8.2 Camouflagers

13.8.1 Sunscreen preparations

Solar ultraviolet irradiation can be harmful to the skin. It is responsible for disorders such as *polymorphic light eruption, solar urticaria*, and it provokes the various *cutaneous porphyrias*. It also provokes (or at least aggravates) skin lesions of *lupus erythematosus* and may aggravate *rosacea* and some other *dermatoses*. Certain drugs such as demeclocycline, phenothiazines, or amiodarone can cause photosensitivity. All these conditions (as well as *sunburn*) may occur after relatively short periods of exposure to the sun. Solar ultraviolet irradiation may provoke attacks of recurrent herpes labialis (but it is not known whether the effect of sunlight exposure is local or systemic).

The effects of exposure over longer periods include *ageing changes* and more importantly the initiation of *skin cancer*.

Solar ultraviolet radiation is approximately 200–400 nm in wavelength. The medium wavelengths (290–320 nm, known as UVB) cause sunburn and contribute to the long-term changes responsible for skin cancer and ageing. The long wavelengths (320–400 nm, known as UVA) do not cause sunburn but are responsible for many *photosensitivity reactions* and *photodermatoses*. Both UVA and UVB contribute to long-term *photodamage* and to the pathogenesis of *skin cancer*.

Sunscreen preparations contain substances that protect the skin against UVB and hence against sunburn, but they are no substitute for covering the skin and avoiding sunlight. The sun protection factor (SPF, usually indicated in the preparation title) provides guidance on the degree of protection offered against UVB; it indicates the multiples of protection provided against burning, compared with unprotected skin; for example, an SPF of 8 should enable a person to remain 8 times longer in the sun without burning. However, in practice users do not apply sufficient sunscreen product and the protection is lower than that found in experimental studies. Sunscreen preparations, do not prevent long-term damage associated with UVA, which might not become apparent for 10 to 20 years. Preparations that also contain reflective substances, such as titanium dioxide, provide the most effective protection against UVA. Some products use a star rating system to indicate the protection against UVA relative to protection against UVB for the same product. Four stars indicate that the product offers balanced UVA and UVB protection; products with 3, 2, or 1 star rating indicate that greater protection is offered against UVB than against UVA. However, the usefulness of the star rating system remains controversial.

Sunscreen preparations, may rarely cause allergic reactions.

> For optimum photoprotection, sunscreen preparations should be applied **thickly** and **frequently** (approximately 2 hourly). In photodermatoses, they should be used from spring to autumn. As maximum protection from sunlight is desirable, preparations with the highest SPF should be prescribed.

Borderline substances The preparations marked 'ACBS' are regarded as drugs when prescribed for skin protection against ultraviolet radiation in abnormal cutaneous photosensitivity resulting from genetic disorders or photodermatoses, including vitiligo and those resulting from radiotherapy; chronic or recurrent herpes simplex labialis. Preparations with SPF less than 30 should not normally be prescribed. See also Appendix 7.

Delph® (Fenton)
Lotion, (UVA and UVB protection; UVB-SPF 30), avobenzone 4%, octinoxate 4.8%, oxybenzone 1.5%, titanium dioxide 2.5%, net price 200 mL = £2.85. ACBS
Excipients include cetostearyl alcohol, fragrance, hydroxybenzoates (parabens), imidurea

E45 Sun® (Crookes)
Reflective Sunscreen (UVA and UVB protection; UVB-SPF 50), waterproof, titanium dioxide 6.4%, zinc oxide 16%, net price 150 mL = £7.09. ACBS
Excipients include hydroxybenzoates (parabens), isopropyl palmitate

SpectraBan® (Stiefel)
Ultra lotion (UVA and UVB protection; UVB-SPF 28), water resistant, avobenzone 2%, oxybenzone 3%, padimate-O 8%, titanium dioxide 2%, net price 150 mL = £6.54. ACBS
Excipients include benzyl alcohol, disodium edetate, sorbic acid, fragrance

Sunsense® Ultra (Crawford)
Lotion (UVA and UVB protection; UVB-SPF 60), octinoxate 7.5% oxybenzone 3%, titanium dioxide 3.5%, net price 50-mL bottle with roll-on applicator = £3.11, 125 mL = £5.10. ACBS
Excipients include butylated hydroxytoluene, cetyl alcohol, fragrance, hydroxybenzoates (parabens), propylene glycol

Uvistat® (LPC)
Cream (UVA and UVB protection; UVB-SPF 30), avobenzone 5%, bisoctrizole 1.5%, octinoxate 7.5%, octocrilene 4%, titanium dioxide 5.2%, net price 125 mL = £7.45. ACBS
Excipients include disodium edetate, hydroxybenzoates (parabens), propylene glycol

Cream (UVA and UVB protection; UVB-SPF 50), amiloxate 2%, avobenzone 5%, bisoctrizole 6%, octinoxate 10%, octocrilene 4%, titanium dioxide 4.8%, net price 125 mL = £8.45. ACBS
Excipients include disodium edetate, polysorbate 60, propylene glycol

Lipscreen (UVA and UVB protection; UVB-SPF 50), avobenzone 5%, bemotrizinol 3%, octinoxate 10%, octocrilene 4%, titanium dioxide 3%, net price 5 g = £2.99. ACBS
Excipients include butylated hydroxytoluene, hydroxybenzoates (parabens)

Photodamage

Patients should be advised to use a high-SPF sunscreen and to minimise exposure of the skin to direct sunlight or sun lamps.

Topical treatments are used for non-hypertrophic *actinic keratosis*. An **emollient** may be sufficient for mild lesions. **Diclofenac** gel is suitable for the treatment of superficial lesions in mild disease. **Fluorouracil** cream is effective against most types of non-hypertrophic actinic keratosis. **Imiquimod** (section 13.7) is used for lesions on the face and scalp when cryotherapy or other topical treatments cannot be used. Fluorouracil and imiquimod produce a more marked inflammatory reaction than diclofenac but lesions resolve faster. **Photodynamic therapy** in combination with methyl-5-aminolevulinate cream (*Metvix®*, available from Galderma) is used in specialist centres for treating superficial and confluent, non-hypertrophic actinic keratosis when other treatments are inadequate or unsuitable; it is particularly suitable for multiple lesions, for periorbital lesions, or for lesions located at sites of poor healing.

Imiquimod or topical fluorouracil is used for treating superficial *basal cell carcinomas*. Photodynamic therapy in combination with methyl-5-aminolevulinate cream is used in specialist centres for treating superficial, nodular basal cell carcinomas when other treatments are unsuitable.

DICLOFENAC SODIUM

Indications actinic keratosis

Cautions as for topical NSAIDs, see section 10.3.2

Contra-indications as for topical NSAIDs, see section 10.3.2

Side-effects as for topical NSAIDs, see section 10.3.2; also paraesthesia; application of large amounts may result in systemic effects, see section 10.1

Dose

- Apply thinly twice daily for 60–90 days; max. 8 g daily

Solaraze® (Shire) PoM
Gel, diclofenac sodium 3% in a sodium hyaluronate basis, net price 25 g = £16.65
Excipients include benzyl alcohol

FLUOROURACIL

Indications superficial malignant and pre-malignant skin lesions; other malignant disease (section 8.1.3)

Cautions avoid contact with mucous membranes; caution in handling—irritant to tissues

Contra-indications pregnancy (Appendix 4); breast-feeding

Side-effects local irritation (use a topical corticosteroid for severe discomfort associated with inflammatory reactions), photosensitivity; *rarely* erythema multiforme

Dose

- Apply thinly to the affected area once or twice daily; if possible, cover malignant lesions with occlusive dressing; max. area of skin treated at one time, 500 cm^2; usual duration of initial therapy, 3–4 weeks

Note Alternative regimens may be in use in some settings

Efudix® (Valeant) PoM
Cream, fluorouracil 5%, net price 20 g = £17.72, 40 g = £35.44
Excipients include hydroxybenzoates (parabens), polysorbate 60, propylene glycol, stearyl alcohol

13.8.2 Camouflagers

Disfigurement of the skin can be very distressing to patients and may have a marked psychological effect. In skilled hands, or with experience, camouflage cosmetics can be very effective in concealing scars and birthmarks. The depigmented patches in vitiligo are also very disfiguring and camouflage creams are of great cosmetic value.

Borderline substances The preparations marked 'ACBS' are regarded as drugs when prescribed for post-operative scars and other deformities and as an adjunctive therapy in the relief of emotional disturbances due to disfiguring skin disease, such as vitiligo. See also Appendix 7.

Covermark® (Epiderm)
Classic foundation (masking cream), net price 15 mL (10 shades) = £10.75. ACBS
Excipients include beeswax, hydroxybenzoates (parabens), fragrance
Finishing powder, net price 60 g = £10.55. ACBS
Excipients include beeswax, hydroxybenzoates (parabens), fragrance

Dermacolor® (Fox)
Camouflage creme, (100 shades), net price 25 g = £9.05. ACBS
Excipients include beeswax, butylated hydroxytoluene, fragrance, propylene glycol, stearyl alcohol, wool fat
Fixing powder, (7 shades), net price 60 g = £7.68. ACBS
Excipients include fragrance

Keromask® (Network)
Masking cream, (2 shades), net price 15 mL = £5.67. ACBS
Excipients include butylated hydroxyanisole, hydroxybenzoates (parabens), wool fat, propylene glycol
Finishing powder, net price 20 g = £5.67. ACBS
Excipients include butylated hydroxytoluene, hydroxybenzoates (parabens)

Veil® (Blake)
Cover cream, (27 shades), net price 19 g = £10.69, 44 g = £17.41, 70 g = £24.38. ACBS
Excipients include hydroxybenzoates (parabens), wool fat derivative
Finishing powder, translucent, net price 35 g = £11.51. ACBS
Excipients include butylated hydroxyanisole, hydroxybenzoates (parabens)

13.9 Shampoos and other preparations for scalp and hair conditions

Dandruff is considered to be a mild form of seborrhoeic dermatitis (see also section 13.5.1). Shampoos containing antimicrobial agents such as **pyrithione zinc** (which are widely available) and **selenium sulphide** may have beneficial effects. Shampoos containing **tar** extracts may be useful and they are also used in *psoriasis*. **Ketoconazole** shampoo should be considered for more persistent or severe dandruff or for seborrhoeic dermatitis of the scalp.

Corticosteroid gels and lotions (section 13.4) can also be used.

Shampoos containing **coal tar** and **salicylic acid** may also be useful. A cream or an ointment containing coal tar and salicylic acid is very helpful in *psoriasis* that affects the scalp (section 13.5.2). Patients who do not respond to these treatments may need to be referred to exclude the possibility of other skin conditions.

Cradle cap in infants may be treated with **coconut oil** or **olive oil** applications followed by shampooing.

See below for male-pattern baldness and also section 13.5 (psoriasis and eczema), section 13.10.4 (lice), and section 13.10.2 (ringworm).

Shampoos

[1]**Ketoconazole** (Non-proprietary) PoM
Cream—section 13.10.2
Shampoo, ketoconazole 2%, net price 120 mL = £4.60
Excipients include imidurea
Brands include *Dandrazol® 2% Shampoo, Nizoral®*
Dose treatment of seborrhoeic dermatitis and dandruff apply twice weekly for 2–4 weeks (prophylaxis apply once every 1–2 weeks); treatment of pityriasis versicolor apply once daily for max. 5 days (prophylaxis apply once daily for up to 3 days before sun exposure); leave preparation on for 3–5 minutes before rinsing

1. Can be sold to the public for the prevention and treatment of dandruff and seborrhoeic dermatitis of the scalp as a shampoo formulation containing ketoconazole max. 2%, in a pack containing max. 120 mL and labelled to show a max. frequency of application of once every 3 days

Alphosyl 2 in 1® (GSK Consumer Healthcare)
Shampoo, alcoholic coal tar extract 5%, net price 125 mL = £1.81, 250 mL = £3.43
Excipients include hydroxybenzoates (parabens), fragrance
Dose dandruff, use once or twice weekly as necessary; psoriasis, seborrhoeic dermatitis, scaling and itching, use every 2–3 days

Capasal® (Dermal)
Shampoo, coal tar 1%, coconut oil 1%, salicylic acid 0.5%, net price 250 mL = £4.91
Excipients none as listed in section 13.1.3
Dose scaly scalp disorders including psoriasis, seborrhoeic dermatitis, dandruff, and cradle cap, apply daily as necessary

Ceanel Concentrate® (Ferndale)
Shampoo, cetrimide 10%, undecenoic acid 1%, phenylethyl alcohol 7.5%, net price 150 mL = £3.40, 500 mL = £9.80
Excipients none as listed in section 13.1.3
Dose scalp psoriasis, seborrhoeic dermatitis, dandruff, apply 3 times in first week then twice weekly

Clinitar® (CHS)
Shampoo, coal tar extract 2%, net price 100 g = £2.50
Excipients include polysorbates, fragrance
Dose scalp psoriasis, seborrhoeic dermatitis, and dandruff, apply up to 3 times weekly

Dermax® (Dermal)
Shampoo, benzalkonium chloride 0.5%, net price 250 mL = £5.95
Excipients none as listed in section 13.1.3
Dose seborrhoeic scalp conditions associated with dandruff and scaling, apply as necessary

Meted® (Alliance)
Shampoo, salicylic acid 3%, sulphur 5%, net price 120 mL = £3.80
Excipients include fragrance
Dose scaly scalp disorders including psoriasis, seborrhoeic dermatitis, and dandruff, apply at least twice weekly

Pentrax® (Alliance)
Shampoo, coal tar 4.3%, net price 120 mL = £3.80
Excipients none as listed in section 13.1.3
Dose scaly scalp disorders including psoriasis, seborrhoeic dermatitis, and dandruff, apply at least twice weekly

Polytar AF® (Stiefel)
Shampoo, arachis (peanut) oil extract of coal tar 0.3%, cade oil 0.3%, coal tar solution 0.1%, pine tar 0.3%, pyrithione zinc 1%, net price 250 mL = £6.52
Excipients include fragrance, imidurea
Dose scaly scalp disorders including psoriasis, seborrhoeic dermatitis, and dandruff, apply 2–3 times weekly for at least 3 weeks

Psoriderm® (Dermal)
Scalp lotion (= shampoo), coal tar 2.5%, lecithin 0.3%, net price 250 mL = £4.96
Excipients include disodium edetate
Dose scalp psoriasis, use as necessary

Selsun® (Chattem UK)
Shampoo, selenium sulphide 2.5%, net price 50 mL = £1.44, 100 mL = £1.96, 150 mL = £2.75
Excipients include fragrance
Cautions avoid using 48 hours before or after applying hair colouring, straightening or waving preparations
Dose seborrhoeic dermatitis and dandruff, apply twice weekly for 2 weeks then once weekly for 2 weeks and then as necessary; CHILD under 5 years not recommended; pityriasis versicolor, section 13.10.2 [unlicensed indication]

T/Gel® (Neutrogena)
Shampoo, coal tar extract 2%, net price 125 mL = £3.18, 250 mL = £4.78
Excipients include fragrance, hydroxybenzoates (parabens), imidurea, tetrasodium edetate
Dose scalp psoriasis, seborrhoeic dermatitis, dandruff, apply as necessary

Other scalp preparations

Cocois®
Section 13.5.2

Etrivex®
Section 13.4

Polytar® (Stiefel)
Liquid, arachis (peanut) oil extract of coal tar 0.3%, cade oil 0.3%, coal tar solution 0.1%, oleyl alcohol 1%, tar 0.3%, net price 250 mL = £2.23
Excipients include fragrance, imidurea, polysorbate 80
Dose scalp disorders including psoriasis, seborrhoea, eczema, pruritus, and dandruff, apply 1–2 times weekly

Polytar Plus® (Stiefel)
Liquid, ingredients as *Polytar®* liquid with hydrolysed animal protein 3%, net price 500 mL = £3.91
Excipients include fragrance, imidurea, polysorbate 80
Dose scalp disorders including psoriasis, seborrhoea, eczema, pruritus, and dandruff, apply 1–2 times weekly

Hirsutism

Hirsutism may result from hormonal disorders or as a side-effect of drugs such as minoxidil, corticosteroids, anabolic steroids, androgens, danazol, and progestogens.

Weight loss can reduce hirsutism in obese women.

Women should be advised about local methods of hair removal, and in the mildest cases this may be all that is required.

Eflornithine, an antiprotozoal drug, inhibits the enzyme ornithine decarboxylase in hair follicles. Topical eflornithine can be used as an adjunct to laser therapy for facial hirsutism in women. Eflornithine should be discontinued in the absence of improvement after treatment for 4 months.

Co-cyprindiol (section 13.6.2) may be effective for moderately severe hirsutism. **Metformin** (section 6.1.2.2) is an alternative in women with polycystic ovary syndrome. Systemic treatment is required for 6–12 months before benefit is seen.

EFLORNITHINE

Indications see notes above
Contra-indications pregnancy (Appendix 4); breast-feeding (Appendix 5)
Side-effects acne, application site reactions including burning and stinging sensation, rash; *less commonly* abnormal hair texture and growth
Dose
- Apply thinly twice daily; CHILD under 12 years not recommended

Note Preparation must be rubbed in thoroughly; cosmetics may be applied over treated area 5 minutes after eflornithine; do not wash treated area for 4 hours after application

Vaniqa® (Shire) ▼ PoM
Cream, eflornithine (as hydrochloride) 11.5%, net price 30 g = £26.04
Excipients include cetostearyl alcohol, hydroxybenzoates, stearyl alcohol
Note The *Scottish Medicines Consortium* has advised (September 2005) that eflornithine for facial hirsutism be restricted for use in women in whom alternative drug treatment cannot be used

Male-pattern baldness

Finasteride is licensed for the treatment of male-pattern baldness in men. Continuous use for 3–6 months is required before benefit is seen, and effects are reversed 6–12 months after treatment is discontinued.

Topical application of **minoxidil** may stimulate limited hair growth in a small proportion of adults but only for as long as it is used.

FINASTERIDE

Indications male-pattern baldness in men
Cautions see section 6.4.2
Side-effects see section 6.4.2
Dose
- By mouth 1 mg daily

Propecia® (MSD) PoM NHS
Tablets, f/c, beige, finasteride 1 mg, net price 28-tab pack = £26.99, 84-tab pack = £81.55

MINOXIDIL

Indications male-pattern baldness (men and women)
Cautions section 2.5.1 (only about 1.4–1.7% absorbed); avoid contact with eyes, mouth and mucous membranes, broken, infected, shaved, or inflamed skin; avoid inhalation of spray mist; avoid occlusive dressings and topical drugs which enhance absorption
Contra-indications section 2.5.1
Side-effects section 2.5.1; irritant dermatitis, allergic contact dermatitis, changes in hair colour or texture, discontinue if increased hair loss persists for more than 2 weeks
Dose
- Apply 1 mL twice daily to dry hair and scalp (discontinue if no improvement after 1 year); 5% strength for use in men only

Regaine® (Pharmacia) NHS
Regaine® Regular Strength topical solution, minoxidil 2% in an aqueous alcoholic basis, net price 60-mL bottle with applicators = £14.16
Excipients include propylene glycol
Cautions flammable; wash hands after application
Regaine® Extra Strength topical solution, minoxidil 5% in an aqueous alcoholic basis, net price 60-mL bottle with applicators = £17.00, 3 × 60-mL bottles = £34.03
Excipients include propylene glycol
Cautions flammable; wash hands after application

13.10 Anti-infective skin preparations

13.10.1 Antibacterial preparations
13.10.2 Antifungal preparations
13.10.3 Antiviral preparations
13.10.4 Parasiticidal preparations
13.10.5 Preparations for minor cuts and abrasions

13.10.1 Antibacterial preparations

13.10.1.1 Antibacterial preparations only used topically
13.10.1.2 Antibacterial preparations also used systemically

Cellulitis, a rapidly spreading deeply seated inflammation of the skin and subcutaneous tissue, requires systemic antibacterial treatment (see Table 1, section 5.1); it often involves staphylococcal infection. Lower leg infections or infections spreading around wounds are almost always cellulitis. *Erysipelas*, a superficial infection with clearly defined edges (and often affecting the face), is also treated with a systemic antibacterial (see Table 1, section 5.1); it usually involves streptococcal infection.

In the community acute *impetigo* on small areas of the skin may be treated by short-term topical application of **fusidic acid**; **mupirocin** should be used only to treat methicillin-resistant *Staphylococcus aureus*. If the impetigo is extensive or longstanding, an oral antibacterial such as **flucloxacillin** (or **erythromycin** in penicillin-allergy) (Table 1, section 5.1) should be used. Mild antiseptics such as **povidone–iodine** (section 13.11.4) are used to soften crusts and exudate.

Although there are a great many antibacterial drugs presented in topical preparations some are potentially hazardous and frequently their use is not necessary if adequate hygienic measures can be taken. Moreover, not all skin conditions that are oozing, crusted, or characterised by pustules are actually infected. Topical antibacterials should be **avoided** on *leg ulcers* unless used in short courses for defined infections; treatment of bacterial colonisation is generally inappropriate.

To minimise the development of resistant organisms it is advisable to limit the choice of antibacterials applied topically to those not used systemically. Unfortunately some of these, for example neomycin, may cause sensitisation, and there is cross-sensitivity with other aminoglycoside antibiotics, such as gentamicin. If *large areas of skin* are being treated, ototoxicity may also be a hazard with aminoglycoside antibiotics (and also with polymyxins), particularly in children, in the elderly, and in those with renal impairment. *Resistant organisms* are more common in hospitals, and whenever possible swabs should be taken for bacteriological examination before beginning treatment.

Mupirocin is not related to any other antibacterial in use; it is effective for skin infections, particularly those due to Gram-positive organisms but it is not indicated for pseudomonal infection. Although *Staphylococcus aureus* strains with low-level resistance to mupirocin are emerging, it is generally useful in infections resistant to other antibacterials. To avoid the development of resistance, mupirocin or fusidic acid should not be used for longer than 10 days and local microbiology advice should be sought before using it in hospital. In the presence of mupirocin-resistant MRSA infection, an antiseptic like povidone–iodine, chlorhexidine, or alcohol can be used; their use should be discussed with the local microbiologist.

Silver sulfadiazine (silver sulphadiazine) is used in the treatment of infected burns.

13.10.1.1 Antibacterial preparations only used topically

MUPIROCIN

Indications bacterial skin infections (see also notes above)
Side-effects local reactions including urticaria, pruritus, burning sensation, rash
Dose
- ADULT and CHILD over 1 year, apply up to 3 times daily for up to 10 days; CHILD under 1 year see *BNF for Children*

Bactroban® (GSK) PoM

Cream, mupirocin (as mupirocin calcium) 2%, net price 15 g = £4.38

Excipients include benzyl alcohol, cetyl alcohol, stearyl alcohol

Ointment, mupirocin 2%, net price 15 g = £4.38

Excipients none as listed in section 13.1.3

Note Contains macrogol and manufacturer advises caution in renal impairment; may sting

Nasal ointment—section 12.2.3

NEOMYCIN SULPHATE

Indications bacterial skin infections

Cautions large areas, see below

Large areas If large areas of skin are being treated ototoxicity may be a hazard, particularly in children, in the elderly, and in those with renal impairment

Contra-indications neonates

Side-effects sensitisation (see also notes above)

Neomycin Cream BPC PoM

Cream, neomycin sulphate 0.5%, cetomacrogol emulsifying ointment 30%, chlorocresol 0.1%, disodium edetate 0.01%, in freshly boiled and cooled purified water, net price 15 g = £2.17

Excipients include cetostearyl alcohol, edetic acid (EDTA)

Dose apply up to 3 times daily (short-term use)

Graneodin® (Squibb) PoM

Ointment, neomycin sulphate 0.25%, gramicidin 0.025%, net price 25 g = £1.37

Excipients none as listed in section 13.1.3

Dose superficial bacterial infection of skin, apply 2–4 times daily (for max. 7 days—possibly longer for sycosis barbae)

POLYMYXINS

Indications bacterial skin infections

Cautions large areas, see below

Large areas If large areas of skin are being treated nephrotoxicity and neurotoxicity may be a hazard, particularly in children, in the elderly, and in those with renal impairment

Side-effects sensitisation (see also notes above)

Polyfax® (PLIVA) PoM

Ointment, polymyxin B sulphate 10 000 units, bacitracin zinc 500 units/g, net price 4 g = £3.26, 20 g = £4.62

Excipients none as listed in section 13.1.3

Dose apply twice daily or more frequently if required

SILVER SULFADIAZINE
(Silver sulphadiazine)

Indications prophylaxis and treatment of infection in burn wounds; as an adjunct to short-term treatment of infection in leg ulcers and pressure sores; as an adjunct to prophylaxis of infection in skin graft donor sites and extensive abrasions; for conservative management of finger-tip injuries

Cautions hepatic and renal impairment; G6PD deficiency; pregnancy and breast-feeding (avoid in late pregnancy and in neonate—see also Appendix 4); may inactivate enzymatic debriding agents—concomitant use may be inappropriate; for large amounts see also **interactions:** Appendix 1 (sulphonamides)

Large areas Plasma-sulfadiazine concentrations may approach therapeutic levels with *side-effects* and *interactions* as for sulphonamides (see section 5.1.8) if large areas of skin are treated. Owing to the association of sulphonamides with severe blood and skin disorders treatment should be stopped immediately if blood disorders or rashes develop—but leucopenia developing 2–3 days after starting treatment of burns patients is reported usually to be self-limiting and silver sulfadiazine need not usually be discontinued provided blood counts are monitored carefully to ensure return to normality within a few days. Argyria may also occur if large areas of skin are treated (or if application is prolonged).

Contra-indications pregnancy (Appendix 4) and breast-feeding (Appendix 5); sensitivity to sulphonamides; not recommended for neonates (see also Appendix 4)

Side-effects allergic reactions including burning, itching and rashes; argyria reported following prolonged use; leucopenia reported (monitor blood levels)

Flamazine® (S&N Hlth.) PoM

Cream, silver sulfadiazine 1%, net price 20 g = £2.91, 50 g = £3.85, 250 g = £10.32, 500 g = £18.27

Excipients include cetyl alcohol, polysorbates, propylene glycol

Dose burns, apply daily or more frequently if very exudative; leg ulcers or pressure sores, apply daily or on alternate days (not recommended if ulcer very exudative); finger-tip injuries, apply every 2–3 days; consult product literature for details

Note Apply with sterile applicator

13.10.1.2 Antibacterial preparations also used systemically

Sodium fusidate is a narrow-spectrum antibacterial used for staphylococcal infections. For the role of sodium fusidate in the treatment of impetigo see p. 628.

Metronidazole is used topically for acne rosacea and to reduce the odour associated with anaerobic infections; oral metronidazole (section 5.1.11) is used to treat wounds infected with anaerobic bacteria.

Angular cheilitis An ointment containing sodium fusidate is used in the fissures of angular cheilitis when associated with staphylococcal infection. For further information on angular cheilitis, see section 12.3.2.

FUSIDIC ACID

Indications staphylococcal skin infections; penicillin-resistant staphylococcal infections (section 5.1.7); staphylococcal eye infections (section 11.3.1)

Cautions see notes above; avoid contact with eyes

Side-effects rarely hypersensitivity reactions

Dose

- Apply 3–4 times daily

Fucidin® (LEO) PoM

Cream, fusidic acid 2%, net price 15 g = £2.00, 30 g = £3.79

Excipients include butylated hydroxyanisole, cetyl alcohol

Ointment, sodium fusidate 2%, net price 15 g = £2.23, 30 g = £3.79

Excipients include cetyl alcohol, wool fat

Dental prescribing on NHS May be prescribed as Sodium Fusidate ointment

METRONIDAZOLE

Indications see preparations; rosacea (see also section 13.6); *Helicobacter pylori* eradication (section 1.3); anaerobic infections (section 5.1.11 and section 7.2.2); protozoal infections (section 5.4.2)

Cautions avoid exposure to strong sunlight or UV light

Side-effects skin irritation

Dose

- See preparations

Acea® (Ferndale) PoM
Gel, metronidazole 0.75%, net price 40 g = £9.95
Excipients include disodium edetate, hydroxybenzoates (parabens)
Dose acute inflammatory exacerbation of rosacea, apply thinly twice daily for 8 weeks

Anabact® (CHS) PoM
Gel, metronidazole 0.75%, net price 15 g = £4.47, 30 g = £7.89
Excipients include hydroxybenzoates (parabens), propylene glycol
Dose malodorous fungating tumours and malodorous gravitational and decubitus ulcers, apply to clean wound 1–2 times daily and cover with non-adherent dressing

Metrogel® (Galderma) PoM
Gel, metronidazole 0.75%, net price 40 g = £19.90
Excipients include hydroxybenzoates (parabens), propylene glycol
Dose acute inflammatory exacerbations of acne rosacea, apply thinly twice daily for 8–9 weeks
Malodorous fungating tumours, apply to clean wound 1–2 times daily and cover with non-adherent dressing

Metrosa® (Linderma) PoM
Gel, metronidazole 0.75%, net price 40 g = £19.90
Excipients include propylene glycol
Dose acute exacerbation of acne rosacea, apply thinly twice daily for up to 8 weeks

Metrotop® (Medlock) PoM
Gel, metronidazole 0.8%, net price 15 g = £4.59, 30 g = £8.10, 60 g = £14.30
Excipients none as listed in section 13.1.3
Dose malodorous fungating tumours and malodorous gravitational and decubitus ulcers, apply to clean wound 1–2 times daily and cover (flat wounds, apply liberally; cavities, smear on paraffin gauze and pack loosely)

Noritate® (Aventis Pharma) PoM
Cream, metronidazole 1%, net price 30 g = £19.08
Excipients include hydroxybenzoates (parabens)
Dose acne rosacea, apply once daily for 8 weeks

Rozex® (Galderma) PoM
Cream, metronidazole 0.75%, net price 40 g = £15.28
Excipients include benzyl alcohol, isopropyl palmitate

Gel, metronidazole 0.75%, net price 40 g = £15.28
Excipients include disodium edetate, hydroxybenzoates (parabens), propylene glycol
Dose inflammatory papules, pustules and erythema of acne rosacea, apply twice daily for 3–4 months

Zyomet® (Goldshield) PoM
Gel, metronidazole 0.75%, net price 30 g = £12.00
Excipients include benzyl alcohol, disodium edetate, propylene glycol
Dose acute inflammatory exacerbations of acne rosacea, apply thinly twice daily for 8–9 weeks

13.10.2 Antifungal preparations

Most localised fungal infections are treated with topical preparations. To prevent relapse, local antifungal treatment should be continued for 1–2 weeks after the disappearance of all signs of infection. Systemic therapy (section 5.2) is necessary for nail or scalp infection or if the skin infection is widespread, disseminated, or intractable. Skin scrapings should be examined if systemic therapy is being considered or where there is doubt about the diagnosis.

Dermatophytoses Ringworm infection can affect the scalp (tinea capitis), body (tinea corporis), groin (tinea cruris), hand (tinea manuum), foot (tinea pedis, athlete's foot), or nail (tinea unguium). Scalp infection requires systemic treatment (section 5.2); additional topical application of an antifungal may reduce the risk of transmission. Most other local ringworm infections can be treated adequately with topical antifungal preparations (including shampoos, section 13.9). The imidazole antifungals **clotrimazole, econazole, ketoconazole, miconazole**, and **sulconazole** are all effective. **Terbinafine** cream is also effective but it is more expensive. Other topical antifungals include **amorolfine, griseofulvin**, and the **undecenoates. Compound benzoic acid ointment** (Whitfield's ointment) has been used for ringworm infections but it is cosmetically less acceptable than proprietary preparations. Topical preparations for athlete's foot containing **tolnaftate** are on sale to the public.

Antifungal dusting powders are of little therapeutic value in the treatment of fungal skin infections and may cause skin irritation; they may have some role in preventing re-infection.

Tinea infection of the nail is almost always treated systemically (section 5.2); topical application of **amorolfine** or **tioconazole** may be effective for treating early onychomycosis when involvement is limited to mild distal disease in up to 2 nails.

Pityriasis versicolor Pityriasis (tinea) versicolor may be treated with **ketoconazole** shampoo (section 13.9). Alternatively, **selenium sulphide** shampoo [unlicensed indication] (section 13.9) may be used as a lotion (diluted with water to reduce irritation) and left on for at least 30 minutes or overnight; it is applied 2–7 times over a fortnight and the course repeated if necessary.

Topical imidazole antifungals **clotrimazole, econazole, ketoconazole, miconazole**, and **sulconazole** and topical **terbinafine** are alternatives but large quantities may be required.

If topical therapy fails, or if the infection is widespread, pityriasis versicolor is treated systemically with a triazole antifungal (section 5.2). Relapse is common, especially in the immunocompromised.

Candidiasis Candidal skin infections may be treated with topical imidazole antifungals **clotrimazole, econazole, ketoconazole, miconazole**, and **sulconazole**; topical terbinafine is an alternative. Topical application of **nystatin** is also effective for candidiasis but it is ineffective against dermatophytosis. Refractory candidiasis requires systemic treatment (section 5.2) generally with a triazole such as fluconazole; systemic treatment with terbinafine is **not appropriate** for refractory candidiasis.

Angular cheilitis Miconazole cream or nystatin ointment are used in the fissures of angular cheilitis when associated with *Candida*. For further information on angular cheilitis, see p. 593.

Compound topical preparations Combination of an imidazole and a mild corticosteroid (such as hydrocortisone 1%) (section 13.4) may be of value in the treatment of eczematous intertrigo and, in the first few days only, of a severely inflamed patch of ringworm. Combination of a mild corticosteroid with either an imidazole or nystatin may be of use in the treatment of intertrigo associated with candida.

Cautions Contact with eyes and mucous membranes should be avoided.

Side-effects Occasional local irritation and hypersensitivity reactions include mild burning sensation, erythema, and itching. Treatment should be discontinued if these are severe.

AMOROLFINE

Indications see under preparations
Cautions see notes above; also avoid contact with ears; pregnancy and breast-feeding
Side-effects see notes above

Loceryl® (Galderma) PoM
Cream, amorolfine (as hydrochloride) 0.25%, net price 20 g = £4.83. Label: 10, patient information leaflet
Excipients include cetostearyl alcohol, disodium edetate
Dose fungal skin infections, apply once daily after cleansing in the evening for at least 2–3 weeks (up to 6 weeks for foot infection) continuing for 3–5 days after lesions have healed

Nail lacquer, amorolfine (as hydrochloride) 5%, net price 5-mL pack (with nail files, spatulas and cleansing swabs) = £18.71. Label: 10, patient information leaflet
Excipients none as listed in section 13.1.3
Dose fungal nail infections, apply to infected nails 1–2 times weekly after filing and cleansing; allow to dry (approx. 3 minutes); treat finger nails for 6 months, toe nails for 9–12 months (review at intervals of 3 months); avoid nail varnish or artificial nails during treatment
Note Amorolfine nail lacquer can be sold to the public if supplied for the treatment of mild cases of distal and lateral subungual onychomycoses caused by dermatophytes, yeasts and moulds; subject to treatment of max. 2 nails, max. strength of nail lacquer amorolfine 5% and a pack size of 3 mL

BENZOIC ACID

Indications ringworm (tinea), but see notes above

Benzoic Acid Ointment, Compound, BP (Whitfield's ointment)
Ointment, benzoic acid 6%, salicylic acid 3%, in emulsifying ointment
Excipients include cetostearyl alcohol
Dose apply twice daily

CLOTRIMAZOLE

Indications fungal skin infections; vaginal candidiasis (section 7.2.2); otitis externa (section 12.1.1)
Cautions see notes above
Side-effects see notes above
Dose
- Apply 2–3 times daily

Clotrimazole (Non-proprietary)
Cream, clotrimazole 1%, net price 20 g = £2.83

Canesten® (Bayer Consumer Care)
Cream, clotrimazole 1%, net price 20 g = £2.14, 50 g = £3.80
Excipients include benzyl alcohol, cetostearyl alcohol, polysorbate 60

Powder, clotrimazole 1%, net price 30 g = £1.52
Excipients none as listed in section 13.1.3

Solution, clotrimazole 1% in macrogol 400 (polyethylene glycol 400), net price 20 mL = £2.43. For hairy areas
Excipients none as listed in section 13.1.3

Spray, clotrimazole 1%, in 30% isopropyl alcohol, net price 40-mL atomiser = £4.99. Label: 15. For large or hairy areas
Excipients include propylene glycol

ECONAZOLE NITRATE

Indications fungal skin infections; vaginal candidiasis (section 7.2.2)
Cautions see notes above
Side-effects see notes above
Dose
- Skin infections apply twice daily; nail infections, apply once daily under occlusive dressing

Ecostatin® (Squibb)
Cream, econazole nitrate 1%, net price 15 g = £1.49; 30 g = £2.75
Excipients include butylated hydroxyanisole, fragrance

Pevaryl® (Janssen-Cilag)
Cream, econazole nitrate 1%, net price 30 g = £2.65
Excipients include butylated hydroxyanisole, fragrance

GRISEOFULVIN

Indications tinea pedis; resistant fungal infections (section 5.2)
Cautions see notes above
Side-effects see notes above
Dose
- Apply 400 micrograms (1 spray) to an area approx. 13 cm² once daily, increased to 1.2 mg (3 sprays, allowing each spray to dry between applications) once daily if necessary; max. treatment duration 4 weeks

Grisol AF® (Transdermal)
Spray, griseofulvin 400 micrograms/metered spray, net price 20-mL (400-dose) spray = £4.00. Label: 15
Excipients include benzyl alcohol

KETOCONAZOLE

Indications fungal skin infections; systemic or resistant fungal infections (section 5.2); vulval candidiasis (section 7.2.2)
Cautions see notes above; do **not** use within 2 weeks of a topical corticosteroid for seborrhoeic dermatitis—risk of skin sensitisation
Side-effects see notes above
Dose
- Tinea pedis, apply twice daily; other fungal infections, apply 1–2 times daily

Nizoral® (Janssen-Cilag) PoM
[1]Cream, ketoconazole 2%, net price 30 g = £3.54
Excipients include cetyl alcohol, polysorbates, propylene glycol, stearyl alcohol
Note A 15-g tube is available for sale to the public for the treatment of tinea pedis, tinea cruris, and candidal intertrigo

Shampoo—section 13.9

1. NHS except for seborrhoeic dermatitis and pityriasis versicolor and endorsed 'SLS'

13 Skin

MICONAZOLE NITRATE

Indications fungal skin infections; oral and intestinal fungal infections (section 12.3.2); vaginal candidiasis (section 7.2.2)

Cautions see notes above

Side-effects see notes above

Dose

- Apply twice daily continuing for 10 days after lesions have healed; nail infections, apply 1–2 times daily

Miconazole (Non-proprietary)
Cream, miconazole nitrate 2%, net price 20 g = £2.05, 45 g = £1.97
Dental prescribing on NHS Miconazole cream may be prescribed

Daktarin® (Janssen-Cilag)
Cream, miconazole nitrate 2%, net price 30 g = £1.93
Excipients include butylated hydroxyanisole
Note A 15-g tube [NHS] is on sale to the public

Powder [NHS], miconazole nitrate 2%, net price 20 g = £1.81
Excipients include none as listed in section 13.1.3

Dual Action Spray powder, miconazole nitrate 0.16%, in an aerosol basis, net price 100 g = £2.27
Excipients none as listed in section 13.1.3

NYSTATIN

Indications skin infections due to *Candida* spp.; intestinal candidiasis (section 5.2); vaginal candidiasis (section 7.2.2); oral fungal infections (section 12.3.2)

Cautions see notes above

Side-effects see notes above

Nystaform® (Typharm) [PoM]
Cream, nystatin 100 000 units/g, chlorhexidine hydrochloride 1%, net price 30 g = £2.62
Excipients include benzyl alcohol, cetostearyl alcohol, polysorbate 60
Dose apply 2–3 times daily continuing for 7 days after lesions have healed.

Nystan® (Squibb) [PoM]
Cream, nystatin 100 000 units/g, net price 30 g = £2.03
Excipients include benzyl alcohol, propylene glycol, fragrance
Dose apply 2–4 times daily

Ointment, nystatin 100 000 units/g, in *Plastibase®*, net price 30 g = £1.63
Excipients none as listed in section 13.1.3
Dose apply 2–4 times daily
Dental prescribing on NHS May be prescribed as Nystatin Ointment

Tinaderm-M® (Schering-Plough) [PoM]
Cream, nystatin 100 000 units/g, tolnaftate 1%, net price 20 g = £1.83
Excipients include butylated hydroxytoluene, cetostearyl alcohol, hydroxybenzoates (parabens), fragrance
Dose apply 2–3 times daily

SALICYLIC ACID

Indications fungal nail infections, particularly tinea; hyperkeratotic skin disorders (section 13.5.2); acne vulgaris (section 13.6.1); warts and calluses (section 13.7)

Cautions avoid broken or inflamed skin

Salicylate toxicity Salicylate toxicity can occur particularly if applied on large areas of skin

Contra-indications pregnancy

Side-effects see notes above

Dose

- ADULT and CHILD over 5 years, apply twice daily and after washing

Phytex® (Wynlit)
Paint, salicylic acid 1.46% (total combined), tannic acid 4.89% and boric acid 3.12% (as borotannic complex), in a vehicle containing alcohol and ethyl acetate, net price 25 mL (with brush) = £1.56
Excipients none as listed in section 13.1.3
Note Flammable

SULCONAZOLE NITRATE

Indications fungal skin infections

Cautions see notes above

Side-effects see notes above; also blistering

Dose

- Apply 1–2 times daily continuing for 2–3 weeks after lesions have healed

Exelderm® (Centrapharm)
Cream, sulconazole nitrate 1%, net price 30 g = £3.90
Excipients include cetyl alcohol, polysorbates, propylene glycol, stearyl alcohol

TERBINAFINE

Indications fungal skin infections

Cautions pregnancy, breast-feeding; avoid contact with eyes

Side-effects see notes above

Lamisil® (Novartis Consumer Health) [PoM]
Cream, terbinafine hydrochloride 1%, net price 15 g = £4.86, 30 g = £8.76
Excipients include benzyl alcohol, cetyl alcohol, polysorbate 60, stearyl alcohol
Dose apply thinly 1–2 times daily for up to 1 week in tinea pedis, 1–2 weeks in tinea corporis and tinea cruris, 2 weeks in cutaneous candidiasis and pityriasis versicolor; review after 2 weeks; CHILD see *BNF for Children*
Note Preparations of terbinafine hydrochloride (max. 1%) can be sold to the public for external use for the treatment of tinea pedis as a cutaneous solution in a pack containing max. 15 g, *or* for the treatment of tinea pedis and cruris as a cream in a pack containing max. 15 g, *or* for the treatment of tinea pedis, cruris, and corporis as a spray in a pack containing max. 30 mL spray or as a gel in a pack containing max. 30 g gel

Tablets—section 5.2

TIOCONAZOLE

Indications fungal nail infections

Cautions see notes above

Contra-indications pregnancy

Side-effects see notes above; also local oedema, dry skin, nail discoloration, periungual inflammation, nail pain, rash, exfoliation

Dose

- Apply to nails and surrounding skin twice daily usually for up to 6 months (may be extended to 12 months)

Trosyl® (Pfizer) [PoM]
Cutaneous solution, tioconazole 28%, net price 12 mL (with applicator brush) = £27.38
Excipients none as listed in section 13.1.3

UNDECENOATES

Indications see under preparations below

Side-effects see notes above

Dose

- See under preparations below

Monphytol® (LAB)
Paint, methyl undecenoate 5%, propyl undecenoate 0.7%, salicylic acid 3%, methyl salicylate 25%, propyl salicylate 5%, chlorobutanol 3%, net price 18 mL (with brush) = £1.95
Excipients none as listed in section 13.1.3
Dose fungal skin and nail infections, apply twice daily

Mycota® (Thornton & Ross)
Cream, zinc undecenoate 20%, undecenoic acid 5%, net price 25 g = £1.37
Excipients include fragrance
Dose treatment of athlete's foot, apply twice daily continuing for 7 days after lesions have healed
Prevention of athlete's foot, apply once daily

Powder, zinc undecenoate 20%, undecenoic acid 2%, net price 70 g = £1.93
Excipients include fragrance
Dose treatment of athlete's foot, apply twice daily continuing for 7 days after lesions have healed
Prevention of athlete's foot, apply once daily

Spray application, undecenoic acid 3.9%, dichlorophen 0.4% (pressurised aerosol pack), net price 100 mL = £2.19
Excipients include fragrance
Dose treatment of athlete's foot, apply twice daily continuing for 7 days after lesions have healed
Prevention of athlete's foot, apply once daily

13.10.3 Antiviral preparations

Aciclovir cream is licensed for the treatment of initial and recurrent labial and genital *herpes simplex infections*; treatment should begin as early as possible. Systemic treatment is necessary for buccal or vaginal infections and for *herpes zoster (shingles)* (for details of systemic use see section 5.3.2.1).

Idoxuridine solution (5% in dimethyl sulfoxide) is of little value.

Herpes labialis Aciclovir cream can be used for the treatment of initial and recurrent labial herpes simplex infections (cold sores). It is best applied at the earliest possible stage, usually when prodromal changes of sensation are felt in the lip and before vesicles appear.

Penciclovir cream is also licensed for the treatment of herpes labialis; it needs to be applied more frequently than aciclovir cream. These creams should not be used in the mouth.

Systemic treatment is necessary if cold sores recur frequently or for infections in the mouth (see p. 335).

ACICLOVIR
(Acyclovir)

Indications see notes above; herpes simplex and varicella–zoster infections (section 5.3.2.1); eye infections (section 11.3.3)
Cautions avoid contact with eyes and mucous membranes
Side-effects transient stinging or burning; occasionally erythema, itching or drying of the skin
Dose
- Apply to lesions every 4 hours (5 times daily) for 5–10 days, starting at first sign of attack

[1]**Aciclovir** (Non-proprietary) PoM
Cream, aciclovir 5%, net price 2 g = £1.09, 10 g = £1.49
Excipients include propylene glycol
Brands include *Zuvogen®* (*excipients* also include cetyl alcohol, propylene glycol)
Dental prescribing on NHS Aciclovir Cream may be prescribed

1. A 2-g tube and a pump pack are on sale to the public for the treatment of cold sores

Zovirax® (GSK) PoM
Cream, aciclovir 5%, net price 2 g = £3.98, 10 g = £14.82
Excipients include cetostearyl alcohol, propylene glycol

Eye ointment—section 11.3.3

Tablets—section 5.3.2.1

PENCICLOVIR

Indications see notes above
Cautions avoid contact with eyes and mucous membranes
Side-effects transient stinging, burning, numbness

Vectavir® (Novartis Consumer Health) PoM
Cream, penciclovir 1%, net price 2 g = £4.20
Excipients include cetostearyl alcohol, propylene glycol
Dose herpes labialis, apply to lesions every 2 hours during waking hours for 4 days starting at first sign of attack; CHILD under 12 years, not recommended
Dental prescribing on NHS May be prescribed as Penciclovir Cream

IDOXURIDINE IN DIMETHYL SULFOXIDE

Indications herpes simplex and herpes zoster infection but of little value
Cautions avoid contact with the eyes, mucous membranes, and textiles; breast-feeding (Appendix 5)
Contra-indications pregnancy (Appendix 4); **not** to be used in mouth
Side-effects stinging on application, changes in taste; overuse may cause maceration

Herpid® (Astellas) PoM
Application, idoxuridine 5% in dimethyl sulfoxide, net price 5 mL (with applicator) = £6.33
Dose apply to lesions 4 times daily for 4 days, starting at first sign of attack; CHILD under 12 years, not recommended

13.10.4 Parasiticidal preparations

Suitable quantities of parasiticidal preparations

	Skin creams	Lotions	Cream rinses
Scalp (head lice)	—	50–100 mL	50–100 mL
Body (scabies)	30–60 g	100 mL	—
Body (crab lice)	30–60 g	100 mL	—

These amounts are usually suitable for an adult for single application.

Scabies

Permethrin is effective for the treatment of *scabies* (*Sarcoptes scabiei*); **malathion** can be used if permethrin is inappropriate.

Aqueous preparations are preferable to alcoholic lotions, which are not recommended owing to irritation of excoriated skin and the genitalia.

Older preparations include **benzyl benzoate,** which is an irritant and should be avoided in children; it is less effective than malathion and permethrin.

Ivermectin (available on a named patient basis from specialist importing companies, see p. 888) in a single dose of 200 micrograms/kg by mouth has been used, in combination with topical drugs, for the treatment of hyperkeratotic (crusted or 'Norwegian') scabies that does not respond to topical treatment alone.

Application Although acaricides have traditionally been applied after a hot bath, this is **not** necessary and there is even evidence that a hot bath may increase absorption into the blood, removing them from their site of action on the skin.

All members of the affected household should be treated simultaneously. Treatment should be applied to the whole body including the scalp, neck, face, and ears. Particular attention should be paid to the webs of the fingers and toes and lotion brushed under the ends of nails. It is now recommended that malathion and permethrin should be applied twice, one week apart; in the case of benzyl benzoate up to 3 applications on consecutive days may be needed. It is important to warn users to reapply treatment to the hands if they are washed. Patients with hyperkeratotic scabies may require 2 or 3 applications of acaricide on consecutive days to ensure that enough penetrates the skin crusts to kill all the mites.

Itching The *itch* and *eczema* of scabies persists for some weeks after the infestation has been eliminated and treatment for pruritus and eczema (section 13.5.1) may be required. Application of **crotamiton** can be used to control itching after treatment with more effective acaricides. A topical corticosteroid may help to reduce itch and inflammation after scabies has been treated successfully; however, persistent symptoms suggest that scabies eradication was not successful. Oral administration of a **sedating antihistamine** (section 3.4.1) at night may also be useful.

Head lice

Carbaryl, **malathion**, and the **pyrethroids** (permethrin and phenothrin) are effective against head lice (*Pediculus humanus capitis*) but lice in some districts have developed resistance; resistance to two or more parasiticidal preparations has also been reported. Careful application of **dimeticone,** which acts on the surface of head lice, is also effective. Benzyl benzoate is licensed for the treatment of head lice but it is less effective than other drugs.

Head lice infestation (pediculosis) should be treated using lotion or liquid formulations. Shampoos are diluted too much in use to be effective. Alcoholic formulations are effective but aqueous formulations are preferred in severe eczema, for patients with asthma, and small children. A contact time of 12 hours or overnight treatment is recommended for lotions and liquids; a 2-hour treatment is not sufficient to kill eggs.

In general, a course of treatment for head lice should be 2 applications of product 7 days apart to prevent lice emerging from any eggs that survive the first application.

The policy of rotating insecticides on a district-wide basis is now considered outmoded. To overcome the development of resistance, a mosaic strategy is required whereby, if a course of treatment fails to cure, a different insecticide is used for the next course. If a course of treatment with either permethrin or phenothrin fails, then a non-pyrethroid parasiticidal product should be used for the next course.

Wet combing methods Head lice may be mechanically removed by combing wet hair meticulously with a plastic detection comb (probably for at least 30 minutes each time) over the whole scalp at 4-day intervals for a minimum of 2 weeks; hair conditioner or vegetable oil may be used to facilitate the process. Several products are available and some are prescribable on the NHS.

Crab lice

Carbaryl [unlicensed for crab lice], **permethrin, phenothrin**, and **malathion** are effective for *crab lice* (*Pthirus pubis*). An aqueous preparation should be applied, allowed to dry naturally and washed off after 12 hours; a second treatment is needed after 7 days to kill lice emerging from surviving eggs. All surfaces of the body should be treated, including the scalp, neck, ears, and face (paying particular attention to the eyebrows and any beard). A different insecticide should be used if a course of treatment fails. Alcoholic lotions are not recommended (owing to irritation of excoriated skin and the genitalia).

Benzyl benzoate

Benzyl benzoate is effective for *scabies* but is not a first-choice for *scabies* (see notes above).

BENZYL BENZOATE

Indications scabies (but see notes above)

Cautions children (not recommended, see also under Dose, below), avoid contact with eyes and mucous membranes; do not use on broken or secondarily infected skin; breast-feeding (suspend feeding until product has been washed off)

Side-effects skin irritation, burning sensation especially on genitalia and excoriations, occasionally rashes

Dose

- Apply over the whole body; repeat without bathing on the following day and wash off 24 hours later; a third application may be required in some cases

  Note Not recommended for children—dilution to reduce irritant effect also reduces efficacy. Some manufacturers recommend application to the body but to exclude the head and neck. However, application should be extended to the scalp, neck, face, and ears

Benzyl Benzoate Application, BP (Non-proprietary)

Application, benzyl benzoate 25% in an emulsion basis, net price 500 mL = £2.50

Brands include *Ascabiol®* (*excipients: include* triethanolamine)

Carbaryl

Carbaryl is recommended for *head lice*; an aqueous preparation is recommended for *crab lice* (see notes above) but a suitable product is not currently licensed for this indication. In the light of experimental data in *animals* it would be prudent to consider carbaryl as a potential human carcinogen and it has been restricted to prescription only use. The Department of Health has emphasised that the risk is a theoretical one and that any risk from the intermittent use of head lice preparations is likely to be exceedingly small.

CARBARYL
(Carbaril)

Indications see notes above and under preparations
Cautions avoid contact with eyes; do not use on broken or secondarily infected skin; do not use more than once a week for 3 consecutive weeks; children under 6 months, medical supervision required; alcoholic lotion **not** recommended for pediculosis in asthma, in severe eczema or in small children
Side-effects skin irritation
Dose
- Head lice, rub into dry hair and scalp, allow to dry naturally, shampoo after 12 hours, and comb wet hair (see also notes above); repeat application after 7 days [unlicensed use]
- Crab lice [unlicensed indication], apply aqueous solution over whole body (see notes above), allow to dry naturally and wash off after 12 hours or overnight; repeat application after 7 days

Carylderm® (SSL) PoM
Liquid, carbaryl 1% in an aqueous basis, net price 50 mL = £2.28
Excipients include cetostearyl alcohol, hydroxybenzoates (parabens)

Dimeticone

Dimeticone coats head lice and interferes with water balance in lice by preventing the excretion of water; it is less active against eggs and treatment should be repeated after 7 days.

DIMETICONE

Indications head lice
Cautions avoid contact with eyes; children under 6 months, medical supervision required
Side-effects skin irritation
Dose
- Rub into dry hair and scalp, allow to dry naturally, shampoo after minimum 8 hours (or overnight); repeat application after 7 days

Hedrin® (Thornton & Ross)
Lotion, dimeticone 4%, net price 50 mL = £2.98, 150 mL = £6.83

Malathion

Malathion is recommended for *scabies, head lice* and *crab lice* (for details see notes above).

The risk of systemic effects associated with 1–2 applications of malathion is considered to be very low; however, applications of lotion repeated at intervals of less than 1 week *or* application for more than 3 consecutive weeks should be **avoided** since the likelihood of eradication of lice is not increased.

MALATHION

Indications see notes above and under preparations
Cautions avoid contact with eyes; do not use on broken or secondarily infected skin; do not use lotion more than once a week for 3 consecutive weeks; children under 6 months, medical supervision required; alcoholic lotions **not** recommended for head lice in severe eczema, asthma or in small children, or for scabies or crab lice
Side-effects skin irritation
Dose
- Head lice, rub 0.5% preparation into dry hair and scalp, allow to dry naturally, remove by washing after 12 hours (see also notes above); repeat application after 7 days
- Crab lice, apply 0.5% aqueous preparation over whole body, allow to dry naturally, wash off after 12 hours or overnight; repeat application after 7 days
- Scabies, apply 0.5% preparation over whole body, and wash off after 24 hours; if hands are washed with soap within 24 hours, they should be retreated; see also notes above; repeat application after 7 days

Note For scabies, manufacturer recommends application to the body but not necessarily to the head and neck. However, application should be extended to the scalp, neck, face, and ears

Derbac-M® (SSL)
Liquid, malathion 0.5% in an aqueous basis, net price 50 mL = £2.27, 200 mL = £5.70
Excipients include cetostearyl alcohol, fragrance, hydroxybenzoates (parabens)
For crab lice, head lice, and scabies

Prioderm® (SSL)
Lotion, malathion 0.5%, in an alcoholic basis, net price 50 mL = £2.22, 200 mL = £5.70. Label: 15
Excipients include fragrance
For head lice (alcoholic formulation, see notes above)

Cream shampoo NHS, malathion 1%, net price 40 g = £2.77
Excipients include cetostearyl alcohol, fragrance, hydroxybenzoates (parabens), sodium edetate, wool fat
Dose head and crab lice, not recommended, therefore no dose stated (product too diluted in use and insufficient contact time)

Quellada M® (GSK Consumer Healthcare)
Liquid, malathion 0.5% in an aqueous basis, net price 50 mL = £1.85, 200 mL = £4.62
Excipients include cetostearyl alcohol, fragrance, hydroxybenzoates (parabens)
For crab lice, head lice, and scabies

Cream shampoo, malathion 1%, net price 40 g = £2.18
Excipients include cetostearyl alcohol, fragrance, hydroxybenzoates (parabens), sodium edetate, wool fat
Dose head and crab lice, not recommended, therefore no dose stated (product too diluted in use and insufficient contact time)

Permethrin

Permethrin is effective for *scabies* and *crab lice* (for details see notes above). Permethrin is active against *head lice* but the formulation and licensed methods of application of the current products make them unsuitable for the treatment of head lice.

PERMETHRIN

Indications see notes above and under Dose

Cautions avoid contact with eyes; do not use on broken or secondarily infected skin; children under 6 months, medical supervision required for cream rinse (head lice); children aged 2 months–2 years, medical supervision required for dermal cream (scabies)

Side-effects pruritus, erythema, and stinging; rarely rashes and oedema

Dose

- Scabies, apply 5% preparation over whole body and wash off after 8–12 hours; CHILD (see also Cautions, above) apply over whole body including face, neck, scalp and ears; if hands washed with soap within 8 hours of application, they should be treated again with cream (see notes above); repeat application after 7 days

  Note Manufacturer recommends application to the body but to exclude head and neck. However, application should be extended to the scalp, neck, face, and ears

  Larger patients may require up to two 30-g packs for adequate treatment

- Crab lice, ADULT over 18 years, apply 5% cream over whole body, allow to dry naturally and wash off after 12 hours or after leaving on overnight; repeat application after 7 days

Permethrin (Non-proprietary)
Cream, permethrin 5%, net price 30 g = £5.52

Lyclear® Creme Rinse (Chefaro UK)
Cream rinse, permethrin 1% in basis containing isopropyl alcohol 20%, net price 59 mL = £2.38, 2 × 59-mL pack = £4.32
Excipients include cetyl alcohol
Dose head lice, not recommended, therefore no dose stated (insufficient contact time)

Lyclear® Dermal Cream (Chefaro UK)
Dermal cream, permethrin 5%, net price 30 g = £5.71. Label: 10, patient information leaflet
Excipients include butylated hydroxytoluene, wool fat derivative

Phenothrin

Phenothrin is recommended for *head lice* and *crab lice* (for details see notes above).

PHENOTHRIN

Indications see notes above and under preparations

Cautions avoid contact with eyes; do not use on broken or secondarily infected skin; do not use more than once a week for 3 weeks at a time; children under 6 months, medical supervision required; alcoholic preparations **not** recommended for head lice in severe eczema, in asthma, in small children, or for crab lice (see notes above)

Side-effects skin irritation

Dose

- See under preparations

Full Marks® (SSL)
Liquid, phenothrin 0.5% in an aqueous basis, net price 50 mL = £2.22, 200 mL = £5.70
Excipients include cetostearyl alcohol, fragrance, hydroxybenzoates (parabens)
Dose head lice, apply to dry hair, allow to dry naturally; shampoo after 12 hours or next day, comb wet hair; repeat application after 7 days [unlicensed use]

Lotion, phenothrin 0.2% in basis containing isopropyl alcohol 69.3%, net price 50 mL = £2.22, 200 mL = £5.70. Label: 15
Excipients include fragrance
Dose crab lice and head lice (alcoholic formulation, see notes above), apply to dry hair, allow to dry naturally; shampoo after 12 hours [unlicensed contact duration], comb wet hair; repeat application after 7 days [unlicensed use]

Mousse (= foam application), phenothrin 0.5% in an alcoholic basis, net price 50 g = £2.53, 150 g = £6.11. Label: 15
Excipients include cetostearyl alcohol
Dose head lice (alcoholic formulation, see notes above), apply to dry hair, shampoo after 30 minutes, comb wet hair—but product not recommended because contact time insufficient (longer contact time not recommended because of risk of irritation)

13.10.5 Preparations for minor cuts and abrasions

Some of the preparations listed are used in minor burns, and abrasions. They are applied as necessary but should not be used on large wounds or for prolonged periods because of the possibility of hypersensitivity. The effervescent effect of hydrogen peroxide (section 13.11.6) is used to clean minor cuts and abrasions. Preparations containing camphor and sulphonamides should be **avoided**. Preparations such as magnesium sulphate paste are also listed but are now rarely used to treat carbuncles and boils as these are best treated with antibiotics (section 5.1.1.2).

Cetrimide Cream, BP
Cream, cetrimide 0.5% in a suitable water-miscible basis such as cetostearyl alcohol 5%, liquid paraffin 50% in freshly boiled and cooled purified water, net price 50 g = £1.11

Proflavine Cream, BPC
Cream, proflavine hemisulphate 0.1%, yellow beeswax 2.5%, chlorocresol 0.1%, liquid paraffin 67.3%, freshly boiled and cooled purified water 25%, wool fat 5%, net price 100 mL = 95p
Excipients include beeswax, wool fat
Note Stains clothing

Preparations for boils

Magnesium Sulphate Paste, BP
Paste, dried magnesium sulphate 45 g, glycerol 55 g, phenol 500 mg, net price 25 g = 63p, 50 g = 77p
Note Should be stirred before use
Dose apply under dressing

Collodion

Flexible collodion may be used to seal minor cuts and wounds that have partially healed.

Collodion, Flexible, BP
Collodion, castor oil 2.5%, colophony 2.5% in a collodion basis, prepared by dissolving pyroxylin (10%) in a mixture of 3 volumes of ether and 1 volume of alcohol (90%), net price 10 mL = 25p. Label: 15
Contra-indications allergy to colophony in elastic adhesive plasters and tape

13 Skin

Skin tissue adhesive

Tissue adhesives are used for closure of minor skin wounds and for additional suture support. They should be applied by an appropriately trained healthcare professional. Skin tissue adhesives may cause skin sensitisation.

Dermabond ProPen® (Ethicon)
Topical Skin Adhesive, sterile, octyl 2-cyanoacrylate, net price 0.5 mL = £18.38

Epiglu® (Schuco)
Tissue adhesive, sterile, ethyl-2-cyanoacrylate 954.5 mg/g, polymethylmethacrylate, net price 4 × 3-g vials = £149.50 (with dispensing pipettes and pallete)

Indermil® (Tyco)
Tissue adhesive, sterile, enbucrilate, net price 5 × 500-mg units = £32.50, 20 × 500-mg units = £130.00

Histoacryl® (Braun)
Tissue adhesive, sterile, enbucrilate, net price 5 × 200-mg unit (blue) = £32.00, 10 × 200-mg unit (blue) = £67.20, 5 × 500-mg unit (clear or blue) = £34.65, 10 × 500-mg unit (blue) = £69.30

LiquiBand® (MedLogic)
Tissue adhesive, sterile, enbucrilate, net price 0.5-g amp = £5.50

13.11 Skin cleansers and antiseptics

13.11.1 Alcohols and saline
13.11.2 Chlorhexidine salts
13.11.3 Cationic surfactants and soaps
13.11.4 Iodine
13.11.5 Phenolics
13.11.6 Oxidisers and dyes
13.11.7 Preparations for promotion of wound healing

Soap or detergent is used with water to cleanse intact skin; emollient preparations such as aqueous cream or emulsifying ointment (section 13.2.1) that do not irritate the skin are best used for cleansing dry skin.

An antiseptic is used for skin that is infected or that is susceptible to recurrent infection. Detergent preparations containing **chlorhexidine**, **triclosan**, or **povidone–iodine**, which should be thoroughly rinsed off, are used. Emollients may also contain antiseptics (section 13.2.1).

Antiseptics such as **chlorhexidine** or **povidone–iodine** are used on intact skin before surgical procedures; their antiseptic effect is enhanced by an alcoholic solvent. **Cetrimide** solution may be used if a detergent effect is also required.

For irrigating ulcers or wounds, lukewarm sterile sodium chloride 0.9% solution is used but tap water is often appropriate.

Potassium permanganate solution 1 in 10 000, a mild antiseptic with astringent properties, can be used for exudative eczematous areas; treatment should be stopped when the skin becomes dry. It can stain skin and nails especially with prolonged use.

13.11.1 Alcohols and saline

ALCOHOL

Indications skin preparation before injection

Cautions flammable; avoid broken skin; patients have suffered severe burns when diathermy has been preceded by application of alcoholic skin disinfectants

Industrial Methylated Spirit, BP
Solution, 19 volumes of ethanol and 1 volume approved wood naphtha, net price '66 OP' (containing 95% by volume alcohol) 100 mL = 39p; '74 OP' (containing 99% by volume alcohol) 100 mL = 39p. Label: 15

Surgical Spirit, BP
Spirit, methyl salicylate 0.5 mL, diethyl phthalate 2%, castor oil 2.5%, in industrial methylated spirit, net price 100 mL = 20p. Label: 15

SODIUM CHLORIDE

Indications see notes above; nebuliser diluent (section 3.1.5); sodium depletion (section 9.2.1.2); electrolyte imbalance (section 9.2.2.1); eye (section 11.8.1); oral hygiene (section 12.3.4)

Sodium Chloride (Non-proprietary)
Solution (sterile), sodium chloride 0.9%, net price 25 × 20-mL unit = £5.50, 200-mL can = £2.65, 1 litre = 95p

Flowfusor® (Fresenius Kabi)
Solution (sterile), sodium chloride 0.9%, net price 120-mL Bellows Pack = £1.50

Irriclens® (ConvaTec)
Solution in aerosol can (sterile), sodium chloride 0.9%, net price 240-mL can = £3.18

Irripod® (C D Medical)
Solution (sterile), sodium chloride 0.9%, net price 25 × 20-mL sachet = £5.50

Miniversol® (Aguettant)
Solution (sterile), sodium chloride 0.9%, net price 30 × 45-mL unit = £13.20; 30 × 100-mL unit = £19.50

Normasol® (Medlock)
Solution (sterile), sodium chloride 0.9%, net price 25 × 25-mL sachet = £5.86; 10 × 100-mL sachet = £7.13

Stericlens® (C D Medical)
Solution in aerosol can (sterile), sodium chloride 0.9%, net price 100-mL can = £1.94, 240-mL can = £2.95

Steripod® Sodium Chloride (Medlock)
Solution (sterile), sodium chloride 0.9%, net price 25 × 20-mL sachet = £7.08

13.11.2 Chlorhexidine salts

CHLORHEXIDINE

Indications see under preparations; bladder irrigation and catheter patency solutions (see section 7.4.4)

Cautions avoid contact with eyes, brain, meninges and middle ear; not for use in body cavities; alcoholic solutions not suitable before diathermy
Side-effects occasional sensitivity

Chlorhexidine 0.05% (Baxter)
2000 Solution (sterile), pink, chlorhexidine acetate 0.05%, net price 500 mL = 72p, 1000 mL = 77p
For cleansing and disinfecting wounds and burns

Cepton® (LPC)
Skin wash (= solution), red, chlorhexidine gluconate 1%, net price 150 mL = £2.48
For use as skin wash in acne
Lotion, blue, chlorhexidine gluconate 0.1%, net price 150 mL = £2.48
For skin disinfection in acne

ChloraPrep® (Enturia)
Cutaneous solution, sterile, chlorhexidine gluconate 2% in isopropyl alcohol 70%, net price (single applicator) 0.67 mL = 30p, 1.5 mL = 55p, 3 mL = 85p, 10.5 mL = £2.92, 6 mL = £6.50
For skin disinfection before invasive procedures; CHILD under 2 months, not recommended
Note Flammable

CX Antiseptic Dusting Powder® (Adams Hlth.)
Dusting powder, sterile, chlorhexidine acetate 1%, net price 15 g = £2.68
For skin disinfection

Hibiscrub® (Regent Medical)
Cleansing solution, red, chlorhexidine gluconate 4%, perfumed, in a surfactant solution, net price 250 mL = £4.25, 500 mL = £5.25, 5 litres = £16.20
Excipients include fragrance
Use instead of soap for pre-operative hand and skin preparation and for general hand and skin disinfection

Hibisol® (Regent Medical)
Solution, chlorhexidine gluconate 0.5%, in isopropyl alcohol 70% with emollients, net price 500 mL = £5.25
To be used undiluted for hand and skin disinfection

Hibitane Obstetric® (Centrapharm)
Cream, chlorhexidine gluconate solution 5% (≡ 1% chlorhexidine gluconate), in a pourable water-miscible basis, net price 250 mL = £3.46
For use in obstetrics and gynaecology as an antiseptic and lubricant (for application to skin around vulva and perineum and to hands of midwife or doctor)

Hydrex® (Adams Hlth.)
Solution, chlorhexidine gluconate solution 2.5% (≡ chlorhexidine gluconate 0.5%), in an alcoholic solution, net price 600 mL (clear) = £2.06; 600 mL (pink) = £2.06, 200-mL spray = £1.77, 500-mL spray = £3.01; 600 mL (blue) = £2.26
For pre-operative skin disinfection
Note Flammable
Surgical scrub, chlorhexidine gluconate 4% in a surfactant solution, net price 250 mL = £1.93, 500 mL = £2.05
For pre-operative hand and skin preparation and for general hand disinfection

Unisept® (Medlock)
Solution (sterile), pink, chlorhexidine gluconate 0.05%, net price 25 × 25-mL sachet = £5.40; 10 × 100-mL sachet = £6.67
For cleansing and disinfecting wounds and burns and swabbing in obstetrics

◢With cetrimide

Tisept® (Medlock)
Solution (sterile), yellow, chlorhexidine gluconate 0.015%, cetrimide 0.15%, net price 25 × 25-mL sachet = £5.20; 10 × 100-mL sachet = £6.68
To be used undiluted for general skin disinfection and wound cleansing

Travasept 100® (Baxter)
Solution (sterile), yellow, chlorhexidine acetate 0.015%, cetrimide 0.15%, net price 500 mL = 72p, 1 litre = 77p
To be used undiluted in skin disinfection such as wound cleansing and obstetrics

◢Concentrates

Hibitane 5% Concentrate® (Regent Medical)
Solution, red, chlorhexidine gluconate 5%, in a perfumed aqueous solution, net price 5 litres = £14.50
Dose to be used diluted 1 in 10 (0.5%) with alcohol 70% for pre-operative skin preparation, or 1 in 100 (0.05%) with water for general skin disinfection
Note Alcoholic solutions not suitable before diathermy (see Alcohol, p. 637)

13.11.3 Cationic surfactants and soaps

CETRIMIDE

Indications skin disinfection
Cautions avoid contact with eyes; avoid use in body cavities
Side-effects skin irritation and occasionally sensitisation

◢Preparations
Ingredient of *Tisept®* and *Travasept® 100*, see above

13.11.4 Iodine

POVIDONE–IODINE

Indications skin disinfection
Cautions pregnancy (Appendix 4), breast-feeding (Appendix 5); broken skin (see below); renal impairment (Appendix 3)
Large open wounds The application of povidone–iodine to large wounds or severe burns may produce systemic adverse effects such as metabolic acidosis, hypernatraemia and impairment of renal function.
Contra-indications preterm neonate gestational age under 32 weeks; avoid regular use in patients with thyroid disorders or those receiving lithium therapy
Side-effects rarely sensitivity; may interfere with thyroid function tests

Betadine® (Mölnlycke)
Dry powder spray, povidone–iodine 2.5% in a pressurised aerosol unit, net price 150-g unit = £2.63
For skin disinfection, particularly minor wounds and infections; CHILD under 2 years not recommended
Note Not for use in serous cavities

13 Skin

Ointment, povidone–iodine 10%, in a water-miscible basis, net price 20 g = £1.33, 80 g = £2.66
Excipients none as listed in section 13.1.3
For skin disinfection, particularly minor wounds and infections; CHILD under 2 years not recommended

Savlon® Dry Antiseptic (Novartis Consumer Health)
Powder spray, povidone–iodine 1.14% in a pressurised aerosol unit, net price 50-mL unit = £2.39
For minor wounds

Videne® (Adams Hlth.)
Alcoholic tincture, povidone–iodine 10%, net price 500 mL = £2.50
To be applied undiluted in pre-operative skin disinfection

Antiseptic solution, povidone–iodine 10% in aqueous solution, net price 500 mL = £2.50
To be applied undiluted in pre-operative skin disinfection and general antisepsis

Surgical scrub, povidone–iodine 7.5% in aqueous solution, net price 500 mL = £2.50
To be used as a pre-operative scrub for hand and skin disinfection

13.11.5 Phenolics

TRICLOSAN

Indications skin disinfection
Cautions avoid contact with eyes

Aquasept® (Medlock)
Skin cleanser, blue, triclosan 2%, net price 250 mL = £1.08, 500 mL = £1.67
Excipients include chlorocresol, propylene glycol, fragrance, tetrasodium edetate
For disinfection and pre-operative hand preparation

Manusept® (Medlock)
Antibacterial hand rub, triclosan 0.5%, isopropyl alcohol 70%, net price 250 mL = £1.04
Excipients none as listed in section 13.1.3
For disinfection and pre-operative hand preparation
Note Flammable

Ster-Zac Bath Concentrate® (Medlock)
Solution, triclosan 2%, net price 28.5 mL = 40p, 500 mL = £2.24
Dose for prevention of cross-infection use 28.5 mL/bath
Excipients include trisodium edetate

13.11.6 Oxidisers and dyes

HYDROGEN PEROXIDE

Indications see under preparations below
Cautions large or deep wounds; avoid on healthy skin and eyes; bleaches fabric; incompatible with products containing iodine or potassium permanganate

Hydrogen Peroxide Solution, BP
Solution 6% (20 vols), net price 200 mL = £1.18
Solution 3% (10 vols), net price 200 mL = 39p
For skin disinfection, particularly cleansing and deodorising wounds and ulcers
Note The BP directs that when hydrogen peroxide is prescribed, hydrogen peroxide solution 6% (20 vols) should be dispensed.
Important Strong solutions of hydrogen peroxide which contain 27% (90 vols) and 30% (100 vols) are only for the preparation of weaker solutions

Crystacide® (GP Pharma)
Cream, hydrogen peroxide 1%, net price 10 g = £4.82, 25 g = £8.07, 40 g = £11.62
Dose superficial bacterial skin infection, apply 2-3 times daily for up to 3 weeks
Excipients include edetic acid (EDTA), propylene glycol

POTASSIUM PERMANGANATE

Indications cleansing and deodorising suppurating eczematous reactions and wounds
Cautions irritant to mucous membranes
Dose
- Wet dressings or baths, approx. 0.01% solution
Note Stains skin and clothing

Potassium Permanganate Solution
Solution, potassium permanganate 0.1% (1 in 1000) in water
Dose to be diluted 1 in 10 to provide a 0.01% (1 in 10 000) solution

Permitabs® (Alliance)
Solution tablets, for preparation of topical solution, potassium permanganate 400 mg, net price 30-tab pack = £6.22
Note 1 tablet dissolved in 4 litres of water provides a 0.01% (1 in 10 000) solution

13.11.7 Preparations for promotion of wound healing

Desloughing agents

Alginate, hydrogel and hydrocolloid dressings (Appendix 8) are effective at wound debridement. Sterile larvae (maggots) (*LarvE®*, Zoobiotic) are also used for managing sloughing wounds and are prescribable on the NHS.

Desloughing solutions and creams are of little clinical value. Substances applied to an open area are easily absorbed and perilesional skin is easily sensitised; gravitational dermatitis may be complicated by superimposed contact sensitivity to substances such as neomycin or lanolin.

For further information on wound management products see Appendix 8, p. 850.

Growth factor

A topical preparation of **becaplermin** (recombinant human platelet-derived growth factor) is licensed as an adjunct treatment of full-thickness, neuropathic, diabetic ulcers. It enhances the formation of granulation tissue, thereby promoting wound healing.

BECAPLERMIN
(Recombinant human platelet-derived growth factor)

Indications see notes above
Cautions malignant disease; avoid on sites with infection, malignancy or peripheral arteriopathy

13 Skin

Side-effects pain; infections including cellulitis and osteomyelitis; local reactions including erythema; *rarely* bullous eruption, oedema, and hypertrophic granulation

Dose

- Full-thickness, neuropathic, diabetic ulcers (no larger than 5 cm^2), apply thin layer daily and cover with gauze dressing moistened with physiological saline; max. duration of treatment 20 weeks (reassess if no healing after first 10 weeks); CHILD under 18 years see *BNF for Children*

Regranex® (Janssen-Cilag) PoM

Gel, becaplermin (recombinant human platelet-derived growth factor) 0.01%, net price 15 g = £255.75

Excipients include hydroxybenzoates

13.12 Antiperspirants

Aluminium chloride is a potent antiperspirant used in the treatment of hyperhidrosis. Aluminium salts are also incorporated in preparations used for minor fungal skin infections associated with hyperhidrosis.

In more severe cases specialists use **glycopyrronium bromide** as a 0.05% solution in the iontophoretic treatment of hyperhidrosis of plantar and palmar areas. **Botulinum A toxin-haemagglutinin complex** (section 4.9.3) is licensed for use intradermally for severe hyperhidrosis of the axillae unresponsive to topical antiperspirant or other antihidrotic treatment.

ALUMINIUM SALTS

Indications see under Dose below

Cautions avoid contact with eyes or mucous membranes; avoid use on broken or irritated skin; do not shave axillae or use depilatories within 12 hours of application; avoid contact with clothing

Side-effects skin irritation

Dose

- Hyperhidrosis affecting axillae, hands or feet, apply liquid formulation at night to dry skin, wash off the following morning, initially daily then reduce frequency as condition improves—do not bathe immediately before use
- Hyperhidrosis, bromidrosis, intertrigo, and prevention of tinea pedis and related conditions, apply powder to dry skin

Anhydrol® Forte (Dermal)

Solution (= application), aluminium chloride hexahydrate 20% in an alcoholic basis, net price 60-mL bottle with roll-on applicator = £2.62. Label: 15

Excipients none as listed in section 13.1.3

Driclor®[1] (Stiefel)

Application, aluminium chloride hexahydrate 20% in an alcoholic basis, net price 60-mL bottle with roll-on applicator = £2.82. Label: 15

Excipients none as listed in section 13.1.3

1. A 30-mL pack is on sale to the public

ZeaSORB® (Stiefel)

Dusting powder, aldioxa 0.22%, chloroxylenol 0.5%, net price 50 g = £2.61

Excipients include fragrance

GLYCOPYRRONIUM BROMIDE

Indications iontophoretic treatment of hyperhidrosis; other indications section 15.1.3

Cautions see section 15.1.3 (but poorly absorbed and systemic effects unlikely)

Contra-indications see section 15.1.3 (but poorly absorbed and systemic effects unlikely), infections affecting the treatment site

Side-effects see section 15.1.3 (but poorly absorbed and systemic effects unlikely), tingling at administration site

Dose

- Consult product literature; only 1 site to be treated at a time, max. 2 sites treated in any 24 hours, treatment not to be repeated within 7 days

Robinul® (Antigen) PoM

Powder, glycopyrronium bromide, net price 3 g = £110.00

13.13 Topical circulatory preparations

These preparations are used to improve circulation in conditions such as bruising, superficial thrombophlebitis, chilblains and varicose veins but are of little value. Chilblains are best managed by avoidance of exposure to cold; neither systemic nor topical vasodilator therapy is established as being effective. Sclerotherapy of varicose veins is described in section 2.13.

Rubefacients are described in section 10.3.2.

Hirudoid® (Genus)

Cream, heparinoid 0.3% in a vanishing-cream basis, net price 50 g = £3.99

Excipients include cetostearyl alcohol, hydroxybenzoates (parabens)

Gel, heparinoid 0.3%, net price 50 g = £3.99

Excipients include propylene glycol, fragrance

Dose apply up to 4 times daily in superficial soft-tissue injuries and superficial thrombophlebitis

14 Immunological products and vaccines

14.1	**Active immunity**	**641**
14.2	**Passive immunity**	**643**
14.3	**Storage and use**	**643**
14.4	**Vaccines and antisera**	**643**
14.5	**Immunoglobulins**	**659**
14.6	**International travel**	**663**

14.1 Active immunity

Vaccines may consist of:

1. a *live attenuated* form of a virus (e.g. measles, mumps and rubella vaccine) or bacteria (e.g. BCG vaccine)
2. *inactivated* preparations of the virus (e.g. influenza vaccine) or bacteria, or
3. *extracts of* or *detoxified exotoxins* produced by a micro-organism (e.g. tetanus vaccine).

They stimulate production of antibodies and other components of the immune mechanism.

Live attenuated vaccines usually produce a durable immunity but not always as long-lasting as that of the natural infection. When two live virus vaccines are required (and are not available as a combined preparation) they should be given either simultaneously at different sites or separated by an interval of at least 4 weeks.

Inactivated vaccines may require a primary series of injections of vaccine to produce adequate antibody response and in most cases booster (reinforcing) injections are required; the duration of immunity varies from months to many years. Some inactivated vaccines are adsorbed onto an adjuvant (such as aluminium hydroxide) to enhance the antibody response.

> Advice in this chapter reflects that in the handbook *Immunisation against Infectious Disease* (2006), which in turn reflects the guidance of the Joint Committee on Vaccination and Immunisation (JCVI).
> Chapters from the handbook are available at www.dh.gov.uk
> The advice incorporates changes announced by the Chief Medical Officer and Health Department Updates.

Side-effects Some vaccines (e.g. poliomyelitis) produce very few reactions, while others (e.g. measles, mumps and rubella) may produce a very mild form of the disease. Some vaccines may produce discomfort at the site of injection and mild fever and malaise. Occasionally there are more serious untoward reactions and these should always be reported to the CHM (see Adverse Reactions to Drugs, p. 11). Anaphylactic reactions are very rare but can be fatal (see section 3.4.3 for management). The product literature should be consulted for full details of side-effects.

> **Post-immunisation pyrexia in infants**
> The parent should be advised that if pyrexia develops after childhood immunisation, the infant can be given a dose of paracetamol and, if necessary, a second dose given 6 hours later; ibuprofen may be used if paracetamol is unsuitable. The parent should be warned to seek medical advice if the pyrexia persists.
> For post-immunisation pyrexia in an infant aged 2–3 months, the dose of paracetamol is 60 mg; the dose of ibuprofen is 50 mg (on doctor's advice). An oral syringe can be obtained from any pharmacy to give the small volume required.

Contra-indications Most vaccines have some basic contra-indication to their use, and the product literature and *Immunisation against Infectious Disease* should be consulted for details. In general, vaccination should be postponed if the individual is suffering from an *acute illness*. Minor illnesses without fever or systemic upset are not contra-indications. Anaphylaxis with a preceding dose of a vaccine (or vaccine component) is a contra-indication to further doses.

Hypersensitivity to egg with evidence of previous anaphylactic reaction, contra-indicates influenza vaccine, tick-borne encephalitis vaccine, and yellow fever vaccine. Some viral vaccines contain small quantities of antibacterials; such vaccines may need to be withheld from individuals who are *extremely sensitive to the antibacterial*. Other excipients in vaccines may also rarely cause allergic reactions. The presence of the following excipients in vaccines and immunological products has been noted under the relevant entries:

Gelatin	Penicillins
Gentamicin	Polymyxin B
Kanamycin	Streptomycin
Neomycin	Thiomersal

Live vaccines should not be administered routinely to *pregnant women* because of possible harm to the fetus but where there is a significant risk of exposure (e.g. to yellow fever), the need for vaccination usually outweighs any possible risk to the fetus. Without specialist advice, live vaccines should not be given to individuals with *impaired immune response*, whether caused by disease (for special reference to *HIV infection*, see below) or treatment with high doses of systemic corticosteroids (dose equivalents of prednisolone: **adults** at least 40 mg daily for more than 1 week; **children** 2 mg/kg daily for at least 1 week or 1 mg/kg daily for 1 month), or other immunosuppressive drugs[1]. They should not be given to those being treated for *malignant conditions* with chemotherapy or generalised radiotherapy[1,2]. The response to vaccines may be reduced and there is risk of generalised infection with live vaccines.

The Royal College of Paediatrics and Child Health has produced a statement, *Immunisation of the Immunocompromised Child (2002)* (available at www.rcpch.ac.uk).

The intramuscular route should not be used in patients with bleeding disorders such as haemophilia or thrombocytopenia. Vaccines that are usually given by the intramuscular route may be given by subcutaneous injection in those with bleeding disorders.

Note The Department of Health has advised *against the use of jet guns* for vaccination owing to the risk of transmitting blood-borne infections, such as HIV.

Vaccines and HIV infection HIV-positive individuals with or without symptoms can receive the following live vaccines:

MMR (but not whilst severely immunosuppressed), varicella-zoster (but avoid if immunity significantly impaired—consult product literature);[2,3]

and the following inactivated vaccines:

anthrax, cholera (oral), diphtheria, haemophilus influenzae type b, hepatitis A, hepatitis B, influenza, meningococcal, pertussis, pneumococcal, poliomyelitis[4], rabies, tetanus, tick-borne encephalitis, typhoid (injection).

HIV-positive individuals should **not** receive:

BCG, typhoid (oral), yellow fever[5]

Note The above advice differs from that for other immunocompromised patients.

Vaccines and asplenia The following vaccines are recommended for asplenic patients or those with splenic dysfunction:

haemophilus influenzae type b, influenza, meningococcal group C, pneumococcal.

For antibiotic prophylaxis in asplenia see p. 282.

Immunisation schedule

Vaccines for the childhood immunisation schedule should be obtained from **local health organisations** or **direct from Movianto**—not to be prescribed on FP10 (HS21 in Northern Ireland; GP10 in Scotland; WP10 in Wales).

During first year of life

Diphtheria, Tetanus, Pertussis (Acellular, Component), Poliomyelitis (Inactivated) and Haemophilus Type b Conjugate Vaccine (Adsorbed)

3 doses; first dose at 2 months of age, second dose at 3 months, and third dose at 4 months

plus

Pneumococcal Polysaccharide Conjugate Vaccine (Adsorbed)

2 doses; first dose at 2 months of age, second dose at 4 months (further dose during second year of life)

plus

Meningococcal Group C Conjugate Vaccine

2 doses; first dose at 3 months of age, second dose at 4 months

BCG Vaccine (for neonates at risk only)

See section 14.4, BCG Vaccines

During second year of life

Haemophilus Type b Conjugate Vaccine and Meningococcal Group C Conjugate Vaccine

Single dose at 12 months of age

plus

Measles, Mumps and Rubella Vaccine, Live (MMR)

Single dose at 13 months of age

plus

Pneumococcal Polysaccharide Conjugate Vaccine (Adsorbed)

Single dose at 13 months of age

Before school or nursery school entry

Adsorbed Diphtheria [low dose], **Tetanus, Pertussis (Acellular, Component) and Inactivated Poliomyelitis Vaccine**

or

Adsorbed Diphtheria, Tetanus, Pertussis (Acellular, Component) and Inactivated Poliomyelitis Vaccine

or

Diphtheria, Tetanus, Pertussis (Acellular, Component), Poliomyelitis (Inactivated) and Haemophilus Influenzae Type b Conjugate Vaccine (Adsorbed)[6]

Single dose

Preferably allow interval of at least 3 years after completing primary course; can be given at same session as MMR Vaccine but use separate syringe and needle, and give in different limb

plus

Measles, Mumps and Rubella Vaccine, Live (MMR)

Single booster dose

Before leaving school or before employment or further education

Adsorbed Diphtheria [low dose], **Tetanus and Inactivated Poliomyelitis Vaccine**

Single booster dose

1. Live vaccines should be postponed until at least 3 months after stopping high-dose systemic corticosteroids and at least 6 months after stopping other immunosuppressive drugs or generalised radiotherapy (at least 12 months after discontinuing immunosuppressants following bone-marrow transplantation).
2. Use of normal immunoglobulin should be considered after exposure to measles (see p. 660) and varicella–zoster immunoglobulin considered after exposure to chickenpox or herpes zoster (see p. 661).
3. The Royal College of Paediatrics and Child Health recommends that MMR is not given to a child with HIV infection whilst severely immunosuppressed.
4. Inactivated poliomyelitis vaccine is now used instead of oral poliomyelitis vaccine for routine immunisation of children.
5. If yellow fever risk is unavoidable, specialist advice should be sought.
6. For children born between 13 March 2003 and 3 September 2005 who have not received a booster dose of Haemophilus Type b Conjugate Vaccine at 12 months of age; see also p. 646.

During adult life

Measles, Mumps and Rubella Vaccine, Live (MMR) (for women of child-bearing age susceptible to rubella)

Single dose

Women of child-bearing age who have not received 2 doses of a rubella-containing vaccine or who do not have a positive antibody test for rubella should be offered rubella immunisation (using the MMR vaccine)—exclude pregnancy before immunisation, but see also section 14.4, Measles, Mumps and Rubella Vaccine

Adsorbed Diphtheria [low dose], **Tetanus and Inactivated Poliomyelitis Vaccine** (if not previously immunised)

3 doses at intervals of 4 weeks

Booster dose at least 1 year after primary course and again 5–10 years later

High-risk groups

For information on high-risk groups, see section 14.4 under individual vaccines

BCG Vaccines

Hepatitis A Vaccine

Hepatitis B Vaccine

Influenza Vaccine

Pneumococcal Vaccines

Tetanus Vaccines

14.2 Passive immunity

Immunity with immediate protection against certain infective organisms can be obtained by injecting preparations made from the plasma of immune individuals with adequate levels of antibody to the disease for which protection is sought (see under Immunoglobulins, section 14.5). The duration of this passive immunity varies according to the dose and the type of immunoglobulin. Passive immunity may last only a few weeks; where necessary, passive immunisation can be repeated.

Antibodies of human origin are usually termed *immunoglobulins*. The term *antiserum* is applied to material prepared in animals. Because of serum sickness and other allergic-type reactions that may follow injections of antisera, this therapy has been replaced wherever possible by the use of immunoglobulins. Reactions are theoretically possible after injection of human immunoglobulins but reports of such reactions are very rare.

14.3 Storage and use

Care must be taken to store all vaccines and other immunological products under the conditions recommended in the product literature, otherwise the preparation may become ineffective. **Refrigerated storage** is usually necessary; many vaccines and immunoglobulins need to be stored at 2–8°C and not allowed to freeze. Vaccines and immunoglobulins should be protected from light. Reconstituted vaccines and opened multidose vials must be used within the period recommended in the product literature. Unused vaccines should be disposed of by incineration at a registered disposal contractor.

Particular attention must be paid to instructions on the use of diluents. Vaccines which are liquid suspensions or are reconstituted before use should be adequately mixed to ensure uniformity of the material to be injected.

14.4 Vaccines and antisera

Availability Anthrax and yellow fever vaccines, botulism antitoxin, diphtheria antitoxin, and snake and spider venom antitoxins are available from local designated holding centres.

For antivenom, see Emergency Treatment of Poisoning, p. 36.

Enquiries for vaccines not available commercially can also be made to:

Immunisation Policy, Monitoring and Surveillance
Department of Health
Wellington House
133–155 Waterloo Road
London, SE1 8UG
Tel: (020) 7972 4047

In Scotland information about availability of vaccines can be obtained from a Specialist in Pharmaceutical Public Health. In Wales enquiries for vaccines not available commercially should be directed to:

Welsh Medicines Information Centre
University Hospital of Wales
Cardiff, CF14 4XW
Tel: (029) 2074 2979

and in Northern Ireland:

Regional Pharmacist (procurement co-ordination) United Hospitals Trust Pharmacy Dept
Whiteabbey Hospital
Doagh Road
Newtownabbey, BT37 9RH
Tel: (028) 9086 5181 ext 2386

For further details of availability, see under individual vaccines.

Anthrax vaccine

Anthrax immunisation is indicated for individuals who handle infected animals, for those exposed to imported infected animal products, and for laboratory staff who work with *Bacillus anthracis*.

In the event of possible contact with *B. anthracis*, post-exposure immunisation may be indicated, in addition to antimicrobial prophylaxis (section 5.1.12). Advice on the use of anthrax vaccine must be obtained from the Centre for Infections, Health Protection Agency (tel. 020 8200 6868).

The vaccine is derived from antigens from *B. anthracis* and, following the primary course of injections, booster doses should be given at about yearly intervals.

Anthrax Vaccine PoM

Dose initial course 3 doses of 0.5 mL *by intramuscular injection* at intervals of 3 weeks followed by a fourth dose after an interval of 6 months

Booster doses: 0.5 mL annually

Note Advice on post-exposure prophylaxis must be obtained from Centre for Infections

Available from Centre for Infections (*excipients include* thiomersal)

BCG vaccines

BCG (Bacillus Calmette-Guérin) is a live attenuated strain derived from *Mycobacterium bovis* which stimulates the development of hypersensitivity to *M. tuberculosis.* BCG vaccine should be given intradermally by operators skilled in the technique (see below).

The expected reaction to successful BCG vaccination is induration at the site of injection followed by a local lesion which starts as a papule 2 or more weeks after vaccination; the lesion may ulcerate then subside over several weeks or months, leaving a small, flat scar. A dry dressing may be used if the ulcer discharges, but air should **not** be excluded.

Serious reactions with BCG are uncommon and most often consist of prolonged ulceration or subcutaneous abscess formation due to faulty injection technique. Anaphylaxis and disseminated BCG complications, such as osteitis or osteomyelitis, are rare.

Apart from children under 6 years, any person being considered for BCG immunisation must first be given a skin test for hypersensitivity to tuberculoprotein (see under Diagnostic Agents, below). A skin test is not necessary for a child under 6 years provided that the child has not stayed for longer than 1 month in a country with an incidence of tuberculosis greater than 40 per 100 000, the child has not had contact with a person with tuberculosis, and there is no family history of tuberculosis within the last 5 years.

BCG is recommended for the following groups if BCG immunisation has not previously been carried out:

- all neonates and infants (0–12 months) born in areas where the incidence[1] of tuberculosis is greater than 40 per 100 000;
- neonates, infants, and children under 16 years with a parent or grandparent born in a country with an incidence[1] of tuberculosis greater than 40 per 100 000;
- new immigrants aged under 16 years who were born in, or lived for more than 3 months in a country with an incidence[1] of tuberculosis greater than 40 per 100 000;
- new immigrants aged 16–35 years from Sub-Saharan Africa or a country with an incidence[1] of tuberculosis greater than 500 per 100 000
- contacts aged under 36 years of those with active respiratory tuberculosis (for healthcare or laboratory workers who have had contact with clinical materials or patients with tuberculosis, age limit does not apply);
- healthcare workers and laboratory staff (irrespective of age) who are likely to have contact with patients, clinical materials, or derived isolates; other individuals under 35 years[2] at occupational risk including veterinary and other staff who handle animal species susceptible to tuberculosis, and staff working directly with prisoners, in care homes for the elderly, or in hostels or facilities for the homeless or refugees;
- individuals under 16 years intending to live with local people for more than 3 months in a country with an incidence[1] of tuberculosis greater than 40 per 100 000 (section 14.6).

BCG vaccine may be given simultaneously with another live vaccine (see also section 14.1), but if they are not given at the same time, an interval of 4 weeks should normally be allowed between them. When BCG is given to infants, there is no need to delay routine primary immunisations. No further vaccination should be given in the arm used for BCG vaccination for at least 3 months because of the risk of regional lymphadenitis.

See section 14.1 for general contra-indications. BCG is also contra-indicated in individuals with generalised septic skin conditions (in the case of eczema, a vaccination site free from lesions should be chosen).

Bladder instillations of BCG are licensed for the management of bladder carcinoma (section 8.2.4).

For advice on chemoprophylaxis against tuberculosis, see section 5.1.9.

Intradermal

Bacillus Calmette-Guérin Vaccine ▼ PoM

BCG Vaccine, Dried/Tub/BCG

A freeze-dried preparation of live bacteria of a strain derived from the bacillus of Calmette and Guérin.

Dose by intradermal injection, 0.1 mL (NEONATE and INFANT under 12 months 0.05 mL)

Available from health organisations or direct from Movianto (SSI brand, multidose vial with diluent)

Intradermal injection technique Skin is stretched between thumb and forefinger and needle (size 25G or 26G) inserted (bevel upwards) for about 3 mm into superficial layers of dermis (almost parallel with surface). Needle should be short with short bevel (can usually be seen through epidermis during insertion). Tense raised blanched bleb showing tips of hair follicles is sign of correct injection; 7 mm bleb ≡ 0.1 mL injection, 3 mm bleb ≡ 0.05 mL injection; if considerable resistance not felt, needle too deep and should be removed and reinserted before giving more vaccine.

To be injected at insertion of deltoid muscle onto humerus (keloid formation more likely with sites higher on arm); tip of shoulder should be **avoided**.

Diagnostic agents

The *Mantoux test* is recommended for tuberculin skin testing, but no licensed preparation is currently available. Guidance for healthcare professionals is available at www.immunisation.nhs.uk.

In the Mantoux test, the diagnostic dose is by intradermal injection of Tuberculin Purified Protein Derivative (PPD).

The *Heaf test* (involving the use of multiple-puncture apparatus) is no longer available.

Note Response to tuberculin may be suppressed by live viral vaccines, viral infection, sarcoidosis, corticosteroid therapy, or immunosuppression due to disease or treatment. Tuberculin testing should not be carried out within 4 weeks of receiving a live viral vaccine.

1. List of countries or primary care trusts where the incidence of tuberculosis is greater than 40 cases per 100 000 is available at www.hpa.org.uk

2. There is inadequate evidence of protection by BCG vaccine in adults aged over 35 years; however, vaccination is recommended for healthcare workers irrespective of age because of the increased risk to them or their patients

Tuberculin Purified Protein Derivative (PoM)
(Tuberculin PPD)

Injection, heat-treated products of growth and lysis of appropriate *Mycobacterium* spp. 20 units/mL (2 units/0.1-mL dose) (for routine use), 1.5-mL vial; 100 units/mL (10 units/0.1-mL dose), 1.5-mL vial

Dose by intradermal injection, 2 units (0.1 mL of 20 units/mL strength) for routine Mantoux test; if first test is negative and a further test is considered appropriate 10 units (0.1 mL of 100 units/mL strength)

Available on a named patient basis from Movianto (SSI brand)

Note The strength of tuberculin PPD in this product may be different to the strengths of products used previously for the Mantoux test; care is required to select the correct strength

Botulism antitoxin

A polyvalent botulism antitoxin is available for the post-exposure prophylaxis of botulism and for the treatment of persons thought to be suffering from botulism. It specifically neutralises the toxins produced by *Clostridium botulinum* types A, B, and E. It is not effective against infantile botulism as the toxin (type A) is seldom, if ever, found in the blood in this type of infection.

Hypersensitivity reactions are a problem. It is essential to read the contra-indications, warnings, and details of sensitivity tests on the package insert. Prior to treatment checks should be made regarding previous administration of any antitoxin and history of any allergic condition, e.g. asthma, hay fever, etc. All patients should be tested for sensitivity (diluting the antitoxin if history of allergy).

Botulism Antitoxin (PoM)

A preparation containing the specific antitoxic globulins that have the power of neutralising the toxins formed by types A, B, and E of *Clostridium botulinum*.

Note The BP title Botulinum Antitoxin is not used because the preparation currently in use may have a different specification.

Dose prophylaxis, consult product literature

Available from local designated centres, for details see TOXBASE (requires registration) www.toxbase.org. For supplies outside working hours apply to other designated centres and, as a last resort, to the duty doctor at the Health Protection Agency (Tel (020) 8200 6868). For major incidents, obtain supplies from the local blood bank

Cholera vaccine

Cholera vaccine (oral) contains inactivated Inaba (including El-Tor biotype) and Ogawa strains of *Vibrio cholerae*, serotype O1 together with recombinant B-subunit of the cholera toxin produced in Inaba strains of *V.cholerae*, serotype O1.

Oral cholera vaccine is licensed for travellers to endemic or epidemic areas on the basis of current recommendations (see also section 14.6). Immunisation should be completed at least 1 week before potential exposure. However, there is no requirement for cholera vaccination for international travel.

Immunisation with cholera vaccine does not provide complete protection and all travellers to a country where cholera exists should be warned that scrupulous attention to food, water, and personal hygiene is **essential**.

Cautions and side-effects Food, drink, and other oral medicines should be avoided 1 hour before and after vaccination. Side-effects of oral cholera vaccine include diarrhoea, abdominal pain, headache; rarely nausea, vomiting, loss of appetite, dizziness, fever, and respiratory symptoms can also occur.

See section 14.1 for general contra-indications.

Injectable cholera vaccine provides unreliable protection and is no longer available in the UK.

Dukoral® (Novartis Vaccines) ▼ (PoM)

Oral suspension, for dilution with solution of effervescent sodium bicarbonate granules, heat- and formaldehyde-inactivated Inaba (including El-Tor biotype) and Ogawa strains of *Vibrio cholerae* bacteria and recombinant cholera toxin B-subunit produced in *V. cholerae*, net price 2-dose pack = £23.42

Dose ADULT and CHILD over 6 years 2 doses separated by an interval of 1–6 weeks; CHILD 2–6 years 3 doses each separated by an interval of 1–6 weeks (consult product literature for dilution and administration)

Note If more than 6 weeks have elapsed between doses, the primary course should be restarted

A single booster dose can be given 2 years after primary course for adults and children over 6 years, and 6 months after primary course for children 2–6 years. If more than 2 years have elapsed since the last vaccination, the primary course should be repeated

Diphtheria vaccines

Diphtheria vaccines are prepared from the toxin of *Corynebacterium diphtheriae* and adsorption on aluminium hydroxide or aluminium phosphate improves antigenicity. The vaccine stimulates the production of the protective antitoxin. Single-antigen diphtheria vaccine is not available and adsorbed diphtheria vaccine is given as a combination product containing other vaccines.

For primary immunisation *of children aged between 2 months and 10 years* vaccination is recommended usually in the form of 3 doses (separated by 1-month intervals) of **diphtheria, tetanus, pertussis (acellular, component), poliomyelitis (inactivated) and haemophilus type b conjugate vaccine (adsorbed)** (see schedule, section 14.1). In unimmunised individuals aged *over 10 years* the primary course comprises of 3 doses of **adsorbed diphtheria** [low dose], **tetanus and inactivated poliomyelitis vaccine**.

A booster dose should be given 3 years after the primary course (this interval can be reduced to a minimum of 1 year if the primary course was delayed). Children *under 10 years* should receive *either* **adsorbed diphtheria, tetanus, pertussis (acellular, component) and inactivated poliomyelitis vaccine** *or* **adsorbed diphtheria** [low dose], **tetanus, pertussis (acellular, component) and inactivated poliomyelitis vaccine**; for children requiring a booster dose of haemophilus influenzae type b vaccine as part of a 'catch-up' programme see p. 646. Individuals aged *over 10 years* should receive **adsorbed diphtheria** [low dose], **tetanus, and inactivated poliomyelitis vaccine**.

A second booster dose of adsorbed diphtheria [low dose], tetanus and inactivated poliomyelitis vaccine should be given 10 years after the previous booster dose (this interval can be reduced to a minimum of 5 years if previous doses were delayed).

Those intending to travel to areas with a risk of diphtheria infection should be fully immunised according to the UK schedule. If more than 10 years have lapsed since completion of the UK schedule, a dose of **adsorbed diphtheria** [low dose], **tetanus and inactivated poliomyelitis vaccine** should be administered.

Staff in contact with diphtheria patients or with potentially pathogenic clinical specimens or working directly with *C. diphtheriae* or *C. ulcerans* should receive a booster dose if fully immunised (with 5 doses of diphtheria-containing vaccine given at appropriate intervals); further doses should be given at 10-year intervals if risk persists. Individuals at risk who are not fully immunised should complete the primary course; a booster dose should be given after 5 years and then at 10-year intervals. **Adsorbed diphtheria** [low dose], **tetanus and inactivated poliomyelitis vaccine** is used for this purpose; immunity should be checked by antibody testing at least 3 months after completion of immunisation.

Advice on the management of cases, carriers, contacts and outbreaks must be sought from health protection units. The immunisation history of infected individuals and their contacts should be determined; those who have been incompletely immunised should complete their immunisation and fully immunised individuals should receive a reinforcing dose. For advice on antibacterial treatment to prevent a secondary case of diphtheria in a non-immune individual, see Table 2, section 5.1.

See section 14.1 for general contra-indications.

See also Predisposition to Neurological Problems, p. 654.

Diphtheria vaccines for children under 10 years

Important Not recommended for persons *aged 10 years or over* (see Diphtheria Vaccines for Children over 10 years and Adults, below)

Diphtheria, Tetanus, Pertussis (Acellular, Component), Poliomyelitis (Inactivated) and Haemophilus Type b Conjugate Vaccine (Adsorbed) PoM

Injection, suspension of diphtheria toxoid, tetanus toxoid, acellular pertussis, inactivated poliomyelitis and *Haemophilus influenzae* type b (conjugated to tetanus protein), net price 0.5-mL vial = £19.94

Excipients may include neomycin, polymyxin B and streptomycin

Dose CHILD up to 10 years, by intramuscular injection 0.5 mL (see schedule, section 14.1)

Brands include ▼*Infanrix-IPV+Hib*®, ▼*Pediacel*®; available as part of childhood immunisation schedule, from health organisations or Movianto

Adsorbed Diphtheria, Tetanus, Pertussis (Acellular, Component) and Inactivated Poliomyelitis Vaccine PoM

Injection, suspension of diphtheria toxoid, tetanus toxoid, acellular pertussis and inactivated poliomyelitis vaccine components adsorbed on a mineral carrier, net price 0.5-mL prefilled syringe = £17.56

Excipients include neomycin and polymyxin B

Dose CHILD 3–10 years, by intramuscular injection, 0.5 mL (see schedule, section 14.1)

Brands include ▼*Infanrix-IPV*®; available as part of childhood immunisation schedule, from health organisations or Movianto

Adsorbed Diphtheria [low dose], Tetanus, Pertussis (Acellular, Component) and Inactivated Poliomyelitis Vaccine PoM

Injection, suspension of diphtheria toxoid [low dose], tetanus toxoid, acellular pertussis and inactivated poliomyelitis vaccine components adsorbed on a mineral carrier, net price 0.5-mL prefilled syringe = £11.98

Excipients include neomycin, polymyxin B and streptomycin

Dose CHILD 3–10 years, by intramuscular injection, 0.5 mL (see schedule, section 14.1)

Brands include ▼*Repevax*®; available as part of childhood immunisation schedule, from health organisations or Movianto

Diphtheria vaccines for children over 10 years and adults

A low dose of diphtheria toxoid is sufficient to recall immunity in individuals previously immunised against diphtheria but whose immunity may have diminished with time; it is insufficient to cause serious reactions that may occur when a higher-dose vaccine is used in an individual who is already immune. Preparations containing low dose diphtheria should be used for adults and children *over 10 years*, whether for primary immunisation or for booster doses.

Adsorbed Diphtheria [low dose], Tetanus and Inactivated Poliomyelitis Vaccine PoM

Injection, suspension of diphtheria toxoid [low dose], tetanus toxoid and inactivated poliomyelitis vaccine components adsorbed on a mineral carrier, net price 0.5-mL prefilled syringe = £6.74

Excipients include neomycin, polymyxin B and streptomycin

Dose primary immunisation in ADULT and CHILD over 10 years, by intramuscular injection, 3 doses each of 0.5 mL separated by intervals of 4 weeks; booster, 0.5 mL after 5 years, repeated 10 years later (see schedule, section 14.1)

Brands include *Revaxis*®; available as part of childhood schedule, from health organisations or Movianto

Diphtheria antitoxin

Diphtheria antitoxin is used for passive immunisation. It is derived from horse serum and reactions are common after administration; resuscitation facilities should be available immediately.

It is now only used in suspected cases of diphtheria (without waiting for bacteriological confirmation); tests for hypersensitivity should be first carried out.

It is no longer used for prophylaxis because of the risk of hypersensitivity; unimmunised contacts should be promptly investigated and given antibacterial prophylaxis (section 5.1, table 2) and vaccine (see notes above).

Diphtheria Antitoxin PoM

Dip/Ser

Dose prophylaxis, not recommended therefore no dose stated (see notes above)

Treatment, consult product literature

Available from Centre for Infections (Tel (020) 8200 6868) or in Northern Ireland from Public Health Laboratory, Belfast City Hospital (Tel (028) 9032 9241)

Haemophilus type B conjugate vaccine

Haemophilus influenzae type b (Hib) vaccine is made from capsular polysaccharide; it is conjugated with a protein such as tetanus toxoid to increase immunogenicity, especially in young children. Haemophilus influenzae type b vaccine is a component of the primary course of childhood immunisation (see schedule, section 14.1); it is combined with diphtheria, tetanus, pertussis (acellular, component) and inactivated poliomyelitis vaccine (see under Diphtheria Vaccines). For infants under 1 year, the course consists of 3 doses of a vaccine containing haemophilus influenzae type b component with an interval of 1 month between doses. A booster dose of haemophilus influenzae type b vaccine (combined with meningococcal group C conjugate vaccine) should be given at around 12 months of age (see schedule, section 14.1).

'Catch-up' programme

Children born between 13 March 2003 and 3 September 2005 who have not received a booster dose of haemophilus influenzae type b vaccine at 12 months of age will be offered combined diphtheria, tetanus, pertussis (acellular, component), poliomyelitis (inactivated) and haemophilus type b conjugate vaccine (adsorbed) as part of a 'catch-up' programme before school entry; children who have already received their pre-school immunisation without the Hib component will be offered haemophilus influenzae type b vaccine combined with meningococcal group C conjugate vaccine. The 'catch-up' dose should be given 3 years after the primary course (this interval can be reduced to a minimum of 1 year if the primary course was delayed).

Unimmunised children over 12 months need receive only 1 dose of Haemophilus influenzae type b vaccine, but for full protection against other diseases, 3 doses should be given of diphtheria, tetanus, pertussis (acellular, component), poliomyelitis (inactivated) and haemophilus type b conjugate vaccine (adsorbed). The risk of infection falls sharply in older children and the vaccine is not normally required for children over 10 years.

Haemophilus influenzae type b vaccine may be given to those over 10 years who are considered to be at increased risk of invasive *H. influenzae* type b disease (such as those with sickle-cell disease and those receiving treatment for malignancy).

Asplenia or splenic dysfunction Haemophilus influenzae type b vaccine is recommended for patients with asplenia or splenic dysfunction. Immunised adults and children over 1 year, who develop splenic dysfunction, should be given 1 additional dose of haemophilus influenzae type b vaccine (combined with meningococcal group C conjugate vaccine). For elective splenectomy, the vaccine should ideally be given at least 2 weeks before surgery. Adults and children over 1 year, who are not immunised against haemophilus influenzae type b, should be given 2 doses of haemophilus influenzae type b vaccine (usually combined with meningococcal group C conjugate vaccine) with an interval of 2 months between doses. However, children under 10 years, who are not immunised against diphtheria, tetanus, pertussis, poliomyelitis, and haemophilus influenzae type b should be given 3 doses (with an interval of 1 month between doses) of combined diphtheria, tetanus, pertussis (acellular component), poliomyelitis (inactivated) and haemophilus type b conjugate vaccine.

Side-effects of haemophilus influenzae type b vaccine include fever, restlessness, prolonged crying, loss of appetite, vomiting, and diarrhoea; hypersensitivity reactions (including anaphylaxis) and collapse have been reported.

See section 14.1 for general contra-indications.

◢Combined vaccines

See also under Diphtheria vaccines

Menitorix® (GSK) ▼ PoM

Injection, powder for reconstitution, capsular polysaccharide of *Haemophilus influenzae* type b and capsular polysaccharide of *Neisseria meningitidis* group C (both conjugated to tetanus protein), net price single-dose vial (with syringe containing 0.5 mL diluent) = £39.87

Dose by intramuscular injection, 0.5 mL (but see notes above and also schedule, section 14.1)

Available as part of the childhood immunisation schedule from Movianto

Hepatitis A vaccine

Hepatitis A vaccine is prepared from formaldehyde-inactivated hepatitis A virus grown in human diploid cells.

Immunisation is recommended for:

- laboratory staff who work directly with the virus;
- staff and residents of homes for those with severe learning difficulties;
- workers at risk of exposure to untreated sewage;
- individuals who work with primates;
- patients with haemophilia treated with plasma-derived clotting factors;
- patients with severe liver disease;
- travellers to high-risk areas (see p. 663);
- individuals who are at risk due to their sexual behaviour;
- parenteral drug abusers.

Immunisation should be considered for :

- patients with chronic liver disease including chronic hepatitis B or chronic hepatitis C;
- prevention of secondary cases in close contacts of confirmed cases of hepatitis A, within 7 days of onset of disease in the primary case.

A booster dose is usually given 6–12 months after the initial dose. A second booster dose can be given 20 years after the previous booster dose to those who continue to be at risk. Specialist advice should be sought on re-immunisation of immunocompromised individuals.

Side-effects of hepatitis A vaccine, usually mild, include transient soreness, erythema, and induration at the injection site. Less common effects include fever, malaise, fatigue, headache, nausea, diarrhoea, and loss of appetite; arthralgia, myalgia, and, generalised rashes are occasionally reported.

See section 14.1 for general contra-indications.

◢Single component

Avaxim® (Sanofi Pasteur) PoM

Injection, suspension of formaldehyde-inactivated hepatitis A virus (GBM grown in human diploid cells) 320 antigen units/mL adsorbed onto aluminium hydroxide, net price 0.5-mL prefilled syringe = £19.19

Excipients include neomycin

Dose by intramuscular injection (see note below), 0.5 mL as a single dose; booster dose 0.5 mL 6–12 months after initial dose; CHILD under 16 years, not recommended

Note Booster dose may be delayed by up to 3 years if not given after recommended interval following primary dose with *Avaxim®*. The deltoid region is the preferred site of injection. The subcutaneous route may be used for patients with bleeding disorders

Epaxal® (MASTA) PoM

Injection, suspension of formaldehyde-inactivated hepatitis A virus (RG-SB grown in human diploid cells)

at least 48 units/mL, net price 0.5-mL prefilled syringe = £23.81

Dose by intramuscular injection (see note below), ADULT and CHILD over 1 year, 0.5 mL as a single dose; booster dose 0.5 mL 6–12 months after initial dose (1–6 months if splenectomised)

Note Booster dose may be delayed by up to 4 years in adults if not given after recommended interval following primary dose. The deltoid region is the preferred site of injection. The subcutaneous route may be used for patients with bleeding disorders

Important *Epaxal®* contains influenza virus haemagglutinin grown in the allantoic cavity of chick embryos, therefore contra-indicated in those hypersensitive to eggs or chicken protein.

Havrix Monodose® (GSK) PoM

Injection, suspension of formaldehyde-inactivated hepatitis A virus (HM 175 grown in human diploid cells) 1440 ELISA units/mL adsorbed onto aluminium hydroxide, net price 1-mL prefilled syringe = £22.14, 0.5-mL (720 ELISA units) prefilled syringe (*Havrix Junior Monodose®*) = £16.77

Excipients include neomycin

Dose by intramuscular injection (see note below), 1 mL as a single dose; booster dose, 1 mL 6–12 months after initial dose; CHILD 1–15 years 0.5 mL; booster dose, 0.5 mL 6–12 months after initial dose

Note Booster dose may be delayed by up to 3 years if not given after recommended interval following primary dose with *Havrix Monodose®*. The deltoid region is the preferred site of injection. The subcutaneous route may be used for patients with bleeding disorders

Vaqta® Paediatric (Sanofi Pasteur) PoM

Injection, suspension of formaldehyde-inactivated hepatitis A virus (grown in human diploid cells) 50 antigen units/mL adsorbed onto aluminium hydroxyphosphate sulphate, net price 0.5-mL prefilled syringe = £15.65

Excipients include neomycin

Dose by intramuscular injection (see note below) CHILD and ADOLESCENT 1–17 years, 0.5 mL as a single dose; booster dose 0.5 mL 6–18 months after initial dose; under 1 year, not recommended

Note The deltoid region is the preferred site of injection. The subcutaneous route may be used for patients with bleeding disorders

With hepatitis B vaccine

Twinrix® (GSK) PoM

Injection, inactivated hepatitis A virus 720 ELISA units and recombinant (DNA) hepatitis B surface antigen 20 micrograms/mL adsorbed onto aluminium hydroxide and aluminium phosphate, net price 1-mL prefilled syringe (*Twinrix® Adult*) = £27.76, 0.5-mL prefilled syringe (*Twinrix® Paediatric*) = £20.79

Excipients include neomycin and thiomersal

Dose by intramuscular injection (see note below); primary course of 3 doses of 1 mL, the second 1 month and the third 6 months after the first dose; CHILD 1–15 years by intramuscular injection, 3 doses of 0.5 mL

Accelerated schedule (e.g. for travellers departing within 1 month), ADULT, second dose 7 days after first dose, third dose after further 14 days and a fourth dose after 12 months

Note Primary course should be completed with *Twinrix®* (single component vaccines given at appropriate intervals may be used for booster dose); the deltoid region is the preferred site of injection in adults and older children; anterolateral thigh is preferred site in infants; not to be injected into the buttock (vaccine efficacy reduced); subcutaneous route used for patients with bleeding disorders (but immune response may be reduced).

Important *Twinrix®* **not** recommended for post-exposure prophylaxis following percutaneous (needle-stick), ocular or mucous membrane exposure to hepatitis B virus.

With typhoid vaccine

Hepatyrix® (GSK) PoM

Injection, suspension of inactivated hepatitis A virus (grown in human diploid cells) 1440 ELISA units/mL adsorbed onto aluminium hydroxide, combined with typhoid vaccine containing 25 micrograms/mL virulence polysaccharide antigen of *Salmonella typhi*, net price 1-mL prefilled syringe = £32.08

Excipients include neomycin

Dose by intramuscular injection (see note below), ADULT and ADOLESCENT over 15 years, 1 mL as a single dose; booster doses, see under single component hepatitis A vaccine and under polysaccharide typhoid vaccine

Note The deltoid region is the preferred site of injection. The subcutaneous route may be used for patients with bleeding disorders

ViATIM® (Sanofi Pasteur) PoM

Injection, suspension of inactivated hepatitis A virus (grown in human diploid cells) 160 antigen units/mL adsorbed onto aluminium hydroxide, combined with typhoid vaccine containing 25 micrograms/mL virulence polysaccharide antigen of *Salmonella typhi*, net price 1-mL prefilled syringe = £30.22

Excipients include neomycin

Dose by intramuscular injection (see note below), ADULT and ADOLESCENT over 16 years, 1 mL as a single dose; booster doses, see under single component hepatitis A vaccine and under polysaccharide typhoid vaccine

Note The deltoid region is the preferred site of injection. The subcutaneous route may be used for patients with bleeding disorders

Hepatitis B vaccine

Hepatitis B vaccine contains inactivated hepatitis B virus surface antigen (HBsAg) adsorbed on aluminium hydroxide adjuvant. It is made biosynthetically using recombinant DNA technology. The vaccine is used in individuals at high risk of contracting hepatitis B.

In the UK, groups at high-risk of hepatitis B include:

- parenteral drug misusers, their sexual partners, and household contacts; other drug misusers who are likely to 'progress' to injecting;
- individuals who change sexual partners frequently;
- close family contacts of a case or carrier;
- babies whose mothers have had acute hepatitis B during pregnancy *or* are positive for hepatitis B surface antigen (regardless of e-antigen markers); hepatitis B vaccination is started immediately on delivery and *hepatitis B immunoglobulin* (see p. 661) given at the same time (but preferably at a different site). Babies whose mothers are positive for hepatitis B surface antigen and for e-antigen antibody should receive the vaccine only (but babies weighing 1.5 kg or less should also receive the immunoglobulin regardless of the mother's e-antigen antibody status);
- individuals with haemophilia, those receiving regular blood transfusions or blood products, and carers responsible for the administration of such products;
- patients with chronic renal failure including those on haemodialysis. Haemodialysis patients should be monitored for antibodies annually and re-immunised if necessary. Home carers (of dialysis patients) should be vaccinated;
- individuals with chronic liver disease;
- healthcare personnel (including trainees) who have direct contact with blood or blood-stained body fluids or with patients' tissues;

- other occupational risk groups such as morticians and embalmers;
- staff and patients of day-care or residential accommodation for those with severe learning difficulties;
- staff and inmates of custodial institutions;
- those travelling to areas of high or intermediate prevalence who are at increased risk or who plan to remain there for lengthy periods (see p. 663);
- families adopting children from countries with a high or intermediate prevalence of hepatitis B;
- foster carers and their families.

Immunisation may take up to 6 months to confer adequate protection; the duration of immunity is not known precisely, but a single booster 5 years after the primary course may be sufficient to maintain immunity for those who continue to be at risk.

More detailed guidance is given in the memorandum *Immunisation against Infectious Disease*. Immunisation does not eliminate the need for commonsense precautions for avoiding the risk of infection from known carriers by the routes of infection which have been clearly established, consult *Guidance for Clinical Health Care Workers: Protection against Infection with Blood-borne Viruses* (available at www.dh.gov.uk). Accidental inoculation of hepatitis B virus-infected blood into a wound, incision, needle-prick, or abrasion may lead to infection, whereas it is unlikely that indirect exposure to a carrier will do so.

Specific **hepatitis B immunoglobulin** ('HBIG') is available for use with the vaccine in those accidentally inoculated and in neonates at special risk of infection (section 14.5).

A combined hepatitis A and hepatitis B vaccine is also available.

See section 14.1 for general contra-indications.

Single component

Engerix B® (GSK) PoM

Injection, suspension of hepatitis B surface antigen (rby, prepared from yeast cells by recombinant DNA technique) 20 micrograms/mL adsorbed onto aluminium hydroxide, net price 0.5-mL (paediatric) vial = £9.16, 0.5-mL (paediatric) prefilled syringe = £9.67, 1-mL vial = £12.34, 1-mL prefilled syringe = £12.99

Excipients include traces of thiomersal

Dose by intramuscular injection (see note below), 3 doses of 20 micrograms, the second 1 month and the third 6 months after the first dose; NEONATE (except if born to hepatitis B surface antigen positive mother, see below) and CHILD 1 month–16 years, 3 doses of 10 micrograms

Accelerated schedule, second dose 1 month after first dose, third dose 2 months after first dose and fourth dose 12 months after first dose; exceptionally (e.g. for travellers departing within 1 month), ADULT over 18 years, second dose 7 days after first dose, third dose 21 days after first dose, and fourth dose 12 months after first dose

Alternative schedule for CHILD 11–15 years, 2 doses of 20 micrograms, the second dose 6 months after the first dose (this schedule not suitable if high risk of infection between doses or if compliance with second dose uncertain)

NEONATE born to hepatitis B surface antigen-positive mother (see also notes above), 4 doses of 10 micrograms, first dose at birth with hepatitis B immunoglobulin injection (separate site) the second 1 month, the third 2 months and the fourth 12 months after the first dose

Renal insufficiency (including haemodialysis patients), by intramuscular injection (see note below) 4 doses of 40 micrograms, the second 1 month, the third 2 months and the fourth 6 months after the first dose; immunisation schedule and booster doses may need to be adjusted in those with low antibody concentration; NEONATE (except if born to hepatitis B surface antigen positive mother, see above) and CHILD 1 month–16 years 3 doses of 10 micrograms, second dose 1 month and third dose 6 months after first dose *or* accelerated schedule, 4 doses of 10 micrograms, second dose 1 month, third dose 2 months and fourth dose 12 months after first dose; immunisation schedule and booster doses may need to be adjusted in those with low antibody concentration

Note Deltoid muscle is preferred site of injection in adults and older children; anterolateral thigh is preferred site in neonates, infants and young children; not to be injected into the buttock (vaccine efficacy reduced); subcutaneous route used for patients with bleeding disorders

Fendrix® (GSK) ▼ PoM

Injection, suspension of hepatitis B surface antigen (prepared from yeast cells by recombinant DNA technique) 40 micrograms/mL adsorbed onto aluminium phosphate, net price 0.5-mL prefilled syringe = £38.10

Dose ADULT and CHILD over 15 years with renal insufficiency (including pre-haemodialysis and haemodialysis patients), by intramuscular injection (see note below) 4 doses of 20 micrograms, the second 1 month, the third 2 months and the fourth 6 months after the first dose; immunisation schedule and booster doses may need to be adjusted in those with low antibody concentration

Note Deltoid muscle is preferred site of injection; not to be injected into the buttock (vaccine efficacy reduced); subcutaneous route used for patients with bleeding disorders

HBvaxPRO® (Sanofi Pasteur) PoM

Injection, suspension of hepatitis B surface antigen (prepared from yeast cells by recombinant DNA technique) 10 micrograms/mL adsorbed onto aluminium hydroxyphosphate sulphate, net price 0.5-mL (5-microgram) vial = £9.02, 1-mL (10-microgram) vial = £12.00; 40 micrograms/mL, 1-mL (40-microgram) vial = £29.30

Dose by intramuscular injection (see note below), ADULT and ADOLESCENT over 16 years, 3 doses of 10 micrograms, the second 1 month and the third 6 months after the first dose; CHILD under 16 years, 3 doses of 5 micrograms

Accelerated schedule, second dose 1 month after first dose, third dose 2 months after first dose with fourth dose at 12 months

Booster doses may be required in immunocompromised patients with low antibody concentration

NEONATE born to hepatitis B surface antigen-positive mother (see also notes above), 5 micrograms, first dose at birth with hepatitis B immunoglobulin injection (separate site), the second 1 month, the third 2 months and the fourth 12 months after the first dose

Chronic haemodialysis patients, by intramuscular injection (see note below) 3 doses of 40 micrograms, the second 1 month and the third 6 months after the first dose; booster doses may be required in those with low antibody concentration

Note Deltoid muscle is preferred site of injection in adults and older children; anterolateral thigh is preferred site in neonates and infants; not to be injected into the buttock (vaccine efficacy reduced); subcutaneous route used for patients with bleeding disorders

With hepatitis A vaccine

See Hepatitis A Vaccine

Human papilloma virus vaccine

Human papilloma virus vaccine is available as a bivalent vaccine (*Cervarix®*) or a quadrivalent vaccine (*Gardasil®*). Both vaccines are licensed for use in females for the prevention of cervical cancer and other pre-cancerous lesions caused by human papilloma virus types 16 and 18. In addition, *Gardasil®* is licensed for use in females for the prevention of genital warts and pre-cancerous lesions caused by human papilloma virus types 6, 11, 16, and 18.

Human papilloma virus vaccine will be most effective if given before sexual activity starts. The duration of protection has not been established, but sustained immunity has been observed in women who have been followed up for 4.5 years after completion of the primary course.

As the vaccines do not protect against all strains of human papilloma virus, routine cervical screening should continue.

See section 14.1 for general contra-indications and side-effects. Injection-site reactions are *very common* with human papilloma virus vaccine. Other side-effects include gastro-intestinal disturbances and dizziness. Headache, myalgia, and arthralgia have been reported frequently with *Cervarix*®.

> From autumn 2008, human papilloma virus vaccine will be offered to girls aged 12–13 years as part of the immunisation schedule.

Note To avoid confusion, prescribers should specify the brand to be dispensed

Cervarix® (GSK) ▼ PoM

Injection, suspension of virus-like particles of human papilloma virus type 16 (40 micrograms/mL), type 18 (40 micrograms/mL) capsid protein (prepared by recombinant DNA technique using a Baculovirus expression system) in monophosphoryl lipid A adjuvant adsorbed onto aluminium hydroxide, net price 0.5-mL prefilled syringe = £80.50

Dose by intramuscular injection into deltoid region, ADULT and CHILD 10–25 years, 3 doses of 0.5 mL, the second 1 month and the third 6 months after the first dose

Gardasil® (Sanofi Pasteur) ▼ PoM

Injection, suspension of virus-like particles of human papilloma virus type 6 (40 micrograms/mL), type 11 (80 micrograms/mL), type 16 (80 micrograms/mL), type 18 (40 micrograms/mL) capsid protein (prepared from yeast cells by recombinant DNA technique) adsorbed onto aluminium hydroxyphosphate sulphate, net price 0.5-mL prefilled syringe = £80.50

Dose by intramuscular injection preferably into deltoid region or higher anterolateral thigh, ADULT and CHILD 9–26 years, 3 doses of 0.5 mL, the second 2 months and the third 6 months after the first dose

Alternative schedule for ADULT and CHILD 9–26 years, 3 doses of 0.5 mL, the second at least 1 month, and the third at least 4 months after the first dose; schedule should be completed within 12 months

Influenza vaccine

While most viruses are antigenically stable, the influenza viruses A and B (especially A) are constantly altering their antigenic structure as indicated by changes in the haemagglutinins (H) and neuraminidases (N) on the surface of the viruses. It is essential that influenza vaccines in use contain the H and N components of the prevalent strain or strains. Every year the World Health Organization recommends which strains should be included.

The recommended strains are grown in the allantoic cavity of chick embryos (therefore **contra-indicated** in those with anaphylactic hypersensitivity to eggs).

Since **influenza vaccines** will not control epidemics they are recommended *only for persons at high risk*. Annual immunisation is strongly recommended for individuals aged over 6 months with the following conditions:

- chronic respiratory disease (includes asthma treated with continuous or repeated use of inhaled or systemic corticosteroids or asthma with previous exacerbations requiring hospital admission);
- chronic heart disease;
- chronic liver disease;
- chronic renal disease;
- diabetes mellitus requiring insulin or oral hypoglycaemic drugs;
- immunosuppression because of disease (including asplenia or splenic dysfunction) or treatment (including prolonged corticosteroid treatment);
- HIV infection (regardless of immune status).

Influenza immunisation is also recommended for all persons aged over 65 years, for residents of nursing or residential homes for the elderly and other long-stay facilities, and for carers of persons whose welfare may be at risk if the carer falls ill.

As part of winter planning, NHS employers should offer vaccination to healthcare workers who are directly involved in patient care. Employers of social care workers should consider similar action. Influenza immunisation should also be considered for household contacts of immunocompromised individuals.

Interactions: Appendix 1 (vaccines).

See section 14.1 for general contra-indications. Where possible, pregnant women and children should receive a thiomersal-free influenza vaccine; if this is not available, a thiomersal-containing influenza vaccine should be given.

Information on pandemic influenza and avian influenza may be found at www.dh.gov.uk/pandemicflu and at www.hpa.org.uk.

Inactivated Influenza Vaccine (Split Virion) (Non-proprietary) PoM

Flu

Injection, suspension of formaldehyde-inactivated influenza virus (split virion), net price 0.25-mL prefilled syringe = £6.29; 0.5-mL prefilled syringe = £6.29

Excipients may include neomycin and polymyxin

Dose by intramuscular injection, ADULT and CHILD over 13 years 0.5 mL as a single dose; CHILD 6–35 months 0.25–0.5 mL, 3–13 years 0.5 mL, in children dose repeated after 4–6 weeks if not previously vaccinated

Note Subcutaneous route used for patients with bleeding disorders

Inactivated Influenza Vaccine (Surface Antigen) (Non-proprietary) PoM

Flu or Flu(adj)

Injection, suspension of propiolactone-inactivated influenza virus (surface antigen), net price 0.5-mL prefilled syringe = £3.98

Excipients may include neomycin, polymyxin B and thiomersal

Dose by intramuscular injection, ADULT and CHILD over 13 years 0.5 mL as a single dose; CHILD 6–35 months 0.25–0.5 mL, 3–13 years 0.5 mL, in children dose repeated after 4–6 weeks if not previously vaccinated

Note Subcutaneous route used for patients with bleeding disorders

Agrippal® (Wyeth) PoM

Injection, suspension of formaldehyde-inactivated influenza virus (surface antigen), net price 0.5-mL prefilled syringe = £5.85

Excipients include kanamycin, neomycin

Dose by intramuscular injection, ADULT and CHILD over 13 years 0.5 mL as a single dose; CHILD 6–35 months 0.25–0.5 mL, 3–13 years 0.5 mL, in children dose repeated after 4–6 weeks if not previously vaccinated

Note Subcutaneous route used for patients with bleeding disorders

Begrivac® (Wyeth) PoM

Injection, suspension of formaldehyde-inactivated influenza virus (split virion), net price 0.5-mL prefilled syringe = £5.85

Excipients include polymyxin B

Dose by intramuscular injection, ADULT and CHILD over 13 years 0.5 mL as a single dose; CHILD 6–35 months 0.25–0.5 mL, 3–13 years 0.5 mL, in children dose repeated after 4–6 weeks if not previously vaccinated

Note Subcutaneous route used for patients with bleeding disorders

Enzira® (Novartis Vaccines) PoM

Injection, suspension of inactivated influenza virus (split virion), net price 0.5-mL prefilled syringe = £6.59

Excipients include neomycin and polymyxin B

Dose by intramuscular injection, ADULT and CHILD over 13 years 0.5 mL as a single dose; CHILD 6–35 months 0.25–0.5 mL, 3–13 years 0.5 mL, in children dose repeated after 4–6 weeks if not previously vaccinated

Note Subcutaneous route used for patients with bleeding disorders

Fluarix® (GSK) PoM

Injection, suspension of formaldehyde-inactivated influenza virus (split virion), net price 0.5-mL prefilled syringe = £4.49

Excipients include gentamicin and traces of thiomersal

Dose by intramuscular injection, ADULT and CHILD over 13 years 0.5 mL as a single dose; CHILD 6–35 months 0.25–0.5 mL, 3–13 years 0.5 mL, in children dose repeated after 4–6 weeks if not previously vaccinated

Note Subcutaneous route used for patients with bleeding disorders

Imuvac® (Solvay) PoM

Injection, suspension of formaldehyde-inactivated influenza virus (surface antigen), net price 0.5-mL prefilled syringe = £6.59

Excipients include gentamicin

Dose by intramuscular injection, ADULT and CHILD over 13 years, 0.5 mL as a single dose; CHILD 6–35 months 0.25–0.5 mL, 3–13 years 0.5 mL, in children dose repeated after 4–6 weeks if not previously vaccinated

Note Subcutaneous route used for patients with bleeding disorders

Influvac Sub-unit® (Solvay) PoM

Injection, suspension of formaldehyde-inactivated influenza virus (surface antigen), net price 0.5-mL prefilled syringe = £5.22

Excipients include gentamicin

Dose by intramuscular injection, ADULT and CHILD over 13 years 0.5 mL as a single dose; CHILD 6–35 months 0.25–0.5 mL, 3–13 years 0.5 mL, in children dose repeated after 4–6 weeks if not previously vaccinated

Note Subcutaneous route used for patients with bleeding disorders

Mastaflu® (MASTA) PoM

Injection, suspension of formaldehyde-inactivated influenza virus (surface antigen), net price 0.5-mL prefilled syringe = £6.50

Excipients include gentamicin

Dose by intramuscular injection, ADULT and CHILD over 13 years 0.5 mL as a single dose; CHILD 6–35 months 0.25–0.5 mL, 3–13 years 0.5 mL, in children dose repeated after 4–6 weeks if not previously vaccinated

Note Subcutaneous route used for patients with bleeding disorders

Viroflu® (Sanofi Pasteur) PoM

Injection, suspension of inactivated influenza virus (surface antigen, virosome), net price 0.5-mL prefilled syringe = £6.59

Excipients include neomycin and polymixin B

Dose by intramuscular injection, ADULT and CHILD over 13 years 0.5 mL as a single dose; CHILD 6–35 months 0.25–0.5 mL, 3–13 years 0.5 mL, in children dose repeated after 4–6 weeks if not previously vaccinated

Note Subcutaneous route used for patients with bleeding disorders

Measles vaccine

Measles vaccine has been replaced by a combined live measles, mumps and rubella vaccine (MMR vaccine) for all eligible children.

MMR vaccine may be used in the control of outbreaks of measles (see under MMR Vaccine).

◢Single antigen vaccine

No longer available in the UK

◢Combined vaccines

See MMR vaccine

Measles, Mumps and Rubella (MMR) vaccine

A combined live **measles, mumps, and rubella vaccine** (MMR vaccine) aims to eliminate measles, mumps, and rubella (and congenital rubella syndrome). Every child should receive two doses of MMR vaccine by entry to primary school, unless there is a valid contra-indication (see below). MMR vaccine should be given irrespective of previous measles, mumps or rubella infection.

The first dose of MMR vaccine is given to children aged 13 months. A second dose is given before starting school at 3–5 years of age (see schedule, section 14.1). When protection against measles is required urgently (e.g. during a measles outbreak), the second dose of MMR vaccine can be given 1 month after the first dose; if the second dose is given before 18 months of age, then children should still receive the routine dose before starting school at 3–5 years of age.

Children presenting for pre-school booster who have not received the first dose of MMR vaccine should be given a dose of MMR vaccine followed 3 months later by a second dose. At school-leaving age or at entry into further education, MMR immunisation should be offered to individuals of both sexes who have not received both doses. In a young adult who has received only a single dose of MMR in childhood, a second dose is recommended to achieve full protection.

MMR vaccine should be used to protect against rubella in *seronegative women of child-bearing age* (see schedule, section 14.1); unimmunised healthcare workers who might put pregnant women at risk of rubella (or measles) should be vaccinated. MMR vaccine may also be offered to previously *unimmunised and seronegative post-partum women*. Vaccination a few days after delivery is important because about 60% of congenital abnormalities from rubella infection occur in babies of women who have borne more than one child. Immigrants arriving after the age of school immunisation are particularly likely to require immunisation.

MMR vaccine may also be used in the control of outbreaks of measles and should be offered to susceptible children aged over 6 months who are contacts of a case, within 3 days of exposure to infection; these children should still receive routine MMR vaccinations at the recommended ages. Household contacts of a case, aged between 6 and 9 months may receive normal immunoglobulin (section 14.5). MMR vaccine is **not suitable** for prophylaxis following exposure to mumps or rubella since the antibody response to the mumps and rubella components is too slow for effective prophylaxis.

Children and adults with impaired immune response should not receive live vaccines (for advice on HIV see section 14.1). If they have been exposed to measles infection they should be given normal immunoglobulin (section 14.5).

Unimmunised travellers, including children over 6 months, to areas where measles is endemic or epidemic should receive MMR vaccine. Children immunised before 12 months of age should still receive two doses of MMR at the recommended ages.

Malaise, fever, or a rash may occur after the first dose of MMR vaccine, most commonly about a week after vaccination and lasting about 2 to 3 days (section 14.1). Leaflets are available for parents on advice for reducing fever (including the use of paracetamol). Febrile seizures occur less commonly 6 to 11 days after MMR vaccination; the incidence of febrile seizures is lower than that following measles infection. Parotid swelling occurs occasionally, usually in the third week, and rarely, arthropathy 2 to 3 weeks after immunisation. Adverse reactions are considerably less frequent after the second dose of MMR vaccine than after the first dose.

Idiopathic thrombocytopenic purpura has occurred rarely following MMR vaccination, usually within 6 weeks of the first dose. The risk of developing idiopathic thrombocytopenic purpura after MMR vaccine is much less than the risk of developing it after infection with wild measles or rubella virus. The CSM has recommended that children who develop idiopathic thrombocytopenic purpura within 6 weeks of the first dose of MMR should undergo serological testing before the second dose is due; if the results suggest incomplete immunity against measles, mumps or rubella then a second dose of MMR is recommended. The Specialist and Reference Microbiology Division, Health Protection Agency offers free serological testing for children who develop idiopathic thrombocytopenic purpura *within 6 weeks* of the first dose of MMR.

Post-vaccination aseptic meningitis was reported (rarely and with complete recovery) following vaccination with MMR vaccine containing Urabe mumps vaccine, which has now been discontinued; no cases have been confirmed in association with the currently used Jeryl Lynn mumps vaccine. Children with post-vaccination symptoms are not infectious.

> Reviews undertaken on behalf of the CSM, the Medical Research Council, and the Cochrane Collaboration, have not found any evidence of a link between MMR vaccination and bowel disease or autism. The Chief Medical Officers have advised that the MMR vaccine is the safest and best way to protect children against measles, mumps, and rubella. Information (including fact sheets and a list of references) may be obtained from:
> www.immunisation.nhs.uk and
> www.mmrthefacts.nhs.uk

Contra-indications to MMR include:

- children with severe immunosuppression (for advice on vaccines and HIV see section 14.1);
- children who have received another live vaccine by injection within 4 weeks;
- children who have had an anaphylactic reaction to excipients such as gelatin and neomycin;
- if given to women, pregnancy should be avoided for 1 month.

The Department of Health recommends avoiding rubella vaccination during pregnancy. However, if given inadvertently during pregnancy, then termination is not recommended because extensive studies have failed to link rubella vaccination in early pregnancy with fetal damage.

MMR vaccine should not be given within 3 months of an immunoglobulin injection because response to the measles component may be reduced.

Note Children with a personal or close family history of convulsions should be given MMR vaccine, provided the parents understand that there may be a febrile response. If the neurological condition is deteriorating, vaccination should be deferred until the condition is stable. Doctors should seek specialist paediatric advice rather than withhold vaccination. There is increasing evidence that MMR vaccine can be given safely even when the child has had an anaphylactic reaction to food containing egg (dislike of egg or refusal to eat egg is not a contra-indication).

See section 14.1 for general contra-indications.

Measles, Mumps and Rubella Vaccine, Live (PoM) **MMR(live)**

Live measles, mumps, and rubella vaccine

Dose by intramuscular injection, 0.5 mL (see schedule, section 14.1)

Available from health organisations or direct from Movianto as *MMR II*® (*excipients include* gelatin and neomycin) or *Priorix*® (*excipients include* neomycin)

Note Subcutaneous route used for patients with bleeding disorders

Meningococcal vaccines

Almost all childhood meningococcal disease in the UK is caused by *Neisseria meningitidis* serogroups B and C. **Meningococcal group C conjugate vaccine** protects only against infection by serogroup C. After early adulthood the risk of meningococcal disease declines, and immunisation is not generally recommended after the age of 25 years.

Childhood immunisation **Meningococcal group C conjugate vaccine** provides long-term protection against infection by serogroup C of *Neisseria meningitidis* in children from 3 months of age. Immunisation (see schedule, section 14.1) consists of 2 doses given at 3 months and 4 months of age; a booster should be given at 12 months of age, usually combined with haemophilus influenzae type b vaccine. It is recommended that meningococcal group C conjugate vaccine be given to anyone aged under 25 years who has not been vaccinated previously with this vaccine; those over 1 year receive a single dose.

A single dose of meningococcal group C conjugate vaccine is also recommended for unimmunised individuals attending university, irrespective of age.

Meningococcal group C conjugate vaccine in patients with asplenia or splenic dysfunction Meningococcal group C conjugate vaccine is recommended for patients with asplenia or splenic dysfunction. Children under 1 year should be vaccinated according to the Immunisation Schedule (section 14.1). Unimmunised adults and children over 1 year should be given 2 doses of meningococcal group C conjugate vaccine (usually combined with haemophilus influenzae type b vaccine) with an interval of 2 months between doses. Immunised adults and children who develop splenic dysfunction should be given 1 additional dose of meningococcal group C conjugate vaccine (usually combined with haemophilus influenzae type b vaccine).

Immunisation for travellers Individuals travelling to countries of risk (see below) should be immunised with a meningococcal polysaccharide vaccine that covers serotypes **A, C, W135 and Y**. Vaccination is particularly important for those living or working with local people or visiting an area of risk during outbreaks.

Countries with risk in Africa are listed below but outbreaks may also occur in countries not listed:

> Angola, Benin, Burkina Faso, Burundi, Cameroon, Central African Republic, Chad, Côte d'Ivoire, Democratic Republic of Congo, Eritrea, Ethiopia, Gambia, Ghana, Guinea, Kenya, Mali, Niger, Nigeria, Rwanda, Senegal, Somalia, Sudan, Tanzania, Togo, Uganda, and Zambia

Proof of vaccination with the tetravalent (A, C, W135 and Y) meningococcal vaccine is required for those travelling to Saudi Arabia during the Hajj and Umrah pilgrimages (where outbreaks of the W135 strain have occurred).

Travellers should be immunised with the meningococcal polysaccharide vaccine that covers serogroups A, C, W135 and Y, even if they have already received meningococcal group C conjugate vaccine. The response to serotype C in unconjugated meningococcal polysaccharide vaccines given to children aged under 18 months is not as good as in adults.

Contacts of infected individuals and laboratory workers For advice on the immunisation of *close contacts* of cases of meningococcal disease in the UK and on the role of the vaccine in the control of *local outbreaks*, consult Guidance for Public Health Management of Meningococcal Disease in the UK at www.hpa.org.uk. See Table 2, section 5.1 for antibacterial prophylaxis to prevent a secondary case of meningococcal meningitis

The need for immunisation of laboratory staff who work directly with *Neisseria meningitidis* should be considered.

Side-effects Side-effects of meningococcal group C conjugate vaccine include redness, swelling, and pain at the site of the injection, mild fever, irritability, drowsiness, dizziness, nausea, vomiting, diarrhoea, anorexia in children, headache, myalgia, rash, urticaria, pruritus, malaise, lymphadenopathy, hypotonia, paraesthesia, hypoaesthesia, and syncope. Hypersensitivity reactions (including anaphylaxis, bronchospasm, and angioedema) and seizures have been reported rarely. Symptoms of meningism have also been reported rarely, but there is no evidence that the vaccine causes meningococcal C meningitis. There have been very rare reports of Stevens-Johnson syndrome.

Meningococcal polysaccharide A, C, W135 and Y vaccine is associated with injection-site reactions and very rarely headache, fatigue, fever, and drowsiness. Hypersensitivity reactions including anaphylaxis have been reported.

See section 14.1 for general contra-indications.

◢Meningococcal group C conjugate vaccine

Meningitec® (Wyeth) PoM

Injection, suspension of capsular polysaccharide antigen of *Neisseria meningitidis* group C (conjugated to *Corynebacterium diphtheriae* protein), adsorbed onto aluminium phosphate, net price 0.5-mL vial = £17.95

Dose by intramuscular injection, ADULT and CHILD over 1 year 0.5 mL as a single dose; for routine immunisation in INFANT, 0.5 mL, see notes above and schedule, section 14.1

Note Subcutaneous route used for patients with bleeding disorders

Available as part of childhood immunisation schedule from Healthcare Logistics

Menjugate Kit® (Sanofi Pasteur, Novartis Vaccines) PoM

Injection, powder for reconstitution, capsular polysaccharide antigen of *Neisseria meningitidis* group C (conjugated to *Corynebacterium diphtheriae* protein), adsorbed onto aluminium hydroxide, single-dose vial with diluent

Dose by intramuscular injection, ADULT and CHILD over 1 year 0.5 mL as a single dose; for routine immunisation in INFANT, 0.5 mL, see notes above and schedule, section 14.1

Note Subcutaneous route used for patients with bleeding disorders

NeisVac-C® (Baxter) PoM

Injection, suspension of polysaccharide antigen of *Neisseria meningitidis* group C (conjugated to tetanus toxoid protein), adsorbed onto aluminium hydroxide, 0.5-mL prefilled syringe

Dose by intramuscular injection, ADULT and CHILD over 1 year 0.5 mL as a single dose; for routine immunisation in INFANT, 0.5 mL, see notes above and schedule, section 14.1

Note Subcutaneous route used for patients with bleeding disorders

Available from Healthcare Logistics

◢Meningococcal polysaccharide A, C, W135 and Y vaccine

ACWY Vax® (GSK) PoM

Injection, powder for reconstitution, capsular polysaccharide antigens of *Neisseria meningitidis* groups A, C, W135 and Y, net price single-dose vial (with syringe containing diluent) = £16.73

Dose by deep subcutaneous injection, ADULT and CHILD over 2 years 0.5 mL as a single dose

Note Two doses of 0.5 mL separated by an interval of 3 months can be given to INFANT 3 months–2 years [unlicensed] but antibody response may be suboptimal

◢Meningococcal Group C conjugate vaccine with Haemophilus Influenzae type B vaccine

See Haemophilus Influenzae type B vaccine

Mumps vaccine

Single antigen vaccine

No longer available in the UK

Combined vaccine

See MMR Vaccine

Pertussis vaccine

Pertussis vaccine is usually given as a combination preparation containing other vaccines (see under Diphtheria Vaccines). Acellular vaccines are derived from highly purified components of *Bordetella pertussis.*

For the routine immunisation of infants, primary immunisation with pertussis (whooping cough) vaccine is recommended in the form of 3 doses (separated by 1-month intervals) of **diphtheria, tetanus, pertussis (acellular, component), poliomyelitis (inactivated) and haemophilus type b conjugate vaccine (adsorbed)** (see schedule, section 14.1).

A booster dose should be given 3 years after the primary course; children *under 10 years* should receive *either* **adsorbed diphtheria, tetanus, pertussis (acellular, component) and inactivated poliomyelitis vaccine** *or* **adsorbed diphtheria** [low dose], **tetanus, pertussis (acellular, component) and inactivated poliomyelitis vaccine**; for children requiring a booster dose of haemophilus influenzae type b vaccine as part of a 'catch-up' programme see p. 646.

The incidence of local and systemic effects is generally lower with vaccines containing acellular pertussis components than with the whole-cell pertussis vaccine used previously. However, compared with primary vaccination, booster doses with vaccines containing acellular pertussis are reported to increase the risk of injection-site reactions (some of which affect the entire limb); local reactions do not contra-indicate further doses (see below).

The vaccine should not be withheld from children with a history to a preceding dose of:

- fever, irrespective of severity;
- persistent crying or screaming for more than 3 hours;
- severe local reaction, irrespective of extent.

These side-effects were associated with whole-cell pertussis vaccine.

Predisposition to neurological problems When there is a personal or family history of *febrile* convulsions, there is an increased risk of these occurring during fever from any cause including immunisation. In such children, immunisation is *recommended* but advice on the *prevention of fever* (see Post-immunisation pyrexia, p. 641) should be given before immunisation.

When a child has had a convulsion not associated with fever and the neurological condition is not deteriorating, immunisation is *recommended.*

Where there is a *still evolving neurological problem* including poorly controlled epilepsy, immunisation should be *deferred* and the child referred to a specialist. Immunisation is recommended if a cause for the neurological disorder is found. If a cause is not found, immunisation should be deferred until the condition is stable.

Children with stable neurological disorders (e.g. spina bifida, congenital brain abnormality, and perinatal hypoxic ischaemic encephalopathy) should be immunised according to the recommended schedule.

Older children All children up to the age of 10 years should receive primary immunisation with diphtheria, tetanus, pertussis (acellular, component), poliomyelitis (inactivated) and haemophilus type b conjugate vaccine (adsorbed). Primary immunisation against pertussis is not currently recommended in individuals over 10 years of age.

Combined vaccines

Combined vaccines, see under Diphtheria vaccines

Pneumococcal vaccines

Pneumococcal vaccines are directed against *Streptococcus pneumoniae* (pneumococcus); the vaccines contain polysaccharide from capsular pneumococci. **Pneumococcal polysaccharide vaccine** contains purified polysaccharide from 23 capsular types of pneumococci whereas **pneumococcal polysaccharide conjugate vaccine (adsorbed)** contains polysaccharide from 7 capsular types, the polysaccharide being conjugated to protein. The conjugate vaccine is effective in young children and is now part of the childhood immunisation schedule (see Choice of Vaccine below, and schedule, section 14.1).

Pneumococcal vaccination is recommended for individuals at increased risk of pneumococcal infection as follows:

- age over 65 years;
- asplenia or splenic dysfunction (including homozygous sickle cell disease and coeliac disease which could lead to splenic dysfunction);
- chronic respiratory disease (includes asthma treated with continuous or frequent use of a systemic corticosteroid);
- chronic heart disease;
- chronic renal disease;
- chronic liver disease;
- diabetes mellitus requiring insulin or oral hypoglycaemic drugs;
- immune deficiency because of disease (e.g. HIV infection) or treatment (including prolonged systemic corticosteroid treatment);
- presence of cochlear implant;
- conditions where leakage of cerebrospinal fluid may occur;
- child under 5 years with a history of invasive pneumococcal disease.

Where possible, the vaccine should be given at least 2 weeks before splenectomy, cochlear implant surgery, and chemotherapy; patients should be given advice about increased risk of pneumococcal infection. A

14 Immunological products and vaccines

patient card and information leaflet for patients with asplenia are available from the Department of Health or in Scotland from the Scottish Executive, Public Health Division 1 (Tel (0131) 244 2501). Prophylactic antibacterial therapy against pneumococcal infection should not be stopped after immunisation.

Choice of vaccine The 7-valent **pneumococcal polysaccharide conjugate vaccine (adsorbed)** is now a component of the primary course of childhood immunisation. The recommended schedule consists of 3 doses, the first at 2 months of age, the second at 4 months, and the third at 13 months (see schedule, section 14.1).

Children at increased risk of pneumococcal infection (see list above) should receive **pneumococcal polysaccharide conjugate vaccine (adsorbed)** at the recommended ages, followed by a single dose of the 23-valent pneumococcal polysaccharide vaccine after their second birthday (see below). Children at increased risk of pneumococcal infection presenting late for vaccination should receive 2 doses (separated by at least 1 month) of pneumococcal polysaccharide conjugate vaccine (adsorbed) before the age of 12 months, and a third dose at 13 months. Children over 12 months and under 5 years (who have not been vaccinated or not completed the primary course) should receive a single dose of pneumococcal polysaccharide conjugate vaccine (adsorbed) (2 doses separated by an interval of 2 months in the immunocompromised or those with asplenia or splenic dysfunction). All children under 5 years at increased risk of pneumococcal infection should receive a single dose of the 23-valent **pneumococcal polysaccharide vaccine** after their second birthday (and at least 2 months after the final dose of the 7-valent pneumococcal polysaccharide conjugate vaccine (adsorbed)).

Children over 5 years and adults who are at increased risk of pneumococcal disease should receive a single dose of the 23-valent unconjugated **pneumococcal polysaccharide vaccine**.

Revaccination In individuals with higher concentrations of antibodies to pneumococcal polysaccharides, revaccination with the 23-valent pneumococcal polysaccharide vaccine more commonly produces adverse reactions. Revaccination is therefore not recommended, except every 5 years in individuals in whom the antibody concentration is likely to decline rapidly (e.g. asplenia, splenic dysfunction and nephrotic syndrome). If there is doubt, the need for revaccination should be discussed with a haematologist, immunologist, or microbiologist.

See section 14.1 for general contra-indications.

◢Pneumococcal polysaccharide vaccines

Pneumovax® II (Sanofi Pasteur) PoM

Polysaccharide from each of 23 capsular types of pneumococcus, net price 0.5-mL vial = £8.83

Dose by intramuscular injection, 0.5 mL; revaccination, see notes above; INFANT under 2 years, not recommended (suboptimal response and also safety and efficacy not established)

◢Pneumococcal polysaccharide conjugate vaccine (adsorbed)

Prevenar® (Wyeth) ▼ PoM

Polysaccharide from each of 7 capsular types of pneumococcus (conjugated to diphtheria toxoid) adsorbed onto aluminium phosphate, net price 0.5-mL prefilled syringe = £34.50

Dose by intramuscular injection, 0.5 mL (see notes above and schedule, section 14.1)

Note Deltoid muscle is preferred site of injection in young children; anterolateral thigh is preferred site in infants

The dose in the BNF may differ from that in product literature

Poliomyelitis vaccines

There are two types of poliomyelitis vaccine, inactivated poliomyelitis vaccine and live (oral) poliomyelitis vaccine. **Inactivated poliomyelitis vaccine** is now recommended for routine immunisation; it is given by injection and contains inactivated strains of human poliovirus types 1, 2 and 3.

A course of primary immunisation consists of 3 doses of a combined preparation containing inactivated poliomyelitis vaccine (see under Diphtheria Vaccines), starting at 2 months of age with intervals of 1 month between doses (see schedule, section 14.1). A course of 3 doses should also be given to all unimmunised adults; no adult should remain unimmunised against poliomyelitis.

Two booster doses of a preparation containing inactivated poliomyelitis vaccine are recommended, the first before school entry and the second before leaving school (see schedule, section 14.1). Further booster doses are only necessary for adults at special risk, such as travellers to endemic areas, or laboratory staff likely to be exposed to the viruses, or healthcare workers in possible contact with cases; booster doses should be given to such individuals every 10 years.

Preparations containing inactivated poliomyelitis vaccine may be used to complete an immunisation course initiated with the live (oral) poliomyelitis vaccine. Live (oral) poliomyelitis vaccine is available only for use during outbreaks. The live (oral) vaccine poses a very rare risk of vaccine-associated paralytic polio because the attenuated strain of the virus can revert to a virulent form. For this reason the live (oral) vaccine must **not** be used for immunosuppressed individuals or their household contacts. The use of inactivated poliomyelitis vaccine removes the risk of vaccine-associated paralytic polio altogether.

Travellers Unimmunised travellers to areas with a high incidence of poliomyelitis should receive a full course of a preparation containing inactivated poliomyelitis vaccine. Those who have not been vaccinated in the last 10 years should receive a booster dose of adsorbed diphtheria [low dose], tetanus and inactivated poliomyelitis vaccine. A list of countries with a high incidence of poliomyelitis can be obtained from www.travax.nhs.uk or by contacting the National Travel Health Network and Centre.

Inactivated (Salk)

Combined vaccines, see under Diphtheria Vaccines

Inactivated Poliomyelitis Vaccine (Non-proprietary) PoM

IPV

Injection, inactivated suspension of suitable strains of poliomyelitis virus, types 1, 2, and 3, net price 0.5-mL prefilled syringe = £10.35

Excipients may include neomycin, polymyxin B and streptomycin

Note Not recommended for routine use—combination vaccines are recommended for primary immunisation and for boosters (see schedule, section 14.1)

Live (oral) (Sabin)

Poliomyelitis Vaccine, Live (Oral) (GSK) PoM

OPV

A suspension of suitable live attenuated strains of poliomyelitis virus, types 1, 2, and 3. Available in single-dose and 10-dose containers

Excipients include neomycin and polymyxin B

Dose control of outbreaks, 3 drops; may be given on a lump of sugar; not to be given with foods which contain preservatives

Note Live poliomyelitis vaccine loses potency once the container has been opened—any vaccine remaining at the end of an immunisation session should be discarded; whenever possible sessions should be arranged to avoid undue wastage.

Rabies vaccine

The licensed rabies vaccines, the human diploid cell vaccine and the purified chick embryo cell vaccine are both cell-derived.

Pre-exposure prophylaxis Immunisation should be offered to those at high risk of exposure to rabies—laboratory staff who handle the rabies virus, those working in quarantine stations, animal handlers, veterinary surgeons and field workers who are likely to be bitten by infected wild animals, certain port officials, and bat handlers. Transmission of rabies by humans has not been recorded but it is advised that those caring for patients with the disease should be vaccinated.

Immunisation against rabies is also recommended where there is limited access to prompt medical care for those living in areas where rabies is enzootic, for those travelling to such areas for longer than 1 month, and for those on shorter visits who may be exposed to unusual risk.

Immunisation against rabies is indicated during pregnancy if there is substantial risk of exposure to rabies and rapid access to post-exposure prophylaxis is likely to be limited.

Up-to-date country-by-country information on the incidence of rabies can be obtained from the National Travel Health Network and Centre (www.nathnac.org) and, in Scotland, from Health Protection Scotland (www.hps.scot.nhs.uk).

Immunisation against rabies requires 3 doses of rabies vaccine, with further booster doses for those who remain at continued risk (see under preparations below for details of regimens). To ensure protection in persons at high risk (e.g. laboratory workers), the concentration of antirabies antibodies in plasma is used to determine the intervals between doses.

Post-exposure management Following potential exposure to rabies, the wound or site of exposure (e.g. mucous membrane) should be cleansed under running water and washed for several minutes with soapy water as soon as possible after exposure. Disinfectant and a simple dressing may be applied, but suturing should be delayed because it may increase the risk of introducing rabies virus into the nerves.

Post-exposure prophylaxis against rabies depends on the level of risk in the country, the nature of exposure, and the individual's immunity. In each case, expert risk assessment and advice on appropriate management should be obtained from the Health Protection Agency Virus Reference Department, Colindale, London (tel. (020) 8200 4400) or the Centre for Infections (tel. (020) 8200 6868), in Scotland from Health Protection Scotland (tel. (0141) 300 1100), in Northern Ireland from the Public Health Laboratory, Belfast City Hospital (tel. (028) 9032 9241).

There are no specific contra-indications to the use of rabies vaccine for post-exposure prophylaxis and its use should be considered whenever a patient has been attacked by an animal in a country where rabies is enzootic, even if there is no direct evidence of rabies in the attacking animal. Because of the potential consequences of untreated rabies exposure and because rabies vaccination has not been associated with fetal abnormalities, pregnancy is not considered a contra-indication to post-exposure prophylaxis.

For post-exposure prophylaxis of *fully immunised* individuals (who have previously received pre-exposure or post-exposure prophylaxis with cell-derived rabies vaccine), 2 doses of cell-derived vaccine, separated by 3 days, are likely to be sufficient. Rabies immunoglobulin is not necessary in such cases.

Post-exposure treatment for *unimmunised individuals* (or those whose prophylaxis is possibly incomplete) comprises 5 doses of rabies vaccine given over 1 month (on days 0, 3, 7, 14, and 30); also, depending on the level of risk (determined by factors such as the nature of the bite and the country where it was sustained), rabies immunoglobulin is given on day 0 (section 14.5). The course may be discontinued if it is proved that the individual was not at risk.

Rabies Vaccine (Sanofi Pasteur) PoM

Rab

Freeze-dried inactivated Wistar rabies virus strain PM/WI 38 1503-3M cultivated in human diploid cells, net price single-dose vial with syringe containing diluent = £24.40

Excipients include neomycin

Dose prophylactic, by deep subcutaneous *or* intramuscular injection in the deltoid region, 1 mL on days 0, 7, and 28; also booster doses every 2–3 years to those at continued risk

Post-exposure, by deep subcutaneous *or* intramuscular injection in the deltoid region, 1 mL, see notes above

Also available from local designated centres (special workers and post-exposure treatment)

Rabipur® (Novartis Vaccines) PoM

Freeze-dried inactivated Flury LEP rabies virus strain cultivated in chick embryo cells, net price single-dose vial = £24.40

Excipients include neomycin

Dose prophylactic, by intramuscular injection in the deltoid muscle or anterolateral thigh in small children, 1 mL on days 0, 7 and 21 or 28; also booster doses every 2–5 years for those at continued risk

Post-exposure, by intramuscular injection in the deltoid muscle or anterolateral thigh in small children, 1 mL, see notes above

Rotavirus vaccine

Rotavirus vaccine (live, oral) is licensed for immunisation of infants over 6 weeks of age for protection against gastro-enteritis caused by rotavirus infection.

Rotavirus vaccine is contra-indicated in individuals with immunodeficiency and in those predisposed to, or with a history of, intussusception. The administration of rotavirus vaccine should be postponed in infants with diarrhoea or vomiting.

The rotavirus vaccine virus is excreted in the stool and may be transmitted to close contacts; the vaccine should be used with caution in those with immunosuppressed close contacts. Carers of a recently vaccinated baby should be advised of the need to wash their hands after changing the baby's nappies.

Side-effects of rotavirus vaccine include diarrhoea, vomiting, anorexia, abdominal pain, fever, and irritability; *rarely* muscle cramps and rash.

Rotarix® (GSK) ▼ PoM

Oral suspension, powder for reconstitution, live attenuated rotavirus (RIX4414 strain), net price single-dose vial (with syringe containing diluent) = £41.38

Dose by mouth INFANT over 6 weeks, 2 doses of 1 mL separated by an interval of at least 4 weeks; course should be completed before 24 weeks of age (preferably before 16 weeks)

Rubella vaccine

A combined measles, mumps and rubella vaccine (MMR vaccine) aims to eliminate rubella (German measles) and congenital rubella syndrome. MMR vaccine is used for childhood vaccination as well as for vaccinating adults (including women of child-bearing age) who do not have immunity against rubella.

◢Single antigen vaccine

No longer available in the UK; the combined live measles, mumps and rubella vaccine is a suitable alternative (see MMR vaccine, p. 651)

◢Combined vaccines

see MMR vaccine

Smallpox vaccine

Limited supplies of **smallpox vaccine** are held at the Specialist and Reference Microbiology Division, Health Protection Agency (Tel. (020) 8200 4400) for the exclusive use of workers in laboratories where pox viruses (such as vaccinia) are handled.

If a wider use of the vaccine is being considered, *Guidelines for smallpox response and management in the post-eradication era* should be consulted at www.dh.gov.uk

Tetanus vaccines

Tetanus vaccines stimulate production of a protective antitoxin. In general, adsorption on aluminium hydroxide or aluminium phosphate improves antigenicity.

Primary immunisation for children under 10 years consists of 3 doses of a combined preparation containing adsorbed tetanus vaccine, with an interval of 1 month between doses (see schedule, section 14.1).

The recommended schedule of tetanus vaccination not only gives protection against tetanus in childhood but also gives the basic immunity for subsequent booster doses (see schedule, section 14.1).

For primary immunisation of adults and children over 10 years previously unimmunised against tetanus, 3 doses of adsorbed diphtheria [low dose], tetanus and inactivated poliomyelitis vaccine are given with an interval of 1 month between doses (see under Diphtheria Vaccines).

Following routine childhood vaccination, 2 booster doses of a preparation containing adsorbed tetanus vaccine are recommended, the first before school entry and the second before leaving school.

If an individual presents for a booster dose but has been vaccinated following a tetanus-prone wound, the vaccine preparation administered at the time of injury should be determined. If this is not possible, the booster should still be given to ensure adequate protection against all antigens in the booster vaccine. An adult who has received 5 doses of tetanus vaccine is likely to have life-long immunity. Active immunisation is important for individuals who may not have completed a course of immunisation. Adults and children over 10 years may be given a course of adsorbed diphtheria [low dose], tetanus and inactivated poliomyelitis vaccine.

Very rarely, tetanus has developed after abdominal surgery; patients awaiting elective surgery should be asked about tetanus immunisation and immunised if necessary. Parenteral drug abuse is also associated with tetanus; those abusing drugs by injection should be vaccinated if unimmunised. Booster doses should be given if there is any doubt about the immunisation status. All laboratory staff should be offered a primary course if unimmunised.

For travel recommendations see section 14.6.

Wounds Wounds are considered to be tetanus-prone if they are sustained more than 6 hours before surgical treatment *or* at any interval after injury and are puncture-type (particularly if contaminated with soil or manure) *or* show much devitalised tissue *or* are septic *or* are compound fractures *or* contain foreign bodies. All wounds should receive thorough cleansing.

- For *clean wounds*, fully immunised individuals (those who have received a total of 5 doses of a tetanus-containing vaccine at appropriate intervals) and those whose primary immunisation is complete (with boosters up to date), do not require tetanus vaccine; individuals whose primary immunisation is incomplete or whose boosters are not up to date require a reinforcing dose of a tetanus-containing vaccine (followed by further doses as required to complete the schedule); non-immunised individuals (or whose immunisation status is not known or who have been fully immunised but are now immunocompromised) should be given a dose of the appropriate tetanus-containing vaccine immediately (followed by completion of the full course of the vaccine if records confirm the need).
- For *tetanus-prone wounds*, management is as for clean wounds with the addition of a dose of tetanus immunoglobulin (section 14.5) given at a different site; in fully immunised individuals and those whose primary immunisation is complete (see above) the immunoglobulin is needed only if the risk of infec-

tion is especially high (e.g. contamination with manure). Antibacterial prophylaxis (with benzylpenicillin, co-amoxiclav, or metronidazole) may also be required for tetanus-prone wounds.

See section 14.1 for general contra-indications.

See also Predisposition to Neurological Problems, p. 654.

Combined vaccines

See Diphtheria Vaccines

Tick-borne encephalitis vaccine

Tick-borne encephalitis vaccine is licensed for immunisation of those in high-risk areas based on official recommendations (see section 14.6). Those working, walking or camping in warm forested areas of Central and Eastern Europe and Scandinavia, particularly from April to October when ticks are most prevalent, are at greatest risk of tick-borne encephalitis. Ideally, immunisation should be completed at least one month before travel.

Fever exceeding 40°C may occur, particularly after the first dose of tick-borne encephalitis vaccine. Tick-borne encephalitis vaccine is **contra-indicated** in those with acute febrile infection and severe hypersensitivity to egg protein. See section 14.1 for general contra-indications and side-effects.

TicoVac® (MASTA) PoM

Injection, suspension, inactivated Neudörfl tick-borne encephalitis virus strain (cultivated in chick embryo cells) adsorbed onto hydrated aluminium hydroxide, net price 0.25-mL prefilled syringe (*TicoVac Junior®*) = £32.00, 0.5-mL prefilled syringe = £32.00

Excipients include gentamicin and neomycin

Dose ADULT and ADOLESCENT over 16 years by intramuscular injection in deltoid muscle, 3 doses each of 0.5 mL, second dose after 1–3 months and third dose after further 5–12 months; CHILD 1–16 years 3 doses of 0.25 mL, second dose after 1–3 months and third dose after further 5–12 months; ELDERLY over 60 years and immunocompromised (including those receiving immunosuppressants), antibody concentration may be measured 4 weeks after second dose and dose repeated if protective levels not achieved

Note To achieve more rapid protection, second dose may be given 14 days after first dose

First booster dose given within 3 years after third dose, subsequent boosters after 3–5 years

Typhoid vaccines

Typhoid immunisation is advised for travellers to areas where sanitation standards may be poor, although it is not a substitute for scrupulous personal hygiene (see p. 663). Immunisation is also advised for laboratory workers handling specimens from suspected cases.

Capsular **polysaccharide typhoid vaccine** is usually given by *intramuscular injection*. Young children may respond suboptimally to the vaccine, but children aged between 12 and 18 months should be immunised if the risk of typhoid fever is considered high (immunisation is not recommended for infants under 12 months). Booster doses are needed every 3 years on continued exposure. Local reactions, including pain, swelling or erythema, may appear 48–72 hours after administration.

An **oral typhoid vaccine** is also available. It is a **live attenuated** vaccine contained in an enteric-coated capsule. It is taken by mouth as 3 doses of one capsule on alternate days, providing protection 7–10 days after the last dose. Protection may persist for up to 3 years in those constantly (or repeatedly) exposed to *Salmonella typhi*, but occasional travellers require further courses at intervals of 1 year. Oral typhoid vaccine is **contra-indicated** in individuals who are immunosuppressed (whether due to a disease or its treatment) and in acute gastro-intestinal illness; it is inactivated by concomitant administration of antibacterials. Administration of a dose of oral typhoid vaccine should be coordinated so that *mefloquine* is not taken for at least 12 hours before or after a dose; vaccination with oral typhoid vaccine should preferably be completed at least 3 days before the first dose of mefloquine or other antimalarials (except proguanil hydrochloride with atovaquone, which may be given concomitantly). Side-effects to oral typhoid vaccine include nausea, vomiting, abdominal pain, diarrhoea, headache, fever, and hypersensitivity reactions including, rarely, anaphylaxis.

For general contra-indications to vaccines, see section 14.1.

Polysaccharide vaccine for injection

Typherix® (GSK) PoM

Injection, Vi capsular polysaccharide typhoid vaccine, 50 micrograms/mL virulence polysaccharide antigen of *Salmonella typhi*, net price 0.5-mL prefilled syringe = £9.93

Dose by intramuscular injection, 0.5 mL; CHILD under 2 years may show suboptimal response (see notes above)

Note Subcutaneous route used for patients with bleeding disorders

Typhim Vi® (Sanofi Pasteur) PoM

Injection, Vi capsular polysaccharide typhoid vaccine, 50 micrograms/mL virulence polysaccharide antigen of formaldehyde-inactivated *Salmonella typhi*, net price 0.5-mL prefilled syringe = £9.49

Dose by intramuscular injection, 0.5 mL; CHILD under 18 months may show suboptimal response (see notes above)

Note Subcutaneous route used for patients with bleeding disorders

Polysaccharide vaccine with hepatitis A vaccine

See Hepatitis A Vaccine

Live Oral vaccine

Vivotif® (MASTA) PoM

Capsules, e/c, live attenuated *Salmonella typhi* (Ty21a), net price 3-cap pack = £8.00. Label: 23, 25, counselling, administration

Dose ADULT and CHILD over 6 years, 1 capsule on days 1, 3, and 5

Counselling Swallow as soon as possible after placing in mouth with a cold or lukewarm drink; it is important to store capsules in a refrigerator

Varicella–zoster vaccine

Varicella–zoster vaccine (live) is licensed for immunisation against varicella in seronegative individuals. It is not recommended for routine use in children but can be given to seronegative healthy children over 1 year who come into close contact with individuals at high risk of severe varicella infections. The Department of Health recommends varicella–zoster vaccine for seronegative healthcare workers who come into direct contact with patients. Those with a history of chickenpox or shingles can be considered immune, but healthcare workers with a negative or uncertain history should be tested.

Varicella–zoster vaccine is contra-indicated in pregnancy (avoid pregnancy for 3 months after vaccination). It must not be given to individuals with primary or acquired immunodeficiency or to individuals receiving immunosuppressive therapy. For further contra-indications, see section 14.1.

Rarely, the varicella–zoster vaccine virus has been transmitted from the vaccinated individual to close contacts. Therefore, contact with the following should be avoided if a vaccine-related cutaneous rash develops within 4–6 weeks of the first or second dose:

- varicella-susceptible pregnant women;
- individuals at high risk of severe varicella, including those with immunodeficiency or those receiving immunosuppressive therapy.

Healthcare workers who develop a generalised papular or vesicular rash on vaccination should avoid contact with patients until the lesions have crusted. Those who develop a localised rash after vaccination should cover the lesions and be allowed to continue working unless in contact with patients at high risk of severe varicella.

For reference to specific **varicella–zoster immunoglobulin** see section 14.5.

Varilrix® (GSK) ▼ PoM
Injection, powder for reconstitution, live attenuated varicella–zoster virus (Oka strain) propagated in human diploid cells, net price 0.5-mL vial (with diluent) = £27.31
Excipients include neomycin
Dose by subcutaneous injection preferably into deltoid region, ADULT and ADOLESCENT over 13 years (see notes above), 2 doses of 0.5 mL separated by an interval of 8 weeks (minimum 6 weeks); CHILD 1–12 years (but see notes above), 0.5 mL as a single dose

Varivax® (Sanofi Pasteur) ▼ PoM
Injection powder for reconstitution, live attenuated varicella-zoster virus (Oka/Merck strain) propagated in human diploid cells, net price 0.5-mL vial (with diluent) = £32.14
Excipients include gelatin and neomycin
Dose by subcutaneous injection into deltoid region or higher anterolateral thigh, ADULT and ADOLESCENT over 13 years (see notes above), 2 doses of 0.5 mL separated by 4–8 weeks; CHILD 1–12 years (but see notes above), 0.5 mL as a single dose (2 doses separated by 12 weeks in children with asymptomatic HIV infection)

Yellow fever vaccine

Live yellow fever vaccine is indicated for those travelling or living in areas where infection is endemic (see p. 663) and for laboratory staff who handle the virus or who handle clinical material from suspected cases. Infants under 6 months of age should not be vaccinated because there is a small risk of encephalitis; infants aged 6–9 months should be vaccinated only if the risk of yellow fever is high and unavoidable. The immunity which probably lasts for life is officially accepted for 10 years starting from 10 days after primary immunisation and for a further 10 years immediately after revaccination.

The vaccine should not be given to those with impaired immune responsiveness, or who have had an anaphylactic reaction to egg; it should not be given during pregnancy but if a significant risk of exposure cannot be avoided then vaccination should be delayed to the third trimester if possible (but the need for immunisation usually outweighs risk to the fetus). See section 14.1 for further contra-indications.

Headache, fever, tiredness, and stiffness may occur 4–7 days after vaccination. Other side-effects include myalgia, asthenia, lymphadenopathy, rash, urticaria, and injection-site reactions, *very rarely*, neurological disorders (such as meningoencephalitis) and viscerotropic disease have been reported.

Yellow Fever Vaccine, Live PoM
Yel(live)
Injection, powder for reconstitution, preparation of 17D strain of yellow fever virus grown in fertilized hens eggs
Dose by deep subcutaneous injection, 0.5 mL
Available (only to designated Yellow Fever Vaccination centres) as *Arilvax®* (*excipients include* gelatin) and *Stamaril®*

14.5 Immunoglobulins

Human immunoglobulins have replaced immunoglobulins of animal origin (antisera) which were frequently associated with hypersensitivity. Injection of immunoglobulins produces immediate protection lasting for several weeks.

Immunoglobulins are produced from pooled human plasma or serum, and are tested and found non-reactive for hepatitis B surface antigen and for antibodies against hepatitis C virus and human immunodeficiency virus (types 1 and 2)

The two types of human immunoglobulin preparation are **normal immunoglobulin** and **specific immunoglobulins**.

Further information about immunoglobulins is included in *Immunisation against Infectious Disease* (see section 14.1) and in the Health Protection Agency's *Immunoglobulin Handbook* www.hpa.org.uk.

Availability **Normal immunoglobulin** is available from Health Protection and microbiology laboratories only for contacts and the control of outbreaks. It is available commercially for other purposes.

Specific immunoglobulins are available from Health Protection and microbiology laboratories with the exception of **tetanus immunoglobulin** which is distributed through BPL to hospital pharmacies or blood transfusion departments and is also available to general medical practitioners. **Rabies immunoglobulin** is available from the Specialist and Reference Microbiology Division, Health Protection Agency. The large amounts of **hepatitis B immunoglobulin** required by transplant centres should be obtained commercially.

In Scotland all immunoglobulins are available from the *Blood Transfusion Service*. **Tetanus immunoglobulin** is distributed by the *Blood Transfusion Service* to hospitals and general medical practitioners on demand.

Normal immunoglobulin

Human **normal immunoglobulin** ('HNIG') is prepared from pools of at least 1000 donations of human plasma; it contains antibody to measles, mumps, varicella, hepatitis A, and other viruses that are currently prevalent in the general population.

Cautions and side-effects Normal immunoglobulin is **contra-indicated** in patients with known class-specific antibody to immunoglobulin A (IgA).

> **CHM advice**
> Intravenous normal immunoglobulin may very rarely induce thromboembolic events and should be used with caution in those with risk factors for arterial or venous thrombotic events and in obese individuals.

Normal immunoglobulin may **interfere with the immune response to live virus vaccines** which should therefore only be given **at least 3 weeks before or 3 months after** an injection of normal immunoglobulin (this does not apply to yellow fever vaccine since normal immunoglobulin does not contain antibody to this virus).

Side-effects of immunoglobulins include malaise, chills, fever, and rarely anaphylaxis.

Uses Normal immunoglobulin is administered by intramuscular injection for the protection of susceptible contacts against **hepatitis A** virus (infectious hepatitis), **measles** and, to a lesser extent, **rubella**.

Special formulations of immunoglobulins for intravenous administration are available for *replacement therapy* for patients with congenital agammaglobulinaemia and hypogammaglobulinaemia, for the treatment of idiopathic thrombocytopenic purpura and Kawasaki syndrome, and for the prophylaxis of infection following bone-marrow transplantation and in children with symptomatic HIV infection who have recurrent bacterial infections. Normal immunoglobulin may also be given intramuscularly or subcutaneously for replacement therapy, but intravenous formulations are normally preferred.

Intravenous immunoglobulin is also used in the treatment of Guillain-Barré syndrome in preference to plasma exchange.

Hepatitis A **Hepatitis A vaccine** is preferred for individuals at risk of infection (see p. 647) including those visiting areas where the disease is highly endemic (all countries excluding Northern and Western Europe, North America, Japan, Australia, and New Zealand). In unimmunised individuals, transmission of hepatitis A is reduced by good hygiene. Intramuscular normal immunoglobulin is no longer recommended for routine prophylaxis in travellers but it may be indicated for immunocompromised patients if their antibody response to vaccine is unlikely to be adequate.

Intramuscular normal immunoglobulin is of value in the prevention of infection in close contacts of confirmed cases of hepatitis A where there has been a delay of more than 7 days in identifying contacts, or for close contacts at high risk of severe disease.

Measles Intramuscular normal immunoglobulin may be given to prevent or attenuate an attack of measles in individuals who do not have adequate immunity. Children and adults with compromised immunity who have come into contact with measles should receive intramuscular normal immunoglobulin as soon as possible after exposure. It is most effective if given within 72 hours but can be effective if given within 6 days. For individuals receiving intravenous immunoglobulin, 100 mg/kg given within 3 weeks before measles exposure should prevent measles. Intramuscular normal immunoglobulin should also be considered for the following individuals if they have been in contact with a confirmed case of measles or with a person associated with a local outbreak:

- non-immune pregnant women;
- infants under 9 months.

Further advice should be sought from the Centre for Infections, Health Protection Agency (tel. (020) 8200 6868).

Individuals with normal immunity who are not in the above categories and who have not been fully immunised against measles, can be given MMR vaccine (section 14.4) for prophylaxis following exposure to measles.

Rubella Intramuscular immunoglobulin after exposure to rubella does **not** prevent infection in non-immune contacts and is **not** recommended for protection of pregnant women exposed to rubella. It may, however, reduce the likelihood of a clinical attack which may possibly reduce the risk to the fetus. It should be used only if termination of pregnancy would be unacceptable to the pregnant woman, when it should be given as soon as possible after exposure. Serological follow-up of recipients is essential. For routine prophylaxis, see MMR vaccine (p. 651).

For intramuscular use

Normal Immunoglobulin PoM

Normal immunoglobulin injection. 250-mg vial; 750-mg vial

Dose by deep intramuscular injection, to control outbreaks of hepatitis A (see notes above), 500 mg; CHILD under 10 years 250 mg

Measles prophylaxis, CHILD under 1 year 250 mg, 1–2 years 500 mg, 3 years and over 750 mg

Rubella in pregnancy, prevention of clinical attack, 750 mg

Available from the Centre for Infections and other regional Health Protection Agency offices (for contacts and control of outbreaks only, see above)

For subcutaneous use

Subcuvia® (Baxter BioScience) PoM

Normal immunoglobulin injection, net price 5-mL vial = £32.56, 10-mL vial = £65.12

Dose by subcutaneous injection, antibody deficiency syndromes, consult product literature

Note May be administered by intramuscular injection (if subcutaneous route not possible) but **not** for patients with thrombocytopenia or other bleeding disorders

Subgam® (BPL) PoM

Normal immunoglobulin injection, net price 250-mg vial = £11.20, 750-mg vial = £28.50, 1500-mg vial = £57.00

Dose by subcutaneous injection, antibody deficiency syndromes, consult product literature

Note May be administered by intramuscular injection (if subcutaneous route not possible) but **not** for patients with thrombocytopenia or other bleeding disorders

Vivaglobin® (CSL Behring) PoM

Normal immunoglobulin injection, net price 3-mL vial = £17.76, 10-mL vial = £59.20

Dose by subcutaneous injection, antibody deficiency syndromes, consult product literature

For intravenous use

Normal Immunoglobulin for Intravenous Use PoM
Brands include *Flebogamma® 5%* (0.5 g, 2.5 g, 5 g, 10 g); *Gammagard® S/D* (0.5 g, 2.5 g, 5 g, 10 g); *Octagam®* (2.5 g, 5 g, 10 g); *Sandoglobulin®* NF Liquid (6 g, 12 g); *Vigam® S* (2.5 g, 5 g); *Vigam® Liquid* (2.5 g, 5 g, 10 g)
Dose consult product literature

Specific immunoglobulins

Specific immunoglobulins are prepared by pooling the plasma of selected donors with high levels of the specific antibody required.

Although a hepatitis B vaccine is now available for those at high risk of infection, specific **hepatitis B immunoglobulin** ('HBIG') is available for use in association with hepatitis B vaccine for the prevention of infection in laboratory and other personnel who have been accidentally inoculated with hepatitis B virus, and in infants born to mothers who have become infected with this virus in pregnancy or who are high-risk carriers (see Hepatitis B Vaccine, p. 648).

Following exposure of an unimmunised individual to an animal in or from a high-risk country, the site of the bite should be washed with soapy water and specific **rabies immunoglobulin** of human origin administered; as much of the dose as possible should be injected in and around the cleansed wound. Rabies vaccine should also be given (for details see Rabies Vaccine, p. 656).

For the management of tetanus-prone wounds, **tetanus immunoglobulin** of human origin ('HTIG') should be used in addition to wound cleansing and, where appropriate, antibacterial prophylaxis and a tetanus-containing vaccine (section 14.4). Tetanus immunoglobulin, together with metronidazole (section 5.1.11) and wound cleansing, should also be used for the treatment of established cases of tetanus.

Varicella–zoster immunoglobulin (VZIG) is recommended for individuals who are at increased risk of severe varicella *and* who have no antibodies to varicella–zoster virus *and* who have significant exposure to chickenpox or herpes zoster. Those at increased risk include:

- neonates whose mothers develop chickenpox in the period 7 days before to 7 days after delivery;
- susceptible neonates exposed in the first 7 days of life;
- susceptible neonates or infants exposed whilst requiring intensive or prolonged special care nursing;
- susceptible women exposed at any stage of pregnancy (but when supplies of VZIG are short, may only be issued to those exposed in the first 20 weeks' gestation or to those near term) providing VZIG is given within 10 days of contact;
- immunosuppressed individuals including those who have received corticosteroids in the previous 3 months at the following dose equivalents of prednisolone; *children* 2 mg/kg daily for at least 1 week or 1 mg/kg daily for 1 month; *adults* about 40 mg daily for more than 1 week.

Important: for full details consult *Immunisation against Infectious Disease*. **Varicella–zoster vaccine** is available—see section 14.4.

Hepatitis B

Hepatitis B Immunoglobulin PoM
See notes above
Dose by intramuscular injection (as soon as possible after exposure; ideally within 12 hours, but no later than 7 days after exposure), ADULT and CHILD over 10 years 500 units; CHILD under 5 years 200 units, 5–9 years 300 units; NEONATE 200 units as soon as possible after birth; for full details consult *Immunisation against Infectious Disease*
Available from selected Health Protection Agency and NHS laboratories (except for Transplant Centres, see p. 659), also available from BPL
Note Hepatitis B immunoglobulin for intravenous use is available from BPL on a named-patient basis

Rabies

Rabies Immunoglobulin PoM
(Antirabies Immunoglobulin Injection)
See notes above
Dose 20 units/kg by infiltration in and around the cleansed wound; if wound not visible or healed or if infiltration of whole volume not possible, give remainder by intramuscular injection into anterolateral thigh (remote from vaccination site)
Available from Specialist and Reference Microbiology Division, Health Protection Agency (also from BPL)

Tetanus

Tetanus Immunoglobulin PoM
(Antitetanus Immunoglobulin Injection)
See notes above
Dose by intramuscular injection, prophylactic 250 units, increased to 500 units if more than 24 hours have elapsed or there is risk of heavy contamination or following burns
Therapeutic, 150 units/kg (multiple sites)
Available from BPL
Note May be difficult to obtain

Tetanus Immunoglobulin for Intravenous Use PoM
Used for proven or suspected clinical tetanus
Dose by intravenous infusion, 5000–10 000 units
Available from BPL on a named-patient basis and from the Northern Ireland Blood Transfusion Service

Varicella–zoster

Varicella–Zoster Immunoglobulin PoM
(Antivaricella–zoster Immunoglobulin)
See notes above
Dose by deep intramuscular injection, prophylaxis (as soon as possible—not later than 10 days after exposure), NEONATE, INFANT and CHILD up to 5 years 250 mg, 6–10 years 500 mg, 11–14 years 750 mg, over 15 years 1 g; give second dose if further exposure occurs more than 3 weeks after first dose
Note No evidence that effective in treatment of severe disease. Normal immunoglobulin for intravenous use may be used in those unable to receive intramuscular injections
Available from selected Health Protection Agency and NHS laboratories (also from BPL)

Anti-D (Rh_0) immunoglobulin

Anti-D (Rh_0) immunoglobulin is available to prevent a rhesus-negative mother from forming antibodies to fetal rhesus-positive cells which may pass into the maternal circulation. The objective is to protect any subsequent child from the hazard of haemolytic disease of the newborn.

Anti-D immunoglobulin should be administered following any sensitising episode (e.g. abortion, miscarriage and birth); it should be injected within 72 hours of the episode but even if a longer period has elapsed it may still give protection and should be administered. The dose of anti-D immunoglobulin is determined according to the level of exposure to rhesus-positive blood.

For routine antenatal prophylaxis (see also NICE guidance below), two doses of at least 500 units of anti-D immunoglobulin should be given, the first at 28 weeks' gestation and the second at 34 weeks.

> **NICE guidance**
> **Routine antenatal anti-D prophylaxis for rhesus-negative women (May 2002)**
> Routine antenatal anti-D prophylaxis should be offered to all non-sensitised pregnant women who are rhesus negative.
> Use of routine *antenatal* anti-D prophylaxis should not be affected by previous anti-D prophylaxis for a sensitising event early in the same pregnancy. Similarly, *postpartum* anti-D prophylaxis should not be affected by previous routine antenatal anti-D prophylaxis or by antenatal anti-D prophylaxis for a sensitising event.

> **Note**
> MMR vaccine may be given in the postpartum period with anti-D (Rh_0) immunoglobulin injection provided that separate syringes are used and the products are administered into different limbs. If blood is transfused, the antibody response to the vaccine may be inhibited—measure rubella antibodies after 6–8 weeks and revaccinate if necessary.

Anti-D (Rh_0) Immunoglobulin (Non-proprietary) PoM

Injection, anti-D (Rh_0) immunoglobulin, net price 250-unit vial = £19.00, 500-unit vial = £27.00, 1500-unit vial = £58.00, 2500-unit vial = £94.40

Dose by deep intramuscular injection, to rhesus-negative woman for prevention of Rh_0(D) sensitisation:

Following birth of rhesus-positive infant, 500 units immediately or within 72 hours; for transplacental bleed of over 4 mL fetal red cells, extra 100–125 units per mL fetal red cells

Following any potentially sensitising episode (e.g. stillbirth, abortion, amniocentesis) up to 20 weeks' gestation 250 units per episode (after 20 weeks, 500 units) immediately or within 72 hours

Antenatal prophylaxis, 500 units given at weeks 28 and 34 of pregnancy; a further dose is still needed immediately or within 72 hours of delivery

Note Some UK authorities recommend different doses for antenatal prophylaxis (see notes above)

Following Rh_0(D) incompatible blood transfusion, 100–125 units per mL transfused rhesus-positive red cells

Available from Blood Centres and from BPL (*D-Gam®*)

Partobulin SDF® (Baxter BioScience) PoM

Injection, anti-D (Rh_0) immunoglobulin 1250 units/mL (250 micrograms/mL), net price 1-mL prefilled syringe = £35.00

Dose by intramuscular injection, to rhesus-negative woman for prevention of Rh_0 (D) sensitisation:

Following birth of rhesus-positive infant, 1000–1650 units immediately or within 72 hours; for large transplacental blood loss, 50–125 units per mL of fetal red cells

Antenatal prophylaxis, 1000–1650 units given at weeks 28 and 34 of pregnancy; if infant rhesus-positive, further dose is needed immediately or within 72 hours of delivery

Note Some UK authorities recommend different doses for antenatal prophylaxis (see notes above)

Following abortion, ectopic pregnancy or hydatidiform mole up to 12 weeks' gestation, 600–750 units (after 12 weeks, 1250–1650 units) immediately or within 72 hours

Following amniocentesis or chorionic villous sampling, 1250–1650 units immediately or within 72 hours

Following Rh_0 (D) incompatible blood or red cell transfusion, 1250 units per 10 mL of transfused rhesus-positive red cells immediately or within 72 hours

Rhophylac® (CSL Behring) PoM

Injection, anti-D (Rh_0) immunoglobulin 750 units/mL (150 micrograms/mL), net price 2-mL (1500-unit) prefilled syringe = £46.50.

Dose by intramuscular *or* intravenous injection, to rhesus-negative woman for prevention of Rh_0(D) sensitisation:

Following birth of rhesus-positive infant, 1000–1500 units immediately or within 72 hours; for large transplacental bleed, extra 100 units per mL fetal red cells (preferably by intravenous injection)

Following any potentially sensitising episode (e.g. abortion, amniocentesis, chorionic villous sampling) up to 12 weeks' gestation 1000 units per episode (after 12 weeks, higher doses may be required) immediately or within 72 hours

Antenatal prophylaxis, 1500 units given between weeks 28–30 of pregnancy; a further dose is still needed immediately or within 72 hours of delivery

Note Some UK authorities recommend different doses for antenatal prophylaxis (see notes above)

Following Rh_0(D) incompatible blood transfusion, by intravenous injection, 50 units per mL transfused rhesus-positive blood (or 100 units per mL of erythrocyte concentrate)

WinRho SDF® (Baxter BioScience) PoM

Injection, anti-D (Rh_0) immunoglobulin, powder for reconstitution, net price 1500-unit (300-microgram) vial (with diluent) = £313.50, 5000-unit (1-mg) vial (with diluent) = £1045.00

Dose to rhesus-negative woman for prevention of Rh_0(D) sensitisation:

Following birth of rhesus-positive infant, by intramuscular injection, 1500 units *or* by intravenous injection, 600 units immediately or within 72 hours; for transplacental bleed of over 25 mL fetal blood, by intramuscular *or* intravenous injection, extra 50 units per mL fetal blood (further doses required for large bleed)

Following any potentially sensitising episode (e.g. abortion, amniocentesis, chorionic villous sampling) up to 12 weeks' gestation, by intramuscular *or* intravenous injection, 600 units per episode (after 12 weeks, 1500 units) immediately or within 72 hours

Antenatal prophylaxis, by intramuscular *or* intravenous injection, 1500 units given at week 28 of pregnancy; a further dose is still needed immediately or within 72 hours of delivery

Note Some UK authorities recommend different doses for antenatal prophylaxis (see notes above)

Following Rh_0(D) incompatible blood transfusion, by intravenous injection, 50 units per mL transfused rhesus-positive blood (or 100 units per mL of erythrocyte concentrate); if intramuscular route used give in divided doses over several days

Following Rh_0(D) incompatible thrombocyte transfusion in rhesus-negative female child or woman of child-bearing age, by intravenous injection, 600 units

Autoimmune (idiopathic) thrombocytopenic purpura, consult product literature

Interferons

Interferon gamma-1b is licensed to reduce the frequency of serious infection in chronic granulomatous disease and in severe malignant osteopetrosis.

INTERFERON GAMMA-1b
(Immune interferon)

Indications see notes above

Cautions severe hepatic impairment (Appendix 2) or severe renal impairment (Appendix 3); seizure disorders (including seizures associated with fever); cardiac disease (including ischaemia, congestive heart failure, and arrhythmias); monitor before and during treatment: haematological tests (including full blood count, differential white cell count, and platelet count), blood chemistry tests (including renal and liver function tests) and urinalysis; avoid simultaneous administration of foreign proteins including immunological products (risk of exaggerated immune response); pregnancy (Appendix 4); breast-feeding (Appendix 5); **interactions:** Appendix 1 (interferons)

Driving May impair ability to drive or operate machinery; effects may be enhanced by alcohol

Side-effects nausea, vomiting; headache, fatigue, fever; myalgia, arthralgia; rash, injection-site reactions; *rarely* confusion and systemic lupus erythematosus; also reported, neutropenia, thrombocytopenia, and raised liver enzymes

Dose

- See under Preparations

Immukin® (Boehringer Ingelheim) PoM

Injection, recombinant human interferon gamma-1b 200 micrograms/mL, net price 0.5-mL vial = £88.00

Dose by subcutaneous injection, 50 micrograms/m² 3 times a week; patients with body surface area of 0.5 m² or less, 1.5 micrograms/kg 3 times a week; not yet recommended for children under 6 months with chronic granulomatous disease

14.6 International travel

Note For advice on **malaria chemoprophylaxis**, see section 5.4.1.

No special immunisation is required for travellers to the United States, Europe, Australia, or New Zealand although all travellers should have immunity to tetanus and poliomyelitis (and childhood immunisations should be up to date). Certain special precautions are required in non-European areas surrounding the Mediterranean, in Africa, the Middle East, Asia, and South America.

Travellers to areas that have a high incidence of **poliomyelitis** or **tuberculosis** should be immunised with the appropriate vaccine; in the case of poliomyelitis previously immunised adults may be given a booster dose of a preparation containing inactivated poliomyelitis vaccine. BCG immunisation is recommended for travellers aged under 35 years[1] proposing to stay for longer than 3 months (or in close contact with the local population) in countries with an incidence of tuberculosis greater than 40 per 100 000[2]; it should preferably be given three months or more before departure.

Yellow fever immunisation is recommended for travel to the endemic zones of Africa and South America. Many countries require an International Certificate of Vaccination from individuals arriving from, or who have been travelling through, endemic areas, whilst other countries require a certificate from all entering travellers (consult the Department of Health handbook, *Health Information for Overseas Travel*, www.dh.gov.uk).

Immunisation against **meningococcal meningitis** is recommended for a number of areas of the world (for details, see p. 653).

Protection against **hepatitis A** is recommended for travellers to high-risk areas outside Northern and Western Europe, North America, Japan, Australia and New Zealand. Hepatitis A vaccine (see p. 647) is preferred and it is likely to be effective even if given shortly before departure; normal immunoglobulin is no longer given routinely but may be indicated in the immunocompromised (see p. 660). Special care must also be taken with food hygiene (see below).

Hepatitis B vaccine (see p. 648) is recommended for those travelling to areas of high or intermediate prevalence who intend to seek employment as healthcare workers or who plan to remain there for lengthy periods and who may therefore be at increased risk of acquiring infection as the result of medical or dental procedures carried out in those countries. Short-term tourists or business travellers are not generally at increased risk of infection but may place themselves at risk by their sexual behaviour when abroad.

Prophylactic immunisation against **rabies** (see p. 656) is recommended for travellers to enzootic areas on long journeys or to areas out of reach of immediate medical attention.

Travellers who have not had a **tetanus** booster in the last 10 years and are visiting areas where medical attention may not be accessible should receive a booster dose of adsorbed diphtheria [low dose], tetanus and inactivated poliomyelitis vaccine (see p. 645), even if they have received 5 doses of a tetanus-containing vaccine previously.

Typhoid vaccine is indicated for travellers to those countries where typhoid is endemic but the vaccine is no substitute for personal precautions (see below).

There is no requirement for cholera vaccination as a condition for entry into any country, but **oral cholera vaccine** (see p. 645) may be considered for backpackers and those travelling to situations where the risk is greatest (e.g. refugee camps). Regardless of vaccination, travellers to areas where cholera is endemic should take special care with food hygiene (see below).

Advice on **diphtheria**, on **Japanese encephalitis**[3] (vaccine available on named-patient basis from Sanofi Pasteur and MASTA) and on **tick-borne encephalitis** is included in *Health Information for Overseas Travel*, see below.

Food hygiene In areas where sanitation is poor, good food hygiene is important to help prevent hepatitis A, typhoid, cholera, and other diarrhoeal diseases (including travellers' diarrhoea). Food should be freshly prepared and hot, and uncooked vegetables (including green salads) should be avoided; only fruits which can be peeled should be eaten. Only suitable bottled water, or tap water that has been boiled, or treated with sterilising tablets should be used for drinking.

1. There is inadequate evidence of protection by BCG vaccine in adults aged over 35 years; however, vaccination is recommended for healthcare workers irrespective of age because of the increased risk to them or their patients

2. List of countries where the incidence of tuberculosis is greater than 40 cases per 100 000 is available at www.hpa.org.uk

3. Japanese encephalitis vaccine not prescribable on the NHS; health authorities may investigate circumstances under which vaccine prescribed

Information on health advice for travellers

The Department of Health booklet, *Health Advice For Travellers* (code: T7.1) includes information on immunisation requirements (or recommendations) around the world. The booklet can be obtained from travel agents, post-offices or by telephoning 0800 555 777 (24-hour service); also available on the Internet at:
www.dh.gov.uk

The Department of Health handbook, *Health Information for Overseas Travel* (2001), which draws together essential information *for healthcare professionals* regarding health advice for travellers, can be obtained from
The Stationery Office
PO Box 29, Norwich NR3 1GN
Telephone orders, 0870 600 5522
Fax: 0870 600 5533
www.tso.co.uk

Immunisation requirements change from time to time, and information on the current requirements for any particular country may be obtained from the embassy or legation of the appropriate country or from:

National Travel Health Network and Centre
Hospital for Tropical Diseases
Mortimer Market Centre
Capper Street, off Tottenham Court Road
London, WC1E 6AU
Tel: 0845 602 6712
(9 a.m.–noon, 2–4.30 p.m. weekdays for healthcare professionals **only**)
www.nathnac.org

Travel Medicine Team
Health Protection Scotland
Clifton House
Clifton Place
Glasgow, G3 7LN
Tel: (0141) 300 1100
(2 p.m.–4 p.m. weekdays)
www.travax.nhs.uk (registration required. Annual fee may be payable for users outside NHS Scotland)

Welsh Medicines Information Centre
University Hospital of Wales
Cardiff, CF14 4XW
Tel: (029) 2074 2979 (8.30 a.m.–5.p.m. weekdays for health professionals in Wales **only**)

Department of Health and Social Services
Castle Buildings
Stormont
Belfast, BT4 3PP
Tel: (028) 9052 0000

15 Anaesthesia

15.1 General anaesthesia 665
15.1.1 Intravenous anaesthetics 666
15.1.2 Inhalational anaesthetics 668
15.1.3 Antimuscarinic drugs 670
15.1.4 Sedative and analgesic peri-operative drugs 671
15.1.4.1 Anxiolytics and neuroleptics 672
15.1.4.2 Non-opioid analgesics 673
15.1.4.3 Opioid analgesics 674
15.1.5 Neuromuscular blocking drugs 676
15.1.6 Anticholinesterases used in anaesthesia 679
15.1.7 Antagonists for central and respiratory depression 679
15.1.8 Drugs for malignant hyperthermia 680
15.2 Local anaesthesia 680

15.1 General anaesthesia

15.1.1 Intravenous anaesthetics
15.1.2 Inhalational anaesthetics
15.1.3 Antimuscarinic drugs
15.1.4 Sedative and analgesic peri-operative drugs
15.1.5 Neuromuscular blocking drugs
15.1.6 Anticholinesterases used in anaesthesia
15.1.7 Antagonists for central and respiratory depression
15.1.8 Drugs for malignant hyperthermia

Note The drugs in section 15.1 should be used only by experienced personnel and where adequate resuscitation equipment is available.

Several different types of drug are given together during general anaesthesia. Anaesthesia is induced with either a volatile drug given by inhalation (section 15.1.2) or with an intravenously administered drug (section 15.1.1); anaesthesia is maintained with an intravenous or inhalational anaesthetic. Analgesics (section 15.1.4), usually short-acting opioids, are also used. The use of neuromuscular blocking drugs (section 15.1.5) necessitates intermittent positive-pressure ventilation. Following surgery, anticholinesterases (section 15.1.6) can be given to reverse the effects of neuromuscular blocking drugs; specific antagonists (section 15.1.7) can be used to reverse central and respiratory depression caused by some drugs used in surgery. A local anaesthetic (section 15.2) can be used to reduce pain at the injection site.

The required dose of induction agent may be less if the patient has been premedicated with a sedative agent or an opioid analgesic has been used.

Surgery and long-term medication The risk of losing disease control on stopping long-term medication before surgery is often greater than the risk posed by continuing it during surgery. It is vital that the anaesthetist knows about **all** drugs that a patient is (or has been) taking.

Patients with adrenal atrophy resulting from long-term corticosteroid use (section 6.3.2) may suffer a precipitous fall in blood pressure unless corticosteroid cover is provided during anaesthesia and in the immediate post-operative period. Anaesthetists must therefore know whether a patient is, or has been, receiving corticosteroids (including high-dose inhaled corticosteroids).

Other drugs that should normally not be stopped before surgery include antiepileptics, antiparkinsonian drugs, antipsychotics, anxiolytics, bronchodilators, cardiovascular drugs (but see potassium-sparing diuretics, angiotensin-converting enzyme inhibitors, and angiotensin-II receptor antagonists below), glaucoma drugs, immunosuppressants, drugs of dependence, and thyroid or antithyroid drugs. Expert advice is required for patients receiving antivirals for HIV infection. For general advice on surgery in diabetic patients see section 6.1.1.

Patients taking aspirin or an oral anticoagulant present an increased risk for surgery. In these circumstances, the anaesthetist and surgeon should assess the relative risks and decide jointly whether aspirin or the anticoagulant should be stopped or replaced with heparin therapy.

before surgery include combined oral contraceptives (see Surgery, section 7.3.1 for details); for advice on hormone replacement therapy, see section 6.4.1.1. If antidepressants need to be stopped, they should be withdrawn gradually to avoid withdrawal symptoms. In view of their hazardous interactions MAOIs should normally be stopped 2 weeks before surgery. Tricyclic antidepressants need not be stopped, but there may be an increased risk of arrhythmias and hypotension (and dangerous interactions with vasopressor drugs); therefore, the anaesthetist should be informed if they are not stopped. Lithium should be stopped 24 hours before major surgery but the normal dose can be continued for minor surgery (with careful monitoring of fluids and electrolytes). Potassium-sparing diuretics may need to be withheld on the morning of surgery because hyperkalaemia may develop if renal perfusion is impaired or if there is tissue damage. Angiotensin-converting enzyme (ACE) inhibitors and angiotensin-II receptor antagonists can be associated with severe hypotension after induction of anaesthesia; these drugs may need to be discontinued 24 hours before surgery.

Anaesthesia and driving Patients given sedatives and analgesics during minor outpatient procedures should be very carefully warned about the risk of driving afterwards. For intravenous benzodiazepines and for a short general anaesthetic the risk extends to **at least 24 hours** after administration. Responsible persons should be available to take patients home. The dangers of taking **alcohol** should also be emphasised.

Prophylaxis of acid aspiration Regurgitation and aspiration of gastric contents (Mendelson's syndrome) is an important complication of general anaesthesia, particularly in obstetrics and during emergency surgery, and requires prophylaxis against acid aspiration. Prophylaxis is also needed in those with gastro-oesophageal reflux disease and in circumstances where gastric emptying may be delayed.

An **H_2-receptor antagonist** (section 1.3.1) or a **proton pump inhibitor** (section 1.3.5) such as omeprazole may be used before surgery to increase the pH and reduce the volume of gastric fluid. They do not affect the pH of fluid already in the stomach and this limits their value in emergency procedures; oral H_2-receptor antagonists can be given 1–2 hours before the procedure but omeprazole must be given at least 12 hours earlier. Antacids are frequently used to neutralise the acidity of the fluid already in the stomach; 'clear' (non-particulate) antacids such as sodium citrate are preferred. Sodium citrate 300 mmol/litre (88.2 mg/mL) oral solution is licensed for use before general anaesthesia for caesarean section (available from Viridian).

Gas cylinders

Each gas cylinder bears a label with the name of the gas contained in the cylinder. The name or chemical symbol of the gas appears on the shoulder of the cylinder and is also clearly and indelibly stamped on the cylinder valve.

The colours on the valve end of the cylinder extend down to the shoulder; in the case of mixed gases the colours for the individual gases are applied in four segments, two for each colour.

Gas cylinders should be stored in a cool well-ventilated room, free from flammable materials.

No lubricant of any description should be used on the cylinder valves.

Anaesthesia, sedation, and resuscitation in dental practice

For details see *A Conscious Decision: A review of the use of general anaesthesia and conscious sedation in primary dental care*; report by a group chaired by the Chief Medical Officer and Chief Dental Officer, July 2000 and associated documents. Further details can also be found in *Conscious Sedation in the Provision of Dental Care*; report of an Expert Group on Sedation for Dentistry (commissioned by the Department of Health), 2003. Both documents are available at www.dh.gov.uk.

Guidance is also included in *Standards for Dental Professionals*, London, General Dental Council, May 2005 (and as amended subsequently), and *Conscious Sedation in Dentistry: Dental Clinical Guidance*, Scottish Dental Effectiveness Programme, May 2006.

15.1.1 Intravenous anaesthetics

Intravenous anaesthetics may be used either to induce anaesthesia or for maintenance of anaesthesia throughout surgery. Intravenous anaesthetics nearly all produce their effect in one arm-brain circulation time and can cause apnoea and hypotension, and so adequate resuscitative facilities **must** be available. They are **contra-indicated** if the anaesthetist is not confident of being able to maintain the airway (e.g. in the presence of a tumour in the pharynx or larynx). Extreme care is required in surgery of the mouth, pharynx, or larynx and in patients with acute circulatory failure (shock) or fixed cardiac output.

Individual requirements vary considerably and the recommended doses are only a guide. Smaller doses are indicated in ill, shocked, or debilitated patients and in significant hepatic impairment, while robust individuals may require larger doses. To facilitate tracheal intubation, induction is usually followed by a neuromuscular blocking drug (section 15.1.5).

Total intravenous anaesthesia This is a technique in which major surgery is carried out with all drugs given intravenously. Respiration can be spontaneous, or controlled with oxygen-enriched air. Neuromuscular blocking drugs can be used to provide relaxation and prevent reflex muscle movements. The main problem to be overcome is the assessment of depth of anaesthesia. Target Controlled Infusion (TCI) systems can be used to titrate intravenous anaesthetic infusions to predicted plasma-drug concentrations in ventilated adult patients.

Anaesthesia and driving See section 15.1.

Barbiturates

Thiopental sodium (thiopentone sodium) is used widely for induction of anaesthesia, but it has no analgesic properties. Induction is generally smooth and rapid, but dose-related cardiorespiratory depression can occur.

Awakening from a moderate dose of thiopental is rapid because the drug redistributes into other tissues, particularly fat. However, metabolism is slow and sedative effects can persist for 24 hours. Repeated doses have a cumulative effect and recovery is much slower.

THIOPENTAL SODIUM
(Thiopentone sodium)

Indications induction of general anaesthesia; anaesthesia of short duration; reduction of raised intracranial pressure if ventilation controlled; status epilepticus (see also section 4.8.2)

Cautions see notes above; cardiovascular disease; hepatic impairment (Appendix 2); reconstituted solution is highly alkaline—extravasation causes tissue necrosis and severe pain; avoid intra-arterial injection; pregnancy (Appendix 4); **interactions**: Appendix 1 (anaesthetics, general)

Contra-indications see notes above; porphyria (section 9.8.2); myotonic dystrophy; breast-feeding (Appendix 5)

Side-effects arrhythmias, myocardial depression, laryngeal spasm, cough, sneezing, hypersensitivity reactions, rash, injection-site reactions; excessive doses associated with hypothermia and profound cerebral impairment

Dose

- Induction of general anaesthesia, by intravenous injection usually as a 2.5% (25 mg/mL) solution, in fit premedicated adults, initially 100–150 mg (reduced in elderly or debilitated) over 10–15 seconds (longer in elderly or debilitated), followed by further quantity if necessary according to response after 30–60 seconds; *or* up to 4 mg/kg (max. 500mg); CHILD induction 2–7 mg/kg
- Raised intracranial pressure, by intravenous injection, 1.5–3 mg/kg, repeated as required
- Status epilepticus (only if other measures fail, see section 4.8.2), by intravenous injection as a 2.5% (25 mg/mL) solution, 75–125 mg as a single dose

Thiopental (Link) PoM
Injection, powder for reconstitution, thiopental sodium, net price 500-mg vial = £3.06

Other intravenous anaesthetics

Propofol is associated with rapid recovery without a hangover effect and it is very widely used. There is sometimes pain on intravenous injection which can be reduced by intravenous lidocaine. Significant extraneous muscle movements may occur. Convulsions, anaphylaxis, and delayed recovery from anaesthesia can occur after propofol administration; since the onset of convulsions can be delayed the CSM has advised special caution after day surgery. Propofol is associated with bradycardia, occasionally profound; intravenous administration of an antimuscarinic drug may prevent this.

Etomidate is an induction agent associated with rapid recovery without a hangover effect. It causes less hypotension than thiopental and propofol during induction. It produces a high incidence of extraneous muscle movement, which can be minimised by an opioid analgesic or a short-acting benzodiazepine given just before induction. Pain on injection can be reduced by injecting into a larger vein or by giving an opioid analgesic just before induction. Etomidate can suppress adrenocortical function, particularly during continuous administration, and it should not be used for maintenance of anaesthesia.

Ketamine is used very rarely now. It has good analgesic properties at sub-anaesthetic dosage. It causes less hypotension than thiopental and propofol during induction. It is used mainly for paediatric anaesthesia, particularly when repeated administration is required; recovery is relatively slow and there is a high incidence of extraneous muscle movements. The main disadvantage of ketamine is the high incidence of hallucinations, nightmares, and other transient psychotic effects; these can be reduced by drugs such as diazepam or midazolam. Ketamine also has abuse potential and can itself cause dependence.

ETOMIDATE

Indications induction of anaesthesia

Cautions see notes above; avoid in porphyria (section 9.8.2); pregnancy (Appendix 4); breast-feeding (Appendix 5); **interactions**: Appendix 1 (anaesthetics, general)

Contra-indications see notes above

Side-effects see notes above

Dose

- See under preparations

Etomidate-Lipuro® (Braun) PoM
Injection (emulsion), etomidate 2 mg/mL, net price 10-mL amp = £1.53
Dose ADULT and CHILD, by slow intravenous injection, 150–300 micrograms/kg; CHILD under 10 years may need up to 400 micrograms/kg; ELDERLY 150–200 micrograms/kg

Hypnomidate® (Janssen-Cilag) PoM
Injection, etomidate 2 mg/mL, net price 10-mL amp = £1.50
Excipients include propylene glycol (see Excipients, p. 2)
Dose ADULT and CHILD, by slow intravenous injection, 300 micrograms/kg; ELDERLY 150–200 micrograms/kg; max. total dose 60 mg

KETAMINE

Indications induction and maintenance of anaesthesia (but rarely used)

Cautions see notes above; increased cerebrospinal fluid pressure; predisposition to hallucinations or nightmares; pregnancy (Appendix 4); **interactions**: Appendix 1 (anaesthetics, general)

15 Anaesthesia

Contra-indications hypertension, pre-eclampsia or eclampsia, severe cardiac disease, stroke; raised intracranial pressure; head trauma; porphyria (section 9.8.2)

Side-effects see notes above; also tachycardia, hypertension, arrhythmias, hypotension, bradycardia; increased salivation, laryngospasm; anxiety, insomnia; diplopia, nystagmus, raised intra-ocular pressure; rashes, injection-site reactions; anaphylaxis also reported

Dose

- By intramuscular injection, short procedures, initially 6.5–13 mg/kg, adjusted according to response (10 mg/kg usually produces 12–25 minutes of surgical anaesthesia)

  Diagnostic manoeuvres and procedures not involving intense pain, initially 4 mg/kg
- By intravenous injection over at least 60 seconds, short procedures, initially 1–4.5 mg/kg, adjusted according to response (2 mg/kg usually produces 5–10 minutes of surgical anaesthesia)
- By intravenous infusion of a solution containing 1 mg/mL, longer procedures, induction, total dose of 0.5–2 mg/kg; maintenance, 10–45 micrograms/kg/minute, rate adjusted according to response

Ketalar® (Pfizer) PoM

Injection, ketamine (as hydrochloride) 10 mg/mL, net price 20-mL vial = £4.22; 50 mg/mL, 10-mL vial = £8.77; 100 mg/mL, 10-mL vial = £16.10

Note For *intravenous injection*, dilute 100 mg/mL strength to a concentration of not more than 50 mg/mL with Glucose 5% *or* Sodium Chloride 0.9% *or* Water for Injections

PROPOFOL

Indications see under dose

Cautions see notes above; cardiac impairment; respiratory impairment; elderly; hypovolaemia; epilepsy; hypotension; patients with high intracranial pressure; monitor blood-lipid concentration if risk of fat overload or if sedation longer than 3 days; hepatic impairment; renal impairment; pregnancy (Appendix 4); breast-feeding (Appendix 5); **interactions**: Appendix 1 (anaesthetics, general)

Contra-indications see notes above; not to be used for sedation of ventilated children and adolescents under 17 years (risk of potentially fatal effects including metabolic acidosis, cardiac failure, rhabdomyolysis, hyperlipidaemia, and hepatomegaly)

Side-effects see notes above; also hypotension, tachycardia, flushing; transient apnoea, hyperventilation, coughing, and hiccup during induction; *less commonly* thrombosis, phlebitis; *rarely* arrhythmia, headache, vertigo, shivering, euphoria; *very rarely* pancreatitis, pulmonary oedema, sexual disinhibition, and discoloration of urine; serious and sometimes fatal side-effects reported with prolonged infusion of doses exceeding 5 mg/kg/hour, including metabolic acidosis, rhabdomyolysis, hyperkalaemia, and cardiac failure; dystonia and dyskinesia also reported

Dose

- *1% injection*
- Induction of anaesthesia, by intravenous injection *or* infusion, 1.5–2.5 mg/kg (1–1.5 mg in those over 55 years) at a rate of 20–40 mg every 10 seconds until response; CHILD over 1 month, administer slowly until response (usual dose in child over 8 years 2.5 mg/kg, may need more in younger child e.g. 2.5–4 mg/kg)
- Maintenance of anaesthesia, by intravenous infusion, 4–12 mg/kg/hour *or* by intravenous injection, 25–50 mg repeated according to response; CHILD over 3 years, by intravenous infusion, 9–15 mg/kg/hour

  Note *Propofol-Lipuro®* and *Propoven®* may be used for maintenance of anaesthesia in CHILD over 1 month, by intravenous infusion, 9–15 mg/kg/hour
- Sedation in intensive care, by intravenous infusion, ADULT over 17 years, 0.3–4 mg/kg/hour; CHILD and ADOLESCENT under 17 years contra-indicated
- Sedation for surgical and diagnostic procedures, initially by intravenous injection over 1–5 minutes, 0.5–1 mg/kg; maintenance, by intravenous infusion, 1.5–4.5 mg/kg/hour (additionally, if rapid increase in sedation required, by intravenous injection, 10–20 mg); those over 55 years may require lower dose; CHILD and ADOLESCENT under 17 years contra-indicated

- *2% injection*
- Induction of anaesthesia, by intravenous infusion, 1.5–2.5 mg/kg (1–1.5 mg in those over 55 years) at a rate of 20–40 mg every 10 seconds; CHILD over 3 years, administer slowly until response (usual dose in child over 8 years 2.5 mg/kg, may need more in younger child e.g. 2.5–4 mg/kg)
- Maintenance of anaesthesia, by intravenous infusion, 4–12 mg/kg/hour; CHILD over 3 years, by intravenous infusion, 9–15 mg/kg/hour
- Sedation in intensive care, by intravenous infusion, ADULT over 17 years, 0.3–4 mg/kg/hour; CHILD and ADOLESCENT under 17 years contra-indicated

Propofol (Non-proprietary) PoM

1% injection (emulsion), propofol 10 mg/mL, net price 20-mL amp = £2.33, 50-mL bottle = £5.82, 100-mL bottle = £11.64

2% injection (emulsion), propofol 20 mg/mL, net price 50-mL vial = £11.64

Brands include *Propofol-Lipuro®*, *Propoven*

Diprivan® (AstraZeneca) PoM

1% injection (emulsion), propofol 10 mg/mL, net price 20-mL amp = £3.88, 50-mL prefilled syringe (for use with *Diprifusor® TCI* system) = £10.67

2% injection (emulsion), propofol 20 mg/mL, net price 50-mL prefilled syringe (for use with *Diprifusor® TCI* system) = £20.37

Note *Diprifusor® TCI* ('target controlled infusion') system is for use **only** for induction and maintenance of general anaesthesia in adults

15.1.2 Inhalational anaesthetics

Inhalational anaesthetics may be gases or volatile liquids. They can be used both for induction and maintenance of anaesthesia and can also be used following induction with an intravenous anaesthetic (section 15.1.1).

Gaseous anaesthetics require suitable equipment for storage and administration. They may be supplied via hospital pipelines or from metal cylinders. *Volatile liquid anaesthetics* are administered using calibrated vaporisers, using air, oxygen, or nitrous oxide–oxygen mixtures as the carrier gas; all can trigger malignant hyperthermia (section 15.1.8) and are contra-indicated in those susceptible to malignant hyperthermia.

To prevent hypoxia inhalational anaesthetics must be given with concentrations of oxygen greater than 21%.

Anaesthesia and driving See section 15.1.

Volatile liquid anaesthetics

Isoflurane is a volatile liquid anaesthetic. Heart rhythm is generally stable during isoflurane anaesthesia, but heart-rate can rise, particularly in younger patients. Systemic arterial pressure can fall and cardiac output can decrease, owing to a decrease in systemic vascular resistance. Respiration is depressed. Muscle relaxation occurs and the effects of muscle relaxant drugs are potentiated. Isoflurane may also cause hepatotoxicity in those sensitised to halogenated anaesthetics.

Desflurane is a rapid acting volatile liquid anaesthetic; it is reported to have about one-fifth the potency of isoflurane.Emergence and recovery from anaesthesia are particularly rapid because of its low solubility. Desflurane is not recommended for induction of anaesthesia as it is irritant to the upper respiratory tract; cough, breath-holding, apnoea, laryngospasm, and increased secretions can occur. The risk of hepatotoxicity with desflurane in those sensitised to halogenated anaesthetics appears to be remote.

Sevoflurane is a rapid acting volatile liquid anaesthetic and is more potent than desflurane. Emergence and recovery are particularly rapid, but slower than desflurane. Sevoflurane is non-irritant and is therefore often used for inhalational induction of anaesthesia. Sevoflurane can interact with carbon dioxide absorbents to form compound A, a potentially nephrotoxic vinyl ether. However, in spite of extensive use, no cases of sevoflurane-induced permanent renal injury have been reported and the carbon dioxide absorbents used in the UK produce very low concentrations of compound A, even in low-flow anaesthetic systems.

Halothane is a volatile liquid anaesthetic. Its advantages are that it is potent, induction is smooth, and the vapour is non-irritant and seldom induces coughing or breath-holding. Despite these advantages, halothane is not widely used because of its association with *severe hepatotoxicity* (**important**: see CSM advice, below).

Halothane causes cardiorespiratory depression. Respiratory depression results in raised arterial carbon dioxide tension and perhaps ventricular arrhythmias. Halothane also depresses the cardiac muscle fibres and can cause bradycardia resulting in diminished cardiac output and fall of arterial pressure. Adrenaline (epinephrine) infiltrations should be avoided in patients anaesthetised with halothane because ventricular arrhythmias may result.

Halothane produces moderate muscle relaxation, but this may be inadequate for major abdominal surgery and specific muscle relaxants are then used.

CSM advice (halothane hepatotoxicity)

Severe hepatotoxicity can follow halothane anaesthesia. The CSM has reported that this occurs more frequently after repeated exposure to halothane and has a high mortality. The risk of severe hepatotoxicity appears to be increased by repeated exposures within a short time interval, but even after a long interval (sometimes of several years), susceptible patients have been reported to develop jaundice. Since there is no reliable way of identifying susceptible patients, the CSM recommends the following precautions prior to use of halothane:

1. a careful anaesthetic history should be taken to determine previous exposure and previous reactions to halothane;
2. repeated exposure to halothane within a period of **at least** 3 months should be **avoided** unless there are **overriding** clinical circumstances;
3. a history of unexplained jaundice or pyrexia in a patient following exposure to halothane is an absolute **contra-indication** to its future use in that patient.

DESFLURANE

Indications see notes above

Cautions see notes above; hepatic impairment (Appendix 2); renal impairment (Appendix 3); pregnancy (Appendix 4); **interactions:** Appendix 1 (anaesthetics, general)

Contra-indications see notes above; susceptibility to malignant hyperthermia

Side-effects see notes above

Dose

- Using a specifically calibrated vaporiser, *induction*, 4–11%; CHILD not recommended for induction
  Maintenance, 2–6% in nitrous oxide; 2.5–8.5% in oxygen or oxygen-enriched air

Suprane® (Baxter) PoM

Desflurane, net price 240 mL = £44.41

HALOTHANE

Indications see notes above

Cautions see notes above (**important**: CSM advice, see notes above); avoid for dental procedures in those under 18 years unless treated in hospital (high risk of arrhythmia); avoid in porphyria (section 9.8.2); hepatic impairment (Appendix 2); pregnancy (Appendix 4); breast-feeding (Appendix 5); **interactions:** Appendix 1 (anaesthetics, general)

Contra-indications see notes above; susceptibility to malignant hyperthermia

Side-effects see notes above

Dose

- Using specifically calibrated vaporiser, *induction*, increased gradually to 2–4% in oxygen or nitrous oxide–oxygen; CHILD (see cautions) 1.5–2%
  Maintenance, 0.5–2%

Halothane (Non-proprietary)

Available on a named-patient basis from specialist importing companies, see p. 888

ISOFLURANE

Indications see notes above

Cautions see notes above; pregnancy (Appendix 4); **interactions**: Appendix 1 (anaesthetics, general)

Contra-indications susceptibility to malignant hyperthermia

Side-effects see notes above

Dose

- Using a specifically calibrated vaporiser, *induction*, increased gradually from 0.5% to 3%, in oxygen or nitrous oxide–oxygen

  Maintenance, 1–2.5% in nitrous oxide–oxygen; an additional 0.5–1% may be required when given with oxygen alone; caesarean section, 0.5–0.75% in nitrous oxide–oxygen

Isoflurane (Abbott)

Isoflurane, net price 250 mL = £47.50

AErrane® (Baxter)

Isoflurane, net price 100 mL = £7.98, 250 mL = £30.00

SEVOFLURANE

Indications see notes above

Cautions see notes above; renal impairment (Appendix 3); pregnancy (Appendix 4); **interactions**: Appendix 1 (anaesthetics, general)

Contra-indications susceptibility to malignant hyperthermia

Side-effects see notes above; also agitation occurs frequently in children

Dose

- Induction of anaesthesia, using a specifically calibrated vaporiser, in oxygen or nitrous oxide–oxygen, adjusted according to response, ADULT up to 5%; CHILD 1 month–18 years up to 8%
- Maintenance of anaesthesia, using a specifically calibrated vaporiser, in oxygen or nitrous oxide–oxygen, adjusted according to response, ADULT and CHILD over 1 month 0.5–3%

Sevoflurane (Non-proprietary) PoM

Sevoflurane, net price 250 mL = £123.00

Available from Abbott, Baxter

Nitrous oxide

Nitrous oxide is used for maintenance of anaesthesia and, in sub-anaesthetic concentrations, for analgesia. For *anaesthesia* it is commonly used in a concentration of 50 to 66% in oxygen as part of a balanced technique in association with other inhalational or intravenous agents. Nitrous oxide is unsatisfactory as a sole anaesthetic owing to lack of potency, but is useful as part of a combination of drugs since it allows a significant reduction in dosage.

For *analgesia* (without loss of consciousness) a mixture of nitrous oxide and oxygen containing 50% of each gas (*Entonox®*, *Equanox®*) is used. Self-administration using a demand valve is popular in obstetric practice, for changing painful dressings, as an aid to postoperative physiotherapy, and in emergency ambulances.

Nitrous oxide may have a deleterious effect if used in patients with an air-containing closed space since nitrous oxide diffuses into such a space with a resulting increase in pressure. This effect may be dangerous in the presence of a pneumothorax which may enlarge to compromise respiration, or in the presence of intracranial air after head injury.

Special care is needed to avoid hypoxia if an anaesthetic machine is being used; machines should incorporate an anti-hypoxia device. Exposure of patients to nitrous oxide for prolonged periods, either by continuous or by intermittent administration, may result in megaloblastic anaemia owing to interference with the action of vitamin B_{12}. For the same reason, exposure of theatre staff to nitrous oxide should be minimised. Depression of white cell formation may also occur.

NITROUS OXIDE

Indications see notes above

Cautions see notes above; pregnancy (Appendix 4); **interactions**: Appendix 1 (anaesthetics, general)

Side-effects see notes above

Dose

- Maintenance of light anaesthesia (using suitable anaesthetic apparatus), up to 66% in oxygen
- Analgesia, up to 50% in oxygen, according to the patient's needs

15.1.3 Antimuscarinic drugs

Antimuscarinic drugs are used (less commonly nowadays) as premedicants to dry bronchial and salivary secretions which are increased by intubation, by surgery to the upper airways, and by some inhalational anaesthetics. They are also used before or with neostigmine (section 15.1.6) to prevent bradycardia, excessive salivation, and other muscarinic actions of neostigmine. They also prevent bradycardia and hypotension associated with drugs such as propofol and suxamethonium.

Atropine sulphate is now rarely used for premedication but still has an emergency role in the treatment of vagotonic side-effects. For its role in acute arrhythmias after myocardial infarction, see section 2.3.1; see also cardiopulmonary resuscitation, section 2.7.3.

Hyoscine hydrobromide reduces secretions and also provides a degree of amnesia, sedation and anti-emesis. Unlike atropine it may produce bradycardia rather than tachycardia. In some patients, especially the elderly, hyoscine may cause the central anticholinergic syndrome (excitement, ataxia, hallucinations, behavioural abnormalities, and drowsiness).

Glycopyrronium bromide reduces salivary secretions. When given intravenously it produces less tachycardia than atropine. It is widely used with neostigmine for reversal of non-depolarising neuromuscular blocking drugs (section 15.1.5).

Phenothiazines do not effectively reduce secretions when used alone.

ATROPINE SULPHATE

Indications drying secretions; reversal of excessive bradycardia; with anticholinesterases for reversal of non-depolarising neuromuscular block; antidote to organophosphorous poisoning (see Emergency Treatment of Poisoning p. 36), antispasmodic (section

1.2); bradycardia (section 2.3.1); cardiopulmonary resuscitation (section 2.7.3); eye (section 11.5)

Cautions paralytic ileus; pyloric stenosis; cardiovascular disease; myasthenia gravis; prostatic enlargement; see also section 1.2; **interactions:** Appendix 1 (antimuscarinics)

Duration of action Since atropine has a shorter duration of action than neostigmine, late unopposed bradycardia may result; close monitoring of the patient is necessary

Side-effects see section 1.2

Dose

- Premedication, by intravenous injection, 300–600 micrograms immediately before induction of anaesthesia; CHILD 20 micrograms/kg (max. 600 micrograms)

  By subcutaneous or intramuscular injection, 300–600 micrograms 30–60 minutes before induction; CHILD 20 micrograms/kg (max. 600 micrograms)
- Intra-operative bradycardia, by intravenous injection, 300–600 micrograms (larger doses in emergencies); CHILD [unlicensed indication] 1–12 years 10–20 micrograms/kg
- Control of muscarinic side-effects of neostigmine or edrophonium in reversal of competitive neuromuscular block (but rarely used), by intravenous injection, 0.6–1.2 mg; CHILD under 12 years 20 micrograms/kg (max. 600 micrograms)
- Arrhythmias after myocardial infarction, see section 2.3.1 and 2.7.3; see also cardiopulmonary resuscitation algorithm, inside back cover

[1]**Atropine** (Non-proprietary) PoM

Injection, atropine sulphate 600 micrograms/mL, net price 1-mL amp = 50p

Note Other strengths also available

Injection, prefilled disposable syringe, atropine sulphate 100 micrograms/mL, net price 5 mL = £4.58, 10 mL = £5.39, 30 mL = £8.95

Injection, prefilled disposable syringe, atropine sulphate 200 micrograms/mL, net price 5 mL = £4.67; 300 micrograms/mL, 10 mL = £4.67; 600 micrograms/mL, 1 mL = £4.67

1. PoM restriction does not apply where administration is for saving life in emergency

[1]**Minijet® Atropine** (UCB Pharma) PoM

Injection, atropine sulphate 100 micrograms/mL, net price 5 mL = £4.58, 10 mL = £5.39, 30 mL = £8.95

1. PoM restriction does not apply where administration is for saving life in emergency

GLYCOPYRRONIUM BROMIDE
(Glycopyrrolate)

Indications drying secretions (see Prescribing in Palliative Care, p. 16); reversal of excessive bradycardia; with neostigmine for reversal of non-depolarising neuromuscular block; hyperhidrosis (section 13.12)

Cautions paralytic ileus, pyloric stenosis; cardiovascular disease; myasthenia gravis; prostatic enlargement; see also section 1.2; **interactions:** Appendix 1 (antimuscarinics)

Side-effects see section 1.2

Dose

- Premedication, by intramuscular *or* intravenous injection, 200–400 micrograms *or* 4–5 micrograms/kg (max. 400 micrograms); CHILD by intramuscular *or* by intravenous injection, 4–8 micrograms/kg (max. 200 micrograms)
- Intra-operative use, by intravenous injection, 200–400 micrograms *or* 4–5 micrograms/kg (max. 400 micrograms), repeated if necessary; CHILD under 18 years 4–8 micrograms/kg (max. 200 micrograms), repeated if necessary
- Control of muscarinic side-effects of neostigmine in reversal of non-depolarising neuromuscular block, by intravenous injection, 200 micrograms per 1 mg of neostigmine, *or* 10–15 micrograms/kg; CHILD 10 micrograms/kg

Robinul® (Anpharm) PoM

Injection, glycopyrronium bromide 200 micrograms/mL, net price 1-mL amp = 60p; 3-mL amp = £1.01

Note May be difficult to obtain

With neostigmine metilsulphate

Section 15.1.6

HYOSCINE HYDROBROMIDE
(Scopolamine hydrobromide)

Indications drying secretions (see Prescribing in Palliative Care, p. 16), amnesia; other indications (section 4.6)

Cautions see under Hyoscine Hydrobromide (section 4.6); also paralytic ileus, myasthenia gravis, epilepsy, prostatic enlargement; avoid in the elderly (see notes above)

Side-effects see under Atropine Sulphate; bradycardia

Dose

- Premedication, by subcutaneous *or* intramuscular injection, 200–600 micrograms 30–60 minutes before induction of anaesthesia; CHILD 15 micrograms/kg

Hyoscine (Non-proprietary) PoM

Injection, hyoscine hydrobromide 400 micrograms/mL, net price 1-mL amp = £2.68; 600 micrograms/mL, 1-mL amp = £2.81

With papaveretum

See under papaveretum (section 4.7.2)

15.1.4 Sedative and analgesic peri-operative drugs

15.1.4.1 Anxiolytics and neuroleptics
15.1.4.2 Non-opioid analgesics
15.1.4.3 Opioid analgesics

These drugs are given to allay fear and anxiety in the pre-operative period (including the night before an operation), to relieve pain and discomfort when present, and to augment the action of subsequent anaesthetic agents. A number of the drugs used also provide some degree of pre-operative amnesia. The choice will vary with the individual patient, the nature of the operative procedure, the anaesthetic to be used, and other prevailing circumstances such as outpatients, obstetrics, and recovery facilities. The choice also varies between elective and emergency operations.

Premedication in children Oral administration is preferred where possible but it is not altogether satisfactory; the rectal route should only be used in exceptional circumstances. For further details consult *BNF for Children*.

Application of a local anaesthetic (section 15.2) to the injection site can help to prevent pain.

Anaesthesia and driving See section 15.1.

15.1.4.1 Anxiolytics and neuroleptics

Anxiolytic benzodiazepines are widely used for premedication; neuroleptics such as **chlorpromazine** are rarely used.

Benzodiazepines

Benzodiazepines possess useful properties for premedication including relief of anxiety, sedation, and amnesia; short-acting benzodiazepines taken by mouth are the most common premedicants. They have no analgesic effect so an opioid analgesic may sometimes be required for pain.

Benzodiazepines can alleviate anxiety at doses that do not necessarily cause excessive sedation and they are of particular value during short procedures or during operations under local anaesthesia (including dentistry). Amnesia reduces the likelihood of any unpleasant memories of the procedure (although benzodiazepines, particularly when used for more profound sedation, can sometimes induce sexual fantasies). Benzodiazepines are also used in intensive care units for sedation, particularly in those receiving assisted ventilation.

Benzodiazepines may occasionally cause marked respiratory depression and facilities for its treatment are essential; flumazenil (section 15.1.7) is used to antagonise the effects of benzodiazepines. They are best avoided in myasthenia gravis, especially peri-operatively.

Diazepam is used to produce mild sedation with amnesia. It is a long-acting drug with active metabolites and a second period of drowsiness can occur several hours after its administration. Peri-operative use of diazepam in children is not generally recommended; its effect and timing of response are unreliable and paradoxical effects may occur.

Diazepam is relatively insoluble in water and preparations formulated in organic solvents are painful on intravenous injection and give rise to a high incidence of venous thrombosis (which may not be noticed for several days after the injection). Intramuscular injection of diazepam is painful and absorption is erratic. An emulsion preparation for intravenous injection is less irritant and reduces the risk of venous thrombosis; it is not suitable for intramuscular injection. Diazepam is also available as a rectal solution but this preparation is not used for premedication or sedation.

Temazepam is given by mouth and has a shorter duration of action and a more rapid onset than diazepam given by mouth. It has been used as a premedicant in inpatient and day-case surgery; anxiolytic and sedative effects last about 90 minutes although there may be residual drowsiness.

Lorazepam produces more prolonged sedation than temazepam and it has marked amnesic effects. It is used as a premedicant the night before major surgery; a further, smaller dose may be required the following morning if any delay in starting surgery is anticipated. Alternatively the first dose may be given early in the morning on the day of operation.

Midazolam is a water-soluble benzodiazepine which is often used in preference to intravenous diazepam; recovery is faster than from diazepam. Midazolam is associated with profound sedation when high doses are given intravenously or when used with certain other drugs.

Dental procedures Anxiolytics diminish tension, anxiety and panic, and may benefit anxious patients. However, their use is no substitute for sympathy and reassurance.

Diazepam and temazepam are effective anxiolytics for dental treatment in adults, but they are less suitable for children. Diazepam has a longer duration of action than temazepam. When given at night diazepam is associated with more residual effects the following day; patients should be very carefully warned **not** to drive (**important**: for general advice on anaesthesia and driving see p. 666). For further information on hypnotics and anxiolytics, see section 4.1. For further information on hypnotics used for dental procedures, see section 4.1.1.

DIAZEPAM

Indications premedication; sedation with amnesia, and in conjunction with local anaesthesia; other indications (section 4.1.2, section 4.8.2, and section 10.2.2)

Cautions see notes above and section 4.1.2 and section 4.8.2

Contra-indications see notes above and section 4.1.2

Side-effects see notes above and section 4.1.2

Dose

- By mouth, 5 mg on night before minor or dental surgery then 5 mg 2 hours before procedure; ELDERLY (or debilitated), half adult dose
- By intravenous injection, into a large vein 10–20 mg over 2–4 minutes as sedative cover for minor surgical and medical procedures; premedication 100–200 micrograms/kg

Preparations

Section 4.1.2

LORAZEPAM

Indications sedation with amnesia; premedication; other indications (section 4.1.2 and section 4.8.2)

Cautions see notes above and section 4.1.2; **interactions**: Appendix 1 (anxiolytics and hypnotics)

Contra-indications see notes above and under Diazepam (section 4.1.2)

Side-effects see notes above and under Diazepam (section 4.1.2)

Dose

- By mouth, 2–3 mg the night before operation; 2–4 mg 1–2 hours before operation

- By slow intravenous injection, preferably diluted with an equal volume of sodium chloride intravenous infusion 0.9% or water for injections, 50 micrograms/kg 30–45 minutes before operation
- By intramuscular injection, diluted as above, 50 micrograms/kg 60–90 minutes before operation

Preparations
Section 4.1.2

MIDAZOLAM

Indications sedation with amnesia; sedation in intensive care; premedication, induction of anaesthesia; status epilepticus [unlicensed use], section 4.8.2

Cautions cardiac disease; respiratory disease; myasthenia gravis; neonates; children (particularly if cardiovascular impairment); history of drug or alcohol abuse; reduce dose in elderly and debilitated; avoid prolonged use (and abrupt withdrawal thereafter); concentration of midazolam in children under 15 kg not to exceed 1 mg/mL; hepatic impairment (Appendix 2); renal impairment (Appendix 3); pregnancy (Appendix 4) and breast-feeding (Appendix 5); **interactions:** Appendix 1 (anxiolytics and hypnotics)

Contra-indications marked neuromuscular respiratory weakness including unstable myasthenia gravis; severe respiratory depression; acute pulmonary insufficiency

Side-effects gastro-intestinal disturbances, increased appetite, jaundice; hypotension, cardiac arrest, heart rate changes, anaphylaxis, thrombosis; laryngospasm, bronchospasm, respiratory depression and respiratory arrest (particularly with high doses or on rapid injection); drowsiness, confusion, ataxia, amnesia, headache, euphoria, hallucinations, convulsions (more common in neonates), dizziness, vertigo, involuntary movements, paradoxical excitement and aggression (especially in children and elderly), dysarthria; urinary retention, incontinence, changes in libido; blood disorders; muscle weakness; visual disturbances; salivation changes; skin reactions; injection-site reactions

Dose

- Conscious sedation, by slow intravenous injection (approx. 2 mg/minute) 5–10 minutes before procedure, initially 2–2.5 mg (ELDERLY 0.5–1 mg), increased if necessary in steps of 1 mg (ELDERLY 0.5–1 mg); usual total dose 3.5–5 mg (max. 7.5 mg), ELDERLY max. 3.5 mg; CHILD by intravenous injection over 2–3 minutes, 6 months–5 years initially 50–100 micrograms/kg, dose increased if necessary in small steps (max. total dose 6 mg), 6–12 years initially 25–50 micrograms/kg, dose increased if necessary in small steps (max. total dose 10 mg)
  By intramuscular injection, CHILD 1–15 years 50–150 micrograms/kg; max. 10 mg
- Sedative in combined anaesthesia, by intravenous injection, 30–100 micrograms/kg repeated as required or by continuous intravenous infusion, 30–100 micrograms/kg/hour (ELDERLY lower doses needed); CHILD not recommended
- Premedication, by deep intramuscular injection, 70–100 micrograms/kg (ELDERLY and debilitated 25–50 micrograms/kg) 20–60 minutes before induction; CHILD 1–15 years 80–200 micrograms/kg
- Induction (but rarely used), by slow intravenous injection, 150–200 micrograms/kg (ELDERLY and debilitated 100–200 micrograms/kg) given in divided doses (max. 5 mg) at intervals of 2 minutes; max. total dose 600 micrograms/kg; CHILD 7–18 years 150 micrograms/kg (max. 7.5 mg) given in steps of 50 micrograms/kg (max. 2.5 mg) over 2–5 minutes; wait for 2–5 minutes then give additional doses of 50 micrograms/kg (max. 2.5 mg) every 2 minutes if necessary, max. total dose 500 micrograms/kg (not exceeding 25 mg)
- Sedation of patients receiving intensive care, by slow intravenous injection, initially 30–300 micrograms/kg given in steps of 1–2.5 mg every 2 minutes, then by slow intravenous injection *or* by continuous intravenous infusion, 30–200 micrograms/kg/hour; reduce dose (or reduce or omit initial dose) in hypovolaemia, vasoconstriction, or hypothermia; lower doses may be adequate if opioid analgesic also used; NEONATE under 32 weeks gestational age by continuous intravenous infusion, 30 micrograms/kg/hour, NEONATE over 32 weeks gestational age and CHILD under 6 months 60 micrograms/kg/hour, CHILD over 6 months by slow intravenous injection, initially 50–200 micrograms/kg, then by continuous intravenous infusion, 60–120 micrograms/kg/hour, adjusted according to response

Midazolam (Non-proprietary) CD
Injection, midazolam (as hydrochloride) 1 mg/mL, net price 50-mL vial = £6.30; 5 mg/mL, 2-mL amp = 79p, 5-mL amp = 91p, 10-mL amp = £4.70, 18-mL amp = £6.80

Hypnovel® (Roche) CD
Injection, midazolam (as hydrochloride) 2 mg/mL, net price 5-mL amp = 75p; 5 mg/mL, 2-mL amp = 90p

TEMAZEPAM

Indications premedication before surgery; anxiety before investigatory procedures; hypnotic (section 4.1.1)

Cautions see notes above and under Diazepam (section 4.1.2; **interactions:** Appendix 1 (anxiolytics and hypnotics)

Contra-indications see notes above and under Diazepam (section 4.1.2)

Side-effects see notes above and under Diazepam (section 4.1.2)

Dose

- By mouth, premedication, 20–40 mg (elderly, 10–20 mg) 1 hour before operation; CHILD 1 mg/kg (max. 30 mg)

Preparations
Section 4.1.1

15.1.4.2 Non-opioid analgesics

Since non-steroidal anti-inflammatory drugs (NSAIDs) do not depress respiration, do not impair gastro-intestinal motility, and do not cause dependence, they may be useful alternatives (or adjuncts) to the use of opioids for the relief of postoperative pain. NSAIDs may be inadequate for the relief of severe pain.

Acemetacin, **diclofenac**, **flurbiprofen**, **ibuprofen**, **ketoprofen**, (section 10.1.1), **paracetamol** (section 4.7.1), **parecoxib**, and **ketorolac** are licensed for postoperative use. Diclofenac, ketoprofen, ketorolac, and paracetamol can be given by injection as well as by mouth. Intramuscular injections of diclofenac and ketoprofen are given deep into the gluteal muscle to minimise pain and tissue damage; diclofenac can also be given by intravenous infusion for the treatment or prevention of postoperative pain. Ketorolac is less irritant on intramuscular injection but pain has been reported; it can also be given by intravenous injection.

Parecoxib (a selective inhibitor of cyclo-oxygenase-2) can be given by intramuscular or intravenous injection (but see also NSAIDs and Cardiovascular Events, section 10.1.1). The *Scottish Medicines Consortium* has advised (January 2003) that parecoxib should **not** be used because there is no evidence of a reduction in postoperative haemorrhagic or gastro-intestinal complications compared with non-selective NSAIDs.

Suppositories of diclofenac and ketoprofen may be effective alternatives to the parenteral use of these drugs. Flurbiprofen is also available as suppositories.

KETOROLAC TROMETAMOL

Indications short-term management of moderate to severe acute postoperative pain **only**

Cautions see section 10.1.1; avoid in porphyria (section 9.8.2); **interactions**: Appendix 1 (NSAIDs)

Contra-indications see section 10.1.1; also complete or partial syndrome of nasal polyps; haemorrhagic diatheses (including coagulation disorders) and following operations with high risk of haemorrhage or incomplete haemostasis; confirmed or suspected cerebrovascular bleeding; hypovolaemia or dehydration

Side-effects see section 10.1.1; also gastro-intestinal disturbances; flushing, bradycardia, palpitation, chest pain; dyspnoea, asthma; malaise, euphoria, psychosis, paraesthesia, convulsions, abnormal dreams, hyperkinesia; urinary frequency, thirst; hyponatraemia, hyperkalaemia, myalgia; visual disturbances (including optic neuritis); pallor, purpura, pain at injection site

Dose

- ADULT and CHILD over 16 years, by mouth, 10 mg every 4–6 hours (ELDERLY every 6–8 hours) as required; max. 40 mg daily; max. duration of treatment 7 days
- ADULT and CHILD over 16 years, by intramuscular injection *or* by intravenous injection over at least 15 seconds, initially 10 mg, then 10–30 mg every 4–6 hours as required (up to every 2 hours during initial postoperative period); max. 90 mg daily (ELDERLY and patients weighing less than 50 kg max. 60 mg daily); max. duration of treatment 2 days

  Note When converting from parenteral to oral administration, total combined dose on the day of converting should not exceed 90 mg (60 mg in the elderly and patients weighing less than 50 kg) of which the oral component should not exceed 40 mg

Toradol® (Roche) PoM

Tablets, ivory, f/c, ketorolac trometamol 10 mg, net price 20-tab pack = £5.79. Label: 17, 21

Injection, ketorolac trometamol 10 mg/mL, net price 1-mL amp = 94p; 30 mg/mL, 1-mL amp = £1.14

PARECOXIB

Indications short-term management of acute postoperative pain

Cautions see section 10.1.1; dehydration; following coronary artery bypass graft surgery; **interactions:** Appendix 1 (NSAIDs)

Contra-indications see section 10.1.1; history of allergic drug reactions including sulphonamide hypersensitivity; inflammatory bowel disease

Side-effects see section 10.1.1; also flatulence; hypertension, hypotension, peripheral oedema; pharyngitis, respiratory insufficiency; hypoaesthesia; alveolar osteitis; oliguria; postoperative anaemia, hypokalaemia; back pain; pruritus; *less commonly* bradycardia, cardiovascular events, increased blood urea nitrogen, ecchymosis, thrombocytopenia, *rarely* vomiting, tachycardia, rash (discontinue—risk of serious reactions including Stevens-Johnson syndrome and toxic epidermal necrolysis), anaphylaxis

Dose

- By deep intramuscular injection *or* by intravenous injection, initially 40 mg, then 20–40 mg every 6–12 hours when required; max. 80 mg daily; ELDERLY weighing less than 50 kg, initially 20 mg, then max. 40 mg daily; CHILD and ADOLESCENT under 18 years, not recommended

Dynastat® (Pharmacia) ▼ PoM

Injection, powder for reconstitution, parecoxib (as sodium salt), net price 40-mg vial = £4.96, 40-mg vial (with solvent) = £5.67

15.1.4.3 Opioid analgesics

Opioid analgesics are now rarely used as premedicants; they are more likely to be administered at induction. Pre-operative use of opioid analgesics is generally limited to those patients who require control of existing pain. The main side-effects of opioid analgesics are respiratory depression, cardiovascular depression, nausea, and vomiting; for general notes on opioid analgesics and their use in postoperative pain, see section 4.7.2.

For the management of opioid-induced respiratory depression, see section 15.1.7.

Intra-operative analgesia Opioid analgesics given in small doses before or with induction reduce the dose requirement of some drugs used during anaesthesia.

Alfentanil, **fentanyl**, and **remifentanil** are particularly useful because they act within 1–2 minutes and have short durations of action. The initial doses of alfentanil or fentanyl are followed either by successive intravenous injections or by an intravenous infusion; prolonged infusions increase the duration of effect. Repeated intra-operative doses of alfentanil or fentanyl should be given with care since the resulting respiratory depression can persist postoperatively and occasionally it may become apparent for the first time postoperatively when monitoring of the patient might be less intensive. Alfentanil, fentanyl, and remifentanil can cause muscle rigidity, particularly of the chest wall or jaw; this can be managed by the use of neuromuscular blocking drugs.

In contrast to other opioids which are metabolised in the liver, remifentanil undergoes rapid metabolism by non-specific blood and tissue esterases; its short duration of action allows prolonged administration at high dosage, without accumulation, and with little risk of residual postoperative respiratory depression. Remifentanil should not be given by intravenous injection intra-operatively, but it is well suited to continuous infusion; a supplementary analgesic is given before stopping the infusion of remifentanil.

ALFENTANIL

Indications analgesia especially during short operative procedure and outpatient surgery; enhancement of anaesthesia; analgesia and suppression of respiratory activity in patients receiving intensive care, with assisted ventilation, for up to 4 days

Cautions see section 4.7.2 and notes above

Contra-indications see section 4.7.2

Side-effects see section 4.7.2 and notes above; also hypertension, myoclonic movements; *less commonly* arrhythmias, cough, hiccup, laryngospasm, visual disturbances

Dose

> To avoid excessive dosage in obese patients, dose may need to be calculated on the basis of ideal body-weight

- By intravenous injection, spontaneous respiration, ADULT, initially up to 500 micrograms over 30 seconds; supplemental, 250 micrograms

  With assisted ventilation, ADULT over 18 years, initially 30–50 micrograms/kg; supplemental, 15 micrograms/kg; CHILD 1 month–18 years, initially 10–20 micrograms/kg; supplemental doses up to 10 micrograms/kg
- By intravenous infusion, with assisted ventilation, ADULT and CHILD, initially 50–100 micrograms/kg over 10 minutes *or* as a bolus, followed by maintenance of 0.5–1 micrograms/kg/minute

  Analgesia and suppression of respiratory activity during intensive care, with assisted ventilation, by intravenous infusion, initially 2 mg/hour subsequently adjusted according to response (usual range 0.5–10 mg/hour); more rapid initial control may be obtained with an intravenous dose of 5 mg given in divided portions over 10 minutes (slowing if hypotension or bradycardia occur); additional doses of 0.5–1 mg may be given by intravenous injection during short painful procedures

Rapifen® (Janssen-Cilag) CD

Injection, alfentanil (as hydrochloride) 500 micrograms/mL. Net price 2-mL amp = 67p; 10-mL amp = £3.08

Intensive care injection, alfentanil (as hydrochloride) 5 mg/mL. To be diluted before use. Net price 1-mL amp = £2.46

FENTANYL

Indications analgesia during operation, enhancement of anaesthesia; respiratory depressant in assisted respiration; analgesia in other situations (section 4.7.2)

Cautions see section 4.7.2 and notes above

Contra-indications see section 4.7.2

Side-effects see section 4.7.2 and notes above; also myoclonic movements; *less commonly* laryngospasm; *rarely* asystole, insomnia

Dose

> To avoid excessive dosage in obese patients dose may need to be calculated on the basis of ideal body-weight

- By slow intravenous injection, with spontaneous respiration, 50–100 micrograms (max. 200 micrograms on specialist advice), then 50 micrograms as required; CHILD 1–5 micrograms/kg, then 1 microgram/kg as required

  With assisted ventilation, 0.3–3.5 mg, then 100–200 micrograms as required; CHILD 5–10 micrograms/kg, then 1–3 micrograms/kg as required
- By intravenous infusion, with spontaneous respiration, ADULT and CHILD, 50–80 nanograms/kg/minute adjusted according to response

  With assisted ventilation, ADULT and CHILD, initially 10 micrograms/kg over 10 minutes then 100 nanograms/kg/minute adjusted according to response; ADULTS may require up to 3 micrograms/kg/minute in cardiac surgery

Note Fentanyl doses in BNF may differ from those in product literature

Fentanyl (Non-proprietary) CD

Injection, fentanyl (as citrate) 50 micrograms/mL, net price 2-mL amp = 54p, 10-mL amp = £1.65

Sublimaze® (Janssen-Cilag) CD

Injection, fentanyl (as citrate) 50 micrograms/mL, net price 2-mL amp = 22p, 10-mL amp = £1.11

REMIFENTANIL

Indications supplementation of general anaesthesia during induction and analgesia during maintenance of anaesthesia (consult product literature for use in patients undergoing cardiac surgery); analgesia and sedation in ventilated, intensive care patients

Cautions see section 4.7.2 (but no dose adjustment necessary in renal impairment) and notes above

Contra-indications see section 4.7.2 and notes above; left ventricular dysfunction

Side-effects see section 4.7.2 and notes above; also hypertension, hypoxia; *very rarely* asystole and anaphylaxis

Dose

> To avoid excessive dosage in obese patients, dose should be calculated on the basis of ideal body-weight

- Induction of anaesthesia, ADULT and CHILD over 12 years, by intravenous infusion, 0.5–1 micrograms/kg/minute, *with or without* an initial dose by intravenous injection of 0.25–1 microgram/kg over at least 30 seconds

  Note If patient to be intubated more than 8 minutes after start of intravenous infusion, initial intravenous injection dose is not necessary
- Maintenance of anaesthesia in ventilated patients, ADULT and CHILD over 12 years, by intravenous infusion, 0.05–2 micrograms/kg/minute (*with or without* an initial dose by intravenous injection of 0.25–

1 micrograms/kg over at least 30 seconds) according to anaesthetic technique and adjusted according to response; in light anaesthesia supplemental doses by intravenous injection every 2–5 minutes

- Maintenance of anaesthesia with spontaneous respiration, ADULT and CHILD over 12 years, by intravenous infusion, initially 40 nanograms/kg/minute adjusted according to response, usual range 25–100 nanograms/kg/minute
- Maintenance of anaesthesia, CHILD 1–12 years, by intravenous infusion, 0.05–1.3 micrograms/kg/minute (*with or without* an initial dose by intravenous injection of 0.1–1 microgram/kg over at least 30 seconds) according to anaesthetic technique and adjusted according to response
- Analgesia and sedation in ventilated, intensive-care patients, by intravenous infusion, ADULT over 18 years initially 100–150 nanograms/kg/minute adjusted according to response in steps of 25 nanograms/kg/minute (allow at least 5 minutes between dose adjustments); usual range 6–740 nanograms/kg/minute; if an infusion rate of 200 nanograms/kg/minute does not produce adequate sedation add another sedative (consult product literature for details)
- Additional analgesia during stimulating or painful procedures in ventilated, intensive-care patients, by intravenous infusion, ADULT over 18 years maintain infusion rate of at least 100 nanograms/kg/minute for at least 5 minutes before procedure and adjust every 2–5 minutes according to requirements, usual range 250–750 nanograms/kg/minute
- Cardiac surgery, consult product literature

Note Remifentanil doses in BNF may differ from those in product literature

Ultiva® (GSK) CD

Injection, powder for reconstitution, remifentanil (as hydrochloride), net price 1-mg vial = £5.12; 2-mg vial = £10.23; 5-mg vial = £25.58

15.1.5 Neuromuscular blocking drugs

Neuromuscular blocking drugs used in anaesthesia are also known as **muscle relaxants**. By specific blockade of the neuromuscular junction they enable light levels of anaesthesia to be employed with adequate relaxation of the muscles of the abdomen and diaphragm. They also relax the vocal cords and allow the passage of a tracheal tube. Their action differs from the muscle relaxants acting on the spinal cord or brain which are used in musculoskeletal disorders (section 10.2.2).

Patients who have received a neuromuscular blocking drug should **always** have their respiration assisted or controlled until the drug has been inactivated or antagonised (section 15.1.6). They should also receive sufficient concomitant inhalational or intravenous anaesthetic, or sedative drugs to prevent awareness.

Non-depolarising neuromuscular blocking drugs

Non-depolarising neuromuscular blocking drugs (also known as competitive muscle relaxants) compete with acetylcholine for receptor sites at the neuromuscular junction and their action may be reversed with anticholinesterases such as neostigmine (section 15.1.6). Non-depolarising neuromuscular blocking drugs may be divided into the **aminosteroid** group comprising pancuronium, rocuronium, and vecuronium, and the **benzylisoquinolinium** group comprising atracurium, cisatracurium, and mivacurium.

Non-depolarising neuromuscular blocking drugs have a slower onset of action than suxamethonium. These drugs can be classified by their duration of action as short-acting (15–30 minutes), intermediate-acting (30–40 minutes) and long-acting (60–120 minutes), although duration of action is dose-dependent. Drugs with a shorter or intermediate duration of action, such as atracurium and vecuronium, are more widely employed than those with a longer duration of action such as pancuronium.

Non-depolarising neuromuscular blocking drugs have no sedative or analgesic effects and are not considered to be a triggering factor for malignant hyperthermia.

For patients receiving intensive care and who require tracheal intubation and mechanical ventilation, a non-depolarising neuromuscular blocking drug is chosen according to its onset of effect, duration of action and side-effects. Rocuronium, with a rapid onset of effect, may facilitate intubation. Atracurium or cisatracurium may be suitable for long-term neuromuscular blockade since their duration of action is not dependent on elimination by the liver or the kidneys.

Cautions Allergic cross-reactivity between neuromuscular blocking drugs has been reported; caution is advised in cases of hypersensitivity to these drugs. Their activity is prolonged in patients with myasthenia gravis and in hypothermia, therefore lower doses are required. Non-depolarising neuromuscular blocking drugs should be used with great care in those with other neuromuscular disorders and those with fluid and electrolyte disturbances, as response is unpredictable. Resistance may develop in patients with burns who may require increased doses; low plasma cholinesterase activity in these patients requires dose titration for mivacurium. **Interactions**: Appendix 1 (muscle relaxants).

Side-effects Benzylisoquinolinium non-depolarising neuromuscular blocking drugs (except cisatracurium) are associated with histamine release which can cause skin flushing, hypotension, tachycardia, bronchospasm and very rarely, anaphylactoid reactions. Most aminosteroid neuromuscular blocking drugs produce minimal histamine release. Drugs possessing vagolytic activity can counteract any bradycardia that occurs during surgery. Acute myopathy has also been reported after prolonged use in intensive care.

Atracurium, a mixture of 10 isomers, is a benzylisoquinolinium neuromuscular blocking drug with an intermediate duration of action. It undergoes non-enzymatic metabolism which is independent of liver and kidney function, thus allowing its use in patients with hepatic or renal impairment. Cardiovascular effects are associated with significant histamine release.

Cisatracurium is a single isomer of atracurium. It is more potent and has a slightly longer duration of action than atracurium and provides greater cardiovascular stability because cisatracurium lacks histamine-releasing effects.

Mivacurium, a benzylisoquinolinium neuromuscular blocking drug, has a short duration of action. It is metabolised by plasma cholinesterase and muscle paralysis is prolonged in individuals deficient in this enzyme. It is not associated with vagolytic activity or ganglionic blockade although histamine release may occur, particularly with rapid injection.

Pancuronium, an aminosteroid neuromuscular blocking drug, has a long duration of action and is often used in patients receiving long-term mechanical ventilation in intensive care units. It lacks a histamine-releasing effect, but vagolytic and sympathomimetic effects can cause tachycardia and hypertension.

Rocuronium exerts an effect within 2 minutes and has the most rapid onset of any of the non-depolarising neuromuscular blocking drugs. It is an aminosteroid neuromuscular blocking drug with an intermediate duration of action. It is reported to have minimal cardiovascular effects; high doses produce mild vagolytic activity.

Vecuronium, an aminosteroid neuromuscular blocking drug, has an intermediate duration of action. It does not generally produce histamine release and lacks cardiovascular effects.

ATRACURIUM BESILATE
(Atracurium besylate)

Indications neuromuscular blockade (short to intermediate duration) for surgery or during intensive care

Cautions see notes above; pregnancy (Appendix 4); breast-feeding (Appendix 5)

Side-effects see notes above

Dose

> To avoid excessive dosage in obese patients, dose should be calculated on the basis of ideal body-weight

- Surgery or intubation, ADULT and CHILD over 1 month, by intravenous injection, initially 300–600 micrograms/kg; maintenance, by intravenous injection, 100–200 micrograms/kg as required *or* by intravenous infusion, 5–10 micrograms/kg/minute (300–600 micrograms/kg/hour)
- Intensive care, ADULT and CHILD over 1 month, by intravenous injection, initially 300–600 micrograms/kg (optional) then by intravenous infusion 4.5–29.5 micrograms/kg/minute (usual dose 11–13 micrograms/kg/minute)

Atracurium (Non-proprietary) PoM
Injection, atracurium besilate 10 mg/mL, net price 2.5-mL amp = £1.85; 5-mL amp = £3.37; 25-mL amp = £14.45

Tracrium® (GSK) PoM
Injection, atracurium besilate 10 mg/mL, net price 2.5-mL amp = £1.66; 5-mL amp = £3.00; 25-mL amp = £12.91

CISATRACURIUM

Indications neuromuscular blockade (intermediate duration) for surgery or during intensive care

Cautions see notes above; pregnancy (Appendix 4); breast-feeding

Side-effects see notes above

Dose

> To avoid excessive dosage in obese patients, dose should be calculated on the basis of ideal body-weight

- Intubation, by intravenous injection ADULT and CHILD over 1 month, initially 150 micrograms/kg; maintenance, by intravenous injection, 30 micrograms/kg approx. every 20 minutes; CHILD 2–12 years, 20 micrograms/kg approx. every 9 minutes; or maintenance, by intravenous infusion, ADULT and CHILD over 2 years, initially, 3 micrograms/kg/minute, *then after stabilisation*, 1–2 micrograms/kg/minute; dose reduced by up to 40% if used with isoflurane
- Intensive care, by intravenous infusion, ADULT 0.5–10.2 micrograms/kg/minute (usual dose 3 micrograms/kg/minute)

Note Lower doses can be used for children over 2 years when *not* for intubation

Nimbex® (GSK) PoM
Injection, cisatracurium (as besilate) 2 mg/mL, net price 10-mL amp = £7.55
Forte injection, cisatracurium (as besilate) 5 mg/mL, net price 30-mL vial = £31.09

MIVACURIUM

Indications neuromuscular blockade (short duration) for surgery

Cautions see notes above; low plasma cholinesterase activity; elderly; hepatic impairment (Appendix 2); renal impairment (Appendix 3); pregnancy (Appendix 4)

Side-effects see notes above

Dose

> To avoid excessive dosage in obese patients, dose should be calculated on the basis of ideal body-weight

- By intravenous injection, 70–250 micrograms/kg; maintenance 100 micrograms/kg every 15 minutes; CHILD 2–6 months initially 150 micrograms/kg, 7 months–12 years initially 200 micrograms/kg; maintenance (CHILD 2 months–12 years) 100 micrograms/kg every 6–9 minutes

Note Doses up to 150 micrograms/kg may be given over 5–15 seconds, higher doses should be given over 30 seconds. In patients with asthma, cardiovascular disease or those who are sensitive to falls in arterial blood pressure give over 60 seconds

- By intravenous infusion, maintenance of block, 8–10 micrograms/kg/minute, adjusted if necessary every 3 minutes by 1 microgram/kg/minute to usual dose of 6–7 micrograms/kg/minute; CHILD 2 months–12 years, usual dose 11–14 micrograms/kg/minute

Mivacron® (GSK) PoM
Injection, mivacurium (as chloride) 2 mg/mL, net price 5-mL amp = £2.79; 10-mL amp = £4.51

PANCURONIUM BROMIDE

Indications neuromuscular blockade (long duration) for surgery or during intensive care

Cautions see notes above; hepatic impairment (Appendix 2); renal impairment (Appendix 3); pregnancy (Appendix 4) and breast-feeding (Appendix 5)

Side-effects see notes above

Dose

> To avoid excessive dosage in obese patients, dose should be calculated on the basis of ideal body-weight

- Intubation, by intravenous injection, initially 50–100 micrograms/kg then 10–20 micrograms/kg as required; CHILD initially 60–100 micrograms/kg, then 10–20 micrograms/kg, NEONATE 30–40 micrograms/kg initially then 10–20 micrograms/kg
- Intensive care, by intravenous injection, 60 micrograms/kg every 60–90 minutes

Pancuronium (Non-proprietary) PoM
Injection, pancuronium bromide 2 mg/mL, net price 2-mL amp = £1.20

ROCURONIUM BROMIDE

Indications neuromuscular blockade (intermediate duration) for surgery or during intensive care
Cautions see notes above; hepatic impairment (Appendix 2); renal impairment (Appendix 3); pregnancy (Appendix 4) and breast-feeding (Appendix 5)
Side-effects see notes above
Dose

> To avoid excessive dosage in obese patients, dose should be calculated on the basis of ideal body-weight

- Intubation, ADULT and CHILD over 1 month, by intravenous injection, initially 600 micrograms/kg; maintenance by intravenous injection, 150 micrograms/kg (ELDERLY 75–100 micrograms/kg) *or* maintenance by intravenous infusion, 300–600 micrograms/kg/hour (ELDERLY up to 400 micrograms/kg/hour)
- Intensive care, by intravenous injection, ADULT initially 600 micrograms/kg; maintenance by intravenous infusion, 300–600 micrograms/kg/hour for first hour, then adjusted according to response

Esmeron® (Organon) PoM
Injection, rocuronium bromide 10 mg/mL, net price 5-mL vial = £3.01, 10-mL vial = £6.01

VECURONIUM BROMIDE

Indications neuromuscular blockade (intermediate duration) for surgery
Cautions see notes above; pregnancy (Appendix 4)
Side-effects see notes above
Dose

> To avoid excessive dosage in obese patients, dose should be calculated on the basis of ideal body-weight

- By intravenous injection, intubation, ADULT and CHILD over 5 months, 80–100 micrograms/kg (CHILD under 1 year, onset more rapid and high intubation dose may not be required); maintenance 20–30 micrograms/kg adjusted according to response; NEONATE and CHILD up to 4 months, initial test dose 10–20 micrograms/kg then incremental doses to achieve response
- By intravenous infusion, 0.8–1.4 micrograms/kg/minute (after initial intravenous injection of 40–100 micrograms/kg)

Norcuron® (Organon) PoM
Injection, powder for reconstitution, vecuronium bromide, net price 10-mg vial = £3.95 (with water for injections)

Depolarising neuromuscular blocking drugs

Suxamethonium has the most rapid onset of action of any of the neuromuscular blocking drugs and is ideal if fast onset and brief duration of action are required e.g. with tracheal intubation. Its duration of action is about 2 to 6 minutes following intravenous doses of about 1 mg/kg; repeated doses can be used for longer procedures.

Suxamethonium acts by mimicking acetylcholine at the neuromuscular junction but hydrolysis is much slower than for acetylcholine; depolarisation is therefore prolonged, resulting in neuromuscular blockade. Unlike the non-depolarising neuromuscular blocking drugs, its action cannot be reversed and recovery is spontaneous; anticholinesterases such as neostigmine potentiate the neuromuscular block.

Suxamethonium should be given after anaesthetic induction because paralysis is usually preceded by painful muscle fasciculations. While tachycardia occurs with single use, bradycardia may occur with repeated doses in adults and with the first dose in children. Premedication with atropine reduces bradycardia as well as the excessive salivation associated with suxamethonium use.

Prolonged paralysis may occur in **dual block**, which occurs with high or repeated doses of suxamethonium and is caused by the development of a non-depolarising block following the initial depolarising block; edrophonium (section 15.1.6) may be used to confirm the diagnosis of dual block. Individuals with myasthenia gravis are resistant to suxamethonium but can develop dual block resulting in delayed recovery. Prolonged paralysis may also occur in those with low or atypical plasma cholinesterase. Assisted ventilation should be continued until muscle function is restored.

SUXAMETHONIUM CHLORIDE

Indications neuromuscular blockade (rapid onset, short duration)
Cautions see notes above; pregnancy (Appendix 4); patients with cardiac, respiratory or neuromuscular disease; raised intra-ocular pressure (avoid in penetrating eye injury); severe sepsis (risk of hyperkalaemia); **interactions**: Appendix 1 (muscle relaxants)
Contra-indications family history of malignant hyperthermia, low plasma cholinesterase activity (including severe liver disease) (Appendix 2), hyperkalaemia; major trauma, severe burns, neurological disease involving acute wasting of major muscle, prolonged immobilisation—risk of hyperkalaemia, personal or family history of congenital myotonic disease, Duchenne muscular dystrophy
Side-effects see notes above; also postoperative muscle pain, myoglobinuria, myoglobinaemia; tachycardia, arrhythmias, cardiac arrest, hypertension, hypotension; bronchospasm, apnoea, prolonged respiratory depression, anaphylactic reactions; hyperkalaemia; hyperthermia; increased gastric pressure; rash, flushing

Dose

- By intravenous injection, initially 1 mg/kg; maintenance, usually 0.5–1 mg/kg at 5–10 minute intervals; max. 500 mg/hour; NEONATE and INFANT under 1 year, 2 mg/kg; CHILD over 1 year, 1 mg/kg
- By intravenous infusion of a solution containing 1–2 mg/mL (0.1–0.2%), 2.5–4 mg/minute; max. 500 mg/hour; CHILD reduce infusion rate according to body-weight
- By intramuscular injection, INFANT under 1 year, up to 4–5 mg/kg; CHILD over 1 year, up to 4 mg/kg; max. 150 mg

Suxamethonium Chloride (Non-proprietary) PoM
Injection, suxamethonium chloride 50 mg/mL, net price 2-mL amp = 70p, 2-mL prefilled syringe = £7.35

Anectine® (GSK) PoM
Injection, suxamethonium chloride 50 mg/mL, net price 2-mL amp = 71p

15.1.6 Anticholinesterases used in anaesthesia

Anticholinesterases reverse the effects of the non-depolarising (competitive) neuromuscular blocking drugs such as pancuronium but they prolong the action of the depolarising neuromuscular blocking drug suxamethonium.

Edrophonium has a transient action and may be used in the diagnosis of suspected dual block due to suxamethonium. Atropine (section 15.1.3) is given before or with edrophonium to prevent muscarinic effects when given for reversal of non-depolarising neuromuscular blockade.

Neostigmine has a longer duration of action than edrophonium. It is the specific drug for reversal of non-depolarising (competitive) blockade. It acts within one minute of intravenous injection and its effects last for 20 to 30 minutes; a second dose may then be necessary. Glycopyrronium or alternatively atropine (section 15.1.3), given before or with neostigmine, prevent bradycardia, excessive salivation, and other muscarinic effects of neostigmine.

EDROPHONIUM CHLORIDE

Indications see under Dose; myasthenia gravis (section 10.2.1)

Cautions see section 10.2.1; atropine should also be given

Contra-indications see section 10.2.1

Side-effects see section 10.2.1

Dose

- Brief reversal of non-depolarising neuromuscular blockade, by intravenous injection over several minutes, 500–700 micrograms/kg (after or with atropine)
- Diagnosis of dual block, by intravenous injection, 10 mg

Edrophonium (Cambridge) PoM
Injection, edrophonium chloride 10 mg/mL, net price 1-mL amp = £6.55

NEOSTIGMINE METILSULFATE
(Neostigmine methylsulphate)

Indications see under Dose

Cautions see section 10.2.1 and notes above; glycopyrronium or atropine should also be given

Contra-indications see section 10.2.1 and notes above

Side-effects see section 10.2.1 and notes above

Dose

- Reversal of non-depolarising neuromuscular blockade, by intravenous injection over 1 minute, 50–70 micrograms/kg (max. 5 mg) after or with glycopyrronium or atropine
- Myasthenia gravis, see section 10.2.1

Neostigmine (Non-proprietary) PoM
Injection, neostigmine metilsulfate 2.5 mg/mL, net price 1-mL amp = 58p

With glycopyrronium

Robinul-Neostigmine® (Anpharm) PoM
Injection, neostigmine metilsulfate 2.5 mg, glycopyrronium bromide 500 micrograms/mL, net price 1-mL amp = £1.01
Dose reversal of non-depolarising neuromuscular blockade by intravenous injection over 10–30 seconds, 1–2 mL *or* 0.02 mL/kg, dose may be repeated if required (total max. 2 mL); CHILD 0.02 mL/kg (*or* 0.2 mL/kg of a 1 in 10 dilution using water for injections or sodium chloride injection 0.9%), dose may be repeated if required (total max. 2 mL)
Note May be difficult to obtain

15.1.7 Antagonists for central and respiratory depression

Respiratory depression is a major concern with opioid analgesics and it may be treated by artificial ventilation or be reversed by **naloxone**. Naloxone will immediately reverse opioid-induced respiratory depression but the dose may have to be repeated because of the short duration of action of naloxone; however, naloxone will also antagonise the analgesic effect.

Flumazenil is a benzodiazepine antagonist for the reversal of the central sedative effects of benzodiazepines after anaesthetic and similar procedures. Flumazenil has a shorter half-life and duration of action than diazepam or midazolam so patients may become resedated.

Doxapram (section 3.5.1) is a central and respiratory stimulant but is of limited value in anaesthesia.

FLUMAZENIL

Indications reversal of sedative effects of benzodiazepines in anaesthetic, intensive care, and diagnostic procedures

Cautions short-acting (repeat doses may be necessary—benzodiazepine effects may persist for at least 24 hours); benzodiazepine dependence (may precipitate withdrawal symptoms); prolonged benzodiazepine therapy for epilepsy (risk of convulsions); history of panic disorders (risk of recurrence); ensure neuromuscular blockade cleared before giving; avoid rapid injection in high-risk or anxious patients and following major surgery; hepatic impairment (Appendix 2);

head injury (rapid reversal of benzodiazepine sedation may cause convulsions); elderly, children, pregnancy (Appendix 4), breast-feeding

Contra-indications life-threatening condition (e.g. raised intracranial pressure, status epilepticus) controlled by benzodiazepines

Side-effects nausea, vomiting, and flushing; if wakening too rapid, agitation, anxiety, and fear; transient increase in blood pressure and heart-rate in intensive care patients; *very rarely* convulsions (particularly in those with epilepsy), hypersensitivity reactions including anaphylaxis

Dose

- By intravenous injection, 200 micrograms over 15 seconds, then 100 micrograms at 60-second intervals if required; usual dose range, 300–600 micrograms; max. total dose 1 mg (2 mg in intensive care); question aetiology if no response to repeated doses
- By intravenous infusion, if drowsiness recurs after injection, 100–400 micrograms/hour, adjusted according to level of arousal

Flumazenil (Non-proprietary) PoM
Injection, flumazenil 100 micrograms/mL, net price 5-mL amp = £14.49

Anexate® (Roche) PoM
Injection, flumazenil 100 micrograms/mL, net price 5-mL amp = £14.49

NALOXONE HYDROCHLORIDE

Indications reversal of opioid-induced respiratory depression; reversal of neonatal respiratory depression resulting from opioid administration to mother during labour; overdosage with opioids (see Emergency Treatment of Poisoning)

Cautions cardiovascular disease or those receiving cardiotoxic drugs (serious adverse cardiovascular effects reported); physical dependence on opioids (precipitates withdrawal); pain (see also under Titration of Dose, below); has short duration of action (repeated doses or infusion may be necessary to reverse effects of opioids with longer duration of action); pregnancy (Appendix 4)

Titration of dose In postoperative use, the dose should be titrated for each patient in order to obtain sufficient respiratory response; however, naloxone antagonises analgesia

Side-effects hypotension, hypertension, ventricular tachycardia and fibrillation, cardiac arrest; hyperventilation, dyspnoea, pulmonary oedema; *less commonly* agitation, excitement, paraesthesia

Dose

- By intravenous injection, 100–200 micrograms (1.5–3 micrograms/kg); if response inadequate, increments of 100 micrograms every 2 minutes; further doses by intramuscular injection after 1–2 hours if required; CHILD by intravenous injection, 10 micrograms/kg; subsequent dose of 100 micrograms/kg if no response; if intravenous route not possible, may be given in divided doses by intramuscular *or* subcutaneous injection
- NEONATE, reversal of respiratory and CNS depression resulting from opioid administration to mother during labour, by subcutaneous, intramuscular, *or* intravenous injection, 10 micrograms/kg, repeated every 2–3 minutes; alternatively by intramuscular injection, 200 micrograms (60 micrograms/kg) as a single dose at birth

Naloxone PoM
See under Emergency Treatment of Poisoning p. 31

15.1.8 Drugs for malignant hyperthermia

Malignant hyperthermia is a rare but potentially lethal complication of anaesthesia. It is characterised by a rapid rise in temperature, increased muscle rigidity, tachycardia, and acidosis. The most common triggers of malignant hyperthermia are the volatile anaesthetics. Suxamethonium has also been implicated, but malignant hyperthermia is more likely if it is given following a volatile anaesthetic. Volatile anaesthetics and suxamethonium should be avoided during anaesthesia in patients at high risk of malignant hyperthermia.

Dantrolene is used in the treatment of malignant hyperthermia. It acts on skeletal muscle cells by interfering with calcium efflux, thereby stopping the contractile process.

DANTROLENE SODIUM

Indications malignant hyperthermia; chronic severe spasticity of voluntary muscle (section 10.2.2)

Cautions avoid extravasation; pregnancy (Appendix 4); **interactions**: Appendix 1 (muscle relaxants)

Contra-indications breast-feeding (Appendix 5)

Dose

- By rapid intravenous injection, 1 mg/kg, repeated as required to a cumulative max. of 10 mg/kg

Dantrium Intravenous® (Procter & Gamble Pharm.) PoM
Injection, powder for reconstitution, dantrolene sodium, net price 20-mg vial = £15.08 (hosp. only)

15.2 Local anaesthesia

The use of local anaesthetics by injection or by application to mucous membranes to produce local analgesia is discussed in this section.

See also section 1.7 (anus), section 11.7 (eye), section 12.3 (oropharynx), and section 13.3 (skin).

Use of local anaesthetics Local anaesthetic drugs act by causing a reversible block to conduction along nerve fibres. The drugs used vary widely in their potency, toxicity, duration of action, stability, solubility in water, and ability to penetrate mucous membranes. These variations determine their suitability for use by various routes, e.g. topical (surface), infiltration, peripheral nerve block, intravenous regional anaesthesia (Bier's block), plexus, epidural (extradural) or spinal block. Local anaesthetics may also be used for postoperative pain relief, thereby reducing the need for analgesics such as opioids.

Administration In estimating the safe dosage of these drugs it is important to take account of the rate at which they are absorbed and excreted as well as their potency. The patient's age, weight, physique, and clinical condition, the degree of vascularity of the area to which the drug is to be applied, and the duration of administration are other factors which must be taken into account.

Local anaesthetics do not rely on the circulation to transport them to their sites of action, but uptake into the systemic circulation is important in terminating their action and producing toxicity. Following most regional anaesthetic procedures, maximum arterial plasma concentrations of anaesthetic develop within about 10 to 25 minutes, so **careful surveillance** for toxic effects is necessary during the first 30 minutes after injection. Great care must be taken to avoid accidental intravascular injection. Local anaesthesia around the oral cavity may impair swallowing and therefore increase the risk of aspiration.

Epidural anaesthesia is commonly used during surgery, often combined with general anaesthesia, because of its protective effect against the stress response of surgery. It is often used when good postoperative pain relief is essential (e.g. aortic aneurysm surgery or major gut surgery).

Toxicity Toxic effects associated with local anaesthetics usually result from excessively high plasma concentrations; single application of topical lidocaine preparations does not generally cause systemic side-effects. Effects initially include a feeling of inebriation and lightheadedness followed by sedation, circumoral paraesthesia and twitching; convulsions can occur in severe reactions. On intravenous injection convulsions and cardiovascular collapse may occur very rapidly. Hypersensitivity reactions occur mainly with the ester-type local anaesthetics such as benzocaine, cocaine, procaine, and tetracaine (amethocaine); reactions are less frequent with the amide types such as lidocaine (lignocaine), bupivacaine, levobupivacaine, prilocaine, and ropivacaine. Local anaesthetics may be associated with methaemoglobinaemia; prilocaine and benzocaine have been implicated.

When prolonged analgesia is required, a long-acting local anaesthetic is preferred to minimise the likelihood of cumulative systemic toxicity. Local anaesthetic injections should be given slowly in order to detect inadvertent intravascular administration. Local anaesthetics should **not** be injected into inflamed or infected tissues nor should they be applied to the traumatised urethra. In such cases absorption into the blood may increase the possibility of systemic side-effects. The local anaesthetic effect may also be reduced by the altered local pH.

Use of vasoconstrictors Most local anaesthetics, with the exception of cocaine, cause dilation of blood vessels. The addition of a vasoconstrictor such as **adrenaline (epinephrine)** diminishes local blood flow, slows the rate of absorption of the local anaesthetic, and prolongs its local effect. Adrenaline must be used in a low concentration (e.g. 1 in 200 000) for this purpose and it should **not** be given with a local anaesthetic injection in digits and appendages; it may produce ischaemic necrosis.

When adrenaline is included the final concentration should be 1 in 200 000 (5 micrograms/mL), but see also Dental Anaesthesia below.

The total dose of adrenaline should **not** exceed 500 micrograms and it is essential not to exceed a concentration of 1 in 200 000 (5 micrograms/mL) if more than 50 mL of the mixture is to be injected. For general cautions associated with the use of adrenaline, see section 2.7.3. For drug interactions, see Appendix 1 (sympathomimetics).

Dental anaesthesia **Lidocaine** (lignocaine) is widely used in dental procedures; it is most often used in combination with **adrenaline** (epinephrine). Lidocaine 2% combined with adrenaline 1 in 80 000 (12.5 micrograms/mL) is a safe and effective preparation; there is no justification for using higher concentrations of adrenaline.

The local anaesthetics **articaine** (carticaine) and **mepivacaine** are also used in dentistry; they are available in cartridges suitable for dental use. Mepivacaine is available with or without adrenaline (as *Scandonest®*) and articaine is available with adrenaline (as *Septanest®*).

In patients with severe hypertension or unstable cardiac rhythm, the use of adrenaline in a local anaesthetic may be hazardous. For these patients **prilocaine** with or without felypressin can be used but there is no evidence that it is any safer. Felypressin can cause coronary vasoconstriction when used at high doses; limit dose in patients with coronary artery disease.

Great care should be taken to avoid inadvertent intravenous administration of a preparation containing adrenaline.

There is no clinical evidence of dangerous interactions between adrenaline-containing local anaesthetics and monoamine-oxidase inhibitors (MAOIs) or tricyclic antidepressants.

Lidocaine

Lidocaine (lignocaine) is effectively absorbed from mucous membranes and is a useful surface anaesthetic in concentrations up to 10%. Except for surface anaesthesia and dental anaesthesia, solutions should **not** usually exceed 1% in strength. The duration of the block (with adrenaline) is about 90 minutes.

LIDOCAINE HYDROCHLORIDE
(Lignocaine hydrochloride)

Indications see under Dose; also dental anaesthesia (see p. 682); ventricular arrhythmias (section 2.3.2)

Cautions epilepsy, respiratory impairment, impaired cardiac conduction, bradycardia, severe shock; porphyria (section 9.8.2); myasthenia gravis; reduce dose in elderly or debilitated; resuscitative equipment should be available; see section 2.3.2 for effects on heart; hepatic impairment (Appendix 2); renal impairment (Appendix 3); pregnancy (Appendix 4); **interactions**: Appendix 1 (lidocaine)

Contra-indications hypovolaemia, complete heart block; do not use solutions containing adrenaline for anaesthesia in appendages

Side-effects CNS effects include confusion, respiratory depression and convulsions; hypotension and bradycardia (may lead to cardiac arrest); *rarely* hypersensitivity reported; see also notes above and section 2.3.2

Dose

- Infiltration anaesthesia, by injection, according to patient's weight and nature of procedure, max. 200 mg (or 500 mg if given in solutions containing adrenaline)—see also Administration on p. 681 and see also **important** warning below
- Intravenous regional anaesthesia and nerve blocks, seek expert advice
- Surface anaesthesia, usual strengths 2–4%, see preparations below

> **Important**
> The licensed doses stated above may not be appropriate in some settings and expert advice should be sought

Lidocaine hydrochloride injections

Lidocaine (Non-proprietary) PoM

Injection 0.5%, lidocaine hydrochloride 5 mg/mL, net price 10-mL amp = 35p

Injection 1%, lidocaine hydrochloride 10 mg/mL, net price 2-mL amp = 21p; 5-mL amp = 23p; 10-mL amp = 35p; 10-mL prefilled syringe = £4.53; 20-mL amp = 62p

Injection 2%, lidocaine hydrochloride 20 mg/mL, net price 2-mL amp = 27p; 5-mL amp = 26p

Xylocaine® (AstraZeneca) PoM

Injection 1% with adrenaline 1 in 200 000, anhydrous lidocaine hydrochloride 10 mg/mL, adrenaline 1 in 200 000 (5 micrograms/mL), net price 20-mL vial = 99p

Injection 2% with adrenaline 1 in 200 000, anhydrous lidocaine hydrochloride 20 mg/mL, adrenaline 1 in 200 000 (5 micrograms/mL), net price 20-mL vial = £1.04

Lidocaine injections for dental use

Note Consult expert dental sources for specific advice in relation to dose of lidocaine for dental anaesthesia

A variety of lidocaine injections with adrenaline is available in dental cartridges; brands include *Lignospan Special®*, *Rexocaine®* and *Xylocaine®*

Lidocaine for surface anaesthesia

Important. Rapid and extensive absorption may result in systemic side-effects

Lidocaine (Non-proprietary)

Ointment, lidocaine hydrochloride 5%, net price 15 g = 88p

Dose dental practice, rub gently into dry gum

Sore nipples from breast-feeding, apply using gauze and wash off immediately before feed

Pain relief (in anal fissures, haemorrhoids, pruritus ani, pruritus vulvae, herpes zoster, or herpes labialis), 1–2 mL applied when necessary; avoid long-term use

Solution, lidocaine hydrochloride 4%, net price 25 mL = £1.35

Dose biopsy in mouth, 3–4 mL with suitable spray *or* swab (with adrenaline if necessary); max. 5 mL, ELDERLY lower max. dose, CHILD max. 3 mg/kg

Puncture of maxillary sinus or polypectomy, apply with swab for 2–3 minutes (with adrenaline); max. 5 mL, ELDERLY lower max. dose, CHILD max. 3 mg/kg

Bronchoscopy and bronchography, 2–3 mL with suitable spray; max. 5 mL, ELDERLY lower max. dose, CHILD max. 3 mg/kg

Lidocaine and chlorhexidine (Non-proprietary)

Gel, lidocaine hydrochloride 1%, chlorhexidine gluconate solution 0.25%, net price 15 mL = 70p; lidocaine hydrochloride 2%, chlorhexidine gluconate solution 0.25%, 15 mL = 70p

Dose urethral catheterisation, into urethra at least 5 minutes before catheter insertion, MEN 10 mL followed by further 3–5 mL; WOMEN 3–5 mL; CHILD 1–5 mL

Mucocutaneous anaesthesia, 2–3 mL applied when necessary; CHILD 1–2 mL

Major aphthous ulcers in immunocompromised patients, 2–3 mL applied when necessary, max. 15 mL in 24 hours; CHILD 1–2 mL, max. 8 mL in 24 hours

EMLA® (AstraZeneca)

Drug Tariff cream, lidocaine 2.5%, prilocaine 2.5%, net price 5-g tube = £1.73

Surgical pack cream, lidocaine 2.5%, prilocaine 2.5%, net price 30-g tube = £10.25

Premedication pack cream, lidocaine 2.5%, prilocaine 2.5%, net price 5 × 5-g tube with 12 occlusive dressings = £9.75

Cautions not for wounds, mucous membranes (except genital warts in adults), or atopic dermatitis; avoid use near eyes or middle ear; although systemic absorption low, caution in anaemia, in congenital or acquired methaemoglobinaemia or in G6PD deficiency (see also Prilocaine, p. 684)

Side-effects include transient paleness, redness, and oedema

Dose anaesthesia before minor skin procedures including venepuncture, apply thick layer under occlusive dressing 1–5 hours before procedure (2–5 hours before procedures on large areas e.g. split skin grafting); INFANT 1–12 months [unlicensed use] single application on intact skin under specialist supervision, under 1 month not recommended (risk of methaemoglobinaemia, see Cautions above)

Removal of warts from genital mucosa in adults, apply up to 10 g 5–10 minutes before removal

Instillagel® (CliniMed)

Gel, lidocaine hydrochloride 2%, chlorhexidine gluconate solution 0.25%, in a sterile lubricant basis in disposable syringe, net price 6-mL syringe = £1.41, 11-mL syringe = £1.58

Excipients include hydroxybenzoates (parabens)

Dose 6–11 mL into urethra

Laryngojet® (Celltech) PoM

Jet spray 4% (disposable kit for laryngotracheal anaesthesia), lidocaine hydrochloride 40 mg/mL, net price per unit (4-mL vial and disposable sterile cannula with cover and vial injector) = £7.81

Cautions may be rapidly and almost completely absorbed from respiratory tract and systemic side-effects may occur; extreme caution if mucosa has been traumatised or if sepsis present

Dose usually 160 mg (4 mL) as a single dose instilled as jet spray to larynx and trachea or applied with a swab (reduce dose according to size, age and condition of patient), max. 200 mg (5 mL); CHILD up to 3 mg/kg

Versatis® (Grünenthal) PoM

Medicated plasters, lidocaine 5% (700 mg/medicated plaster), net price 10 = £24.13, 30 = £72.40

Excipients include hydroxybenzoates (parabens), propylene glycol

Dose postherpetic neuralgia, ADULT over 18 years, apply to intact, dry, non-hairy, non-irritated skin once daily for up to 12

hours, followed by a 12-hour plaster-free period; discontinue if no response after 4 weeks

Note Up to 3 plasters may be used to cover large areas; plasters may be cut

Note The *Scottish Medicines Consortium* has advised (December 2006) that *Versatis®* is not recommended for the treatment of postherpetic neuralgia

Xylocaine® (AstraZeneca)
Spray (= pump spray), lidocaine 10% (100 mg/g) supplying 10 mg lidocaine/dose; 500 spray doses per container. Net price 50-mL bottle = £3.13

Dose dental practice, 1–5 doses
Maxillary sinus puncture, 3 doses
During delivery in obstetrics, up to 20 doses
Bronchoscopy, laryngoscopy, oesophagoscopy, endotracheal intubation, up to 20 doses; CHILD up to 3 mg/kg

Note Lidocaine can damage plastic cuffs of endotracheal tubes

Lidocaine for ear, nose, and oropharyngeal use

Lidocaine with Phenylephrine (Non-proprietary)
Topical solution, lidocaine hydrochloride 5%, phenylephrine hydrochloride 0.5%, net price 2.5 mL (with nasal applicator) = £8.73. For cautions, contra-indications and side-effects of phenylephrine, see section 2.7.2

Bupivacaine

The advantage of bupivacaine over other local anaesthetics is its longer duration of action. It has a slow onset of action, taking up to 30 minutes for full effect. It is often used in lumbar epidural blockade and is particularly suitable for continuous epidural analgesia in labour, or for postoperative pain relief. It is the principal drug used for spinal anaesthesia.

BUPIVACAINE HYDROCHLORIDE

Indications see under Dose

Cautions see under Lidocaine Hydrochloride and notes above; myocardial depression may be more severe and more resistant to treatment; **interactions:** Appendix 1 (bupivacaine)

Contra-indications see under Lidocaine Hydrochloride and notes above; intravenous regional anaesthesia (Bier's block)

Side-effects see under Lidocaine Hydrochloride and notes above

Dose

Note Doses should be adjusted according to patient's physical status and nature of procedure—**important**: see also under Administration, p. 681

- Local infiltration, max. 60 mL, using a 2.5 mg/mL (0.25%) solution
- Peripheral nerve block, max. 60 mL, using a 2.5 mg/mL (0.25%) solution; max. 30 mL, using a 5 mg/mL (0.5%) solution
- Epidural block

  Surgery, *lumbar*, max. 20 mL, using a 5 mg/mL (0.5%) solution

  Surgery, *caudal*, max. 30 mL, using a 5 mg/mL (0.5%) solution; CHILD (up to 10 years) using a 2.5 mg/mL (0.25%) solution, up to lower-thoracic (T10) 0.3–0.4 mL/kg, up to mid-thoracic (T6) 0.4–0.8 mL/kg

  Labour, *lumbar*, max. 12 mL using a 2.5 mg/mL (0.25%) or 5 mg/mL (0.5%) solution; *caudal* (but rarely used) max. 20 mL using a 2.5 mg/mL (0.25%) or 5 mg/mL (0.5%) solution
- Sympathetic block, max. 50 mL, using a 2.5 mg/mL (0.25%) solution
- Intrathecal anaesthesia, see under preparations

> **Important**
> The licensed doses stated above may not be appropriate in some settings and expert advice should be sought

Bupivacaine (Non-proprietary) PoM
Injection, anhydrous bupivacaine hydrochloride 2.5 mg/mL (0.25%) net price 10 mL = 82p; 5 mg/mL (0.5%), 10 mL = 94p

Note Bupivacaine hydrochloride injection 0.25% and 0.5% are available in glass or plastic ampoules, and sterile-wrapped glass ampoules

Infusion, anhydrous bupivacaine hydrochloride 1 mg/mL (0.1%), net price 100 mL = £8.41, 250 mL = £10.59; 1.25 mg/mL (0.125%), 250 mL = £10.80

Dose Continuous lumbar epidural infusion during labour (once epidural block established), 10–15 mg/hour of 0.1% or 0.125% solution; max. 2 mg/kg over 4 hours and total of 400 mg in 24 hours
Continuous thoracic, upper abdominal, or lower abdominal epidural infusion for post-operative pain (once epidural block established), 4–15 mg/hour of 0.1% or 0.125% solution; max. 2 mg/kg over 4 hours and total of 400 mg in 24 hours; not recommended for use in children

Marcain® (AstraZeneca) PoM
Injection, anhydrous bupivacaine hydrochloride 2.5 mg/mL (*Marcain® 0.25%*), net price 10-mL *Polyamp®* = £1.06; 5 mg/mL (*Marcain® 0.5%*), 10-mL *Polyamp®* = £1.21

Marcain Heavy® (AstraZeneca) PoM
Injection, anhydrous bupivacaine hydrochloride 5 mg, glucose 80 mg/mL, net price 4-mL amp = £1.21

Dose intrathecal anaesthesia for surgery, 2–4 mL (dose may need to be reduced in elderly and in late pregnancy)

With adrenaline

Bupivacaine and Adrenaline (Non-proprietary) PoM
Injection, anhydrous bupivacaine hydrochloride 2.5 mg/mL (0.25%), adrenaline 1 in 200 000 (5 micrograms/mL), net price 10-mL amp = £1.23

Injection, anhydrous bupivacaine hydrochloride 5 mg/mL (0.5%), adrenaline 1 in 200 000 (5 micrograms/mL), net price 10-mL amp = £1.40

Levobupivacaine

Levobupivacaine, an isomer of bupivacaine, has anaesthetic and analgesic properties similar to bupivacaine, but is thought to have fewer adverse effects.

LEVOBUPIVACAINE

Note Levobupivacaine is an isomer of bupivacaine

Indications see under Dose

Cautions see under Lidocaine Hydrochloride and notes above; **interactions:** Appendix 1 (levobupivacaine)

Contra-indications see under Lidocaine Hydrochloride and notes above; intravenous regional anaesthesia (Bier's block); paracervical block in obstetrics; do not use 7.5 mg/mL strength in obstetrics

Side-effects see under Lidocaine Hydrochloride and notes above

Dose

Note Doses should be adjusted according to patient's physical status and nature of procedure—**important**: see also under Administration, p. 681

- Surgical anaesthesia

  Lumbar epidural, 10–20 mL (50–150 mg) of 5 mg/mL or 7.5 mg/mL solution over 5 minutes; caesarean section, 15–30 mL (75–150 mg) of 5 mg/mL solution over 15–20 minutes

  Intrathecal, 3 mL (15 mg) of 5 mg/mL solution

  Peripheral nerve block, 1–40 mL of 2.5 mg/mL or 5 mg/mL solution (max. 150 mg)

  Ilioinguinal/iliohypogastric block, CHILD under 12 years 0.25–0.5 mL/kg (0.625–2.5 mg/kg) of a 2.5 mg/mL or 5 mg/mL solution

  Peribulbar block, 5–15 mL (37.5–112.5 mg) of 7.5 mg/mL solution

  Local infiltration, 1–60 mL (max. 150 mg) of 2.5 mg/mL solution
- Acute pain

  Lumbar epidural, labour pain, 6–10 mL (15–25 mg) of 2.5 mg/mL solution at intervals of at least 15 minutes *or* 5–12.5 mg/hour as a continuous epidural infusion, postoperative pain, 12.5–18.75 mg/hour as a continuous epidural infusion; max. 400 mg in 24 hours

> **Important**
> The licensed doses stated above may not be appropriate in some settings and expert advice should be sought

Chirocaine® (Abbott) PoM

Injection, levobupivacaine (as hydrochloride) 2.5 mg/mL, net price 10-mL amp = £1.66; 5 mg/mL, 10-mL amp = £1.90; 7.5 mg/mL, 10-mL amp = £2.85

Note For 1.25 mg/mL concentration dilute standard solutions with sodium chloride 0.9%

Infusion, levobupivacaine (as hydrochloride) 625 micrograms/mL, net price 100 mL = £7.80, 200 mL = £10.40; 1.25 mg/mL, net price 100 mL = £8.54, 200 mL = £12.20

Prilocaine

Prilocaine is a local anaesthetic of low toxicity which is similar to lidocaine (lignocaine). If used in high doses, methaemoglobinaemia may occur which can be treated with intravenous injection of methylthioninium chloride (methylene blue) 1% using a dose of 1 mg/kg. Infants under 6 months are particularly susceptible to methaemoglobinaemia.

PRILOCAINE HYDROCHLORIDE

Indications infiltration anaesthesia (higher strengths for dental use only), nerve block

Cautions see under Lidocaine Hydrochloride and notes above; severe or untreated hypertension, severe heart disease; concomitant drugs which cause methaemoglobinaemia; reduce dose in elderly or debilitated; pregnancy (Appendix 4); **interactions:** Appendix 1 (prilocaine)

Contra-indications see under Lidocaine Hydrochloride and notes above; anaemia or congenital or acquired methaemoglobinaemia

Side-effects see under Lidocaine Hydrochloride and notes above; ocular toxicity (including blindness) reported with excessively high strengths used for ophthalmic procedures

Dose

- See under preparations—**important**: see also under Administration, p. 681

Citanest® (AstraZeneca) PoM

Injection 1%, prilocaine hydrochloride 10 mg/mL, net price 50-mL multidose vial = £2.01

Dose adjusted according to site of administration and response, 100–200 mg/minute, or in incremental doses, to max. total dose 400 mg; CHILD over 6 months up to 5 mg/kg

For dental use

Note Consult expert dental sources for specific advice in relation to dose of prilocaine for dental anaesthesia.

Citanest® (Dentsply) PoM

Injection 4%, prilocaine hydrochloride 40 mg/mL, net price 2-mL cartridge = 17p

Citanest with Octapressin® (Dentsply) PoM

Injection 3%, prilocaine hydrochloride 30 mg/mL, felypressin 0.03 unit/mL, net price 2-mL cartridge and self-aspirating cartridge (both) = 15p

Procaine

Procaine is now seldom used. It is as potent as lidocaine (lignocaine) but has a shorter duration of action. It provides less intense analgesia because of reduced spread through the tissues. It is of no value as a surface anaesthetic.

PROCAINE HYDROCHLORIDE

Indications local anaesthesia by infiltration and regional routes (but see notes above)

Cautions see notes above; pregnancy (Appendix 4)

Side-effects see notes above

Dose

Note Doses should be adjusted according to patient's physical status and nature of procedure—**important**: see also under Administration, p. 681

- By injection, up to 1 g (200 mL of 0.5% solution or 100 mL of 1%) with adrenaline 1 in 200 000

Procaine (Martindale) PoM

Injection, procaine hydrochloride 2% (20 mg/mL) in sodium chloride intravenous infusion, net price 2-mL amp = £1.27

Ropivacaine

Ropivacaine is an amide-type local anaesthetic agent similar to bupivacaine. It is less cardiotoxic than bupivacaine, but also less potent.

ROPIVACAINE HYDROCHLORIDE

Indications see under Dose

Cautions see Lidocaine Hydrochloride and notes above; **interactions:** Appendix 1 (ropivacaine)

Contra-indications see Lidocaine Hydrochloride and notes above; intravenous regional anaesthesia (Bier's block); paracervical block in obstetrics

Side-effects see Lidocaine Hydrochloride and notes above; also nausea, vomiting; hypertension, tachycardia; headache, rigors, impaired temperature regulation; urinary retention; back pain; *less commonly* syncope, dyspnoea, anxiety; *rarely* arrhythmia

Dose

Note Doses should be adjusted according to patient's physical status and nature of procedure—**important** see also under Administration on p. 681

- Surgical anaesthesia

  Lumbar epidural, ADULT and CHILD over 12 years, 15–20 mL of 10 mg/mL solution *or* 15–25 mL of 7.5 mg/mL solution (max. total dose 200 mg); caesarean section, 15–20 mL of 7.5 mg/mL solution in incremental doses (max. total dose 150 mg)

  Thoracic epidural (to establish block for postoperative pain), ADULT and CHILD over 12 years, 5–15 mL of 7.5 mg/mL solution

  Major nerve block (brachial plexus block), ADULT and CHILD over 12 years, 30–40 mL of 7.5 mg/mL solution

  Field block, ADULT and CHILD over 12 years, 1–30 mL of 7.5 mg/mL solution

- Acute pain

  Lumbar epidural, ADULT and CHILD over 12 years, 10–20 mL of 2 mg/mL solution followed by 10–15 mL of 2 mg/mL solution at intervals of at least 30 minutes *or* 6–10 mL/hour of 2 mg/mL solution as a continuous epidural infusion for labour pain *or* 6–14 mL/hour of 2 mg/mL solution as a continuous epidural infusion for postoperative pain

  Thoracic epidural, ADULT and CHILD over 12 years, 6–14 mL/hour of 2 mg/mL solution as a continuous infusion

  Field block, ADULT and CHILD over 12 years, 1–100 mL of 2 mg/mL solution

  Peripheral nerve block, ADULT and CHILD over 12 years, 5–10 mL/hour of 2 mg/mL solution as a continuous infusion *or* by intermittent injection

  CHILD under 12 years, consult product literature

Naropin® (AstraZeneca) PoM

Injection, ropivacaine hydrochloride 2 mg/mL, net price 10-mL *Polyamp®* = £1.78; 7.5 mg/mL, 10-mL *Polyamp®* = £2.65; 10 mg/mL, 10-mL *Polyamp®* = £3.20

Electrolytes Na^+ <0.5 mmol/mL

Infusion, ropivacaine hydrochloride 2 mg/mL, net price 200-mL *Polybag®* = £14.45

Electrolytes Na^+ <0.5 mmol/mL

Tetracaine

Tetracaine (amethocaine) is an effective local anaesthetic for topical application; a 4% gel is indicated for anaesthesia prior to venepuncture or venous cannulation. It is rapidly absorbed from mucous membranes and should **never** be applied to inflamed, traumatised, or highly vascular surfaces. It should **never** be used to provide anaesthesia for bronchoscopy or cystoscopy, as lidocaine (lignocaine) is a safer alternative. It is used in ophthalmology (section 11.7) and in skin preparations (section 13.3). Hypersensitivity to tetracaine has been reported.

TETRACAINE
(Amethocaine)

Indications see under preparation below

Cautions see notes above

Contra-indications see notes above

Side-effects see notes above; also erythema, oedema and pruritus; very rarely blistering

Important. Rapid and extensive absorption may result in systemic side-effects (see also notes above)

Ametop® (S&N Hlth.)

Gel, tetracaine 4%, net price 1.5-g tube = £1.08

Dose ADULT and CHILD over 1 month, apply contents of tube to site of venepuncture or venous cannulation and cover with occlusive dressing; remove gel and dressing after 30 minutes for venepuncture and after 45 minutes for venous cannulation; NEONATE see *BNF for Children*

Other local anaesthetics

Benzocaine is a local anaesthetic of low potency and toxicity. It is used in concentrations of up to 20% for topical anaesthesia of the oral mucosa before injection. It is an ingredient of some proprietary topical preparations for musculoskeletal conditions (section 10.3.2), mouth-ulcer preparations (section 12.3.1), and throat lozenges (section 12.3.3). Benzocaine sprays used in the mouth and throat have been associated with methaemoglobinaemia.

Cocaine readily penetrates mucous membranes and is an effective surface anaesthetic with an intense vasoconstrictor action. However, apart from its use in otolaryngology (see below), it has now been replaced by less toxic alternatives. It has marked sympathomimetic activity and should **never** be given by injection because of its toxicity. As a result of its intense stimulant effect it is a drug of addiction. In otolaryngology cocaine is applied to the nasal mucosa in concentrations of 4 to 10% (40–100 mg/mL); an oromucosal solution and nasal spray both containing cocaine hydrochloride 10% are available (Aurum). In order to avoid systemic effects, the maximum dose recommended for application to the nasal mucosa in fit adults is a total of 1.5 mg/kg, which is equivalent to a total topical dose of approximately 100 mg for an adult male; this dose relates to direct application of cocaine (application on gauze may reduce systemic absorption). It should be used only by those skilled in the precautions needed to *minimise absorption* and the *consequent risk of arrhythmias*. Although cocaine interacts with other drugs liable to induce arrhythmias, including adrenaline, some otolaryngologists consider that combined use of topical cocaine with topical adrenaline (in the form of a paste or a solution) improves the operative field and may possibly reduce absorption. Cocaine is a mydriatic as well as a local anaesthetic but owing to corneal toxicity it is now little used in ophthalmology. Cocaine should be avoided in porphyria (section 9.8.2).

A1 Interactions

Two or more drugs given at the same time may exert their effects independently or may interact. The interaction may be potentiation or antagonism of one drug by another, or occasionally some other effect. Adverse drug interactions should be reported to the CHM as for other adverse drug reactions.

Drug interactions may be **pharmacodynamic** or **pharmacokinetic**.

Pharmacodynamic interactions

These are interactions between drugs which have similar or antagonistic pharmacological effects or side-effects. They may be due to competition at receptor sites, or occur between drugs acting on the same physiological system. They are usually predictable from a knowledge of the pharmacology of the interacting drugs; in general, those demonstrated with one drug are likely to occur with related drugs. They occur to a greater or lesser extent in most patients who receive the interacting drugs.

Pharmacokinetic interactions

These occur when one drug alters the absorption, distribution, metabolism, or excretion of another, thus increasing or reducing the amount of drug available to produce its pharmacological effects. They are not easily predicted and many of them affect only a small proportion of patients taking the combination of drugs. Pharmacokinetic interactions occurring with one drug cannot be assumed to occur with related drugs unless their pharmacokinetic properties are known to be similar.

Pharmacokinetic interactions are of several types:

Affecting absorption The rate of absorption or the total amount absorbed can both be altered by drug interactions. Delayed absorption is rarely of clinical importance unless high peak plasma concentrations are required (e.g. when giving an analgesic). Reduction in the total amount absorbed, however, may result in ineffective therapy.

Due to changes in protein binding To a variable extent most drugs are loosely bound to plasma proteins. Protein-binding sites are non-specific and one drug can displace another thereby increasing its proportion free to diffuse from plasma to its site of action. This only produces a detectable increase in effect if it is an extensively bound drug (more than 90%) that is not widely distributed throughout the body. Even so displacement rarely produces more than transient potentiation because this increased concentration of free drug results in an increased rate of elimination.

Displacement from protein binding plays a part in the potentiation of warfarin by sulphonamides and tolbutamide but the importance of these interactions is due mainly to the fact that warfarin metabolism is also inhibited.

Affecting metabolism Many drugs are metabolised in the liver. Induction of the hepatic microsomal enzyme system by one drug can gradually increase the rate of metabolism of another, resulting in lower plasma concentrations and a reduced effect. On withdrawal of the inducer plasma concentrations increase and toxicity may occur. Barbiturates, griseofulvin, many antiepileptics, and rifampicin are the most important enzyme inducers. Drugs affected include warfarin and the oral contraceptives.

Conversely when one drug inhibits the metabolism of another higher plasma concentrations are produced, rapidly resulting in an increased effect with risk of toxicity. Some drugs which potentiate warfarin and phenytoin do so by this mechanism.

Isoenzymes of the hepatic cytochrome P450 system interact with a wide range of drugs. Drugs may be substrates, inducers or inhibitors of the different isoenzymes. A great deal of *in-vitro* information is available on the effect of drugs on the isoenzymes; however, since drugs are eliminated by a number of different metabolic routes as well as renal excretion, the clinical effects of interactions cannot be predicted accurately from laboratory data on the cytochrome P450 isoenzymes. Except where a combination of drugs is specifically contra-indicated, the BNF presents only interactions that have been reported in clinical practice. In all cases the possibility of an interaction must be considered if toxic effects occur or if the activity of a drug diminishes.

Affecting renal excretion Drugs are eliminated through the kidney both by glomerular filtration and by active tubular secretion. Competition occurs between those which share active transport mechanisms in the proximal tubule. For example, salicylates and some other NSAIDs delay the excretion of methotrexate; serious methotrexate toxicity is possible.

Relative importance of interactions

Many drug interactions are harmless and many of those which are potentially harmful only occur in a small proportion of patients; moreover, the severity of an interaction varies from one patient to another. Drugs with a small therapeutic ratio (e.g. phenytoin) and those which require careful control of dosage (e.g. anticoagulants, antihypertensives, and antidiabetics) are most often involved.

Patients at increased risk from drug interactions include the elderly and those with impaired renal or liver function.

Hazardous interactions The symbol • has been placed against interactions that are **potentially hazardous** and where combined administration of the drugs involved should be **avoided** (or only undertaken with caution and appropriate monitoring).

Interactions that have no symbol do not usually have serious consequences.

List of drug interactions

The following is an alphabetical list of drugs and their interactions; to avoid excessive cross-referencing each drug or group is listed twice: in the alphabetical list and also against the drug or group with which it interacts; changes in the interactions lists since BNF No. 54 (September 2007) are underlined.

For explanation of symbol • see above

Abacavir
- Analgesics: abacavir possibly reduces plasma concentration of methadone
- Antibacterials: plasma concentration of abacavir possibly reduced by rifampicin
- Antiepileptics: plasma concentration of abacavir possibly reduced by phenytoin
- • Antivirals: plasma concentration of abacavir reduced by •tipranavir
- Barbiturates: plasma concentration of abacavir possibly reduced by phenobarbital

Abatacept
- Adalimumab: increased risk of side-effects when abatacept given with adalimumab
- Etanercept: increased risk of side-effects when abatacept given with etanercept
- Infliximab: increased risk of side-effects when abatacept given with infliximab
- • Vaccines: avoid concomitant use of abatacept with live •vaccines (see p. 641)

Acarbose *see* Antidiabetics

ACE Inhibitors
- Alcohol: enhanced hypotensive effect when ACE inhibitors given with alcohol
- Aldesleukin: enhanced hypotensive effect when ACE inhibitors given with aldesleukin
- Allopurinol: increased risk of toxicity when captopril given with allopurinol especially in renal impairment
- Alpha-blockers: enhanced hypotensive effect when ACE inhibitors given with alpha-blockers
- Anaesthetics, General: enhanced hypotensive effect when ACE inhibitors given with general anaesthetics
- Analgesics: increased risk of renal impairment when ACE inhibitors given with NSAIDs, also hypotensive effect antagonised
- <u>Angiotensin-II Receptor Antagonists</u>: increased risk of hyperkalaemia when ACE inhibitors given with angiotensin-II receptor antagonists
- Antacids: absorption of ACE inhibitors possibly reduced by antacids; absorption of captopril, enalapril and fosinopril reduced by antacids
- Anti-arrhythmics: increased risk of toxicity when captopril given with procainamide especially in renal impairment
- Antibacterials: plasma concentration of active metabolite of imidapril reduced by rifampicin (reduced antihypertensive effect); quinapril tablets reduce absorption of tetracyclines (quinapril tablets contain magnesium carbonate)
- Anticoagulants: increased risk of hyperkalaemia when ACE inhibitors given with heparins
- Antidepressants: hypotensive effect of ACE inhibitors possibly enhanced by MAOIs
- Antidiabetics: ACE inhibitors possibly enhance hypoglycaemic effect of insulin, metformin and sulphonylureas
- Antipsychotics: enhanced hypotensive effect when ACE inhibitors given with antipsychotics
- Anxiolytics and Hypnotics: enhanced hypotensive effect when ACE inhibitors given with anxiolytics and hypnotics
- Beta-blockers: enhanced hypotensive effect when ACE inhibitors given with beta-blockers
- Calcium-channel Blockers: enhanced hypotensive effect when ACE inhibitors given with calcium-channel blockers
- Cardiac Glycosides: captopril possibly increases plasma concentration of digoxin
- • Ciclosporin: increased risk of hyperkalaemia when ACE inhibitors given with •ciclosporin

ACE Inhibitors *(continued)*
- Clonidine: enhanced hypotensive effect when ACE inhibitors given with clonidine; antihypertensive effect of captopril possibly delayed by previous treatment with clonidine
- Corticosteroids: hypotensive effect of ACE inhibitors antagonised by corticosteroids
- Cytotoxics: increased risk of leucopenia when captopril given with azathioprine
- Diazoxide: enhanced hypotensive effect when ACE inhibitors given with diazoxide
- • Diuretics: enhanced hypotensive effect when ACE inhibitors given with •diuretics; increased risk of severe hyperkalaemia when ACE inhibitors given with •potassium-sparing diuretics and aldosterone antagonists (monitor potassium concentration with low-dose spironolactone in heart failure)
- Dopaminergics: enhanced hypotensive effect when ACE inhibitors given with levodopa
- Epoetin: antagonism of hypotensive effect and increased risk of hyperkalaemia when ACE inhibitors given with epoetin
- • Lithium: ACE inhibitors reduce excretion of •lithium (increased plasma concentration)
- Methyldopa: enhanced hypotensive effect when ACE inhibitors given with methyldopa
- Moxisylyte (thymoxamine): enhanced hypotensive effect when ACE inhibitors given with moxisylyte
- Moxonidine: enhanced hypotensive effect when ACE inhibitors given with moxonidine
- Muscle Relaxants: enhanced hypotensive effect when ACE inhibitors given with baclofen or tizanidine
- Nitrates: enhanced hypotensive effect when ACE inhibitors given with nitrates
- Oestrogens: hypotensive effect of ACE inhibitors antagonised by oestrogens
- • Potassium Salts: increased risk of severe hyperkalaemia when ACE inhibitors given with •potassium salts
- Probenecid: excretion of captopril reduced by probenecid
- Progestogens: risk of hyperkalaemia when ACE inhibitors given with drospirenone (monitor serum potassium during first cycle)
- Prostaglandins: enhanced hypotensive effect when ACE inhibitors given with alprostadil
- Vasodilator Antihypertensives: enhanced hypotensive effect when ACE inhibitors given with hydralazine, minoxidil or sodium nitroprusside

Acebutolol *see* Beta-blockers

Aceclofenac *see* NSAIDs

Acemetacin *see* NSAIDs

Acenocoumarol (nicoumalone) *see* Coumarins

Acetazolamide *see* Diuretics

Aciclovir

Note Interactions do not apply to topical aciclovir preparations

Note Valaciclovir interactions as for aciclovir
- Ciclosporin: increased risk of nephrotoxicity when aciclovir given with ciclosporin
- Cytotoxics: plasma concentration of aciclovir increased by mycophenolate, also plasma concentration of inactive metabolite of mycophenolate increased
- Probenecid: excretion of aciclovir reduced by probenecid (increased plasma concentration)
- Tacrolimus: possible increased risk of nephrotoxicity when aciclovir given with tacrolimus

Acitretin *see* Retinoids

Adalimumab
- Abatacept: increased risk of side-effects when adalimumab given with abatacept
- • Anakinra: avoid concomitant use of adalimumab with •anakinra
- • Vaccines: avoid concomitant use of adalimumab with live •vaccines (see p. 641)

Adefovir
- Antivirals: monitoring of renal function with adefovir recommended by manufacturer of tenofovir

Adenosine

Note Possibility of interaction with drugs tending to impair myocardial conduction

Anaesthetics, Local: increased myocardial depression when anti-arrhythmics given with bupivacaine, levobupivacaine, prilocaine or ropivacaine

• Anti-arrhythmics: increased myocardial depression when anti-arrhythmics given with other •anti-arrhythmics

• Antipsychotics: increased risk of ventricular arrhythmias when anti-arrhythmics that prolong the QT interval given with •antipsychotics that prolong the QT interval

• Beta-blockers: increased myocardial depression when anti-arrhythmics given with •beta-blockers

• Dipyridamole: effect of adenosine enhanced and extended by •dipyridamole (important risk of toxicity)

$5HT_3$ Antagonists: caution with anti-arrhythmics advised by manufacturer of tropisetron (risk of ventricular arrhythmias)

Theophylline: anti-arrhythmic effect of adenosine antagonised by theophylline

Adrenaline (epinephrine) *see* Sympathomimetics

Adrenergic Neurone Blockers

Alcohol: enhanced hypotensive effect when adrenergic neurone blockers given with alcohol

Alpha-blockers: enhanced hypotensive effect when adrenergic neurone blockers given with alpha-blockers

• Anaesthetics, General: enhanced hypotensive effect when adrenergic neurone blockers given with •general anaesthetics

Analgesics: hypotensive effect of adrenergic neurone blockers antagonised by NSAIDs

Angiotensin-II Receptor Antagonists: enhanced hypotensive effect when adrenergic neurone blockers given with angiotensin-II receptor antagonists

Antidepressants: enhanced hypotensive effect when adrenergic neurone blockers given with MAOIs; hypotensive effect of adrenergic neurone blockers antagonised by tricyclics

Antipsychotics: hypotensive effect of adrenergic neurone blockers antagonised by haloperidol; hypotensive effect of adrenergic neurone blockers antagonised by higher doses of chlorpromazine; enhanced hypotensive effect when adrenergic neurone blockers given with phenothiazines

Anxiolytics and Hypnotics: enhanced hypotensive effect when adrenergic neurone blockers given with anxiolytics and hypnotics

Beta-blockers: enhanced hypotensive effect when adrenergic neurone blockers given with beta-blockers

Calcium-channel Blockers: enhanced hypotensive effect when adrenergic neurone blockers given with calcium-channel blockers

Clonidine: enhanced hypotensive effect when adrenergic neurone blockers given with clonidine

Corticosteroids: hypotensive effect of adrenergic neurone blockers antagonised by corticosteroids

Diazoxide: enhanced hypotensive effect when adrenergic neurone blockers given with diazoxide

Diuretics: enhanced hypotensive effect when adrenergic neurone blockers given with diuretics

Dopaminergics: enhanced hypotensive effect when adrenergic neurone blockers given with levodopa

Methyldopa: enhanced hypotensive effect when adrenergic neurone blockers given with methyldopa

Moxisylyte (thymoxamine): enhanced hypotensive effect when adrenergic neurone blockers given with moxisylyte

Moxonidine: enhanced hypotensive effect when adrenergic neurone blockers given with moxonidine

Muscle Relaxants: enhanced hypotensive effect when adrenergic neurone blockers given with baclofen or tizanidine

Nitrates: enhanced hypotensive effect when adrenergic neurone blockers given with nitrates

Oestrogens: hypotensive effect of adrenergic neurone blockers antagonised by oestrogens

Adrenergic Neurone Blockers *(continued)*

Pizotifen: hypotensive effect of adrenergic neurone blockers antagonised by pizotifen

Prostaglandins: enhanced hypotensive effect when adrenergic neurone blockers given with alprostadil

• Sympathomimetics: hypotensive effect of adrenergic neurone blockers antagonised by •ephedrine, •isometheptene, •metaraminol, •methylphenidate, •noradrenaline (norepinephrine), •oxymetazoline, •phenylephrine, •phenylpropanolamine, •pseudoephedrine and •xylometazoline

Vasodilator Antihypertensives: enhanced hypotensive effect when adrenergic neurone blockers given with hydralazine, minoxidil or sodium nitroprusside

Adsorbents *see* Kaolin

Agalsidase Beta

Anti-arrhythmics: effects of agalsidase beta possibly inhibited by amiodarone (manufacturer of agalsidase beta advises avoid concomitant use)

Antibacterials: effects of agalsidase beta possibly inhibited by gentamicin (manufacturer of agalsidase beta advises avoid concomitant use)

Antimalarials: effects of agalsidase beta possibly inhibited by chloroquine and hydroxychloroquine (manufacturer of agalsidase beta advises avoid concomitant use)

Alcohol

ACE Inhibitors: enhanced hypotensive effect when alcohol given with ACE inhibitors

Adrenergic Neurone Blockers: enhanced hypotensive effect when alcohol given with adrenergic neurone blockers

Alpha-blockers: increased sedative effect when alcohol given with indoramin; enhanced hypotensive effect when alcohol given with alpha-blockers

Analgesics: enhanced hypotensive and sedative effects when alcohol given with opioid analgesics

Angiotensin-II Receptor Antagonists: enhanced hypotensive effect when alcohol given with angiotensin-II receptor antagonists

• Antibacterials: disulfiram-like reaction when alcohol given with metronidazole; possibility of disulfiram-like reaction when alcohol given with tinidazole; increased risk of convulsions when alcohol given with •cycloserine

• Anticoagulants: major changes in consumption of alcohol may affect anticoagulant control with •coumarins or •phenindione

• Antidepressants: some beverages containing alcohol and some dealcoholised beverages contain tyramine which interacts with •MAOIs (hypertensive crisis)—if no tyramine, enhanced hypotensive effect; sedative effects possibly increased when alcohol given with SSRIs; increased sedative effect when alcohol given with •mirtazapine, •tricyclic-related antidepressants or •tricyclics

Antidiabetics: alcohol enhances hypoglycaemic effect of antidiabetics; increased risk of lactic acidosis when alcohol given with metformin; flushing, in susceptible subjects, when alcohol given with chlorpropamide

Antiepileptics: alcohol possibly increases CNS side-effects of carbamazepine; increased sedative effect when alcohol given with primidone

Antifungals: effects of alcohol possibly enhanced by griseofulvin

Antihistamines: increased sedative effect when alcohol given with antihistamines (possibly less effect with non-sedating antihistamines)

Antimuscarinics: increased sedative effect when alcohol given with hyoscine

Antipsychotics: increased sedative effect when alcohol given with antipsychotics

Anxiolytics and Hypnotics: increased sedative effect when alcohol given with anxiolytics and hypnotics

Barbiturates: increased sedative effect when alcohol given with barbiturates

Beta-blockers: enhanced hypotensive effect when alcohol given with beta-blockers

Calcium-channel Blockers: enhanced hypotensive effect when alcohol given with calcium-channel

Alcohol

Calcium-channel Blockers *(continued)*
blockers; plasma concentration of alcohol possibly increased by verapamil

Clonidine: enhanced hypotensive effect when alcohol given with clonidine

Cytotoxics: disulfiram-like reaction when alcohol given with procarbazine

Diazoxide: enhanced hypotensive effect when alcohol given with diazoxide

Disulfiram: disulfiram reaction when alcohol given with disulfiram (see p. 270)

Diuretics: enhanced hypotensive effect when alcohol given with diuretics

Dopaminergics: alcohol reduces tolerance to bromocriptine

Levamisole: possibility of disulfiram-like reaction when alcohol given with levamisole

Lofexidine: increased sedative effect when alcohol given with lofexidine

Methyldopa: enhanced hypotensive effect when alcohol given with methyldopa

Moxonidine: enhanced hypotensive effect when alcohol given with moxonidine

Muscle Relaxants: increased sedative effect when alcohol given with baclofen, methocarbamol or tizanidine

Nabilone: increased sedative effect when alcohol given with nabilone

Nicorandil: alcohol possibly enhances hypotensive effect of nicorandil

Nitrates: enhanced hypotensive effect when alcohol given with nitrates

• Paraldehyde: increased sedative effect when alcohol given with •paraldehyde

Retinoids: presence of alcohol causes etretinate to be formed from acitretin

Vasodilator Antihypertensives: enhanced hypotensive effect when alcohol given with hydralazine, minoxidil or sodium nitroprusside

Aldesleukin

ACE Inhibitors: enhanced hypotensive effect when aldesleukin given with ACE inhibitors

Alpha-blockers: enhanced hypotensive effect when aldesleukin given with alpha-blockers

Angiotensin-II Receptor Antagonists: enhanced hypotensive effect when aldesleukin given with angiotensin-II receptor antagonists

Beta-blockers: enhanced hypotensive effect when aldesleukin given with beta-blockers

Calcium-channel Blockers: enhanced hypotensive effect when aldesleukin given with calcium-channel blockers

Clonidine: enhanced hypotensive effect when aldesleukin given with clonidine

Diazoxide: enhanced hypotensive effect when aldesleukin given with diazoxide

Diuretics: enhanced hypotensive effect when aldesleukin given with diuretics

Methyldopa: enhanced hypotensive effect when aldesleukin given with methyldopa

Moxonidine: enhanced hypotensive effect when aldesleukin given with moxonidine

Nitrates: enhanced hypotensive effect when aldesleukin given with nitrates

Vasodilator Antihypertensives: enhanced hypotensive effect when aldesleukin given with hydralazine, minoxidil or sodium nitroprusside

Alendronic Acid *see* Bisphosphonates

Alfentanil *see* Opioid Analgesics

Alfuzosin *see* Alpha-blockers

Alimemazine (trimeprazine) *see* Antihistamines

Aliskiren

Angiotensin-II Receptor Antagonists: plasma concentration of aliskiren possibly reduced by irbesartan

Anticoagulants: increased risk of hyperkalaemia when aliskiren given with heparins

Antifungals: plasma concentration of aliskiren increased by ketoconazole

Aliskiren *(continued)*

Diuretics: aliskiren reduces plasma concentration of furosemide (frusemide); increased risk of hyperkalaemia when aliskiren given with potassium-sparing diuretics and aldosterone antagonists

Potassium Salts: increased risk of hyperkalaemia when aliskiren given with potassium salts

Alkylating Drugs *see* Busulfan, Cyclophosphamide, Ifosfamide, Melphalan, and Thiotepa

Allopurinol

ACE Inhibitors: increased risk of toxicity when allopurinol given with captopril especially in renal impairment

Antibacterials: increased risk of rash when allopurinol given with amoxicillin or ampicillin

Anticoagulants: allopurinol possibly enhances anticoagulant effect of coumarins

Antivirals: allopurinol possibly increases plasma concentration of didanosine

Ciclosporin: allopurinol possibly increases plasma concentration of ciclosporin (risk of nephrotoxicity)

• Cytotoxics: allopurinol enhances effects and increases toxicity of •azathioprine and •mercaptopurine (reduce dose of azathioprine and mercaptopurine to one quarter of usual dose); avoidance of allopurinol advised by manufacturer of •capecitabine

Diuretics: increased risk of hypersensitivity when allopurinol given with thiazides and related diuretics especially in renal impairment

Theophylline: allopurinol possibly increases plasma concentration of theophylline

Almotriptan *see* $5HT_1$ Agonists

Alpha$_2$-adrenoceptor Stimulants

Antidepressants: manufacturer of apraclonidine and brimonidine advises avoid concomitant use with MAOIs; manufacturer of apraclonidine and brimonidine advises avoid concomitant use with tricyclic-related antidepressants; manufacturer of apraclonidine and brimonidine advises avoid concomitant use with tricyclics

Alpha-blockers

ACE Inhibitors: enhanced hypotensive effect when alpha-blockers given with ACE inhibitors

Adrenergic Neurone Blockers: enhanced hypotensive effect when alpha-blockers given with adrenergic neurone blockers

Alcohol: enhanced hypotensive effect when alpha-blockers given with alcohol; increased sedative effect when indoramin given with alcohol

Aldesleukin: enhanced hypotensive effect when alpha-blockers given with aldesleukin

• Anaesthetics, General: enhanced hypotensive effect when alpha-blockers given with •general anaesthetics

Analgesics: hypotensive effect of alpha-blockers antagonised by NSAIDs

Angiotensin-II Receptor Antagonists: enhanced hypotensive effect when alpha-blockers given with angiotensin-II receptor antagonists

• Antidepressants: enhanced hypotensive effect when alpha-blockers given with MAOIs; manufacturer of indoramin advises avoid concomitant use with •MAOIs

Antipsychotics: enhanced hypotensive effect when alpha-blockers given with antipsychotics

• Antivirals: plasma concentration of alfuzosin possibly increased by •ritonavir—avoid concomitant use

Anxiolytics and Hypnotics: enhanced hypotensive and sedative effects when alpha-blockers given with anxiolytics and hypnotics

• Beta-blockers: enhanced hypotensive effect when alpha-blockers given with •beta-blockers, also increased risk of first-dose hypotension with post-synaptic alpha-blockers such as prazosin

• Calcium-channel Blockers: enhanced hypotensive effect when alpha-blockers given with •calcium-channel blockers, also increased risk of first-dose hypotension with post-synaptic alpha-blockers such as prazosin

Cardiac Glycosides: prazosin increases plasma concentration of digoxin

Alpha-blockers *(continued)*
Clonidine: enhanced hypotensive effect when alpha-blockers given with clonidine
Corticosteroids: hypotensive effect of alpha-blockers antagonised by corticosteroids
Diazoxide: enhanced hypotensive effect when alpha-blockers given with diazoxide
• Diuretics: enhanced hypotensive effect when alpha-blockers given with •diuretics, also increased risk of first-dose hypotension with post-synaptic alpha-blockers such as prazosin
Dopaminergics: enhanced hypotensive effect when alpha-blockers given with levodopa
Methyldopa: enhanced hypotensive effect when alpha-blockers given with methyldopa
• Moxisylyte (thymoxamine): possible severe postural hypotension when alpha-blockers given with •moxisylyte
Moxonidine: enhanced hypotensive effect when alpha-blockers given with moxonidine
Muscle Relaxants: enhanced hypotensive effect when alpha-blockers given with baclofen or tizanidine
Nitrates: enhanced hypotensive effect when alpha-blockers given with nitrates
Oestrogens: hypotensive effect of alpha-blockers antagonised by oestrogens
Prostaglandins: enhanced hypotensive effect when alpha-blockers given with alprostadil
• Sildenafil: enhanced hypotensive effect when alpha-blockers given with •sildenafil (avoid alpha-blockers for 4 hours after sildenafil)
• Sympathomimetics: avoid concomitant use of tolazoline with •adrenaline (epinephrine) or •dopamine
• Tadalafil: enhanced hypotensive effect when alpha-blockers given with •tadalafil—avoid concomitant use
• Ulcer-healing Drugs: effects of tolazoline antagonised by •cimetidine and •ranitidine
• Vardenafil: enhanced hypotensive effect when alpha-blockers (excludes tamsulosin) given with •vardenafil—avoid vardenafil for 6 hours after alpha-blockers
Vasodilator Antihypertensives: enhanced hypotensive effect when alpha-blockers given with hydralazine, minoxidil or sodium nitroprusside

Alpha-blockers (post-synaptic) *see* Alpha-blockers
Alprazolam *see* Anxiolytics and Hypnotics
Alprostadil *see* Prostaglandins
Aluminium Hydroxide *see* Antacids

Amantadine
Antimuscarinics: increased risk of antimuscarinic side-effects when amantadine given with antimuscarinics
Antipsychotics: increased risk of extrapyramidal side-effects when amantadine given with antipsychotics
Bupropion: increased risk of side-effects when amantadine given with bupropion
Domperidone: increased risk of extrapyramidal side-effects when amantadine given with domperidone
• Memantine: increased risk of CNS toxicity when amantadine given with •memantine (manufacturer of memantine advises avoid concomitant use); effects of dopaminergics possibly enhanced by memantine
Methyldopa: increased risk of extrapyramidal side-effects when amantadine given with methyldopa; antiparkinsonian effect of dopaminergics antagonised by methyldopa
Metoclopramide: increased risk of extrapyramidal side-effects when amantadine given with metoclopramide
Tetrabenazine: increased risk of extrapyramidal side-effects when amantadine given with tetrabenazine

Amikacin *see* Aminoglycosides
Amiloride *see* Diuretics

Aminoglycosides
Agalsidase Beta: gentamicin possibly inhibits effects of agalsidase beta (manufacturer of agalsidase beta advises avoid concomitant use)
Analgesics: plasma concentration of amikacin and gentamicin in neonates possibly increased by indometacin
Antibacterials: neomycin reduces absorption of phenoxymethylpenicillin; increased risk of nephrotoxicity when aminoglycosides given with colistin or polymyxins; increased risk of nephrotoxicity and ototoxicity when aminoglycosides given with capreomycin, teicoplanin or vancomycin
• Anticoagulants: experience in anticoagulant clinics suggests that INR possibly altered when neomycin (given for local action on gut) is given with •coumarins or •phenindione
Antidiabetics: neomycin possibly enhances hypoglycaemic effect of acarbose, also severity of gastro-intestinal effects increased
Antifungals: increased risk of nephrotoxicity when aminoglycosides given with amphotericin
Bisphosphonates: increased risk of hypocalcaemia when aminoglycosides given with bisphosphonates
Cardiac Glycosides: gentamicin possibly increases plasma concentration of digoxin; neomycin reduces absorption of digoxin
• Ciclosporin: increased risk of nephrotoxicity when aminoglycosides given with •ciclosporin
• Cytotoxics: neomycin possibly reduces absorption of methotrexate; increased risk of nephrotoxicity and possibly of ototoxicity when aminoglycosides given with •platinum compounds
• Diuretics: increased risk of otoxicity when aminoglycosides given with •loop diuretics
• Muscle Relaxants: aminoglycosides enhance effects of •non-depolarising muscle relaxants and •suxamethonium
Oestrogens: antibacterials that do not induce liver enzymes possibly reduce contraceptive effect of oestrogens (risk probably small, see p. 428)
• Parasympathomimetics: aminoglycosides antagonise effects of •neostigmine and •pyridostigmine
• Tacrolimus: increased risk of nephrotoxicity when aminoglycosides given with •tacrolimus
Vitamins: neomycin possibly reduces absorption of vitamin A

Aminophylline *see* Theophylline

Aminosalicylates
Cardiac Glycosides: sulfasalazine possibly reduces absorption of digoxin
Cytotoxics: possible increased risk of leucopenia when aminosalicylates given with azathioprine or mercaptopurine
Folates: sulfasalazine possibly reduces absorption of folic acid

Amiodarone
Note Amiodarone has a long half-life; there is a potential for drug interactions to occur for several weeks (or even months) after treatment with it has been stopped
Agalsidase Beta: amiodarone possibly inhibits effects of agalsidase beta (manufacturer of agalsidase beta advises avoid concomitant use)
Anaesthetics, Local: increased myocardial depression when anti-arrhythmics given with bupivacaine, levobupivacaine, prilocaine or ropivacaine
• Anti-arrhythmics: increased myocardial depression when anti-arrhythmics given with other •anti-arrhythmics; increased risk of ventricular arrhythmias when amiodarone given with •disopyramide—avoid concomitant use; amiodarone increases plasma concentration of •flecainide (halve dose of flecainide); amiodarone increases plasma concentration of •procainamide (increased risk of ventricular arrhythmias—avoid concomitant use)
• Antibacterials: increased risk of ventricular arrhythmias when amiodarone given with parenteral •erythromycin—avoid concomitant use; increased risk of ventricular arrhythmias when amiodarone given with •moxifloxacin—avoid concomitant use; increased risk of ventricular arrhythmias when amiodarone given with •sulfamethoxazole and •trimethoprim (as co-trimoxazole)—avoid concomitant use of co-trimoxazole
• Anticoagulants: amiodarone inhibits metabolism of •coumarins and •phenindione (enhanced anti-coagulant effect)

Amiodarone *(continued)*
- Antidepressants: increased risk of ventricular arrhythmias when amiodarone given with •tricyclics—avoid concomitant use
- Antiepileptics: amiodarone inhibits metabolism of •phenytoin (increased plasma concentration)
- Antihistamines: increased risk of ventricular arrhythmias when amiodarone given with •mizolastine—avoid concomitant use
- Antimalarials: avoidance of amiodarone advised by manufacturer of •artemether/lumefantrine (risk of ventricular arrhythmias); increased risk of ventricular arrhythmias when amiodarone given with •chloroquine and hydroxychloroquine, •mefloquine or •quinine—avoid concomitant use
- Antipsychotics: increased risk of ventricular arrhythmias when anti-arrhythmics that prolong the QT interval given with •antipsychotics that prolong the QT interval; increased risk of ventricular arrhythmias when amiodarone given with •amisulpride, •haloperidol, •phenothiazines, •pimozide or •sertindole—avoid concomitant use
- Antivirals: plasma concentration of amiodarone possibly increased by •amprenavir (increased risk of ventricular arrhythmias—avoid concomitant use); plasma concentration of amiodarone possibly increased by •atazanavir; plasma concentration of amiodarone possibly increased by •indinavir—avoid concomitant use; increased risk of ventricular arrhythmias when amiodarone given with •nelfinavir—avoid concomitant use; plasma concentration of amiodarone increased by •ritonavir (increased risk of ventricular arrhythmias—avoid concomitant use)
- Atomoxetine: increased risk of ventricular arrhythmias when amiodarone given with •atomoxetine
- Beta-blockers: increased risk of bradycardia, AV block and myocardial depression when amiodarone given with •beta-blockers; increased myocardial depression when anti-arrhythmics given with •beta-blockers; increased risk of ventricular arrhythmias when amiodarone given with •sotalol—avoid concomitant use
- Calcium-channel Blockers: increased risk of bradycardia, AV block and myocardial depression when amiodarone given with •diltiazem or •verapamil
- Cardiac Glycosides: amiodarone increases plasma concentration of •digoxin (halve dose of digoxin)

Ciclosporin: amiodarone possibly increases plasma concentration of ciclosporin

Diuretics: increased cardiac toxicity with amiodarone if hypokalaemia occurs with acetazolamide, loop diuretics or thiazides and related diuretics; amiodarone increases plasma concentration of eplerenone (reduce dose of eplerenone)

Grapefruit Juice: plasma concentration of amiodarone increased by grapefruit juice

- $5HT_3$ Antagonists: increased risk of ventricular arrhythmias when amiodarone given with •dolasetron—avoid concomitant use; caution with anti-arrhythmics advised by manufacturer of tropisetron (risk of ventricular arrhythmias)
- Ivabradine: increased risk of ventricular arrhythmias when amiodarone given with •ivabradine
- Lipid-regulating Drugs: increased risk of myopathy when amiodarone given with •simvastatin
- Lithium: manufacturer of amiodarone advises avoid concomitant use with •lithium (risk of ventricular arrhythmias)

Orlistat: plasma concentration of amiodarone possibly reduced by orlistat

- Pentamidine Isetionate: increased risk of ventricular arrhythmias when amiodarone given with •pentamidine isetionate—avoid concomitant use

Thyroid Hormones: for concomitant use of amiodarone and thyroid hormones see p. 80

Ulcer-healing Drugs: plasma concentration of amiodarone increased by cimetidine

Amisulpride *see* Antipsychotics
Amitriptyline *see* Antidepressants, Tricyclic
Amlodipine *see* Calcium-channel Blockers
Amobarbital *see* Barbiturates
Amoxicillin *see* Penicillins

Amphotericin

Note Close monitoring required with concomitant administration of nephrotoxic drugs or cytotoxics

Antibacterials: increased risk of nephrotoxicity when amphotericin given with aminoglycosides or polymyxins; possible increased risk of nephrotoxicity when amphotericin given with vancomycin

Antifungals: amphotericin reduces renal excretion and increases cellular uptake of flucytosine (toxicity possibly increased); effects of amphotericin possibly antagonised by imidazoles and triazoles

- Cardiac Glycosides: hypokalaemia caused by amphotericin increases cardiac toxicity with •cardiac glycosides
- Ciclosporin: increased risk of nephrotoxicity when amphotericin given with •ciclosporin
- Corticosteroids: increased risk of hypokalaemia when amphotericin given with •corticosteroids—avoid concomitant use unless corticosteroids needed to control reactions

Diuretics: increased risk of hypokalaemia when amphotericin given with loop diuretics or thiazides and related diuretics

Pentamidine Isetionate: possible increased risk of nephrotoxicity when amphotericin given with pentamidine isetionate

- Tacrolimus: increased risk of nephrotoxicity when amphotericin given with •tacrolimus

Ampicillin *see* Penicillins

Amprenavir

Note Fosamprenavir is a prodrug of amprenavir

Analgesics: amprenavir reduces plasma concentration of methadone

Antacids: absorption of amprenavir possibly reduced by antacids

- Anti-arrhythmics: amprenavir possibly increases plasma concentration of •amiodarone, •flecainide and •propafenone (increased risk of ventricular arrhythmias—avoid concomitant use); amprenavir possibly increases plasma concentration of •lidocaine (lignocaine)—avoid concomitant use
- Antibacterials: plasma concentration of both drugs increased when amprenavir given with erythromycin; amprenavir increases plasma concentration of •rifabutin (reduce dose of rifabutin); plasma concentration of amprenavir significantly reduced by •rifampicin—avoid concomitant use; amprenavir possibly increases plasma concentration of dapsone; avoidance of concomitant amprenavir in severe renal and hepatic impairment advised by manufacturer of •telithromycin

Anticoagulants: amprenavir may enhance or reduce anticoagulant effect of coumarins

- Antidepressants: amprenavir possibly reduces plasma concentration of paroxetine; plasma concentration of amprenavir reduced by •St John's wort—avoid concomitant use; amprenavir possibly increases side-effects of tricyclics

Antiepileptics: plasma concentration of amprenavir possibly reduced by carbamazepine and phenytoin

Antifungals: amprenavir increases plasma concentration of ketoconazole; amprenavir possibly increases plasma concentration of itraconazole

Antihistamines: amprenavir possibly increases plasma concentration of loratadine

- Antimalarials: avoid concomitant use of amprenavir with •artemether/lumefantrine

Antimuscarinics: avoidance of amprenavir advised by manufacturer of darifenacin and tolterodine

- Antipsychotics: amprenavir possibly inhibits metabolism of •aripiprazole (reduce dose of aripiprazole); amprenavir possibly increases plasma concentration of clozapine; amprenavir increases plasma concentration of •pimozide and •sertindole (increased risk of ventricular arrhythmias—avoid concomitant use)
- Antivirals: plasma concentration of amprenavir reduced by efavirenz and •tipranavir; plasma concentration of amprenavir reduced by lopinavir, effect on lopinavir plasma concentration not predictable; plasma con-

Amprenavir

- Antivirals *(continued)*
  centration of amprenavir possibly reduced by nevirapine; plasma concentration of amprenavir increased by ritonavir
- Anxiolytics and Hypnotics: increased risk of prolonged sedation and respiratory depression when amprenavir given with •alprazolam, clonazepam, •diazepam, •flurazepam or •midazolam

  Barbiturates: plasma concentration of amprenavir possibly reduced by phenobarbital
- Cilostazol: amprenavir possibly increases plasma concentration of •cilostazol—avoid concomitant use
- Ergot Alkaloids: increased risk of ergotism when amprenavir given with •ergotamine and methysergide—avoid concomitant use
- Lipid-regulating Drugs: possible increased risk of myopathy when amprenavir given with atorvastatin; possible increased risk of myopathy when amprenavir given with •simvastatin—avoid concomitant use

  Oestrogens: amprenavir increases plasma concentration of oestrogens, also plasma concentration of amprenavir reduced—alternative contraception recommended

  Progestogens: amprenavir increases plasma concentration of progestogens, also plasma concentration of amprenavir reduced—alternative contraception recommended

  Sildenafil: amprenavir possibly increases plasma concentration of sildenafil—reduce initial dose of sildenafil

  Tadalafil: amprenavir possibly increases plasma concentration of tadalafil

  Ulcer-healing Drugs: amprenavir possibly increases plasma concentration of cimetidine

  Vardenafil: amprenavir possibly increases plasma concentration of vardenafil

Anabolic Steroids

- Anticoagulants: anabolic steroids enhance anticoagulant effect of •coumarins and •phenindione

  Antidiabetics: anabolic steroids possibly enhance hypoglycaemic effect of antidiabetics

Anaesthetics, General

Note *See also* Surgery and Long-term Medication, p. 665

ACE Inhibitors: enhanced hypotensive effect when general anaesthetics given with ACE inhibitors
- Adrenergic Neurone Blockers: enhanced hypotensive effect when general anaesthetics given with •adrenergic neurone blockers
- Alpha-blockers: enhanced hypotensive effect when general anaesthetics given with •alpha-blockers

  Angiotensin-II Receptor Antagonists: enhanced hypotensive effect when general anaesthetics given with angiotensin-II receptor antagonists

  Antibacterials: general anaesthetics possibly potentiate hepatotoxicity of isoniazid; effects of thiopental enhanced by sulphonamides; hypersensitivity-like reactions can occur when general anaesthetics given with intravenous vancomycin
- Antidepressants: Because of hazardous interactions between general anaesthetics and •MAOIs, MAOIs should normally be stopped 2 weeks before surgery; increased risk of arrhythmias and hypotension when general anaesthetics given with tricyclics
- Antipsychotics: enhanced hypotensive effect when general anaesthetics given with •antipsychotics

  Anxiolytics and Hypnotics: increased sedative effect when general anaesthetics given with anxiolytics and hypnotics

  Beta-blockers: enhanced hypotensive effect when general anaesthetics given with beta-blockers
- Calcium-channel Blockers: enhanced hypotensive effect when general anaesthetics or isoflurane given with calcium-channel blockers; general anaesthetics enhance hypotensive effect of •verapamil (also AV delay)

  Clonidine: enhanced hypotensive effect when general anaesthetics given with clonidine

Anaesthetics, General *(continued)*

- Cytotoxics: nitrous oxide increases antifolate effect of •methotrexate—avoid concomitant use

  Diazoxide: enhanced hypotensive effect when general anaesthetics given with diazoxide

  Diuretics: enhanced hypotensive effect when general anaesthetics given with diuretics
- Dopaminergics: increased risk of arrhythmias when volatile liquid general anaesthetics given with •levodopa

  Ergot Alkaloids: halothane reduces effects of ergometrine on the parturient uterus
- Memantine: increased risk of CNS toxicity when ketamine given with •memantine (manufacturer of memantine advises avoid concomitant use)

  Methyldopa: enhanced hypotensive effect when general anaesthetics given with methyldopa

  Moxonidine: enhanced hypotensive effect when general anaesthetics given with moxonidine
- Muscle Relaxants: increased risk of myocardial depression and bradycardia when propofol given with •suxamethonium; volatile liquid general anaesthetics enhance effects of non-depolarising muscle relaxants and suxamethonium

  Nitrates: enhanced hypotensive effect when general anaesthetics given with nitrates

  Oxytocin: oxytocic effect possibly reduced, also enhanced hypotensive effect and risk of arrhythmias when volatile liquid general anaesthetics given with oxytocin
- Sympathomimetics: increased risk of arrhythmias when volatile liquid general anaesthetics given with •adrenaline (epinephrine); increased risk of hypertension when volatile liquid general anaesthetics given with •methylphenidate

  Theophylline: increased risk of convulsions when ketamine given with theophylline; increased risk of arrhythmias when halothane given with theophylline

  Vasodilator Antihypertensives: enhanced hypotensive effect when general anaesthetics given with hydralazine, minoxidil or sodium nitroprusside

Anaesthetics, General (intravenous) *see* Anaesthetics, General

Anaesthetics, General (volatile liquids) *see* Anaesthetics, General

Anaesthetics, Local *see* Bupivacaine, Levobupivacaine, Lidocaine (lignocaine), Prilocaine, and Ropivacaine

Anagrelide

- Cilostazol: manufacturer of anagrelide advises avoid concomitant use with •cilostazol
- Phosphodiesterase Inhibitors: manufacturer of anagrelide advises avoid concomitant use with •enoximone and •milrinone

Anakinra

- Adalimumab: avoid concomitant use of anakinra with •adalimumab
- Etanercept: increased risk of side-effects when anakinra given with •etanercept—avoid concomitant use
- Infliximab: avoid concomitant use of anakinra with •infliximab
- Vaccines: avoid concomitant use of anakinra with live •vaccines (see p. 641)

Analgesics *see* Aspirin, Nefopam, NSAIDs, Opioid Analgesics, and Paracetamol

Angiotensin-II Receptor Antagonists

ACE Inhibitors: increased risk of hyperkalaemia when angiotensin-II receptor antagonists given with ACE inhibitors

Adrenergic Neurone Blockers: enhanced hypotensive effect when angiotensin-II receptor antagonists given with adrenergic neurone blockers

Alcohol: enhanced hypotensive effect when angiotensin-II receptor antagonists given with alcohol

Aldesleukin: enhanced hypotensive effect when angiotensin-II receptor antagonists given with aldesleukin

Aliskiren: irbesartan possibly reduces plasma concentration of aliskiren

Alpha-blockers: enhanced hypotensive effect when angiotensin-II receptor antagonists given with alpha-blockers

Angiotensin-II Receptor Antagonists *(continued)*
Anaesthetics, General: enhanced hypotensive effect when angiotensin-II receptor antagonists given with general anaesthetics
Analgesics: increased risk of renal impairment when angiotensin-II receptor antagonists given with NSAIDs, also hypotensive effect antagonised
Anticoagulants: increased risk of hyperkalaemia when angiotensin-II receptor antagonists given with heparin
Antidepressants: hypotensive effect of angiotensin-II receptor antagonists possibly enhanced by MAOIs
Antipsychotics: enhanced hypotensive effect when angiotensin-II receptor antagonists given with antipsychotics
Anxiolytics and Hypnotics: enhanced hypotensive effect when angiotensin-II receptor antagonists given with anxiolytics and hypnotics
Beta-blockers: enhanced hypotensive effect when angiotensin-II receptor antagonists given with beta-blockers
Calcium-channel Blockers: enhanced hypotensive effect when angiotensin-II receptor antagonists given with calcium-channel blockers
• Ciclosporin: increased risk of hyperkalaemia when angiotensin-II receptor antagonists given with •ciclosporin
Clonidine: enhanced hypotensive effect when angiotensin-II receptor antagonists given with clonidine
Corticosteroids: hypotensive effect of angiotensin-II receptor antagonists antagonised by corticosteroids
Diazoxide: enhanced hypotensive effect when angiotensin-II receptor antagonists given with diazoxide
• Diuretics: enhanced hypotensive effect when angiotensin-II receptor antagonists given with •diuretics; increased risk of hyperkalaemia when angiotensin-II receptor antagonists given with •potassium-sparing diuretics and aldosterone antagonists
Dopaminergics: enhanced hypotensive effect when angiotensin-II receptor antagonists given with levodopa
Epoetin: antagonism of hypotensive effect and increased risk of hyperkalaemia when angiotensin-II receptor antagonists given with epoetin
• Lithium: angiotensin-II receptor antagonists reduce excretion of •lithium (increased plasma concentration)
Methyldopa: enhanced hypotensive effect when angiotensin-II receptor antagonists given with methyldopa
Moxisylyte (thymoxamine): enhanced hypotensive effect when angiotensin-II receptor antagonists given with moxisylyte
Moxonidine: enhanced hypotensive effect when angiotensin-II receptor antagonists given with moxonidine
Muscle Relaxants: enhanced hypotensive effect when angiotensin-II receptor antagonists given with baclofen or tizanidine
Nitrates: enhanced hypotensive effect when angiotensin-II receptor antagonists given with nitrates
Oestrogens: hypotensive effect of angiotensin-II receptor antagonists antagonised by oestrogens
• Potassium Salts: increased risk of hyperkalaemia when angiotensin-II receptor antagonists given with •potassium salts
Progestogens: risk of hyperkalaemia when angiotensin-II receptor antagonists given with drospirenone (monitor serum potassium during first cycle)
Prostaglandins: enhanced hypotensive effect when angiotensin-II receptor antagonists given with alprostadil
Tacrolimus: increased risk of hyperkalaemia when angiotensin-II receptor antagonists given with tacrolimus
Vasodilator Antihypertensives: enhanced hypotensive effect when angiotensin-II receptor antagonists given with hydralazine, minoxidil or sodium nitroprusside

Antacids
Note Antacids should preferably not be taken at the same time as other drugs since they may impair absorption
ACE Inhibitors: antacids possibly reduce absorption of ACE inhibitors; antacids reduce absorption of captopril, enalapril and fosinopril
Analgesics: alkaline urine due to some antacids increases excretion of aspirin
Antibacterials: antacids reduce absorption of azithromycin, cefaclor, cefpodoxime, ciprofloxacin, isoniazid, levofloxacin, moxifloxacin, norfloxacin, ofloxacin, rifampicin and tetracyclines; oral magnesium salts (as magnesium trisilicate) reduce absorption of nitrofurantoin
Antiepileptics: antacids reduce absorption of gabapentin and phenytoin
Antifungals: antacids reduce absorption of itraconazole and ketoconazole
Antihistamines: antacids reduce absorption of fexofenadine
Antimalarials: antacids reduce absorption of chloroquine and hydroxychloroquine; oral magnesium salts (as magnesium trisilicate) reduce absorption of proguanil
Antipsychotics: antacids reduce absorption of phenothiazines and sulpiride
Antivirals: antacids possibly reduce absorption of amprenavir; antacids possibly reduce plasma concentration of atazanavir; antacids reduce absorption of tipranavir
Bile Acids: antacids possibly reduce absorption of bile acids
Bisphosphonates: antacids reduce absorption of bisphosphonates
Cardiac Glycosides: antacids possibly reduce absorption of digoxin
Corticosteroids: antacids reduce absorption of deflazacort
Cytotoxics: antacids reduce absorption of mycophenolate
Deferasirox: antacids containing aluminium possibly reduce absorption of deferasirox (manufacturer of deferasirox advises avoid concomitant use)
Dipyridamole: antacids possibly reduce absorption of dipyridamole
Iron: oral magnesium salts (as magnesium trisilicate) reduce absorption of *oral* iron
Lipid-regulating Drugs: antacids reduce absorption of rosuvastatin
Lithium: sodium bicarbonate increases excretion of lithium (reduced plasma concentration)
Penicillamine: antacids reduce absorption of penicillamine
Thyroid Hormones: antacids possibly reduce absorption of levothyroxine (thyroxine)
Ulcer-healing Drugs: antacids possibly reduce absorption of lansoprazole

Antazoline *see* Antihistamines
Anti-arrhythmics *see* Adenosine, Amiodarone, Disopyramide, Flecainide, Lidocaine (lignocaine), Mexiletine, Procainamide, and Propafenone
Antibacterials *see* individual drugs
Antibiotics (cytotoxic) *see* Bleomycin, Doxorubicin, Epirubicin, Mitomycin
Anticoagulants *see* Coumarins, Heparins, and Phenindione
Antidepressants *see* Antidepressants, SSRI; Antidepressants, Tricyclic; Antidepressants, Tricyclic (related); MAOIs; Mirtazapine; Moclobemide; Reboxetine; St John's Wort; Tryptophan; Venlafaxine
Antidepressants, Noradrenaline Re-uptake Inhibitors *see* Reboxetine

Antidepressants, SSRI
Alcohol: sedative effects possibly increased when SSRIs given with alcohol
Anaesthetics, Local: fluvoxamine inhibits metabolism of ropivacaine—avoid prolonged administration of ropivacaine
• Analgesics: increased risk of bleeding when SSRIs given with •NSAIDs or •aspirin; fluvoxamine possibly

Antidepressants, SSRI
- Analgesics *(continued)*
  increases plasma concentration of methadone; increased risk of CNS toxicity when SSRIs given with •tramadol
- Anti-arrhythmics: fluoxetine increases plasma concentration of flecainide; fluvoxamine inhibits metabolism of •mexiletine (increased risk of toxicity); paroxetine possibly inhibits metabolism of propafenone (increased risk of toxicity)
- Anticoagulants: SSRIs possibly enhance anticoagulant effect of •coumarins
- Antidepressants: avoidance of fluvoxamine advised by manufacturer of •reboxetine; possible increased serotonergic effects when SSRIs given with duloxetine; fluvoxamine inhibits metabolism of •duloxetine—avoid concomitant use; citalopram, escitalopram, fluvoxamine or paroxetine should not be started until 2 weeks after stopping •MAOIs, also MAOIs should not be started until at least 1 week after stopping citalopram, escitalopram, fluvoxamine or paroxetine; CNS effects of SSRIs increased by •MAOIs (risk of serious toxicity); sertraline should not be started until 2 weeks after stopping •MAOIs, also MAOIs should not be started until at least 2 weeks after stopping sertraline; fluoxetine should not be started until 2 weeks after stopping •MAOIs, also MAOIs should not be started until at least 5 weeks after stopping fluoxetine; increased risk of CNS toxicity when escitalopram given with •moclobemide, preferably avoid concomitant use; after stopping citalopram, fluvoxamine or paroxetine do not start •moclobemide for at least 1 week; after stopping fluoxetine do not start •moclobemide for 5 weeks; after stopping sertraline do not start •moclobemide for 2 weeks; increased serotonergic effects when SSRIs given with •St John's wort—avoid concomitant use; SSRIs increase plasma concentration of some •tricyclics; agitation and nausea may occur when SSRIs given with •tryptophan
- Antiepileptics: SSRIs antagonise anticonvulsant effect of •antiepileptics (convulsive threshold lowered); fluoxetine and fluvoxamine increase plasma concentration of •carbamazepine; plasma concentration of paroxetine reduced by carbamazepine, phenytoin and primidone; fluoxetine and fluvoxamine increase plasma concentration of •phenytoin

  Antihistamines: antidepressant effect of SSRIs possibly antagonised by cyproheptadine
- Antimalarials: avoidance of antidepressants advised by manufacturer of •artemether/lumefantrine

  Antimuscarinics: paroxetine increases plasma concentration of darifenacin and procyclidine
- Antipsychotics: fluoxetine increases plasma concentration of •clozapine, •haloperidol, risperidone, •sertindole and •zotepine; paroxetine inhibits metabolism of perphenazine (reduce dose of perphenazine); fluoxetine and paroxetine possibly inhibit metabolism of •aripiprazole (reduce dose of aripiprazole); fluvoxamine, paroxetine and sertraline increase plasma concentration of •clozapine; citalopram possibly increases plasma concentration of clozapine (increased risk of toxicity); fluvoxamine increases plasma concentration of olanzapine; paroxetine possibly increases plasma concentration of •pimozide—avoid concomitant use; sertraline increases plasma concentration of •pimozide (increased risk of ventricular arrhythmias—avoid concomitant use); paroxetine possibly increases plasma concentration of risperidone (increased risk of toxicity); paroxetine increases plasma concentration of •sertindole
- Antivirals: plasma concentration of paroxetine possibly reduced by amprenavir, darunavir and ritonavir; plasma concentration of sertraline possibly reduced by darunavir; plasma concentration of sertraline reduced by efavirenz; plasma concentration of SSRIs possibly increased by •ritonavir

  Anxiolytics and Hypnotics: fluvoxamine increases plasma concentration of some benzodiazepines;

Antidepressants, SSRI

Anxiolytics and Hypnotics *(continued)*
sedative effects possibly increased when sertraline given with zolpidem

Atomoxetine: possible increased risk of convulsions when antidepressants given with atomoxetine; fluoxetine and paroxetine possibly inhibit metabolism of atomoxetine

Barbiturates: SSRIs antagonise anticonvulsant effect of barbiturates (convulsive threshold lowered); plasma concentration of paroxetine reduced by phenobarbital

Beta-blockers: citalopram and escitalopram increase plasma concentration of metoprolol; paroxetine possibly increases plasma concentration of metoprolol (enhanced effect); fluvoxamine increases plasma concentration of propranolol

Bupropion: plasma concentration of citalopram possibly increased by bupropion
- Dopaminergics: caution with paroxetine advised by manufacturer of entacapone; increased risk of CNS toxicity when SSRIs given with •rasagiline; fluvoxamine should not be started until 2 weeks after stopping •rasagiline; fluoxetine should not be started until 2 weeks after stopping •rasagiline, also rasagiline should not be started until at least 5 weeks after stopping fluoxetine; increased risk of hypertension and CNS excitation when paroxetine or sertraline given with •selegiline (selegiline should not be started until 2 weeks after stopping paroxetine or sertraline, avoid paroxetine or sertraline for 2 weeks after stopping selegiline); increased risk of hypertension and CNS excitation when fluvoxamine given with •selegiline (selegiline should not be started until 1 week after stopping fluvoxamine, avoid fluvoxamine for 2 weeks after stopping selegiline); increased risk of hypertension and CNS excitation when fluoxetine given with •selegiline (selegiline should not be started until 5 weeks after stopping fluoxetine, avoid fluoxetine for 2 weeks after stopping selegiline); theoretical risk of serotonin syndrome if citalopram given with selegiline (especially if dose of selegiline exceeds 10 mg daily); manufacturer of escitalopram advises caution with selegiline
- $5HT_1$ Agonists: fluvoxamine inhibits the metabolism of frovatriptan; possible increased serotonergic effects when SSRIs given with frovatriptan; increased risk of CNS toxicity when citalopram, escitalopram, fluoxetine, fluvoxamine or paroxetine given with •sumatriptan; increased risk of CNS toxicity when sertraline given with •sumatriptan (manufacturer of sertraline advises avoid concomitant use); fluvoxamine possibly inhibits metabolism of zolmitriptan (reduce dose of zolmitriptan)
- Lithium: Increased risk of CNS effects when SSRIs given with •lithium (lithium toxicity reported)
- Muscle Relaxants: fluvoxamine increases plasma concentration of •tizanidine (increased risk of toxicity)—avoid concomitant use

  Parasympathomimetics: paroxetine increases plasma concentration of galantamine
- Sibutramine: increased risk of CNS toxicity when SSRIs given with •sibutramine (manufacturer of sibutramine advises avoid concomitant use)

  Sympathomimetics: metabolism of SSRIs possibly inhibited by methylphenidate
- Theophylline: fluvoxamine increases plasma concentration of •theophylline (concomitant use should usually be avoided, but where not possible halve theophylline dose and monitor plasma-theophylline concentration)

  Ulcer-healing Drugs: plasma concentration of citalopram, escitalopram and sertraline increased by cimetidine; plasma concentration of escitalopram increased by omeprazole

Antidepressants, SSRI (related) *see* Duloxetine and Venlafaxine

Antidepressants, Tricyclic

Adrenergic Neurone Blockers: tricyclics antagonise hypotensive effect of adrenergic neurone blockers

Antidepressants, Tricyclic *(continued)*

- Alcohol: increased sedative effect when tricyclics given with •alcohol
- Alpha$_2$-adrenoceptor Stimulants: avoidance of tricyclics advised by manufacturer of apraclonidine and brimonidine
- Anaesthetics, General: increased risk of arrhythmias and hypotension when tricyclics given with general anaesthetics
- • Analgesics: increased risk of CNS toxicity when tricyclics given with •tramadol; side-effects possibly increased when tricyclics given with nefopam; sedative effects possibly increased when tricyclics given with opioid analgesics
- • Anti-arrhythmics: increased risk of ventricular arrhythmias when tricyclics given with •amiodarone—avoid concomitant use; increased risk of ventricular arrhythmias when tricyclics given with •disopyramide, •flecainide or •procainamide; increased risk of arrhythmias when tricyclics given with •propafenone
- • Antibacterials: increased risk of ventricular arrhythmias when tricyclics given with •moxifloxacin—avoid concomitant use; plasma concentration of tricyclics possibly reduced by rifampicin
- • Anticoagulants: tricyclics may enhance or reduce anticoagulant effect of •coumarins
- • Antidepressants: possible increased serotonergic effects when amitriptyline or clomipramine given with duloxetine; increased risk of hypertension and CNS excitation when tricyclics given with •MAOIs, tricyclics should not be started until 2 weeks after stopping MAOIs (3 weeks if starting clomipramine or imipramine), also MAOIs should not be started for at least 1–2 weeks after stopping tricyclics (3 weeks in the case of clomipramine or imipramine); after stopping tricyclics do not start •moclobemide for at least 1 week; plasma concentration of some tricyclics increased by •SSRIs; plasma concentration of amitriptyline reduced by St John's wort
- • Antiepileptics: tricyclics antagonise anticonvulsant effect of •antiepileptics (convulsive threshold lowered); metabolism of tricyclics accelerated by •carbamazepine (reduced plasma concentration and reduced effect); plasma concentration of tricyclics possibly reduced by •phenytoin; tricyclics antagonises anticonvulsant effect of •primidone (convulsive threshold lowered), also metabolism of tricyclics possibly accelerated (reduced plasma concentration)
- Antifungals: plasma concentration of imipramine and nortriptyline possibly increased by terbinafine
- Antihistamines: increased antimuscarinic and sedative effects when tricyclics given with antihistamines
- • Antimalarials: avoidance of antidepressants advised by manufacturer of •artemether/lumefantrine
- Antimuscarinics: increased risk of antimuscarinic side-effects when tricyclics given with antimuscarinics
- • Antipsychotics: plasma concentration of tricyclics increased by •antipsychotics—possibly increased risk of ventricular arrhythmias; possibly increased antimuscarinic side-effects when tricyclics given with clozapine; increased risk of antimuscarinic side-effects when tricyclics given with phenothiazines; increased risk of ventricular arrhythmias when tricyclics given with •pimozide—avoid concomitant use
- • Antivirals: side-effects of tricyclics possibly increased by amprenavir; plasma concentration of tricyclics possibly increased by •ritonavir
- Anxiolytics and Hypnotics: increased sedative effect when tricyclics given with anxiolytics and hypnotics
- • Atomoxetine: increased risk of ventricular arrhythmias when tricyclics given with •atomoxetine; possible increased risk of convulsions when antidepressants given with atomoxetine
- • Barbiturates: tricyclics antagonises anticonvulsant effect of •barbiturates (convulsive threshold lowered), also metabolism of tricyclics possibly accelerated (reduced plasma concentration)
- • Beta-blockers: plasma concentration of imipramine increased by labetalol and propranolol; increased risk of ventricular arrhythmias when tricyclics given with •sotalol
- Calcium-channel Blockers: plasma concentration of tricyclics possibly increased by diltiazem and verapamil; plasma concentration of imipramine increased by diltiazem and verapamil
- • Clonidine: tricyclics antagonise hypotensive effect of •clonidine, also increased risk of hypertension on clonidine withdrawal
- Disulfiram: metabolism of tricyclics inhibited by disulfiram (increased plasma concentration); concomitant amitriptyline reported to increase disulfiram reaction with alcohol
- Diuretics: increased risk of postural hypotension when tricyclics given with diuretics
- • Dopaminergics: caution with tricyclics advised by manufacturer of entacapone; increased risk of CNS toxicity when tricyclics given with •rasagiline; CNS toxicity reported when tricyclics given with •selegiline
- Lithium: risk of toxicity when tricyclics given with lithium
- Muscle Relaxants: tricyclics enhance muscle relaxant effect of baclofen
- Nicorandil: tricyclics possibly enhance hypotensive effect of nicorandil
- Nitrates: tricyclics reduce effects of sublingual tablets of nitrates (failure to dissolve under tongue owing to dry mouth)
- Oestrogens: antidepressant effect of tricyclics antagonised by oestrogens (but side-effects of tricyclics possibly increased due to increased plasma concentration)
- • Pentamidine Isetionate: increased risk of ventricular arrhythmias when tricyclics given with •pentamidine isetionate
- • Sibutramine: increased risk of CNS toxicity when tricyclics given with •sibutramine (manufacturer of sibutramine advises avoid concomitant use)
- Sodium Oxybate: increased risk of side-effects when tricyclics given with sodium oxybate
- • Sympathomimetics: increased risk of hypertension and arrhythmias when tricyclics given with •adrenaline (epinephrine) (but local anaesthetics with adrenaline appear to be safe); metabolism of tricyclics possibly inhibited by methylphenidate; increased risk of hypertension and arrhythmias when tricyclics given with •noradrenaline (norepinephrine)
- Thyroid Hormones: effects of tricyclics possibly enhanced by thyroid hormones; effects of amitriptyline and imipramine enhanced by thyroid hormones
- Ulcer-healing Drugs: plasma concentration of tricyclics possibly increased by cimetidine; metabolism of amitriptyline, doxepin, imipramine and nortriptyline inhibited by cimetidine (increased plasma concentration)

Antidepressants, Tricyclic (related)

- • Alcohol: increased sedative effect when tricyclic-related antidepressants given with •alcohol
- Alpha$_2$-adrenoceptor Stimulants: avoidance of tricyclic-related antidepressants advised by manufacturer of apraclonidine and brimonidine
- • Antidepressants: tricyclic-related antidepressants should not be started until 2 weeks after stopping •MAOIs, also MAOIs should not be started until at least 1–2 weeks after stopping tricyclic-related antidepressants; after stopping tricyclic-related antidepressants do not start •moclobemide for at least 1 week
- • Antiepileptics: tricyclic-related antidepressants possibly antagonise anticonvulsant effect of •antiepileptics (convulsive threshold lowered); plasma concentration of mianserin reduced by •carbamazepine and •phenytoin; metabolism of mianserin accelerated by •primidone (reduced plasma concentration)

Antidepressants, Tricyclic (related) *(continued)*

Antihistamines: possible increased antimuscarinic and sedative effects when tricyclic-related antidepressants given with antihistamines

• Antimalarials: avoidance of antidepressants advised by manufacturer of •artemether/lumefantrine

Antimuscarinics: possibly increased antimuscarinic side-effects when tricyclic-related antidepressants given with antimuscarinics

Antivirals: side-effects possibly increased when trazodone given with ritonavir

Anxiolytics and Hypnotics: increased sedative effect when tricyclic-related antidepressants given with anxiolytics and hypnotics

Atomoxetine: possible increased risk of convulsions when antidepressants given with atomoxetine

• Barbiturates: tricyclic-related antidepressants possibly antagonise anticonvulsant effect of •barbiturates (convulsive threshold lowered); metabolism of mianserin accelerated by •phenobarbital (reduced plasma concentration)

Diazoxide: enhanced hypotensive effect when tricyclic-related antidepressants given with diazoxide

Nitrates: tricyclic-related antidepressants possibly reduce effects of sublingual tablets of nitrates (failure to dissolve under tongue owing to dry mouth)

• Sibutramine: increased risk of CNS toxicity when tricyclic-related antidepressants given with •sibutramine (manufacturer of sibutramine advises avoid concomitant use)

Vasodilator Antihypertensives: enhanced hypotensive effect when tricyclic-related antidepressants given with hydralazine or sodium nitroprusside

Antidiabetics

Note Other oral drugs may be taken at least 1 hour before or 4 hours after exenatide injection, or taken with a meal when exenatide is not administered, to minimise possible interference with absorption

ACE Inhibitors: hypoglycaemic effect of insulin, metformin and sulphonylureas possibly enhanced by ACE inhibitors

Alcohol: hypoglycaemic effect of antidiabetics enhanced by alcohol; increased risk of lactic acidosis when metformin given with alcohol; flushing, in susceptible subjects, when chlorpropamide given with alcohol

Anabolic Steroids: hypoglycaemic effect of antidiabetics possibly enhanced by anabolic steroids

• Analgesics: effects of sulphonylureas possibly enhanced by •NSAIDs; effects of tolbutamide enhanced by •azapropazone (avoid concomitant use)

Anti-arrhythmics: hypoglycaemic effect of gliclazide, insulin and metformin possibly enhanced by disopyramide

• Antibacterials: hypoglycaemic effect of acarbose possibly enhanced by neomycin, also severity of gastro-intestinal effects increased; effects of repaglinide enhanced by clarithromycin; effects of glibenclamide possibly enhanced by ciprofloxacin and norfloxacin; plasma concentration of nateglinide reduced by rifampicin; hypoglycaemic effect of repaglinide possibly antagonised by rifampicin; plasma concentration of rosiglitazone reduced by •rifampicin—consider increasing dose of rosiglitazone; effects of sulphonylureas enhanced by •chloramphenicol; metabolism of sulphonylureas possibly accelerated by •rifamycins (reduced effect); metabolism of chlorpropamide and tolbutamide accelerated by •rifamycins (reduced effect); effects of sulphonylureas rarely enhanced by sulphonamides and trimethoprim; hypoglycaemic effect of repaglinide possibly enhanced by trimethoprim—manufacturer advises avoid concomitant use

• Anticoagulants: exenatide possibly enhances anticoagulant effect of warfarin; hypoglycaemic effect of sulphonylureas possibly enhanced by •coumarins, also possible changes to anticoagulant effect

Antidepressants: hypoglycaemic effect of insulin, metformin and sulphonylureas enhanced by MAOIs; hypoglycaemic effect of antidiabetics possibly enhanced by MAOIs

Antidiabetics *(continued)*

Antiepileptics: tolbutamide transiently increases plasma concentration of phenytoin (possibility of toxicity)

• Antifungals: plasma concentration of sulphonylureas increased by •fluconazole and •miconazole; hypoglycaemic effect of gliclazide and glipizide enhanced by •miconazole—avoid concomitant use; hypoglycaemic effect of nateglinide possibly enhanced by fluconazole; hypoglycaemic effect of repaglinide possibly enhanced by itraconazole; hypoglycaemic effect of glipizide possibly enhanced by posaconazole; plasma concentration of sulphonylureas possibly increased by voriconazole

Antihistamines: thrombocyte count depressed when metformin given with ketotifen (manufacturer of ketotifen advises avoid concomitant use)

Antipsychotics: hypoglycaemic effect of sulphonylureas possibly antagonised by phenothiazines

Antivirals: plasma concentration of tolbutamide possibly increased by ritonavir

Aprepitant: plasma concentration of tolbutamide reduced by aprepitant

Beta-blockers: warning signs of hypoglycaemia (such as tremor) with antidiabetics may be masked when given with beta-blockers; hypoglycaemic effect of insulin enhanced by beta-blockers

• Bosentan: increased risk of hepatotoxicity when glibenclamide given with •bosentan—avoid concomitant use

Calcium-channel Blockers: glucose tolerance occasionally impaired when insulin given with nifedipine

Cardiac Glycosides: sitagliptin increases plasma concentration of digoxin; acarbose possibly reduces plasma concentration of digoxin

Ciclosporin: hypoglycaemic effect of repaglinide possibly enhanced by ciclosporin

Corticosteroids: hypoglycaemic effect of antidiabetics antagonised by corticosteroids

Cytotoxics: metabolism of rosiglitazone possibly inhibited by paclitaxel

Diazoxide: hypoglycaemic effect of antidiabetics antagonised by diazoxide

Diuretics: hypoglycaemic effect of antidiabetics antagonised by loop diuretics and thiazides and related diuretics; increased risk of hyponatraemia when chlorpropamide given with potassium-sparing diuretics and aldosterone antagonists plus thiazide; increased risk of hyponatraemia when chlorpropamide given with thiazides and related diuretics plus potassium-sparing diuretic

Hormone Antagonists: requirements for insulin, metformin, repaglinide and sulphonylureas possibly reduced by lanreotide; requirements for insulin, metformin, repaglinide and sulphonylureas possibly reduced by octreotide

Leflunomide: hypoglycaemic effect of tolbutamide possibly enhanced by leflunomide

• Lipid-regulating Drugs: hypoglycaemic effect of acarbose possibly enhanced by colestyramine; hypoglycaemic effect of nateglinide possibly enhanced by gemfibrozil; increased risk of severe hypoglycaemia when repaglinide given with •gemfibrozil—avoid concomitant use; plasma concentration of rosiglitazone increased by •gemfibrozil (consider reducing dose of rosiglitazone); may be improved glucose tolerance and an additive effect when insulin or sulphonylureas given with fibrates

Oestrogens: hypoglycaemic effect of antidiabetics antagonised by oestrogens

Orlistat: avoidance of acarbose advised by manufacturer of orlistat

Pancreatin: hypoglycaemic effect of acarbose antagonised by pancreatin

Probenecid: hypoglycaemic effect of chlorpropamide possibly enhanced by probenecid

Progestogens: hypoglycaemic effect of antidiabetics antagonised by progestogens

• Sulfinpyrazone: effects of sulphonylureas enhanced by •sulfinpyrazone

Antidiabetics *(continued)*
Testosterone: hypoglycaemic effect of antidiabetics possibly enhanced by testosterone
Ulcer-healing Drugs: excretion of metformin reduced by cimetidine (increased plasma concentration); hypoglycaemic effect of sulphonylureas enhanced by cimetidine

Antiepileptics *see* Carbamazepine, Ethosuximide, Gabapentin, Lamotrigine, Levetiracetam, Oxcarbazepine, Phenytoin, Primidone, Rufinamide, Tiagabine, Topiramate, Valproate, Vigabatrin, and Zonisamide

Antifungals *see* Amphotericin; Antifungals, Imidazole; Antifungals, Triazole; Caspofungin; Flucytosine; Griseofulvin; Terbinafine

Antifungals, Imidazole
Aliskiren: ketoconazole increases plasma concentration of aliskiren
• Analgesics: ketoconazole inhibits metabolism of •buprenorphine (reduce dose of buprenorphine)
Antacids: absorption of ketoconazole reduced by antacids
• Anti-arrhythmics: increased risk of ventricular arrhythmias when ketoconazole given with •disopyramide—avoid concomitant use
• Antibacterials: metabolism of ketoconazole accelerated by •rifampicin (reduced plasma concentration), also plasma concentration of rifampicin may be reduced by ketoconazole; plasma concentration of ketoconazole possibly reduced by isoniazid; avoidance of concomitant ketoconazole in severe renal and hepatic impairment advised by manufacturer of •telithromycin
• Anticoagulants: ketoconazole enhances anticoagulant effect of •coumarins; miconazole enhances anticoagulant effect of •coumarins (miconazole oral gel and possibly vaginal formulations absorbed)
• Antidepressants: avoidance of imidazoles advised by manufacturer of •reboxetine; ketoconazole increases plasma concentration of mirtazapine
• Antidiabetics: miconazole enhances hypoglycaemic effect of •gliclazide and •glipizide—avoid concomitant use; miconazole increases plasma concentration of •sulphonylureas
• Antiepileptics: ketoconazole and miconazole possibly increase plasma concentration of carbamazepine; plasma concentration of ketoconazole reduced by •phenytoin; miconazole enhances anticonvulsant effect of •phenytoin (plasma concentration of phenytoin increased)
Antifungals: imidazoles possibly antagonise effects of amphotericin
• Antihistamines: manufacturer of loratadine advises ketoconazole possibly increases plasma concentration of loratadine; imidazoles possibly inhibit metabolism of •mizolastine (avoid concomitant use); ketoconazole inhibits metabolism of •mizolastine—avoid concomitant use
• Antimalarials: avoidance of imidazoles advised by manufacturer of •artemether/lumefantrine
Antimuscarinics: absorption of ketoconazole reduced by antimuscarinics; ketoconazole increases plasma concentration of darifenacin—avoid concomitant use; ketoconazole increases plasma concentration of solifenacin; avoidance of ketoconazole advised by manufacturer of tolterodine
• Antipsychotics: ketoconazole inhibits metabolism of •aripiprazole (reduce dose of aripiprazole); increased risk of ventricular arrhythmias when imidazoles given with •pimozide—avoid concomitant use; imidazoles possibly increase plasma concentration of quetiapine (reduce dose of quetiapine); possible increased risk of ventricular arrhythmias when imidazoles given with •sertindole—avoid concomitant use; increased risk of ventricular arrhythmias when ketoconazole given with •sertindole—avoid concomitant use
• Antivirals: plasma concentration of ketoconazole increased by amprenavir; plasma concentration of both drugs increased when ketoconazole given with darunavir; ketoconazole inhibits the metabolism of indinavir; ketoconazole increases plasma concentration of •maraviroc (consider reducing dose of maraviroc); plasma concentration of ketoconazole reduced by •nevirapine—avoid concomitant use; combination of ketoconazole with •ritonavir may increase plasma concentration of either drug (or both); imidazoles possibly increase plasma concentration of saquinavir; ketoconazole increases plasma concentration of saquinavir
• Anxiolytics and Hypnotics: ketoconazole increases plasma concentration of alprazolam; ketoconazole increases plasma concentration of •midazolam (risk of prolonged sedation)
Aprepitant: ketoconazole increases plasma concentration of aprepitant
Bosentan: ketoconazole increases plasma concentration of bosentan
• Calcium-channel Blockers: ketoconazole inhibits metabolism of •felodipine (increased plasma concentration); avoidance of ketoconazole advised by manufacturer of lercanidipine and nisoldipine; ketoconazole possibly inhibits metabolism of dihydropyridines (increased plasma concentration)
• Ciclosporin: ketoconazole inhibits metabolism of •ciclosporin (increased plasma concentration); miconazole possibly inhibits metabolism of •ciclosporin (increased plasma concentration)
• Cilostazol: ketoconazole possibly increases plasma concentration of •cilostazol—avoid concomitant use
Cinacalcet: ketoconazole inhibits metabolism of cinacalcet (increased plasma concentration)
Corticosteroids: ketoconazole possibly inhibits metabolism of corticosteroids; ketoconazole increases plasma concentration of inhaled and oral budesonide; ketoconazole inhibits the metabolism of methylprednisolone; ketoconazole increases plasma concentration of inhaled mometasone
• Cytotoxics: ketoconazole inhibits metabolism of erlotinib and sunitinib (increased plasma concentration); ketoconazole increases plasma concentration of imatinib; *in vitro* studies suggest a possible interaction between ketoconazole and docetaxel (consult docetaxel product literature); ketoconazole reduces plasma concentration of •irinotecan (but concentration of active metabolite of irinotecan increased)—avoid concomitant use
• Diuretics: ketoconazole increases plasma concentration of •eplerenone—avoid concomitant use
• Domperidone: ketoconazole possibly increases risk of arrhythmias with •domperidone
• Ergot Alkaloids: increased risk of ergotism when imidazoles given with •ergotamine and methysergide—avoid concomitant use
• $5HT_1$ Agonists: ketoconazole increases plasma concentration of almotriptan (increased risk of toxicity); ketoconazole increases plasma concentration of •eletriptan (risk of toxicity)—avoid concomitant use
• Ivabradine: ketoconazole increases plasma concentration of •ivabradine—avoid concomitant use
Lanthanum: absorption of ketoconazole possibly reduced by lanthanum (give at least 2 hours apart)
• Lipid-regulating Drugs: possible increased risk of myopathy when imidazoles given with atorvastatin or simvastatin; increased risk of myopathy when ketoconazole given with •simvastatin (avoid concomitant use); possible increased risk of myopathy when miconazole given with •simvastatin—avoid concomitant use
Oestrogens: anecdotal reports of contraceptive failure when imidazoles or ketoconazole given with oestrogens
Parasympathomimetics: ketoconazole increases plasma concentration of galantamine
Rimonabant: ketoconazole increases plasma concentration of rimonabant
Sildenafil: ketoconazole increases plasma concentration of sildenafil—reduce initial dose of sildenafil

Antifungals, Imidazole *(continued)*
- Sirolimus: ketoconazole increases plasma concentration of •sirolimus—avoid concomitant use; miconazole increases plasma concentration of •sirolimus
- Tacrolimus: imidazoles possibly increase plasma concentration of •tacrolimus; ketoconazole increases plasma concentration of •tacrolimus

Tadalafil: ketoconazole increases plasma concentration of tadalafil
- Theophylline: ketoconazole possibly increases plasma concentration of •theophylline

Ulcer-healing Drugs: absorption of ketoconazole reduced by histamine H_2-antagonists, proton pump inhibitors and sucralfate
- Vardenafil: ketoconazole increases plasma concentration of •vardenafil—avoid concomitant use

Vitamins: ketoconazole possibly increases plasma concentration of paricalcitol

Antifungals, Polyene *see* Amphotericin

Antifungals, Triazole

Note In general, fluconazole interactions relate to multiple-dose treatment
- Analgesics: fluconazole increases plasma concentration of celecoxib (halve dose of celecoxib); fluconazole increases plasma concentration of parecoxib (reduce dose of parecoxib); fluconazole inhibits metabolism of alfentanil (risk of prolonged or delayed respiratory depression); itraconazole possibly inhibits metabolism of alfentanil; voriconazole increases plasma concentration of •methadone (consider reducing dose of methadone)

Antacids: absorption of itraconazole reduced by antacids
- Antibacterials: plasma concentration of itraconazole increased by clarithromycin; triazoles possibly increase plasma concentration of •rifabutin (increased risk of uveitis—reduce rifabutin dose); posaconazole increases plasma concentration of •rifabutin (also plasma concentration of posaconazole reduced); voriconazole increases plasma concentration of •rifabutin, also rifabutin reduces plasma concentration of voriconazole (increase dose of voriconazole and also monitor for rifabutin toxicity); fluconazole increases plasma concentration of •rifabutin (increased risk of uveitis—reduce rifabutin dose); plasma concentration of itraconazole reduced by •rifabutin—avoid concomitant use; plasma concentration of posaconazole reduced by •rifampicin; plasma concentration of voriconazole reduced by •rifampicin—avoid concomitant use; metabolism of fluconazole and itraconazole accelerated by •rifampicin (reduced plasma concentration)
- Anticoagulants: fluconazole, itraconazole and voriconazole enhance anticoagulant effect of •coumarins
- <u>Antidepressants</u>: avoidance of triazoles advised by manufacturer of •reboxetine; plasma concentration of voriconazole reduced by •St John's wort—avoid concomitant use
- Antidiabetics: posaconazole possibly enhances hypoglycaemic effect of glipizide; fluconazole possibly enhances hypoglycaemic effect of nateglinide; itraconazole possibly enhances hypoglycaemic effect of repaglinide; fluconazole increases plasma concentration of •sulphonylureas; voriconazole possibly increases plasma concentration of sulphonylureas
- Antiepileptics: plasma concentration of itraconazole and posaconazole possibly reduced by •carbamazepine; fluconazole possibly increases plasma concentration of carbamazepine; plasma concentration of voriconazole possibly reduced by •carbamazepine and •primidone—avoid concomitant use; fluconazole increases plasma concentration of •phenytoin (consider reducing dose of phenytoin); voriconazole increases plasma concentration of •phenytoin, also phenytoin reduces plasma concentration of voriconazole (increase dose of voriconazole and also monitor for phenytoin toxicity); plasma concentration of posaconazole reduced by •phenytoin; plasma concentration of itraconazole reduced by •phenytoin—

Antifungals, Triazole
- Antiepileptics *(continued)* avoid concomitant use; plasma concentration of posaconazole possibly reduced by •primidone

Antifungals: triazoles possibly antagonise effects of amphotericin
- Antihistamines: itraconazole inhibits metabolism of •mizolastine—avoid concomitant use
- Antimalarials: avoidance of triazoles advised by manufacturer of •artemether/lumefantrine

Antimuscarinics: avoidance of itraconazole advised by manufacturer of darifenacin and tolterodine; itraconazole increases plasma concentration of solifenacin
- Antipsychotics: itraconazole possibly inhibits metabolism of •aripiprazole (reduce dose of aripiprazole); increased risk of ventricular arrhythmias when triazoles given with •pimozide—avoid concomitant use; triazoles possibly increase plasma concentration of quetiapine (reduce dose of quetiapine); possible increased risk of ventricular arrhythmias when triazoles given with •sertindole—avoid concomitant use; increased risk of ventricular arrhythmias when itraconazole given with •sertindole—avoid concomitant use
- Antivirals: plasma concentration of itraconazole possibly increased by amprenavir; plasma concentration of voriconazole reduced by •efavirenz, also plasma concentration of efavirenz increased (consider increasing voriconazole dose and reducing efavirenz dose); plasma concentration of itraconazole reduced by efavirenz; itraconazole increases plasma concentration of •indinavir (consider reducing dose of indinavir); fluconazole increases plasma concentration of •nevirapine, ritonavir and tipranavir; plasma concentration of voriconazole reduced by •ritonavir—avoid concomitant use; combination of itraconazole with •ritonavir may increase plasma concentration of either drug (or both); triazoles possibly increase plasma concentration of saquinavir; fluconazole increases plasma concentration of •zidovudine (increased risk of toxicity)
- Anxiolytics and Hypnotics: itraconazole increases plasma concentration of alprazolam; posaconazole increases plasma concentration of •midazolam; fluconazole and itraconazole increase plasma concentration of •midazolam (risk of prolonged sedation); itraconazole increases plasma concentration of buspirone (reduce dose of buspirone)
- Barbiturates: plasma concentration of itraconazole and posaconazole possibly reduced by •phenobarbital; plasma concentration of voriconazole possibly reduced by •phenobarbital—avoid concomitant use
- Bosentan: fluconazole possibly increases plasma concentration of •bosentan—avoid concomitant use; itraconazole possibly increases plasma concentration of bosentan
- Calcium-channel Blockers: negative inotropic effect possibly increased when itraconazole given with calcium-channel blockers; itraconazole inhibits metabolism of •felodipine (increased plasma concentration); avoidance of itraconazole advised by manufacturer of lercanidipine and nisoldipine; avoidance of fluconazole advised by manufacturer of nisoldipine; itraconazole possibly inhibits metabolism of dihydropyridines (increased plasma concentration)
- Cardiac Glycosides: itraconazole increases plasma concentration of •digoxin
- Ciclosporin: fluconazole, itraconazole, posaconazole and voriconazole inhibit metabolism of •ciclosporin (increased plasma concentration)

Corticosteroids: itraconazole possibly inhibits metabolism of corticosteroids and methylprednisolone; itraconazole increases plasma concentration of inhaled budesonide
- Cytotoxics: itraconazole inhibits metabolism of busulfan (increased risk of toxicity); itraconazole possibly increases side-effects of cyclophosphamide; posaconazole possibly inhibits metabolism of •vinblastine and •vincristine (increased risk of neurotoxicity); itracon-

Antifungals, Triazole
- Cytotoxics *(continued)*
  azole possibly inhibits metabolism of •vincristine (increased risk of neurotoxicity)
- Diuretics: fluconazole increases plasma concentration of eplerenone (reduce dose of eplerenone); itraconazole increases plasma concentration of •eplerenone—avoid concomitant use; plasma concentration of fluconazole increased by hydrochlorothiazide
- Ergot Alkaloids: increased risk of ergotism when triazoles given with •ergotamine and methysergide—avoid concomitant use
- $5HT_1$ Agonists: itraconazole increases plasma concentration of •eletriptan (risk of toxicity)—avoid concomitant use
- Ivabradine: fluconazole increases plasma concentration of ivabradine—reduce initial dose of ivabradine; itraconazole possibly increases plasma concentration of •ivabradine—avoid concomitant use
- Lipid-regulating Drugs: possible increased risk of myopathy when triazoles given with atorvastatin or simvastatin; increased risk of myopathy when itraconazole or posaconazole given with •atorvastatin (avoid concomitant use); increased risk of myopathy when itraconazole or posaconazole given with •simvastatin (avoid concomitant use)

Oestrogens: anecdotal reports of contraceptive failure when fluconazole or itraconazole given with oestrogens

Sildenafil: itraconazole increases plasma concentration of sildenafil—reduce initial dose of sildenafil
- Sirolimus: posaconazole possibly increases plasma concentration of sirolimus; itraconazole and voriconazole increase plasma concentration of •sirolimus—avoid concomitant use
- Tacrolimus: triazoles possibly increase plasma concentration of •tacrolimus; posaconazole increases plasma concentration of •tacrolimus (reduce dose of tacrolimus); fluconazole, itraconazole and voriconazole increase plasma concentration of •tacrolimus

Tadalafil: itraconazole possibly increases plasma concentration of tadalafil
- Theophylline: fluconazole possibly increases plasma concentration of •theophylline
- Ulcer-healing Drugs: plasma concentration of posaconazole reduced by •cimetidine; voriconazole increases plasma concentration of omeprazole (reduce dose of omeprazole); absorption of itraconazole reduced by histamine H_2-antagonists and proton pump inhibitors
- Vardenafil: itraconazole possibly increases plasma concentration of •vardenafil—avoid concomitant use

Antihistamines

Note Sedative interactions apply to a lesser extent to the non-sedating antihistamines. Interactions do not generally apply to antihistamines used for topical action (including inhalation)

Alcohol: increased sedative effect when antihistamines given with alcohol (possibly less effect with non-sedating antihistamines)

Antacids: absorption of fexofenadine reduced by antacids
- Anti-arrhythmics: increased risk of ventricular arrhythmias when mizolastine given with •amiodarone, •disopyramide, •flecainide, •mexiletine, •procainamide or •propafenone—avoid concomitant use
- Antibacterials: manufacturer of loratadine advises plasma concentration possibly increased by erythromycin; metabolism of mizolastine inhibited by •erythromycin—avoid concomitant use; increased risk of ventricular arrhythmias when mizolastine given with •moxifloxacin—avoid concomitant use; metabolism of mizolastine possibly inhibited by •macrolides (avoid concomitant use)

Antidepressants: increased antimuscarinic and sedative effects when antihistamines given with MAOIs or tricyclics; cyproheptadine possibly antagonises antidepressant effect of SSRIs; possible increased antimuscarinic and sedative effects when antihistamines given with tricyclic-related antidepressants

Antihistamines *(continued)*

Antidiabetics: thrombocyte count depressed when ketotifen given with metformin (manufacturer of ketotifen advises avoid concomitant use)
- Antifungals: manufacturer of loratadine advises plasma concentration possibly increased by ketoconazole; metabolism of mizolastine inhibited by •itraconazole or •ketoconazole—avoid concomitant use; metabolism of mizolastine possibly inhibited by •imidazoles (avoid concomitant use)

Antimuscarinics: increased risk of antimuscarinic side-effects when antihistamines given with antimuscarinics

Antivirals: plasma concentration of loratadine possibly increased by amprenavir; plasma concentration of chlorphenamine (chlorpheniramine) possibly increased by lopinavir; plasma concentration of non-sedating antihistamines possibly increased by ritonavir

Anxiolytics and Hypnotics: increased sedative effect when antihistamines given with anxiolytics and hypnotics
- Beta-blockers: increased risk of ventricular arrhythmias when mizolastine given with •sotalol—avoid concomitant use

Betahistine: antihistamines theoretically antagonise effect of betahistine

Ulcer-healing Drugs: manufacturer of loratadine advises plasma concentration possibly increased by cimetidine

Antihistamines, Non-sedating *see* Antihistamines

Antihistamines, Sedating *see* Antihistamines

Antimalarials *see* Artemether with Lumefantrine, Chloroquine and Hydroxychloroquine, Mefloquine, Primaquine, Proguanil, and Quinine

Antimetabolites *see* Cytarabine, Fludarabine, Fluorouracil, Mercaptopurine, Methotrexate, and Tioguanine

Antimuscarinics

Note Many drugs have antimuscarinic effects; concomitant use of two or more such drugs can increase side-effects such as dry mouth, urine retention, and constipation; concomitant use can also lead to confusion in the elderly. Interactions do not generally apply to antimuscarinics used by inhalation

Alcohol: increased sedative effect when hyoscine given with alcohol

Analgesics: increased risk of antimuscarinic side-effects when antimuscarinics given with nefopam

Anti-arrhythmics: increased risk of antimuscarinic side-effects when antimuscarinics given with disopyramide; atropine delays absorption of mexiletine

Antibacterials: manufacturer of tolterodine advises avoid concomitant use with clarithromycin and erythromycin; plasma concentration of darifenacin possibly increased by erythromycin

Antidepressants: plasma concentration of darifenacin and procyclidine increased by paroxetine; increased risk of antimuscarinic side-effects when antimuscarinics given with MAOIs or tricyclics; possibly increased antimuscarinic side-effects when antimuscarinics given with tricyclic-related antidepressants

Antifungals: antimuscarinics reduce absorption of ketoconazole; plasma concentration of darifenacin increased by ketoconazole—avoid concomitant use; plasma concentration of solifenacin increased by itraconazole and ketoconazole; manufacturer of tolterodine advises avoid concomitant use with itraconazole and ketoconazole; manufacturer of darifenacin advises avoid concomitant use with itraconazole

Antihistamines: increased risk of antimuscarinic side-effects when antimuscarinics given with antihistamines

Antipsychotics: antimuscarinics possibly reduce effects of haloperidol; increased risk of antimuscarinic side-effects when antimuscarinics given with clozapine; antimuscarinics reduce plasma concentration of phenothiazines, but risk of antimuscarinic side-effects increased

Antimuscarinics *(continued)*

Antivirals: manufacturer of darifenacin and tolterodine advises avoid concomitant use with amprenavir; manufacturer of darifenacin advises avoid concomitant use with atazanavir, indinavir, lopinavir, nelfinavir, ritonavir, saquinavir and tipranavir; manufacturer of tolterodine advises avoid concomitant use with indinavir, lopinavir, nelfinavir, ritonavir and saquinavir; plasma concentration of solifenacin increased by nelfinavir and ritonavir

Calcium-channel Blockers: manufacturer of darifenacin advises avoid concomitant use with verapamil

Cardiac Glycosides: darifenacin possibly increases plasma concentration of digoxin

Ciclosporin: manufacturer of darifenacin advises avoid concomitant use with ciclosporin

Domperidone: antimuscarinics antagonise effects of domperidone on gastro-intestinal activity

Dopaminergics: increased risk of antimuscarinic side-effects when antimuscarinics given with amantadine; antimuscarinics possibly reduce absorption of levodopa

Memantine: effects of antimuscarinics possibly enhanced by memantine

Metoclopramide: antimuscarinics antagonise effects of metoclopramide on gastro-intestinal activity

Nitrates: antimuscarinics possibly reduce effects of sublingual tablets of nitrates (failure to dissolve under tongue owing to dry mouth)

Parasympathomimetics: antimuscarinics antagonise effects of parasympathomimetics

Antipsychotics

Note Increased risk of toxicity with myelosuppressive drugs

Note Avoid concomitant use of clozapine with drugs that have a substantial potential for causing agranulocytosis

ACE Inhibitors: enhanced hypotensive effect when antipsychotics given with ACE inhibitors

Adrenergic Neurone Blockers: enhanced hypotensive effect when phenothiazines given with adrenergic neurone blockers; higher doses of chlorpromazine antagonise hypotensive effect of adrenergic neurone blockers; haloperidol antagonises hypotensive effect of adrenergic neurone blockers

Adsorbents: absorption of phenothiazines possibly reduced by kaolin

Alcohol: increased sedative effect when antipsychotics given with alcohol

Alpha-blockers: enhanced hypotensive effect when antipsychotics given with alpha-blockers

• Anaesthetics, General: enhanced hypotensive effect when antipsychotics given with •general anaesthetics

• Analgesics: avoid concomitant use of clozapine with •azapropazone (increased risk of agranulocytosis); possible severe drowsiness when haloperidol given with indometacin; increased risk of convulsions when antipsychotics given with tramadol; enhanced hypotensive and sedative effects when antipsychotics given with opioid analgesics

Angiotensin-II Receptor Antagonists: enhanced hypotensive effect when antipsychotics given with angiotensin-II receptor antagonists

Antacids: absorption of phenothiazines and sulpiride reduced by antacids

• Anti-arrhythmics: increased risk of ventricular arrhythmias when antipsychotics that prolong the QT interval given with •anti-arrhythmics that prolong the QT interval; increased risk of ventricular arrhythmias when amisulpride, haloperidol, phenothiazines, pimozide or sertindole given with •amiodarone—avoid concomitant use; increased risk of ventricular arrhythmias when amisulpride, pimozide or sertindole given with •disopyramide—avoid concomitant use; increased risk of ventricular arrhythmias when phenothiazines given with •disopyramide or •procainamide; increased risk of arrhythmias when clozapine given with •flecainide; increased risk of ventricular arrhythmias when amisulpride, pimozide or sertindole given with •procainamide—avoid concomitant use

Antipsychotics *(continued)*

• Antibacterials: increased risk of ventricular arrhythmias when pimozide given with •clarithromycin, •moxifloxacin or •telithromycin—avoid concomitant use; increased risk of ventricular arrhythmias when sertindole given with •erythromycin or •moxifloxacin—avoid concomitant use; increased risk of ventricular arrhythmias when amisulpride given with parenteral •erythromycin—avoid concomitant use; plasma concentration of clozapine possibly increased by •erythromycin (possible increased risk of convulsions); possible increased risk of ventricular arrhythmias when pimozide given with •erythromycin—avoid concomitant use; plasma concentration of clozapine increased by ciprofloxacin; plasma concentration of olanzapine possibly increased by ciprofloxacin; increased risk of ventricular arrhythmias when haloperidol or phenothiazines given with •moxifloxacin—avoid concomitant use; plasma concentration of aripiprazole possibly reduced by •rifabutin and •rifampicin—increase dose of aripiprazole; plasma concentration of clozapine possibly reduced by rifampicin; metabolism of haloperidol accelerated by •rifampicin (reduced plasma concentration); avoid concomitant use of clozapine with •chloramphenicol or •sulphonamides (increased risk of agranulocytosis); possible increased risk of ventricular arrhythmias when sertindole given with •macrolides—avoid concomitant use; plasma concentration of quetiapine possibly increased by macrolides (reduce dose of quetiapine)

• Antidepressants: plasma concentration of clozapine possibly increased by citalopram (increased risk of toxicity); metabolism of aripiprazole possibly inhibited by •fluoxetine and •paroxetine (reduce dose of aripiprazole); plasma concentration of clozapine, haloperidol, risperidone, sertindole and zotepine increased by •fluoxetine; plasma concentration of clozapine and olanzapine increased by •fluvoxamine; plasma concentration of clozapine and sertindole increased by •paroxetine; plasma concentration of pimozide possibly increased by •paroxetine—avoid concomitant use; plasma concentration of risperidone possibly increased by paroxetine (increased risk of toxicity); metabolism of perphenazine inhibited by paroxetine (reduce dose of perphenazine); plasma concentration of clozapine increased by •sertraline and •venlafaxine; plasma concentration of pimozide increased by •sertraline (increased risk of ventricular arrhythmias—avoid concomitant use); plasma concentration of haloperidol increased by venlafaxine; clozapine possibly increases CNS effects of •MAOIs; plasma concentration of aripiprazole possibly reduced by •St John's wort—increase dose of aripiprazole; antipsychotics increase plasma concentration of •tricyclics—possibly increased risk of ventricular arrhythmias; increased risk of antimuscarinic side-effects when phenothiazines given with tricyclics; increased risk of ventricular arrhythmias when pimozide given with •tricyclics—avoid concomitant use; possibly increased antimuscarinic side-effects when clozapine given with tricyclics

Antidiabetics: phenothiazines possibly antagonise hypoglycaemic effect of sulphonylureas

• Antiepileptics: metabolism of clozapine accelerated by •carbamazepine (reduced plasma concentration), also avoid concomitant use of drugs with substantial potential for causing agranulocytosis; metabolism of haloperidol, olanzapine, quetiapine, risperidone and sertindole accelerated by carbamazepine (reduced plasma concentration); plasma concentration of aripiprazole reduced by •carbamazepine—increase dose of aripiprazole; antipsychotics antagonise anticonvulsant effect of •carbamazepine, •ethosuximide, •oxcarbazepine, •phenytoin, •primidone and •valproate (convulsive threshold lowered); plasma concentration of aripiprazole possibly reduced by •phenytoin and •primidone—increase dose of aripiprazole; metabolism of clozapine, quetiapine and sertindole accelerated by phenytoin (reduced plasma

Antipsychotics

- Antiepileptics *(continued)* concentration); metabolism of haloperidol accelerated by primidone (reduced plasma concentration); increased risk of neutropenia when olanzapine given with •valproate
- Antifungals: metabolism of aripiprazole inhibited by •ketoconazole (reduce dose of aripiprazole); increased risk of ventricular arrhythmias when sertindole given with •itraconazole or •ketoconazole—avoid concomitant use; metabolism of aripiprazole possibly inhibited by •itraconazole (reduce dose of aripiprazole); increased risk of ventricular arrhythmias when pimozide given with •imidazoles or •triazoles—avoid concomitant use; possible increased risk of ventricular arrhythmias when sertindole given with •imidazoles or •triazoles—avoid concomitant use; plasma concentration of quetiapine possibly increased by imidazoles and triazoles (reduce dose of quetiapine)
- Antimalarials: avoidance of antipsychotics advised by manufacturer of •artemether/lumefantrine; increased risk of ventricular arrhythmias when pimozide given with •mefloquine or •quinine—avoid concomitant use

Antimuscarinics: increased risk of antimuscarinic side-effects when clozapine given with antimuscarinics; plasma concentration of phenothiazines reduced by antimuscarinics, but risk of antimuscarinic side-effects increased; effects of haloperidol possibly reduced by antimuscarinics

- Antipsychotics: avoid concomitant use of clozapine with depot formulation of •flupentixol, •fluphenazine, •haloperidol, •pipotiazine, •risperidone or •zuclopenthixol as cannot be withdrawn quickly if neutropenia occurs; increased risk of ventricular arrhythmias when sertindole given with •amisulpride—avoid concomitant use; increased risk of ventricular arrhythmias when pimozide given with •phenothiazines—avoid concomitant use
- Antivirals: plasma concentration of pimozide and sertindole increased by •amprenavir (increased risk of ventricular arrhythmias—avoid concomitant use); plasma concentration of clozapine possibly increased by amprenavir; metabolism of aripiprazole possibly inhibited by •amprenavir, •atazanavir, •indinavir, •lopinavir, •nelfinavir, •ritonavir and •saquinavir (reduce dose of aripiprazole); plasma concentration of pimozide possibly increased by •atazanavir—avoid concomitant use; plasma concentration of aripiprazole possibly reduced by •efavirenz and •nevirapine—increase dose of aripiprazole; plasma concentration of pimozide possibly increased by •efavirenz, •indinavir, •nelfinavir and •saquinavir (increased risk of ventricular arrhythmias—avoid concomitant use); plasma concentration of sertindole increased by •indinavir, •lopinavir, •nelfinavir, •ritonavir and •saquinavir (increased risk of ventricular arrhythmias—avoid concomitant use); plasma concentration of antipsychotics possibly increased by •ritonavir; plasma concentration of pimozide increased by •ritonavir (increased risk of ventricular arrhythmias—avoid concomitant use); plasma concentration of olanzapine reduced by ritonavir—consider increasing dose of olanzapine; plasma concentration of clozapine increased by •ritonavir (increased risk of toxicity)—avoid concomitant use
- Anxiolytics and Hypnotics: increased sedative effect when antipsychotics given with anxiolytics and hypnotics; plasma concentration of zotepine increased by diazepam; increased risk of hypotension, bradycardia and respiratory depression when intramuscular olanzapine given with parenteral •benzodiazepines; plasma concentration of haloperidol increased by buspirone
- Aprepitant: avoidance of pimozide advised by manufacturer of •aprepitant
- Atomoxetine: increased risk of ventricular arrhythmias when antipsychotics that prolong the QT interval given with •atomoxetine

Antipsychotics *(continued)*

- Barbiturates: antipsychotics antagonise anticonvulsant effect of •barbiturates (convulsive threshold lowered); plasma concentration of aripiprazole possibly reduced by •phenobarbital—increase dose of aripiprazole; metabolism of haloperidol accelerated by phenobarbital (reduced plasma concentration); plasma concentration of both drugs reduced when chlorpromazine given with phenobarbital
- Beta-blockers: enhanced hypotensive effect when phenothiazines given with beta-blockers; plasma concentration of both drugs may increase when chlorpromazine given with •propranolol; increased risk of ventricular arrhythmias when amisulpride, phenothiazines, pimozide or sertindole given with •sotalol

Calcium-channel Blockers: enhanced hypotensive effect when antipsychotics given with calcium-channel blockers

Clonidine: enhanced hypotensive effect when phenothiazines given with clonidine

- Cytotoxics: avoid concomitant use of clozapine with •cytotoxics (increased risk of agranulocytosis)

Desferrioxamine: manufacturer of levomepromazine (methotrimeprazine) advises avoid concomitant use with desferrioxamine; avoidance of prochlorperazine advised by manufacturer of desferrioxamine

Diazoxide: enhanced hypotensive effect when phenothiazines given with diazoxide

- Diuretics: risk of ventricular arrhythmias with amisulpride or sertindole increased by hypokalaemia caused by •diuretics; risk of ventricular arrhythmias with pimozide increased by hypokalaemia caused by •diuretics (avoid concomitant use); enhanced hypotensive effect when phenothiazines given with diuretics

Dopaminergics: increased risk of extrapyramidal side-effects when antipsychotics given with amantadine; antipsychotics antagonise effects of apomorphine, levodopa and pergolide; antipsychotics antagonise hypoprolactinaemic and antiparkinsonian effects of bromocriptine and cabergoline; manufacturer of amisulpride advises avoid concomitant use of levodopa (antagonism of effect); avoidance of antipsychotics advised by manufacturer of pramipexole, ropinirole and rotigotine (antagonism of effect)

- Ivabradine: increased risk of ventricular arrhythmias when pimozide or sertindole given with •ivabradine
- Lithium: increased risk of ventricular arrhythmias when sertindole given with •lithium—avoid concomitant use; increased risk of extrapyramidal side-effects and possibly neurotoxicity when clozapine, haloperidol or phenothiazines given with lithium; increased risk of extrapyramidal side-effects when sulpiride given with lithium

Memantine: effects of antipsychotics possibly reduced by memantine

Methyldopa: enhanced hypotensive effect when antipsychotics given with methyldopa (also increased risk of extrapyramidal effects)

Metoclopramide: increased risk of extrapyramidal side-effects when antipsychotics given with metoclopramide

Moxonidine: enhanced hypotensive effect when phenothiazines given with moxonidine

Muscle Relaxants: promazine possibly enhances effects of suxamethonium

Nitrates: enhanced hypotensive effect when phenothiazines given with nitrates

- Penicillamine: avoid concomitant use of clozapine with •penicillamine (increased risk of agranulocytosis)
- Pentamidine Isetionate: increased risk of ventricular arrhythmias when amisulpride given with •pentamidine isetionate—avoid concomitant use; increased risk of ventricular arrhythmias when phenothiazines given with •pentamidine isetionate
- Sibutramine: increased risk of CNS toxicity when antipsychotics given with •sibutramine (manufacturer of sibutramine advises avoid concomitant use)

Antipsychotics *(continued)*

Sodium Benzoate: haloperidol possibly reduces effects of sodium benzoate

Sodium Oxybate: antipsychotics possibly enhance effects of sodium oxybate

Sodium Phenylbutyrate: haloperidol possibly reduces effects of sodium phenylbutyrate

Sympathomimetics: antipsychotics antagonise hypertensive effect of sympathomimetics

Tetrabenazine: increased risk of extrapyramidal side-effects when antipsychotics given with tetrabenazine

• Ulcer-healing Drugs: effects of antipsychotics, chlorpromazine and clozapine possibly enhanced by cimetidine; increased risk of ventricular arrhythmias when sertindole given with •cimetidine—avoid concomitant use; plasma concentration of clozapine possibly reduced by omeprazole; absorption of sulpiride reduced by sucralfate

Vasodilator Antihypertensives: enhanced hypotensive effect when phenothiazines given with hydralazine, minoxidil or sodium nitroprusside

Antivirals *see* Abacavir, Aciclovir, Adefovir, Amprenavir, Atazanavir, Cidofovir, Darunavir, Didanosine, Efavirenz, Emtricitabine, Famciclovir, Foscarnet, Ganciclovir, Indinavir, Lamivudine, Lopinavir, Maraviroc, Nelfinavir, Nevirapine, Ribavirin, Ritonavir, Saquinavir, Stavudine, Tenofovir, Tipranavir, Valaciclovir, and Zidovudine

Anxiolytics and Hypnotics

ACE Inhibitors: enhanced hypotensive effect when anxiolytics and hypnotics given with ACE inhibitors

Adrenergic Neurone Blockers: enhanced hypotensive effect when anxiolytics and hypnotics given with adrenergic neurone blockers

Alcohol: increased sedative effect when anxiolytics and hypnotics given with alcohol

Alpha-blockers: enhanced hypotensive and sedative effects when anxiolytics and hypnotics given with alpha-blockers

Anaesthetics, General: increased sedative effect when anxiolytics and hypnotics given with general anaesthetics

Analgesics: increased sedative effect when anxiolytics and hypnotics given with opioid analgesics

Angiotensin-II Receptor Antagonists: enhanced hypotensive effect when anxiolytics and hypnotics given with angiotensin-II receptor antagonists

• Antibacterials: metabolism of midazolam inhibited by •clarithromycin, •erythromycin, •quinupristin/dalfopristin and •telithromycin (increased plasma concentration with increased sedation); plasma concentration of buspirone increased by erythromycin (reduce dose of buspirone); metabolism of zopiclone inhibited by erythromycin and quinupristin/dalfopristin; metabolism of benzodiazepines possibly accelerated by rifampicin (reduced plasma concentration); metabolism of diazepam accelerated by rifampicin (reduced plasma concentration); metabolism of buspirone and zaleplon possibly accelerated by rifampicin; metabolism of zolpidem accelerated by rifampicin (reduced plasma concentration and reduced effect); plasma concentration of zopiclone significantly reduced by rifampicin; metabolism of diazepam inhibited by isoniazid

Anticoagulants: chloral and triclofos may transiently enhance anticoagulant effect of coumarins

Antidepressants: plasma concentration of some benzodiazepines increased by fluvoxamine; sedative effects possibly increased when zolpidem given with sertraline; manufacturer of buspirone advises avoid concomitant use with MAOIs; increased sedative effect when anxiolytics and hypnotics given with mirtazapine, tricyclic-related antidepressants or tricyclics

Antiepileptics: plasma concentration of clonazepam often reduced by carbamazepine, phenytoin and primidone; diazepam increases or decreases plasma concentration of phenytoin; benzodiazepines possibly increase or decrease plasma concentration of phenytoin; plasma concentration of diazepam and lorazepam possibly increased by valproate; increased risk of side-effects when clonazepam given with valproate; clobazam possibly increases plasma concentration of valproate

• Antifungals: plasma concentration of alprazolam increased by itraconazole and ketoconazole; plasma concentration of midazolam increased by •fluconazole, •itraconazole and •ketoconazole (risk of prolonged sedation); plasma concentration of buspirone increased by itraconazole (reduce dose of buspirone); plasma concentration of midazolam increased by •posaconazole

Antihistamines: increased sedative effect when anxiolytics and hypnotics given with antihistamines

• Antipsychotics: increased sedative effect when anxiolytics and hypnotics given with antipsychotics; buspirone increases plasma concentration of haloperidol; increased risk of hypotension, bradycardia and respiratory depression when parenteral benzodiazepines given with intramuscular •olanzapine; diazepam increases plasma concentration of zotepine

• Antivirals: increased risk of prolonged sedation and respiratory depression when alprazolam, clonazepam, diazepam, flurazepam or midazolam given with •amprenavir; plasma concentration of midazolam possibly increased by •atazanavir—avoid concomitant use of oral midazolam; increased risk of prolonged sedation when midazolam given with •efavirenz—avoid concomitant use; plasma concentration of midazolam possibly increased by •indinavir, •nelfinavir and •ritonavir (risk of prolonged sedation—avoid concomitant use of oral midazolam); increased risk of prolonged sedation when alprazolam given with •indinavir—avoid concomitant use; plasma concentration of alprazolam, diazepam, flurazepam and zolpidem possibly increased by •ritonavir (risk of extreme sedation and respiratory depression —avoid concomitant use); plasma concentration of buspirone increased by ritonavir (increased risk of toxicity); plasma concentration of anxiolytics and hypnotics possibly increased by •ritonavir; plasma concentration of midazolam increased by •saquinavir (risk of prolonged sedation—avoid concomitant use of oral midazolam)

Barbiturates: plasma concentration of clonazepam often reduced by phenobarbital

Beta-blockers: enhanced hypotensive effect when anxiolytics and hypnotics given with beta-blockers

Calcium-channel Blockers: enhanced hypotensive effect when anxiolytics and hypnotics given with calcium-channel blockers; midazolam increases absorption of lercanidipine; plasma concentration of buspirone increased by diltiazem and verapamil (reduce dose of buspirone); metabolism of midazolam inhibited by diltiazem and verapamil (increased plasma concentration with increased sedation)

Cardiac Glycosides: alprazolam increases plasma concentration of digoxin (increased risk of toxicity)

Clonidine: enhanced hypotensive effect when anxiolytics and hypnotics given with clonidine

Diazoxide: enhanced hypotensive effect when anxiolytics and hypnotics given with diazoxide

Disulfiram: metabolism of benzodiazepines inhibited by disulfiram (increased sedative effects); increased risk of temazepam toxicity when given with disulfiram

Diuretics: enhanced hypotensive effect when anxiolytics and hypnotics given with diuretics; administration of chloral or triclofos with parenteral furosemide (frusemide) may displace thyroid hormone from binding sites

Dopaminergics: benzodiazepines possibly antagonise effects of levodopa

Grapefruit Juice: plasma concentration of buspirone increased by grapefruit juice

Lofexidine: increased sedative effect when anxiolytics and hypnotics given with lofexidine

Anxiolytics and Hypnotics *(continued)*
Methyldopa: enhanced hypotensive effect when anxiolytics and hypnotics given with methyldopa
Moxonidine: enhanced hypotensive effect when anxiolytics and hypnotics given with moxonidine; sedative effects possibly increased when benzodiazepines given with moxonidine
Muscle Relaxants: increased sedative effect when anxiolytics and hypnotics given with baclofen or tizanidine
Nabilone: increased sedative effect when anxiolytics and hypnotics given with nabilone
Nitrates: enhanced hypotensive effect when anxiolytics and hypnotics given with nitrates
• Sodium Oxybate: benzodiazepines enhance effects of •sodium oxybate (avoid concomitant use)
Theophylline: effects of benzodiazepines possibly reduced by theophylline
Ulcer-healing Drugs: metabolism of benzodiazepines, clomethiazole and zaleplon inhibited by cimetidine (increased plasma concentration); metabolism of diazepam possibly inhibited by esomeprazole and omeprazole (increased plasma concentration)
Vasodilator Antihypertensives: enhanced hypotensive effect when anxiolytics and hypnotics given with hydralazine, minoxidil or sodium nitroprusside

Apomorphine
Antipsychotics: effects of apomorphine antagonised by antipsychotics
Dopaminergics: effects of apomorphine possibly enhanced by entacapone
Memantine: effects of dopaminergics possibly enhanced by memantine
Methyldopa: antiparkinsonian effect of dopaminergics antagonised by methyldopa

Apraclonidine *see* Alpha$_2$-adrenoceptor Stimulants

Aprepitant
Antibacterials: plasma concentration of aprepitant possibly increased by clarithromycin and telithromycin; plasma concentration of aprepitant reduced by rifampicin
Anticoagulants: aprepitant possibly reduces anticoagulant effect of warfarin
• Antidepressants: manufacturer of aprepitant advises avoid concomitant use with •St John's wort
Antidiabetics: aprepitant reduces plasma concentration of tolbutamide
Antiepileptics: plasma concentration of aprepitant possibly reduced by carbamazepine and phenytoin
Antifungals: plasma concentration of aprepitant increased by ketoconazole
• Antipsychotics: manufacturer of aprepitant advises avoid concomitant use with •pimozide
Antivirals: plasma concentration of aprepitant possibly increased by ritonavir
Barbiturates: plasma concentration of aprepitant possibly reduced by phenobarbital
Corticosteroids: aprepitant inhibits metabolism of dexamethasone and methylprednisolone (reduce dose of dexamethasone and methylprednisolone)
• Oestrogens: aprepitant possibly causes contraceptive failure of hormonal contraceptives containing •oestrogens (alternative contraception recommended)
• Progestogens: aprepitant possibly causes contraceptive failure of hormonal contraceptives containing •progestogens (alternative contraception recommended)

Aripiprazole *see* Antipsychotics

Artemether with Lumefantrine
• Anti-arrhythmics: manufacturer of artemether/lumefantrine advises avoid concomitant use with •amiodarone, •disopyramide, •flecainide or •procainamide (risk of ventricular arrhythmias)
• Antibacterials: manufacturer of artemether/lumefantrine advises avoid concomitant use with •macrolides and •quinolones
• Antidepressants: manufacturer of artemether/lumefantrine advises avoid concomitant use with •antidepressants

Artemether with Lumefantrine *(continued)*
• Antifungals: manufacturer of artemether/lumefantrine advises avoid concomitant use with •imidazoles and •triazoles
• Antimalarials: manufacturer of artemether/lumefantrine advises avoid concomitant use with •antimalarials; increased risk of ventricular arrhythmias when artemether/lumefantrine given with •quinine
• Antipsychotics: manufacturer of artemether/lumefantrine advises avoid concomitant use with •antipsychotics
• Antivirals: avoid concomitant use of artemether/lumefantrine with •amprenavir, •atazanavir, •darunavir, •indinavir, •lopinavir, •nelfinavir, •ritonavir, •saquinavir or •tipranavir
• Beta-blockers: manufacturer of artemether/lumefantrine advises avoid concomitant use with •metoprolol and •sotalol
• Grapefruit Juice: metabolism of artemether/lumefantrine possibly inhibited by •grapefruit juice (avoid concomitant use)
• Ulcer-healing Drugs: manufacturer of artemether/lumefantrine advises avoid concomitant use with •cimetidine

Ascorbic acid *see* Vitamins

Aspirin
Adsorbents: absorption of aspirin possibly reduced by kaolin
• Analgesics: avoid concomitant use of aspirin with •NSAIDs (increased side-effects); antiplatelet effect of aspirin possibly reduced by ibuprofen
Antacids: excretion of aspirin increased by alkaline urine due to some antacids
• Anticoagulants: increased risk of bleeding when aspirin given with •coumarins or •phenindione (due to antiplatelet effect); aspirin enhances anticoagulant effect of •heparins
• Antidepressants: increased risk of bleeding when aspirin given with •SSRIs or •venlafaxine
Antiepileptics: aspirin enhances effects of phenytoin and valproate
Cilostazol: manufacturer of cilostazol recommends dose of aspirin should not exceed 80 mg daily when given with cilostazol
Clopidogrel: increased risk of bleeding when aspirin given with clopidogrel
Corticosteroids: increased risk of gastro-intestinal bleeding and ulceration when aspirin given with corticosteroids, also corticosteroids reduce plasma concentration of salicylate
• Cytotoxics: aspirin reduces excretion of •methotrexate (increased risk of toxicity)—but for concomitant use in rheumatic disease see p. 551
Diuretics: aspirin antagonises diuretic effect of spironolactone; increased risk of toxicity when high-dose aspirin given with carbonic anhydrase inhibitors
Iloprost: increased risk of bleeding when aspirin given with iloprost
Leukotriene Antagonists: aspirin increases plasma concentration of zafirlukast
Metoclopramide: rate of absorption of aspirin increased by metoclopramide (enhanced effect)
Mifepristone: avoidance of aspirin advised by manufacturer of mifepristone
Probenecid: aspirin antagonises effects of probenecid
Sibutramine: increased risk of bleeding when aspirin given with sibutramine
Sulfinpyrazone: aspirin antagonises effects of sulfinpyrazone

Atazanavir
Antacids: plasma concentration of atazanavir possibly reduced by antacids
• Anti-arrhythmics: atazanavir possibly increases plasma concentration of •amiodarone and •lidocaine (lignocaine)
• Antibacterials: plasma concentration of both drugs increased when atazanavir given with clarithromycin; atazanavir increases plasma concentration of •rifabutin (reduce dose of rifabutin); plasma concentration of atazanavir reduced by •rifampicin—avoid concomi-

Atazanavir

- Antibacterials *(continued)* tant use; avoidance of concomitant atazanavir in severe renal and hepatic impairment advised by manufacturer of •telithromycin
- Anticoagulants: atazanavir may enhance or reduce anticoagulant effect of warfarin
- Antidepressants: plasma concentration of atazanavir reduced by •St John's wort—avoid concomitant use
- Antimalarials: avoid concomitant use of atazanavir with •artemether/lumefantrine
- Antimuscarinics: avoidance of atazanavir advised by manufacturer of darifenacin
- Antipsychotics: atazanavir possibly inhibits metabolism of •aripiprazole (reduce dose of aripiprazole); atazanavir possibly increases plasma concentration of •pimozide—avoid concomitant use
- Antivirals: plasma concentration of atazanavir reduced by efavirenz—increase dose of atazanavir; avoid concomitant use of atazanavir with •indinavir; atazanavir increases plasma concentration of •maraviroc (consider reducing dose of maraviroc); plasma concentration of atazanavir possibly reduced by •nevirapine—avoid concomitant use; atazanavir increases plasma concentration of saquinavir; plasma concentration of atazanavir reduced by tenofovir, also plasma concentration of tenofovir possibly increased; atazanavir increases plasma concentration of tipranavir (also plasma concentration of atazanavir reduced)
- Anxiolytics and Hypnotics: atazanavir possibly increases plasma concentration of •midazolam—avoid concomitant use of oral midazolam
- Calcium-channel Blockers: atazanavir increases plasma concentration of •diltiazem (reduce dose of diltiazem); atazanavir possibly increases plasma concentration of verapamil
- Ciclosporin: atazanavir possibly increases plasma concentration of •ciclosporin
- Cytotoxics: atazanavir possibly inhibits metabolism of •irinotecan (increased risk of toxicity)
- Ergot Alkaloids: atazanavir possibly increases plasma concentration of •ergot alkaloids—avoid concomitant use
- Lipid-regulating Drugs: possible increased risk of myopathy when atazanavir given with atorvastatin; increased risk of myopathy when atazanavir given with •simvastatin (avoid concomitant use)
- Oestrogens: atazanavir increases plasma concentration of •ethinylestradiol—avoid concomitant use
- Sildenafil: atazanavir possibly increases side-effects of •sildenafil
- Sirolimus: atazanavir possibly increases plasma concentration of •sirolimus
- Tacrolimus: atazanavir possibly increases plasma concentration of •tacrolimus
- Ulcer-healing Drugs: plasma concentration of atazanavir significantly reduced by •esomeprazole and •omeprazole—avoid concomitant use; plasma concentration of atazanavir possibly reduced by histamine H_2-antagonists; plasma concentration of atazanavir possibly reduced by •proton pump inhibitors—avoid concomitant use

Atenolol *see* Beta-blockers

Atomoxetine

- Analgesics: increased risk of ventricular arrhythmias when atomoxetine given with •methadone; possible increased risk of convulsions when atomoxetine given with tramadol
- Anti-arrhythmics: increased risk of ventricular arrhythmias when atomoxetine given with •amiodarone, •disopyramide or •procainamide
- Antibacterials: increased risk of ventricular arrhythmias when atomoxetine given with parenteral •erythromycin; increased risk of ventricular arrhythmias when atomoxetine given with •moxifloxacin
- Antidepressants: metabolism of atomoxetine possibly inhibited by fluoxetine and paroxetine; possible increased risk of convulsions when atomoxetine given with antidepressants; atomoxetine should not be started until 2 weeks after stopping •MAOIs, also MAOIs should not be started until at least 2 weeks after stopping atomoxetine; increased risk of ventricular arrhythmias when atomoxetine given with •tricyclics
- Antimalarials: increased risk of ventricular arrhythmias when atomoxetine given with •mefloquine
- Antipsychotics: increased risk of ventricular arrhythmias when atomoxetine given with •antipsychotics that prolong the QT interval
- Beta-blockers: increased risk of ventricular arrhythmias when atomoxetine given with •sotalol
- Bupropion: possible increased risk of convulsions when atomoxetine given with bupropion
- Diuretics: risk of ventricular arrhythmias with atomoxetine increased by hypokalaemia caused by •diuretics
- Sympathomimetics, $Beta_2$: Increased risk of cardiovascular side-effects when atomoxetine given with parenteral salbutamol

Atorvastatin *see* Statins

Atovaquone

- Antibacterials: plasma concentration of atovaquone reduced by •rifabutin and •rifampicin (possible therapeutic failure of atovaquone); plasma concentration of atovaquone reduced by tetracycline
- Antivirals: atovaquone possibly reduces plasma concentration of indinavir; atovaquone possibly inhibits metabolism of zidovudine (increased plasma concentration)
- Metoclopramide: plasma concentration of atovaquone reduced by metoclopramide

Atracurium *see* Muscle Relaxants

Atropine *see* Antimuscarinics

Azapropazone *see* NSAIDs

Azathioprine

- ACE Inhibitors: increased risk of leucopenia when azathioprine given with captopril
- Allopurinol: enhanced effects and increased toxicity of azathioprine when given with •allopurinol (reduce dose of azathioprine to one quarter of usual dose)
- Aminosalicylates: possible increased risk of leucopenia when azathioprine given with aminosalicylates
- Antibacterials: increased risk of haematological toxicity when azathioprine given with •sulfamethoxazole (as co-trimoxazole); increased risk of haematological toxicity when azathioprine given with •trimethoprim (also with co-trimoxazole)
- Anticoagulants: azathioprine possibly reduces anticoagulant effect of •coumarins
- Antiepileptics: cytotoxics possibly reduce absorption of phenytoin
- Antipsychotics: avoid concomitant use of cytotoxics with •clozapine (increased risk of agranulocytosis)
- Cardiac Glycosides: cytotoxics reduce absorption of digoxin tablets

Azelastine *see* Antihistamines

Azithromycin *see* Macrolides

Aztreonam

- Anticoagulants: aztreonam possibly enhances anticoagulant effect of •coumarins
- Oestrogens: antibacterials that do not induce liver enzymes possibly reduce contraceptive effect of oestrogens (risk probably small, see p. 428)

Baclofen *see* Muscle Relaxants

Balsalazide *see* Aminosalicylates

Bambuterol *see* Sympathomimetics, $Beta_2$

Barbiturates

- Alcohol: increased sedative effect when barbiturates given with alcohol
- Anti-arrhythmics: barbiturates accelerate metabolism of disopyramide (reduced plasma concentration)
- Antibacterials: barbiturates accelerate metabolism of •chloramphenicol, doxycycline and metronidazole (reduced plasma concentration); phenobarbital possibly reduces plasma concentration of rifampicin; phenobarbital reduces plasma concentration of •teli-

Barbiturates
- Antibacterials *(continued)*
  thromycin (avoid during and for 2 weeks after phenobarbital)
- Anticoagulants: barbiturates accelerate metabolism of •coumarins (reduced anticoagulant effect)
- Antidepressants: phenobarbital reduces plasma concentration of paroxetine; phenobarbital accelerates metabolism of •mianserin (reduced plasma concentration); anticonvulsant effect of barbiturates possibly antagonised by MAOIs and •tricyclic-related antidepressants (convulsive threshold lowered); anticonvulsant effect of barbiturates antagonised by SSRIs (convulsive threshold lowered); avoid concomitant use of phenobarbital with •St John's wort; anticonvulsant effect of barbiturates antagonised by •tricyclics (convulsive threshold lowered), also metabolism of tricyclics possibly accelerated (reduced plasma concentration)
- Antiepileptics: phenobarbital reduces plasma concentration of carbamazepine, lamotrigine, tiagabine and zonisamide; phenobarbital possibly reduces plasma concentration of ethosuximide; plasma concentration of phenobarbital increased by oxcarbazepine, also plasma concentration of an active metabolite of oxcarbazepine reduced; plasma concentration of phenobarbital often increased by phenytoin, plasma concentration of phenytoin often reduced but may be increased; increased sedative effect when barbiturates given with primidone; plasma concentration of phenobarbital increased by valproate (also plasma concentration of valproate reduced); plasma concentration of phenobarbital possibly reduced by vigabatrin
- Antifungals: phenobarbital possibly reduces plasma concentration of itraconazole and •posaconazole; phenobarbital possibly reduces plasma concentration of •voriconazole—avoid concomitant use; phenobarbital reduces absorption of griseofulvin (reduced effect)
- Antipsychotics: anticonvulsant effect of barbiturates antagonised by •antipsychotics (convulsive threshold lowered); phenobarbital accelerates metabolism of haloperidol (reduced plasma concentration); plasma concentration of both drugs reduced when phenobarbital given with chlorpromazine; phenobarbital possibly reduces plasma concentration of •aripiprazole—increase dose of aripiprazole
- Antivirals: phenobarbital possibly reduces plasma concentration of abacavir, amprenavir, darunavir and •lopinavir; barbiturates possibly reduce plasma concentration of •indinavir, •nelfinavir and •saquinavir
- Anxiolytics and Hypnotics: phenobarbital often reduces plasma concentration of clonazepam
- Aprepitant: phenobarbital possibly reduces plasma concentration of aprepitant
- Beta-blockers: barbiturates reduce plasma concentration of metoprolol and timolol; barbiturates possibly reduce plasma concentration of propranolol
- Calcium-channel Blockers: barbiturates reduce effects of •felodipine and •isradipine; barbiturates probably reduce effects of •dihydropyridines, •diltiazem and •verapamil
- Cardiac Glycosides: barbiturates accelerate metabolism of digitoxin (reduced effect)
- Ciclosporin: barbiturates accelerate metabolism of •ciclosporin (reduced effect)
- Corticosteroids: barbiturates accelerate metabolism of •corticosteroids (reduced effect)
- Cytotoxics: phenobarbital possibly reduces plasma concentration of etoposide; phenobarbital reduces plasma concentration of irinotecan and its active metabolite
- Diuretics: phenobarbital reduces plasma concentration of •eplerenone—avoid concomitant use; increased risk of osteomalacia when phenobarbital given with carbonic anhydrase inhibitors
- Folates: plasma concentration of phenobarbital possibly reduced by folates

Barbiturates *(continued)*
- Hormone Antagonists: barbiturates accelerate metabolism of gestrinone (reduced plasma concentration); barbiturates possibly accelerate metabolism of toremifene (reduced plasma concentration)
- $5HT_3$ Antagonists: phenobarbital reduces plasma concentration of tropisetron
- Leukotriene Antagonists: phenobarbital reduces plasma concentration of montelukast
- Lofexidine: increased sedative effect when barbiturates given with lofexidine
- Memantine: effects of barbiturates possibly reduced by memantine
- Oestrogens: barbiturates accelerate metabolism of •oestrogens (reduced contraceptive effect—see p. 428)
- Progestogens: barbiturates accelerate metabolism of •progestogens (reduced contraceptive effect—see p. 428)
- Sodium Oxybate: barbiturates enhance effects of •sodium oxybate (avoid concomitant use)
- Sympathomimetics: plasma concentration of phenobarbital possibly increased by methylphenidate
- Tacrolimus: phenobarbital reduces plasma concentration of •tacrolimus
- Theophylline: barbiturates accelerate metabolism of theophylline (reduced effect)
- Thyroid Hormones: barbiturates accelerate metabolism of thyroid hormones (may increase requirements for thyroid hormones in hypothyroidism)
- Tibolone: barbiturates accelerate metabolism of tibolone (reduced plasma concentration)
- Vitamins: barbiturates possibly increase requirements for vitamin D

Beclometasone *see* Corticosteroids
Belladonna Alkaloids *see* Antimuscarinics
Bemiparin *see* Heparins
Bendroflumethiazide (bendrofluazide) *see* Diuretics
Benperidol *see* Antipsychotics
Benzatropine (benztropine) *see* Antimuscarinics
Benzodiazepines *see* Anxiolytics and Hypnotics
Benzthiazide *see* Diuretics
Benzylpenicillin *see* Penicillins

Beta-blockers

Note Since systemic absorption may follow topical application of beta-blockers to the eye the possibility of interactions, in particular, with drugs such as verapamil should be borne in mind

- ACE Inhibitors: enhanced hypotensive effect when beta-blockers given with ACE inhibitors
- Adrenergic Neurone Blockers: enhanced hypotensive effect when beta-blockers given with adrenergic neurone blockers
- Alcohol: enhanced hypotensive effect when beta-blockers given with alcohol
- Aldesleukin: enhanced hypotensive effect when beta-blockers given with aldesleukin
- Alpha-blockers: enhanced hypotensive effect when beta-blockers given with •alpha-blockers, also increased risk of first-dose hypotension with post-synaptic alpha-blockers such as prazosin
- Anaesthetics, General: enhanced hypotensive effect when beta-blockers given with general anaesthetics
- Anaesthetics, Local: propranolol increases risk of •bupivacaine toxicity
- Analgesics: hypotensive effect of beta-blockers antagonised by NSAIDs; plasma concentration of esmolol possibly increased by morphine
- Angiotensin-II Receptor Antagonists: enhanced hypotensive effect when beta-blockers given with angiotensin-II receptor antagonists
- Anti-arrhythmics: increased myocardial depression when beta-blockers given with •anti-arrhythmics; increased risk of ventricular arrhythmias when sotalol given with •amiodarone, •disopyramide or •procainamide—avoid concomitant use; increased risk of bradycardia, AV block and myocardial depression when beta-blockers given with •amiodarone; increased risk of myocardial depression and bradycardia when beta-blockers given with •flecainide;

Beta-blockers
- Anti-arrhythmics *(continued)*
  propranolol increases risk of •lidocaine (lignocaine) toxicity; plasma concentration of metoprolol and propranolol increased by propafenone
- Antibacterials: increased risk of ventricular arrhythmias when sotalol given with •moxifloxacin—avoid concomitant use; metabolism of bisoprolol and propranolol accelerated by rifampicin (plasma concentration significantly reduced); plasma concentration of carvedilol, celiprolol and metoprolol reduced by rifampicin
- Antidepressants: plasma concentration of metoprolol increased by citalopram and escitalopram; plasma concentration of propranolol increased by fluvoxamine; plasma concentration of metoprolol possibly increased by paroxetine (enhanced effect); labetalol and propranolol increase plasma concentration of imipramine; enhanced hypotensive effect when beta-blockers given with MAOIs; increased risk of ventricular arrhythmias when sotalol given with •tricyclics

  Antidiabetics: beta-blockers may mask warning signs of hypoglycaemia (such as tremor) with antidiabetics; beta-blockers enhance hypoglycaemic effect of insulin
- Antihistamines: increased risk of ventricular arrhythmias when sotalol given with •mizolastine—avoid concomitant use
- Antimalarials: avoidance of metoprolol and sotalol advised by manufacturer of •artemether/lumefantrine; increased risk of bradycardia when beta-blockers given with mefloquine
- Antipsychotics: plasma concentration of both drugs may increase when propranolol given with •chlorpromazine; increased risk of ventricular arrhythmias when sotalol given with •amisulpride, •phenothiazines, •pimozide or •sertindole; enhanced hypotensive effect when beta-blockers given with phenothiazines
- Antivirals: avoidance of metoprolol for heart failure advised by manufactuer of •tipranavir

  Anxiolytics and Hypnotics: enhanced hypotensive effect when beta-blockers given with anxiolytics and hypnotics
- Atomoxetine: increased risk of ventricular arrhythmias when sotalol given with •atomoxetine

  Barbiturates: plasma concentration of metoprolol and timolol reduced by barbiturates; plasma concentration of propranolol possibly reduced by barbiturates
- Calcium-channel Blockers: enhanced hypotensive effect when beta-blockers given with calcium-channel blockers; possible severe hypotension and heart failure when beta-blockers given with •nifedipine or •nisoldipine; increased risk of AV block and bradycardia when beta-blockers given with •diltiazem; asystole, severe hypotension and heart failure when beta-blockers given with •verapamil (see p. 117)

  Cardiac Glycosides: increased risk of AV block and bradycardia when beta-blockers given with cardiac glycosides
- Ciclosporin: carvedilol increases plasma concentration of •ciclosporin
- Clonidine: increased risk of withdrawal hypertension when beta-blockers given with •clonidine (withdraw beta-blockers several days before slowly withdrawing clonidine)

  Corticosteroids: hypotensive effect of beta-blockers antagonised by corticosteroids

  Diazoxide: enhanced hypotensive effect when beta-blockers given with diazoxide
- Diuretics: enhanced hypotensive effect when beta-blockers given with diuretics; risk of ventricular arrhythmias with sotalol increased by hypokalaemia caused by •loop diuretics or •thiazides and related diuretics

  Dopaminergics: enhanced hypotensive effect when beta-blockers given with levodopa

Beta-blockers *(continued)*

  Ergot Alkaloids: increased peripheral vasoconstriction when beta-blockers given with ergotamine and methysergide

  $5HT_1$ Agonists: propranolol increases plasma concentration of rizatriptan (manufacturer of rizatriptan advises halve dose and avoid within 2 hours of propranolol)
- $5HT_3$ Antagonists: increased risk of ventricular arrhythmias when sotalol given with •dolasetron—avoid concomitant use; caution with beta-blockers advised by manufacturer of tropisetron (risk of ventricular arrhythmias)
- Ivabradine: increased risk of ventricular arrhythmias when sotalol given with •ivabradine

  Methyldopa: enhanced hypotensive effect when beta-blockers given with methyldopa
- Moxisylyte (thymoxamine): possible severe postural hypotension when beta-blockers given with •moxisylyte

  Moxonidine: enhanced hypotensive effect when beta-blockers given with moxonidine

  Muscle Relaxants: propranolol enhances effects of muscle relaxants; enhanced hypotensive effect when beta-blockers given with baclofen; possible enhanced hypotensive effect and bradycardia when beta-blockers given with tizanidine

  Nitrates: enhanced hypotensive effect when beta-blockers given with nitrates

  Oestrogens: hypotensive effect of beta-blockers antagonised by oestrogens

  Parasympathomimetics: propranolol antagonises effects of neostigmine and pyridostigmine; increased risk of arrhythmias when beta-blockers given with pilocarpine

  Prostaglandins: enhanced hypotensive effect when beta-blockers given with alprostadil
- Sympathomimetics: increased risk of severe hypertension and bradycardia when non-cardioselective beta-blockers given with •adrenaline (epinephrine), also reponse to adrenaline (epinephrine) may be reduced; increased risk of severe hypertension and bradycardia when non-cardioselective beta-blockers given with •dobutamine; possible increased risk of severe hypertension and bradycardia when non-cardioselective beta-blockers given with •noradrenaline (norepinephrine)

  Thyroid Hormones: metabolism of propranolol accelerated by levothyroxine (thyroxine)

  Ulcer-healing Drugs: plasma concentration of labetalol, metoprolol and propranolol increased by cimetidine

  Vasodilator Antihypertensives: enhanced hypotensive effect when beta-blockers given with hydralazine, minoxidil or sodium nitroprusside

Betahistine

  Antihistamines: effect of betahistine theoretically antagonised by antihistamines

Betamethasone *see* Corticosteroids

Betaxolol *see* Beta-blockers

Bethanechol *see* Parasympathomimetics

Bexarotene

  Antiepileptics: cytotoxics possibly reduce absorption of phenytoin
- Antipsychotics: avoid concomitant use of cytotoxics with •clozapine (increased risk of agranulocytosis)

  Cardiac Glycosides: cytotoxics reduce absorption of digoxin tablets
- Lipid-regulating Drugs: plasma concentration of bexarotene increased by •gemfibrozil—avoid concomitant use

Bezafibrate *see* Fibrates

Bicalutamide

  Anticoagulants: bicalutamide possibly enhances anticoagulant effect of coumarins

Biguanides *see* Antidiabetics

Bile Acid Sequestrants *see* Colesevelam, Colestipol, and Colestyramine

Bile Acids *see* Ursodeoxycholic Acid

Bisoprolol *see* Beta-blockers

Bisphosphonates
Analgesics: bioavailability of tiludronic acid increased by indometacin
Antacids: absorption of bisphosphonates reduced by antacids
Antibacterials: increased risk of hypocalcaemia when bisphosphonates given with aminoglycosides
Calcium Salts: absorption of bisphosphonates reduced by calcium salts
Iron: absorption of bisphosphonates reduced by *oral* iron

Bleomycin
Antiepileptics: cytotoxics possibly reduce absorption of phenytoin
• Antipsychotics: avoid concomitant use of cytotoxics with •clozapine (increased risk of agranulocytosis)
Cardiac Glycosides: cytotoxics reduce absorption of digoxin tablets
• Cytotoxics: increased pulmonary toxicity when bleomycin given with •cisplatin

Bosentan
• Antibacterials: plasma concentration of bosentan reduced by •rifampicin—avoid concomitant use
Anticoagulants: manufacturer of bosentan recommends monitoring anticoagulant effect of coumarins
• Antidiabetics: increased risk of hepatotoxicity when bosentan given with •glibenclamide—avoid concomitant use
• Antifungals: plasma concentration of bosentan increased by ketoconazole; plasma concentration of bosentan possibly increased by •fluconazole—avoid concomitant use; plasma concentration of bosentan possibly increased by itraconazole
Antivirals: plasma concentration of bosentan possibly increased by ritonavir
• Ciclosporin: plasma concentration of bosentan increased by •ciclosporin (also plasma concentration of ciclosporin reduced—avoid concomitant use)
Lipid-regulating Drugs: bosentan reduces plasma concentration of simvastatin
• Oestrogens: bosentan possibly causes contraceptive failure of hormonal contraceptives containing •oestrogens (alternative contraception recommended)
• Progestogens: bosentan possibly causes contraceptive failure of hormonal contraceptives containing •progestogens (alternative contraception recommended)
Sildenafil: bosentan reduces plasma concentration of sildenafil

Brimonidine *see* Alpha$_2$-adrenoceptor Stimulants

Brinzolamide *see* Diuretics

Bromocriptine
Alcohol: tolerance of bromocriptine reduced by alcohol
Antibacterials: plasma concentration of bromocriptine increased by erythromycin (increased risk of toxicity); plasma concentration of bromocriptine possibly increased by macrolides (increased risk of toxicity)
Antipsychotics: hypoprolactinaemic and antiparkinsonian effects of bromocriptine antagonised by antipsychotics
Domperidone: hypoprolactinaemic effect of bromocriptine possibly antagonised by domperidone
Hormone Antagonists: plasma concentration of bromocriptine increased by octreotide
Memantine: effects of dopaminergics possibly enhanced by memantine
Methyldopa: antiparkinsonian effect of dopaminergics antagonised by methyldopa
Metoclopramide: hypoprolactinaemic effect of bromocriptine antagonised by metoclopramide
• Sympathomimetics: risk of toxicity when bromocriptine given with •isometheptene or •phenylpropanolamine

Buclizine *see* Antihistamines

Budesonide *see* Corticosteroids

Bumetanide *see* Diuretics

Bupivacaine
Anti-arrhythmics: increased myocardial depression when bupivacaine given with anti-arrhythmics
• Beta-blockers: increased risk of bupivacaine toxicity when given with •propranolol

Buprenorphine *see* Opioid Analgesics

Bupropion
Note Bupropion should be administered with extreme caution to patients receiving other medication known to lower the seizure threshold—see CSM advice p. 270 and Cautions, Contra-indications and Side-effects of individual drugs
• Antidepressants: bupropion possibly increases plasma concentration of citalopram; manufacturer of bupropion advises avoid for 2 weeks after stopping •MAOIs; manufacturer of bupropion advises avoid concomitant use with •moclobemide
Antiepileptics: plasma concentration of bupropion reduced by carbamazepine and phenytoin; metabolism of bupropion inhibited by valproate
• Antivirals: plasma concentration of bupropion increased by •ritonavir (risk of toxicity)—avoid concomitant use
Atomoxetine: possible increased risk of convulsions when bupropion given with atomoxetine
Dopaminergics: increased risk of side-effects when bupropion given with amantadine or levodopa

Buspirone *see* Anxiolytics and Hypnotics

Busulfan
Analgesics: metabolism of *intravenous* busulfan possibly inhibited by paracetamol (manufacturer of *intravenous* busulfan advises caution within 72 hours of paracetamol)
• Antibacterials: plasma concentration of busulfan increased by •metronidazole (increased risk of toxicity)
Antiepileptics: cytotoxics possibly reduce absorption of phenytoin; plasma concentration of busulfan possibly reduced by phenytoin
Antifungals: metabolism of busulfan inhibited by itraconazole (increased risk of toxicity)
• Antipsychotics: avoid concomitant use of cytotoxics with •clozapine (increased risk of agranulocytosis)
Cardiac Glycosides: cytotoxics reduce absorption of digoxin tablets
Cytotoxics: increased risk of hepatotoxicity when busulfan given with tioguanine

Butobarbital *see* Barbiturates

Butyrophenones *see* Antipsychotics

Cabergoline
Antibacterials: plasma concentration of cabergoline increased by erythromycin (increased risk of toxicity); plasma concentration of cabergoline possibly increased by macrolides (increased risk of toxicity)
Antipsychotics: hypoprolactinaemic and antiparkinsonian effects of cabergoline antagonised by antipsychotics
Domperidone: hypoprolactinaemic effect of cabergoline possibly antagonised by domperidone
Memantine: effects of dopaminergics possibly enhanced by memantine
Methyldopa: antiparkinsonian effect of dopaminergics antagonised by methyldopa
Metoclopramide: hypoprolactinaemic effect of cabergoline antagonised by metoclopramide

Calcium Salts
Note *see also* Antacids
Antibacterials: calcium salts reduce absorption of ciprofloxacin and tetracycline
Bisphosphonates: calcium salts reduce absorption of bisphosphonates
Cardiac Glycosides: large intravenous doses of calcium salts can precipitate arrhythmias when given with cardiac glycosides
Corticosteroids: absorption of calcium salts reduced by corticosteroids
Diuretics: increased risk of hypercalcaemia when calcium salts given with thiazides and related diuretics
Fluorides: calcium salts reduce absorption of fluorides
Iron: calcium salts reduce absorption of *oral* iron
Thyroid Hormones: calcium salts reduce absorption of levothyroxine (thyroxine)
Zinc: calcium salts reduce absorption of zinc

Calcium-channel Blockers

Note Dihydropyridine calcium-channel blockers include amlodipine, felodipine, isradipine, lacidipine, lercanidipine, nicardipine, nifedipine, nimodipine, and nisoldipine

ACE Inhibitors: enhanced hypotensive effect when calcium-channel blockers given with ACE inhibitors

Adrenergic Neurone Blockers: enhanced hypotensive effect when calcium-channel blockers given with adrenergic neurone blockers

Alcohol: enhanced hypotensive effect when calcium-channel blockers given with alcohol; verapamil possibly increases plasma concentration of alcohol

Aldesleukin: enhanced hypotensive effect when calcium-channel blockers given with aldesleukin

• Alpha-blockers: enhanced hypotensive effect when calcium-channel blockers given with •alpha-blockers, also increased risk of first-dose hypotension with post-synaptic alpha-blockers such as prazosin

• Anaesthetics, General: enhanced hypotensive effect when calcium-channel blockers given with general anaesthetics or isoflurane; hypotensive effect of verapamil enhanced by •general anaesthetics (also AV delay)

Analgesics: hypotensive effect of calcium-channel blockers antagonised by NSAIDs; diltiazem inhibits metabolism of alfentanil (risk of prolonged or delayed respiratory depression)

Angiotensin-II Receptor Antagonists: enhanced hypotensive effect when calcium-channel blockers given with angiotensin-II receptor antagonists

• Anti-arrhythmics: increased risk of bradycardia, AV block and myocardial depression when diltiazem or verapamil given with •amiodarone; increased risk of myocardial depression and asystole when verapamil given with •disopyramide or •flecainide

• Antibacterials: metabolism of verapamil possibly inhibited by •clarithromycin and •erythromycin (increased risk of toxicity); metabolism of felodipine possibly inhibited by erythromycin (increased plasma concentration); manufacturer of lercanidipine advises avoid concomitant use with erythromycin; metabolism of diltiazem, nifedipine, nimodipine and verapamil accelerated by •rifampicin (plasma concentration significantly reduced); metabolism of isradipine, nicardipine and nisoldipine possibly accelerated by •rifampicin (possible significantly reduced plasma concentration); plasma concentration of nifedipine increased by •quinupristin/dalfopristin

Antidepressants: diltiazem and verapamil increase plasma concentration of imipramine; enhanced hypotensive effect when calcium-channel blockers given with MAOIs; plasma concentration of amlodipine possibly reduced by St John's wort; diltiazem and verapamil possibly increase plasma concentration of tricyclics

Antidiabetics: glucose tolerance occasionally impaired when nifedipine given with insulin

• Antiepileptics: effects of dihydropyridines, nicardipine and nifedipine probably reduced by carbamazepine; diltiazem and verapamil enhance effects of •carbamazepine; effects of felodipine and isradipine reduced by carbamazepine; plasma concentration of nisoldipine reduced by phenytoin; effects of dihydropyridines, nicardipine and nifedipine probably reduced by •phenytoin; effects of felodipine, isradipine and verapamil reduced by phenytoin; diltiazem increases plasma concentration of •phenytoin but also effect of diltiazem reduced; effects of dihydropyridines, diltiazem and verapamil probably reduced by •primidone; effects of felodipine and isradipine reduced by •primidone

• Antifungals: metabolism of dihydropyridines possibly inhibited by itraconazole and ketoconazole (increased plasma concentration); metabolism of felodipine inhibited by •itraconazole and •ketoconazole (increased plasma concentration); manufacturer of lercanidipine and nisoldipine advises avoid concomitant use with ketoconazole; manufacturer of nisoldipine advises avoid concomitant use with fluconazole and itraconazole; negative inotropic effect possibly increased when calcium-channel blockers given with itraconazole; manufacturer of lercanidipine advises avoid concomitant use with itraconazole

Antimalarials: possible increased risk of bradycardia when calcium-channel blockers given with mefloquine

Antimuscarinics: avoidance of verapamil advised by manufacturer of darifenacin

Antipsychotics: enhanced hypotensive effect when calcium-channel blockers given with antipsychotics

• Antivirals: plasma concentration of verapamil possibly increased by atazanavir; plasma concentration of diltiazem increased by •atazanavir (reduce dose of diltiazem); plasma concentration of diltiazem reduced by efavirenz; manufacturer of lercanidipine advises avoid concomitant use with ritonavir; plasma concentration of calcium-channel blockers possibly increased by •ritonavir

Anxiolytics and Hypnotics: enhanced hypotensive effect when calcium-channel blockers given with anxiolytics and hypnotics; diltiazem and verapamil inhibit metabolism of midazolam (increased plasma concentration with increased sedation); absorption of lercanidipine increased by midazolam; diltiazem and verapamil increase plasma concentration of buspirone (reduce dose of buspirone)

• Barbiturates: effects of dihydropyridines, diltiazem and verapamil probably reduced by •barbiturates; effects of felodipine and isradipine reduced by •barbiturates

• Beta-blockers: enhanced hypotensive effect when calcium-channel blockers given with beta-blockers; increased risk of AV block and bradycardia when diltiazem given with •beta-blockers; asystole, severe hypotension and heart failure when verapamil given with •beta-blockers (see p. 117); possible severe hypotension and heart failure when nifedipine or nisoldipine given with •beta-blockers

Calcium-channel Blockers: plasma concentration of both drugs may increase when diltiazem given with nifedipine

• Cardiac Glycosides: diltiazem, lercanidipine and nicardipine increase plasma concentration of •digoxin; nifedipine possibly increases plasma concentration of •digoxin; verapamil increases plasma concentration of •digoxin, also increased risk of AV block and bradycardia

• Ciclosporin: diltiazem, nicardipine and verapamil increase plasma concentration of •ciclosporin; combination of lercanidipine with •ciclosporin may increase plasma concentration of either drug (or both)—avoid concomitant use; plasma concentration of nifedipine possibly increased by ciclosporin (increased risk of toxicity including gingival hyperplasia)

• Cilostazol: diltiazem increases plasma concentration of •cilostazol—avoid concomitant use

Clonidine: enhanced hypotensive effect when calcium-channel blockers given with clonidine

Corticosteroids: hypotensive effect of calcium-channel blockers antagonised by corticosteroids

Cytotoxics: nifedipine possibly inhibits metabolism of vincristine

Diazoxide: enhanced hypotensive effect when calcium-channel blockers given with diazoxide

Diuretics: enhanced hypotensive effect when calcium-channel blockers given with diuretics; diltiazem and verapamil increase plasma concentration of eplerenone (reduce dose of eplerenone)

Dopaminergics: enhanced hypotensive effect when calcium-channel blockers given with levodopa

Grapefruit Juice: plasma concentration of felodipine, isradipine, lacidipine, lercanidipine, nicardipine, nifedipine, nimodipine, nisoldipine and verapamil increased by grapefruit juice

Hormone Antagonists: diltiazem and verapamil increase plasma concentration of dutasteride

Calcium-channel Blockers *(continued)*
- Ivabradine: diltiazem and verapamil increase plasma concentration of •ivabradine—avoid concomitant use
- Lipid-regulating Drugs: diltiazem increases plasma concentration of atorvastatin; possible increased risk of myopathy when diltiazem given with simvastatin; increased risk of myopathy when verapamil given with •simvastatin

Lithium: neurotoxicity may occur when diltiazem or verapamil given with lithium without increased plasma concentration of lithium
- Magnesium (parenteral): profound hypotension reported with concomitant use of nifedipine and •parenteral magnesium in pre-eclampsia

Methyldopa: enhanced hypotensive effect when calcium-channel blockers given with methyldopa

Moxisylyte (thymoxamine): enhanced hypotensive effect when calcium-channel blockers given with moxisylyte

Moxonidine: enhanced hypotensive effect when calcium-channel blockers given with moxonidine

Muscle Relaxants: verapamil enhances effects of non-depolarising muscle relaxants and suxamethonium; enhanced hypotensive effect when calcium-channel blockers given with baclofen or tizanidine; hypotension, myocardial depression, and hyperkalaemia when verapamil given with intravenous dantrolene; risk of arrhythmias when diltiazem given with intravenous dantrolene; nifedipine enhances effects of non-depolarising muscle relaxants

Nitrates: enhanced hypotensive effect when calcium-channel blockers given with nitrates

Oestrogens: hypotensive effect of calcium-channel blockers antagonised by oestrogens

Prostaglandins: enhanced hypotensive effect when calcium-channel blockers given with alprostadil

Sildenafil: enhanced hypotensive effect when amlodipine given with sildenafil
- Sirolimus: diltiazem increases plasma concentration of •sirolimus; plasma concentration of both drugs increased when verapamil given with •sirolimus
- Tacrolimus: diltiazem and nifedipine increase plasma concentration of •tacrolimus; felodipine, nicardipine and verapamil possibly increase plasma concentration of tacrolimus
- Theophylline: calcium-channel blockers possibly increase plasma concentration of •theophylline (enhanced effect); diltiazem increases plasma concentration of theophylline; verapamil increases plasma concentration of •theophylline (enhanced effect)

Ulcer-healing Drugs: metabolism of calcium-channel blockers possibly inhibited by cimetidine (increased plasma concentration)

Vardenafil: enhanced hypotensive effect when nifedipine given with vardenafil

Vasodilator Antihypertensives: enhanced hypotensive effect when calcium-channel blockers given with hydralazine, minoxidil or sodium nitroprusside

Calcium-channel Blockers (dihydropyridines) *see* Calcium-channel Blockers

Candesartan *see* Angiotensin-II Receptor Antagonists

Capecitabine *see* Fluorouracil

Capreomycin

Antibacterials: increased risk of nephrotoxicity when capreomycin given with colistin or polymyxins; increased risk of nephrotoxicity and ototoxicity when capreomycin given with aminoglycosides or vancomycin

Cytotoxics: increased risk of nephrotoxicity and ototoxicity when capreomycin given with platinum compounds

Oestrogens: antibacterials that do not induce liver enzymes possibly reduce contraceptive effect of oestrogens (risk probably small, see p. 428)

Captopril *see* ACE Inhibitors

Carbamazepine

Alcohol: CNS side-effects of carbamazepine possibly increased by alcohol
- Analgesics: effects of carbamazepine enhanced by •dextropropoxyphene; carbamazepine reduces plasma concentration of methadone; carbamazepine reduces effects of tramadol
- Antibacterials: plasma concentration of carbamazepine increased by •clarithromycin and •erythromycin; plasma concentration of carbamazepine reduced by •rifabutin; carbamazepine accelerates metabolism of doxycycline (reduced effect); plasma concentration of carbamazepine increased by •isoniazid (also possibly increased isoniazid hepatotoxicity); carbamazepine reduces plasma concentration of •telithromycin (avoid during and for 2 weeks after carbamazepine)
- Anticoagulants: carbamazepine accelerates metabolism of •coumarins (reduced anticoagulant effect)
- Antidepressants: plasma concentration of carbamazepine increased by •fluoxetine and •fluvoxamine; carbamazepine reduces plasma concentration of •mianserin, mirtazapine and paroxetine; anticonvulsant effect of antiepileptics possibly antagonised by MAOIs and •tricyclic-related antidepressants (convulsive threshold lowered); manufacturer of carbamazepine advises avoid for 2 weeks after stopping •MAOIs, also antagonism of anticonvulsant effect; anticonvulsant effect of antiepileptics antagonised by •SSRIs and •tricyclics (convulsive threshold lowered); avoid concomitant use of antiepileptics with •St John's wort; carbamazepine accelerates metabolism of •tricyclics (reduced plasma concentration and reduced effect)

Antiepileptics: carbamazepine possibly reduces plasma concentration of ethosuximide; carbamazepine often reduces plasma concentration of lamotrigine, also plasma concentration of an active metabolite of carbamazepine sometimes raised (but evidence is conflicting); plasma concentration of carbamazepine sometimes reduced by oxcarbazepine (but concentration of an active metabolite of carbamazepine may be increased), also plasma concentration of an active metabolite of oxcarbazepine often reduced; plasma concentration of both drugs often reduced when carbamazepine given with phenytoin, also plasma concentration of phenytoin may be increased; plasma concentration of carbamazepine often reduced by primidone, also plasma concentration of primidone sometimes reduced (but concentration of an active metabolite of primidone often increased); carbamazepine reduces plasma concentration of tiagabine and zonisamide; carbamazepine often reduces plasma concentration of topiramate; carbamazepine reduces plasma concentration of valproate, also plasma concentration of active metabolite of carbamazepine increased
- Antifungals: plasma concentration of carbamazepine possibly increased by fluconazole, ketoconazole and miconazole; carbamazepine possibly reduces plasma concentration of itraconazole and •posaconazole; carbamazepine possibly reduces plasma concentration of •voriconazole—avoid concomitant use; carbamazepine possibly reduces plasma concentration of caspofungin—consider increasing dose of caspofungin
- Antimalarials: possible increased risk of convulsions when antiepileptics given with chloroquine and hydroxychloroquine; anticonvulsant effect of antiepileptics and carbamazepine antagonised by •mefloquine
- Antipsychotics: anticonvulsant effect of carbamazepine antagonised by •antipsychotics (convulsive threshold lowered); carbamazepine accelerates metabolism of haloperidol, olanzapine, quetiapine, risperidone and sertindole (reduced plasma concentration); carbamazepine reduces plasma concentration of •aripiprazole—increase dose of aripiprazole; carbamazepine accelerates metabolism of •clozapine (reduced plasma concentration), also avoid concomitant use of drugs with substantial potential for causing agranulocytosis
- Antivirals: carbamazepine possibly reduces plasma concentration of amprenavir, darunavir, indinavir,

Carbamazepine
- Antivirals *(continued)*
lopinavir, nelfinavir, saquinavir and tipranavir; plasma concentration of both drugs reduced when carbamazepine given with efavirenz; plasma concentration of carbamazepine possibly increased by •ritonavir

Anxiolytics and Hypnotics: carbamazepine often reduces plasma concentration of clonazepam

Aprepitant: carbamazepine possibly reduces plasma concentration of aprepitant

Barbiturates: plasma concentration of carbamazepine reduced by phenobarbital

Bupropion: carbamazepine reduces plasma concentration of bupropion

- Calcium-channel Blockers: carbamazepine reduces effects of felodipine and isradipine; carbamazepine probably reduces effects of dihydropyridines, nicardipine and nifedipine; effects of carbamazepine enhanced by •diltiazem and •verapamil

Cardiac Glycosides: carbamazepine accelerates metabolism of digitoxin (reduced effect)

- Ciclosporin: carbamazepine accelerates metabolism of •ciclosporin (reduced plasma concentration)
- Corticosteroids: carbamazepine accelerates metabolism of •corticosteroids (reduced effect)

Cytotoxics: carbamazepine reduces plasma concentration of irinotecan and its active metabolite

- Diuretics: increased risk of hyponatraemia when carbamazepine given with diuretics; plasma concentration of carbamazepine increased by •acetazolamide; carbamazepine reduces plasma concentration of •eplerenone—avoid concomitant use
- Hormone Antagonists: metabolism of carbamazepine inhibited by •danazol (increased risk of toxicity); carbamazepine accelerates metabolism of gestrinone (reduced plasma concentration); carbamazepine possibly accelerates metabolism of toremifene (reduced plasma concentration)

$5HT_3$ Antagonists: carbamazepine accelerates metabolism of ondansetron (reduced effect)

Lithium: neurotoxicity may occur when carbamazepine given with lithium without increased plasma concentration of lithium

Muscle Relaxants: carbamazepine antagonises muscle relaxant effect of non-depolarising muscle relaxants (accelerated recovery from neuromuscular blockade)

- Oestrogens: carbamazepine accelerates metabolism of •oestrogens (reduced contraceptive effect—see p. 428)
- Progestogens: carbamazepine accelerates metabolism of •progestogens (reduced contraceptive effect—see p. 428)

Retinoids: plasma concentration of carbamazepine possibly reduced by isotretinoin

Theophylline: carbamazepine accelerates metabolism of theophylline (reduced effect)

Thyroid Hormones: carbamazepine accelerates metabolism of thyroid hormones (may increase requirements for thyroid hormones in hypothyroidism)

Tibolone: carbamazepine accelerates metabolism of tibolone (reduced plasma concentration)

- Ulcer-healing Drugs: metabolism of carbamazepine inhibited by •cimetidine (increased plasma concentration)

Vitamins: carbamazepine possibly increases requirements for vitamin D

Carbapenems *see* Ertapenem, Imipenem with Cilastatin, and Meropenem

Carbonic Anhydrase Inhibitors *see* Diuretics

Carboplatin *see* Platinum Compounds

Carboprost *see* Prostaglandins

Cardiac Glycosides

ACE Inhibitors: plasma concentration of digoxin possibly increased by captopril

Alpha-blockers: plasma concentration of digoxin increased by prazosin

Aminosalicylates: absorption of digoxin possibly reduced by sulfasalazine

Cardiac Glycosides *(continued)*

Analgesics: plasma concentration of cardiac glycosides possibly increased by NSAIDs, also possible exacerbation of heart failure and reduction of renal function

Antacids: absorption of digoxin possibly reduced by antacids

- Anti-arrhythmics: plasma concentration of digoxin increased by •amiodarone and •propafenone (halve dose of digoxin)

Antibacterials: plasma concentration of digoxin possibly increased by gentamicin, telithromycin and trimethoprim; absorption of digoxin reduced by neomycin; plasma concentration of digoxin possibly reduced by rifampicin; plasma concentration of digoxin increased by macrolides (increased risk of toxicity); metabolism of digitoxin accelerated by rifamycins (reduced effect)

- Antidepressants: plasma concentration of digoxin reduced by •St John's wort—avoid concomitant use

Antidiabetics: plasma concentration of digoxin possibly reduced by acarbose; plasma concentration of digoxin increased by sitagliptin

Antiepileptics: metabolism of digitoxin accelerated by carbamazepine, phenytoin and primidone (reduced effect); plasma concentration of digoxin possibly reduced by phenytoin

- Antifungals: increased cardiac toxicity with cardiac glycosides if hypokalaemia occurs with •amphotericin; plasma concentration of digoxin increased by •itraconazole
- Antimalarials: plasma concentration of digoxin possibly increased by •chloroquine and hydroxychloroquine; possible increased risk of bradycardia when digoxin given with mefloquine; plasma concentration of digoxin increased by •quinine

Antimuscarinics: plasma concentration of digoxin possibly increased by darifenacin

Antivirals: plasma concentration of digoxin possibly increased by ritonavir

Anxiolytics and Hypnotics: plasma concentration of digoxin increased by alprazolam (increased risk of toxicity)

Barbiturates: metabolism of digitoxin accelerated by barbiturates (reduced effect)

Beta-blockers: increased risk of AV block and bradycardia when cardiac glycosides given with beta-blockers

Calcium Salts: arrhythmias can be precipitated when cardiac glycosides given with large intravenous doses of calcium salts

- Calcium-channel Blockers: plasma concentration of digoxin increased by •diltiazem, •lercanidipine and •nicardipine; plasma concentration of digoxin possibly increased by •nifedipine; plasma concentration of digoxin increased by •verapamil, also increased risk of AV block and bradycardia
- Ciclosporin: plasma concentration of digoxin increased by •ciclosporin (increased risk of toxicity)

Corticosteroids: increased risk of hypokalaemia when cardiac glycosides given with corticosteroids

Cytotoxics: absorption of digoxin tablets reduced by cytotoxics

- Diuretics: increased cardiac toxicity with cardiac glycosides if hypokalaemia occurs with •acetazolamide, •loop diuretics or •thiazides and related diuretics; plasma concentration of digitoxin possibly affected by spironolactone; plasma concentration of digoxin increased by •spironolactone

Lenalidomide: plasma concentration of digoxin possibly increased by lenalidomide

Lipid-regulating Drugs: absorption of cardiac glycosides possibly reduced by colestipol and colestyramine; plasma concentration of digoxin possibly increased by atorvastatin

Muscle Relaxants: risk of ventricular arrhythmias when cardiac glycosides given with suxamethonium; possible increased risk of bradycardia when cardiac glycosides given with tizanidine

Penicillamine: plasma concentration of digoxin possibly reduced by penicillamine

Cardiac Glycosides *(continued)*
Sympathomimetics, $Beta_2$: plasma concentration of digoxin possibly reduced by salbutamol
Ulcer-healing Drugs: plasma concentration of digoxin possibly slightly increased by proton pump inhibitors; absorption of cardiac glycosides possibly reduced by sucralfate

Carisoprodol *see* Muscle Relaxants
Carteolol *see* Beta-blockers
Carvedilol *see* Beta-blockers
Caspofungin
Antibacterials: plasma concentration of caspofungin initially increased and then reduced by rifampicin (consider increasing dose of caspofungin)
Antiepileptics: plasma concentration of caspofungin possibly reduced by carbamazepine and phenytoin—consider increasing dose of caspofungin
Antivirals: plasma concentration of caspofungin possibly reduced by efavirenz and nevirapine—consider increasing dose of caspofungin
• Ciclosporin: plasma concentration of caspofungin increased by •ciclosporin (manufacturer of caspofungin recommends monitoring liver enzymes)
Corticosteroids: plasma concentration of caspofungin possibly reduced by dexamethasone—consider increasing dose of caspofungin
• Tacrolimus: caspofungin reduces plasma concentration of •tacrolimus

Cefaclor *see* Cephalosporins
Cefadroxil *see* Cephalosporins
Cefalexin *see* Cephalosporins
Cefixime *see* Cephalosporins
Cefotaxime *see* Cephalosporins
Cefpodoxime *see* Cephalosporins
Cefradine *see* Cephalosporins
Ceftazidime *see* Cephalosporins
Ceftriaxone *see* Cephalosporins
Cefuroxime *see* Cephalosporins
Celecoxib *see* NSAIDs
Celiprolol *see* Beta-blockers
Cephalosporins
Antacids: absorption of cefaclor and cefpodoxime reduced by antacids
• Anticoagulants: cephalosporins possibly enhance anticoagulant effect of •coumarins
Oestrogens: antibacterials that do not induce liver enzymes possibly reduce contraceptive effect of oestrogens (risk probably small, see p. 428)
Probenecid: excretion of cephalosporins reduced by probenecid (increased plasma concentration)
Ulcer-healing Drugs: absorption of cefpodoxime reduced by histamine H_2-antagonists

Cetirizine *see* Antihistamines
Chloral *see* Anxiolytics and Hypnotics
Chloramphenicol
Antibacterials: metabolism of chloramphenicol accelerated by rifampicin (reduced plasma concentration)
• Anticoagulants: chloramphenicol enhances anticoagulant effect of •coumarins
• Antidiabetics: chloramphenicol enhances effects of •sulphonylureas
• Antiepileptics: chloramphenicol increases plasma concentration of •phenytoin (increased risk of toxicity); metabolism of chloramphenicol accelerated by •primidone (reduced plasma concentration)
• Antipsychotics: avoid concomitant use of chloramphenicol with •clozapine (increased risk of agranulocytosis)
• Barbiturates: metabolism of chloramphenicol accelerated by •barbiturates (reduced plasma concentration)
• Ciclosporin: chloramphenicol possibly increases plasma concentration of •ciclosporin
Hydroxocobalamin: chloramphenicol reduces response to hydroxocobalamin
Oestrogens: antibacterials that do not induce liver enzymes possibly reduce contraceptive effect of oestrogens (risk probably small, see p. 428)
• Tacrolimus: chloramphenicol possibly increases plasma concentration of •tacrolimus

Chlordiazepoxide *see* Anxiolytics and Hypnotics
Chloroquine and Hydroxychloroquine
Adsorbents: absorption of chloroquine and hydroxychloroquine reduced by kaolin
Agalsidase Beta: chloroquine and hydroxychloroquine possibly inhibit effects of agalsidase beta (manufacturer of agalsidase beta advises avoid concomitant use)
Antacids: absorption of chloroquine and hydroxychloroquine reduced by antacids
• Anti-arrhythmics: increased risk of ventricular arrhythmias when chloroquine and hydroxychloroquine given with •amiodarone—avoid concomitant use
• Antibacterials: increased risk of ventricular arrhythmias when chloroquine and hydroxychloroquine given with •moxifloxacin—avoid concomitant use
Antiepileptics: possible increased risk of convulsions when chloroquine and hydroxychloroquine given with antiepileptics
• Antimalarials: avoidance of antimalarials advised by manufacturer of •artemether/lumefantrine; increased risk of convulsions when chloroquine and hydroxychloroquine given with •mefloquine
• Cardiac Glycosides: chloroquine and hydroxychloroquine possibly increase plasma concentration of •digoxin
• Ciclosporin: chloroquine and hydroxychloroquine increase plasma concentration of •ciclosporin (increased risk of toxicity)
Lanthanum: absorption of chloroquine and hydroxychloroquine possibly reduced by lanthanum (give at least 2 hours apart)
Laronidase: chloroquine and hydroxychloroquine possibly inhibit effects of laronidase (manufacturer of laronidase advises avoid concomitant use)
Parasympathomimetics: chloroquine and hydroxychloroquine have potential to increase symptoms of myasthenia gravis and thus diminish effect of neostigmine and pyridostigmine
Ulcer-healing Drugs: metabolism of chloroquine and hydroxychloroquine inhibited by cimetidine (increased plasma concentration)

Chlorothiazide *see* Diuretics
Chlorphenamine (chlorpheniramine) *see* Antihistamines
Chlorpromazine *see* Antipsychotics
Chlorpropamide *see* Antidiabetics
Chlortalidone *see* Diuretics
Chlortetracycline *see* Tetracyclines
Ciclesonide *see* Corticosteroids
Ciclosporin
• ACE Inhibitors: increased risk of hyperkalaemia when ciclosporin given with •ACE inhibitors
Allopurinol: plasma concentration of ciclosporin possibly increased by allopurinol (risk of nephrotoxicity)
• Analgesics: increased risk of nephrotoxicity when ciclosporin given with •NSAIDs; ciclosporin increases plasma concentration of •diclofenac (halve dose of diclofenac)
• Angiotensin-II Receptor Antagonists: increased risk of hyperkalaemia when ciclosporin given with •angiotensin-II receptor antagonists
Anti-arrhythmics: plasma concentration of ciclosporin possibly increased by amiodarone and propafenone
• Antibacterials: metabolism of ciclosporin inhibited by •clarithromycin and •erythromycin (increased plasma concentration); metabolism of ciclosporin accelerated by •rifampicin (reduced plasma concentration); plasma concentration of ciclosporin possibly reduced by •sulfadiazine; plasma concentration of ciclosporin possibly increased by •chloramphenicol, •doxycycline and •telithromycin; increased risk of nephrotoxicity when ciclosporin given with •aminoglycosides, •polymyxins, •quinolones, •sulphonamides or •vancomycin; increased risk of myopathy when ciclosporin given with •daptomycin (preferably avoid concomitant use); metabolism of ciclosporin possibly inhibited by •macrolides (increased plasma concentration); plasma concentration of ciclosporin increased by •quinupristin/dalfo-

Ciclosporin

- Antibacterials *(continued)* pristin; increased risk of nephrotoxicity when ciclosporin given with •trimethoprim, also plasma concentration of ciclosporin reduced by intravenous trimethoprim
- Antidepressants: plasma concentration of ciclosporin reduced by •St John's wort—avoid concomitant use

Antidiabetics: ciclosporin possibly enhances hypoglycaemic effect of repaglinide

- Antiepileptics: metabolism of ciclosporin accelerated by •carbamazepine and •phenytoin (reduced plasma concentration); plasma concentration of ciclosporin possibly reduced by oxcarbazepine; metabolism of ciclosporin accelerated by •primidone (reduced effect)
- Antifungals: metabolism of ciclosporin inhibited by •fluconazole, •itraconazole, •ketoconazole, •posaconazole and •voriconazole (increased plasma concentration); metabolism of ciclosporin possibly inhibited by •miconazole (increased plasma concentration); increased risk of nephrotoxicity when ciclosporin given with •amphotericin; ciclosporin increases plasma concentration of •caspofungin (manufacturer of caspofungin recommends monitoring liver enzymes); plasma concentration of ciclosporin possibly reduced by griseofulvin
- Antimalarials: plasma concentration of ciclosporin increased by •chloroquine and hydroxychloroquine (increased risk of toxicity)

Antimuscarinics: avoidance of ciclosporin advised by manufacturer of darifenacin

- Antivirals: increased risk of nephrotoxicity when ciclosporin given with aciclovir; plasma concentration of ciclosporin possibly increased by •atazanavir, •nelfinavir and •ritonavir; plasma concentration of both drugs increased when ciclosporin given with •saquinavir
- Barbiturates: metabolism of ciclosporin accelerated by •barbiturates (reduced effect)
- Beta-blockers: plasma concentration of ciclosporin increased by •carvedilol
- Bile Acids: absorption of ciclosporin increased by •ursodeoxycholic acid
- Bosentan: ciclosporin increases plasma concentration of •bosentan (also plasma concentration of ciclosporin reduced—avoid concomitant use)
- Calcium-channel Blockers: combination of ciclosporin with •lercanidipine may increase plasma concentration of either drug (or both)—avoid concomitant use; plasma concentration of ciclosporin increased by •diltiazem, •nicardipine and •verapamil; ciclosporin possibly increases plasma concentration of nifedipine (increased risk of toxicity including gingival hyperplasia)
- Cardiac Glycosides: ciclosporin increases plasma concentration of •digoxin (increased risk of toxicity)
- Colchicine: possible increased risk of nephrotoxicity and myotoxicity when ciclosporin given with •colchicine (increased plasma concentration of ciclosporin)
- Corticosteroids: plasma concentration of ciclosporin increased by high-dose •methylprednisolone (risk of convulsions); ciclosporin increases plasma concentration of prednisolone
- Cytotoxics: increased risk of nephrotoxicity when ciclosporin given with •melphalan; increased risk of neurotoxicity when ciclosporin given with •doxorubicin; risk of toxicity when ciclosporin given with •methotrexate; *in vitro* studies suggest a possible interaction between ciclosporin and docetaxel (consult docetaxel product literature); ciclosporin possibly increases plasma concentration of etoposide (increased risk of toxicity)
- Diuretics: increased risk of hyperkalaemia when ciclosporin given with •potassium-sparing diuretics and aldosterone antagonists; increased risk of nephrotoxicity and possibly hypermagnesaemia when ciclosporin given with thiazides and related diuretics

Ciclosporin *(continued)*

- Grapefruit Juice: plasma concentration of ciclosporin increased by •grapefruit juice (increased risk of toxicity)
- Hormone Antagonists: metabolism of ciclosporin inhibited by •danazol (increased plasma concentration); plasma concentration of ciclosporin reduced by lanreotide and •octreotide
- Lipid-regulating Drugs: increased risk of renal impairment when ciclosporin given with bezafibrate or fenofibrate; increased risk of myopathy when ciclosporin given with •rosuvastatin (avoid concomitant use); plasma concentration of both drugs may increase when ciclosporin given with •ezetimibe; increased risk of myopathy when ciclosporin given with •statins
- Metoclopramide: plasma concentration of ciclosporin increased by •metoclopramide
- Modafinil: plasma concentration of ciclosporin reduced by •modafinil

Oestrogens: plasma concentration of ciclosporin possibly increased by oestrogens

- Orlistat: absorption of ciclosporin possibly reduced by •orlistat
- Potassium Salts: increased risk of hyperkalaemia when ciclosporin given with •potassium salts
- Progestogens: metabolism of ciclosporin inhibited by •progestogens (increased plasma concentration)

Sirolimus: ciclosporin increases plasma concentration of sirolimus

- Sitaxentan: ciclosporin increases plasma concentration of •sitaxentan—avoid concomitant use
- Tacrolimus: plasma concentration of ciclosporin increased by •tacrolimus (increased risk of nephrotoxicity)—avoid concomitant use
- Ulcer-healing Drugs: plasma concentration of ciclosporin possibly increased by •cimetidine; plasma concentration of ciclosporin possibly affected by omeprazole

Cidofovir

Antivirals: combination of cidofovir with tenofovir may increase plasma concentration of either drug (or both)

Cilazapril *see* ACE Inhibitors

Cilostazol

- Anagrelide: avoidance of cilostazol advised by manufacturer of •anagrelide

Analgesics: manufacturer of cilostazol recommends dose of concomitant aspirin should not exceed 80 mg daily

- Antibacterials: plasma concentration of cilostazol increased by •erythromycin (also plasma concentration of erythromycin reduced)—avoid concomitant use
- Antifungals: plasma concentration of cilostazol possibly increased by •ketoconazole—avoid concomitant use
- Antivirals: plasma concentration of cilostazol possibly increased by •amprenavir, •indinavir, •lopinavir, •nelfinavir, •ritonavir and •saquinavir—avoid concomitant use
- Calcium-channel Blockers: plasma concentration of cilostazol increased by •diltiazem—avoid concomitant use
- Ulcer-healing Drugs: plasma concentration of cilostazol possibly increased by •cimetidine and •lansoprazole—avoid concomitant use; plasma concentration of cilostazol increased by •omeprazole (risk of toxicity)—avoid concomitant use

Cimetidine *see* Histamine H_2-antagonists

Cinacalcet

Antifungals: metabolism of cinacalcet inhibited by ketoconazole (increased plasma concentration)

Tobacco: metabolism of cinacalcet increased by tobacco smoking (reduced plasma concentration)

Cinnarizine *see* Antihistamines

Ciprofibrate *see* Fibrates

Ciprofloxacin *see* Quinolones

Cisatracurium *see* Muscle Relaxants

Cisplatin *see* Platinum Compounds

Citalopram *see* Antidepressants, SSRI

Clarithromycin *see* Macrolides

Clemastine *see* Antihistamines

Clindamycin

- Muscle Relaxants: clindamycin enhances effects of •non-depolarising muscle relaxants and •suxamethonium

Oestrogens: antibacterials that do not induce liver enzymes possibly reduce contraceptive effect of oestrogens (risk probably small, see p. 428)

Parasympathomimetics: clindamycin antagonises effects of neostigmine and pyridostigmine

Clobazam *see* Anxiolytics and Hypnotics

Clomethiazole *see* Anxiolytics and Hypnotics

Clomipramine *see* Antidepressants, Tricyclic

Clonazepam *see* Anxiolytics and Hypnotics

Clonidine

ACE Inhibitors: enhanced hypotensive effect when clonidine given with ACE inhibitors; previous treatment with clonidine possibly delays antihypertensive effect of captopril

Adrenergic Neurone Blockers: enhanced hypotensive effect when clonidine given with adrenergic neurone blockers

Alcohol: enhanced hypotensive effect when clonidine given with alcohol

Aldesleukin: enhanced hypotensive effect when clonidine given with aldesleukin

Alpha-blockers: enhanced hypotensive effect when clonidine given with alpha-blockers

Anaesthetics, General: enhanced hypotensive effect when clonidine given with general anaesthetics

Analgesics: hypotensive effect of clonidine antagonised by NSAIDs

Angiotensin-II Receptor Antagonists: enhanced hypotensive effect when clonidine given with angiotensin-II receptor antagonists

- Antidepressants: enhanced hypotensive effect when clonidine given with MAOIs; hypotensive effect of clonidine antagonised by •tricyclics, also increased risk of hypertension on clonidine withdrawal

Antipsychotics: enhanced hypotensive effect when clonidine given with phenothiazines

Anxiolytics and Hypnotics: enhanced hypotensive effect when clonidine given with anxiolytics and hypnotics

- Beta-blockers: increased risk of withdrawal hypertension when clonidine given with •beta-blockers (withdraw beta-blockers several days before slowly withdrawing clonidine)

Calcium-channel Blockers: enhanced hypotensive effect when clonidine given with calcium-channel blockers

Corticosteroids: hypotensive effect of clonidine antagonised by corticosteroids

Diazoxide: enhanced hypotensive effect when clonidine given with diazoxide

Diuretics: enhanced hypotensive effect when clonidine given with diuretics

Dopaminergics: enhanced hypotensive effect when clonidine given with levodopa

Methyldopa: enhanced hypotensive effect when clonidine given with methyldopa

Moxisylyte (thymoxamine): enhanced hypotensive effect when clonidine given with moxisylyte

Moxonidine: enhanced hypotensive effect when clonidine given with moxonidine

Muscle Relaxants: enhanced hypotensive effect when clonidine given with baclofen or tizanidine

Nitrates: enhanced hypotensive effect when clonidine given with nitrates

Oestrogens: hypotensive effect of clonidine antagonised by oestrogens

Prostaglandins: enhanced hypotensive effect when clonidine given with alprostadil

- Sympathomimetics: possible risk of hypertension when clonidine given with adrenaline (epinephrine) or noradrenaline (norepinephrine); serious adverse events reported with concomitant use of clonidine and •methylphenidate (causality not established)

Clonidine *(continued)*

Vasodilator Antihypertensives: enhanced hypotensive effect when clonidine given with hydralazine, minoxidil or sodium nitroprusside

Clopamide *see* Diuretics

Clopidogrel

Analgesics: increased risk of bleeding when clopidogrel given with NSAIDs or aspirin

- Anticoagulants: manufacturer of clopidogrel advises avoid concomitant use with •warfarin; antiplatelet action of clopidogrel enhances anticoagulant effect of •coumarins and •phenindione; increased risk of bleeding when clopidogrel given with heparins

Dipyridamole: increased risk of bleeding when clopidogrel given with dipyridamole

Iloprost: increased risk of bleeding when clopidogrel given with iloprost

Clotrimazole *see* Antifungals, Imidazole

Clozapine *see* Antipsychotics

Co-amoxiclav *see* Penicillins

Co-beneldopa *see* Levodopa

Co-careldopa *see* Levodopa

Codeine *see* Opioid Analgesics

Co-fluampicil *see* Penicillins

Colchicine

- Antibacterials: increased risk of colchicine toxicity when given with •clarithromycin or •erythromycin
- Ciclosporin: possible increased risk of nephrotoxicity and myotoxicity when colchicine given with •ciclosporin (increased plasma concentration of ciclosporin)

Colesevelam

Note Other drugs should be taken at least 1 hour before or 4 hours after colesevelam to reduce possible interference with absorption

Colestipol

Note Other drugs should be taken at least 1 hour before or 4-6 hours after colestipol to reduce possible interference with absorption

Antibacterials: colestipol possibly reduces absorption of tetracycline

Bile Acids: colestipol possibly reduces absorption of bile acids

Cardiac Glycosides: colestipol possibly reduces absorption of cardiac glycosides

Diuretics: colestipol reduces absorption of thiazides and related diuretics (give at least 2 hours apart)

Thyroid Hormones: colestipol reduces absorption of thyroid hormones

Colestyramine

Note Other drugs should be taken at least 1 hour before or 4-6 hours after colestyramine to reduce possible interference with absorption

Analgesics: colestyramine increases the excretion of meloxicam; colestyramine reduces absorption of paracetamol

Antibacterials: colestyramine possibly reduces absorption of tetracycline; colestyramine antagonises effects of oral vancomycin

- Anticoagulants: colestyramine may enhance or reduce anticoagulant effect of •coumarins and •phenindione

Antidiabetics: colestyramine possibly enhances hypoglycaemic effect of acarbose

Antiepileptics: colestyramine possibly reduces absorption of valproate

Bile Acids: colestyramine possibly reduces absorption of bile acids

Cardiac Glycosides: colestyramine possibly reduces absorption of cardiac glycosides

Cytotoxics: colestyramine reduces absorption of mycophenolate

Diuretics: colestyramine reduces absorption of thiazides and related diuretics (give at least 2 hours apart)

Leflunomide: colestyramine significantly decreases effect of leflunomide (enhanced elimination)—avoid unless drug elimination desired

Raloxifene: colestyramine reduces absorption of raloxifene (manufacturer of raloxifene advises avoid concomitant administration)

Thyroid Hormones: colestyramine reduces absorption of thyroid hormones

Colistin *see* Polymyxins
Contraceptives, oral *see* Oestrogens and Progestogens
Corticosteroids
Note Interactions do not generally apply to corticosteroids used for topical action (including inhalation) unless specified
ACE Inhibitors: corticosteroids antagonise hypotensive effect of ACE inhibitors
Adrenergic Neurone Blockers: corticosteroids antagonise hypotensive effect of adrenergic neurone blockers
Alpha-blockers: corticosteroids antagonise hypotensive effect of alpha-blockers
Analgesics: increased risk of gastro-intestinal bleeding and ulceration when corticosteroids given with NSAIDs; increased risk of gastro-intestinal bleeding and ulceration when corticosteroids given with aspirin, also corticosteroids reduce plasma concentration of salicylate
Angiotensin-II Receptor Antagonists: corticosteroids antagonise hypotensive effect of angiotensin-II receptor antagonists
Antacids: absorption of deflazacort reduced by antacids
• Antibacterials: plasma concentration of methylprednisolone possibly increased by clarithromycin; metabolism of corticosteroids possibly inhibited by erythromycin; metabolism of methylprednisolone inhibited by erythromycin; corticosteroids possibly reduce plasma concentration of isoniazid; metabolism of corticosteroids accelerated by •rifamycins (reduced effect)
• Anticoagulants: corticosteroids may enhance or reduce anticoagulant effect of •coumarins (high-dose corticosteroids enhance anticoagulant effect)
Antidiabetics: corticosteroids antagonise hypoglycaemic effect of antidiabetics
• Antiepileptics: metabolism of corticosteroids accelerated by •carbamazepine, •phenytoin and •primidone (reduced effect)
• Antifungals: metabolism of corticosteroids possibly inhibited by itraconazole and ketoconazole; plasma concentration of inhaled mometasone increased by ketoconazole; plasma concentration of inhaled and oral budesonide increased by ketoconazole; metabolism of methylprednisolone inhibited by ketoconazole; increased risk of hypokalaemia when corticosteroids given with •amphotericin—avoid concomitant use unless corticosteroids needed to control reactions; plasma concentration of inhaled budesonide increased by itraconazole; metabolism of methylprednisolone possibly inhibited by itraconazole; dexamethasone possibly reduces plasma concentration of caspofungin—consider increasing dose of caspofungin
• Antivirals: dexamethasone possibly reduces plasma concentration of indinavir, lopinavir and saquinavir; plasma concentration of corticosteroids, dexamethasone and prednisolone possibly increased by ritonavir; plasma concentration of inhaled and intranasal budesonide and fluticasone increased by •ritonavir
Aprepitant: metabolism of dexamethasone and methylprednisolone inhibited by aprepitant (reduce dose of dexamethasone and methylprednisolone)
• Barbiturates: metabolism of corticosteroids accelerated by •barbiturates (reduced effect)
Beta-blockers: corticosteroids antagonise hypotensive effect of beta-blockers
Calcium Salts: corticosteroids reduce absorption of calcium salts
Calcium-channel Blockers: corticosteroids antagonise hypotensive effect of calcium-channel blockers
Cardiac Glycosides: increased risk of hypokalaemia when corticosteroids given with cardiac glycosides
• Ciclosporin: high-dose methylprednisolone increases plasma concentration of •ciclosporin (risk of convulsions); plasma concentration of prednisolone increased by ciclosporin
Clonidine: corticosteroids antagonise hypotensive effect of clonidine
• Cytotoxics: increased risk of haematological toxicity when corticosteroids given with •methotrexate

Corticosteroids *(continued)*
Diazoxide: corticosteroids antagonise hypotensive effect of diazoxide
Diuretics: corticosteroids antagonise diuretic effect of diuretics; increased risk of hypokalaemia when corticosteroids given with acetazolamide, loop diuretics or thiazides and related diuretics
Methyldopa: corticosteroids antagonise hypotensive effect of methyldopa
Mifepristone: effect of corticosteroids (including inhaled corticosteroids) may be reduced for 3–4 days after mifepristone
Moxonidine: corticosteroids antagonise hypotensive effect of moxonidine
Muscle Relaxants: corticosteroids possibly antagonise effects of pancuronium and vecuronium
Nitrates: corticosteroids antagonise hypotensive effect of nitrates
Oestrogens: plasma concentration of corticosteroids increased by oral contraceptives containing oestrogens
Sodium Benzoate: corticosteroids possibly reduce effects of sodium benzoate
Sodium Phenylbutyrate: corticosteroids possibly reduce effects of sodium phenylbutyrate
Somatropin: corticosteroids may inhibit growth-promoting effect of somatropin
Sympathomimetics: metabolism of dexamethasone accelerated by ephedrine
Sympathomimetics, Beta$_2$: increased risk of hypokalaemia when corticosteroids given with high doses of beta$_2$ sympathomimetics—for CSM advice (hypokalaemia) see p. 150
Theophylline: increased risk of hypokalaemia when corticosteroids given with theophylline
• Vaccines: high doses of corticosteroids impair immune response to •vaccines, avoid concomitant use with live vaccines (see p. 641)
Vasodilator Antihypertensives: corticosteroids antagonise hypotensive effect of hydralazine, minoxidil and sodium nitroprusside

Cortisone *see* Corticosteroids
Co-trimoxazole *see* Trimethoprim and Sulfamethoxazole
Coumarins
Note Change in patient's clinical condition, particularly associated with liver disease, intercurrent illness, or drug administration, necessitates more frequent testing. Major changes in diet (especially involving salads and vegetables) and in alcohol consumption may also affect anticoagulant control
• Alcohol: anticoagulant control with coumarins may be affected by major changes in consumption of •alcohol
Allopurinol: anticoagulant effect of coumarins possibly enhanced by allopurinol
• Anabolic Steroids: anticoagulant effect of coumarins enhanced by •anabolic steroids
• Analgesics: anticoagulant effect of coumarins possibly enhanced by •NSAIDs, •celecoxib, •dextropropoxyphene, •etodolac, •etoricoxib, •flurbiprofen, •ibuprofen, •mefenamic acid, •meloxicam, •parecoxib, •piroxicam and •sulindac; anticoagulant effect of coumarins enhanced by •azapropazone (avoid concomitant use); anticoagulant effect of coumarins possibly enhanced by •diclofenac, also increased risk of haemorrhage with intravenous diclofenac (avoid concomitant use); increased risk of bleeding when coumarins given with •ketorolac (avoid concomitant use); anticoagulant effect of coumarins enhanced by •tramadol; increased risk of bleeding when coumarins given with •aspirin (due to antiplatelet effect); anticoagulant effect of coumarins possibly enhanced by prolonged regular use of paracetamol
• Anti-arrhythmics: metabolism of coumarins inhibited by •amiodarone (enhanced anticoagulant effect); anticoagulant effect of coumarins enhanced by •propafenone
• Antibacterials: experience in anticoagulant clinics suggests that INR possibly altered when coumarins are given with •neomycin (given for local action on gut); anticoagulant effect of coumarins enhanced by

Coumarins

- Antibacterials *(continued)*
  •chloramphenicol, •ciprofloxacin, •clarithromycin, •erythromycin, •metronidazole, •nalidixic acid, •norfloxacin, •ofloxacin and •sulphonamides; anticoagulant effect of coumarins possibly enhanced by •aztreonam, •cephalosporins, levofloxacin, •macrolides, •tetracyclines, tigecycline and trimethoprim; studies have failed to demonstrate an interaction with coumarins, but common experience in anticoagulant clinics is that INR can be altered by a course of broad-spectrum penicillins such as ampicillin; metabolism of coumarins accelerated by •rifamycins (reduced anticoagulant effect)
- Antidepressants: anticoagulant effect of warfarin possibly enhanced by •venlafaxine; anticoagulant effect of coumarins possibly enhanced by •SSRIs; anticoagulant effect of coumarins reduced by •St John's wort (avoid concomitant use); anticoagulant effect of warfarin enhanced by mirtazapine; anticoagulant effect of coumarins may be enhanced or reduced by •tricyclics
- Antidiabetics: anticoagulant effect of warfarin possibly enhanced by exenatide; coumarins possibly enhance hypoglycaemic effect of •sulphonylureas, also possible changes to anticoagulant effect
- Antiepileptics: metabolism of coumarins accelerated by •carbamazepine and •primidone (reduced anticoagulant effect); metabolism of coumarins accelerated by •phenytoin (possibility of reduced anticoagulant effect, but enhancement also reported); anticoagulant effect of coumarins possibly enhanced by valproate
- Antifungals: anticoagulant effect of coumarins enhanced by •fluconazole, •itraconazole, •ketoconazole and •voriconazole; anticoagulant effect of coumarins enhanced by •miconazole (miconazole oral gel and possibly vaginal formulations absorbed); anticoagulant effect of coumarins reduced by •griseofulvin

  Antimalarials: isolated reports that anticoagulant effect of warfarin may be enhanced by proguanil
- Antivirals: anticoagulant effect of coumarins may be enhanced or reduced by amprenavir; anticoagulant effect of warfarin may be enhanced or reduced by atazanavir, •nevirapine and •ritonavir; anticoagulant effect of coumarins possibly enhanced by •ritonavir; anticoagulant effect of warfarin possibly enhanced by saquinavir

  Anxiolytics and Hypnotics: anticoagulant effect of coumarins may transiently be enhanced by chloral and triclofos

  Aprepitant: anticoagulant effect of warfarin possibly reduced by aprepitant
- Barbiturates: metabolism of coumarins accelerated by •barbiturates (reduced anticoagulant effect)

  Bosentan: monitoring anticoagulant effect of coumarins recommended by manufacturer of bosentan
- Clopidogrel: anticoagulant effect of coumarins enhanced due to antiplatelet action of •clopidogrel; avoidance of warfarin advised by manufacturer of •clopidogrel
- Corticosteroids: anticoagulant effect of coumarins may be enhanced or reduced by •corticosteroids (high-dose corticosteroids enhance anticoagulant effect)
- Cranberry Juice: anticoagulant effect of coumarins possibly enhanced by •cranberry juice—avoid concomitant use
- Cytotoxics: anticoagulant effect of coumarins possibly enhanced by •etoposide, •ifosfamide and •sorafenib; anticoagulant effect of coumarins enhanced by •fluorouracil; anticoagulant effect of coumarins possibly reduced by •azathioprine, •mercaptopurine and •mitotane; increased risk of bleeding when coumarins given with •erlotinib; replacement of warfarin with a heparin advised by manufacturer of imatinib (possibility of enhanced warfarin effect)
- Dipyridamole: anticoagulant effect of coumarins enhanced due to antiplatelet action of •dipyridamole

Coumarins *(continued)*

- Disulfiram: anticoagulant effect of coumarins enhanced by •disulfiram
- Dopaminergics: anticoagulant effect of warfarin enhanced by •entacapone
- Enteral Foods: anticoagulant effect of coumarins antagonised by vitamin K (present in some •enteral feeds)
- Glucosamine: anticoagulant effect of warfarin enhanced by •glucosamine (avoid concomitant use)
- Hormone Antagonists: anticoagulant effect of coumarins possibly enhanced by bicalutamide and •toremifene; metabolism of coumarins inhibited by •danazol (enhanced anticoagulant effect); anticoagulant effect of coumarins enhanced by •flutamide and •tamoxifen

  Iloprost: anticoagulant effect of coumarins possibly enhanced by iloprost

  Lactulose: anticoagulant effect of coumarins possibly enhanced by lactulose

  Leflunomide: anticoagulant effect of warfarin possibly enhanced by leflunomide

  Leukotriene Antagonists: anticoagulant effect of warfarin enhanced by zafirlukast
- Levamisole: anticoagulant effect of warfarin possibly enhanced by •levamisole
- Lipid-regulating Drugs: anticoagulant effect of coumarins may be enhanced or reduced by •colestyramine; anticoagulant effect of warfarin may be transiently reduced by atorvastatin; anticoagulant effect of coumarins enhanced by •fibrates, •fluvastatin and simvastatin; anticoagulant effect of coumarins possibly enhanced by ezetimibe and •rosuvastatin

  Memantine: anticoagulant effect of warfarin possibly enhanced by memantine
- Oestrogens: anticoagulant effect of coumarins may be enhanced or reduced by •oestrogens

  Orlistat: monitoring anticoagulant effect of coumarins recommended by manufacturer of orlistat
- Progestogens: anticoagulant effect of coumarins may be enhanced or reduced by •progestogens

  Raloxifene: anticoagulant effect of coumarins antagonised by raloxifene
- Retinoids: anticoagulant effect of coumarins possibly reduced by •acitretin

  Sibutramine: increased risk of bleeding when anticoagulants given with sibutramine
- Sitaxentan: anticoagulant effect of coumarins enhanced by •sitaxentan
- Sulfinpyrazone: anticoagulant effect of coumarins enhanced by •sulfinpyrazone
- Sympathomimetics: anticoagulant effect of coumarins possibly enhanced by •methylphenidate

  Terpene Mixture: anticoagulant effect of coumarins possibly reduced by Rowachol®
- Testolactone: anticoagulant effect of coumarins enhanced by •testolactone
- Testosterone: anticoagulant effect of coumarins enhanced by •testosterone
- Thyroid Hormones: anticoagulant effect of coumarins enhanced by •thyroid hormones

  Ubidecarenone: anticoagulant effect of warfarin may be enhanced or reduced by ubidecarenone
- Ulcer-healing Drugs: metabolism of coumarins inhibited by •cimetidine (enhanced anticoagulant effect); anticoagulant effect of coumarins possibly enhanced by •esomeprazole, •omeprazole and pantoprazole; absorption of coumarins possibly reduced by •sucralfate (reduced anticoagulant effect)

  Vaccines: anticoagulant effect of warfarin possibly enhanced by influenza vaccine
- Vitamins: anticoagulant effect of coumarins antagonised by •vitamin K

Cranberry Juice

- Anticoagulants: cranberry juice possibly enhances anticoagulant effect of •coumarins—avoid concomitant use

Cyclizine *see* Antihistamines

Cyclopenthiazide *see* Diuretics

Cyclopentolate *see* Antimuscarinics

Cyclophosphamide

Antiepileptics: cytotoxics possibly reduce absorption of phenytoin

Antifungals: side-effects of cyclophosphamide possibly increased by itraconazole

• Antipsychotics: avoid concomitant use of cytotoxics with •clozapine (increased risk of agranulocytosis)

Cardiac Glycosides: cytotoxics reduce absorption of digoxin tablets

• Cytotoxics: increased toxicity when high-dose cyclophosphamide given with •pentostatin—avoid concomitant use

Muscle Relaxants: cyclophosphamide enhances effects of suxamethonium

Cycloserine

• Alcohol: increased risk of convulsions when cycloserine given with •alcohol

Antibacterials: increased risk of CNS toxicity when cycloserine given with isoniazid

Oestrogens: antibacterials that do not induce liver enzymes possibly reduce contraceptive effect of oestrogens (risk probably small, see p. 428)

Cyproheptadine *see* Antihistamines

Cytarabine

Antiepileptics: cytotoxics possibly reduce absorption of phenytoin

Antifungals: cytarabine possibly reduces plasma concentration of flucytosine

• Antipsychotics: avoid concomitant use of cytotoxics with •clozapine (increased risk of agranulocytosis)

Cardiac Glycosides: cytotoxics reduce absorption of digoxin tablets

Cytotoxics: intracellular concentration of cytarabine increased by fludarabine

Cytotoxics *see* individual drugs

Dairy Products

Antibacterials: dairy products reduces absorption of ciprofloxacin and norfloxacin; dairy products reduces absorption of tetracyclines (except doxycycline and minocycline)

Dalteparin *see* Heparins

Danazol

• Anticoagulants: danazol inhibits metabolism of •coumarins (enhanced anticoagulant effect)

• Antiepileptics: danazol inhibits metabolism of •carbamazepine (increased risk of toxicity)

• Ciclosporin: danazol inhibits metabolism of •ciclosporin (increased plasma concentration)

• Lipid-regulating Drugs: possible increased risk of myopathy when danazol given with •simvastatin

Tacrolimus: danazol possibly increases plasma concentration of tacrolimus

Dantrolene *see* Muscle Relaxants

Dapsone

Antibacterials: plasma concentration of dapsone reduced by rifamycins; plasma concentration of both drugs may increase when dapsone given with trimethoprim

Antivirals: plasma concentration of dapsone possibly increased by amprenavir

Oestrogens: antibacterials that do not induce liver enzymes possibly reduce contraceptive effect of oestrogens (risk probably small, see p. 428)

Probenecid: excretion of dapsone reduced by probenecid (increased risk of side-effects)

Daptomycin

• Ciclosporin: increased risk of myopathy when daptomycin given with •ciclosporin (preferably avoid concomitant use)

• Lipid-regulating Drugs: increased risk of myopathy when daptomycin given with •fibrates or •statins (preferably avoid concomitant use)

Oestrogens: antibacterials that do not induce liver enzymes possibly reduce contraceptive effect of oestrogens (risk probably small, see p. 428)

Darbepoetin *see* Epoetin

Darifenacin *see* Antimuscarinics

Darunavir

Anti-arrhythmics: darunavir possibly increases plasma concentration of lidocaine (lignocaine)—avoid concomitant use

• Antibacterials: darunavir increases plasma concentration of •rifabutin (reduce dose of rifabutin); plasma concentration of darunavir significantly reduced by •rifampicin—avoid concomitant use

• Antidepressants: darunavir possibly reduces plasma concentration of paroxetine and sertraline; plasma concentration of darunavir reduced by •St John's wort—avoid concomitant use

Antiepileptics: plasma concentration of darunavir possibly reduced by carbamazepine and phenytoin

Antifungals: plasma concentration of both drugs increased when darunavir given with ketoconazole

• Antimalarials: avoid concomitant use of darunavir with •artemether/lumefantrine

• Antivirals: plasma concentration of darunavir reduced by efavirenz and saquinavir; plasma concentration of both drugs increased when darunavir given with indinavir; darunavir increases plasma concentration of lopinavir (also plasma concentration of darunavir reduced); darunavir increases plasma concentration of •maraviroc (consider reducing dose of maraviroc)

Barbiturates: plasma concentration of darunavir possibly reduced by phenobarbital

Lipid-regulating Drugs: darunavir possibly increases plasma concentration of pravastatin

Dasatinib

• Antibacterials: metabolism of dasatinib accelerated by •rifampicin (reduced plasma concentration—avoid concomitant use)

Antiepileptics: cytotoxics possibly reduce absorption of phenytoin

• Antipsychotics: avoid concomitant use of cytotoxics with •clozapine (increased risk of agranulocytosis)

Cardiac Glycosides: cytotoxics reduce absorption of digoxin tablets

Lipid-regulating Drugs: dasatinib possibly increases plasma concentration of simvastatin

Ulcer-healing Drugs: plasma concentration of dasatinib possibly reduced by famotidine

Deferasirox

Antacids: absorption of deferasirox possibly reduced by antacids containing aluminium (manufacturer of deferasirox advises avoid concomitant use)

Deflazacort *see* Corticosteroids

Demeclocycline *see* Tetracyclines

Desferrioxamine

Antipsychotics: avoidance of desferrioxamine advised by manufacturer of levomepromazine (methotrimeprazine); manufacturer of desferrioxamine advises avoid concomitant use with prochlorperazine

Desflurane *see* Anaesthetics, General

Desloratadine *see* Antihistamines

Desmopressin

Analgesics: effects of desmopressin enhanced by indometacin

Loperamide: plasma concentration of *oral* desmopressin increased by loperamide

Desogestrel *see* Progestogens

Dexamethasone *see* Corticosteroids

Dexamfetamine *see* Sympathomimetics

Dexibuprofen *see* NSAIDs

Dexketoprofen *see* NSAIDs

Dextromethorphan *see* Opioid Analgesics

Dextropropoxyphene *see* Opioid Analgesics

Diamorphine *see* Opioid Analgesics

Diazepam *see* Anxiolytics and Hypnotics

Diazoxide

ACE Inhibitors: enhanced hypotensive effect when diazoxide given with ACE inhibitors

Adrenergic Neurone Blockers: enhanced hypotensive effect when diazoxide given with adrenergic neurone blockers

Alcohol: enhanced hypotensive effect when diazoxide given with alcohol

Diazoxide *(continued)*
Aldesleukin: enhanced hypotensive effect when diazoxide given with aldesleukin
Alpha-blockers: enhanced hypotensive effect when diazoxide given with alpha-blockers
Anaesthetics, General: enhanced hypotensive effect when diazoxide given with general anaesthetics
Analgesics: hypotensive effect of diazoxide antagonised by NSAIDs
Angiotensin-II Receptor Antagonists: enhanced hypotensive effect when diazoxide given with angiotensin-II receptor antagonists
Antidepressants: enhanced hypotensive effect when diazoxide given with MAOIs or tricyclic-related antidepressants
Antidiabetics: diazoxide antagonises hypoglycaemic effect of antidiabetics
Antiepileptics: diazoxide reduces plasma concentration of phenytoin, also effect of diazoxide may be reduced
Antipsychotics: enhanced hypotensive effect when diazoxide given with phenothiazines
Anxiolytics and Hypnotics: enhanced hypotensive effect when diazoxide given with anxiolytics and hypnotics
Beta-blockers: enhanced hypotensive effect when diazoxide given with beta-blockers
Calcium-channel Blockers: enhanced hypotensive effect when diazoxide given with calcium-channel blockers
Clonidine: enhanced hypotensive effect when diazoxide given with clonidine
Corticosteroids: hypotensive effect of diazoxide antagonised by corticosteroids
Diuretics: enhanced hypotensive effect when diazoxide given with diuretics
Dopaminergics: enhanced hypotensive effect when diazoxide given with levodopa
Methyldopa: enhanced hypotensive effect when diazoxide given with methyldopa
Moxisylyte (thymoxamine): enhanced hypotensive effect when diazoxide given with moxisylyte
Moxonidine: enhanced hypotensive effect when diazoxide given with moxonidine
Muscle Relaxants: enhanced hypotensive effect when diazoxide given with baclofen or tizanidine
Nitrates: enhanced hypotensive effect when diazoxide given with nitrates
Oestrogens: hypotensive effect of diazoxide antagonised by oestrogens
Prostaglandins: enhanced hypotensive effect when diazoxide given with alprostadil
Vasodilator Antihypertensives: enhanced hypotensive effect when diazoxide given with hydralazine, minoxidil or sodium nitroprusside

Diclofenac *see* NSAIDs
Dicycloverine (dicyclomine) *see* Antimuscarinics
Didanosine
Note Antacids in tablet formulation may affect absorption of other drugs
Allopurinol: plasma concentration of didanosine possibly increased by allopurinol
• Antivirals: plasma concentration of didanosine possibly increased by ganciclovir; increased risk of side-effects when didanosine given with •ribavirin or •stavudine; plasma concentration of didanosine increased by •tenofovir (increased risk of toxicity)—avoid concomitant use; plasma concentration of didanosine reduced by •tipranavir
• Cytotoxics: increased risk of toxicity when didanosine given with •hydroxycarbamide—avoid concomitant use

Digitoxin *see* Cardiac Glycosides
Digoxin *see* Cardiac Glycosides
Dihydrocodeine *see* Opioid Analgesics
Diltiazem *see* Calcium-channel Blockers
Dimercaprol
• Iron: avoid concomitant use of dimercaprol with •iron

Dinoprostone *see* Prostaglandins
Diphenoxylate *see* Opioid Analgesics
Diphenylpyraline *see* Antihistamines
Dipipanone *see* Opioid Analgesics
Dipivefrine *see* Sympathomimetics
Dipyridamole
Antacids: absorption of dipyridamole possibly reduced by antacids
• Anti-arrhythmics: dipyridamole enhances and extends the effects of •adenosine (important risk of toxicity)
• Anticoagulants: antiplatelet action of dipyridamole enhances anticoagulant effect of •coumarins and •phenindione; dipyridamole enhances anticoagulant effect of heparins
Clopidogrel: increased risk of bleeding when dipyridamole given with clopidogrel
Cytotoxics: dipyridamole possibly reduces effects of fludarabine

Disodium Etidronate *see* Bisphosphonates
Disodium Pamidronate *see* Bisphosphonates
Disopyramide
Anaesthetics, Local: increased myocardial depression when anti-arrhythmics given with bupivacaine, levobupivacaine, prilocaine or ropivacaine
• Anti-arrhythmics: increased myocardial depression when anti-arrhythmics given with other •anti-arrhythmics; increased risk of ventricular arrhythmias when disopyramide given with •amiodarone—avoid concomitant use
• Antibacterials: plasma concentration of disopyramide possibly increased by •clarithromycin (increased risk of toxicity); plasma concentration of disopyramide increased by •erythromycin (increased risk of toxicity); increased risk of ventricular arrhythmias when disopyramide given with •moxifloxacin or •quinupristin/dalfopristin—avoid concomitant use; metabolism of disopyramide accelerated by •rifamycins (reduced plasma concentration)
• Antidepressants: increased risk of ventricular arrhythmias when disopyramide given with •tricyclics
Antidiabetics: disopyramide possibly enhances hypoglycaemic effect of gliclazide, insulin and metformin
Antiepileptics: plasma concentration of disopyramide reduced by phenytoin; metabolism of disopyramide accelerated by primidone (reduced plasma concentration)
• Antifungals: increased risk of ventricular arrhythmias when disopyramide given with •ketoconazole—avoid concomitant use
• Antihistamines: increased risk of ventricular arrhythmias when disopyramide given with •mizolastine—avoid concomitant use
• Antimalarials: avoidance of disopyramide advised by manufacturer of •artemether/lumefantrine (risk of ventricular arrhythmias)
Antimuscarinics: increased risk of antimuscarinic side-effects when disopyramide given with antimuscarinics
• Antipsychotics: increased risk of ventricular arrhythmias when anti-arrhythmics that prolong the QT interval given with •antipsychotics that prolong the QT interval; increased risk of ventricular arrhythmias when disopyramide given with •amisulpride, •pimozide or •sertindole—avoid concomitant use; increased risk of ventricular arrhythmias when disopyramide given with •phenothiazines
• Antivirals: plasma concentration of disopyramide possibly increased by •ritonavir (increased risk of toxicity)
• Atomoxetine: increased risk of ventricular arrhythmias when disopyramide given with •atomoxetine
Barbiturates: metabolism of disopyramide accelerated by barbiturates (reduced plasma concentration)
• Beta-blockers: increased myocardial depression when anti-arrhythmics given with •beta-blockers; increased risk of ventricular arrhythmias when disopyramide given with •sotalol—avoid concomitant use
• Calcium-channel Blockers: increased risk of myocardial depression and asystole when disopyramide given with •verapamil
• Diuretics: increased cardiac toxicity with disopyramide if hypokalaemia occurs with •acetazolamide, •loop diuretics or •thiazides and related diuretics
• $5HT_3$ Antagonists: increased risk of ventricular arrhythmias when disopyramide given with •dolasetron—

Disopyramide
- 5HT$_3$ Antagonists *(continued)* avoid concomitant use; caution with anti-arrhythmics advised by manufacturer of tropisetron (risk of ventricular arrhythmias)
- Ivabradine: increased risk of ventricular arrhythmias when disopyramide given with •ivabradine

Nitrates: disopyramide reduces effects of sublingual tablets of nitrates (failure to dissolve under tongue owing to dry mouth)

Distigmine *see* Parasympathomimetics

Disulfiram

Alcohol: disulfiram reaction when disulfiram given with alcohol (see p. 270)

Antibacterials: psychotic reaction reported when disulfiram given with metronidazole
- Anticoagulants: disulfiram enhances anticoagulant effect of •coumarins

Antidepressants: increased disulfiram reaction with alcohol reported with concomitant amitriptyline; disulfiram inhibits metabolism of tricyclics (increased plasma concentration)
- Antiepileptics: disulfiram inhibits metabolism of •phenytoin (increased risk of toxicity)

Anxiolytics and Hypnotics: disulfiram increases risk of temazepam toxicity; disulfiram inhibits metabolism of benzodiazepines (increased sedative effects)
- Paraldehyde: risk of toxicity when disulfiram given with •paraldehyde

Theophylline: disulfiram inhibits metabolism of theophylline (increased risk of toxicity)

Diuretics

Note Since systemic absorption may follow topical application of brinzolamide to the eye, the possibility of interactions should be borne in mind

Note Since systemic absorption may follow topical application of dorzolamide to the eye, the possibility of interactions should be borne in mind
- ACE Inhibitors: enhanced hypotensive effect when diuretics given with •ACE inhibitors; increased risk of severe hyperkalaemia when potassium-sparing diuretics and aldosterone antagonists given with •ACE inhibitors (monitor potassium concentration with low-dose spironolactone in heart failure)

Adrenergic Neurone Blockers: enhanced hypotensive effect when diuretics given with adrenergic neurone blockers

Alcohol: enhanced hypotensive effect when diuretics given with alcohol

Aldesleukin: enhanced hypotensive effect when diuretics given with aldesleukin

Aliskiren: plasma concentration of furosemide (frusemide) reduced by aliskiren; increased risk of hyperkalaemia when potassium-sparing diuretics and aldosterone antagonists given with aliskiren

Allopurinol: increased risk of hypersensitivity when thiazides and related diuretics given with allopurinol especially in renal impairment
- Alpha-blockers: enhanced hypotensive effect when diuretics given with •alpha-blockers, also increased risk of first-dose hypotension with post-synaptic alpha-blockers such as prazosin

Anaesthetics, General: enhanced hypotensive effect when diuretics given with general anaesthetics
- Analgesics: diuretics increase risk of nephrotoxicity of NSAIDs, also antagonism of diuretic effect; possibly increased risk of hyperkalaemia when potassium-sparing diuretics and aldosterone antagonists given with NSAIDs; effects of diuretics antagonised by indometacin and ketorolac; increased risk of hyperkalaemia when potassium-sparing diuretics and aldosterone antagonists given with indometacin; occasional reports of reduced renal function when triamterene given with •indometacin—avoid concomitant use; diuretic effect of spironolactone antagonised by aspirin; increased risk of toxicity when carbonic anhydrase inhibitors given with high-dose aspirin
- Angiotensin-II Receptor Antagonists: enhanced hypotensive effect when diuretics given with •angiotensin-II receptor antagonists; increased risk of hyperkalaemia when potassium-sparing diuretics and aldosterone antagonists given with •angiotensin-II receptor antagonists
- Anti-arrhythmics: hypokalaemia caused by acetazolamide, loop diuretics or thiazides and related diuretics increases cardiac toxicity with amiodarone; plasma concentration of eplerenone increased by amiodarone (reduce dose of eplerenone); hypokalaemia caused by acetazolamide, loop diuretics or thiazides and related diuretics increases cardiac toxicity with •disopyramide; hypokalaemia caused by acetazolamide, loop diuretics or thiazides and related diuretics increases cardiac toxicity with •flecainide; hypokalaemia caused by acetazolamide, loop diuretics or thiazides and related diuretics antagonises action of •lidocaine (lignocaine); hypokalaemia caused by acetazolamide, loop diuretics or thiazides and related diuretics antagonises action of •mexiletine
- Antibacterials: plasma concentration of eplerenone increased by •clarithromycin and •telithromycin—avoid concomitant use; plasma concentration of eplerenone increased by erythromycin (reduce dose of eplerenone); plasma concentration of eplerenone reduced by •rifampicin—avoid concomitant use; avoidance of diuretics advised by manufacturer of lymecycline; increased risk of otoxicity when loop diuretics given with •aminoglycosides, •polymyxins or •vancomycin; acetazolamide antagonises effects of •methenamine; increased risk of hyperkalaemia when eplerenone given with trimethoprim
- Antidepressants: possible increased risk of hypokalaemia when loop diuretics or thiazides and related diuretics given with reboxetine; enhanced hypotensive effect when diuretics given with MAOIs; plasma concentration of eplerenone reduced by •St John's wort—avoid concomitant use; increased risk of postural hypotension when diuretics given with tricyclics

Antidiabetics: loop diuretics and thiazides and related diuretics antagonise hypoglycaemic effect of antidiabetics; increased risk of hyponatraemia when thiazides and related diuretics plus potassium-sparing diuretic given with chlorpropamide; increased risk of hyponatraemia when potassium-sparing diuretics and aldosterone antagonists plus thiazide given with chlorpropamide
- Antiepileptics: acetazolamide increases plasma concentration of •carbamazepine; plasma concentration of eplerenone reduced by •carbamazepine and •phenytoin—avoid concomitant use; increased risk of hyponatraemia when diuretics given with carbamazepine; increased risk of osteomalacia when carbonic anhydrase inhibitors given with phenytoin or primidone; effects of furosemide (frusemide) antagonised by phenytoin; acetazolamide possibly reduces plasma concentration of primidone
- Antifungals: plasma concentration of eplerenone increased by •itraconazole and •ketoconazole—avoid concomitant use; increased risk of hypokalaemia when loop diuretics or thiazides and related diuretics given with amphotericin; hydrochlorothiazide increases plasma concentration of fluconazole; plasma concentration of eplerenone increased by fluconazole (reduce dose of eplerenone)
- Antipsychotics: hypokalaemia caused by diuretics increases risk of ventricular arrhythmias with •amisulpride or •sertindole; enhanced hypotensive effect when diuretics given with phenothiazines; hypokalaemia caused by diuretics increases risk of ventricular arrhythmias with •pimozide (avoid concomitant use)
- Antivirals: plasma concentration of eplerenone increased by •nelfinavir and •ritonavir—avoid concomitant use; plasma concentration of eplerenone increased by saquinavir (reduce dose of eplerenone)

Diuretics *(continued)*

Anxiolytics and Hypnotics: enhanced hypotensive effect when diuretics given with anxiolytics and hypnotics; administration of parenteral furosemide (frusemide) with chloral or triclofos may displace thyroid hormone from binding sites

- Atomoxetine: hypokalaemia caused by diuretics increases risk of ventricular arrhythmias with •atomoxetine
- Barbiturates: plasma concentration of eplerenone reduced by •phenobarbital—avoid concomitant use; increased risk of osteomalacia when carbonic anhydrase inhibitors given with phenobarbital
- Beta-blockers: enhanced hypotensive effect when diuretics given with beta-blockers; hypokalaemia caused by loop diuretics or thiazides and related diuretics increases risk of ventricular arrhythmias with •sotalol

Calcium Salts: increased risk of hypercalcaemia when thiazides and related diuretics given with calcium salts

Calcium-channel Blockers: enhanced hypotensive effect when diuretics given with calcium-channel blockers; plasma concentration of eplerenone increased by diltiazem and verapamil (reduce dose of eplerenone)

- Cardiac Glycosides: hypokalaemia caused by acetazolamide, loop diuretics or thiazides and related diuretics increases cardiac toxicity with •cardiac glycosides; spironolactone possibly affects plasma concentration of digitoxin; spironolactone increases plasma concentration of •digoxin
- Ciclosporin: increased risk of nephrotoxicity and possibly hypermagnesaemia when thiazides and related diuretics given with ciclosporin; increased risk of hyperkalaemia when potassium-sparing diuretics and aldosterone antagonists given with •ciclosporin

Clonidine: enhanced hypotensive effect when diuretics given with clonidine

Corticosteroids: diuretic effect of diuretics antagonised by corticosteroids; increased risk of hypokalaemia when acetazolamide, loop diuretics or thiazides and related diuretics given with corticosteroids

Cytotoxics: avoidance of spironolactone advised by manufacturer of mitotane (antagonism of effect); increased risk of nephrotoxicity and ototoxicity when diuretics given with platinum compounds

Diazoxide: enhanced hypotensive effect when diuretics given with diazoxide

Diuretics: increased risk of hypokalaemia when loop diuretics or thiazides and related diuretics given with acetazolamide; profound diuresis possible when metolazone given with furosemide (frusemide); increased risk of hypokalaemia when thiazides and related diuretics given with loop diuretics

Dopaminergics: enhanced hypotensive effect when diuretics given with levodopa

Hormone Antagonists: increased risk of hypercalcaemia when thiazides and related diuretics given with toremifene; increased risk of hyperkalaemia when potassium-sparing diuretics and aldosterone antagonists given with trilostane

Lipid-regulating Drugs: absorption of thiazides and related diuretics reduced by colestipol and colestyramine (give at least 2 hours apart)

- Lithium: loop diuretics and thiazides and related diuretics reduce excretion of •lithium (increased plasma concentration and risk of toxicity)—loop diuretics safer than thiazides; potassium-sparing diuretics and aldosterone antagonists reduce excretion of •lithium (increased plasma concentration and risk of toxicity); acetazolamide increases the excretion of •lithium

Methyldopa: enhanced hypotensive effect when diuretics given with methyldopa

Moxisylyte (thymoxamine): enhanced hypotensive effect when diuretics given with moxisylyte

Moxonidine: enhanced hypotensive effect when diuretics given with moxonidine

Muscle Relaxants: enhanced hypotensive effect when diuretics given with baclofen or tizanidine

Diuretics *(continued)*

Nitrates: enhanced hypotensive effect when diuretics given with nitrates

Oestrogens: diuretic effect of diuretics antagonised by oestrogens

- Potassium Salts: increased risk of hyperkalaemia when potassium-sparing diuretics and aldosterone antagonists given with •potassium salts

Progestogens: risk of hyperkalaemia when potassium-sparing diuretics and aldosterone antagonists given with drospirenone (monitor serum potassium during first cycle)

Prostaglandins: enhanced hypotensive effect when diuretics given with alprostadil

Sympathomimetics, Beta$_2$: increased risk of hypokalaemia when acetazolamide, loop diuretics or thiazides and related diuretics given with high doses of beta$_2$ sympathomimetics—for CSM advice (hypokalaemia) see p. 150

- Tacrolimus: increased risk of hyperkalaemia when potassium-sparing diuretics and aldosterone antagonists given with •tacrolimus

Theophylline: increased risk of hypokalaemia when acetazolamide, loop diuretics or thiazides and related diuretics given with theophylline

Vasodilator Antihypertensives: enhanced hypotensive effect when diuretics given with hydralazine, minoxidil or sodium nitroprusside

Vitamins: increased risk of hypercalcaemia when thiazides and related diuretics given with vitamin D

Diuretics, Loop *see* Diuretics

Diuretics, Potassium-sparing and Aldosterone Antagonists *see* Diuretics

Diuretics, Thiazide and related *see* Diuretics

Dobutamine *see* Sympathomimetics

Docetaxel

Antibacterials: *in vitro* studies suggest a possible interaction between docetaxel and erythromycin (consult docetaxel product literature)

Antiepileptics: cytotoxics possibly reduce absorption of phenytoin

Antifungals: *in vitro* studies suggest a possible interaction between docetaxel and ketoconazole (consult docetaxel product literature)

- Antipsychotics: avoid concomitant use of cytotoxics with •clozapine (increased risk of agranulocytosis)

Cardiac Glycosides: cytotoxics reduce absorption of digoxin tablets

Ciclosporin: *in vitro* studies suggest a possible interaction between docetaxel and ciclosporin (consult docetaxel product literature)

Cytotoxics: plasma concentration of docetaxel increased by sorafenib

Dolasetron *see* 5HT$_3$ Antagonists

Domperidone

Analgesics: effects of domperidone on gastro-intestinal activity antagonised by opioid analgesics

- Antifungals: risk of arrhythmias with domperidone possibly increased by •ketoconazole

Antimuscarinics: effects of domperidone on gastro-intestinal activity antagonised by antimuscarinics

Dopaminergics: increased risk of extrapyramidal side-effects when domperidone given with amantadine; domperidone possibly antagonises hypoprolactinaemic effects of bromocriptine and cabergoline

Donepezil *see* Parasympathomimetics

Dopamine *see* Sympathomimetics

Dopaminergics *see* Amantadine, Apomorphine, Bromocriptine, Cabergoline, Entacapone, Levodopa, Pergolide, Pramipexole, Quinagolide, Rasagiline, Ropinirole, Rotigotine, Selegiline, and Tolcapone

Dopexamine *see* Sympathomimetics

Dorzolamide *see* Diuretics

Dosulepin (dothiepin) *see* Antidepressants, Tricyclic

Doxapram

Antidepressants: effects of doxapram enhanced by MAOIs

Sympathomimetics: increased risk of hypertension when doxapram given with sympathomimetics

Doxapram *(continued)*
Theophylline: increased CNS stimulation when doxapram given with theophylline
Doxazosin *see* Alpha-blockers
Doxepin *see* Antidepressants, Tricyclic
Doxorubicin
Antiepileptics: cytotoxics possibly reduce absorption of phenytoin
• Antipsychotics: avoid concomitant use of cytotoxics with •clozapine (increased risk of agranulocytosis)
Antivirals: doxorubicin possibly inhibits effects of stavudine
Cardiac Glycosides: cytotoxics reduce absorption of digoxin tablets
• Ciclosporin: increased risk of neurotoxicity when doxorubicin given with •ciclosporin
Cytotoxics: plasma concentration of doxorubicin possibly increased by sorafenib
Doxycycline *see* Tetracyclines
Drospirenone *see* Progestogens
Drotrecogin Alfa
• Anticoagulants: manufacturer of drotrecogin alfa advises avoid concomitant use with high doses of •heparin—consult product literature
Duloxetine
Analgesics: possible increased serotonergic effects when duloxetine given with pethidine or tramadol
• Antibacterials: metabolism of duloxetine inhibited by •ciprofloxacin—avoid concomitant use
• Antidepressants: metabolism of duloxetine inhibited by •fluvoxamine—avoid concomitant use; possible increased serotonergic effects when duloxetine given with SSRIs, St John's wort, amitriptyline, clomipramine, •moclobemide, tryptophan or venlafaxine; duloxetine should not be started until 2 weeks after stopping •MAOIs, also MAOIs should not be started until at least 5 days after stopping duloxetine; after stopping SSRI-related antidepressants do not start •moclobemide for at least 1 week
• Antimalarials: avoidance of antidepressants advised by manufacturer of •artemether/lumefantrine
Atomoxetine: possible increased risk of convulsions when antidepressants given with atomoxetine
$5HT_1$ Agonists: possible increased serotonergic effects when duloxetine given with $5HT_1$ agonists
• Sibutramine: increased risk of CNS toxicity when SSRI-related antidepressants given with •sibutramine (manufacturer of sibutramine advises avoid concomitant use)
Dutasteride
Calcium-channel Blockers: plasma concentration of dutasteride increased by diltiazem and verapamil
Dydrogesterone *see* Progestogens
Edrophonium *see* Parasympathomimetics
Efalizumab
• Vaccines: discontinue efalizumab 8 weeks before and until 2 weeks after vaccination with live or live-attenuated •vaccines
Efavirenz
Analgesics: efavirenz reduces plasma concentration of methadone
Antibacterials: increased risk of rash when efavirenz given with clarithromycin; efavirenz reduces plasma concentration of rifabutin—increase dose of rifabutin; plasma concentration of efavirenz reduced by rifampicin—increase dose of efavirenz
• Antidepressants: efavirenz reduces plasma concentration of sertraline; plasma concentration of efavirenz reduced by •St John's wort—avoid concomitant use
Antiepileptics: plasma concentration of both drugs reduced when efavirenz given with carbamazepine
• Antifungals: efavirenz reduces plasma concentration of itraconazole; efavirenz reduces plasma concentration of •voriconazole, also plasma concentration of efavirenz increased (consider increasing voriconazole dose and reducing efavirenz dose); efavirenz possibly reduces plasma concentration of caspofungin—consider increasing dose of caspofungin

Efavirenz *(continued)*
• Antipsychotics: efavirenz possibly reduces plasma concentration of •aripiprazole—increase dose of aripiprazole; efavirenz possibly increases plasma concentration of •pimozide (increased risk of ventricular arrhythmias—avoid concomitant use)
• Antivirals: efavirenz reduces plasma concentration of amprenavir, darunavir, indinavir and lopinavir; efavirenz reduces plasma concentration of atazanavir—increase dose of atazanavir; efavirenz possibly reduces plasma concentration of •maraviroc—consider increasing dose of maraviroc; plasma concentration of efavirenz reduced by nevirapine; toxicity of efavirenz increased by ritonavir, monitor liver function tests; efavirenz significantly reduces plasma concentration of saquinavir
• Anxiolytics and Hypnotics: increased risk of prolonged sedation when efavirenz given with •midazolam—avoid concomitant use
Calcium-channel Blockers: efavirenz reduces plasma concentration of diltiazem
• Ergot Alkaloids: increased risk of ergotism when efavirenz given with •ergot alkaloids—avoid concomitant use
Grapefruit Juice: plasma concentration of efavirenz possibly increased by grapefruit juice
Lipid-regulating Drugs: efavirenz reduces plasma concentration of atorvastatin, pravastatin and simvastatin
Oestrogens: efavirenz possibly reduces contraceptive effect of oestrogens
Eletriptan *see* $5HT_1$ Agonists
Emtricitabine
Antivirals: manufacturer of emtricitabine advises avoid concomitant use with lamivudine
Enalapril *see* ACE Inhibitors
Enoxaparin *see* Heparins
Enoximone *see* Phosphodiesterase Inhibitors
Entacapone
• Anticoagulants: entacapone enhances anticoagulant effect of •warfarin
• Antidepressants: manufacturer of entacapone advises caution with moclobemide, paroxetine, tricyclics and venlafaxine; avoid concomitant use of entacapone with non-selective •MAOIs
Dopaminergics: entacapone possibly enhances effects of apomorphine; entacapone possibly reduces plasma concentration of rasagiline; manufacturer of entacapone advises max. dose of 10 mg selegiline if used concomitantly
Iron: absorption of entacapone reduced by *oral* iron
Memantine: effects of dopaminergics possibly enhanced by memantine
Methyldopa: entacapone possibly enhances effects of methyldopa; antiparkinsonian effect of dopaminergics antagonised by methyldopa
Sympathomimetics: entacapone possibly enhances effects of adrenaline (epinephrine), dobutamine, dopamine and noradrenaline (norepinephrine)
Enteral Foods
• Anticoagulants: the presence of vitamin K in some enteral feeds can antagonise the anticoagulant effect of •coumarins and •phenindione
Antiepileptics: enteral feeds possibly reduce absorption of phenytoin
Ephedrine *see* Sympathomimetics
Epinephrine (adrenaline) *see* Sympathomimetics
Epirubicin
Antiepileptics: cytotoxics possibly reduce absorption of phenytoin
• Antipsychotics: avoid concomitant use of cytotoxics with •clozapine (increased risk of agranulocytosis)
Cardiac Glycosides: cytotoxics reduce absorption of digoxin tablets
• Ulcer-healing Drugs: plasma concentration of epirubicin increased by •cimetidine
Eplerenone *see* Diuretics

Epoetin

ACE Inhibitors: antagonism of hypotensive effect and increased risk of hyperkalaemia when epoetin given with ACE inhibitors

Angiotensin-II Receptor Antagonists: antagonism of hypotensive effect and increased risk of hyperkalaemia when epoetin given with angiotensin-II receptor antagonists

Eprosartan *see* Angiotensin-II Receptor Antagonists

Eptifibatide

Iloprost: increased risk of bleeding when eptifibatide given with iloprost

Ergometrine *see* Ergot Alkaloids

Ergot Alkaloids

Anaesthetics, General: effects of ergometrine on the parturient uterus reduced by halothane

• Antibacterials: increased risk of ergotism when ergotamine and methysergide given with •macrolides or •telithromycin—avoid concomitant use; avoidance of ergotamine and methysergide advised by manufacturer of •quinupristin/dalfopristin; increased risk of ergotism when ergotamine and methysergide given with tetracyclines

Antidepressants: possible risk of hypertension when ergotamine and methysergide given with reboxetine

• Antifungals: increased risk of ergotism when ergotamine and methysergide given with •imidazoles or •triazoles—avoid concomitant use

• Antivirals: increased risk of ergotism when ergotamine and methysergide given with •amprenavir, •indinavir, •nelfinavir, •ritonavir or •saquinavir—avoid concomitant use; plasma concentration of ergot alkaloids possibly increased by •atazanavir—avoid concomitant use; increased risk of ergotism when ergot alkaloids given with •efavirenz—avoid concomitant use

Beta-blockers: increased peripheral vasoconstriction when ergotamine and methysergide given with beta-blockers

• $5HT_1$ Agonists: increased risk of vasospasm when ergotamine and methysergide given with •almotriptan, •rizatriptan, •sumatriptan or •zolmitriptan (avoid ergotamine and methysergide for 6 hours after almotriptan, rizatriptan, sumatriptan or zolmitriptan, avoid almotriptan, rizatriptan, sumatriptan or zolmitriptan for 24 hours after ergotamine and methysergide); increased risk of vasospasm when ergotamine and methysergide given with •eletriptan or •frovatriptan (avoid ergotamine and methysergide for 24 hours after eletriptan or frovatriptan, avoid eletriptan or frovatriptan for 24 hours after ergotamine and methysergide)

Sympathomimetics: increased risk of ergotism when ergotamine and methysergide given with sympathomimetics

• Ulcer-healing Drugs: increased risk of ergotism when ergotamine and methysergide given with •cimetidine—avoid concomitant use

Ergotamine and Methysergide *see* Ergot Alkaloids

Erlotinib

• Analgesics: increased risk of bleeding when erlotinib given with •NSAIDs

Antibacterials: metabolism of erlotinib accelerated by rifampicin (reduced plasma concentration)

• Anticoagulants: increased risk of bleeding when erlotinib given with •coumarins

Antiepileptics: cytotoxics possibly reduce absorption of phenytoin

Antifungals: metabolism of erlotinib inhibited by ketoconazole (increased plasma concentration)

• Antipsychotics: avoid concomitant use of cytotoxics with •clozapine (increased risk of agranulocytosis)

Cardiac Glycosides: cytotoxics reduce absorption of digoxin tablets

Cytotoxics: plasma concentration of erlotinib possibly increased by capecitabine

Tobacco: plasma concentration of erlotinib reduced by tobacco smoking

Ertapenem

Antiepileptics: ertapenem possibly reduces plasma concentration of valproate

Oestrogens: antibacterials that do not induce liver enzymes possibly reduce contraceptive effect of oestrogens (risk probably small, see p. 428)

Erythromycin *see* Macrolides

Erythropoietin *see* Epoetin

Escitalopram *see* Antidepressants, SSRI

Esmolol *see* Beta-blockers

Esomeprazole *see* Proton Pump Inhibitors

Estradiol *see* Oestrogens

Estriol *see* Oestrogens

Estrone *see* Oestrogens

Estropipate *see* Oestrogens

Etanercept

Abatacept: increased risk of side-effects when etanercept given with abatacept

• Anakinra: increased risk of side-effects when etanercept given with •anakinra—avoid concomitant use

• Vaccines: avoid concomitant use of etanercept with live •vaccines (see p. 641)

Ethinylestradiol *see* Oestrogens

Ethosuximide

• Antibacterials: metabolism of ethosuximide inhibited by •isoniazid (increased plasma concentration and risk of toxicity)

• Antidepressants: anticonvulsant effect of antiepileptics possibly antagonised by MAOIs and •tricyclic-related antidepressants (convulsive threshold lowered); anticonvulsant effect of antiepileptics antagonised by •SSRIs and •tricyclics (convulsive threshold lowered); avoid concomitant use of antiepileptics with •St John's wort

• Antiepileptics: plasma concentration of ethosuximide possibly reduced by carbamazepine and primidone; plasma concentration of ethosuximide possibly reduced by •phenytoin, also plasma concentration of phenytoin possibly increased; plasma concentration of ethosuximide possibly increased by valproate

• Antimalarials: possible increased risk of convulsions when antiepileptics given with chloroquine and hydroxychloroquine; anticonvulsant effect of antiepileptics antagonised by •mefloquine

• Antipsychotics: anticonvulsant effect of ethosuximide antagonised by •antipsychotics (convulsive threshold lowered)

Barbiturates: plasma concentration of ethosuximide possibly reduced by phenobarbital

Etodolac *see* NSAIDs

Etomidate *see* Anaesthetics, General

Etonogestrel *see* Progestogens

Etoposide

• Anticoagulants: etoposide possibly enhances anticoagulant effect of •coumarins

Antiepileptics: plasma concentration of etoposide possibly reduced by phenytoin; cytotoxics possibly reduce absorption of phenytoin

• Antipsychotics: avoid concomitant use of cytotoxics with •clozapine (increased risk of agranulocytosis)

Barbiturates: plasma concentration of etoposide possibly reduced by phenobarbital

Cardiac Glycosides: cytotoxics reduce absorption of digoxin tablets

Ciclosporin: plasma concentration of etoposide possibly increased by ciclosporin (increased risk of toxicity)

Etoricoxib *see* NSAIDs

Etynodiol *see* Progestogens

Exemestane

Antibacterials: plasma concentration of exemestane possibly reduced by rifampicin

Ezetimibe

Anticoagulants: ezetimibe possibly enhances anticoagulant effect of coumarins

• Ciclosporin: plasma concentration of both drugs may increase when ezetimibe given with •ciclosporin

Lipid-regulating Drugs: increased risk of cholelithiasis and gallbladder disease when ezetimibe given with fibrates—discontinue if suspected

Famciclovir
Probenecid: excretion of famciclovir possibly reduced by probenecid (increased plasma concentration)

Famotidine *see* Histamine H_2-antagonists
Felodipine *see* Calcium-channel Blockers
Fenbufen *see* NSAIDs
Fenofibrate *see* Fibrates
Fenoprofen *see* NSAIDs
Fenoterol *see* Sympathomimetics, $Beta_2$
Fentanyl *see* Opioid Analgesics
Ferrous Salts *see* Iron
Fexofenadine *see* Antihistamines

Fibrates
- Antibacterials: increased risk of myopathy when fibrates given with •daptomycin (preferably avoid concomitant use)
- Anticoagulants: fibrates enhance anticoagulant effect of •coumarins and •phenindione
- Antidiabetics: gemfibrozil increases plasma concentration of •rosiglitazone (consider reducing dose of rosiglitazone); fibrates may improve glucose tolerance and have an additive effect with insulin or sulphonylureas; gemfibrozil possibly enhances hypoglycaemic effect of nateglinide; increased risk of severe hypoglycaemia when gemfibrozil given with •repaglinide—avoid concomitant use

Ciclosporin: increased risk of renal impairment when bezafibrate or fenofibrate given with ciclosporin
- Cytotoxics: gemfibrozil increases plasma concentration of •bexarotene—avoid concomitant use
- Lipid-regulating Drugs: increased risk of cholelithiasis and gallbladder disaese when fibrates given with ezetimibe—discontinue if suspected; increased risk of myopathy when fibrates given with •statins; increased risk of myopathy when gemfibrozil given with •statins (preferably avoid concomitant use)

Filgrastim
Note Pegfilgrastim interactions as for filgrastim
Cytotoxics: neutropenia possibly exacerbated when filgrastim given with fluorouracil

Flavoxate *see* Antimuscarinics

Flecainide
Anaesthetics, Local: increased myocardial depression when anti-arrhythmics given with bupivacaine, levobupivacaine, prilocaine or ropivacaine
- Anti-arrhythmics: increased myocardial depression when anti-arrhythmics given with other •anti-arrhythmics; plasma concentration of flecainide increased by •amiodarone (halve dose of flecainide)
- Antidepressants: plasma concentration of flecainide increased by fluoxetine; increased risk of ventricular arrhythmias when flecainide given with •tricyclics
- Antihistamines: increased risk of ventricular arrhythmias when flecainide given with •mizolastine—avoid concomitant use
- Antimalarials: avoidance of flecainide advised by manufacturer of •artemether/lumefantrine (risk of ventricular arrhythmias); plasma concentration of flecainide increased by •quinine
- Antipsychotics: increased risk of ventricular arrhythmias when anti-arrhythmics that prolong the QT interval given with •antipsychotics that prolong the QT interval; increased risk of arrhythmias when flecainide given with •clozapine
- Antivirals: plasma concentration of flecainide possibly increased by •amprenavir (increased risk of ventricular arrhythmias—avoid concomitant use); plasma concentration of flecainide increased by •ritonavir (increased risk of ventricular arrhythmias—avoid concomitant use)
- Beta-blockers: increased risk of myocardial depression and bradycardia when flecainide given with •beta-blockers; increased myocardial depression when anti-arrhythmics given with •beta-blockers
- Calcium-channel Blockers: increased risk of myocardial depression and asystole when flecainide given with •verapamil

Flecainide *(continued)*
- Diuretics: increased cardiac toxicity with flecainide if hypokalaemia occurs with •acetazolamide, •loop diuretics or •thiazides and related diuretics
- $5HT_3$ Antagonists: increased risk of ventricular arrhythmias when flecainide given with •dolasetron—avoid concomitant use; caution with anti-arrhythmics advised by manufacturer of tropisetron (risk of ventricular arrhythmias)

Ulcer-healing Drugs: metabolism of flecainide inhibited by cimetidine (increased plasma concentration)

Flucloxacillin *see* Penicillins
Fluconazole *see* Antifungals, Triazole

Flucytosine
Antifungals: renal excretion of flucytosine decreased and cellular uptake increased by amphotericin (toxicity possibly increased)
Cytotoxics: plasma concentration of flucytosine possibly reduced by cytarabine

Fludarabine
Antiepileptics: cytotoxics possibly reduce absorption of phenytoin
- Antipsychotics: avoid concomitant use of cytotoxics with •clozapine (increased risk of agranulocytosis)

Cardiac Glycosides: cytotoxics reduce absorption of digoxin tablets
- Cytotoxics: fludarabine increases intracellular concentration of cytarabine; increased pulmonary toxicity when fludarabine given with •pentostatin (unacceptably high incidence of fatalities)

Dipyridamole: effects of fludarabine possibly reduced by dipyridamole

Fludrocortisone *see* Corticosteroids
Flunisolide *see* Corticosteroids

Fluorides
Calcium Salts: absorption of fluorides reduced by calcium salts

Fluorouracil
Note Capecitabine is a prodrug of fluorouracil
Note Tegafur is a prodrug of fluorouracil
- Allopurinol: manufacturer of capecitabine advises avoid concomitant use with •allopurinol

Antibacterials: metabolism of fluorouracil inhibited by metronidazole (increased toxicity)
- Anticoagulants: fluorouracil enhances anticoagulant effect of •coumarins

Antiepileptics: fluorouracil possibly inhibits metabolism of phenytoin (increased risk of toxicity); cytotoxics possibly reduce absorption of phenytoin
- Antipsychotics: avoid concomitant use of cytotoxics with •clozapine (increased risk of agranulocytosis)

Cardiac Glycosides: cytotoxics reduce absorption of digoxin tablets
Cytotoxics: capecitabine possibly increases plasma concentration of erlotinib
Filgrastim: neutropenia possibly exacerbated when fluorouracil given with filgrastim
- Temoporfin: increased skin photosensitivity when topical fluorouracil used with •temoporfin

Ulcer-healing Drugs: metabolism of fluorouracil inhibited by cimetidine (increased plasma concentration)

Fluoxetine *see* Antidepressants, SSRI
Flupentixol *see* Antipsychotics
Fluphenazine *see* Antipsychotics
Flurazepam *see* Anxiolytics and Hypnotics
Flurbiprofen *see* NSAIDs

Flutamide
- Anticoagulants: flutamide enhances anticoagulant effect of •coumarins

Fluticasone *see* Corticosteroids
Fluvastatin *see* Statins
Fluvoxamine *see* Antidepressants, SSRI

Folates
Aminosalicylates: absorption of folic acid possibly reduced by sulfasalazine
Antiepileptics: folates possibly reduce plasma concentration of phenytoin and primidone
Barbiturates: folates possibly reduce plasma concentration of phenobarbital

Folic Acid *see* Folates
Folinic Acid *see* Folates
Formoterol (eformoterol) *see* Sympathomimetics, $Beta_2$
Fosamprenavir *see* Amprenavir
Foscarnet
Antivirals: avoidance of foscarnet advised by manufacturer of lamivudine
Fosinopril *see* ACE Inhibitors
Fosphenytoin *see* Phenytoin
Framycetin *see* Aminoglycosides
Frovatriptan *see* $5HT_1$ Agonists
Furosemide (frusemide) *see* Diuretics
Fusidic Acid
• Antivirals: plasma concentration of both drugs increased when fusidic acid given with •ritonavir—avoid concomitant use
Lipid-regulating Drugs: possible increased risk of myopathy when fusidic acid given with atorvastatin or simvastatin
Oestrogens: antibacterials that do not induce liver enzymes possibly reduce contraceptive effect of oestrogens (risk probably small, see p. 428)
Gabapentin
Antacids: absorption of gabapentin reduced by antacids
• Antidepressants: anticonvulsant effect of antiepileptics possibly antagonised by MAOIs and •tricyclic-related antidepressants (convulsive threshold lowered); anticonvulsant effect of antiepileptics antagonised by •SSRIs and •tricyclics (convulsive threshold lowered); avoid concomitant use of antiepileptics with •St John's wort
• Antimalarials: possible increased risk of convulsions when antiepileptics given with chloroquine and hydroxychloroquine; anticonvulsant effect of antiepileptics antagonised by •mefloquine
Galantamine *see* Parasympathomimetics
Ganciclovir
Note Increased risk of myelosuppression with other myelosuppressive drugs—consult product literature
Note Valganciclovir interactions as for ganciclovir
• Antibacterials: increased risk of convulsions when ganciclovir given with •imipenem with cilastatin
• Antivirals: ganciclovir possibly increases plasma concentration of didanosine; avoidance of intravenous ganciclovir advised by manufacturer of lamivudine; profound myelosuppression when ganciclovir given with •zidovudine (if possible avoid concomitant administration, particularly during initial ganciclovir therapy)
Cytotoxics: plasma concentration of ganciclovir possibly increased by mycophenolate, also plasma concentration of inactive metabolite of mycophenolate possibly increased
Probenecid: excretion of ganciclovir reduced by probenecid (increased plasma concentration and risk of toxicity)
Tacrolimus: possible increased risk of nephrotoxicity when ganciclovir given with tacrolimus
Gemeprost *see* Prostaglandins
Gemfibrozil *see* Fibrates
Gentamicin *see* Aminoglycosides
Gestodene *see* Progestogens
Gestrinone
Antibacterials: metabolism of gestrinone accelerated by rifampicin (reduced plasma concentration)
Antiepileptics: metabolism of gestrinone accelerated by carbamazepine, phenytoin and primidone (reduced plasma concentration)
Barbiturates: metabolism of gestrinone accelerated by barbiturates (reduced plasma concentration)
Glibenclamide *see* Antidiabetics
Gliclazide *see* Antidiabetics
Glimepiride *see* Antidiabetics
Glipizide *see* Antidiabetics
Glucosamine
• Anticoagulants: glucosamine enhances anticoagulant effect of •warfarin (avoid concomitant use)
Glyceryl Trinitrate *see* Nitrates
Glycopyrronium *see* Antimuscarinics
Grapefruit Juice
Anti-arrhythmics: grapefruit juice increases plasma concentration of amiodarone
• Antimalarials: grapefruit juice possibly inhibits metabolism of •artemether/lumefantrine (avoid concomitant use)
Antivirals: grapefruit juice possibly increases plasma concentration of efavirenz
Anxiolytics and Hypnotics: grapefruit juice increases plasma concentration of buspirone
Calcium-channel Blockers: grapefruit juice increases plasma concentration of felodipine, isradipine, lacidipine, lercanidipine, nicardipine, nifedipine, nimodipine, nisoldipine and verapamil
• Ciclosporin: grapefruit juice increases plasma concentration of •ciclosporin (increased risk of toxicity)
Ivabradine: grapefruit juice increases plasma concentration of ivabradine
• Lipid-regulating Drugs: grapefruit juice possibly increases plasma concentration of atorvastatin; grapefruit juice increases plasma concentration of •simvastatin—avoid concomitant use
Sildenafil: grapefruit juice possibly increases plasma concentration of sildenafil
• Sirolimus: grapefruit juice increases plasma concentration of •sirolimus—avoid concomitant use
• Tacrolimus: grapefruit juice increases plasma concentration of •tacrolimus
Tadalafil: grapefruit juice possibly increases plasma concentration of tadalafil
• Vardenafil: grapefruit juice possibly increases plasma concentration of •vardenafil—avoid concomitant use
Griseofulvin
Alcohol: griseofulvin possibly enhances effects of alcohol
• Anticoagulants: griseofulvin reduces anticoagulant effect of •coumarins
Antiepileptics: absorption of griseofulvin reduced by primidone (reduced effect)
Barbiturates: absorption of griseofulvin reduced by phenobarbital (reduced effect)
Ciclosporin: griseofulvin possibly reduces plasma concentration of ciclosporin
• Oestrogens: griseofulvin accelerates metabolism of •oestrogens (reduced contraceptive effect—see p. 428)
• Progestogens: griseofulvin accelerates metabolism of •progestogens (reduced contraceptive effect—see p. 428)
Guanethidine *see* Adrenergic Neurone Blockers
Haloperidol *see* Antipsychotics
Halothane *see* Anaesthetics, General
Heparin *see* Heparins
Heparins
ACE Inhibitors: increased risk of hyperkalaemia when heparins given with ACE inhibitors
Aliskiren: increased risk of hyperkalaemia when heparins given with aliskiren
• Analgesics: possible increased risk of bleeding when heparins given with NSAIDs; increased risk of haemorrhage when heparins given with intravenous •diclofenac (avoid concomitant use, including low-dose heparin); increased risk of haemorrhage when heparins given with •ketorolac (avoid concomitant use, including low-dose heparin); anticoagulant effect of heparins enhanced by •aspirin
Angiotensin-II Receptor Antagonists: increased risk of hyperkalaemia when heparin given with angiotensin-II receptor antagonists
Clopidogrel: increased risk of bleeding when heparins given with clopidogrel
Dipyridamole: anticoagulant effect of heparins enhanced by dipyridamole
• Drotrecogin Alfa: avoidance of concomitant use of high doses of heparin with drotrecogin alfa advised by manufacturer of •drotrecogin alfa—consult product literature
Iloprost: anticoagulant effect of heparins possibly enhanced by iloprost

Heparins *(continued)*
- • Nitrates: anticoagulant effect of heparins reduced by infusion of •glyceryl trinitrate
- Sibutramine: increased risk of bleeding when anticoagulants given with sibutramine

Histamine H_2-antagonists
- • Alpha-blockers: cimetidine and ranitidine antagonise effects of •tolazoline
- Analgesics: cimetidine possibly increases plasma concentration of azapropazone; cimetidine inhibits metabolism of opioid analgesics (increased plasma concentration)
- • Anti-arrhythmics: cimetidine increases plasma concentration of amiodarone, •procainamide and •propafenone; cimetidine inhibits metabolism of flecainide (increased plasma concentration); cimetidine increases plasma concentration of •lidocaine (lignocaine) (increased risk of toxicity)
- Antibacterials: histamine H_2-antagonists reduce absorption of cefpodoxime; cimetidine increases plasma concentration of erythromycin (increased risk of toxicity, including deafness); cimetidine inhibits metabolism of metronidazole (increased plasma concentration); metabolism of cimetidine accelerated by rifampicin (reduced plasma concentration)
- • Anticoagulants: cimetidine inhibits metabolism of •coumarins (enhanced anticoagulant effect)
- Antidepressants: cimetidine increases plasma concentration of citalopram, escitalopram, mirtazapine and sertraline; cimetidine inhibits metabolism of amitriptyline, doxepin, imipramine and nortriptyline (increased plasma concentration); cimetidine increases plasma concentration of moclobemide (halve dose of moclobemide); cimetidine possibly increases plasma concentration of tricyclics
- Antidiabetics: cimetidine reduces excretion of metformin (increased plasma concentration); cimetidine enhances hypoglycaemic effect of sulphonylureas
- • Antiepileptics: cimetidine inhibits metabolism of •carbamazepine, •phenytoin and •valproate (increased plasma concentration)
- • Antifungals: histamine H_2-antagonists reduce absorption of itraconazole and ketoconazole; cimetidine reduces plasma concentration of •posaconazole; cimetidine increases plasma concentration of terbinafine
- Antihistamines: manufacturer of loratadine advises cimetidine possibly increases plasma concentration of loratadine
- • Antimalarials: avoidance of cimetidine advised by manufacturer of •artemether/lumefantrine; cimetidine inhibits metabolism of chloroquine and hydroxychloroquine and quinine (increased plasma concentration)
- • Antipsychotics: cimetidine possibly enhances effects of antipsychotics, chlorpromazine and clozapine; increased risk of ventricular arrhythmias when cimetidine given with •sertindole—avoid concomitant use
- Antivirals: plasma concentration of cimetidine possibly increased by amprenavir; histamine H_2-antagonists possibly reduce plasma concentration of atazanavir
- Anxiolytics and Hypnotics: cimetidine inhibits metabolism of benzodiazepines, clomethiazole and zaleplon (increased plasma concentration)
- Beta-blockers: cimetidine increases plasma concentration of labetalol, metoprolol and propranolol
- Calcium-channel Blockers: cimetidine possibly inhibits metabolism of calcium-channel blockers (increased plasma concentration)
- • Ciclosporin: cimetidine possibly increases plasma concentration of •ciclosporin
- • Cilostazol: cimetidine possibly increases plasma concentration of •cilostazol—avoid concomitant use
- • Cytotoxics: cimetidine increases plasma concentration of •epirubicin; cimetidine inhibits metabolism of fluorouracil (increased plasma concentration); famotidine possibly reduces plasma concentration of dasatinib
- Dopaminergics: cimetidine reduces excretion of pramipexole (increased plasma concentration)

Histamine H_2-antagonists *(continued)*
- • Ergot Alkaloids: increased risk of ergotism when cimetidine given with •ergotamine and methysergide—avoid concomitant use
- Hormone Antagonists: absorption of cimetidine possibly delayed by octreotide
- $5HT_1$ Agonists: cimetidine inhibits metabolism of zolmitriptan (reduce dose of zolmitriptan)
- Mebendazole: cimetidine possibly inhibits metabolism of mebendazole (increased plasma concentration)
- Sildenafil: cimetidine increases plasma concentration of sildenafil (reduce initial dose of sildenafil)
- • Theophylline: cimetidine inhibits metabolism of •theophylline (increased plasma concentration)
- Thyroid Hormones: cimetidine reduces absorption of levothyroxine (thyroxine)

Homatropine *see* Antimuscarinics

Hormone Antagonists *see* Bicalutamide, Danazol, Dutasteride, Exemestane, Flutamide, Gestrinone, Lanreotide, Octreotide, Tamoxifen, Toremifene, and Trilostane

$5HT_1$ Agonists
- • Antibacterials: plasma concentration of eletriptan increased by •clarithromycin and •erythromycin (risk of toxicity)—avoid concomitant use; metabolism of zolmitriptan possibly inhibited by quinolones (reduce dose of zolmitriptan)
- • Antidepressants: increased risk of CNS toxicity when sumatriptan given with •citalopram, •escitalopram, •fluoxetine, •fluvoxamine or •paroxetine; metabolism of frovatriptan inhibited by fluvoxamine; metabolism of zolmitriptan possibly inhibited by fluvoxamine (reduce dose of zolmitriptan); increased risk of CNS toxicity when sumatriptan given with •sertraline (manufacturer of sertraline advises avoid concomitant use); possible increased serotonergic effects when $5HT_1$ agonists given with duloxetine; risk of CNS toxicity when rizatriptan or sumatriptan given with •MAOIs (avoid rizatriptan or sumatriptan for 2 weeks after MAOIs); increased risk of CNS toxicity when zolmitriptan given with •MAOIs; risk of CNS toxicity when rizatriptan or sumatriptan given with •moclobemide (avoid rizatriptan or sumatriptan for 2 weeks after moclobemide); risk of CNS toxicity when zolmitriptan given with •moclobemide (reduce dose of zolmitriptan); possible increased serotonergic effects when frovatriptan given with SSRIs; increased serotonergic effects when $5HT_1$ agonists given with •St John's wort—avoid concomitant use
- • Antifungals: plasma concentration of eletriptan increased by •itraconazole and •ketoconazole (risk of toxicity)—avoid concomitant use; plasma concentration of almotriptan increased by ketoconazole (increased risk of toxicity)
- • Antivirals: plasma concentration of eletriptan increased by •indinavir, •nelfinavir and •ritonavir (risk of toxicity)—avoid concomitant use
- Beta-blockers: plasma concentration of rizatriptan increased by propranolol (manufacturer of rizatriptan advises halve dose and avoid within 2 hours of propranolol)
- • Ergot Alkaloids: increased risk of vasospasm when eletriptan or frovatriptan given with •ergotamine and methysergide (avoid ergotamine and methysergide for 24 hours after eletriptan or frovatriptan, avoid eletriptan or frovatriptan for 24 hours after ergotamine and methysergide); increased risk of vasospasm when almotriptan, rizatriptan, sumatriptan or zolmitriptan given with •ergotamine and methysergide (avoid ergotamine and methysergide for 6 hours after almotriptan, rizatriptan, sumatriptan or zolmitriptan, avoid almotriptan, rizatriptan, sumatriptan or zolmitriptan for 24 hours after ergotamine and methysergide)
- Ulcer-healing Drugs: metabolism of zolmitriptan inhibited by cimetidine (reduce dose of zolmitriptan)

$5HT_3$ Antagonists
- Analgesics: ondansetron possibly antagonises effects of tramadol

5HT$_3$ Antagonists *(continued)*

- • Anti-arrhythmics: manufacturer of tropisetron advises caution with anti-arrhythmics (risk of ventricular arrhythmias); increased risk of ventricular arrhythmias when dolasetron given with •amiodarone, •disopyramide, •flecainide, •lidocaine (lignocaine), •mexiletine, •procainamide or •propafenone—avoid concomitant use
- Antibacterials: plasma concentration of tropisetron reduced by rifampicin; metabolism of ondansetron accelerated by rifampicin (reduced effect)
- Antiepileptics: metabolism of ondansetron accelerated by carbamazepine and phenytoin (reduced effect); plasma concentration of tropisetron reduced by primidone
- Barbiturates: plasma concentration of tropisetron reduced by phenobarbital
- • Beta-blockers: manufacturer of tropisetron advises caution with beta-blockers (risk of ventricular arrhythmias); increased risk of ventricular arrhythmias when dolasetron given with •sotalol—avoid concomitant use

Hydralazine *see* Vasodilator Antihypertensives

Hydrochlorothiazide *see* Diuretics

Hydrocortisone *see* Corticosteroids

Hydroflumethiazide *see* Diuretics

Hydromorphone *see* Opioid Analgesics

Hydrotalcite *see* Antacids

Hydroxocobalamin

- Antibacterials: response to hydroxocobalamin reduced by chloramphenicol

Hydroxycarbamide

- Antiepileptics: cytotoxics possibly reduce absorption of phenytoin
- • Antipsychotics: avoid concomitant use of cytotoxics with •clozapine (increased risk of agranulocytosis)
- • Antivirals: increased risk of toxicity when hydroxycarbamide given with •didanosine and •stavudine—avoid concomitant use
- Cardiac Glycosides: cytotoxics reduce absorption of digoxin tablets

Hydroxychloroquine *see* Chloroquine and Hydroxychloroquine

Hydroxyzine *see* Antihistamines

Hyoscine *see* Antimuscarinics

Ibandronic Acid *see* Bisphosphonates

Ibuprofen *see* NSAIDs

Ifosfamide

- • Anticoagulants: ifosfamide possibly enhances anticoagulant effect of •coumarins
- Antiepileptics: cytotoxics possibly reduce absorption of phenytoin
- • Antipsychotics: avoid concomitant use of cytotoxics with •clozapine (increased risk of agranulocytosis)
- Cardiac Glycosides: cytotoxics reduce absorption of digoxin tablets

Iloprost

- Analgesics: increased risk of bleeding when iloprost given with NSAIDs or aspirin
- Anticoagulants: iloprost possibly enhances anticoagulant effect of coumarins and heparins; increased risk of bleeding when iloprost given with phenindione
- Clopidogrel: increased risk of bleeding when iloprost given with clopidogrel
- Eptifibatide: increased risk of bleeding when iloprost given with eptifibatide
- Tirofiban: increased risk of bleeding when iloprost given with tirofiban

Imatinib

- • Antibacterials: plasma concentration of imatinib reduced by •rifampicin—avoid concomitant use
- Anticoagulants: manufacturer of imatinib advises replacement of warfarin with a heparin (possibility of enhanced warfarin effect)
- • Antiepileptics: plasma concentration of imatinib reduced by •phenytoin—avoid concomitant use; cytotoxics possibly reduce absorption of phenytoin
- Antifungals: plasma concentration of imatinib increased by ketoconazole

Imatinib *(continued)*

- • Antipsychotics: avoid concomitant use of cytotoxics with •clozapine (increased risk of agranulocytosis)
- Cardiac Glycosides: cytotoxics reduce absorption of digoxin tablets
- Lipid-regulating Drugs: imatinib increases plasma concentration of simvastatin
- Thyroid Hormones: imatinib possibly reduces plasma concentration of levothyroxine (thyroxine)

Imidapril *see* ACE Inhibitors

Imipenem with Cilastatin

- • Antivirals: increased risk of convulsions when imipenem with cilastatin given with •ganciclovir
- Oestrogens: antibacterials that do not induce liver enzymes possibly reduce contraceptive effect of oestrogens (risk probably small, see p. 428)

Imipramine *see* Antidepressants, Tricyclic

Immunoglobulins

Note For advice on immunoglobulins and live virus vaccines, see under Normal Immunoglobulin, p. 660

Immunosuppressants (antiproliferative) *see* Azathioprine and Mycophenolate Mofetil

Indapamide *see* Diuretics

Indinavir

- • Anti-arrhythmics: indinavir possibly increases plasma concentration of •amiodarone—avoid concomitant use
- • Antibacterials: indinavir increases plasma concentration of •rifabutin, also plasma concentration of indinavir decreased (reduce dose of rifabutin and increase dose of indinavir); metabolism of indinavir accelerated by •rifampicin (reduced plasma concentration—avoid concomitant use); avoidance of concomitant indinavir in severe renal and hepatic impairment advised by manufacturer of •telithromycin
- • Antidepressants: plasma concentration of indinavir reduced by •St John's wort—avoid concomitant use
- • Antiepileptics: plasma concentration of indinavir possibly reduced by carbamazepine, phenytoin and •primidone
- • Antifungals: metabolism of indinavir inhibited by ketoconazole; plasma concentration of indinavir increased by •itraconazole (consider reducing dose of indinavir)
- • Antimalarials: avoid concomitant use of indinavir with •artemether/lumefantrine
- Antimuscarinics: avoidance of indinavir advised by manufacturer of darifenacin and tolterodine
- • Antipsychotics: indinavir possibly inhibits metabolism of •aripiprazole (reduce dose of aripiprazole); indinavir possibly increases plasma concentration of •pimozide (increased risk of ventricular arrhythmias—avoid concomitant use); indinavir increases plasma concentration of •sertindole (increased risk of ventricular arrhythmias—avoid concomitant use)
- • <u>Antivirals</u>: avoid concomitant use of indinavir with •atazanavir; plasma concentration of both drugs increased when indinavir given with darunavir; plasma concentration of indinavir reduced by efavirenz and nevirapine; indinavir increases plasma concentration of •maraviroc (consider reducing dose of maraviroc); combination of indinavir with nelfinavir may increase plasma concentration of either drug (or both); plasma concentration of indinavir increased by ritonavir; indinavir increases plasma concentration of saquinavir
- • <u>Anxiolytics and Hypnotics</u>: increased risk of prolonged sedation when indinavir given with •alprazolam—avoid concomitant use; indinavir possibly increases plasma concentration of •midazolam (risk of prolonged sedation—avoid concomitant use of oral midazolam)
- Atovaquone: plasma concentration of indinavir possibly reduced by atovaquone
- • Barbiturates: plasma concentration of indinavir possibly reduced by •barbiturates
- • Cilostazol: indinavir possibly increases plasma concentration of •cilostazol—avoid concomitant use
- Corticosteroids: plasma concentration of indinavir possibly reduced by dexamethasone

Indinavir *(continued)*
- • Ergot Alkaloids: increased risk of ergotism when indinavir given with •ergotamine and methysergide—avoid concomitant use
- • $5HT_1$ Agonists: indinavir increases plasma concentration of •eletriptan (risk of toxicity)—avoid concomitant use
- • Lipid-regulating Drugs: possible increased risk of myopathy when indinavir given with atorvastatin; increased risk of myopathy when indinavir given with •simvastatin (avoid concomitant use)
- Sildenafil: indinavir increases plasma concentration of sildenafil—reduce initial dose of sildenafil
- • Vardenafil: indinavir increases plasma concentration of •vardenafil—avoid concomitant use

Indometacin *see* NSAIDs
Indoramin *see* Alpha-blockers
Infliximab
- Abatacept: increased risk of side-effects when infliximab given with abatacept
- • Anakinra: avoid concomitant use of infliximab with •anakinra
- • Vaccines: avoid concomitant use of infliximab with live •vaccines (see p. 641)

Influenza Vaccine *see* Vaccines
Insulin *see* Antidiabetics
Interferon Alfa *see* Interferons
Interferon Gamma *see* Interferons
Interferons
- Note Peginterferon alfa interactions as for interferon alfa
- Theophylline: interferon alfa inhibits metabolism of theophylline (increased plasma concentration)
- Vaccines: manufacturer of interferon gamma advises avoid concomitant use with vaccines

Ipratropium *see* Antimuscarinics
Irbesartan *see* Angiotensin-II Receptor Antagonists
Irinotecan
- • Antidepressants: metabolism of irinotecan accelerated by •St John's wort (reduced plasma concentration—avoid concomitant use)
- Antiepileptics: plasma concentration of irinotecan and its active metabolite reduced by carbamazepine and phenytoin; cytotoxics possibly reduce absorption of phenytoin
- • Antifungals: plasma concentration of irinotecan reduced by •ketoconazole (but concentration of active metabolite of irinotecan increased)—avoid concomitant use
- • Antipsychotics: avoid concomitant use of cytotoxics with •clozapine (increased risk of agranulocytosis)
- • Antivirals: metabolism of irinotecan possibly inhibited by •atazanavir (increased risk of toxicity)
- Barbiturates: plasma concentration of irinotecan and its active metabolite reduced by phenobarbital
- Cardiac Glycosides: cytotoxics reduce absorption of digoxin tablets
- Cytotoxics: plasma concentration of irinotecan possibly increased by sorafenib

Iron
- Antacids: absorption of *oral* iron reduced by oral magnesium salts (as magnesium trisilicate)
- Antibacterials: *oral* iron reduces absorption of ciprofloxacin, levofloxacin, moxifloxacin, norfloxacin and ofloxacin; *oral* iron reduces absorption of tetracyclines, also absorption of *oral* iron reduced by tetracyclines
- Bisphosphonates: *oral* iron reduces absorption of bisphosphonates
- Calcium Salts: absorption of *oral* iron reduced by calcium salts
- Cytotoxics: *oral* iron reduces absorption of mycophenolate
- • Dimercaprol: avoid concomitant use of iron with •dimercaprol
- Dopaminergics: *oral* iron reduces absorption of entacapone; *oral* iron possibly reduces absorption of levodopa
- Methyldopa: *oral* iron antagonises hypotensive effect of methyldopa

Iron *(continued)*
- Penicillamine: *oral* iron reduces absorption of penicillamine
- Thyroid Hormones: *oral* iron reduces absorption of levothyroxine (thyroxine) (give at least 2 hours apart)
- Trientine: absorption of *oral* iron reduced by trientine
- Zinc: *oral* iron reduces absorption of zinc, also absorption of *oral* iron reduced by zinc

Isocarboxazid *see* MAOIs
Isoflurane *see* Anaesthetics, General
Isometheptene *see* Sympathomimetics
Isoniazid
- Anaesthetics, General: hepatotoxicity of isoniazid possibly potentiated by general anaesthetics
- Antacids: absorption of isoniazid reduced by antacids
- Antibacterials: increased risk of CNS toxicity when isoniazid given with cycloserine
- • Antiepileptics: isoniazid increases plasma concentration of •carbamazepine (also possibly increased isoniazid hepatotoxicity); isoniazid inhibits metabolism of •ethosuximide (increased plasma concentration and risk of toxicity); isoniazid inhibits metabolism of •phenytoin (increased plasma concentration)
- Antifungals: isoniazid possibly reduces plasma concentration of ketoconazole
- Anxiolytics and Hypnotics: isoniazid inhibits the metabolism of diazepam
- Corticosteroids: plasma concentration of isoniazid possibly reduced by corticosteroids
- Oestrogens: antibacterials that do not induce liver enzymes possibly reduce contraceptive effect of oestrogens (risk probably small, see p. 428)
- Theophylline: isoniazid possibly increases plasma concentration of theophylline

Isosorbide Dinitrate *see* Nitrates
Isosorbide Mononitrate *see* Nitrates
Isotretinoin *see* Retinoids
Isradipine *see* Calcium-channel Blockers
Itraconazole *see* Antifungals, Triazole
Ivabradine
- • Anti-arrhythmics: increased risk of ventricular arrhythmias when ivabradine given with •amiodarone or •disopyramide
- • Antibacterials: plasma concentration of ivabradine possibly increased by •clarithromycin and •telithromycin—avoid concomitant use; increased risk of ventricular arrhythmias when ivabradine given with •erythromycin—avoid concomitant use
- Antidepressants: plasma concentration of ivabradine reduced by St John's wort—avoid concomitant use
- • Antifungals: plasma concentration of ivabradine increased by •ketoconazole—avoid concomitant use; plasma concentration of ivabradine increased by fluconazole—reduce initial dose of ivabradine; plasma concentration of ivabradine possibly increased by •itraconazole—avoid concomitant use
- • Antimalarials: increased risk of ventricular arrhythmias when ivabradine given with •mefloquine
- • Antipsychotics: increased risk of ventricular arrhythmias when ivabradine given with •pimozide or •sertindole
- • Antivirals: plasma concentration of ivabradine possibly increased by •nelfinavir and •ritonavir—avoid concomitant use
- • Beta-blockers: increased risk of ventricular arrhythmias when ivabradine given with •sotalol
- • Calcium-channel Blockers: plasma concentration of ivabradine increased by •diltiazem and •verapamil—avoid concomitant use
- Grapefruit Juice: plasma concentration of ivabradine increased by grapefruit juice
- • Pentamidine Isetionate: increased risk of ventricular arrhythmias when ivabradine given with •pentamidine isetionate

Kaolin
- Analgesics: kaolin possibly reduces absorption of aspirin
- Antibacterials: kaolin possibly reduces absorption of tetracyclines

Kaolin *(continued)*

Antimalarials: kaolin reduces absorption of chloroquine and hydroxychloroquine

Antipsychotics: kaolin possibly reduces absorption of phenothiazines

Ketamine *see* Anaesthetics, General

Ketoconazole *see* Antifungals, Imidazole

Ketoprofen *see* NSAIDs

Ketorolac *see* NSAIDs

Ketotifen *see* Antihistamines

Labetalol *see* Beta-blockers

Lacidipine *see* Calcium-channel Blockers

Lactulose

Anticoagulants: lactulose possibly enhances anticoagulant effect of coumarins

Lamivudine

Antibacterials: plasma concentration of lamivudine increased by trimethoprim (as co-trimoxazole)—avoid concomitant use of high-dose co-trimoxazole

Antivirals: avoidance of lamivudine advised by manufacturer of emtricitabine; manufacturer of lamivudine advises avoid concomitant use with foscarnet; manufacturer of lamivudine advises avoid concomitant use of intravenous ganciclovir

Lamotrigine

• Antibacterials: plasma concentration of lamotrigine reduced by •rifampicin

• Antidepressants: anticonvulsant effect of antiepileptics possibly antagonised by MAOIs and •tricyclic-related antidepressants (convulsive threshold lowered); anticonvulsant effect of antiepileptics antagonised by •SSRIs and •tricyclics (convulsive threshold lowered); avoid concomitant use of antiepileptics with •St John's wort

Antiepileptics: plasma concentration of lamotrigine often reduced by carbamazepine, also plasma concentration of an active metabolite of carbamazepine sometimes raised (but evidence is conflicting); plasma concentration of lamotrigine reduced by phenytoin and primidone; plasma concentration of lamotrigine increased by valproate

• Antimalarials: possible increased risk of convulsions when antiepileptics given with chloroquine and hydroxychloroquine; anticonvulsant effect of antiepileptics antagonised by •mefloquine

Barbiturates: plasma concentration of lamotrigine reduced by phenobarbital

• Oestrogens: plasma concentration of lamotrigine reduced by •oestrogens

• Progestogens: plasma concentration of lamotrigine reduced by •progestogens

Lanreotide

Antidiabetics: lanreotide possibly reduces requirements for insulin, metformin, repaglinide and sulphonylureas

Ciclosporin: lanreotide reduces plasma concentration of ciclosporin

Lansoprazole *see* Proton Pump Inhibitors

Lanthanum

Antifungals: lanthanum possibly reduces absorption of ketoconazole (give at least 2 hours apart)

Antimalarials: lanthanum possibly reduces absorption of chloroquine and hydroxychloroquine (give at least 2 hours apart)

Laronidase

Anaesthetics, Local: effects of laronidase possibly inhibited by procaine (manufacturer of laronidase advises avoid concomitant use)

Antimalarials: effects of laronidase possibly inhibited by chloroquine and hydroxychloroquine (manufacturer of laronidase advises avoid concomitant use)

Leflunomide

Note Increased risk of toxicity with other haematotoxic and hepatotoxic drugs

Anticoagulants: leflunomide possibly enhances anticoagulant effect of warfarin

Antidiabetics: leflunomide possibly enhances hypoglycaemic effect of tolbutamide

Antiepileptics: leflunomide possibly increases plasma concentration of phenytoin

Leflunomide *(continued)*

Lipid-regulating Drugs: the effect of leflunomide is significantly decreased by colestyramine (enhanced elimination)—avoid unless drug elimination desired

• Vaccines: avoid concomitant use of leflunomide with live •vaccines (see p. 641)

Lenalidomide

Cardiac Glycosides: lenalidomide possibly increases plasma concentration of digoxin

Lercanidipine *see* Calcium-channel Blockers

Leukotriene Antagonists

Analgesics: plasma concentration of zafirlukast increased by aspirin

Antibacterials: plasma concentration of zafirlukast reduced by erythromycin

Anticoagulants: zafirlukast enhances anticoagulant effect of warfarin

Antiepileptics: plasma concentration of montelukast reduced by primidone

Barbiturates: plasma concentration of montelukast reduced by phenobarbital

Theophylline: zafirlukast possibly increases plasma concentration of theophylline, also plasma concentration of zafirlukast reduced

Levamisole

Alcohol: possibility of disulfiram-like reaction when levamisole given with alcohol

• Anticoagulants: levamisole possibly enhances anticoagulant effect of •warfarin

Antiepileptics: levamisole possibly increases plasma concentration of phenytoin

Levetiracetam

• Antidepressants: anticonvulsant effect of antiepileptics possibly antagonised by MAOIs and •tricyclic-related antidepressants (convulsive threshold lowered); anticonvulsant effect of antiepileptics antagonised by •SSRIs and •tricyclics (convulsive threshold lowered); avoid concomitant use of antiepileptics with •St John's wort

• Antimalarials: possible increased risk of convulsions when antiepileptics given with chloroquine and hydroxychloroquine; anticonvulsant effect of antiepileptics antagonised by •mefloquine

Levobunolol *see* Beta-blockers

Levobupivacaine

Anti-arrhythmics: increased myocardial depression when levobupivacaine given with anti-arrhythmics

Levocetirizine *see* Antihistamines

Levodopa

ACE Inhibitors: enhanced hypotensive effect when levodopa given with ACE inhibitors

Adrenergic Neurone Blockers: enhanced hypotensive effect when levodopa given with adrenergic neurone blockers

Alpha-blockers: enhanced hypotensive effect when levodopa given with alpha-blockers

• Anaesthetics, General: increased risk of arrhythmias when levodopa given with •volatile liquid general anaesthetics

Angiotensin-II Receptor Antagonists: enhanced hypotensive effect when levodopa given with angiotensin-II receptor antagonists

• Antidepressants: risk of hypertensive crisis when levodopa given with •MAOIs, avoid levodopa for at least 2 weeks after stopping MAOIs; increased risk of side-effects when levodopa given with moclobemide

Antiepileptics: effects of levodopa possibly reduced by phenytoin

Antimuscarinics: absorption of levodopa possibly reduced by antimuscarinics

Antipsychotics: effects of levodopa antagonised by antipsychotics; avoidance of levodopa advised by manufacturer of amisulpride (antagonism of effect)

Anxiolytics and Hypnotics: effects of levodopa possibly antagonised by benzodiazepines

Beta-blockers: enhanced hypotensive effect when levodopa given with beta-blockers

Bupropion: increased risk of side-effects when levodopa given with bupropion

Levodopa *(continued)*
Calcium-channel Blockers: enhanced hypotensive effect when levodopa given with calcium-channel blockers
Clonidine: enhanced hypotensive effect when levodopa given with clonidine
Diazoxide: enhanced hypotensive effect when levodopa given with diazoxide
Diuretics: enhanced hypotensive effect when levodopa given with diuretics
Dopaminergics: enhanced effects and increased toxicity of levodopa when given with selegiline (reduce dose of levodopa)
Iron: absorption of levodopa possibly reduced by *oral* iron
Memantine: effects of dopaminergics possibly enhanced by memantine
Methyldopa: enhanced hypotensive effect when levodopa given with methyldopa; antiparkinsonian effect of dopaminergics antagonised by methyldopa
Moxonidine: enhanced hypotensive effect when levodopa given with moxonidine
Muscle Relaxants: possible agitation, confusion and hallucinations when levodopa given with baclofen
Nitrates: enhanced hypotensive effect when levodopa given with nitrates
Vasodilator Antihypertensives: enhanced hypotensive effect when levodopa given with hydralazine, minoxidil or sodium nitroprusside
Vitamins: effects of levodopa reduced by pyridoxine when given without dopa-decarboxylase inhibitor

Levofloxacin *see* Quinolones
Levomepromazine (methotrimeprazine) *see* Antipsychotics
Levonorgestrel *see* Progestogens
Levothyroxine (thyroxine) *see* Thyroid Hormones
Lidocaine (lignocaine)
Note Interactions less likely when lidocaine used topically
Anaesthetics, Local: increased myocardial depression when anti-arrhythmics given with bupivacaine, levobupivacaine, prilocaine or ropivacaine
• Anti-arrhythmics: increased myocardial depression when anti-arrhythmics given with other •anti-arrhythmics
• Antibacterials: increased risk of ventricular arrhythmias when lidocaine (lignocaine) given with •quinupristin/dalfopristin—avoid concomitant use
• Antipsychotics: increased risk of ventricular arrhythmias when anti-arrhythmics that prolong the QT interval given with •antipsychotics that prolong the QT interval
• Antivirals: plasma concentration of lidocaine (lignocaine) possibly increased by •amprenavir and darunavir—avoid concomitant use; plasma concentration of lidocaine (lignocaine) possibly increased by •atazanavir and lopinavir
• Beta-blockers: increased myocardial depression when anti-arrhythmics given with •beta-blockers; increased risk of lidocaine (lignocaine) toxicity when given with •propranolol
• Diuretics: action of lidocaine (lignocaine) antagonised by hypokalaemia caused by •acetazolamide, •loop diuretics or •thiazides and related diuretics
• $5HT_3$ Antagonists: increased risk of ventricular arrhythmias when lidocaine (lignocaine) given with •dolasetron—avoid concomitant use; caution with anti-arrhythmics advised by manufacturer of tropisetron (risk of ventricular arrhythmias)
Muscle Relaxants: neuromuscular blockade enhanced and prolonged when lidocaine (lignocaine) given with suxamethonium
• Ulcer-healing Drugs: plasma concentration of lidocaine (lignocaine) increased by •cimetidine (increased risk of toxicity)

Linezolid
Note Linezolid is a reversible, non-selective MAO inhibitor—see interactions of MAOIs
Oestrogens: antibacterials that do not induce liver enzymes possibly reduce contraceptive effect of oestrogens (risk probably small, see p. 428)

Liothyronine *see* Thyroid Hormones
Lipid-regulating Drugs *see* Colestipol, Colestyramine, Ezetimibe, Fibrates, Nicotinic Acid, and Statins
Lisinopril *see* ACE Inhibitors
Lithium
• ACE Inhibitors: excretion of lithium reduced by •ACE inhibitors (increased plasma concentration)
• Analgesics: excretion of lithium probably reduced by •NSAIDs (increased risk of toxicity); excretion of lithium reduced by •diclofenac, •ibuprofen, •indometacin, •mefenamic acid, •naproxen, •parecoxib and •piroxicam (increased risk of toxicity); excretion of lithium reduced by •ketorolac (increased risk of toxicity)—avoid concomitant use
• Angiotensin-II Receptor Antagonists: excretion of lithium reduced by •angiotensin-II receptor antagonists (increased plasma concentration)
Antacids: excretion of lithium increased by sodium bicarbonate (reduced plasma concentration)
• Anti-arrhythmics: avoidance of lithium advised by manufacturer of •amiodarone (risk of ventricular arrhythmias)
Antibacterials: increased risk of lithium toxicity when given with metronidazole
• Antidepressants: possible increased serotonergic effects when lithium given with venlafaxine; increased risk of CNS effects when lithium given with •SSRIs (lithium toxicity reported); risk of toxicity when lithium given with tricyclics
Antiepileptics: neurotoxicity may occur when lithium given with carbamazepine or phenytoin without increased plasma concentration of lithium
• Antipsychotics: increased risk of extrapyramidal side-effects and possibly neurotoxicity when lithium given with clozapine, haloperidol or phenothiazines; increased risk of ventricular arrhythmias when lithium given with •sertindole—avoid concomitant use; increased risk of extrapyramidal side-effects when lithium given with sulpiride
Calcium-channel Blockers: neurotoxicity may occur when lithium given with diltiazem or verapamil without increased plasma concentration of lithium
• Diuretics: excretion of lithium increased by •acetazolamide; excretion of lithium reduced by •loop diuretics and •thiazides and related diuretics (increased plasma concentration and risk of toxicity)—loop diuretics safer than thiazides; excretion of lithium reduced by •potassium-sparing diuretics and aldosterone antagonists (increased plasma concentration and risk of toxicity)
• Methyldopa: neurotoxicity may occur when lithium given with •methyldopa without increased plasma concentration of lithium
Muscle Relaxants: lithium enhances effects of muscle relaxants; hyperkinesis caused by lithium possibly aggravated by baclofen
Parasympathomimetics: lithium antagonises effects of neostigmine and pyridostigmine
Theophylline: excretion of lithium increased by theophylline (reduced plasma concentration)

Lofepramine *see* Antidepressants, Tricyclic
Lofexidine
Alcohol: increased sedative effect when lofexidine given with alcohol
Anxiolytics and Hypnotics: increased sedative effect when lofexidine given with anxiolytics and hypnotics
Barbiturates: increased sedative effect when lofexidine given with barbiturates

Loperamide
Desmopressin: loperamide increases plasma concentration of *oral* desmopressin

Lopinavir
Note In combination with ritonavir as *Kaletra*® (ritonavir is present to inhibit lopinavir metabolism and increase plasma-lopinavir concentration)—see also Ritonavir
Anti-arrhythmics: lopinavir possibly increases plasma concentration of lidocaine (lignocaine)
• Antibacterials: plasma concentration of lopinavir reduced by •rifampicin—avoid concomitant use; avoidance of concomitant lopinavir in severe renal

Lopinavir

- Antibacterials *(continued)*
  and hepatic impairment advised by manufacturer of •telithromycin
- Antidepressants: plasma concentration of lopinavir reduced by •St John's wort—avoid concomitant use
- Antiepileptics: plasma concentration of lopinavir possibly reduced by carbamazepine, phenytoin and •primidone

Antihistamines: lopinavir possibly increases plasma concentration of chlorphenamine (chlorpheniramine)

- Antimalarials: avoid concomitant use of lopinavir with •artemether/lumefantrine

Antimuscarinics: avoidance of lopinavir advised by manufacturer of darifenacin and tolterodine

- Antipsychotics: lopinavir possibly inhibits metabolism of •aripiprazole (reduce dose of aripiprazole); lopinavir increases plasma concentration of •sertindole (increased risk of ventricular arrhythmias—avoid concomitant use)
- Antivirals: lopinavir reduces plasma concentration of amprenavir, effect on lopinavir plasma concentration not predictable; plasma concentration of lopinavir increased by darunavir (also plasma concentration of darunavir reduced); plasma concentration of lopinavir reduced by efavirenz and •tipranavir; lopinavir increases plasma concentration of •maraviroc (consider reducing dose of maraviroc); plasma concentration of lopinavir reduced by nelfinavir, also plasma concentration of active metabolite of nelfinavir increased; plasma concentration of lopinavir reduced by nevirapine—increase dose of lopinavir; lopinavir increases plasma concentration of saquinavir and tenofovir
- Barbiturates: plasma concentration of lopinavir possibly reduced by •phenobarbital
- Cilostazol: lopinavir possibly increases plasma concentration of •cilostazol—avoid concomitant use

Corticosteroids: plasma concentration of lopinavir possibly reduced by dexamethasone

- Lipid-regulating Drugs: possible increased risk of myopathy when lopinavir given with atorvastatin; possible increased risk of myopathy when lopinavir given with •simvastatin—avoid concomitant use

Sirolimus: lopinavir possibly increases plasma concentration of sirolimus

Loprazolam *see* Anxiolytics and Hypnotics
Loratadine *see* Antihistamines
Lorazepam *see* Anxiolytics and Hypnotics
Lormetazepam *see* Anxiolytics and Hypnotics
Losartan *see* Angiotensin-II Receptor Antagonists
Lumefantrine *see* Artemether with Lumefantrine
Lymecycline *see* Tetracyclines

Macrolides

Note *See also* Telithromycin

Note Interactions do not apply to small amounts of erythromycin used topically

Analgesics: erythromycin increases plasma concentration of alfentanil

Antacids: absorption of azithromycin reduced by antacids

- Anti-arrhythmics: increased risk of ventricular arrhythmias when parenteral erythromycin given with •amiodarone—avoid concomitant use; clarithromycin possibly increases plasma concentration of •disopyramide (increased risk of toxicity); erythromycin increases plasma concentration of •disopyramide (increased risk of toxicity)
- Antibacterials: increased risk of ventricular arrhythmias when parenteral erythromycin given with •moxifloxacin—avoid concomitant use; macrolides possibly increase plasma concentration of •rifabutin (increased risk of uveitis—reduce rifabutin dose); clarithromycin increases plasma concentration of •rifabutin (increased risk of uveitis—reduce rifabutin dose); plasma concentration of clarithromycin reduced by rifamycins
- Anticoagulants: macrolides possibly enhance anticoagulant effect of •coumarins; clarithromycin and erythromycin enhance anticoagulant effect of •coumarins

Macrolides

- Antidepressants: avoidance of macrolides advised by manufacturer of •reboxetine

Antidiabetics: clarithromycin enhances effects of repaglinide

- Antiepileptics: clarithromycin and erythromycin increase plasma concentration of •carbamazepine; clarithromycin inhibits metabolism of phenytoin (increased plasma concentration); erythromycin possibly inhibits metabolism of valproate (increased plasma concentration)

Antifungals: clarithromycin increases plasma concentration of itraconazole

- Antihistamines: manufacturer of loratadine advises erythromycin possibly increases plasma concentration of loratadine; macrolides possibly inhibit metabolism of •mizolastine (avoid concomitant use); erythromycin inhibits metabolism of •mizolastine—avoid concomitant use
- Antimalarials: avoidance of macrolides advised by manufacturer of •artemether/lumefantrine

Antimuscarinics: erythromycin possibly increases plasma concentration of darifenacin; avoidance of clarithromycin and erythromycin advised by manufacturer of tolterodine

- Antipsychotics: increased risk of ventricular arrhythmias when parenteral erythromycin given with •amisulpride—avoid concomitant use; erythromycin possibly increases plasma concentration of •clozapine (possible increased risk of convulsions); possible increased risk of ventricular arrhythmias when erythromycin given with •pimozide—avoid concomitant use; increased risk of ventricular arrhythmias when clarithromycin given with •pimozide—avoid concomitant use; macrolides possibly increase plasma concentration of quetiapine (reduce dose of quetiapine); increased risk of ventricular arrhythmias when erythromycin given with •sertindole—avoid concomitant use; possible increased risk of ventricular arrhythmias when macrolides given with •sertindole—avoid concomitant use
- Antivirals: plasma concentration of both drugs increased when erythromycin given with amprenavir; plasma concentration of both drugs increased when clarithromycin given with atazanavir; increased risk of rash when clarithromycin given with efavirenz; clarithromycin possibly increases plasma concentration of •maraviroc (consider reducing dose of maraviroc); plasma concentration of azithromycin and erythromycin possibly increased by ritonavir; plasma concentration of clarithromycin increased by •ritonavir (reduce dose of clarithromycin in renal impairment); plasma concentration of clarithromycin increased by •tipranavir (reduce dose of clarithromycin in renal impairment), also clarithromycin increases plasma concentration of tipranavir; clarithromycin tablets reduce absorption of zidovudine
- Anxiolytics and Hypnotics: clarithromycin and erythromycin inhibit metabolism of •midazolam (increased plasma concentration with increased sedation); erythromycin increases plasma concentration of buspirone (reduce dose of buspirone); erythromycin inhibits the metabolism of zopiclone

Aprepitant: clarithromycin possibly increases plasma concentration of aprepitant

- Atomoxetine: increased risk of ventricular arrhythmias when parenteral erythromycin given with •atomoxetine
- Calcium-channel Blockers: erythromycin possibly inhibits metabolism of felodipine (increased plasma concentration); avoidance of erythromycin advised by manufacturer of lercanidipine; clarithromycin and erythromycin possibly inhibit metabolism of •verapamil (increased risk of toxicity)

Macrolides *(continued)*

Cardiac Glycosides: macrolides increase plasma concentration of digoxin (increased risk of toxicity)

• Ciclosporin: macrolides possibly inhibit metabolism of •ciclosporin (increased plasma concentration); clarithromycin and erythromycin inhibit metabolism of •ciclosporin (increased plasma concentration)

• Cilostazol: erythromycin increases plasma concentration of •cilostazol (also plasma concentration of erythromycin reduced)—avoid concomitant use

• Colchicine: clarithromycin or erythromycin increase risk of •colchicine toxicity

Corticosteroids: erythromycin possibly inhibits metabolism of corticosteroids; clarithromycin possibly increases plasma concentration of methylprednisolone; erythromycin inhibits the metabolism of methylprednisolone

• Cytotoxics: *in vitro* studies suggest a possible interaction between erythromycin and docetaxel (consult docetaxel product literature); erythromycin increases toxicity of •vinblastine—avoid concomitant use

• Diuretics: clarithromycin increases plasma concentration of •eplerenone—avoid concomitant use; erythromycin increases plasma concentration of eplerenone (reduce dose of eplerenone)

Dopaminergics: erythromycin increases plasma concentration of bromocriptine and cabergoline (increased risk of toxicity); macrolides possibly increase plasma concentration of bromocriptine and cabergoline (increased risk of toxicity)

• Ergot Alkaloids: increased risk of ergotism when macrolides given with •ergotamine and methysergide—avoid concomitant use

• $5HT_1$ Agonists: clarithromycin and erythromycin increase plasma concentration of •eletriptan (risk of toxicity)—avoid concomitant use

• Ivabradine: clarithromycin possibly increases plasma concentration of •ivabradine—avoid concomitant use; increased risk of ventricular arrhythmias when erythromycin given with •ivabradine—avoid concomitant use

Leukotriene Antagonists: erythromycin reduces plasma concentration of zafirlukast

• Lipid-regulating Drugs: clarithromycin increases plasma concentration of •atorvastatin; possible increased risk of myopathy when erythromycin given with atorvastatin; erythromycin reduces plasma concentration of rosuvastatin; increased risk of myopathy when clarithromycin or erythromycin given with •simvastatin (avoid concomitant use)

Oestrogens: antibacterials that do not induce liver enzymes possibly reduce contraceptive effect of oestrogens (risk probably small, see p. 428)

Parasympathomimetics: erythromycin increases plasma concentration of galantamine

• Pentamidine Isetionate: increased risk of ventricular arrhythmias when parenteral erythromycin given with •pentamidine isetionate

Sildenafil: clarithromycin possibly increases plasma concentration of sildenafil—reduce initial dose of sildenafil; erythromycin increases plasma concentration of sildenafil—reduce initial dose of sildenafil

• Sirolimus: clarithromycin increases plasma concentration of •sirolimus—avoid concomitant use; plasma concentration of both drugs increased when erythromycin given with •sirolimus

• Tacrolimus: clarithromycin and erythromycin increase plasma concentration of •tacrolimus

Tadalafil: clarithromycin and erythromycin possibly increase plasma concentration of tadalafil

• Theophylline: azithromycin possibly increases plasma concentration of theophylline; clarithromycin inhibits metabolism of •theophylline (increased plasma concentration); erythromycin inhibits metabolism of •theophylline (increased plasma concentration), if erythromycin given by mouth, also decreased plasma-erythromycin concentration

Ulcer-healing Drugs: plasma concentration of erythromycin increased by cimetidine (increased risk of toxicity, including deafness); plasma concentration of both drugs increased when clarithromycin given with omeprazole

Vardenafil: erythromycin increases plasma concentration of vardenafil (reduce dose of vardenafil)

Magnesium (parenteral)

• Calcium-channel Blockers: profound hypotension reported with concomitant use of parenteral magnesium and •nifedipine in pre-eclampsia

Muscle Relaxants: parenteral magnesium enhances effects of non-depolarising muscle relaxants and suxamethonium

Magnesium Salts (oral) *see* Antacids

MAOIs

Note For interactions of reversible MAO-A inhibitors (RIMAs) see Moclobemide, and for interactions of MAO-B inhibitors see Rasagiline and Selegiline; the antibacterial Linezolid is a reversible, non-selective MAO inhibitor

ACE Inhibitors: MAOIs possibly enhance hypotensive effect of ACE inhibitors

Adrenergic Neurone Blockers: enhanced hypotensive effect when MAOIs given with adrenergic neurone blockers

• Alcohol: MAOIs interact with tyramine found in some beverages containing •alcohol and some dealcoholised beverages (hypertensive crisis)—if no tyramine, enhanced hypotensive effect

$Alpha_2$-adrenoceptor Stimulants: avoidance of MAOIs advised by manufacturer of apraclonidine and brimonidine

• Alpha-blockers: avoidance of MAOIs advised by manufacturer of •indoramin; enhanced hypotensive effect when MAOIs given with alpha-blockers

• Anaesthetics, General: Because of hazardous interactions between MAOIs and •general anaesthetics, MAOIs should normally be stopped 2 weeks before surgery

• Analgesics: CNS excitation or depression (hypertension or hypotension) when MAOIs given with •pethidine—avoid concomitant use and for 2 weeks after stopping MAOIs; avoidance of MAOIs advised by manufacturer of •nefopam; possible CNS excitation or depression (hypertension or hypotension) when MAOIs given with •opioid analgesics—avoid concomitant use and for 2 weeks after stopping MAOIs

Angiotensin-II Receptor Antagonists: MAOIs possibly enhance hypotensive effect of angiotensin-II receptor antagonists

• Antidepressants: increased risk of hypertension and CNS excitation when MAOIs given with •reboxetine (MAOIs should not be started until 1 week after stopping reboxetine, avoid reboxetine for 2 weeks after stopping MAOIs); after stopping MAOIs do not start •citalopram, •escitalopram, •fluvoxamine or •paroxetine for 2 weeks, also MAOIs should not be started until at least 1 week after stopping citalopram, escitalopram, fluvoxamine or paroxetine; after stopping MAOIs do not start •fluoxetine for 2 weeks, also MAOIs should not be started until at least 5 weeks after stopping fluoxetine; after stopping MAOIs do not start •mirtazapine or •sertraline for 2 weeks, also MAOIs should not be started until at least 2 weeks after stopping mirtazapine or sertraline; after stopping MAOIs do not start •duloxetine for 2 weeks, also MAOIs should not be started until at least 5 days after stopping duloxetine; enhanced CNS effects and toxicity when MAOIs given with •venlafaxine (venlafaxine should not be started until 2 weeks after stopping MAOIs, avoid MAOIs for 1 week after stopping venlafaxine); increased risk of hypertension and CNS excitation when MAOIs given with other •MAOIs (avoid for at least 2 weeks after stopping previous MAOIs and then start at a reduced dose); after stopping MAOIs do not start •moclobemide for at least 1 week; MAOIs increase CNS effects of •SSRIs (risk of serious toxicity); after stopping MAOIs do not start •tricyclic-related antidepressants for 2 weeks, also MAOIs should not be started until at least 1–2 weeks after stopping tricyclic-related antidepressants;

MAOIs

- Antidepressants *(continued)* increased risk of hypertension and CNS excitation when MAOIs given with •tricyclics, tricyclics should not be started until 2 weeks after stopping MAOIs (3 weeks if starting clomipramine or imipramine), also MAOIs should not be started for at least 1–2 weeks after stopping tricyclics (3 weeks in the case of clomipramine or imipramine); CNS excitation and confusion when MAOIs given with •tryptophan (reduce dose of tryptophan)
- Antidiabetics: MAOIs possibly enhance hypoglycaemic effect of antidiabetics; MAOIs enhance hypoglycaemic effect of insulin, metformin and sulphonylureas
- • Antiepileptics: MAOIs possibly antagonise anticonvulsant effect of antiepileptics (convulsive threshold lowered); avoidance for 2 weeks after stopping MAOIs advised by manufacturer of •carbamazepine, also antagonism of anticonvulsant effect
- Antihistamines: increased antimuscarinic and sedative effects when MAOIs given with antihistamines
- • Antimalarials: avoidance of antidepressants advised by manufacturer of •artemether/lumefantrine
- Antimuscarinics: increased risk of antimuscarinic side-effects when MAOIs given with antimuscarinics
- • Antipsychotics: CNS effects of MAOIs possibly increased by •clozapine
- Anxiolytics and Hypnotics: avoidance of MAOIs advised by manufacturer of buspirone
- • Atomoxetine: after stopping MAOIs do not start •atomoxetine for 2 weeks, also MAOIs should not be started until at least 2 weeks after stopping atomoxetine; possible increased risk of convulsions when antidepressants given with atomoxetine
- Barbiturates: MAOIs possibly antagonise anticonvulsant effect of barbiturates (convulsive threshold lowered)
- Beta-blockers: enhanced hypotensive effect when MAOIs given with beta-blockers
- • Bupropion: avoidance of bupropion for 2 weeks after stopping MAOIs advised by manufacturer of •bupropion
- Calcium-channel Blockers: enhanced hypotensive effect when MAOIs given with calcium-channel blockers
- Clonidine: enhanced hypotensive effect when MAOIs given with clonidine
- Diazoxide: enhanced hypotensive effect when MAOIs given with diazoxide
- Diuretics: enhanced hypotensive effect when MAOIs given with diuretics
- • Dopaminergics: avoid concomitant use of non-selective MAOIs with •entacapone; risk of hypertensive crisis when MAOIs given with •levodopa, avoid levodopa for at least 2 weeks after stopping MAOIs; risk of hypertensive crisis when MAOIs given with •rasagiline, avoid MAOIs for at least 2 weeks after stopping rasagiline; enhanced hypotensive effect when MAOIs given with selegiline; avoid concomitant use of MAOIs with tolcapone
- Doxapram: MAOIs enhance effects of doxapram
- • $5HT_1$ Agonists: risk of CNS toxicity when MAOIs given with •rizatriptan or •sumatriptan (avoid rizatriptan or sumatriptan for 2 weeks after MAOIs); increased risk of CNS toxicity when MAOIs given with •zolmitriptan
- • Methyldopa: avoidance of MAOIs advised by manufacturer of •methyldopa
- Moxonidine: enhanced hypotensive effect when MAOIs given with moxonidine
- Muscle Relaxants: phenelzine enhances effects of suxamethonium
- Nicorandil: enhanced hypotensive effect when MAOIs given with nicorandil
- Nitrates: enhanced hypotensive effect when MAOIs given with nitrates
- • Sibutramine: increased CNS toxicity when MAOIs given with •sibutramine (manufacturer of sibutramine advises avoid concomitant use), also avoid sibutramine for 2 weeks after stopping MAOIs
- • Sympathomimetics: risk of hypertensive crisis when MAOIs given with •dexamfetamine, •dopamine, •dopexamine, •ephedrine, •isometheptene, •phenylephrine, •phenylpropanolamine, •pseudoephedrine or •sympathomimetics; risk of hypertensive crisis when MAOIs given with •methylphenidate, some manufacturers advise avoid methylphenidate for at least 2 weeks after stopping MAOIs
- • Tetrabenazine: risk of CNS excitation and hypertension when MAOIs given with •tetrabenazine
- Vasodilator Antihypertensives: enhanced hypotensive effect when MAOIs given with hydralazine, minoxidil or sodium nitroprusside

MAOIs, reversible *see* Moclobemide

Maraviroc

- • <u>Antibacterials</u>: plasma concentration of maraviroc possibly increased by •clarithromycin and •telithromycin (consider reducing dose of maraviroc); plasma concentration of maraviroc reduced by •rifampicin—consider increasing dose of maraviroc
- • <u>Antidepressants</u>: plasma concentration of maraviroc possibly reduced by •St John's wort—avoid concomitant use
- • <u>Antifungals</u>: plasma concentration of maraviroc increased by •ketoconazole (consider reducing dose of maraviroc)
- • <u>Antivirals</u>: plasma concentration of maraviroc increased by •atazanavir, •darunavir, •indinavir, •lopinavir and •saquinavir (consider reducing dose of maraviroc); plasma concentration of maraviroc possibly reduced by •efavirenz—consider increasing dose of maraviroc; plasma concentration of maraviroc possibly increased by •nelfinavir (consider reducing dose of maraviroc)

Mebendazole

- Ulcer-healing Drugs: metabolism of mebendazole possibly inhibited by cimetidine (increased plasma concentration)

Medroxyprogesterone *see* Progestogens

Mefenamic Acid *see* NSAIDs

Mefloquine

- • Anti-arrhythmics: increased risk of ventricular arrhythmias when mefloquine given with •amiodarone—avoid concomitant use
- • <u>Antibacterials</u>: increased risk of ventricular arrhythmias when mefloquine given with •moxifloxacin—avoid concomitant use; plasma concentration of mefloquine reduced by •rifampicin—avoid concomitant use
- • Antiepileptics: mefloquine antagonises anticonvulsant effect of •antiepileptics, •carbamazepine and •valproate
- • Antimalarials: avoidance of antimalarials advised by manufacturer of •artemether/lumefantrine; increased risk of convulsions when mefloquine given with •chloroquine and hydroxychloroquine; increased risk of convulsions when mefloquine given with •quinine (but should not prevent the use of intravenous quinine in severe cases)
- • Antipsychotics: increased risk of ventricular arrhythmias when mefloquine given with •pimozide—avoid concomitant use
- • Atomoxetine: increased risk of ventricular arrhythmias when mefloquine given with •atomoxetine
- Beta-blockers: increased risk of bradycardia when mefloquine given with beta-blockers
- Calcium-channel Blockers: possible increased risk of bradycardia when mefloquine given with calcium-channel blockers
- Cardiac Glycosides: possible increased risk of bradycardia when mefloquine given with digoxin
- • Ivabradine: increased risk of ventricular arrhythmias when mefloquine given with •ivabradine

Megestrol *see* Progestogens

Meloxicam *see* NSAIDs

Melphalan

Antibacterials: increased risk of melphalan toxicity when given with nalidixic acid

Antiepileptics: cytotoxics possibly reduce absorption of phenytoin

• Antipsychotics: avoid concomitant use of cytotoxics with •clozapine (increased risk of agranulocytosis)

Cardiac Glycosides: cytotoxics reduce absorption of digoxin tablets

• Ciclosporin: increased risk of nephrotoxicity when melphalan given with •ciclosporin

Memantine

• Anaesthetics, General: increased risk of CNS toxicity when memantine given with •ketamine (manufacturer of memantine advises avoid concomitant use)

• Analgesics: increased risk of CNS toxicity when memantine given with •dextromethorphan (manufacturer of memantine advises avoid concomitant use)

Anticoagulants: memantine possibly enhances anticoagulant effect of warfarin

Antiepileptics: memantine possibly reduces effects of primidone

Antimuscarinics: memantine possibly enhances effects of antimuscarinics

Antipsychotics: memantine possibly reduces effects of antipsychotics

Barbiturates: memantine possibly reduces effects of barbiturates

• Dopaminergics: memantine possibly enhances effects of dopaminergics and selegiline; increased risk of CNS toxicity when memantine given with •amantadine (manufacturer of memantine advises avoid concomitant use)

Muscle Relaxants: memantine possibly modifies effects of baclofen and dantrolene

Mepacrine

Antimalarials: mepacrine increases plasma concentration of primaquine (increased risk of toxicity)

Meprobamate *see* Anxiolytics and Hypnotics

Meptazinol *see* Opioid Analgesics

Mercaptopurine

• Allopurinol: enhanced effects and increased toxicity of mercaptopurine when given with •allopurinol (reduce dose of mercaptopurine to one quarter of usual dose)

Aminosalicylates: possible increased risk of leucopenia when mercaptopurine given with aminosalicylates

• Antibacterials: increased risk of haematological toxicity when mercaptopurine given with •sulfamethoxazole (as co-trimoxazole); increased risk of haematological toxicity when mercaptopurine given with •trimethoprim (also with co-trimoxazole)

• Anticoagulants: mercaptopurine possibly reduces anticoagulant effect of •coumarins

Antiepileptics: cytotoxics possibly reduce absorption of phenytoin

• Antipsychotics: avoid concomitant use of cytotoxics with •clozapine (increased risk of agranulocytosis)

Cardiac Glycosides: cytotoxics reduce absorption of digoxin tablets

Meropenem

Antiepileptics: meropenem reduces plasma concentration of valproate

Oestrogens: antibacterials that do not induce liver enzymes possibly reduce contraceptive effect of oestrogens (risk probably small, see p. 428)

Probenecid: excretion of meropenem reduced by probenecid (manufacturers of meropenem advise avoid concomitant use)

Mesalazine *see* Aminosalicylates

Mestranol *see* Oestrogens

Metaraminol *see* Sympathomimetics

Metformin *see* Antidiabetics

Methadone *see* Opioid Analgesics

Methenamine

• Antibacterials: increased risk of crystalluria when methenamine given with •sulphonamides

• Diuretics: effects of methenamine antagonised by •acetazolamide

Methenamine *(continued)*

Oestrogens: antibacterials that do not induce liver enzymes possibly reduce contraceptive effect of oestrogens (risk probably small, see p. 428)

Potassium Salts: avoid concomitant use of methenamine with potassium citrate

Methocarbamol *see* Muscle Relaxants

Methotrexate

• Anaesthetics, General: antifolate effect of methotrexate increased by •nitrous oxide—avoid concomitant use

• Analgesics: excretion of methotrexate probably reduced by •NSAIDs (increased risk of toxicity)—but for concomitant use in rheumatic disease see p. 551; excretion of methotrexate reduced by •azapropazone (avoid concomitant use); excretion of methotrexate reduced by •aspirin, •diclofenac, •ibuprofen, •indometacin, •ketoprofen, •meloxicam and •naproxen (increased risk of toxicity)—but for concomitant use in rheumatic disease see p. 551

• Antibacterials: absorption of methotrexate possibly reduced by neomycin; excretion of methotrexate possibly reduced by ciprofloxacin (increased risk of toxicity); increased risk of haematological toxicity when methotrexate given with •sulfamethoxazole (as co-trimoxazole); increased risk of methotrexate toxicity when given with doxycycline, sulphonamides or tetracycline; excretion of methotrexate reduced by penicillins (increased risk of toxicity); increased risk of haematological toxicity when methotrexate given with •trimethoprim (also with co-trimoxazole)

Antiepileptics: antifolate effect of methotrexate increased by phenytoin; cytotoxics possibly reduce absorption of phenytoin

• Antimalarials: antifolate effect of methotrexate increased by •pyrimethamine

• Antipsychotics: avoid concomitant use of cytotoxics with •clozapine (increased risk of agranulocytosis)

Cardiac Glycosides: cytotoxics reduce absorption of digoxin tablets

• Ciclosporin: risk of toxicity when methotrexate given with •ciclosporin

• Corticosteroids: increased risk of haematological toxicity when methotrexate given with •corticosteroids

• Cytotoxics: increased pulmonary toxicity when methotrexate given with •cisplatin

• Probenecid: excretion of methotrexate reduced by •probenecid (increased risk of toxicity)

• Retinoids: plasma concentration of methotrexate increased by •acitretin (also increased risk of hepatotoxicity)—avoid concomitant use

Theophylline: methotrexate possibly increases plasma concentration of theophylline

Ulcer-healing Drugs: excretion of methotrexate possibly reduced by omeprazole (increased risk of toxicity)

Methoxamine *see* Sympathomimetics

Methyldopa

ACE Inhibitors: enhanced hypotensive effect when methyldopa given with ACE inhibitors

Adrenergic Neurone Blockers: enhanced hypotensive effect when methyldopa given with adrenergic neurone blockers

Alcohol: enhanced hypotensive effect when methyldopa given with alcohol

Aldesleukin: enhanced hypotensive effect when methyldopa given with aldesleukin

Alpha-blockers: enhanced hypotensive effect when methyldopa given with alpha-blockers

Anaesthetics, General: enhanced hypotensive effect when methyldopa given with general anaesthetics

Analgesics: hypotensive effect of methyldopa antagonised by NSAIDs

Angiotensin-II Receptor Antagonists: enhanced hypotensive effect when methyldopa given with angiotensin-II receptor antagonists

• Antidepressants: manufacturer of methyldopa advises avoid concomitant use with •MAOIs

Antipsychotics: enhanced hypotensive effect when methyldopa given with antipsychotics (also increased risk of extrapyramidal effects)

Methyldopa *(continued)*
Anxiolytics and Hypnotics: enhanced hypotensive effect when methyldopa given with anxiolytics and hypnotics
Beta-blockers: enhanced hypotensive effect when methyldopa given with beta-blockers
Calcium-channel Blockers: enhanced hypotensive effect when methyldopa given with calcium-channel blockers
Clonidine: enhanced hypotensive effect when methyldopa given with clonidine
Corticosteroids: hypotensive effect of methyldopa antagonised by corticosteroids
Diazoxide: enhanced hypotensive effect when methyldopa given with diazoxide
Diuretics: enhanced hypotensive effect when methyldopa given with diuretics
Dopaminergics: methyldopa antagonises antiparkinsonian effect of dopaminergics; increased risk of extrapyramidal side-effects when methyldopa given with amantadine; effects of methyldopa possibly enhanced by entacapone; enhanced hypotensive effect when methyldopa given with levodopa
Iron: hypotensive effect of methyldopa antagonised by *oral* iron
• Lithium: neurotoxicity may occur when methyldopa given with •lithium without increased plasma concentration of lithium
Moxisylyte (thymoxamine): enhanced hypotensive effect when methyldopa given with moxisylyte
Moxonidine: enhanced hypotensive effect when methyldopa given with moxonidine
Muscle Relaxants: enhanced hypotensive effect when methyldopa given with baclofen or tizanidine
Nitrates: enhanced hypotensive effect when methyldopa given with nitrates
Oestrogens: hypotensive effect of methyldopa antagonised by oestrogens
Prostaglandins: enhanced hypotensive effect when methyldopa given with alprostadil
• Sympathomimetics, $Beta_2$: acute hypotension reported when methyldopa given with infusion of •salbutamol
Vasodilator Antihypertensives: enhanced hypotensive effect when methyldopa given with hydralazine, minoxidil or sodium nitroprusside

Methylphenidate *see* Sympathomimetics
Methylprednisolone *see* Corticosteroids
Methysergide *see* Ergot Alkaloids
Metipranolol *see* Beta-blockers

Metoclopramide
Analgesics: metoclopramide increases rate of absorption of aspirin (enhanced effect); effects of metoclopramide on gastro-intestinal activity antagonised by opioid analgesics; metoclopramide increases rate of absorption of paracetamol
Antimuscarinics: effects of metoclopramide on gastro-intestinal activity antagonised by antimuscarinics
Antipsychotics: increased risk of extrapyramidal side-effects when metoclopramide given with antipsychotics
Atovaquone: metoclopramide reduces plasma concentration of atovaquone
• Ciclosporin: metoclopramide increases plasma concentration of •ciclosporin
Dopaminergics: increased risk of extrapyramidal side-effects when metoclopramide given with amantadine; metoclopramide antagonises hypoprolactinaemic effects of bromocriptine and cabergoline; metoclopramide antagonises antiparkinsonian effect of pergolide; avoidance of metoclopramide advised by manufacturer of ropinirole and rotigotine (antagonism of effect)
Muscle Relaxants: metoclopramide enhances effects of suxamethonium
Tetrabenazine: increased risk of extrapyramidal side-effects when metoclopramide given with tetrabenazine

Metolazone *see* Diuretics
Metoprolol *see* Beta-blockers

Metronidazole
Note Interactions do not apply to topical metronidazole preparations
Alcohol: disulfiram-like reaction when metronidazole given with alcohol
• Anticoagulants: metronidazole enhances anticoagulant effect of •coumarins
• Antiepileptics: metronidazole inhibits metabolism of •phenytoin (increased plasma concentration); metabolism of metronidazole accelerated by primidone (reduced plasma concentration)
Barbiturates: metabolism of metronidazole accelerated by barbiturates (reduced plasma concentration)
• Cytotoxics: metronidazole increases plasma concentration of •busulfan (increased risk of toxicity); metronidazole inhibits metabolism of fluorouracil (increased toxicity); metronidazole possibly reduces bioavailability of mycophenolate
Disulfiram: psychotic reaction reported when metronidazole given with disulfiram
Lithium: metronidazole increases risk of lithium toxicity
Oestrogens: antibacterials that do not induce liver enzymes possibly reduce contraceptive effect of oestrogens (risk probably small, see p. 428)
Ulcer-healing Drugs: metabolism of metronidazole inhibited by cimetidine (increased plasma concentration)

Mexiletine
Anaesthetics, Local: increased myocardial depression when anti-arrhythmics given with bupivacaine, levobupivacaine, prilocaine or ropivacaine
Analgesics: absorption of mexiletine delayed by opioid analgesics
• Anti-arrhythmics: increased myocardial depression when anti-arrhythmics given with other •anti-arrhythmics
Antibacterials: metabolism of mexiletine accelerated by rifampicin (reduced plasma concentration)
• Antidepressants: metabolism of mexiletine inhibited by •fluvoxamine (increased risk of toxicity)
Antiepileptics: metabolism of mexiletine accelerated by phenytoin (reduced plasma concentration)
• Antihistamines: increased risk of ventricular arrhythmias when mexiletine given with •mizolastine—avoid concomitant use
Antimuscarinics: absorption of mexiletine delayed by atropine
• Antipsychotics: increased risk of ventricular arrhythmias when anti-arrhythmics that prolong the QT interval given with •antipsychotics that prolong the QT interval
• Antivirals: plasma concentration of mexiletine possibly increased by •ritonavir (increased risk of toxicity)
• Beta-blockers: increased myocardial depression when anti-arrhythmics given with •beta-blockers
• Diuretics: action of mexiletine antagonised by hypokalaemia caused by •acetazolamide, •loop diuretics or •thiazides and related diuretics
• $5HT_3$ Antagonists: increased risk of ventricular arrhythmias when mexiletine given with •dolasetron—avoid concomitant use; caution with anti-arrhythmics advised by manufacturer of tropisetron (risk of ventricular arrhythmias)
Theophylline: mexiletine increases plasma concentration of theophylline

Mianserin *see* Antidepressants, Tricyclic (related)
Miconazole *see* Antifungals, Imidazole
Midazolam *see* Anxiolytics and Hypnotics

Mifepristone
Analgesics: manufacturer of mifepristone advises avoid concomitant use with NSAIDs and aspirin
Corticosteroids: mifepristone may reduce effect of corticosteroids (including inhaled corticosteroids) for 3–4 days

Milrinone *see* Phosphodiesterase Inhibitors
Minocycline *see* Tetracyclines
Minoxidil *see* Vasodilator Antihypertensives

Mirtazapine
• Alcohol: increased sedative effect when mirtazapine given with •alcohol

Mirtazapine *(continued)*

Anticoagulants: mirtazapine enhances anticoagulant effect of warfarin

• Antidepressants: mirtazapine should not be started until 2 weeks after stopping •MAOIs, also MAOIs should not be started until at least 2 weeks after stopping mirtazapine; after stopping mirtazapine do not start •moclobemide for at least 1 week

Antiepileptics: plasma concentration of mirtazapine reduced by carbamazepine and phenytoin

Antifungals: plasma concentration of mirtazapine increased by ketoconazole

• Antimalarials: avoidance of antidepressants advised by manufacturer of •artemether/lumefantrine

Anxiolytics and Hypnotics: increased sedative effect when mirtazapine given with anxiolytics and hypnotics

Atomoxetine: possible increased risk of convulsions when antidepressants given with atomoxetine

• Sibutramine: increased risk of CNS toxicity when mirtazapine given with •sibutramine (manufacturer of sibutramine advises avoid concomitant use)

Ulcer-healing Drugs: plasma concentration of mirtazapine increased by cimetidine

Mitomycin

Antiepileptics: cytotoxics possibly reduce absorption of phenytoin

• Antipsychotics: avoid concomitant use of cytotoxics with •clozapine (increased risk of agranulocytosis)

Cardiac Glycosides: cytotoxics reduce absorption of digoxin tablets

Mitotane

• Anticoagulants: mitotane possibly reduces anticoagulant effect of •coumarins

Antiepileptics: cytotoxics possibly reduce absorption of phenytoin

• Antipsychotics: avoid concomitant use of cytotoxics with •clozapine (increased risk of agranulocytosis)

Cardiac Glycosides: cytotoxics reduce absorption of digoxin tablets

Diuretics: manufacturer of mitotane advises avoid concomitant use of spironolactone (antagonism of effect)

Mivacurium *see* Muscle Relaxants

Mizolastine *see* Antihistamines

Moclobemide

• Analgesics: possible CNS excitation or depression (hypertension or hypotension) when moclobemide given with •dextromethorphan or •pethidine—avoid concomitant use; possible CNS excitation or depression (hypertension or hypotension) when moclobemide given with •opioid analgesics

• Antidepressants: moclobemide should not be started for at least 1 week after stopping •MAOIs, •SSRI-related antidepressants, •citalopram, •fluvoxamine, •mirtazapine, •paroxetine, •tricyclic-related antidepressants or •tricyclics; increased risk of CNS toxicity when moclobemide given with •escitalopram, preferably avoid concomitant use; moclobemide should not be started until 5 weeks after stopping •fluoxetine; moclobemide should not be started until 2 weeks after stopping •sertraline; possible increased serotonergic effects when moclobemide given with •duloxetine

• Antimalarials: avoidance of antidepressants advised by manufacturer of •artemether/lumefantrine

Atomoxetine: possible increased risk of convulsions when antidepressants given with atomoxetine

• Bupropion: avoidance of moclobemide advised by manufacturer of •bupropion

• Dopaminergics: caution with moclobemide advised by manufacturer of entacapone; increased risk of side-effects when moclobemide given with levodopa; avoid concomitant use of moclobemide with •selegiline

• $5HT_1$ Agonists: risk of CNS toxicity when moclobemide given with •rizatriptan or •sumatriptan (avoid rizatriptan or sumatriptan for 2 weeks after moclobemide); risk of CNS toxicity when moclobemide given with •zolmitriptan (reduce dose of zolmitriptan)

Moclobemide *(continued)*

• Sibutramine: increased CNS toxicity when moclobemide given with •sibutramine (manufacturer of sibutramine advises avoid concomitant use), also avoid sibutramine for 2 weeks after stopping moclobemide

• Sympathomimetics: risk of hypertensive crisis when moclobemide given with •dexamfetamine, •dopamine, •dopexamine, •ephedrine, •isometheptene, •methylphenidate, •phenylephrine, •phenylpropanolamine, •pseudoephedrine or •sympathomimetics

Ulcer-healing Drugs: plasma concentration of moclobemide increased by cimetidine (halve dose of moclobemide)

Modafinil

Antiepileptics: modafinil possibly increases plasma concentration of phenytoin

• Ciclosporin: modafinil reduces plasma concentration of •ciclosporin

• Oestrogens: modafinil accelerates metabolism of •oestrogens (reduced contraceptive effect—see p. 428)

Moexipril *see* ACE Inhibitors

Mometasone *see* Corticosteroids

Monobactams *see* Aztreonam

Montelukast *see* Leukotriene Antagonists

Morphine *see* Opioid Analgesics

Moxifloxacin *see* Quinolones

Moxisylyte (thymoxamine)

ACE Inhibitors: enhanced hypotensive effect when moxisylyte given with ACE inhibitors

Adrenergic Neurone Blockers: enhanced hypotensive effect when moxisylyte given with adrenergic neurone blockers

• Alpha-blockers: possible severe postural hypotension when moxisylyte given with •alpha-blockers

Angiotensin-II Receptor Antagonists: enhanced hypotensive effect when moxisylyte given with angiotensin-II receptor antagonists

• Beta-blockers: possible severe postural hypotension when moxisylyte given with •beta-blockers

Calcium-channel Blockers: enhanced hypotensive effect when moxisylyte given with calcium-channel blockers

Clonidine: enhanced hypotensive effect when moxisylyte given with clonidine

Diazoxide: enhanced hypotensive effect when moxisylyte given with diazoxide

Diuretics: enhanced hypotensive effect when moxisylyte given with diuretics

Methyldopa: enhanced hypotensive effect when moxisylyte given with methyldopa

Moxonidine: enhanced hypotensive effect when moxisylyte given with moxonidine

Nitrates: enhanced hypotensive effect when moxisylyte given with nitrates

Vasodilator Antihypertensives: enhanced hypotensive effect when moxisylyte given with hydralazine, minoxidil or sodium nitroprusside

Moxonidine

ACE Inhibitors: enhanced hypotensive effect when moxonidine given with ACE inhibitors

Adrenergic Neurone Blockers: enhanced hypotensive effect when moxonidine given with adrenergic neurone blockers

Alcohol: enhanced hypotensive effect when moxonidine given with alcohol

Aldesleukin: enhanced hypotensive effect when moxonidine given with aldesleukin

Alpha-blockers: enhanced hypotensive effect when moxonidine given with alpha-blockers

Anaesthetics, General: enhanced hypotensive effect when moxonidine given with general anaesthetics

Analgesics: hypotensive effect of moxonidine antagonised by NSAIDs

Angiotensin-II Receptor Antagonists: enhanced hypotensive effect when moxonidine given with angiotensin-II receptor antagonists

Moxonidine *(continued)*
- Antidepressants: enhanced hypotensive effect when moxonidine given with MAOIs
- Antipsychotics: enhanced hypotensive effect when moxonidine given with phenothiazines
- Anxiolytics and Hypnotics: enhanced hypotensive effect when moxonidine given with anxiolytics and hypnotics; sedative effects possibly increased when moxonidine given with benzodiazepines
- Beta-blockers: enhanced hypotensive effect when moxonidine given with beta-blockers
- Calcium-channel Blockers: enhanced hypotensive effect when moxonidine given with calcium-channel blockers
- Clonidine: enhanced hypotensive effect when moxonidine given with clonidine
- Corticosteroids: hypotensive effect of moxonidine antagonised by corticosteroids
- Diazoxide: enhanced hypotensive effect when moxonidine given with diazoxide
- Diuretics: enhanced hypotensive effect when moxonidine given with diuretics
- Dopaminergics: enhanced hypotensive effect when moxonidine given with levodopa
- Methyldopa: enhanced hypotensive effect when moxonidine given with methyldopa
- Moxisylyte (thymoxamine): enhanced hypotensive effect when moxonidine given with moxisylyte
- Muscle Relaxants: enhanced hypotensive effect when moxonidine given with baclofen or tizanidine
- Nitrates: enhanced hypotensive effect when moxonidine given with nitrates
- Oestrogens: hypotensive effect of moxonidine antagonised by oestrogens
- Prostaglandins: enhanced hypotensive effect when moxonidine given with alprostadil
- Vasodilator Antihypertensives: enhanced hypotensive effect when moxonidine given with hydralazine, minoxidil or sodium nitroprusside

Muscle Relaxants
- ACE Inhibitors: enhanced hypotensive effect when baclofen or tizanidine given with ACE inhibitors
- Adrenergic Neurone Blockers: enhanced hypotensive effect when baclofen or tizanidine given with adrenergic neurone blockers
- Alcohol: increased sedative effect when baclofen, methocarbamol or tizanidine given with alcohol
- Alpha-blockers: enhanced hypotensive effect when baclofen or tizanidine given with alpha-blockers
- • Anaesthetics, General: increased risk of myocardial depression and bradycardia when suxamethonium given with •propofol; effects of non-depolarising muscle relaxants and suxamethonium enhanced by volatile liquid general anaesthetics
- Analgesics: excretion of baclofen possibly reduced by NSAIDs (increased risk of toxicity); excretion of baclofen reduced by ibuprofen (increased risk of toxicity)
- Angiotensin-II Receptor Antagonists: enhanced hypotensive effect when baclofen or tizanidine given with angiotensin-II receptor antagonists
- • Anti-arrhythmics: neuromuscular blockade enhanced and prolonged when suxamethonium given with lidocaine (lignocaine); effects of muscle relaxants enhanced by •procainamide
- • Antibacterials: effects of non-depolarising muscle relaxants and suxamethonium enhanced by piperacillin; plasma concentration of tizanidine increased by •ciprofloxacin (increased risk of toxicity)—avoid concomitant use; effects of non-depolarising muscle relaxants and suxamethonium enhanced by •aminoglycosides; effects of non-depolarising muscle relaxants and suxamethonium enhanced by •clindamycin; effects of non-depolarising muscle relaxants and suxamethonium enhanced by •polymyxins; effects of suxamethonium enhanced by •vancomycin
- • <u>Antidepressants</u>: plasma concentration of tizanidine increased by •fluvoxamine (increased risk of toxicity)—avoid concomitant use; effects of suxamethonium enhanced by phenelzine; muscle relaxant effect of baclofen enhanced by tricyclics
- Antiepileptics: muscle relaxant effect of non-depolarising muscle relaxants antagonised by carbamazepine and phenytoin (accelerated recovery from neuromuscular blockade)
- Antimalarials: effects of suxamethonium possibly enhanced by quinine
- Antipsychotics: effects of suxamethonium possibly enhanced by promazine
- Anxiolytics and Hypnotics: increased sedative effect when baclofen or tizanidine given with anxiolytics and hypnotics
- Beta-blockers: enhanced hypotensive effect when baclofen given with beta-blockers; possible enhanced hypotensive effect and bradycardia when tizanidine given with beta-blockers; effects of muscle relaxants enhanced by propranolol
- Calcium-channel Blockers: enhanced hypotensive effect when baclofen or tizanidine given with calcium-channel blockers; effects of non-depolarising muscle relaxants enhanced by nifedipine and verapamil; risk of arrhythmias when intravenous dantrolene given with diltiazem; hypotension, myocardial depression, and hyperkalaemia when intravenous dantrolene given with verapamil; effects of suxamethonium enhanced by verapamil
- Cardiac Glycosides: possible increased risk of bradycardia when tizanidine given with cardiac glycosides; risk of ventricular arrhythmias when suxamethonium given with cardiac glycosides
- Clonidine: enhanced hypotensive effect when baclofen or tizanidine given with clonidine
- <u>Corticosteroids</u>: effects of pancuronium and vecuronium possibly antagonised by corticosteroids
- Cytotoxics: effects of suxamethonium enhanced by cyclophosphamide and thiotepa
- Diazoxide: enhanced hypotensive effect when baclofen or tizanidine given with diazoxide
- Diuretics: enhanced hypotensive effect when baclofen or tizanidine given with diuretics
- Dopaminergics: possible agitation, confusion and hallucinations when baclofen given with levodopa
- Lithium: effects of muscle relaxants enhanced by lithium; baclofen possibly aggravates hyperkinesis caused by lithium
- Magnesium (parenteral): effects of non-depolarising muscle relaxants and suxamethonium enhanced by parenteral magnesium
- Memantine: effects of baclofen and dantrolene possibly modified by memantine
- Methyldopa: enhanced hypotensive effect when baclofen or tizanidine given with methyldopa
- Metoclopramide: effects of suxamethonium enhanced by metoclopramide
- Moxonidine: enhanced hypotensive effect when baclofen or tizanidine given with moxonidine
- Nitrates: enhanced hypotensive effect when baclofen or tizanidine given with nitrates
- <u>Oestrogens</u>: plasma concentration of tizanidine possibly increased by oestrogens (increased risk of toxicity)
- Parasympathomimetics: effects of non-depolarising muscle relaxants possibly antagonised by donepezil; effects of suxamethonium possibly enhanced by donepezil, effects of non-depolarising muscle relaxants antagonised by edrophonium, neostigmine, pyridostigmine and rivastigmine; effects of suxamethonium enhanced by edrophonium, galantamine, neostigmine, pyridostigmine and rivastigmine
- <u>Progestogens</u>: plasma concentration of tizanidine possibly increased by progestogens (increased risk of toxicity)
- Sympathomimetics, Beta$_2$: effects of suxamethonium enhanced by bambuterol
- Vasodilator Antihypertensives: enhanced hypotensive effect when baclofen or tizanidine given with hydralazine; enhanced hypotensive effect when baclofen or

Muscle Relaxants
Vasodilator Antihypertensives *(continued)*
tizanidine given with minoxidil; enhanced hypotensive effect when baclofen or tizanidine given with sodium nitroprusside

Muscle Relaxants, depolarising *see* Muscle Relaxants
Muscle Relaxants, non-depolarising *see* Muscle Relaxants

Mycophenolate
Antacids: absorption of mycophenolate reduced by antacids
• Antibacterials: bioavailability of mycophenolate possibly reduced by metronidazole and norfloxacin; plasma concentration of active metabolite of mycophenolate reduced by •rifampicin
Antiepileptics: cytotoxics possibly reduce absorption of phenytoin
• Antipsychotics: avoid concomitant use of cytotoxics with •clozapine (increased risk of agranulocytosis)
Antivirals: mycophenolate increases plasma concentration of aciclovir, also plasma concentration of inactive metabolite of mycophenolate increased; mycophenolate possibly increases plasma concentration of ganciclovir, also plasma concentration of inactive metabolite of mycophenolate possibly increased
Cardiac Glycosides: cytotoxics reduce absorption of digoxin tablets
Iron: absorption of mycophenolate reduced by *oral* iron
Lipid-regulating Drugs: absorption of mycophenolate reduced by colestyramine
Sevelamer: plasma concentration of mycophenolate possibly reduced by sevelamer

Mycophenolate Mofetil *see* Mycophenolate
Mycophenolate Sodium *see* Mycophenolate
Mycophenolic Acid *see* Mycophenolate

Nabilone
Alcohol: increased sedative effect when nabilone given with alcohol
Anxiolytics and Hypnotics: increased sedative effect when nabilone given with anxiolytics and hypnotics

Nabumetone *see* NSAIDs
Nadolol *see* Beta-blockers
Nalidixic Acid *see* Quinolones
Nandrolone *see* Anabolic Steroids
Naproxen *see* NSAIDs
Naratriptan *see* $5HT_1$ Agonists
Nateglinide *see* Antidiabetics
Nebivolol *see* Beta-blockers

Nefopam
• Antidepressants: manufacturer of nefopam advises avoid concomitant use with •MAOIs; side-effects possibly increased when nefopam given with tricyclics
Antimuscarinics: increased risk of antimuscarinic side-effects when nefopam given with antimuscarinics

Nelfinavir
Analgesics: nelfinavir reduces plasma concentration of methadone
• Anti-arrhythmics: increased risk of ventricular arrhythmias when nelfinavir given with •amiodarone—avoid concomitant use
• Antibacterials: nelfinavir increases plasma concentration of •rifabutin (halve dose of rifabutin); plasma concentration of nelfinavir significantly reduced by •rifampicin—avoid concomitant use; avoidance of concomitant nelfinavir in severe renal and hepatic impairment advised by manufacturer of •telithromycin
• Antidepressants: plasma concentration of nelfinavir reduced by •St John's wort—avoid concomitant use
• Antiepileptics: plasma concentration of nelfinavir possibly reduced by carbamazepine and •primidone; nelfinavir reduces plasma concentration of phenytoin
• Antimalarials: avoid concomitant use of nelfinavir with •artemether/lumefantrine
Antimuscarinics: avoidance of nelfinavir advised by manufacturer of darifenacin and tolterodine; nelfinavir increases plasma concentration of solifenacin
• Antipsychotics: nelfinavir possibly inhibits metabolism of •aripiprazole (reduce dose of aripiprazole); nelfinavir possibly increases plasma concentration of •pimozide (increased risk of ventricular arrhythmias—avoid concomitant use); nelfinavir increases plasma concentration of •sertindole (increased risk of ventricular arrhythmias—avoid concomitant use)
• Antivirals: combination of nelfinavir with indinavir, ritonavir or saquinavir may increase plasma concentration of either drug (or both); nelfinavir reduces plasma concentration of lopinavir, also plasma concentration of active metabolite of nelfinavir increased; nelfinavir possibly increases plasma concentration of •maraviroc (consider reducing dose of maraviroc)
• Anxiolytics and Hypnotics: nelfinavir possibly increases plasma concentration of •midazolam (risk of prolonged sedation—avoid concomitant use of oral midazolam)
• Barbiturates: plasma concentration of nelfinavir possibly reduced by •barbiturates
• Ciclosporin: nelfinavir possibly increases plasma concentration of •ciclosporin
• Cilostazol: nelfinavir possibly increases plasma concentration of •cilostazol—avoid concomitant use
Cytotoxics: nelfinavir increases plasma concentration of paclitaxel
• Diuretics: nelfinavir increases plasma concentration of •eplerenone—avoid concomitant use
• Ergot Alkaloids: increased risk of ergotism when nelfinavir given with •ergotamine and methysergide—avoid concomitant use
• $5HT_1$ Agonists: nelfinavir increases plasma concentration of •eletriptan (risk of toxicity)—avoid concomitant use
• Ivabradine: nelfinavir possibly increases plasma concentration of •ivabradine—avoid concomitant use
• Lipid-regulating Drugs: possible increased risk of myopathy when nelfinavir given with atorvastatin; increased risk of myopathy when nelfinavir given with •simvastatin (avoid concomitant use)
• Oestrogens: nelfinavir accelerates metabolism of •oestrogens (reduced contraceptive effect—see p. 428)
Progestogens: nelfinavir possibly reduces contraceptive effect of progestogens
Sildenafil: nelfinavir possibly increases plasma concentration of sildenafil—reduce initial dose of sildenafil
• Tacrolimus: nelfinavir possibly increases plasma concentration of •tacrolimus
• Ulcer-healing Drugs: plasma concentration of nelfinavir reduced by •omeprazole—avoid concomitant use

Neomycin *see* Aminoglycosides
Neostigmine *see* Parasympathomimetics

Nevirapine
Analgesics: nevirapine possibly reduces plasma concentration of methadone
• Antibacterials: nevirapine possibly increases plasma concentration of rifabutin; plasma concentration of nevirapine reduced by •rifampicin—avoid concomitant use
• Anticoagulants: nevirapine may enhance or reduce anticoagulant effect of •warfarin
• Antidepressants: plasma concentration of nevirapine reduced by •St John's wort—avoid concomitant use
• Antifungals: nevirapine reduces plasma concentration of •ketoconazole—avoid concomitant use; plasma concentration of nevirapine increased by •fluconazole; nevirapine possibly reduces plasma concentration of caspofungin—consider increasing dose of caspofungin
• Antipsychotics: nevirapine possibly reduces plasma concentration of •aripiprazole—increase dose of aripiprazole
• Antivirals: nevirapine possibly reduces plasma concentration of amprenavir; nevirapine possibly reduces plasma concentration of •atazanavir—avoid concomitant use; nevirapine reduces plasma concentration

Nevirapine

- Antivirals *(continued)* of efavirenz and indinavir; nevirapine reduces plasma concentration of lopinavir—increase dose of lopinavir
- Oestrogens: nevirapine accelerates metabolism of •oestrogens (reduced contraceptive effect—see p. 428)
- Progestogens: nevirapine accelerates metabolism of •progestogens (reduced contraceptive effect—see p. 428)

Nicardipine *see* Calcium-channel Blockers

Nicorandil

Alcohol: hypotensive effect of nicorandil possibly enhanced by alcohol

Antidepressants: enhanced hypotensive effect when nicorandil given with MAOIs; hypotensive effect of nicorandil possibly enhanced by tricyclics

- Sildenafil: hypotensive effect of nicorandil significantly enhanced by •sildenafil (avoid concomitant use)
- Tadalafil: hypotensive effect of nicorandil significantly enhanced by •tadalafil (avoid concomitant use)
- Vardenafil: possible increased hypotensive effect when nicorandil given with •vardenafil—avoid concomitant use

Vasodilator Antihypertensives: possible enhanced hypotensive effect when nicorandil given with hydralazine, minoxidil or sodium nitroprusside

Nicotinic Acid

Note Interactions apply to lipid-regulating doses of nicotinic acid

- Lipid-regulating Drugs: increased risk of myopathy when nicotinic acid given with •statins (applies to lipid regulating doses of nicotinic acid)

Nifedipine *see* Calcium-channel Blockers

Nimodipine *see* Calcium-channel Blockers

Nisoldipine *see* Calcium-channel Blockers

Nitrates

ACE Inhibitors: enhanced hypotensive effect when nitrates given with ACE inhibitors

Adrenergic Neurone Blockers: enhanced hypotensive effect when nitrates given with adrenergic neurone blockers

Alcohol: enhanced hypotensive effect when nitrates given with alcohol

Aldesleukin: enhanced hypotensive effect when nitrates given with aldesleukin

Alpha-blockers: enhanced hypotensive effect when nitrates given with alpha-blockers

Anaesthetics, General: enhanced hypotensive effect when nitrates given with general anaesthetics

Analgesics: hypotensive effect of nitrates antagonised by NSAIDs

Angiotensin-II Receptor Antagonists: enhanced hypotensive effect when nitrates given with angiotensin-II receptor antagonists

Anti-arrhythmics: effects of sublingual tablets of nitrates reduced by disopyramide (failure to dissolve under tongue owing to dry mouth)

- Anticoagulants: infusion of glyceryl trinitrate reduces anticoagulant effect of •heparins

Antidepressants: enhanced hypotensive effect when nitrates given with MAOIs; effects of sublingual tablets of nitrates possibly reduced by tricyclic-related antidepressants (failure to dissolve under tongue owing to dry mouth); effects of sublingual tablets of nitrates reduced by tricyclics (failure to dissolve under tongue owing to dry mouth)

Antimuscarinics: effects of sublingual tablets of nitrates possibly reduced by antimuscarinics (failure to dissolve under tongue owing to dry mouth)

Antipsychotics: enhanced hypotensive effect when nitrates given with phenothiazines

Anxiolytics and Hypnotics: enhanced hypotensive effect when nitrates given with anxiolytics and hypnotics

Beta-blockers: enhanced hypotensive effect when nitrates given with beta-blockers

Nitrates *(continued)*

Calcium-channel Blockers: enhanced hypotensive effect when nitrates given with calcium-channel blockers

Clonidine: enhanced hypotensive effect when nitrates given with clonidine

Corticosteroids: hypotensive effect of nitrates antagonised by corticosteroids

Diazoxide: enhanced hypotensive effect when nitrates given with diazoxide

Diuretics: enhanced hypotensive effect when nitrates given with diuretics

Dopaminergics: enhanced hypotensive effect when nitrates given with levodopa

Methyldopa: enhanced hypotensive effect when nitrates given with methyldopa

Moxisylyte (thymoxamine): enhanced hypotensive effect when nitrates given with moxisylyte

Moxonidine: enhanced hypotensive effect when nitrates given with moxonidine

Muscle Relaxants: enhanced hypotensive effect when nitrates given with baclofen or tizanidine

Oestrogens: hypotensive effect of nitrates antagonised by oestrogens

Prostaglandins: enhanced hypotensive effect when nitrates given with alprostadil

- Sildenafil: hypotensive effect of nitrates significantly enhanced by •sildenafil (avoid concomitant use)
- Tadalafil: hypotensive effect of nitrates significantly enhanced by •tadalafil (avoid concomitant use)
- Vardenafil: possible increased hypotensive effect when nitrates given with •vardenafil—avoid concomitant use

Vasodilator Antihypertensives: enhanced hypotensive effect when nitrates given with hydralazine, minoxidil or sodium nitroprusside

Nitrazepam *see* Anxiolytics and Hypnotics

Nitrofurantoin

Antacids: absorption of nitrofurantoin reduced by oral magnesium salts (as magnesium trisilicate)

Oestrogens: antibacterials that do not induce liver enzymes possibly reduce contraceptive effect of oestrogens (risk probably small, see p. 428)

Probenecid: excretion of nitrofurantoin reduced by probenecid (increased risk of side-effects)

Sulfinpyrazone: excretion of nitrofurantoin reduced by sulfinpyrazone (increased risk of toxicity)

Nitroimidazoles *see* Metronidazole and Tinidazole

Nitrous Oxide *see* Anaesthetics, General

Nizatidine *see* Histamine H_2-antagonists

Noradrenaline (norepinephrine) *see* Sympathomimetics

Norelgestromin *see* Progestogens

Norepinephrine (noradrenaline) *see* Sympathomimetics

Norethisterone *see* Progestogens

Norfloxacin *see* Quinolones

Norgestimate *see* Progestogens

Norgestrel *see* Progestogens

Nortriptyline *see* Antidepressants, Tricyclic

NSAIDs

Note *See also* Aspirin. Interactions do not generally apply to topical NSAIDs

ACE Inhibitors: increased risk of renal impairment when NSAIDs given with ACE inhibitors, also hypotensive effect antagonised

Adrenergic Neurone Blockers: NSAIDs antagonise hypotensive effect of adrenergic neurone blockers

Alpha-blockers: NSAIDs antagonise hypotensive effect of alpha-blockers

- Analgesics: avoid concomitant use of NSAIDs with •NSAIDs or •aspirin (increased side-effects); avoid concomitant use of NSAIDs with •ketorolac (increased side-effects and haemorrhage); ibuprofen possibly reduces antiplatelet effect of aspirin

Angiotensin-II Receptor Antagonists: increased risk of renal impairment when NSAIDs given with angiotensin-II receptor antagonists, also hypotensive effect antagonised

- Antibacterials: indometacin possibly increases plasma concentration of amikacin and gentamicin in neonates; plasma concentration of etoricoxib reduced by

NSAIDs

- Antibacterials *(continued)*
  rifampicin; possible increased risk of convulsions when NSAIDs given with •quinolones
- Anticoagulants: NSAIDs possibly enhance anticoagulant effect of •coumarins and •phenindione; celecoxib, etodolac, etoricoxib, flurbiprofen, ibuprofen, mefenamic acid, meloxicam, parecoxib, piroxicam and sulindac possibly enhance anticoagulant effect of •coumarins; increased risk of bleeding when ketorolac given with •coumarins (avoid concomitant use); diclofenac possibly enhances anticoagulant effect of •coumarins, also increased risk of haemorrhage with intravenous diclofenac (avoid concomitant use); azapropazone enhances anticoagulant effect of •coumarins (avoid concomitant use); increased risk of haemorrhage when intravenous diclofenac given with •heparins (avoid concomitant use, including low-dose heparin); possible increased risk of bleeding when NSAIDs given with heparins; increased risk of haemorrhage when ketorolac given with •heparins (avoid concomitant use, including low-dose heparin); ketorolac enhances anticoagulant effect of •phenindione (increased risk of haemorrhage—avoid concomitant use); diclofenac enhances anticoagulant effect of •phenindione, also increased risk of haemorrhage with intravenous diclofenac (avoid concomitant use)
- Antidepressants: increased risk of bleeding when NSAIDs given with •SSRIs or •venlafaxine
- Antidiabetics: azapropazone enhances effects of •tolbutamide (avoid concomitant use); NSAIDs possibly enhance effects of •sulphonylureas
- Antiepileptics: NSAIDs possibly enhance effects of •phenytoin; azapropazone significantly increases plasma concentration of •phenytoin—avoid concomitant use

Antifungals: plasma concentration of parecoxib increased by fluconazole (reduce dose of parecoxib); plasma concentration of celecoxib increased by fluconazole (halve dose of celecoxib)

- Antipsychotics: possible severe drowsiness when indometacin given with haloperidol; avoid concomitant use of azapropazone with •clozapine (increased risk of agranulocytosis)
- Antivirals: plasma concentration of piroxicam increased by •ritonavir (risk of toxicity)—avoid concomitant use; plasma concentration of NSAIDs possibly increased by ritonavir; increased risk of haematological toxicity when NSAIDs given with zidovudine

Beta-blockers: NSAIDs antagonise hypotensive effect of beta-blockers

Bisphosphonates: indometacin increases bioavailability of tiludronic acid

Calcium-channel Blockers: NSAIDs antagonise hypotensive effect of calcium-channel blockers

Cardiac Glycosides: NSAIDs possibly increase plasma concentration of cardiac glycosides, also possible exacerbation of heart failure and reduction of renal function

- Ciclosporin: increased risk of nephrotoxicity when NSAIDs given with •ciclosporin; plasma concentration of diclofenac increased by •ciclosporin (halve dose of diclofenac)

Clonidine: NSAIDs antagonise hypotensive effect of clonidine

Clopidogrel: increased risk of bleeding when NSAIDs given with clopidogrel

Corticosteroids: increased risk of gastro-intestinal bleeding and ulceration when NSAIDs given with corticosteroids

- Cytotoxics: NSAIDs probably reduce excretion of •methotrexate (increased risk of toxicity)—but for concomitant use in rheumatic disease see p. 551; azapropazone reduces excretion of •methotrexate (avoid concomitant use); diclofenac, ibuprofen, indometacin, ketoprofen, meloxicam and naproxen reduce excretion of •methotrexate (increased risk of toxicity)—but for concomitant use in rheumatic disease

NSAIDs

- Cytotoxics *(continued)*
  see p. 551; increased risk of bleeding when NSAIDs given with •erlotinib

Desmopressin: indometacin enhances effects of desmopressin

Diazoxide: NSAIDs antagonise hypotensive effect of diazoxide

- Diuretics: risk of nephrotoxicity of NSAIDs increased by diuretics, also antagonism of diuretic effect; indometacin and ketorolac antagonise effects of diuretics; occasional reports of reduced renal function when indometacin given with •triamterene—avoid concomitant use; possibly increased risk of hyperkalaemia when NSAIDs given with potassium-sparing diuretics and aldosterone antagonists; increased risk of hyperkalaemia when indometacin given with potassium-sparing diuretics and aldosterone antagonists

Iloprost: increased risk of bleeding when NSAIDs given with iloprost

Lipid-regulating Drugs: excretion of meloxicam increased by colestyramine

- Lithium: NSAIDs probably reduce excretion of •lithium (increased risk of toxicity); diclofenac, ibuprofen, indometacin, mefenamic acid, naproxen, parecoxib and piroxicam reduce excretion of •lithium (increased risk of toxicity); ketorolac reduces excretion of •lithium (increased risk of toxicity)—avoid concomitant use

Methyldopa: NSAIDs antagonise hypotensive effect of methyldopa

Mifepristone: avoidance of NSAIDs advised by manufacturer of mifepristone

Moxonidine: NSAIDs antagonise hypotensive effect of moxonidine

Muscle Relaxants: ibuprofen reduces excretion of baclofen (increased risk of toxicity); NSAIDs possibly reduce excretion of baclofen (increased risk of toxicity)

Nitrates: NSAIDs antagonise hypotensive effect of nitrates

Oestrogens: etoricoxib increases plasma concentration of ethinylestradiol

Penicillamine: possible increased risk of nephrotoxicity when NSAIDs given with penicillamine

- Pentoxifylline (oxpentifylline): possible increased risk of bleeding when NSAIDs given with pentoxifylline (oxpentifylline); increased risk of bleeding when ketorolac given with •pentoxifylline (oxpentifylline) (avoid concomitant use)
- Probenecid: excretion of indometacin, ketoprofen and naproxen reduced by •probenecid (increased plasma concentration); excretion of ketorolac reduced by •probenecid (increased plasma concentration)—avoid concomitant use

Progestogens: risk of hyperkalaemia when NSAIDs given with drospirenone (monitor serum potassium during first cycle)

Sibutramine: increased risk of bleeding when NSAIDs given with sibutramine

- Tacrolimus: possible increased risk of nephrotoxicity when NSAIDs given with tacrolimus; increased risk of nephrotoxicity when ibuprofen given with •tacrolimus

Ulcer-healing Drugs: plasma concentration of azapropazone possibly increased by cimetidine

Vasodilator Antihypertensives: NSAIDs antagonise hypotensive effect of hydralazine, minoxidil and sodium nitroprusside

Octreotide

Antidiabetics: octreotide possibly reduces requirements for insulin, metformin, repaglinide and sulphonylureas

- Ciclosporin: octreotide reduces plasma concentration of •ciclosporin

Dopaminergics: octreotide increases plasma concentration of bromocriptine

Ulcer-healing Drugs: octreotide possibly delays absorption of cimetidine

Oestrogens

Note Interactions of combined oral contraceptives may also apply to combined contraceptive patches; in case of hormone replacement therapy low dose unlikely to induce interactions

ACE Inhibitors: oestrogens antagonise hypotensive effect of ACE inhibitors

Adrenergic Neurone Blockers: oestrogens antagonise hypotensive effect of adrenergic neurone blockers

Alpha-blockers: oestrogens antagonise hypotensive effect of alpha-blockers

Analgesics: plasma concentration of ethinylestradiol increased by etoricoxib

Angiotensin-II Receptor Antagonists: oestrogens antagonise hypotensive effect of angiotensin-II receptor antagonists

• Antibacterials: contraceptive effect of oestrogens possibly reduced by antibacterials that do not induce liver enzymes (risk probably small, see p. 428); metabolism of oestrogens accelerated by •rifamycins (reduced contraceptive effect—see p. 428)

• Anticoagulants: oestrogens may enhance or reduce anticoagulant effect of •coumarins; oestrogens antagonise anticoagulant effect of •phenindione

• Antidepressants: contraceptive effect of oestrogens reduced by •St John's wort (avoid concomitant use); oestrogens antagonise antidepressant effect of tricyclics (but side-effects of tricyclics possibly increased due to increased plasma concentration)

Antidiabetics: oestrogens antagonise hypoglycaemic effect of antidiabetics

• Antiepileptics: metabolism of oestrogens accelerated by •carbamazepine, •oxcarbazepine, •phenytoin, •primidone, •rufinamide and •topiramate (reduced contraceptive effect—see p. 428); oestrogens reduce plasma concentration of •lamotrigine

• Antifungals: anecdotal reports of contraceptive failure when oestrogens given with fluconazole, imidazoles, itraconazole or ketoconazole; metabolism of oestrogens accelerated by •griseofulvin (reduced contraceptive effect—see p. 428); occasional reports of breakthrough bleeding when oestrogens (used for contraception) given with terbinafine

• Antivirals: plasma concentration of oestrogens increased by amprenavir, also plasma concentration of amprenavir reduced—alternative contraception recommended; plasma concentration of ethinylestradiol increased by •atazanavir—avoid concomitant use; contraceptive effect of oestrogens possibly reduced by efavirenz; metabolism of oestrogens accelerated by •nelfinavir, •nevirapine and •ritonavir (reduced contraceptive effect—see p. 428)

• Aprepitant: possible contraceptive failure of hormonal contraceptives containing oestrogens when given with •aprepitant (alternative contraception recommended)

• Barbiturates: metabolism of oestrogens accelerated by •barbiturates (reduced contraceptive effect—see p. 428)

Beta-blockers: oestrogens antagonise hypotensive effect of beta-blockers

Bile Acids: elimination of cholesterol in bile increased when oestrogens given with bile acids

• Bosentan: possible contraceptive failure of hormonal contraceptives containing oestrogens when given with •bosentan (alternative contraception recommended)

Calcium-channel Blockers: oestrogens antagonise hypotensive effect of calcium-channel blockers

Ciclosporin: oestrogens possibly increase plasma concentration of ciclosporin

Clonidine: oestrogens antagonise hypotensive effect of clonidine

Corticosteroids: oral contraceptives containing oestrogens increase plasma concentration of corticosteroids

Diazoxide: oestrogens antagonise hypotensive effect of diazoxide

Diuretics: oestrogens antagonise diuretic effect of diuretics

Dopaminergics: oestrogens increase plasma concentration of ropinirole; oestrogens increase plasma concentration of selegiline (increased risk of toxicity)

Oestrogens *(continued)*

Lipid-regulating Drugs: plasma concentration of ethinylestradiol increased by atorvastatin and rosuvastatin

Methyldopa: oestrogens antagonise hypotensive effect of methyldopa

• Modafinil: metabolism of oestrogens accelerated by •modafinil (reduced contraceptive effect—see p. 428)

Moxonidine: oestrogens antagonise hypotensive effect of moxonidine

Muscle Relaxants: oestrogens possibly increase plasma concentration of tizanidine (increased risk of toxicity)

Nitrates: oestrogens antagonise hypotensive effect of nitrates

Sitaxentan: plasma concentration of oestrogens increased by sitaxentan

Somatropin: oestrogens (when used as oral replacement therapy) may increase dose requirements of somatropin

Tacrolimus: metabolism of oestrogens possibly inhibited by tacrolimus; ethinylestradiol possibly increases plasma concentration of tacrolimus

Theophylline: oestrogens reduce excretion of theophylline (increased plasma concentration)

Vasodilator Antihypertensives: oestrogens antagonise hypotensive effect of hydralazine, minoxidil and sodium nitroprusside

Oestrogens, conjugated *see* Oestrogens

Ofloxacin *see* Quinolones

Olanzapine *see* Antipsychotics

Olmesartan *see* Angiotensin-II Receptor Antagonists

Olsalazine *see* Aminosalicylates

Omeprazole *see* Proton Pump Inhibitors

Ondansetron *see* $5HT_3$ Antagonists

Opioid Analgesics

Alcohol: enhanced hypotensive and sedative effects when opioid analgesics given with alcohol

Anti-arrhythmics: opioid analgesics delay absorption of mexiletine

Antibacterials: plasma concentration of alfentanil increased by erythromycin; avoidance of premedication with opioid analgesics advised by manufacturer of ciprofloxacin (reduced plasma concentration of ciprofloxacin) when ciprofloxacin used for surgical prophylaxis; metabolism of methadone accelerated by rifampicin (reduced effect)

• Anticoagulants: tramadol enhances anticoagulant effect of •coumarins; dextropropoxyphene possibly enhances anticoagulant effect of •coumarins

• Antidepressants: plasma concentration of methadone possibly increased by fluvoxamine; possible increased serotonergic effects when pethidine or tramadol given with duloxetine; CNS excitation or depression (hypertension or hypotension) when pethidine given with •MAOIs—avoid concomitant use and for 2 weeks after stopping MAOIs; possible CNS excitation or depression (hypertension or hypotension) when opioid analgesics given with •MAOIs—avoid concomitant use and for 2 weeks after stopping MAOIs; possible CNS excitation or depression (hypertension or hypotension) when opioid analgesics given with •moclobemide; possible CNS excitation or depression (hypertension or hypotension) when dextromethorphan or pethidine given with •moclobemide—avoid concomitant use; increased risk of CNS toxicity when tramadol given with •SSRIs or •tricyclics; sedative effects possibly increased when opioid analgesics given with tricyclics

• Antiepileptics: dextropropoxyphene enhances effects of •carbamazepine; effects of tramadol reduced by carbamazepine; plasma concentration of methadone reduced by carbamazepine; metabolism of methadone accelerated by phenytoin (reduced effect and risk of withdrawal effects)

• Antifungals: metabolism of buprenorphine inhibited by •ketoconazole (reduce dose of buprenorphine); metabolism of alfentanil inhibited by fluconazole (risk of prolonged or delayed respiratory depression); metabolism of alfentanil possibly inhibited by itraconazole; plasma concentration of methadone

Opioid Analgesics
- • Antifungals *(continued)*
  increased by •voriconazole (consider reducing dose of methadone)
- Antipsychotics: enhanced hypotensive and sedative effects when opioid analgesics given with antipsychotics; increased risk of convulsions when tramadol given with antipsychotics
- • Antivirals: plasma concentration of methadone possibly reduced by abacavir and nevirapine; plasma concentration of methadone reduced by amprenavir, efavirenz, nelfinavir and ritonavir; plasma concentration of dextropropoxyphene increased by •ritonavir (risk of toxicity)—avoid concomitant use; plasma concentration of pethidine reduced by •ritonavir, but plasma concentration of toxic pethidine metabolite increased (avoid concomitant use); plasma concentration of morphine possibly reduced by ritonavir; plasma concentration of fentanyl increased by •ritonavir; methadone possibly increases plasma concentration of zidovudine
- Anxiolytics and Hypnotics: increased sedative effect when opioid analgesics given with anxiolytics and hypnotics
- • Atomoxetine: increased risk of ventricular arrhythmias when methadone given with •atomoxetine; possible increased risk of convulsions when tramadol given with atomoxetine
- Beta-blockers: morphine possibly increases plasma concentration of esmolol
- Calcium-channel Blockers: metabolism of alfentanil inhibited by diltiazem (risk of prolonged or delayed respiratory depression)
- Domperidone: opioid analgesics antagonise effects of domperidone on gastro-intestinal activity
- • Dopaminergics: risk of CNS toxicity when pethidine given with •rasagiline (avoid pethidine for 2 weeks after rasagiline); avoid concomitant use of dextromethorphan with •rasagiline; hyperpyrexia and CNS toxicity reported when pethidine given with •selegiline (avoid concomitant use); caution with tramadol advised by manufacturer of selegiline
- $5HT_3$ Antagonists: effects of tramadol possibly antagonised by ondansetron
- • Memantine: increased risk of CNS toxicity when dextromethorphan given with •memantine (manufacturer of memantine advises avoid concomitant use)
- Metoclopramide: opioid analgesics antagonise effects of metoclopramide on gastro-intestinal activity
- • Sodium Oxybate: opioid analgesics enhance effects of •sodium oxybate (avoid concomitant use)
- Ulcer-healing Drugs: metabolism of opioid analgesics inhibited by cimetidine (increased plasma concentration)

Orciprenaline *see* Sympathomimetics

Orlistat
- Anti-arrhythmics: orlistat possibly reduces plasma concentration of amiodarone
- Anticoagulants: manufacturer of orlistat recommends monitoring anticoagulant effect of coumarins
- Antidiabetics: manufacturer of orlistat advises avoid concomitant use with acarbose
- • Ciclosporin: orlistat possibly reduces absorption of •ciclosporin

Orphenadrine *see* Antimuscarinics

Oxaliplatin *see* Platinum Compounds

Oxandrolone *see* Anabolic Steroids

Oxazepam *see* Anxiolytics and Hypnotics

Oxcarbazepine
- • Antidepressants: anticonvulsant effect of antiepileptics possibly antagonised by MAOIs and •tricyclic-related antidepressants (convulsive threshold lowered); anticonvulsant effect of antiepileptics antagonised by •SSRIs and •tricyclics (convulsive threshold lowered); avoid concomitant use of antiepileptics with •St John's wort
- Antiepileptics: oxcarbazepine sometimes reduces plasma concentration of carbamazepine (but concentration of an active metabolite of carbamazepine may be increased), also plasma concentration of an active metabolite of oxcarbazepine often reduced; oxcarbazepine increases plasma concentration of phenytoin, also plasma concentration of an active metabolite of oxcarbazepine reduced; plasma concentration of an active metabolite of oxcarbazepine sometimes reduced by valproate
- • Antimalarials: possible increased risk of convulsions when antiepileptics given with chloroquine and hydroxychloroquine; anticonvulsant effect of antiepileptics antagonised by •mefloquine
- • Antipsychotics: anticonvulsant effect of oxcarbazepine antagonised by •antipsychotics (convulsive threshold lowered)
- Barbiturates: oxcarbazepine increases plasma concentration of phenobarbital, also plasma concentration of an active metabolite of oxcarbazepine reduced
- Ciclosporin: oxcarbazepine possibly reduces plasma concentration of ciclosporin
- • Oestrogens: oxcarbazepine accelerates metabolism of •oestrogens (reduced contraceptive effect—see p. 428)
- • Progestogens: oxcarbazepine accelerates metabolism of •progestogens (reduced contraceptive effect—see p. 428)

Oxprenolol *see* Beta-blockers

Oxybutynin *see* Antimuscarinics

Oxycodone *see* Opioid Analgesics

Oxymetazoline *see* Sympathomimetics

Oxytetracycline *see* Tetracyclines

Oxytocin
- Anaesthetics, General: oxytocic effect possibly reduced, also enhanced hypotensive effect and risk of arrhythmias when oxytocin given with volatile liquid general anaesthetics
- Prostaglandins: uterotonic effect of oxytocin potentiated by prostaglandins
- Sympathomimetics: risk of hypertension when oxytocin given with vasoconstrictor sympathomimetics (due to enhanced vasopressor effect)

Paclitaxel
- Antidiabetics: paclitaxel possibly inhibits metabolism of rosiglitazone
- Antiepileptics: cytotoxics possibly reduce absorption of phenytoin
- • Antipsychotics: avoid concomitant use of cytotoxics with •clozapine (increased risk of agranulocytosis)
- Antivirals: plasma concentration of paclitaxel increased by nelfinavir and ritonavir
- Cardiac Glycosides: cytotoxics reduce absorption of digoxin tablets

Paliperidone *see* Antipsychotics

Pancreatin
- Antidiabetics: pancreatin antagonises hypoglycaemic effect of acarbose

Pancuronium *see* Muscle Relaxants

Pantoprazole *see* Proton Pump Inhibitors

Papaveretum *see* Opioid Analgesics

Paracetamol
- Anticoagulants: prolonged regular use of paracetamol possibly enhances anticoagulant effect of coumarins
- Cytotoxics: paracetamol possibly inhibits metabolism of *intravenous* busulfan (manufacturer of *intravenous* busulfan advises caution within 72 hours of paracetamol)
- Lipid-regulating Drugs: absorption of paracetamol reduced by colestyramine
- Metoclopramide: rate of absorption of paracetamol increased by metoclopramide

Paraldehyde
- • Alcohol: increased sedative effect when paraldehyde given with •alcohol
- • Disulfiram: risk of toxicity when paraldehyde given with •disulfiram

Parasympathomimetics
- Anti-arrhythmics: effects of neostigmine and pyridostigmine antagonised by procainamide; effects of

Parasympathomimetics

Anti-arrhythmics *(continued)*
neostigmine and pyridostigmine possibly antagonised by propafenone

- Antibacterials: plasma concentration of galantamine increased by erythromycin; effects of neostigmine and pyridostigmine antagonised by •aminoglycosides; effects of neostigmine and pyridostigmine antagonised by clindamycin; effects of neostigmine and pyridostigmine antagonised by •polymyxins

Antidepressants: plasma concentration of galantamine increased by paroxetine

Antifungals: plasma concentration of galantamine increased by ketoconazole

Antimalarials: effects of neostigmine and pyridostigmine may be diminished because of potential for chloroquine and hydroxychloroquine to increase symptoms of myasthenia gravis

Antimuscarinics: effects of parasympathomimetics antagonised by antimuscarinics

Beta-blockers: increased risk of arrhythmias when pilocarpine given with beta-blockers; effects of neostigmine and pyridostigmine antagonised by propranolol

Lithium: effects of neostigmine and pyridostigmine antagonised by lithium

Muscle Relaxants: donepezil possibly enhances effects of suxamethonium; edrophonium, galantamine, neostigmine, pyridostigmine and rivastigmine enhance effects of suxamethonium; donepezil possibly antagonises effects of non-depolarising muscle relaxants ; edrophonium, neostigmine, pyridostigmine and rivastigmine antagonise effects of non-depolarising muscle relaxants

Parecoxib *see* NSAIDs
Paricalcitol *see* Vitamins
Paroxetine *see* Antidepressants, SSRI
Pegfilgrastim *see* Filgrastim
Peginterferon Alfa *see* Interferons

Penicillamine

Analgesics: possible increased risk of nephrotoxicity when penicillamine given with NSAIDs

Antacids: absorption of penicillamine reduced by antacids

- Antipsychotics: avoid concomitant use of penicillamine with •clozapine (increased risk of agranulocytosis)

Cardiac Glycosides: penicillamine possibly reduces plasma concentration of digoxin

Iron: absorption of penicillamine reduced by *oral* iron

Zinc: penicillamine reduces absorption of zinc, also absorption of penicillamine reduced by zinc

Penicillins

Allopurinol: increased risk of rash when amoxicillin or ampicillin given with allopurinol

Antibacterials: absorption of phenoxymethylpenicillin reduced by neomycin

Anticoagulants: common experience in anticoagulant clinics is that INR can be altered by a course of broad-spectrum penicillins such as ampicillin, although studies have failed to demonstrate an interaction with coumarins or phenindione

Cytotoxics: penicillins reduce excretion of methotrexate (increased risk of toxicity)

Muscle Relaxants: piperacillin enhances effects of non-depolarising muscle relaxants and suxamethonium

Oestrogens: antibacterials that do not induce liver enzymes possibly reduce contraceptive effect of oestrogens (risk probably small, see p. 428)

Probenecid: excretion of penicillins reduced by probenecid (increased plasma concentration)

Sulfinpyrazone: excretion of penicillins reduced by sulfinpyrazone

Pentamidine Isetionate

- Anti-arrhythmics: increased risk of ventricular arrhythmias when pentamidine isetionate given with •amiodarone—avoid concomitant use
- Antibacterials: increased risk of ventricular arrhythmias when pentamidine isetionate given with parenteral •erythromycin; increased risk of ventricular arrhythmias when pentamidine isetionate given with •moxifloxacin—avoid concomitant use
- Antidepressants: increased risk of ventricular arrhythmias when pentamidine isetionate given with •tricyclics

Antifungals: possible increased risk of nephrotoxicity when pentamidine isetionate given with amphotericin

- Antipsychotics: increased risk of ventricular arrhythmias when pentamidine isetionate given with •amisulpride—avoid concomitant use; increased risk of ventricular arrhythmias when pentamidine isetionate given with •phenothiazines
- Ivabradine: increased risk of ventricular arrhythmias when pentamidine isetionate given with •ivabradine

Pentazocine *see* Opioid Analgesics

Pentostatin

Antiepileptics: cytotoxics possibly reduce absorption of phenytoin

- Antipsychotics: avoid concomitant use of cytotoxics with •clozapine (increased risk of agranulocytosis)

Cardiac Glycosides: cytotoxics reduce absorption of digoxin tablets

- Cytotoxics: increased toxicity when pentostatin given with high-dose •cyclophosphamide—avoid concomitant use; increased pulmonary toxicity when pentostatin given with •fludarabine (unacceptably high incidence of fatalities)

Pentoxifylline (oxpentifylline)

- Analgesics: possible increased risk of bleeding when pentoxifylline (oxpentifylline) given with NSAIDs; increased risk of bleeding when pentoxifylline (oxpentifylline) given with •ketorolac (avoid concomitant use)

Theophylline: pentoxifylline (oxpentifylline) increases plasma concentration of theophylline

Pergolide

Antipsychotics: effects of pergolide antagonised by antipsychotics

Memantine: effects of dopaminergics possibly enhanced by memantine

Methyldopa: antiparkinsonian effect of dopaminergics antagonised by methyldopa

Metoclopramide: antiparkinsonian effect of pergolide antagonised by metoclopramide

Pericyazine *see* Antipsychotics
Perindopril *see* ACE Inhibitors
Perphenazine *see* Antipsychotics
Pethidine *see* Opioid Analgesics
Phenazocine *see* Opioid Analgesics
Phenelzine *see* MAOIs

Phenindione

Note Change in patient's clinical condition particularly associated with liver disease, intercurrent illness, or drug administration, necessitates more frequent testing. Major changes in diet (especially involving salads and vegetables) and in alcohol consumption may also affect anticoagulant control

- Alcohol: anticoagulant control with phenindione may be affected by major changes in consumption of •alcohol
- Anabolic Steroids: anticoagulant effect of phenindione enhanced by •anabolic steroids
- Analgesics: anticoagulant effect of phenindione possibly enhanced by •NSAIDs; anticoagulant effect of phenindione enhanced by •diclofenac, also increased risk of haemorrhage with intravenous diclofenac (avoid concomitant use); anticoagulant effect of phenindione enhanced by •ketorolac (increased risk of haemorrhage—avoid concomitant use); increased risk of bleeding when phenindione given with •aspirin (due to antiplatelet effect)
- Anti-arrhythmics: metabolism of phenindione inhibited by •amiodarone (enhanced anticoagulant effect)
- Antibacterials: experience in anticoagulant clinics suggests that INR possibly altered when phenindione is given with •neomycin (given for local action on gut); anticoagulant effect of phenindione possibly enhanced by levofloxacin and •tetracyclines; studies have failed to demonstrate an interaction with phenindione, but

Phenindione
- Antibacterials *(continued)*
  common experience in anticoagulant clinics is that INR can be altered by a course of broad-spectrum penicillins such as ampicillin
- Antivirals: anticoagulant effect of phenindione possibly enhanced by •ritonavir
- Clopidogrel: anticoagulant effect of phenindione enhanced due to antiplatelet action of •clopidogrel
- Dipyridamole: anticoagulant effect of phenindione enhanced due to antiplatelet action of •dipyridamole
- Enteral Foods: anticoagulant effect of phenindione antagonised by vitamin K (present in some •enteral feeds)

Iloprost: increased risk of bleeding when phenindione given with iloprost
- Lipid-regulating Drugs: anticoagulant effect of phenindione may be enhanced or reduced by •colestyramine; anticoagulant effect of phenindione possibly enhanced by •rosuvastatin; anticoagulant effect of phenindione enhanced by •fibrates
- Oestrogens: anticoagulant effect of phenindione antagonised by •oestrogens
- Progestogens: anticoagulant effect of phenindione antagonised by •progestogens

Sibutramine: increased risk of bleeding when anticoagulants given with sibutramine
- Testolactone: anticoagulant effect of phenindione enhanced by •testolactone
- Testosterone: anticoagulant effect of phenindione enhanced by •testosterone
- Thyroid Hormones: anticoagulant effect of phenindione enhanced by •thyroid hormones
- Vitamins: anticoagulant effect of phenindione antagonised by •vitamin K

Phenobarbital *see* Barbiturates
Phenoperidine *see* Opioid Analgesics
Phenothiazines *see* Antipsychotics
Phenoxybenzamine *see* Alpha-blockers
Phenoxymethylpenicillin *see* Penicillins
Phentolamine *see* Alpha-blockers
Phenylephrine *see* Sympathomimetics
Phenylpropanolamine *see* Sympathomimetics
Phenytoin
- Analgesics: effects of phenytoin possibly enhanced by •NSAIDs; plasma concentration of phenytoin significantly increased by •azapropazone—avoid concomitant use; phenytoin accelerates metabolism of methadone (reduced effect and risk of withdrawal effects); effects of phenytoin enhanced by aspirin

Antacids: absorption of phenytoin reduced by antacids
- Anti-arrhythmics: metabolism of phenytoin inhibited by •amiodarone (increased plasma concentration); phenytoin reduces plasma concentration of disopyramide; phenytoin accelerates metabolism of mexiletine (reduced plasma concentration)
- Antibacterials: metabolism of phenytoin inhibited by clarithromycin, •isoniazid and •metronidazole (increased plasma concentration); plasma concentration of phenytoin increased or decreased by ciprofloxacin; phenytoin accelerates metabolism of doxycycline (reduced plasma concentration); plasma concentration of phenytoin increased by •chloramphenicol (increased risk of toxicity); metabolism of phenytoin accelerated by •rifamycins (reduced plasma concentration); plasma concentration of phenytoin possibly increased by sulphonamides; phenytoin reduces plasma concentration of •telithromycin (avoid during and for 2 weeks after phenytoin); plasma concentration of phenytoin increased by •trimethoprim (also increased antifolate effect)
- Anticoagulants: phenytoin accelerates metabolism of •coumarins (possibility of reduced anticoagulant effect, but enhancement also reported)
- Antidepressants: plasma concentration of phenytoin increased by •fluoxetine and •fluvoxamine; phenytoin reduces plasma concentration of •mianserin, mirtazapine and paroxetine; anticonvulsant effect of antiepileptics possibly antagonised by MAOIs and

Phenytoin
- Antidepressants *(continued)*
  •tricyclic-related antidepressants (convulsive threshold lowered); anticonvulsant effect of antiepileptics antagonised by •SSRIs and •tricyclics (convulsive threshold lowered); avoid concomitant use of antiepileptics with •St John's wort; phenytoin possibly reduces plasma concentration of •tricyclics

Antidiabetics: plasma concentration of phenytoin transiently increased by tolbutamide (possibility of toxicity)
- Antiepileptics: plasma concentration of both drugs often reduced when phenytoin given with carbamazepine, also plasma concentration of phenytoin may be increased; plasma concentration of phenytoin possibly increased by •ethosuximide, also plasma concentration of ethosuximide possibly reduced; phenytoin reduces plasma concentration of lamotrigine, tiagabine and zonisamide; plasma concentration of phenytoin increased by oxcarbazepine, also plasma concentration of an active metabolite of oxcarbazepine reduced; phenytoin possibly reduces plasma concentration of primidone (but concentration of an active metabolite increased), plasma concentration of phenytoin often reduced but may be increased; plasma concentration of phenytoin possibly increased by rufinamide; plasma concentration of phenytoin increased by •topiramate (also plasma concentration of topiramate reduced); plasma concentration of phenytoin increased or possibly reduced when given with valproate, also plasma concentration of valproate reduced; plasma concentration of phenytoin reduced by vigabatrin
- Antifungals: phenytoin reduces plasma concentration of •ketoconazole and •posaconazole; anticonvulsant effect of phenytoin enhanced by •miconazole (plasma concentration of phenytoin increased); plasma concentration of phenytoin increased by •fluconazole (consider reducing dose of phenytoin); phenytoin reduces plasma concentration of •itraconazole—avoid concomitant use; plasma concentration of phenytoin increased by •voriconazole, also phenytoin reduces plasma concentration of voriconazole (increase dose of voriconazole and also monitor for phenytoin toxicity); phenytoin possibly reduces plasma concentration of caspofungin—consider increasing dose of caspofungin
- Antimalarials: possible increased risk of convulsions when antiepileptics given with chloroquine and hydroxychloroquine; anticonvulsant effect of antiepileptics antagonised by •mefloquine; anticonvulsant effect of phenytoin antagonised by •pyrimethamine, also increased antifolate effect
- Antipsychotics: anticonvulsant effect of phenytoin antagonised by •antipsychotics (convulsive threshold lowered); phenytoin possibly reduces plasma concentration of •aripiprazole—increase dose of aripiprazole; phenytoin accelerates metabolism of clozapine, quetiapine and sertindole (reduced plasma concentration)

Antivirals: phenytoin possibly reduces plasma concentration of abacavir, amprenavir, darunavir, indinavir, lopinavir and saquinavir; plasma concentration of phenytoin reduced by nelfinavir; plasma concentration of phenytoin possibly increased by ritonavir, also plasma concentration of ritonavir possibly reduced; plasma concentration of phenytoin increased or decreased by zidovudine

Anxiolytics and Hypnotics: phenytoin often reduces plasma concentration of clonazepam; plasma concentration of phenytoin increased or decreased by diazepam; plasma concentration of phenytoin possibly increased or decreased by benzodiazepines

Aprepitant: phenytoin possibly reduces plasma concentration of aprepitant

Barbiturates: phenytoin often increases plasma concentration of phenobarbital, plasma concentration of phenytoin often reduced but may be increased

Bupropion: phenytoin reduces plasma concentration of bupropion

Phenytoin *(continued)*
- Calcium-channel Blockers: phenytoin reduces effects of felodipine, isradipine and verapamil; phenytoin probably reduces effects of dihydropyridines, nicardipine and •nifedipine; phenytoin reduces plasma concentration of nisoldipine; plasma concentration of phenytoin increased by •diltiazem but also effect of diltiazem reduced

Cardiac Glycosides: phenytoin accelerates metabolism of digitoxin (reduced effect); phenytoin possibly reduces plasma concentration of digoxin
- Ciclosporin: phenytoin accelerates metabolism of •ciclosporin (reduced plasma concentration)
- Corticosteroids: phenytoin accelerates metabolism of •corticosteroids (reduced effect)
- Cytotoxics: phenytoin possibly reduces plasma concentration of busulfan and etoposide; metabolism of phenytoin possibly inhibited by fluorouracil (increased risk of toxicity); phenytoin increases antifolate effect of methotrexate; absorption of phenytoin possibly reduced by cytotoxics; phenytoin reduces plasma concentration of •imatinib—avoid concomitant use; phenytoin reduces plasma concentration of irinotecan and its active metabolite

Diazoxide: plasma concentration of phenytoin reduced by diazoxide, also effect of diazoxide may be reduced
- Disulfiram: metabolism of phenytoin inhibited by •disulfiram (increased risk of toxicity)
- Diuretics: phenytoin antagonises effects of furosemide (frusemide); phenytoin reduces plasma concentration of •eplerenone—avoid concomitant use; increased risk of osteomalacia when phenytoin given with carbonic anhydrase inhibitors

Dopaminergics: phenytoin possibly reduces effects of levodopa
Enteral Foods: absorption of phenytoin possibly reduced by enteral feeds
Folates: plasma concentration of phenytoin possibly reduced by folates
Hormone Antagonists: phenytoin accelerates metabolism of gestrinone (reduced plasma concentration); phenytoin possibly accelerates metabolism of toremifene
$5HT_3$ Antagonists: phenytoin accelerates metabolism of ondansetron (reduced effect)
Leflunomide: plasma concentration of phenytoin possibly increased by leflunomide
Levamisole: plasma concentration of phenytoin possibly increased by levamisole
Lipid-regulating Drugs: combination of phenytoin with fluvastatin may increase plasma concentration of either drug (or both)
Lithium: neurotoxicity may occur when phenytoin given with lithium without increased plasma concentration of lithium
Modafinil: plasma concentration of phenytoin possibly increased by modafinil
Muscle Relaxants: phenytoin antagonises muscle relaxant effect of non-depolarising muscle relaxants (accelerated recovery from neuromuscular blockade)
- Oestrogens: phenytoin accelerates metabolism of •oestrogens (reduced contraceptive effect—see p. 428)
- Progestogens: phenytoin accelerates metabolism of •progestogens (reduced contraceptive effect—see p. 428)
- Sulfinpyrazone: plasma concentration of phenytoin increased by •sulfinpyrazone

Sympathomimetics: plasma concentration of phenytoin increased by methylphenidate
Tacrolimus: phenytoin reduces plasma concentration of tacrolimus, also plasma concentration of phenytoin possibly increased
- Theophylline: plasma concentration of both drugs reduced when phenytoin given with •theophylline

Thyroid Hormones: phenytoin accelerates metabolism of thyroid hormones (may increase requirements in hypothyroidism), also plasma concentration of phenytoin possibly increased
Tibolone: phenytoin accelerates metabolism of tibolone

Phenytoin *(continued)*
- Ulcer-healing Drugs: metabolism of phenytoin inhibited by •cimetidine (increased plasma concentration); effects of phenytoin enhanced by •esomeprazole; effects of phenytoin possibly enhanced by omeprazole; absorption of phenytoin reduced by •sucralfate

Vaccines: effects of phenytoin enhanced by influenza vaccine
Vitamins: phenytoin possibly increases requirements for vitamin D

Phosphodiesterase Inhibitors
- Anagrelide: avoidance of enoximone and milrinone advised by manufacturer of •anagrelide

Physostigmine *see* Parasympathomimetics
Pilocarpine *see* Parasympathomimetics
Pimozide *see* Antipsychotics
Pindolol *see* Beta-blockers
Pioglitazone *see* Antidiabetics
Piperacillin *see* Penicillins
Pipotiazine *see* Antipsychotics
Piroxicam *see* NSAIDs
Pivmecillinam *see* Penicillins
Pizotifen
Adrenergic Neurone Blockers: pizotifen antagonises hypotensive effect of adrenergic neurone blockers
Platinum Compounds
- Antibacterials: increased risk of nephrotoxicity and possibly of ototoxicity when platinum compounds given with •aminoglycosides or •polymyxins; increased risk of nephrotoxicity and ototoxicity when platinum compounds given with capreomycin; increased risk of nephrotoxicity and possibly of ototoxicity when cisplatin given with vancomycin

Antiepileptics: cytotoxics possibly reduce absorption of phenytoin
- Antipsychotics: avoid concomitant use of cytotoxics with •clozapine (increased risk of agranulocytosis)

Cardiac Glycosides: cytotoxics reduce absorption of digoxin tablets
- Cytotoxics: increased pulmonary toxicity when cisplatin given with •bleomycin and •methotrexate

Diuretics: increased risk of nephrotoxicity and ototoxicity when platinum compounds given with diuretics
Polymyxin B *see* Polymyxins
Polymyxins
Antibacterials: increased risk of nephrotoxicity when colistin or polymyxins given with aminoglycosides; increased risk of nephrotoxicity when colistin or polymyxins given with capreomycin; increased risk of nephrotoxicity and ototoxicity when colistin given with teicoplanin or vancomycin; increased risk of nephrotoxicity when polymyxins given with vancomycin
Antifungals: increased risk of nephrotoxicity when polymyxins given with amphotericin
- Ciclosporin: increased risk of nephrotoxicity when polymyxins given with •ciclosporin
- Cytotoxics: increased risk of nephrotoxicity and possibly of ototoxicity when polymyxins given with •platinum compounds
- Diuretics: increased risk of otoxicity when polymyxins given with •loop diuretics
- Muscle Relaxants: polymyxins enhance effects of •non-depolarising muscle relaxants and •suxamethonium

Oestrogens: antibacterials that do not induce liver enzymes possibly reduce contraceptive effect of oestrogens (risk probably small, see p. 428)
- Parasympathomimetics: polymyxins antagonise effects of •neostigmine and •pyridostigmine

Posaconazole *see* Antifungals, Triazole
Potassium Aminobenzoate
Antibacterials: potassium aminobenzoate inhibits effects of sulphonamides
Potassium Bicarbonate *see* Potassium Salts
Potassium Chloride *see* Potassium Salts
Potassium Citrate *see* Potassium Salts

Potassium Salts

Note Includes salt substitutes

- ACE Inhibitors: increased risk of severe hyperkalaemia when potassium salts given with •ACE inhibitors

Aliskiren: increased risk of hyperkalaemia when potassium salts given with aliskiren

- Angiotensin-II Receptor Antagonists: increased risk of hyperkalaemia when potassium salts given with •angiotensin-II receptor antagonists

Antibacterials: avoid concomitant use of potassium citrate with methenamine

- Ciclosporin: increased risk of hyperkalaemia when potassium salts given with •ciclosporin
- Diuretics: increased risk of hyperkalaemia when potassium salts given with •potassium-sparing diuretics and aldosterone antagonists
- Tacrolimus: increased risk of hyperkalaemia when potassium salts given with •tacrolimus

Pramipexole

Antipsychotics: manufacturer of pramipexole advises avoid concomitant use of antipsychotics (antagonism of effect)

Memantine: effects of dopaminergics possibly enhanced by memantine

Methyldopa: antiparkinsonian effect of dopaminergics antagonised by methyldopa

Ulcer-healing Drugs: excretion of pramipexole reduced by cimetidine (increased plasma concentration)

Pravastatin *see* Statins

Prazosin *see* Alpha-blockers

Prednisolone *see* Corticosteroids

Prilocaine

Anti-arrhythmics: increased myocardial depression when prilocaine given with anti-arrhythmics

Antibacterials: increased risk of methaemoglobinaemia when prilocaine given with sulphonamides

Primaquine

- Antimalarials: avoidance of antimalarials advised by manufacturer of •artemether/lumefantrine

Mepacrine: plasma concentration of primaquine increased by mepacrine (increased risk of toxicity)

Primidone

Alcohol: increased sedative effect when primidone given with alcohol

Anti-arrhythmics: primidone accelerates metabolism of disopyramide (reduced plasma concentration)

- Antibacterials: primidone accelerates metabolism of •chloramphenicol, doxycycline and metronidazole (reduced plasma concentration); primidone reduces plasma concentration of •telithromycin (avoid during and for 2 weeks after primidone)
- Anticoagulants: primidone accelerates metabolism of •coumarins (reduced anticoagulant effect)
- Antidepressants: primidone reduces plasma concentration of paroxetine; primidone accelerates metabolism of •mianserin (reduced plasma concentration); anticonvulsant effect of antiepileptics possibly antagonised by MAOIs and •tricyclic-related antidepressants (convulsive threshold lowered); anticonvulsant effect of antiepileptics antagonised by •SSRIs and •tricyclics (convulsive threshold lowered); avoid concomitant use of antiepileptics with •St John's wort; anticonvulsant effect of primidone antagonised by •tricyclics (convulsive threshold lowered), also metabolism of tricyclics possibly accelerated (reduced plasma concentration)
- Antiepileptics: primidone often reduces plasma concentration of carbamazepine, also plasma concentration of primidone sometimes reduced (but concentration of an active metabolite of primidone often increased); primidone possibly reduces plasma concentration of ethosuximide; primidone reduces plasma concentration of lamotrigine and tiagabine; plasma concentration of primidone possibly reduced by phenytoin (but concentration of an active metabolite increased), plasma concentration of phenytoin often reduced but may be increased; plasma concentration of primidone possibly increased by •valproate (plasma concentration of active metabolite of primidone increased), also plasma concentration of valproate reduced; plasma concentration of primidone possibly reduced by vigabatrin

Primidone

- Antiepileptics *(continued)*
- Antifungals: primidone possibly reduces plasma concentration of •posaconazole; primidone possibly reduces plasma concentration of •voriconazole—avoid concomitant use; primidone reduces absorption of griseofulvin (reduced effect)
- Antimalarials: possible increased risk of convulsions when antiepileptics given with chloroquine and hydroxychloroquine; anticonvulsant effect of antiepileptics antagonised by •mefloquine
- Antipsychotics: anticonvulsant effect of primidone antagonised by •antipsychotics (convulsive threshold lowered); primidone accelerates metabolism of haloperidol (reduced plasma concentration); primidone possibly reduces plasma concentration of •aripiprazole—increase dose of aripiprazole
- Antivirals: primidone possibly reduces plasma concentration of •indinavir, •lopinavir, •nelfinavir and •saquinavir

Anxiolytics and Hypnotics: primidone often reduces plasma concentration of clonazepam

Barbiturates: increased sedative effect when primidone given with barbiturates

- Calcium-channel Blockers: primidone reduces effects of •felodipine and •isradipine; primidone probably reduces effects of •dihydropyridines, •diltiazem and •verapamil

Cardiac Glycosides: primidone accelerates metabolism of digitoxin (reduced effect)

- Ciclosporin: primidone accelerates metabolism of •ciclosporin (reduced effect)
- Corticosteroids: primidone accelerates metabolism of •corticosteroids (reduced effect)

Diuretics: plasma concentration of primidone possibly reduced by acetazolamide; increased risk of osteomalacia when primidone given with carbonic anhydrase inhibitors

Folates: plasma concentration of primidone possibly reduced by folates

Hormone Antagonists: primidone accelerates metabolism of gestrinone and toremifene (reduced plasma concentration)

$5HT_3$ Antagonists: primidone reduces plasma concentration of tropisetron

Leukotriene Antagonists: primidone reduces plasma concentration of montelukast

Memantine: effects of primidone possibly reduced by memantine

- Oestrogens: primidone accelerates metabolism of •oestrogens (reduced contraceptive effect—see p. 428)
- Progestogens: primidone accelerates metabolism of •progestogens (reduced contraceptive effect—see p. 428)

Sympathomimetics: plasma concentration of primidone possibly increased by methylphenidate

Theophylline: primidone accelerates metabolism of theophylline (reduced effect)

Thyroid Hormones: primidone accelerates metabolism of thyroid hormones (may increase requirements for thyroid hormones in hypothyroidism)

Tibolone: primidone accelerates metabolism of tibolone (reduced plasma concentration)

Vitamins: primidone possibly increases requirements for vitamin D

Probenecid

ACE Inhibitors: probenecid reduces excretion of captopril

- Analgesics: probenecid reduces excretion of •indometacin, •ketoprofen and •naproxen (increased plasma concentration); probenecid reduces excretion of •ketorolac (increased plasma concentration)—avoid concomitant use; effects of probenecid antagonised by aspirin

Probenecid *(continued)*

Antibacterials: probenecid reduces excretion of meropenem (manufacturers of meropenem advise avoid concomitant use); probenecid reduces excretion of cephalosporins, ciprofloxacin, nalidixic acid, norfloxacin and penicillins (increased plasma concentration); probenecid reduces excretion of dapsone and nitrofurantoin (increased risk of side-effects); effects of probenecid antagonised by pyrazinamide

Antidiabetics: probenecid possibly enhances hypoglycaemic effect of chlorpropamide

Antivirals: probenecid reduces excretion of aciclovir (increased plasma concentration); probenecid possibly reduces excretion of famciclovir (increased plasma concentration); probenecid reduces excretion of ganciclovir and zidovudine (increased plasma concentration and risk of toxicity)

• Cytotoxics: probenecid reduces excretion of •methotrexate (increased risk of toxicity)

Sodium Benzoate: probenecid possibly reduces excretion of conjugate formed by sodium benzoate

Sodium Phenylbutyrate: probenecid possibly reduces excretion of conjugate formed by sodium phenylbutyrate

Procainamide

ACE Inhibitors: increased risk of toxicity when procainamide given with captopril especially in renal impairment

Anaesthetics, Local: increased myocardial depression when anti-arrhythmics given with bupivacaine, levobupivacaine, prilocaine or ropivacaine

• Anti-arrhythmics: increased myocardial depression when anti-arrhythmics given with other •anti-arrhythmics; plasma concentration of procainamide increased by •amiodarone (increased risk of ventricular arrhythmias—avoid concomitant use)

• Antibacterials: increased risk of ventricular arrhythmias when procainamide given with •moxifloxacin—avoid concomitant use; plasma concentration of procainamide increased by trimethoprim

• Antidepressants: increased risk of ventricular arrhythmias when procainamide given with •tricyclics

• Antihistamines: increased risk of ventricular arrhythmias when procainamide given with •mizolastine—avoid concomitant use

• Antimalarials: avoidance of procainamide advised by manufacturer of •artemether/lumefantrine (risk of ventricular arrhythmias)

• Antipsychotics: increased risk of ventricular arrhythmias when anti-arrhythmics that prolong the QT interval given with •antipsychotics that prolong the QT interval; increased risk of ventricular arrhythmias when procainamide given with •amisulpride, •pimozide or •sertindole—avoid concomitant use; increased risk of ventricular arrhythmias when procainamide given with •phenothiazines

• Atomoxetine: increased risk of ventricular arrhythmias when procainamide given with •atomoxetine

• Beta-blockers: increased myocardial depression when anti-arrhythmics given with •beta-blockers; increased risk of ventricular arrhythmias when procainamide given with •sotalol—avoid concomitant use

• $5HT_3$ Antagonists: increased risk of ventricular arrhythmias when procainamide given with •dolasetron—avoid concomitant use; caution with anti-arrhythmics advised by manufacturer of tropisetron (risk of ventricular arrhythmias)

• Muscle Relaxants: procainamide enhances effects of •muscle relaxants

Parasympathomimetics: procainamide antagonises effects of neostigmine and pyridostigmine

• Ulcer-healing Drugs: plasma concentration of procainamide increased by •cimetidine

Procaine

Laronidase: procaine possibly inhibits effects of laronidase (manufacturer of laronidase advises avoid concomitant use)

Procarbazine

Alcohol: disulfiram-like reaction when procarbazine given with alcohol

Antiepileptics: cytotoxics possibly reduce absorption of phenytoin

• Antipsychotics: avoid concomitant use of cytotoxics with •clozapine (increased risk of agranulocytosis)

Cardiac Glycosides: cytotoxics reduce absorption of digoxin tablets

Prochlorperazine *see* Antipsychotics

Procyclidine *see* Antimuscarinics

Progesterone *see* Progestogens

Progestogens

Note Interactions of combined oral contraceptives may also apply to combined contraceptive patches

ACE Inhibitors: risk of hyperkalaemia when drospirenone given with ACE inhibitors (monitor serum potassium during first cycle)

Analgesics: risk of hyperkalaemia when drospirenone given with NSAIDs (monitor serum potassium during first cycle)

Angiotensin-II Receptor Antagonists: risk of hyperkalaemia when drospirenone given with angiotensin-II receptor antagonists (monitor serum potassium during first cycle)

• Antibacterials: metabolism of progestogens accelerated by •rifamycins (reduced contraceptive effect—see p. 428)

• Anticoagulants: progestogens may enhance or reduce anticoagulant effect of •coumarins; progestogens antagonise anticoagulant effect of •phenindione

• Antidepressants: contraceptive effect of progestogens reduced by •St John's wort (avoid concomitant use)

Antidiabetics: progestogens antagonise hypoglycaemic effect of antidiabetics

• Antiepileptics: metabolism of progestogens accelerated by •carbamazepine, •oxcarbazepine, •phenytoin, •primidone, •rufinamide and •topiramate (reduced contraceptive effect—see p. 428); progestogens reduce plasma concentration of •lamotrigine

• Antifungals: metabolism of progestogens accelerated by •griseofulvin (reduced contraceptive effect—see p. 428); occasional reports of breakthrough bleeding when progestogens (used for contraception) given with terbinafine

• Antivirals: plasma concentration of progestogens increased by amprenavir, also plasma concentration of amprenavir reduced—alternative contraception recommended; contraceptive effect of progestogens possibly reduced by nelfinavir; metabolism of progestogens accelerated by •nevirapine (reduced contraceptive effect—see p. 428)

• Aprepitant: possible contraceptive failure of hormonal contraceptives containing progestogens when given with •aprepitant (alternative contraception recommended)

• Barbiturates: metabolism of progestogens accelerated by •barbiturates (reduced contraceptive effect—see p. 428)

• Bosentan: possible contraceptive failure of hormonal contraceptives containing progestogens when given with •bosentan (alternative contraception recommended)

• Ciclosporin: progestogens inhibit metabolism of •ciclosporin (increased plasma concentration)

Diuretics: risk of hyperkalaemia when drospirenone given with potassium-sparing diuretics and aldosterone antagonists (monitor serum potassium during first cycle)

Dopaminergics: progestogens increase plasma concentration of selegiline (increased risk of toxicity)

Lipid-regulating Drugs: plasma concentration of norethisterone increased by atorvastatin; plasma concentration of norgestrel increased by rosuvastatin

Muscle Relaxants: progestogens possibly increase plasma concentration of tizanidine (increased risk of toxicity)

Sitaxentan: plasma concentration of progestogens increased by sitaxentan

Progestogens *(continued)*

Tacrolimus: metabolism of progestogens possibly inhibited by tacrolimus

Proguanil

Antacids: absorption of proguanil reduced by oral magnesium salts (as magnesium trisilicate)

Anticoagulants: isolated reports that proguanil may enhance anticoagulant effect of warfarin

• Antimalarials: avoidance of antimalarials advised by manufacturer of •artemether/lumefantrine; increased antifolate effect when proguanil given with pyrimethamine

Promazine *see* Antipsychotics

Promethazine *see* Antihistamines

Propafenone

Anaesthetics, Local: increased myocardial depression when anti-arrhythmics given with bupivacaine, levobupivacaine, prilocaine or ropivacaine

• Anti-arrhythmics: increased myocardial depression when anti-arrhythmics given with other •anti-arrhythmics

• Antibacterials: metabolism of propafenone accelerated by •rifampicin (reduced effect)

• Anticoagulants: propafenone enhances anticoagulant effect of •coumarins

• Antidepressants: metabolism of propafenone possibly inhibited by paroxetine (increased risk of toxicity); increased risk of arrhythmias when propafenone given with •tricyclics

• Antihistamines: increased risk of ventricular arrhythmias when propafenone given with •mizolastine—avoid concomitant use

• Antipsychotics: increased risk of ventricular arrhythmias when anti-arrhythmics that prolong the QT interval given with •antipsychotics that prolong the QT interval

• Antivirals: plasma concentration of propafenone possibly increased by •amprenavir (increased risk of ventricular arrhythmias—avoid concomitant use); plasma concentration of propafenone increased by •ritonavir (increased risk of ventricular arrhythmias—avoid concomitant use)

• Beta-blockers: increased myocardial depression when anti-arrhythmics given with •beta-blockers; propafenone increases plasma concentration of metoprolol and propranolol

• Cardiac Glycosides: propafenone increases plasma concentration of •digoxin (halve dose of digoxin)

Ciclosporin: propafenone possibly increases plasma concentration of ciclosporin

• $5HT_3$ Antagonists: increased risk of ventricular arrhythmias when propafenone given with •dolasetron—avoid concomitant use; caution with anti-arrhythmics advised by manufacturer of tropisetron (risk of ventricular arrhythmias)

Parasympathomimetics: propafenone possibly antagonises effects of neostigmine and pyridostigmine

Theophylline: propafenone increases plasma concentration of theophylline

• Ulcer-healing Drugs: plasma concentration of propafenone increased by •cimetidine

Propantheline *see* Antimuscarinics

Propiverine *see* Antimuscarinics

Propofol *see* Anaesthetics, General

Propranolol *see* Beta-blockers

Prostaglandins

ACE Inhibitors: enhanced hypotensive effect when alprostadil given with ACE inhibitors

Adrenergic Neurone Blockers: enhanced hypotensive effect when alprostadil given with adrenergic neurone blockers

Alpha-blockers: enhanced hypotensive effect when alprostadil given with alpha-blockers

Angiotensin-II Receptor Antagonists: enhanced hypotensive effect when alprostadil given with angiotensin-II receptor antagonists

Beta-blockers: enhanced hypotensive effect when alprostadil given with beta-blockers

Prostaglandins *(continued)*

Calcium-channel Blockers: enhanced hypotensive effect when alprostadil given with calcium-channel blockers

Clonidine: enhanced hypotensive effect when alprostadil given with clonidine

Diazoxide: enhanced hypotensive effect when alprostadil given with diazoxide

Diuretics: enhanced hypotensive effect when alprostadil given with diuretics

Methyldopa: enhanced hypotensive effect when alprostadil given with methyldopa

Moxonidine: enhanced hypotensive effect when alprostadil given with moxonidine

Nitrates: enhanced hypotensive effect when alprostadil given with nitrates

Oxytocin: prostaglandins potentiate uterotonic effect of oxytocin

Vasodilator Antihypertensives: enhanced hypotensive effect when alprostadil given with hydralazine, minoxidil or sodium nitroprusside

Protein Kinase Inhibitors *see* Dasatinib, Erlotinib, Imatinib, Sorafenib, and Sunitinib

Proton Pump Inhibitors

Antacids: absorption of lansoprazole possibly reduced by antacids

Antibacterials: plasma concentration of both drugs increased when omeprazole given with clarithromycin

• Anticoagulants: esomeprazole, omeprazole and pantoprazole possibly enhance anticoagulant effect of •coumarins

Antidepressants: omeprazole increases plasma concentration of escitalopram

• Antiepileptics: omeprazole possibly enhances effects of phenytoin; esomeprazole enhances effects of •phenytoin

Antifungals: proton pump inhibitors reduce absorption of itraconazole and ketoconazole; plasma concentration of omeprazole increased by voriconazole (reduce dose of omeprazole)

Antipsychotics: omeprazole possibly reduces plasma concentration of clozapine

• Antivirals: esomeprazole and omeprazole significantly reduce plasma concentration of •atazanavir—avoid concomitant use; proton pump inhibitors possibly reduce plasma concentration of •atazanavir—avoid concomitant use; omeprazole reduces plasma concentration of •nelfinavir—avoid concomitant use; omeprazole possibly increases plasma concentration of saquinavir

Anxiolytics and Hypnotics: esomeprazole and omeprazole possibly inhibit metabolism of diazepam (increased plasma concentration)

Cardiac Glycosides: proton pump inhibitors possibly slightly increase plasma concentration of digoxin

Ciclosporin: omeprazole possibly affects plasma concentration of ciclosporin

• Cilostazol: omeprazole increases plasma concentration of •cilostazol (risk of toxicity)—avoid concomitant use; lansoprazole possibly increases plasma concentration of •cilostazol—avoid concomitant use

Cytotoxics: omeprazole possibly reduces excretion of methotrexate (increased risk of toxicity)

Tacrolimus: omeprazole possibly increases plasma concentration of tacrolimus

Ulcer-healing Drugs: absorption of lansoprazole possibly reduced by sucralfate

Pseudoephedrine *see* Sympathomimetics

Pyrazinamide

Oestrogens: antibacterials that do not induce liver enzymes possibly reduce contraceptive effect of oestrogens (risk probably small, see p. 428)

Probenecid: pyrazinamide antagonises effects of probenecid

Sulfinpyrazone: pyrazinamide antagonises effects of sulfinpyrazone

Pyridostigmine *see* Parasympathomimetics

Pyridoxine *see* Vitamins

Pyrimethamine
- Antibacterials: increased antifolate effect when pyrimethamine (includes Fansidar®) given with •sulphonamides; increased antifolate effect when pyrimethamine given with •trimethoprim
- Antiepileptics: pyrimethamine antagonises anticonvulsant effect of •phenytoin, also increased antifolate effect
- Antimalarials: avoidance of antimalarials advised by manufacturer of •artemether/lumefantrine; increased antifolate effect when pyrimethamine given with proguanil

Antivirals: increased antifolate effect when pyrimethamine given with zidovudine
- Cytotoxics: pyrimethamine increases antifolate effect of •methotrexate

Quetiapine *see* Antipsychotics
Quinagolide

Memantine: effects of dopaminergics possibly enhanced by memantine

Methyldopa: antiparkinsonian effect of dopaminergics antagonised by methyldopa

Quinapril *see* ACE Inhibitors
Quinine
- Anti-arrhythmics: increased risk of ventricular arrhythmias when quinine given with •amiodarone—avoid concomitant use; quinine increases plasma concentration of •flecainide
- Antibacterials: increased risk of ventricular arrhythmias when quinine given with •moxifloxacin—avoid concomitant use
- Antimalarials: avoidance of antimalarials advised by manufacturer of •artemether/lumefantrine; increased risk of ventricular arrhythmias when quinine given with •artemether/lumefantrine; increased risk of convulsions when quinine given with •mefloquine (but should not prevent the use of intravenous quinine in severe cases)
- Antipsychotics: increased risk of ventricular arrhythmias when quinine given with •pimozide—avoid concomitant use
- Cardiac Glycosides: quinine increases plasma concentration of •digoxin

Muscle Relaxants: quinine possibly enhances effects of suxamethonium

Ulcer-healing Drugs: metabolism of quinine inhibited by cimetidine (increased plasma concentration)

Quinolones
- Analgesics: possible increased risk of convulsions when quinolones given with •NSAIDs; manufacturer of ciprofloxacin advises avoid premedication with opioid analgesics (reduced plasma concentration of ciprofloxacin) when ciprofloxacin used for surgical prophylaxis

Antacids: absorption of ciprofloxacin, levofloxacin, moxifloxacin, norfloxacin and ofloxacin reduced by antacids
- Anti-arrhythmics: increased risk of ventricular arrhythmias when moxifloxacin given with •amiodarone, •disopyramide or •procainamide—avoid concomitant use
- Antibacterials: increased risk of ventricular arrhythmias when moxifloxacin given with parenteral •erythromycin—avoid concomitant use
- Anticoagulants: ciprofloxacin, nalidixic acid, norfloxacin and ofloxacin enhance anticoagulant effect of •coumarins; levofloxacin possibly enhances anticoagulant effect of coumarins and phenindione
- Antidepressants: ciprofloxacin inhibits metabolism of •duloxetine—avoid concomitant use; increased risk of ventricular arrhythmias when moxifloxacin given with •tricyclics—avoid concomitant use

Antidiabetics: ciprofloxacin and norfloxacin possibly enhance effects of glibenclamide

Antiepileptics: ciprofloxacin increases or decreases plasma concentration of phenytoin
- Antihistamines: increased risk of ventricular arrhythmias when moxifloxacin given with •mizolastine—avoid concomitant use

Quinolones *(continued)*
- Antimalarials: avoidance of quinolones advised by manufacturer of •artemether/lumefantrine; increased risk of ventricular arrhythmias when moxifloxacin given with •chloroquine and hydroxychloroquine, •mefloquine or •quinine—avoid concomitant use
- Antipsychotics: increased risk of ventricular arrhythmias when moxifloxacin given with •haloperidol, •phenothiazines, •pimozide or •sertindole—avoid concomitant use; ciprofloxacin increases plasma concentration of clozapine; ciprofloxacin possibly increases plasma concentration of olanzapine
- Atomoxetine: increased risk of ventricular arrhythmias when moxifloxacin given with •atomoxetine
- Beta-blockers: increased risk of ventricular arrhythmias when moxifloxacin given with •sotalol—avoid concomitant use

Calcium Salts: absorption of ciprofloxacin reduced by calcium salts
- Ciclosporin: increased risk of nephrotoxicity when quinolones given with •ciclosporin

Cytotoxics: nalidixic acid increases risk of melphalan toxicity; ciprofloxacin possibly reduces excretion of methotrexate (increased risk of toxicity); norfloxacin possibly reduces bioavailability of mycophenolate

Dairy Products: absorption of ciprofloxacin and norfloxacin reduced by dairy products

Dopaminergics: ciprofloxacin inhibits metabolism of ropinirole (increased plasma concentration)

$5HT_1$ Agonists: quinolones possibly inhibit metabolism of zolmitriptan (reduce dose of zolmitriptan)

Iron: absorption of ciprofloxacin, levofloxacin, moxifloxacin, norfloxacin and ofloxacin reduced by *oral* iron
- Muscle Relaxants: ciprofloxacin increases plasma concentration of •tizanidine (increased risk of toxicity)—avoid concomitant use

Oestrogens: antibacterials that do not induce liver enzymes possibly reduce contraceptive effect of oestrogens (risk probably small, see p. 428)
- Pentamidine Isetionate: increased risk of ventricular arrhythmias when moxifloxacin given with •pentamidine isetionate—avoid concomitant use

Probenecid: excretion of ciprofloxacin, nalidixic acid and norfloxacin reduced by probenecid (increased plasma concentration)

Sevelamer: bioavailability of ciprofloxacin reduced by sevelamer

Strontium Ranelate: absorption of quinolones reduced by strontium ranelate (manufacturer of strontium ranelate advises avoid concomitant use)
- Theophylline: possible increased risk of convulsions when quinolones given with •theophylline; ciprofloxacin and norfloxacin increase plasma concentration of •theophylline

Ulcer-healing Drugs: absorption of ciprofloxacin, levofloxacin, moxifloxacin, norfloxacin and ofloxacin reduced by sucralfate

Zinc: absorption of ciprofloxacin, levofloxacin, moxifloxacin, norfloxacin and ofloxacin reduced by zinc

Quinupristin with Dalfopristin
- Anti-arrhythmics: increased risk of ventricular arrhythmias when quinupristin/dalfopristin given with •disopyramide or •lidocaine (lignocaine)—avoid concomitant use

Antibacterials: manufacturer of quinupristin/dalfopristin recommends monitoring liver function when given with rifampicin

Antivirals: quinupristin/dalfopristin possibly increases plasma concentration of saquinavir
- Anxiolytics and Hypnotics: quinupristin/dalfopristin inhibits metabolism of •midazolam (increased plasma concentration with increased sedation); quinupristin/dalfopristin inhibits the metabolism of zopiclone
- Calcium-channel Blockers: quinupristin/dalfopristin increases plasma concentration of •nifedipine
- Ciclosporin: quinupristin/dalfopristin increases plasma concentration of •ciclosporin

Quinupristin with Dalfopristin *(continued)*

- Ergot Alkaloids: manufacturer of quinupristin/dalfopristin advises avoid concomitant use with •ergotamine and methysergide
  Oestrogens: antibacterials that do not induce liver enzymes possibly reduce contraceptive effect of oestrogens (risk probably small, see p. 428)
- Tacrolimus: quinupristin/dalfopristin increases plasma concentration of •tacrolimus

Rabeprazole *see* Proton Pump Inhibitors

Raloxifene

Anticoagulants: raloxifene antagonises anticoagulant effect of coumarins

Lipid-regulating Drugs: absorption of raloxifene reduced by colestyramine (manufacturer of raloxifene advises avoid concomitant administration)

Ramipril *see* ACE Inhibitors

Ranitidine *see* Histamine H_2-antagonists

Rasagiline

Note Rasagiline is a MAO-B inhibitor

- Analgesics: avoid concomitant use of rasagiline with •dextromethorphan; risk of CNS toxicity when rasagiline given with •pethidine (avoid pethidine for 2 weeks after rasagiline)
- Antidepressants: after stopping rasagiline do not start •fluoxetine for 2 weeks, also rasagiline should not be started until at least 5 weeks after stopping fluoxetine; after stopping rasagiline do not start •fluvoxamine for 2 weeks; risk of hypertensive crisis when rasagiline given with •MAOIs, avoid MAOIs for at least 2 weeks after stopping rasagiline; increased risk of CNS toxicity when rasagiline given with •SSRIs or •tricyclics
  Dopaminergics: plasma concentration of rasagiline possibly reduced by entacapone
  Memantine: effects of dopaminergics possibly enhanced by memantine
  Methyldopa: antiparkinsonian effect of dopaminergics antagonised by methyldopa
- Sympathomimetics: avoid concomitant use of rasagiline with •sympathomimetics

Reboxetine

- Antibacterials: manufacturer of reboxetine advises avoid concomitant use with •macrolides
- Antidepressants: manufacturer of reboxetine advises avoid concomitant use with •fluvoxamine; increased risk of hypertension and CNS excitation when reboxetine given with •MAOIs (MAOIs should not be started until 1 week after stopping reboxetine, avoid reboxetine for 2 weeks after stopping MAOIs)
- Antifungals: manufacturer of reboxetine advises avoid concomitant use with •imidazoles and •triazoles
- Antimalarials: avoidance of antidepressants advised by manufacturer of •artemether/lumefantrine
  Atomoxetine: possible increased risk of convulsions when antidepressants given with atomoxetine
  Diuretics: possible increased risk of hypokalaemia when reboxetine given with loop diuretics or thiazides and related diuretics
  Ergot Alkaloids: possible risk of hypertension when reboxetine given with ergotamine and methysergide
- Sibutramine: increased risk of CNS toxicity when noradrenaline re-uptake inhibitors given with •sibutramine (manufacturer of sibutramine advises avoid concomitant use)

Remifentanil *see* Opioid Analgesics

Repaglinide *see* Antidiabetics

Retinoids

Alcohol: etretinate formed from acitretin in presence of alcohol

- Antibacterials: possible increased risk of benign intracranial hypertension when retinoids given with •tetracyclines (avoid concomitant use)
- Anticoagulants: acitretin possibly reduces anticoagulant effect of •coumarins
  Antiepileptics: isotretinoin possibly reduces plasma concentration of carbamazepine
- Cytotoxics: acitretin increases plasma concentration of •methotrexate (also increased risk of hepatotoxicity)—avoid concomitant use

Retinoids *(continued)*

Vitamins: risk of hypervitaminosis A when retinoids given with vitamin A

Ribavirin

- Antivirals: increased risk of side-effects when ribavirin given with •didanosine; ribavirin possibly inhibits effects of •stavudine

Rifabutin *see* Rifamycins

Rifampicin *see* Rifamycins

Rifamycins

ACE Inhibitors: rifampicin reduces plasma concentration of active metabolite of imidapril (reduced antihypertensive effect)

Analgesics: rifampicin reduces plasma concentration of etoricoxib; rifampicin accelerates metabolism of methadone (reduced effect)

Antacids: absorption of rifampicin reduced by antacids

- Anti-arrhythmics: rifamycins accelerate metabolism of •disopyramide (reduced plasma concentration); rifampicin accelerates metabolism of mexiletine (reduced plasma concentration); rifampicin accelerates metabolism of •propafenone (reduced effect)
- Antibacterials: rifamycins reduce plasma concentration of clarithromycin and dapsone; plasma concentration of rifabutin increased by •clarithromycin (increased risk of uveitis—reduce rifabutin dose); rifampicin accelerates metabolism of chloramphenicol (reduced plasma concentration); plasma concentration of rifabutin possibly increased by •macrolides (increased risk of uveitis—reduce rifabutin dose); monitoring of liver function with rifampicin recommended by manufacturer of quinupristin/dalfopristin; rifampicin reduces plasma concentration of •telithromycin (avoid during and for 2 weeks after rifampicin); rifampicin possibly reduces plasma concentration of trimethoprim
- Anticoagulants: rifamycins accelerate metabolism of •coumarins (reduced anticoagulant effect)
  Antidepressants: rifampicin possibly reduces plasma concentration of tricyclics
- Antidiabetics: rifamycins accelerate metabolism of •chlorpropamide and •tolbutamide (reduced effect); rifampicin reduces plasma concentration of •rosiglitazone—consider increasing dose of rosiglitazone; rifampicin reduces plasma concentration of nateglinide; rifampicin possibly antagonises hypoglycaemic effect of repaglinide; rifamycins possibly accelerate metabolism of •sulphonylureas (reduced effect)
- Antiepileptics: rifabutin reduces plasma concentration of •carbamazepine; rifampicin reduces plasma concentration of •lamotrigine; rifamycins accelerate metabolism of •phenytoin (reduced plasma concentration)
- Antifungals: rifampicin accelerates metabolism of •ketoconazole (reduced plasma concentration), also plasma concentration of rifampicin may be reduced by ketoconazole; plasma concentration of rifabutin increased by •fluconazole (increased risk of uveitis—reduce rifabutin dose); rifampicin accelerates metabolism of •fluconazole and •itraconazole (reduced plasma concentration); rifabutin reduces plasma concentration of •itraconazole—avoid concomitant use; plasma concentration of rifabutin increased by •posaconazole (also plasma concentration of posaconazole reduced); rifampicin reduces plasma concentration of •posaconazole and terbinafine; plasma concentration of rifabutin increased by •voriconazole, also rifabutin reduces plasma concentration of voriconazole (increase dose of voriconazole and also monitor for rifabutin toxicity); rifampicin reduces plasma concentration of •voriconazole—avoid concomitant use; rifampicin initially increases and then reduces plasma concentration of caspofungin (consider increasing dose of caspofungin); plasma concentration of rifabutin possibly increased by •triazoles (increased risk of uveitis—reduce rifabutin dose)
- Antimalarials: rifampicin reduces plasma concentration of •mefloquine—avoid concomitant use
- Antipsychotics: rifampicin accelerates metabolism of •haloperidol (reduced plasma concentration);

Rifamycins

- Antipsychotics *(continued)*
  rifabutin and rifampicin possibly reduce plasma concentration of •aripiprazole—increase dose of aripiprazole; rifampicin possibly reduces plasma concentration of clozapine
- Antivirals: rifampicin possibly reduces plasma concentration of abacavir; plasma concentration of rifabutin increased by •amprenavir, •atazanavir, •darunavir and •tipranavir (reduce dose of rifabutin); rifampicin significantly reduces plasma concentration of •amprenavir, •darunavir and •nelfinavir—avoid concomitant use; rifampicin reduces plasma concentration of •atazanavir, •lopinavir and •nevirapine—avoid concomitant use; rifampicin reduces plasma concentration of efavirenz—increase dose of efavirenz; plasma concentration of rifabutin reduced by efavirenz—increase dose of rifabutin; plasma concentration of rifabutin increased by •indinavir, also plasma concentration of indinavir decreased (reduce dose of rifabutin and increase dose of indinavir); rifampicin accelerates metabolism of •indinavir (reduced plasma concentration—avoid concomitant use); rifampicin reduces plasma concentration of •maraviroc—consider increasing dose of maraviroc; plasma concentration of rifabutin increased by •nelfinavir (halve dose of rifabutin); plasma concentration of rifabutin possibly increased by nevirapine; plasma concentration of rifabutin increased by •ritonavir (increased risk of toxicity); rifampicin significantly reduces plasma concentration of •saquinavir, also risk of hepatotoxicity—avoid concomitant use; rifabutin reduces plasma concentration of •saquinavir; rifampicin possibly reduces plasma concentration of •tipranavir—avoid concomitant use; avoidance of rifampicin advised by manufacturer of zidovudine

Anxiolytics and Hypnotics: rifampicin accelerates metabolism of diazepam (reduced plasma concentration); rifampicin possibly accelerates metabolism of benzodiazepines (reduced plasma concentration); rifampicin possibly accelerates metabolism of buspirone and zaleplon; rifampicin accelerates metabolism of zolpidem (reduced plasma concentration and reduced effect); rifampicin significantly reduces plasma concentration of zopiclone

Aprepitant: rifampicin reduces plasma concentration of aprepitant

- Atovaquone: rifabutin and rifampicin reduce plasma concentration of •atovaquone (possible therapeutic failure of atovaquone)

Barbiturates: plasma concentration of rifampicin possibly reduced by phenobarbital

Beta-blockers: rifampicin accelerates metabolism of bisoprolol and propranolol (plasma concentration significantly reduced); rifampicin reduces plasma concentration of carvedilol, celiprolol and metoprolol

- Bosentan: rifampicin reduces plasma concentration of •bosentan—avoid concomitant use
- Calcium-channel Blockers: rifampicin possibly accelerates metabolism of •isradipine, •nicardipine and •nisoldipine (possible significantly reduced plasma concentration); rifampicin accelerates metabolism of •diltiazem, •nifedipine, •nimodipine and •verapamil (plasma concentration significantly reduced)

Cardiac Glycosides: rifamycins accelerate metabolism of digitoxin (reduced effect); rifampicin possibly reduces plasma concentration of digoxin

- Ciclosporin: rifampicin accelerates metabolism of •ciclosporin (reduced plasma concentration)
- Corticosteroids: rifamycins accelerate metabolism of •corticosteroids (reduced effect)
- Cytotoxics: rifampicin reduces plasma concentration of active metabolite of •mycophenolate; rifampicin accelerates metabolism of •dasatinib (reduced plasma concentration—avoid concomitant use); rifampicin accelerates metabolism of erlotinib and sunitinib (reduced plasma concentration); rifampicin reduces plasma concentration of •imatinib—avoid concomitant use; rifampicin reduces plasma concentration of sorafenib
- Diuretics: rifampicin reduces plasma concentration of •eplerenone—avoid concomitant use

Hormone Antagonists: rifampicin possibly reduces plasma concentration of exemestane; rifampicin accelerates metabolism of gestrinone (reduced plasma concentration)

$5HT_3$ Antagonists: rifampicin accelerates metabolism of ondansetron (reduced effect); rifampicin reduces plasma concentration of tropisetron

Lipid-regulating Drugs: rifampicin possibly reduces plasma concentration of atorvastatin and simvastatin; rifampicin accelerates metabolism of fluvastatin (reduced effect)

- Oestrogens: rifamycins accelerate metabolism of •oestrogens (reduced contraceptive effect—see p. 428); antibacterials that do not induce liver enzymes possibly reduce contraceptive effect of oestrogens (risk probably small, see p. 428)
- Progestogens: rifamycins accelerate metabolism of •progestogens (reduced contraceptive effect—see p. 428)
- Sirolimus: rifabutin and rifampicin reduce plasma concentration of •sirolimus—avoid concomitant use
- Tacrolimus: rifampicin reduces plasma concentration of •tacrolimus

Tadalafil: rifampicin reduces plasma concentration of tadalafil

Theophylline: rifampicin accelerates metabolism of theophylline (reduced plasma concentration)

Thyroid Hormones: rifampicin accelerates metabolism of levothyroxine (thyroxine) (may increase requirements for levothyroxine (thyroxine) in hypothyroidism)

Tibolone: rifampicin accelerates metabolism of tibolone (reduced plasma concentration)

Ulcer-healing Drugs: rifampicin accelerates metabolism of cimetidine (reduced plasma concentration)

Rimonabant

Antifungals: plasma concentration of rimonabant increased by ketoconazole

Risedronate Sodium *see* Bisphosphonates

Risperidone *see* Antipsychotics

Ritodrine *see* Sympathomimetics, $Beta_2$

Ritonavir

- Alpha-blockers: ritonavir possibly increases plasma concentration of •alfuzosin—avoid concomitant use
- Analgesics: ritonavir possibly increases plasma concentration of NSAIDs; ritonavir increases plasma concentration of •dextropropoxyphene and •piroxicam (risk of toxicity)—avoid concomitant use; ritonavir increases plasma concentration of •fentanyl; ritonavir reduces plasma concentration of methadone; ritonavir possibly reduces plasma concentration of morphine; ritonavir reduces plasma concentration of •pethidine, but increases plasma concentration of toxic metabolite of pethidine (avoid concomitant use)
- Anti-arrhythmics: ritonavir increases plasma concentration of •amiodarone, •flecainide and •propafenone (increased risk of ventricular arrhythmias—avoid concomitant use); ritonavir possibly increases plasma concentration of •disopyramide and •mexiletine (increased risk of toxicity)
- Antibacterials: ritonavir possibly increases plasma concentration of azithromycin and erythromycin; ritonavir increases plasma concentration of •clarithromycin (reduce dose of clarithromycin in renal impairment); ritonavir increases plasma concentration of •rifabutin (increased risk of toxicity); plasma concentration of both drugs increased when ritonavir given with •fusidic acid—avoid concomitant use; avoidance of concomitant ritonavir in severe renal and hepatic impairment advised by manufacturer of •telithromycin
- Anticoagulants: ritonavir may enhance or reduce anticoagulant effect of •warfarin; ritonavir possibly

Ritonavir

- Anticoagulants *(continued)*
  enhances anticoagulant effect of •coumarins and •phenindione
- Antidepressants: ritonavir possibly reduces plasma concentration of paroxetine; side-effects possibly increased when ritonavir given with trazodone; ritonavir possibly increases plasma concentration of •SSRIs and •tricyclics; plasma concentration of ritonavir reduced by •St John's wort—avoid concomitant use

  Antidiabetics: ritonavir possibly increases plasma concentration of tolbutamide
- Antiepileptics: ritonavir possibly increases plasma concentration of •carbamazepine; plasma concentration of ritonavir possibly reduced by phenytoin, also plasma concentration of phenytoin possibly increased
- Antifungals: combination of ritonavir with •itraconazole or •ketoconazole may increase plasma concentration of either drug (or both); plasma concentration of ritonavir increased by fluconazole; ritonavir reduces plasma concentration of •voriconazole—avoid concomitant use

  Antihistamines: ritonavir possibly increases plasma concentration of non-sedating antihistamines
- Antimalarials: avoid concomitant use of ritonavir with •artemether/lumefantrine

  Antimuscarinics: avoidance of ritonavir advised by manufacturer of darifenacin and tolterodine; ritonavir increases plasma concentration of solifenacin
- Antipsychotics: ritonavir possibly increases plasma concentration of •antipsychotics; ritonavir possibly inhibits metabolism of •aripiprazole (reduce dose of aripiprazole); ritonavir increases plasma concentration of •clozapine (increased risk of toxicity)—avoid concomitant use; ritonavir reduces plasma concentration of olanzapine—consider increasing dose of olanzapine; ritonavir increases plasma concentration of •pimozide and •sertindole (increased risk of ventricular arrhythmias—avoid concomitant use)
- Antivirals: ritonavir increases plasma concentration of amprenavir, indinavir and •saquinavir; ritonavir increases toxicity of efavirenz, monitor liver function tests; combination of ritonavir with nelfinavir may increase plasma concentration of either drug (or both)
- Anxiolytics and Hypnotics: ritonavir possibly increases plasma concentration of •anxiolytics and hypnotics; ritonavir possibly increases plasma concentration of •alprazolam, •diazepam, •flurazepam and •zolpidem (risk of extreme sedation and respiratory depression—avoid concomitant use); ritonavir possibly increases plasma concentration of •midazolam (risk of prolonged sedation—avoid concomitant use of oral midazolam); ritonavir increases plasma concentration of buspirone (increased risk of toxicity)

  Aprepitant: ritonavir possibly increases plasma concentration of aprepitant

  Bosentan: ritonavir possibly increases plasma concentration of bosentan
- Bupropion: ritonavir increases plasma concentration of •bupropion (risk of toxicity)—avoid concomitant use
- Calcium-channel Blockers: ritonavir possibly increases plasma concentration of •calcium-channel blockers; avoidance of ritonavir advised by manufacturer of lercanidipine

  Cardiac Glycosides: ritonavir possibly increases plasma concentration of digoxin
- Ciclosporin: ritonavir possibly increases plasma concentration of •ciclosporin
- Cilostazol: ritonavir possibly increases plasma concentration of •cilostazol—avoid concomitant use
- Corticosteroids: ritonavir possibly increases plasma concentration of corticosteroids, dexamethasone and prednisolone; ritonavir increases plasma concentration of inhaled and intranasal budesonide and •fluticasone

  Cytotoxics: ritonavir increases plasma concentration of paclitaxel

Ritonavir *(continued)*

- Diuretics: ritonavir increases plasma concentration of •eplerenone—avoid concomitant use
- Ergot Alkaloids: increased risk of ergotism when ritonavir given with •ergotamine and methysergide—avoid concomitant use
- $5HT_1$ Agonists: ritonavir increases plasma concentration of •eletriptan (risk of toxicity)—avoid concomitant use
- Ivabradine: ritonavir possibly increases plasma concentration of •ivabradine—avoid concomitant use
- Lipid-regulating Drugs: possible increased risk of myopathy when ritonavir given with atorvastatin; increased risk of myopathy when ritonavir given with •simvastatin (avoid concomitant use)
- Oestrogens: ritonavir accelerates metabolism of •oestrogens (reduced contraceptive effect—see p. 428)
- Sildenafil: ritonavir significantly increases plasma concentration of •sildenafil—avoid concomitant use

  Sympathomimetics: ritonavir possibly increases plasma concentration of dexamfetamine
- Tacrolimus: ritonavir possibly increases plasma concentration of •tacrolimus

  Tadalafil: ritonavir increases plasma concentration of tadalafil
- Theophylline: ritonavir accelerates metabolism of •theophylline (reduced plasma concentration)
- Vardenafil: ritonavir possibly increases plasma concentration of •vardenafil—avoid concomitant use

Rivastigmine *see* Parasympathomimetics

Rizatriptan *see* $5HT_1$ Agonists

Rocuronium *see* Muscle Relaxants

Ropinirole

Antibacterials: metabolism of ropinirole inhibited by ciprofloxacin (increased plasma concentration)

Antipsychotics: manufacturer of ropinirole advises avoid concomitant use of antipsychotics (antagonism of effect)

Memantine: effects of dopaminergics possibly enhanced by memantine

Methyldopa: antiparkinsonian effect of dopaminergics antagonised by methyldopa

Metoclopramide: manufacturer of ropinirole advises avoid concomitant use of metoclopramide (antagonism of effect)

Oestrogens: plasma concentration of ropinirole increased by oestrogens

Ropivacaine

Anti-arrhythmics: increased myocardial depression when ropivacaine given with anti-arrhythmics

Antidepressants: metabolism of ropivacaine inhibited by fluvoxamine—avoid prolonged administration of ropivacaine

Rosiglitazone *see* Antidiabetics

Rosuvastatin *see* Statins

Rotigotine

Antipsychotics: manufacturer of rotigotine advises avoid concomitant use of antipsychotics (antagonism of effect)

Memantine: effects of dopaminergics possibly enhanced by memantine

Methyldopa: antiparkinsonian effect of dopaminergics antagonised by methyldopa

Metoclopramide: manufacturer of rotigotine advises avoid concomitant use of metoclopramide (antagonism of effect)

Rowachol®

Anticoagulants: Rowachol® possibly reduces anticoagulant effect of coumarins

Rufinamide

- Antidepressants: anticonvulsant effect of antiepileptics possibly antagonised by MAOIs and •tricyclic-related antidepressants (convulsive threshold lowered); anticonvulsant effect of antiepileptics antagonised by •SSRIs and •tricyclics (convulsive threshold lowered); avoid concomitant use of antiepileptics with •St John's wort

  Antiepileptics: rufinamide possibly increases plasma concentration of phenytoin; plasma concentration of

Rufinamide

Antiepileptics *(continued)*
rufinamide possibly increased by valproate (reduce dose of rufinamide)
- Antimalarials: possible increased risk of convulsions when antiepileptics given with chloroquine and hydroxychloroquine; anticonvulsant effect of antiepileptics antagonised by •mefloquine
- Oestrogens: rufinamide accelerates metabolism of •oestrogens (reduced contraceptive effect—see p. 428)
- Progestogens: rufinamide accelerates metabolism of •progestogens (reduced contraceptive effect—see p. 428)

St John's Wort
- Antibacterials: St John's wort reduces plasma concentration of •telithromycin (avoid during and for 2 weeks after St John's wort)
- Anticoagulants: St John's wort reduces anticoagulant effect of •coumarins (avoid concomitant use)
- Antidepressants: possible increased serotonergic effects when St John's wort given with duloxetine; St John's wort reduces plasma concentration of amitriptyline; increased serotonergic effects when St John's wort given with •SSRIs—avoid concomitant use
- Antiepileptics: avoid concomitant use of St John's wort with •antiepileptics
- Antifungals: St John's wort reduces plasma concentration of •voriconazole—avoid concomitant use
- Antimalarials: avoidance of antidepressants advised by manufacturer of •artemether/lumefantrine
- Antipsychotics: St John's wort possibly reduces plasma concentration of •aripiprazole—increase dose of aripiprazole
- Antivirals: St John's wort reduces plasma concentration of •amprenavir, •atazanavir, •darunavir, •efavirenz •indinavir, •lopinavir, •nelfinavir, •nevirapine, •ritonavir and •saquinavir—avoid concomitant use; St John's wort possibly reduces plasma concentration of •maraviroc and •tipranavir—avoid concomitant use
- Aprepitant: avoidance of St John's wort advised by manufacturer of •aprepitant

Atomoxetine: possible increased risk of convulsions when antidepressants given with atomoxetine
- Barbiturates: avoid concomitant use of St John's wort with •phenobarbital

Calcium-channel Blockers: St John's wort possibly reduces plasma concentration of amlodipine
- Cardiac Glycosides: St John's wort reduces plasma concentration of •digoxin—avoid concomitant use
- Ciclosporin: St John's wort reduces plasma concentration of •ciclosporin—avoid concomitant use
- Cytotoxics: St John's wort accelerates metabolism of •irinotecan (reduced plasma concentration—avoid concomitant use)
- Diuretics: St John's wort reduces plasma concentration of •eplerenone—avoid concomitant use
- $5HT_1$ Agonists: increased serotonergic effects when St John's wort given with •$5HT_1$ agonists—avoid concomitant use

Ivabradine: St John's wort reduces plasma concentration of ivabradine—avoid concomitant use

Lipid-regulating Drugs: St John's wort reduces plasma concentration of simvastatin
- Oestrogens: St John's wort reduces contraceptive effect of •oestrogens (avoid concomitant use)
- Progestogens: St John's wort reduces contraceptive effect of •progestogens (avoid concomitant use)
- Tacrolimus: St John's wort reduces plasma concentration of •tacrolimus—avoid concomitant use
- Theophylline: St John's wort reduces plasma concentration of •theophylline—avoid concomitant use

Salbutamol *see* Sympathomimetics, $Beta_2$

Salmeterol *see* Sympathomimetics, $Beta_2$

Saquinavir
- Antibacterials: plasma concentration of saquinavir reduced by •rifabutin; plasma concentration of saquinavir significantly reduced by •rifampicin, also risk of

Saquinavir
- Antibacterials *(continued)*
hepatotoxicity—avoid concomitant use; plasma concentration of saquinavir possibly increased by quinupristin/dalfopristin; avoidance of concomitant saquinavir in severe renal and hepatic impairment advised by manufacturer of •telithromycin

Anticoagulants: saquinavir possibly enhances anticoagulant effect of warfarin
- Antidepressants: plasma concentration of saquinavir reduced by •St John's wort—avoid concomitant use
- Antiepileptics: plasma concentration of saquinavir possibly reduced by carbamazepine, phenytoin and •primidone

Antifungals: plasma concentration of saquinavir increased by ketoconazole; plasma concentration of saquinavir possibly increased by imidazoles and triazoles
- Antimalarials: avoid concomitant use of saquinavir with •artemether/lumefantrine

Antimuscarinics: avoidance of saquinavir advised by manufacturer of darifenacin and tolterodine
- Antipsychotics: saquinavir possibly inhibits metabolism of •aripiprazole (reduce dose of aripiprazole); saquinavir possibly increases plasma concentration of •pimozide (increased risk of ventricular arrhythmias—avoid concomitant use); saquinavir increases plasma concentration of •sertindole (increased risk of ventricular arrhythmias—avoid concomitant use)
- Antivirals: plasma concentration of saquinavir increased by atazanavir, indinavir, lopinavir and •ritonavir; saquinavir reduces plasma concentration of darunavir; plasma concentration of saquinavir significantly reduced by efavirenz; saquinavir increases plasma concentration of •maraviroc (consider reducing dose of maraviroc); combination of saquinavir with nelfinavir may increase plasma concentration of either drug (or both); plasma concentration of saquinavir reduced by •tipranavir
- Anxiolytics and Hypnotics: saquinavir increases plasma concentration of •midazolam (risk of prolonged sedation—avoid concomitant use of oral midazolam)
- Barbiturates: plasma concentration of saquinavir possibly reduced by •barbiturates
- Ciclosporin: plasma concentration of both drugs increased when saquinavir given with •ciclosporin
- Cilostazol: saquinavir possibly increases plasma concentration of •cilostazol—avoid concomitant use

Corticosteroids: plasma concentration of saquinavir possibly reduced by dexamethasone

Diuretics: saquinavir increases plasma concentration of eplerenone (reduce dose of eplerenone)
- Ergot Alkaloids: increased risk of ergotism when saquinavir given with •ergotamine and methysergide—avoid concomitant use
- Lipid-regulating Drugs: possible increased risk of myopathy when saquinavir given with atorvastatin; increased risk of myopathy when saquinavir given with •simvastatin (avoid concomitant use)

Sildenafil: saquinavir possibly increases plasma concentration of sildenafil—reduce initial dose of sildenafil
- Tacrolimus: saquinavir increases plasma concentration of •tacrolimus (consider reducing dose of tacrolimus)

Tadalafil: saquinavir possibly increases plasma concentration of tadalafil—reduce initial dose of tadalafil

Ulcer-healing Drugs: plasma concentration of saquinavir possibly increased by omeprazole

Vardenafil: saquinavir possibly increases plasma concentration of vardenafil—reduce initial dose of vardenafil

Secobarbital *see* Barbiturates

Selegiline

Note Selegiline is a MAO-B inhibitor
- Analgesics: hyperpyrexia and CNS toxicity reported when selegiline given with •pethidine (avoid concomitant use); manufacturer of selegiline advises caution with tramadol

Selegiline *(continued)*
- Antidepressants: theoretical risk of serotonin syndrome if selegiline given with citalopram (especially if dose of selegiline exceeds 10 mg daily); caution with selegiline advised by manufacturer of escitalopram; increased risk of hypertension and CNS excitation when selegiline given with •fluoxetine (selegiline should not be started until 5 weeks after stopping fluoxetine, avoid fluoxetine for 2 weeks after stopping selegiline); increased risk of hypertension and CNS excitation when selegiline given with •fluvoxamine or •venlafaxine (selegiline should not be started until 1 week after stopping fluvoxamine or venlafaxine, avoid fluvoxamine or venlafaxine for 2 weeks after stopping selegiline); increased risk of hypertension and CNS excitation when selegiline given with •paroxetine or •sertraline (selegiline should not be started until 2 weeks after stopping paroxetine or sertraline, avoid paroxetine or sertraline for 2 weeks after stopping selegiline); enhanced hypotensive effect when selegiline given with MAOIs; avoid concomitant use of selegiline with •moclobemide; CNS toxicity reported when selegiline given with •tricyclics

Dopaminergics: max. dose of 10 mg selegiline advised by manufacturer of entacapone if used concomitantly; selegiline enhances effects and increases toxicity of levodopa (reduce dose of levodopa)

Memantine: effects of dopaminergics and selegiline possibly enhanced by memantine

Methyldopa: antiparkinsonian effect of dopaminergics antagonised by methyldopa

Oestrogens: plasma concentration of selegiline increased by oestrogens (increased risk of toxicity)

Progestogens: plasma concentration of selegiline increased by progestogens (increased risk of toxicity)
- Sympathomimetics: risk of hypertensive crisis when selegiline given with •dopamine

Selenium

Vitamins: absorption of selenium possibly reduced by ascorbic acid (give at least 4 hours apart)

Sertindole *see* Antipsychotics

Sertraline *see* Antidepressants, SSRI

Sevelamer

Antibacterials: sevelamer reduces bioavailability of ciprofloxacin

Cytotoxics: sevelamer possibly reduces plasma concentration of mycophenolate

Sevoflurane *see* Anaesthetics, General

Sibutramine

Analgesics: increased risk of bleeding when sibutramine given with NSAIDs or aspirin

Anticoagulants: increased risk of bleeding when sibutramine given with anticoagulants
- Antidepressants: increased CNS toxicity when sibutramine given with •MAOIs or •moclobemide (manufacturer of sibutramine advises avoid concomitant use), also avoid sibutramine for 2 weeks after stopping MAOIs or moclobemide; increased risk of CNS toxicity when sibutramine given with •SSRI-related antidepressants, •SSRIs, •mirtazapine, •noradrenaline re-uptake inhibitors, •tricyclic-related antidepressants, •tricyclics or •tryptophan (manufacturer of sibutramine advises avoid concomitant use)
- Antipsychotics: increased risk of CNS toxicity when sibutramine given with •antipsychotics (manufacturer of sibutramine advises avoid concomitant use)

Sildenafil
- Alpha-blockers: enhanced hypotensive effect when sildenafil given with •alpha-blockers (avoid alpha-blockers for 4 hours after sildenafil)

Antibacterials: plasma concentration of sildenafil possibly increased by clarithromycin and telithromycin—reduce initial dose of sildenafil; plasma concentration of sildenafil increased by erythromycin—reduce initial dose of sildenafil

Antifungals: plasma concentration of sildenafil increased by itraconazole and ketoconazole—reduce initial dose of sildenafil
- Antivirals: plasma concentration of sildenafil possibly increased by amprenavir, nelfinavir and saquinavir—

Sildenafil
- Antivirals *(continued)* reduce initial dose of sildenafil; side-effects of sildenafil possibly increased by •atazanavir; plasma concentration of sildenafil increased by indinavir—reduce initial dose of sildenafil; plasma concentration of sildenafil significantly increased by •ritonavir—avoid concomitant use

Bosentan: plasma concentration of sildenafil reduced by bosentan

Calcium-channel Blockers: enhanced hypotensive effect when sildenafil given with amlodipine

Grapefruit Juice: plasma concentration of sildenafil possibly increased by grapefruit juice
- Nicorandil: sildenafil significantly enhances hypotensive effect of •nicorandil (avoid concomitant use)
- Nitrates: sildenafil significantly enhances hypotensive effect of •nitrates (avoid concomitant use)

Ulcer-healing Drugs: plasma concentration of sildenafil increased by cimetidine (reduce initial dose of sildenafil)

Simvastatin *see* Statins

Sirolimus
- Antibacterials: plasma concentration of sirolimus increased by •clarithromycin and •telithromycin—avoid concomitant use; plasma concentration of both drugs increased when sirolimus given with •erythromycin; plasma concentration of sirolimus reduced by •rifabutin and •rifampicin—avoid concomitant use
- Antifungals: plasma concentration of sirolimus increased by •itraconazole, •ketoconazole and •voriconazole—avoid concomitant use; plasma concentration of sirolimus increased by •miconazole; plasma concentration of sirolimus possibly increased by posaconazole
- Antivirals: plasma concentration of sirolimus possibly increased by •atazanavir and lopinavir
- Calcium-channel Blockers: plasma concentration of sirolimus increased by •diltiazem; plasma concentration of both drugs increased when sirolimus given with •verapamil

Ciclosporin: plasma concentration of sirolimus increased by ciclosporin
- Grapefruit Juice: plasma concentration of sirolimus increased by •grapefruit juice—avoid concomitant use

Sitaxentan
- Anticoagulants: sitaxentan enhances anticoagulant effect of •coumarins
- Ciclosporin: plasma concentration of sitaxentan increased by •ciclosporin—avoid concomitant use

Oestrogens: sitaxentan increases plasma concentration of oestrogens

Progestogens: sitaxentan increases plasma concentration of progestogens

Sodium Nitroprusside *see* Vasodilator Antihypertensives

Sodium Benzoate

Antiepileptics: effects of sodium benzoate possibly reduced by valproate

Antipsychotics: effects of sodium benzoate possibly reduced by haloperidol

Corticosteroids: effects of sodium benzoate possibly reduced by corticosteroids

Probenecid: excretion of conjugate formed by sodium benzoate possibly reduced by probenecid

Sodium Bicarbonate *see* Antacids

Sodium Clodronate *see* Bisphosphonates

Sodium Oxybate
- Analgesics: effects of sodium oxybate enhanced by •opioid analgesics (avoid concomitant use)

Antidepressants: increased risk of side-effects when sodium oxybate given with tricyclics

Antipsychotics: effects of sodium oxybate possibly enhanced by antipsychotics
- Anxiolytics and Hypnotics: effects of sodium oxybate enhanced by •benzodiazepines (avoid concomitant use)
- Barbiturates: effects of sodium oxybate enhanced by •barbiturates (avoid concomitant use)

Sodium Phenylbutyrate

Antiepileptics: effects of sodium phenylbutyrate possibly reduced by valproate

Antipsychotics: effects of sodium phenylbutyrate possibly reduced by haloperidol

Corticosteroids: effects of sodium phenylbutyrate possibly reduced by corticosteroids

Probenecid: excretion of conjugate formed by sodium phenylbutyrate possibly reduced by probenecid

Sodium Polystyrene Sulphonate

Thyroid Hormones: sodium polystyrene sulphonate reduces absorption of levothyroxine (thyroxine)

Sodium Valproate *see* Valproate

Solifenacin *see* Antimuscarinics

Somatropin

Corticosteroids: growth-promoting effect of somatropin may be inhibited by corticosteroids

Oestrogens: increased doses of somatropin may be needed when given with oestrogens (when used as oral replacement therapy)

Sorafenib

Antibacterials: plasma concentration of sorafenib reduced by rifampicin

• Anticoagulants: sorafenib possibly enhances anticoagulant effect of •coumarins

Antiepileptics: cytotoxics possibly reduce absorption of phenytoin

• Antipsychotics: avoid concomitant use of cytotoxics with •clozapine (increased risk of agranulocytosis)

Cardiac Glycosides: cytotoxics reduce absorption of digoxin tablets

Cytotoxics: sorafenib possibly increases plasma concentration of doxorubicin and irinotecan; sorafenib increases plasma concentration of docetaxel

Sotalol *see* Beta-blockers

Spironolactone *see* Diuretics

Statins

Antacids: absorption of rosuvastatin reduced by antacids

• Anti-arrhythmics: increased risk of myopathy when simvastatin given with •amiodarone

• Antibacterials: plasma concentration of atorvastatin increased by •clarithromycin; increased risk of myopathy when simvastatin given with •clarithromycin, •erythromycin or •telithromycin (avoid concomitant use); plasma concentration of rosuvastatin reduced by erythromycin; possible increased risk of myopathy when atorvastatin given with erythromycin or fusidic acid; plasma concentration of atorvastatin and simvastatin possibly reduced by rifampicin; metabolism of fluvastatin accelerated by rifampicin (reduced effect); increased risk of myopathy when statins given with •daptomycin (preferably avoid concomitant use); possible increased risk of myopathy when simvastatin given with fusidic acid; increased risk of myopathy when atorvastatin given with •telithromycin (avoid concomitant use)

• Anticoagulants: atorvastatin may transiently reduce anticoagulant effect of warfarin; fluvastatin and simvastatin enhance anticoagulant effect of •coumarins; rosuvastatin possibly enhances anticoagulant effect of •coumarins and •phenindione

Antidepressants: plasma concentration of simvastatin reduced by St John's wort

Antiepileptics: combination of fluvastatin with phenytoin may increase plasma concentration of either drug (or both)

• Antifungals: increased risk of myopathy when simvastatin given with •itraconazole, •ketoconazole or •posaconazole (avoid concomitant use); possible increased risk of myopathy when simvastatin given with •miconazole—avoid concomitant use; increased risk of myopathy when atorvastatin given with •itraconazole or •posaconazole (avoid concomitant use); possible increased risk of myopathy when atorvastatin or simvastatin given with imidazoles; possible increased risk of myopathy when atorvastatin or simvastatin given with triazoles

Statins *(continued)*

• Antivirals: possible increased risk of myopathy when simvastatin given with •amprenavir or •lopinavir—avoid concomitant use; possible increased risk of myopathy when atorvastatin given with amprenavir, atazanavir, indinavir, lopinavir, nelfinavir, ritonavir or saquinavir; increased risk of myopathy when simvastatin given with •atazanavir, •indinavir, •nelfinavir, •ritonavir or •saquinavir (avoid concomitant use); plasma concentration of pravastatin possibly increased by darunavir; plasma concentration of atorvastatin, pravastatin and simvastatin reduced by efavirenz

Bosentan: plasma concentration of simvastatin reduced by bosentan

• Calcium-channel Blockers: plasma concentration of atorvastatin increased by diltiazem; possible increased risk of myopathy when simvastatin given with diltiazem; increased risk of myopathy when simvastatin given with •verapamil

Cardiac Glycosides: atorvastatin possibly increases plasma concentration of digoxin

• Ciclosporin: increased risk of myopathy when statins given with •ciclosporin; increased risk of myopathy when rosuvastatin given with •ciclosporin (avoid concomitant use)

Cytotoxics: plasma concentration of simvastatin possibly increased by dasatinib; plasma concentration of simvastatin increased by imatinib

• Grapefruit Juice: plasma concentration of atorvastatin possibly increased by grapefruit juice; plasma concentration of simvastatin increased by •grapefruit juice—avoid concomitant use

• Hormone Antagonists: possible increased risk of myopathy when simvastatin given with •danazol

• Lipid-regulating Drugs: increased risk of myopathy when statins given with •gemfibrozil (preferably avoid concomitant use); increased risk of myopathy when statins given with •fibrates; increased risk of myopathy when statins given with •nicotinic acid (applies to lipid regulating doses of nicotinic acid)

Oestrogens: atorvastatin and rosuvastatin increase plasma concentration of ethinylestradiol

Progestogens: atorvastatin increases plasma concentration of norethisterone; rosuvastatin increases plasma concentration of norgestrel

Stavudine

• Antivirals: increased risk of side-effects when stavudine given with •didanosine; effects of stavudine possibly inhibited by •ribavirin; effects of stavudine possibly inhibited by •zidovudine (manufacturers advise avoid concomitant use)

• Cytotoxics: effects of stavudine possibly inhibited by doxorubicin; increased risk of toxicity when stavudine given with •hydroxycarbamide—avoid concomitant use

Streptomycin *see* Aminoglycosides

Strontium Ranelate

Antibacterials: strontium ranelate reduces absorption of quinolones and tetracyclines (manufacturer of strontium ranelate advises avoid concomitant use)

Sucralfate

Antibacterials: sucralfate reduces absorption of ciprofloxacin, levofloxacin, moxifloxacin, norfloxacin, ofloxacin and tetracyclines

• Anticoagulants: sucralfate possibly reduces absorption of •coumarins (reduced anticoagulant effect)

• Antiepileptics: sucralfate reduces absorption of •phenytoin

Antifungals: sucralfate reduces absorption of ketoconazole

Antipsychotics: sucralfate reduces absorption of sulpiride

Cardiac Glycosides: sucralfate possibly reduces absorption of cardiac glycosides

Theophylline: sucralfate possibly reduces absorption of theophylline (give at least 2 hours apart)

Thyroid Hormones: sucralfate reduces absorption of levothyroxine (thyroxine)

Sucralfate *(continued)*
Ulcer-healing Drugs: sucralfate possibly reduces absorption of lansoprazole
Sulfadiazine *see* Sulphonamides
Sulfadoxine *see* Sulphonamides
Sulfamethoxazole *see* Sulphonamides
Sulfasalazine *see* Aminosalicylates
Sulfinpyrazone
Analgesics: effects of sulfinpyrazone antagonised by aspirin
Antibacterials: sulfinpyrazone reduces excretion of nitrofurantoin (increased risk of toxicity); sulfinpyrazone reduces excretion of penicillins; effects of sulfinpyrazone antagonised by pyrazinamide
• Anticoagulants: sulfinpyrazone enhances anticoagulant effect of •coumarins
• Antidiabetics: sulfinpyrazone enhances effects of •sulphonylureas
• Antiepileptics: sulfinpyrazone increases plasma concentration of •phenytoin
Theophylline: sulfinpyrazone reduces plasma concentration of theophylline
Sulindac *see* NSAIDs
Sulphonamides
Anaesthetics, General: sulphonamides enhance effects of thiopental
Anaesthetics, Local: increased risk of methaemoglobinaemia when sulphonamides given with prilocaine
• Anti-arrhythmics: increased risk of ventricular arrhythmias when sulfamethoxazole (as co-trimoxazole) given with •amiodarone—avoid concomitant use of co-trimoxazole
• Antibacterials: increased risk of crystalluria when sulphonamides given with •methenamine
• Anticoagulants: sulphonamides enhance anticoagulant effect of •coumarins
Antidiabetics: sulphonamides rarely enhance the effects of sulphonylureas
Antiepileptics: sulphonamides possibly increase plasma concentration of phenytoin
• Antimalarials: increased antifolate effect when sulphonamides given with •pyrimethamine (includes Fansidar®)
• Antipsychotics: avoid concomitant use of sulphonamides with •clozapine (increased risk of agranulocytosis)
• Ciclosporin: increased risk of nephrotoxicity when sulphonamides given with •ciclosporin; sulfadiazine possibly reduces plasma concentration of •ciclosporin
• Cytotoxics: increased risk of haematological toxicity when sulfamethoxazole (as co-trimoxazole) given with •azathioprine, •mercaptopurine or •methotrexate; sulphonamides increase risk of methotrexate toxicity
Oestrogens: antibacterials that do not induce liver enzymes possibly reduce contraceptive effect of oestrogens (risk probably small, see p. 428)
Potassium Aminobenzoate: effects of sulphonamides inhibited by potassium aminobenzoate
Sulphonylureas *see* Antidiabetics
Sulpiride *see* Antipsychotics
Sumatriptan *see* $5HT_1$ Agonists
Sunitinib
Antibacterials: metabolism of sunitinib accelerated by rifampicin (reduced plasma concentration)
Antiepileptics: cytotoxics possibly reduce absorption of phenytoin
Antifungals: metabolism of sunitinib inhibited by ketoconazole (increased plasma concentration)
• Antipsychotics: avoid concomitant use of cytotoxics with •clozapine (increased risk of agranulocytosis)
Cardiac Glycosides: cytotoxics reduce absorption of digoxin tablets
Suxamethonium *see* Muscle Relaxants
Sympathomimetics
• Adrenergic Neurone Blockers: ephedrine, isometheptene, metaraminol, methylphenidate, noradrenaline (norepinephrine), oxymetazoline, phenylephrine, phenylpropanolamine, pseudoephedrine and xylometazoline antagonise hypotensive effect of •adrenergic neurone blockers
• Alpha-blockers: avoid concomitant use of adrenaline (epinephrine) or dopamine with •tolazoline
• Anaesthetics, General: increased risk of arrhythmias when adrenaline (epinephrine) given with •volatile liquid general anaesthetics; increased risk of hypertension when methylphenidate given with •volatile liquid general anaesthetics
• Anticoagulants: methylphenidate possibly enhances anticoagulant effect of •coumarins
• Antidepressants: risk of hypertensive crisis when dexamfetamine, dopamine, dopexamine, ephedrine, isometheptene, phenylephrine, phenylpropanolamine, pseudoephedrine or sympathomimetics given with •MAOIs; risk of hypertensive crisis when methylphenidate given with •MAOIs, some manufacturers advise avoid methylphenidate for at least 2 weeks after stopping MAOIs; risk of hypertensive crisis when dexamfetamine, dopamine, dopexamine, ephedrine, isometheptene, methylphenidate, phenylephrine, phenylpropanolamine, pseudoephedrine or sympathomimetics given with •moclobemide; methylphenidate possibly inhibits metabolism of SSRIs and tricyclics; increased risk of hypertension and arrhythmias when noradrenaline (norepinephrine) given with •tricyclics; increased risk of hypertension and arrhythmias when adrenaline (epinephrine) given with •tricyclics (but local anaesthetics with adrenaline appear to be safe)
Antiepileptics: methylphenidate increases plasma concentration of phenytoin; methylphenidate possibly increases plasma concentration of primidone
Antipsychotics: hypertensive effect of sympathomimetics antagonised by antipsychotics
Antivirals: plasma concentration of dexamfetamine possibly increased by ritonavir
Barbiturates: methylphenidate possibly increases plasma concentration of phenobarbital
• Beta-blockers: increased risk of severe hypertension and bradycardia when adrenaline (epinephrine) given with non-cardioselective •beta-blockers, also response to adrenaline (epinephrine) may be reduced; increased risk of severe hypertension and bradycardia when dobutamine given with non-cardioselective •beta-blockers; possible increased risk of severe hypertension and bradycardia when noradrenaline (norepinephrine) given with non-cardioselective •beta-blockers
• Clonidine: possible risk of hypertension when adrenaline (epinephrine) or noradrenaline (norepinephrine) given with clonidine; serious adverse events reported with concomitant use of methylphenidate and •clonidine (causality not established)
Corticosteroids: ephedrine accelerates metabolism of dexamethasone
• Dopaminergics: risk of toxicity when isometheptene or phenylpropanolamine given with •bromocriptine; effects of adrenaline (epinephrine), dobutamine, dopamine and noradrenaline (norepinephrine) possibly enhanced by entacapone; avoid concomitant use of sympathomimetics with •rasagiline; risk of hypertensive crisis when dopamine given with •selegiline
Doxapram: increased risk of hypertension when sympathomimetics given with doxapram
Ergot Alkaloids: increased risk of ergotism when sympathomimetics given with ergotamine and methysergide
Oxytocin: risk of hypertension when vasoconstrictor sympathomimetics given with oxytocin (due to enhanced vasopressor effect)
• Sympathomimetics: effects of adrenaline (epinephrine) possibly enhanced by •dopexamine; dopexamine possibly enhances effects of •noradrenaline (norepinephrine)
Theophylline: avoidance of ephedrine in children advised by manufacturer of theophylline

Sympathomimetics, Beta$_2$

Atomoxetine: Increased risk of cardiovascular side-effects when parenteral salbutamol given with atomoxetine

Cardiac Glycosides: salbutamol possibly reduces plasma concentration of digoxin

Corticosteroids: increased risk of hypokalaemia when high doses of beta$_2$ sympathomimetics given with corticosteroids—for CSM advice (hypokalaemia) see p. 150

Diuretics: increased risk of hypokalaemia when high doses of beta$_2$ sympathomimetics given with acetazolamide, loop diuretics or thiazides and related diuretics—for CSM advice (hypokalaemia) see p. 150

• Methyldopa: acute hypotension reported when infusion of salbutamol given with •methyldopa

Muscle Relaxants: bambuterol enhances effects of suxamethonium

Theophylline: increased risk of hypokalaemia when high doses of beta$_2$ sympathomimetics given with theophylline—for CSM advice (hypokalaemia) see p. 150

Tacrolimus

Note Interactions do not generally apply to tacrolimus used topically; risk of facial flushing and skin irritation with alcohol consumption (p. 618) does not apply to tacrolimus taken systemically

• Analgesics: possible increased risk of nephrotoxicity when tacrolimus given with NSAIDs; increased risk of nephrotoxicity when tacrolimus given with •ibuprofen

Angiotensin-II Receptor Antagonists: increased risk of hyperkalaemia when tacrolimus given with angiotensin-II receptor antagonists

• Antibacterials: plasma concentration of tacrolimus increased by •clarithromycin, •erythromycin and •quinupristin/dalfopristin; plasma concentration of tacrolimus reduced by •rifampicin; increased risk of nephrotoxicity when tacrolimus given with •aminoglycosides; plasma concentration of tacrolimus possibly increased by •chloramphenicol and •telithromycin; possible increased risk of nephrotoxicity when tacrolimus given with vancomycin

• Antidepressants: plasma concentration of tacrolimus reduced by •St John's wort—avoid concomitant use

Antiepileptics: plasma concentration of tacrolimus reduced by phenytoin, also plasma concentration of phenytoin possibly increased

• Antifungals: plasma concentration of tacrolimus increased by •fluconazole, •itraconazole, •ketoconazole and •voriconazole; increased risk of nephrotoxicity when tacrolimus given with •amphotericin; plasma concentration of tacrolimus increased by •posaconazole (reduce dose of tacrolimus); plasma concentration of tacrolimus reduced by •caspofungin; plasma concentration of tacrolimus possibly increased by •imidazoles and •triazoles

• Antivirals: possible increased risk of nephrotoxicity when tacrolimus given with aciclovir or ganciclovir, plasma concentration of tacrolimus possibly increased by •atazanavir, •nelfinavir and •ritonavir; plasma concentration of tacrolimus increased by •saquinavir (consider reducing dose of tacrolimus)

• Barbiturates: plasma concentration of tacrolimus reduced by •phenobarbital

• Calcium-channel Blockers: plasma concentration of tacrolimus possibly increased by felodipine, nicardipine and verapamil; plasma concentration of tacrolimus increased by •diltiazem and •nifedipine

• Ciclosporin: tacrolimus increases plasma concentration of •ciclosporin (increased risk of nephrotoxicity)—avoid concomitant use

• Diuretics: increased risk of hyperkalaemia when tacrolimus given with •potassium-sparing diuretics and aldosterone antagonists

• Grapefruit Juice: plasma concentration of tacrolimus increased by •grapefruit juice

Hormone Antagonists: plasma concentration of tacrolimus possibly increased by danazol

Oestrogens: tacrolimus possibly inhibits metabolism of oestrogens; plasma concentration of tacrolimus possibly increased by ethinylestradiol

Tacrolimus *(continued)*

• Potassium Salts: increased risk of hyperkalaemia when tacrolimus given with •potassium salts

Progestogens: tacrolimus possibly inhibits metabolism of progestogens

Ulcer-healing Drugs: plasma concentration of tacrolimus possibly increased by omeprazole

Tadalafil

• Alpha-blockers: enhanced hypotensive effect when tadalafil given with •alpha-blockers—avoid concomitant use

Antibacterials: plasma concentration of tadalafil possibly increased by clarithromycin and erythromycin; plasma concentration of tadalafil reduced by rifampicin

Antifungals: plasma concentration of tadalafil increased by ketoconazole; plasma concentration of tadalafil possibly increased by itraconazole

Antivirals: plasma concentration of tadalafil possibly increased by amprenavir; plasma concentration of tadalafil increased by ritonavir; plasma concentration of tadalafil possibly increased by saquinavir—reduce initial dose of tadalafil

Grapefruit Juice: plasma concentration of tadalafil possibly increased by grapefruit juice

• Nicorandil: tadalafil significantly enhances hypotensive effect of •nicorandil (avoid concomitant use)

• Nitrates: tadalafil significantly enhances hypotensive effect of •nitrates (avoid concomitant use)

Tamoxifen

• Anticoagulants: tamoxifen enhances anticoagulant effect of •coumarins

Tamsulosin *see* Alpha-blockers

Taxanes *see* Docetaxel and Paclitaxel

Tegafur with uracil *see* Fluorouracil

Teicoplanin

Antibacterials: increased risk of nephrotoxicity and ototoxicity when teicoplanin given with aminoglycosides or colistin

Oestrogens: antibacterials that do not induce liver enzymes possibly reduce contraceptive effect of oestrogens (risk probably small, see p. 428)

Telithromycin

• Antibacterials: plasma concentration of telithromycin reduced by •rifampicin (avoid during and for 2 weeks after rifampicin)

• Antidepressants: plasma concentration of telithromycin reduced by •St John's wort (avoid during and for 2 weeks after St John's wort)

• Antiepileptics: plasma concentration of telithromycin reduced by •carbamazepine, •phenytoin and •primidone (avoid during and for 2 weeks after carbamazepine, phenytoin and primidone)

• Antifungals: manufacturer of telithromycin advises avoid concomitant use with •ketoconazole in severe renal and hepatic impairment

• Antipsychotics: increased risk of ventricular arrhythmias when telithromycin given with •pimozide—avoid concomitant use

• Antivirals: manufacturer of telithromycin advises avoid concomitant use with •amprenavir, •atazanavir, •indinavir, •lopinavir, •nelfinavir, •ritonavir, •saquinavir and •tipranavir in severe renal and hepatic impairment; telithromycin possibly increases plasma concentration of •maraviroc (consider reducing dose of maraviroc)

• Anxiolytics and Hypnotics: telithromycin inhibits metabolism of •midazolam (increased plasma concentration with increased sedation)

Aprepitant: telithromycin possibly increases plasma concentration of aprepitant

• Barbiturates: plasma concentration of telithromycin reduced by •phenobarbital (avoid during and for 2 weeks after phenobarbital)

Cardiac Glycosides: telithromycin possibly increases plasma concentration of digoxin

• Ciclosporin: telithromycin possibly increases plasma concentration of •ciclosporin

• Diuretics: telithromycin increases plasma concentration of •eplerenone—avoid concomitant use

Telithromycin *(continued)*
- Ergot Alkaloids: increased risk of ergotism when telithromycin given with •ergotamine and methysergide—avoid concomitant use
- Ivabradine: telithromycin possibly increases plasma concentration of •ivabradine—avoid concomitant use
- Lipid-regulating Drugs: increased risk of myopathy when telithromycin given with •atorvastatin or •simvastatin (avoid concomitant use)

Oestrogens: antibacterials that do not induce liver enzymes possibly reduce contraceptive effect of oestrogens (risk probably small, see p. 428)

Sildenafil: telithromycin possibly increases plasma concentration of sildenafil—reduce initial dose of sildenafil
- Sirolimus: telithromycin increases plasma concentration of •sirolimus—avoid concomitant use
- Tacrolimus: telithromycin possibly increases plasma concentration of •tacrolimus

Telmisartan *see* Angiotensin-II Receptor Antagonists
Temazepam *see* Anxiolytics and Hypnotics
Temocillin *see* Penicillins
Temoporfin
- Cytotoxics: increased skin photosensitivity when temoporfin given with topical •fluorouracil

Temozolomide

Antiepileptics: cytotoxics possibly reduce absorption of phenytoin; plasma concentration of temozolomide increased by valproate
- Antipsychotics: avoid concomitant use of cytotoxics with •clozapine (increased risk of agranulocytosis)

Cardiac Glycosides: cytotoxics reduce absorption of digoxin tablets

Tenofovir
- Antivirals: manufacturer of tenofovir recommends monitoring of renal function when given with adefovir; tenofovir reduces plasma concentration of atazanavir, also plasma concentration of tenofovir possibly increased; combination of tenofovir with cidofovir may increase plasma concentration of either drug (or both); tenofovir increases plasma concentration of •didanosine (increased risk of toxicity)—avoid concomitant use; plasma concentration of tenofovir increased by lopinavir

Tenoxicam *see* NSAIDs
Terazosin *see* Alpha-blockers
Terbinafine

Antibacterials: plasma concentration of terbinafine reduced by rifampicin

Antidepressants: terbinafine possibly increases plasma concentration of imipramine and nortriptyline

Oestrogens: occasional reports of breakthrough bleeding when terbinafine given with oestrogens (when used for contraception)

Progestogens: occasional reports of breakthrough bleeding when terbinafine given with progestogens (when used for contraception)

Ulcer-healing Drugs: plasma concentration of terbinafine increased by cimetidine

Terbutaline *see* Sympathomimetics, $Beta_2$
Terpene Mixture *see* Rowachol®
Testolactone
- Anticoagulants: testolactone enhances anticoagulant effect of •coumarins and •phenindione

Testosterone
- Anticoagulants: testosterone enhances anticoagulant effect of •coumarins and •phenindione

Antidiabetics: testosterone possibly enhances hypoglycaemic effect of antidiabetics

Tetrabenazine
- Antidepressants: risk of CNS excitation and hypertension when tetrabenazine given with •MAOIs

Antipsychotics: increased risk of extrapyramidal side-effects when tetrabenazine given with antipsychotics

Dopaminergics: increased risk of extrapyramidal side-effects when tetrabenazine given with amantadine

Metoclopramide: increased risk of extrapyramidal side-effects when tetrabenazine given with metoclopramide

Tetracosactide *see* Corticosteroids
Tetracycline *see* Tetracyclines
Tetracyclines

ACE Inhibitors: absorption of tetracyclines reduced by quinapril tablets (quinapril tablets contain magnesium carbonate)

Adsorbents: absorption of tetracyclines possibly reduced by kaolin

Antacids: absorption of tetracyclines reduced by antacids
- Anticoagulants: tetracyclines possibly enhance anticoagulant effect of •coumarins and •phenindione

Antiepileptics: metabolism of doxycycline accelerated by carbamazepine (reduced effect); metabolism of doxycycline accelerated by phenytoin and primidone (reduced plasma concentration)

Atovaquone: tetracycline reduces plasma concentration of atovaquone

Barbiturates: metabolism of doxycycline accelerated by barbiturates (reduced plasma concentration)

Calcium Salts: absorption of tetracycline reduced by calcium salts
- Ciclosporin: doxycycline possibly increases plasma concentration of •ciclosporin

Cytotoxics: doxycycline or tetracycline increase risk of methotrexate toxicity

Dairy Products: absorption of tetracyclines (except doxycycline and minocycline) reduced by dairy products

Diuretics: manufacturer of lymecycline advises avoid concomitant use with diuretics

Ergot Alkaloids: increased risk of ergotism when tetracyclines given with ergotamine and methysergide

Iron: absorption of tetracyclines reduced by *oral* iron, also absorption of *oral* iron reduced by tetracyclines

Lipid-regulating Drugs: absorption of tetracycline possibly reduced by colestipol and colestyramine

Oestrogens: antibacterials that do not induce liver enzymes possibly reduce contraceptive effect of oestrogens (risk probably small, see p. 428)
- Retinoids: possible increased risk of benign intracranial hypertension when tetracyclines given with •retinoids (avoid concomitant use)

Strontium Ranelate: absorption of tetracyclines reduced by strontium ranelate (manufacturer of strontium ranelate advises avoid concomitant use)

Ulcer-healing Drugs: absorption of tetracyclines reduced by sucralfate and tripotassium dicitratobismuthate

Zinc: absorption of tetracyclines reduced by zinc, also absorption of zinc reduced by tetracyclines

Theophylline

Allopurinol: plasma concentration of theophylline possibly increased by allopurinol

Anaesthetics, General: increased risk of convulsions when theophylline given with ketamine; increased risk of arrhythmias when theophylline given with halothane

Anti-arrhythmics: theophylline antagonises anti-arrhythmic effect of adenosine; plasma concentration of theophylline increased by mexiletine and propafenone
- Antibacterials: plasma concentration of theophylline possibly increased by azithromycin and isoniazid; metabolism of theophylline inhibited by •clarithromycin (increased plasma concentration); metabolism of theophylline inhibited by •erythromycin (increased plasma concentration), if erythromycin given by mouth, also decreased plasma-erythromycin concentration; plasma concentration of theophylline increased by •ciprofloxacin and •norfloxacin; metabolism of theophylline accelerated by rifampicin (reduced plasma concentration); possible increased risk of convulsions when theophylline given with •quinolones
- Antidepressants: plasma concentration of theophylline increased by •fluvoxamine (concomitant use should usually be avoided, but where not possible halve theophylline dose and monitor plasma-theophylline concentration); plasma concentration of theophylline reduced by •St John's wort—avoid concomitant use

Appendix 1: Interactions

Theophylline *(continued)*
- • Antiepileptics: metabolism of theophylline accelerated by carbamazepine and primidone (reduced effect); plasma concentration of both drugs reduced when theophylline given with •phenytoin
- • Antifungals: plasma concentration of theophylline possibly increased by •fluconazole and •ketoconazole
- • Antivirals: metabolism of theophylline accelerated by •ritonavir (reduced plasma concentration)
- Anxiolytics and Hypnotics: theophylline possibly reduces effects of benzodiazepines
- Barbiturates: metabolism of theophylline accelerated by barbiturates (reduced effect)
- • Calcium-channel Blockers: plasma concentration of theophylline possibly increased by •calcium-channel blockers (enhanced effect); plasma concentration of theophylline increased by diltiazem; plasma concentration of theophylline increased by •verapamil (enhanced effect)
- Corticosteroids: increased risk of hypokalaemia when theophylline given with corticosteroids
- Cytotoxics: plasma concentration of theophylline possibly increased by methotrexate
- Disulfiram: metabolism of theophylline inhibited by disulfiram (increased risk of toxicity)
- Diuretics: increased risk of hypokalaemia when theophylline given with acetazolamide, loop diuretics or thiazides and related diuretics
- Doxapram: increased CNS stimulation when theophylline given with doxapram
- Interferons: metabolism of theophylline inhibited by interferon alfa (increased plasma concentration)
- Leukotriene Antagonists: plasma concentration of theophylline possibly increased by zafirlukast, also plasma concentration of zafirlukast reduced
- Lithium: theophylline increases excretion of lithium (reduced plasma concentration)
- Oestrogens: excretion of theophylline reduced by oestrogens (increased plasma concentration)
- Pentoxifylline (oxpentifylline): plasma concentration of theophylline increased by pentoxifylline (oxpentifylline)
- Sulfinpyrazone: plasma concentration of theophylline reduced by sulfinpyrazone
- Sympathomimetics: manufacturer of theophylline advises avoid concomitant use with ephedrine in children
- Sympathomimetics, Beta$_2$: increased risk of hypokalaemia when theophylline given with high doses of beta$_2$ sympathomimetics—for CSM advice (hypokalaemia) see p. 150
- Tobacco: metabolism of theophylline increased by tobacco smoking (reduced plasma concentration)
- • Ulcer-healing Drugs: metabolism of theophylline inhibited by •cimetidine (increased plasma concentration); absorption of theophylline possibly reduced by sucralfate (give at least 2 hours apart)
- Vaccines: plasma concentration of theophylline possibly increased by influenza vaccine

Thiazolidinediones *see* Antidiabetics

Thiopental *see* Anaesthetics, General

Thiotepa
- Antiepileptics: cytotoxics possibly reduce absorption of phenytoin
- • Antipsychotics: avoid concomitant use of cytotoxics with •clozapine (increased risk of agranulocytosis)
- Cardiac Glycosides: cytotoxics reduce absorption of digoxin tablets
- Muscle Relaxants: thiotepa enhances effects of suxamethonium

Thioxanthenes *see* Antipsychotics

Thyroid Hormones
- Antacids: absorption of levothyroxine (thyroxine) possibly reduced by antacids
- Anti-arrhythmics: for concomitant use of thyroid hormones and amiodarone see p. 80
- Antibacterials: metabolism of levothyroxine (thyroxine) accelerated by rifampicin (may increase requirements for levothyroxine (thyroxine) in hypothyroidism)

Thyroid Hormones *(continued)*
- • Anticoagulants: thyroid hormones enhance anticoagulant effect of •coumarins and •phenindione
- Antidepressants: thyroid hormones enhance effects of amitriptyline and imipramine; thyroid hormones possibly enhance effects of tricyclics
- Antiepileptics: metabolism of thyroid hormones accelerated by carbamazepine and primidone (may increase requirements for thyroid hormones in hypothyroidism); metabolism of thyroid hormones accelerated by phenytoin (may increase requirements in hypothyroidism), also plasma concentration of phenytoin possibly increased
- Barbiturates: metabolism of thyroid hormones accelerated by barbiturates (may increase requirements for thyroid hormones in hypothyroidism)
- Beta-blockers: levothyroxine (thyroxine) accelerates metabolism of propranolol
- Calcium Salts: absorption of levothyroxine (thyroxine) reduced by calcium salts
- Cytotoxics: plasma concentration of levothyroxine (thyroxine) possibly reduced by imatinib
- Iron: absorption of levothyroxine (thyroxine) reduced by *oral* iron (give at least 2 hours apart)
- Lipid-regulating Drugs: absorption of thyroid hormones reduced by colestipol and colestyramine
- Sodium Polystyrene Sulphonate: absorption of levothyroxine (thyroxine) reduced by sodium polystyrene sulphonate
- Ulcer-healing Drugs: absorption of levothyroxine (thyroxine) reduced by cimetidine and sucralfate

Tiagabine
- • Antidepressants: anticonvulsant effect of antiepileptics possibly antagonised by MAOIs and •tricyclic-related antidepressants (convulsive threshold lowered); anticonvulsant effect of antiepileptics antagonised by •SSRIs and •tricyclics (convulsive threshold lowered); avoid concomitant use of antiepileptics with •St John's wort
- Antiepileptics: plasma concentration of tiagabine reduced by carbamazepine, phenytoin and primidone
- • Antimalarials: possible increased risk of convulsions when antiepileptics given with chloroquine and hydroxychloroquine; anticonvulsant effect of antiepileptics antagonised by •mefloquine
- Barbiturates: plasma concentration of tiagabine reduced by phenobarbital

Tiaprofenic Acid *see* NSAIDs

Tibolone
- Antibacterials: metabolism of tibolone accelerated by rifampicin (reduced plasma concentration)
- Antiepileptics: metabolism of tibolone accelerated by carbamazepine and primidone (reduced plasma concentration); metabolism of tibolone accelerated by phenytoin
- Barbiturates: metabolism of tibolone accelerated by barbiturates (reduced plasma concentration)

Ticarcillin *see* Penicillins

Tigecycline
- Anticoagulants: tigecycline possibly enhances anticoagulant effect of coumarins
- Oestrogens: antibacterials that do not induce liver enzymes possibly reduce contraceptive effect of oestrogens (risk probably small, see p. 428)

Tiludronic Acid *see* Bisphosphonates

Timolol *see* Beta-blockers

Tinidazole
- Alcohol: possibility of disulfiram-like reaction when tinidazole given with alcohol
- Oestrogens: antibacterials that do not induce liver enzymes possibly reduce contraceptive effect of oestrogens (risk probably small, see p. 428)

Tinzaparin *see* Heparins

Tioguanine
- Antiepileptics: cytotoxics possibly reduce absorption of phenytoin
- • Antipsychotics: avoid concomitant use of cytotoxics with •clozapine (increased risk of agranulocytosis)

Tioguanine *(continued)*
Cardiac Glycosides: cytotoxics reduce absorption of digoxin tablets
Cytotoxics: increased risk of hepatotoxicity when tioguanine given with busulfan

Tiotropium *see* Antimuscarinics

Tipranavir
Antacids: absorption of tipranavir reduced by antacids
• Antibacterials: tipranavir increases plasma concentration of •clarithromycin (reduce dose of clarithromycin in renal impairment), also plasma concentration of tipranavir increased by clarithromycin; tipranavir increases plasma concentration of •rifabutin (reduce dose of rifabutin); plasma concentration of tipranavir possibly reduced by •rifampicin—avoid concomitant use; avoidance of concomitant tipranavir in severe renal and hepatic impairment advised by manufacturer of •telithromycin
• Antidepressants: plasma concentration of tipranavir possibly reduced by •St John's wort—avoid concomitant use
Antiepileptics: plasma concentration of tipranavir possibly reduced by carbamazepine
Antifungals: plasma concentration of tipranavir increased by fluconazole
• Antimalarials: avoid concomitant use of tipranavir with •artemether/lumefantrine
Antimuscarinics: avoidance of tipranavir advised by manufacturer of darifenacin
• Antivirals: tipranavir reduces plasma concentration of •abacavir, •amprenavir, •didanosine, •lopinavir, •saquinavir and •zidovudine; plasma concentration of tipranavir increased by atazanavir (also plasma concentration of atazanavir reduced)
• Beta-blockers: manufacturer of tipranavir advises avoid concomitant use with •metoprolol for heart failure

Tirofiban
Iloprost: increased risk of bleeding when tirofiban given with iloprost

Tizanidine *see* Muscle Relaxants

Tobacco
Cinacalcet: tobacco smoking increases cinacalcet metabolism (reduced plasma concentration)
Cytotoxics: tobacco smoking reduces plasma concentration of erlotinib
Theophylline: tobacco smoking increases theophylline metabolism (reduced plasma concentration)

Tobramycin *see* Aminoglycosides

Tolazoline *see* Alpha-blockers

Tolbutamide *see* Antidiabetics

Tolcapone
Antidepressants: avoid concomitant use of tolcapone with MAOIs
Memantine: effects of dopaminergics possibly enhanced by memantine
Methyldopa: antiparkinsonian effect of dopaminergics antagonised by methyldopa

Tolfenamic Acid *see* NSAIDs

Tolterodine *see* Antimuscarinics

Topiramate
• Antidepressants: anticonvulsant effect of antiepileptics possibly antagonised by MAOIs and •tricyclic-related antidepressants (convulsive threshold lowered); anticonvulsant effect of antiepileptics antagonised by •SSRIs and •tricyclics (convulsive threshold lowered); avoid concomitant use of antiepileptics with •St John's wort
• Antiepileptics: plasma concentration of topiramate often reduced by carbamazepine; topiramate increases plasma concentration of •phenytoin (also plasma concentration of topiramate reduced)
• Antimalarials: possible increased risk of convulsions when antiepileptics given with chloroquine and hydroxychloroquine; anticonvulsant effect of antiepileptics antagonised by •mefloquine
• Oestrogens: topiramate accelerates metabolism of •oestrogens (reduced contraceptive effect—see p. 428)

Topiramate *(continued)*
• Progestogens: topiramate accelerates metabolism of •progestogens (reduced contraceptive effect—see p. 428)

Torasemide *see* Diuretics

Toremifene
• Anticoagulants: toremifene possibly enhances anticoagulant effect of •coumarins
Antiepileptics: metabolism of toremifene possibly accelerated by carbamazepine (reduced plasma concentration); metabolism of toremifene possibly accelerated by phenytoin; metabolism of toremifene accelerated by primidone (reduced plasma concentration)
Barbiturates: metabolism of toremifene possibly accelerated by barbiturates (reduced plasma concentration)
Diuretics: increased risk of hypercalcaemia when toremifene given with thiazides and related diuretics

Trabectedin
Antiepileptics: cytotoxics possibly reduce absorption of phenytoin
• Antipsychotics: avoid concomitant use of cytotoxics with •clozapine (increased risk of agranulocytosis)
Cardiac Glycosides: cytotoxics reduce absorption of digoxin tablets

Tramadol *see* Opioid Analgesics

Trandolapril *see* ACE Inhibitors

Tranylcypromine *see* MAOIs

Trazodone *see* Antidepressants, Tricyclic (related)

Tretinoin *see* Retinoids

Triamcinolone *see* Corticosteroids

Triamterene *see* Diuretics

Triclofos *see* Anxiolytics and Hypnotics

Trientine
Iron: trientine reduces absorption of *oral* iron
Zinc: trientine reduces absorption of zinc, also absorption of trientine reduced by zinc

Trifluoperazine *see* Antipsychotics

Trihexyphenidyl (benzhexol) *see* Antimuscarinics

Trilostane
Diuretics: increased risk of hyperkalaemia when trilostane given with potassium-sparing diuretics and aldosterone antagonists

Trimethoprim
• Anti-arrhythmics: increased risk of ventricular arrhythmias when trimethoprim (as co-trimoxazole) given with •amiodarone—avoid concomitant use of co-trimoxazole; trimethoprim increases plasma concentration of procainamide
Antibacterials: plasma concentration of trimethoprim possibly reduced by rifampicin; plasma concentration of both drugs may increase when trimethoprim given with dapsone
Anticoagulants: trimethoprim possibly enhances anticoagulant effect of coumarins
Antidiabetics: trimethoprim possibly enhances hypoglycaemic effect of repaglinide—manufacturer advises avoid concomitant use; trimethoprim rarely enhances the effects of sulphonylureas
• Antiepileptics: trimethoprim increases plasma concentration of •phenytoin (also increased antifolate effect)
• Antimalarials: increased antifolate effect when trimethoprim given with •pyrimethamine
Antivirals: trimethoprim (as co-trimoxazole) increases plasma concentration of lamivudine—avoid concomitant use of high-dose co-trimoxazole
Cardiac Glycosides: trimethoprim possibly increases plasma concentration of digoxin
• Ciclosporin: increased risk of nephrotoxicity when trimethoprim given with •ciclosporin, also plasma concentration of ciclosporin reduced by intravenous trimethoprim
• Cytotoxics: increased risk of haematological toxicity when trimethoprim (also with co-trimoxazole) given with •azathioprine, •mercaptopurine or •methotrexate
Diuretics: increased risk of hyperkalaemia when trimethoprim given with eplerenone

Trimethoprim *(continued)*
Oestrogens: antibacterials that do not induce liver enzymes possibly reduce contraceptive effect of oestrogens (risk probably small, see p. 428)
Trimipramine *see* Antidepressants, Tricyclic
Tripotassium Dicitratobismuthate
Antibacterials: tripotassium dicitratobismuthate reduces absorption of tetracyclines
Tropicamide *see* Antimuscarinics
Tropisetron *see* $5HT_3$ Antagonists
Trospium *see* Antimuscarinics
Tryptophan
• Antidepressants: possible increased serotonergic effects when tryptophan given with duloxetine; CNS excitation and confusion when tryptophan given with •MAOIs (reduce dose of tryptophan); agitation and nausea may occur when tryptophan given with •SSRIs
• Antimalarials: avoidance of antidepressants advised by manufacturer of •artemether/lumefantrine
Atomoxetine: possible increased risk of convulsions when antidepressants given with atomoxetine
• Sibutramine: increased risk of CNS toxicity when tryptophan given with •sibutramine (manufacturer of sibutramine advises avoid concomitant use)
Typhoid Vaccine *see* Vaccines
Ubidecarenone
Anticoagulants: ubidecarenone may enhance or reduce anticoagulant effect of warfarin
Ulcer-healing Drugs *see* Histamine H_2-antagonists, Proton Pump Inhibitors, Sucralfate, and Tripotassium Dicitratobismuthate
Ursodeoxycholic Acid
Antacids: absorption of bile acids possibly reduced by antacids
• Ciclosporin: ursodeoxycholic acid increases absorption of •ciclosporin
Lipid-regulating Drugs: absorption of bile acids possibly reduced by colestipol and colestyramine
Oestrogens: elimination of cholesterol in bile increased when bile acids given with oestrogens
Vaccines
Note For a general warning on live vaccines and high doses of corticosteroids or other immunosuppressive drugs, see p. 641 ; for advice on live vaccines and immunoglobulins, see under Normal Immunoglobulin, p. 660
Note For interactions of oral typhoid vaccine see p. 658
• Abatacept: avoid concomitant use of live vaccines with •abatacept (see p. 641)
• Adalimumab: avoid concomitant use of live vaccines with •adalimumab (see p. 641)
• Anakinra: avoid concomitant use of live vaccines with •anakinra (see p. 641)
Anticoagulants: influenza vaccine possibly enhances anticoagulant effect of warfarin
Antiepileptics: influenza vaccine enhances effects of phenytoin
• Corticosteroids: immune response to vaccines impaired by high doses of •corticosteroids, avoid concomitant use with live vaccines (see p. 641)
• Efalizumab: live or live-attenuated vaccines should be given 2 weeks before •efalizumab or withheld until 8 weeks after discontinuation
• Etanercept: avoid concomitant use of live vaccines with •etanercept (see p. 641)
• Infliximab: avoid concomitant use of live vaccines with •infliximab (see p. 641)
Interferons: avoidance of vaccines advised by manufacturer of interferon gamma
• Leflunomide: avoid concomitant use of live vaccines with •leflunomide (see p. 641)
Theophylline: influenza vaccine possibly increases plasma concentration of theophylline
Valaciclovir *see* Aciclovir
Valganciclovir *see* Ganciclovir
Valproate
Analgesics: effects of valproate enhanced by aspirin
Antibacterials: plasma concentration of valproate possibly reduced by ertapenem; plasma concentration of valproate reduced by meropenem; metabolism of

Valproate
Antibacterials *(continued)*
valproate possibly inhibited by erythromycin (increased plasma concentration)
Anticoagulants: valproate possibly enhances anticoagulant effect of coumarins
• Antidepressants: anticonvulsant effect of antiepileptics possibly antagonised by MAOIs and •tricyclic-related antidepressants (convulsive threshold lowered); anticonvulsant effect of antiepileptics antagonised by •SSRIs and •tricyclics (convulsive threshold lowered); avoid concomitant use of antiepileptics with •St John's wort
• Antiepileptics: plasma concentration of valproate reduced by carbamazepine, also plasma concentration of active metabolite of carbamazepine increased; valproate possibly increases plasma concentration of ethosuximide; valproate increases plasma concentration of lamotrigine; valproate sometimes reduces plasma concentration of an active metabolite of oxcarbazepine; valproate increases or possibly decreases plasma concentration of phenytoin, also plasma concentration of valproate reduced; valproate possibly increases plasma concentration of •primidone (plasma concentration of active metabolite of primidone increased), also plasma concentration of valproate reduced; valproate possibly increases plasma concentration of rufinamide (reduce dose of rufinamide)
• Antimalarials: possible increased risk of convulsions when antiepileptics given with chloroquine and hydroxychloroquine; anticonvulsant effect of antiepileptics and valproate antagonised by •mefloquine
• Antipsychotics: anticonvulsant effect of valproate antagonised by •antipsychotics (convulsive threshold lowered); increased risk of neutropenia when valproate given with •olanzapine
Antivirals: valproate possibly increases plasma concentration of zidovudine (increased risk of toxicity)
Anxiolytics and Hypnotics: plasma concentration of valproate possibly increased by clobazam; increased risk of side-effects when valproate given with clonazepam; valproate possibly increases plasma concentration of diazepam and lorazepam
Barbiturates: valproate increases plasma concentration of phenobarbital (also plasma concentration of valproate reduced)
Bupropion: valproate inhibits the metabolism of bupropion
Cytotoxics: valproate increases plasma concentration of temozolomide
Lipid-regulating Drugs: absorption of valproate possibly reduced by colestyramine
Sodium Benzoate: valproate possibly reduces effects of sodium benzoate
Sodium Phenylbutyrate: valproate possibly reduces effects of sodium phenylbutyrate
• Ulcer-healing Drugs: metabolism of valproate inhibited by •cimetidine (increased plasma concentration)
Valsartan *see* Angiotensin-II Receptor Antagonists
Vancomycin
Anaesthetics, General: hypersensitivity-like reactions can occur when intravenous vancomycin given with general anaesthetics
Antibacterials: increased risk of nephrotoxicity and ototoxicity when vancomycin given with aminoglycosides, capreomycin or colistin; increased risk of nephrotoxicity when vancomycin given with polymyxins
Antifungals: possible increased risk of nephrotoxicity when vancomycin given with amphotericin
• Ciclosporin: increased risk of nephrotoxicity when vancomycin given with •ciclosporin
Cytotoxics: increased risk of nephrotoxicity and possibly of ototoxicity when vancomycin given with cisplatin
• Diuretics: increased risk of otoxicity when vancomycin given with •loop diuretics

Vancomycin *(continued)*

Lipid-regulating Drugs: effects of oral vancomycin antagonised by colestyramine

• Muscle Relaxants: vancomycin enhances effects of •suxamethonium

Oestrogens: antibacterials that do not induce liver enzymes possibly reduce contraceptive effect of oestrogens (risk probably small, see p. 428)

Tacrolimus: possible increased risk of nephrotoxicity when vancomycin given with tacrolimus

Vardenafil

• Alpha-blockers: enhanced hypotensive effect when vardenafil given with •alpha-blockers (exludes tamsulosin)—avoid vardenafil for 6 hours after alpha-blockers

Antibacterials: plasma concentration of vardenafil increased by erythromycin (reduce dose of vardenafil)

• Antifungals: plasma concentration of vardenafil increased by •ketoconazole—avoid concomitant use; plasma concentration of vardenafil possibly increased by •itraconazole—avoid concomitant use

• Antivirals: plasma concentration of vardenafil possibly increased by amprenavir; plasma concentration of vardenafil increased by •indinavir—avoid concomitant use; plasma concentration of vardenafil possibly increased by •ritonavir—avoid concomitant use; plasma concentration of vardenafil possibly increased by saquinavir—reduce initial dose of vardenafil

Calcium-channel Blockers: enhanced hypotensive effect when vardenafil given with nifedipine

• Grapefruit Juice: plasma concentration of vardenafil possibly increased by •grapefruit juice—avoid concomitant use

• Nicorandil: possible increased hypotensive effect when vardenafil given with •nicorandil—avoid concomitant use

• Nitrates: possible increased hypotensive effect when vardenafil given with •nitrates—avoid concomitant use

Vasodilator Antihypertensives

ACE Inhibitors: enhanced hypotensive effect when hydralazine, minoxidil or sodium nitroprusside given with ACE inhibitors

Adrenergic Neurone Blockers: enhanced hypotensive effect when hydralazine, minoxidil or sodium nitroprusside given with adrenergic neurone blockers

Alcohol: enhanced hypotensive effect when hydralazine, minoxidil or sodium nitroprusside given with alcohol

Aldesleukin: enhanced hypotensive effect when hydralazine, minoxidil or sodium nitroprusside given with aldesleukin

Alpha-blockers: enhanced hypotensive effect when hydralazine, minoxidil or sodium nitroprusside given with alpha-blockers

Anaesthetics, General: enhanced hypotensive effect when hydralazine, minoxidil or sodium nitroprusside given with general anaesthetics

Analgesics: hypotensive effect of hydralazine, minoxidil and sodium nitroprusside antagonised by NSAIDs

Angiotensin-II Receptor Antagonists: enhanced hypotensive effect when hydralazine, minoxidil or sodium nitroprusside given with angiotensin-II receptor antagonists

Antidepressants: enhanced hypotensive effect when hydralazine, minoxidil or sodium nitroprusside given with MAOIs; enhanced hypotensive effect when hydralazine or sodium nitroprusside given with tricyclic-related antidepressants

Antipsychotics: enhanced hypotensive effect when hydralazine, minoxidil or sodium nitroprusside given with phenothiazines

Anxiolytics and Hypnotics: enhanced hypotensive effect when hydralazine, minoxidil or sodium nitroprusside given with anxiolytics and hypnotics

Beta-blockers: enhanced hypotensive effect when hydralazine, minoxidil or sodium nitroprusside given with beta-blockers

Vasodilator Antihypertensives *(continued)*

Calcium-channel Blockers: enhanced hypotensive effect when hydralazine, minoxidil or sodium nitroprusside given with calcium-channel blockers

Clonidine: enhanced hypotensive effect when hydralazine, minoxidil or sodium nitroprusside given with clonidine

Corticosteroids: hypotensive effect of hydralazine, minoxidil and sodium nitroprusside antagonised by corticosteroids

Diazoxide: enhanced hypotensive effect when hydralazine, minoxidil or sodium nitroprusside given with diazoxide

Diuretics: enhanced hypotensive effect when hydralazine, minoxidil or sodium nitroprusside given with diuretics

Dopaminergics: enhanced hypotensive effect when hydralazine, minoxidil or sodium nitroprusside given with levodopa

Methyldopa: enhanced hypotensive effect when hydralazine, minoxidil or sodium nitroprusside given with methyldopa

Moxisylyte (thymoxamine): enhanced hypotensive effect when hydralazine, minoxidil or sodium nitroprusside given with moxisylyte

Moxonidine: enhanced hypotensive effect when hydralazine, minoxidil or sodium nitroprusside given with moxonidine

Muscle Relaxants: enhanced hypotensive effect when hydralazine, minoxidil or sodium nitroprusside given with baclofen; enhanced hypotensive effect when hydralazine, minoxidil or sodium nitroprusside given with tizanidine

Nicorandil: possible enhanced hypotensive effect when hydralazine, minoxidil or sodium nitroprusside given with nicorandil

Nitrates: enhanced hypotensive effect when hydralazine, minoxidil or sodium nitroprusside given with nitrates

Oestrogens: hypotensive effect of hydralazine, minoxidil and sodium nitroprusside antagonised by oestrogens

Prostaglandins: enhanced hypotensive effect when hydralazine, minoxidil or sodium nitroprusside given with alprostadil

Vasodilator Antihypertensives: enhanced hypotensive effect when hydralazine given with minoxidil or sodium nitroprusside; enhanced hypotensive effect when minoxidil given with sodium nitroprusside

Vecuronium *see* Muscle Relaxants

Venlafaxine

• Analgesics: increased risk of bleeding when venlafaxine given with •NSAIDs or •aspirin

• Anticoagulants: venlafaxine possibly enhances anticoagulant effect of •warfarin

• Antidepressants: possible increased serotonergic effects when venlafaxine given with duloxetine; enhanced CNS effects and toxicity when venlafaxine given with •MAOIs (venlafaxine should not be started until 2 weeks after stopping MAOIs, avoid MAOIs for 1 week after stopping venlafaxine); after stopping SSRI-related antidepressants do not start •moclobemide for at least 1 week

• Antimalarials: avoidance of antidepressants advised by manufacturer of •artemether/lumefantrine

• Antipsychotics: venlafaxine increases plasma concentration of •clozapine and haloperidol

Atomoxetine: possible increased risk of convulsions when antidepressants given with atomoxetine

• Dopaminergics: caution with venlafaxine advised by manufacturer of entacapone; increased risk of hypertension and CNS excitation when venlafaxine given with •selegiline (selegiline should not be started until 1 week after stopping venlafaxine, avoid venlafaxine for 2 weeks after stopping selegiline)

Lithium: possible increased serotonergic effects when venlafaxine given with lithium

• Sibutramine: increased risk of CNS toxicity when SSRI-related antidepressants given with •sibutramine

Venlafaxine
- Sibutramine *(continued)*
 (manufacturer of sibutramine advises avoid concomitant use)

Verapamil *see* Calcium-channel Blockers
Vigabatrin
- Antidepressants: anticonvulsant effect of antiepileptics possibly antagonised by MAOIs and •tricyclic-related antidepressants (convulsive threshold lowered); anticonvulsant effect of antiepileptics antagonised by •SSRIs and •tricyclics (convulsive threshold lowered); avoid concomitant use of antiepileptics with •St John's wort

Antiepileptics: vigabatrin reduces plasma concentration of phenytoin; vigabatrin possibly reduces plasma concentration of primidone
- Antimalarials: possible increased risk of convulsions when antiepileptics given with chloroquine and hydroxychloroquine; anticonvulsant effect of antiepileptics antagonised by •mefloquine

Barbiturates: vigabatrin possibly reduces plasma concentration of phenobarbital

Vinblastine
- Antibacterials: toxicity of vinblastine increased by •erythromycin—avoid concomitant use

Antiepileptics: cytotoxics possibly reduce absorption of phenytoin
- Antifungals: metabolism of vinblastine possibly inhibited by •posaconazole (increased risk of neurotoxicity)
- Antipsychotics: avoid concomitant use of cytotoxics with •clozapine (increased risk of agranulocytosis)

Cardiac Glycosides: cytotoxics reduce absorption of digoxin tablets

Vincristine

Antiepileptics: cytotoxics possibly reduce absorption of phenytoin
- Antifungals: metabolism of vincristine possibly inhibited by •itraconazole and •posaconazole (increased risk of neurotoxicity)
- Antipsychotics: avoid concomitant use of cytotoxics with •clozapine (increased risk of agranulocytosis)

Calcium-channel Blockers: metabolism of vincristine possibly inhibited by nifedipine

Cardiac Glycosides: cytotoxics reduce absorption of digoxin tablets

Vinorelbine

Antiepileptics: cytotoxics possibly reduce absorption of phenytoin
- Antipsychotics: avoid concomitant use of cytotoxics with •clozapine (increased risk of agranulocytosis)

Cardiac Glycosides: cytotoxics reduce absorption of digoxin tablets

Vitamin A *see* Vitamins
Vitamin D *see* Vitamins
Vitamin K (Phytomenadione) *see* Vitamins
Vitamins

Antibacterials: absorption of vitamin A possibly reduced by neomycin
- Anticoagulants: vitamin K antagonises anticoagulant effect of •coumarins and •phenindione

Antiepileptics: vitamin D requirements possibly increased when given with carbamazepine, phenytoin or primidone

Antifungals: plasma concentration of paricalcitol possibly increased by ketoconazole

Barbiturates: vitamin D requirements possibly increased when given with barbiturates

Diuretics: increased risk of hypercalcaemia when vitamin D given with thiazides and related diuretics

Dopaminergics: pyridoxine reduces effects of levodopa when given without dopa-decarboxylase inhibitor

Retinoids: risk of hypervitaminosis A when vitamin A given with retinoids

Selenium: ascorbic acid possibly reduces absorption of selenium (give at least 4 hours apart)

Voriconazole *see* Antifungals, Triazole
Warfarin *see* Coumarins
Xipamide *see* Diuretics
Xylometazoline *see* Sympathomimetics
Zafirlukast *see* Leukotriene Antagonists
Zaleplon *see* Anxiolytics and Hypnotics
Zidovudine

Note Increased risk of toxicity with nephrotoxic and myelosuppressive drugs—for further details consult product literature

Analgesics: increased risk of haematological toxicity when zidovudine given with NSAIDs; plasma concentration of zidovudine possibly increased by methadone

Antibacterials: absorption of zidovudine reduced by clarithromycin tablets; manufacturer of zidovudine advises avoid concomitant use with rifampicin

Antiepileptics: zidovudine increases or decreases plasma concentration of phenytoin; plasma concentration of zidovudine possibly increased by valproate (increased risk of toxicity)
- Antifungals: plasma concentration of zidovudine increased by •fluconazole (increased risk of toxicity)

Antimalarials: increased antifolate effect when zidovudine given with pyrimethamine
- Antivirals: profound myelosuppression when zidovudine given with •ganciclovir (if possible avoid concomitant administration, particularly during initial ganciclovir therapy); zidovudine possibly inhibits effects of •stavudine (manufacturers advise avoid concomitant use); plasma concentration of zidovudine reduced by •tipranavir

Atovaquone: metabolism of zidovudine possibly inhibited by atovaquone (increased plasma concentration)

Probenecid: excretion of zidovudine reduced by probenecid (increased plasma concentration and risk of toxicity)

Zinc

Antibacterials: zinc reduces absorption of ciprofloxacin, levofloxacin, moxifloxacin, norfloxacin and ofloxacin; zinc reduces absorption of tetracyclines, also absorption of zinc reduced by tetracyclines

Calcium Salts: absorption of zinc reduced by calcium salts

Iron: absorption of zinc reduced by *oral* iron, also absorption of *oral* iron reduced by zinc

Penicillamine: absorption of zinc reduced by penicillamine, also absorption of penicillamine reduced by zinc

Trientine: absorption of zinc reduced by trientine, also absorption of trientine reduced by zinc

Zoledronic Acid *see* Bisphosphonates
Zolmitriptan *see* $5HT_1$ Agonists
Zolpidem *see* Anxiolytics and Hypnotics
Zonisamide
- Antidepressants: anticonvulsant effect of antiepileptics possibly antagonised by MAOIs and •tricyclic-related antidepressants (convulsive threshold lowered); anticonvulsant effect of antiepileptics antagonised by •SSRIs and •tricyclics (convulsive threshold lowered); avoid concomitant use of antiepileptics with •St John's wort

Antiepileptics: plasma concentration of zonisamide reduced by carbamazepine and phenytoin
- Antimalarials: possible increased risk of convulsions when antiepileptics given with chloroquine and hydroxychloroquine; anticonvulsant effect of antiepileptics antagonised by •mefloquine

Barbiturates: plasma concentration of zonisamide reduced by phenobarbital

Zopiclone *see* Anxiolytics and Hypnotics
Zotepine *see* Antipsychotics
Zuclopenthixol *see* Antipsychotics

A2 Liver disease

Liver disease may alter the response to drugs in several ways as indicated below, and drug prescribing should be kept to a minimum in all patients with severe liver disease. The main problems occur in patients with jaundice, ascites, or evidence of encephalopathy.

Impaired drug metabolism Metabolism by the liver is the main route of elimination for many drugs, but hepatic reserve is large and liver disease has to be severe before important changes in drug metabolism occur. Routine liver-function tests are a poor guide to the capacity of the liver to metabolise drugs, and in the individual patient it is not possible to predict the extent to which the metabolism of a particular drug may be impaired.

A few drugs, e.g. rifampicin and fusidic acid, are excreted in the bile unchanged and can accumulate in patients with intrahepatic or extrahepatic obstructive jaundice.

Hypoproteinaemia The hypoalbuminaemia in severe liver disease is associated with reduced protein binding and increased toxicity of some highly protein-bound drugs such as phenytoin and prednisolone.

Reduced clotting Reduced hepatic synthesis of blood-clotting factors, indicated by a prolonged prothrombin time, increases the sensitivity to oral anticoagulants such as warfarin and phenindione.

Hepatic encephalopathy In severe liver disease many drugs can further impair cerebral function and may precipitate hepatic encephalopathy. These include all sedative drugs, opioid analgesics, those diuretics that produce hypokalaemia, and drugs that cause constipation.

Fluid overload Oedema and ascites in chronic liver disease may be exacerbated by drugs that give rise to fluid retention, e.g. NSAIDs, and corticosteroids.

Hepatotoxic drugs Hepatotoxicity is either dose-related or unpredictable (idiosyncratic). Drugs that cause dose-related toxicity may do so at lower doses in the presence of hepatic impairment than in individuals with normal liver function, and some drugs that produce reactions of the idiosyncratic kind do so more frequently in patients with liver disease. These drugs should be avoided or used very carefully in patients with liver disease.

Table of drugs to be avoided or used with caution in liver disease

The list of drugs given below is not comprehensive and is based on current information concerning the use of prescribed drugs in therapeutic dosage. Products introduced or amended since publication of BNF No. 54 (September 2007) are underlined.

Drug	Comment
Abacavir	Avoid in moderate hepatic impairment unless essential; avoid in severe hepatic impairment
Abciximab	Avoid in severe liver disease—increased risk of bleeding
Acamprosate	Avoid in severe liver disease
Acarbose	Avoid
ACE inhibitors	Use of prodrugs such as cilazapril, enalapril, fosinopril, imidapril, moexipril, perindopril, quinapril, ramipril, and trandolapril requires close monitoring in patients with impaired liver function
Aceclofenac	*see* NSAIDs
Acemetacin	*see* NSAIDs
Acenocoumarol (nicoumalone)	*see* Anticoagulants, Oral
Acitretin	Avoid—further impairment of liver function may occur
Alfentanil	*see* Opioid Analgesics
Alfuzosin	Reduce dose in mild to moderate liver disease; avoid if severe
Alimemazine (trimeprazine)	Avoid—may precipitate coma in severe liver disease; hepatotoxic
Allopurinol	Reduce dose
Almotriptan	Manufacturer advises caution in mild to moderate liver disease; avoid in severe liver disease
Alprazolam	*see* Anxiolytics and Hypnotics
Alteplase	*see* Fibrinolytics
Amfebutamone	*see* Bupropion
Aminophylline	*see* Theophylline
Amitriptyline	*see* Antidepressants, Tricyclic (and related)
Amlodipine	Half-life prolonged—may need dose reduction
Amprenavir	Avoid oral solution due to high propylene glycol content; without low-dose ritonavir, reduce dose of amprenavir capsules to 450 mg every 12 hours in moderate hepatic impairment and reduce dose to 300 mg every 12 hours in severe impairment
Amsacrine	Reduce dose
Anabolic steroids	Preferably avoid—dose-related toxicity
Anagrelide	Manufacturer advises caution in mild hepatic impairment; avoid in moderate to severe impairment
Analgesics	*see* Aspirin, NSAIDs, Opioid Analgesics and Paracetamol

Drug	Comment
Anastrozole	Avoid in moderate to severe liver disease
Androgens	Preferably avoid—dose-related toxicity with some, and produce fluid retention
Antacids	In patients with fluid retention, avoid those containing large amounts of sodium Avoid those causing constipation—can precipitate coma
Anticoagulants, oral	Avoid in severe liver disease, especially if prothrombin time already prolonged
Antidepressants, MAOI	May cause idiosyncratic hepatotoxicity; see also Moclobemide
Antidepressants, SSRI	Reduce dose or avoid; *see also* Escitalopram
Antidepressants, tricyclic (and related)	Tricyclics preferable to MAOIs but sedative effects increased (avoid in severe liver disease)
Antihistamines	*see* individual entries
Antipsychotics	All can precipitate coma; phenothiazines are hepatotoxic; *see also* Aripiprazole, Clozapine, Olanzapine, Paliperidone, Quetiapine, Risperidone and Sertindole
Anxiolytics and hypnotics	All can precipitate coma; small dose of oxazepam or temazepam probably safest; reduce oral dose of clomethiazole; reduce dose of zaleplon to 5 mg (avoid if severe); reduce dose of zolpidem to 5 mg (avoid if severe); reduce dose of zopiclone (avoid if severe); *see also* Chloral Hydrate and Clonazepam
Apomorphine	Manufacturer of *APO-go*® advises avoid
Aprepitant	Manufacturer advises caution in moderate to severe hepatic impairment
Aripiprazole	Manufacturer advises use with caution in severe impairment
Artemether [ingredient]	*see Riamet*®
Aspirin	Avoid in severe hepatic impairment—increased risk of gastro-intestinal bleeding
Atazanavir	Manufacturer advises caution in mild hepatic impairment; avoid in moderate to severe hepatic impairment
Atomoxetine	Halve dose in moderate liver disease; quarter dose in severe liver disease
Atorvastatin	*see* Statins
Atosiban	No information available
Atovaquone	Manufacturer advises caution—monitor more closely
Auranofin	Caution in mild to moderate liver disease; avoid in severe liver disease
Azapropazone	*see* NSAIDs
Azathioprine	May need dose reduction
Azithromycin	Manufacturer advises avoid in severe liver disease—no information available
Bambuterol	Avoid in severe liver disease
Beclometasone dipropionate	Manufacturer advises avoid tablets in severe hepatic impairment—no information available
Bemiparin	Manufacturer advises avoid in severe liver disease
Bendrofluazide	*see* Thiazides and Related Diuretics
Bendroflumethiazide (bendrofluazide)	*see* Thiazides and Related Diuretics
Benperidol	*see* Antipsychotics
Benzthiazide	*see* Thiazides and Related Diuretics
Bexarotene	Avoid
Bezafibrate	Avoid in severe liver disease
Bicalutamide	Increased accumulation possible in moderate to severe hepatic impairment
Bisoprolol	Max. 10 mg daily in severe liver impairment
Bortezomib	Manufacturer advises caution in mild to moderate hepatic impairment—consider dose reduction; avoid in severe hepatic impairment
Bosentan	Avoid in moderate and severe hepatic impairment
Bromocriptine	Dose reduction may be necessary
Buclizine	Sedation inappropriate in severe liver disease—avoid
Budesonide	Plasma-budesonide concentration may increase on oral administration
Bumetanide	*see* Loop Diuretics
Bupivacaine	Manufacturer advises caution in severe hepatic impairment
Buprenorphine	*see* Opioid Analgesics
Bupropion	Manufacturer recommends 150 mg daily; avoid in severe hepatic cirrhosis
Buspirone	Reduce dose in mild to moderate liver disease; avoid in severe liver disease
Busulfan	Manufacturer advises monitor liver function—no information available
Cabergoline	Reduce dose in severe hepatic impairment
Calcitriol	Manufacturer of topical calcitriol advises avoid in severe liver disease
Candesartan	For hypertension, initially 2 mg once daily in mild or moderate hepatic impairment (no initial dose adjustment necessary in heart failure); avoid in severe hepatic impairment
Capecitabine	Manufacturer advises avoid in severe hepatic impairment
Carbamazepine	Metabolism impaired in advanced liver disease
Carvedilol	Avoid
Caspofungin	70 mg on first day then 35 mg once daily in moderate hepatic impairment; no information available for severe hepatic impairment

Drug	Comment
Ceftriaxone	Reduce dose and monitor plasma concentration if both hepatic and severe renal impairment
Celecoxib	*see* NSAIDs
Cetrorelix	Manufacturer advises avoid in moderate or severe liver impairment
Chloral hydrate	Reduce dose in mild to moderate hepatic impairment; avoid in severe impairment; *see also* Anxiolytics and Hypnotics
Chlorambucil	Manufacturer advises consider dose reduction in severe hepatic impairment—limited information available
Chloramphenicol	Avoid if possible—increased risk of bone-marrow depression; reduce dose and monitor plasma-chloramphenicol concentration
Chlordiazepoxide	*see* Anxiolytics and Hypnotics
Chlorphenamine (chlorpheniramine)	Sedation inappropriate in severe liver disease—avoid
Chlorpheniramine	*see* Chlorphenamine
Chlorpromazine	*see* Antipsychotics
Chlorpropamide	*see* Sulphonylureas
Chlortalidone	*see* Thiazides and Related Diuretics
Ciclosporin	May need dose adjustment
Cilazapril	*see* ACE Inhibitors
Cilostazol	Avoid in moderate or severe liver disease
Cimetidine	Increased risk of confusion; reduce dose
Cinacalcet	Manufacturer advises caution in moderate to severe hepatic impairment—monitor closely especially when increasing dose
Cinnarizine	Sedation inappropriate in severe liver disease—avoid
Ciprofibrate	Avoid in severe liver disease
Citalopram	Use doses at lower end of range
Cladribine	Regular monitoring recommended
Clarithromycin	Hepatic dysfunction including jaundice reported
Clavulanic acid [ingredient]	*see* Co-amoxiclav, below and *Timentin®*, p. 771
Clemastine	Sedation inappropriate in severe liver disease—avoid
Clobazam	*see* Anxiolytics and Hypnotics
Clofarabine	Manufacturer advises caution in mild to moderate hepatic impairment; avoid in severe hepatic impairment
Clomethiazole	*see* Anxiolytics and Hypnotics
Clomifene	Avoid in severe liver disease
Clomipramine	*see* Antidepressants, Tricyclic (and related)
Clonazepam	Reduce dose in mild to moderate impairment; avoid in severe liver impairment; *see also* Anxiolytics and Hypnotics
Clopamide	*see* Thiazides and Related Diuretics
Clopidogrel	Manufacturer advises caution (risk of bleeding); avoid in severe hepatic impairment
Clozapine	Monitor hepatic function regularly; avoid in symptomatic or progressive liver disease or hepatic failure
Co-amoxiclav	Monitor liver function in liver disease. Cholestatic jaundice, *see* p. 288
Codeine	*see* Opioid Analgesics
Colesevelam	Manufacturer advises caution
Contraceptives, oral	Avoid in active liver disease and if history of pruritus or cholestasis during pregnancy
Co-trimoxazole	Manufacturer advises avoid in severe liver disease
Cyclizine	Sedation inappropriate in severe liver disease—avoid
Cyclopenthiazide	*see* Thiazides and Related Diuretics
Cyclophosphamide	Reduce dose
Cyclosporin	*see* Ciclosporin
Cyproheptadine	Sedation inappropriate in severe liver disease—avoid
Cyproterone acetate	Dose-related toxicity; *see also* side-effects of cyproterone, section 8.3.4.2
Cytarabine	Reduce dose
Dacarbazine	Dose reduction may be required in mild to moderate liver disease; avoid if severe
Dalfopristin [ingredient]	*see Synercid®*
Dalteparin	*see* Heparin
Danaparoid	Use with caution in moderate hepatic impairment (increased risk of bleeding); avoid in severe hepatic impairment unless patient has heparin-induced thrombocytopenia and no alternative
Dantrolene	Avoid oral use—may cause severe liver damage; injection may be used in emergency for malignant hyperthermia
Daptomycin	Manufacturer advises caution in severe hepatic impairment—no information available
Darbepoetin	Manufacturer advises caution
Darifenacin	Max. 7.5 mg daily in moderate hepatic impairment; avoid in severe hepatic impairment
Darunavir	Manufacturer advises caution in mild to moderate hepatic impairment; avoid in severe hepatic impairment—no information available
Dasatinib	Manufacturer advises caution in moderate to severe hepatic impairment—no information available
Daunorubicin	Reduce dose
Deferasirox	Manufacturer advises caution—no information available; avoid in severe hepatic impairment

Drug	Comment
Deferiprone	Manufacturer advises monitor liver function—interrupt treatment if persistent elevation in serum alanine aminotransferase
Demeclocycline	*see* Tetracyclines
Desflurane	Reduce dose
Desogestrel	Avoid; *see also* Contraceptives, Oral
Dexibuprofen	*see* NSAIDs
Dexketoprofen	*see* NSAIDs
Dexrazoxane	Monitor liver function in patients with liver disease
Dextromethorphan	*see* Opioid Analgesics
Diamorphine	*see* Opioid Analgesics
Diazepam	*see* Anxiolytics and Hypnotics
Diclofenac	*see* NSAIDs
Didanosine	Insufficient information but monitor for toxicity
Diethylstilbestrol	Avoid; *see also* Contraceptives, Oral
Dihydrocodeine	*see* Opioid Analgesics
Diltiazem	Reduce dose
Diphenoxylate	*see* Opioid Analgesics
Dipipanone	*see* Opioid Analgesics
Disodium pamidronate	Manufacturer advises caution in severe hepatic impairment—no information available
Disopyramide	Half-life prolonged—may need dose reduction
Docetaxel	Monitor liver function—reduce dose according to liver enzymes; avoid in severe hepatic impairment
Domperidone	Avoid
Donepezil	Manufacturer advises caution in mild to moderate hepatic impairment
Dosulepin (dothiepin)	*see* Antidepressants, Tricyclic (and related)
Dothiepin	*see* Antidepressants, Tricyclic (and related)
Doxazosin	No information—manufacturer advises caution
Doxepin	*see* Antidepressants, Tricyclic (and related)
Doxorubicin	Reduce dose according to bilirubin concentration
Doxycycline	*see* Tetracyclines
Drotrecogin alfa (activated)	Avoid in chronic severe liver disease
Duloxetine	Manufacturer advises avoid
Dutasteride	Manufacturer advises avoid in severe liver impairment—no information available
Dydrogesterone	Avoid; *see also* Contraceptives, Oral
Efavirenz	In mild to moderate liver disease, monitor for dose related side-effects (e.g. CNS effects) and monitor liver function; avoid in severe hepatic impairment
Eletriptan	Manufacturer advises avoid in severe hepatic impairment
Enalapril	*see* ACE Inhibitors
Enfuvirtide	Manufacturer advises caution—no information available
Enoxaparin	*see* Heparin
Entacapone	Avoid
Epirubicin	Reduce dose according to bilirubin concentration
Eplerenone	Avoid in severe liver disease
Epoetin	Manufacturers advise caution in chronic hepatic failure
Eprosartan	Halve initial dose in mild or moderate liver disease; avoid if severe
Eptifibatide	Avoid in severe liver disease—increased risk of bleeding
Erdosteine	Manufacturer advises max. 300 mg daily in mild to moderate hepatic impairment; avoid in severe hepatic impairment
Ergometrine	Avoid in severe liver disease
Ergotamine	Avoid in severe liver disease—risk of toxicity increased
Erlotinib	Manufacturer advises caution in mild to moderate impairment; avoid in severe impairment
Erythromycin	May cause idiosyncratic hepatotoxicity
Escitalopram	Initial dose 5 mg daily in mild to moderate hepatic impairment (for 2 weeks), increased to 10 mg daily according to response; manufacturer advises caution in severe hepatic impairment
Esomeprazole	In severe liver disease dose should not exceed 20 mg daily
Estradiol	Avoid; *see also* Contraceptives, Oral
Estramustine	Manufacturer advises caution and regular liver function tests; avoid in severe liver disease
Estriol	Avoid; *see also* Contraceptives, Oral
Estrone	Avoid; *see also* Contraceptives, Oral
Estropipate	Avoid; *see also* Contraceptives, Oral
Ethinylestradiol	Avoid; *see also* Contraceptives, Oral
Etodolac	*see* NSAIDs
Etoposide	Avoid in severe hepatic impairment
Etoricoxib	Max. 60 mg daily in mild hepatic impairment; max. 60 mg on alternate days in moderate hepatic impairment; avoid in severe hepatic impairment; *see also* NSAIDs
Etynodiol diacetate	Avoid; *see also* Contraceptives, Oral
Exemestane	Manufacturer advises caution
Ezetimibe	Avoid in moderate and severe hepatic impairment—may accumulate
Famciclovir	Usual dose in well compensated liver disease (information not available on decompensated)

Drug	Comment
Felodipine	Reduce dose
Fenbufen	*see* NSAIDs
Fenofibrate	Avoid in severe liver disease
Fenoprofen	*see* NSAIDs
Fentanyl	*see* Opioid Analgesics
Fibrinolytics	Avoid in severe hepatic impairment—increased risk of bleeding
Flecainide	Avoid (or reduce dose) in severe liver disease
Flucloxacillin	Caution in hepatic impairment (risk of cholestatic jaundice and hepatitis, *see* p. 286)
Fluconazole	Toxicity with related drugs
Flumazenil	Carefully titrate dose
Fluorouracil	Manufacturer advises caution
Fluoxetine	*see* Antidepressants, SSRI
Flupentixol	*see* Antipsychotics
Fluphenazine	*see* Antipsychotics
Flurazepam	*see* Anxiolytics and Hypnotics
Flurbiprofen	*see* NSAIDs
Flutamide	Use with caution (hepatotoxic)
Fluvastatin	*see* Statins
Fluvoxamine	*see* Antidepressants, SSRI
Fondaparinux sodium	Caution in severe hepatic impairment (increased risk of bleeding)
Formoterol (eformoterol)	Metabolism possibly reduced in severe cirrhosis
Fosamprenavir	Manufacturer advises caution in mild hepatic impairment; reduce dose to 450 mg twice daily in moderate hepatic impairment; avoid in severe hepatic impairment
Fosinopril	*see* ACE Inhibitors
Fosphenytoin	Consider 10–25% reduction in dose or infusion rate (except initial dose for status epilepticus)
Frovatriptan	Avoid in severe hepatic impairment
Frusemide	*see* Loop Diuretics
Fulvestrant	Manufacturer advises caution in mild to moderate hepatic impairment; avoid in severe hepatic impairment
Furosemide (frusemide)	*see* Loop Diuretics
Fusidic acid	*see* Sodium Fusidate
Galantamine	Reduce dose in moderate hepatic impairment; avoid in severe impairment
Ganirelix	Manufacturer advises avoid in moderate or severe hepatic impairment
Gemcitabine	Manufacturer advises caution
Gemfibrozil	Avoid in liver disease
Gestodene	Avoid; *see also* Contraceptives, Oral
Gestrinone	Avoid in severe liver disease
Glibenclamide	*see* Sulphonylureas
Gliclazide	*see* Sulphonylureas
Glimepiride	Manufacturer advises avoid in severe hepatic impairment
Glipizide	*see* Sulphonylureas
Glyceryl trinitrate	*see* Nitrates
Griseofulvin	Avoid in severe liver disease

Drug	Comment
Haloperidol	*see* Antipsychotics
Halothane	Avoid if history of unexplained pyrexia or jaundice following previous exposure to halothane
Heparin	Reduce dose in severe liver disease
Hydralazine	Reduce dose
Hydrochlorothiazide	*see* Thiazides and Related Diuretics
Hydroflumethiazide	*see* Thiazides and Related Diuretics
Hydromorphone	*see* Opioid Analgesics
Hydroxyzine	Sedation inappropriate in severe liver disease—avoid
Hyoscine hydrobromide	Manufacturer advises caution
Hypnotics	*see* Anxiolytics and Hypnotics
Ibuprofen	*see* NSAIDs
Idarubicin	Reduce dose according to bilirubin concentration
Ifosfamide	Avoid
Iloprost	Elimination reduced in hepatic impairment—initially 2.5 micrograms no more frequently than every 3 hours (max. 6 times daily), adjusted according to response (consult product literature)
Imatinib	Max. 400 mg daily; reduce dose further if not tolerated
Imidapril	*see* ACE Inhibitors
Imipramine	*see* Antidepressants, Tricyclic (and related)
Indapamide	*see* Thiazides and Related Diuretics
Indinavir	Increased risk of nephrolithiasis; reduce dose to 600 mg every 8 hours in mild to moderate hepatic impairment; not studied in severe impairment
Indometacin	*see* NSAIDs
Indoramin	Manufacturer advises caution
Interferon alfa	Close monitoring in mild to moderate hepatic impairment; avoid if severe
Interferon beta	Avoid in decompensated liver disease
Interferon gamma-1b	Manufacturer advises caution in severe liver disease
Irinotecan	Monitor closely for neutropenia if plasma-bilirubin concentration 1.5–3 times upper limit of normal range; avoid if plasma-bilirubin concentration greater than 3 times upper limit of normal range
Iron dextran	Avoid in severe hepatic impairment
Iron sucrose	Avoid
Isocarboxazid	*see* Antidepressants, MAOI
Isometheptene [ingredient]	*see Midrid®*
Isoniazid	Use with caution; monitor liver function regularly and particularly frequently in first 2 months; *see also* p. 312
Isosorbide dinitrate	*see* Nitrates

Drug	Comment
Isosorbide mononitrate	*see* Nitrates
Isotretinoin	Avoid—further impairment of liver function may occur
Isradipine	Reduce dose
Itraconazole	Use only if potential benefit outweighs risk of hepatotoxicity (*see* p. 324); dose reduction may be necessary
Ivabradine	Manufacturer advises caution in moderate hepatic impairment; avoid in severe hepatic impairment
Kaletra®	Avoid oral solution because of propylene glycol content; manufacturer advises avoid capsules and tablets in severe hepatic impairment
Ketoconazole	Avoid; *see also* p. 325
Ketoprofen	*see* NSAIDs
Ketorolac	*see* NSAIDs
Ketotifen	Sedation inappropriate in severe liver disease—avoid
Labetalol	Avoid—severe hepatocellular injury reported
Lacidipine	Antihypertensive effect possibly increased
Lamotrigine	Halve dose in moderate hepatic impairment; quarter dose in severe hepatic impairment
Lansoprazole	In severe liver disease dose should not exceed 30 mg daily
Leflunomide	Avoid—active metabolite may accumulate
Lepirudin	No information—manufacturer advises that cirrhosis may affect renal excretion
Lercanidipine	Avoid in severe liver disease
Levetiracetam	Halve dose in severe hepatic impairment if creatinine clearance less than 70 mL/minute
Levobupivacaine	Manufacturer advises caution in liver disease
Levomepromazine (methotrimeprazine)	*see* Antipsychotics
Levonorgestrel	Avoid (however levonorgestrel emergency contraception can be used); *see also* Contraceptives, Oral
Lidocaine (lignocaine)	Manufacturer advises caution—increased risk of side-effects
Lignocaine	*see* Lidocaine
Linezolid	In severe hepatic impairment manufacturer advises use only if potential benefit outweighs risk
Lofepramine	*see* Antidepressants, Tricyclic (and related)
Loop diuretics	Hypokalaemia may precipitate coma (use potassium-sparing diuretic to prevent this); increased risk of hypomagnesaemia in alcoholic cirrhosis
Lopinavir [ingredient]	*see Kaletra*®
Loprazolam	*see* Anxiolytics and Hypnotics
Lorazepam	*see* Anxiolytics and Hypnotics
Lormetazepam	*see* Anxiolytics and Hypnotics
Losartan	Consider lower dose
Lumefantrine [ingredient]	*see Riamet*®
Lymecycline	*see* Tetracyclines
Magnesium salts	Avoid in hepatic coma if risk of renal failure
Maraviroc	Manufacturer advises caution
Medroxyprogesterone	Avoid; *see also* Contraceptives, Oral
Mefenamic acid	*see* NSAIDs
Mefloquine	Avoid for prophylaxis in severe liver disease
Megestrol	Avoid; *see also* Contraceptives, Oral
Meloxicam	*see* NSAIDs
Meprobamate	*see* Anxiolytics and Hypnotics
Meptazinol	*see* Opioid Analgesics
Mercaptopurine	May need dose reduction
Meropenem	Monitor transaminase and bilirubin concentrations
Mesalazine	Avoid in severe hepatic impairment
Mesterolone	*see* Androgens
Mestranol	Avoid; *see also* Contraceptives, Oral
Metformin	Withdraw if tissue hypoxia likely—manufacturers advise avoid
Methadone	*see* Opioid Analgesics
Methenamine	Avoid
Methionine	May precipitate coma
Methocarbamol	Manufacturer advises caution; half-life may be prolonged
Methotrexate	Dose-related toxicity—avoid in non-malignant conditions (e.g. psoriasis); avoid for all indications in severe hepatic impairment
Methotrimeprazine	*see* Antipsychotics
Methoxy polyethylene glycol epoetin beta	Manufacturer advises caution in severe liver disease—no information available
Methyldopa	Manufacturer advises caution in history of liver disease; avoid in active liver disease
Methysergide	Avoid
Metoclopramide	Reduce dose
Metolazone	*see* Thiazides and Related Diuretics
Metoprolol	Reduce dose in severe hepatic impairment
Metronidazole	In severe liver disease reduce total daily dose to one-third, and give once daily
Mexiletine	May need dose reduction in moderate to severe liver impairment
Mianserin	*see* Antidepressants, Tricyclic (and related)
Miconazole	Avoid
Midazolam	*see* Anxiolytics and Hypnotics
Midrid®	Avoid in severe liver disease; *see also* Paracetamol
Miglustat	No information available—manufacturer advises caution
Minocycline	*see* Tetracyclines
Mirtazapine	Manufacturer advises caution

Drug	Comment
Mitotane	Manufacturer advises caution in mild to moderate impairment—monitoring of plasma-mitotane concentration recommended; avoid in severe impairment
Mitoxantrone	Manufacturer advises caution in severe hepatic impairment
Mivacurium	Reduce dose in severe liver impairment
Mizolastine	Manufacturer recommends avoid in significant hepatic impairment
Moclobemide	Reduce dose in severe liver disease
Modafinil	Halve dose in severe liver disease
Moexipril	*see* ACE Inhibitors
Morphine	*see* Opioid Analgesics
Moxifloxacin	Manufacturer advises avoid in severe hepatic impairment
Moxonidine	Avoid in severe liver disease
Nabilone	Avoid in severe liver disease
Nabumetone	*see* NSAIDs
Nadolol	Manufacturer advises caution
Nalidixic acid	Manufacturer advises caution in liver disease
Naltrexone	Manufacturer advises caution; avoid in acute hepatitis or hepatic failure
Nandrolone	*see* Anabolic Steroids
Naproxen	*see* NSAIDs
Naratriptan	Max. 2.5 mg in 24 hours in moderate hepatic impairment; avoid if severe
Nateglinide	Manufacturer advises caution in moderate hepatic impairment; avoid in severe impairment—no information available
Nebivolol	No information available—manufacturer advises avoid
Nelfinavir	No information available—manufacturer advises caution
Neomycin	Absorbed from gastro-intestinal tract in liver disease—increased risk of ototoxicity
Nevirapine	Manufacturer advises caution in moderate hepatic impairment; avoid in severe hepatic impairment; *see also* p. 334
Nicardipine	Half-life prolonged in severe hepatic impairment—may need dose reduction
Nicotine	Manufacturers advise caution in moderate to severe hepatic impairment
Nicotinic acid	Manufacturer advises monitor liver function in mild to moderate hepatic impairment and avoid in severe impairment; discontinue if severe abnormalities in liver function tests
Nicoumalone	*see* Anticoagulants, Oral
Nifedipine	Reduce dose in severe liver disease
Nimodipine	Elimination reduced in cirrhosis—monitor blood pressure
Nisoldipine	Formulation not suitable in hepatic impairment
Nitrates	Caution in severe hepatic impairment
Nitrazepam	*see* Anxiolytics and Hypnotics
Nitrofurantoin	Cholestatic jaundice and chronic active hepatitis reported
Nitroprusside	*see* Sodium Nitroprusside
Nizatidine	Manufacturer advises caution
Norethisterone	Avoid; *see also* Contraceptives, Oral
Norgestimate	Avoid; *see also* Contraceptives, Oral
Norgestrel	Avoid; *see also* Contraceptives, Oral
Nortriptyline	*see* Antidepressants, Tricyclic (and related)
NSAIDs	Increased risk of gastro-intestinal bleeding and can cause fluid retention; avoid in severe liver disease; aceclofenac, initially 100 mg daily; celecoxib, halve initial dose in moderate liver disease; parecoxib, halve dose in moderate hepatic impairment (max. 40 mg daily); tiaprofenic acid, reduce dose in mild or moderate hepatic impairment; *see also* Etoricoxib
Oestrogens	Avoid; *see also* Contraceptives, Oral
Ofloxacin	Elimination may be reduced in severe hepatic impairment
Olanzapine	Consider initial dose of 5 mg daily
Olmesartan	Dose should not exceed 20 mg daily in moderate impairment; manufacturer advises avoid in severe impairment—no information available
Omalizumab	Manufacturer advises caution—no information available
Omega-3-acid ethyl esters	Monitor liver function
Omeprazole	In liver disease not more than 20 mg daily should be needed
Ondansetron	Max. 8 mg daily in moderate or severe hepatic impairment
Opioid analgesics	Avoid or reduce dose—may precipitate coma
Oral contraceptives	*see* Contraceptives, Oral
Oxazepam	*see* Anxiolytics and Hypnotics
Oxcarbazepine	Manufacturer advises caution in severe hepatic impairment—no information available
Oxprenolol	Reduce dose
Oxybutynin	Manufacturer advises caution
Oxycodone	*see* Opioid Analgesics
Oxytetracycline	*see* Tetracyclines
Paclitaxel	Avoid in severe liver disease
Paliperidone	Manufacturer advises caution in severe hepatic impairment—no information available

Drug	Comment
Pancuronium	Possibly slower onset, higher dose requirement and prolonged recovery time
Pantoprazole	Max. 20 mg daily in severe hepatic impairment and cirrhosis—monitor liver function (discontinue if deterioration)
Papaveretum	*see* Opioid Analgesics
Paracetamol	Dose-related toxicity—avoid large doses
Parathyroid hormone	Avoid
Parecoxib	*see* NSAIDs
Paroxetine	*see* Antidepressants, SSRI
Peginterferon alfa	Avoid in severe hepatic impairment
Pentazocine	*see* Opioid Analgesics
Pericyazine	*see* Antipsychotics
Perindopril	*see* ACE Inhibitors
Perphenazine	*see* Antipsychotics
Pethidine	*see* Opioid Analgesics
Phenelzine	*see* Antidepressants, MAOI
Phenindione	*see* Anticoagulants, Oral
Phenobarbital	May precipitate coma; avoid in severe hepatic impairment
Phenothiazines	*see* Antipsychotics
Phenytoin	Reduce dose to avoid toxicity
Pholcodine	*see* Opioid Analgesics
Pilocarpine	Reduce initial oral dose in moderate or severe cirrhosis
Pimozide	*see* Antipsychotics
Pioglitazone	Avoid
Piperazine	Manufacturer advises avoid
Pipotiazine	*see* Antipsychotics
Piracetam	Avoid
Piroxicam	*see* NSAIDs
Posaconazole	Monitor liver function; use with caution in severe hepatic impairment
Pravastatin	*see* Statins
Prazosin	Initially 500 micrograms daily; increased with caution
Prednisolone	Side-effects more common
Prilocaine	Manufacturer advises caution
Primidone	Reduce dose; may precipitate coma
Procainamide	Avoid or reduce dose
Procarbazine	Avoid in severe hepatic impairment
Prochlorperazine	*see* Antipsychotics
Progesterone	Avoid; *see also* Contraceptives, Oral
Progestogens	Avoid; *see also* Contraceptives, Oral
Promazine	*see* Antipsychotics
Promethazine	Avoid—may precipitate coma in severe liver disease; hepatotoxic
Propafenone	Reduce dose
Propantheline	Manufacturer advises caution
Propiverine	Avoid in moderate to severe hepatic impairment
Propofol	Use with caution
Propranolol	Reduce oral dose
Propylthiouracil	Reduce dose
Pyrazinamide	Monitor hepatic function—idiosyncratic hepatotoxicity more common; avoid in severe hepatic impairment; *see also* p. 313
Pyrimethamine	Manufacturer advises caution
Quetiapine	Manufacturer advises initially 25 mg daily, increased daily in steps of 25–50 mg
Quinagolide	Manufacturer advises avoid—no information available
Quinapril	*see* ACE Inhibitors
Quinupristin [ingredient]	*see Synercid®*
Rabeprazole	Manufacturer advises caution in severe hepatic dysfunction
Raloxifene	Manufacturer advises avoid
Raltitrexed	Caution in mild or moderate disease; avoid if severe
Ramipril	*see* ACE Inhibitors
Rasagiline	Manufacturer advises caution in mild hepatic impairment; avoid in moderate to severe impairment
Reboxetine	Initial dose 2 mg twice daily, increased according to tolerance
Remifentanil	*see* Opioid Analgesics
Repaglinide	Manufacturer advises avoid in severe liver disease
Reteplase	*see* Fibrinolytics
Riamet®	Manufacturer advises caution in severe hepatic impairment—monitor ECG and plasma potassium concentration
Ribavirin	No dosage adjustment required; avoid oral administration in severe hepatic dysfunction or decompensated cirrhosis
Rifabutin	Reduce dose in severe hepatic impairment
Rifampicin	Impaired elimination; monitor liver function; avoid or do not exceed 8 mg/kg daily; *see also* p. 313
Riluzole	Avoid
Rimonabant	Manufacturer advises caution in moderate hepatic impairment; avoid in severe impairment
Risperidone	Manufacturer advises initial oral dose of 500 micrograms twice daily increased in steps of 500 micrograms twice daily to 1–2 mg twice daily; if an oral dose of at least 2 mg daily tolerated, 25 mg as a depot injection can be given every 2 weeks
Ritonavir	Avoid in decompensated liver disease; in severe hepatic impairment without decompensation, use 'booster' doses with caution (avoid treatment doses)
Rivastigmine	No information available—manufacturer advises avoid in severe liver disease

Drug	Comment
Rizatriptan	Reduce dose to 5 mg in mild to moderate liver disease; avoid in severe liver disease
Rocuronium	Reduce dose
Ropinirole	Manufacturer advises caution in moderate hepatic impairment; avoid in severe hepatic impairment
Ropivacaine	Manufacturer advises caution in severe liver disease
Rosiglitazone	Avoid
Rosuvastatin	*see* Statins
Rotigotine	Manufacturer advises caution in severe hepatic impairment—no information available
Rufinamide	Manufacturer advises caution and careful dose titration in mild to moderate hepatic impairment; avoid in severe impairment
Saquinavir	Manufacturer advises caution in moderate hepatic impairment; avoid in severe impairment
Sertindole	Slower titration and lower maintenance dose in mild to moderate hepatic impairment; avoid in severe hepatic impairment; *see also* Antipsychotics
Sertraline	*see* Antidepressants, SSRI
Sibutramine	Increased plasma-sibutramine concentration; manufacturer advises caution in mild to moderate hepatic impairment; avoid if severe impairment
Sildenafil	For erectile dysfunction, initial dose 25 mg; for pulmonary hypertension reduce to 20 mg twice daily if usual dose not tolerated; manufacturer advises avoid in severe hepatic impairment
Simvastatin	*see* Statins
Sirolimus	Monitor blood-sirolimus trough concentration
Sitaxentan sodium	Avoid
Sodium aurothiomalate	Caution in mild to moderate liver disease; avoid in severe liver disease
Sodium bicarbonate	*see* Antacids
Sodium fusidate	Impaired biliary excretion; possibly increased risk of hepatotoxicity; avoid or reduce dose
Sodium nitroprusside	Avoid in severe liver disease
Sodium oxybate	Halve initial dose
Sodium phenylbutyrate	Manufacturer advises caution
Sodium valproate	*see* Valproate
Solifenacin	Max. 5 mg daily in moderate liver disease; avoid if severe
Sorafenib	Manufacturer advises caution in severe hepatic impairment—no information available
Statins	Avoid in active liver disease or unexplained persistent elevations in serum transaminases
Stilboestrol (diethylstilbestrol)	Avoid; *see also* Contraceptives, Oral
Streptokinase	*see* Fibrinolytics
Sulindac	*see* NSAIDs
Sulphonylureas	Increased risk of hypoglycaemia in severe liver disease; avoid or use small dose; can produce jaundice; *see also* Glimepiride
Sulpiride	*see* Antipsychotics
Sumatriptan	Manufacturer advises 50 mg oral dose in hepatic impairment; avoid in severe hepatic impairment
Suxamethonium	Prolonged apnoea may occur in severe liver disease because of reduced hepatic synthesis of pseudocholinesterase
Synercid®	Consider reducing dose to 5 mg/kg every 8 hours in moderate hepatic impairment, adjusted according to clinical response; avoid in severe hepatic impairment or if plasma-bilirubin concentration greater than 3 times upper limit of reference range
Tacrolimus	Dose reduction may be necessary in severe hepatic impairment
Tadalafil	Max. dose 10 mg; manufacturer advises monitor patient in severe hepatic impairment
Tamsulosin	Avoid in severe hepatic impairment
Tegafur with uracil	*see Uftoral®*
Telithromycin	Manufacturer advises caution; *see also* p. 303
Telmisartan	20–40 mg once daily in mild or moderate impairment; avoid in severe hepatic impairment or biliary obstruction
Temazepam	*see* Anxiolytics and Hypnotics
Tenecteplase	*see* Fibrinolytics
Tenoxicam	*see* NSAIDs
Terbinafine	Manufacturer advises avoid—elimination reduced
Testosterone and esters	*see* Androgens
Tetracyclines	Avoid (or use with caution); tetracycline and demeclocycline max. 1 g daily in divided doses; *see also* Tigecycline
Theophylline	Reduce dose
Thiazides and related diuretics	Avoid in severe liver disease; hypokalaemia may precipitate coma (potassium-sparing diuretic can prevent); increased risk of hypomagnesaemia in alcoholic cirrhosis
Thiopental	Reduce dose for induction in severe liver disease
Tiagabine	Maintenance dose 5–10 mg 1–2 times daily initially in mild to moderate hepatic impairment; avoid in severe impairment

Drug	Comment
Tiaprofenic acid	*see* NSAIDs
Tibolone	Avoid in severe liver disease
Ticarcillin [ingredient]	*see Timentin®*
Tigecycline	Initially 100 mg then 25 mg every 12 hours in severe hepatic impairment
Timentin®	Cholestatic jaundice, *see* under Co-amoxiclav p. 288
Timolol	Dose reduction may be necessary
Tinzaparin	*see* Heparin
Tioguanine	Reduce dose in hepatic impairment
Tipranavir	Manufacturer advises monitor liver function in mild hepatic impairment (*see* p. 334); avoid in moderate or severe hepatic impairment—no information available
Tirofiban	Caution in mild to moderate liver disease; avoid in severe liver disease—increased risk of bleeding
Tizanidine	Avoid in severe liver disease
Tolbutamide	*see* Sulphonylureas
Tolcapone	Avoid
Tolfenamic acid	*see* NSAIDs
Tolterodine	Reduce dose to 1 mg twice daily
Topiramate	Use with caution in hepatic impairment—clearance may be decreased
Topotecan	Avoid in severe hepatic impairment
Torasemide	*see* Loop Diuretics
Toremifene	Elimination decreased in hepatic impairment—avoid if severe
Trabectedin	Manufacturer advises caution in liver impairment—consider dose reduction; avoid in patients with raised bilirubin
Tramadol	*see* Opioid Analgesics
Trandolapril	*see* ACE Inhibitors
Tranylcypromine	*see* Antidepressants, MAOI
Trazodone	*see* Antidepressants, Tricyclic (and related)
Tretinoin (oral)	Reduce dose
Tribavirin	*see* Ribavirin
Triclofos	*see* Anxiolytics and Hypnotics
Trifluoperazine	*see* Antipsychotics
Trimeprazine	*see* Alimemazine
Trimetrexate	Manufacturer advises caution; interrupt treatment if severe abnormalities in liver function tests (consult product literature)
Trimipramine	*see* Antidepressants, Tricyclic (and related)
Trospium	Manufacturer advises avoid—no information available
Uftoral®	Manufacturer advises monitor liver function in mild to moderate hepatic impairment and avoid in severe impairment
Urokinase	*see* Fibrinolytics
Ursodeoxycholic acid	Avoid in chronic liver disease (but used in primary biliary cirrhosis)
Valaciclovir	Manufacturer advises caution with high doses used for preventing cytomegalovirus disease—no information available
Valproate	Avoid if possible—hepatotoxicity and hepatic failure may occasionally occur (usually in first 6 months); *see also* p. 252
Valproic acid	*see* Valproate
Valsartan	Halve dose in mild to moderate hepatic impairment; avoid if severe
Vardenafil	Initial dose 5 mg in mild to moderate hepatic impairment, increased subsequently according to response (max. 10 mg in moderate hepatic impairment); manufacturer advises avoid in severe hepatic impairment
Venlafaxine	Halve dose in moderate hepatic impairment; avoid if severe
Verapamil	Reduce oral dose
Verteporfin	Avoid in severe hepatic impairment
Vinblastine	Dose reduction may be necessary
Vincristine	Dose reduction may be necessary
Vindesine	Dose reduction may be necessary
Vinorelbine	Dose reduction may be required in significant hepatic impairment
Voriconazole	In mild to moderate hepatic cirrhosis use usual initial dose then halve subsequent doses; no information available for severe hepatic cirrhosis—manufacturer advises use only if potential benefit outweighs risk
Warfarin	*see* Anticoagulants, Oral
Xipamide	*see* Thiazides and Related Diuretics
Zafirlukast	Manufacturer advises avoid
Zaleplon	*see* Anxiolytics and Hypnotics
Zidovudine	Accumulation may occur
Zoledronic acid	Manufacturer advises caution in severe hepatic impairment—limited information available
Zolmitriptan	Max. 5 mg in 24 hours in moderate or severe hepatic impairment
Zolpidem	*see* Anxiolytics and Hypnotics
Zonisamide	Initially, increase dose at 2-week intervals if mild or moderate hepatic impairment; avoid in severe impairment
Zopiclone	*see* Anxiolytics and Hypnotics
Zotepine	Initial dose 25 mg twice daily, increased gradually according to response (max. 75 mg twice daily); monitor liver function at weekly intervals for first 3 months
Zuclopenthixol	*see* Antipsychotics

A3 Renal impairment

The use of drugs in patients with reduced renal function can give rise to problems for several reasons:

- reduced renal excretion of a drug or its metabolites may cause toxicity;
- sensitivity to some drugs is increased even if elimination is unimpaired;
- many side-effects are tolerated poorly by patients with renal impairment;
- some drugs are not effective when renal function is reduced.

Many of these problems can be avoided by reducing the dose or by using alternative drugs.

Principles of dose adjustment in renal impairment

The level of renal function below which the dose of a drug must be reduced depends on the proportion of the drug eliminated by renal excretion and its toxicity.

For many drugs with only minor or no dose-related side-effects very precise modification of the dose regimen is unnecessary and a simple scheme for dose reduction is sufficient.

For more toxic drugs with a small safety margin dose regimens based on glomerular filtration rate should be used. When both efficacy and toxicity are closely related to plasma-drug concentration, recommended regimens should be regarded only as a guide to initial treatment; subsequent doses must be adjusted according to clinical response and plasma-drug concentration.

Renal function declines with age; many elderly patients have renal impairment but, because of reduced muscle mass, this may not be indicated by a raised serum creatinine. It is wise to assume at least mild impairment of renal function when prescribing for the elderly.

The total daily maintenance dose of a drug can be reduced either by reducing the size of the individual doses or by increasing the interval between doses. For some drugs, although the size of the maintenance dose is reduced it is important to give a loading dose if an immediate effect is required. This is because it takes about five times the half-life of the drug to achieve steady-state plasma concentrations. Because the plasma half-life of drugs excreted by the kidney is prolonged in renal impairment it can take many doses for the reduced dosage to achieve a therapeutic plasma concentration. The loading dose should usually be the same size as the initial dose for a patient with normal renal function.

Nephrotoxic drugs should, if possible, be avoided in patients with renal disease because the consequences of nephrotoxicity are likely to be more serious when renal reserve is already reduced.

Use of dosage table

Dose recommendations are based on the severity of renal impairment.

Renal function is measured either in terms of **glomerular filtration rate** (GFR) estimated from a formula derived from the Modification of Diet in Renal Disease study ('MDRD formula' that uses serum creatinine, age, sex, and race) or it can be expressed as **creatinine clearance** (best derived from a 24-hour urine collection but often calculated from a formula or a nomogram that uses serum creatinine, weight, sex, and age).

The serum-creatinine concentration is sometimes used instead as a measure of renal function but it is only a **rough guide** to drug dosing.

> **Important**
>
> The information on dosage adjustment in the BNF is based on creatinine clearance. This is because published information on the effects of renal impairment on drug elimination is usually given in terms of creatinine clearance as a surrogate for glomerular filtration rate (GFR).
>
> Special care is required when interpreting advice on dosage adjustment based on creatinine clearance (e.g. calculated from the Cockcroft and Gault formula) because renal function is increasingly being reported on the basis of estimated glomerular filtration rate (eGFR) normalised to a body surface area of 1.73 m^2 and derived from the MDRD (Modification of Diet in Renal Disease) formula. Although, the two measures of renal function are not interchangeable, in practice, for most drugs and for most patients of average build and height, eGFR (MDRD) can be used to determine dosage adjustments in place of creatinine clearance. For potentially toxic drugs with a small safety margin and in some patients (e.g. those at both extremes of weight) the absolute glomerular filtration rate or creatinine clearance should be used or dosage should be adjusted according to plasma-drug concentration and clinical response.
>
> An individual's absolute glomerular filtration rate can be calculated from the eGFR as follows:
>
> $GFR_{Absolute}$ = eGFR × (individual's body surface area/1.73)

Previously in the BNF, renal impairment was arbitrarily divided into 3 grades (mild, moderate, and severe). This grading system has been removed and where possible values for creatinine clearance or another measure of renal function are included. However, where such values are not available, the BNF reflects the terms used in the published information.

> **Dialysis**
>
> For prescribing in patients on continuous ambulatory peritoneal dialysis (CAPD) or haemodialysis, consult specialist literature.

The following table can be used as a guide to drugs which require a reduction in dose in renal impairment, and to those which are potentially harmful or are ineffective. Drug prescribing should be kept to the minimum in all patients with severe renal disease.

If even mild renal impairment is considered likely on clinical grounds, renal function should be checked before prescribing **any** drug which requires dose modification.

For adjusting drug doses in renal impairment, see Important on p. 772.

Table of drugs to be avoided or used with caution in renal impairment

The list of drugs given below may not be comprehensive and is based on current information concerning the use of prescribed drugs in therapeutic dosage.

Products introduced or amended since publication of BNF No. 54 (September 2007) are underlined.

Drug	Comment
Abacavir	Manufacturer advises avoid in end-stage renal disease
Abciximab	Use with caution in severe renal impairment—increased risk of bleeding
Acamprosate	Avoid if serum-creatinine greater than 120 micromol/litre
Acarbose	Manufacturer advises avoid if creatinine clearance less than 25 mL/minute
ACE inhibitors	Use with caution and monitor response (*see also* p. 100); hyperkalaemia and other side-effects more common; *see also* individual drugs
Acebutolol	Halve dose if creatinine clearance 25–50 mL/minute; use quarter dose if creatinine clearance less than 25 mL/minute; do not administer more than once daily
Aceclofenac	*see* NSAIDs; avoid if creatinine clearance less than 20 mL/minute
Acemetacin	*see* NSAIDs
Acenocoumarol (nicoumalone)	*see* Anticoagulants, Oral
Acetazolamide	Avoid; metabolic acidosis
Aciclovir	Use normal intravenous dose every 12 hours if creatinine clearance 25–50 mL/minute (every 24 hours if creatinine clearance 10–25 mL/minute); consult product literature for intravenous dose if creatinine clearance less than 10 mL/minute; for herpes zoster, use normal oral dose every 8 hours if creatinine clearance 10–25 mL/minute (every 12 hours if creatinine clearance less than 10 mL/minute); for herpes simplex, use normal oral dose every 12 hours if creatinine clearance less than 10 mL/minute
Acipimox	Reduce dose if creatinine clearance 30–60 mL/minute; avoid if creatinine clearance less than 30 mL/minute
Acitretin	Avoid; increased risk of toxicity
Adefovir dipivoxil	10 mg every 48 hours if creatinine clearance 30–50 mL/minute; 10 mg every 72 hours if creatinine clearance 10–30 mL/minute; no information available if creatinine clearance less than 10 mL/minute
Alendronic acid	Manufacturer advises avoid if glomerular filtration rate less than 35 mL/minute
Alfentanil	*see* Opioid Analgesics
Alfuzosin	Start at 2.5 mg twice daily and adjust according to response
Alimemazine (trimeprazine)	Avoid
Aliskiren	Manufacturer advises caution if estimated glomerular filtration rate less than 30mL/minute—no information available
Allopurinol	Max. 100 mg daily, increased only if response inadequate; if creatinine clearance less than 10 mL/minute, reduce daily dose below 100 mg, or increase dose interval; if facilities available, adjust dose to maintain plasma-oxipurinol concentration below 100 micromol/litre
Almotriptan	Max. 12.5 mg in 24 hours if creatinine clearance less than 30 mL/minute
Alprazolam	*see* Anxiolytics and Hypnotics
Aluminium salts	Risk of accumulation and aluminium toxicity **Note** Absorption of aluminium from aluminium salts is increased by citrates, which are contained in many effervescent preparations (such as effervescent analgesics)
Amantadine	Reduce dose; avoid if creatinine clearance less than 15 mL/minute
Amfebutamone	*see* Bupropion
Amikacin	*see* Aminoglycosides
Amiloride	*see* Potassium-sparing Diuretics
Aminoglycosides	Reduce dose; monitor serum concentrations; *see also* Neomycin and section 5.1.4
Amisulpride	Halve dose if creatinine clearance 30–60 mL/minute; use one-third dose if creatinine clearance 10–30 mL/minute; manufacturers advise intermittent treatment with a reduced dose if creatinine clearance less than 10 mL/minute
Amoxicillin	Reduce dose; risk of crystalluria with high doses (particularly during parenteral therapy); by mouth, max. 500 mg every 12 hours if creatinine clearance 10–30 mL/minute, max. 500 mg daily if creatinine clearance less than 10 mL/minute

Drug	Comment
Amphotericin	Use only if no alternative; nephrotoxicity may be reduced with use of lipid formulations
Ampicillin	Reduce dose if creatinine clearance less than 10 mL/minute; rashes more common
Amprenavir	Use oral solution with caution in renal impairment due to high propylene glycol content; avoid oral solution in renal failure
Amsacrine	Reduce dose
Anagrelide	Manufacturer advises avoid if creatinine clearance less than 50 mL/minute but usual doses have been used
Anakinra	Manufacturer advises caution if creatinine clearance 30–50 mL/minute; avoid if creatinine clearance less than 30 mL/minute
Analgesics	*see* Opioid Analgesics and NSAIDs
Anastrozole	Avoid if creatinine clearance less than 20 mL/minute
Angeliq®	Manufacturer advises avoid if creatinine clearance less than 30 mL/minute
Anticoagulants, oral	Avoid if creatinine clearance less than 10 mL/minute
Antipsychotics	Start with small doses in severe impairment; increased cerebral sensitivity; *see also* Amisulpride, Clozapine, Flupentixol, Fluphenazine, Haloperidol, Olanzapine, Paliperidone, Pericyazine, Quetiapine, Risperidone, Sulpiride, and Zotepine
Anxiolytics and hypnotics	Start with small doses in severe impairment; increased cerebral sensitivity; *see also* Buspirone, Chloral Hydrate, and Sodium Oxybate
Arsenic trioxide	Manufacturer advises caution
Artemether [ingredient]	*see Riamet*®
Aspirin	Avoid if creatinine clearance less than 10 mL/minute; sodium and water retention; deterioration in renal function; increased risk of gastro-intestinal bleeding
Atenolol	Max. 50 mg daily (10 mg on alternate days *intravenously*) if creatinine clearance 15–35 mL/minute; max. 25 mg daily or 50 mg on alternate days (10 mg every 4 days *intravenously*) if creatinine clearance less than 15 mL/minute
Atosiban	No information available
Atovaquone	Manufacturer advises caution—monitor more closely
Auranofin	*see* Sodium Aurothiomalate
Azapropazone	Reduce dose (max. 600 mg daily) in rheumatoid arthritis and ankylosing spondylitis; avoid in severe impairment (avoid in gout if creatinine clearance less than 60 mL/minute)
Azathioprine	Reduce dose and monitor full blood count
Aztreonam	If creatinine clearance 10–30 mL/minute, usual initial dose, then half normal dose; if creatinine clearance less than 10 mL/minute usual initial dose, then one-quarter normal dose

For adjusting drug doses in renal impairment, see Important on p. 772.

Drug	Comment
Baclofen	Use smaller doses (e.g. 5 mg daily by mouth); excreted by kidney
Balsalazide	Avoid if creatinine clearance less than 20 mL/minute
Bambuterol	Reduce initial dose by half if creatinine clearance less than 50 mL/minute
Barbiturates	Reduce dose if creatinine clearance less than 10 mL/minute; *see also* Phenobarbital
Bemiparin	*see* Heparin
Bendrofluazide	*see* Thiazides and Related Diuretics
Bendroflumethiazide (bendrofluazide)	*see* Thiazides and Related Diuretics
Benperidol	*see* Antipsychotics
Benzodiazepines	Use with caution; reduce dose
Benzylpenicillin	Reduce dose—consult product literature; high doses may cause cerebral irritation, convulsions, or coma
Beta-blockers	*see under* individual drugs
Bezafibrate	Reduce dose to 400 mg daily if creatinine clearance 40–60 mL/minute; reduce dose to 200 mg every 1–2 days if creatinine clearance 15–40 mL/minute; avoid if creatinine clearance less than 15 mL/minute; avoid modified-release preparations in renal impairment
Bisoprolol	Reduce dose if creatinine clearance less than 20 mL/minute (max. 10 mg daily)
Bivalirudin	Reduce dose of infusion to 1.4 mg/kg/hour if creatinine clearance 30–60 mL/minute; avoid if creatinine clearance less than 30 mL/minute
Bleomycin	Reduce dose by half if serum-creatinine 177–354 micromol/litre; reduce dose further if serum-creatinine greater than 354 micromol/litre
Bortezomib	Manufacturer advises caution—consider dose reduction
Bupivacaine	Manufacturer advises caution
Buprenorphine	*see* Opioid Analgesics

Drug	Comment
Bupropion	Manufacturer recommends 150 mg daily
Buspirone	Reduce dose; avoid if creatinine clearance less than 20 mL/minute
Calcitriol	Manufacturer of topical calcitriol advises avoid—no information available
Candesartan	Initially 4 mg daily
Capecitabine	Reduce starting dose of 1250 mg/m² to 75% if creatinine clearance 30–50 mL/minute; avoid if creatinine clearance less than 30 mL/minute
Capreomycin	Reduce dose—consult product literature; nephrotoxic; ototoxic
Captopril	*see* ACE inhibitors; reduce dose; max. initial dose 25 mg daily (do not exceed 100 mg daily) if creatinine clearance 20–40 mL/minute; max. initial dose 12.5 mg daily (do not exceed 70 mg daily) if creatinine clearance 10–20 mL/minute; max. initial dose 6.25 mg daily (do not exceed 37.5 mg daily) if creatinine clearance less than 10 mL/minute
Carbamazepine	Manufacturer advises caution
Carboplatin	Reduce dose and monitor haematological parameters and renal function; avoid if creatinine clearance less than 20 mL/minute
Cefaclor	No dose adjustment required—manufacturer advises caution
Cefadroxil	Reduce dose if creatinine clearance less than 50 mL/minute—consult product literature
Cefalexin	Max. 3 g daily if creatinine clearance 40–50 mL/minute; max. 1.5 g daily if creatinine clearance 10–40 mL/minute; max. 750 mg daily if creatinine clearance less than 10 mL/minute
Cefixime	Reduce dose if creatinine clearance less than 20 mL/minute (max. 200 mg once daily)
Cefotaxime	If creatinine clearance less than 5 mL/minute, initial dose of 1 g then use half normal dose
Cefpodoxime	Reduce dose if creatinine clearance less than 40 mL/minute—consult product literature
Cefradine	Use half normal dose if creatinine clearance 5–20 mL/minute; use one-quarter normal dose if creatinine clearance less than 5 mL/minute
Ceftazidime	Reduce dose if creatinine clearance less than 50 mL/minute—consult product literature
Ceftriaxone	Reduce dose if creatinine clearance less than 10 mL/minute (max. 2 g daily); monitor plasma concentration if both hepatic and severe renal impairment
Cefuroxime	Use parenteral dose of 750 mg twice daily if creatinine clearance 10–20 mL/minute; use parenteral dose of 750 mg once daily if creatinine clearance less than 10 mL/minute
Celecoxib	*see* NSAIDs; avoid if creatinine clearance less than 30 mL/minute
Celiprolol	Reduce dose by half if creatinine clearance 15–40 mL/minute; avoid if creatinine clearance less than 15 mL/minute
Cetirizine	Use half normal dose if creatinine clearance less than 30 mL/minute
Cetrorelix	Manufacturer advises avoid in moderate or severe renal impairment
Chloral hydrate	Avoid if creatinine clearance less than 10 mL/minute
Chloramphenicol	Avoid unless no alternative; reduce dose; also monitor serum concentration—dose-related depression of haematopoiesis
Chlordiazepoxide	*see* Anxiolytics and Hypnotics
Chloroquine	Manufacturer advises caution; reduce dose (but for malaria prophylaxis *see* p. 346)
Chlorpromazine	*see* Antipsychotics
Chlorpropamide	Avoid
Chlortalidone	*see* Thiazides and Related Diuretics
Ciclosporin	*see* p. 475 (*see also* p. 616 if used in atopic dermatitis or psoriasis and p. 549 if used in rheumatoid arthritis)
Cidofovir	Avoid if creatinine clearance less than 55 mL/minute; nephrotoxic
Cilastatin [ingredient]	*see Primaxin®*
Cilazapril	*see* ACE inhibitors; reduce dose; max. initial dose 500 micrograms once daily (do not exceed 2.5 mg once daily) if creatinine clearance 10–40 mL/minute; avoid if creatinine clearance less than 10 mL/minute
Cilostazol	Avoid if creatinine clearance less than 25 mL/minute

Drug	Comment
Cimetidine	Reduce dose; 200 mg 4 times daily if creatinine clearance 30–50 mL/minute; 200 mg 3 times daily if creatinine clearance 15–30 mL/minute; 200 mg twice daily if creatinine clearance less than 15 mL/minute; occasional risk of confusion
Ciprofibrate	100 mg on alternate days if creatinine clearance 10–20 mL/minute; avoid if creatinine clearance less than 10 mL/minute
Ciprofloxacin	Use half normal dose if creatinine clearance less than 20 mL/minute
Cisplatin	Avoid if possible; nephrotoxic
Citalopram	No information available for creatinine clearance less than 20 mL/minute
CitraFleet®	Manufacturer advises avoid in severe renal impairment—risk of hypermagnesaemia
Citramag®	Caution—risk of hypermagnesaemia; avoid if creatinine clearance less than 10 mL/minute
Citrates	Absorption of aluminium from aluminium salts is increased by citrates, which are contained in many effervescent preparations (such as effervescent analgesics)
Cladribine	Regular monitoring recommended
Clarithromycin	Use half normal dose if creatinine clearance less than 30 mL/minute; avoid *Klaricid XL®* if creatinine clearance less than 30 mL/minute
Clavulanic acid [ingredient]	*see* Co-amoxiclav and *Timentin®*
Clobazam	*see* Anxiolytics and Hypnotics
Clodronate sodium	*see* Sodium Clodronate
Clofarabine	Manufacturer advises caution in mild to moderate renal impairment; avoid in severe renal impairment
Clomethiazole	*see* Anxiolytics and Hypnotics
Clopamide	*see* Thiazides and Related Diuretics
Clopidogrel	Manufacturer advises caution
Clozapine	Avoid if creatinine clearance less than 10 mL/minute
Co-amoxiclav	Risk of crystalluria with high doses (particularly during parenteral therapy); reduce dose if creatinine clearance less than 30 mL/minute
Codeine	*see* Opioid Analgesics
Colchicine	Reduce dose by up to 50% if creatinine clearance less than 50 mL/minute; avoid if creatinine clearance less than 10 mL/minute
Colistin	Reduce dose and monitor plasma-colistin concentration during parenteral or nebulised treatment—consult product literature
Co-trimoxazole	Use half normal dose if creatinine clearance 15–30 mL/minute; avoid if creatinine clearance less than 15 mL/minute and if plasma-sulfamethoxazole concentration cannot be monitored
Cyclopenthiazide	*see* Thiazides and Related Diuretics
Cyclophosphamide	Reduce dose

For adjusting drug doses in renal impairment, see Important on p. 772.

Drug	Comment
Cycloserine	Reduce dose (see also p. 312); avoid if creatinine clearance less than 10 mL/minute
Cyclosporin	*see* Ciclosporin
Dacarbazine	Dose reduction may be required in combined renal and hepatic impairment; avoid if creatinine clearance less than 10 mL/minute
Dalteparin	*see* Heparin
Danaparoid	Caution if creatinine clearance 10–20 mL/minute; increased risk of bleeding (monitor anti-Factor Xa activity); avoid if creatinine clearance less than 10 ml/minute unless patient has heparin-induced thrombocytopenia and no alternative
Daptomycin	Monitor renal function if creatinine clearance less than 80 mL/minute; for complicated skin and soft-tissue infections without bacteraemia use 4 mg/kg every 48 hours if creatinine clearance less than 30 mL/minute; for other indications, consult product literature if creatinine clearance less than 50 mL/minute
Daunorubicin	Reduce dose by 25% if serum creatinine 105–265 micromol/litre and by 50% if serum creatinine greater than 265 micromol/litre
Deferasirox	Reduce dose by 10 mg/kg if creatinine clearance 60–90 mL/minute and if serum creatinine increased by more than 33% of baseline measurement on 2 consecutive occasions—interrupt treatment if deterioration in renal function persists after dose reduction; avoid if creatinine clearance less than 60 mL/minute
Deferiprone	Manufacturer advises caution—no information available
Demeclocycline	Avoid
Desflurane	Reduce dose if creatinine clearance less than 20 mL/minute

Drug	Comment
Desloratadine	Manufacturer advises caution in severe renal insufficiency
Desmopressin	Antidiuretic effect may be reduced
Dexibuprofen	*see* NSAIDs; reduce initial dose; avoid if glomerular filtration rate less than 30 mL/minute
Dexketoprofen	*see* NSAIDs; reduce initial dose to 50 mg daily if creatinine clearance 20–50 mL/minute; avoid if creatinine clearance less than 20 mL/minute
Dexrazoxane	Manufacturer of *Cardioxane*® advises reduce dose by 50% if creatinine clearance less than 40 mL/minute
Dextromethorphan	*see* Opioid Analgesics
Diamorphine	*see* Opioid Analgesics
Diazepam	*see* Anxiolytics and Hypnotics
Diazoxide	Increased sensitivity to hypotensive and hyperglycaemic effect; dose reduction may be required
Diclofenac	*see* NSAIDs; avoid if creatinine clearance less than 10 mL/minute
Didanosine	Reduce dose if creatinine clearance less than 60 mL/minute; consult product literature
Digoxin	Reduce dose; toxicity increased by electrolyte disturbances
Dihydrocodeine	*see* Opioid Analgesics
Diltiazem	Start with smaller dose
Diphenoxylate	*see* Opioid Analgesics
Dipipanone	*see* Opioid Analgesics
Disodium etidronate	Reduce dose if creatinine clearance 20–50 mL/minute; avoid if creatinine clearance less than 20 mL/minute
Disodium pamidronate	Max. infusion rate 20 mg/hour; except in life-threatening hypercalcaemia, manufacturer advises avoid if creatinine clearance less than 30 mL/minute; if renal function deteriorates in patients with bone metastases, withhold dose until serum creatinine returns to within 10% of baseline value
Disopyramide	Reduce dose by increasing dose interval; adjust according to response; avoid sustained release preparation
Diuretics, potassium-sparing	*see* Potassium-sparing Diuretics
Domperidone	Manufacturer advises reduce dose
Dorzolamide	Manufacturer advises avoid if creatinine clearance less than 30 mL/minute
Doxycycline	Use with caution (avoid excessive doses)
Drospirenone [ingredient]	*see Angeliq*® and *Yasmin*®
Duloxetine	Avoid if creatinine clearance less than 30 mL/minute
Efavirenz	Manufacturer advises caution in severe renal failure—no information available
Eletriptan	Reduce initial dose to 20 mg; max. 40 mg in 24 hours; avoid if creatinine clearance less than 30 mL/minute
Emtricitabine	Reduce dose if creatinine clearance less than 50 mL/minute; consult product literature; *see also Truvada*®
Enalapril	*see* ACE inhibitors; max. initial dose 2.5 mg daily if creatinine clearance less than 30 mL/minute
Enoxaparin	Consider switching to heparin if creatinine clearance less than 30 mL/minute; alternatively adjust dose according to plasma concentration of anti-factor Xa
Enoximone	Consider dose reduction
Entecavir	Reduce dose if creatinine clearance less than 50 mL/minute; consult product literature
Ephedrine	Use with caution
Eplerenone	Increased risk of hyperkalaemia—close monitoring required; avoid if creatinine clearance less than 50 mL/minute
Eprosartan	Halve initial dose if creatinine clearance less than 60 mL/minute
Eptifibatide	Reduce infusion to 1 microgram/kg/minute if creatinine clearance 30–50 mL/minute; avoid if creatinine clearance less than 30 mL/minute
Erdosteine	Manufacturer advises avoid if creatinine clearance less than 25 mL/minute—no information available
Ergometrine	Manufacturer advises caution in mild or moderate renal impairment and avoid in severe renal impairment
Ergotamine	Avoid; risk of renal vasoconstriction
Erlotinib	Manufacturer advises avoid if creatinine clearance less than 15 mL/minute—no information available
Ertapenem	Risk of seizures; max. 500 mg daily if creatinine clearance less than 30 mL/minute
Erythromycin	Max. 1.5 g daily in severe renal impairment (ototoxicity)
Escitalopram	Manufacturer advises caution if creatinine clearance less than 30 mL/minute
Esmolol	Manufacturer advises caution
Esomeprazole	Manufacturer advises caution in severe renal insufficiency
Estramustine	Manufacturer advises caution

Drug	Comment
Ethambutol	Reduce dose; if creatinine clearance less than 30 mL/minute monitor plasma-ethambutol concentration; optic nerve damage
Etidronate disodium	*see* Disodium Etidronate
Etodolac	*see* NSAIDs
Etoposide	Consider dose reduction
Etoricoxib	Avoid if creatinine clearance less than 30 mL/minute; *see also* NSAIDs
Exemestane	Manufacturer advises caution

For adjusting drug doses in renal impairment, see Important on p. 772.

Drug	Comment
Exenatide	Manufacturer advises caution if creatinine clearance 30–50 mL/minute; avoid if creatinine clearance less than 30 mL/minute
Famciclovir	Reduce dose; consult product literature
Famotidine	Reduce dose to 20 mg at night if creatinine clearance less than 10 mL/minute
Fenbufen	*see* NSAIDs
Fenofibrate	Reduce dose to 134 mg daily if creatinine less than 60 mL/minute; reduce dose to 67 mg daily if creatinine clearance less than 20 mL/minute; avoid if creatinine clearance less than 10 mL/minute
Fenoprofen	*see* NSAIDs
Fentanyl	*see* Opioid Analgesics
Flecainide	Reduce initial oral dose to max. 100 mg daily or reduce intravenous dose by 50% if creatinine clearance less than 35 mL/minute
Fleet Phospho-soda®	Manufacturer advises caution; avoid in renal failure
Flucloxacillin	Reduce dose if creatinine clearance less than 10 mL/minute
Fluconazole	Usual initial dose then halve subsequent doses if creatinine clearance less than 50 mL/minute
Flucytosine	Reduce dose and monitor plasma-flucytosine concentration—consult product literature
Fludarabine	Reduce dose by up to 50% if creatinine clearance 30–70 mL/minute; avoid if creatinine clearance less than 30 mL/minute
Flupentixol	*see* Antipsychotics; manufacturer advises caution; avoid in renal failure
Fluphenazine	*see* Antipsychotics; manufacturer advises caution; avoid in renal failure
Flurazepam	*see* Anxiolytics and Hypnotics
Flurbiprofen	*see* NSAIDs
Fluvoxamine	Start with smaller dose
Fondaparinux	Increased risk of bleeding; for treatment of acute coronary syndromes avoid if creatinine clearance less than 20 mL/minute; for treatment of venous thromboembolism use with caution if creatinine clearance 30–50 mL/minute, avoid if creatinine clearance less than 30 mL/minute; for prophylaxis of venous thromboembolism reduce dose to 1.5 mg daily if creatinine clearance 20–50 mL/minute, avoid if less than 20 mL/minute
Foscarnet	Reduce dose; consult product literature
Fosinopril	*see* ACE inhibitors
Fosphenytoin	Consider 10–25% reduction in dose or infusion rate (except initial dose for status epilepticus)
Frusemide	*see* Furosemide
Furosemide (frusemide)	May need high doses; deafness may follow rapid i/v injection
Fybogel Mebeverine®	Contains 2.5 mmol potassium per sachet
Gabapentin	Reduce dose if creatinine clearance less than 80 mL/minute; consult product literature
Galantamine	Avoid if creatinine clearance less than 9 mL/minute
Ganciclovir	Reduce dose if creatinine clearance less than 70 mL/minute; consult product literature
Ganirelix	Avoid if creatinine clearance less than 20 mL/minute
Gemcitabine	Manufacturer advises caution
Gemeprost	Manufacturer advises avoid
Gemfibrozil	Initially 900 mg daily if creatinine clearance 30–80 mL/minute; avoid if creatinine clearance less than 30 mL/minute
Gentamicin	*see* Aminoglycosides
Gestrinone	Avoid if creatinine clearance less than 10 mL/minute
Glatiramer	No information available—manufacturer advises caution
Glibenclamide	Avoid if creatinine clearance less than 10 mL/minute
Gliclazide	Reduce initial dose and monitor closely; avoid if creatinine clearance less than 10 mL/minute
Glimepiride	Avoid if creatinine clearance less than 10 mL/minute
Glipizide	Increased risk of hypoglycaemia; avoid if creatinine clearance less than 10 mL/minute or if hepatic impairment also present
Glyceryl trinitrate	*see* Nitrates

Drug	Comment
Guanethidine	Reduce dose if creatinine clearance less than 65 mL/minute, avoid if creatinine clearance less than 40 mL/minute
Haloperidol	*see* Antipsychotics; manufacturer advises caution in renal impairment
Heparin	Risk of bleeding increased if creatinine clearance less than 10 mL/minute—dose may need to be reduced
Hetastarch	Avoid if creatinine clearance less than 10 mL/minute; excreted by kidney
Hydralazine	Reduce dose if creatinine clearance less than 30 mL/minute
Hydrochlorothiazide	*see* Thiazides and Related Diuretics
Hydroflumethiazide	*see* Thiazides and Related Diuretics
Hydromorphone	*see* Opioid Analgesics
Hydroxychloroquine	Manufacturer advises caution and monitoring of plasma-hydroxychloroquine concentration in severe renal impairment
Hydroxyzine	Use half normal dose
Hyoscine hydrobromide	Manufacturer advises caution
Hypnotics	*see* Anxiolytics and Hypnotics
Ibandronic acid	For repeated doses, if creatinine clearance less than 30 mL/minute, reduce intravenous dose to 2 mg every 3–4 weeks and in bone metastasis, change oral dose to 50 mg once weekly
Ibuprofen	*see* NSAIDs
Idarubicin	Reduce dose; avoid if creatinine clearance less than 10 mL/minute
Ifosfamide	Avoid if serum creatinine concentration greater than 120 micromol/litre
Imatinib	Max. starting dose 400 mg daily if creatinine clearance less than 60 mL/minute
Imidapril	*see* ACE inhibitors; max. initial dose 2.5 mg daily if creatinine clearance 30–80 mL/minute; avoid if creatinine clearance less than 30 mL/minute
Imipenem [ingredient]	*see Primaxin®*
Indapamide	*see* Thiazides and Related Diuretics
Indometacin	*see* NSAIDs; avoid if creatinine clearance less than 10 mL/minute
Indoramin	Manufacturer advises caution
Inosine pranobex	Manufacturer advises caution; metabolised to uric acid
Insulin	May need dose reduction; insulin requirements fall; compensatory response to hypoglycaemia is impaired
Interferon alfa	Close monitoring required; avoid if creatinine clearance less than 10 mL/minute
Interferon beta	Manufacturers advise caution and close monitoring in severe renal impairment
Interferon gamma-1b	Manufacturer advises caution if creatinine clearance less than 10 mL/minute
Irinotecan	Manufacturer advises avoid—no information available
Iron dextran	Avoid in acute renal failure
Isometheptene [ingredient]	*see Midrid®*
Isoniazid	Max. 200 mg daily if creatinine clearance less than 10 mL/minute; peripheral neuropathy
Isosorbide dinitrate	*see* Nitrates
Isosorbide mononitrate	*see* Nitrates
Isotretinoin	Reduce initial dose (e.g. 10 mg daily) and increase gradually up to 1 mg/kg daily as tolerated
Itraconazole	Risk of congestive heart failure; bioavailability of oral formulations possibly reduced; use intravenous infusion with caution if creatinine clearance 30–50 mL/minute (monitor renal function); avoid intravenous infusion if creatinine clearance less than 30 mL/minute
Ivabradine	Manufacturer advises caution if creatinine clearance less than 15 mL/minute
Kaletra®	Avoid oral solution due to propylene glycol content; use capsules and tablets with caution if creatinine clearance less than 10 mL/minute
Ketoprofen	*see* NSAIDs; avoid if creatinine clearance less than 10 mL/minute
Ketorolac	*see* NSAIDs; use lowest effective dose (max. 60 mg daily when given by intramuscular or intravenous injection); avoid if serum creatinine more than 160 micromol/litre
Labetalol	Dose reduction may be required
Lamivudine	Reduce dose if creatinine clearance less than 50 mL/minute; consult product literature
Lamotrigine	Manufacturer advises caution in renal failure; metabolite may accumulate
Leflunomide	Manufacturer advises avoid in moderate or severe impairment—no information available
Lenalidomide	Starting dose 10 mg once daily if creatinine clearance 30–50 mL/minute; starting dose 15 mg on alternate days if creatinine clearance less than 30 mL/minute

Drug	Comment
Lepirudin	Reduce initial intravenous injection dose to 200 micrograms/kg and reduce subsequent infusion dose by 50–85% if creatinine clearance less than 60 mL/minute; but avoid or stop infusion if creatinine clearance less than 15 mL/minute (consult product literature)
Lercanidipine	Avoid if creatinine clearance less than 30 mL/minute
Letrozole	Manufacturer advises caution if creatinine clearance less than 10 mL/minute
Levetiracetam	Max. 2 g daily if creatinine clearance 50–80 mL/minute; max. 1.5 g daily if creatinine clearance 30–50 mL/minute; max. 1 g daily if creatinine clearance less than 30 mL/minute
Levocetirizine	5 mg on alternate days if creatinine clearance 30–50 mL/minute; 5 mg every 3 days if creatinine clearance 10–30 mL/minute; avoid if creatinine clearance less than 10 mL/minute
Levofloxacin	Usual initial dose then reduce subsequent doses (consult product literature) if creatinine clearance less than 50 mL/minute
Levomepromazine (methotrimeprazine)	*see* Antipsychotics
Lidocaine	Caution if creatinine clearance less than 10 mL./minute
Linezolid	Manufacturer advises metabolites may accumulate if creatinine clearance less than 30 mL/minute
Lisinopril	see ACE inhibitors; max. initial doses 5–10 mg daily if creatinine clearance 30–80 mL/minute (max. 40 mg daily); 2.5–5 mg daily if creatinine clearance 10–30 mL/minute (max. 40 mg daily); 2.5 mg daily if creatinine clearance less than 10 mL/minute
Lithium salts	Avoid if possible or reduce dose and monitor plasma concentration carefully
Lofepramine	Manufacturer advises avoid in severe impairment
Lofexidine	Manufacturer advises caution in chronic renal impairment
Lopinavir [ingredient]	*see Kaletra®*
Loprazolam	*see* Anxiolytics and Hypnotics
Lorazepam	*see* Anxiolytics and Hypnotics
Lormetazepam	*see* Anxiolytics and Hypnotics
Losartan	Start with 25 mg once daily if creatinine clearance less than 20 mL/minute
Lumefantrine [ingredient]	*see Riamet®*
Lymecycline	Avoid
Magnesium salts	Avoid or reduce dose; increased risk of toxicity; magnesium carbonate mixture and magnesium trisilicate mixture also have high sodium content
Malarone®	Avoid for malaria prophylaxis (and if possible for malaria treatment) if creatinine clearance less than 30 mL/minute
Maraviroc	If creatinine clearance less than 80 mL/minute, consult product literature
Mefenamic acid	*see* NSAIDs; avoid if creatinine clearance less than 10 mL/minute
Meloxicam	*see* NSAIDs; avoid if creatinine clearance less than 25 mL/minute
Melphalan	Reduce dose initially (consult product literature)
Memantine	Reduce dose to 10 mg daily if creatinine clearance 30–49 mL/minute, if well tolerated after at least 7 days dose can be increased in steps to 20 mg daily; reduce dose to 10 mg daily if creatinine clearance 5–29 mL/minute; manufacturer advises avoid if creatinine clearance less than 5 mL/minute
Meprobamate	*see* Anxiolytics and Hypnotics
Meptazinol	*see* Opioid Analgesics
Mercaptopurine	Reduce dose
Meropenem	Increase dose interval to every 12 hours if creatinine clearance 26–50 mL/minute; use half normal dose every 12 hours if creatinine clearance 10–25 mL/minute; use half normal dose every 24 hours if creatinine clearance less than 10 mL/minute
Mesalazine	Use with caution; avoid if creatinine clearance less than 20 mL/minute
Metformin	Avoid if creatinine clearance less than 60 mL/minute; increased risk of lactic acidosis
Methadone	*see* Opioid Analgesics
Methenamine	Avoid if creatinine clearance less than 10 mL/minute—risk of hippurate crystalluria
Methocarbamol	Manufacturer advises caution
Methotrexate	Reduce dose; nephrotoxic and accumulates; avoid if creatinine clearance less than 20 mL/minute
Methotrimeprazine	*see* Antipsychotics
Methyldopa	Start with small dose; increased sensitivity to hypotensive and sedative effect
Methysergide	Avoid
Metoclopramide	Avoid or use small dose if creatinine clearance less than 10 mL/minute; increased risk of extrapyramidal reactions
Metolazone	*see* Thiazides and Related Diuretics

Drug	Comment
Mexiletine	May need dose reduction if creatinine clearance less than 10 mL/minute
Midazolam	*see* Anxiolytics and Hypnotics
Midrid®	Avoid if creatinine clearance less than 10 mL/minute
Miglustat	Initially 100 mg twice daily if creatinine clearance 50–70 mL/minute; initially 100 mg once daily if creatinine clearance 30–50 mL/minute; avoid if creatinine clearance less than 30 mL/minute
Milrinone	Reduce dose and monitor response if creatinine clearance less than 50 mL/minute—consult product literature for details
Minocycline	Use with caution (avoid excessive doses)
Mirtazapine	Manufacturer advises caution
Mitotane	Manufacturer advises caution if creatinine clearance 30–80 mL/minute—monitoring of plasma-mitotane concentration recommended; avoid if creatinine clearance less than 30 mL/minute
Mivacurium	Clinical effect prolonged in end-stage renal failure—reduce dose according to response
Modafinil	Use half normal dose if creatinine clearance less than 10 mL/minute
Moexipril	*see* ACE inhibitors; initial dose 3.75 mg once daily if creatinine clearance less than 40 mL/minute
Morphine	*see* Opioid Analgesics
Moxonidine	Max. single dose 200 micrograms and max. daily dose 400 micrograms if creatinine clearance 30–60 mL/minute; avoid if creatinine clearance less than 30 mL/minute

For adjusting drug doses in renal impairment, see Important on p. 772.

Drug	Comment
Nabumetone	*see* NSAIDs; avoid if creatinine clearance less than 30 mL/minute
Nadolol	Increase dosage interval if creatinine clearance less than 50 mL/minute
Nalidixic acid	Use with caution; avoid if creatinine clearance less than 20 mL/minute
Naltrexone	Manufacturers advise caution
Naproxen	*see* NSAIDs; avoid if creatinine clearance less than 20 mL/minute
Naratriptan	Max. 2.5 mg in 24 hours; avoid if creatinine clearance less than 15 mL/minute
Narcotic analgesics	*see* Opioid Analgesics
Nebivolol	For hypertension, initially 2.5 mg once daily, increased to 5 mg once daily if required; for heart failure, manufacturer advises avoid if serum creatinine greater than 250 micromol/litre
Nelfinavir	No information available—manufacturer advises caution
Neomycin	Avoid; ototoxic; nephrotoxic
Neostigmine	May need dose reduction
Nicardipine	Start with small dose
Nicotine	Manufacturers advise caution in severe renal impairment
Nicoumalone	*see* Acenocoumarol
Nimodipine	Manufacturer advises caution with intravenous administration
Nitrates	Use with caution if creatinine clearance less than 10 mL/minute
Nitrazepam	*see* Anxiolytics and Hypnotics
Nitrofurantoin	Avoid if creatinine clearance less than 60 mL/minute; ineffective because of inadequate urine concentrations
Nitroprusside	*see* Sodium Nitroprusside
Nizatidine	Use half normal dose if creatinine clearance 20–50 mL/minute; use one-quarter normal dose if creatinine clearance less than 20 mL/minute
Norfloxacin	Use half normal dose if creatinine clearance less than 30 mL/minute
NSAIDs	Use lowest effective dose and monitor renal function; sodium and water retention; deterioration in renal function possibly leading to renal failure; deterioration also reported after topical use; avoid if possible creatinine clearance less than 20 mL/minute; *see also* individual drugs
Ofloxacin	Usual initial dose, then use half normal dose if creatinine clearance 20–50 mL/minute; 100 mg every 24 hours if creatinine clearance less than 20 mL/minute
Olanzapine	Consider lower initial dose of 5 mg daily
Olmesartan	Max. 20 mg daily if creatinine clearance 20–60 mL/minute; avoid if creatinine clearance less than 20 mL/minute
Olsalazine	Use with caution; manufacturer advises avoid in significant renal impairment
Omalizumab	Manufacturer advises caution—no information available
Opioid analgesics	Reduce doses or avoid; increased and prolonged effect; increased cerebral sensitivity

Drug	Comment
Oseltamivir	Reduce dose if creatinine clearance 10–30 mL/minute; avoid if creatinine clearance less than 10 mL/minute
Oxaliplatin	Manufacturer advises avoid if creatinine clearance less than 30 mL/minute
Oxazepam	*see* Anxiolytics and Hypnotics
Oxcarbazepine	Use half initial dose if creatinine clearance less than 30 mL/minute; increase according to response at intervals of at least 1 week
Oxpentifylline	*see* Pentoxifylline
Oxybutynin	Manufacturer advises caution
Oxycodone	*see* Opioid Analgesics
Oxytetracycline	Avoid
Paliperidone	Initially 3 mg daily if creatinine clearance 30–80 mL/minute; initially 3 mg on alternate days if creatinine clearance 10–30 mL/minute; manufacturer advises avoid if creatinine clearance less than 10 mL/minute
Pamidronate disodium	*see* Disodium Pamidronate
Pancuronium	Manufacturer advises caution; prolonged duration of block
Pantoprazole	Max. oral dose 40 mg daily
Papaveretum	*see* Opioid Analgesics
Paracetamol	Increase *infusion* dose interval to every 6 hours if creatinine clearance less than 30 mL/minute
Parathyroid hormone	Avoid if creatinine clearance less than 30 mL/minute
Parecoxib	*see* NSAIDs; manufacturer advises caution
Paroxetine	Reduce dose if creatinine clearance less than 30 mL/minute
Peginterferon alfa	Close monitoring required—reduce dose if necessary
Penicillamine	Reduce dose and monitor renal function or avoid (consult product literature)
Pentamidine	Reduce dose for pneumocystis pneumonia if creatinine clearance less than 10 mL/minute—consult product literature
Pentazocine	*see* Opioid Analgesics
Pentoxifylline (oxpentifylline)	Reduce dose by 30–50% if creatinine clearance less than 30 mL/minute
Pericyazine	Manufacturer advises avoid
Perindopril	see ACE inhibitors; max. initial doses 2 mg once daily if creatinine clearance 30–60 mL/minute; 2 mg once daily on alternate days if creatinine clearance 15–30 mL/minute
Perphenazine	*see* Antipsychotics
Pethidine	*see* Opioid Analgesics
Phenindione	*see* Anticoagulants, Oral
Phenobarbital	Use with caution
Phenothiazines	*see* Antipsychotics
Pholcodine	*see* Opioid Analgesics
Picolax®	Manufacturer advises avoid in severe renal impairment—risk of hypermagnesaemia
Pilocarpine	Manufacturer advises caution with tablets
Pimozide	*see* Antipsychotics
Pindolol	May adversely affect renal function in severe impairment—manufacturer advises avoid
Piperacillin [ingredient]	*see Tazocin®*
Piperazine	Use with caution; avoid if creatinine clearance less than 10 mL/minute
Pipotiazine	*see* Antipsychotics
Piracetam	Use two-thirds of normal dose if creatinine clearance 50–80 mL/minute; use one-third of normal dose in 2 divided doses if creatinine clearance 30–50 mL/minute; use one-sixth normal dose as a single dose if creatinine clearance 20–30 mL/minute; avoid if creatinine clearance less than 20 mL/minute
Piroxicam	*see* NSAIDs
Potassium salts	Close monitoring required—high risk of hyperkalaemia; avoid if creatinine clearance less than 10 mL/minute
Potassium-sparing diuretics	Monitor plasma K^+; high risk of hyperkalaemia in renal impairment; avoid if creatinine clearance less than 20 mL/minute; *see also* Eplerenone
Povidone–iodine	Avoid regular application to inflamed or broken mucosa
Pramipexole	In Parkinson's disease, initially 88 micrograms twice daily if creatinine clearance 20–50 mL/minute (88 micrograms once daily if creatinine clearance less than 20 mL/minute); if renal function declines during treatment, reduce dose by the same percentage as the decline in creatinine clearance; in restless legs syndrome, reduce dose if creatinine clearance less than 20 mL/minute
Pravastatin	Start at lower end of dosage range if creatinine clearance less than 20 mL/minute
Prazosin	Initially 500 micrograms daily in moderate to severe renal impairment; increased with caution
Pregabalin	Initially 75 mg daily and max. 300 mg daily in 2–3 divided doses if creatinine clearance 30–60 mL/minute; initially 25–50 mg daily and max. 150 mg daily in 1–2 divided doses if creatinine clearance 15–30 mL/minute; initially 25 mg once daily and max. 75 mg once daily if creatinine clearance less than 15 mL/minute

Drug	Comment
Prilocaine	Manufacturer advises caution
Primaxin®	Reduce dose if creatinine clearance less than 70 mL/minute—consult product literature
Primidone	*see* Phenobarbital
Probenecid	Avoid if creatinine clearance less than 30 mL/minute
Procainamide	Avoid or reduce dose
Procarbazine	Use with caution; avoid if creatinine clearance less than 10 mL/minute
Prochlorperazine	*see* Antipsychotics
Proguanil	100 mg once daily if creatinine clearance 20–60 mL/minute; 50 mg on alternate days if creatinine clearance 10–20 mL/minute; 50 mg once weekly if creatinine clearance less than 10 mL/minute (increased risk of haematological toxicity)
Promazine	*see* Antipsychotics
Propantheline	Manufacturer advises caution
Propiverine	Doses above 30 mg daily should be used with caution if creatinine clearance less than 30 mL/minute
Propofol	Use with caution
Propranolol	Manufacturer advises caution—dose reduction may be required
Propylthiouracil	Use three-quarters normal dose if creatinine clearance 10–50 mL/minute; use half normal dose if creatinine clearance less than 10 mL/minute
Pseudoephedrine	Manufacturer advises caution in moderate to severe renal impairment
Pyridostigmine	Reduce dose; excreted by kidney
Pyrimethamine	Manufacturer advises caution
Quetiapine	Manufacturer advises initial dose of 25 mg daily, increased daily in steps of 25–50 mg
Quinagolide	Manufacturer advises avoid—no information available
Quinapril	*see* ACE inhibitors; max. initial dose 2.5 mg once daily if creatinine clearance less than 40 mL/minute
Quinine	For treatment of falciparum malaria, reduce parenteral maintenance dose to 5–7 mg/kg of salt

For adjusting drug doses in renal impairment, see Important on p. 772.

Drug	Comment
Raloxifene	Avoid if creatinine clearance less than 10 mL/minute
Raltitrexed	Reduce dose and increase dosing interval if creatinine clearance less than 65 mL/minute (consult product literature); avoid if creatinine clearance less than 25 mL/minute
Ramipril	*see* ACE inhibitors; max. initial dose 1.25 mg once daily (do not exceed 5 mg once daily) if creatinine clearance less than 30 mL/minute; max. initial dose 1.25 mg once daily (do not exceed 2.5 mg once daily) if creatinine clearance less than 10 mL/minute
Ranitidine	Use half normal dose; occasional risk of confusion
Reboxetine	Initial dose 2 mg twice daily, increased according to tolerance
Riamet®	Manufacturer advises caution in severe renal impairment—monitor ECG and plasma potassium concentration
Ribavirin	Plasma-ribavirin concentration increased; manufacturer advises avoid oral ribavirin unless essential if creatinine clearance less than 50 mL/minute—monitor haemoglobin concentration closely
Rifabutin	Use half normal dose if creatinine clearance less than 30 mL/minute
Riluzole	No information available—manufacturer advises avoid
Rimonabant	Manufacturer advises avoid in severe impairment—no information available
Risedronate sodium	Manufacturer advises avoid if creatinine clearance less than 30 mL/minute
Risperidone	Manufacturer advises initial oral dose of 500 micrograms twice daily increased in steps of 500 micrograms twice daily to 1–2 mg twice daily; if an oral dose of at least 2 mg daily tolerated, 25 mg as a depot injection can be given every 2 weeks
Ritonavir [ingredient]	*see Kaletra*®
Rivastigmine	Manufacturer advises caution
Rizatriptan	Reduce dose to 5 mg if creatinine clearance 10–60 mL/minute; avoid if creatinine clearance less than 10 mL/minute
Rocuronium	Reduce maintenance dose; prolonged paralysis
Ropinirole	Manufacturers advise avoid if creatinine clearance less than 30 mL/minute
Ropivacaine	Manufacturer advises caution in severe renal impairment
Rosiglitazone	Manufacturer advises caution, if creatinine clearance less than 30 mL/minute
Rosuvastatin	Initially 5 mg once daily and avoid dose of 40 mg daily if creatinine clearance less than 60 mL/minute; avoid if creatinine clearance less than 30 mL/minute

Drug	Comment
Saquinavir	Dose adjustment possibly required if creatinine clearance less than 10 mL/minute—no information available
Sertraline	Manufacturer advises caution
Sevoflurane	Manufacturer advises caution
Sibutramine	Manufacturer advises caution if creatinine clearance 30–80 mL/minute; avoid if creatinine clearance less than 30 mL/minute
Sildenafil	For erectile dysfunction initial dose 25 mg if creatinine clearance less than 30 mL/minute; for pulmonary hypertension reduce to 20 mg twice daily if usual dose not tolerated
Simvastatin	Doses above 10 mg daily should be used with caution if creatinine clearance less than 30 mL/minute
Sirolimus	Adjust immunosuppressant regimen in patients with raised serum creatinine
Sitagliptin	Manufacturer advises avoid if creatinine clearance less than 50 mL/minute
Sodium aurothiomalate	Caution; nephrotoxic
Sodium bicarbonate	Avoid; specialised role in some forms of renal disease
Sodium clodronate	Use half normal oral dose if creatinine clearance 10–30 mL/minute; use three quarters of normal injection dose if creatinine clearance 50–80 mL/minute, use half if creatinine clearance 10–50 mL/minute; avoid if creatinine clearance less than 10 mL/minute
Sodium nitroprusside	Metabolite may accumulate; avoid prolonged use
Sodium oxybate	Caution—*Xyrem*® oral solution contains 2.98 mmol Na^+/mL
Sodium valproate	*see* Valproate
Solifenacin	Max. 5 mg daily if creatinine clearance less than 30 mL/minute
Solpadol®	Avoid effervescent tablets; contains 16.9 mmol sodium per tablet; *see also* Opioid Analgesics
Sotalol	Use half normal dose if creatinine clearance 30–60 mL/minute; use one-quarter normal dose if creatinine clearance 10–30 mL/minute; avoid if creatinine clearance less than 10 mL/minute
Spironolactone	*see* Potassium-sparing Diuretics
Stavudine	Use half normal dose every 12 hours if creatinine clearance 25–50 mL/minute; use half normal dose every 24 hours if creatinine clearance less than 25 mL/minute
Streptomycin	*see* Aminoglycosides
Strontium ranelate	Manufacturer advises no dose adjustment required if creatinine clearance 30–70 mL/minute; avoid if creatinine clearance less than 30 mL/minute
Sucralfate	Use with caution; aluminium is absorbed and may accumulate
Sulfadiazine	Use with caution; avoid if creatinine clearance less than 10 mL/minute; high risk of crystalluria
Sulfasalazine	Risk of toxicity including crystalluria—ensure high fluid intake; avoid if creatinine clearance less than 15 mL/minute
Sulfinpyrazone	Reduce dose; avoid if creatinine clearance less than 10 mL/minute
Sulindac	*see* NSAIDs; reduce dose; avoid if creatinine clearance less than 10 mL/minute
Sulphonamides	Ensure high fluid intake; rashes and blood disorders; crystalluria a risk; *see* also individual drugs
Sulphonylureas	*see under* individual drugs
Sulpiride	Reduce dose; avoid if creatinine clearance less than 10 mL/minute
Sumatriptan	Manufacturer advises caution
Tacalcitol	Monitor serum calcium concentration
Tadalafil	Max. dose 10 mg if creatinine clearance less than 30 mL/minute
Tamsulosin	Manufacturer advises caution if creatinine clearance less than 10 mL/minute
Tazobactam [ingredient]	*see Tazocin*®
Tazocin®	Max. 4.5 g every 8 hours if creatinine clearance 20–80 mL/minute; max. 4.5 g every 12 hours if creatinine clearance less than 20 mL/minute; child under 12 years: Consult product literature
Teicoplanin	On day 4 use half normal dose if creatinine clearance is 40–60 mL/minute and use one-third normal dose if creatinine clearance is less than 40 mL/minute
Telbivudine	Use normal dose every 48 hours if creatinine clearance 30–49 mL/minute; use normal dose every 72 hours if creatinine clearance less than 30 mL/minute
Telithromycin	Manufacturer advises avoid if possible if creatinine clearance less than 30 mL/minute—if no alternative, use alternating daily doses of 800 mg and 400 mg, starting with 800 mg dose
Telmisartan	Initially 20 mg once daily if creatinine clearance less than 10 mL/minute

Drug	Comment
Temazepam	*see* Anxiolytics and Hypnotics
Temocillin	Use normal dose every 24 hours if creatinine clearance 10–30 mL/minute; use normal dose every 48 hours if creatinine clearance less than 10 mL/minute
Tenofovir	Monitor renal function — interrupt treatment if further deterioration; 245 mg every 2 days if creatinine clearance 30–50 mL/minute; 245 mg every 3–4 days if creatinine clearance 10–30 mL/minute; *see also Truvada®*
Tenoxicam	*see* NSAIDs
Terbinafine	Use half normal dose if creatinine clearance less than 50 mL/minute
Tetracyclines	Avoid tetracyclines except doxycycline or minocycline which may be used cautiously (avoid excessive doses)
Thiazides and related diuretics	Avoid if creatinine clearance less than 30 mL/minute—ineffective (metolazone remains effective but risk of excessive diuresis)
Tiaprofenic acid	*see* NSAIDs; reduce dose; avoid if creatinine clearance less than 10 mL/minute
Ticarcillin [ingredient]	*see Timentin®*
Tiludronic acid	Manufacturer advises caution if creatinine clearance 30–90 mL/minute; avoid if creatinine clearance less than 30 mL/minute
Timentin®	Reduce dose to 3.2 g every eight hours if creatinine clearance 30–60 mL/minute; 1.6 g every eight hours if creatinine clearance 10–30 mL/minute; 1.6 g every twelve hours if creatinine clearance less than 10 mL/minute
Timolol	Manufacturer advises caution—dose reduction may be required
Tinzaparin	May need dose reduction if creatinine clearance less than 10 mL/minute
Tioguanine	Reduce dose
Tiotropium	Plasma-tiotropium concentration raised; manufacturer advises caution if creatinine clearance less than 50 mL/minute
Tirofiban	Use half normal dose if creatinine clearance less than 30 mL/minute
Tizanidine	Initially 2 mg once daily if creatinine clearance less than 25 mL/minute; increase once-daily dose gradually according to response before increasing frequency
Tobramycin	*see* Aminoglycosides
Tolbutamide	Avoid if possible; if no alternative reduce dose and monitor closely
Tolcapone	Caution if creatinine clearance less than 30 mL/minute
Tolfenamic acid	*see* NSAIDs
Tolterodine	Reduce dose to 1 mg twice daily if creatinine clearance less than 30 mL/minute
Topiramate	Longer time to steady-state plasma concentrations
Topotecan	Reduce dose; avoid if creatinine clearance less than 20 mL/minute
Torasemide	May need high doses
Trabectedin	Avoid if creatinine clearance less than 30 mL/minute
Tramadol	*see* Opioid Analgesics
Trandolapril	*see* ACE Inhibitors; max. 2 mg daily if creatinine clearance less than 10 mL/minute
Tranexamic acid	Reduce dose—consult product literature for details
Tretinoin (oral)	Reduce dose to 25 mg/m^2
Triamterene	*see* Potassium-sparing Diuretics
Tribavirin	*see* Ribavirin
Triclofos	*see* Anxiolytics and Hypnotics
Trifluoperazine	*see* Antipsychotics
Trimeprazine	*see* Alimemazine
Trimethoprim	Use half normal dose after 3 days if creatinine clearance 15–30 mL/minute; use half normal dose if creatinine clearance less than 15 mL/minute (monitor plasma-trimethoprim concentration if creatinine clearance less than 10 mL/minute)
Tripotassium dicitratobismuthate	Avoid if creatinine clearance less than 10 mL/minute
Trospium	Reduce dose to 20 mg once daily or 20 mg on alternate days if creatinine clearance less than 30 mL/minute
Truvada®	Monitor renal function; use normal dose every 48 hours if creatinine clearance 30–50 mL/minute; avoid if creatinine clearance less than 30 mL/minute
Tylex®	Manufacturer advises caution in severe impairment; effervescent tablets contain 13.6 mmol sodium per tablet; *see also* Opioid Analgesics

For adjusting drug doses in renal impairment, see Important on p. 772.

Drug	Comment
Valaciclovir	For herpes zoster, 1 g every 12 hours if creatinine clearance 15–30 mL/minute (every 24 hours if creatinine clearance less than 15 mL/minute); for treatment of herpes simplex, 500 mg every 24 hours if creatinine clearance less than 15 mL/minute; for suppression of herpes simplex, 250 mg (500 mg in immunocompromised) every 24 hours if creatinine clearance less than 15 mL/minute; for reduction of genital herpes transmission, 250 mg every 24 hours if creatinine clearance less than 15 mL/minute; reduce dose according to creatinine clearance for cytomegalovirus prophylaxis following renal transplantation (consult product literature)
Valganciclovir	Reduce dose; consult product literature
Valproate	Reduce dose; adjust dosage according to free serum valproic acid concentration
Valproic acid	*see* Valproate
Valsartan	Initially 40 mg once daily if creatinine clearance less than 20 mL/minute
Vancomycin	Reduce dose—monitor plasma-vancomycin concentration and renal function regularly
Vardenafil	Initial dose 5 mg if creatinine clearance less than 30 mL/minute; avoid in endstage renal disease requiring dialysis
Varenicline	If creatinine clearance less than 30 mL/minute initial dose 500 micrograms once daily, increased after 3 days to 1 mg once daily
Venlafaxine	Use half normal dose if creatinine clearance 10–30 mL/minute; avoid if creatinine clearance less than 10 mL/minute
Vigabatrin	Manufacturer advises caution if creatinine clearance less than 60 mL/minute; consider dose reduction; monitor for sedation or confusion
Voriconazole	Intravenous vehicle may accumulate if creatinine clearance less than 50 mL/minute—manufacturer advises use intravenous infusion only if potential benefit outweighs risk, and monitor renal function; alternatively, use tablets or oral suspension (no dose adjustment required)
Warfarin	*see* Anticoagulants, Oral
Xipamide	*see* Thiazides and Related Diuretics
Yasmin®	Manufacturer advises avoid if creatinine clearance less than 30 mL/minute
Zafirlukast	Manufacturer advises caution in moderate to severe impairment
Zidovudine	Reduce oral dose to 300–400 mg daily in divided doses or intravenous dose to 1 mg/kg 3–4 times daily if creatinine clearance less than 10 mL/minute
Zoledronic acid	Avoid if serum creatinine above 400 micromol/litre in tumour-induced hypercalcaemia; in cancer and bone metastases, if creatinine clearance 50–60 mL/minute reduce dose to 3.5 mg every 3–4 weeks, if creatinine clearance 40–50 mL/minute reduce dose to 3.3 mg every 3–4 weeks, if creatinine clearance 30–40 mL/minute reduce dose to 3 mg every 3–4 weeks, and avoid if creatinine clearance less than 30 mL/minute (or if serum creatinine greater than 265 micromol/litre); if renal function deteriorates in patients with bone metastases, withhold dose until serum creatinine returns to within 10% of baseline value; avoid in Paget's disease and treatment of postmenopausal osteoporosis if creatinine clearance less than 40 mL/minute
Zonisamide	Initially increase dose at 2-week intervals; discontinue if renal function deteriorates
Zopiclone	*see* Anxiolytics and Hypnotics
Zotepine	Initial dose 25 mg twice daily, increased gradually according to response (max. 75 mg twice daily)
Zuclopenthixol	*see* Antipsychotics

A4 Pregnancy

Drugs can have harmful effects on the fetus at any time during pregnancy. It is important to bear this in mind when prescribing for a woman of *childbearing age* or for men *trying* to *father* a child.

During the *first trimester* drugs can produce congenital malformations (teratogenesis), and the period of greatest risk is from the third to the eleventh week of pregnancy.

During the *second* and *third trimesters* drugs can affect the growth and functional development of the fetus or have toxic effects on fetal tissues. Drugs given shortly before term or during labour can have adverse effects on labour or on the neonate after delivery.

The following list includes drugs which:

- may have harmful effects in pregnancy and indicates the trimester of risk
- are not known to be harmful in pregnancy

The list is based on human data, but information on *animal* studies has been included for some drugs when its omission might be misleading.

> Drugs should be prescribed in pregnancy only if the expected benefit to the mother is thought to be greater than the risk to the fetus, and all drugs should be avoided if possible during the first trimester. Drugs which have been extensively used in pregnancy and appear to be usually safe should be prescribed in preference to new or untried drugs; and the smallest effective dose should be used.
> Few drugs have been shown conclusively to be teratogenic in man, but no drug is safe beyond all doubt in early pregnancy. Screening procedures are available when there is a known risk of certain defects.
> Absence of a drug from the list does not imply safety.
> It should be noted that the BNF provides independent advice and may not always agree with the product literature.
> Information on drugs and pregnancy is also available from the National Teratology Information Service Telephone: (0191) 232 1525
> (0191) 223 1307 (out of hours emergency only)
> www.nyrdtc.nhs.uk/Services/teratology/teratology.html

Table of drugs to be avoided or used with caution in pregnancy

Products introduced or amended since publication of BNF No. 54 (September 2007) are underlined.

Drug (trimester of risk)	Comment
Abacavir	Manufacturer advises avoid (toxicity in *animal* studies); *see also* p. 328
Abatacept	Manufacturer advises avoid unless essential—no information available; effective contraception required during treatment and for 14 weeks after last dose
Abciximab	Manufacturer advises use only if potential benefit outweighs risk—no information available
Acamprosate	Manufacturer advises avoid
Acarbose	Manufacturer advises avoid; insulin is normally substituted during pregnancy in all diabetics
ACE inhibitors (1, 2, 3)	Avoid; may adversely affect fetal and neonatal blood pressure control and renal function; also possible skull defects and oligohydramnios; toxicity in *animal* studies
Acebutolol	*see* Beta-blockers
Aceclofenac	*see* NSAIDs
Acemetacin	*see* NSAIDs
Acenocoumarol (nicoumalone)	*see* Anticoagulants, Oral
Acetazolamide	*see* Diuretics
Aciclovir	Not known to be harmful—manufacturers advise use only when potential benefit outweighs risk; limited absorption from topical aciclovir preparations
Acipimox	Manufacturer advises avoid
Acitretin (1, 2, 3)	Teratogenic; effective contraception must be used for at least 1 month before treatment, during treatment, and for at least 2 years after stopping (oral progestogen-only contraceptives not considered effective)
Adalimumab	Avoid; manufacturer advises adequate contraception during and for at least 5 months after last dose
Adapalene	Manufacturer advises teratogenicity in *animal* studies and recommends effective contraception during treatment

Drug (trimester of risk)	Comment
Adefovir dipivoxil	Toxicity in *animal* studies—manufacturer advises use only if potential benefit outweighs risk; effective contraception required during treatment
Agalsidase	Use with caution—no information available
Alclometasone	*see* Corticosteroids
Alcohol	
(1, 2)	Regular daily drinking is teratogenic (fetal alcohol syndrome) and may cause growth restriction; occasional single drinks are probably safe
(3)	Withdrawal syndrome may occur in babies of alcoholic mothers
Alemtuzumab	Avoid; manufacturer advises effective contraception during and for 6 months after treatment in men or women
Alendronic acid	*see* Bisphosphonates
Alfentanil	*see* Opioid Analgesics
Alglucosidase alfa	Manufacturer advises avoid unless essential—no information available
Alimemazine (trimeprazine)	*see* Antihistamines
Aliskiren	Manufacturer advises avoid—no information available; other drugs acting on the renin-angiotensin system have been associated with fetal malformations and neonatal death
Allopurinol	Toxicity not reported; manufacturer advises use only if no safer alternative and disease carries risk for mother or child
Almotriptan	*see* $5HT_1$ Agonists
Alpha-blockers, post-synaptic	No evidence of teratogenicity; manufacturers advise use only when potential benefit outweighs risk
Alprazolam	*see* Benzodiazepines
Alprostadil (urethral application only)	Manufacturer advises barrier contraception if partner pregnant
Alteplase	*see* Fibrinolytics
Amantadine	Avoid; toxicity in *animal* studies
Amfebutamone	*see* Bupropion
Amikacin	*see* Aminoglycosides
Amiloride	*see* Diuretics
Aminoglycosides	
(2, 3)	Auditory or vestibular nerve damage; risk greatest with streptomycin; probably very small with gentamicin and tobramycin, but avoid unless essential (if given, serum-aminoglycoside concentration monitoring essential)
Aminophylline	*see* Theophylline
Amiodarone	
(2, 3)	Possible risk of neonatal goitre; use only if no alternative
Amisulpride	Manufacturer advises avoid
Amitriptyline	*see* Antidepressants, Tricyclic (and related)
Amlodipine	No information available—manufacturer advises avoid, but risk to fetus should be balanced against risk of uncontrolled maternal hypertension
Amobarbital	*see* Barbiturates
Amorolfine	Systemic absorption very low, but manufacturer advises avoid—no information available
Amoxicillin	*see* Penicillins
Amphotericin	Not known to be harmful but manufacturers advise avoid unless potential benefit outweighs risk
Ampicillin	*see* Penicillins
Amprenavir	Avoid oral solution due to high propylene glycol content; manufacturer advises use capsules only if potential benefit outweighs risk
Amsacrine	Avoid (teratogenic and toxic in *animal* studies); may reduce fertility; *see also* section 8.1
Anabolic steroids	
(1, 2, 3)	Masculinisation of female fetus
Anaesthetics, general	
(3)	Depress neonatal respiration; for maintenance of anaesthesia, doses of propofol should not exceed 6 mg/kg/hour; dose of thiopental should not exceed 250 mg
Anaesthetics, local	
(3)	With large doses, neonatal respiratory depression, hypotonia, and bradycardia after paracervical or epidural block; neonatal methaemoglobinaemia with prilocaine and procaine; use lower doses of bupivacaine for intrathecal use during late pregnancy; *see also* Levobupivacaine and Ropivacaine
Anagrelide	Manufacturer advises avoid (toxicity in *animal* studies)
Anakinra	Manufacturer advises avoid; effective contraception must be used during treatment
Analgesics	*see* Opioid Analgesics, Nefopam, NSAIDs, and Paracetamol
Androgens	
(1, 2, 3)	Masculinisation of female fetus
Anidulafungin	Manufacturer advises avoid—no information available
Anticoagulants, oral	
(1, 2, 3)	Congenital malformations; fetal and neonatal haemorrhage; *see also* section 2.8.2
Antidepressants, MAOI	
(1, 2, 3)	No evidence of harm but manufacturers advise avoid unless compelling reasons

Drug (trimester of risk)	Comment
Antidepressants, SSRI	Manufacturers advise use only if potential benefit outweighs risk; risk of neonatal withdrawal, particularly with fluoxetine and paroxetine; toxicity in *animal* studies with escitalopram and paroxetine
Antidepressants, tricyclic (and related) (3)	Tachycardia, irritability, and muscle spasms in neonate reported with imipramine
Antiepileptics	Benefit of treatment outweighs risk to fetus; risk of teratogenicity greater if more than one drug used; **important**: *see also* Carbamazepine, Ethosuximide, Gabapentin, Lamotrigine, Levetiracetam, Oxcarbazepine, Phenobarbital, Phenytoin, Pregabalin, Primidone, Rufinamide, Topiramate, Valproate, Vigabatrin, Zonisamide, and p. 245
Antihistamines	No evidence of teratogenicity; embryotoxicity in *animal* studies with high doses of hydroxyzine and loratadine; manufacturers of cetirizine, cinnarizine, desloratadine, dimenhydrinate, hydroxyzine, ketotifen, loratadine, and mizolastine advise avoid
Antimalarials	
(1, 3)	Benefit of prophylaxis and treatment in malaria outweighs risk; **important**: *see also* individual drugs and p. 345 and p. 346
Antipsychotics	*See also* Amisulpride, Clozapine, Olanzapine, Paliperidone, Quetiapine, Risperidone, Sertindole, Zotepine
(3)	Extrapyramidal effects in neonate occasionally reported
Apomorphine	Caution
Aprepitant	
(1, 2, 3)	Manufacturer advises avoid unless potential benefit outweighs risk—no information available
Aripiprazole	
(1, 2, 3)	Manufacturer advises use only if potential benefit outweighs risk—no information available
Arsenic trioxide	Avoid (teratogenic and embryotoxic in *animal* studies); manufacturer advises effective contraception during treatment in men or women; *see also* section 8.1
Artemether [ingredient]	*see Riamet®*

Drug (trimester of risk)	Comment
Aspirin	
(3)	Impaired platelet function and risk of haemorrhage; delayed onset and increased duration of labour with increased blood loss; avoid analgesic doses if possible in last few weeks (low doses probably not harmful); with high doses, closure of fetal ductus arteriosus *in utero* and possibly persistent pulmonary hypertension of newborn; kernicterus in jaundiced neonates
Atazanavir	Manufacturer advises use only if potential benefit outweighs risk; theoretical risk of hyperbilirubinaemia in neonate if used at term
Atenolol	*see* Beta-blockers
Atomoxetine	Manufacturer advises avoid unless potential benefit outweighs risk—no information available
Atorvastatin	*see* Statins
Atosiban	For use in premature labour *see* section 7.1.3
Atovaquone	Manufacturer advises avoid unless potential benefit outweighs risk—no information available
Atracurium	Does not cross placenta in significant amounts but manufacturer advises use only if potential benefit outweighs risk
Atropine	Not known to be harmful; manufacturer advises caution
Auranofin	Manufacturer advises avoid (effective contraception should be used during and for at least 6 months after treatment) but limited data suggests usually not necessary to withdraw if condition well controlled—consider reducing dose and frequency
Azapropazone	*see* NSAIDs
Azathioprine	*see* p. 473
Azelastine	*see* Antihistamines
Azithromycin	Manufacturer advises use only if adequate alternatives not available
Aztreonam	Manufacturer advises avoid—no information available
Baclofen	Manufacturer advises use only if potential benefit outweighs risk (toxicity in *animal* studies)
Balsalazide	Manufacturer advises avoid
Bambuterol	*see* section 3.1
Barbiturates	
(1, 2, 3)	Fetal abnormalities reported
(3)	Withdrawal effects in neonate; respiratory depression in neonate if used during labour; *see also* Phenobarbital
Basiliximab	Avoid; adequate contraception must be used during treatment and for 8 weeks after last dose

Drug (trimester of risk)	Comment
Beclometasone	*see* Corticosteroids
Bemiparin	Manufacturer advises avoid unless essential—no information available
Bendrofluazide	*see* Diuretics
Bendroflumethiazide (bendrofluazide)	*see* Diuretics
Benperidol	*see* Antipsychotics
Benzatropine	Manufacturer advises use only if essential
Benzodiazepines	Avoid regular use (risk of neonatal withdrawal symptoms); use only if clear indication such as seizure control (high doses during late pregnancy or labour may cause neonatal hypothermia, hypotonia and respiratory depression)
Benzylpenicillin	*see* Penicillins
Beta-blockers	May cause intra-uterine growth restriction, neonatal hypoglycaemia, and bradycardia; risk greater in severe hypertension; *see also* section 2.5
Betamethasone	*see* Corticosteroids
Bethanechol	Manufacturer advises avoid—no information available
Bevacizumab	Manufacturer advises avoid—toxicity in *animal* studies; effective contraception required during and for at least 6 months after treatment in women (*see also* section 8.1)
Bexarotene	Avoid; manufacturer advises effective contraception during and for at least 1 month after treatment in men or women; *see also* section 8.1
Bezafibrate	*see* Fibrates
Bimatoprost	Manufacturer advises use only if potential benefit outweighs risk
Bisoprolol	*see* Beta-blockers
Bisphosphonates	Manufacturers advise avoid
Bivalirudin	Manufacturer advises avoid unless potential benefit outweighs risk—no information available
Bleomycin	Avoid (teratogenic and carcinogenic in *animal* studies); *see also* section 8.1
Bortezomib	Manufacturer advises effective contraception during and for 3 months after treatment in men or women—no information available; *see also* section 8.1
Bosentan	Avoid (teratogenic in *animal* studies); effective contraception required during and for at least 3 months after administration (hormonal contraception not considered effective); monthly pregnancy tests advised
Botulinum toxin	Manufacturers advise avoid unless essential—toxicity in *animal* studies
Brinzolamide	Manufacturer advises avoid unless essential
Buclizine	*see* Anthistamines
Budesonide	*see* Corticosteroids
Bumetanide	*see* Diuretics
Bupivacaine	*see* Anaesthetics, Local
Buprenorphine	*see* Opioid Analgesics
Bupropion	Manufacturer advises avoid—no information available
Buserelin	Avoid
Buspirone	Manufacturer advises avoid
Busulfan	Avoid (teratogenic in *animals*); manufacturers advise effective contraception during and for 6 months after treatment in men or women; *see also* section 8.1
Cabergoline	No evidence of harm; manufacturer advises discontinuation one month before intended conception and avoidance during pregnancy; *see also* section 6.7.1
Calcipotriol	Manufacturer advises avoid if possible; *see also* Vitamin D
Calcitonin (salmon) (salcatonin)	Manufacturer advises avoid unless potential benefit outweighs risk (toxicity in *animal* studies)
Calcitriol	*see* Vitamin D
Calcium folinate	Manufacturer advises use only if potential benefit outweighs risk
Calcium levofolinate	*see* Calcium Folinate
Candesartan	*As for* ACE Inhibitors
Capecitabine	Avoid (teratogenic in animal studies); *see also* section 8.1
Capreomycin	Manufacturer advises use only if potential benefit outweighs risk—teratogenic in *animal* studies
Captopril	*see* ACE Inhibitors
Carbamazepine	Risk of teratogenesis including increased risk of neural tube defects; *see also* Antiepileptics
Carbimazole (2, 3)	Neonatal goitre and hypothyroidism; has been associated with aplasia cutis of the neonate
Carbocisteine (1)	Manufacturer advises avoid
Carboplatin	Avoid (teratogenic and embryotoxic in *animal* studies); *see also* section 8.1
Carglumic acid	Manufacturer advises avoid unless essential—no information available
Carmustine	Avoid (teratogenic and embryotoxic in *animals*); manufacturer advises effective contraception during treatment in men or women; *see also* section 8.1
Carnitine	Appropriate to use; no evidence of teratogenicity in *animal* studies
Carvedilol	*see* Beta-blockers

Drug (trimester of risk)	Comment
Caspofungin	Manufacturer advises avoid unless essential—toxicity in *animal* studies
Cefaclor	Not known to be harmful
Cefadroxil	Not known to be harmful
Cefalexin	Not known to be harmful
Cefixime	Not known to be harmful
Cefotaxime	Not known to be harmful
Cefpodoxime	Not known to be harmful
Cefradine	Not known to be harmful
Ceftazidime	Not known to be harmful
Ceftriaxone	Not known to be harmful
Cefuroxime	Not known to be harmful
Celecoxib	Manufacturer advises avoid (teratogenic in *animal* studies); *see also* NSAIDs
Celiprolol	*see* Beta-blockers
Cetirizine	*see* Antihistamines
Cetrorelix	Manufacturer advises avoid in confirmed pregnancy
Cetuximab	Manufacturer advises use only if potential benefit outweighs risk—no information available
Chloral hydrate	Avoid
Chlorambucil	Avoid; manufacturer advises effective contraception during treatment in men or women; *see also* section 8.1
Chloramphenicol (3)	Neonatal 'grey' syndrome
Chlordiazepoxide	*see* Benzodiazepines
Chloroquine	*see* Antimalarials
Chlorphenamine (chlorpheniramine)	*see* Anthistamines
Chlorpheniramine	*see* Antihistamines
Chlorpromazine	*see* Antipsychotics
Chlorpropamide	*see* Sulphonylureas
Chlortalidone	*see* Diuretics
Ciclesonide	*see* Corticosteroids
Ciclosporin	*see* p. 473
Cidofovir	Avoid (toxicity in *animal* studies); effective contraception required during and for 1 month after treatment; also men should avoid fathering a child during and for 3 months after treatment
Cilastatin [ingredient]	*see Primaxin®*
Cilazapril	*see* ACE Inhibitors
Cilostazol	Avoid—toxicity in *animal* studies
Cimetidine	Manufacturer advises avoid unless essential
Cinacalcet	Manufacturer advises use only if potential benefit outweighs risk—no information available
Cinnarizine	*see* Anthistamines
Ciprofibrate	*see* Fibrates
Ciprofloxacin	*see* Quinolones
Cisatracurium	Manufacturer advises avoid—no information available
Cisplatin	Avoid (teratogenic and toxic in *animal* studies); *see also* section 8.1
Citalopram	*see* Antidepressants, SSRI
Cladribine	Avoid (teratogenic in *animal* studies); manufacturer advises that men should not father children during and for 6 months after treatment; *see also* section 8.1
Clarithromycin	Manufacturer advises avoid unless potential benefit outweighs risk
Clavulanic acid [ingredient]	*see* Co-amoxiclav, *Timentin®*
Clemastine	*see* Anthistamines
Clindamycin	Not known to be harmful
Clobazam	*see* Benzodiazepines
Clobetasol	*see* Corticosteroids
Clobetasone	*see* Corticosteroids
Clodronate sodium	*see* Bisphosphonates
Clofarabine	Manufacturer advises avoid (teratogenic in *animal* studies); *see also* section 8.1
Clomethiazole	Avoid if possible—especially during first and third trimesters
Clomifene	Possible effects on fetal development
Clomipramine	*see* Antidepressants, Tricyclic (and related)
Clonazepam	*see* Benzodiazepines
Clonidine	May lower fetal heart rate, but risk should be balanced against risk of uncontrolled maternal hypertension; avoid intravenous injection
Clopidogrel	Manufacturer advises avoid—no information available
Clozapine	Manufacturer advises caution
Co-amoxiclav	*see* Penicillins
Co-beneldopa	*see* Levodopa
Co-careldopa	*see* Levodopa
Co-cyprindiol (1, 2, 3)	Feminisation of male fetus (due to cyproterone)
Co-danthramer	Manufacturer advises avoid—no information available
Co-danthrusate	Manufacturer advises avoid—no information available
Codeine	*see* Opioid Analgesics
Co-fluampicil	*see* Penicillins
Colchicine	Avoid—teratogenicity in animal studies
Colesevelam	Use with caution—drug not absorbed but may cause fat-soluble vitamin deficiency on prolonged use
Colestipol	Use with caution—drug not absorbed but may cause fat-soluble vitamin deficiency on prolonged use
Colestyramine	Use with caution—drug not absorbed but may cause fat-soluble vitamin deficiency on prolonged use
Colistin (2, 3)	Avoid—possible risk of fetal toxicity
Contraceptives, oral	Epidemiological evidence suggests no harmful effects on fetus

Drug (trimester of risk)	Comment
Corticosteroids	Benefit of treatment, e.g. in asthma, outweighs risk (*see also* CSM advice, section 6.3.2); risk of intra-uterine growth restriction on prolonged or repeated systemic treatment; corticosteroid cover required by mother during labour; monitor closely if fluid retention
Co-trimoxazole	
(1)	Teratogenic risk (trimethoprim a folate antagonist)
(3)	Neonatal haemolysis and methaemoglobinaemia; fear of increased risk of kernicterus in neonates appears to be unfounded
Crisantaspase	Avoid; *see also* section 8.1
Cromoglicate	*see* Sodium Cromoglicate
Cyclizine	*see* Antihistamines
Cyclopenthiazide	*see* Diuretics
Cyclophosphamide	Avoid (manufacturer advises effective contraception during and for at least 3 months after treatment in men or women); *see also* section 8.1
Cycloserine	Manufacturer advises use only if potential benefit outweighs risk—crosses the placenta
Cyclosporin	*see* p. 473
Cyproheptadine	*see* Antihistamines
Cyproterone [ingredient]	*see* Co-cyprindiol
Cytarabine	Avoid (teratogenic in *animal* studies); *see also* section 8.1
Dacarbazine	Avoid (carcinogenic and teratogenic in *animal* studies); ensure effective contraception during and for at least 6 months after treatment in men or women; *see also* section 8.1
Daclizumab	Avoid
Dactinomycin	Avoid (teratogenic in *animal* studies); *see also* section 8.1
Dalfopristin [ingredient]	*see Synercid®*
Dalteparin	Not known to be harmful
Danaparoid	Limited information available but not known to be harmful—manufacturer advises avoid
Danazol	
(1, 2, 3)	Avoid; has weak androgenic effects and virilisation of female fetus reported
Dantrolene	Use only for malignant hyperthermia if potential benefit outweighs risk; avoid use in chronic spasticity—embryotoxic in *animal* studies
Dantron (danthron)	*see* Co-danthramer, Co-danthrusate
Dapsone	Folic acid 5 mg daily should be given to mother throughout pregnancy
(3)	Neonatal haemolysis and methaemoglobinaemia reported
Daptomycin	Manufacturer advises use only if potential benefit outweighs risk—no information available
Darbepoetin	No evidence of harm in *animal* studies—manufacturer advises caution
Darifenacin	Manufacturer advises avoid—toxicity in *animal* studies
Darunavir	Manufacturer advises use only if potential benefit outweighs risk—no information available
Dasatinib	Manufacturer advises avoid unless potential benefit outweighs risk—toxicity in *animal* studies; effective contraception required during treatment
Daunorubicin	Avoid (teratogenic and carcinogenic in *animal* studies); *see also* section 8.1
Deferasirox	Manufacturer advises avoid unless potential benefit outweighs risk—toxicity in *animal* studies
Deferiprone	Manufacturer advises avoid before intended conception and during pregnancy—teratogenic and embryotoxic in *animal* studies; contraception advised in women of child-bearing potential
Deflazacort	*see* Corticosteroids
Demeclocycline	*see* Tetracyclines
Desferrioxamine	Teratogenic in *animal* studies; manufacturer advises use only if potential benefit outweighs risk
Desflurane	*see* Anaesthetics, General
Desloratadine	*see* Antihistamines
Desmopressin	
(3)	Small oxytocic effect in third trimester; increased risk of pre-eclampsia
Desogestrel	*see* Contraceptives, Oral
Dexamethasone	*see* Corticosteroids
Dexamfetamine	Manufacturer advises avoid (retrospective evidence of uncertain significance suggesting possible embryotoxicity)
Dexibuprofen	*see* NSAIDs
Dexketoprofen	*see* NSAIDs
Dexrazoxane	Manufacturer advises avoid unless essential; ensure effective contraception during and for 3 months after treatment in men and women
Dextran	Avoid—reports of anaphylaxis in mother causing fetal anoxia, neurological damage and death
Dextromethorphan	*see* Opioid Analgesics
Diamorphine	*see* Opioid Analgesics
Diazepam	*see* Benzodiazepines
Diazoxide	
(2, 3)	Prolonged use may produce alopecia and impaired glucose tolerance in neonate; inhibits uterine activity during labour

Drug (trimester of risk)	Comment
Diclofenac	*see* NSAIDs
Didanosine	Manufacturer advises use only if potential benefit outweighs risk—no information available
Diethylstilbestrol	
(1)	High doses associated with vaginal carcinoma, urogenital abnormalities, and reduced fertility in female offspring; increased risk of hypospadias in male offspring
Diflucortolone	*see* Corticosteroids
Digoxin	May need dosage adjustment
Dihydrocodeine	*see* Opioid Analgesics
Diloxanide	Manufacturer advises avoid—no information available
Diltiazem	Avoid
Dimenhydrinate	*see* Antihistamines
Diphenoxylate	*see* Opioid Analgesics
Dipipanone	*see* Opioid Analgesics
Dipyridamole	Not known to be harmful
Disodium etidronate	*see* Bisphosphonates
Disodium pamidronate	*see* Bisphosphonates
Disopyramide	
(3)	May induce labour
Distigmine	Manufacturer advises avoid (may stimulate uterine contractions)
Disulfiram	
(1)	High concentrations of acetaldehyde which occur in presence of alcohol may be teratogenic
Diuretics	Not used to treat hypertension in pregnancy
(1)	Manufacturers advise avoid acetazolamide and torasemide (toxicity in *animal* studies)
(3)	Thiazides may cause neonatal thrombocytopenia
Dobutamine	No information available
Docetaxel	Avoid (toxicity and reduced fertility in *animal* studies); manufacturer advises effective contraception during and for at least 3 months after treatment; *see also* section 8.1
Docusate sodium	Not known to be harmful—manufacturer advises caution
Dolasetron	Not known to be harmful but manufacturer advises avoid unless potential benefit outweighs risk
Domperidone	Manufacturer advises avoid
Donepezil	Manufacturer advises use only if potential benefit outweighs risk
Dopamine	Manufacturer advises use only if potential benefit outweighs risk
Dopexamine	No information available—manufacturer advises avoid
Dornase alfa	No evidence of teratogenicity; manufacturer advises use only if potential benefit outweighs risk

Drug (trimester of risk)	Comment
Dosulepin (dothiepin)	*see* Antidepressants, Tricyclic (and related)
Dothiepin	*see* Antidepressants, Tricyclic (and related)
Doxazosin	*see* Alpha-blockers, Post-synaptic
Doxepin	*see* Antidepressants, Tricyclic (and related)
Doxorubicin	Avoid (teratogenic and toxic in *animal* studies); manufacturer of liposomal product advises effective contraception during and for at least 6 months after treatment in men or women; *see also* section 8.1
Doxycycline	*see* Tetracyclines
Drotrecogin alfa (activated)	Manufacturer advises avoid unless benefit outweighs risk—no information available
Duloxetine	Toxicity in *animal* studies—manufacturer advises avoid in patients with stress urinary incontinence and use only if potential benefit outweighs risk in depression; risk of neonatal withdrawal symptoms if used near term
Dutasteride	
(1, 2, 3)	Avoid unprotected intercourse (*see* section 6.4.2). May cause feminisation of male fetus
Dydrogesterone	Not known to be harmful
Econazole	Not known to be harmful
Eculizumab	No information available—use only if potential benefit outweighs risk; human IgG antibodies known to cross placenta; manufacturer advises effective contraception during and for 5 months after treatment
Edrophonium	Manufacturer advises use only if potential benefit outweighs risk
Efalizumab	Manufacturer advises avoid
Efavirenz	Manufacturer advises avoid unless no alternative available
Eflornithine	Toxicity in *animal* studies—manufacturer advises avoid
Eletriptan	*see* $5HT_1$ Agonists
Emtricitabine	No information available—manufacturer advises use only if essential
Enalapril	*see* ACE Inhibitors
Enfuvirtide	Manufacturer advises use only if potential benefit outweighs risk
Enoxaparin	Not known to be harmful
Enoximone	Manufacturer advises use only if potential benefit outweighs risk
Entacapone	Manufacturer advises avoid—no information available
Entecavir	Toxicity in *animal* studies—manufacturer advises use only if potential benefit outweighs risk; effective contraception required during treatment

Drug (trimester of risk)	Comment
Ephedrine	Increased fetal heart rate reported with parenteral ephedrine
Epinastine	*see* Antihistamines
Epirubicin	Avoid (carcinogenic in *animal* studies); *see also* section 8.1
Eplerenone	Manufacturer advises caution—no information available
Epoetin	No evidence of harm; benefits probably outweigh risk of anaemia and of transfusion in pregnancy
Epoprostenol	Manufacturer advises use with caution—no information available
Eprosartan	*As for* ACE Inhibitors
Eptifibatide	Manufacturer advises use only if potential benefit outweighs risk—no information available
Erdosteine	Manufacturer advises avoid—no information available
Ergotamine (1, 2, 3)	Oxytocic effects on the pregnant uterus
Erlotinib	Manufacturer advises avoid—toxicity in *animal* studies; effective contraception required during and for at least 2 weeks after treatment; *see also* section 8.1
Ertapenem	Manufacturer advises avoid unless potential benefit outweighs risk
Erythromycin	Not known to be harmful
Escitalopram	*see* Antidepressants, SSRI
Esmolol	*see* Beta-blockers
Esomeprazole	Manufacturer advises caution—no information available
Etanercept	Manufacturer advises avoid—no information available
Ethambutol	Not known to be harmful; *see also* p. 310
Ethinylestradiol	*see* Contraceptives, Oral
Ethosuximide (1)	May possibly be teratogenic; *see also* Antiepileptics
Etidronate disodium	*see* Bisphosphonates
Etodolac	*see* NSAIDs
Etomidate	*see* Anaesthetics, General
Etoposide	Avoid (teratogenic in *animal* studies); *see also* section 8.1
Etoricoxib	*see* NSAIDs
Etynodiol	*see* Contraceptives, Oral
Exenatide	Manufacturer advises avoid—toxicity in *animal* studies; insulin is normally substituted during pregnancy in all diabetics
Ezetimibe	Manufacturer advises use only if potential benefit outweighs risk—no information available
Famciclovir	*see* Aciclovir
Famotidine	Manufacturer advises avoid unless potential benefit outweighs risk
Fansidar® (1)	Possible teratogenic risk (pyrimethamine a folate antagonist)
(3)	Neonatal haemolysis and methaemoglobinaemia; fear of increased risk of kernicterus in neonates appears to be unfounded
	see also Antimalarials
Felodipine	Avoid; toxicity in *animal* studies; may inhibit labour
Fenbufen	*see* NSAIDs
Fenofibrate	*see* Fibrates
Fenoprofen	*see* NSAIDs
Fenoterol	*see* section 3.1
Fentanyl	*see* Opioid Analgesics
Fexofenadine	*see* Antihistamines
Fibrates	Embryotoxicity in *animal* studies—manufacturers advise avoid
Fibrinolytics (1, 2, 3)	Possibility of premature separation of placenta in first 18 weeks; risk of maternal haemorrhage throughout pregnancy and on post-partum; theoretical risk of fetal haemorrhage throughout pregnancy
Filgrastim	Toxicity in *animal* studies; manufacturer advises use only if potential benefit outweighs risk
Finasteride (1, 2, 3)	Avoid unprotected intercourse (*see* section 6.4.2). May cause feminisation of male fetus
Flavoxate	Manufacturer advises avoid unless no safer alternative
Flecainide	Used in pregnancy to treat maternal and fetal arrhythmias in specialist centres; toxicity reported in *animal* studies; infant hyperbilirubinaemia also reported
Flucloxacillin	*see* Penicillins
Fluconazole	Manufacturer advises avoid—multiple congenital abnormalities reported with long-term high doses
Flucytosine	Teratogenic in *animal* studies; manufacturer advises use only if potential benefit outweighs risk
Fludarabine	Avoid (embryotoxic and teratogenic in *animal* studies); manufacturer advises effective contraception during and for at least 6 months after treatment in men or women; *see also* section 8.1
Fludrocortisone	*see* Corticosteroids
Fludroxycortide (flurandrenolone)	*see* Corticosteroids
Flumazenil	May cross placenta in small amounts—manufacturer advises avoid unless potential benefit outweighs risk

Drug (trimester of risk)	Comment
Flunisolide	*see* Corticosteroids
Fluocinolone	*see* Corticosteroids
Fluocinonide	*see* Corticosteroids
Fluocortolone	*see* Corticosteroids
Fluorometholone	*see* Corticosteroids
Fluorouracil	Avoid (teratogenic); *see also* section 8.1
Fluoxetine	*see* Antidepressants, SSRI
Flupentixol	*see* Antipsychotics
Fluphenazine	*see* Antipsychotics
Flurandrenolone	*see* Corticosteroids
Flurazepam	*see* Benzodiazepines
Flurbiprofen	*see* NSAIDs
Fluticasone	*see* Corticosteroids
Fluvastatin	*see* Statins
Fluvoxamine	*see* Antidepressants, SSRI
Follitropin alfa and beta	Avoid
Fondaparinux	Manufacturer advises avoid unless potential benefit outweighs possible risk—no information available
Formoterol (eformoterol)	Manufacturers advise use only if potential benefit outweighs risk; *see also* section 3.1
Fosamprenavir	Toxicity in *animal* studies; manufacturer advises use only if potential benefit outweighs risk
Foscarnet	Manufacturer advises avoid
Fosinopril	*see* ACE Inhibitors
Fosphenytoin	*see* Phenytoin
Framycetin	*see* Aminoglycosides
Frovatriptan	*see* $5HT_1$ Agonists
Frusemide	*see* Diuretics
Fulvestrant	Manufacturer advises avoid—increased incidence of fetal abnormalities and death in *animal* studies
Furosemide (frusemide)	*see* Diuretics
Fusidic acid	*see* Sodium Fusidate
Gabapentin	Toxicity in *animal* studies; *see also* Antiepileptics
Galantamine	Developmental delay in *animal* studies
Galsulfase	Manufacturer advises avoid unless essential
Ganciclovir	Avoid—teratogenic risk; *see also* p. 338
Ganirelix	Manufacturer advises avoid in confirmed pregnancy—toxicity in *animal* studies
Gemcitabine	Avoid (teratogenic in *animal* studies); *see also* section 8.1
Gemfibrozil	*see* Fibrates
Gentamicin	*see* Aminoglycosides
Gestodene	*see* Contraceptives, Oral
Gestrinone (1, 2, 3)	Avoid
Glatiramer	Manufacturer advises avoid—no information available
Glibenclamide	*see* Sulphonylureas
Gliclazide	*see* Sulphonylureas
Glimepiride	*see* Sulphonylureas
Glipizide	*see* Sulphonylureas
Glucosamine	Manufacturer advises avoid—no information available
Glyceryl trinitrate	Not known to be harmful but most manufacturers advise avoid unless potential benefit outweighs risk
Gonadorelin analogues	*see* individual entries
Goserelin	Manufacturer advises avoid in pregnancy—exclude pregnancy before treatment and use non-hormonal contraceptives during treatment
Granisetron	Manufacturer advises use only when compelling reasons—no information available
Griseofulvin	Avoid (fetotoxicity and teratogenicity in *animals*); effective contraception required during and for at least 1 month after administration (**important**: effectiveness of oral contraceptives reduced, see p. 428); also men should avoid fathering a child during and for at least 6 months after administration
Guanethidine (3)	Postural hypotension and reduced uteroplacental perfusion; should not be used to treat hypertension in pregnancy
Haem arginate	Manufacturer advises avoid unless essential
Haloperidol	*see* Antipsychotics
Halothane	*see* Anaesthetics, General
Heparin (1, 2, 3)	Does not cross the placenta; maternal osteoporosis reported after prolonged use; multidose vials may contain benzyl alcohol—some manufacturers advise avoid; *see also* Bemiparin, Dalteparin, Enoxaparin, and Tinzaparin
$5HT_1$ agonists	Limited experience—manufacturers advise avoid unless potential benefit outweighs risk
Human menopausal gonadotrophins	Avoid
Hydralazine (1, 2)	Manufacturer advises avoid before third trimester; no reports of serious harm following use in third trimester
Hydrochlorothiazide	*see* Diuretics
Hydrocortisone	*see* Corticosteroids
Hydroflumethiazide	*see* Diuretics
Hydromorphone	*see* Opioid Analgesics
Hydroxycarbamide (hydroxyurea)	Avoid (teratogenic in *animal* studies); manufacturer advises effective contraception before and during treatment *see also* section 8.1
Hydroxychloroquine	Manufacturer advises avoid but see p. 548

Drug (trimester of risk)	Comment
Hydroxyurea	*see* Hydroxycarbamide
Hydroxyzine	*see* Antihistamines
Hyoscine butylbromide	Manufacturer advises use only if potential benefit outweighs risk
Hyoscine hydrobromide	Manufacturer advises use only if potential benefit outweighs risk; injection may depress neonatal respiration
Ibandronic acid	*see* Bisphosphonates
Ibuprofen	*see* NSAIDs
Idarubicin	Avoid (teratogenic and toxic in *animal* studies); *see also* section 8.1
Idoxuridine	Teratogenic in *animal* studies—manufacturer advises avoid
Idursulfase	Manufacturer advises avoid—no information available
Ifosfamide	Avoid (teratogenic and carcinogenic in *animals*); manufacturer advises adequate contraception during and for at least 6 months after treatment in men or women; *see also* section 8.1
Iloprost	Manufacturer advises avoid (toxicity in *animal* studies); effective contraception must be used during treatment
Imatinib	Manufacturer advises avoid unless potential benefit outweighs risk; *see also* section 8.1
Imidapril	*see* ACE Inhibitors
Imiglucerase	Manufacturer advises use only if potential benefit outweighs risk—no information available
Imipenem [ingredient]	*see Primaxin*®
Imipramine	*see* Antidepressants, Tricyclic (and related)
Imiquimod	No evidence of teratogenicity or toxicity in *animal* studies; manufacturer advises caution
Indapamide	*see* Diuretics
Indinavir	Toxicity in *animal* studies; manufacturer advises use only if potential benefit outweighs risk; theoretical risk of hyperbilirubinaemia and renal stones in neonate if used at term
Indometacin	*see* NSAIDs
Infliximab	Avoid; manufacturer advises adequate contraception during and for at least 6 months after last dose
Influenza vaccine	Not known to be harmful
Inosine pranobex	Manufacturer advises avoid
Inositol nicotinate	No information available—manufacturer advises avoid unless potential benefit outweighs risk
Insulin (1, 2, 3)	Insulin requirements should be assessed frequently by an experienced diabetes physician; limited evidence of safety of newer insulin analogues
Interferon beta	Manufacturers advise avoid—increased risk of spontaneous abortion; effective contraception required during treatment
Interferons	Manufacturers recommend avoid unless compelling reasons; effective contraception to be used by men and women receiving treatment; *see also* Interferon Beta
Iodine and iodides (2, 3)	Neonatal goitre and hypothyroidism; *see also* Iodine, Radioactive and Povidone–iodine
Iodine, radioactive (1, 2, 3)	Permanent hypothyroidism—avoid
Iodoform	*see* Povidone–iodine
Ipratropium	Not known to be harmful; *see* section 3.1
Irbesartan	*As for* ACE Inhibitors
Irinotecan	Avoid (teratogenic and toxic in *animal* studies); manufacturer advises effective contraception during and for at least 3 months after treatment; *see also* section 8.1
Iron (parenteral)	Avoid in first trimester
Iron dextran	*see* Iron (parenteral)
Iron sucrose	*see* Iron (parenteral)
Isocarboxazid	*see* Antidepressants, MAOI
Isoflurane	*see* Anaesthetics, General
Isometheptene [ingredient]	*see Midrid*®
Isoniazid	Not known to be harmful; *see also* p. 310
Isosorbide dinitrate	May cross placenta—manufacturers advise avoid unless potential benefit outweighs risk
Isosorbide mononitrate	Manufacturers advise avoid unless potential benefit outweighs risk
Isotretinoin (1, 2, 3)	Teratogenic; effective contraception must be used for at least 1 month before oral treatment, during treatment and for at least 1 month after stopping (oral progestogen-only contraceptives not considered effective); also avoid topical treatment
Isradipine	May inhibit labour; risk to fetus should be balanced against risk of uncontrolled maternal hypertension

Drug (trimester of risk)	Comment
Itraconazole	Manufacturer advises use only in life-threatening situations (toxicity at high doses in *animal* studies); ensure effective contraception during treatment and until the next menstrual period following end of treatment
Ivabradine	Manufacturer advises avoid—toxicity in *animal* studies
Kaletra®	Avoid oral solution due to high propylene glycol content; manufacturer advises use capsules and tablets only if potential benefit outweighs risk (toxicity in *animal* studies)
Ketamine	*see* Anaesthetics, General
Ketoconazole	Manufacturer advises avoid unless potential benefit outweighs risk (teratogenicity in *animal* studies)
Ketoprofen	*see* NSAIDs
Ketorolac	*see* NSAIDs
Ketotifen	*see* Antihistamines
Labetalol	*see* Beta-blockers
Lacidipine	Manufacturer advises avoid; may inhibit labour
Lactulose	Not known to be harmful
Lamivudine	
(1)	Manufacturer advises avoid during first trimester; *see also* p. 328
Lamotrigine	Risk of teratogenesis; *see also* Antiepileptics
Lanreotide	Manufacturer advises use only if potential benefit outweighs risk
Lansoprazole	Manufacturer advises avoid
Lanthanum	Manufacturer advises avoid—toxicity in *animal* studies
Laronidase	Manufacturer advises avoid unless essential—no information available
Latanoprost	Manufacturer advises avoid
Leflunomide	Avoid—active metabolite teratogenic in *animal* studies; effective contraception essential during treatment and for at least 2 years after treatment in women and at least 3 months after treatment in men (*see also* Leflunomide section 10.1.3)
Lenalidomide	Teratogenic risk; effective contraception must be used for at least 1 month before, during, and for at least 1 month after treatment (oral combined hormonal contraceptives and copper-releasing intrauterine devices not recommended); men should use condoms during treatment and for at least 1 week after stopping
Lenograstim	Toxicity in *animal* studies; manufacturer advises use only if potential benefit outweighs risk
Lepirudin	Avoid
Lercanidipine	Manufacturer advises avoid—no information available
Letrozole	Avoid (toxicity in *animal* studies); manufacturer advises effective contraception required until postmenopausal status fully established
Leuprorelin	Avoid—teratogenic in *animal* studies
Levetiracetam	Toxicity in *animal* studies—manufacturer advises use only if potential benefit outweighs risk; *see also* Antiepileptics
Levobupivacaine	
(1)	Manufacturer advises avoid if possible—toxicity in *animal* studies; *see also* Anaesthetics, Local
Levocetirizine	*see* Antihistamines
Levodopa	Manufacturers advise toxicity in *animal* studies
Levofloxacin	*see* Quinolones
Levomepromazine (methotrimeprazine)	*see* Antipsychotics
Levonorgestrel	*see* Contraceptives, Oral
Levothyroxine (thyroxine)	Monitor maternal serum-thyrotrophin concentration—levothyroxine may cross the placenta and excessive maternal concentration can be detrimental to fetus
Lidocaine (lignocaine)	*see* Anaesthetics, Local
Lignocaine	*see* Anaesthetics, Local
Linezolid	Manufacturer advises use only if potential benefit outweighs risk—no information available
Liothyronine	Does not cross the placenta in significant amounts; monitor maternal thyroid function tests—dosage adjustment may be necessary
Lisinopril	*see* ACE Inhibitors
Lithium salts	
(1)	Avoid if possible (risk of teratogenicity, including cardiac abnormalities)
(2, 3)	Dose requirements increased (but on delivery return to normal abruptly); close monitoring of serum-lithium concentration advised (risk of toxicity in neonate)
Lofepramine	*see* Antidepressants, Tricyclic (and related)
Lofexidine	Manufacturer advises use only if benefit outweighs risk—no information available
Lomustine	Avoid (manufacturer advises effective contraception during and for at least 6 months after treatment in men or women); *see also* section 8.1
Loperamide	Manufacturers advise avoid—no information available
Lopinavir [ingredient]	*see Kaletra®*
Loprazolam	*see* Benzodiazepines

Appendix 4: Pregnancy

Drug (trimester of risk)	Comment
Loratadine	Embryotoxic in *animal* studies; *see also* Antihistamines
Lorazepam	*see* Benzodiazepines
Lormetazepam	*see* Benzodiazepines
Losartan	*As for* ACE Inhibitors
Lumefantrine [ingredient]	*see Riamet®*
Lymecycline	*see* Tetracyclines
Macrogols (oral)	Manufacturers advise use only if essential—no information available
Magnesium sulphate (3)	Not known to be harmful for short-term intravenous administration in eclampsia but excessive doses cause neonatal respiratory depression
Malarone®	Manufacturer advises avoid unless essential
Maraviroc	Manufacturer advises use only if potential benefit outweighs risk—toxicity in *animal* studies
Mebendazole	Manufacturer advises toxicity in *animal* studies
Mebeverine	Not known to be harmful; manufacturers advise caution
Mecasermin	Manufacturer advises avoid unless essential; contraception advised in women of child-bearing potential
Mecysteine	Manufacturer advises avoid
Medroxyprogesterone	Avoid—genital malformations and cardiac defects reported with high doses; no evidence of adverse effect with depot injection for contraception
Mefenamic acid	*see* NSAIDs
Mefloquine (1)	Manufacturer advises teratogenicity in *animal* studies, but *see* p. 346
Meloxicam	*see* NSAIDs
Melphalan	Avoid (manufacturer advises adequate contraception during treatment in men or women); *see also* section 8.1
Memantine	Manufacturer advises avoid unless essential—intra-uterine growth restriction in *animal* studies
Menadiol (3)	Neonatal haemolytic anaemia, hyperbilirubinaemia and increased risk of kernicterus in jaundiced infants
Menotrophin	Avoid
Meprobamate	Manufacturer advises avoid if possible
Meptazinol	*see* Opioid Analgesics
Mercaptamine	Manufacturer advises avoid
Mercaptopurine	Avoid (teratogenic); *see also* section 8.1
Meropenem	Manufacturer advises use only if potential benefit outweighs risk—no information available
Mesalazine	Negligible quantities cross placenta
Mesna	Not known to be harmful; *see also* section 8.1
Mesterolone	*see* Androgens
Mestranol	*see* Contraceptives, Oral
Metaraminol	May reduce placental perfusion—manufacturer advises use only if potential benefit outweighs risk
Metformin (1, 2, 3)	Avoid; insulin is normally substituted during pregnancy in all diabetics
Methadone	*see* Opioid Analgesics
Methocarbamol	Manufacturer advises avoid unless potential benefit outweighs risk
Methotrexate	Avoid (teratogenic; fertility may be reduced during therapy but this may be reversible); manufacturer advises effective contraception during and for at least 3 months after treatment in men or women; *see also* section 8.1
Methotrimeprazine	*see* Antipsychotics
Methoxy polyethylene glycol-epoetin beta	No evidence of harm in *animal* studies—manufacturer advises caution
Methyldopa	Not known to be harmful
Methylphenidate	Limited experience—manufacturer advises avoid unless potential benefit outweighs risk; toxicity in *animals*
Methylprednisolone	*see* Corticosteroids
Methysergide	Manufacturer advises avoid
Metoclopramide	Not known to be harmful but manufacturer advises use only when compelling reasons
Metolazone	*see* Diuretics
Metoprolol	*see* Beta-blockers
Metronidazole	Manufacturer advises avoidance of high-dose regimens
Metyrapone	Avoid (may impair biosynthesis of fetal-placental steroids)
Mexiletine	Manufacturer advises avoid unless potential benefit outweighs risk
Mianserin	*see* Antidepressants, Tricyclic (and related)
Miconazole	Manufacturer advises avoid if possible—toxicity at high doses in *animal* studies
Midazolam	*see* Benzodiazepines
Midrid®	Manufacturer advises avoid
Mifepristone	Manufacturer advises that if treatment fails, essential that pregnancy be terminated by another method
Miglustat	Manufacturer advises avoid (toxicity in *animal* studies)—effective contraception must be used during treatment; also men should avoid fathering a child during and for 3 months after treatment

Drug (trimester of risk)	Comment
Milrinone	Manufacturer advises use only if potential benefit outweighs risk
Minocycline	*see* Tetracyclines
Minoxidil (3)	Neonatal hirsutism reported
Mirtazapine	Manufacturers advise avoid—toxicity in *animal* studies
Misoprostol (1, 2, 3)	Avoid—potent uterine stimulant (has been used to induce abortion) and may be teratogenic
Mitomycin	Avoid (teratogenic in *animal* studies); *see also* section 8.1
Mitotane	Manufacturer advises avoid—women of childbearing age should use effective contraception during and after treatment; *see also* section 8.1
Mitoxantrone (mitozantrone)	Avoid; manufacturer advises effective contraception during and for at least 6 months after treatment in men or women; *see also* section 8.1
Mitozantrone	*see* Mitoxantrone
Mivacurium	Manufacturer advises avoid—no information available
Mizolastine	Manufacturer advises avoid; *see also* Antihistamines
Moclobemide	*see* Antidepressants, MAOI
Modafinil	Manufacturer advises avoid
Moexipril	*see* ACE Inhibitors
Montelukast	Manufacturer advises avoid unless essential
Morphine	*see* Opioid Analgesics
Moxifloxacin	*see* Quinolones
Moxisylyte (thymoxamine)	Manufacturer advises avoid
Moxonidine	Manufacturer advises avoid—no information available
Mupirocin	Manufacturer advises avoid unless potential benefit outweighs risk—no information available
Mycophenolate mofetil	Manufacturer advises avoid—congenital malformations reported; effective contraception required during and for 6 weeks after discontinuation of treatment
Nabilone	Manufacturer advises avoid unless essential
Nabumetone	*see* NSAIDs
Nadolol	*see* Beta-blockers
Nafarelin	Avoid
Nalidixic acid	*see* Quinolones
Naloxone	Manufacturer advises use only if potential benefit outweighs risk
Naltrexone	Manufacturers advise use only if potential benefit outweighs risk
Nandrolone	*see* Anabolic Steroids
Naproxen	*see* NSAIDs
Naratriptan	*see* $5HT_1$ Agonists
Narcotic analgesics	*see* Opioid Analgesics
Natalizumab	Manufacturer advises avoid unless essential—toxicity in *animal* studies
Nateglinide	Manufacturer advises avoid—toxicity in *animal* studies; insulin is normally substituted during pregnancy in all diabetics
Nebivolol	*see* Beta-blockers
Nedocromil	*see* section 3.1
Nefopam	No information available—manufacturer advises avoid unless no safer treatment
Nelarabine	Avoid (toxicity in *animal* studies); manufacturer advises effective contraception during and for at least 3 months after treatment in men and women; see also Section 8.1
Nelfinavir	No information available—manufacturer advises use only if potential benefit outweighs risk
Neomycin	*see* Aminoglycosides
Neostigmine	Manufacturer advises use only if potential benefit outweighs risk
Nevirapine	Although manufacturers advise avoid, may be appropriate to use if clearly indicated; *see also* p. 328
Nicardipine	May inhibit labour; manufacturer advises avoid, but risk to fetus should be balanced against risk of uncontrolled maternal hypertension
Nicorandil	Manufacturer advises use only if potential benefit outweighs risk—no information available
Nicotine	Use only if smoking cessation without nicotine replacement fails; intermittent therapy preferable but avoid liquorice-flavoured nicotine products
Nicotinic acid	No information available—manufacturer advises avoid unless potential benefit outweighs risk
Nicoumalone	*see* Anticoagulants, Oral
Nifedipine	May inhibit labour; manufacturer advises avoid, but risk to fetus should be balanced against risk of uncontrolled maternal hypertension
Nimodipine	Manufacturer advises use only if potential benefit outweighs risk
Nisoldipine	Avoid (toxicity in *animal* studies)
Nitisinone	Manufacturer advises avoid unless potential benefit outweighs risk—toxicity in *animal* studies
Nitrazepam	*see* Benzodiazepines
Nitrofurantoin (3)	May produce neonatal haemolysis if used at term
Nitroprusside	*see* Sodium Nitroprusside

Drug (trimester of risk)	Comment
Nitrous oxide	*see* Anaesthetics, General
Nizatidine	Manufacturer advises avoid unless essential
Noradrenaline (norepinephrine) (1, 2, 3)	Avoid—may reduce placental perfusion
Norethisterone	Masculinisation of female fetuses and other defects reported; *see also* Contraceptives, Oral
Norfloxacin	*see* Quinolones
Norgestimate	*see* Contraceptives, Oral
Norgestrel	*see* Contraceptives, Oral
Nortriptyline	*see* Antidepressants, Tricyclic (and related)
NSAIDs	Most manufacturers advise avoid (or avoid unless potential benefit outweighs risk); ketorolac contra-indicated during pregnancy, labour and delivery
(3)	With regular use closure of fetal ductus arteriosus *in utero* and possibly persistent pulmonary hypertension of the newborn. Delayed onset and increased duration of labour
Nystatin	No information available, but absorption from gastro-intestinal tract negligible
Octreotide (1, 2, 3)	Possible effect on fetal growth; manufacturer advises use only if potential benefit outweighs risk
Oestrogens	*see* Contraceptives, Oral
Ofloxacin	*see* Quinolones
Olanzapine (3)	Manufacturer advises use only if potential benefit outweighs risk; neonatal lethargy, tremor, and hypertonia reported
Olmesartan	*As for* ACE inhibitors
Olsalazine	Manufacturer advises avoid unless potential benefit outweighs risk
Omalizumab	Manufacturer advises avoid unless essential; no evidence of teratogenicity in *animal* studies
Omega-3-acid ethyl esters	Manufacturer advises use only if potential benefit outweighs risk—no information available
Omeprazole	Not known to be harmful
Ondansetron	No information available; manufacturer advises avoid unless potential benefit outweighs risk
Opioid analgesics (3)	Depress neonatal respiration; withdrawal effects in neonates of dependent mothers; gastric stasis and risk of inhalation pneumonia in mother during labour; *see also* Tramadol
Oral contraceptives	*see* Contraceptives, Oral
Orlistat	Manufacturer advises caution
Orphenadrine	Manufacturer advises caution

Drug (trimester of risk)	Comment
Oseltamivir	Manufacturer advises avoid unless potential benefit outweighs risk
Oxaliplatin	Manufacturer advises avoid—toxicity in *animal* studies; effective contraception required during and for 4 months after treatment in women and 6 months after treatment in men; *see also* section 8.1
Oxazepam	*see* Benzodiazepines
Oxcarbazepine	Risk of teratogenesis including increased risk of neural tube defects; *see also* Antiepileptics
Oxprenolol	*see* Beta-blockers
Oxybutynin	Manufacturer advises avoid unless potential benefit outweighs risk—toxicity in *animal* studies
Oxycodone	*see* Opioid Analgesics
Oxytetracycline	*see* Tetracyclines
Paclitaxel	Avoid (toxicity in *animal* studies); ensure effective contraception during and for at least 6 months after treatment in men or women; *see also* section 8.1
Palifermin	Manufacturer advises avoid unless potential benefit outweighs risk—toxicity in *animal* studies
Paliperidone	Manufacturer advises use only if potential benefit outweighs risk—toxicity in *animal* studies
Palonosetron	Manufacturer advises avoid—no information available
Pamidronate disodium	*see* Bisphosphonates
Pancreatin	Not known to be harmful
Pancuronium	Manufacturer advises avoid unless potential benefit outweighs risk—no information available
Pantoprazole	Manufacturer advises avoid unless potential benefit outweighs risk—fetotoxic in *animals*
Papaveretum	*see* Opioid Analgesics
Paracetamol	Not known to be harmful
Paraldehyde	Manufacturer advises avoid unless essential—crosses the placenta
Parecoxib	*see* NSAIDS
Paricalcitol	Toxicity in *animal* studies—manufacturer advises avoid unless potential benefit outweighs risk; *see also* Vitamin D
Paroxetine	*see* Antidepressants, SSRI
Pegaptinib	Manufacturer advises avoid unless potential benefit outweighs risk
Pegfilgrastim	Toxicity in *animal* studies; manufacturer advises use only if potential benefit ouweighs risk

Appendix 4: Pregnancy

Drug (trimester of risk)	Comment
Pemetrexed	Avoid (toxicity in *animal* studies); manufacturer advises effective contraception during treatment; men must avoid fathering a child during and for at least 6 months after treatment; *see also* section 8.1
Penicillamine (1, 2, 3)	Fetal abnormalities reported rarely; avoid if possible
Penicillins	Not known to be harmful
Pentamidine isetionate	Manufacturer advises avoid unless essential
Pentazocine	*see* Opioid Analgesics
Pentostatin	Avoid (teratogenic in *animal* studies); manufacturer advises that men should not father children during and for 6 months after treatment; *see also* section 8.1
Pergolide	Manufacturer advises use only if potential benefit outweighs risk
Pericyazine	*see* Antipsychotics
Perindopril	*see* ACE Inhibitors
Perphenazine	*see* Antipsychotics
Pethidine	*see* Opioid Analgesics
Phenelzine	*see* Antidepressants, MAOI
Phenindione	*see* Anticoagulants, Oral
Phenobarbital	Congenital malformations; *see also* Antiepileptics
Phenothiazines	*see* Antipsychotics
Phenoxybenzamine	Hypotension may occur in newborn
Phenoxymethylpenicillin	*see* Penicillins
Phentolamine	Use with caution—may cause marked decrease in maternal blood pressure with resulting fetal anoxia
Phenylephrine	
(1)	Malformations reported
(3)	Avoid if possible—fetal hypoxia and bradycardia reported in late pregnancy and labour
Phenytoin	Congenital malformations; caution in interpreting plasma concentrations—bound may be reduced but free (i.e. effective) unchanged; *see also* Antiepileptics
Pholcodine	*see* Opioid Analgesics
Phytomenadione	Manufacturer advises use only if potential benefit outweighs risk—no specific information available
Pilocarpine	Avoid—smooth muscle stimulant; toxicity in *animal* studies
Pimozide	*see* Antipsychotics
Pindolol	*see* Beta-blockers
Pioglitazone	Manufacturer advises avoid—toxicity in *animal* studies; insulin is normally substituted during pregnancy in all diabetics
Piperacillin [ingredient]	*see Tazocin®*
Piperazine	Not known to be harmful but manufacturer advises avoid in first trimester
Pipotiazine	*see* Antipsychotics
Piracetam	Manufacturer advises avoid
Piroxicam	*see* NSAIDs
Pivmecillinam	*see* Penicillins
Pizotifen	Manufacturer advises avoid unless potential benefit outweighs risk
Podophyllum	Avoid—neonatal death and teratogenesis have been reported
Polystyrene sulphonate resins	Manufacturers advise use only if potential benefit outweighs risk—no information available
Porfimer	Manufacturer advises avoid unless essential
Posaconazole	Manufacturer advises avoid unless potential benefit outweighs risk and recommends effective contraception during treatment; toxicity in *animal* studies
Povidone–iodine (2, 3)	Sufficient iodine may be absorbed to affect the fetal thyroid
Pramipexole	Manufacturer advises use only if potential benefit outweighs risk—no information available
Pravastatin	*see* Statins
Prazosin	*see* Alpha-blockers, Post-synaptic
Prednisolone	*see* Corticosteroids
Pregabalin	Toxicity in *animal* studies—manufacturer advises use only if potential benefit outweighs risk; *see also* Antiepileptics
Prilocaine (3)	Neonatal methaemoglobinaemia reported after paracervical block or pudendal block; *see also* Anaesthetics, Local
Primaquine (3)	Neonatal haemolysis and methaemoglobinaemia; *see also* Antimalarials
Primaxin®	Manufacturer advises avoid unless potential benefit outweighs risk (toxicity in *animal* studies)
Primidone	*see* Phenobarbital
Procainamide	Manufacturer advises avoid unless potential benefit outweighs risk
Procaine (3)	Neonatal methaemoglobinaemia; *see also* Anaesthetics, Local
Procarbazine	Avoid (teratogenic in *animal* studies and isolated reports in humans); *see also* section 8.1
Prochlorperazine	*see* Antipsychotics

Drug (trimester of risk)	Comment
Procyclidine	Manufacturers advise use only if potential benefit outweighs risk
Progesterone	Not known to be harmful
Proguanil	Adequate folate supplements should be given to mother; *see also* Antimalarials
Promazine	*see* Antipsychotics
Promethazine	*see* Antihistamines
Propafenone	Manufacturer advises avoid—no information available
Propantheline	Manufacturer advises avoid—no information available
Propiverine	Manufacturer advises avoid (restriction of skeletal development in *animals*)
Propofol	*see* Anaesthetics, General
Propranolol	*see* Beta-blockers
Propylthiouracil	
(2, 3)	Neonatal goitre and hypothyroidism
Protionamide	
(1)	May be teratogenic
Pseudoephedrine	Defective closure of the abdominal wall (gastroschisis) reported very rarely in newborns after first trimester exposure
Pyrazinamide	Manufacturer advises use only if potential benefit outweighs risk; see also p. 310
Pyridostigmine	Manufacturer advises use only if potential benefit outweighs risk
Pyrimethamine	
(1)	Theoretical teratogenic risk (folate antagonist); adequate folate supplements should be given to mother; *see also* Antimalarials
Quetiapine	Manufacturer advises use only if potential benefit outweighs risk
Quinagolide	Manufacturer advises discontinue when pregnancy confirmed unless medical reason for continuing
Quinapril	*see* ACE Inhibitors
Quinine	
(1)	High doses are teratogenic; but in malaria benefit of treatment outweighs risk
Quinolones	
(1, 2, 3)	Avoid—arthropathy in *animal* studies; safer alternatives available
Quinupristin [ingredient]	*see Synercid®*
Rabeprazole	Manufacturer advises avoid—no information available
Raltitrexed	Pregnancy must be excluded before treatment; ensure effective contraception during and for at least 6 months after treatment in men or women; *see also* section 8.1
Ramipril	*see* ACE Inhibitors
Ranibizumab	Manufacturer advises avoid unless potential benefit outweighs risk and recommends effective contraception during treatment
Ranitidine	Manufacturer advises avoid unless essential, but not known to be harmful
Rasagiline	Manufacturer advises caution
Rasburicase	Manufacturer advises avoid—no information available
Reboxetine	Manufacturer advises avoid (and discontinue if pregnancy occurs)—no information available
Remifentanil	No information available; *see also* Opioid Analgesics
Repaglinide	Manufacturer advises avoid; insulin is normally substituted during pregnancy in all diabetics
Reteplase	*see* Fibrinolytics
Riamet®	Toxicity in *animal* studies with artemether; manufacturer advises use only if potential benefit outweighs risk
Ribavirin	Avoid; teratogenicity in *animal* studies; ensure effective contraception during oral administration and for 4 months after treatment in women and for 7 months after treatment in men; *see also* Ribavirin section 5.3.5
Rifabutin	Manufacturer advises avoid—no information available
Rifampicin	
(1)	Manufacturers advise very high doses teratogenic in *animal* studies; *see also* p. 310
(3)	Risk of neonatal bleeding may be increased
Riluzole	No information available; manufacturer advises avoid
Rimonabant	Manufacturer advises avoid
Risedronate sodium	*see* Bisphosphonates
Risperidone	Manufacturer advises use only if potential benefit outweighs risk.
(3)	Extrapyramidal effects reported in neonates
Ritodrine	For use in premature labour *see* section 7.1.3
Ritonavir	Manufacturer advises use only if potential benefit outweighs risk—no information available
Rituximab	Avoid unless potential benefit to mother outweighs risk of B-lymphocyte depletion in fetus—effective contraception required during and for 12 months after treatment
Rivastigmine	Manufacturer advises use only if potential benefit outweighs risk
Rizatriptan	*see* $5HT_1$ Agonists

Drug (trimester of risk)	Comment
Rocuronium	Manufacturer advises avoid unless potential benefit outweighs risk
Ropinirole (1)	Manufacturer advises avoid unless potential benefit outweighs risk—toxicity in *animal* studies
Ropivacaine	Safety not established but not known to be harmful
Rosiglitazone	Manufacturer advises avoid—toxicity in *animal* studies; insulin is normally substituted during pregnancy in all diabetics
Rosuvastatin	*see* Statins
Rotigotine	Manufacturer advises avoid—no information available
Rufinamide	Manufacturer advises avoid unless potential benefit outweighs risk—fetotoxic in *animal* studies; effective contraception must be used during treatment; *see also* Antiepileptics
Salbutamol	For use in asthma *see* section 3.1
(3)	For use in premature labour *see* section 7.1.3
Salcatonin	*see* Calcitonin (salmon)
Salmeterol	*see* section 3.1
Saquinavir	Manufacturer advises use only if potential benefit outweighs risk
Selegiline	Manufacturer advises avoid—no information available
Sertindole	Manufacturer advises avoid
Sertraline	*see* Antidepressants, SSRI
Sevelamer	Manufacturer advises use only if potential benefit outweighs risk
Sevoflurane	*see* Anaesthetics, General
Sibutramine	Manufacturer advises avoid—toxicity in *animal* studies
Sildenafil	Manufacturer advises use only if potential benefit outweighs risk—toxicity in *animal* studies
Silver sulfadiazine	*see* Sulphonamides
Simvastatin	*see* Statins
Sirolimus	Manufacturer advises avoid (toxicity in *animal* studies); effective contraception must be used during treatment and for 12 weeks after stopping
Sitagliptin	Manufacturer advises avoid—toxicity in *animal* studies; insulin is normally substituted during pregnancy in all diabetics
Sitaxentan sodium	Avoid unless essential—toxicity in *animal* studies; manufacturer advises effective contraception during treatment
Sodium aurothiomalate	Manufacturer advises avoid but limited data suggests usually not necessary to withdraw if condition well controlled—consider reducing dose and frequency
Sodium clodronate	*see* Bisphosphonates
Sodium cromoglicate	Not known to be harmful; *see also* section 3.1
Sodium fusidate	Not known to be harmful; manufacturer advises use only if potential benefit outweighs risk
Sodium nitroprusside	Potential for accumulation of cyanide in fetus—avoid prolonged use
Sodium oxybate	Manufacturer advises avoid
Sodium phenylbutyrate	Avoid (toxicity in *animal* studies); manufacturer advises adequate contraception during administration
Sodium stibogluconate	Manufacturer advises use only if potential benefit outweighs risk
Sodium valproate	*see* Valproate
Solifenacin	Manufacturer advises caution—no information available
Somatropin	Discontinue if pregnancy occurs—no information available but theoretical risk
Sorafenib	Manufacturer advises avoid unless essential—toxicity in *animal* studies; *see also* section 8.1
Sotalol	*see* Beta-blockers
Spironolactone	Manufacturers advise toxicity in *animal* studies
Statins	Avoid—congenital anomalies reported; decreased synthesis of cholesterol possibly affects fetal development
Stavudine	Manufacturer advises use only if potential benefit outweighs risk
Streptokinase	*see* Fibrinolytics
Streptomycin	*see* Aminoglycosides
Strontium ranelate	Avoid—toxicity in *animal* studies
Sulfadiazine	*see* Sulphonamides
Sulfadoxine	*see* Sulphonamides
Sulfasalazine (3)	Theoretical risk of neonatal haemolysis; adequate folate supplements should be given to mother
Sulindac	*see* NSAIDs
Sulphonamides (3)	Neonatal haemolysis and methaemoglobinaemia; fear of increased risk of kernicterus in neonates appears to be unfounded

Drug (trimester of risk)	Comment
Sulphonylureas	
(3)	Neonatal hypoglycaemia; insulin is normally substituted during pregnancy in all diabetics; if oral drugs are used therapy should be stopped at least 2 days before delivery
Sulpiride	*see* Antipsychotics
Sumatriptan	*see* $5HT_1$ Agonists
Sunitinib	Manufacturer advises avoid unless potential benefit outweighs risk—toxicity in *animal* studies; *see also* section 8.1
Suxamethonium	Mildly prolonged maternal paralysis may occur
Synercid®	Manufacturer advises avoid unless potential benefit outweighs risk—no information available
Tacalcitol	Manufacturer advises avoid unless no safer alternative—no information available; *see also* Vitamin D
Tacrolimus	Avoid; manufacturer advises toxicity in *animal* studies following systemic administration
Tamoxifen	Avoid—possible effects on fetal development; effective contraception must be used during treatment and for 2 months after stopping
Tazarotene	Avoid; effective contraception required (oral progestogen-only contraceptives not considered effective)
Tazobactam [ingredient]	*see Tazocin*®
Tazocin®	Manufacturer advises use only if potential benefit outweighs risk
Tegafur with uracil	*see Uftoral*®
Teicoplanin	Manufacturer advises use only if potential benefit outweighs risk
Telbivudine	Manufacturer advises use only if potential benefit outweighs risk
Telithromycin	Toxicity in animal studies—manufacturer advises use only if potential benefit outweighs risk
Telmisartan	*As for* ACE Inhibitors
Temazepam	*see* Benzodiazepines
Temocillin	Temocillin *see* Penicillins
Temoporfin	Toxicity in *animal* studies—manufacturer advises avoid pregnancy for at least 3 months after treatment
Temozolomide	Avoid (teratogenic and embryotoxic in *animal* studies); manufacturer advises adequate contraception during treatment; *see also* section 8.1; also men should avoid fathering a child during and for at least 6 months after treatment
Tenecteplase	*see* Fibrinolytics
Tenofovir	No information available—manufacturer advises use only if potential benefit outweighs risk
Tenoxicam	*see* NSAIDs
Terazosin	*see* Alpha-blockers, Post-synaptic
Terbinafine	Manufacturer advises use only if potential benefit outweighs risk—no information available
Terbutaline	For use in asthma *see* section 3.1
(3)	For use in premature labour *see* section 7.1.3
Testosterone	*see* Androgens
Tetrabenazine	Inadequate information but no evidence of harm
Tetracyclines	
(1)	Effects on skeletal development in *animal* studies
(2, 3)	Dental discoloration; maternal hepatotoxicity with large parenteral doses
Theophylline	
(3)	Neonatal irritability and apnoea have been reported
Thiazides and related diuretics	*see* Diuretics
Thiopental	*see* Anaesthetics, General
Thiotepa	Avoid (teratogenic and embryotoxic in *animals*); *see also* section 8.1
Thymoxamine	*see* Moxisylyte
Thyroxine	*see* Levothyroxine
Tiagabine	Manufacturer advises avoid unless potential benefit outweighs risk; *see also* Antiepileptics
Tiaprofenic acid	*see* NSAIDs
Ticarcillin [ingredient]	*see* Penicillins
Tigecycline	*see* Tetracyclines
Tiludronic acid	*see* Bisphosphonates
Timentin®	*see* Penicillins
Timolol	*see* Beta-blockers
Tinidazole	Manufacturer advises avoid in first trimester
Tinzaparin	Not known to be harmful
Tioconazole	Manufacturer advises avoid
Tioguanine	Avoid (teratogenicity reported when men receiving tioguanine have fathered children); ensure effective contraception during treatment in men or women; *see also* section 8.1
Tiotropium	Toxicity in *animal* studies—manufacturer advises use only if potential benefit outweighs risk
Tipranavir	Manufacturer advises use only if potential benefit outweighs risk—toxicity in *animal* studies
Tirofiban	Manufacturer advises use only if potential benefit outweighs risk—no information available
Tizanidine	Manufacturer advises use only if potential benefit outweighs risk—no information available

Drug (trimester of risk)	Comment
Tobramycin	*see* Aminoglycosides
Tocopheryl acetate (1, 2, 3)	No evidence of safety of high doses
Tolbutamide	*see* Sulphonylureas
Tolcapone	Toxicity in *animal* studies—manufacturer advises use only if potential benefit outweighs risk
Tolfenamic acid	*see* NSAIDs
Tolterodine	Manufacturer advises avoid—toxicity in *animal* studies
Topiramate	Manufacturer advises avoid unless potential benefit outweighs risk—toxicity in *animal* studies; *see also* Antiepileptics
Topotecan	Avoid (teratogenicity and fetal loss in *animal* studies); *see also* section 8.1
Torasemide	*see* Diuretics
Trabectedin	Effective contraception recommended during and for at least 3 months after treatment in women and at least 5 months after treatment in men; *see also* section 8.1
Tramadol	Embryotoxic in animal studies—manufacturers advise avoid; *see also* Opioid Analgesics
Trandolapril	*see* ACE Inhibitors
Tranexamic acid	No evidence of teratogenicity in *animal* studies; manufacturer advises use only if potential benefit outweighs risk—crosses the placenta
Tranylcypromine	*see* Antidepressants, MAOI
Trastuzumab	Avoid unless potential benefit outweighs risk
Travoprost	Manufacturer advises use only if potential benefit outweighs risk
Trazodone	*see* Antidepressants, Tricyclic (and related)
Treosulfan	Avoid; *see also* section 8.1
Tretinoin (1, 2, 3)	Teratogenic; effective contraception must be used for at least 1 month before oral treatment, during treatment and for at least 1 month after stopping (oral progestogen-only contraceptives not considered effective); also avoid topical treatment
Triamcinolone	*see* Corticosteroids
Triamterene	*see* Diuretics
Tribavirin	*see* Ribavirin
Triclofos	Avoid
Trientine	Manufacturer advises use only if potential benefit outweighs risk; monitor maternal and neonatal serum-copper concentration; teratogenic in *animal* studies
Trifluoperazine	*see* Antipsychotics
Trihexyphenidyl	Manufacturer advises use only if potential benefit outweighs risk
Trilostane (1, 2, 3)	Interferes with placental sex hormone production
Trimeprazine	*see* Antihistamines
Trimethoprim (1)	Teratogenic risk (folate antagonist); manufacturers advise avoid
Trimipramine	*see* Antidepressants, Tricyclic (and related)
Tripotassium dicitratobismuthate	Manufacturer advises avoid on theoretical grounds
Triptorelin	Manufacturers advise avoid
Tropisetron	Manufacturer advises toxicity in *animal* studies
Trospium	Manufacturer advises caution—no information available
Uftoral®	Avoid; manufacturer advises effective contraception during and for 3 months after treatment in men or women
Urokinase	*see* Fibrinolytics
Ursodeoxycholic acid	No evidence of harm but manufacturer advises avoid
Vaccines (live) (1)	Theoretical risk of congenital malformations, but need for vaccination may outweigh possible risk to fetus (*see also* p. 641); avoid MMR vaccine but *see* p. 657
Valaciclovir	*see* Aciclovir
Valganciclovir	*see* Ganciclovir
Valproate (1, 3)	Increased risk of congenital malformations and developmental delay (counselling and screening advised—**important:** *see also* Antiepileptics and p. 245); neonatal bleeding (related to hypofibrinaemia) and neonatal hepatotoxicity also reported
Valproic acid	*see* Valproate
Valsartan	*As for* ACE Inhibitors
Vancomycin	Manufacturer advises use only if potential benefit outweighs risk—plasma-vancomycin concentration monitoring essential to reduce risk of fetal toxicity
Varenicline	Manufacturer advises avoid—toxicity in *animal* studies
Vasopressin	Oxytocic effect in third trimester
Vecuronium	Manufacturer advises avoid unless potential benefit outweighs risk—no information available
Venlafaxine	Manufacturer advises avoid unless potential benefit outweighs risk; risk of withdrawal effects in neonate

Drug (trimester of risk)	Comment
Verapamil	May reduce uterine blood flow with fetal hypoxia; manufacturer advises avoid in first trimester unless absolutely necessary; may inhibit labour
Verteporfin	Manufacturer advises use only if potential benefit outweighs risk (teratogenic in *animal* studies)
Vigabatrin	Congenital anomalies reported—manufacturer advises avoid unless potential benefit outweighs risk; *see also* Antiepileptics
Vinblastine	Avoid (limited experience suggests fetal harm; teratogenic in *animal* studies); *see also* section 8.1
Vincristine	Avoid (teratogenicity and fetal loss in *animal* studies); *see also* section 8.1
Vindesine	Avoid (teratogenic in *animal* studies); *see also* section 8.1
Vinorelbine	Avoid (teratogenicity and fetal loss in *animal* studies); *see also* section 8.1
Vitamin A (1)	Excessive doses may be teratogenic; *see also* p. 523
Vitamin D	High systemic doses teratogenic in *animals* but therapeutic doses unlikely to be harmful; avoid *topical* calcitriol—use in restricted amounts if clearly necessary (significant systemic absorption; monitor urine and plasma-calcium concentration); *see also* Calcipotriol, Paricalcitol, and Tacalcitol
Voriconazole	Toxicity in *animal* studies—manufacturer advises avoid unless potential benefit outweighs risk; effective contraception required during treatment
Warfarin	*see* Anticoagulants, Oral
Xipamide	*see* Diuretics
Zafirlukast	Manufacturer advises use only if potential benefit outweighs risk
Zaleplon	Use only if necessary and restrict to occasional short-term use; risk of withdrawal symptoms in neonate if used in late pregnancy
Zanamivir	Manufacturer advises use only if potential benefit outweighs risk—no information available
Zidovudine	Limited information available; manufacturer advises use only if clearly indicated; *see also* p. 328
Zinc acetate	Usual dose 25 mg 3 times daily adjusted according to plasma-copper concentration and urinary copper excretion
Zinc sulphate	Safety not established—crosses placenta
Zoledronic acid	Manufacturer advises avoid—toxicity in *animal* studies
Zolmitriptan	*see* $5HT_1$ Agonists
Zolpidem	*see* Benzodiazepines
Zonisamide	Toxicity in *animal* studies; manufacturer advises use only if potential benefit outweighs risk—effective contraception required during and for 4 weeks after treatment; *see also* Antiepileptics
Zopiclone	*see* Benzodiazepines
Zotepine	Manufacturer advises avoid unless potential benefit outweighs risk
Zuclopenthixol	*see* Antipsychotics

A5 Breast-feeding

Breast-feeding is beneficial; the immunological and nutritional value of breast milk to the infant is greater than that of formula feeds.

Although there is concern that drugs taken by the mother might affect the infant, there is very little information on this. In the absence of evidence of an effect, the potential for harm to the infant can be inferred from:

- the amount of drug or active metabolite of the drug delivered to the infant (dependent on the pharmacokinetic characteristics of the drug in the mother);
- the efficiency of absorption, distribution and elimination of the drug by the infant (infant pharmacokinetics);
- the nature of the effect of the drug on the infant (pharmacodynamic properties of the drug in the infant).

The amount of drug transferred in breast milk is rarely sufficient to produce a discernible effect on the infant. This applies particularly to drugs that are poorly absorbed and need to be given parenterally. However, there is a theoretical possibility that the small amount of drug present in breast milk can induce a hypersensitivity reaction.

A clinical effect can occur in the infant if a pharmacologically significant quantity of the drug is present in milk. For some drugs (e.g. fluvastatin), the ratio between the concentration in milk and that in maternal plasma may be high enough to expose the infant to adverse effects. Some infants, such at those born prematurely or who have jaundice, are at a slightly higher risk of toxicity.

Some drugs inhibit the infant's sucking reflex (e.g. phenobarbital) while others can affect lactation (e.g. bromocriptine)

The following table identifies drugs:

- that should be used with caution or are contra-indicated in breast-feeding;
- which can be given to the mother during breast-feeding because they are present in milk in amounts which are too small to be harmful to the infant;
- which might be present in milk in significant amount but are not known to be harmful.

> For many drugs insufficient evidence is available to provide guidance and it is advisable to use only essential drugs to a mother during breast-feeding. Because of the inadequacy of information on drugs in breast-feeding, absence from the table does not imply safety.

Table of drugs present in breast milk

Products introduced or amended since publication of BNF No. 54 (September 2007) are underlined.

Drug	Comment
Abacavir	Breast-feeding not advised in HIV infection
Abatacept	Present in milk in *animal* studies—manufacturer advises avoid breast-feeding during treatment and for 14 weeks after last dose
Abciximab	Manufacturer advises avoid—no information available
Acamprosate	Manufacturer advises avoid
Acarbose	Manufacturer advises avoid
Acebutolol	*see* Beta-blockers
Aceclofenac	Manufacturer advises avoid—no information available
Acemetacin	Manufacturer advises avoid
Acenocoumarol (nicoumalone)	*see* Anticoagulants, Oral
Acetazolamide	Amount too small to be harmful
Aciclovir	Significant amount in milk after systemic administration—not known to be harmful but manufacturer advises caution
Acipimox	Manufacturer advises avoid
Acitretin	Avoid
Adalimumab	Avoid; manufacturer advises avoid for at least 5 months after last dose
Adapalene	Manufacturer advises avoid (if used, avoid application to chest)—no information available
Adefovir dipivoxil	Manufacturer advises avoid—no information available
Agalsidase	Use with caution—no information available
Alcohol	Large amounts may affect infant and reduce milk consumption
Alemtuzumab	Avoid; manufacturer advises avoid breast-feeding for at least 4 weeks after administration
Alendronic acid	No information available
Alfacalcidol	*see* Vitamin D
Alfentanil	Present in milk—manufacturer advises withhold breast-feeding for 24 hours
Alglucosidase alfa	Manufacturer advises avoid—no information available
Alimemazine (trimeprazine)	*see* Antihistamines
<u>Aliskiren</u>	Present in milk in *animal* studies—manufacturer advises avoid
Allopurinol	Present in milk—not known to be harmful

Drug	Comment
Almotriptan	Present in milk in *animal* studies—withhold breast-feeding for 24 hours
Alprazolam	*see* Benzodiazepines
Alverine	Manufacturer advises avoid—little information available
Amantadine	Avoid; present in milk; toxicity in infant reported
Amfebutamone	*see* Bupropion
Amiloride	Manufacturer advises avoid—no information available
Aminophylline	*see* Theophylline
Amiodarone	Avoid; present in milk in significant amounts; theoretical risk from release of iodine; *see also* Iodine
Amisulpride	Manufacturer advises avoid—no information available
Amitriptyline	*see* Antidepressants, Tricyclic (and related)
Amlodipine	Manufacturer advises avoid—no information available
Amobarbital	*see* Barbiturates
Amorolfine	Manufacturer advises avoid—no information available
Amoxicillin	*see* Penicillins
Amphetamines	Significant amount in milk. Avoid
Amphotericin	No information available
Ampicillin	*see* Penicillins
Amprenavir	Breast-feeding not advised in HIV infection
Amsacrine	*see* Cytotoxic Drugs
Anagrelide	Manufacturer advises avoid—no information available
Anakinra	Manufacturer advises avoid—no information available
Analgesics	*see* Aspirin, NSAIDs, Opioid Analgesics and Paracetamol
Androgens	Avoid; may cause masculinisation in the female infant or precocious development in the male infant; high doses suppress lactation
Anidulafungin	Manufacturer advises avoid unless potential benefit outweighs risk—present in milk in *animal* studies
Anticoagulants, oral	Risk of haemorrhage; increased by vitamin-K deficiency; warfarin appears safe but phenindione should be avoided; manufacturer of acenocoumarol (nicoumalone) recommends prophylactic vitamin K for the infant (consult product literature)
Antidepressants, SSRI	*see* individual entries
Antidepressants, tricyclic (and related)	Amount of tricyclic antidepressants (including related drugs such as mianserin and trazodone) too small to be harmful but most manufacturers advise avoid; accumulation of doxepin metabolite may cause sedation and respiratory depression
Antihistamines	Significant amount of some antihistamines present in milk; although not known to be harmful, manufacturers of alimemazine, cetirizine, cinnarizine, cyproheptadine, desloratadine, dimenhydrinate, fexofenadine, hydroxyzine, loratadine, and mizolastine advise avoid; manufacturer of ketotifen advises avoid; adverse effects in infant reported with clemastine
Antipsychotics	Although amount present in milk probably too small to be harmful, *animal* studies indicate possible adverse effects of these drugs on developing nervous system therefore avoid unless absolutely necessary; *see also* Amisulpride, Chlorpromazine, Clozapine, Olanzapine, Paliperidone, Quetiapine, Risperidone, Sertindole, Sulpiride, Zotepine
Apomorphine	Manufacturer advises avoid—no information available
Aprepitant	Manufacturer advises avoid—present in milk in *animal* studies
Aripiprazole	Manufacturer advises avoid—present in milk in *animal* studies
Arsenic trioxide	*see* Cytotoxic Drugs
Artemether [ingredient]	*see Riamet*®
Aspirin	Avoid—possible risk of Reye's syndrome; regular use of high doses could impair platelet function and produce hypoprothrombinaemia in infant if neonatal vitamin K stores low
Atazanavir	Breast-feeding not advised in HIV infection
Atenolol	*see* Beta-blockers
Atomoxetine	Manufacturer advises avoid—present in milk in *animal* studies
Atorvastatin	*see* Statins
Atosiban	Small amounts present in milk
Atovaquone	Manufacturer advises avoid; for malaria prophylaxis or treatment *see Malarone*®
Atracurium	Breast-feeding unlikely to be harmful following recovery from neuromuscular block; some manufacturers advise avoiding breast-feeding for 24 hours after administration
Atropine	Small amount present in milk—manufacturer advises caution
Auranofin	Present in milk; manufacturer advises avoid
Azapropazone	Small amount present in milk—manufacturer advises avoid
Azathioprine	*see* Cytotoxic Drugs
Azithromycin	Present in milk; use only if no suitable alternative

Drug	Comment
Aztreonam	Amount probably too small to be harmful—manufacturer advises avoid
Baclofen	Amount too small to be harmful
Balsalazide	Manufacturer advises avoid
Barbiturates	Avoid if possible (*see also* Phenobarbital); large doses may produce drowsiness
Basiliximab	Avoid
Beclometasone	*see* Corticosteroids
Bemiparin	Manufacturer advises avoid—no information available
Bendrofluazide	*see* Thiazides and Related Diuretics
Bendroflumethiazide (bendrofluazide)	*see* Thiazides and Related Diuretics
Benperidol	*see* Antipsychotics
Benzatropine	Manufacturer advises caution—no information available
Benzodiazepines	Present in milk—avoid if possible; *see also* Midazolam
Benzylpenicillin	*see* Penicillins
Beta-blockers	Monitor infant; possible toxicity due to beta-blockade but amount of most beta-blockers present in milk too small to affect infant; acebutolol, atenolol, nadolol, and sotalol are present in greater amounts than other beta-blockers; manufacturers advise avoid celiprolol and nebivolol
Betamethasone	*see* Corticosteroids
Bethanechol	Manufacturer advises avoid
Bevacizumab	Manufacturer advises avoid breast-feeding during and for at least 6 months after treatment
Bexarotene	*see* Cytotoxic Drugs
Bezafibrate	Manufacturer advises avoid—no information available
Bimatoprost	Manufacturer advises avoid
Bisoprolol	*see* Beta-blockers
Bivalirudin	Manufacturer advises caution—no information available
Bleomycin	*see* Cytotoxic Drugs
Bortezomib	*see* Cytotoxic Drugs
Bosentan	Manufacturer advises avoid—no information available
Botulinum toxin	Manufacturers advise avoid (or avoid unless essential)—no information available
Bromocriptine	Suppresses lactation
Buclizine	*see* Antihistamines
Budesonide	*see* Corticosteroids
Bumetanide	Manufacturer advises avoid if possible—no information available
Bupivacaine	Amount too small to be harmful
Buprenorphine	Avoid unless essential—may inhibit lactation; manufacturer advises contra-indicated in the treatment of opioid dependence
Bupropion	Present in milk—manufacturer advises avoid
Buserelin	Small amount present in milk—manufacturer advises avoid
Buspirone	Manufacturer advises avoid
Busulfan	*see* Cytotoxic Drugs
Butobarbital	*see* Barbiturates
Cabergoline	Suppresses lactation
Caffeine	Regular intake of large amounts can affect infant
Calciferol	*see* Vitamin D
Calcipotriol	No information available; *see also* Vitamin D
Calcitonin (salmon) (salcatonin)	Avoid; inhibits lactation in *animals*
Calcitriol	*see* Vitamin D
Calcium folinate	Manufacturer advises caution—no information available
Calcium levofolinate	*see* Calcium Folinate
Candesartan	Manufacturer advises avoid—no information available
Capecitabine	Discontinue breast-feeding
Capreomycin	Manufacturer advises caution—no information available
Captopril	Present in milk—manufacturers advise avoid
Carbamazepine	Amount probably too small to be harmful
Carbimazole	Amounts in milk may be sufficient to affect neonatal thyroid function therefore lowest effective dose should be used (*see also* section 6.2.2)
Carbocisteine	No information available
Carboplatin	*see* Cytotoxic Drugs
Carglumic acid	Manufacturer advises avoid unless essential—no information available
Carisoprodol	Concentrated in milk; no adverse effects reported but best avoided
Carmustine	*see* Cytotoxic Drugs
Carvedilol	*see* Beta-blockers
Caspofungin	Present in milk in *animal* studies—manufacturer advises avoid
Cefaclor	Present in milk in low concentration
Cefadroxil	Present in milk in low concentration
Cefalexin	Present in milk in low concentration
Cefixime	Manufacturer advises avoid—no information available
Cefotaxime	Present in milk in low concentration
Cefpodoxime	Present in milk in low concentration
Cefradine	Present in milk in low concentration
Ceftazidime	Present in milk in low concentration
Ceftriaxone	Present in milk in low concentration
Cefuroxime	Present in milk in low concentration
Celecoxib	Manufacturer advises avoid—no information available
Celiprolol	*see* Beta-blockers

Drug	Comment
Cetirizine	*see* Antihistamines
Cetrorelix	Manufacturer advises avoid
Cetuximab	Manufacturer advises avoid breast-feeding during and for 2 months after treatment—no information available
Chloral hydrate	Sedation in infant—manufacturer advises avoid
Chlorambucil	*see* Cytotoxic Drugs
Chloramphenicol	Use another antibiotic; may cause bone-marrow toxicity in infant; concentration in milk usually insufficient to cause 'grey syndrome'
Chlordiazepoxide	*see* Benzodiazepines
Chloroquine	Amount probably too small to be harmful when used for malaria prophylaxis; inadequate for reliable protection against malaria, *see* section 5.4.1; avoid breast-feeding when used for rheumatic diseases
Chlorphenamine (chlorpheniramine)	*see* Antihistamines
Chlorpheniramine	*see* Antihistamines
Chlorpromazine	Drowsiness in infant reported; *see* Antipsychotics
Chlorpropamide	*see* Sulphonylureas
Chlortalidone	*see* Thiazides and Related Diuretics
Ciclesonide	*see* Corticosteroids
Ciclosporin	Present in milk—manufacturer advises avoid
Cidofovir	Manufacturer advises avoid
Cilastatin [ingredient]	*see Primaxin®*
Cilazapril	No information available—manufacturer advises avoid
Cilostazol	Present in milk in *animal* studies—manufacturer advises avoid
Cimetidine	Significant amount—not known to be harmful but manufacturer advises avoid
Cinacalcet	Manufacturer advises avoid—present in milk in *animal* studies
Cinnarizine	*see* Antihistamines
Ciprofibrate	Manufacturer advises avoid—present in milk in *animal* studies
Ciprofloxacin	Amount probably too small to be harmful but manufacturer advises avoid
Cisatracurium	No information available
Cisplatin	*see* Cytotoxic Drugs
Citalopram	Present in milk—manufacturer advises avoid
Cladribine	*see* Cytotoxic Drugs
Clarithromycin	Manufacturer advises avoid unless potential benefit outweighs risk—present in milk
Clavulanic acid [ingredient]	see Co-amoxiclav, *Timentin®*
Clemastine	*see* Antihistamines
Clindamycin	Amount probably too small to be harmful but bloody diarrhoea reported in 1 infant
Clobazam	*see* Benzodiazepines
Clodronate sodium	*see* Sodium Clodronate
Clofarabine	*see* Cytotoxic Drugs
Clomethiazole	Amount too small to be harmful
Clomifene	May inhibit lactation
Clomipramine	*see* Antidepressants, Tricyclic (and related)
Clonazepam	*see* Benzodiazepines
Clonidine	Present in milk—manufacturer advises avoid
Clopidogrel	Manufacturer advises avoid
Clozapine	Manufacturer advises avoid
Co-amoxiclav	*see* Penicillins
Co-beneldopa	*see* Levodopa
Co-careldopa	*see* Levodopa
Co-danthramer	Manufacturer advises avoid—limited information available
Co-danthrusate	Manufacturer advises avoid—limited information available
Codeine	Amount usually too small to be harmful; however mothers vary considerably in their capacity to metabolise codeine—fatal morphine toxicity reported in infant
Co-fluampicil	*see* Penicillins
Colchicine	Present in milk but no adverse effects reported; manufacturers advise avoid because of risk of cytotoxicity
Colecalciferol	*see* Vitamin D
Colesevelam	Use with caution—drug not absorbed but may cause fat-soluble vitamin deficiency on prolonged use
Colestipol	Use with caution—drug not absorbed but may cause fat-soluble vitamin deficiency on prolonged use
Colestyramine	Use with caution—drug not absorbed but may cause fat-soluble vitamin deficiency on prolonged use
Colistin	Present in milk but poorly absorbed from gut; manufacturers advise avoid (or use only if potential benefit outweighs risk)
Contraceptives, oral	Avoid combined oral contraceptives until weaning or for 6 months after birth (adverse effects on lactation); progestogen-only contraceptives do not affect lactation (start 3 weeks after birth or later)
Corticosteroids	Systemic effects in infant unlikely with maternal dose of prednisolone up to 40 mg daily; monitor infant's adrenal function with higher doses—the amount of inhaled drugs in breast milk is probably too small to be harmful
Cortisone acetate	*see* Corticosteroids
Co-trimoxazole	Small risk of kernicterus in jaundiced infants and of haemolysis in G6PD-deficient infants (due to sulfamethoxazole)
Crisantaspase	*see* Cytotoxic Drugs

Drug	Comment
Cromoglicate	*see* Sodium Cromoglicate
Cyclopenthiazide	*see* Thiazides and Related Diuretics
Cyclophosphamide	Discontinue breast-feeding during and for 36 hours after stopping treatment
Cycloserine	Amount too small to be harmful
Cyclosporin	*see* Ciclosporin
Cyproheptadine	*see* Antihistamines
Cyproterone	Caution; possibility of anti-androgen effects in neonate
Cytarabine	*see* Cytotoxic Drugs
Cytotoxic drugs	Discontinue breast-feeding; *see also* Natalizumab, Rituximab, and Trabectedin
Dacarbazine	*see* Cytotoxic Drugs
Daclizumab	Avoid
Dactinomycin	*see* Cytotoxic Drugs
Dalfopristin [ingredient]	*see Synercid®*
Dalteparin	No information available
Danaparoid	Amount probably too small to be harmful but manufacturer advises avoid
Danazol	No data available but avoid because of possible androgenic effects in infant
Dantrolene	Present in milk—manufacturer advises avoid
Dantron (danthron)	*see* Co-danthramer, Co-danthrusate
Dapsone	Haemolytic anaemia; although significant amount in milk, risk to infant very small unless infant is G6PD deficient
Daptomycin	Manufacturer advises avoid—no information available
Darbepoetin	Manufacturer advises avoid—no information available
Darifenacin	Present in milk in *animal* studies—manufacturer advises caution
Darunavir	Breast-feeding not advised in HIV infection
Dasatinib	*see* Cytotoxic Drugs
Daunorubicin	*see* Cytotoxic Drugs
Deferasirox	Manufacturer advises avoid—present in milk in *animal* studies
Deferiprone	Manufacturer advises avoid—no information available
Deflazacort	*see* Corticosteroids
Demeclocycline	*see* Tetracyclines
Desferrioxamine	Manufacturer advises use only if potential benefit outweighs risk—no information available
Desloratadine	*see* Antihistamines
Desmopressin	Not known to be harmful
Desogestrel	*see* Contraceptives, Oral
Dexamethasone	*see* Corticosteroids
Dexamfetamine	*see* Amphetamines
Dexibuprofen	Present in milk—but risk to infant minimal
Dexketoprofen	Manufacturer advises avoid—no information available
Dexrazoxane	*see* Cytotoxic Drugs
Diamorphine	Therapeutic doses unlikely to affect infant; withdrawal symptoms in infants of dependent mothers; breast-feeding not best method of treating dependence in offspring
Diazepam	*see* Benzodiazepines
Diclofenac	Amount too small to be harmful
Dicycloverine	Present in milk—one report of apnoea
Didanosine	Breast-feeding not advised in HIV infection
Digoxin	Amount too small to be harmful
Dihydrocodeine	Manufacturer advises use only if potential benefit outweighs risk
Dihydrotachysterol	*see* Vitamin D
Diloxanide	Manufacturer advises avoid
Diltiazem	Significant amount present in milk—no evidence of harm but avoid unless no safer alternative
Dimenhydrinate	*see* Antihistamines
Dipyridamole	Small amount present in milk—manufacturer advises caution
Disodium etidronate	No information available
Disodium pamidronate	Manufacturer advises avoid
Disopyramide	Present in milk—use only if essential and monitor infant for antimuscarinic effects
Distigmine	Manufacturer advises avoid—no information available
Disulfiram	Manufacturer advises avoid—no information available
Docetaxel	*see* Cytotoxic Drugs
Docusate sodium	Present in milk following oral administration—manufacturer advises caution; rectal administration not known to be harmful
Dolasetron	Not known to be harmful but manufacturer advises avoid
Domperidone	Amount probably too small to be harmful
Donepezil	Manufacturer advises avoid—no information available
Dornase alfa	Amount probably too small to be harmful—manufacturer advises caution
Dosulepin (dothiepin)	*see* Antidepressants, Tricyclic (and related)
Dothiepin	*see* Antidepressants, Tricyclic (and related)
Doxazosin	Accumulates in milk—manufacturer advises avoid
Doxepin	*see* Antidepressants, Tricyclic (and related)
Doxorubicin	*see* Cytotoxic Drugs
Doxycycline	*see* Tetracyclines
Drotrecogin alfa (activated)	Manufacturer advises avoid—no information available
Duloxetine	Present in milk—manufacturer advises avoid
Dydrogesterone	Present in milk—no adverse effects reported

Drug	Comment
Eculizumab	No information available—manufacturer advises avoid breast-feeding during and for 5 months after treatment
Edrophonium	Amount probably too small to be harmful
Efalizumab	May be present in milk—manufacturer advises avoid
Efavirenz	Breast-feeding not advised in HIV infection
Eflornithine	Manufacturer advises avoid—no information available
Eletriptan	Present in milk—avoid breast-feeding for 24 hours
Emtricitabine	Breast-feeding not advised in HIV infection
Enalapril	Amount probably too small to be harmful
Enfuvirtide	Breast-feeding not advised in HIV infection
Enoxaparin	Manufacturer advises avoid—no information available
Enoximone	Manufacturer advises caution—no information available
Entacapone	Manufacturer advises avoid—present in milk in *animal* studies
Entecavir	Manufacturer advises avoid—present in milk in *animal* studies
Ephedrine	Irritability and disturbed sleep reported
Epinastine	Present in milk in *animal* studies—manufacturer advises caution
Epirubicin	*see* Cytotoxic Drugs
Eplerenone	Manufacturer advises use only if potential benefit outweighs risk
Epoetin	Unlikely to be present in milk; minimal effect on infant
Eprosartan	Manufacturer advises avoid—no information available
Eptifibatide	No information available—manufacturer advises avoid
Erdosteine	Manufacturer advises avoid—no information available
Ergocalciferol	*see* Vitamin D
Ergotamine	Avoid; ergotism may occur in infant; repeated doses may inhibit lactation
Erlotinib	Manufacturer advises avoid—no information available
Ertapenem	Present in milk—manufacturer advises avoid
Erythromycin	Only small amounts in milk—not known to be harmful
Escitalopram	Manufacturer advises avoid—no information available
Esmolol	*see* Beta-blockers
Esomeprazole	Manufacturer advises avoid—no information available
Etamsylate	Significant amount but not known to be harmful
Etanercept	Manufacturer advises avoid—present in milk in *animal* studies
Ethambutol	Amount too small to be harmful
Ethinylestradiol	*see* Oestrogens
Ethosuximide	Present in milk but unlikely to be harmful; manufacturer advises avoid
Etidronate disodium	*see* Disodium Etidronate
Etodolac	Manufacturer advises avoid—no information available
Etomidate	Avoid breast-feeding for 24 hours after administration
Etoposide	*see* Cytotoxic Drugs
Etoricoxib	Manufacturer advises avoid—present in milk in *animal* studies
Etynodiol	*see* Contraceptives, Oral
Exenatide	Manufacturer advises avoid—no information available
Ezetimibe	Present in milk in *animal* studies—manufacturer advises avoid
Famciclovir	Manufacturer advises avoid unless potential benefit outweighs risk—present in milk in *animal* studies
Famotidine	Present in milk—not known to be harmful but manufacturer advises avoid
Fansidar®	Small risk of kernicterus in jaundiced infants and of haemolysis in G6PD-deficient infants (due to sulfadoxine)
Felodipine	Present in milk
Fenbufen	Small amount present in milk—manufacturer advises avoid
Fenofibrate	Manufacturer advises avoid—no information available
Fenoprofen	Amount too small to be harmful
Fentanyl	Amount too small to be harmful
Fexofenadine	*see* Antihistamines
Filgrastim	No information available—manufacturer advises avoid
Flavoxate	Manufacturer advises caution—no information available
Flecainide	Significant amount but not known to be harmful
Flucloxacillin	*see* Penicillins
Fluconazole	Present in milk but amount probably too small to be harmful
Flucytosine	Manufacturer advises avoid
Fludarabine	*see* Cytotoxic Drugs
Fluorouracil	*see* Cytotoxic Drugs
Fluoxetine	Present in milk—manufacturer advises avoid
Flupentixol	*see* Antipsychotics
Fluphenazine	*see* Antipsychotics
Flurazepam	*see* Benzodiazepines
Flurbiprofen	Amount too small to be harmful
Fluticasone	*see* Corticosteroids
Fluvastatin	*see* Statins
Fluvoxamine	Present in milk—manufacturer advises avoid
Follitropin alfa and beta	Avoid

Drug	Comment
Fomepizole	Manufacturer advises caution—no information available
Fondaparinux	Present in milk in *animal* studies—manufacturer advises avoid
Formoterol (eformoterol)	Amount in milk probably too small to be harmful but manufacturers advise avoid
Fosamprenavir	Breast-feeding not advised in HIV infection
Foscarnet	Avoid—present in milk in *animal* studies
Fosinopril	Present in milk—manufacturer advises avoid
Fosphenytoin	*see* Phenytoin
Frovatriptan	Present in milk in *animal* studies—withhold breast-feeding for 24 hours
Frusemide	*see* Furosemide
Fulvestrant	Manufacturer advises avoid—present in milk in *animal* studies
Furosemide (frusemide)	Amount too small to be harmful; may inhibit lactation
Fusidic acid	*see* Sodium Fusidate
Gabapentin	Present in milk—manufacturer advises use only if potential benefit outweighs risk
Galantamine	Manufacturer advises avoid—no information available
Galsulfase	Manufacturer advises avoid—no information available
Ganciclovir	Avoid—no information available
Ganirelix	Manufacturer advises avoid—no information available
Gemcitabine	*see* Cytotoxic Drugs
Gemfibrozil	Manufacturer advises avoid—no information available
Gestodene	*see* Contraceptives, Oral
Gestrinone	Manufacturer advises avoid
Glatiramer	Manufacturer advises caution—no information available
Glibenclamide	*see* Sulphonylureas
Gliclazide	*see* Sulphonylureas
Glimepiride	*see* Sulphonylureas
Glipizide	*see* Sulphonylureas
Glucosamine	Manufacturer advises avoid—no information available
Glyceryl trinitrate	No information available—manufacturers advise use only if potential benefit outweighs risk
Goserelin	Manufacturer advises avoid
Granisetron	Not known to be harmful but manufacturer advises avoid
Griseofulvin	Avoid—no information available
Haem arginate	Manufacturer advises avoid unless essential—no information available
Haloperidol	*see* Antipsychotics
Halothane	Present in milk
Hepatitis A vaccine	No information available
Human menopausal gonadotrophins	Avoid
Hydralazine	Present in milk but not known to be harmful; monitor infant
Hydrochlorothiazide	*see* Thiazides and Related Diuretics
Hydrocortisone	*see* Corticosteroids
Hydroflumethiazide	*see* Thiazides and Related Diuretics
Hydromorphone	Manufacturer advises avoid—no information available
Hydroxocobalamin	Present in milk but not known to be harmful
Hydroxycarbamide (hydroxyurea)	*see* Cytotoxic Drugs
Hydroxychloroquine	Avoid—risk of toxicity in infant
Hydroxyurea	*see* Cytotoxic Drugs
Hydroxyzine	*see* Antihistamines
Hyoscine	Amount too small to be harmful
Ibandronic acid	Manufacturer advises avoid—present in milk in *animal* studies
Ibuprofen	Amount too small to be harmful but some manufacturers advise avoid (including topical use)
Idarubicin	*see* Cytotoxic Drugs
Idoxuridine	May make milk taste unpleasant
Idursulfase	No information available
Ifosfamide	*see* Cytotoxic Drugs
Iloprost	Manufacturer advises avoid—no information available
Imatinib	*see* Cytotoxic Drugs
Imidapril	Manufacturer advises avoid—no information available
Imiglucerase	No information available
Imipenem [ingredient]	*see Primaxin®*
Imipramine	*see* Antidepressants, Tricyclic (and related)
Imiquimod	Manufacturer advises no information available
Indapamide	No information available—manufacturer advises avoid
Indinavir	Breast-feeding not advised in HIV infection
Indometacin	Amount probably too small to be harmful but convulsions reported in one infant—manufacturers advise avoid
Infliximab	Avoid; manufacturer advises avoid for at least 6 months after last dose
Influenza vaccine	Not known to be harmful
Interferons	Manufacturers advise avoid—no information available
Iodine and iodides	Stop breast-feeding; danger of neonatal hypothyroidism or goitre; appears to be concentrated in milk; *see also* Povidone–iodine
Iodine, radioactive	Breast-feeding contra-indicated after therapeutic doses. With diagnostic doses withhold breast-feeding for at least 24 hours
Ipratropium	Amount probably too small to be harmful
Irbesartan	Manufacturer advises avoid—no information available
Irinotecan	*see* Cytotoxic Drugs

Drug	Comment
Isoniazid	Monitor infant for possible toxicity; theoretical risk of convulsions and neuropathy; prophylactic pyridoxine advisable in mother and infant
Isosorbide dinitrate	No information available—manufacturers advise use only if potential benefit outweighs risk
Isosorbide mononitrate	No information available—manufacturers advise use only if potential benefit outweighs risk
Isotretinoin	Avoid
Isradipine	Manufacturer advises avoid—present in milk in *animal* studies
Itraconazole	Small amounts present in milk—may accumulate; manufacturer advises avoid unless potential benefit outweighs risk
Ivabradine	Present in milk in *animal* studies—manufacturer advises avoid
Kaletra®	Breast-feeding not advised in HIV infection
Ketoconazole	Manufacturer advises avoid
Ketoprofen	Amount probably too small to be harmful but manufacturer advises avoid unless essential
Ketorolac	Amount too small to be harmful but manufacturer advises avoid
Ketotifen	*see* Antihistamines
Labetalol	*see* Beta-blockers
Lacidipine	Manufacturer advises avoid—no information available
Lamivudine	Present in milk—manufacturer advises avoid; breast-feeding not advised in HIV infection
Lamotrigine	Present in milk but limited data suggest no harmful effects on infants
Lanreotide	Manufacturer advises avoid unless potential benefit outweighs risk—no information available
Lansoprazole	Manufacturer advises avoid unless essential—present in milk in *animal* studies
Lanthanum	Manufacturer advises caution—no information available
Laronidase	Manufacturer advises avoid—no information available
Latanoprost	May be present in milk—manufacturer advises avoid
Leflunomide	Present in milk—manufacturer advises avoid
Lenalidomide	Manufacturer advises discontinue breast-feeding—no information available
Lenograstim	Manufacturer advises avoid—no information available
Lepirudin	Avoid
Lercanidipine	Manufacturer advises avoid
Letrozole	Manufacturer advises avoid
Leuprorelin	Manufacturer advises avoid
Levetiracetam	Present in milk—manufacturer advises avoid
Levobupivacaine	Likely to be present in milk but risk to infant minimal
Levocetirizine	*see* Antihistamines
Levodopa	May suppress lactation; present in milk—manufacturers advise avoid
Levofloxacin	Manufacturer advises avoid
Levomepromazine (methotrimeprazine)	*see* Antipsychotics
Levonorgestrel	*see* Contraceptives, Oral
Levothyroxine (thyroxine)	Amount too small to affect tests for neonatal hypothyroidism
Lidocaine (lignocaine)	Amount too small to be harmful
Lignocaine	*see* Lidocaine
Linezolid	Manufacturer advises avoid—present in milk in *animal* studies
Liothyronine	Amount too small to affect tests for neonatal hypothyroidism
Lisinopril	No information available—manufacturer advises avoid
Lithium salts	Present in milk and risk of toxicity in infant—manufacturers advise avoid
Lofepramine	*see* Antidepressants, Tricyclic (and related)
Lofexidine	Manufacturer advises use only if potential benefit outweighs risk—no information available
Loperamide	Amount probably too small to be harmful
Lopinavir [ingredient]	*see Kaletra®*
Loprazolam	*see* Benzodiazepines
Loratadine	*see* Antihistamines
Lorazepam	*see* Benzodiazepines
Lormetazepam	*see* Benzodiazepines
Losartan	Manufacturer advises avoid—no information available
Lumefantrine [ingredient]	*see Riamet®*
Lymecycline	*see* Tetracyclines
Macrogols	Manufacturers advise use only if essential—no information available
Malarone®	Use only if no suitable alternative available; *see also* p. 346
Maraviroc	Breast-feeding not advised in HIV infection
Mebendazole	Amount too small to be harmful but manufacturer advises avoid
Mecysteine	Manufacturer advises avoid
Medroxyprogesterone	Present in milk—no adverse effects reported
Mefenamic acid	Amount too small to be harmful but manufacturer advises avoid
Mefloquine	Present in milk but risk to infant minimal
Meloxicam	No information available—manufacturer advises avoid
Melphalan	*see* Cytotoxic Drugs
Memantine	Manufacturer advises avoid—no information available
Menotrophin	Avoid

Drug	Comment
Meprobamate	Avoid; concentration in milk may exceed maternal plasma concentrations fourfold and may cause drowsiness in infant
Meptazinol	Manufacturer advises use only if potential benefit outweighs risk
Mercaptamine	Manufacturer advises avoid
Mercaptopurine	*see* Cytotoxic Drugs
Meropenem	Unlikely to be absorbed (however, manufacturer advises avoid unless potential benefit justifies potential risk)
Mesalazine	Diarrhoea reported but manufacturers advise negligible amounts detected in breast milk
Mesterolone	*see* Androgens
Mestranol	*see* Oestrogens
Metaraminol	Manufacturer advises caution—no information available
Metformin	Manufacturer advises avoid; present in milk
Methadone	Withdrawal symptoms in infant; breast-feeding permissible during maintenance but dose should be as low as possible and infant monitored to avoid sedation
Methenamine	Amount too small to be harmful
Methocarbamol	Present in milk in *animal* studies—manufacturer advises caution
Methotrexate	*see* Cytotoxic Drugs
Methotrimeprazine	*see* Antipsychotics
Methoxy polyethylene glycol-epoetin beta	Manufacturer advises use only if potential benefit outweighs risk—present in milk in *animal* studies
Methyldopa	Amount too small to be harmful
Methylphenidate	No information available—manufacturer advises avoid
Methylprednisolone	*see* Corticosteroids
Methysergide	Manufacturer advises avoid
Metoclopramide	Small amount present in milk; manufacturer advises avoid
Metolazone	*see* Thiazides and Related Diuretics
Metoprolol	*see* Beta-blockers
Metronidazole	Significant amount in milk; manufacturer advises avoid large single doses
Metyrapone	Manufacturer advises avoid—no information available
Mexiletine	Amount too small to be harmful
Mianserin	*see* Antidepressants, Tricyclic (and related)
Miconazole	Manufacturer advises caution—no information available
Midazolam	Present in milk—manufacturer advises avoid breast-feeding for 24 hours after administration
Mifepristone	No information available—manufacturer advises stop breast-feeding for 14 days after administration
Miglustat	Manufacturer advises avoid—no information available
Milrinone	Manufacturer advises caution—no information available
Minocycline	*see* Tetracyclines
Minoxidil	Present in milk but not known to be harmful
Mirtazapine	Manufacturer advises avoid—present in milk in *animal* studies
Misoprostol	No information available—manufacturer advises avoid
Mitomycin	*see* Cytotoxic Drugs
Mitotane	*see* Cytotoxic Drugs
Mitoxantrone (mitozantrone)	*see* Cytotoxic Drugs
Mitozantrone	*see* Cytotoxic Drugs
Mizolastine	*see* Antihistamines
Moclobemide	Amount too small to be harmful, but patient leaflet advises avoid
Modafinil	Manufacturer advises avoid—no information available
Moexipril	Manufacturer advises avoid—no information available
Montelukast	Manufacturer advises avoid unless essential
Morphine	Therapeutic doses unlikely to affect infant; withdrawal symptoms in infants of dependent mothers; breast-feeding not best method of treating dependence in offspring
Moxifloxacin	Manufacturer advises avoid—present in milk in *animal* studies
Moxonidine	Present in milk—manufacturer advises avoid
Mupirocin	Manufacturer advises avoid unless potential benefit outweighs risk—no information available
Mycophenolate mofetil	Manufacturer advises avoid—present in milk in *animal* studies
Nabilone	Manufacturer advises avoid—no information available
Nabumetone	No information available—manufacturer advises avoid
Nadolol	*see* Beta-blockers
Nafarelin	Manufacturer advises avoid—no information available
Nalidixic acid	Risk to infant very small but one case of haemolytic anaemia reported
Naloxone	No information available
Naltrexone	Manufacturers advise avoid—present in milk in *animal* studies
Naproxen	Amount too small to be harmful but manufacturer advises avoid
Naratriptan	Manufacturer advises caution—no information available

Drug	Comment
Natalizumab	Present in milk in *animal* studies—manufacturer advises avoid
Nateglinide	Manufacturer advises avoid—present in milk in *animal* studies
Nebivolol	*see* Beta-blockers
Nedocromil	Unlikely to be present in milk
Nelarabine	*see* Cytotoxic Drugs
Nelfinavir	Breast-feeding not advised in HIV infection
Neostigmine	Amount probably too small to be harmful; monitor infant
Nevirapine	Breast-feeding not advised in HIV infection
Nicardipine	Manufacturer advises avoid—no information available
Nicorandil	No information available—manufacturer advises avoid
Nicotine	Present in milk; intermittent therapy preferable
Nicotinic acid	Present in milk—avoid
Nicoumalone	*see* Anticoagulants, Oral
Nifedipine	Amount too small to be harmful but manufacturers advise avoid
Nimodipine	No information available
Nisoldipine	Manufacturer advises avoid—no information available
Nitisinone	Manufacturer advises avoid—adverse effects in *animal* studies
Nitrazepam	*see* Benzodiazepines
Nitrofurantoin	Only small amounts in milk but could be enough to produce haemolysis in G6PD-deficient infants
Nitroprusside	*see* Sodium Nitroprusside
Nizatidine	Amount too small to be harmful
Nonoxinol 9	Present in milk in *animal* studies
Norethisterone	Higher doses may suppress lactation and alter milk composition—use lowest effective dose; *see also* Contraceptives, Oral
Norfloxacin	No information available—manufacturer advises avoid
Norgestimate	*see* Contraceptives, Oral
Norgestrel	*see* Contraceptives, Oral
Nortriptyline	*see* Antidepressants, Tricyclic (and related)
NSAIDs	*see* individual entries
Nystatin	No information available, but absorption from gastro-intestinal tract negligible
Octreotide	Manufacturer advises avoid unless essential—no information available
Oestrogens	Avoid; adverse effects on lactation; *see also* Contraceptives, Oral
Ofloxacin	Amount probably too small to be harmful but manufacturer advises avoid
Olanzapine	Manufacturer advises avoid—present in milk
Olmesartan	Manufacturer advises avoid—present in milk in *animal* studies
Olsalazine	Manufacturer advises avoid
Omalizumab	Manufacturer advises avoid—present in milk in *animal* studies
Omega-3-acid ethyl esters	Manufacturer advises avoid—no information available
Omeprazole	Present in milk but not known to be harmful
Ondansetron	Not known to be harmful but manufacturer advises avoid
Opioid analgesics	*see* individual entries
Oral contraceptives	*see* Contraceptives, Oral
Orlistat	Manufacturer advises avoid—no information available
Orphenadrine	Manufacturers advise caution
Oseltamivir	Manufacturer advises use only if potential benefit outweighs risk—present in milk in *animal* studies
Oxaliplatin	*see* Cytotoxic Drugs
Oxazepam	*see* Benzodiazepines
Oxcarbazepine	Present in milk—manufacturer advises avoid
Oxprenolol	*see* Beta-blockers
Oxybutynin	Present in milk—manufacturers advise avoid
Oxycodone	Present in milk—manufacturer advises avoid
Oxytetracycline	*see* Tetracyclines
Paclitaxel	*see* Cytotoxic Drugs
Palifermin	Manufacturer advises avoid—no information available
Paliperidone	Manufacturer advises avoid—present in milk
Palonosetron	Manufacturer advises avoid—no information available
Pamidronate disodium	*see* Disodium Pamidronate
Pancuronium	Manufacturer advises avoid unless potential benefit outweighs possble risk—no information available
Pantoprazole	Manufacturer advises avoid unless potential benefit outweighs risk—small amount present in milk in *animal* studies
Papaveretum	*see* Morphine
Paracetamol	Amount too small to be harmful
Paraldehyde	Manufacturer advises avoid unless essential—present in milk
Parecoxib	Manufacturer advises avoid—present in milk in animal studies
Paricalcitol	Manufacturer advises caution—no information available; *see also* Vitamin D
Paroxetine	Present in milk but amount too small to be harmful
Pegaptinib	Manufacturer advises avoid—no information available
Pegfilgrastim	No information available—manufacturer advises avoid
Peginterferon alfa	*see* Interferons

Appendix 5: Breast-feeding

Drug	Comment
Pemetrexed	*see* Cytotoxic Drugs
Penicillamine	Manufacturer advises avoid unless potential benefit outweighs risk—no information available
Penicillins	Trace amounts in milk
Pentamidine isetionate	Manufacturer advises avoid unless essential
Pentazocine	Small amount present in milk—manufacturer advises caution
Pentostatin	*see* Cytotoxic Drugs
Pergolide	May suppress lactation
Pericyazine	*see* Antipsychotics
Perindopril	Manufacturer advises avoid—no information available
Perphenazine	*see* Antipsychotics
Pethidine	Present in milk but not known to be harmful
Phenindione	*see* Anticoagulants, Oral
Phenobarbital	Avoid when possible; drowsiness may occur but risk probably small; one report of methaemoglobinaemia with phenobarbital and phenytoin
Phenoxybenzamine	May be present in milk
Phenoxymethylpenicillin	*see* Penicillins
Phentolamine	Manufacturer advises avoid—no information available
Phenytoin	Small amount present in milk; manufacturer advises avoid—but *see* section 4.8.1
Phytomenadione	Present in milk
Pilocarpine	Manufacturer advises avoid—no information available
Pimozide	*see* Antipsychotics
Pindolol	*see* Beta-blockers
Pioglitazone	Manufacturer advises avoid—present in milk in *animal* studies
Piperacillin [ingredient]	*see Tazocin®*
Piperazine	Present in milk—manufacturer advises avoid breast-feeding for 8 hours after dose (express and discard milk during this time)
Piracetam	Manufacturer advises avoid
Piroxicam	Amount too small to be harmful
Pivmecillinam	*see* Penicillins
Pizotifen	Amount probably too small to be harmful, but manufacturer advises avoid
Podophyllum	Avoid
Porfimer	No information available—manufacturer advises avoid
Posaconazole	Manufacturer advises avoid—present in milk in *animal* studies
Povidone–iodine	Avoid; iodine absorbed from vaginal preparations is concentrated in milk
Pramipexole	May suppress lactation; manufacturer advises avoid—present in milk in *animal* studies
Pravastatin	Small amount present in milk—manufacturer advises avoid
Prazosin	Amount probably too small to be harmful
Prednisolone	*see* Corticosteroids
Pregabalin	Present in milk in *animal* studies—manufacturer advises avoid
Prilocaine	Present in milk but not known to be harmful
Primaxin®	Present in milk but unlikely to be absorbed (however, manufacturer advises avoid)
Primidone	*see* Phenobarbital
Probenecid	No information available
Procainamide	Present in milk—manufacturer advises avoid
Procarbazine	*see* Cytotoxic Drugs
Prochlorperazine	*see* Antipsychotics
Procyclidine	No information available
Progesterone	Manufacturers advise avoid—present in milk
Proguanil	Amount probably too small to be harmful when used for malaria prophylaxis; inadequate for reliable protection against malaria in breast-fed infant, *see* p. 346; for Proguanil with Atovaquone *see Malarone®*
Promazine	*see* Antipsychotics
Promethazine	*see* Antihistamines
Propafenone	Manufacturer advises avoid—no information available
Propantheline	May suppress lactation
Propiverine	Manufacturer advises avoid—present in milk in *animal* studies
Propofol	Present in milk but amount probably too small to be harmful
Propranolol	*see* Beta-blockers
Propylthiouracil	Monitor infant's thyroid status but amounts in milk probably too small to affect infant; high doses might affect neonatal thyroid function
Protirelin	Breast enlargement and leaking of milk reported
Pseudoephedrine	Amount too small to be harmful
Pyrazinamide	Amount too small to be harmful
Pyridostigmine	Amount probably too small to be harmful
Pyrimethamine	Significant amount—avoid administration of other folate antagonists to infant; avoid breast-feeding during toxoplasmosis treatment
Quetiapine	Manufacturer advises avoid—no information available
Quinagolide	Suppresses lactation
Quinapril	Present in milk—manufacturers advise avoid
Quinupristin [ingredient]	*see Synercid®*

Drug	Comment
Rabeprazole	Manufacturer advises avoid—no information available
Raltitrexed	*see* Cytotoxic Drugs
Ramipril	Manufacturer advises avoid—no information available
Ranibizumab	Manufacturer advises avoid—no information available
Ranitidine	Significant amount but not known to be harmful
Rasagiline	Manufacturer advises caution—may suppress lactation
Rasburicase	Manufacturer advises avoid—no information available
Reboxetine	Manufacturer advises avoid—no information available
Remifentanil	Manufacturer advises caution—present in milk in *animal* studies
Repaglinide	Manufacturer advises avoid—present in milk in *animal* studies
Reteplase	Manufacturer advises avoid breast-feeding for 24 hours after dose (express and discard milk during this time)
Riamet®	Manufacturer advises avoid breast-feeding for at least 1 week after last dose; present in milk in *animal* studies
Ribavirin	Avoid—no information available
Rifabutin	Manufacturer advises avoid—no information available
Rifampicin	Amount too small to be harmful
Riluzole	Manufacturer advises avoid—no information available
Rimonabant	Manufacturer advises avoid—present in milk in *animal* studies
Risedronate sodium	Manufacturer advises avoid
Risperidone	Present in milk—manufacturer advises avoid
Ritonavir	Breast-feeding not advised in HIV infection
Rituximab	Avoid breast-feeding during and for 12 months after treatment
Rivastigmine	Present in milk in *animal* studies—manufacturer advises avoid
Rizatriptan	Present in milk in *animal* studies—withhold breast-feeding for 24 hours
Rocuronium	Manufacturer advises avoid unless potential benefit outweighs risk—present in milk in *animal* studies
Ropinirole	May suppress lactation—manufacturer advises avoid
Ropivacaine	Not known to be harmful
Rosiglitazone	Manufacturer advises avoid—present in milk in *animal* studies
Rosuvastatin	*see* Statins
Rotigotine	May suppress lactation; manufacturer advises avoid—present in milk in *animal* studies
Rufinamide	Manufacturer advises avoid—no information available
Salbutamol	Probably present in milk; manufacturer advises avoid unless potential benefit outweighs risk—the amount of inhaled drugs in breast milk is probably too small to be harmful
Salcatonin	*see* Calcitonin (salmon)
Saquinavir	Breast-feeding not advised in HIV infection
Secobarbital	*see* Barbiturates
Selegiline	Manufacturer advises avoid—no information available
Senna	Not known to be harmful
Sertindole	Manufacturer advises avoid—no information available
Sertraline	Present in milk but not known to be harmful in short-term use
Sevelamer	Manufacturer advises use only if potential benefit outweighs risk
Sibutramine	Manufacturer advises avoid—no information available
Sildenafil	Manufacturer advises avoid—no information available
Silver sulfadiazine	*see* Sulphonamides
Simvastatin	*see* Statins
Sirolimus	Discontinue breast-feeding
Sitagliptin	Manufacturer advises avoid—present in milk in *animal* studies
Sitaxentan sodium	Manufacturer advises avoid—present in milk in *animal* studies
Sodium aurothiomalate	Caution—present in milk; theoretical possibility of rashes and idiosyncratic reactions
Sodium clodronate	No information available
Sodium cromoglicate	Unlikely to be present in milk
Sodium fusidate	Present in milk—manufacturer advises caution
Sodium nitroprusside	Manufacturer advises caution—no information available
Sodium oxybate	No information available
Sodium phenylbutyrate	Manufacturer advises avoid—no information available
Sodium picosulfate	Not known to be present in milk but manufacturer advises avoid
Sodium stibogluconate	Amount probably too small to be harmful
Sodium valproate	*see* Valproate
Solifenacin	Manufacturer advises avoid—present in milk in *animal* studies
Somatropin	No information available
Sorafenib	*see* Cytotoxic Drugs
Sotalol	*see* Beta-blockers
Spironolactone	Amount probably too small to be harmful but manufacturer advises avoid
Statins	Manufacturers of atorvastatin, fluvastatin, rosuvastatin and simvastatin advise avoid—no information available; *see also* pravastatin

Drug	Comment
Stavudine	Breast-feeding not advised in HIV infection
Strontium ranelate	Avoid
Sulfadiazine	*see* Sulphonamides
Sulfasalazine	Small amounts in milk (1 report of bloody diarrhoea and rashes); theoretical risk of neonatal haemolysis especially in G6PD-deficient infants
Sulfinpyrazone	No information available
Sulindac	No information available
Sulphonamides	Small risk of kernicterus in jaundiced infants particularly with long-acting sulphonamides, and of haemolysis in G6PD-deficient infants
Sulphonylureas	Theoretical possibility of hypoglycaemia in infant
Sulpiride	Best avoided; present in milk; *see also* Antipsychotics
Sumatriptan	Present in milk—withhold breast-feeding for 12 hours
Sunitinib	*see* Cytotoxic Drugs
Suxamethonium	No information available
Synercid®	Manufacturer advises avoid—no information available
Tacalcitol	Manufacturer advises avoid application to breast area—no information available; *see also* Vitamin D
Tacrolimus	Avoid—present in milk following systemic administration
Tamoxifen	Supresses lactation; manufacturer advises avoid unless potential benefit outweighs risk
Tazarotene	Manufacturer advises avoid—present in milk in *animal* studies
Tazobactam [ingredient]	*see Tazocin®*
Tazocin®	Present in milk—manufacturer advises use only if potential benefit outweighs risk
Tegafur with uracil	*see* Cytotoxic Drugs
Teicoplanin	No information available
Telbivudine	Manufacturer advises avoid—present in milk in *animal* studies
Telithromycin	Manufacturer advises avoid—present in milk in *animal* studies
Telmisartan	Manufacturer advises avoid—no information available
Temazepam	*see* Benzodiazepines
Temocillin	*see* Penicillins
Temoporfin	Manufacturer advises avoid breast-feeding for at least 1 month after treatment—no information available
Temozolomide	*see* Cytotoxic Drugs
Tenecteplase	Manufacturer advises avoid breast-feeding for 24 hours after dose (express and discard milk during this time)
Tenofovir	Breast-feeding not advised in HIV infection
Tenoxicam	No information available
Terazosin	No information available
Terbinafine	Present in milk—manufacturer advises avoid
Terbutaline	Amount too small to be harmful
Terlipressin	Not known to be harmful
Testosterone	*see* Androgens
Tetrabenazine	Manufacturer advises avoid
Tetracyclines	Avoid (although absorption and therefore discoloration of teeth in infant probably usually prevented by chelation with calcium in milk); *see also* tigecycline
Theophylline	Present in milk—irritability in infant reported; modified-release preparations preferable
Thiamine	Severely thiamine-deficient mothers should avoid breast-feeding as toxic methyl-glyoxal present in milk
Thiazides and related diuretics	Amount too small to be harmful; large doses may suppress lactation
Thiopental	Present in milk—manufacturer advises avoid
Thiotepa	*see* Cytotoxic Drugs
Thyroxine	*see* Levothyroxine
Tiagabine	Manufacturer advises avoid unless potential benefit outweighs risk
Tiaprofenic acid	Amount too small to be harmful
Ticarcillin [ingredient]	*see* Penicillins
Tigecycline	Manufacturer advises caution—present in milk in *animal* studies
Tiludronic acid	Manufacturer advises avoid—no information available
Timentin®	*see* Penicillins
Timolol	*see* Beta-blockers
Tinidazole	Present in milk—manufacturer advises avoid breast-feeding during and for 3 days after stopping treatment
Tinzaparin	Manufacturer advises avoid—no information available
Tioguanine	*see* Cytotoxic Drugs
Tiotropium	Amount in milk probably too small to be harmful (present in milk in *animal* studies)—manufacturer advises use only if potential benefit outweighs risk
Tipranavir	Breast-feeding not advised in HIV infection
Tirofiban	Manufacturer advises avoid—no information available
Tizanidine	Manufacturer advises use only if potential benefit outweighs risk—no information available
Tolbutamide	*see* Sulphonylureas
Tolcapone	Manufacturer advises avoid—present in milk in *animal* studies
Tolfenamic acid	Amount too small to be harmful
Tolterodine	Manufacturer advises avoid—no information available
Topiramate	Manufacturer advises avoid—present in milk

Drug	Comment
Topotecan	*see* Cytotoxic Drugs
Torasemide	No information available
Trabectedin	Manufacturer advises avoid breast-feeding during and for 3 months after treatment
Tramadol	Amount probably too small to be harmful, but manufacturer advises avoid
Trandolapril	Manufacturers advise avoid
Tranexamic acid	Small amount present in milk—antifibrinolytic effect in infant unlikely
Trastuzumab	Avoid breast-feeding during treatment and for six months after
Travoprost	Present in milk in animal studies; manufacturer advises avoid
Trazodone	*see* Antidepressants, Tricyclic (and related)
Treosulfan	*see* Cytotoxic Drugs
Tretinoin	Avoid
Triamcinolone	*see* Corticosteroids
Triamterene	Present in milk—manufacturer advises avoid
Tribavirin	*see* Ribavirin
Triclofos	Avoid
Trifluoperazine	*see* Antipsychotics
Trihexyphenidyl	Manufacturer advises avoid
Trimeprazine	*see* Antihistamines
Trimethoprim	Present in milk—short-term use not known to be harmful
Trimipramine	*see* Antidepressants, Tricyclic (and related)
Triptorelin	Manufacturers advise avoid
Tropisetron	No information available
Trospium	Manufacturer advises caution—no information available
Urokinase	Manufacturer advises avoid—no information available
Ursodeoxycholic acid	Not known to be harmful but manufacturer advises avoid
Valaciclovir	No information available; *see also* Aciclovir
Valganciclovir	*see* Ganciclovir
Valproate	Amount too small to be harmful
Valproic acid	*see* Valproate
Valsartan	Manufacturer advises avoid—no information available
Vancomycin	Present in milk—significant absorption following oral administration unlikely
Varenicline	Present in milk in *animal* studies
Vasopressin	Not known to be harmful
Vecuronium	No information available
Venlafaxine	Present in milk—manufacturer advises avoid
Verapamil	Amount too small to be harmful
Verteporfin	No information available—manufacturer advises avoid breast-feeding for 48 hours after administration
Vigabatrin	Present in milk—manufacturer advises avoid
Vinblastine	*see* Cytotoxic Drugs
Vincristine	*see* Cytotoxic Drugs
Vindesine	*see* Cytotoxic Drugs
Vinorelbine	*see* Cytotoxic Drugs
Vitamin A	Theoretical risk of toxicity in infants of mothers taking large doses
Vitamin D	Caution with high systemic doses; may cause hypercalcaemia in infant; manufacturer of *topical* calcitriol advises avoid; *see also* Calcipotriol, Paricalcitol, and Tacalcitol
Voriconazole	Manufacturer advises avoid—no information available
Warfarin	*see* Anticoagulants, Oral
Xipamide	No information available
Zafirlukast	Present in milk—manufacturer advises avoid
Zaleplon	Present in milk but amount probably too small to be harmful
Zanamivir	Manufacturer advises avoid—present in milk in *animal* studies
Zidovudine	Breast-feeding not advised in HIV infection
Zoledronic acid	Manufacturer advises avoid—no information available
Zolmitriptan	Manufacturer advises caution—present in milk in *animal* studies
Zolpidem	Small amounts present in milk—manufacturer advises avoid
Zonisamide	Avoid; manufacturer advises avoid breast-feeding for 4 weeks after administration
Zopiclone	Present in milk—manufacturer advises avoid
Zotepine	Manufacturer advises avoid
Zuclopenthixol	*see* Antipsychotics

A6 Intravenous additives

Intravenous additives policies A local policy on the addition of drugs to intravenous fluids should be drawn up by a multi-disciplinary team in each Strategic Health Authority (or equivalent) and issued as a document to the members of staff concerned.

Centralised additive services are provided in a number of hospital pharmacy departments and should be used in preference to making additions on wards.

The information that follows should be read in conjunction with local policy documents.

Guidelines

1. Drugs should only be added to infusion containers when constant plasma concentrations are needed or when the administration of a more concentrated solution would be harmful.
2. In general, only one drug should be added to any infusion container and the components should be compatible. Ready-prepared solutions should be used whenever possible. Drugs should not normally be added to blood products, mannitol, or sodium bicarbonate. Only specially formulated additives should be used with fat emulsions or amino-acid solutions (section 9.3).
3. Solutions should be thoroughly mixed by shaking and checked for absence of particulate matter before use.
4. Strict asepsis should be maintained throughout and in general the giving set should not be used for more than 24 hours (for drug admixtures).
5. The infusion container should be labelled with the patient's name, the name and quantity of additives, and the date and time of addition (and the new expiry date or time). Such additional labelling should not interfere with information on the manufacturer's label that is still valid. When possible, containers should be retained for a period after use in case they are needed for investigation.
6. It is good practice to examine intravenous infusions from time to time while they are running. If cloudiness, crystallisation, change of colour, or any other sign of interaction or contamination is observed the infusion should be discontinued.

Problems

Microbial contamination The accidental entry and subsequent growth of micro-organisms converts the infusion fluid pathway into a potential vehicle for infection with micro-organisms, particularly species of Candida, Enterobacter, and Klebsiella. Ready-prepared infusions containing the additional drugs, or infusions prepared by an additive service (when available) should therefore be used in preference to making extemporaneous additions to infusion containers on wards etc. However, when this is necessary strict aseptic procedure should be followed.

Incompatibility Physical and chemical incompatibilities may occur with loss of potency, increase in toxicity, or other adverse effect. The solutions may become opalescent or precipitation may occur, but in many instances there is no visual indication of incompatibility. Interaction may take place at any point in the infusion fluid pathway, and the potential for incompatibility is increased when more than one substance is added to the infusion fluid.

Common incompatibilities. Precipitation reactions are numerous and varied and may occur as a result of pH, concentration changes, 'salting-out' effects, complexation or other chemical changes. Precipitation or other particle formation must be avoided since, apart from lack of control of dosage on administration, it may initiate or exacerbate adverse effects. This is particularly important in the case of drugs which have been implicated in either thrombophlebitis (e.g. diazepam) or in skin sloughing or necrosis caused by extravasation (e.g. sodium bicarbonate and certain cytotoxic drugs). It is also especially important to effect solution of colloidal drugs and to prevent their subsequent precipitation in order to avoid a pyrogenic reaction (e.g. amphotericin).

It is considered undesirable to mix beta-lactam antibiotics, such as semi-synthetic penicillins and cephalosporins, with proteinaceous materials on the grounds that immunogenic and allergenic conjugates could be formed.

A number of preparations undergo significant loss of potency when added singly or in combination to large volume infusions. Examples include ampicillin in infusions that contain glucose or lactates. The breakdown products of dacarbazine have been implicated in adverse effects.

Blood. Because of the large number of incompatibilities, drugs should not normally be added to blood and blood products for infusion purposes. Examples of incompatibility with blood include hypertonic mannitol solutions (irreversible crenation of red cells), dextrans (rouleaux formation and interference with cross-matching), glucose (clumping of red cells), and oxytocin (inactivated).

If the giving set is not changed after the administration of blood, but used for other infusion fluids, a fibrin clot may form which, apart from blocking the set, increases the likelihood of microbial growth.

Intravenous fat emulsions may break down with coalescence of fat globules and separation of phases when additions such as antibacterials or electrolytes are made, thus increasing the possibility of embolism. Only specially formulated products such as *Vitlipid N®* (section 9.3) may be added to appropriate intravenous fat emulsions.

Other infusions that frequently give rise to incompatibility include amino acids, mannitol, and sodium bicarbonate.

Bactericides such as chlorocresol 0.1% or phenylmercuric nitrate 0.001% are present in some injection solutions. The total volume of such solutions added to a container for infusion on one occasion should not exceed 15 mL.

Method

Ready-prepared infusions should be used whenever available. **Potassium chloride** is usually available in concentrations of 20, 27, and 40 mmol/litre in sodium chloride intravenous infusion (0.9%), glucose intravenous infusion (5%) or sodium chloride and glucose intravenous infusion. **Lidocaine hydrochloride** (lignocaine hydrochloride) is usually available in concentrations of 0.1 or 0.2% in glucose intravenous infusion (5%).

When addition is required to be made extemporaneously, any product reconstitution instructions such as those relating to concentration, vehicle, mixing, and handling precautions should be strictly followed using an aseptic technique throughout. Once the product has been reconstituted, addition to the infusion fluid should be made immediately in order to minimise microbial contamination and, with certain products, to prevent degradation or other formulation change which may occur; e.g. reconstituted ampicillin injection degrades rapidly on standing, and also may form polymers which could cause sensitivity reactions.

It is also important in certain instances that an infusion fluid of specific pH be used (e.g. **furosemide** (frusemide) injection requires dilution in infusions of pH greater than 5.5).

When drug additions are made it is important to mix thoroughly; additions should not be made to an infusion container that has been connected to a giving set, as mixing is hampered. If the solutions are not thoroughly mixed a concentrated layer of the additive may form owing to differences in density. **Potassium chloride** is particularly prone to this 'layering' effect when added without adequate mixing to infusions packed in non-rigid infusion containers; if such a mixture is administered it may have a serious effect on the heart.

A time limit between addition and completion of administration must be imposed for certain admixtures to guarantee satisfactory drug potency and compatibility. For admixtures in which degradation occurs without the formation of toxic substances, an acceptable limit is the time taken for 10% decomposition of the drug. When toxic substances are produced stricter limits may be imposed. Because of the risk of microbial contamination a maximum time limit of 24 hours may be appropriate for additions made elsewhere than in hospital pharmacies offering central additive service.

Certain injections must be protected from light during continuous infusion to minimise oxidation, e.g. amphotericin, dacarbazine, and sodium nitroprusside.

Dilution with a small volume of an appropriate vehicle and administration using a motorised infusion pump is advocated for preparations such as heparin where strict control over administration is required. In this case the appropriate dose may be dissolved in a convenient volume (e.g. 24 to 48 mL) of sodium chloride intravenous infusion (0.9%).

Use of table

The table lists preparations given by three methods:

continuous infusion,

intermittent infusion, and

addition via the drip tubing.

Drugs for **continuous infusion** must be diluted in a large volume infusion. Penicillins and cephalosporins are not usually given by continuous infusion because of stability problems and because adequate plasma and tissue concentrations are best obtained by intermittent infusion. Where it is necessary to administer them by continuous infusion, detailed literature should be consulted.

Drugs that are both compatible and clinically suitable may be given by **intermittent infusion** in a relatively small volume of infusion over a short period of time, e.g. 100 mL in 30 minutes. The method is used if the product is incompatible or unstable over the period necessary for continuous infusion; the limited stability of ampicillin or amoxicillin in large volume glucose or lactate infusions may be overcome in this way.

Intermittent infusion is also used if adequate plasma and tissue concentrations are not produced by continuous infusion as in the case of drugs such as dacarbazine, gentamicin, and ticarcillin.

An in-line burette may be used for intermittent infusion techniques in order to achieve strict control over the time and rate of administration, especially for infants and children and in intensive care units. Intermittent infusion may also make use of the 'piggy-back' technique provided that no additions are made to the primary infusion. In this method the drug is added to a small secondary container connected to a Y-type injection site on the primary infusion giving set; the secondary solution is usually infused within 30 minutes.

Addition *via the drip tubing* is indicated for a number of cytotoxic drugs in order to minimise extravasation. The preparation is added aseptically *via* the rubber septum of the injection site of a fast-running infusion. In general, drug preparations intended for a bolus effect should be given directly into a separate vein where possible. Failing this, administration may be made *via* the drip tubing provided that the preparation is compatible with the infusion fluid when given in this manner.

Table of drugs given by intravenous infusion

Covers addition to *Glucose intravenous infusion* 5 and 10%, *Sodium chloride intravenous infusion* 0.9%, *Compound sodium chloride intravenous infusion* (Ringer's solution), and *Compound sodium lactate intravenous infusion* (Hartmann's solution). Compatibility with glucose 5% and with sodium chloride 0.9% indicates compatibility with *Sodium chloride and glucose intravenous infusion*. Infusion of a large volume of hypotonic solution should be avoided therefore care should be taken if water for injections is used. The information in the Table relates to the proprietary preparations indicated; for other preparations suitability should be checked with the manufacturer

Abatacept (*Orencia®*)

Intermittent *in* Sodium chloride 0.9%

Reconstitute each vial with 10 mL water for injections using the silicone-free syringe provided; dilute requisite dose in infusion fluid to 100 mL (using the same silicone-free syringe); give over 30 minutes through a low protein-binding filter (pore size 0.2–1.2 micron)

Abciximab (*ReoPro®*)

Continuous *in* Glucose 5% *or* Sodium chloride 0.9%

Dilute requisite dose in infusion fluid and give *via* infusion pump; filter upon dilution with infusion fluid through a non-pyrogenic low protein-binding 0.2, 0.22, or 5 micron filter *or* upon administration through an in-line non-pyrogenic low protein-binding 0.2 or 0.22 micron filter

Acetylcysteine (*Parvolex®*)

Continuous *in* Glucose 5% or Sodium chloride 0.9%

Glucose 5% is preferable—see Emergency Treatment of Poisoning

Aciclovir (as sodium salt) (*Zovirax IV®*; *Aciclovir IV*, Mayne; *Aciclovir IV*, Genus; *Aciclovir Sodium*, Zurich)

Intermittent *in* Sodium chloride 0.9% *or* Sodium chloride and glucose *or* Compound sodium lactate

For *Zovirax IV®*, *Aciclovir IV* (Genus) initially reconstitute to 25 mg/mL in water for injections or sodium chloride 0.9% then dilute to not more than 5 mg/mL with the infusion fluid; to be given over 1 hour; alternatively, may be administered in a concentration of 25 mg/mL using a suitable infusion pump and given over 1 hour; for *Aciclovir IV* (Mayne) dilute to not more than 5 mg/mL with infusion fluid; give over 1 hour

Agalsidase alfa (*Replagal®*)

Intermittent *in* Sodium chloride 0.9%

Dilute requisite dose with 100 mL infusion fluid and give over 40 minutes; use within 3 hours of dilution

Agalsidase beta (*Fabrazyme®*)

Intermittent *in* Sodium chloride 0.9%

Reconstitute with water for injections (35 mg in 7.2 mL, 5 mg in 1.1 mL) to give 5 mg/mL solution; dilute requisite dose to 500 mL with infusion fluid and give through an in-line low-protein binding 0.2 micron filter at an initial rate of no more than 15 mg/hour; infusion rate may be increased gradually for subsequent infusions

Alemtuzumab (*MabCampath®*)

Intermittent in Glucose 5% *or* Sodium chloride 0.9%

Add requisite dose to 100 mL infusion fluid; infuse over 2 hours

Alfentanil (as hydrochloride) (*Rapifen®*)

Continuous *or* intermittent *in* Glucose 5% *or* Sodium chloride 0.9% *or* Compound sodium lactate

Alglucosidase alfa (*Myozyme®*)

Intermittent *in* Sodium chloride 0.9%

Reconstitute 50 mg with 10.3 mL water for injections to produce 5 mg/mL solution; gently rotate vial without shaking; dilute requisite dose with infusion fluid to give a final concentration of 0.5–4 mg/mL; give through a low protein-binding in-line filter (0.2 micron) at an initial rate of 1 mg/kg/hour increased by 2 mg/kg/hour every 30 minutes to max. 7 mg/kg/hour

Alprostadil (*Prostin VR®*)

Continuous *in* Glucose 5% *or* Sodium chloride 0.9%

Add directly to the infusion solution avoiding contact with the walls of plastic containers

Alteplase (*Actilyse®*)

Continuous *or* intermittent *in* Sodium chloride 0.9%

Dissolve in water for injections to a concentration of 1 mg/mL or 2 mg/mL and infuse intravenously; alternatively dilute the solution further in the infusion fluid to a concentration of not less than 200 micrograms/mL; not to be infused in glucose solution

Amikacin sulphate (*Amikin®*)

Intermittent *in* Glucose 5% *or* Sodium chloride 0.9% *or* Compound sodium lactate

To be given over 30 minutes

Aminophylline

Continuous *in* Glucose 5% *or* Sodium chloride 0.9% *or* Compound sodium lactate

Amiodarone hydrochloride (*Cordarone X®*)

Continuous *or* intermittent *in* Glucose 5%

Suggested initial infusion volume 250 mL given over 20–120 minutes; for repeat infusions up to 1.2 g in max. 500 mL; infusion in extreme emergency see section 2.7.3; should not be diluted to less than 600 micrograms/mL; incompatible with sodium chloride infusion; avoid equipment containing the plasticizer di-2-ethylhexyphthalate (DEHP)

Amoxicillin (as sodium salt) (*Amoxil®*)

Intermittent *in* Glucose 5% *or* Sodium chloride 0.9%

Reconstituted solutions diluted and given without delay; suggested volume 100 mL given over 30–60 minutes

via drip tubing *in* Glucose 5% *or* Sodium chloride 0.9%

Continuous infusion not usually recommended

Amphotericin (colloidal) (*Amphocil®*)

Intermittent *in* Glucose 5%

Initially reconstitute with water for injections (50 mg in 10 mL, 100 mg in 20 mL), shaking gently to dissolve (fluid may be opalescent) then dilute to a concentration of 625 micrograms/mL (1 volume of reconstituted solution with 7 volumes of infusion fluid); give at a rate of 1–2 mg/kg/hour or slower if not tolerated (initial test dose 2 mg of a 100 microgram/mL solution over 10 minutes); incompatible with sodium chloride or other electrolyte solutions, flush existing intravenous line with glucose 5% or use separate line

Amphotericin (lipid complex) (*Abelcet®*)

Intermittent *in* Glucose 5%

Allow suspension to reach room temperature, shake gently to ensure no yellow settlement, withdraw requisite dose (using 17–19 gauge needle) into one or more 20-mL syringes; replace needle on syringe with a 5-micron filter needle provided (fresh needle for each syringe) and dilute to a concentration of 1 mg/mL (2 mg/mL can be used in fluid restriction and in children); preferably give *via* an infusion pump at a rate of 2.5 mg/kg/hour (initial test dose of 1 mg given over 15 minutes); an in-line filter (pore size no less than 15 micron) may be used; do not use sodium chloride or other electrolyte solutions, flush existing intravenous line with glucose 5% or use separate line

Amphotericin (liposomal) (*AmBisome®*)

Intermittent *in* Glucose 5%

Reconstitute each vial with 12 mL water for injections and shake vigorously to produce a preparation containing 4 mg/mL; withdraw requisite dose from vial and introduce into infusion fluid through the 5 micron filter provided to produce a final concentration of 0.2–2 mg/mL; infuse over 30–60 minutes (initial test dose 1 mg over 10 minutes); incompatible with sodium chloride solutions, flush existing intravenous line with glucose 5% or use separate line

Amphotericin (as sodium deoxycholate complex) (*Fungizone®*)

Intermittent *in* Glucose 5%

Reconstitute each vial with 10 mL water for injections and shake immediately to produce a 5 mg/mL colloidal solution; dilute further in infusion fluid to a concentration of 100 micrograms/mL; pH of the glucose must not be below 4.2 (check each container—consult product literature for details of buffer); infuse over 2–4 hours, or longer if not tolerated (initial test dose 1 mg over 20–30 minutes); begin infusion immediately after dilution and protect from light; incompatible with sodium chloride solutions, flush existing intravenous line with glucose 5% or use separate line; an in-line filter (pore size no less than 1 micron) may be used

Ampicillin sodium (*Penbritin®*)

Intermittent *in* Glucose 5% *or* Sodium chloride 0.9%

Reconstituted solutions diluted and given without delay; suggested volume 100 mL given over 30–60 minutes

via drip tubing *in* Glucose 5% *or* Sodium chloride 0.9% *or* Ringer's solution *or* Compound sodium lactate

Continuous infusion not usually recommended

Amsacrine (*Amsidine®*)
Intermittent in Glucose 5%
Reconstitute with diluent provided and dilute to suggested volume 500 mL; give over 60–90 minutes; use glass syringes; incompatible with sodium chloride infusion

Anidulafungin (*Ecalta®*)
Intermittent *in* Glucose 5% *or* Sodium chloride 0.9%
Reconstitute each 100 mg with solvent provided, allow up to 5 minutes for reconstitution; dilute dose in infusion fluid to a concentration of 360 micrograms/mL; give at a rate not exceeding 1.1 mg/minute

Arsenic trioxide (*Trisenox®*)
Intermittent *in* Glucose 5% *or* Sodium chloride 0.9%
Dilute requisite dose with 100–250 mL infusion fluid; infuse over 1–2 hours (up to 4 hours if vasomotor reactions observed)

Atenolol (*Tenormin®*)
Intermittent *in* Glucose 5% *or* Sodium chloride 0.9%
Suggested infusion time 20 minutes

Atosiban (*Tractocile®*)
Continuous *in* Glucose 5% *or* Sodium chloride 0.9% *or* Compound sodium lactate
Withdraw 10 mL infusion fluid from 100-mL bag and replace with 10 mL atosiban concentrate (7.5 mg/mL) to produce a final concentration of 750 micrograms/mL

Atracurium besilate (*Tracrium®*; *Atracurium besilate injection*, Mayne; *Atracurium injection/infusion*, Genus)
Continuous *in* Glucose 5% *or* Sodium chloride 0.9% *or* Compound sodium lactate
Stability varies with diluent; dilute requisite dose with infusion fluid to a concentration of 0.5–5 mg/mL

Azathioprine (as sodium salt) (*Imuran®*)
Intermittent *in* Sodium chloride 0.9% *or* Sodium chloride and glucose
Reconstitute 50 mg with 5–15 mL water for injections; dilute with 20–200 mL infusion fluid

Aztreonam (*Azactam®*)
Intermittent *in* Glucose 5% *or* Sodium chloride 0.9% *or* Ringer's solution *or* Compound sodium lactate
Dissolve initially in water for injections (1 g per 3 mL) then dilute to a concentration of less than 20 mg/mL; to be given over 20–60 minutes

Basiliximab (*Simulect®*)
Intermittent in Glucose 5% or Sodium chloride 0.9%
Reconstitute 10 mg with 5 mL water for injections then dilute to at least 25 mL with infusion fluid; reconstitute 20 mg with 10 mL water for injections then dilute to at least 50 mL with infusion fluid; give over 20–30 minutes

Benzylpenicillin sodium (*Crystapen®*)
Intermittent *in* Glucose 5% *or* Sodium chloride 0.9%
Suggested volume 100 mL given over 30–60 minutes
Continuous infusion not usually recommended

Betamethasone (as sodium phosphate) (*Betnesol®*)
Continuous *or* intermittent *or via* drip tubing *in* Glucose 5% *or* Sodium chloride 0.9%

Bevacizumab (*Avastin®*)
Intermittent in Sodium chloride 0.9%
Dilute requisite dose in infusion fluid to 100 mL and give over 90 minutes; if initial dose well tolerated give second dose over 60 minutes; if second dose well tolerated give subsequent doses over 30 minutes; incompatible with glucose solutions

Bivalirudin (*Angiox®*)
Continuous *in* Glucose 5% *or* Sodium chloride 0.9%
Reconstitute each 250-mg vial with 5 mL water for injections then withdraw 5 mL and dilute to 50 mL with infusion fluid

Bleomycin sulphate
Intermittent *in* Sodium chloride 0.9%
To be given slowly; suggested volume 200 mL

Bumetanide (*Burinex®*)
Intermittent *in* Glucose 5% *or* Sodium chloride 0.9%
Suggested volume 500 mL given over 30–60 minutes

Busulfan (*Busilvex®*)
Intermittent in Glucose 5% or Sodium chloride 0.9%
Dilute to a concentration of 500 micrograms/mL; give through a central venous catheter over 2 hours

Calcitonin (salmon)/Salcatonin (*Miacalcic®*)
Intermittent *in* Sodium chloride 0.9%
Diluted solution given without delay; dilute in 500 mL and give over at least 6 hours; glass or hard plastic containers should not be used; some loss of potency on dilution and administration

Calcium folinate (*Calcium Leucovorin®*, *Refolinon®*)
Intermittent *in* Sodium chloride 0.9%
Calcium Leucovorin® can also be infused in Glucose 5 and 10% or Compound sodium lactate
Protect from light

Calcium gluconate
Continuous *in* Glucose 5% *or* Sodium chloride 0.9%
Avoid bicarbonates, phosphates, or sulphates

Calcium levofolinate (*Isovorin®*)
Intermittent *in* Glucose 5 and 10% *or* Sodium chloride 0.9% *or* Compound sodium lactate
Protect from light

Carboplatin (*Paraplatin®*)
Intermittent *in* Glucose 5% *or* Sodium chloride 0.9%
Final concentration as low as 500 micrograms/mL; give over 15–60 minutes

Carmustine (*BiCNU®*)
Intermittent *in* Glucose 5% *or* Sodium chloride 0.9%
Reconstitute with solvent provided; give over 1–2 hours

Caspofungin (*Cancidas®*)
Intermittent *in* Sodium chloride 0.9% *or* Compound sodium lactate
Allow vial to reach room temperature; initially reconstitute each vial with 10.5 mL water for injections, mixing gently to dissolve then dilute requisite dose in 250 mL infusion fluid (35- or 50-mg doses may be diluted in 100 mL infusion fluid if necessary); give over 60 minutes; incompatible with glucose solutions

Cefotaxime (as sodium salt) (*Claforan®*; *Cefotaxime Injection*, Genus)
Intermittent *in* Glucose 5% *or* Sodium chloride 0.9% *or* Compound sodium lactate *or* Water for injections
Suggested volume 40–100 mL given over 20–60 minutes

Cefradine (*Velosef®*)
Continuous *or* intermittent *in* Glucose 5 and 10% *or* Sodium chloride 0.9% *or* Ringer's solution *or* Compound sodium lactate
Reconstitute 500 mg with 5 mL water for injections or glucose 5% or sodium chloride 0.9% then dilute with infusion fluid

Ceftazidime (as pentahydrate) (*Fortum®*, *Kefadim®*)
Intermittent *or via* drip tubing *in* Glucose 5 and 10% *or* Sodium chloride 0.9% *or* Compound sodium lactate
Dissolve 2 g initially in 10 mL (3 g in 15 mL) infusion fluid; for *Fortum®* dilute further to a concentration of 40 mg/mL; for *Kefadim®* dilute further to a concentration of 20 mg/mL; give over up to 30 minutes

Ceftriaxone (as sodium salt) (*Rocephin®*; *Ceftriaxone Injection*, Genus)

Intermittent *or via* drip tubing *in* Glucose 5 and 10% *or* Sodium chloride 0.9%

Reconstitute 2-g vial with 40 mL infusion fluid; give intermittent infusion over at least 30 minutes (60 minutes in neonates); not to be given with total parenteral nutrition or infusion fluids containing calcium, even by different infusion lines

Cefuroxime (as sodium salt) (*Zinacef®*)

Intermittent *or via* drip tubing *in* Glucose 5% *or* Sodium chloride 0.9% *or* Compound sodium lactate

Dissolve initially in water for injections (at least 2 mL for each 250 mg, 15 mL for 1.5 g); suggested volume 50–100 mL given over 30 minutes

Chloramphenicol (as sodium succinate) (*Kemicetine®*)

Intermittent *or via* drip tubing *in* Glucose 5% *or* Sodium chloride 0.9%

Ciclosporin (*Sandimmun®*)

Continuous *in* Glucose 5% *or* Sodium chloride 0.9%

Dilute to a concentration of 50 mg in 20–100 mL; give over 2–6 hours; not to be used with PVC equipment

Cidofovir (*Vistide®*)

Intermittent *in* Sodium chloride 0.9%

Dilute requisite dose with 100 mL infusion fluid; infuse over 1 hour

Cimetidine (*Tagamet®*)

Continuous *or* intermittent *in* Glucose 5% *or* Sodium chloride 0.9%

For intermittent infusion suggested volume 100 mL given over 30–60 minutes

Cisatracurium (*Nimbex®*, *Nimbex Forte®*)

Continuous *in* Glucose 5% *or* Sodium chloride 0.9%

Solutions of 2 mg/mL and 5 mg/mL may be infused undiluted; alternatively dilute with infusion fluid to a concentration of 0.1–2 mg/mL

Cisplatin (*Cisplatin*, Pharmacia; *Cisplatin injection solution*, Mayne)

Intermittent *in* Sodium chloride 0.9% *or* Sodium chloride and glucose

Reconstitute initially with water for injections to produce 1 mg/mL solution then dilute in 2 litres infusion fluid; give over 6–8 hours

Cladribine (*Leustat®*)

Continuous *in* Sodium chloride 0.9%

Dilute with 100–500 mL; glucose solutions are unsuitable

Clarithromycin (*Klaricid® I.V.*)

Intermittent *in* Glucose 5% *or* Sodium chloride 0.9% *or* Ringer's solution *or* Compound sodium lactate

Dissolve initially in water for injections (500 mg in 10 mL) then dilute to a concentration of 2 mg/mL; give over 60 minutes

Clindamycin (as phosphate) (*Dalacin® C Phosphate*)

Continuous *or* intermittent *in* Glucose 5% *or* Sodium chloride 0.9%

Dilute to not more than 18 mg/mL and give over 10–60 minutes at a rate not exceeding 30 mg/minute (1.2 g over at least 60 minutes; higher doses by continuous infusion)

Clofarabine (*Evoltra®*)

Intermittent *in* Sodium chloride 0.9%

Filter requisite dose through a 0.2 micron filter and dilute with infusion fluid; give over 2 hours

Clonazepam (*Rivotril®*)

Intermittent *in* Glucose 5 and 10% *or* Sodium chloride 0.9%

Suggested volume 250 mL

Co-amoxiclav (*Augmentin®*; *Co-amoxiclav Injection*, Wockhardt)

Intermittent *in* Sodium chloride 0.9% *or* Water for injections; see also package leaflet

Suggested volume 50–100 mL given over 30–40 minutes and completed within 4 hours of reconstitution

via drip tubing *in* Glucose 5% *or* Sodium chloride 0.9%

Co-fluampicil (as sodium salts) (*Magnapen®*)

Intermittent *in* Glucose 5% *or* Sodium chloride 0.9%

Reconstituted solutions diluted and given without delay; suggested volume 100 mL given over 30–60 minutes

via drip tubing *in* Glucose 5% *or* Sodium chloride 0.9% *or* Ringer's solution *or* Compound sodium lactate

Colistimethate sodium (*Colomycin®*)

Intermittent *in* Sodium chloride 0.9% *or* Water for injections

Dilute with 50 mL infusion fluid and give over 30 minutes

Co-trimoxazole (*Septrin® for infusion*)

Intermittent *in* Glucose 5 and 10% *or* Sodium chloride 0.9% *or* Ringer's solution

Dilute contents of 1 ampoule (5 mL) to 125 mL, 2 ampoules (10 mL) to 250 mL or 3 ampoules (15 mL) to 500 mL; suggested duration of infusion 60–90 minutes (but may be adjusted according to fluid requirements); if fluid restriction necessary, 1 ampoule (5 mL) may be diluted with 75 mL glucose 5% and infused over max. 60 minutes

Cyclophosphamide (*Endoxana®*)

via drip tubing *in* Glucose 5% *or* Sodium chloride 0.9%

Reconstitute with sodium chloride 0.9%

Cyclosporin *see* Ciclosporin

Cytarabine (*Cytarabine injection solution*, Pharmacia, Mayne)

Continuous *or* intermittent *in* Glucose 5% *or* Sodium chloride 0.9%

For *Cytarabine injection solution* 100 mg/mL (Pharmacia) before use, vials should be warmed to 55°C for 30 minutes, with adequate shaking, and allowed to cool to room temperature

Dacarbazine (*Dacarbazine*, Medac)

Intermittent *in* Glucose 5% *or* Sodium chloride 0.9%

Reconstitute initially with water for injections then dilute in 200–300 mL infusion fluid; give over 15–30 minutes; protect infusion from light

Daclizumab (*Zenapax®*)

Intermittent *in* Sodium chloride 0.9%

Dilute requisite dose in 50 mL infusion fluid; infuse over 15 minutes

Dactinomycin (*Cosmegen Lyovac®*)

Intermittent *or via* drip tubing *in* Glucose 5% *or* Sodium chloride 0.9%

Reconstitute with water for injections

Danaparoid sodium (*Orgaran®*)

Continuous *in* Glucose 5% *or* Sodium chloride 0.9%

Daptomycin (*Cubicin®*)

Intermittent *in* Sodium chloride 0.9%

Reconstitute with water for injections or sodium chloride 0.9% (350 mg in 7 mL, 500 mg in 10 mL); gently rotate vial without shaking; allow to stand for at least 10 minutes then rotate gently to dissolve; dilute requisite dose in 50 mL infusion fluid and give over 30 minutes

Daunorubicin (as hydrochloride) (*Cerubidin®*)

via drip tubing *in* Sodium chloride 0.9%

Reconstitute vial with 4 mL water for injections to give 5 mg/mL solution; dilute requisite dose with infusion fluid to a concentration of 1 mg/mL; give over 20 minutes

Daunorubicin (liposomal) (*DaunoXome®*)
Intermittent *in* Glucose 5%
Dilute to a concentration of 0.2–1 mg/mL; give over 30–60 minutes; incompatible with sodium chloride solutions; in-line filter not recommended (if used, pore size should be no less than 5 micron)

Desferrioxamine mesilate (*Desferal®*)
Continuous *or* intermittent *in* Glucose 5% *or* Sodium chloride 0.9%
Reconstitute with water for injections to a concentration of 100 mg/mL; dilute with infusion fluid

Desmopressin (*DDAVP®*, *Octim®*)
Intermittent *in* Sodium chloride 0.9%
Dilute with 50 mL and give over 20 minutes

Dexamethasone sodium phosphate (*Dexamethasone*, Mayne; *Dexamethasone*, Organon)
Continuous *or* intermittent *or via* drip tubing *in* Glucose 5% *or* Sodium chloride 0.9%
Dexamethasone (Organon) can also be infused in Ringer's solution *or* Compound sodium lactate

Dexrazoxane (*Savene®*)
Intermittent *in Savene®* diluent
Reconstitute 500 mg with 25 mL of Water for Injections then dilute in 500 mL *Savene®* diluent; give over 1–2 hours into a large vein in an area other than the one affected

Diamorphine hydrochloride (*Diamorphine Injection*, Wockhardt)
Continuous *in* Glucose 5% *or* Sodium chloride 0.9%
Glucose is preferred as infusion fluid

Diazepam (solution) (*Diazepam*, Wockhardt)
Continuous *in* Glucose 5% *or* Sodium chloride 0.9%
Dilute to a concentration of not more than 10 mg in 200 mL; adsorbed to some extent by the plastics of bags and infusion sets

Diazepam (emulsion) (*Diazemuls®*)
Continuous *in* Glucose 5 and 10%
May be diluted to a max. concentration of 200 mg in 500 mL; max. 6 hours between addition and completion of administration; adsorbed to some extent by the plastics of the infusion set
via drip tubing *in* Glucose 5 and 10% *or* Sodium chloride 0.9%
Adsorbed to some extent by the plastics of the infusion set

Diclofenac sodium (*Voltarol®*)
Continuous *or* intermittent *in* Glucose 5% *or* Sodium chloride 0.9%
Dilute 75 mg with 100–500 mL infusion fluid (previously buffered with 0.5 mL sodium bicarbonate 8.4% solution *or* with 1 mL sodium bicarbonate 4.2% solution); for intermittent infusion give 25–50 mg over 15–60 minutes or 75 mg over 30–120 minutes; for continuous infusion give at a rate of 5 mg/hour

Digoxin (*Lanoxin®*)
Intermittent *in* Glucose 5% *or* Sodium chloride 0.9%
To be given over at least 2 hours

Digoxin-specific antibody fragments (*Digibind®*)
Intermittent *in* Sodium chloride 0.9%
Dissolve initially in water for injections (4 mL/vial) then dilute with the sodium chloride 0.9% and give through a 0.22 micron sterile, disposable filter over 30 minutes

Dinoprostone (*Prostin E2®*)
Continuous *or* intermittent *in* Glucose 5% *or* Sodium chloride 0.9%

Disodium folinate (*Sodiofolin®*)
Intermittent *in* Sodium chloride 0.9%
Protect from light
Avoid bicarbonate containing infusions

Disodium pamidronate (*Aredia®*; *Disodium pamidronate*, Britannia, Mayne, Medac)
Intermittent *in* Glucose 5% *or* Sodium chloride 0.9%
For *Aredia®* and *Pamidronate disodium* (Britannia), reconstitute initially with water for injections (15 mg in 5 mL, 30 mg or 90 mg in 10 mL); for *Aredia®*, *Pamidronate disodium* (Britannia), *Disodium pamidronate* (Mayne), dilute with infusion fluid to a concentration of not more than 60 mg in 250 mL; for *Disodium pamidronate* (Medac) dilute with infusion fluid to a concentration of not more than 90 mg in 250 mL; give at a rate not exceeding 1 mg/minute; not to be given with infusion fluids containing calcium

Disopyramide (as phosphate) (*Rythmodan®*)
Continuous *or* intermittent *in* Glucose 5% *or* Sodium chloride 0.9% *or* Ringer's solution *or* Compound sodium lactate
Max. rate by continuous infusion 20–30 mg/hour (or 400 micrograms/kg/hour)

Dobutamine (as hydrochloride) (*Dobutrex®*, *Posiject®*)
Continuous *in* Glucose 5% *or* Sodium chloride 0.9%
Dilute to a concentration of 0.5–1 mg/mL and give *via* a controlled infusion device; give higher concentration (max. 5 mg/mL) with infusion pump; incompatible with bicarbonate

Docetaxel (*Taxotere®*)
Intermittent *in* Glucose 5% *or* Sodium chloride 0.9%
Stand docetaxel vials and diluent at room temperature for 5 minutes; add diluent to produce a concentrate containing 10 mg/mL and allow to stand for a further 5 minutes; dilute the requisite dose with at least 250 mL infusion fluid to a final concentration not exceeding 740 micrograms/mL; infuse over 1 hour

Dolasetron mesilate (*Anzemet®*)
Intermittent *in* Glucose 5% *or* Sodium chloride 0.9% *or* Compound sodium lactate
Suggested volume 50 mL given over 30 seconds–15 minutes

Dopamine hydrochloride
Continuous *in* Glucose 5% *or* Sodium chloride 0.9% *or* Compound sodium lactate
Dilute to max concentration of 3.2 mg/mL; incompatible with bicarbonate

Dopexamine hydrochloride (*Dopacard®*)
Continuous *in* Glucose 5% *or* Sodium chloride 0.9%
Dilute to a concentration of 400 or 800 micrograms/mL; max. concentration *via* large peripheral vein 1 mg/mL, concentrations up to 4 mg/mL may be infused *via* central vein; give *via* infusion pump or other device which provides accurate control of rate; contact with metal should be minimised; incompatible with bicarbonate

Doxorubicin hydrochloride
Continuous *or via* drip tubing *in* Glucose 5% *or* Sodium chloride 0.9%
Reconstitute with water for injections or sodium chloride 0.9% (10 mg in 5 mL, 50 mg in 25 mL); give over 3–5 minutes; for continuous infusion over 24 hours (*Doxorubicin*, Medac and *Doxorubicin*, Teva UK only), consult local protocol

Doxorubicin hydrochloride (liposomal) (*Caelyx®*)
via drip tubing *in* Glucose 5%
Dilute up to 90 mg in 250 mL infusion fluid and over 90 mg in 500 mL infusion fluid

Eculizumab (*Soliris®*)
Intermittent *in* Glucose 5% *or* Sodium chloride 0.9%
Dilute requisite dose to a concentration of 5 mg/mL and mix gently; give over 25–45 minutes (infusion time may be increased to 2 hours if infusion-related reactions occur)

Enoximone (*Perfan®*)
Continuous *or* intermittent *in* Sodium chloride 0.9% *or* Water for injections
Dilute to a concentration of 2.5 mg/mL; incompatible with glucose solutions; use only plastic containers or syringes

Epirubicin hydrochloride (*Pharmorubicin® Rapid Dissolution, Pharmorubicin® Solution*)
via drip tubing *in* Sodium chloride 0.9%
Reconstitute *Pharmorubicin® Rapid Dissolution* with sodium chloride 0.9% or with water for injections (10 mg in 5 mL, 20 mg in 10 mL, 50 mg in 25 mL); give over 3–5 minutes

Epoprostenol (*Flolan®*)
Continuous *in* Sodium chloride 0.9% (but see also below)
Reconstitute using the filter and solvent (glycine buffer diluent) provided to make a concentrate; may be diluted further (consult product literature); for *pulmonary hypertension* dilute further with glycine buffer diluent only, for *renal dialysis* may be diluted further with sodium chloride 0.9%

Ertapenem (*Invanz®*)
Intermittent *in* Sodium chloride 0.9%
Reconstitute 1 g with 10 mL water for injections or sodium chloride 0.9%; dilute requisite dose in infusion fluid to a final concentration not exceeding 20 mg/mL; give over 30 minutes; incompatible with glucose solutions

Erythromycin (as lactobionate)
Continuous *or* intermittent *in* Glucose 5% (neutralised with sodium bicarbonate) *or* Sodium chloride 0.9%
Dissolve initially in water for injections (1 g in 20 mL) then dilute to a concentration of 1 mg/mL for continuous infusion and 1–5 mg/mL for intermittent infusion; give intermittent infusion over 20–60 minutes

Esmolol hydrochloride (*Brevibloc®*)
Continuous *or* intermittent *in* Glucose 5% *or* Sodium chloride 0.9%
Dilute to a concentration of 10 mg/mL; for continuous infusion use a suitable infusion control device; incompatible with bicarbonate

Esomeprazole (as sodium salt) (*Nexium®*)
Intermittent *in* Sodium chloride 0.9%
Reconstitute 40 mg with 5 mL sodium chloride 0.9% then dilute with up to 100 mL infusion fluid, give requisite dose over 10–30 minutes

Ethanol
Continuous *in* Glucose 5% *or* Sodium chloride 0.9% *or* Ringer's solution *or* Compound sodium lactate
Dilute to a concentration of 5–10%

Etoposide (*Eposin®*; *Etoposide*, TEVA UK and Mayne)
Intermittent *in* Sodium chloride 0.9%
For *Etoposide* (TEVA UK) dilute with either sodium chloride 0.9% or glucose 5% to a concentration of 200 micrograms/mL and give over 30–60 minutes; for *Etoposide* (Mayne) dilute with either sodium chloride 0.9% or glucose 5% to a concentration of not more than 250 micrograms/mL and give over not less than 30 minutes; for *Eposin®* dilute with either sodium chloride 0.9% or glucose 5% to a concentration of 200–400 micrograms/mL and give over at least 30 minutes; check container for haze or precipitate during infusion

Etoposide (as phosphate) (*Etopophos®*)
Intermittent *in* Glucose 5% *or* Sodium chloride 0.9%
Reconstitute with 5–10 mL of either water for injections *or* with infusion fluid then dilute further with infusion fluid to a concentration as low as 100 micrograms/mL and give over 5 minutes to 3.5 hours

Fentanyl (*Sublimaze®*)
Continuous *or* intermittent *in* Glucose 5% *or* Sodium chloride 0.9%

Filgrastim (*Neupogen®*)
Continuous *or* intermittent *in* Glucose 5%
For a filgrastim concentration of less than 1 500 000 units/mL (15 micrograms/mL) albumin solution (human serum albumin) is added to produce a final albumin concentration of 2 mg/mL; should not be diluted to a filgrastim concentration of less than 200 000 units/mL (2 micrograms/mL) and should not be diluted with sodium chloride solution

Flecainide acetate (*Tambocor®*)
Continuous *or* intermittent *in* Glucose 5% *or* Sodium chloride 0.9% *or* Compound sodium lactate
Minimum volume in infusion fluids containing chlorides 500 mL

Flucloxacillin (as sodium salt) (*Floxapen®*)
Intermittent *in* Glucose 5% *or* Sodium chloride 0.9%
Suggested volume 100 mL given over 30–60 minutes
via drip tubing *in* Glucose 5% *or* Sodium chloride 0.9% *or* Ringer's solution *or* Compound sodium lactate
Continuous infusion not usually recommended

Fludarabine phosphate (*Fludara®*)
Intermittent *in* Sodium chloride 0.9%
Reconstitute each 50 mg with 2 mL water for injections and dilute requisite dose in 100 mL; give over 30 minutes

Flumazenil (*Anexate®*)
Continuous *in* Glucose 5% *or* Sodium chloride 0.9%

Fluorouracil (as sodium salt)
Continuous *or* intermittent *or via* drip tubing *in* Glucose 5% *or* Sodium chloride 0.9%
Give intermittent infusion over 30–60 minutes or over 4 hours

Fondaparinux (*Arixtra®*)
Intermittent *in* Sodium chloride 0.9%
For ST-segment elevation myocardial infarction, add requisite dose to 25–50 mL infusion fluid and give over 1–2 minutes

Foscarnet sodium (*Foscavir®*)
Intermittent *in* Glucose 5% *or* Sodium chloride 0.9%
Dilute to a concentration of 12 mg/mL for infusion into peripheral vein (undiluted solution *via* central venous line only); infuse over at least 1 hour

Fosphenytoin Sodium (*Pro-Epanutin®*)
Intermittent *in* Glucose 5% *or* Sodium chloride 0.9%
Dilute to a concentration of 1.5–25 mg (phenytoin sodium equivalent)/mL

Furosemide/Frusemide (as sodium salt) (*Lasix®*)
Continuous *in* Sodium chloride 0.9% *or* Ringer's solution
Infusion pH must be above 5.5 and rate should not exceed 4 mg/minute; glucose solutions are unsuitable

Fusidic acid (as sodium salt)
Continuous *in* Glucose 5% (but see below) *or* Sodium chloride 0.9%
Reconstitute with the buffer solution provided and dilute to 500 mL; give through central venous line over 2 hours (or over 6 hours if superficial vein used); incompatible in solution of pH less than 7.4

Galsulfase (*Naglazyme®*)
Intermittent *in* Sodium chloride 0.9%
Dilute requisite dose with infusion fluid to final volume of 250 mL and mix gently; infuse through a 0.2 micron in-line filter; give approx. 2.5% of the total volume over 1 hour, then infuse remaining volume over next 3 hours; if patient under 20 kg and at risk of fluid overload, dilute requisite dose in 100 mL infusion fluid and give over at least 4 hours

Ganciclovir (as sodium salt) (*Cymevene®*)
Intermittent *in* Glucose 5% *or* Sodium chloride 0.9% *or* Ringer's solution *or* Compound sodium lactate
Reconstitute initially in water for injections (500 mg/10 mL) then dilute to not more than 10 mg/mL with infusion fluid (usually 100 mL); give over 1 hour

Gemcitabine (*Gemzar®*)
Intermittent *in* Sodium chloride 0.9%
Reconstitute initially with sodium chloride 0.9% (200 mg in at least 5 mL, 1 g in at least 25 mL); may be diluted further with infusion fluid; give over 30 minutes

Gentamicin (as sulphate) (*Cidomycin®*; *Gentamicin Paediatric Injection*, Beacon; *Gentamicin Injection*, Mayne)
Intermittent *or via* drip tubing *in* Glucose 5% *or* Sodium chloride 0.9%
Suggested volume for intermittent infusion 50–100 mL given over 20–30 minutes

Glyceryl trinitrate (*Nitrocine®*, *Nitronal®*)
Continuous *in* Glucose 5% *or* Sodium chloride 0.9%
For *Nitrocine®* suggested infusion concentration 100 micrograms/mL; incompatible with polyvinyl chloride infusion containers such as *Viaflex®* or *Steriflex®*; use glass or polyethylene containers or give *via* a syringe pump

Granisetron (as hydrochloride) (*Kytril®*)
Intermittent *in* Glucose 5% *or* Sodium chloride 0.9% *or* Compound sodium lactate
Dilute 3 mL in 20–50 mL infusion fluid (up to 3 mL in 10–30 mL for children); give over 5 minutes

Haem arginate (*Normosang®*)
Intermittent *in* Sodium chloride 0.9%
Dilute requisite dose in 100 mL infusion fluid in glass bottle and give over at least 30 minutes *via* large antebrachial vein; administer within 1 hour after dilution

Heparin sodium
Continuous *in* Glucose 5% *or* Sodium chloride 0.9%
Administration with a motorised pump advisable

Hydralazine hydrochloride (*Apresoline®*)
Continuous *in* Sodium chloride 0.9% *or* Ringer's solution
Suggested infusion volume 500 mL

Hydrocortisone (as sodium phosphate) (*Efcortesol®*)
Continuous *or* intermittent *or via* drip tubing *in* Glucose 5% *or* Sodium chloride 0.9%

Hydrocortisone (as sodium succinate) (*SoluCortef®*)
Continuous *or* intermittent *or via* drip tubing *in* Glucose 5% *or* Sodium chloride 0.9%

Ibandronic acid (*Bondronat®*)
Intermittent *in* Glucose 5% *or* Sodium chloride 0.9%
Dilute requisite dose in 500 mL infusion fluid and give over 1–2 hours

Idarubicin hydrochloride (*Zavedos®*)
via drip tubing *in* Sodium chloride 0.9%
Reconstitute with water for injections; give over 5–10 minutes

Idursulfase (*Elaprase®*)
Intermittent *in* Sodium chloride 0.9%
Dilute requisite dose in 100 mL infusion fluid and mix gently (do not shake); give over 3 hours (gradually reduced to 1 hour if no infusion-related reactions)

Ifosfamide (*Mitoxana®*)
Continuous *or* intermittent *or via* drip tubing *in* Glucose 5% *or* Sodium chloride 0.9%
For continuous infusion, suggested volume 3 litres given over 24 hours; for intermittent infusion, give over 30–120 minutes

Imiglucerase (*Cerezyme®*)
Intermittent *in* Sodium chloride 0.9%
Initially reconstitute with water for injections (200 units in 5.1 mL, 400 units in 10.2 mL) to give 40 units/mL solution; dilute requisite dose with infusion fluid to a final volume of 100–200 mL and give over 1–2 hours *or* at a rate not exceeding 1 unit/kg/minute; administer within 3 hours after reconstitution

Imipenem with cilastatin (as sodium salt) (*Primaxin®*)
Intermittent *in* Sodium chloride 0.9% *or* Sodium chloride and Glucose
Dilute to a concentration of 5 mg (as imipenem)/mL; infuse 250–500 mg (as imipenem) over 20–30 minutes, 1 g over 40–60 minutes
Continuous infusion not usually recommended

Infliximab (*Remicade®*)
Intermittent *in* Sodium chloride 0.9%
Reconstitute each 100-mg vial with 10 mL water for injections using a 21-gauge or smaller needle; gently swirl vial without shaking to dissolve; allow to stand for 5 minutes; dilute requisite dose with infusion fluid to a final volume of 250 mL and give through a low protein-binding filter (1.2 micron or less) over at least 2 hours (patients being treated for rheumatoid arthritis who have tolerated 3 initial 2-hour infusions may be given subsequent infusions of up to 6 mg/kg over at least 1 hour); start infusion within 3 hours of reconstitution

Insulin (soluble)
Continuous *in* Sodium chloride 0.9% *or* Compound sodium lactate
Adsorbed to some extent by plastics of infusion set; see also section 6.1.3; ensure insulin is not injected into 'dead space' of injection port of the infusion bag

Insulin aspart
Continuous *in* Sodium chloride 0.9% *or* Glucose 5%
Dilute to 0.05–1 unit/mL with infusion fluid; adsorbed to some extent by plastics of infusion set

Insulin lispro
Continuous *in* Sodium chloride 0.9% *or* Glucose 5%

Interferon alfa-2b (*IntronA®*)
Intermittent *in* Sodium chloride 0.9%
For *IntronA®* solution, dilute requisite dose in 50 mL infusion fluid and administer over 20 minutes; not to be diluted to less than 300 000 units/mL
For *IntronA®* powder, reconstitute with 1 mL water for injections; dilute requisite dose in 100 mL infusion fluid and administer over 20 minutes; not to be diluted to less than 100 000 units/mL

Irinotecan hydrochloride (*Campto®*)
Intermittent *in* Glucose 5% *or* Sodium chloride 0.9%
Dilute requisite dose in 250 mL infusion fluid; give over 30–90 minutes

Iron dextran (*Cosmofer®*)
Intermittent *in* Glucose 5% *or* Sodium chloride 0.9%
Dilute 100–200 mg in 100 mL infusion fluid; give 25 mg over 15 minutes as a test dose initially, then give at a rate not exceeding 6.67 mg/minute; *total dose infusion* diluted in 500 mL infusion fluid and given over 4–6 hours (initial test dose 25 mg over 15 minutes)

Iron sucrose (*Venofer®*)
Intermittent *in* Sodium chloride 0.9%
Dilute 100 mg in up to 100 mL infusion fluid; give 25 mg over 15 minutes as a test dose initially, then give at a rate not exceeding 3.33 mg/minute

Isosorbide dinitrate (*Isoket 0.05%®*, *Isoket 0.1%®*)
Continuous *in* Glucose 5% *or* Sodium chloride 0.9%
Adsorbed to some extent by polyvinyl chloride infusion containers; preferably use glass or polyethylene containers or give *via* a syringe pump; *Isoket 0.05%®* can alternatively be administered undiluted using a syringe pump with a glass or rigid plastic syringe

Itraconazole (*Sporanox®*)
Intermittent *in* Sodium chloride 0.9%
Dilute 250 mg in 50 mL infusion fluid and infuse only **60 mL** through an in-line filter (0.2 micron) over 60 minutes

Ketamine (as hydrochloride) (*Ketalar®*)
Continuous *in* Glucose 5% *or* Sodium chloride 0.9%
Dilute to 1 mg/mL; microdrip infusion for maintenance of anaesthesia

Labetalol hydrochloride (*Trandate*®)

Intermittent *in* Glucose 5% *or* Sodium chloride and glucose

Dilute to a concentration of 1 mg/mL; suggested volume 200 mL; adjust rate with in-line burette

Laronidase (*Aldurazyme*®)

Intermittent *in* Sodium chloride 0.9%

Body-weight under 20 kg, use 100 mL infusion fluid; body-weight over 20 kg use 250 mL infusion fluid; withdraw volume of infusion fluid equivalent to volume of laronidase concentrate being added; give through an in-line filter (0.22 micron) at an initial rate of 2 units/kg/hour then increasing gradually every 15 minutes to max. 43 units/kg/hour

Lenograstim (*Granocyte*®)

Intermittent *in* Sodium chloride 0.9%

Initially reconstitute with 1 mL water for injection provided (do not shake vigorously) then dilute with up to 50 mL infusion fluid for each vial of *Granocyte-13* or up to 100 mL infusion fluid for *Granocyte-34*; give over 30 minutes

Lepirudin (*Refludan*®)

Continuous *in* Glucose 5% *or* Sodium chloride 0.9%

Reconstitute initially with water for injections *or* sodium chloride 0.9% then dilute to a concentration of 2 mg/mL with infusion fluid

Levetiracetam (*Keppra*®)

Intermittent *in* Glucose 5% *or* Sodium chloride 0.9% *or* Compound sodium lactate

Dilute requisite dose with at least 100 mL of infusion fluid; give over 15 minutes

Magnesium sulphate

Continuous *in* Glucose 5% *or* Sodium chloride 0.9%

Suggested concentration up to 200 mg/mL; max. rate 150 mg/minute

Melphalan (*Alkeran*®)

Intermittent *or via* drip tubing *in* Sodium chloride 0.9%

Reconstitute with the solvent provided then dilute with infusion fluid; max. 90 minutes between addition and completion of administration; incompatible with glucose infusion

Meropenem (*Meronem*®)

Intermittent *in* Glucose 5 and 10% *or* Sodium chloride 0.9%

Dilute in 50–200 mL infusion fluid and give over 15–30 minutes

Mesna (*Uromitexan*®)

Continuous *or via* drip tubing *in* Glucose 5% *or* Sodium chloride 0.9%

Metaraminol (as tartrate) (*Aramine*®)

Continuous *or via* drip tubing *in* Glucose 5% *or* Sodium chloride 0.9%

Suggested volume 500 mL

Methotrexate (as sodium salt) (*Methotrexate*, Lederle)

Continuous *or via* drip tubing *in* Glucose 5% *or* Sodium chloride 0.9% *or* Compound sodium lactate *or* Ringer's solution

Dilute in a large-volume infusion; max. 24 hours between addition and completion of administration

Methylprednisolone (as sodium succinate) (*Solu-Medrone*®)

Continuous *or* intermittent *or via* drip tubing *in* Glucose 5% *or* Sodium chloride 0.9%

Reconstitute initially with water for injections; doses up to 250 mg should be given over at least 5 minutes, high doses over at least 30 minutes

Metoclopramide hydrochloride (*Maxolon High Dose*®)

Continuous *or* intermittent *in* Glucose 5% *or* Sodium chloride 0.9% *or* Compound sodium lactate

Continuous infusion recommended; loading dose, dilute with 50–100 mL and give over 15–20 minutes; maintenance dose, dilute with 500 mL and give over 8–12 hours; for intermittent infusion dilute with at least 50 mL and give over at least 15 minutes

Mexiletine hydrochloride (*Mexitil*®)

Continuous *in* Glucose 5% *or* Sodium chloride 0.9%

For loading dose, dilute to a concentration of 1 mg/mL; for maintenance dose, dilute to a concentration of 500 micrograms/mL; discard after 8 hours from preparation

Midazolam (*Hypnovel*®)

Continuous *in* Glucose 5% *or* Sodium chloride 0.9%

For neonates and children under 15 kg dilute to a max. concentration of 1 mg/mL

Milrinone (*Primacor*®)

Continuous *in* Glucose 5% *or* Sodium chloride 0.9%

Dilute to a suggested concentration of 200 micrograms/mL

Mitoxantrone/Mitozantrone (as hydrochloride) (*Novantrone*®, *Onkotrone*®)

Intermittent *or via* drip tubing *in* Glucose 5% *or* Sodium chloride 0.9%

For administration *via* drip tubing suggested volume at least 50 mL given over at least 3–5 minutes; for intermittent infusion (*Onkotrone*® only), dilute with 50–100 mL and give over 15–30 minutes

Mivacurium (as chloride) (*Mivacron*®)

Continuous *in* Glucose 5% *or* Sodium chloride 0.9%

Dilute to a concentration of 500 micrograms/mL; may also be given undiluted

Mycophenolate mofetil (as hydrochloride) (*CellCept*®)

Intermittent *in* Glucose 5%

Reconstitute each 500-mg vial with 14 mL glucose 5% and dilute the contents of 2 vials in 140 mL infusion fluid; give over 2 hours

Naloxone (*Min-I-Jet*® *Naloxone Hydrochloride*)

Continuous *in* Glucose 5% *or* Sodium chloride 0.9%

Reversal of opioid-induced respiratory depression, dilute to a concentration of 4 micrograms/mL; opioid overdose only, dilute 10 mg in 50 mL glucose 5%, see Emergency Treatment of Poisoning

Natalizumab (*Tysabri*®)

Intermittent *in* Sodium chloride 0.9%

Dilute 300 mg in 100 mL infusion fluid; gently invert to mix, do not shake. Use within 8 hours of dilution and give over 1 hour

Nimodipine (*Nimotop*®)

via drip tubing *in* Glucose 5% *or* Sodium chloride 0.9% *or* Compound sodium lactate

Not to be added to infusion container; administer *via* an infusion pump through a Y-piece into a central catheter; incompatible with polyvinyl chloride giving sets or containers; protect infusion from light

Nizatidine (*Axid*®)

Continuous *or* intermittent *in* Glucose 5% *or* Sodium chloride 0.9% *or* Compound sodium lactate

For continuous infusion, dilute 300 mg in 150 mL and give at a rate of 10 mg/hour; for intermittent infusion, dilute 100 mg in 50 mL and give over 15 minutes

Noradrenaline acid tartrate/Norepinephrine bitartrate

Continuous *in* Glucose 5% *or* Sodium chloride and glucose

Give *via* controlled infusion device; for administration *via* syringe pump, dilute 4 mg noradrenaline acid tartrate (2 mL solution) with 48 mL; for administration *via* drip counter dilute 40 mg (20 mL solution) with 480 mL give through a central venous catheter; incompatible with alkalis

Omeprazole (as sodium salt) (*Losec*®)
Intermittent *in* Glucose 5% *or* Sodium chloride 0.9%
Reconstitute with infusion fluid and dilute to 100 mL; give over 20–30 minutes

Ondansetron (as hydrochloride) (*Zofran*®)
Continuous *or* intermittent *in* Glucose 5% *or* Sodium chloride 0.9% *or* Ringer's solution
For intermittent infusion, dilute 32 mg in 50–100 mL and give over at least 15 minutes

Oxaliplatin (*Eloxatin*®)
Continuous *in* Glucose 5%
Dilute requisite dose to a concentration of 200–700 micrograms/mL and give over 2–6 hours; incompatible with alkaline or chloride-containing fluids; avoid equipment containing aluminium

Oxycodone hydrochloride (*OxyNorm*®)
Continuous *or* intermittent *in* Glucose 5% *or* Sodium chloride 0.9%
Dilute to a concentration of 1 mg/mL

Oxytocin (*Syntocinon*®)
Continuous *in* Glucose 5% *or* Sodium chloride 0.9% or Compound sodium lactate *or* Ringer's solution
Preferably given *via* a variable-speed infusion pump in a concentration appropriate to the pump; if given by drip infusion for *induction or enhancement of labour*, dilute 10 units in 500 mL infusion fluid or for higher doses, 30 units in 500 mL; for *treatment of postpartum uterine haemorrhage* dilute 5–30 units in 500 mL; if high doses given for prolonged period (e.g. for inevitable or missed abortion or for postpartum haemorrhage), use low volume of an electrolyte-containing infusion fluid (not Glucose 5%) given at higher concentration than for induction or enhancement of labour; close attention to patient's fluid and electrolyte status essential

Paclitaxel (*Taxol*®)
Continuous *in* Glucose 5% *or* Sodium chloride 0.9%
Dilute to a concentration of 0.3–1.2 mg/mL and give through an in-line filter (0.22 micron or less) over 3 hours; not to be used with PVC equipment (short PVC inlet or outlet on filter may be acceptable)

Pantoprazole (as sodium sesquihydrate) (*Protium*®)
Intermittent *in* Glucose 5 and 10% *or* Sodium chloride 0.9%
Reconstitute 40 mg with 10 mL sodium chloride 0.9% and dilute to 100 mL with infusion fluid

Paracetamol (*Perfalgan*®)
Intermittent *in* Sodium chloride 0.9% *or* Glucose 5%
Dilute to a concentration of 1 mg/mL and use within 1 hour; may also be given undiluted

Pemetrexed (*Alimta*®)
Intermittent *in* Sodium chloride 0.9%
Reconstitute 500-mg vial with 20 mL sodium chloride 0.9% to produce a 25 mg/mL solution; dilute requisite dose with infusion fluid to 100 mL; give over 10 minutes

Pentamidine isetionate (*Pentacarinat*®)
Intermittent *in* Glucose 5% *or* Sodium chloride 0.9%
Dissolve initially in water for injections (300 mg in 3–5 mL) then dilute in 50–250 mL; give over at least 60 minutes

Pentostatin (*Nipent*®)
Intermittent *in* Glucose 5% *or* Sodium chloride 0.9%
Reconstitute initially with 5 mL water for injections to produce a 2 mg/mL solution; dilute requisite dose in 25–50 mL infusion fluid (final concentration 180–330 micrograms/mL) and give over 20–30 minutes

Phenoxybenzamine hydrochloride
Intermittent *in* Sodium chloride 0.9%
Dilute in 200–500 mL infusion; give over at least 2 hours; max. 4 hours between dilution and completion of administration

Phenylephrine hydrochloride
Intermittent *in* Glucose 5% *or* Sodium chloride 0.9%
Dilute 10 mg in 500 mL infusion fluid

Phenytoin sodium (*Epanutin*®)
Intermittent *in* Sodium chloride 0.9%
Flush intravenous line with Sodium chloride 0.9% before and after infusion; dilute in 50–100 mL infusion fluid (final concentration not to exceed 10 mg/mL) and give through an in-line filter (0.22–0.50 micron) at a rate not exceeding 50 mg/minute (neonates, give at a rate of 1–3 mg/kg/minute); complete administration within 1 hour of preparation

Phytomenadione (in mixed micelles vehicle) (*Konakion*® *MM*)
Intermittent *in* Glucose 5%
Dilute with 55 mL; may be injected into lower part of infusion apparatus

Piperacillin with tazobactam (as sodium salts) (*Tazocin*®)
Intermittent *in* Glucose 5% *or* Sodium chloride 0.9% *or* Water for injections
Reconstitute initially with water for injections or sodium chloride infusion 0.9% (2.25 g in 10 mL, 4.5 g in 20 mL) then dilute to at least 50 mL with infusion fluid; give over 20–30 minutes

Potassium chloride
Continuous *in* Glucose 5% *or* Sodium chloride 0.9%
Dilute in a large-volume infusion; mix thoroughly to avoid 'layering', especially in non-rigid infusion containers; use ready-prepared solutions when possible

Procainamide hydrochloride (*Pronestyl*®)
Continuous *or* intermittent *in* Glucose 5%
For maintenance, dilute to a concentration of *either* 2 mg/mL and give at a rate of 1–3 mL/minute *or* 4 mg/mL and give at a rate of 0.5–1.5 mL/minute

Propofol (emulsion) (*Diprivan*®; Abbott; Baxter; *Propofol-Lipuro*®, *Propofen*®, Braun; Mayne; Fresenius Kabi; Zurich)

1% or 2% emulsion
via drip tubing *in* Glucose 5% *or* Sodium chloride 0.9%
To be administered *via* a Y-piece close to injection site; microbiological filter not recommended

1% emulsion only
Continuous *in* Glucose 5% (*or* Sodium chloride 0.9% for *Propofol-Lipuro*®, *Propofen*®, Braun, Fresenius Kabi, and Zurich brands only)
Dilute to a concentration not less than 2 mg/mL; microbiological filter not recommended; administer using suitable device to control infusion rate; use glass or PVC containers (if PVC bag used it should be full—withdraw volume of infusion fluid equal to that of propofol to be added); give within 6 hours of preparation; propofol may alternatively be infused undiluted using a suitable infusion pump

Quinine dihydrochloride
Continuous *in* Glucose 5% *or* Sodium chloride 0.9%
To be given over 4 hours; see also section 5.4.1

Quinupristin with dalfopristin (*Synercid*®)
Intermittent *in* Glucose 5%
Reconstitute 500 mg with 5 mL water for injections or glucose 5%; gently swirl vial without shaking to dissolve; allow to stand for at least 2 minutes until foam disappears; dilute requisite dose in 100 mL infusion fluid and give over 60 minutes *via* central venous catheter (in an emergency, first dose may be diluted in 250 mL infusion fluid and given over 60 minutes *via* peripheral line); flush line with glucose 5% before and after infusion; incompatible with sodium chloride solutions

Raltitrexed (*Tomudex*®)
Intermittent *in* Glucose 5% *or* Sodium chloride 0.9%
Reconstitute with water for injections; dilute requisite dose in 50–250 mL infusion fluid and give over 15 minutes

Ranitidine (as hydrochloride) (*Zantac®*)
Intermittent *in* Glucose 5% *or* Sodium chloride 0.9% *or* Compound sodium lactate

Rasburicase (*Fasturtec®*)
Intermittent *in* Sodium chloride 0.9%
Reconstitute with solvent provided; gently swirl vial without shaking to dissolve; dilute requisite dose to 50 mL with infusion fluid and give over 30 minutes

Remifentanil (*Ultiva®*)
Continuous *in* Glucose 5% *or* Sodium chloride 0.9% *or* Water for injections
Reconstitute with infusion fluid to a concentration of 1 mg/mL then dilute further to a concentration of 20–250 micrograms/mL (50 micrograms/mL recommended for general anaesthesia, 20–25 micrograms/mL recommended for children 1–12 years; 20–50 micrograms/mL recommended when used with target controlled infusion (TCI) device)

Rifampicin (*Rifadin®*, *Rimactane®*)
Intermittent *in* Glucose 5 and 10% *or* Sodium chloride 0.9% *or* Ringer's solution
Reconstitute with solvent provided then dilute with 250 mL (*Rimactane®*) or 500 mL (*Rifadin®*) infusion fluid; give over 2–3 hours

Ritodrine hydrochloride (*Yutopar®*)
Continuous *in* Glucose 5%
Give *via* controlled infusion device, preferably a syringe pump; if syringe pump available dilute to a concentration of 3 mg/mL; if syringe pump not available dilute to a concentration of 300 micrograms/mL; close attention to patient's fluid and electrolyte status essential

Rituximab (*MabThera®*)
Intermittent *in* Glucose 5% *or* Sodium chloride 0.9%
Dilute to 1–4 mg/mL and gently invert bag to avoid foaming

Rocuronium bromide (*Esmeron®*)
Continuous *or via* drip tubing *in* Glucose 5% *or* Sodium chloride 0.9%

Salbutamol (as sulphate) (*Ventolin® For Intravenous Infusion*)
Continuous *in* Glucose 5%
For *bronchodilatation* dilute to a concentration of 200 micrograms/mL with glucose 5%, sodium chloride 0.9%, or water for injections; for *premature labour* dilute with glucose 5% to a concentration of 200 micrograms/mL for use in a syringe pump *or* for other infusion methods (preferably *via* controlled infusion device), dilute to a concentration of 20 micrograms/mL; close attention to patient's fluid and electrolyte status essential

Sodium calcium edetate (*Ledclair®*)
Continuous *in* Glucose 5% *or* Sodium chloride 0.9%
Dilute to a concentration of not more than 3%; suggested volume 250–500 mL given over at least 1 hour

Sodium clodronate (*Bonefos® Concentrate*)
Continuous *in* Glucose 5% *or* Sodium chloride 0.9%
Dilute 300 mg in 500 mL and give over at least 2 hours or 1.5 g in 500 mL and give over at least 4 hours

Sodium nitroprusside (Mayne)
Continuous *in* Glucose 5%
Reconstitute 50 mg with 2–3 mL glucose 5% then dilute immediately with 250–1000 mL infusion fluid; preferably infuse *via* infusion device to allow precise control; protect infusion from light

Sodium valproate (*Epilim®*, *Episenta®*)
Continuous *or* intermittent *in* Glucose 5% *or* Sodium chloride 0.9%
Reconstitute *Epilim®* with solvent provided then dilute with infusion fluid

Sotalol hydrochloride (*Sotacor®*)
Continuous *or* intermittent *in* Glucose 5% *or* Sodium chloride 0.9%
Dilute to a concentration of between 0.01–2 mg/mL

Streptokinase (*Streptase®*; *Streptokinase*, Braun)
Continuous *or* intermittent *in* Glucose 5% *or* Sodium chloride 0.9%
Reconstitute *Streptase®* with sodium chloride 0.9%, and *Streptokinase* (Braun) with either water for injections or sodium chloride 0.9% then dilute further with infusion fluid

Sulfadiazine sodium
Continuous *in* Sodium chloride 0.9%
Suggested volume 500 mL; ampoule solution has a pH of over 10

Suxamethonium chloride (*Anectine®*)
Continuous *in* Glucose 5% *or* Sodium chloride 0.9%

Tacrolimus (*Prograf®*)
Continuous *in* Glucose 5% *or* Sodium chloride 0.9%
Dilute concentrate in infusion fluid to a final concentration of 4–100 micrograms/mL; give over 24 hours; incompatible with PVC

Teicoplanin (*Targocid®*)
Intermittent *in* Glucose 5% *or* Sodium chloride 0.9% *or* Compound sodium lactate
Reconstitute initially with water for injections provided; infuse over 30 minutes
Continuous infusion not usually recommended

Temocillin (*Negaban®*)
Intermittent *in* Glucose 5% or 10% *or* Sodium chloride 0.9% *or* Ringer's solution *or* Compound sodium lactate
Reconstitute 1 g with 20 mL water for injections then dilute with 50–150 mL infusion fluid; give over 30–40 minutes

Terbutaline sulphate (*Bricanyl®*)
Continuous *in* Glucose 5%
For *bronchodilatation* dilute 1.5–2.5 mg with 500 mL glucose 5% or sodium chloride 0.9% and give over 8–10 hours; for *premature labour* dilute in glucose 5% and give *via* controlled infusion device preferably a syringe pump; if syringe pump available dilute to a concentration of 100 micrograms/mL; if syringe pump not available dilute to a concentration of 10 micrograms/mL; close attention to patient's fluid and electrolyte status essential

Ticarcillin sodium with clavulanic acid (*Timentin®*)
Intermittent *in* Glucose 5% *or* Water for injections
Suggested volume (depending on dose) glucose 5% 100–150 mL or water for injections 50–100 mL; given over 30–40 minutes

Tigecycline (*Tygacil®*)
Intermittent *in* Glucose 5% *or* Sodium chloride 0.9%
Reconstitute each vial with 5.3 mL infusion fluid to produce a 10 mg/mL solution; dilute requisite dose in 100 mL infusion fluid; give over 30–60 minutes

Tirofiban (*Aggrastat®*)
Continuous *in* Glucose 5% *or* Sodium chloride 0.9%
Withdraw 50 mL infusion fluid from 250-mL bag and replace with 50 mL tirofiban concentrate (250 micrograms/mL) to give a final concentration of 50 micrograms/mL

Tobramycin (as sulphate) (*Nebcin®*)
Intermittent *or via* drip tubing *in* Glucose 5% *or* Sodium chloride 0.9%
For adult intermittent infusion suggested volume 50–100 mL (children proportionately smaller volume) given over 20–60 minutes

Topotecan (as hydrochloride) (*Hycamtin®*)
Intermittent *in* Glucose 5% *or* Sodium chloride 0.9%
Reconstitute 4 mg with 4 mL water for injections then dilute to a final concentration of 25–50 micrograms/mL; give over 30 minutes

Tramadol hydrochloride (*Zydol®*)
Continuous *or* intermittent *in* Glucose 5% *or* Sodium chloride 0.9% *or* Ringer's solution *or* Compound sodium lactate

Tranexamic acid (*Cyklokapron®*)
Continuous *in* Glucose 5% *or* Sodium chloride 0.9% *or* Ringer's solution

Trastuzumab (*Herceptin®*)
Intermittent *in* Sodium chloride 0.9%
Reconstitute each 150-mg vial with 7.2 mL water for injections to produce 21 mg/mL solution, swirl vial gently to avoid excessive foaming and allow to stand for approximately 5 minutes; dilute requisite dose in 250 mL infusion fluid

Treosulfan (*Treosulfan*) (Medac)
Intermittent *in* Water for injections
Infusion suggested for doses above 5 g; dilute to a concentration of 5 g in 100 mL

Tropisetron (as hydrochloride) (*Navoban®*)
Intermittent *or via* drip tubing *in* Glucose 5% *or* Sodium chloride 0.9% *or* Ringer's solution
Suggested concentration for infusion 50 micrograms/mL

Urokinase (*Syner-KINASE®*)
Continuous *or* intermittent *in* Sodium chloride 0.9%

Vancomycin (as hydrochloride) (*Vancocin®*)
Intermittent *in* Glucose 5% *or* Sodium chloride 0.9%
Reconstitute each 500 mg with 10 mL water for injections and dilute with infusion fluid to a concentration of up to 5 mg/mL (10 mg/mL in fluid restriction but increased risk of infusion-related effects); give over at least 60 minutes (rate not to exceed 10 mg/minute for doses over 500 mg); use continuous infusion only if intermittent not feasible

Vasopressin, synthetic (*Pitressin®*)
Intermittent *in* Glucose 5%
Suggested concentration 20 units/100 mL given over 15 minutes

Vecuronium bromide (*Norcuron®*)
Continuous *or* via drip tubing *in* Glucose 5% *or* Sodium chloride 0.9% *or* Ringer's solution
Reconstitute each vial with 5 mL water for injections to give 2 mg/mL solution; *alternatively* reconstitute with up to 10 mL glucose 5% *or* sodium chloride 0.9% *or* water for injections—unsuitable for further dilution if not reconstituted with water for injections. For *continuous intravenous infusion*, dilute to a concentration of not less than 40 micrograms/mL

Verteporfin (*Visudyne®*)
Intermittent *in* Glucose 5%
Reconstitute each 15 mg with 7 mL water for injections to produce a 2 mg/mL solution then dilute requisite dose with infusion fluid to a final volume of 30 mL and give over 10 minutes; protect from light and administer within 4 hours of reconstitution. Incompatible with sodium chloride infusion

Vinblastine sulphate (*Velbe®*)
via drip tubing *in* Sodium chloride 0.9%
Reconstitute with sodium chloride 0.9%; give over approx. 1 minute

Vincristine sulphate (*Oncovin®*)
via drip tubing *in* Glucose 5% *or* Sodium chloride 0.9%

Vindesine sulphate (*Eldisine®*)
via drip tubing *in* Glucose 5% *or* Sodium chloride 0.9%
Reconstitute with sodium chloride 0.9%; give over 1–3 minutes

Vinorelbine (*Navelbine®*)
Intermittent *in* Glucose 5% *or* Sodium chloride 0.9%
Dilute in 125 mL infusion fluid; give over 20–30 minutes

Vitamins B & C (*Pabrinex® I/V High potency*)
Intermittent *or via* drip tubing *in* Glucose 5% *or* Sodium chloride 0.9%
Ampoule contents should be mixed, diluted, and administered without delay; give over 30 minutes (see MHRA/CHM advice, section 9.6.2)

Vitamins, multiple
(*Cernevit®*)
Intermittent *in* Glucose 5% *or* Sodium chloride 0.9%
Dissolve initially in 5 mL water for injections (or infusion fluid)
(*Solivito N®*)
Intermittent *in* Glucose 5 and 10%
Suggested volume 500–1000 mL given over 2–3 hours; see also section 9.3

Voriconazole (*Vfend®*)
Intermittent *in* Glucose 5% *or* Sodium chloride 0.9% *or* Compound sodium lactate
Reconstitute each 200 mg with 19 mL water for injections to produce a 10 mg/mL solution; dilute dose in infusion fluid to concentration of 0.5–5 mg/mL; give at a rate not exceeding 3 mg/kg/hour

Zidovudine (*Retrovir®*)
Intermittent *in* Glucose 5%
Dilute to a concentration of 2 mg/mL or 4 mg/mL and give over 1 hour

Zoledronic acid (*Zometa®*)
Intermittent *in* Glucose 5% *or* Sodium chloride 0.9%
Dilute requisite dose with 100 mL infusion fluid; infuse over at least 15 minutes

A7 Borderline substances

In certain conditions some foods (and toilet preparations) have characteristics of drugs and the Advisory Committee on Borderline Substances advises as to the circumstances in which such substances may be regarded as drugs. Prescriptions issued in accordance with the Committee's advice and endorsed 'ACBS' will normally not be investigated.

> General Practitioners are reminded that the ACBS recommends products on the basis that they may be regarded as drugs for the management of specified conditions. Doctors should satisfy themselves that the products can safely be prescribed, that patients are adequately monitored and that, where necessary, expert hospital supervision is available.

Foods which may be prescribed on FP10, GP10 (Scotland), or when available WP10 (Wales)

Note This is a list of food products which the ACBS has approved. The clinical condition for which the product has approval follows each entry.

Foods included in this Appendix may contain cariogenic sugars and patients should be advised to take appropriate oral hygiene measures.

Note Feeds containing more than 6 g/100 mL protein or 2 g/100 mL fibre should be avoided in children unless recommended by an appropriate specialist or dietician.

Enteral foods and supplements

> **Standard ACBS indications:** short-bowel syndrome, intractable malabsorption, pre-operative preparation of undernourished patients, proven inflammatory bowel disease, following total gastrectomy, bowel fistulas, or disease-related malnutrition.

Calogen® (Nutricia Clinical)
Emulsion, vegetable oils in water, net price 200 mL = £4.59; 500 mL = £9.00 (neutral, banana, strawberry flavour).
For disease-related malnutrition, malabsorption states or other conditions requiring fortification with a high-fat supplement with or without fluid and electrolyte restrictions

Caloreen® (Nestlé)
Powder, water-soluble dextrins, 390 kcal/100 g, with less than 1.8 mmol of Na^+ and 0.3 mmol of K^+/100 g. Gluten-, lactose-, and fructose-free. Net price 500 g = £3.02.
For disease-related malnutrition, malabsorption states or other conditions requiring fortification with a high or readily available carbohydrate supplement

Calshake® (Fresenius Kabi)
Powder, protein 4 g, carbohydrate 58 g, fat 20.4 g, energy 1809 kJ (432 kcal)/87 g. Gluten-free. Strawberry, vanilla, neutral, and banana flavours, net price 87-g sachet = £1.82; also available chocolate flavour (protein 4 g, carbohydrate 58 g, fat 20.4 g, fibre 1.6 g, energy 1809 kJ (432 kcal)/90 g = £1.82.
For disease-related malnutrition, malabsorption states or other conditions requiring fortification with a fat/carbohydrate supplement

Clinutren® 1.5 (Nestlé)
Liquid, protein 11 g, carbohydrate 42 g, fat 10 g, energy 1260 kJ (300 kcal)/200 mL with vitamins and minerals. Gluten-free; clinically lactose-free. Flavours: apricot, banana, chocolate, coffee, strawberry-raspberry or vanilla, net price 4 × 200-mL bottle = £6.40.
For indications see *Clinutren Fruit*

Clinutren® 1.5 Fibre (Nestlé)
Liquid, protein 5.7 g, carbohydrate 19 g, fat 5.9 g, fibre 2.6 g, energy 630 kJ (150 kcal)/100 mL with vitamins, minerals and trace elements. Gluten-free; clinically lactose-free. Flavours: vanilla or plum, net price 4 × 200-mL pot = £6.40.
A sole source of nutrition or nutritional supplement for standard ACBS indications (see above) and dysphagia. Not suitable for any child under 3 years; not suitable as a sole source of nutrition for children under 6 years

Clinutren® Dessert (Nestlé)
Semi-solid, protein 12 g, carbohydrate 19 g, fat 3.3 g, energy 650 kJ (160 kcal)/125 g with vitamins and minerals. Gluten-free. Flavours: caramel, chocolate, peach or vanilla, net price 4 × 125-g pot = £5.40.
Nutritional supplement for standard ACBS indications (see above) and dysphagia, continuous ambulatory peritoneal dialysis (CAPD), or haemodialysis. Not suitable for any child under 3 years; maximum of 3 units daily for children aged 3 to 6 years

Clinutren® Fruit (Nestlé)
Liquid, protein 8 g, carbohydrate 54 g, fat less than 0.4 g, energy 1050 kJ (250 kcal)/200 mL with vitamins and minerals. Gluten-free. Low-lactose. Flavours: grapefruit, orange, pear-cherry, or raspberry-blackcurrant, net price 4 × 200-mL cup = £6.44.
Nutritional supplement for standard ACBS indications (see above) and dysphagia. Not suitable for any child under 3 years; maximum of 3 units daily for children aged 3 to 6 years

Clinutren® ISO (Nestlé)
Liquid, protein 7.6 g, carbohydrate 28 g, fat 6.6 g, energy 840 kJ (200 kcal)/200 mL with vitamins and minerals. Gluten-free. Flavours: chocolate or vanilla, net price 4 × 200-mL pot = £6.40.
A sole source of nutrition or nutritional supplement for standard ACBS indications (see above) and dysphagia. Not suitable for any child under 3 years; not suitable as a sole source of nutrition for children under 6 years; maximum of 3 units daily for children aged 3 to 6 years

Clinutren Junior® (Nestlé)
Powder, protein 13.9 g, carbohydrate 62.2 g, fat 18.3 g, energy 1950 kJ (467 kcal)/100 g with vitamins, minerals and trace elements. Gluten-free; clinically lactose-free. Flavour: vanilla, net price 400 g = £9.72.
A sole source of nutrition or nutritional supplement for standard ACBS indications (see above), growth failure, and dysphagia in children 1 to 10 years.

Complan® Shake (Complan Foods)
Powder, protein 15.6 g, carbohydrate 44.17 g, fat 16.43 g, fibre 200 mg, energy 1619 kJ (387 kcal)/serving (serving = 1 × 57-g sachet reconstituted with 200 mL whole milk (can be reconstituted with water which will significantly decrease nutritional content) with vitamins, minerals and trace elements. Flavours: banana, vanilla, chocolate, strawberry, milk, net price 4 × 57-g sachet = £3.26.
Nutritional supplement for standard ACBS indications (see above) and dysphagia. Not suitable for patients with cows' milk intolerance or galactosaemia. Not to be prescribed for any child under 1 year; use with caution for children up to 5 years

Duobar® (SHS)
Bar, protein-free (phenylalanine nil added), carbohydrate 49.9 g, fat 49.9 g, energy 2692 kJ (648 kcal)/100 g. Low sodium and potassium. Strawberry, toffee, or neutral flavours. Net price 45-g bar = £1.48.
For disease-related malnutrition, malabsorption states or other conditions requiring fortification with fat/carbohydrate supplement

Duocal® (SHS)

Liquid, emulsion providing carbohydrate 23.4 g, fat 7.1 g, energy 661 kJ (158 kcal)/100 mL. Low-electrolyte, gluten-, lactose-, and protein-free. Net price 250 mL = £3.02; 1 litre = £10.37

MCT Powder, carbohydrate 74 g, fat 23.2 g (of which MCT 83%), energy 2042 kJ (486 kcal)/100 g. Low electrolyte, gluten-, protein- and lactose-free. Net price 400 g = £16.19

Super Soluble Powder, carbohydrate 72.7 g, fat 22.3 g, energy 2061 kJ (492 kcal)/100 g. Low electrolyte, gluten-, protein-, and lactose-free. Net price 400 g = £13.62

All for disease-related malnutrition, malabsorption states or other conditions requiring fortification with fat/carbohydrate supplement

Elemental 028® (SHS)

028 Powder, amino acids 12%, carbohydrate 70.5–72%, fat 6.64%, energy 1544–1568 kJ (364–370 kcal)/100 g with vitamins and minerals. For preparation with water before use. Net price 100-g box (orange flavoured or plain) = £4.28

For use as the sole source of nutrition or as a nutritional supplement prescribed on medical grounds for: short-bowel syndrome, intractable malabsorption, proven inflammatory bowel disease, bowel fistulas. Not to be prescribed for any child under 1 year; use with caution for children up to 5 years

Note See also Flavour Sachets, for use with unflavoured amino acid and peptide products from SHS

Elemental 028® Extra (SHS)

Liquid, amino acids 3 g, carbohydrate 11 g, fat 3.48 g, energy 358 kJ (86 kcal)/100 mL, with vitamins, minerals, and trace elements. Flavours: grapefruit, orange and pineapple, summer fruits. Net price 250-mL carton = £2.77

Powder, amino acids 15%, carbohydrate 59%, fat 17.45%, energy 1860 kJ (443 kcal)/100 g, with vitamins, minerals, and trace elements. For preparation with water before use. Net price 100 g (plain) = £5.19; also available in banana, citrus, or orange flavours (carbohydrate 55%, energy 1793 kJ (427 kcal)/100 g), 100 g = £5.38

All for use as the sole source of nutrition or as a nutritional supplement prescribed on medical grounds for: short-bowel syndrome, intractable malabsorption, proven inflammatory bowel disease, bowel fistulas. Not to be prescribed for any child under 1 year; use with caution for children up to 5 years

NOTE see also Flavour Sachets, for use with unflavoured amino acid and peptide products from SHS

Emsogen® (SHS)

Powder, amino acids 15%, carbohydrate 60%, fat 16.4%, energy 1839 kJ (438 kcal)/100 g, with vitamins, minerals, and trace elements. For preparation with water before use. Net price 100 g = £5.54; also available orange-flavoured (carbohydrate 55%, energy 1754 kJ (418 kcal)/100 g), 100 g = £5.54.

For use as the sole source of nutrition or as a nutritional supplement prescribed on medical grounds for short-bowel syndrome, intractable malabsorption, proven inflammatory bowel disease, bowel fistulas. Not to be prescribed for any child under 1 year; use with caution for children up to 5 years

Enlive Plus® (Abbott)

Liquid, protein 4.8 g, carbohydrate 32.7 g, energy 638 kJ (150 kcal)/100 mL, with vitamins, minerals and trace elements Fat- and gluten-free; clinically lactose-free. Flavours: apple, fruit punch, grapefruit, lemon and lime, orange, peach, pineapple, strawberry, net price 220-mL Tetrapak® = £1.69.

Nutritional supplement for standard ACBS indications (see p. 833) and dysphagia. Not for use in galactosaemia. Not to be prescribed for any child under 1 year; use with caution for children up to 5 years

Enmix Plus Commence® (Abbott)

Starter pack, contains: *Ensure Plus* milkshake-style (4 flavours), yoghurt-style (2 flavours); *Enlive Plus* (4 flavours) – see *Ensure Plus®* and *Enlive Plus®* for product information, net price 1 pack (10 × 220 mL) = £16.90

Intended as an initial 5- to 10-day supply to establish patient preferences Nutritional supplement for standard ACBS indications (see p. 833) and dysphagia. Not to be prescribed for any child under 1 year; use with caution for children up to 5 years

Enrich® (Abbott)

Liquid with dietary fibre, providing protein 3.8 g, carbohydrate 14 g, fat 3.5 g, fibre 1.4 g, energy 432 kJ (102 kcal)/100 mL with vitamins and minerals. Lactose- and gluten-free. Vanilla flavour. Net price 250-mL can = £2.24.

For use as the sole source of nutrition or as a nutritional supplement prescribed on medical grounds for: short-bowel syndrome, intractable malabsorption, pre-operative preparation of patients who are undernourished, proven inflammatory bowel disease, following total gastrectomy, dysphagia, disease-related malnutrition. Not to be prescribed for any child under 1 year; use with caution for children up to 5 years

Enshake® (Abbott)

Powder, protein 16 g, carbohydrate 78.4 g, fat 24.7 g, energy 2519 kJ (600 kcal)/310 mL serving (serving = 1 sachet reconstituted with 240mL whole milk), with vitamins, minerals and trace elements. Gluten-free. Flavours: banana, chocolate, strawberry, vanilla, net price 96.5-g sachet = £1.87.

Nutritional supplement for disease-related malnutrition, malabsorption states or other conditions requiring fortification with a fat/carbohydrate supplement. Not suitable for children under 1 year

Ensure® (Abbott)

Liquid, protein 4 g, fat 3.4 g, carbohydrate 13.6 g, energy 423 kJ (100 kcal)/100 mL with minerals and vitamins, lactose- and gluten-free. Flavours: chocolate, vanilla, coffee, eggnog, nut, chicken, mushroom, and asparagus, net price 250-mL can = £1.96; 500-mL ready-to-hang (vanilla) = £3.74

A sole source of nutrition or nutritional supplement for standard ACBS indications (see p. 833) and dysphagia. Not to be prescribed for any child under 1 year; use with caution for children up to 5 years

Ensure Plus® (Abbott)

Liquid, protein 6.3 g, fat 4.9 g, carbohydrate 20.2 g, with vitamins and minerals, lactose- and gluten-free, energy 632 kJ (150 kcal)/100 mL. Vanilla flavour, (formulations may vary slightly). Net price 220-mL Tetrapak® = £1.69; 250-mL can = £2.16; 500-mL ready-to-hang (unflavoured) = £4.03; 1-litre ready-to-hang (unflavoured) = £7.86; 1.5-litre ready-to-hang (unflavoured) = £11.78. Caramel, chocolate, strawberry, banana, fruits of the forest, raspberry, orange, coffee, blackcurrant, peach, vanilla, or neutral flavours. Net price 220-mL Tetrapak® = £1.69.

Yoghurt Style, protein 6.3 g, fat 4.9 g, carbohydrate 20.2 g, with vitamins, minerals and trace elements, gluten-free, clinically lactose-free, energy 632 kJ (150 kcal)/100 mL. Orange, peach, pineapple, or strawberry flavour, net price 220-mL Tetrapak® = £1.69.

Nutritional supplement for standard ACBS indications (see p. 833) and dysphagia, continuous ambulatory peritoneal dialysis (CAPD), or haemodialysis. Not to be prescribed for any child under 1 year; use with caution for children up to 5 years

Ensure Plus Commence® (Abbott)

Starter pack, contains: *Ensure Plus* (various flavours) see *Ensure Plus* for product information, net price 1 pack (10 × 220-mL) = £16.90.

Intended as an initial 5 - 10 day supply to establish patient preferences.

Ensure Plus Fibre® (Abbott)

Liquid with dietary fibre, providing protein 6.25 g, carbohydrate 20.2 g, fat 4.92 g, fibre 1.25 g, energy 642 kJ (153 kcal)/100 mL with vitamins and minerals. Lactose- and gluten-free. Vanilla, chocolate, fruits of the forest, raspberry, strawberry and banana flavours. Net price 200-mL Tetrapak® = £1.74.

Nutritional supplement for standard ACBS indications (see p. 833) and dysphagia or continuous ambulatory peritoneal dialysis (CAPD). Not to be prescribed for any child under 1 year; use with caution for children up to 5 years

Foodlink Complete (Foodlink)

Powder, protein 21.9 g, carbohydrate 57.3 g, fat 13.3 g, energy 1838 kJ (436.5 kcal)/100 g with vitamins and minerals, Flavours: banana, chocolate, natural, or strawberry, net price 450-g carton = £3.19; also available, vanilla with fibre, protein 19.5 g, carbohydrate 60.2 g, fat 12.3 g, fibre 8 g, energy 1804 kJ (428 kcal)/100 g = £3.75.

Nutritional supplement for standard ACBS indications (see p. 833) and dysphagia. Not to be prescribed for any child under 1 year; use with caution for children up to 5 years

Forticare® (Nutricia Clinical)
Liquid, protein 9 g, carbohydrate 19.1 g, fat 5.3 g, fibre 2.1 g, energy 675 kJ (160 kcal)/100 mL, with vitamins, minerals, and trace elements. Gluten- and lactose-free. Flavours: cappuccino, orange and lemon, or peach and ginger. Net price 125-mL carton = £1.86.

As a nutritional supplement for patients with pancreatic cancer

Forticreme® Complete (Nutricia Clinical)
Semi-solid, protein 9.5 g, carbohydrate 19.3 g, fat 5 g, energy 675 kJ (160 kcal)/100 g with vitamins and minerals. Gluten-free. Vanilla, chocolate, banana, and forest fruit flavours, net price 4 × 125-g pot = £6.75.

Nutritional supplement for standard ACBS indications (see p. 833) and dysphagia, continuous ambulatory peritoneal dialysis (CAPD), or haemodialysis. Not to be prescribed for any child under 3 years; use with caution for children aged 3 to 5 years

Fortifresh® (Nutricia Clinical)
Liquid, protein 6 g, carbohydrate 18.7 g, fat 5.8 g, energy 630 kJ (150 kcal)/100 mL with vitamins, minerals and trace elements. Gluten-free. Flavours: blackcurrant, peach and orange, pineapple, raspberry, and vanilla and lemon, net price 200 mL carton = £1.74

A sole source of nutrition or nutritional supplement for standard ACBS indications (see p. 833) and dysphagia. Not to be prescribed for any child under 3 years; use with caution for children aged 3 to 5 years; not suitable as a sole source of nutrition in children under 6 years

Fortijuce® (Nutricia Clinical)
Liquid, protein 4 g, carbohydrate 33.5 g, energy 630 kJ (150 kcal)/100 mL, with vitamins, minerals and trace elements. Fat-free. Flavours: apple, apricot, blackcurrant, forest fruits, lemon, orange, strawberry, tropical, net price 200-mL carton = £1.74; 4 × 200 mL starter pack = £6.76.

Nutritional supplement for standard ACBS indications (see p. 833) and dysphagia. Not to be prescribed for any child under 3 years; use with caution for children up to 5 years

Fortimel® (Nutricia Clinical)
Liquid, protein 10 g, carbohydrate 10.3 g (chocolate flavour 10.4 g), fat 2.1 g, energy 420 kJ (100 kcal)/100 mL with vitamins and minerals. Gluten-free. Vanilla, strawberry, chocolate, and forest fruits flavours. Net price 200-mL = £1.47.

Nutritional supplement for standard ACBS indications (see p. 833) and dysphagia. Not to be prescribed for any child under 3 years; use with caution for children up to 5 years

Fortini® (Nutricia Clinical)
Liquid, protein 3.4 g, carbohydrate 18.8 g, fat 6.8 g, energy 630 kJ (150 kcal)/100 mL with vitamins, minerals, and trace elements. Gluten- and lactose-free. Flavours: strawberry or vanilla, net price 200 mL = £2.52.

A sole source of nutrition or as a nutritional supplement prescribed on medical grounds for disease-related malnutrition, and growth failure. For children aged 1–6 years (8–20 kg body-weight)

Fortini Multifibre® (Nutricia Clinical)
Liquid, protein 3.4 g, carbohydrate 18.8 g, fat 6.8 g, fibre 1.5 g, energy 630 kJ (150 kcal)/ 100 mL with vitamins, minerals, and trace elements. Gluten- and lactose-free. Flavours: banana, chocolate, strawberry, and vanilla, net price 200-mL = £2.65.

For indications see Fortini liquid

Fortisip® Bottle (Nutricia Clinical)
Liquid, protein 6 g, carbohydrate 18.4 g, fat 5.8 g, energy 630 kJ (150 kcal)/100 mL, with vitamins, minerals and trace elements. Gluten-free; clinically lactose-free. Vanilla, banana, chocolate, orange, strawberry, tropical fruits, toffee, and neutral flavours, net price 200 mL = £1.74.

Nutritional supplement for standard ACBS indications (see p. 833) and dysphagia. Not to be prescribed for any child under 3 years; use with caution for children aged 3 to 5 years

Fortisip® Fruit Dessert (Nutricia Clinical)
Semi-Solid, protein 7 g, carbohydrate 16.7 g, fat 4 g, fibre 2.6 g, energy 560 kJ (133 kcal)/100 g, with vitamins, minerals, and trace elements. Lactose-free. Apple flavour, net price 3 x 150-g pots = £6.09.

A sole source of nutrition or nutritional supplement for standard ACBS indications (see p. 833) and dysphagia, continuous ambulatory peritoneal dialysis (CAPD), or haemodialysis. Not suitable for patients with galactosaemia. Not suitable for children under 3 years; caution in children under 6 years

Fortisip® Multi Fibre (Nutricia Clinical)
Liquid, protein 6 g, carbohydrate 18.4 g, fat 5.8 g, fibre 2.3 g, energy 630 kJ (150 kcal)/100 mL, with vitamins, minerals and trace elements. Gluten-free, clinically lactose-free. Banana, chicken, orange, strawberry, tomato, vanilla flavours; also available chocolate flavour (protein 5 g, carbohydrate 18 g, fat 6.5 g, fibre 2.25 g, energy 630 kJ (150 kcal)/ 100 mL, net price 200 mL = £1.79.

As a sole source of nutrition or as a nutritional supplement prescribed on medical grounds for: short-bowel syndrome, intractable malabsorption, pre-operative preparation of undernourished patients, proven inflammatory bowel disease, following total gastrectomy, dysphagia, disease-related malnutrition. Not to be prescribed for any child under 3 years; use with caution for children aged 3 to 5 years

Fortisip® Protein (Nutricia Clinical)
Liquid, protein 10 g, carbohydrate 14.7 g, fat 3.5 g, energy 630 kJ (150 kcal)/100 mL, with vitamins, minerals and trace elements. Gluten-free. Apricot, chocolate, forest fruits, mocha, strawberry, and vanilla flavour, net price 200 mL = £1.69; starter pack 4 × 200mL = £6.76

Nutritional supplement for standard ACBS indications (see p. 833) and dysphagia. Not to be prescribed for any child under 3 years

Fortisip® Range (Nutricia Clinical)
Starter pack contains 1 × Fortisip® Bottle, 4 × Fortijuce®, 2 × Fortifresh®, see separate entries for details, net price 1 pack (10 × 200 mL) = £16.87.

Fortisip® Yoghurt Style (Nutricia Clinical)
Yoghurt, protein 6 g, carbohydrate 18.7 g, fat 5.8 g, fibre 0.2 g, energy 630 kJ (150 kcal)/100 mL, with vitamins, minerals, and trace elements. Gluten-free. Peach and orange, raspberry, vanilla and lemon flavours, net price 200-mL bottle =£1.74.

A sole source of nutrition or nutritional supplement for standard ACBS indications (see p. 833) and dysphagia. Not suitable for children under 3 years; not suitable as a sole source of nutrition for children under 6 years

Frebini® Energy (Fresenius Kabi)
Sip feed, protein 3.75 g, carbohydrate 18.8 g, fat 6.65 g, energy 630 kJ (150 kcal)/100 mL, with vitamins, minerals and trace elements. Gluten-free; clinically lactose-free. Flavours: banana or strawberry. Net price 200-mL carton = £2.16.

Tube feed, protein 3.75 g, carbohydrate 18.75 g, fat 6.7 g, energy 630 kJ (150 kcal)/100 mL, with vitamins, minerals and trace elements. Gluten-free; clinically lactose-free. Flavour: neutral, net price 500-mL EasyBag® = £5.70.

A sole source of nutrition or nutritional supplement for standard ACBS indications (see p. 833) and dysphagia in children 1–10 years, or body-weight 8–30 kg. Not suitable for children under 1 year.

Frebini® Energy Fibre (Fresenius Kabi)
Sip feed, protein 3.75 g, carbohydrate 18.8 g, fat 6.65 g, fibre 1.1 g, energy 630 kJ (150 kcal)/100 mL, with vitamins, minerals and trace elements. Gluten-free; clinically lactose-free. Chocolate flavour, net price 200-mL carton = £2.21.

Tube feed, protein 3.75 g, carbohydrate 18.75 g, fat 6.7 g, fibre 1.13 g, energy 630 kJ (150 kcal)/100 mL, with vitamins, minerals and trace elements. Gluten-free, clinically lactose-free. Flavour: neutral, net price 500-mL EasyBag® = £6.10.

For indications see *Frebini Energy®*

Frebini® Original (Fresenius Kabi)
Liquid, tube feed, protein 2.5 g, carbohydrate 13.5 g, fat 4 g, energy 420 kJ (100 kcal)/100 mL, with vitamins, minerals and trace elements. Flavour: neutral, net price 500-mL EasyBag® = £4.55

For indications see *Frebini Energy®*.

Frebini® Original Fibre (Fresenius Kabi)
Tube feed, protein 2.5 g, carbohydrate 12.5 g, fat 4.4 g, fibre 750 mg, energy 420 kJ (100 kcal)/100 mL, with vitamins, minerals and trace elements. Gluten-free, clinically lactose-free. Neutral flavour, net price 500-mL EasyBag® = £5.05

For indications see *Frebini Energy®*

Fresubin® Energy (Fresenius Kabi)
Liquid, protein 5.65 g, carbohydrate 18.8 g, fat 5.83 g, energy 630 kJ (150 kcal)/100 mL, with vitamins and minerals. Net price 200-mL carton = £1.60 (flavours: vanilla, strawberry, blackcurrant, banana, cappuccino, tropical fruits, chocolate, lemon, and neutral): 500-mL bottle = £3.80 (flavour: neutral); 500-mL EasyBag® = £3.91; 1-litre EasyBag® = £7.70; 1.5-litre EasyBag® = £9.92.

A sole source of nutrition or nutritional supplement for standard ACBS indications (see p. 833) and dysphagia. Not to be prescribed for any child under 1 year; use with caution for children under 5 years

Fresubin® Energy Fibre (Fresenius Kabi)
Sip feed, protein 5.65 g, carbohydrate 18.8 g, fat 5.83 g, fibre 2.5 g, energy 630 kJ (150 kcal)/100 mL, with vitamins, minerals and trace elements. Gluten-free; clinically lactose-free. Flavours: banana, caramel, chocolate, cherry, strawberry, vanilla. Net price 200-mL carton = £1.70.

For indications see *Fresubin® Energy*

Tube feed, protein 5.6 g, carbohydrate 18.8 g, fat 5.8 g, fibre 2 g, energy 630 kJ (150 kcal)/100 mL, with vitamins, minerals and trace elements. Gluten-free; clinically lactose-free. Unflavoured, net price 500-mL EasyBag® = £4.13; 1-litre EasyBag® = £8.20; 1.5-litre EasyBag® = £10.95.

For indications see *Fresubin® Energy*

Fresubin HP Energy® (Fresenius Kabi)
Liquid, protein 7.5 g, carbohydrate 17 g, fat 6 g, energy 630 kJ (150 kcal)/100 mL with vitamins, minerals, and trace elements. Gluten-free and low lactose. Vanilla flavour. Net price 500-mL bottle = £3.67; 500-mL EasyBag® = £3.84; 1-litre EasyBag® = £7.69.

Nutritional supplement for standard ACBS indications (see p. 833) and dysphagia, continuous ambulatory peritoneal dialysis (CAPD), or haemodialysis. Not to be prescribed for any child under 1 year; use with caution for children up to 5 years

Fresubin® 1000 Complete (Fresenius Kabi)
Liquid, tube feed, protein 5.5 g, carbohydrate 12.5 g, fat 3.1 g, fibre 2 g, energy 420 kJ (100 kcal)/100mL with vitamins, minerals and trace elements. Gluten-free, clinically lactose-free, net price 1-litre EasyBag® = £8.20.

For indications see *Fresubin Energy®*

Fresubin® 1200 Complete (Fresenius Kabi)
Liquid, tube feed, protein 6 g, carbohydrate 15 g, fat 4.1 g, fibre 2 g, energy 500 kJ (120 kcal)/100 mL with vitamins, minerals and trace elements. Gluten-free, clinically lactose-free, net price 1-litre EasyBag® = £10.20.

A sole source of nutrition or nutritional supplement for standard ACBS indications (see p. 833). Not suitable for children under 5 years

Fresubin® Original (Fresenius Kabi)
Liquid, protein 3.8 g, carbohydrate 13.8 g, fat 3.4 g, energy 420 kJ (100 kcal)/100 mL with vitamins and minerals. Gluten-free, low lactose and cholesterol. Net price 200-mL carton (nut, peach, blackcurrant, chocolate, mocha, and vanilla flavours) = £1.60; 500-mL bottle (neutral flavour) = £3.08; 500-mL EasyBag® = £3.09; 1-litre EasyBag® = £6.09; 1.5-litre EasyBag® = £9.14

For indications see *Fresubin Energy®*

Fresubin® Original Fibre (Fresenius Kabi)
Liquid with dietary fibre, protein 3.8 g, carbohydrate 13.8 g, fat 3.4 g, energy 420 kJ (100 kcal)/100 mL, with vitamins and minerals. Flavour: neutral. Net price 500-mL bottle = £3.48; 500-mL EasyBag® = £3.62; 1-litre EasyBag® = £7.24; 1.5-litre EasyBag® = £10.20.

A sole source of nutrition or nutritional supplement for standard ACBS indications (see p. 833) and dysphagia. Not to be prescribed for any child under 2 years; use with caution for children up to 5 years

Fresubin Protein Energy Drink (Fresenius Kabi)
Liquid, protein 10 g, carbohydrate 12.4 g, fat 6.7 g, energy 630 kJ (150 kcal)/100 mL, with vitamins, minerals and trace elements. Gluten- and lactose-free. Chocolate, strawberry, and vanilla flavours, net price 200-mL = £1.63.

Nutritional supplement for standard ACBS indications (see p. 833) and dysphagia, continuous ambulatory peritoneal dialysis (CAPD), or haemodialysis. Not to be prescribed for any child under 1 year; use with caution for children up to 5 years of age

Infatrini® (Nutricia Clinical)
Liquid, protein 2.6 g, carbohydrate 10.3 g, fat 5.4 g, energy 420 kJ (100 kcal)/100 mL with vitamins, minerals and trace elements. Gluten-free. Net price 100-mL bottle = 91p, 200-mL Tetrapak® = £1.82

For use as a sole source of nutrition or as a nutritional supplement prescribed on medical grounds for: failure to thrive, disease-related malnutrition and malabsorption. Manufacturer advises suitable for infants up to 8 kg body-weight (0–12 months of age)

Isosource® Energy (Nestlé)
Liquid, protein 5.7 g, carbohydrate 20 g, fat 6.2 g, energy 660 kJ (160 kcal)/100 mL with vitamins, minerals and trace elements. Gluten-free; clinically lactose-free. Net price 500-mL flexible pouch = £3.55, 1-litre flexible pouch = £7.10.

For indications see *Isosource Standard*

Isosource® Energy Fibre (Nestlé)
Liquid, tube feed, protein 4.9 g, carbohydrate 20.2 g, fat 5.5 g, fibre, 1.5 g, energy 630 kJ (150 kcal)/100 mL with vitamins, minerals and trace elements. Gluten-free; clinically lactose-free. Net price 500-mL flexible pouch = £3.85, 1-litre flexible pouch = £7.70.

For indications see *Isosource Standard®*

Isosource® Fibre (Nestlé)
Liquid , protein 3.8 g, carbohydrate 13.6 g, fat 3.4 g, fibre 1.4 g, energy 422 kJ (100 kcal)/100 mL with vitamins, minerals and trace elements. Gluten-free; clinically lactose-free. Net price 500-mL flexible pouch = £3.29, 1-litre flexible pouch = £6.58.

For indications see *Isosource Standard*

Isosource® Junior (Nestlé)
Liquid, protein 2.7 g, carbohydrate 17 g, fat 4.7 g, energy 512 kJ (122 kcal)/100 mL with vitamins, minerals and trace elements. Gluten-free; clinically lactose-free. Net price 500-mL flexible pouch = £5.17.

A sole source of nutrition or nutritional supplement for standard ACBS indications (see p. 833), dysphagia and growth failure in children 1 to 6 years or body-weight 8 to 20 kg

Isosource® Standard (Nestlé)
Liquid, protein 4 g, carbohydrate 13.6 g, fat 3.3 g, energy 420 kJ (100 kcal)/100 mL with vitamins, minerals and trace elements. Gluten-free; clinically lactose-free. Net price 500-mL flexible pouch = £2.89, 1-litre flexible pouch = £5.78.

A sole source of nutrition or nutritional supplement for standard ACBS indications (see p. 833) and dysphagia. Not to be prescribed for any child under 1 year; use with caution for children up to 5 years

Jevity® (Abbott)
Liquid, protein 4 g, fat 3.5 g, carbohydrate 14.1 g, dietary fibre 1.8 g, energy 441 kJ (106 kcal)/100 mL, with vitamins and minerals. Gluten-, lactose-, and sucrose-free. Net price 500-mL ready-to-hang = £3.74, 1-litre ready-to-hang = £7.02, 1.5-litre ready-to-hang = £10.54.

A sole source of nutrition or nutritional supplement for standard ACBS indications (see p. 833) and dysphagia. Not to be prescribed for any child under 2 years; use with caution for children up to 5 years

Jevity 1.5 kcal® (Abbott)
Liquid, tube feed, protein 6.38 g, carbohydrate 20.1 g, fat 4.9 g, fibre 2.2 g, energy 640 kJ (152 kcal)/100 mL, with vitamins, minerals and trace elements. Gluten- and lactose-free. Net price 500-mL ready-to-hang = £4.55, 1-litre ready-to-hang = £8.45, 1.5-litre ready-to-hang = £13.18.

A sole source of nutrition or nutritional supplement for standard ACBS indications (see p. 833) and dysphagia. Not to be prescribed for any child under 2 years; use with caution for children up to 10 years

Jevity Plus® (Abbott)
Liquid, protein 5.6 g, carbohydrate 15.1 g, fat 3.9 g, dietary fibre 2.2 g, energy 504 kJ (120 kcal)/100 mL, with vitamins and minerals. Gluten- and lactose-free. Net price 500-mL ready-to-hang = £4.12, 1-litre ready-to-hang = £8.43, 1.5-litre ready-to-hang = £12.65.

For indications see under *Jevity®*.

Jevity Promote® (Abbott)
Liquid, protein 5.55 g, carbohydrate 11.98 g, fat 3.32 g, dietary fibre 1.7 g, energy 427 kJ (101 kcal)/100 mL, with vitamins and minerals. Gluten-free, clinically lactose-free. Net price 1-litre ready-to-hang = £8.24.

For indications see *Jevity 1.5 kcal®*

Kindergen® (SHS)
Powder, protein 7.5 g, carbohydrate 60.5 g, fat 26.1 g, energy 2060 kJ (492 kcal)/100 g with vitamins and minerals. Net price 400 g = £21.89.

For complete nutritional support or supplementary feeding for infants and children with chronic renal failure who are receiving peritoneal rapid overnight dialysis

Maxijul® (SHS)
Liquid, carbohydrate 50%, with potassium 0.004%, sodium 0.023%. Gluten-, lactose-, and fructose-free. Flavours: blackcurrant, lemon and lime, orange, and natural. Net price 200 mL = £1.23

Super Soluble Powder, glucose polymer, potassium 0.004%, sodium 0.046%. Gluten-, lactose-, and fructose-free. Net price 4 × 132-g sachet pack = £4.84, 200 g = £1.96, 2.5 kg = £17.25, 25 kg = £117.16

All for disease-related malnutrition; malabsorption states or other conditions requiring fortification with high or readily available carbohydrate supplement

Modulen IBD® (Nestlé)
Powder, protein 18 g, carbohydrate 54 g, fat 23 g, energy 2040 kJ (500 kcal)/100 g with vitamins, minerals and trace elements. Net price 400 g = £13.20.

For use as the sole source of nutrition during the active phase of Crohn's disease and for nutritional support during the remission phase in patients who are malnourished. Not to be prescribed for any child under one year; use with caution for children up to 5 years

May be flavoured with Nestlé Nutrition Flavour Mix (see under *Peptamen*)

Novasource® GI Forte (Nestlé)
Liquid, protein 6 g, carbohydrate 18.3 g, fat 5.9 g, fibre 2.2 g, energy 631 kJ (150 kcal)/100 mL with vitamins, minerals and trace elements. Gluten-free; low-lactose, net price 500-mL flexible pouch = £4.36, 1-litre flexible pouch = £8.72.

A sole source of nutrition or nutritional supplement for standard ACBS indications (see p. 833) and dysphagia. Not to be prescribed for any child under 1 year; use with caution for children up to 5 years

Novasource GI Control® (Nestlé)
Liquid, protein 4.1 g, carbohydrate 14.2 g, fat 3.5 g, fibre 2.2 g, energy 440 kJ (100 kcal)/100 mL with vitamins minerals and trace elements. Gluten-free; clinically lactose-free, net price 500-mL bottle = £4.39, 500-mL flexible pouch = £4.39.

For indications see *Novasource GI Forte®*

Nutrini® (Nutricia Clinical)
Liquid, protein 2.75 g, carbohydrate 12.3 g, fat 4.4 g, energy 420 kJ (100 kcal)/100 mL. Gluten- and sucrose-free; clinically lactose-free. Net price 200-mL bottle = £2.11, 500-mL = £5.28.

A sole source of nutrition or nutritional supplement for standard ACBS indications (see p. 833) and dysphagia in children 1–6 years or 8–20 kg body-weight

Nutrini® Energy (Nutricia Clinical)
Liquid, protein 4.1 g, carbohydrate 18.5 g, fat 6.7 g, energy 630 kJ (150 kcal)/100 mL. Gluten- and sucrose-free; clinically lactose-free. Net price 200-mL bottle = £2.59, 500-mL = £6.62.

For indications see *Nutrini®*

Nutrini® Energy Multi Fibre (Nutricia Clinical)
Liquid, tube feed, protein 4.1 g, carbohydrate 18.5 g, fat 6.7 g, fibre 0.75 g, energy 630 kJ (150 kcal)/100 mL with vitamins, minerals and trace elements. Gluten- and lactose-free, net price 200-mL bottle = £2.74, 500-mL pack = £6.82.

For short-bowel syndrome, intractable malabsorption, pre-operative preparation of undernourished patients, total gastrectomy, dysphagia, disease-related malnutrition, and growth failure. For children 1 to 6 years or 8–20 kg body-weight

Nutrini® Low Energy Multi Fibre (Nutricia Clinical)
Liquid, tube feed, protein 2.06 g, carbohydrate 9.3 g, fat 3.3 g, fibre 0.75 g, energy 315 kJ (75 kcal)/100 mL with vitamins, minerals and trace elements. Gluten- and lactose-free, net price 200-mL bottle = £1.98 500-mL pack = £5.00

For indications see *Nutrini*

Nutrini® Multi Fibre (Nutricia Clinical)
Liquid, protein 2.75 g, carbohydrate 12.3 g, fat 4.4 g, fibre 750 mg, energy 420 kJ (100 kcal)/100 mL. Gluten- and sucrose-free; clinically lactose-free. Net price 200-mL bottle = £2.35, 500-mL pack = £5.87.

For use as a sole source of nutrition or as a nutritional supplement prescribed on medical grounds for: short-bowel syndrome, intractable malabsorption, pre-operative preparation of undernourished patients, total gastrectomy, dysphagia, disease-related malnutrition and growth failure. For children 1 to 6 years or 8–20 kg body-weight

Nutriprem 2® (Cow & Gate)
Liquid, protein 2 g, carbohydrate 7.5 g, fat 4.1 g, energy 310 kJ (75 kcal)/100 mL, with vitamins, minerals, and trace elements, net price 200-mL Tetrapak® = £1.36. Also available to hospitals-only as a sterilised prepared feed in 100-mL bottles

Powder, protein 2 g, carbohydrate 7.4 g, fat 4.1 g, energy 310 kJ (75 kcal) per 100 mL when reconstituted, with vitamins and minerals. Net price 900 g = £9.06.

For catch-up growth in pre-term infants (less than 35 weeks at birth), and small-for-gestational-age infants, until 6 months corrected age

Nutrison® Energy (Nutricia Clinical)
Liquid, protein 6 g, carbohydrate 18.5 g, fat 5.8 g, energy 630 kJ (150 kcal)/100 mL with vitamins, minerals and trace elements. Gluten- and sucrose-free; clinically lactose-free. Net price 500-mL bottle = £4.11; 500-mL pack = £4.56; 1-litre pack = £8.26; 1.5-litre pack = £12.37.

Nutritional supplement for standard ACBS indications (see p. 833) and dysphagia. Not to be prescribed for any child under 1 year; use with caution for children aged 1 to 6 years

Nutrison® Energy Multi Fibre (Nutricia Clinical)
Liquid, protein 6 g, carbohydrate 18.5 g, fat 5.8 g, fibre 1.5 g, energy 630 kJ (150 kcal)/100 mL with vitamins, minerals, and trace elements. Gluten-free and clinically lactose-free. Net price 500-mL bottle = £4.60; 500-mL pack = £5.05; 1-litre pack = £9.17; 1.5-litre pack = £14.69.

For use as the sole source of nutrition or as a nutritional supplement prescribed on medical grounds for: short-bowel syndrome, intractable malabsorption, pre-operative preparation of undernourished patients, proven inflammatory bowel disease, following total gastrectomy, dysphagia, disease-related malnutrition. Not to be prescribed for any child under 1 year; use with caution for children aged 1 to 6 years

Nutrison MCT® (Nutricia Clinical)
Liquid, protein 5 g, carbohydrate 12.6 g, fat 3.3 g, energy 420 kJ (100 kcal)/100 mL with vitamins, minerals and trace elements. Gluten- and fructose-free, clinically lactose-free. Net price 1-Litre pack = £7.47.

For indications see *Nutrison Energy®*

Nutrison® Multi Fibre (Nutricia Clinical)
Liquid, protein 4 g, carbohydrate 12.3 g, fat 3.9 g, fibre 1.5 g, energy 420 kJ (100 kcal)/100 mL with vitamins, minerals and trace elements. Gluten- and sucrose-free; clinically lactose-free. Net price 500-mL bottle = £3.84; 500-mL pack = £4.23; 1-litre pack = £7.65, 1.5-litre pack = £11.49.

For indications, excluding bowel fistulas, see *Nutrison Standard*

Nutrison® Protein Plus (Nutricia Clinical)
Liquid, protein 6.3 g, carbohydrate 14.2 g, fat 4.9 g, energy 525 kJ (125 kcal)/100 mL, with vitamins, minerals and trace elements. Gluten- and lactose-free. Net price 1-litre pack = £7.68.

For use in the dietary management of disease-related malnutrition. Not suitable for children under 1 year; caution in children 1–6 years

Nutrison® Protein Plus Multi Fibre (Nutricia Clinical)
Liquid, protein 6.3 g, carbohydrate 14.2 g, fat 4.9 g, fibre 1.5 g, energy 525 kJ (125 kcal)/100 mL, with vitamins, minerals and trace elements. Gluten- and lactose-free. Net price l-litre pack = £8.55.

For use in the dietary management of disease-related malnutrition. Not suitable for children under 1 year; caution in children 1–6 years

Nutrison® Soya (Nutricia Clinical)
Liquid, protein 4 g, carbohydrate 12.3 g, fat 3.9 g, energy 420 kJ (100 kcal)/100 mL, with vitamins, minerals and trace elements. Gluten- and sucrose-free; clinically lactose-free. Net price 500-mL bottle = £3.98; 1-litre pack = £7.96.

A sole source of nutrition or nutritional supplement for standard ACBS indications (see p. 833) and cow's milk protein and lactose intolerance. Not to be prescribed for any child under 1 year; use with caution for children aged 1 to 6 years

Nutrison® Standard (Nutricia Clinical)
Liquid, protein 4 g, carbohydrate 12.3 g, fat 3.9 g, energy 425 kJ (100 kcal)/100 mL, with vitamins, minerals and trace elements. Gluten- and sucrose-free; clinically lactose-free. Net price 500-mL bottle = £3.53; 500-mL pack = £3.91; 1-litre pack = £6.87; 1.5-litre pack = £10.29.

A sole source of nutrition or nutritional supplement for standard ACBS indications (see p. 833) and dysphagia. Not to be prescribed for any child under 1 year; use with caution for children aged 1 to 6 years

Nutrison® 1000 Complete Multi Fibre (Nutricia Clinical)
Liquid, protein 5.5 g, carbohydrate 11.3 g, fat 3.7 g, fibre 2 g, energy 420 kJ (100 kcal)/100 mL, with vitamins, minerals and trace elements. Gluten- and clinically lactose-free, net price l-litre pack = £8.30.

For use as the sole source of nutrition or as a nutritional supplement for the dietary management of disease-related malnutrition in patients with low-energy and/or low fluid requirements. Not to be prescribed for any child under 1 year; use with caution for children aged 1 to 6 years

Nutrison® 1200 Complete Multi Fibre (Nutricia Clinical)
Liquid, protein 5.5 g, carbohydrate 15 g, fat 4.3 g, fibre 2 g, energy 505 kJ (120 kcal)/100 mL, with vitamins, minerals and trace elements. Gluten-free and clinically lactose-free, net price 500-mL bottle = £4.40; l-litre pack = £8.53; 1.5-litre pack = £13.20.

As a sole source of nutrition or as a nutritional supplement prescribed on medical grounds for: short-bowel syndrome, intractable malabsorption, pre-operative preparation of undernourished patients, proven inflammatory bowel disease, following total gastrectomy, dysphagia, disease-related malnutrition. Not to be prescribed for any child under 1 year; use with caution for children aged 1 to 6 years

Osmolite® (Abbott)
Liquid, protein 4 g, carbohydrate 13.56 g, fat 3.4 g, energy 424 kJ (100 kcal)/100 mL with vitamins and minerals. Gluten- and lactose-free. Net price 250-mL can = £1.74; 500-mL bottle = £3.29, 1-litre bottle = £6.27, 1.5-litre bottle = £9.41

A sole source of nutrition or nutritional supplement for standard ACBS indications (see p. 833) and dysphagia. Not to be prescribed for any child under 1 year; use with caution for children up to 5 years

Osmolite Plus® (Abbott)
Liquid, protein 5.6 g, carbohydrate 15.8 g, fat 3.9 g, energy 508 kJ (121 kcal)/100 mL with vitamins, minerals and trace elements. Gluten-free and clinically lactose-free. Net price 500-mL ready-to-hang = £3.84, 1-litre ready-to-hang = £7.42, 1.5-litre ready-to-hang = £11.11.

For indications see *Osmolite*

Paediasure® (Abbott)
Liquid, protein 2.8 g, carbohydrate 11 g, fat 5 g, energy 422 kJ (101 kcal)/100 mL with vitamins and minerals. Gluten-free, clinically lactose-free. Flavours: vanilla (can, ready-to-hang and Tetrapak®), strawberry, chocolate and banana (Tetrapak®). Net price 250-mL can = £2.41, 500-mL ready-to-hang = £4.83, 200-mL Tetrapak® = £1.94.

For use as the sole source of nutrition or as a nutritional supplement prescribed on medical grounds for children aged 1 to 10 years for short-bowel syndrome, intractable malabsorption, pre-operative preparation of undernourished patients, dysphagia, bowel fistulas, and disease-related malnutrition and/or growth failure. Not to be prescribed for any child under 1 year

Paediasure® Fibre (Abbott)
Liquid, protein 2.8 g, carbohydrate 11.16 g, fat 5 g, fibre 520 mg, energy 422 kJ (101 kcal)/100 mL with vitamins and minerals. Gluten-free, clinically lactose-free. Flavours: vanilla (ready-to-hang and Tetrapak®), banana (Tetrapak®), strawberry (Tetrapak®). Net price 500-mL ready-to-hang = £5.36, 200-mL Tetrapak® = £2.14.

For indications see *Paediasure®*

Paediasure® Plus (Abbott)
Liquid, protein 4.2 g, carbohydrate 16.7 g, fat 7.5 g, energy 632 kJ (151 kcal)/100 mL with vitamins and minerals. Gluten-free, clinically lactose-free. Flavours: vanilla (ready-to-hang and Tetrapak®), strawberry (Tetrapak®). Net price 200-mL Tetrapak® = £2.37, 500-mL ready-to-hang = £6.05.

For indications see *Paediasure®*

Paediasure® Plus Fibre (Abbott)
Sip feed, protein 4.2 g, carbohydrate 16.4 g, fat 7.47 g, fibre 1.1g, energy 626 kJ (150 kcal)/100 mL with vitamins and minerals. Gluten-free, clinically lactose-free, net price 200-mL Tetrapak® = £2.58.

Tube feed, protein 4.2 g, carbohydrate 16.7 g, fat 7.5 g, fibre 1.1g, energy 629 kJ (150 kcal)/100 mL with vitamins and minerals. Gluten-free, clinically lactose-free, net price 500-mL ready-to-hang = £6.44.

As a sole source of nutrition, or as a nutritional supplement for children aged 1 to 10 years, or 8–30 kg body-weight, with disease-related malnutrition and/or growth failure, short-bowel syndrome, intractable malabsorption, dysphagia, bowel fistulas, pre-operative preparation of undernourished patients. Not to be prescribed for any child under 1 year.

Peptamen® (Nestlé)
Liquid, protein 4 g, carbohydrate 12.7 g, fat 3.7 g, energy 420 kJ (100 kcal)/100 mL, with vitamins, minerals and trace elements. Lactose- and gluten-free. Flavours: unflavoured (can), vanilla (cup, see also *Flavour Sachets*). Net price 375-mL can = £4.70, 200-mL cup = £2.60; 500-mL (Dripac-Flex) = £5.38, 1-litre = £10.10.

A sole source of nutrition or nutritional supplement for short-bowel syndrome, intractable malabsorption, proven inflammatory bowel disease, bowel fistulas. Not to be prescribed for any child under 1 year; use with caution for children up to 5 years

Nestlé Nutrition Flavour Mix for use with *Peptamen Liquid* 200-mL cup and *Modulen IBD*. Flavours: banana, chocolate, coffee, lemon and lime, strawberry. Net price 60 g = £5.62

Peptamen Junior® (Nestlé)
Powder, protein 3 g, carbohydrate 13.8 g, fat 3.85 g, energy 420 kJ (100 kcal)/100 mL, with vitamins, minerals and trace elements. Gluten-free and clinically lactose-free. Vanilla flavour, net price 400-g can = £14.10

A sole source of nutrition or nutritional supplement for short-bowel syndrome, intractable malabsorption, proven inflammatory bowel disease, bowel fistulas, in children aged 1 to 10 years

Peptisorb® (Nutricia Clinical)
Liquid, protein 4 g, carbohydrate 17.6 g, fat 1.7 g, energy 425 kJ (100 kcal)/100 mL with vitamins, minerals and trace elements. Gluten-free. Net price 500-mL bottle = £5.32; 500-mL pack = £5.84; 1-litre pack = £10.55.

A sole source of nutrition or nutritional supplement prescribed on medical grounds for short-bowel syndrome, intractable malabsorption, proven inflammatory bowel disease, bowel fistulas. Not to be prescribed for any child under 1 year; use with caution in children up to 5 years

Perative® (Abbott)
Liquid, providing protein 6.7 g, carbohydrate 17.7 g, fat 3.7 g, energy 552 kJ (131 kcal)/100 mL, with vitamins and minerals. Gluten-free, unflavoured. Net price 500-mL ready-to-hang = £5.52, 1-litre ready-to-hang = £11.04.

Nutritional supplement for standard ACBS indications (see p. 833). Not suitable for children under 5 years

Polycal® (Nutricia Clinical)
Powder, glucose, maltose, and polysaccharides, providing 1630 kJ (384 kcal)/100 g. Net price 400 g = £3.43

Liquid, glucose polymers providing carbohydrate 61.9 g/100 mL. Low-electrolyte, protein-free. Flavours: orange and neutral. Net price 200 mL = £1.37

Nutritional supplement for disease-related malnutrition; malabsorption states or other conditions requiring fortification with a high or readily available carbohydrate supplement

Polycose® (Abbott)

Powder, glucose polymers, providing carbohydrate 94 g, energy 1598 kJ (376 kcal)/100 g. Net price 350-g can = £3.30.

Nutritional supplement for disease-related malnutrition; malabsorption states or other conditions requiring fortification with a high or readily available carbohydrate supplement

PremCare® (Heinz)

Powder, protein 1.85 g, carbohydrate 7.24 g, fat 3.96 g, energy 301 kJ (72 kcal) per 100 mL when reconstituted, with vitamins and minerals. Gluten-, sucrose-, and lactose-free. Net price 450 g = £3.29.

Nutritional supplement for catch-up growth in pre-term infants (less than 35 weeks at birth), and small-for-gestational-age infants, until 6 months post-natal age

Pro-Cal® (Vitaflo)

Powder, protein 13.5 g, carbohydrate 26.8 g, fat 56.2 g, energy 2788 kJ (667 kcal)/100 g, net price 25 x 15 g sachets = £12.45, 510 g = £11.53, 1.5 kg = £23.50, 12.5 kg = £167.10, 25 kg = £257.50.

Nutritional supplement for disease-related malnutrition, malabsorption states or other conditions requiring fortification with a fat/carbohydrate supplement. Not suitable for children under 1 year, caution in children 1–5 years

Pro-Cal Shot® (Vitaflo)

Liquid, protein 6.7 g, carbohydrate 13.4 g, fat 28.2 g, energy 1385 kJ (334 kcal)/100 mL, neutral flavour, net price 250-mL sachets = £4.17.

Nutritional supplement for disease-related malnutrition, malabsorption states, or other conditions requiring fortification with a fat/carbohydrate supplement. Not suitable for children under 1 year, caution in children 1–5 years

ProSure® (Abbott)

Liquid, protein 6.65 g, carbohydrate 19.4 g, fat 2.56 g, fibre 0.97 g, energy 528 kJ (125 kcal)/100 mL with vitamins, minerals, and trace elements. Gluten-free, clinically lactose-free. Vanilla, orange, or banana flavour, net price, 240-mL carton = £2.70; 500-mL ready-to-hang = £5.80 (vanilla only).

Nutritional supplement for patients with pancreatic cancer. Not to be prescribed for children under 1 year; use with caution in children under 4 years

Provide Xtra® (Fresenius Kabi)

Liquid, protein 3.75 g, carbohydrate 27.5 g, energy 525 kJ (125 kcal)/100 mL with vitamins, minerals and trace elements. Gluten-free. Apple, blackcurrant, carrot-apple, cherry, citrus cola, lemon & lime, melon, orange & pineapple, or tomato flavour. Net price 200-mL carton = £1.63.

Nutritional supplement for standard ACBS indications (see p. 833) and dysphagia. Not to be prescribed for any child under 1 year; use with caution for children up to 5 years

QuickCal® (Vitaflo)

Powder, protein 4.6 g, carbohydrate 17 g, fat 77 g, energy 3260 kJ (780 kcal)/100 g, net price 25 × 13-g sachets = £11.20.

For disease-related malnutrition, malabsorption states or other conditions requiring fortification with a fat/carbohydrate supplement. Not to be prescribed for any child under 1 year; use with caution for young children up to 5 years

Renilon 7.5® (Nutricia Clinical)

Liquid, protein 7.5 g, carbohydrate 20 g, fat 10 g, energy 840 kJ (200 kcal)/100 mL, with vitamins, minerals and trace elements. Gluten-free. Apricot or caramel flavour, net price 125-mL Tetrapak® = £1.73.

Nutritional supplement for standard ACBS indications (see p. 833). Not to be prescribed for any child under 3 years; use with caution in children under 6 years

Resource® Benefiber® (Nestlé)

Powder, soluble dietary fibre, carbohydrate 19 g, fibre 78 g, energy 323 kJ (76 kcal)/100 g with minerals. Gluten-free; low lactose, net price 250-g pack = £8.76, 16 x 8-g sachets = £5.72.

Nutritional supplement for standard ACBS indications (see p. 833). Not suitable for children under 5 years

Resource® Dessert Energy (Nestlé)

Semi-solid, protein 4.8 g, carbohydrate 21.2 g, fat 6.24 g, energy 671 kJ (160 kcal)/100 g with vitamins, minerals, and trace elements. Gluten-free; low lactose. Flavours: caramel, chocolate, or vanilla, net price 125-g cup = £1.35.

Nutritional supplement for standard ACBS indications (see p. 833) and dysphagia, continuous ambulatory peritoneal dialysis (CAPD), or haemodialysis. Not to be prescribed for any child under 1 year; use with caution for children up to 5 years

Resource® Dessert Fruit (Nestlé)

Semi-solid, protein 5 g, carbohydrate 24 g, fat 5 g, fibre 1.4 g, energy 671 kJ (160 kcal)/100 g with vitamins, minerals, and trace elements. Gluten-free; low lactose. Flavours: apple, apple-strawberry, or apple-peach, net price 3 × 125-g cup = £4.05.

For indications see *Resource® Dessert Energy*

Resource® 2.0 Fibre (Nestlé)

Liquid, protein 9 g, carbohydrate 21.4 g, fat 8.7 g, fibre 2.5 g, energy 836 kJ (200 kcal)/100 mL, with vitamins, minerals, and trace elements. Gluten-free; low lactose. Flavours: summer fruits, strawberry, vanilla, coffee, apricot, or neutral. Net price 200-mL carton = £1.65.

Nutritional supplement for standard ACBS indications (see p. 833) and dysphagia and conditions requiring a high energy and low volume diet. Not to be prescribed for any child under 3 years; use with caution in children up to 5 years

Resource® Fruit Flavour Drink (Nestlé)

Liquid, protein 4 g, carbohydrate 33.5 g, energy 638 kJ (150 kcal)/100 mL with vitamins, minerals, and trace elements. Fat- and gluten-free; low lactose. Flavours: apple, orange, or pineapple, net price 200-mL carton = £1.49.

Nutritional supplement for standard ACBS indications (see p. 833) and dysphagia. Not to be prescribed for any child under 3 years; use with caution for children up to 5 years

Resource® Junior (Nestlé)

Liquid, protein 3 g, carbohydrate 20.6 g, fat 6.2 g, energy 631 kJ (150 kcal)/100 mL with vitamins, minerals, and trace elements. Gluten-free; clinically lactose-free. Flavours: chocolate, strawberry, or vanilla, net price 200-mL carton = £1.69.

A sole source of nutrition or nutritional supplement for standard ACBS indications (see p. 833), and dysphagia. Not to be prescribed for any child under 1 year

Resource® Protein (Nestlé)

Liquid, protein 9.4 g, carbohydrate 14 g, fat 3.5 g, energy 530 kJ (125 kcal)/100 mL with vitamins, minerals and trace elements. Gluten-free; low lactose. Flavours: apricot, chocolate, forest fruits, strawberry, or vanilla. Net price 200-mL bottle = £1.33

For indications see *Resource® Fruit Flavour Drink*. Not to be prescribed for any child under 3 years; use with caution for children up to 5 years

Resource® Shake (Nestlé)

Liquid, protein 5.1 g, carbohydrate 22.6 g, fat 7 g, energy 731 kJ (174 kcal)/100 mL with vitamins, minerals and trace elements. Gluten-free; low lactose. Flavours: banana, chocolate, lemon, strawberry, summer fruits, toffee, or vanilla. Net price 175-mL carton = £1.46.

Nutritional supplement for standard ACBS indications (see p. 833) and dysphagia. Not to be prescribed for any child under 1 year; use with caution for children up to 5 years

Resource® Support (Nestlé)

Liquid, protein 9 g, carbohydrate 17.9 g, fat 5.3 g, fibre 1.6 g, energy 653 kJ (155 kcal)/100 mL, with vitamins, minerals, and trace elements. Gluten-free; low lactose. Flavours: coffee, chocolate, or vanilla. Net price 200-mL carton = £2.25.

A nutritional supplement for patients with pancreatic cancer. Not to be prescribed for any child under 3 years; use with caution for children up to 5 years

Scandishake® Mix (Nutricia Clinical)

Powder, protein 11.7 g, carbohydrate 66.8 g, fat 30.4 g, energy 2457 kJ (588 kcal)/unflavoured serving (serving = 1 sachet reconstituted with 240 mL whole milk; protein, carbohydrate and energy values vary with flavour). Flavours:

Appendix 7: Borderline substances

banana, caramel, chocolate, strawberry, vanilla, and unflavoured. Net price 85-g sachet = £1.95.

Nutritional support for disease-related malnutrition; malabsorption states or other conditions requiring fortification with a fat/carbohydrate supplement

SMA High Energy® (SMA Nutrition)

Liquid, protein 2 g, carbohydrate 9.8 g, fat 4.9 g, energy 382 kJ (91 kcal)/100mL, with vitamins and minerals. Net price 250 mL = £1.84.

For disease-related malnutrition, malabsorption, and growth failure

Survimed OPD® (Fresenius Kabi)

Liquid, protein 4.5 g, carbohydrate 15 g, fat 2.6 g, energy 420 kJ (100 kcal)/100 mL, with vitamins, minerals, and trace elements. Gluten-free, and low lactose. Net price 500-mL EasyBag® = £5.17.

Nutritional supplement for standard ACBS indications (see p. 833) and dysphagia. Not to be prescribed for any child under 1 year; use with caution for children up to 5 years

Tentrini® (Nutricia Clinical)

Liquid, tube feed, protein 3.3 g, carbohydrate 12.3 g, fat 4.2 g, energy 420 kJ (100 kcal)/100 mL, with vitamins, minerals and trace elements. Gluten- and lactose-free. Unflavoured, net price 500-mL bottle or pack = £4.50

For short-bowel syndrome, intractable malabsorption, pre-operative preparation of undernourished patients, inflammatory bowel disease, total gastrectomy, dysphagia, bowel fistulas, disease-related malnutrition, and growth failure. Suitable for child 7–12 years, body-weight 21–45 kg

Tentrini® Energy (Nutricia Clinical)

Liquid, tube feed, protein 4.9 g, carbohydrate 18.5 g, fat 6.3 g, energy 630 kJ (150 kcal)/100 mL, with vitamins, minerals and trace elements. Gluten- and lactose-free. Unflavoured, net price 500-mL bottle or pack = £5.57

For indications see *Tentrini®*

Tentrini® Energy Multi Fibre (Nutricia Clinical)

Liquid, tube feed, protein 4.9 g, carbohydrate 18.5 g, fat 6.3 g, fibre 1.12 g, energy 630 kJ (150 kcal)/100 mL, with vitamins, minerals and trace elements. Gluten- and lactose-free. Unflavoured, net price 500-mL bottle or pack = £6.14

For indications see *Tentrini®*

Tentrini® Multi Fibre (Nutricia Clinical)

Liquid, tube feed, protein 3.3 g, carbohydrate 12.3 g, fat 4.2 g, fibre 1.12 g, energy 420 kJ (100 kcal)/100 mL, with vitamins, minerals and trace elements. Gluten- and lactose-free. Unflavoured, net price 500-mL bottle or pack = £4.95

For short-bowel syndrome, intractable malabsorption, pre-operative preparation of undernourished patients, inflammatory bowel disease, total gastrectomy, dysphagia, disease-related malnutrition, and growth failure. Not suitable for children under 1 year; caution in children under 7 years or body-weight less than 21 kg

TwoCal HN® (Abbott)

Liquid, protein 8.4 g, carbohydrate 21.6 g, fat 8.9 g, fibre 840 mg, energy 850 kJ (202 kcal)/100 mL, with vitamins, minerals, and trace elements. Gluten- and lactose-free. Vanilla flavour, net price 237-mL can = £2.40.

A sole source of nutrition or nutritional supplement for standard ACBS indications (see p. 833) and dysphagia. Not to be prescribed for any child under 6 years; use with caution in children aged up to 10 years

Vegenat®-med (Vegenat)

Powder - high protein varieties, average nutritional content: protein 24.6 g, carbohydrate 59.2 g, fat 16.3 g, fibre 6 g, energy 2020 kJ (480 kcal)/110 g, with vitamins, minerals, and trace elements. Gluten-free, low lactose. Flavours: chicken, fish, veal, ham, winter vegetables, fish and vegetable, lentil, vegetable, chickpea, and curry chicken, net price 12 × 110-g sachets = £46.20; Lemon, or rice with lemon flavours, 12 × 110-g sachets = £43.89; rice with apple, 24 × 55-g sachets = £43.89

Powder - balanced protein varieties, average nutritional content: protein 18.4 g, carbohydrate 63.8 g, fat 15 g, fibre 6 g, energy 1970 kJ (470 kcal)/110 g, with vitamins, minerals, and trace elements. Gluten-free, low lactose. Flavours: apple, chocolate, honey, or orange, net price 12 × 110-g sachets = £33.00

For use as a nutritional supplement prescribed on medical grounds for: short-bowel syndrome, intractable malabsorption, pre-operative preparation of undernourished patients, proven inflammatory bowel disease, following total gastrectomy, dysphagia, disease-related malnutrition. Not suitable for any child under 12 years; use with caution in children under 16 years

Vitajoule® (Vitaflo)

Powder, glucose polymers, providing carbohydrate 96 g, energy 1610 kJ (380 kcal)/100 g. Net price 500 g = £3.48, 2.5 kg = £17.14, 25 kg = £101.97.

For disease-related malnutrition; malabsorption states or other conditions requiring fortification with a high or readily available carbohydrate supplement

Vitasavoury® (Vitaflo)

Powder, protein 12 g, carbohydrate 24 g, fat 54 g, energy 2610 kJ (630 kcal)/100 g, net price 10 x 50-g sachets = £15.52, 24 × 33-g ready cups = £25.76. Flavours: chicken, leek and potato, mushroom, vegetable.

Nutritional supplement for disease-related malnutrition, malabsorption states or other conditions requiring fortification with a fat/carbohydrate supplement. Not to be prescribed for any child under 1 year; use with caution for young children up to 5 years

Feed thickeners and pre-thickened foods

Carobel, Instant® (Cow & Gate)

Powder, carob seed flour. Net price 135 g = £2.72.

For thickening feeds in the treatment of vomiting

Clinutren® Thickened Drinks (Nestlé)

Liquid, modified maize starch, gluten-free. Flavours: orange, peppermint, and tea, net price 4 × 125 g = £2.80.

Thickening of foods and fluids in dysphagia. Not to be used for children under 3 years

Clinutren® Thickener (Nestlé)

Powder, modified maize starch, gluten-free, net price 300 g = £5.30.

Thickening of foods and fluids in dysphagia. Not to be used for children under 3 years

Enfamil AR® (Mead Johnson)

AR (Anti-Reflux), powder, protein 1.7 g, fat 3.5 g, carbohydrate 7.6 g, energy 285 kJ (68 kcal)/100 mL, with vitamins, minerals and trace elements, net price 400 g = £2.76.

For significant reflux disease. For use not in excess of a 6-month period. Not to be used in conjunction with any other thickener or antacid product.

Nestargel® (Nestlé)

Powder, carob seed flour 96.5%, calcium lactate 3.5%. Net price 125 g = £2.99.

For thickening feeds in the treatment of vomiting

Nutilis® (Nutricia Clinical)

Powder, modified maize starch, gluten- and lactose-free, net price 20 × 9-g sachets = £5.52; 225 g = £4.23.

For thickening of foods in dysphagia. Not to be prescribed for children under 3 years

Resource® Thickened Drink (Nestlé)

Liquid, carbohydrate 22 g, energy: orange 383 kJ (89 kcal); apple 375 kJ (89 kcal)/100 mL. Syrup and custard consistencies. Gluten-free; clinically lactose free, net price 12 × 114-mL cups = £7.08.

For dysphagia. Not suitable for children under 1 year

Resource® Thickened Squash (Nestlé)

Liquid, syrup consistency: carbohydrate 16.9 g, energy 287 kJ (68 kcal)/100 mL; custard consistency: carbohydrate 17.8 g, energy 303 kJ (71 kcal)/100 mL. Gluten-free; clinically lactose-free. Orange and lemon flavour, net price 1.89-litre bottle = £3.99.

For dysphagia. Not suitable for children under 1 year

Resource® ThickenUp® (Nestlé)

Powder, modified maize starch. Gluten- and lactose-free, net price 227 g = £3.99; 75 × 4.5-g sachet = £15.75.

For thickening of foods in dysphagia. Not to be prescribed for children under 1 year

SLO Drinks® (SLO Drinks)
Powder, carbohydrate content varies with flavour and chosen consistency (3 consistencies available), see product literature. Flavours: black currant, lemon, orange, or peach, net price 25-cups = £7.50.
For patient hydration in the dietary management of dysphagia. Not suitable as a sole source of nutrition. Not to be used in children under 3 years

SMA Staydown® (SMA Nutrition)
Powder, protein 12.4 g, fat 27.9 g, carbohydrate 54.3 g, energy 2166 kJ (518 kcal)/100g, with vitamins, minerals, and trace elements. Net price 900 g = £5.74.
For significant reflux disease. Not to be used for more than 6 months or in conjunction with any other thickener or antacid product

Thick and Easy® (Fresenius Kabi)
Powder. Modified maize starch, net price 225-g can = £3.99; 100 × 9-g sachets = £26.35; 4.54 kg = £70.53.
Thickened Juices, liquid, modified food starch. Flavours: apple, blackcurrant, cranberry, kiwi-strawberry, and orange, net price 118-mL pot = 52p; 1.42-litre bottle = £3.61.
For thickening of foods in dysphagia. Not to be prescribed for children under 1 year except in cases of failure to thrive

Thixo-D® (Sutherland)
Powder, modified maize starch, gluten-free. Net price 375-g tub = £5.79.
For thickening of foods in dysphagia. Not to be prescribed for children under 1 year except in cases of failure to thrive

Vitaquick® (Vitaflo)
Powder. Modified maize starch. Net price 300 g = £6.40; 2 kg = £32.59; 6 kg = £83.40.
For thickening of foods in dysphagia. Not to be prescribed for children under 1 year except in cases of failure to thrive

Hypoproteinaemia (biochemically proven)

Casilan 90® (Heinz)
Powder, whole protein, containing all essential amino acids, 90% with less than 0.1% Na^+. Net price 250 g = £5.90.
For biochemically proven hypoproteinaemia

Dialamine® (SHS)
Powder, essential amino acids 30%, with carbohydrate 62%, energy 1500 kJ (360 kcal)/100 g, with ascorbic acid, minerals, and trace elements. Flavour: orange. Net price 200 g = £27.66.
For oral feeding where essential amino acid supplements are required; e.g. chronic renal failure, hypoproteinaemia, wound fistula leakage with excessive protein loss, conditions requiring a controlled nitrogen intake, and haemodialysis

Maxisorb® (SHS)
Powder, protein 12 g, carbohydrate 9 g, fat 6 g, energy 579 kJ (138 kcal)/30 g with minerals. Vanilla, strawberry and chocolate flavours. Net price 5 × 30-g sachets = £4.00.
For biochemically proven hypoproteinaemia. Not to be prescribed for any child under 1 year; use with caution for children up to 5 years

Protifar® (Nutricia Clinical)
Powder, protein 88.5%. Low lactose, gluten- and sucrose-free. Net price 225 g = £6.98.
For biochemically proven hypoproteinaemia

Renapro® (KoRa)
Powder, whey protein providing protein 92 g, carbohydrate less than 300 mg, fat 500 mg, 1562 kJ (367 kcal)/100 g. Net price 20-g sachet = £2.32.
For dialysis and hypoproteinaemia. Not suitable for infants under 1 year

Vitapro® (Vitaflo)
Powder, whole milk proteins, containing all essential amino acids, 75%. Net price 250 g = £6.89, 2 kg = £54.00.
For biochemically proven hypoproteinaemia

Foods and supplements for special diets

Alcoholic Beverages
see under Rectified Spirit

Alembicol D® (Alembic Products)
Fractionated coconut oil. Net price 5 kg = £125.55.
For steatorrhoea associated with cystic fibrosis of the pancreas, intestinal lymphangiectasia, surgery of the intestine, chronic liver disease, liver cirrhosis, other proven malabsorption syndromes; in a ketogenic diet in the management of epilepsy; type 1 hyperlipoproteinaemia

Caprilon® (SHS)
Powder, protein 11.8%, carbohydrate 55.1%, fat 28.3% (medium chain triglycerides 21.3%). Low in lactose, gluten- and sucrose-free. Used as a 12.7% solution. Net price 420 g = £13.73.
For disorders in which a high intake of MCT is beneficial

Corn flour and corn starch
For hypoglycaemia associated with glycogen-storage disease

Energivit® (SHS)
Powder, protein-free, carbohydrate 66.7 g, fat 25 g, energy 2059 kJ, (492 kcal)/100 g with vitamins, minerals and trace elements, net price 400 g = £16.57.
For infants requiring additional energy, vitamins, minerals and trace elements following a protein restricted diet

Generaid® (SHS)
Powder, whey protein and additional branched-chain amino acids (protein equivalent 81%). Net price 200 g (unflavoured) = £23.05. See also Flavour Sachets.
For patients with chronic liver disease and/or porto-hepatic encephalopathy

Generaid Plus® (SHS)
Powder, whey protein and additional branched-chain amino acids (protein equivalent 11%) carbohydrate 62%, fat 19% with vitamins, minerals and trace elements. Net price 400 g = £16.49.
For children over 1 year with hepatic disorders

KetoCal® (SHS)
Powder, protein 3.1 g, carbohydrate 600 mg, fat 14.6 g, energy 602 kJ (146 kcal)/100 mL serving (serving = 20 g powder reconstituted with water up to final volume of 100 mL), with vitamins, minerals, and trace elements. Vanilla or unflavoured, net price 300-g can = £23.87.
For use as part of the ketogenic diet in the management of epilepsy resistant to drug therapy. Only to be prescribed on the advice of a secondary care physician with experience of the ketogenic diet; not to be prescribed for children under 1 year

Liquigen® (SHS)
Emulsion, medium chain triglycerides 52%. Net price 250 mL = £6.73; 1 litre = £28.25.
For steatorrhoea associated with cystic fibrosis of the pancreas; intestinal lymphangiectasia, surgery of the intestine; chronic liver disease and liver cirrhosis; other proven malabsorption syndromes; ketogenic diet in the management of epilepsy; type I hyperlipoproteinaemia

MCT Oil
Triglycerides from medium chain fatty acids. For steatorrhoea associated with cystic fibrosis of the pancreas; intestinal lymphangiectasia; surgery of the intestine; chronic liver disease and liver cirrhosis, other proven malabsorption syndromes; in a ketogenic diet in the management of epilepsy; in type I hyperlipoproteinaemia
Available from SHS (net price 500 mL = £11.06)

MCT Pepdite® (SHS)
Powder, essential and non-essential amino acids, peptides, medium chain triglycerides, monoglyceride of sunflower oil, with carbohydrate, fat, vitamins, minerals, and trace elements. Flavour Sachets available.
MCT Pepdite 0–2 Net price 400 g = £15.39
MCT Pepdite 1+. Net price 400 g = £15.39
Both for disorders in which a high intake of medium chain triglyceride is beneficial

Appendix 7: Borderline substances

Metabolic Mineral Mixture® (SHS)
Powder, essential mineral salts. Net price 100 g = £9.56.
For mineral supplementation in synthetic diets

MCT Step 1® (Vitaflo)
Powder, protein 2.1 g, carbohydrate 12 g, fat 2.1 g, energy 310 kJ (74 kcal)/100 mL (when reconstituted), with vitamins, minerals and trace elements. Includes fat high in medium-chain triglycerides and low in long-chain triglycerides. Net price 30 × 87.5-g sachets = £94.04; 400g = £14.33.
For the dietary management of fat malabsorption in disorders of fatty acid oxidation

Monogen® (SHS)
Powder, protein 11.4 g, carbohydrate 68 g, fat 11.4 g (of which MCT 93%), energy 1772 kJ (420 kcal)/100 g, with vitamins, minerals and trace elements. Net price 400 g = £15.30.
For long-chain acyl-CoA dehydrogenase deficiency (LCAD), carnitine palmitoyl transferase deficiency (CPTD), primary and secondary lipoprotin lipase deficiency

Nepro® (Abbott)
Liquid, protein 7 g, carbohydrate 20.6 g, fat 9.6 g, fibre 1.56g, energy 840 kJ (200 kcal)/100 mL with vitamins and minerals. Gluten- and lactose-free. Net price 500-mL ready-to-hang = £4.95 (vanilla); 200-mL Tetrapak® = £2.28 (strawberry or vanilla).
For patients with chronic renal failure who are on haemodialysis or continuous ambulatory peritoneal dialysis (CAPD), or patients with cirrhosis or other conditions requiring a high energy, low fluid, low electrolyte diet

Paediatric Seravit® (SHS)
Powder, vitamins, minerals, low sodium and potassium, and trace elements. Net price 200 g (unflavoured) = £13.49; pineapple flavour, 200 g = £14.37.
For vitamin and mineral supplementation in restrictive therapeutic diets in infants and children

Rectified Spirit
Where the therapeutic qualities of alcohol are required rectified spirit (suitably flavoured and diluted) should be prescribed

Renamil® (KoRa)
Powder, protein 4.7 g, carbohydrate 70.2 g, fat 18.7 g, energy 1984 kJ (468 kcal)/100 g, with vitamins and minerals. Net price 1 kg = £25.40.
For chronic renal failure. Not suitable for infants and children under 1 year

Suplena® (Abbott)
Liquid, protein 3 g, carbohydrate 25.5 g, fat 9.6 g, energy 841 kJ (201 kcal)/100 mL. Flavour: vanilla. Net price 237-mL can = £2.34.
For patients with chronic or acute renal failure who are not undergoing dialysis; chronic or acute liver disease with fluid restriction; other conditions requiring a high-energy, low-protein, low-electrolyte, low-volume enteral feed

Special foods for conditions of intolerance

Colief® (Britannia)
Liquid, lactase 50 000 units/g, net price 7-mL dropper bottle = £7.00
For the relief of symptoms associated with lactose intolerance in infants, provided that lactose intolerance is confirmed by the presence of reducing substances and/or excessive acid in stools, a low concentration of the corresponding disaccharide enzyme on intestinal biopsy or by breath hydrogen test or lactose intolerance test. For dosage and administration details, consult product literature

Comminuted Chicken Meat (SHS)
Suspension (aqueous). Net price 150 g = £2.72.
For carbohydrate intolerance in association with possible or proven intolerance of milk; glucose and galactose intolerance

Cow & Gate Pepti® (Cow & Gate)
Powder, protein equivalent 12.4 g, fat 28.5 g, carbohydrate 54.2 g, energy 2185 kJ (522 kcal)/100 g, with vitamins, minerals, and trace elements. Used as a solution in place of milk, net price 900 g = £17.10.
For the dietary management of established cows' milk protein intolerance with or without proven secondary lactose intolerance

Cow & Gate Pepti-Junior® (Cow & Gate)
Powder, protein 15.3 g, fat 28.3 g, carbohydrate 55.1 g, energy 2140 kJ (507 kcal)/100 g with vitamins and minerals. Used as a 13.1% solution in place of milk. Net price 450 g = £9.42.
For disaccharide and/or whole protein intolerance or where amino acids and peptides are indicated in conjunction with medium chain triglycerides

Enfamil Lactofree® (Mead Johnson)
Powder, protein 1.42 g, fat 3.7 g, carbohydrate 7.2 g, energy 280 kJ (68 kcal)/100 mL with vitamins, minerals and trace elements. Lactose- and sucrose-free, net price 400 g = £2.76.
For proven lactose intolerance

Farley's Soya Formula (Heinz)
Powder, providing protein 2%, carbohydrate 7%, fat 3.8% with vitamins and minerals when reconstituted. Gluten-, sucrose-, and lactose-free. Net price 900 g = £5.43.
For proven lactose and associated sucrose intolerance in preschool children, galactokinase deficiency, galactosaemia, and cow's milk protein intolerance

Fructose (Laevulose)
For proven glucose/galactose intolerance

Galactomin 17® (SHS)
Powder, protein 14.5 g, fat 25.9 g, carbohydrate 56.9 g, mineral salts 3.4 g/100 g. Used as a 13.1% solution with additional vitamins in place of milk. Net price 400 g = £12.95.
For proven lactose intolerance in preschool children, galactosaemia and galactokinase deficiency

Galactomin 19® (SHS)
Powder, protein 14.6 g, fat 30.8 g, carbohydrate 49.7 g (fructose as carbohydrate source), mineral salts 2.1 g/100 g, with vitamins. Used as a 12.9% solution in place of milk. Net price 400 g = £33.32.
For glucose plus galactose intolerance

Glucose (Dextrose monohydrate)
Net price 500 g = £1.05.
For glycogen storage disease and sucrose/isomaltose intolerance

InfaSoy® (Cow & Gate)
Powder, carbohydrate 7.1%, fat 3.6%, and protein 1.8% with vitamins and minerals when used as a 12.7% solution. Net price 450 g = £3.88; 900 g = £7.44.
For proven lactose and associated sucrose intolerance in preschool children, galactokinase deficiency, galactosaemia, and proven whole cow's milk sensitivity

Isomil® (Abbott)
Powder, protein 1.8%, carbohydrate 6.9%, fat 3.7% with vitamins and minerals when reconstituted. Lactose-free. Net price 400 g = £3.38.
For proven lactose intolerance in preschool children, galactokinase deficiency, galactosaemia, and proven whole cow's milk sensitivity

Locasol® (SHS)
Powder, protein 14.6 g, carbohydrate 56.5 g, fat 26.1 g, mineral salts 1.9 g, not more than 55 mg of Ca^{2+}/100 g and vitamins. Used as a 13.1% solution in place of milk. Net price 400 g = £16.95.
For calcium intolerance

Neocate® (SHS)
Powder, essential and non-essential amino acids, maltodextrin, fat, vitamins, minerals, and trace elements. Net price 400 g = £22.02.
For proven whole protein intolerance, short-bowel syndrome, intractable malabsorption, and other gastrointestinal disorders where an elemental diet is specifically indicated; for use in children under 1 year

Neocate Active® (SHS)
Powder, protein equivalent 2.8g (essential and non-essential amino acids), carbohydrate 11.3g, fat 4.8g, energy 418kJ (100kcal)/100mL (when a 63-g sachet is reconstituted with 250mL of water), with vitamins, minerals, and trace elements. Black currant or unflavoured (SHS Flavour sachets compatible), net price 14 × 63-g sachets = £49.12.

As a nutritional supplement in children over 1 year with proven whole protein intolerance, short-bowel syndrome, intractable malabsorption, or other gastrointestinal disorders where an elemental diet is specifically indicated.

Neocate Advance® (SHS)
Powder, essential and non-essential amino acids, carbohydrate, fat, vitamins, minerals and trace elements. Milk protein-, soy- and lactose-free. Net price 100 g = £4.63; banana-vanilla flavour 15 x 50 g = £36.60.

For proven whole protein intolerance, short-bowel syndrome, intractable malabsorption, and other gastrointestinal disorders where an elemental diet is specifically indicated; for use in children over 1 year

Nutramigen® 1 (Mead Johnson)
Powder, protein 1.9 g, carbohydrate 7.5 g, fat 3.4 g, energy 280 kJ (68 kcal)/100 mL with vitamins and minerals. Gluten-, sucrose-, and lactose-free. Net price 400 g = £8.20.

For disaccharide and/or whole protein intolerance where additional medium chain triglyceride is not indicated

Nutramigen® 2 (Mead Johnson)
Powder, protein 1.7 g, carbohydrate 8.6 g, fat 2.9 g energy 285 kJ (68 kcal)/100 mL when normal dilution used, with vitamins, minerals and trace elements. Gluten-, sucrose-, and lactose-free, net price 400 g = £8.20.

For disaccharide and/or whole protein intolerance where additional medium chain triglyceride is not indicated. Not suitable for infants under 6 months

Pepdite® (SHS)
Powder, peptides, essential and non-essential amino acids, with carbohydrate, fat, vitamins, minerals, and trace elements. Flavour Sachets available.

Pepdite (birth to 1 year). Providing 1925 kJ (472 kcal)/100 g. Net price 400 g = £14.13

Pepdite 1+. Providing 1787 kJ (439 kcal)/100 g. Net price 400 g = £14.85; 57 g (banana flavour) = £2.40

Both for disaccharide and/or whole protein intolerance, or where amino acids or peptides are indicated in conjunction with medium chain triglycerides

Pregestimil® (Mead Johnson)
Powder, protein 12.8%, carbohydrate 61.6%, fat 18.3% with vitamins and minerals. Gluten-, sucrose-, and lactose-free. Net price 400 g = £8.91.

For disaccharide and/or whole protein intolerance or where amino acids or peptides are indicated in conjunction with medium chain triglycerides

Prejomin® (Milupa)
Granules, protein 13.5 g, carbohydrate 57 g, fat 24 g, energy 2085 kJ (497 kcal)/100 g, with vitamins and minerals. Gluten-free. For preparation with water before use. Net price 400 g = £9.82.

For disaccharide and/or whole protein intolerance where additional medium chain triglyceride is not indicated

Prosobee® (Mead Johnson)
Powder, protein 1.76 g, carbohydrate 6.8 g, fat 3.7 g, energy 285 kJ (68 kcal)/100 mL with vitamins and minerals. Gluten-, sucrose-, and lactose-free. Net price 400 g = £3.51.

For proven lactose and associated sucrose intolerance in pre-school children, galactokinase deficiency, galactosaemia, and proven whole cow's milk sensitivity

SMA LF® (SMA Nutrition)
Powder, protein 1.5 g, carbohydrate 7.2 g, fat 3.6 g, energy 282 kJ (67 kcal)/100 mL, with vitamins and minerals. Net price 430 g = £4.07.

For proven lactose intolerance

Wysoy® (Wyeth)
Powder, carbohydrate 6.9%, fat 3.6%, and protein 2.1% with vitamins and minerals when reconstituted. Net price 430 g = £3.98; 860 g = £7.58

For proven lactose and associated sucrose intolerance in pre-school children, galactokinase deficiency, galactosaemia and proven whole cow's milk sensitivity

Gluten-sensitive enteropathies

> ACBS indications: gluten-sensitive enteropathies including steatorrhoea due to gluten sensitivity, coeliac disease, and dermatitis herpetiformis.

Aproten® (Ultrapharm)
Gluten-free. Flour. Net price 500 g = £4.99.

Arnott® (Ultrapharm)
Rice Cookies, gluten-free. Net price 200 g = £2.06.

Baker's Delight®
Gluten-free. Bread, net price 100 g = 80p.

Barkat® (Gluten Free Foods Ltd)
Gluten-free. Baguettes (par-baked), net price 200 g = £2.24. Bread (white, par-baked), 550 g = £3.37; country loaf (par-baked, sliced), 250 g = £2.46; rolls (par-baked), 300 g = £2.24. Bread mix, 500 g = £4.12. Multi Grain Bread, 450 g = £2.99. Rice bread (sliced), brown or white, 450 g = £2.99. Pasta, buckwheat (penne or spirals), 250 g = £1.58. Rice pizza crust, brown or white, 150 g = £2.21

Bi-Aglut® (Ultrapharm)
Gluten-free. Bread flour mix or plain flour, net price 500 g = £4.75. Bread rolls, 150 g = £1.77. Bread sticks, 150 g = £1.95.Biscuits, 180 g = £2.89. Crackers, 150 g = £2.36. Cracker toast, 240 g = £4.18. Pasta (fusilli, macaroni, penne, spaghetti), 500 g = £5.23.

Dietary Specials (Nutrition Point)
Gluten-free. Bread. Loaf, sliced (brown, white or multigrain) 400 g = £2.80; bread rolls, long (white) 3 = £1.75. Bread mix, net price 500 g = £4.95; cracker bread, 150 g = £1.80; cake mix (white), 750 g = £4.95; white mix, 500 g = £4.95. Tea biscuits, 220 g = £2.00. Pasta (spaghetti, penne, fusilli), 500 g = £3.20

Ener-G® (General Dietary)
Gluten-free. Cookies (vanilla flavour), net price 435 g = £4.88. Dinner Rolls (× 6), 280 g = £2.90. Rice bread (sliced), brown, 474 g = £4.28; white, 456 g = £4.28. Rice loaf (sliced), 612 g = £4.28. Seattle brown loaf, 600 g = £4.93. Tapioca bread (sliced), 480 g = £4.28. Rice pasta (macaroni, shells, small shells, and lasagne), 454 g = £3.98; spaghetti, 447 g = £3.98; tagliatelle, 400 g = £3.98; vermicelli, 300 g = £3.98; cannelloni, 335 g = £3.98. Brown rice pasta: lasagne, 454 g = £3.98; macaroni, 454 g = £3.98; spaghetti, 447 g = £3.98. Xanthan gum, 170 g = £6.76.

Gadsby's
Gluten-free. White bread flour, net price 1 kg = £4.99. White sliced bread, 400 g = £2.50. White bread rolls, 4 × 75 g = £2.00

Generpharm (Generpharm)
Gluten-free. Bread, (white, sliced), net price 165 g = £2.24; sandwich bread, 155 g = £2.18. Baguettes (part-baked), 2 × 125 g = £2.96. Bread buns, 4 × 50 g = £3.25. Dinner rolls (white, part-baked), 4 × 35 g = £1.91. Flat bread (part-baked), 3 × 40 g = £3.99. Hotdog rolls (white, part-baked) 3 × 35 g = £1.95. Long rolls (white, part-baked), 3 × 83 g = £2.81. Lunch rolls (white), 6 × 45 g = £3.22. Flour (white), 1 kg = £6.88; flour (fibre mix), 500 g = £5.46. Pasta (macaroni, small macaroni, puntini, short spaghetti, spirals), 250 g = £2.99. Pizza bases, 3 × 125 g = £5.99. Rice bread (sandwich loaf), 200 g = £2.32; rice bread (brown), 220 g = £2.32.

Glutafin® (Nutricia Dietary)
Gluten-free. Biscuits, savoury, 125 g = £1.74; 150 g = £2.32. Biscuits, digestive, sweet or tea, 150 g = £1.74. Biscuits, 200 g = £3.40. Biscuits, shortbread, 125 g = £1.47. Cake mix, 500 g = £5.31. Crackers, 200 g = £2.84. High fibre crackers, 200 g =

£2.38. Pasta (penne, shells, spirals, spaghetti), 500 g = £5.52; (lasagne, tagliatelle), 250 g = £2.90. Pizza bases, 2 × 110 g = £3.94.

Select Gluten-free. Fibre loaf (sliced or unsliced), 400 g = £2.81; part-baked, 400 g = £3.15. Fresh Bread, white or brown loaf, (sliced), 400 g = £3.02 Seeded loaf, 400 g = £2.97. White loaf (sliced or unsliced), 400 g = £2.81; part-baked, 400 g = £3.15. Fibre rolls, 4 = £3.15; (part-baked), 4 = £3.15; long, 2 = £3.15. White rolls, 4 = £3.15; (part-baked), 4 = £3.15; long, 2 = £3.15. Mixes (bread, cake, fibre, fibre bread, pastry, and white), 500 g = £5.46

Glutano® (Gluten Free Foods Ltd)
Gluten-free. Tea biscuits, net price 125 g = £1.79; wheat-free digestive biscuit, 200 g = £1.79. Shortcake rings, 125 g = £1.79. Crispbread, 125 g = £1.79. Crackers, 150 g = £1.79. Flour mix, 750 g = £4.72. Pasta (animal shapes, spaghetti, spirals, tagliatelle), 250 g = £1.79; macaroni, 500 g = £3.58. White sliced bread (par-baked), 300 g = £2.00. Wholemeal bread (sliced), 500 g = £2.24. Baguette or rolls (par-baked), 200 g = £1.79.

Innovative Solutions (Innovative)
Gluten-free. Potato flour, net price 500 g = £1.99; rice flour (brown or white), 500 g = £1.25; tapioca flour, 500 g = £1.49.

Juvela® (Juvela)
Gluten-free. Harvest mix, fibre mix, and flour mix, net price 500 g = £5.81. Bread (whole or sliced), 400-g loaf = £2.80; part-baked loaf (with or without fibre), 400g = £3.13. Fibre bread (sliced and unsliced), 400-g loaf = £2.80. Bread rolls, 5 × 85 g = £3.78, fibre bread rolls, 5 × 85 g = £3.78, part-baked rolls (with or without fibre), 5 × 75 g = £3.90. Crispbread, 210 g = £3.66. Pasta (Fibre Linguine, fibre Penne, fusilli, macaroni, spaghetti), 500 g = £5.69; lasagne, 250 g = £2.91; tagliatelle, 250 g = £2.82. Pizza bases, 2 × 180 g = £6.94. Digestive biscuits, 150 g = £2.41. Savoury biscuits, 150 g = £3.01. Sweet biscuits, 150 g = £2.28. Tea biscuits, 150 g = £2.41.

Lifestyle® (Ultrapharm)
Gluten-free. Brown bread (sliced and unsliced), net price 400 g = £2.82. White bread (sliced and unsliced), 400 g = £2.82. High fibre bread (sliced and unsliced), 400 g = £2.82. Bread rolls, (brown, white, or high-fibre) 400 g = £2.82.

Orgran® (Community)
Gluten-free. Pasta: lasagne (corn, rice and maize), 150 g = £2.89; shells (split pea and soya), 200 g = £2.25; spaghetti (corn, rice, rice and maize), 250 g = £2.25; spirals (buckwheat, corn, rice, rice and millet, rice and maize), 250 g = £2.25, spirals (organic brown rice), 250 g = £2.60. Crispbread (corn or rice), 200 g = £2.56. Pizza and pastry mix, 375 g = £3.33.

Pleniday® (TOL)
Gluten-free. Bread: loaf (sliced) net price 350 g = £1.80; country loaf (sliced), 500 g = £2.85; rustic loaf (par-baked baguette), 400 g = £2.09; petit pain, 2 × 150 g = £2.02. Pasta (penne), 250 g = £1.27; (rigate), 250 g = £1.50

Polial® (Ultrapharm)
Biscuits. Gluten- and lactose-free. Net price 200-g pack = £2.85.

Rite-Diet® Gluten-free (Nutricia Dietary)
Gluten-free. White bread (sliced or unsliced), 400 g = £2.83. White loaf (part-baked), 400 g = £3.18. Fibre bread (sliced or unsliced), 400 g = £2.83. Fibre loaf (part-baked), 400 g = £3.18. White rolls, 4 = £2.72; (part-baked) long, 2 = £3.13. Fibre rolls, 4 = £2.72 (part-baked) long, 2 = £2.95. Flour mix (white or fibre), 500 g = £5.22.

Schar® (Nutrition Point)
Gluten-free. Bread.(white, sliced), net price 2 x 200 g = £2.90. Baguette (french bread), 400 g = £3.05. Bread rolls, 150 g = £1.82. Lunch rolls, 150 g = £1.85. White bread buns, 200 g = £2.42. Bread mix, 1 kg = £4.75. Ertha brown bread, 2 x 250 g = £3.10. Cake mix, 500 g = £4.50. Flour mix, 1 kg = £4.75. Breadsticks (Grissini), 150 g = £1.95. Cracker toast, 150 g = £2.10. Crackers, 200 g = £2.55. Crispbread, 250 g = £3.50. Pasta (fusilli, penne), 500 g = £3.30; lasagne, 250 g = £3.30; macaroni pipette, 500 g = £3.30; spaghetti, 500 g = £3.30. Pizza bases, 300 g (2 × 150 g) = £5.10. Biscuits, 200 g = £2.00. Savoy biscuits, 200 g = £2.45.

Sunnyvale® (Everfresh)
Mixed grain bread, gluten-free. Net price 400 g = £1.91.

Tritamyl® (Gluten Free Foods Ltd)
Gluten-free. Flour, net price 1 kg = £5.60. Brown bread mix, 1 kg = £5.60. White bread mix, 1 kg = £5.60.

Ultra® (Ultrapharm)
Gluten-free. Baguette, net price 400 g = £2.46. Bread, net price 400 g = £2.46. High-fibre bread, 500 g = £3.35. Crackerbread, 100 g = £1.77. Pizza base, net price 400 g = £2.65.

Valpiform® (Ultrapharm)
Gluten-free. Bread mix, 2 × 500 g = £6.73; country loaf (sliced), 400 g = £3.75. Crac'form toast, 2 × 125 g = £3.52. Crisp rolls, 220 g = £3.60; Maxi baguettes, 2 × 200 g = £4.49. Pastry mix, 2 × 500 g = £6.73. Petites baguettes, 2 × 160 g = £2.99.

Gluten-sensitive enteropathies with co-existent established wheat sensitivity

ACBS indications: established gluten enteropathy with coexisting established wheat sensitivity only.

Ener-G® (General Dietary)
Gluten-free, wheat-free. Pizza bases, 372 g = £3.75. Six flour bread loaf, 576 g = £3.60. Seattle brown rolls (round or long), 4 x 119 g = £3.00

Glutafin® (Nutricia Dietary)
Gluten-free, wheat-free, crisp bread, 2 × 125 g = £3.82. Fibre loaf (sliced or unsliced), 400 g = £2.81. Fibre rolls, 4 = £2.97. White loaf (sliced or unsliced), 400 g = £3.15. White rolls, 4 = £2.97. Mixes (fibre bread, bread, white or fibre), 500 g = £5.46; cake or pastry mix, 500 g = £5.46.

Low-protein foods

Aminex® (Gluten Free Foods Ltd)
Low-protein. Biscuits, net price 200 g = £3.75. Cookies, 150 g = £3.75. Rusks, 200 g = £3.75.
For inherited metabolic disorders, renal or liver failure requiring a low-protein diet

Aproten® (Ultrapharm)
Low protein. Low Na^+ and K^+. Net prices: biscuits 180 g (36) = £2.88; bread mix 250 g = £2.17; cake mix 300 g = £2.10; crispbread 260 g = £4.06; pasta (anellini, ditalini, rigatini, spaghetti) 500 g = £4.06; tagliatelle 250 g = £2.16.
For inherited metabolic disorders, renal or liver failure requiring a low-protein diet

Ener-G® (General Dietary)
Low protein egg replacer, carbohydrate 94 g, energy 1574 kJ (376 kcal)/100 g. Egg-, gluten- and lactose-free, net price 454 g = £4.05.
For phenylketonuria, similar amino acid abnormalities, renal failure, liver failure and liver cirrhosis.
Low protein rice bread, net price 600 g = £4.39.
For inherited metabolic disorders, renal or liver failure requiring a low-protein diet

Fate® (Fate)
Low protein. All-purpose mix, net price 500 g = £6.15; Cake mix, 2 × 250 g = £6.15; Chocolate-flavour cake mix, 2 × 250 g = £6.15.
For inherited metabolic disorders, renal or liver failure requiring a low-protein diet

Juvela® (SHS)
Low Protein. Mix, net price 500 g = £6.17. Bread (whole or sliced), 400-g loaf = £2.89. Bread rolls, 5 × 70 g = £3.59. Biscuits, orange and cinnamon flavour, 125 g = £6.03; chocolate chip, 130 g = £6.03.
For inherited metabolic disorders, renal or liver failure requiring a low-protein diet

Loprofin® (SHS)
Low protein. Sweet biscuits, net price 150 g = £2.00; chocolate cream-filled biscuits, 125 g = £2.00; cookies (chocolate chip or cinnamon), 100 g = £5.11; crunch bar, 8 × 41 g = £11.09; wafers (orange, vanilla, or chocolate), 100 g = £1.94. Breakfast cereal, 375 g = £6.23. Egg replacer, 500 g = £11.66. Egg-white replacer, 100 g = £7.51. Bread (sliced), 400-g loaf = £3.00. Bread rolls (part-baked), 4 × 65 g = £3.04. Mix, 500 g = £6.36. Crackers, 150 g = £2.73. Herb crackers, 150 g = £2.73. Pasta (macaroni, pasta spirals, spaghetti), 500 g = £6.64. Pasta (lasagne), 250 g = £3.23. Pasta (vermicelli), 250 g = £3.31. Snack Pot (curry or tomato and basil), 47 g = £3.53, Rice, 500 g = £6.45.
For inherited metabolic disorders, renal or liver failure requiring a low-protein diet

Low protein drink (Milupa)
Powder, protein 0.4%, carbohydrate 5.1%, fat 2% when reconstituted. Net price 400 g = £7.23.
For inherited disorders of amino acid metabolism in childhood
Note Termed *Milupa® lpd* by manufacturer

Promin® (Firstplay Dietary)
Low protein. Cous Cous, 500 g = £5.88. Pasta (alphabets, macaroni, shells, shortcut spaghetti, spirals); Pasta tricolour (alphabets, shells, spirals), net price 500 g = £6.05; Lasagne sheets, 200 g = £2.57. Pasta shells in tomato, pepper and herb sauce, 4 x 72-g sachets = £6.65; Pasta elbows in cheese and broccoli sauce, 4 x 66- g sachets = £6.65. Pasta meal, 500 g = £6.05. Pasta imitation rice, 500 g = £6.05. Rice pudding imitation, (apple, banana, strawberry, and original flavours), 4 × 69-g sachets = £5.10.
For inherited metabolic disorders, renal or liver failure requiring a low-protein diet

Rite-Diet® Low-protein (SHS)
Low protein. Baking mix. Net price 500 g = £6.36. Flour mix. 400 g = £5.46.
For inherited metabolic disorders, renal or liver failure requiring a low-protein diet

Sno-Pro® (SHS)
Drink, protein 220 mg (phenylalanine 12.5 mg), carbohydrate 8 g, fat 3.8 g, energy 280 kJ (67 kcal)/100 mL. Net price 200 mL = 94p.
For phenylketonuria, chronic renal failure, and other inborn errors of metabolism

Ultra® (Ultrapharm)
Low protein. PKU bread, 400 g = £2.25. PKU flour, 500 g = £3.07. PKU biscuits, 200 g = £2.21. PKU cookies, 250 g = £2.31. PKU pizza base, 400 g = £2.35. PKU savoy biscuits, 150 g = £2.06.
For inherited metabolic disorders, renal or liver failure requiring a low-protein diet

Vita Bite® (Vitaflo)
Bar, protein 30 mg (less than 2.5 mg phenylalanine), carbohydrate 15.35 g, fat 8.4 g, energy 572 kJ (137 kcal)/25 g. Chocolate flavoured, net price 25 g = 93p.
For inherited metabolic disorders, renal or liver failure requiring a low-protein diet. Not recommended for any child under 1 year

Flavouring preparations

FlavourPac® (Vitaflo)
Powder, flavours: blackcurrant, lemon, orange, tropical or raspberry, net price 4 × 30 × 4-g sachets = £42.56
For use in conjuntion with Vitaflo's Inborn Error range of protein substitutes

Flavour Sachets (SHS)
Powder, flavours: cherry-vanilla, grapefruit, lemon-lime, net price 20 × 5-g sachets = £8.84.
For use with SHS unflavoured amino acid and peptide products

SHS Modjul® Flavour System (SHS)
Powder, blackcurrant, cherry-vanilla, orange, and pineapple flavours. Net price 100 g = £9.17.
For use with any unflavoured products based on peptides or amino acids

Metabolic Diseases

Glutaric aciduria (type 1)

XLYS, Low TRY, Analog (SHS)
Powder, essential and non-essential amino acids 15.5% except lysine, and low tryptophan, with carbohydrate, fat, vitamins, minerals, and trace elements. Net price 400 g = £27.13.
For type 1 glutaric aciduria
Note Analog products are generally intended for use in children up to 1 year

[1]**XLYS, Low TRY, Maxamaid** (SHS)
Powder, essential and non-essential amino acids 30% except lysine, with carbohydrate, fat less than 0.5%, vitamins, minerals, and trace elements. Net price 500 g = £73.98.
For type 1 glutaric aciduria

Homocystinuria or hypermethioninaemia

HCU Express® (Vitaflo)
Powder, protein (essential and non-essential amino acids except methionine) 15 g, carbohydrate 3.8 g, fat 0.03 g, energy 315 kJ (75.3 kcal)/25 g with vitamins, minerals and trace elements. Unflavoured, net price 30 × 25-g sachets = £245.86
A methionine-free protein substitute for use as a nutritional supplement in patients over 8 years of age with homocystinuria

HCU gel® (Vitaflo)
Powder, protein (essential and non-essential amino acids except methionine) 8.4 g, carbohydrate 8.6 g, fat 0.03 g, energy 286 kJ (68 kcal)/20 g with vitamins, minerals and trace elements. Unflavoured, net price 30 × 20-g sachets = £137.39
For the dietary management of homocystinuria in children between 12 months and 10 years of age

HCU LV® (SHS)
Powder, protein (essential and non-essential amino acids except methionine) 20 g, carbohydrate 2.5 g, fat 190 mg, energy 390 kJ (92 kcal)/27.8-g sachet, with vitamins, minerals and trace elements. Unflavoured or tropical flavour (formulation varies slightly), net price 30 × 27.8-g sachets = £371.40
For the dietary management of hypermethioninaemia or vitamin B_6 non-responsive homocystinuria. Not recommended for children under 8 years

XMET Analog (SHS)
Powder essential and non-essential amino acids 15.5% except methionine, with carbohydrate, fat, vitamins, minerals, and trace elements. Net price 400 g = £27.13.
For hypermethioninaemia, homocystinuria
NOTE Analog products are generally intended for use in children up to 1 year

XMET Homidon (SHS)
Powder, essential and non-essential amino acids 93%, except methionine. Net price 500 g = £140.15.
For homocystinuria or hypermethioninaemia

[1]**XMET Maxamaid** (SHS)
Powder, essential and non-essential amino acids 30% except methionine, with carbohydrate, fat less than 0.5%, vitamins, minerals, and trace elements. Net price 500 g = £73.98
For hypermethioninaemia, homocystinuria

[2]**XMET Maxamum®** (SHS)
Powder, essential and non-essential amino acids 47% except methionine, with carbohydrate, fat less than 0.5%, vitamins, minerals, and trace elements. Unflavoured, see also Flavour Sachets. Net price 500 g = £118.60.
For hypermethioninaemia, homocystinuria

1. Maxamaid products are generally intended for use in children aged 1 to 8 years, see also Flavour Sachets, for use with unflavoured amino acid and peptide products from SHS
2. Maxamum products are generally intended for use in children aged over 8 years

Hyperlysinaemia

XLYS Analog (SHS)
Powder, essential and non-essential amino acids 15.5% except lysine, with carbohydrate, fat, vitamins, minerals, and trace elements. Net price 400 g = £27.13.
For hyperlysinaemia
NOTE Analog products are generally intended for use in children up to 1 year

[1]XLYS Maxamaid (SHS)
Powder, essential and non-essential amino acids 30% except lysine, with carbohydrate, fat less than 0.5%, vitamins, minerals, and trace elements. Net price 500 g = £73.98.
For hyperlysinaemia

Isovaleric acidaemia

XLEU Analog (SHS)
Powder, essential and non-essential amino acids 15.5% except leucine, with carbohydrate, fat, vitamins, minerals, and trace elements. Net price 400 g = £27.13.
For isovaleric acidaemia
Ingredients: include arachis oil (peanut oil)
Note Analog products are generally intended for use in children up to 1 year

XLEU Faladon (SHS)
Powder, essential and non-essential amino acids 93%, except leucine. Net price 200 g = £56.05.
For isovaleric acidaemia

[1]XLEU Maxamaid (SHS)
Powder, essential and non-essential amino acids 28.6% except leucine, with carbohydrate, fat less than 0.5%, vitamins, minerals, and trace elements. Net price 500 g = £73.98.
For isovaleric acidaemia

Maple syrup urine disease

Isoleucine Amino Acid Supplement (Vitaflo)
Powder, isoleucine 0.05 g, carbohydrate 4 g, fat nil, energy 64 kJ (15 kcal)/4 g, net price 30 × 4-g sachets = £41.00
For use in conjunction with a protein supplement for maple syrup urine disease in children over 1 year

Mapleflex® (SHS)
Powder, essential and non-essential amino acids 35% except isoleucine, leucine, and valine, with carbohydrate 38%, fat 13.5%, vitamins, minerals, and trace elements. Unflavoured. Net price 30 × 29-g sachets = £156.60.
For maple syrup urine disease in children aged 1–10 years

MSUD Aid III® (SHS)
Powder, containing full range of amino acids except isoleucine, leucine, and valine, with vitamins, minerals, and trace elements. Net price 500 g = £140.15.
For maple syrup urine disease and related conditions where it is necessary to limit the intake of branched chain amino acids

MSUD Analog (SHS)
Powder, essential and non-essential amino acids 15.5% except isoleucine, leucine and valine, with carbohydrate, fat, vitamins, minerals, and trace elements. Net price 400 g = £27.13.
For maple syrup urine disease
NOTE Analog products are generally intended for use in children up to 1 year

MSUD express® (Vitaflo)
Powder, protein equivalent (essential and non-essential amino acids except leucine, isoleucine, and valine) 15 g, carbohydrate 3.8 g, fat less than 0.1 g, energy 315 kJ (75 kcal)/25 g with vitamins, minerals, and trace elements. Unflavoured (see FlavourPac® for available flavouring sachets), net price 30 × 25-g sachets = £245.86.
For maple syrup urine disease in children over 8 years and adults

1. Maxamaid products are generally intended for use in children aged 1 to 8 years, see also Flavour Sachets, for use with unflavoured amino acid and peptide products from SHS

MSUD express cooler® (Vitaflo)
Liquid, protein equivalent 15 g (essential and non-essential amino acids except leucine, isoleucine, and valine), carbohydrate 7.8 g, fat trace, energy 386 kJ (92 kcal)/130-mL pouch, with vitamins, minerals, and trace elements. Orange flavour, net price 30 × 130-mL = £250.64.
For maple syrup urine disease in children over 3 years and adults

MSUD Gel® (Vitaflo)
Powder, protein equivalent (essential and non-essential amino acids except leucine, isoleucine, and valine) 8.4 g, carbohydrate 8.6 g, fat less than 0.1 g, energy 286 kJ (68 kcal)/20 g with vitamins, minerals, and trace elements. Unflavoured (see FlavourPac® for available flavouring sachets), net price 30 × 20-g sachets = £137.39.
For maple syrup urine disease in children aged 1 to 10 years

[1]MSUD Maxamaid® (SHS)
Powder, essential and non-essential amino acids 30% except isoleucine, leucine, and valine, with carbohydrate, fat less than 0.5%, vitamins, minerals, and trace elements. Net price 500 g = £73.98.
For maple syrup urine disease

[2]MSUD Maxamum® (SHS)
Powder, essential and non-essential amino acids 47% except isoleucine, leucine, and valine, with carbohydrate, fat less than 0.5%, vitamins, minerals, and trace elements. Flavours: orange, unflavoured, see also Flavour Sachets. Net price 500 g = £118.60.
For maple syrup urine disease

Valine Amino Acid Supplement (Vitaflo)
Powder, valine 0.05 g, carbohydrate 4 g, fat nil, energy 64 kJ (15 kcal)/4 g, net price 30 × 4-g sachets = £41.00
For use in conjunction with a protein supplement for maple syrup urine disease in children over 1 year

Methylmalonic or propionic acidaemia

XMTVI Analog (SHS)
Powder, essential and non-essential amino acids 15.5% except methionine, threonine, valine and low isoleucine, with carbohydrate, fat, vitamins, minerals, and trace elements. Net price 400 g = £27.13.
For methylmalonic acidaemia or propionic acidaemia
NOTE Analog products are generally intended for use in children up to 1 year

XMTVI Asadon (SHS)
Powder, essential and non-essential amino acids 93%, except methionine, threonine, and valine, with trace amounts of isoleucine. Net price 200 g = £56.05.
For methylmalonic acidaemia or propionic acidaemia

[1]XMTVI Maxamaid (SHS)
Powder, essential and non-essential amino acids 30% except methionine, threonine, valine and low isoleucine, with carbohydrate, fat less than 0.5%, vitamins, minerals, and trace elements. Net price 500 g = £73.98.
For methylmalonic acidaemia or propionic acidaemia

[2]XMTVI Maxamum® (SHS)
Powder, essential and non-essential amino acids 47% except methionine, threonine, valine, and low isoleucine, with carbohydrate, fat less than 0.5%, vitamins, minerals, and trace elements. Unflavoured, see also Flavour Sachets. Net price 500 g = £118.60.
For methylmalonic acidaemia or propionic acidaemia

Other errors of protein metabolism

Cystine Amino Acid Supplement (Vitaflo)
Powder, cystine 0.5 g, carbohydrate 3.4 g, fat nil, energy 63 kJ (15 kcal)/4 g, net price 30 x 4-g sachets = £41.00
For use in the dietary management of inborn errors of protein metabolism

2. Maxamum products are generally intended for use in children aged over 8 years

Leucine Amino Acid Supplement (Vitaflo)
Powder, leucine 0.1 g, carbohydrate 4 g, fat nil, energy 64 kJ (15 kcal)/4 g, net price 30 x 4-g sachets = £41.00
For use in the dietary management of inborn errors of protein metabolism

Phenylketonuria

Add-Ins® (SHS)
Powder, protein equivalent (containing essential and non-essential amino acids, phenylalanine-free) 10 g, carbohydrate 0.01 g. fat 4.8 g, fibre 0.4 g, energy 348 kJ (83 kcal)/serving (serving = 1 × Add-Ins sachet plus 1 × Add-Ins Vits 1.7 g tablet), with vitamins, minerals, and trace elements. Flavourless, net price 60 × 17g = £294.00.
For the dietary management of proven phenylketonuria. Not to be prescribed for children under 11 years

Aminogran® (UCB Pharma)
Food Supplement, powder, containing all essential amino acids except phenylalanine, net price 500 g = £39.78.
Aminogran PKU tablet (≡ 1 g powder), net price 150-tab pack = £30.00.
For the dietary management of phenylketonuria. Tablets not to be prescribed for any child under 8 years

Easiphen® (SHS)
Liquid, protein (containing essential and non-essential amino acids, phenylalanine-free) 6.7 g, carbohydrate 5.1 g, fat 2 g, energy 275 kJ (65 kcal)/100 mL with vitamins, minerals, and trace elements. Forest berries, grapefruit, orange, or tropical flavour, net price 250-mL carton = £7.27.
For the dietary management of proven phenylketonuria. Not to be prescribed for children under 8 years

Lophlex® (SHS)
Powder, (containing essential and non-essential amino acids, phenylalanine-free) protein equivalent 20 g, carbohydrate 1.4 g, fibre 220 mg, energy 366 kJ (86 kcal)/27.8 g with vitamins, minerals, and trace elements. Flavours: berry, orange or unflavoured, net price 30 × 27.8-g sachets = £218.10.
For use in the dietary management of proven phenylketonuria in older children (over 8 years) and adults (includes use in pregnant women)

Lophlex® LQ (SHS)
Liquid, (containing essential and non-essential amino acids, phenylalanine-free) protein equivalent 20 g, carbohydrate 8.8 g, fibre 340 mg, energy 490 kJ (115 kcal)/125 mL, with vitamins, minerals, and trace elements. Flavours: berry, citrus, or orange, net price 3 × 125 mL = £23.34.
For use in the dietary management of phenylketonuria. Not recommended for children under 8 years

Loprofin (SHS)
PKU Drink, protein 0.4 g (phenylalanine 10 mg), lactose 9.4 g, fat 2 g, energy 165 kJ (40 kcal)/100 mL. Net price 200-mL Tetrapak® = 58p.
For phenylketonuria

Minaphlex® (SHS)
Liquid, protein equivalent 8.4 g, carbohydrate 9.9 g, fat 3.9 g, energy 455 (108 kcal)/29-g sachet, with vitamins, minerals, and trace elements. Phenylalanine-free. Chocolate, pineapple, and vanilla. Unflavoured version also available (contains an extra 5 kcal of carbohydrate per sachet), net price 30 × 29 g sachets = £95.10.
For the dietary management of phenylketonuria. Not recommended for children under 1 year

Phlexy-10® Exchange System (SHS)
Bar, essential and non-essential amino acids except phenylalanine 8.33 g, carbohydrate 20.5 g, fat 4.5 g/42-g bar. Citrus fruit flavour. Net price per bar = £4.58
Capsules, essential and non-essential amino acids except phenylalanine 500 mg/capsule. Net price 200-cap pack = £32.05
Tablets, essential and non-essential amino acids except phenylalanine, 1 g tablet. Net price 75-tab pack = £20.76
Drink Mix, powder, containing essential and non-essential amino acids except phenylalanine 10 g, carbohydrate 8.8 g/20-g sachet. Apple and blackcurrant, citrus, or tropical flavour. Net price 30 × 20-g sachet = £96.60
All for phenylketonuria

Phlexy-Vits® (SHS)
Powder, vitamins, minerals, and trace elements, net price 30 × 7-g sachets = £53.70.
For use as a vitamin and mineral component of restricted therapeutic diets in older children from the age of around 11 years and over and adults with phenylketonuria and similar amino acid abnormalities
Tablets, vitamins, minerals, and trace elements, net price 180-tab pack = £63.60.
For use in the dietary management of phenylketonuria. Not suitable for children under 8 years

PK Aid 4® (SHS)
Powder, containing essential and non-essential amino acids except phenylalanine. Net price 500 g = £107.73.
For phenylketonuria

PK Foods (Gluten Free Foods Ltd)
Bread, white (sliced), 550 g = £4.00. Crispbread, 75 g = £2.00. Pasta (spirals), 250 g = £2.00.
For phenylketonuria and similar amino acid abnormalities
Cookies (chocolate chip, orange, or cinnamon), 150 g = £3.75. Egg replacer, 350 g = £3.75. Flour mix, 750 g = £6.99. Jelly (orange or cherry flavour), 4 × 80 g = £5.76.
For phenylketonuria

PKU 2® (Milupa)
Granules, containing essential and non-essential amino acids except phenylalanine; with vitamins, minerals, trace elements, 7.1% sucrose. Flavour: vanilla. Net price 500 g = £44.75.
For phenylketonuria

PKU 3® (Milupa)
Granules, containing essential and non-essential amino acids except phenylalanine, vitamins, minerals, and trace elements, with 3.4% sucrose. Flavour: vanilla. Net price 500 g = £44.75.
For phenylketonuria, not recommended for child under 8 years

PKU cooler10® (Vitaflo)
Liquid, protein equivalent (containing essential and non-essential amino acids, phenylalanine-free) 10 g, carbohydrate 5.1 g, energy 258 kJ (62 kcal)/87-mL pouch, with vitamins, minerals, and trace elements. Orange or purple option. Net price 30 × 87 mL = £102.00.
For the dietary management of phenylketonuria. Not recommended for children under 3 years

PKU cooler15® (Vitaflo)
Liquid, protein equivalent 15 g, carbohydrate 7.8 g, energy 386 kJ (92 kcal)/130-mL pouch, with vitamins, minerals, and trace elements. Phenylalanine-free. Orange or purple option, net price 30 x 130 mL = £151.80.
For the dietary management of phenylketonuria, not recommended for children under 8 years

PKU cooler20® (Vitaflo)
Liquid, protein equivalent (containing essential and non-essential amino acids, phenylalanine-free) 20 g, carbohydrate 10.2 g, energy 517 kJ (124 kcal)/174 mL pouch, with vitamins, minerals, and trace elements. Orange or purple option. Net price 30 × 174 mL = £204.00.
For the dietary management of phenylketonuria. Not recommended for children under 8 years

PKU express® (Vitaflo)
Powder, protein (containing essential and non-essential amino acids, phenylalanine-free) 72 g, carbohydrate 15.1 g, energy 1260 kJ (301.5 kcal)/100 g with vitamins, minerals, and trace elements. Lemon, orange, tropical or unflavoured, net price 30 x 25 g sachets = £149.06.
For phenylketonuria, not recommended for children under 8 years

PKU gel® (Vitaflo)
Powder, protein (containing essential and non-essential amino acids, phenylalanine-free) 8.4 g, carbohydrate 8.6 g, fat 0.03 g, energy 285.5 kJ (68 kcal)/20 g with vitamins, minerals and trace elements. Orange or unflavoured, net price 30 × 20-g sachets = £85.93.
For use as part of the low-protein dietary management of phenylketonuria in children aged 1 to 10 years. Not recommended for children under 1 year

PKU Start® (Vitaflo)
Liquid, ready-to-feed formula, phenylalanine-free containing essential and non-essential amino acids, carbohydrate, fat, vitamins, minerals, and trace elements. Includes long-chain polyunsaturated fatty acids. Net price 500-mL bottle = £5.15
For the dietary management of phenylketonuria in infants under 12 months

L-Tyrosine (SHS)
Powder, net price 100 g = £12.53.
For use as a supplement in maternal phenylketonurics who have low plasma tyrosine concentrations

Tyrosine Amino Acid Supplement (Vitaflo)
Powder, tyrosine 1 g, carbohydrate 2.9 g, energy 62 kJ (15 kcal)/4-g sachet, net price 30 × 4-g sachets = £37.80.
For the dietary management of phenylketonuria. Not suitable as a sole source of nutrition.

XP Analog (SHS)
Powder, essential and non-essential amino acids 15.5% except phenylalanine, with carbohydrate, fat, vitamins, minerals, and trace elements. Net price 400 g = £21.67.
For phenylketonuria
NOTE Analog products are generally intended for use in children up to 1 year

XP LCP Analog (SHS)
Powder, essential and non-essential amino acids except phenylalanine 15.5%, with carbohydrate, fat, vitamins, minerals and trace elements. Gluten- and lactose-free. Net price 400 g = £24.66.
For phenylketonuria in infants and children under 2 years of age

[1]**XP Maxamaid** (SHS)
Powder, essential and non-essential amino acids 30% except phenylalanine, with carbohydrate, vitamins, minerals, and trace elements. Net price powder (unflavoured), 500 g = £43.77; (orange-flavoured), 500 g = £43.77.
For phenylketonuria. Not to be prescribed for children under 2 years

[1]**XP Maxamaid Concentrate** (SHS)
Powder, essential and non-essential amino acids 65% except phenylalanine, with carbohydrate, fat less than 0.5%, vitamins, minerals, and trace elements. Unflavoured. Net price 500 g = £112.07.
For phenylketonuria. Not to be prescribed for children under 2 years
Note See also Flavour Sachets, for use with unflavoured amino acid and peptide products from SHS

[2]**XP Maxamum®** (SHS)
Powder, essential and non-essential amino acids 47% except phenylalanine, with carbohydrates, vitamins, minerals, and trace elements. Flavours: orange, unflavoured, see also Flavour Sachets. Net price 30 × 50-g sachets = £202.80, 500 g = £67.68.
For phenylketonuria. Not to be prescribed for children under 8 years

1. Maxamaid products are generally intended for use in children aged 1 to 8 years, see also Flavour Sachets, for use with unflavoured amino acid and peptide products from SHS
2. Maxamum products are generally intended for use in children aged over 8 years

Tyrosinaemia

TYR express® (Vitaflo)
Powder, essential and non-essential amino acids (except tyrosine and phenylalanine) 18.2 g, protein equivalent 15 g, carbohydrate 3.8 g, fat less than 0.1 g, energy 315 kJ (76 kcal)/25 g, with vitamins, minerals, and trace elements. Unflavoured (see FlavourPac® for available flavouring sachets), net price 30 × 25-g sachets = £245.86
A tyrosine- and phenylalanine-free protein substitute for use in the dietary management of tyrosinaemia. Not recommended for children under 8 years

TYR cooler (Vitaflo)
Liquid, essential and non-essential amino acids (except tyrosine and phenylalanine) 18 g, protein equivalent 15 g, carbohydrate 7.8 g, fat trace, energy 386 kJ (92 kcal)/130 mL, with vitamins, minerals, and trace elements. Orange flavour, net price 30 x 130-mL pouch = £250.64.
A tyrosine- and phenylalanine-free protein substitute for use in the dietary management of tryrosinaemia in children over 3 years

TYR Gel® (Vitaflo)
Gel, essential and non-essential amino acids (except tyrosine and phenylalanine) 10.1 g, protein equivalent 8.4 g, carbohydrate 8.6 g, fat 0.03 g, energy 285.5 kJ (68 kcal)/20 g, with vitamins, minerals and trace elements. Unflavoured, net price 30 × 20-g sachets = £137.39
A tyrosine- and phenylalanine-free protein substitute for use in the dietary management of tyrosinaemia in children between 12 months and 10 years

XPHEN TYR Analog (SHS)
Powder, essential and non-essential amino acids 15.5% except phenylalanine and tyrosine, with carbohydrate, fat, vitamins, minerals and trace elements. Net price 400 g = £27.13.
For tyrosinaemia
Note Analog products are generally intended for use in children up to 1 year

[1]**XPHEN TYR Maxamaid** (SHS)
Powder, essential and non-essential amino acids 30% except phenylalanine and tyrosine, with carbohydrate, fat less than 0.5%, vitamins, minerals, and trace elements. Unflavoured. Net price 500 g = £73.98.
For tyrosinaemia

XPHEN TYR Tyrosidon (SHS)
Powder, essential and non-essential amino acids 93%, except phenylalanine and tyrosine. Net price 500 g = £135.08
For tyrosinaemia where plasma methionine concentrations are normal

XPTM Analog (SHS)
Powder, essential and non-essential amino acids 15.5% except phenylalanine, tyrosine and methionine, with carbohydrate, fat, vitamins, minerals and trace elements. Net price 400 g = £27.13.
For tyrosinaemia
Note Analog products are generally intended for use in children up to 1 year

XPTM Tyrosidon (SHS)
Powder, essential and non-essential amino acids 93%, except methionine, phenylalanine, and tyrosine. Net price 500 g = £140.15.
For tyrosinaemia type I where plasma concentrations are above normal

Urea cycle disorders (other than arginase deficiency)

L-Arginine (SHS)
Powder, net price 100 g = £8.39.
For use as a supplement in urea cycle disorders other than arginase deficiency, such as hyperammonaemia types I and II, citrullaemia, arginosuccinic aciduria, and deficiency of N-acetyl glutamate synthetase

Conditions for which toilet preparations may be prescribed on FP10, GP10 (Scotland), WP10 (Wales)

Note This is a list of clinical conditions for which the ACBS has approved toilet preparations. For details of the preparations see Chapter 13.

Birthmarks
See disfiguring skin lesions.

Dermatitis
Aveeno Bath Oil; Aveeno Cream; Aveeno Colloidal; Aveeno Baby Colloidal ; E45 Emollient Bath Oil; E45 Emollient Wash Cream; E45 Lotion; Vaseline Dermacare Cream and Lotion

Dermatitis herpetiformis
See also gluten-sensitive enteropathies, above.

Disfiguring skin lesions (birthmarks, mutilating lesions, scars, vitiligo)
Covermark classic foundation and finishing powder; Dermacolor Camouflage cream and fixing powder; Keromask masking cream and finishing powder; Veil Cover cream and Finishing Powder. (Cleansing Creams, Cleansing Milks, and Cleansing Lotions are excluded)

Disinfectants (antiseptics)
May be prescribed on an FP10 only when ordered in such quantities and with such directions as are appropriate for the treatment of patients, but not for general hygenic purposes.

Eczema
See dermatitis.

Photodermatoses (skin protection in)
Delph Sun Lotion SPF 30; E45 Sun Block SPF 30+; Spectraban Ultra; Sunsense Ultra; Uvistat Lipscreen SPF 50, Uvistat Suncream SPF 30 and 50.

Pruritus
See dermatitis.

A8 Wound management products and elastic hosiery

A8.1 Wound dressings 850
A8.1.1 Alginate dressings 851
A8.1.2 Foam dressings 852
A8.1.3 Hydrogel dressings 853
A8.1.4 Hydrocolloid dressings 855
A8.1.5 Vapour-permeable films and membranes 856
A8.1.6 Low adherence dressing and wound contact materials 857
A8.1.7 Odour absorbent dressings 859
A8.1.8 Dressing packs 859
A8.1.9 Surgical absorbents 859
A8.1.10 Capillary dressings 860
A8.2 Bandages and adhesives 860
A8.2.1 Non-extensible bandages 860
A8.2.2 Light-weight conforming bandages 861
A8.2.3 Tubular bandages 861
A8.2.4 Support bandages 862
A8.2.5 Compression bandages 862
A8.2.6 Extra-high performance compression bandages 863
A8.2.7 Adhesive bandages 863
A8.2.8 Cohesive bandages 863
A8.2.9 Medicated bandages 864
A8.2.10 Multi-layer compression bandaging 864
A8.2.11 Surgical adhesive tapes 864
A8.2.12 Adhesive dressings 865
A8.2.13 Skin closure dressings 866
A8.3 Elastic hosiery 866
A8.3.1 Graduated compression hosiery 866
A8.3.2 Accessories 866
A8.3.3 Anklets 866
A8.3.4 Knee caps 866
A8.3.5 Lymphoedema garments 866

A8.1 Wound dressings

An overview of the management of *chronic wounds* (including venous ulcers and pressure sores) and the role of different dressings is given below as is the NICE guidance on difficult-to-heal surgical wounds; the notes do not deal with the management of clean surgical wounds which usually heal very rapidly. The correct dressing for wound management depends not only on the type of wound but also on the stage of the healing process. The principal stages of healing are:

- cleansing, removal of debris;
- granulation, vascularisation;
- epithelialisation.

Greater understanding of the requirements of a wound dressing, including recognition of the benefits of maintaining a moist environment for wound healing, has improved the management of chronic wounds.

The ideal dressing needs to ensure that the wound remains:

- moist with exudate, but not macerated;
- free of clinical infection and excessive slough;
- free of toxic chemicals, particles or fibres;
- at the optimum temperature for healing;
- undisturbed by the need for frequent changes;
- at the optimum pH value.

As wound healing passes through its different stages, variations in dressing type may be required to satisfy better one or other of these requirements. The type of dressing depends on the type of wound or the stage of the healing process.

Functions of dressings

Type of wound	Role of dressing
Dry, necrotic, black	Moisture retention or rehydration
Yellow, sloughy	If dry, moisture retention or rehydration If moist, fluid absorption Possibly odour absorption Possibly antimicrobial activity
Clean, exuding (granulating)	Fluid absorption Thermal insulation Possibly odour absorption Possibly antimicrobial activity
Dry, low exudate (epithelialising)	Moisture retention or rehydration Low adherence Thermal insulation

A decrease in pain and reduction in healing time is achieved to a marked extent with **alginate**, **foam**, **hydrogel** and **hydrocolloid** dressings and also to an important extent with **vapour-permeable films** and **membranes**; dressings such as dry gauze have little place. Practices such as the use of irritant cleansers may be harmful and are largely obsolete; removal of debris and dressing remnants should need minimal irrigation with physiological saline.

Alginate, **foam**, **hydrogel** and **hydrocolloid** dressings are designed to absorb wound exudate and thus to control the state of hydration of a wound. All are claimed to be effective, but as yet there have been few trials able to establish a clear advantage for any particular product. The choice between different dressings may therefore often depend not only on the type and stage of the wound, but also on personal experience, availability of the dressing, patient preference or tolerance and site of the wound.

> **NICE guidance**
>
> **Debriding agents for difficult-to-heal surgical wounds (April 2001)**
>
> Alginate, foam, hydrocolloid, hydrogel, and polysaccharide (as beads or paste) dressings as well as maggots may reduce pain from difficult-to-heal surgical wounds. There is insufficient evidence to support one debriding agent over another and choice should be based on patient acceptability (including factors such as comfort and odour control), type and location of the wound, and total cost (including time for changing the dressings).

A8.1.1 Alginate dressings

The gelling characteristics of alginate dressings vary according to the product used. Some products only gel to a limited extent to form a partially gelled sheet that can be lifted off; others form an amorphous gel that can be rinsed off with water or physiological saline. A secondary covering is needed. They are highly absorbent and are therefore suitable for moderately or heavily exuding wounds, but not for eschars or for dry wounds.

Acticoat® Absorbent (S&N Hlth.)

Calcium alginate dressing with a silver coated antimicrobial barrier, 5 cm × 5 cm = £4.81, 10 cm × 12.5 cm = £11.55; cavity dressing, 2 cm × 30 cm = £11.62

Uses moderately to heavily exuding wounds including decubitus ulcers, venous stasis ulcers, surgical wounds, first and second degree burns, grafts and donor sites

ActivHeal® Alginate (MedLogic)

Calcium sodium alginate dressing, sterile, 5 cm × 5 cm = 57p, 10 cm × 10 cm = £1.11, 10 cm × 20 cm = £2.73; cavity dressing, 2 cm × 30 cm = £2.05

Uses moderately to heavily exuding wounds

Algisite® M (S&N Hlth.)

Calcium alginate fibre, sterile, flat non-woven dressing, 5 cm × 5 cm = 83p, 10 cm × 10 cm = £1.72, 15 cm × 20 cm = £4.62

Uses moderately to heavily exuding wounds

Algisite® M Rope, 2 cm × 30 cm = £3.12

Uses moderately to heavily exuding cavity wounds

Algivon® (Advancis)

Absorbent, sterile, non-adherent calcium alginate dressing impregnated with medical grade manuka honey, 5 cm × 5 cm = £2.09, 10 cm × 10 cm = £3.53

Uses leg ulcers, pressure sores, fungating lesions, abrasions, sloughy and sutured wounds

Algosteril® (S&N Hlth.)

Calcium alginate dressing, 5 cm × 5 cm = 83p, 10 cm × 10 cm = £1.88, 10 cm × 20 cm = £3.19; cavity dressing, 2 g, 30 cm = £3.40

Uses moderately to heavily exuding wounds

Curasorb® (Tyco)

Calcium alginate dressing, 5 cm × 5 cm = 69p, 10 cm × 10 cm = £1.46, 10 cm × 14 cm = £2.36, 10 cm × 20 cm = £2.87, 15 cm × 25 cm = £5.05, 30 cm × 61 cm = £26.50 (other sizes (NHS))

Curasorb® Plus, calcium alginate dressing, 10 cm × 10 cm = £2.00

Curasorb® Rope, calcium alginate cavity dressing, 30 cm = £2.78, 61 cm = £4.38, 91 cm = £5.25

Curasorb® Zn, calcium alginate and zinc dressing, 5 cm × 5 cm = 78p, 10 cm × 10 cm = £1.65, 10 cm × 20 cm = £3.24 (other sizes (NHS))

Kaltostat® (ConvaTec)

(Alginate Dressing, BP 1993, type C). Calcium alginate fibre, flat non-woven pads, 5 cm × 5 cm = 86p, 7.5 cm × 12 cm = £1.87, 10 cm × 20 cm = £3.70, 15 cm × 25 cm = £6.36, (NHS) 30 cm × 60 cm = £25.13

Uses moderately to heavily exuding wounds

Kaltostat® Wound Packing, 2 g = £3.47

Uses moderately to heavily exuding cavity wounds

Melgisorb® (Mölnlycke)

Calcium sodium alginate fibre, sterile, highly absorbent, gelling dressing, flat non-woven pads, 5 cm × 5 cm = 82p, 10 cm × 10 cm = £1.71, 10 cm × 20 cm = £3.21

Uses moderately to heavily exuding wounds including leg ulcers, dermal lesions and traumatic wounds

Melgisorb® Cavity, calcium sodium alginate fibre, sterile, highly absorbent, gelling filler ribbon, 32 cm × 2.2 cm, (2 g) = £3.23

Uses moderately to heavily exuding cavity wounds, fistulas, sinuses, pressure sores and deep leg ulcers

SeaSorb® (Coloplast)

SeaSorb® Soft, alginate containing hydrocolloid dressing, sterile, highly absorbent, gelling dressing, 5 cm × 5 cm = 88p, 10 cm × 10 cm = £2.09, 15 cm × 15 cm = £3.97

Uses heavily exuding wounds including leg ulcers and pressure sores

SeaSorb® Soft Filler, calcium sodium alginate fibre, highly absorbent, gelling filler, 44 cm = £2.47

Uses moderately to heavily exuding cavity wounds, fistulas, sinus drainage, decubitus and deep leg ulcers

Sorbalgon® (Hartmann)

Calcium alginate dressing, 5 cm × 5 cm = 73p, 10 cm × 10 cm = £1.52

Uses for medium to heavily exuding wounds

Sorbalgon T®, calcium alginate cavity dressing, net price 2 g, 32 cm = £3.11

Uses for medium to heavily exuding wounds

Sorbsan® (Unomedical)

Sorbsan® Flat, (Alginate Dressing, BP 1993, type A). Calcium alginate fibre, highly absorbent, flat non-woven pads, 5 cm × 5 cm = 77p, 10 cm × 10 cm = £1.61, 10 cm × 20 cm = £3.02; with silver, 5 cm × 5 cm = £1.50, 10 cm × 10 cm = £3.80, 10 cm × 20 cm = £6.94

Uses moderately to heavily exuding wounds; with silver, for infected and exuding wounds

Sorbsan® Plus, alginate dressing bonded to a secondary absorbent viscose pad, 7.5 cm × 10 cm = £1.63, 10 cm × 15 cm = £2.88, 10 cm × 20 cm = £3.67, 15 cm × 20 cm = £5.10

Uses moderately to heavily exuding shallow wounds and ulcers

Sorbsan® Plus SA, sterile, alginate dressing with adhesive border and absorbent backing, 11.5 cm × 14 cm = £2.84, 14 cm × 19 cm = £4.14, 14 cm × 24 cm = £5.00, 19 cm × 24 cm = £6.28

Uses moderately to lightly exuding shallow wounds

Sorbsan® Ribbon, 40 cm (with 12.5-cm probe) = £1.95; with silver, 40 cm (with probe) = £3.97

Sorbsan® Surgical Packing, 30 cm (2 g) = £3.35; with silver, 30 cm (2 g) = £5.55

Uses moderately to heavily exuding cavity wounds; with silver, for, infected and exuding wounds

Suprasorb A® (Vernon-Carus)

Calcium alginate dressing, sterile, 5 cm × 5 cm = 56p, 10 cm × 10 cm = £1.10

Suprasorb A® Rope, 2 g × 30 cm = £2.04

Uses moderate to heavily exuding wounds

Tegaderm® Alginate (3M)

(formerly *Tegagen®*). 5 cm × 5 cm = 76p, 10 cm × 10 cm = £1.61

Uses for leg ulcers, pressure sores, second degree burns, post-operative wounds, fungating carcinomas

(formerly *Tegagen® Rope*) cavity dressing, 2 cm × 30 cm = £2.68

Uses moderately to heavily exuding cavity wounds

Tielle® Packing (J&J)

Tielle® Packing, 9.5 cm × 9.5 cm = £2.04

Urgosorb® (Urgo)

Alginate containing hydrocolloid dressing without adhesive border, sterile, 5 cm × 5 cm = 79p, 10 cm × 10 cm = £1.90, 10 cm × 20 cm = £3.48

Urgosorb® Rope cavity dressing, 30 cm = £2.53; impregnated with silver, 2.5 cm × 30 cm = £3.34

Urgosorb® Silver alginate containing hydrocolloid dressing, impregnated with silver, 5 cm × 5 cm = £1.39, 10 cm × 10 cm = £3.32, 10 cm × 20 cm = £6.26

A8.1.2 Foam dressings

Foam dressings vary from products that are suitable for lightly exuding wounds to highly absorbent structures for heavily exuding wounds. They may also be used as secondary dressings. In hypergranulating (or overgranulating) tissue (which may arise from the use of occlusive dressings such as hydrocolloids), changing to a more permeable product such as a foam dressing may be beneficial.

Polyurethane Foam Dressing, BP 1993

Absorbent foam dressing of low adherence, sterile

Lyofoam®, 7.5 cm × 7.5 cm = £1.00, 10 cm × 10 cm = £1.14, 10 cm × 17.5 cm = £1.85, 15 cm × 20 cm = £2.49, other sizes (NHS) 10 cm × 25 cm = £4.79 (hosp. only), 25 cm × 30 cm = £11.35 (Medlock)

Uses treatment of burns, decubitus ulcers, donor sites, granulating wounds

Polyurethane Foam Film Dressing, Sterile, with Adhesive Border

(Drug Tariff specification 47)

Allevyn® Lite Island, 9.75 cm × 16.5 cm = £1.74; 13.5 cm × 13.5 cm = £2.27; 16 cm × 16 cm = £2.70; 13.5 cm × 23.5 cm = £3.48 (S & N Hlth)

Uses lightly to moderately exuding wounds

Lyofoam® Extra Adhesive, 9 cm × 9 cm = £1.25, 15 cm × 15 cm = £2.34, 22 cm × 22 cm = £4.61; sacral, 15 cm × 13 cm = £1.92; 22 cm × 26 cm = £3.56 (Medlock)

Suprasorb P®, 7.5 cm × 7.5 cm = £1.16, 10 cm × 10 cm = £1.25, 15 cm × 15 cm = £2.24 (Vernon-Carus)

Tielle®, 11 cm × 11 cm = £2.29; 15 cm × 15 cm = £3.74; 18 cm × 18 cm = £4.76; 7 cm × 9 cm = £1.23; 15 cm × 20 cm = £4.68; *Tielle® Sacrum* 18 cm × 18 cm = £3.46 (J&J)

Trufoam®, 7 cm × 9 cm = £1.07; 11 cm × 11 cm = £2.04 (Unomedical)

Uses light to moderately exuding wounds, not recommended for dry superficial wounds

Polyurethane Foam Film Dressing, Sterile, without Adhesive Border

(Drug Tariff specification 47)

Allevyn® Lite, 5 cm × 5 cm = £1.01; 10 cm × 10 cm = £1.84; 10 cm × 20 cm = £3.16; 15 cm × 20 cm = £3.94 (S&N Hlth)

Uses lightly to moderately exuding wounds

Allevyn® Thin (adhesive), net price 5 cm × 6 cm = 96p, 10 cm × 10 cm = £1.94, 15 cm × 15 cm = £3.20, 15 cm × 20 cm = £3.88

Uses lightly to moderately exuding wounds

FlexiPore® (adhesive), 6 cm × 7 cm = 93p; 10 cm × 10 cm = £1.73, 15 cm × 20 cm = £3.70; 20 cm × 20 cm = £5.06; 10 cm × 30 cm = £3.60 (MedLogic)

Lyofoam® Extra, 10 cm × 10 cm = £1.99; 17.5 cm × 17.5 cm = £3.36; 20 cm × 15 cm = £4.35 (Medlock)

Suprasorb M®, 10 cm × 10 cm = £1.72, 10 cm × 20 cm = £3.03, 20 cm × 20 cm = £5.05 (Vernon-Carus)

Suprasorb P®, 5 cm × 5 cm = 90p, 7.5 cm × 7.5 cm = 96p, 10 cm × 10 cm = £1.13, 15 cm × 15 cm = £3.01 (Vernon-Carus)

Transorbent® (adhesive), 5 cm × 7 cm = 98p; 10 cm × 10 cm = £1.85; 15 cm × 15 cm = £3.40; 20 cm × 20 cm = £5.44 (Unomedical)

Uses light to moderately exuding wounds, not recommended for dry superficial wounds

Polyurethane Foam Film Dressing, Sterile, with Adhesive Border

ActivHeal® Foam Island, 10 cm × 10 cm = £1.57, 12.5 cm × 12.5 cm = £1.50, 15 cm × 15 cm = £1.92, 20 cm × 20 cm = £4.34 (MedLogic)

Uses moderate to heavily exuding wounds

Allevyn® Adhesive, 7.5 cm × 7.5 cm = £1.37, 10 cm × 10 cm = £2.00, 12.5 cm × 12.5 cm = £2.45, 17.5 cm × 17.5 cm = £4.83, 12.5 cm × 22.5 cm = £3.81, 22.5 cm × 22.5 cm = £7.04; (sacral) 17 cm x 17 cm = £3.62, 22 cm x 22 cm = £5.22 (S&N Hlth)

Uses moderate to heavily exuding wounds

Allevyn® Plus Adhesive, 12.5 cm × 12.5 cm = £3.02; 17.5 cm × 17.5 cm = £5.82; 12.5 cm × 22.5 cm = £5.34; (sacral) 17 cm x 17 cm = £4.40, 22 cm x 22 cm = £6.36

Uses heavily and extremely heavily exuding wounds

Allevyn® Sacrum shaped, 17 cm × 17 cm = £3.49, 22 cm × 22 cm = £5.02

Uses light to moderately exuding sacral wounds

Biatain® Adhesive, 10 cm × 10 cm = £1.59; 12 cm × 12 cm = £2.34, 18 cm × 18 cm = £4.68, 18 cm × 28 cm = £6.92, 23 cm × 23 cm (sacral) = £4.00, 19 cm × 20 cm (heel) = £4.67; 17 cm diameter (contour) = £4.50 (Coloplast)

Uses moderate to heavily exuding wounds

Comfifoam®, 7.5 cm × 7.5 cm = £1.13, 10 cm × 10 cm = £1.65, 12.5 cm × 12.5 cm = £2.03, 17.5 cm × 17.5 cm = £4.01 (Synergy)

PermaFoam®, concave 16.5 cm × 18 cm = £ 3.60; sacral 18 cm × 18 cm = £2.96, 22 cm × 22 cm = £3.40; *PermaFoam Comfort®* 8 cm × 8 cm = £1.00, 10 cm × 20 cm = £3.00, 11 cm × 11 cm = £1.90, 15 cm × 15 cm = £3.10, 20 cm × 20 cm = £4.50 (Hartmann)

PolyMem®, 5 cm × 5 cm = 48p (for lightly exuding wounds); 5 cm × 7.6 cm = £1.07, 8.8 cm × 12.7 cm = £1.90, 10 cm × 13 cm = £2.02, 15 cm × 15 cm = £2.72, 16.5 cm × 20.9 cm = £6.25, 18.4 cm × 20 cm (sacral) = £4.20 (Unomedical)

Uses moderate to heavily exuding wounds

Tegaderm® Foam Adhesive, 10 cm × 11 cm = £2.28, 14 cm × 14 cm = £3.37, 14 cm × 15 cm = £4.05, 19 cm × 22.5 cm = £6.64, 14 cm × 14 cm (heel) = £4.06 (3M)

Uses moderately to heavily exuding wounds

Tielle® Lite, 11 cm × 11 cm = £2.20; 7 cm × 9 cm = £1.16; 8 cm × 15 cm = £2.70; 8 cm × 20 cm = £2.86 (J&J)

Uses light to non-exuding wounds

Tielle® Plus, 11 cm × 11 cm = £2.53; 15 cm × 15 cm = £4.13; 15 cm × 20 cm = £5.18; 15 cm × 15 cm (sacrum) = £3.01; *Tielle® Plus Heel Hydropolymer Adhesive Dressing* 20 cm × 26.5 cm = £4.28 (J&J)

Uses moderate to heavily exuding wounds

Trufoam®, 11 cm × 11 cm = £2.12, 15 cm × 15 cm = £3.55, 7 cm × 9 cm = £1.11, 15 cm × 20 cm = £4.45 (Unomedical)

Uses moderate to heavily exuding wounds

Polyurethane Foam Film Dressing, Sterile, without Adhesive Border

ActivHeal® Foam Non-Adhesive, 5 cm × 5 cm = 72p, 10 cm × 10 cm = £1.09, 10 cm × 17.8 cm = £2.26, 20 cm × 20 cm = £3.78 (MedLogic)

Uses heavily exuding wounds

Advazorb® Plus, 5 cm × 7.5 cm = 70p, 10 cm × 10 cm = £1.08, 15 cm × 15 cm = £2.10, 20 cm × 20 cm = £3.75 (Advancis)

Uses moderate to heavily exuding wounds

Allevyn®, 5 cm × 5 cm = £1.16, 9 cm × 9 cm = £3.49 (NHS), 10 cm × 10 cm = £2.29, 10 cm × 20 cm = £3.68, 20 cm × 20 cm = £6.14, 10.5 cm × 13.5 cm (heel) = £4.59 (S&N Hlth)

Uses moderate to heavily exuding wounds

Allevyn® Compression, 5 cm × 6 cm = £1.13; 10 cm × 10 cm = £2.32; 15 cm × 15 cm = £3.93, 15 cm × 20 cm = £4.41 (S&N Hlth)

Uses moderate to heavily exuding wounds surrounded by sensitive skin

Askina® Foam, 10 cm × 10 cm = £2.06, 10 cm × 20 cm = £3.25, 20 cm × 20 cm = £5.43, 12 cm × 20 cm (heel) = £4.40 (Braun)

Biatain® Non-Adhesive, 10 cm × 10 cm = £2.16, 10 cm × 20 cm = £3.56, 15 cm × 15 cm = £3.97, 20 cm × 20 cm = £5.90; 5 cm diameter (circular) = £1.11, 8 cm diameter (circular) = £1.56; *Biatain® Soft-Hold* 10 cm × 10 cm = £2.34, 10 cm ×20 cm = £3.56, 15 cm × 15 cm = £3.89 (Coloplast)

Comfifoam®, 5 cm × 5 cm = 96p, 10 cm × 10 cm = £1.90, 10 cm × 20 cm = £3.05, 20 cm × 20 cm = £5.09 (Synergy)

Kerraboot®, (clear or white) extra small = £14.27, small = £14.55, large = £14.55, extra large = £14.27 (Ark)

Uses diabetic foot ulcers

PermaFoam®, 10 cm × 10 cm = £1.90, 10 cm × 20 cm = £3.25, 15 cm × 15 cm = £3.60, 20 cm × 20 cm = £5.50; 6 cm diameter = 98p; *PermaFoam® Cavity®* 10 cm × 10 cm = £1.80 (Hartmann)

PolyMem®, 8 cm × 8 cm = £1.47, 10 cm × 10 cm = £2.29, 13 cm × 13 cm = £3.82, 17 cm × 19 cm = £5.64, 10 cm × 61 cm = £12.15; *PolyMem® Max* 11 cm × 11 cm = £2.75; *PolyMem® Silver* 10.8 cm × 10.8 cm = £8.20 (Unomedical)

Uses moderate to heavily exuding wounds

Tegaderm® Foam, 8.8 cm × 8.8 cm (fenestrated) = £2.13, 10 cm × 10 cm = £2.09, 10 cm × 20 cm = £3.54, 20 cm × 20 cm = £5.65, 10 cm × 60 cm = £11.96 (3M)

Tielle® Plus Borderless, 11 cm × 11 cm = £3.04; 15 cm × 20 cm = £5.51 (J&J)

Trufoam® NA, 5 cm × 5 cm = £1.06, 10 cm × 10 cm = £2.01, 15 cm × 15 cm = £3.70 (Unomedical)

Uses moderate to heavily exuding wounds

Acticoat® Moisture Control (S&N Hlth.)

Three layer polyurethane dressing consisting of a silver coated layer, a foam layer, and a waterproof layer, 5 cm × 5 cm = £6.45, 10 cm × 10 cm = £15.09, 10 cm × 20 cm = £29.40

Uses antimicrobial dressing for light to moderately exuding wounds including decubitus ulcers, diabetic ulcers, first and second degree burns, and donor sites

Allevyn® (S&N Hlth.)

Hydrophilic polyurethane dressing, foam sheets with trilaminate structure, non-adherent wound contact layer, foam based central layer, bacteria- and water-proof outer layer

Allevyn® Cavity, circular, 5 cm diameter = £3.79, 10 cm diameter = £9.03; tubular, 9 cm × 2.5 cm = £3.67, 12 cm × 4 cm = £6.47

Uses moderately to heavily exuding cavity wounds including deep pressure sores and leg ulcers, surgical incisions and excisions such as pilonidal sinus excisions

Allevyn® Plus Cavity Sterile, highly absorbent polyurethane dressing consisting of a vapour-permeable foam matrix, 5 cm × 6 cm = £1.70, 10 cm × 10 cm = £2.84, 15 cm × 20 cm = £5.67

Uses heavily exuding deep wounds, including deep leg ulcers, decubitus ulcers, abscesses; management of post-operative wounds including pilonidal sinus excision

Avance® (Medlock)

Silver impregnated polyurethane foam film dressing

Avance® (without adhesive border), 10 cm × 10 cm = £2.70, 10 cm × 17 cm = £4.29, 15 cm × 20 cm = £5.93

Avance®A (with adhesive border), 9 cm × 9 cm = £2.26, 12 cm × 12 cm = £3.75, 15 cm × 15 cm = £4.60, 15 cm × 13 cm (sacral) = £3.38

Uses antimicrobial dressing for exuding wounds

Cavi-Care® (S&N Hlth)

Soft, conforming cavity wound dressing prepared by mixing thoroughly for 15 seconds immediately before use and allowing to expand its volume within the cavity. 20 g = £17.77

Uses in the management of open post-operative granulating cavity wounds (with no underlying tracts or sinuses) such as pilonidal sinus excision, dehisced surgical wounds, hydradenitis suppurativa wounds, perianal wounds, perineal wounds, pressure sores

Contreet Foam® (Coloplast)

Silver impregnated, polyurethane foam film dressing with adhesive border, 12.5 cm × 12.5 cm = £8.38, 18 cm × 18 cm = £16.81, 19 cm × 20 cm (heel) = £16.58, 23 cm × 23 cm (sacral) = £17.62; without adhesive border 10 cm × 10 cm = £7.32, 10 cm × 20 cm = £13.46, 15 cm × 15 cm = £14.70, 20 cm × 20 cm = £20.74, 5 cm diameter = £3.07; cavity dressing 5 cm × 8 cm = £3.65

Uses antimicrobial dressing for moderate to heavily exuding or malodorous wounds

A8.1.3 Hydrogel dressings

Hydrogel dressings are most commonly supplied as an amorphous, cohesive material that can take up the shape of a wound. A secondary covering is needed. These dressings are generally used to donate liquid to dry sloughy wounds and facilitate autolytic debridement but they may also have the ability to absorb limited amounts of exudate. Hydrogel sheets are also available which have a fixed structure; such products have limited fluid handling capacity. Hydrogel sheets are best avoided in the presence of infection.

ActiFormCool® (Activa)

5 cm × 6.5 cm = £1.62, 10 cm × 10 cm = £2.38, 10 cm × 15 cm = £3.42

ActivHeal® Hydrogel (MedLogic)

15 g = £1.36

Uses pressure sores, cavity wounds, leg ulcers, skin donor sites, diabetic foot ulcers

Aquaform® (Unomedical)

(Drug Tariff specification 50) Hydrogel containing modified starch copolymer, 8 g = £1.54, 15 g = £1.87

Uses for dry, sloughy or necrotic wounds, lightly exuding wounds, granulating wounds

Aquaflo® (Tyco)

7.5 cm diameter = £2.50, 12 cm = £5.16

Askina® Gel (Braun)

15 g = £1.89

Citrugel® (Advancis)

15 g = £1.35

Coolie® (Zeroderma)

Sterile, hydrogel dressing with lint backing, 7 cm diameter = £1.96

Uses for dry, sloughy or necrotic wounds, lightly exuding wounds, granulating wounds

Curagel® (Tyco)

5 cm × 7.5 cm = £1.74, 10 cm × 10 cm = £2.71

Curagel Island (with adhesive border), 7.5 cm × 10 cm = £2.47, 12.5 cm × 12.5 cm = £3.58

Cutinova® Hydro (S&N Hlth.)

5 cm × 6 cm = £1.14, 10 cm × 10 cm = £2.29, 15 cm × 20 cm = £4.84

Uses light to moderately exuding wounds

Flexigran® (A1 Pharmaceuticals)

15 g = £1.90

Gel FX® (Vernon-Carus)

Hydrogel dressing (without adhesive border) 10 cm × 10 cm = £1.60, 10 cm × 15 cm = £2.20, 15 cm × 15 cm = £3.20

Geliperm® (Geistlich)

Gel sheets in wet form, 10 cm × 10 cm = £2.27, 12 cm × 26 cm = £9.31 (NHS)

Uses wound and ulcer dressing, burns, donor sites

GranuGel® (ConvaTec)

(Drug Tariff Specification 50), 15 g = £2.09

Uses dry, sloughy or necrotic wounds, lightly exuding wounds, granulating wounds

Hydrosorb® (Hartmann)

Absorbent, transparent, hydrogel sheets containing polyurethane polymers covered with a semi-permeable film

Hydrosorb®, 5 cm × 7.5 cm = £1.40; 10 cm × 10 cm = £2.00; 20 cm × 20 cm = £6.00

Hydrosorb® comfort (with adhesive border, waterproof), 4.5 cm × 6.5 cm = £1.66; 7.5 cm × 10 cm = £2.20; 12.5 cm × 12.5 cm = £3.20

Uses second degree burns, donor sites; chronic wounds where granulation is unsatisfactory, including leg ulcers, pressure sores

Intrasite Conformable® (S&N Hlth.)

(Drug Tariff specification 50). Soft and easily moulded non-woven dressing impregnated with Intrasite gel, 10 cm × 10 cm = £1.62; 10 cm × 20 cm = £2.19; 10 cm × 40 cm = £3.92

Uses for dry, sloughy or necrotic wounds, lightly exuding wounds; granulating wounds

Intrasite® Gel (S&N Hlth.)

(Drug Tariff specification 50). A ready-mixed hydrogel containing modified carmellose polymer applied directly into the wound, 8-g sachet = £1.62, 15-g sachet = £2.18, 25-g sachet = £3.23

Uses for dry, sloughy or necrotic wounds; lightly exuding wounds; granulating wounds

Iodoflex® (S&N Hlth.)

Paste, iodine 0.9% as cadexomer–iodine in a paste basis with gauze backing, 5-g unit = £3.66; 10 g = £7.31; 17 g = £11.58

Uses for treatment of chronic exuding wounds, such as leg ulcers, apply to wound surface, remove gauze backing and cover; renew when saturated (usually 2–3 times weekly, daily for heavily exuding wounds); max. single application 50 g, max. weekly application 150 g; max. duration up to 3 months in any single course of treatment

Cautions severe renal impairment or history of thyroid disorders; iodine may be absorbed particularly if large wounds treated

Contra-indications avoid in thyroid disorders, in those receiving lithium, in pregnancy and breast-feeding, and in children

Iodosorb® (S&N Hlth.)

Ointment, iodine 0.9% as cadexomer–iodine in an ointment basis, 10 g = £4.04; 20 g = £8.08

Powder, iodine 0.9% as cadexomer–iodine microbeads, 3-g sachet = £1.73

Uses for treatment of chronic exuding wounds, such as leg ulcers, apply to wound surface to depth of approx. 3 mm and cover; renew when saturated (usually 2–3 times weekly, daily for heavily exuding wounds); max. single application 50 g, max. weekly application 150 g; max. duration up to 3 months in any single course of treatment

Cautions severe renal impairment or history of thyroid disorders; iodine may be absorbed particularly if large wounds treated

Contra-indications avoid in thyroid disorders, in those receiving lithium, in pregnancy and breast-feeding, and in children

Mesitran® (Unomedical)

Sterile, absorbent, semi-permeable dressings impregnated with medical grade honey, 10 cm × 10 cm = £2.46, 10 cm × 17.5 cm = £4.43, 15 cm × 20 cm = £5.12

Mesitran® Border, with adhesive border, 10 cm × 10 cm = £2.56, 15 cm × 13 cm (sacral) = £4.33, 15 cm × 15 cm = £4.53

Uses pressure ulcers, diabetic ulcers, fungating wounds, donor sites, surgical wounds, abrasions, and first and second degree burns

Mesitran® Mesh, non-adherent wound contact layer, without adhesive border, 10 cm × 10 cm = £2.37

Uses pressure ulcers, diabetic ulcers, donor sites, abrasions, trauma wounds, post-operative wounds, and first and second degree burns

Novogel® (Ford)

Sterile, glycerol-based hydrogel sheets, 10 cm × 10 cm = £3.01; 30 cm × 30 cm, standard = £12.74, thin = £12.03; 5 cm × 7.5 cm = £1.91; 15 cm × 20 cm = £5.74; 20 cm × 40 cm = £10.94; 7.5 cm diameter = £2.73

Uses diabetic wounds, burns, leg ulcers, decubitus ulcers, donor sites

Nu-Gel® (J&J)

(Drug Tariff Specification 50). A ready-mixed hydrogel containing alginate, applied directly into wound and covered with secondary dressing, 15 g = £2.01

Uses dry, sloughy or necrotic, lightly exuding or granulating wounds

Prontosan® Wound Gel (Braun)

(Drug Tariff Specification 50). A ready-mixed hydrogel containing betaine surfactant and polyhexanide, applied directly into the wound and covered with secondary dressing. 30 mL = £5.85

Purilon® Gel (Coloplast)

(Drug Tariff specification 50), 8 g = £1.58, 15 g = £2.06

Uses for dry, sloughy or necrotic wounds; lightly exuding wounds; granulating wounds

Suprasorb® G (Vernon-Carus)

Hydrogel dressing (without adhesive border) 5 cm × 7.5 cm = £1.73, 10 cm × 10 cm = £2.22, 20 cm × 20 cm = £6.71; (amorphous gel) 6 g = £1.10, 20 g = £1.80

Vacunet® (Protex)

Non-adherent, hydrogel coated polyester net dressing, 10 cm × 10 cm = £1.93, 10 cm × 15 cm = £2.86

Uses lacerations, abrasions, pressure ulcers, burns, surgical and malignant wounds

Protease modulating matrix

Cadesorb® (S&N Hlth.)

Ointment, sterile, starch-based, 10 g = £4.86, 20 g = £8.29

Uses chronic wounds free of necrotic tissue and infection

Flaminal® (Ark Therapeutics)

Gel, alginate, 15 g = £7.13

Uses moderate to heavily exuding wounds

Hydrogel, alginate, 15 g = £7.13

Uses light to moderately exuding wounds

Promogran® (J&J)

Sterile, collagen and oxidised regenerated cellulose matrix, applied directly to wound and covered with secondary dressing, 28 cm² (hexagonal) = £4.99, 123 cm² (hexagonal) = £15.02

Uses chronic wounds free of necrotic tissue and infection, e.g. leg ulcers, pressure sores, diabetic foot ulcers

Promogran® Prisma® Matrix (J&J)

Sterile collagen, silver and oxidised regenerated cellulose matrix, applied directly to wound and covered with secondary dressing, 28 cm² (hexagonal) = £6.07, 123 cm² (hexagonal) = £17.28

Uses chronic wounds free of necrotic tissue, e.g. leg ulcers, pressure sores, diabetic foot ulcers

Suprasorb C® (Vernon-Carus)

Sterile collagen, 4 cm × 6 cm = £2.55, 6 cm × 8 cm = £3.90, 8 cm × 12 cm = £7.65

Tegaderm® Matrix (3M)
(formerly *Epi-Max®*) 5 cm × 6 cm £4.75, 8 cm × 10 cm = £9.75

A8.1.4 Hydrocolloid dressings

Hydrocolloid dressings are usually presented as a hydrocolloid layer on a vapour-permeable film or foam. Because of their impermeable nature, hydrocolloid dressings facilitate rehydration and autolytic debridement of dry, sloughy, or necrotic wounds; they are also suitable for promoting granulation. Fibrous dressings made from modified carmellose fibres resemble alginate dressings (e.g. *Aquacel®*); these are not occlusive.

ActivHeal® Hydrocolloid (MedLogic)
Sterile, semi-permeable polyurethane film backing, hydrocolloid wound contact layer, 5 cm × 7.5 cm = 75p, 10 cm × 10 cm = £1.52, 15 cm × 15 cm = £3.31, 15 cm × 18 cm (sacral) = £3.84; with polyurethane foam layer, 5 cm × 7.5 cm = 94p, 10 cm × 10 cm = £1.49, 15 cm × 15 cm = £2.81, 15 cm × 18 cm (sacral) = £3.24
Uses light to moderately exuding wounds

Alione® (Coloplast)
Sterile, semi-permeable hydrocolloid dressing with adhesive border, 10 cm × 10 cm = £2.90, 12.5 cm × 12.5 cm = £3.99, 12 cm × 20 cm = £5.24, 15 cm × 15 cm = £5.04, 20 cm × 20 cm = £7.52; without adhesive border 10 cm × 10 cm = £2.90, 12.5 cm × 12.5 cm = £3.99, 12 cm × 20 cm = £5.24, 15 cm × 15 cm = £5.04, 20 cm × 20 cm = £7.52
Uses chronic and exuding wounds

Aquacel® (ConvaTec)
Soft sterile non-woven pad containing hydrocolloid fibres, 4 cm × 10 cm = £1.35, 4 cm × 20 cm = £2.00, 4 cm × 30 cm = £2.99, 5 cm × 5 cm = £1.05; 10 cm × 10 cm = £2.49; 15 cm × 15 cm = £4.69
Uses moderately to heavily exuding wounds

Aquacel® Ag (silver impregnated), 4 cm × 10 cm = £2.60, 4 cm × 20 cm = £3.39, 4 cm × 30 cm = £5.07, 5 cm × 5 cm = £1.78, 10 cm × 10 cm = £4.23, 15 cm × 15 cm = £7.97, 20 cm × 30 cm = £19.78
Uses antimicrobial dressing for moderately to heavily exuding wounds

Aquacel® Ag Ribbon (silver impregnated), 2 cm × 45 cm = £4.26
Uses antimicrobial dressing for moderately to heavily exuding cavity wounds

Aquacel® Ribbon, 2 cm × 45 cm = £2.54
Uses moderately to heavily exuding cavity wounds

Askina® Biofilm Transparent (Braun)
Sterile, semi-permeable, polyurethane film dressing with hydrocolloid adhesive, 10 cm × 10 cm = £1.02, 15 cm × 15 cm = £2.31, 20 cm × 20 cm = £3.02

Biofilm S® (Braun) NHS
Hydrocolloid dressing with polyurethane-polyester backing; also in powder form for direct application into wound, 10 cm × 10 cm = £1.65, 20 cm × 20 cm = £5.70

Biofilm® powder, 1 sachet = £1.82

CombiDERM® (ConvaTec)
Dressing with hydrocolloid adhesive border and absorbent wound contact pad, 10 cm × 10 cm = £1.50, 14 cm × 14 cm = £2.08, 15 cm × 18 cm (triangular) = £3.59, 20 cm × 20 cm = £4.00, 20 cm × 23 cm (triangular) = £4.82
Uses chronic exuding wounds such as leg ulcers, pressure sores; postoperative wounds

CombiDERM N® Hydrocolloid absorbent dressing, 7.5 cm × 7.5 cm = £1.17, 14 cm × 14 cm = £2.09, 15 cm × 25 cm = £4.26
Uses chronic wounds (e.g. leg ulcers and diabetic ulcers) and exuding wounds (e.g. biopsies), and surgical wounds

Comfeel® (Coloplast)
Soft elastic pad consisting of carmellose sodium particles embedded in adhesive mass; smooth outer layer and polyurethane film backing; available as sheets, powder in plastic blister units and paste for direct application into the wound: ulcer dressing, 10 cm × 10 cm = £2.41; 15 cm × 15 cm = £4.83; 20 cm × 20 cm = £7.39; other sizes (NHS): 4 cm × 6 cm = £1.19; powder 6 g = £4.04; paste 12-g sachet = £1.61; 50 g = £6.20

Comfeel® Plus (Coloplast)
Hydrocolloid dressings containing carmellose sodium and calcium alginate. Contour dressing, 6 cm × 8 cm = £2.00, 9 cm × 11 cm = £3.47; Ulcer Dressing, 4 cm × 6 cm = 87p, 10 cm × 10 cm = £2.21, 15 cm × 15 cm = £4.73, 18 cm × 20 cm (triangular) = £5.14, 20 cm × 20 cm = £6.81; Transparent Dressing, 5 cm × 7 cm = 60p, 5 cm × 15 cm = £1.43, 5 cm × 25 cm = £2.32, 9 cm × 14 cm = £2.19, 9 cm × 25 cm = £3.11, 10 cm × 10 cm = £1.15, 15 cm × 15 cm = £3.00, 15 cm × 20 cm = £3.05, 17 cm × 17 cm (sacral) = £3.37, 20 cm × 20 cm = £3.07; Pressure Relieving Dressing, 7 cm diameter = £3.12, 10 cm = £4.18, 15 cm = £6.29

Contreet® Hydrocolloid (Coloplast)
Semi-permeable antimicrobial barrier dressing with ionic silver (silver sodium thiosulphate), 10 cm × 10 cm = £6.59, 15 cm × 15 cm = £13.17
Uses low to moderate exuding venous leg ulcers

DuoDERM® Extra Thin (ConvaTec)
5 cm × 10 cm = 68p, 7.5 cm × 7.5 cm = 72p, 10 cm × 10 cm = £1.19, 9 cm × 15 cm = £1.60, 9 cm × 25 cm = £2.56, 9 cm × 35 cm = £3.58, 15 cm × 15 cm = £2.56, NHS 5 cm × 20 cm = £1.38
Uses minimally exuding wounds, such as abrasions, minor burns or minor surgery

DuoDERM® Signal, hydrocolloid dressing with 'Time to change' indicator, 10 cm × 10 cm = £1.93, 14 cm × 14 cm = £3.38, 20 cm × 20 cm = £6.72, 11 cm × 19 cm (oval) = £2.93, 18.5 cm × 19.5 cm (heel) = £4.73, 22.5 cm × 20 cm (sacral) = £5.53
Uses leg ulcers, pressure sores, diabetic ulcers, burns, post-operative wounds

Flexigran® (A1 Pharmaceuticals)
Sterile, semi-permeable hydrocolloid dressing without adhesive border, 10 cm × 10 cm = £2.19

Flexigran® Thin, 10 cm × 10 cm = £1.08

Granuflex® (ConvaTec)
Hydrocolloid wound contact layer bonded to plastic foam layer, with outer semi-permeable polyurethane film, 10 cm × 10 cm = £2.51, 15 cm × 15 cm = £4.77, 15 cm × 20 cm = £5.17, 20 cm × 20 cm = £7.18, NHS 20 cm × 30 cm = £11.78

Granuflex® Bordered Dressing, 6 cm × 6 cm = £1.59, 10 cm × 10 cm = £3.00, 15 cm × 15 cm = £5.77, triangular dressing, 10 cm × 13 cm = £3.54, 15 cm × 18 cm = £5.51
Uses chronic ulcers, pressure sores, open wounds, debridement of wounds; powders, gel, and pastes used with sheet dressings to fill deep or heavily exuding wounds

Granuflex® Paste (NHS), 30 g = £2.73

Hydrocoll® (Hartmann)
Hydrocolloid dressing with adhesive border and absorbent wound contact pad, 5 cm × 5 cm = 90p, 7.5 cm × 7.5 cm = £1.48, 10 cm × 10 cm = £2.15, 15 cm × 15 cm = £4.05; Concave dressing 8 cm × 12 cm = £1.90; Sacral dressing, 12 cm × 18 cm = £3.22; Basic dressing without adhesive border, 10 cm × 10 cm = £2.19; Thin film dressing, 7.5 cm × 7.5 cm = 62p, 10 cm × 10 cm = £1.03, 15 cm × 15 cm = £2.32
Uses light to medium exuding wounds

NU DERM® (J&J)
Sterile, semi-permeable hydrocolloid dressing without adhesive border, 5 cm × 5 cm = 82p, 10 cm × 10 cm = £1.50, 15 cm × 15 cm = £3.06, 20 cm × 20 cm = £6.12, 8 cm × 12 cm (heel/elbow) = £3.06, 15 cm × 18 cm (sacral) = £4.28; without adhesive border, thin, 10 cm × 10 cm = £1.02

Replicare Ultra® (S&N Hlth.)
Sterile, adhesive hydrocolloid dressing with outer semi-permeable polyurethane film backing, 10 cm × 10 cm = £2.29, 15 cm × 15 cm = £4.56, 20 cm × 20 cm = £6.73; Sacral dressing, 15 cm × 18 cm = £4.32
Uses lightly to moderately exuding wounds such as leg ulcers, pressure sores; postoperative wounds; superficial burns

Silvercel® (J&J)

Sterile, hydrocolloid and alginate dressing impregnated with silver, 2.5 cm × 30.5 cm = £4.28, 5 cm × 5 cm = £1.61, 10 cm × 20 cm = £7.38, 11 cm × 11 cm = £3.98

Uses antimicrobial dressing for moderate to heavily exuding wounds

Suprasorb H® (Vernon-Carus)

Sterile, semi permeable hydrocolloid dressing, with adhesive border, 14 cm × 14 cm = £2.23; without adhesive border 10 cm × 10 cm = £1.51, 15 cm × 15 cm = £3.30; without adhesive border, thin 5 cm × 10 cm = 65p, 10 cm × 10 cm = 99p, 15 cm × 15 cm = £2.26

Uses lightly to moderately exuding wounds

Tegaderm® Hydrocolloid (3M)

(formerly *Tegasorb®*), hydrocolloid dressing with adhesive border, 10 cm × 12 cm (oval) = £2.24; 13 cm × 15 cm (oval) = £4.19; 17.1 cm × 16.1 cm (sacral) = £4.68; without adhesive border, 10 cm × 10 cm = £2.29, 15 cm × 15 cm = £4.42

Uses chronic wounds such as leg ulcers and pressure sores

Tegaderm® Hydrocolloid Thin (formerly *Tegasorb® Thin*), sterile, semi-permeable, clear film dressing with hydrocolloid and adhesive border, 10 cm × 12 cm (oval) = £1.49; 13 cm × 15 cm (oval) = £2.79; without adhesive border, 10 cm × 10 cm = £1.50

Uses low to moderately exuding wounds including leg ulcers, abrasions, burns, and donor sites

Ultec Pro® (Tyco)

Sterile, semi-permeable hydrocolloid dressing with adhesive border, 10.5 cm × 10.5 cm = £1.39, 14 cm × 14 cm = £2.24, 21 cm × 21 cm = £4.49, 15 cm × 18 cm (sacral) = £3.17, 19.5 cm × 23 cm (sacral) = £4.88; without adhesive border 10 cm × 10 cm = £2.19, 15 cm × 15 cm = £4.27, 20 cm × 20 cm = £6.43

Uses lightly to moderately exuding wounds

Versiva® (ConvaTec)

Sterile, semi-permeable hydrocolloid dressing with fibre layer and polyurethane foam backing with adhesive border, 9 cm × 9 cm = £2.39, 11 cm × 19 cm (oval) = £4.16, 14 cm × 14 cm = £4.47, 19 cm × 19 cm = £6.94, 19 cm × 24 cm = £8.39, 19 cm × 17.7 cm (sacral) = £5.80, 21 cm × 22.5 cm (sacral) = £8.39, 19.5 cm × 18.5 cm (heel) = £7.13

Uses chronic and acute exudating wounds

Versiva® XC, hydrocolloid gelling foam dressing, with adhesive border, 10 cm × 10 cm = £2.30, 14 cm × 14 cm = £3.10, 19 cm × 19 cm = £4.95, 22 cm × 22 cm = £5.50, 18.5 cm × 20.5 cm (heel) = £5.50, 21 cm × 25 cm (sacral) = £5.90; without adhesive border, 7.5 cm × 7.5 cm = £1.35, 11 cm × 11 cm = £2.25, 15 cm × 15 cm = £4.15, 20 cm × 20 cm = £6.20

Keloid dressings

Silicone gel and gel sheets are used to reduce or prevent hypertrophic and keloid scarring. They should not be used on open wounds. Application times should be increased gradually. Silicone sheets can be washed and reused.

Advasil® (Advancis)

Self-adhesive silicone gel sheet with polyurethane film backing, 10 cm × 10 cm = £5.20, 10 cm × 15 cm = £9.17

Cica-Care® (S&N Hlth.)

Soft, self-adhesive, semi-occlusive silicone gel sheet with backing. 6 cm × 12 cm = £13.16; 15 cm × 12 cm = £25.65

Dermatix® (Valeant)

(formerly *Oleeva®*) self-adhesive silicone gel sheet (clear- or fabric-backed), 4 cm × 13 cm = £6.61, 13 cm × 13 cm = £15.17, 13 cm × 25 cm = £27.41, 20 cm × 30 cm = £49.92;
Silicone spray, 100 mL = £48.45
Silicone gel, 15 g = £19.00, 60 g = £57.00

Kelo-cote® (ABT Healthcare)

Silicone gel, 15 g = £17.88, 60 g = £51.00
Silicone spray, 100 mL = £51.00

Mepiform® (Mölnlycke)

Self-adhesive silicone gel sheet with polyurethane film backing, 5 cm × 7.5 cm = £3.36, 10 cm × 18 cm = £13.64, 4 cm × 30 cm = £9.60

Silgel® (Nagor)

Silicone gel sheet, 10 cm × 10 cm = £13.50; 20 cm × 20 cm = £40.00; 40 cm × 40 cm = £144.00; 10 cm × 5 cm = £7.50; 15 cm x 10 cm = £19.50; 30 cm × 5 cm = £19.50; 10 cm × 30 cm = £31.50; 25 cm × 15 cm (submammary) = £21.12; 46 cm × 8.5 cm (abdominal) = £39.46; 5.5 cm diameter (circular) = £4.00

Silgel® STC-SE silicone gel, 20-mL tube = £19.00

Hyaluronic acid

Hyalofill® (ConvaTec)

Hyalofill-F, NHS flat, non-woven, absorbent fibrous fleece of *Hyaff* (an ester of hyaluronic acid), 5 cm × 5 cm = £9.98, 10 cm × 10 cm = £27.68

Uses for treatment of chronic or acute wounds, place on surface of lesion and cover with sterile dressing, renew daily or when saturated (at least every 2–3 days)

Hyalofill-R, NHS absorbent fibrous rope of *Hyaff* (an ester of hyaluronic acid), 500 mg = £27.68

Uses for treatment of chronic or acute wounds, position gently inside cavity and cover with sterile dressing, renew daily or when saturated (at least every 2–3 days)

A8.1.5 Vapour-permeable films and membranes

Vapour-permeable films and membranes allow the passage of water vapour and oxygen but not of water or micro-organisms, and are suitable for mildly exuding wounds. They are highly conformable, convenient to use, provide a moist healing environment, and some may permit constant observation of the wound. However, water vapour loss may occur at a slower rate than exudate is generated, so that fluid accumulates under the dressing, which can lead to tissue maceration and to wrinkling at the adhesive contact site (with risk of bacterial entry). Newer versions have increased moisture vapour permeability; some also contain water-soluble antimicrobials. Despite these advances vapour-permeable films and membranes remain less suitable for large heavily exuding wounds and are probably not suitable for chronic leg ulcers. They are most commonly used as secondary dressings over alginates or gels; they are also sometimes used to protect fragile skin of patients at risk of developing minor skin damage.

Vapour-permeable Adhesive Film Dressing, BP 1993 (Semi-permeable Adhesive Dressing)

Sterile, extensible, waterproof, water vapour-permeable polyurethane film coated with synthetic adhesive mass; transparent. Supplied in single-use pieces.

ActivHeal® Film, 6 cm × 7 cm = 31p, 10 cm × 12.7 cm = 73p, 15 cm × 17.8 cm = £1.78 (MedLogic)

Alldress® (with absorbent pad), 10 cm × 10 cm = 86p, 15 cm × 15 cm = £1.88, 15 cm × 20 cm = £2.33 (Mölnlycke)

Bioclusive®, 10.2 cm × 12.7 cm = £1.48 (J&J)

Blisterfilm®, 5 cm × 8 cm = 40p, 9 cm × 10 cm = 70p, 10 cm × 13 cm = 90p, 14 cm × 15 cm = £1.23 (Tyco)

C-View®, 6 cm × 7 cm = 38p, 10 cm × 12 cm = £1.06, 12 cm × 12 cm = £1.22, 15 cm × 20 cm = £2.42, 20 cm × 30 cm = £3.53 (NHS) (Unomedical)

Hydrofilm®, 6 cm × 9 cm = 50p, 10 cm × 15 cm = £1.32, 12 cm × 25 cm = £2.37 (Hartmann)

Mepore® Film (formerly *Mefilm®*), 6 cm × 7 cm = 42p, 10 cm × 12.7 cm = £1.12, 10 cm × 25 cm = £2.19, 15 cm × 21.5 cm = £2.78 (Mölnlycke)

Mepore® Ultra (with absorbent pad), 6 cm × 7 cm = 28p, 9 cm × 10 cm = 60p, 9 cm × 15 cm = 90p, 9 cm × 20 cm = £1.36, 9 cm × 25 cm = £1.51, 9 cm × 30 cm = £2.49 (Mölnlycke)

OpSite® Flexifix, 5 cm × 1 m = £3.52, 10 cm × 1 m = £5.93, *OpSite® Flexigrid*, 6 cm × 7 cm = 36p, 12 cm × 12 cm = £1.01, 15 cm × 20 cm = £2.57, 12 cm × 25 cm = £3.20 (NHS), 10 cm × 12 cm = £2.06 (NHS), *OpSite® Plus* (with absorbent pad), 5 cm × 5 cm = 28p, 9.5 cm × 8.5 cm = 79p, 10 cm × 12 cm = £1.08, 10 cm × 20 cm = £1.82, 35 cm × 10 cm = £3.01 (S&N Hlth)

Pharmapore-PU® (with absorbent pad), 8.5 cm × 15.5 cm = 20p, 10 cm × 25 cm = 38p, 10 cm × 30 cm = 58p (Wallace Cameron)

Polyskin® II, 4 cm × 4 cm = 35p, 5 cm × 7 cm = 38p, 10 cm × 12 cm = 99p, 10 cm × 20 cm = £1.96, 15 cm × 20 cm = £2.26, 20 cm × 25 cm = £3.95 (Tyco)

Polyskin® MR, 5 cm × 7 cm = 40p, 10 cm × 12 cm = £1.08, 15 cm × 20 cm = £2.53 (Tyco)

PremierPore VP®, (with absorbent pad), 5 cm × 7 cm = 13p, 6 cm × 7 cm = 21p, 10 cm × 15 cm = 24p, 10 cm × 20 cm = 36p, 10 cm × 25 cm = 38p, 10 cm × 30 cm = 57p, 10 cm × 35 cm = 69p (Shermond)

ProtectFilm®, 6 cm × 7 cm = 11p, 10 cm × 12 cm = 20p, 15 cm × 20 cm = 40p (Wallace Cameron)

Suprasorb F®, 5 cm × 7 cm = 30p, 10 cm × 12 cm = 72p, 15 cm × 20 cm = £2.25, 10 cm × 25 cm = £3.44 (NHS) (Vernon-Carus)

Tegaderm®, 6 cm × 7 cm = 38p, 12 cm × 12 cm = £1.23, 15 cm × 20 cm = £2.34; with absorbent pad, 5 cm × 7 cm = 24p, 9 cm × 10 cm = 61p, 9 cm × 15 cm = 90p, 9 cm × 20 cm = £1.32, 9 cm × 25 cm = £1.48, 9 cm × 35 cm = £2.50 (3M)

Vacuskin®, 6 cm × 7 cm = 40p, 10 cm × 12 cm = £1.06, 10 cm × 25 cm = £2.06, 15 cm × 20 cm = £2.19 (Protex)

Uses postoperative dressing, donor sites, superficial decubitus ulcers, amputation stumps, stoma care; protective cover to prevent skin breakdown

Omiderm® (Chemical Search) (NHS)

Sterile, water-vapour permeable polyurethane film (plain and meshed versions). 5 cm × 7 cm = £2.00; 8 cm × 10 cm = £3.50, meshed = £4.75; 18 cm × 10 cm = £6.40, meshed = £9.50; 60 cm × 10 cm = £23.50; 21 cm × 31 cm = £24.00, meshed = £32.00; meshed 23 cm × 39 cm = £48.75

Uses ulcers; donor sites; superficial and partial thickness burns; meshed: donor sites, skin grafts

For intravenous and subcutaneous catheter sites

Central Gard® (Unomedical)

16 cm × 7 cm (central venous catheter) = 92p, 16 cm × 8.8 cm (central venous catheter) = £1.01

IV3000® (S&N Hlth.)

5 cm × 6 cm (1-hand) = 38p, 6 cm × 7 cm (non-winged peripheral catheter) = 50p, 7 cm × 9 cm (ported peripheral catheter) = 66p, 9 cm × 12 cm (PICC line) = £1.29, 10 cm × 12 cm (central venous catheter) = £1.26

Mepore® IV (Mölnlycke)

5 cm × 5.5 cm = 28p, 8 cm × 9 cm = 36p, 10 cm × 11 cm = 95p

Niko Fix® IV (Unomedical)

7 cm × 8.5 cm (ported and non-ported peripheral catheter) = 38p

Pharmapore-PU® IV (Wallace Cameron)

8.5 cm × 7 cm = 7p, 6 cm × 7 cm (ported peripheral cannula) = 8p, 7 cm × 9 cm (peripheral cannula, hand) = 17p

Tegaderm® IV (3M)

7 cm × 8.5 cm (peripheral catheter) = 57p, 8.5 cm × 10.5 cm (central venous catheter) = £1.11, 10 cm × 15.5 cm (peripherally inserted central venous catheter) = £1.60

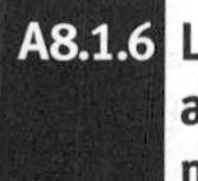

A8.1.6 Low adherence dressing and wound contact materials

Low adherence dressings and wound contact materials are used as interface layers under secondary absorbent dressings.

Tulle dressings are manufactured from cotton or viscose fibres which are impregnated with white or yellow soft paraffin to prevent the fibres from sticking, but this is only partly successful and it may be necessary to change the dressings frequently. The paraffin reduces absorbency of the dressing. Dressings with a reduced content of soft paraffin (i.e. *Paratulle®* and *Unitulle®*) are less liable to interfere with absorption; those containing the traditional amount (such as *Jelonet®*) have been considered more suitable for skin graft transfer.

Medicated tulle dressings are not generally recommended for wound care. Although hypersensitivity is unlikely with **chlorhexidine gauze dressing**, its antibacterial efficacy has not been established.

Povidone–iodine fabric dressing is a knitted viscose dressing with povidone–iodine incorporated in a hydrophilic polyethylene glycol basis; this facilitates diffusion of the iodine into the wound and permits removal of the dressing by irrigation. The iodine has a wide spectrum of antimicrobial activity but it is rapidly deactivated by wound exudate; systemic absorption of iodine may occur.

Perforated film absorbent dressings partially overcome the problems of adherence but they are suitable only for wounds with mild to moderate amounts of exudate; they are **not** appropriate for leg ulcers or for other lesions that produce large quantities of viscous exudate.

Knitted viscose primary dressing is an alternative to tulle dressings for exuding wounds; it is sometimes used as the initial layer of multi-layer compression bandaging.

Absorbent Cellulose Dressing with Fluid Repellent Backing

Eclypse®, 15 cm × 15 cm = 97p, 20 cm × 30 cm = £2.14, 60 cm × 40 cm = £8.15; *Eclypse® Adherent* with silicone wound contact layer, 10 cm × 10 cm = £2.99, 10 cm × 20 cm = £3.75, 15 cm × 15 cm = £4.99, 20 cm × 30 cm = £9.99 (Advancis)

Uses primary or secondary dressing for medium to heavily exuding wounds

Exu-Dry®, 10 cm × 15 cm = £1.01, 15 cm × 23 cm = £2.07, 23 cm × 33 cm = £4.80 (S&N Hlth.)

Uses primary or secondary dressing for medium to heavily exuding wounds

Mesorb® cellulose wadding pad with gauze wound contact layer and non-woven repellent backing, 10 cm × 10 cm = 57p, 10 cm × 15 cm = 74p, 10 cm × 20 cm = 91p, 15 cm × 20 cm = £1.29, 20 cm × 25 cm = £2.04, 20 cm × 30 cm = £2.31 (Mölnlycke)

Uses post-operative use for heavily exuding wounds

Telfa Max®, 15 cm × 22.8 cm = £1.96, 22.8 cm × 38 cm = £4.53, 38 cm × 45.7 cm = £5.50, 38 cm × 60.9 cm = £8.00 (Tyco)

Uses primary or secondary dressing for medium to heavily exuding wounds

Zetuvit® E, *non-sterile*, 10 cm × 10 cm = 6p, 10 cm × 20 cm = 8p, 20 cm × 20 cm = 13p, 20 cm × 40 cm = 25p; *sterile*, 10 cm × 10 cm = 19p, 10 cm × 20 cm = 22p, 20 cm × 20 cm = 35p, 20 cm × 40 cm = 98p (Hartmann)

Uses primary or secondary dressing for medium to heavily exuding wounds

Absorbent Dressing Pads, Sterile

Drisorb®, 10 cm × 20 cm = 17p (Vernon-Carus)

Xupad®, 10 cm × 20 cm = 17p, 20 cm × 20 cm = 28p, 20 cm × 40 cm = 40p (Richardson)

Absorbent Perforated Dressing with Adhesive Border

Low adherence dressing consisting of viscose and rayon absorbent pad with adhesive border.

Cosmopor E®, 5 cm × 7.2 cm = 7p, 6 cm × 10 cm = 13p, 8 cm × 10 cm = 16p, 6 cm × 15 cm = 18p, 8 cm × 15 cm = 25p, 8 cm × 20 cm = 33p, 10 cm × 20 cm = 40p, 10 cm × 25 cm = 50p, 10 cm × 35 cm = 69p (Hartmann)

Medipore® + Pad, 5 cm × 7.2 cm = 7p, 10 cm × 10 cm = 15p, 10 cm × 15 cm = 23p, 10 cm × 20 cm = 36p, 10 cm × 25 cm = 44p, 10 cm × 35 cm = 61p (3M)

Medisafe®, 6 cm × 8 cm = 8p, 8 cm × 10 cm = 13p, 8 cm × 12 cm = 23p, 9 cm × 15 cm = 29p, 9 cm × 20 cm = 34p, 9 cm × 25 cm = 36p (Neomedic)

Mepore®, 7 cm × 8 cm = 10p, 10 cm × 11 cm = 20p, 11 cm × 15 cm = 33p, 9 cm × 20 cm = 40p, 9 cm × 25 cm = 55p, 9 cm × 30 cm = 64p, 9 cm × 35 cm = 69p (Mölnlycke)

Primapore®, 6 cm × 8.3 cm = 16p, 8 cm × 10 cm = 17p, 8 cm × 15 cm = 30p, 10 cm × 20 cm = 39p, 10 cm × 25 cm = 45p, 10 cm × 30 cm = 56p, 10 cm × 35 cm = 87p (S&N Hlth)

Softpore®, 6 cm × 7 cm = 6p, 10 cm × 10 cm = 13p, 10 cm × 15 cm = 20p, 10 cm × 20 cm = 35p, 10 cm × 25 cm = 40p, 10 cm × 30 cm = 49p, 10 cm × 35 cm = 58p (Richardson)

Sterifix®, 5 cm × 7 cm = 18p, 7 cm × 10 cm = 29p, 10 cm × 14 cm = 52p (Hartmann)

Telfa® Island, 5 cm × 10 cm = 8p, 10 cm × 12.5 cm = 26p, 10 cm × 20 cm = 34p, 10 cm × 25.5 cm = 43p, 10 cm × 35 cm = 60p; *Telfa® AMD Island* (with polyhexamethylene biguanide—antimicrobial), 10 cm × 12.5 cm = 57p, 10 cm × 20 cm = 83p, 10 cm × 25.5 cm = 94p, 10 cm × 35 cm = £1.17 (Tyco)

Uses lightly exuding and post-operative wounds

Absorbent Perforated Plastic Film Faced Dressing

(Drug Tariff specification 9). Low-adherence dressing consisting of 3 layers.

Askina® Pad, 5 cm × 5 cm = 13p, 10 cm × 10 cm = 20p, 10 cm × 20 cm = 40p (Braun)

Cutilin®, 5 cm × 5 cm = 13p, 10 cm × 10 cm = 21p, 10 cm × 20 cm = 40p (Beiersdorf)

Interpose®, 5 cm × 5 cm = 9p, 10 cm × 10 cm = 15p, 10 cm × 20 cm = 32p (Frontier)

Melolin®, 5 cm × 5 cm = 15p, 10 cm × 10 cm = 25p, 20 cm × 10 cm = 48p (S&N Hlth)

Release®, 5 cm × 5 cm = 14p, 10 cm × 10 cm = 23p, 20 cm × 10 cm = 43p (J&J)

Skintact®, 5 cm × 5 cm = 10p, 10 cm × 10 cm = 17p, 20 cm × 10 cm = 34p (Robinson)

Solvaline N®, 5 cm × 5 cm = 9p, 10 cm × 10 cm = 16p, 10 cm × 20 cm = 32p (Vernon-Carus)

Telfa®, 5 cm × 7.5 cm = 12p, 10 cm × 7.5 cm = 15p, 15 cm × 7.5 cm = 17p, 20 cm × 7.5 cm = 28p; *Telfa® AMD* (with polyhexamtheylene biguanide—antimicrobial), 7.5 cm × 10 cm = 17p, 7.5 cm × 20 cm = 27p (Tyco)

Where no size specified by the prescriber, the 5 cm × 5 cm size to be supplied

Uses dressing for post-operative and low exudate wounds; low adherence property and low absorption capacity

Chlorhexidine Gauze Dressing, BP 1993

Fabric of leno weave, weft and warp threads of cotton and/or viscose yarn, impregnated with ointment containing chlorhexidine acetate, sterile, 5 cm × 5 cm = 26p; 10 cm × 10 cm = 55p (S&N Hlth.—*Bactigras®*)

Knitted Viscose Primary Dressing, BP 1993

Warp knitted fabric manufactured from a bright viscose monofilament.

Activon Tulle® impregnated with medical grade manuka honey, 5 cm × 5 cm = £1.78, 10 cm × 10 cm = £3.01 (Advancis)

Where no size stated by the prescriber the 5 cm size to be supplied

Uses leg ulcers, pressure sores, malodorous wounds, and dry, sloughy, or necrotic wounds

N-A Dressing®, 9.5 cm × 9.5 cm = 34p, 9.5 cm × 19 cm = 64p (J&J)

N-A Ultra® (silicone-coated), 9.5 cm × 9.5 cm = 32p, 9.5 cm × 19 cm = 61p (J&J)

Paratex®, 9.5 cm × 9.5 cm = 24p (Urgo)

Profore® wound contact layer, 14 cm × 20 cm = 29p (S&N Hlth.)

Robinson Primary®, 12.5 cm × 14.5 cm = 39p (Robinsons)

Setoprime®, 9.5 cm × 9.5 cm = 26p (Mölnlyke)

Tricotex®, 9.5 cm × 9.5 cm = 31p (S&N Hlth)

Uses low adherence wound contact layer for use on ulcerative and other granulating wounds with superimposed absorbent pad

Paraffin Gauze Dressing, BP 1993

(Tulle Gras). Fabric of leno weave, weft and warp threads of cotton and/or viscose yarn, impregnated with white or yellow soft paraffin, sterile, 10 cm × 10 cm, (light loading) = 25p; (normal loading) = 37p (most suppliers including Vernon-Carus—*Paranet®* (light loading); Aventis Pharma—*Unitulle®* (light loading); Neomedic—*Neotulle®* (normal loading); C D Medical—*Paragauze®* (normal loading); S&N Hlth—*Jelonet®* (normal loading))

Uses treatment of abrasions, burns, and other injuries of skin, and ulcerative conditions; postoperatively as penile and vaginal dressing and for sinus packing; heavier loading for skin graft transfer

Povidone–iodine Fabric Dressing

(Drug Tariff specification 43). Knitted viscose primary dressing impregnated with povidone–iodine ointment 10%, 5 cm × 5 cm = 31p; 9.5 cm × 9.5 cm = 46p (J&J—*Inadine®*)

Uses wound contact layer for abrasions and superficial burns

Cautions iodine may be absorbed particularly if large wounds treated; children under 6 months; thyroid disease

Contra-indications severe renal impairment; pregnancy; breast-feeding

Acticoat® (S&N Hlth.)

Three layer antimicrobial barrier dressing consisting of a polyester core between low adherent silver coated high density polyethylene mesh, 5 cm × 5 cm = £3.15, 10 cm × 10 cm =£7.70, 10 cm × 20 cm = £12.04, 20 cm × 40 cm = £41.19

Acticoat® 7 five layer antimicrobial barrier dressing consisting of a polyester core between low adherent silver coated high density polyethylene mesh, 5 cm × 5 cm = £5.48, 10 cm × 12.5 cm = £16.32, 15 cm × 15 cm = £29.34

Uses pressure ulcers, venous ulcers, diabetic ulcers, burns, donor and recipient graft sites; with silver for infected and exuding wounds

Atrauman® (Hartmann)

Non-adherent knitted polyester primary dressing impregnated with neutral triglycerides, 5 cm × 5 cm = 24p, 7.5 cm × 10 cm = 25p, 10 cm × 20 cm = 56p, 20 cm × 30 cm = £1.54

Uses abrasions, burns, and other injuries of skin, and ulcerative conditions; postoperatively for granulating wounds

Atrauman® Ag, non-adherent polyamide fabric impregnated with silver and neutral triglycerides, 5 cm × 5 cm = 46p, 10 cm × 10 cm = £1.12, 10 cm × 20 cm = £2.19

Uses antimicrobial dressing for burns, traumatic or chronic wounds, donor graft sites, diabetic ulcers

Cutisorb® Sorbact (BSN Medical)

Low adherence acetate tissue impregnated with dialkylcarbamoyl chloride.

Cutisorb® Sorbact Dressing Pads 7 cm × 9 cm = £3.20, 10 cm × 10 cm = £5.00, 10 cm × 20 cm = £7.80

Cutisorb® Sorbact Swabs 4 cm × 6 cm = £1.50, 7 cm × 9 cm = £2.50

Cutisorb® Sorbact Tupfer 3 cm, 5 pad pack = £3.00

Uses colonized and infected wounds

Mepilex® (Mölnlycke)

Absorbent soft silicone dressing with polyurethane foam film backing, 10 cm × 10 cm = £2.41, 10 cm × 20 cm = £3.98, 15 cm × 15 cm = £4.49, 20 cm × 20 cm = £6.64

Mepilex® Border, with soft silicone adhesive border, 7.5 cm × 7.5 cm = £1.40, 10 cm × 10 cm = £2.54, 10 cm × 20 cm = £3.40, 10 cm × 30 cm = £5.11, 15 cm × 15 cm = £4.15, 15 cm × 20 cm = £5.21

Mepilex® Border Lite, thin absorbent soft silicone dressing with adhesive border, 4 cm × 5 cm = 87p, 7.5 cm × 7.5 cm = £1.30, 5 cm × 12.5 cm = £1.89, 10 cm × 10 cm = £2.38, 15 cm × 15 cm = £3.87

Mepilex® Border Sacrum, soft silicone dressing with adhesive border, 18 cm × 18 cm = £4.47, 23 cm × 23 cm = £7.29

Mepilex® Heel, soft silicone adhesive dressing, 13 cm × 20 cm = £5.05

Mepilex® Lite, thin absorbent soft silicone dressing, 6 cm × 8.5 cm = £1.66, 10 cm × 10 cm = £1.98, 15 cm × 15 cm = £3.85, 20 cm × 50 cm = £24.28

Mepilex® Transfer, soft silicone exudate transfer dressing, 7.5 cm × 8.5 cm = £2.06, 10 cm × 12 cm = £3.24, 15 cm × 20 cm = £9.70, 20 cm × 50 cm = £24.78

Mepitel® (Mölnlycke)

Soft silicone wound contact dressing. 5 cm × 7 cm = £1.49, 8 cm × 10 cm = £2.99, 12 cm × 15 cm = £6.05, 20 cm × 30 cm = £15.58

Uses leg ulcers, decubitus ulcers, burns, fixation of skin grafts; should be covered with simple absorbent secondary dressing

Physiotulle® (Coloplast)

Non-adherent soft polymer wound contact dressing, 10 cm × 10 cm = £2.05, 15 cm × 20 cm = £6.25

Uses leg ulcers, pressure sores, burns, postoperative wounds, donor sites, skin abrasions

Physiotulle® Ag (silver impregnated), 10 cm × 10 cm = £2.06

Uses antimicrobial dressing for leg ulcers, diabetic ulcers, pressure sores, burns, postoperative wounds, donor sites, skin abrasions

Proguide® (S&N Hlth.)

Non-adherent polyurethane wound contact layer, 10 cm × 10 cm = £1.96

[1]**Surgipad®** (J&J) NHS

Absorbent pad of absorbent cotton and viscose in sleeve of non-woven viscose fabric, sterile, pouch 12 cm × 10 cm = 18p, 20 cm × 10 cm = 25p, 20 cm × 20 cm = 30p, 40 cm × 20 cm = 41p; non-sterile, net price pack 12 cm × 10 cm = 5p, 20 cm × 10 cm = 10p, 20 cm × 20 cm = 17p, 40 cm × 20 cm = 28p

Uses for heavily exuding wounds requiring frequent dressing changes

1. NHS Except in Sterile Dressing Pack with Non-woven Pads

Tegaderm® Contact (3M)

(formerly *Tegapore®*), non-adherent soft polymer wound contact dressing, 7.5 cm × 10 cm = £2.13, 7.5 cm × 20 cm = £4.17, 20 cm × 25 cm = £10.16

Urgotul® (Urgo)

Non-adherent soft polymer wound contact dressing, 11 cm × 11 cm = £2.92, 10 cm × 40 cm = £9.69, 16 cm × 21 cm = £8.26; *Urgotul® Silver*, 10 cm × 12 cm = £3.25, 15 cm × 20 cm = £8.85

Urgotul® Duo, 5 cm × 10 cm = £2.24, 10 cm × 12 cm = £3.47, 15 cm × 20 cm = £8.05; *Urgotul® Duo Silver* 5 cm × 7 cm = £1.90, 11 cm × 11 cm = £3.77, 15 cm × 20 cm = £9.10

Urgotul® SSD (silver impregnated), 11 cm × 11 cm = £2.89, 16 cm × 21 cm = £8.19

UrgoCell® (with polyurethane foam film backing), 10 cm × 12 cm = £4.35, 15 cm × 20 cm = £8.82; with adhesive border 13 cm × 13 cm = £4.35, 15 cm × 20 cm = £8.82; *Urgocell® Silver*, 6 cm × 6 cm = £4.00, 10 cm × 10 cm = £5.50, 15 cm × 20 cm = £9.90

A8.1.7 Odour absorbent dressings

Dressings containing activated charcoal are used to absorb odour from wounds. Wound odour is most effectively reduced by debridement of slough, reduction in bacterial levels, and frequent dressing changes.

Actisorb® Silver 220 (J&J)

(formerly Actisorb® Plus) Knitted fabric of activated charcoal, with one-way stretch, with silver residues, within spun-bonded nylon sleeve. 6.5 cm × 9.5 cm = £1.58, 10.5 cm × 10.5 cm = £2.48, 10.5 cm × 19 cm = £4.51

Askina® Carbosorb (Braun)

Activated charcoal absorbent dressing, 10 cm × 10 cm = £2.72, 10 cm × 20 cm = £5.25

CarboFLEX® (ConvaTec)

Dressing in 5 layers: wound-facing absorbent layer containing alginate and hydrocolloid; water-resistant second layer; third layer containing activated charcoal; non-woven absorbent fourth layer; water-resistant backing layer. 10 cm × 10 cm = £2.90, 8 cm × 15 cm = £3.48, 15 cm × 20 cm = £6.59

Carbonet® (S&N Hlth.) NHS

Activated charcoal dressing, 10 cm × 10 cm = £3.13, 10 cm × 20 cm = £6.10

Carbopad® VC (Vernon-Carus)

Activated charcoal non-absorbent dressing, 10 cm × 10 cm = £1.59, 10 cm × 20 cm = £2.15

CliniSorb® Odour Control Dressings (CliniMed)

Layer of activated charcoal cloth between viscose rayon with outer polyamide coating. 10 cm × 10 cm = £1.72, 10 cm × 20 cm = £2.29, 15 cm × 25 cm = £3.68

Lyofoam C® (Medlock)

Lyofoam sheet with layer of activated charcoal cloth and additional outer envelope of polyurethane foam. 10 cm × 10 cm = £2.79, 15 cm × 20 cm = £6.35

Sorbsan® Plus Carbon (Unomedical)

Alginate dressing with activated carbon, 7.5 cm × 10 cm = £2.37, 10 cm × 15 cm = £4.60, 10 cm × 20 cm = £5.51, 15 cm × 20 cm = £6.34

A8.1.8 Dressing packs

The role of dressing packs is very limited. They are used to provide a clean or sterile working surface; packs shown below include cotton wool balls, but they are not recommended for use on wounds.

Non-Drug Tariff Specification Sterile Dressing Pack

Dress-it® contains vitrex gloves, large apron, disposable bag, paper towel, softswabs, adsorbent pad, sterile field = 60p (Richardson)

Polyfield® Nitrile Patient Pack contains powder-free nitrile gloves, laminate sheet, non-woven swabs, towel, polythene disposable bag, apron = 52p (Shermond)

Polyfield® Soft Vinyl Patient Pack contains powder-free sterile soft vinyl gloves, polythene sheet, non-woven swabs, towel, polythene disposable bag, apron = 52p (Shermond)

Propax® SDP contains paper towel, disposable bag, gauze swabs, dressing pad, sterile field = 45p (BSN Medical)

Sterile Dressing Pack

(Drug Tariff specification 10). Contains gauze and cotton tissue pad, gauze swabs, absorbent cotton wool balls, absorbent paper towel, water repellent inner wrapper. 1 pack = 48p (Vernon-Carus—*Vernaid®*)

Sterile Dressing Pack with Non-woven Pads

(Drug Tariff specification 35). Contains non-woven fabric covered dressing pad, non-woven fabric swabs, absorbent cotton wool balls, absorbent paper towel, water repellent inner wrapper. 1 pack = 47p (Vernon-Carus—*Vernaid®*)

A8.1.9 Surgical absorbents

Surgical absorbent dressings, applied directly to the wound, have many disadvantages, since they adhere to the wound, shed fibres into it, and dehydrate it; they also permit leakage of exudate ('strike through') with an associated risk of infection. Surgical absorbents may be used as secondary absorbent layers in the management of heavily exuding wounds.

Absorbent Cotton, BP

Carded cotton fibres of not less than 10 mm average staple length, available in rolls and balls, 25 g = 68p; 100 g = £1.54; 500 g = £5.20 (most suppliers). 25-g pack to be supplied when weight not stated

Uses general purpose cleansing and swabbing, pre-operative skin preparation, application of medicaments; supplementary absorbent pad to absorb excess wound exudate

Absorbent Cotton, Hospital Quality

As for absorbent cotton but lower quality materials, shorter staple length etc. 100 g = £1.07; 500 g = £3.38 (most suppliers)

Drug Tariff specifies to be supplied only where specifically ordered

Uses suitable only as general purpose absorbent, for swabbing, and routine cleansing of incontinent patients; not for wound cleansing

Absorbent Cotton Gauze, BP 1988

Cotton fabric of plain weave, in rolls and as swabs (see below), usually Type 13 light, sterile, 90 cm (all) × 1 m = £1.02; 3 m = £2.12; 5 m = £3.30; 10 m = £6.33 (most suppliers). 1-m packet supplied when no size stated

Uses pre-operative preparation, for cleansing and swabbing

Note Drug Tariff also includes unsterilised absorbent cotton gauze, 25 m roll = £14.50

Absorbent Cotton Ribbon Gauze, BP 1993 NHS

Cotton fabric of plain weave in ribbon form with fast selvedge edges

Uses post-surgery cavity packing for sinus, dental, throat cavities etc.

Absorbent Cotton and Viscose Ribbon Gauze, BP 1993

Woven fabric in ribbon form with fast selvedge edges, warp threads of cotton, weft threads of viscose or combined cotton and viscose yarn, sterile. 5 m (both) × 1.25 cm = 76p; 2.5 cm = 85p

Uses post-surgery cavity packing for sinus, dental, throat cavities etc.

Gauze and Cotton Tissue, BP 1988

Consists of absorbent cotton enclosed in absorbent cotton gauze type 12 or absorbent cotton and viscose gauze type 2. 500 g = £6.59 (most suppliers, including Robinsons—*Gamgee Tissue®* (blue label))

Uses absorbent and protective pad, as burns dressing on non-adherent layer

Gauze and Cotton Tissue

(Drug Tariff specification 14). Similar to above. 500 g = £4.81 (most suppliers, including Robinsons—*Gamgee Tissue®* (pink label))

Drug Tariff specifies to be supplied only where specifically ordered

Uses absorbent and protective pad, as burns dressing on non-adherent layer

Absorbent Lint, BPC

Cotton cloth of plain weave with nap raised on one side from warp yarns. 25 g = 84p; 100 g = £2.57; 500 g = £10.83 (most suppliers). 25-g pack supplied where no quantity stated

Note Not recommended for wound management

Absorbent Muslin, BP 1988 NHS

Fabric of plain weave, warp threads of cotton, weft threads of cotton and/or viscose

Uses wet dressing, soaked in 0.9% sterile sodium chloride solution

Gauze Swab, BP 1988

Consists of absorbent cotton gauze type 13 light or absorbent cotton and viscose gauze type 1 folded into squares or rectangles of 8-ply with no cut edges exposed, sterile, 7.5 cm × 7.5 cm 5-pad packet = 37p; non-sterile, 10 cm × 10 cm 100-pad packet = £1.28 (most suppliers)

Filmated Gauze Swab, BP 1988

As for Gauze Swab, but with thin layer of Absorbent Cotton enclosed within, non-sterile, 10 cm × 10 cm, 100-pad packet = £3.45 (Vernon-Carus—*Cotfil®*)

Uses general swabbing and cleansing

Non-woven Fabric Swab

(Drug Tariff specification 28). Consists of non-woven fabric folded 4-ply; alternative to gauze swabs, type 13 light, sterile, 7.5 cm × 7.5 cm, 5-pad packet = 24p; non-sterile, 10 cm × 10 cm, 100-pad packet = 74p

Uses general purpose swabbing and cleansing; absorbs more quickly than gauze

Filmated Non-woven Fabric Swab

(Drug Tariff specification 29). Film of viscose fibres enclosed within non-woven viscose fabric folded 8-ply, non-sterile, 10 cm × 10 cm, 100-pad packet = £3.45 (J & J—*Regal®*)

Uses general purpose swabbing and cleansing

A8.1.10 Capillary dressings

Capillary dressings consist of an absorbent core of hydrophilic fibres sandwiched between two low-adherent wound-contact layers. Wound exudate is taken up by the dressing and retained within the highly absorbent central layer.

The dressing may be applied intact to relatively superficial areas, but for deeper wounds or cavities it may be cut to shape to ensure good contact with the wound base. Multiple layers may be applied to heavily exuding wounds to further increase the fluid-absorbing capacity of the dressing.

Capillary dressings can be applied to a variety of wounds but they are contra-indicated for heavily bleeding wounds or arterial bleeding.

Advadraw® (Advancis)

Non-adherent, sterile dressing consisting of a soft viscose and polyester absorbent pad with central wicking layer between two perforated permeable wound contact layers. 5 cm × 7.5 cm = 56p, 10 cm × 10 cm = 87p, 10 cm × 15 cm = £1.17, 15 cm × 20 cm = £1.54

Advadraw Spiral®, 0.5 cm × 40 cm = 81p

Sumar® (Robinsons)

Sumar® Lite, for light to moderately exuding wounds and cavities, 10 cm × 10 cm = £1.59, 10 cm × 15 cm = £2.12

Sumar® Max, for heavily exuding wounds, 10 cm × 10 cm = £1.61, 10 cm × 15 cm = £2.15

Vacutex® (Protex)

Low-adherent dressing consisting of two external polyester wound contact layers with central wicking polyester/cotton mix absorbent layer. 5 cm × 5 cm = 94p, 10 cm × 10 cm = £1.66, 10 cm × 15 cm = £2.23, 10 cm × 20 cm = £2.68, 15 cm × 20 cm = £3.14, 20 cm × 20 cm = £4.28

A8.2 Bandages and adhesives

According to their structure and performance bandages are used for dressing retention, for support, and for compression.

A8.2.1 Non-extensible bandages

Bandages made from non-extensible woven fabrics have generally been replaced by more conformable products, therefore their role is now extremely limited. Triangular calico bandage has a role as a sling.

Domette Bandage, BP 1988 (NHS)

Fabric, plain weave, cotton warp and wool weft (hospital quality also available, all cotton). 5 m (all): 5 cm = 54p; 7.5 cm = 81p; 10 cm = £1.08; 15 cm = £1.61 (Steraid)

Uses protection and support where warmth required

Multiple Pack Dressing No. 1

(Drug Tariff). Contains absorbent cotton, absorbent cotton gauze type 13 light (sterile), open-wove bandages (banded). 1 pack = £3.84

Open-wove Bandage, BP 1988

Cotton cloth, plain weave, warp of cotton, weft of cotton, viscose, or combination, one continuous length. Type 1, 5 m (all): 2.5 cm = 30p; 5 cm = 50p; 7.5 cm = 70p; 10 cm = 92p (most suppliers) 5 m × 5 cm supplied when size not stated

Uses protection and retention of absorbent dressings; support for minor strains, sprains; securing splints

Triangular Calico Bandage, BP 1980

Unbleached calico right-angled triangle, 90 cm × 90 cm × 1.27 m = £1.10 (most suppliers)

Uses sling

A8.2.2 Light-weight conforming bandages

Lightweight conforming bandages are used for dressing retention, with the aim of keeping the dressing close to the wound without inhibiting movement or restricting blood flow. The elasticity of **conforming-stretch bandages** (also termed contour bandages) is greater than that of **cotton conforming bandages**.

Conforming Bandage (Synthetic)

Fabric, plain weave, warp of polyamide, weft of viscose. 4 m stretched (all):

Hospiform® (formerly *Peha Crepp®* E), 6 cm = 12p, 8 cm = 15p, 10 cm = 17p, 12 cm = 21p (Hartmann)

Cotton Conforming Bandage, BP 1988

Cotton fabric, plain weave, treated to impart some elasticity to warp and weft. 3.5 m (all): type A, 5 cm = 67p, 7.5 cm = 83p, 10 cm = £1.02, 15 cm = £1.39 (S&N Hlth— *Easifix Crinx®*)

Knitted Polyamide and Cellulose Contour Bandage, BP 1988

Fabric, knitted warp of polyamide filament, weft of cotton or viscose, fast edges, one continuous length. 4 m stretched (all):

K-Band®, 5 cm = 18p, 7 cm = 23p, 10 cm = 25p, 15 cm = 45p (Urgo)

Knit-Band®, 5 cm = 10p, 7 cm = 15p, 10 cm = 17p, 15 cm = 30p (CliniMed)

Knit Fix®, 5 cm = 12p, 7 cm = 17p, 10 cm = 17p, 15 cm = 33p (Steraid)

Polyamide and Cellulose Contour Bandage, BP 1988 (formerly Nylon and Viscose Stretch Bandage)

Fabric, plain weave, warp of polyamide filament, weft of cotton or viscose, fast edges, one continuous length, 4 m stretched (all):

Acti-Wrap®, cohesive, latex-free, 6 cm = 42p, 8 cm = 61p, 10 cm = 72p (Activa)

Easifix®, 5 cm = 33p, 7.5 cm = 40p, 10 cm = 47p, 15 cm = 80p (S&N Hlth)

Kontour®, cohesive, 5 cm = 28p, 7.5 cm = 35p, 10 cm = 40p, 15 cm = 66p (Easigrip)

Slinky®, 5 cm = 39p, 7.5 cm = 55p, 10 cm = 66p, 15 cm = 95p (Medlock)

Stayform®, 5 cm = 29p, 7.5 cm = 36p, 10 cm = 40p, 15 cm = 68p (Robinsons)

A8.2.3 Tubular bandages

Tubular bandages are available in different forms, according to the function required of them. Some are used under orthopaedic casts and some are suitable for protecting areas to which creams or ointments (other than those containing potent corticosteroids) have been applied. The conformability of the elasticated versions makes them particularly suitable for retaining dressings on difficult parts of the body or for soft tissue injury, but their use as the only means of applying pressure to an oedematous limb or to a varicose ulcer is not appropriate, since the pressure they exert is inadequate. Compression hosiery (section A8.3.1) reduces the recurrence of venous leg ulcers and should be considered after wound healing.

Cotton Stockinette, Bleached, BP 1988

Knitted fabric, cotton yarn, tubular, 1 m × 2.5 cm = 33p; 5 cm = 50p; 7.5 cm = 61p; 6 m × 10 cm = £4.13 (J&J, Medlock)

Uses 1 m lengths, basis (with wadding) for Plaster of Paris bandages etc.; 6 m length, compression bandage

Elasticated Surgical Tubular Stockinette, Foam padded

(Drug Tariff specification 25). Fabric as for Elasticated Tubular Bandage with polyurethane foam lining. Heel, elbow, knee, small = £2.68, medium = £2.83, large = £3.09; sacral, small, medium, and large (all) = £13.82 (Medlock—*Tubipad®*)

Uses relief of pressure and elimination of friction in relevant area; porosity of foam lining allows normal water loss from skin surface

Elasticated Tubular Bandage, BP 1993

(formerly Elasticated Surgical Tubular Stockinette). Knitted fabric, elasticated threads of rubber-cored polyamide or polyester with cotton or cotton and viscose yarn, tubular. Lengths 50 cm and 1 m, widths 6.25 cm, 6.75 cm, 7.5 cm, 8.75 cm, 10 cm, 12 cm (other sizes (NHS)): Synergy—*Comfigrip®*; Easigrip—*EasiGRIP®*; Sallis—*Eesiban®*; Sigma—*Sigma ETB®*; S&N Hlth—*Tensogrip®* (NHS); JLB—*Textube®*; Medlock—*Tubigrip®*. Where no size stated by prescriber the 50 cm length should be supplied and width endorsed

Uses retention of dressings on limbs, abdomen, trunk

Elasticated Viscose Stockinette

(Drug Tariff specification 46). Lightweight plain-knitted elasticated tubular bandage.

Acti-Fast®, 3.5 cm red line (small limb), length 1 m = 62p; 5 cm green line (medium limb), length 1 m = 65p, 3 m = £1.90, 5 m = £3.30; 7.5 cm blue line (large limb), length 1 m = 90p, 3 m = £2.50, 5 m = £4.40; 10.75 cm yellow line (child trunk), length 1 m = £1.45, 3 m = £4.10, 5 m = £7.10; 17.5 cm beige line (adult trunk), length 1 m = £2.15 (Activa)

CliniFast®, 3.5 cm red line (small limb), length 1 m = 56p; 5 cm green line (medium limb), length 1 m = 58p, 3 m = £1.62, 5 m = £2.81; 7.5 cm blue line (large limb), length 1 m = 77p, 3 m = £2.13, 5 m = £3.74 10.75 cm yellow line (child trunk), length 1 m = £1.20, 3 m = £3.49, 5 m = £6.04; 17.5 cm beige line (adult trunk), length 1 m = £1.83; vest 6–24 months = £7.13, 2–5 years = £9.50, 5–8 years = £10.69, 8–11 years = £11.88, 11–14 years = £11.88; tights (pair) 6–24 months = £7.13; leggings (pair) 2–5 years = £9.50, 5–8 years = £10.69, 8–11 years = £11.88, 11–14 years = £11.88; socks (pair) up to 8 years = £2.97, 8–14 years = £2.97; mittens (pair) up to 24 months = £2.97, 2–8 years = £2.97, 8–14 years = £2.97; clava 6 months–5 years = £5.85, 5–14 years = £6.75 (Clinisupplies)

Comfifast® 3.5 cm red line (small limb), length 1 m = 64p; 5 cm green line (medium limb), length 1 m = 68p, 3 m = £1.94, 5 m = £3.33; 7.5 cm blue line (large limb), length 1 m = 92p, 3 m = £2.56, 5 m = £ 4.47; 10.75 cm yellow line (child trunk), length 1 m = £1.46, 3 m = £4.17, 5 m = £7.16; 17.5 cm beige line (adult trunk), length 1 m = £1.84 (Synergy)

Comfifast® Easy Wrap, 6–24 months = £7.92, 2–5 years = £10.56, 5–8 years = £11.88, 8–11 years = £13.20, 11–14 years = £13.20; tights (pair) 6–24 months = £7.92; leggings (pair) 2–5 years = £10.56, 5–8 years = £11.88, 8–11 years = £13.20, 11–14 years = £13.20; socks (pair) up to 8 years = £3.30, 8–14 = £3.30; mittens (pair) up to 24 months = £3.30, 2–8 years =

£3.30, 8–14 years = £3.30; clava 6 months–5 years = £6.50, 5–14 years = £7.50 (Synergy)

Coverflex®, 3.5 cm red line (small limb), length 1 m = 73p; 5 cm green line (medium limb), length 1 m = 76p, 3 m = £2.24, 5 m = £3.87; 7.5 cm blue line (large limb), length 1 m = £1.07, 3 m = £2.54, 5 m = £ 5.04; 10.75 cm yellow line (child trunk), length 1 m = £1.68, 3 m = £4.83, 5 m = £8.50; 17.5 cm beige line (adult trunk), length 1 m = £2.24 (Hartmann)

Easifast®, 3.5 cm red line (small limb), length 1 m = 65p; 5 cm green line (medium limb), length 1 m = 69p, 3 m = £1.95, 5 m = £3.40; 7.5 cm blue line (large limb), length 1 m = 94p, 3 m = £2.60, 5 m = £4.50; 10.75 cm yellow line (child trunk), length 1m = £1.50, 3 m = £4.25, 5 m = £7.20; 17.5 cm beige line (adult trunk), length 1 m = £1.90 (Easigrip)

Tubifast®, 3.5 cm red line (small limb), length 1 m = 84p; 5 cm green line (medium limb), length 1 m = 90p, 3 m = £2.57, 5 m = £4.40; 7.5 cm blue line (large limb), length 1 m = £1.20, 3 m = £3.39, 5 m = £5.90; 10.75 cm yellow line (child trunk), length 1 m = £1.93, 3 m = £5.51, 5 m = £9.47; 17.5 cm beige line (adult trunk), length 1 m = £2.43, 25 cm (large adult trunk) 1 m = £3.98, 25 cm purple line (large adult trunk), 5 m = £19.48; vest, 6–24 months = £10.47, 2–5 years = £13.95, 5–8 years = £15.70, 8–11 years = £17.44, 11–14 years = £17.44; tights (pair) 6–24 months = £10.47; leggings (pair) 2–5 years = £13.95, 5–8 years = £15.70, 8–11 years = £17.44, 11–14 years = £17.44; socks (pair) = £4.37; gloves (small, medium or large adult, medium or large child) = £5.25 (Medlock)

Uses retention of dressings

Ribbed Cotton and Viscose Surgical Tubular Stockinette, BP 1988

Knitted fabric of 1:1 ribbed structure, singles yarn spun from blend of two-thirds cotton and one-third viscose fibres, tubular. Length 5 m (all):

type A (lightweight): arm/leg (child), arm (adult) 5 cm = £2.35; arm (OS adult), leg (adult) 7.5 cm = £3.08; leg (OS adult) 10 cm = £4.09; trunk (child) 15 cm = £5.89; trunk (adult) 20 cm = £6.80; trunk (OS adult) 25 cm = £8.13 (SSL)

type B (heavyweight): sizes as for type A, net price £2.30–£7.97 (Sallis—*Esiban*®)

Drug Tariff specifies various combinations of sizes to provide sufficient material for part or full body coverage

Uses protective dressings with tar-based and other non-steroid ointments

Tubular Gauze Bandage, Seamless NHS

Unbleached cotton yarn, positioned with applicators. 20 m roll (all): 00 = £2.95; 01 = £3.55; 12 = £4.60; 34 = £6.75; 56 = £9.35; 78 = £10.75; T1 = £14.75; T2 = £19.00 (Medlock—*Tubegauz*®)

Uses retention of dressings on limbs, abdomen, trunk

A8.2.4 Support bandages

Light support bandages, which include the various forms of crepe bandage, are used in the prevention of oedema; they are also used to provide support for mild sprains and joints but their effectiveness has not been proven for this purpose. Since they have limited extensibility, they are able to provide light support without exerting undue pressure. For a warning against injudicious compression see section A8.2.5.

Crepe Bandage, BP 1988

Fabric, plain weave, warp of wool threads and crepe-twisted cotton threads, weft of cotton threads; stretch bandage. 4.5 m stretched (all): 5 cm = 88p; 7.5 cm = £1.23; 10 cm = £1.61; 15 cm = £2.33 (most suppliers)

Uses light support system for strains, sprains, compression over paste bandages for varicose veins

Cotton Crepe Bandage

Light support bandage, 4.5 m stretched (all): 5 cm = 48p; 7.5 cm = 67p; 10 cm = 87p; 15 cm = £1.27 (Steraid—*Hospicrepe*® *239*)

Cotton Crepe Bandage, BP 1988

Fabric, plain weave, warp of crepe-twisted cotton threads, weft of cotton and/or viscose threads; stretch bandage. 4.5 m stretched (both): 7.5 cm = £2.75; 10 cm = £3.54; other sizes NHS (most suppliers)

Uses light support system for strains, sprains, compression over paste bandages for varicose ulcers

Cotton, Polyamide and Elastane Bandage

Fabric, cotton, polyamide, and elastane; light support bandage (Type 2), 4.5 m stretched (all): 5 cm = 54p, 7.5 cm = 73p, 10 cm = 91p, 15 cm = £1.12 (Neomedic—*Neosport*®); 5 cm = 63p, 7.5 cm = 89p, 10 cm = £1.14, 15 cm = £1.64 (BSN Medical—*Soffcrepe*®); 10 cm = £1.10 (Medlock—*Setocrepe*®); 10 cm = £1.21, latex-free = £1.28 (S&N Hlth.—*Profore*® *#2*)

Uses light support for sprains and strains; retention of dressings

Cotton Stretch Bandage, BP 1988

Fabric, plain weave, warp of crepe-twisted cotton threads, weft of cotton threads; stretch bandage, lighter than cotton crepe, 4.5 m stretched (all): 5 cm = 52p; 7.5 cm = 72p; 10 cm = 96p; 15 cm = £1.36 (Steraid—*Hospicrepe*® *233*)

Uses light support system for strains, sprains, compression over paste bandages for varicose veins

Cotton Suspensory Bandage

(Drug Tariff). Type 1: cotton net bag with draw tapes and webbing waistband; small, medium, and large (all) = £1.52, extra large = £1.61. Type 2: cotton net bag with elastic edge and webbing waistband; small = £1.68, medium = £1.73, large = £1.79, extra large = £1.87. Type 3: cotton net bag with elastic edge and webbing waistband with elastic insertion; small, medium, and large (all) = £1.81; extra large = £1.88. Type supplied to be endorsed

Uses support of scrotum

Knitted Elastomer and Viscose Bandage

Knitted fabric, viscose and elastomer yarn. Type 2 (light support bandage)

K-Lite®, 4.5 m stretched, 5 cm = 50p, 7 cm = 69p, 10 cm = 91p, 15 cm = £1.32; 5.2 m stretched, 10 cm = £1.04 (Urgo)

Knit-Firm®, 4.5 m stretched, 5 cm = 36p, 7 cm = 51p, 10 cm = 66p, 15 cm = 96p (Steraid)

Uses light support for sprains and strains

Type 3a (light compression bandage):

Elset®, 6 m stretched, 10 cm = £2.39, 15 cm = £2.59; 8 m stretched, 10 cm = £3.06; 12 m stretched, 15 cm = £5.13 (Medlock)

K-Plus®, 8.7 m stretched, 10 cm = £2.04; 10.25 m stretched, 10 cm = £2.36 (Urgo)

K-Plus® Long, 10.25 m stretched, 10 cm = £2.36 (Urgo)

Profore® #3, 8.7 m stretched, 10 cm = £3.53, latex-free = £3.83 (S&N Hlth.)

A8.2.5 Compression bandages

High compression products are used to provide the high compression needed for the management of gross varices, post-thrombotic venous insufficiency, venous leg ulcers, and gross oedema in average-sized limbs. Their use calls for an expert knowledge of the elastic properties of the products and experience in the technique of providing careful graduated compression. Incorrect application can lead to uneven and inadequate pressures or to hazardous levels of pressure. In particular, injudicious use of compression in limbs with arterial disease has been reported to cause severe skin and tissue necrosis (in some instances calling for amputation). Doppler testing is required before treatment with compression. Pentoxifylline (section 2.6.4) may be of benefit if a chronic venous leg ulcer does not respond to compression bandaging [unlicensed indication].

High compression bandages

PEC High Compression Bandage

(Drug Tariff specification 52). Polyamide, elastane, and cotton compression (high) extensible bandage, 3.5 m unstretched (both): 7.5 cm = £2.51; 10 cm = £3.25 (Medlock—*Setopress*®)

VEC High Compression Bandage
(Drug Tariff specification 52). Viscose, elastane, and cotton compression (high) extensible bandage, 3 m unstretched (both); 7.5 cm = £2.48; 10 cm = £3.19 (S&N—*Tensopress*®)

High Compression Bandage
(Drug Tariff specification 52). Cotton, viscose, nylon, and Lycra® extensible bandage, 3 m (unstretched), 10 cm = £3.26 (ConvaTec—*SurePress*®); 3.5 m (unstretched), 10 cm = £1.82 (Advancis—*Adva-Co*®)

ProGuide® #2 (S&N Hlth.)
Woven, elastomer, cohesive, extensible, compression bandage, 3 m (unstretched), 10 cm (red) = £5.26, 10 cm (yellow) = £5.74, 10 cm (green) = £6.22

◢Short stretch compression bandage

Short stretch bandages help to reduce oedema and promote healing of venous leg ulcers. They are also used to reduce swelling associated with lymphoedema. They are applied at full stretch over padding (*see* Sub-compression Wadding Bandage below) which protects areas of high pressure and sites at high risk of pressure damage.

Actiban® (Activa)
All 5 m, 8 cm = £3.02; 10 cm = £3.24; 12 cm = £3.95

Actico® (Activa)
Cohesive, all 6 m, 4 cm = £2.15, 6 cm = £2.52, 8 cm = £2.90, 10 cm = £3.01, 12 cm = £3.83

Comprilan® (BSN Medical)
All 5 m, 6 cm = £2.47; 8 cm = £2.90; 10 cm = £3.12; 12 cm = £3.80

Rosidal K® (Vernon-Carus)
All 5 m, 4cm = £1.70, 6cm = £2.37, 8 cm = £2.83, 10 cm = £3.09, 12 cm = £3.75; 10m x 10cm = £5.38

Silkolan® (Urgo)
All 5 m, 8 cm = £3.00; 10 cm = £3.39

◢Sub-compression wadding bandage

Advasoft® (Advancis)
3.5 m unstretched, 10 cm = 37p

Cellona® Undercast Padding (Vernon-Carus)
2.75 m unstretched (all): 5 cm = 28p, 7.5 cm = 34p; 10 cm = 42p; 15 cm = 54p

Flexi-Ban® (Activa)
Padding, 3.5 m unstretched, 10cm = 45p

K-Soft® (Urgo)
3.5 m unstretched, 10 cm = 41p; 4.5 m unstretched, 10 cm = 51p

K-Tech® (Urgo)
5 m unstretched, 10 cm = £3.66; 6 m unstretched, 10 cm = £4.39

Ortho-Band Plus® (Steraid)
10 cm × 3.5 cm unstretched = 37p

Profore® #1 (S&N Hlth.)
Viscose fleece, 3.5 m unstretched, 10 cm = 63p, latex-free = 68p

ProGuide® #1 (S&N Hlth.)
Polyester and viscose fleece, 4 m unstretched, 10 cm = £1.43

Softexe® (Medlock)
3.5 m unstretched, 10 cm = 58p

SurePress® (ConvaTec)
Absorbent padding, 3 m unstretched, 10 cm = 53p

Ultra Soft® (Robinsons)
Soft absorbent bandage, 3.5 m unstretched, 10 cm = 39p

Velband® (J&J)
Absorbent padding, 4.5 m unstretched, 10 cm = 66p

A8.2.6 Extra-high performance compression bandages

These bandages are capable of applying pressures even higher than those of high compression bandages, therefore the same stringent warnings apply. Their use is reserved for the largest and most oedematous limbs. Extra-high performance compression bandages are poorly tolerated by patients.

Elastic Web Bandage, BP 1993
(Also termed Blue Line Webbing). Characteristic fabric woven ribbon fashion, warp threads of cotton and rubber with mid-line threads coloured blue, weft threads of cotton or combined cotton and viscose; may be dyed skin colour; with or without foot loop. Per m (both) 7.5 cm = 80p; 10 cm = £1.15; with foot loop (Drug Tariff specification 2a) 7.5 cm = £4.62
Uses provision of support and high compression over large surface

Elastic Web Bandage without Foot Loop
(Also termed Red Line Webbing) (Drug Tariff specification 2b) (Scott-Curwen). Characteristic fabric woven ribbon fashion, warp threads of cotton and rubber with mid-line threads coloured red, weft threads of cotton or combined cotton and viscose. 7.5 cm × 2.75 m (2.5 m unstretched) = £3.65; 7.5 cm × 3.75 m (3.5 m unstretched) = £4.41
Uses provision of support and high compression over large surfaces

Heavy Cotton and Rubber Elastic Bandage, BP 1993
Fabric, plain weave, warp of combined cotton and rubber threads, weft of cotton threads with one end folded as foot loop; fastener also supplied. 1.8 m unstretched × 7.5 cm = £12.40 (SSL—*Elastoweb*®).
Uses provision of high even compression over large surface

A8.2.7 Adhesive bandages

Elastic adhesive bandages are used to provide compression in the treatment of varicose veins and for the support of injured joints; they should no longer be used for the support of fractured ribs and clavicles. They have also been used with **zinc paste bandage** in the treatment of venous ulcers, but they can cause skin reactions in susceptible patients and may not produce sufficient pressures for healing (significantly lower than those provided by other compression bandages).

Elastic Adhesive Bandage, BP 1993
Woven fabric, elastic in warp (crepe-twisted cotton threads), weft of cotton and/or viscose threads spread with adhesive mass containing zinc oxide. 4.5 m stretched (all): 5 cm = £3.24; 7.5 cm = £4.59; 10 cm = £6.24 (Robinsons—*Flexoplast*®; S&N Hlth—*Elastoplast*® Bandage). 7.5 cm width supplied when size not stated
Uses compression for chronic leg ulcers; compression and support for swollen or sprained joints

A8.2.8 Cohesive bandages

Cohesive bandages adhere to themselves, but not to the skin, and are useful for providing support for sports use where ordinary stretch bandages might become displaced and adhesive bandages are inappropriate. Care is needed in their application, however, since the loss of ability for movement between turns of the bandage to equalise local areas of high tension carries the potential for creating a tourniquet effect. They should not be used if arterial disease is suspected.

Cohesive extensible bandages

These elastic bandages adhere to themselves and not to skin; this prevents slipping during use.

Uses: support of sprained joints; outer layer of multi-layer compression bandaging

Coban® (3M)

6 m (stretched), 10 cm = £2.76; other sizes [NHS] 4.5 m stretched (all): 2.5 cm = £1.29; 5 cm = £1.81; 7.5 cm = £2.74; 10 cm = £3.61; 15 cm = £5.33

K-Press® (Urgo)

6.5 m × 10 cm = £2.71, 7.5 m × 10 cm = £3.16

Profore® #4 (S&N Hlth.)

2.5 m (unstretched) = £2.92, latex-free = £3.17

Ultra Fast® (Robinsons)

6.3 m (stretched), 10 cm = £2.59

A8.2.9 Medicated bandages

Zinc Paste Bandage has been used with compression bandaging for the treatment of venous leg ulcers. However, zinc paste bandages are associated with hypersensitivity reactions and should be used with caution.

Zinc paste bandages are also used with **coal tar** or **ichthammol** in chronic lichenified skin conditions such as chronic eczema (ichthammol often being preferred since its action is considered to be milder). They are also used with **calamine** in milder eczematous skin conditions.

Zinc Paste Bandage, BP 1993

Cotton fabric, plain weave, impregnated with suitable paste containing zinc oxide; requires additional bandaging, 6 m × 7.5 cm = £3.23 (Medlock—*Zincaband®* (15%), *excipients: include* hydroxybenzoates); £3.28 (S&N Hlth—*Viscopaste PB7®* (10%), *excipients: include* hydroxybenzoates)

Zinc Paste and Calamine Bandage

(Drug Tariff specification 5). Cotton fabric, plain weave, impregnated with suitable paste containing calamine and zinc oxide; requires additional bandaging. 6 m × 7.5 cm = £3.33 (Medlock—*Calaband®*)

Zinc Paste and Ichthammol Bandage, BP 1993

Cotton fabric, plain weave, impregnated with suitable paste containing zinc oxide and ichthammol; requires additional bandaging, 6 m × 7.5 cm = £3.31 (Medlock—*Icthaband®* (15/2%), *excipients: include* hydroxybenzoates; S&N Hlth—*Ichthopaste®* (6/2%)

Excipients none as listed in section 13.1.3

Uses see section 13.5

Steripaste® (Medlock)

Cotton fabric, selvedge weave impregnated with paste containing zinc oxide (requires additional bandaging), 6 m × 7.5 cm = £3.24

Excipients include polysorbate 80

Medicated stocking

Zipzoc® (S&N Hlth.)

Sterile rayon stocking impregnated with ointment containing zinc oxide 20%. 4-pouch carton = £12.52; 10-pouch carton = £31.30

Uses chronic leg ulcers; can be used under appropriate compression bandages or hosiery in chronic venous insufficiency

A8.2.10 Multi-layer compression bandaging

Multi-layer compression bandaging systems are an alternative to High Compression Bandages (section A8.2.5) for the treatment of venous leg ulcers. Compression is achieved by the combined effects of two or three extensible bandages applied over a layer of orthopaedic wadding and a wound contact dressing.

Four layer systems

K-Four® (Urgo)

K-Four® Wound Dressing (*Paratex®*—see Knitted Viscose Primary Dressing, p. 858); *K-Four®* # 1 (*K-Soft®*—see Sub-compression Wadding Bandage, p. 863); *K-Four®* # 2 (*K-Lite®*—see Knitted Elastomer and Viscose Bandage, p. 862); *K-Four®* # 3 (*K-Plus®*—see Knitted Elastomer and Viscose Bandage, p. 862); *K-Four®* # 4 (*Ko-Flex®*), 6 m (stretched), 10 cm = £2.76; 7 m (stretched), 10 cm = £3.16

Multi-layer compression bandaging kit, four layer system, for ankle circumference 18–25 cm = £6.38

Profore® (S&N Hlth.)

Profore® wound contact layer (see Knitted Viscose Primary Dressing, p. 858); *Profore® #1* (see Sub-compression Wadding Bandage, p. 863); *Profore® #2* (see Cotton, Polyamide and Elastane Bandage, p. 862); *Profore® #3* (see Knitted Elastomer and Viscose Bandage, p. 862); *Profore® #4* (see Cohesive bandages, above); *Profore® Plus* 3 m (unstretched), 10 cm = £3.30, latex-free = £3.53

Multi-layer compression bandaging kit, four layer system, for ankle circumference up to 18 cm = £8.96, 18–25 cm = £8.35, 25–30 cm = £6.93, above 30 cm = £10.38, latex-free, 18–25 cm = £9.09; *Profore Lite®* above 18 cm = £4.91, latex-free = £5.34

System 4® (Medlock)

System 4® wound contact layer (*Setoprime®*—see Knitted Viscose Primary Dressing, p. 858); *System 4® #1* (*Softexe®*—see Sub-compression Wadding Bandage, p. 863); *System 4® #2* (*Setocrepe®*—see Cotton, Polyamide and Elastane Bandage, p. 862); *System 4® #3* (*Elset®*—see Knitted Elastomer and Viscose Bandage, p. 862); *System 4® #4* (*Coban®*—see Cohesive Bandages, above)

Multi-layer compression bandaging kit, four layer system, for ankle circumference 18–25 cm = £7.77

Ultra Four® (Robinsons)

Ultra Four® #1 (*Ultra Soft®*—see Sub-compression Wadding Bandage, p. 863); *Ultra Four® #2* (*Ultra Lite®*) 10 cm × 4.5 cm (stretched) = 85p; *Ultra Four® #3* (*Ultra Plus®*), 10 cm × 8.7 cm (stretched) = £1.89; *Ultra Four® #4* (*Ultra Fast®*—see Cohesive Bandages, above)

Multi-layer compression bandaging kit, four layer system, for ankle circumference up to 18 cm = £6.41, 18–25 cm = £5.67; *Ultra Four® RC* (reduced compression) 18–25 cm = £4.14

Two layer systems

Coban® (3M)

Multi-layer compression bandaging kit, two layer system (latex-free, foam bandage and cohesive compression bandage), one size = £8.08

K-Two® (Urgo)

K-Tech® (see Sub-compression Wadding Bandages, p. 863); *K-Press®* (see Cohesive Bandages, above)

Multi-layer compression bandaging kit, two layer system, standard lengths = £6.37, longer lengths = £7.55

ProGuide® (S&N Hlth.)

ProGuide® wound contact layer (see Low Adherence Dressing and Wound Contact Materials, p. 859); *ProGuide®* #1 (see Sub-compression Wadding Bandage, p. 863); *ProGuide®* #2 (see High Compression Bandages, p. 863)

Multi-layer compression bandaging kit, two layer system, for ankle circumference 18–22 cm (red) = £8.81; 22–28 cm (yellow) = £9.30; 28–32 cm (green) = £9.77

A8.2.11 Surgical adhesive tapes

Adhesive tapes are useful for retaining dressings on joints or awkward body parts. These tapes, particularly those containing rubber, can cause irritant and allergic reactions in susceptible patients; synthetic adhesives have been developed to overcome this problem, but they, too, may sometimes be associated with reactions. Adhesive tapes that are occlusive may cause skin maceration. Care is needed not to apply these tapes under tension, to avoid creating a tourniquet effect. If applied over joints they need to be orientated so that the area of maximum extensibility of the fabric is in the direction of movement of the limb.

Permeable adhesive tapes

Elastic Adhesive Tape, BP 1988
(Elastic Adhesive Plaster). Woven fabric, elastic in warp (crepe-twisted cotton threads), weft of cotton and/or viscose threads, spread with adhesive mass containing zinc oxide. 4.5 m stretched × 2.5 cm = £1.61 (Robinsons—*Flexoplast*®; S&N—*Elastoplast*®)

Uses securing dressings

For 5 cm width, see Elastic Adhesive Bandage

Permeable, Apertured Non-Woven Synthetic Adhesive Tape, BP 1988
Non-woven fabric with a polyacrylate adhesive.

Hypafix®, 10 m (all): 2.5 cm = £1.53, 5 cm = £2.44, 10 cm = £4.25, 15 cm = £6.30, 20 cm = £8.35, 30 cm = £12.07 (BSN Medical)

Mefix®, 5 m (all): 2.5 cm = 93p, 5 cm = £1.65; 10 cm = £2.63, 15 cm = £3.59, 20 cm = £4.60, 30 cm = £6.59 (Mölnlycke)

Omnifix®, 10 m (all): 5 cm = £2.15, 10 cm = £3.62, 15 cm = £5.34 (Hartmann)

Uses securing dressings

Permeable Non-woven Synthetic Adhesive Tape, BP 1988
Backing of paper-based or non-woven textile material spread with a polymeric adhesive mass, 5 m (all):

Clinipore®, 1.25 cm = 35p, 2.5 cm = 59p, 5 cm = 99p (Clinisupplies)

Leukofix®, 1.25 cm = 51p, 2.5 cm = 81p, 5 cm = £1.42 (BSN Medical)

Leukopor®, 1.25 cm = 45p, 2.5 cm = 70p, 5 cm = £1.23 (BSN Medical)

Mediplast®, 1.25 cm = 30p, 2.5 cm = 50p (Neomedic)

Micropore®, 1.25 cm = 60p, 2.5 cm = 89p, 5 cm = £1.57 (3M)

Scanpor®, 1.25 cm = 40p, 2.5 cm = 64p, 5 cm = £1.11; 10 m (all), 1.25 cm = 52p, 2.5 cm = 86p, 5 cm = £1.64, 7.5 cm = £2.40 (BioDiagnostics)

Where no brand stated by prescriber, net price of tape supplied not to exceed 35p (1.25 cm), 59p (2.5 cm), 99p (5 cm)

Uses securing dressings; skin closures for small incisions for patients with skin reactions to other plasters and strapping, which require use for long periods

Permeable Woven Synthetic Adhesive Tape, BP 1988
Non-extensible closely woven fabric, spread with a polymeric adhesive. 5 m (all): 1.25 cm = 75p; 2.5 cm = £1.10; 5 cm = £1.91 (Beiersdorf—*Leukosilk*®)

Uses securing dressings for patients with skin reactions to other plasters and strapping, which require use for long periods

Zinc Oxide Adhesive Tape, BP 1988
(Zinc Oxide Plaster). Fabric, plain weave, warp and weft of cotton and/or viscose, spread with an adhesive containing zinc oxide. 5 m (all): 1.25 cm = 91p; 2.5 cm = £1.32; 5 cm = £2.23; 7.5 cm = £3.35 (most suppliers)

Uses securing dressings and immobilising small areas

Mediplast® (Neomedic)
Zinc oxide adhesive tape, 5 m (all), 1.25 cm = 82p, 2.5 cm = £1.19, 5 cm = £1.99, 7.5 cm = £2.99

Mepitac® (Mölnlycke)
Soft silicone, water-resistant, knitted fabric, polyurethane film tape, 2 cm × 3 m = £6.26, 4 cm × 1.5 m = £6.26

Uses securing dressing and appliances, skin protection under devices

Strappal® (BSN Medical)
Zinc oxide adhesive tape. 5 m (all): 1.25 cm = 87p, 2.5 cm = £1.26, 5 cm = £2.13, 7.5 cm = £3.21; other sizes NHS

Occlusive adhesive tapes

Impermeable Plastic Adhesive Tape, BP 1988
Extensible water-impermeable plastic film spread with an adhesive mass. 2.5 cm × 3 m = £1.27; 2.5 cm × 5 m = £1.91; 5 cm × 5 m = £2.41; 7.5 cm × 5 m = £3.51 (Robinsons; Medlock—*Setoplast*®; S&N Hlth)

Uses securing dressings; covering site of infection where exclusion of air, water, and water vapour is required

Impermeable Plastic Synthetic Adhesive Tape, BP 1988
Extensible water-impermeable plastic film spread with a polymeric adhesive mass. 5 m (both): 2.5 cm = £1.72; 5 cm = £3.27 (3M—*Blenderm*®)

Uses isolating wounds from external environment; covering sites where total exclusion of water and water vapour required; securing dressings and appliances

A8.2.12 Adhesive dressings

Adhesive dressings (also termed 'island dressings') have a limited role for minor wounds only. The inclusion of an antiseptic is not particularly useful and may cause skin irritation in susceptible subjects.

Permeable adhesive dressings

Elastic Adhesive Dressing, BP 1993 NHS
Wound dressing or dressing strip, pad attached to piece of extension plaster, leaving suitable adhesive margin; both pad and margin covered with suitable protector; pad may be dyed yellow and may be impregnated with suitable antiseptic (see below); extension plaster may be perforated or ventilated

Uses general purpose wound dressing

Note Permitted antiseptics are aminoacridine hydrochloride (aminacrine hydrochloride) chlorhexidine hydrochloride (both 0.07–0.13%), chlorhexidine gluconate (0.11–0.20%); domiphen bromide (0.05–0.25%)

Permeable Plastic Wound Dressing, BP 1993 NHS
Consisting of an absorbent pad, which may be dyed and impregnated with a suitable antiseptic (see under Elastic Adhesive Dressing), attached to a piece of permeable plastic surgical adhesive tape, to leave a suitable adhesive margin; both pad and margin covered with suitable protector (most suppliers)

Uses general purpose wound dressing, permeable to air and water

Vapour permeable adhesive dressings

Vapour-permeable Waterproof Plastic Wound Dressing, BP 1993
(former Drug Tariff title: Semipermeable Waterproof Plastic Wound Dressing). Consists of absorbent pad, may be dyed and impregnated with suitable antiseptic (see under Elastic Adhesive Dressing), attached to piece of semi-permeable waterproof surgical adhesive tape, to leave suitable adhesive margin; both pad and margin covered with suitable protector.(S&N Hlth—*Elastoplast Airstrip*®)

Uses general purpose waterproof wound dressing, permeable to air and water vapour

Occlusive adhesive dressings

Impermeable Plastic Wound Dressing, BP 1993 NHS
Consists of absorbent pad, may be dyed and impregnated with suitable antiseptic (see under Elastic Adhesive Dressing), attached to piece of impermeable plastic surgical adhesive tape, to leave suitable adhesive margin; both pad and margin covered with suitable protector (most suppliers)

Uses protective covering for wounds requiring an occlusive dressing

A8.2.13 Skin closure dressings

Skin closure strips are used as an alternative to sutures for minor cuts and lacerations.

Skin closure strips, sterile

Leukostrip®, 6.4 mm × 76 mm, 3 strips per envelope. 10 envelopes = £5.68 (S&N Hlth.)

Steri-strip®, 6 mm × 75 mm, 3 strips per envelope. 12 envelopes = £8.52; (NHS) 3 mm × 75 mm, 12 envelopes = £8.32; 12 mm × 100 mm, 12 envelopes = £8.52 (3M)

Drug Tariff specifies that these are specifically for personal administration by the prescriber

A8.3 Elastic hosiery

Before elastic hosiery can be dispensed, the quantity (single or pair), article (including accessories), and compression class (I, II or III)[1] must be specified by the prescriber; all dispensed articles must state on the packaging that they conform with Drug Tariff technical specification No. 40, for further details see Drug Tariff.

Note Graduated compression tights are (NHS)

A8.3.1 Graduated compression hosiery

Class 1[1] Light Support

Hosiery, compression at ankle 14–17 mmHg, thigh length or below knee with knitted in heel. 1 pair, circular knit (standard), thigh length = £7.28, below knee = £6.65; light weight elastic net (made-to-measure), thigh length = £19.49, below knee = £15.21

Uses superficial or early varices, varicosis during pregnancy

Class 2[1] Medium Support

Hosiery, compression at ankle 18–24 mmHg, thigh length or below knee with knitted in heel. 1 pair, circular knit (standard), thigh length = £10.82, below knee = £9.72, (made-to-measure), thigh length = £36.14, below knee = £22.61; net (made-to-measure), thigh length = £19.49, below knee = £15.21; flat bed (made-to-measure, only with closed heel and open toe), thigh length = £36.14, below knee = £22.61

Uses varices of medium severity, ulcer treatment and prophylaxis, mild oedema, varicosis during pregnancy

Class 3[1] Strong Support

Hosiery, compression at ankle 25–35 mmHg, thigh length or below knee with open or knitted in heel. 1 pair, circular knit (standard), thigh length = £12.82, below knee = £11.02, (made-to-measure) thigh length = £36.14, below knee = £22.61; flat bed (made-to-measure, only with open heel and open toe), thigh length = £36.14, below knee = £22.61

Uses gross varices, post thrombotic venous insufficiency, gross oedema, ulcer treatment and prophylaxis

A8.3.2 Accessories

Suspender

Suspender, for thigh stockings = 63p, belt (specification 13), = £4.85, fitted (additional price) = 62p

1. Graduated compression hosiery is classified according to British Standard compression values; these values are different to the compression values used for classification of lymphoedema garments.

A8.3.3 Anklets

Class 2[1] Medium Support

Anklets, compression 18–24 mmHg, circular knit (standard and made-to-measure), 1 pair = £6.37; flat bed (standard and made-to-measure) = £13.23; made-to-measure = £12.52

Uses soft tissue support

Class 3[1] Strong Support

Anklets, compression 25–35 mmHg, circular knit (standard and made-to-measure), 1 pair = £8.72; flat bed (standard) = £8.89; made-to-measure = £13.23

Uses soft tissue support

A8.3.4 Knee caps

Class 2[1] Medium Support

Kneecaps, compression 18–24 mmHg, circular knit (standard and made-to-measure), 1 pair = £6.37; flat bed (standard and made-to-measure) = £13.23; net made-to-measure = £10.40

Uses soft tissue support

Class 3[1] Strong Support

Kneecaps, compression 25–35 mmHg, circular knit (standard and made-to-measure), 1 pair = £8.49; flat bed (standard) = £8.49; made-to-measure = £13.23

Uses soft tissue support

A8.3.5 Lymphoedema garments

Low Compression

Armsleeves (with grip top), compression 12–16 mmHg, small, medium, and large sizes all available short or long, 1 pair = £16.70

Class 1[1] Light support

Hosiery and armsleeves, compression 18–21 mmHg, small, medium, large, and extra large (hosiery only) sizes all available standard length (some available petite), 1 pair below knee closed toe (no top band) = £25.50, thigh closed toe (with top band) = £49.00; 1 piece armsleeve (no top band) = £13.50, armsleeve (with top band) = £18.00, combined armsleeve (no top band) = £24.50, combined armsleeve (with top band) = £29.00

Armsleeves (with grip top), compression 18–22 mmHg, small, medium, and large sizes all available short or long, 1 pair = £16.70

Class 2[1] Medium support

Hosiery and armsleeves, compression 23–32 mmHg, small, medium, large, and extra large (hosiery only) sizes all available standard length (some available petite), 1 pair below knee closed or open toe (no top band) = £25.50, thigh closed or open toe (with top band) = £49.00; 1 piece armsleeve (no top band) = £14.50, armsleeve (with top band) = £19.00, combined armsleeve (no top band) = £25.50, combined armsleeve (with top band) = £30.00

Class 3[1] Strong support

Hosiery, compression 34–46 mmHg, small, medium, large, and extra large sizes all available standard length (some available petite), 1 pair below knee open toe (no top band) = £28.00, thigh open toe (with top band) = £51.00

Note Made-to-measure garments up to compression 90 mmHg and accessories also available; see Drug Tariff for details

A9 Cautionary and advisory labels for dispensed medicines

Numbers following the preparation entries in the BNF correspond to the code numbers of the cautionary labels that pharmacists are recommended to add when dispensing. It is also expected that pharmacists will counsel patients when necessary.

Counselling needs to be related to the age, experience, background, and understanding of the individual patient. The pharmacist should ensure that the patient understands how to take or use the medicine and how to follow the correct dosage schedule. Any effects of the medicine on driving or work, any foods or medicines to be avoided, and what to do if a dose is missed should also be explained. Other matters, such as the possibility of staining of the clothes or skin by a medicine should also be mentioned.

For some preparations there is a special need for counselling, such as an unusual method or time of administration or a potential interaction with a common food or domestic remedy, and this is indicated where necessary.

Original packs Most preparations are now dispensed in unbroken original packs (see Patient Packs, p. x) that include further advice for the patient in the form of patient information leaflets. Label 10 may be of value where appropriate. More general leaflets advising on the administration of preparations such as eye drops, eye ointments, inhalers, and suppositories are also available.

Scope of labels In general no label recommendations have been made for injections on the assumption that they will be administered by a healthcare professional or a well-instructed patient. The labelling is not exhaustive and pharmacists are recommended to use their professional discretion in labelling new preparations and those for which no labels are shown.

Individual labelling advice is not given on the administration of the large variety of antacids. In the absence of instructions from the prescriber, and if on enquiry the patient has had no verbal instructions, the directions given under 'Dose' should be used on the label.

It is recognised that there may be occasions when pharmacists will use their knowledge and professional discretion and decide to omit one or more of the recommended labels for a particular patient. In this case counselling is of the utmost importance. There may also be an occasion when a prescriber does not wish additional cautionary labels to be used, in which case the prescription should be endorsed 'NCL' (no cautionary labels). The exact wording that is required instead should then be specified on the prescription.

Pharmacists label medicines with various wordings in addition to those directions specified on the prescription. Such labels include 'Shake the bottle', 'For external use only', and 'Store in a cool place', as well as 'Discard . . . days after opening' and 'Do not use after . . . .', which apply particularly to antibiotic mixtures, diluted liquid and topical preparations, and to eye-drops. Although not listed in the BNF these labels should continue to be used when appropriate; indeed, 'For external use only' is a legal requirement on external liquid preparations, while 'Keep out of the reach of children' is a legal requirement on all dispensed medicines. Care should be taken not to obscure other relevant information with adhesive labelling.

It is the usual practice for patients to take standard tablets with water or other liquid and for this reason no separate label has been recommended.

The label wordings recommended by the BNF apply to medicines dispensed against a prescription. Patients should be aware that a dispensed medicine should never be taken by, or shared with, anyone other than for whom the prescriber intended it. Therefore, the BNF does not include warnings against the use of a dispensed medicine by persons other than for whom it was specifically prescribed.

The label or labels for each preparation are recommended after careful consideration of the information available. However, it is recognised that in some cases this information may be either incomplete or open to a different interpretation. The Executive Editor will therefore be grateful to receive any constructive comments on the labelling suggested for any preparation.

Recommended label wordings

Wordings which can be given as separate warnings are labels 1-19 and labels 29-33. Wordings which can be incorporated in an appropriate position in the directions for dosage or administration are labels 21-28. A label has been omitted for number 20.

If separate labels are used it is recommended that the wordings be used without modification. If changes are made to suit computer requirements, care should be taken to retain the sense of the original.

1 **Warning. May cause drowsiness**
To be used on *preparations for children* containing antihistamines, or other preparations given to children where the warnings of label 2 on driving or alcohol would not be appropriate.

2 **Warning. May cause drowsiness. If affected do not drive or operate machinery. Avoid alcoholic drink**
To be used on *preparations for adults that can cause drowsiness*, thereby affecting the ability to drive and operate hazardous machinery; label 1 is more appropriate for children. *It is an offence to drive while under the influence of drink or drugs.*

Some of these preparations only cause drowsiness in the first few days of treatment and some only cause drowsiness in higher doses.

In such cases the patient should be told that the advice applies until the effects have worn off. However many of these preparations can produce a slowing of reaction time and a loss of mental concentration that can have the same effects as drowsiness.

Avoidance of alcoholic drink is recommended because the effects of CNS depressants are enhanced by alcohol. Strict prohibition however could lead to some patients not taking the medicine. Pharmacists should therefore explain the risk and encourage compliance, particularly in patients who may think they already tolerate the effects of alcohol (see also label 3).

Queries from patients with epilepsy regarding fitness to drive should be referred back to the patient's doctor.

Side-effects unrelated to drowsiness that may affect a patient's ability to drive or operate machinery safely include *blurred vision, dizziness, or nausea*. In general, no label has been recommended to cover these cases, but the patient should be suitably counselled.

3 Warning. May cause drowsiness. If affected do not drive or operate machinery

To be used on *preparations containing monoamine-oxidase inhibitors*; the warning to avoid alcohol and dealcoholised (low alcohol) drink is covered by the patient information leaflet.

Also to be used as for label 2 but where alcohol is not an issue.

4 Warning. Avoid alcoholic drink

To be used on *preparations where a reaction such as flushing may occur if alcohol is taken* (e.g. metronidazole and chlorpropamide). Alcohol may also enhance the hypoglycaemia produced by some oral antidiabetic drugs but routine application of a warning label is not considered necessary.

5 Do not take indigestion remedies at the same time of day as this medicine

To be used with label 25 on *preparations coated to resist gastric acid* (e.g. enteric-coated tablets). This is to avoid the possibility of premature dissolution of the coating in the presence of an alkaline pH.

Label 5 also applies to drugs such as ketoconazole *where the absorption is significantly affected by antacids*; the usual period of avoidance recommended is 2 to 4 hours.

6 Do not take indigestion remedies or medicines containing iron or zinc at the same time of day as this medicine

To be used on *preparations containing ofloxacin and some other quinolones, doxycycline, lymecycline, minocycline, and penicillamine*. These drugs chelate calcium, iron and zinc and are less well absorbed when taken with calcium-containing antacids or preparations containing iron or zinc. These incompatible preparations should be taken 2-3 hours apart.

7 Do not take milk, indigestion remedies, or medicines containing iron or zinc at the same time of day as this medicine

To be used on *preparations containing ciprofloxacin, norfloxacin or tetracyclines that chelate calcium, iron, magnesium, and zinc* and are thus less available for absorption; these incompatible preparations should be taken 2-3 hours apart. Doxycycline, lymecycline and minocycline are less liable to form chelates and therefore only require label 6 (see above).

8 Do not stop taking this medicine except on your doctor's advice

To be used on *preparations that contain a drug which is required to be taken over long periods without the patient necessarily perceiving any benefit* (e.g. antituberculous drugs).

Also to be used on *preparations that contain a drug whose withdrawal is likely to be a particular hazard* (e.g. clonidine for hypertension). Label 10 (see below) is more appropriate for corticosteroids.

9 Take at regular intervals. Complete the prescribed course unless otherwise directed

To be used on *preparations where a course of treatment should be completed* to reduce the incidence of relapse or failure of treatment.

The preparations are antimicrobial drugs given by mouth. Very occasionally, some may have severe side-effects (e.g. diarrhoea in patients receiving clindamycin) and in such cases the patient may need to be advised of reasons for stopping treatment quickly and returning to the doctor.

10 Warning. Follow the printed instructions you have been given with this medicine

To be used particularly on *preparations containing anticoagulants, lithium and oral corticosteroids*. The appropriate treatment card should be given to the patient and any necessary explanations given.

This label may also be used on other preparations to remind the patient of the instructions that have been given.

11 Avoid exposure of skin to direct sunlight or sun lamps

To be used on *preparations that may cause phototoxic or photoallergic reactions* if the patient is exposed to ultraviolet radiation. Many drugs other than those listed in Appendix 9 (e.g. phenothiazines and sulphonamides) may, on rare occasions, cause reactions in susceptible patients. Exposure to high intensity ultraviolet radiation from sunray lamps and sunbeds is particularly likely to cause reactions.

12 Do not take anything containing aspirin while taking this medicine

To be used on *preparations containing probenecid and sulfinpyrazone* whose activity is reduced by aspirin.

Label 12 should not be used for anticoagulants since label 10 is more appropriate.

13 Dissolve or *mix with water* before taking

To be used on *preparations that are intended to be dissolved in water* (e.g. soluble tablets) or *mixed with water* (e.g. powders, granules) before use. In a few cases other liquids such as fruit juice or milk may be used.

14 This medicine may colour the urine

To be used on *preparations that may cause the patient's urine to turn an unusual colour*. These include phenolphthalein (alkaline urine pink), triamterene (blue under some lights), levodopa (dark reddish), and rifampicin (red).

15 Caution flammable: keep away from fire or flames

To be used on *preparations containing sufficient flammable solvent to render them flammable if exposed to a naked flame*.

16 Allow to dissolve under the tongue. Do not transfer from this container. Keep tightly closed. Discard eight weeks after opening

To be used on *glyceryl trinitrate tablets* to remind the patient not to transfer the tablets to plastic or less suitable containers.

17 Do not take more than . . . in 24 hours

To be used on *preparations for the treatment of acute migraine* except those containing ergotamine, for which label 18 is used. The dose form should be specified, e.g. tablets or capsules.

It may also be used on preparations for which no dose has been specified by the prescriber.

18 Do not take more than . . . in 24 hours or . . . in any one week

To be used on preparations containing ergotamine. The dose form should be specified, e.g. tablets or suppositories.

19 Warning. Causes drowsiness which may continue the next day. If affected do not drive or operate machinery. Avoid alcoholic drink

To be used on *preparations containing hypnotics (or some other drugs with sedative effects) prescribed to be taken at night*. On the rare occasions (e.g. nitrazepam in epilepsy) when hypnotics are prescribed for

daytime administration this label would clearly not be appropriate. Also to be used as an *alternative to the label 2 wording* (the choice being at the discretion of the pharmacist) *for anxiolytics prescribed to be taken at night.*
It is hoped that this wording will convey adequately the problem of residual morning sedation after taking 'sleeping tablets'.

21 . . . with or after food
To be used on *preparations that are liable to cause gastric irritation, or those that are better absorbed with food.*
Patients should be advised that a *small amount of food is sufficient.*

22 . . . half to one hour before food
To be used on some preparations *whose absorption is thereby improved.*
Most oral antibacterials require label 23 instead (see below).

23 . . . an hour before food or on an empty stomach
To be used on *oral preparations whose absorption may be reduced by the presence of food and acid in the stomach.*

24 . . . sucked or chewed
To be used on *preparations that should be sucked or chewed.*
The pharmacist should use discretion as to which of these words is appropriate.

25 . . . swallowed whole, not chewed
To be used on *preparations that are enteric-coated or designed for modified-release.*
Also to be used on *preparations that taste very unpleasant or may damage the mouth* if not swallowed whole.

26 . . . dissolved under the tongue
To be used on *preparations designed for sublingual use.* Patients should be advised to hold under the tongue and avoid swallowing until dissolved. The buccal mucosa between the gum and cheek is occasionally specified by the prescriber.

27 . . . with plenty of water
To be used on *preparations that should be well diluted* (e.g. chloral hydrate), *where a high fluid intake is required* (e.g. sulphonamides), or *where water is required to aid the action* (e.g. methylcellulose). The patient should be advised that 'plenty' means at least 150 mL (about a tumblerful). In most cases fruit juice, tea, or coffee may be used.

28 To be spread thinly . . .
To be used on *external preparations* that should be applied sparingly (e.g. corticosteroids, dithranol).

29 Do not take more than 2 at any one time. Do not take more than 8 in 24 hours
To be used on containers of dispensed *solid dose preparations containing paracetamol for adults when the instruction on the label indicates that the dose can be taken on an 'as required' basis.* The dose form should be specified, e.g. tablets or capsules.
This label has been introduced because of the serious consequences of overdosage with paracetamol.

30 Do not take with any other paracetamol products
To be used on all containers of dispensed *preparations containing paracetamol.*

31 Contains aspirin and paracetamol. Do not take with any other paracetamol products
To be used on all containers of dispensed *preparations containing aspirin and paracetamol.*

32 Contains aspirin
To be used on containers of dispensed *preparations containing aspirin when the name on the label does not include the word 'aspirin'.*

33 Contains an aspirin-like medicine
To be used on containers of dispensed *preparations containing aspirin derivatives.*

Products and their labels

Products introduced or amended since publication of BNF No. 54 (September 2007) are underlined.
Proprietary names are in *italic.*
C = counselling advised; see BNF = consult product entry in BNF

Abacavir, C, hypersensitivity reactions, see BNF
***Abilify*, 2**
Acamprosate, 21, 25
Acarbose, C, administration, see BNF
***Accolate*, 23**
Acebutolol, 8
Aceclofenac, 21
Acemetacin, 21, C, driving
Acenocoumarol, 10, anti-coagulant card
Acetazolamide, 3
Acetazolamide m/r, 3, 25
Aciclovir susp and tabs, 9
Acipimox, 21
Acitretin, 10, patient information leaflet, 21
***Acomplia*, C, depression, see BNF**
***Actinac*, 28**
***Actiq*, 2**
***Actonel*, C, administration, food and calcium, see BNF**
***Acupan*, 2, 14, (urine pink)**
***Adalat LA*, 25**
***Adalat Retard*, 25**
Adalimumab, C, tuberculosis
***Adcal*, 24**
***Adcal-D_3*, 24**
***Adcal-D_3 Dissolve*, 13**
***Adcortyl with Graneodin*, 23**
***Adipine MR*, 21, 25**
***Adipine XL*, 25**
***Adizem preps*, 25**
***Advagraf*, 23, 25, C, driving, see BNF**
***AeroBec*, 8, C, dose**
***AeroBec Forte*, 8, 10, steroid card, C, dose**
***Agenerase caps*, 5**
***Agenerase oral solution*, 4, 5**
***Airomir*, C, dose, change to CFC-free inhaler, see BNF**
Albendazole, 9
Alclometasone external preps, 28
***Aldactone*, 21**
***Aldara*, 10, patient information leaflet**
***Aldomet*, 3, 8**
Alendronic acid, C, administration, see BNF
Alfuzosin, 3, C, dose, see BNF
Alfuzosin m/r, 3, 21, 25, C, dose, see BNF
Alimemazine, 2
Aliskiren, 21
***Allegron*, 2**
Allopurinol, 8, 21, 27
***Almogran*, 3**
Almotriptan, 3
***Alphosyl HC*, 28**
***Alphaderm*, 28**
Alprazolam, 2
***Alvedon*, 30**
***Alvesco*, 8, C, dose**
Amantadine, C, driving
Aminophylline m/r, see preps
Amiodarone, 11
Amisulpride, 2
Amitriptyline, 2
Amitriptyline m/r, 2, 25
Amobarbital sodium, 19

Amorolfine, 10, patient information leaflet
Amoxicillin, 9
Amoxicillin chewable tabs, 9, 10, patient information leaflet
Amoxicillin dispersible sachets, 9, 13
Amoxil, 9
Amoxil dispersible sachets, 9, 13
Amoxil paed susp, 9, C, use of pipette
Amphotericin loz, 9, 24, C, after food
Amphotericin tabs, 9
Ampicillin, 9, 23
Amprenavir caps, 5
Amprenavir oral solution, 4, 5
Anafranil, 2
Anafranil m/r, 2, 25
Anagrelide, C, driving
Anakinra, C, blood disorder symptoms
Androcur, 21
Andropatch, C, administration, see BNF
Angettes-75, 32
Angitil SR, 25
Angitil XL, 25
Anhydrol Forte, 15
Anquil, 2
Antabuse, 2, C, alcohol reaction, see BNF
Antacids, see BNF dose statements
Antepsin, 5
Anthranol preps, 28
Anticoagulants, oral, 10, anticoagulant card
Antihistamines, (see individual preparations)
Anturan, 12, 21
Aptivus, 5, 21
Arava, 4
Aricept Evess, C, administration
Aripiprazole, 2
Arlevert, 2
Aromasin, 21
Arpicolin, C, driving
Artane, C, before or after food, driving, see BNF
Artemether with lumefantrine, 21, C, driving
Arythmol, 21, 25
Arthrotec, 21, 25
Asacol MR tabs, 5, 25, C, blood disorder symptoms, see BNF
Asacol enema and supps, C, blood disorder symptoms, see BNF
Asasantin Retard, 21, 25
Ascorbic acid, effervescent, 13
Ascorbic acid tabs (500mg), 24
Asmabec preps, 8, 10, steroid card (high-dose preparations only), C, dose
Asmanex, 8, 10, steroid card, C, dose
Asmasal, C, dose, see BNF
Aspav, 2, 13, 21, 32
Aspirin and papaveretum dispersible tabs, 2, 13, 21, also 32 (if 'aspirin' not on label)
Aspirin dispersible tabs, 13, 21, also 32 (if 'aspirin' not on label)
Aspirin effervescent, 13, also 32 (if 'aspirin' not on label)
Aspirin e/c, 5, 25, also 32 (if 'aspirin' not on label)
Aspirin m/r, 25, also 32 (if 'aspirin' not on label)
Aspirin supps, 32, (if 'aspirin' not on label)
Aspirin tabs, 21, also 32 (if 'aspirin' not on label)
Aspirin, paracetamol and codeine tabs, 21, 29, also 31 (if 'aspirin' and 'paracetamol' not on label)
Atarax, 2
Atazanavir, 5, 21
Atenolol, 8
Atomoxetine, 3
Atorvastatin, C, muscle effects, see BNF
Atovaquone, 21
Atripla, 23, 25
Atrovent inhalations, C, dose, see BNF
Augmentin susp and tabs, 9
Augmentin Duo, 9
Augmentin dispersible tabs, 9, 13
Auranofin, 21, C, blood disorder symptoms, see BNF
Aureocort, 28
Avandamet, 21
Avelox, 6, 9, C, driving
Avloclor, 5, C, malaria prophylaxis, see BNF
Avodart, 25
Avomine, 2
Azathioprine, 21
Azithromycin caps, 5, 9, 23
Azithromycin susp and tabs, 5, 9

Baclofen, 2, 8
Balsalazide, 21, 25
Baraclude, C, administration
Baratol, 2
Baxan, 9
Beclazone, 8, 10, steroid card (250-microgram only), C, dose
Beclometasone inhalations, 8, 10, steroid card (high-dose preparations only), C, dose
Becodisks, 8, 10, steroid card (high-dose preparation only), C, dose
Benemid, 12, 21, 27
Benperidol, 2
Benzatropine, 2
Benzoin tincture, cpd, 15
Beta-Adalat, 8, 25
Betacap, 15, 28
Beta-Cardone, 8
Betahistine, 21
Betaloc-SA, 8, 25
Betamethasone inj, 10, steroid card
Betamethasone soluble tab, 10, steroid card, 13, 21, (when used as a mouthwash, Label: 10, 13, C, administration)
Betamethasone tab, 10, steroid card, 21
Betamethasone external preps, 28
Betamethasone scalp application, 15, 28
Bethanechol, 22
Betim, 8
Betnelan, 10, steroid card, 21
Betnesol injection, 10, steroid card
Betnesol tabs, 10, steroid card, 13, 21, (when used as a mouthwash, Label: 10, 13, C, administration)
Betnovate external preps, 28
Betnovate scalp application, 15, 28
Betnovate-RD, 28
Bettamousse, 28
Bezafibrate, 21
Bezafibrate m/r, 21, 25
Bezalip, 21
Bezalip-Mono, 21, 25
Biorphen, C, driving
Bisacodyl tabs, 5, 25
Bisoprolol, 8
Bondronat tabs, C, administration, see BNF
Bonefos caps and tabs, C, food and calcium, see BNF
Bonviva tabs, C, administration, see BNF
Brexidol, 21
Bricanyl inhalations, C, dose, see BNF
Bricanyl SA, 25
Britlofex, 2
Broflex, C, driving, see BNF
Bromocriptine, 21, C, hypotensive reactions, see BNF
Brufen, 21
Brufen gran, 13, 21
Brufen Retard, 25, 27
Buccastem, 2, C, administration, see BNF
Budenofalk, 5, 10, steroid card, 22, 25
Budesonide inhalations, 8, 10, steroid card (high-dose preparations only), C, dose
Budesonide caps, 5, 10, steroid card, 22, 25
Budesonide m/r caps, 5, 10, steroid card, 25
Buprenorphine, 2, 26
Bupropion, 25, C, driving
Buserelin nasal spray, C, nasal decongestants, see BNF
Buspar, C, driving
Buspirone, C, driving
Butobarbital, 19
BuTrans, 2
Byetta, C, administration, see BNF

Cabaser, 21, C, driving, hypotensive reactions, see BNF
Cabergoline, 21, C, driving, hypotensive reactions, see BNF
Cacit, 13
Cacit D3, 13
Cafergot, 18, C, dosage
Calceos, 24
Calcicard CR, 25
Calcichew preps, 24
Calcisorb, 13, 21, C, may be sprinkled on food
Calcium-500, 25
Calcium acetate tabs, 21, 25
Calcium carbonate tabs, chewable, 24
Calcium carbonate tabs and gran effervescent, 13
Calcium gluconate tabs, 24
Calcium phosphate sachets, 13
Calcium Resonium, 13
Calcium and ergocalciferol tabs, C, administration, see BNF
Calcort, 5, 10, steroid card
Calfovit D3, 13, 21
Calmurid HC, 28
Calpol susp, 30
Camcolit 250 tabs, 10, lithium card, C, fluid and salt intake, see BNF
Camcolit 400 tabs, 10, lithium card, 25, C, fluid and salt intake, see BNF
Campral EC, 21, 25
Canesten HC, 28
Canesten spray, 15
Capecitabine, 21
Caprin, 5, 25, 32
Carbaglu, 13
Carbamazepine chewable, 3, 8, 21, 24, C, blood, hepatic or skin disorder symptoms (see BNF), driving (see BNF)
Carbamazepine liq, supps and tabs, 3, 8, C, blood, hepatic or skin disorder symptoms (see BNF), driving (see BNF)
Carbamazepine m/r, 3, 8, 25, C, blood, hepatic or skin disorder symptoms (see BNF), driving (see BNF)
Carbimazole, C, blood disorder symptoms, see BNF
Cardene SR, 25
Cardilate MR, 25
Cardinol, 8
Cardura XL, 25
Carglumic acid, 13
Carisoma, 2
Carisoprodol, 2
Carvedilol, 8
Catapres, 3, 8
Cedocard Retard, 25
Cefaclor, 9
Cefaclor m/r, 9, 21, 25
Cefadroxil, 9
Cefalexin, 9
Cefixime, 9
Cefpodoxime, 5, 9, 21

Cefradine, 9
Cefuroxime susp, 9, 21
Cefuroxime sachets, 9, 13, 21
Cefuroxime tab, 9, 21, 25
Celance, C, driving, hypotensive reactions, see BNF
Celectol, 8, 22
Celevac (constipation or diarrhoea), C, administration, see BNF
Celevac tabs (anorectic), C, administration, see BNF
Celiprolol, 8, 22
Centyl K, 25, 27, C, posture, see BNF
Ceporex caps, mixts, and tabs, 9
Cerivastatin, C, muscle effects, see BNF
Cetirizine, C, driving, alcohol, see BNF
Chemydur 60XL, 25
Chloral hydrate, 19, 27
Chloral paed elixir, 1, 27
Chloral mixt, 19, 27
Chlordiazepoxide, 2
Chloroquine, 5, C, malaria prophylaxis, see BNF
Chlorphenamine, 2
Chlorpromazine mixts and supps, 2, 11
Chlorpromazine tabs, 2, 11
Chlorpropamide, 4
Cholera vaccine (oral), C, administration
Cholestagel, 21
Ciclesonide, 8, C, dose
Ciclosporin, C, administration, see BNF
Cimetidine chewable tabs, C, administration, see BNF
Cinacalcet, 21
Cinnarizine, 2
Cipralex drops, C, driving, administration
Cipralex tabs, C, driving
Cipramil drops, C, driving, administration
Cipramil tabs, C, driving
Ciprofloxacin, 7, 9, 25, C, driving
Ciproxin susp and tabs, 7, 9, 25, C, driving
Citalopram drops, C, driving, administration
Citalopram tabs, C, driving
CitraFleet, 10, patient information leaflet, 13, C, administration
Citramag, 10, patient information leaflet, 13, C, administration
Clarelux, 15, 28
Clarithromycin, 9
Clarithromycin m/r, 9, 21, 25
Clarithromycin sachets, 9, 13
Clarithromycin straws, 9, C, administration
Clarosip, 9, C, administration
Clemastine, 2
Clenil Modulite, 8, 10, steroid card (high-dose preparations only), C, dose

Clindamycin, 9, 27, C, diarrhoea, see BNF
Clinoril, 21
Clipper, 25
Clobazam, 2 or 19, 8, C, driving (see BNF)
Clobetasol external preps, 28
Clobetasol scalp application, 15, 28
Clofazimine, 8, 14, (urine red), 21
Clomethiazole, 19
Clomipramine, 2
Clomipramine m/r, 2, 25
Clonazepam, 2, 8, C, driving (see BNF)
Clonidine, *see Catapres*
Clopixol, 2
Clotrimazole spray, 15
Clozapine, 2, 10, patient information leaflet
Clozaril, 2, 10, patient information leaflet
Coal tar paint, 15
Co-amoxiclav, 9
Co-amoxiclav dispersible tabs, 9, 13
Cobadex, 28
Co-beneldopa, 14, (urine reddish), C, driving
Co-beneldopa dispersible tabs, 14, (urine reddish), C, administration, driving, see BNF
Co-beneldopa m/r, 14, (urine reddish), 25, C, driving
Co-careldopa, 14, (urine reddish), C, driving
Co-careldopa intestinal gel, 14, (urine reddish), C, driving
Co-careldopa m/r, 14, (urine reddish), 25, C, driving
Co-codamol, see preps
Co-codaprin dispersible tabs, 13, 21, 32
Codalax, 14, (urine red)
Co-danthramer, 14, (urine red)
Co-danthrusate, 14, (urine red)
Codeine phosphate linctus, syr and tabs, 2
Codipar, 2, 29, 30
Co-dydramol, 21, 29, 30
Co-fluampicil, 9, 22
Cogentin, 2
Colazide, 21, 25
Colesevelam, 21
Colestid, 13, C, avoid other drugs at same time, see BNF
Colestipol preps, 13, C, avoid other drugs at same time, see BNF
Colestyramine, 13, C, avoid other drugs at same time, see BNF
Collodion, flexible, 15
Colofac, C, administration, see BNF
Colofac MR, 25, C, administration, see BNF
Colpermin, 5, 22, 25
Co-methiamol, 29, 30
Competact, 21

Comtess, 14, (urine reddish-brown), C, driving, avoid iron-containing preparations at the same time of day
Concerta XL, 25
Condyline, 15
Convulex, 8, 25, C, blood or hepatic disorder symptoms (see BNF), driving (see BNF)
Copegus, 21
Co-prenozide, 8, 25
Coracten preps, 25
Cordarone X, 11
Corgard, 8
Corticosteroid external preps, 28
Corticosteroid tabs, 10, steroid card, 21
Corticosteroid injections (systemic), 10, steroid card
Cortisone tab, 10, steroid card, 21
Cosalgesic, 2, 10, patient information leaflet, 29, 30
Co-tenidone, 8
Co-triamterzide, 14, (urine blue in some lights), 21
Co-trimoxazole susp and tabs, 9
Co-trimoxazole dispersible tabs, 9, 13
Coversyl, 22
Coversyl Plus, 22
Creon preps, C, administration, see BNF
Crixivan, 27, C, administration, see BNF
Cuplex, 15
Cyclizine, 2
Cyclophosphamide, 23, 25, 27
Cycloserine caps, 2, 8
Cymbalta, 2
Cymevene, 21
Cyproheptadine, 2
Cyprostat, 21
Cyproterone, 21
Cystrin, 3
Cytotec, 21

Daktacort, 28
Daktarin oral gel, 9, C, hold in mouth, after food
Dalacin C, 9, 27, C, diarrhoea, see BNF
Dalmane, 19
Dantrium, 2
Dantrolene, 2
Dapsone, 8
Darifenacin m/r, 3, 25
Darunavir, 21, C, missed dose, see BNF
Dasatinib, 25
DDAVP Melt, 26, C, fluid intake, see BNF
DDAVP tabs and intranasal, C, fluid intake, see BNF
Deferasirox, 13, 22
Deferiprone, 14, C, blood disorders
Deflazacort, 5, 10, steroid card
Deltacortril e/c, 5, 10, steroid card, 25
Deltastab inj, 10, steroid card
Demeclocycline, 7, 9, 11, 23
De-Noltab, C, administration, see BNF
Denzapine, 2, 10, patient information leaflet
Depakote, 25
Depixol, 2
Depo-Medrone (systemic), 10, steroid card
Dermestril, C, administration, see BNF
Dermovate cream and oint, 28
Dermovate scalp application, 15, 28
Deseril, 2, 21
DesmoMelt, 26, C, fluid intake, see BNF
Desmopressin sublingual tabs, 26, C, fluid intake, see BNF
Desmopressin tabs and intranasal, C, fluid intake, see BNF
Desmospray, C, fluid intake, see BNF
Desmotabs, C, fluid intake, see BNF
Destolit, 21
Detrunorm, 3
Detrunorm XL, 3, 25
Detrusitol, 3
Detrusitol XL, 3, 25
Dexamethasone inj, 10, steroid card
Dexamethasone tabs and solution, 10, steroid card, 21
Dexamfetamine, C, driving
Dexedrine, C, driving
Dexibuprofen, 21
Dexketoprofen, 22
DF118 Forte, 2, 21
DHC Continus, 2, 25
Diamicron MR, 25
Diamorphine preps, 2
Diamox tabs, 3
Diamox SR, 3, 25
Diazepam, 2 or 19
Diclofenac dispersible tabs, 13, 21
Diclofenac e/c, 5, 25
Diclofenac m/r, 21, 25
Dicloflex Retard, 21, 25
Diclomax 75 mg SR and Retard, 21, 25
Diconal, 2
Didanosine e/c caps, 25, C, administration
Didronel, C, food and calcium, see BNF
Didronel PMO, 10, patient leaflet, C, food and calcium, see BNF
Diflucan 50 and 200mg, 9
Diflucan susp, 9
Diflucortolone external preps, 28
Digoxin elixir, C, use of pipette
Dihydrocodeine, 2, 21
Dihydrocodeine m/r, 2, 25
Dilcardia SR, 25
Diloxanide, 9
Diltiazem, 25
Dilzem preps, 25
Dindevan, 10, anticoagulant card, 14, (urine pink or orange)
Dioderm, 28
Dipentum, 21, C, blood disorder symptoms, see BNF
Diprosalic, 28
Diprosone, 28
Dipyridamole, 22
Dipyridamole m/r, 21, 25
Disipal, C, driving
Disodium etidronate, C, food and calcium, see BNF
Disopyramide m/r, 25
Disprin CV, 25, 32
Disprol, 30
Distaclor, 9
Distaclor MR, 9, 21, 25
Distalgesic, 2, 10, patient information leaflet, 29, 30
Distamine, 6, 22, C, blood disorder symptoms, see BNF
Distigmine, 22
Disulfiram, 2, C, alcohol reaction, see BNF
Dithranol preps, 28
Dithrocream preps, 28
Dithrolan, 28
Ditropan, 3
Diumide-K Continus, 25, 27
Dolmatil, 2
Dolobid, 21, 25, C, avoid aluminium hydroxide
Doloxene, 2
Doloxene Compound, 2, 21, 32
Donepezil orodispersible tabs, C, administration
Doralese, 2
Dostinex, 21, C, hypotensive reactions, see BNF
Dosulepin, 2
Dovobet, 28
Doxazosin m/r, 25
Doxepin, 2
Doxepin topical, 2, 10, patient information leaflet
Doxycycline caps, 6, 9, 11, 27, C, posture, see BNF
Doxycycline dispersible tabs, 6, 9, 11, 13
Doxycycline tabs, 6, 11, 27, C, posture, see BNF
Dozic, 2
Driclor, 15
Droleptan, 2
Dromadol XL, 2, 25
Dukoral, C, administration
Duloxetine, 2
Dumicoat, 10, patient information leaflet
Duodopa, 14, (urine reddish), C, driving
Duofilm, 15
Duovent inhalations, C, dose
Duraphat toothpaste, C, administration
Durogesic, 2

Dutasteride, 25
Dutonin, 3
Dyazide, 14, (urine blue in some lights), 21
Dytac, 14, (urine blue in some lights), 21
Dytide, 14, (urine blue in some lights), 21

Econacort, 28
Eculizumab, C, meningococcal infection, patient information card
Edronax, C, driving
Efavirenz caps and tabs, 23
Efcortelan external preps, 28
Efcortesol, 10, steroid card
Efexor, 3, C, driving
Efexor XL, 3, 25, C, driving
Elantan preps, 25
Elidel, 4, 28
Elleste Solo MX patches, C, administration, see BNF
Elocon, 28
Emcor preps, 8
Emeside, 8, C, blood disorder symptoms (see BNF), driving (see BNF)
Emflex, 21, C, driving
Emselex, 3, 25
En-De-Kay mouthwash, C, food and drink, see BNF
Endoxana, 23, 25, 27
Enfuvirtide, C, hypersensitivity reactions, see BNF
Entacapone, 14, (urine reddish-brown), C, driving, avoid iron-containing preparations at the same time of day
Entecavir, C, administration
Entocort CR, 5, 10, steroid card, 25
Epanutin caps, 8, C, administration, blood or skin disorder symptoms (see BNF), driving (see BNF)
Epanutin Infatabs, 8, 24, C, blood or skin disorder symptoms (see BNF), driving (see BNF)
Epanutin susp, 8, C, administration, blood or skin disorder symptoms (see BNF), driving (see BNF)
Epilim Chrono, 8, 25, C, blood or hepatic disorder symptoms (see BNF), driving (see BNF)
Epilim e/c tabs, 5, 8, 25, C, blood or hepatic disorder symptoms (see BNF), driving (see BNF)
Epilim crushable tabs, liquid and syrup, 8, C, blood or hepatic disorder symptoms (see BNF), driving (see BNF)
Episenta, 8, 25, C, administration, blood or hepatic disorder symptoms (see BNF), driving (see BNF)
Eprosartan, 21
Equanil, 2
Equasym XL, 25
Ergotamine, 18, C, dosage
Erlotinib, 23
Erymax, 5, 9, 25
Erythrocin, 9
Erythromycin caps, 5, 9, 25
Erythromycin ethyl succinate, 9
Erythromycin ethyl succinate gran, 9, 13
Erythromycin stearate tabs, 9
Erythromycin tabs, 5, 9, 25
Erythroped, 9
Erythroped A tabs, 9
Escitalopram drops, C, driving, administration
Escitalopram tabs, C, driving
Esomeprazole, C, administration, see BNF
Estracombi, C, administration, see BNF
Estracyt, 23, C, dairy products, see BNF
Estraderm MX, C, administration see BNF
Estraderm TTS, C, administration, see BNF
Estradot, C, administration, see BNF
Estrapak-50, C, administration, see BNF
Estramustine, 23, C, dairy products, see BNF
Estring, 10, patient information leaflet
Estriol, 25
Ethambutol, 8
Ethosuximide, 8, C, blood disorder symptoms (see BNF), driving (see BNF)
Etidronate, C, food and calcium, see BNF
Etodolac m/r, 25
Etonogestrel implant, C, see patient information leaflet
Etoposide caps, 23
Etrivex, 28
Eucardic, 8
Eumovate external preps, 28
Eurax-Hydrocortisone, 28
Evorel preps, C, administration, see BNF
Exelon caps, 21, 25
Exelon solution, 21
Exemestane, 21
Exenatide, C, administration, see BNF
Exjade, 13, 22, C, administration, see BNF

Famciclovir, 9
Famvir, 9
Farlutal 500-mg tabs, 27
Fasigyn, 4, 9, 21, 25
Faverin, C, driving, see BNF
Fefol, 25
Fefol-Vit, 25
Felbinac foam, 15
Feldene caps, 21
Feldene Melt, 10, patient information leaflet, 21
Felodipine m/r, 25
Fematrix, C, administration, see BNF
Femapak, C, administration, see BNF
FemSeven, C, administration, see BNF
Fenbid, 25
Fenbufen, 21
Fenofibrate, 21
Fenogal, 21
Fenoprofen, 21
Fenopron, 21
Fentanyl patches and lozenges, 2
Fentazin, 2
Feospan, 25
Ferriprox, 14, C, blood disorders
Ferrograd, 25
Ferrograd C, 25
Ferrograd Folic, 25
Ferrous salts m/r, see preps
Ferrous sulphate paed mixt, 27
Fexofenadine, C, driving, see BNF
Fibrelief, 13, C, administration, see BNF
Flagyl S, 4, 9, 23
Flagyl supps, 4, 9
Flagyl tabs, 4, 9, 21, 25, 27
Flavoxate, 3
Fleet Phospho-soda, 10, patient information leaflet, C, administration
Flixotide, 8, 10, steroid card (high-dose preparations only), C, dose
Flixotide Evohaler, 8, C, dose, change to CFC-free inhaler (see BNF), 10, steroid card (250-*Evohaler* only)
Flomax MR, 25
Florinef, 10, steroid card
Floxapen 9, 23
Fluanxol, 2, C, administration, driving, see BNF
Flucloxacillin, 9, 23
Fluconazole 50 and 200mg, 9
Fluconazole susp, 9
Fludrocortisone, 10, steroid card
Fludroxycortide external preps, 28
Fluocinolone external preps, 28
Fluocinonide external preps, 28
Fluocinonide scalp lotion, 15, 28
Fluocortolone external preps, 28
Fluorigard mouthwash, C, food and drink, see BNF
Fluoxetine, C, driving, see BNF
Flupentixol, see preps
Fluprednidene, 28
Flurazepam, 19
Flurbiprofen, 21
Flurbiprofen m/r, 21, 25
Fluticasone inhalations, 8, 10, steroid card (high-dose preparations only), C, dose

Fluticasone inhalations (CFC-free), 8, C, dose, change to CFC-free inhaler (see BNF), 10, steroid card (high-dose preparations only)
Fluvastatin, C, muscle effects, see BNF
Fluvastatin m/r, 25, C, muscle effects, see BNF
Fluvoxamine, C, driving, see BNF
Foradil, C, dose, see BNF
Forceval caps, 25
Formoterol fumarate, C, dose, see BNF
Fortipine LA 40, 21, 25
Fortral caps and tabs, 2, 21
Fortral supps, 2
Fosamax, C, administration, see BNF
Fosamprenavir susp, 23
Fosavance, C, administration, see BNF
Fostair, 8, C, dose, 10, steroid card
Frisium, 2 or 19, 8, C, driving (see BNF)
Froben, 21
Froben SR, 21, 25
Frovatriptan, 3
Frusene, 14, (urine blue in some lights), 21
Fucibet, 28
Fucidin susp, 9, 21
Fucidin tabs, 9
Fucidin H, 28
Full Marks lotion, mousse, 15
Fungilin loz, 9, 24, C, after food
Furadantin, 9, 14, (urine yellow or brown), 21
Furamide, 9
Fuzeon, C, hypersensitivity reactions, see BNF
Fybogel, 13, C, administration, see BNF
Fybogel Mebeverine, 13, 22, C, administration, see BNF

Gabapentin, 3, 5, 8, C, driving (see BNF)
Gabitril, 21
Galantamine, 3, 21
Galantamine m/r, 3, 21, 25
Ganciclovir, 21
Gemfibrozil, 22
Gliclazide m/r, 25
Glivec, 21, 27
Glucobay, C, administration, see BNF
Glucophage, 21
Glucophage SR, 21, 25
Glyceryl trinitrate patch, see preps
Glyceryl trinitrate m/r, 25
Glyceryl trinitrate tabs, 16
Griseofulvin spray, 15
Griseofulvin tabs, 9, 21, C, driving
Grisol AF, 15
Grisovin, 9, 21, C, driving
GTN 300 mcg, 16

Haelan, 28
Haldol, 2
Half-Inderal LA, 8, 25
Half-Securon SR, 25
Half-Sinemet CR, 14, (urine reddish), 25
Haloperidol, 2
Heminevrin, 19
Hiprex, 9
Humira, C, tuberculosis
Hydrocortisone inj, 10, steroid card
Hydrocortisone external preps, 28
Hydrocortisone tabs, 10, steroid card, 21
Hydrocortisone butyrate external preps, 28
Hydrocortisone butyrate scalp lotion, 15, 28
Hydrocortistab inj, 10, steroid card
Hydrocortone, 10, steroid card, 21
Hydromorphone caps, 2, C, administration, see BNF
Hydromorphone m/r, 2, C, administration, see BNF
Hydroxychloroquine, 5, 21
Hydroxyzine, 2
Hyoscine hydrobromide, 2, (patches 19)
Hypolar Retard, 25
Hypovase, 3, C, initial dose, see BNF
Hytrin, 3, C, dose, see BNF

Ibandronic acid tabs, C, administration, see BNF
Ibumousse, 15
Ibuprofen, 21
Ibuprofen gran, 13, 21
Ibuprofen m/r, 25, 27
Ibuspray, 15
Idarubicin caps, 25
Idrolax, 13
Imatinib, 21, 27
Imdur, 25
Imigran, 3, 10, patient information leaflet
Imigran RADIS, 3, 10, patient information leaflet
Imipramine, 2
Imiquimod, 10, patient information leaflet
Imodium Plus, 24
Implanon, C, see patient information leaflet
Imunovir, 9
Imuran, 21
Increlex, C, administration, see BNF
Indapamide m/r, 25
Inderal-LA, 8, 25
Indinavir, 27, C, administration, see BNF
Indolar SR, 21, 25, C, driving
Indometacin caps and mixt, 21, C, driving
Indometacin m/r, see preps
Indometacin supps, C, driving
Indoramin, 2
Industrial methylated spirit, 15
Inegy, C, muscle effects, see BNF
Infacol, C, use of dropper
Infliximab, 10, Alert card, C, tuberculosis and hypersensitivity reactions
Inosine pranobex, 9
Insulin, C, see BNF
Intal Spincaps, 8
Inovelon, 21, C, driving, see BNF
Invega, 2, 25
Invirase, 21
Iodine Solution, Aqueous, 27
Ionamin, 25, C, driving
Ipocol, 5, 25, C, blood disorder symptoms, see BNF
Ipratropium inhalations, C, dose, see BNF
ISENTRESS, 25
Isib 60XL, 25
Ismo Retard, 25
Ismo tabs, 25
Isocarboxazid, 3, 10, patient information leaflet
Isodur XL, 25
Isogel, 13, C, administration, see BNF
Isoket Retard, 25
Isomide CR, 25
Isoniazid elixir and tabs, 8, 22
Isosorbide dinitrate m/r, 25
Isosorbide mononitrate, 25
Isosorbide mononitrate m/r, 25
Isotard XL, 25
Isotretinoin, 10, patient information leaflet, 11, 21
Isotretinoin gel, 10, patient information leaflet
Isotrex, 10, patient information leaflet
Isotrexin, 10, patient information leaflet
Ispagel, 13, C, administration, see BNF
Ispaghula, 13, C, administration, see BNF
Itraconazole caps, 5, 9, 21, 25, C, hepatotoxicity
Itraconazole liq, 9, 23, C, hepatotoxicity

Junifen, 21

Kaletra caps and solution, 21
Kaletra tabs, 25
Kalspare, 14, (urine blue in some lights), 21
Kalten, 8
Kapake caps and tabs, 2, 29, 30
Kapake effervescent, 2, 13, 29, 30
Kay-Cee-L, 21
Keflex, 9

Kemadrin, C, driving
Kenalog (systemic), 10, steroid card
Kentera, 3, C, administration, see BNF
Keppra, 8
Keral, 22
Ketek, 9, C, driving, hepatic disorders
Ketoconazole tabs, 5, 9, 21, C, hepatotoxicity
Ketoprofen caps, 21
Ketoprofen CR, 21, 25
Ketoprofen m/r caps, 21, 25
Ketotifen, 2, 21
Ketorolac tabs, 17, 21
Ketovail, 21, 25
Kineret, C, blood disorder symptoms
Kivexa, C, hypersensitivity reactions, see BNF
Klaricid, 9
Klaricid sachets, 9, 13
Klaricid XL, 9, 21, 25
Klean-Prep, 10, patient information leaflet, 13, C, administration
Kloref, 13, 21
Konakion tabs, 24

Labetalol, 8, 21
Lamictal dispersible tabs, 8, 13, C, driving (see BNF), skin reactions
Lamictal tabs, 8, C, driving (see BNF), skin reactions
Lamisil, 9
Lamotrigine dispersible tabs, 8, 13, C, driving (see BNF), skin reactions
Lamotrigine tabs, 8, C, driving (see BNF), skin reactions
Lanoxin-PG elixir, C, use of pipette
Lansoprazole caps, 5, 25
Lansoprazole oro-dispersible tabs, 5, C, administration, see BNF
Larapam SR, 2, 25
Largactil, 2, 11
Lariam, 21, 25, 27, C, driving, malaria prophylaxis, see BNF
Lasikal, 25, 27, C, posture, see BNF
Lasix + K, 25, 27, C, posture, see BNF
Lederfen, 21
Ledermycin, 7, 9, 11, 23
Leflunomide, 4
<u>Lenalidomide</u>, 25, C, symptoms of thromboembolism, neutropenia, or thrombocytopenia, patient information leaflet
Lercanidipine, 22
Lescol, C, muscle effects, see BNF
Lescol XL, 25, C, muscle effects, see BNF
Levetiracetam, 8
Levocetirizine, C, driving
Levofloxacin, 6, 9, 25, C, driving
Levomepromazine, 2
Librium, 2
Li-Liquid, 10, lithium card, C, fluid and salt intake, see BNF
Linezolid susp and tabs, 9, 10, patient information leaflet
Lioresal, 2, 8
Lipantil, 21
Lipitor, C, muscle effects, see BNF
Lipostat, C, muscle effects, see BNF
Liquid paraffin, C, administration, see BNF
Liskonum, 10, lithium card, 25, C, fluid and salt intake, see BNF
Litarex, 10, lithium card, 25, C, fluid and salt intake, see BNF
Lithium carbonate, 10, lithium card, C, fluid and salt intake, see BNF
Lithium carbonate m/r, 10, lithium card, 25, C, fluid and salt intake, see BNF
Lithium citrate liq, 10, lithium card, C, fluid and salt intake, see BNF
Lithium citrate m/r, 10, lithium card, 25, C, fluid and salt intake, see BNF
Lithonate, 10, lithium card, 25, C, fluid and salt intake, see BNF
Loceryl, 10, patient information leaflet
Locoid cream, oint, and topical emulsion, 28
Locoid scalp lotion, 15, 28
Locoid C, 28
Lofepramine, 2
Lofexidine, 2
Lopid, 22
Loprazolam, 19
Lopresor, 8
Lopresor SR, 8, 25
Loratadine, C, driving, alcohol, see BNF
Lorazepam, 2 or 19
Lormetazepam, 19
Loron tabs, 10, patient information leaflet, C, food and calcium, see BNF
Losec, C, administration, see BNF
Lotriderm, 28
Lugol's solution, 27
Lustral, C, driving, see BNF
Lyclear Dermal cream, 10, patient information leaflet
Lymecycline, 6, 9
Lyrica, 3, 8, C, driving
Lysodren, 2, 21
Lysovir, C, driving

Mabron, 2, 25
Macrobid, 9, 14, (urine yellow or brown), 21, 25
Macrodantin, 9, 14, (urine yellow or brown), 21
Madopar, 14, (urine reddish), C, driving
Madopar dispersible tabs, 14, (urine reddish), C, administration, driving, see BNF
Madopar CR, 5, 14, (urine reddish), 25, C, driving
Magnapen, 9, 22
Magnesium citrate effervescent pdr, 10, patient information leaflet, 13, C, administration
Magnesium sulphate, 13, 23
Malarivon, 5, C, malaria prophylaxis
Malarone, 21, C, malaria prophylaxis
Manerix, 10, patient information leaflet, 21
Manevac, 25, 27
Marevan, 10, anticoagulant card
Maxalt, 3
Maxalt Melt, 3, C, administration
Maxepa, 21
Maxolon paed liquid, C, use of pipette
Maxolon SR, 25
Maxtrex (methotrexate), C, NSAIDs (see BNF)
Mebeverine, C, administration, see BNF
<u>Mecasermin</u>, C, administration, see BNF
Mecysteine, 5, 22, 25
Medikinet XL, 25
Medrone tabs, 10, steroid card, 21
Mefenamic acid caps, paed susp, and tabs, 21
Mefloquine, 21, 25, 27, C, driving, malaria prophylaxis, see BNF
Meloxicam tabs, 21
Mepacrine, 4, 9, 14, 21
Meprobamate, 2
Meptazinol, 2
Meptid, 2
Mesalazine e/c, see preps
Mesalazine m/r, see preps
Mesalazine enema and supps, C, blood disorder symptoms, see BNF
Mesalazine gran, see preps
Mesren MR, 5, 25, C, blood disorder symptoms, see BNF
Metformin, 21
Metformin m/r, 21, 25
Methadone, 2
Methadose, 2
Methenamine, 9
Methocarbamol, 2
Methotrexate tabs, C, NSAIDs (see BNF)
Methylcellulose (constipation or diarrhoea), C, administration, see BNF
Methylcellulose tabs (anorectic), C, administration, see BNF
Methyldopa, 3, 8
Methylphenidate m/r, 25

Methylprednisolone external preps, 28
Methylprednisolone inj, 10, steroid card
Methylprednisolone tabs, 10, steroid card, 21
Methysergide, 2, 21
Metirosine, 2
Metoclopramide paed liquid, C, use of pipette
Metoclopramide m/r, see preps
Metopirone, 21, C, driving
Metoprolol, 8
Metoprolol m/r, see preps
Metosyn cream and oint, 28
Metosyn scalp lotion, 15, 28
Metrolyl supps, 4, 9
Metronidazole mixt, 4, 9, 23
Metronidazole supps, 4, 9
Metronidazole tabs, 4, 9, 21, 25, 27
Metyrapone, 21, C, driving
Mexiletine caps, 21, 27
Mexitil caps, 21, 27
Mezavant XL, 5, 21, 25, C, blood disorder symptoms, see BNF
Mianserin, 2, 25
Micanol, 28
Miconazole denture lacquer, 10, patient information leaflet
Miconazole oral gel, 9, C, hold in mouth, after food
Miconazole tabs, 9, 21
Midrid, 30, C, dosage
Mifegyne, 10, patient information leaflet
Mifepristone, 10, patient information leaflet
Migard, 3
Migraleve, 2, (pink tablets), 17, 30
Migravess, 13, 17, 32
Migravess Forte, 13, 17, 32
Migril, 2, 18, C, dosage
Mildison, 28
Mimpara, 21
Minocin, 6, 9, C, posture, see BNF
Minocin MR, 6, 25
Minocycline, 6, 9, C, posture, see BNF
Minocycline m/r, 6, 25
Mintec, 5, 22, 25
Mintezol, 3, 21, 24
Mirapexin, C, hypotensive reactions, driving, see BNF
Mirtazapine oral solution, 2
Mirtazapine orodispersible tablets, 2, C, administration, see BNF
Mirtazapine tabs, 2, 25
Misoprostol, 21
Mitotane, 2, 21, C, driving, adrenal suppression
Mizolastine, 25, C, driving
Mizollen, 25, C, driving
Mobic tabs, 21
Mobiflex, 21
Moclobemide, 10, patient information leaflet, 21
Modisal LA, 25
Modisal XL, 25
Modrasone, 28
Modrenal, 21
Moducren, 8
Mogadon, 19
Molipaxin, 2, 21
Mometasone cream, 28
Mometasone inhaler, 8, 10, steroid card, C, dose
Mometasone ointment, 28
Mometasone scalp lotion, 28
Mono-Cedocard, 25
Monomax SR, 25
Monomax XL, 25
Monomil XL, 25
Monosorb XL, 25
Montelukast chewable tabs, 23, 24
Morphine preps, 2
Morphine m/r susp, 2, 13
Morphine m/r caps and tabs, see preps
Motifene, 25
Movicol, 13
Movicol-Half, 13
Moviprep, 10, patient information leaflet, 13, C, administration
Moxifloxacin, 6, 9, C, driving
Moxisylyte, 21
Moxonidine, 3
MST Continus susp, 2, 13
MST Continus tabs, 2, 25
MXL, 2, C, administration, see BNF
Myambutol, 8
Mycobutin, 8, 14, (urine orange-red), C, soft lenses
Mycophenolic acid, 25
Myfortic, 25
Mynah, 8, 23
Myocrisin inj, C, blood disorder symptoms, see BNF
Myotonine Chloride, 22
Mysoline, 2, 8, C, driving (see BNF)

Nabilone, 2, C, behavioural effects, see BNF
Nabumetone, 21
Nabumetone dispersible tabs, 13, 21
Nabumetone susp, 21
Nadolol, 8
Nafarelin spray, 10, patient information leaflet, C, nasal decongestants, see BNF
Naftidrofuryl, 25, 27
Nalcrom, 22, C, administration, see BNF
Nalidixic acid, 9, 11
Naloxone (sublingual), 2, 26
Napratec, 21
Naprosyn EC, 5, 25
Naprosyn tabs and susp, 21
Naproxen e/c, 5, 25
Naproxen tabs and susp, 21
Naramig, 3
Naratriptan, 3
Nardil, 3, 10, patient information leaflet
Natrilix SR, 25
Navelbine caps, 21, 25
Navoban, 23
Nebilet, 8
Nebivolol, 8
Nedocromil sodium inhalation, 8, C, change to CFC-free inhaler
Nefopam, 2, 14, (urine pink)
Nelfinavir tabs, 21
Nelfinavir powder, 21, C, administration, see BNF
Neo-Medrone, 28
Neo-Mercazole, C, blood disorder symptoms, see BNF
Neo-NaClex-K, 25, 27, C, posture, see BNF
Neoral, C, administration, see BNF
Neotigason, 10, patient information leaflet, 21
Nerisone, 28
Nerisone Forte, 28
Neulactil, 2
Neupro, C, hypotensive reactions, driving
Neurontin, 3, 5, 8, C, driving (see BNF)
Nevirapine, C, hypersensitivity reactions, see BNF
Nexavar, 23
Nexium, C, administration, see BNF
Niaspan, 21, 25
Nicardipine m/r, 25
Nicorette Microtab, 26
Nicotine (sublingual), 26
Nicotinic acid m/r, see preps
Nidazol, 4, 9, 21, 25, 27
Nifedipine m/r, see preps
Nifedipress MR, 25
Nifedotard, 25
Nifelease, 25
Niferex elixir, C, infants, use of dropper
Nisoldipine, 22, 25
Nitrazepam, 19, (infantile spasms 1, 8)
Nitrofurantoin, 9, 14, (urine yellow or brown), 21
Nitrofurantoin m/r, 9, 14, (urine yellow or brown), 21, 25
Nivaquine, 5, C, malaria prophylaxis, see BNF
Nizoral, 5, 9, 21, C, hepatotoxicity
Nootropil, 3
Norfloxacin, 7, 9, 23, C, driving
Normacol preps, 25, 27, C, administration, see BNF
Normax, 14, (urine red)
Norprolac, 21, C, hypotensive reactions, see BNF
Nortriptyline, 2

Norvir, 21, C, administration, see BNF
Novoliser, 8, 10, steroid card (high-doses only), C, dose
Noxafil, 9, 21
Nozinan, 2
Nuelin SA preps, 21, 25
Nurofen for children, 21
Nu-Seals Aspirin, 5, 25, 32
Nycopren, 5, 25
Nystadermal, 28
Nystaform-HC, 28
Nystan pastilles, 9, 24, C, after food
Nystan susp (g.i.), 9, C, use of pipette
Nystan susp (mouth), 9, C, use of pipette, hold in mouth, after food
Nystan tabs, 9
Nystatin mixt (g.i.), 9, C, use of pipette
Nystatin mixt (mouth), 9, C, use of pipette, hold in mouth, after food
Nystatin pastilles, 9, 24, C, after food
Nystatin tabs, 9

Occlusal, 15
Octim, C, fluid intake, see BNF
Ocusert Pilo, C, method of use
Oestrogel, C, administration, see BNF
Ofloxacin, 6, 9, 11, C, driving
Olanzapine tabs, 2
Olanzapine orodispersible tabs, 2, C, administration, see BNF
Olbetam, 21
Olsalazine, 21, C, blood disorder symptoms, see BNF
Omacor, 21
Omega-3-acid ethyl esters, 21
Omeprazole caps, C, administration, see BNF
Omeprazole tabs, 25
Ondansetron (freeze-dried tablets), C, administration, see BNF
Opilon, 21
Optimax, 3
Oramorph preps, 2
Oramorph SR, 2, 25
Orap, 2
Orbenin, 9, 23
Orelox, 5, 9, 21
Orovite Complement B6, 25
Orphenadrine, C, driving
Orudis caps, 21
Oruvail, 21, 25
Oseltamivir, 9
Ovestin, 25
Oxazepam, 2
Oxcarbazepine, 3, 8, C, see BNF
Oxerutins, 21
Oxis, C, dose, see BNF
Oxprenolol, 8
Oxprenolol m/r, 8, 25

Oxybutynin tabs and elixir, 3
Oxybutynin patch, 3, C, administration, see BNF
Oxycodone caps and liq, 2
Oxycodone m/r, 2, 25
OxyContin, 2, 25
OxyNorm, 2
Oxytetracycline, 7, 9, 23

Paliperidone, 2, 25
Palladone, 2, C, administration, see BNF
Palladone SR, 2, C, administration, see BNF
Paludrine, 21, C, malaria prophylaxis, see BNF
Panadeine, 29, 30
Panadeine effervescent, 13, 29, 30
Panadol tabs, 29, 30
Panadol Soluble, 13, 29, 30
Panadol susp, 30
Pancrease preps, C, administration, see BNF
Pancreatin, C, administration, see BNF
Pancrex gran, 25, C, dose, see BNF
Pancrex V Forte tabs, 5, 25, C, dose, see BNF
Pancrex V caps, 125 caps and pdr, C, administration, see BNF
Pancrex V tabs, 5, 25, C, dose, see BNF
Pantoprazole, 25
Paracetamol liq and supps, 30
Paracetamol tabs, 29, 30
Paracetamol tabs, soluble, 13, 29, 30
Paracodol, 13, 29, 30
Paradote, 29, 30
Paramax sachets, 13, 17, 30
Paramax tabs, 17, 30
Pariet, 25
Parlodel, 21, C, hypotensive reactions, see BNF
Paroven, 21
Paroxetine tabs, 21, C, driving
Paroxetine susp, 5, 21, C, driving
Penbritin, 9, 23
Penicillamine, 6, 22, C, blood disorder symptoms, see BNF
Pentasa tabs and gran, 25, C, administration, blood disorder symptoms, see BNF
Pentasa enema and supps, C, blood disorder symptoms, see BNF
Pentazocine caps and tabs, 2, 21
Pentazocine supps, 2
Pentoxifylline m/r, 21, 25
Peppermint oil caps, 5, 22, 25
Percutol, C, administration, see BNF
Pergolide, C, driving, hypotensive reactions, see BNF
Periactin, 2
Pericyazine, 2

Perindopril, 22
Periostat, 6, 11, 27, C, posture, see BNF
Permethrin dermal cream, 10, patient information leaflet
Perphenazine, 2
Persantin, 22
Persantin Retard, 21, 25
Pethidine, 2
Phenelzine, 3, 10, patient information leaflet
Phenergan, 2
Phenindione, 10, anticoagulant card, 14, (urine pink or orange)
Phenobarbital elixir and tabs, 2, 8, C, driving (see BNF)
Phenothrin lotion, mousse, 15
Phenoxymethylpenicillin, 9, 23
Phentermine m/r, 25, C, driving
Phenytoin caps and tabs, 8, C, administration, blood or skin disorder symptoms (see BNF), driving (see BNF)
Phenytoin chewable tabs, 8, 24, C, blood or skin disorder symptoms (see BNF), driving (see BNF)
Phenytoin susp, 8, C, administration, blood or skin disorder symptoms (see BNF), driving (see BNF)
Phosex, 21 25
Phosphate-Sandoz, 13
Phyllocontin Continus, 25
Physeptone, 2
Physiotens, 3
Phytomenadione, 24
Picolax, 10, patient information leaflet, 13, C, solution, see BNF
Pilocarpine tabs, 21, 27, C, driving
Pimecrolimus, 4, 28
Pimozide, 2
Pindolol, 8
Piperazine powder, 13
Piracetam, 3
Piriton, 2
Piroxicam caps and tabs, 21
Piroxicam dispersible tabs, 13, 21
Pivmecillinam, 9, 21, 27, C, posture, see BNF
Pizotifen, 2
Plaquenil, 5, 21
Plendil, 25
Podophyllin paint cpd, 15, C, application, see BNF
Ponstan, 21
Posaconazole, 9, 21
Potaba caps and tabs, 21
Potaba Envules, 13, 21
Potassium chloride m/r, see preps
Potassium citrate mixt, 27
Potassium effervescent tabs, 13, 21
Pramipexole, C, hypotensive reactions, driving, see BNF
Pranoxen Continus, 25

Pravastatin, C, muscle effects, see BNF
Praxilene, 25, 27
Prazosin, 3, C, initial dose, see BNF
Prednesol, 10, steroid card, 13, 21
Prednisolone inj, 10, steroid card
Prednisolone tabs, 10, steroid card, 21
Prednisolone e/c, 5, 10, steroid card, 25
Pregabalin, 3, 8, C, driving
Preservex, 21
Prestim, 8
Prezista, 21, C, missed dose, see BNF
Priadel liq, 10, lithium card, C, fluid and salt intake, see BNF
Priadel tabs, 10, lithium card, 25, C, fluid and salt intake, see BNF
Primidone, 2, 8, C, driving (see BNF)
Prioderm lotion, 15
Pripsen, 13
Pro-Banthine, 23
Probenecid, 12, 21, 27
Procarbazine, 4
Prochlorperazine, 2
Prochlorperazine buccal tabs, 2, C, administration, see BNF
Procyclidine, C, driving
Progesterone (micronised), 23
Prograf, 23, C, driving, see BNF
Proguanil, 21, C, malaria prophylaxis, see BNF
Progynova TS preps, C, administration, see BNF
Promazine, 2
Promethazine, 2
Propafenone, 21, 25
Propantheline, 23
Propiverine hydrochloride, 3
Propiverine hydrochloride m/r, 3, 25
Propranolol oral solution and tabs, 8
Propranolol m/r, 8, 25
Protelos, 5, 13, C, administration, see BNF
Prothiaden, 2
Protionamide, 8, 21
Protium, 25
Protopic, 4, 11, 28
Prozac, C, driving, see BNF
Psorin, 28
Pulmicort, 8, 10, steroid card, C, dose
Pulmicort LS, 8, C, dose
Pulmicort Respules, 8, 10, steroid card, C, dose
Pyrazinamide, 8

Questran preps, 13, C, avoid other drugs at same time, see BNF
Quetiapine, 2
Quinagolide, 21, C, hypotensive reactions, see BNF
Quinocort, 28
Quinoderm with Hydrocortisone, 28
Qvar preps, 8, 10, steroid card (high-dose preparations only), C, dose

Rabeprazole, 25
Raltagravir, 25
Ranitidine effervescent tabs, 13
Rapamune, C, administration
Rasilez, 21
Rebetol, 21
Reboxetine, C, driving
Regulan, 13, C, administration, see BNF
Regurin, 23
Relifex, 21
Relifex dispersible tablets, 13, 21
Relifex susp, 21
Remedeine, 2, 21, 29, 30
Remedeine effervescent tabs, 2, 13, 21, 29, 30
Remicade, 10, Alert card, C, tuberculosis and hypersensitivity reactions
Reminyl, 3, 21
Reminyl XL, 3, 21, 25
Renagel, 25, C, with meals
Requip, 21, C, driving, see BNF
Resonium A, 13
Restandol, 21, 25
Retrovir syrup, C, use of oral syringe
Revlimid, 25, C, symptoms of thromboembolism, neutropenia, or thrombocytopenia, patient information leaflet
Reyataz, 5, 21
Rhumalgan, 5, 25
Riamet, 21, C, driving
Ribavirin caps and tabs, 21
Ridaura, 21, C, blood disorder symptoms, see BNF
Rifabutin, 8, 14, (urine orange-red), C, soft lenses
Rifadin, 8, 14, (urine orange-red), 22, C, soft lenses
Rifampicin caps and mixt, 8, 14, (urine orange-red), 22, C, soft lenses
Rifater, 8, 14, (urine orange-red), 22, C, soft lenses
Rifinah, 8, 14, (urine orange-red), 22, C, soft lenses
Rilutek, C, blood disorders, driving
Rimactane, 8, 14, (urine orange-red), 22, C, soft lenses
Rimonabant, C, depression, see BNF
Risedronate sodium, C, administration, food and calcium, see BNF
Risperdal, 2
Risperidone, 2
Ritonavir, 21, C, administration, see BNF
Rivastigmine, 21, 25
Rivotril, 2, 8, C, driving (see BNF)
Rizatriptan tabs, 3
Rizatriptan wafers, 3, C, administration
Roaccutane, 10, patient information leaflet, 11, 21
Robaxin, 2
Ropinirole, 21, C, driving, see BNF
Rotigotine, C, hypotensive reactions, driving
Rowachol, 22
Rowatinex caps, 25
Rufinamide, 21, C, driving (see BNF)
Rythmodan Retard, 25

Sabril sachets, 3, 8, 13, C, driving (see BNF)
Sabril tabs, 3, 8, C, driving (see BNF)
Safapryn, 5, 25
Safapryn-Co, 5, 25
Salactol, 15
Salagen, 21, 27, C, driving
Salatac, 15
Salazopyrin, 14, (urine orange-yellow), C, blood disorder symptoms and soft lenses, see BNF
Salazopyrin EN-tabs, 5, 14, (urine orange-yellow), 25, C, blood disorder symptoms and soft lenses, see BNF
Salbutamol inhalations, C, dose, see BNF
Salbutamol inhalations (CFC-free), C, dose, change to CFC-free inhaler, see BNF
Salbutamol m/r, 25
Salicylic acid collodion, 15
Salicylic acid lotion, 15
Salmeterol, C, dose, see BNF
Salmeterol (CFC-free), C, dose, change to CFC-free inhaler, see BNF
Salofalk enema and supps, C, blood disorder symptoms, see BNF
Salofalk gran, 25, C, administration, blood disorder symptoms, see BNF
Salofalk tabs, 5, 25, C, blood disorder symptoms, see BNF
Sandimmun, C, administration, see BNF
Sandrena, C, administration, see BNF
Sando-K, 13, 21
Sandocal, 13
Sanomigran, 2
Saquinavir, 21
Scopoderm TTS, 19, C, administration, see BNF
Sebivo, C, muscle effects

Sebomin MR, 6, 25
Secobarbital, 19
Seconal, 19
Sectral, 8
Securon SR, 25
Selegiline (freeze-dried tablets), C, administration, see BNF
Selexid, 9, 21, 27, C, posture, see BNF
Septrin susp and tabs, 9
Septrin dispersible tabs, 9, 13
Seractil, 21
Serc, 21
Serenace, 2
Seretide, 8, 10, steroid card (250- and 500-*Accuhaler* only), C, dose
Seretide Evohaler, 8, C, dose, change to CFC-free inhaler (see BNF), 10, steroid card (125- and 250-*Evohaler* only)
Serevent, C, dose, see BNF
Serevent (CFC-free), C, dose, change to CFC-free inhaler, see BNF
Seroquel, 2
Seroxat tabs, 21, C, driving
Seroxat susp, 5, 21, C, driving
Sertraline, C, driving, see BNF
Sevelamer, 21
Sevredol, 2
Simeticone, see paediatric prep
Simvastatin, C, muscle effects, see BNF
Sinemet CR, 14, (urine reddish), 25, C, driving
Sinemet preps, 14, (urine reddish), C, driving
Sinepin, 2
Singulair chewable tabs, 23, 24
Sinthrome, 10, anticoagulant card
Sirolimus, C, administration
Skelid, C, food and calcium
Slo-Indo, 21, 25, C, driving
Slo-Phyllin, 25 or C, administration, see BNF
Sloprolol, 8, 25
Slow Sodium, 25
Slow-Fe, 25
Slow-Fe Folic, 25
Slow-K, 25, 27, C, posture, see BNF
Slow-Trasicor, 8, 25
Slozem, 25
Sodium Amytal, 19
Sodium aurothiomalate, C, blood disorder symptoms, see BNF
Sodium cellulose phosphate, 13, 21, C, may be sprinkled on food
Sodium chloride m/r, 25
Sodium chloride tabs, 13
Sodium chloride and glucose oral pdr, cpd, 13
Sodium chloride solution-tabs, 13
Sodium clodronate, C, food and calcium, see BNF
Sodium cromoglicate (oral), 22, C, administration, see BNF
Sodium cromoglicate inhalations, 8
Sodium fusidate susp, 9, 21
Sodium fusidate tabs, 9
Sodium picosulfate pdr, 10, patient information leaflet, 13, C, see BNF
Sodium valproate e/c, 5, 8, 25, C, blood or hepatic disorder symptoms (see BNF), driving (see BNF)
Sodium valproate m/r and granules, 8, 25, C, blood or hepatic disorder symptoms (see BNF), driving (see BNF)
Sodium valproate crushable tabs, liquid and syrup, 8, C, blood or hepatic disorder symptoms (see BNF), driving (see BNF)
Solian, 2
Solifenacin, 3
Soliris, C, meningococcal infection, patient information card
Solpadol caps and caplets, 2, 29, 30
Solpadol Effervescent, 2, 13, 29, 30
Solu-Cortef, 10, steroid card
Solu-Medrone, 10, steroid card
Solvazinc, 13, 21
Somnite, 19
Sonata, 2
Soneryl, 19
Sorafenib, 23
Sotacor, 8
Sotalol, 8
Spironolactone, 21
Sporanox caps, 5, 9, 21, 25, C, hepatotoxicity
Sporanox liq, 9, 23, C, administration, hepatotoxicity
Sprycel, 25
Stalevo, 14, (urine reddish-brown), C, driving, avoid iron-containing preparations at the same time of day
Stavudine, 23
Stelazine syrup and tabs, 2
Stelazine Spansule, 2, 25
Stemetil, 2
Sterculia, C, administration, see BNF
Stilnoct, 19
Strattera, 3
Striant SR, C, administration, see BNF
Strontium, 5, 13, C, administration, see BNF
Stugeron, 2
Suboxone, 2, 26
Subutex, 2, 26
Sucralfate, 5
Sudafed Plus, 2
Sulfadiazine, 9, 27
Sulfasalazine, 14, (urine orange-yellow), C, blood disorder symptoms and soft lenses, see BNF
Sulfasalazine e/c, 5, 14, (urine orange-yellow), 25, C, blood disorder symptoms and soft lenses, see BNF
Sulfinpyrazone, 12, 21
Sulindac, 21
Sulpiride, 2
Sulpor, 2
Sumatriptan, 3, 10, patient information leaflet
Suprax, 9
Supralip, 21
Suprecur, C, nasal decongestants, see BNF
Suprefact nasal spray, C, nasal decongestants, see BNF
Surgam tabs, 21
Surgical spirit, 15
Surmontil, 2
Suscard Buccal, C, administration, see BNF
Sustiva caps and tabs, 23
Symbicort, 8, C, dose, 10, steroid card (200/6- and 400/12-*Turbohaler* only)
Symmetrel, C, driving
Synalar external preps, 28
Synarel, 10, patient information leaflet, C, nasal decongestants, see BNF
Synflex, 21
Syscor MR, 22, 25

Tacrolimus caps, 23, C, driving, see BNF
Tacrolimus topical, 4, 11, 28
Tamiflu, 9
Tamsulosin m/r, 25
Tarceva, 23
Tarivid, 6, 9, 11, C, driving
Tarka, 25
Tasmar, 14, 25
Tavanic, 5, 9, 25, C, driving
Tavegil, 2
Tegretol Chewtabs, 3, 8, 21, 24, C, blood, hepatic or skin disorder symptoms (see BNF), driving (see BNF)
Tegretol liq, supps and tabs, 3, 8, C, blood, hepatic or skin disorder symptoms (see BNF), driving (see BNF)
Tegretol Retard, 3, 8, 25, C, blood, hepatic or skin disorder symptoms (see BNF), driving (see BNF)
Telbivudine, C, muscle effects
Telfast, C, driving, see BNF
Telithromycin, 9, C, driving, hepatic disorders
Telzir susp, 23
Temazepam, 19
Temgesic, 2, 26
Temodal, 23, 25

Temozolomide, 23, 25
Tenben, 8
Tenif, 8, 25
Tenofovir, 21, C, administration, see BNF
Tenoret 50, 8
Tenoretic, 8
Tenormin, 8
Tenoxicam tabs, 21
Tensipine MR, 21, 25
Terazosin, 3, C, dose, see BNF
Terbinafine, 9
Terbutaline inhalations, C, dose, see BNF
Terbutaline m/r, 25
Testim, C, administration, see BNF
Testogel, C, administration, see BNF
Testosterone buccal tablets, C, administration, see BNF
Testosterone gel, C, administration, see BNF
Testosterone patch, C, administration, see BNF
Testosterone undecanoate caps, 21, 25
Tetrabenazine, 2
Tetracycline, 7, 9, 23, C, posture
Tetracycline mouthwash, see BNF
Tetralysal preps, 6, 9
Teveten, 21
Theophylline, 21
Theophylline m/r, see preps
Tiabendazole, 3, 21, 24
Tiagabine, 21
Tiaprofenic acid m/r, 25
Tiaprofenic acid tabs, 21
Tilade, 8, C, change to CFC-free inhaler
Tildiem preps, 25
Tiludronic acid, C, food and calcium
Timodine, 28
Timolol, 8
Tinidazole tabs, 4, 9, 21, 25
Tipranavir, 5, 21
Tizanidine, 2
Tolcapone, 14, 25
Tolterodine, 3
Tolterodine m/r, 3, 25
Topamax Sprinkle, 3, 8, C, administration, driving (see BNF)
Topamax tabs, 3, 8, C, driving (see BNF)
Topiramate Sprinkle caps, 3, 8, C, administration, driving (see BNF)
Topiramate tabs, 3, 8, C, driving (see BNF)
Toradol tabs, 17, 21
Tostran, C, administration
Tradorec XL, 2, 25
Tramacet, 2, 25, 29, 30
Tramadol, 2
Tramadol m/r, 2, 25
Tramadol sachets, 2, 13
Tramadol soluble, 2, 13
Tramake, 2
Trandate, 8, 21
Trasicor, 8
Trasidrex, 8, 25
Traxam foam, 15
Trazodone, 2, 21
Trazodone m/r, 2, 21, 25
Trental m/r, 21, 25
Treosulfan, 25
Tretinoin caps, 21, 25
Tri-Adcortyl external preps, 28
Triamcinolone inj, 10, steroid card
Triamcinolone tabs, 10, steroid card, 21
Triamterene, 14, (urine blue in some lights), 21
Triapin preps, 25
Triclofos sodium, 19
Trientine, 6, 22
Trifluoperazine, 2
Trihexyphenidyl syrup, C, driving, see BNF
Trihexyphenidyl tabs, C, with or after food, driving, see BNF
Trileptal, 3, 8, C, see BNF
Trilostane, 21
Trimethoprim mixt and tabs, 9
Trimipramine, 2
Trimopan, 9
Trimovate, 28
Tripotassium dicitratobismuthate, C, administration, see BNF
Triprolidine m/r, 2, 25
Triptafen preps, 2
Trizivir, C, hypersensitivity reactions, see BNF
Tropisetron, 23
Tropium, 2
Trospium chloride, 23
Truvada, 21, C, administration, see BNF
Tryptophan, 3
Tuinal, 19
Tylex caps, 2, 29, 30
Tylex effervescent tabs, 2, 13, 29, 30
Typhoid vaccine, oral, 23, 25, C, administration, see BNF

Ubretid, 22
Ucerax, 2
Ultralanum Plain, 28
Uniphyllin Continus, 25
Univer, 25
Urdox, 21
Uriben, 9, 11
Urispas, 3
Ursodeoxycholic acid, 21
Ursogal, 21
Ursofalk, 21
Utinor, 7, 9, 23, C, driving
Utrogestan, 23

Valaciclovir, 9
Valcyte, 21
Valganciclovir, 21
Vallergan, 2
Valoid, 2
Valproic acid, see individual preparations
Valtrex, 9
Vancocin caps, 9
Vancomycin caps, 9
Velosef, 9
Venlafaxine, 3, C, driving
Venlafaxine m/r, 3, 25, C, driving
Ventmax SR, 25
Ventolin Evohaler, C, dose, change to CFC-free inhaler, see BNF
Ventolin inhalations, C, dose, see BNF
Vepesid caps, 23
Verapamil m/r, 25
Verapress, 25
Vertab SR, 25
Vesanoid, 21, 25
Vesicare, 3
Vfend, 9, 11, 23
Viazem XL, 25
Vibramycin caps, 6, 9, 11, 27, C, posture, see BNF
Vibramycin-D, 6, 9, 11, 13
Videx, 23, C, administration, see BNF
Videx e/c caps, 25, C, administration
Videx tabs, 23, C, administration
Vigabatrin sachets, 3, 8, 13, C, driving (see BNF)
Vigabatrin tabs, 3, 8, C, driving (see BNF)
Vinorelbine caps, 21, 25
Vioform-Hydrocortisone, 28
Viracept powder, 21, C, administration, see BNF
Viracept tabs, 21
Viramune, C, hypersensitivity reactions, see BNF
Viread, 21, C, administration, see BNF
Visclair, 5, 22, 25
Viskaldix, 8
Visken, 8
Vivotif, 23, 25, C, administration, see BNF
Volmax, 25
Voltarol dispersible tabs, 13, 21
Voltarol 75mg SR and Retard, 21, 25
Voltarol tabs, 5, 25
Voriconazole, 9, 11, 23

Warfarin, 10, anticoagulant card
Warfarin WBP, 10, anticoagulant card
Warticon, 15
Welldorm, 19, 27
Wellvone, 21

Xagrid, C, driving
Xanax, 2
Xatral, 3, C, dose, see BNF
Xatral XL, 3, 21, 25, C, dose, see BNF

Xeloda, 21
Xepin, 2, 10, patient information leaflet
Xismox XL, 25
Xyzal, C, driving

Yentreve, 2

Zaditen, 2, 21
Zadstat supps, 4, 9
Zafirlukast, 23
Zaleplon, 2
Zamadol, 2
Zamadol 24hr, 2, 25
Zamadol SR, 2, 25
Zanaflex, 2
Zanidip, 22
Zantac effervescent tabs, 13
Zaponex, 2, 10, patient information leaflet
Zarontin, 8, C, blood disorder symptoms (see BNF), driving (see BNF)
Zavedos caps, 25
Zelapar, C, administration, see BNF
Zemon XL, 25
Zemtard XL, 25
Zerit, 23
Ziagen, C, hypersensitivity reactions, see BNF
Zidovudine syrup, C, use of oral syringe
Zimbacol XL, 21, 25
Zimovane, 19
Zinamide, 8
Zinc sulphate, see preps
Zinnat susp, 9, 21
Zinnat tabs, 9, 21, 25
Zispin SolTab, 2
Zithromax caps, 5, 9, 23
Zithromax susp, 5, 9
Zocor, C, muscle effects, see BNF
Zofran Melt, C, administration, see BNF
Zoleptil, 2
Zolmitriptan orodispersible tabs, C, administration, see BNF
Zolpidem, 19
Zomig Rapimelt, C, administration, see BNF
Zomorph, 2, 25
Zonegran, 3
Zonisamide, 3
Zopiclone, 19
Zotepine, 2
Zoton caps, 5, 25
Zoton FasTab, 5, C, administration, see BNF
Zovirax susp and tabs, 9
Zuclopenthixol, 2
Zyban, 25, C, driving
Zydol, 2
Zydol soluble, 2, 13
Zydol SR, 2, 25
Zydol XL, 2, 25
Zyloric, 8, 21, 27
Zyprexa tabs, 2
Zyprexa Velotab, 2, C, administration, see BNF
Zyvox susp and tabs, 9, 10, patient information leaflet

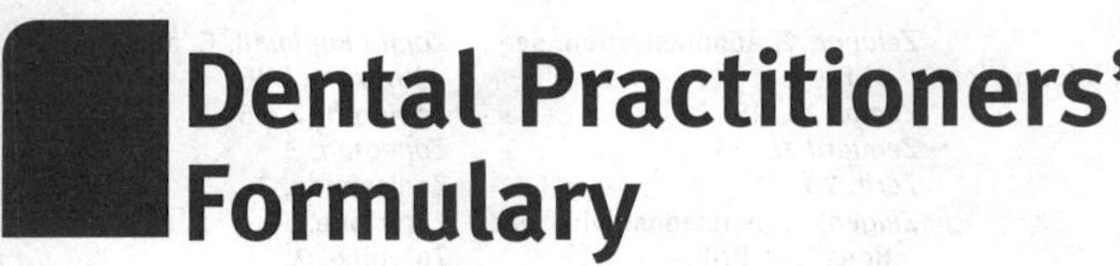

Dental Practitioners' Formulary

List of Dental Preparations

The following list has been approved by the appropriate Secretaries of State, and the preparations therein may be prescribed by dental practitioners on form FP10D (GP14 in Scotland, WP10D in Wales).

Sugar-free versions, where available, are preferred.

Aciclovir Cream, BP
Aciclovir Oral Suspension, BP, 200 mg/5 mL
Aciclovir Tablets, BP, 200 mg
Aciclovir Tablets, BP, 800 mg
Amoxicillin Capsules, BP
Amoxicillin Oral Powder, DPF[1]
Amoxicillin Oral Suspension, BP
Amphotericin Lozenges, BP
Ampicillin Capsules, BP
Ampicillin Oral Suspension, BP
Artificial Saliva, DPF[2]
Artificial Saliva Substitutes as listed below (to be prescribed only for indications approved by ACBS[3]):
- AS Saliva Orthana®
- Glandosane®
- Biotene Oralbalance®
- BioXtra®
- Saliveze®
- Salivix®

Ascorbic Acid Tablets, BP
Aspirin Tablets, Dispersible, BP[4]
Azithromycin Oral Suspension, 200 mg/5 mL, DPF
Beclometasone Dipropionate Aerosol Inhalation 50 micrograms/metered dose, DPF
Benzydamine Mouthwash, BP 0.15%
Benzydamine Oromucosal Spray, BP 0.15%
Betamethasone Soluble Tablets, 500 micrograms, DPF
Carbamazepine Tablets, BP
Carmellose Gelatin Paste, DPF
Cefalexin Capsules, BP
Cefalexin Oral Suspension, BP
Cefalexin Tablets, BP
Cefradine Capsules, BP
Cefradine Oral Solution, DPF
Chlorhexidine Gluconate 1% Gel, DPF
Chlorhexidine Mouthwash, BP
Chlorhexidine Oral Spray, DPF
Chlorphenamine Tablets, BP
Choline Salicylate Dental Gel, BP
Clindamycin Capsules, BP
Diazepam Oral Solution, BP, 2 mg/5 mL
Diazepam Tablets, BP
Diclofenac Sodium Tablets, BP
Dihydrocodeine Tablets, BP, 30 mg
Doxycycline Capsules, BP, 100 mg
Doxycycline Tablets, 20 mg, DPF
Ephedrine Nasal Drops, BP
Erythromycin Ethyl Succinate Oral Suspension, BP
Erythromycin Ethyl Succinate Tablets, BP
Erythromycin Stearate Tablets, BP
Erythromycin Tablets, BP
Fluconazole Capsules, 50 mg, DPF
Fluconazole Oral Suspension, 50 mg/5 mL, DPF
Hydrocortisone Cream, BP, 1%
Hydrocortisone Oromucosal Tablets, BP
Hydrocortisone and Miconazole Cream, DPF
Hydrocortisone and Miconazole Ointment, DPF
Hydrogen Peroxide Mouthwash, BP
Ibuprofen Oral Suspension, BP, sugar-free
Ibuprofen Tablets, BP
Lidocaine 5% Ointment, DPF
Lidocaine Spray 10%, DPF
Menthol and Eucalyptus Inhalation, BP 1980[5]
Metronidazole Oral Suspension, DPF
Metronidazole Tablets, BP
Miconazole Cream, BP
Miconazole Oromucosal Gel, BP
Mouthwash Solution-tablets, DPF
Nitrazepam Tablets, BP
Nystatin Ointment, BP
Nystatin Oral Suspension, BP
Oxytetracycline Tablets, BP
Paracetamol Oral Suspension, BP[6]
Paracetamol Tablets, BP
Paracetamol Tablets, Soluble, BP
Penciclovir Cream, DPF
Pethidine Tablets, BP
Phenoxymethylpenicillin Oral Solution, BP
Phenoxymethylpenicillin Tablets, BP
Promethazine Hydrochloride Tablets, BP
Promethazine Oral Solution, BP
Saliva Stimulating Tablets, DPF
Sodium Chloride Mouthwash, Compound, BP
Sodium Fluoride Mouthwash, BP
Sodium Fluoride Oral Drops, BP
Sodium Fluoride Tablets, BP
Sodium Fluoride Toothpaste 0.619%, DPF
Sodium Fluoride Toothpaste 1.1%, DPF
Sodium Fusidate Ointment, BP
Temazepam Oral Solution, BP
Temazepam Tablets, BP
Tetracycline Tablets, BP
Triamcinolone Dental Paste, BP
Vitamin B Tablets, Compound, Strong, BPC

Preparations in this list which are not included in the BP or BPC are described on p. 883

1. Amoxicillin Dispersible Tablets are no longer available
2. Supplies may be difficult to obtain
3. Indications approved by the ACBS are: patients suffering from dry mouth as a result of having (or having undergone) radiotherapy or sicca syndrome
4. The BP directs that when soluble aspirin tablets are prescribed, dispersible aspirin tablets should be dispensed
5. This preparation does not appear in subsequent editions of the BP
6. The BP directs that when Paediatric Paracetamol Oral Suspension or Paediatric Paracetamol Mixture is prescribed and no strength stated Paracetamol Oral Suspension 120 mg/5 mL should be dispensed

Details of DPF preparations

Preparations on the List of Dental Preparations which are specified as DPF are described as follows in the DPF.

Although brand names have sometimes been included for identification purposes preparations on the list should be prescribed by non-proprietary name.

Amoxicillin Oral Powder PoM

(proprietary product: *Amoxil Sachets SF*), amoxicillin (as trihydrate) 750 mg[1] and 3 g sachet

1. 750-mg sachets are no longer available

Artificial Saliva

(proprietary product: *Luborant*) consists of sorbitol 1.8 g, carmellose sodium (sodium carboxymethylcellulose) 390 mg, dibasic potassium phosphate 48.23 mg, potassium chloride 37.5 mg, monobasic potassium phosphate 21.97 mg, calcium chloride 9.972 mg, magnesium chloride 3.528 mg, sodium fluoride 258 micrograms/60 mL, with preservatives and colouring agents

Azithromycin Oral Suspension 200 mg/5 mL PoM

(proprietary product: *Zithromax*); azithromycin (as dihydrate) 200 mg/5 mL when reconstituted with water

Beclometasone Dipropionate Aerosol Inhalation 50 micrograms/metered dose PoM

beclometasone dipropionate 50 micrograms/metered dose

Betamethasone Soluble Tablets 500 micrograms PoM

(proprietary product: *Betnesol Soluble Tablets*), betamethasone (as sodium phosphate) 500 micrograms

Carmellose Gelatin Paste

(proprietary product: *Orabase Oral Paste*), gelatin, pectin, carmellose sodium, 16.58% of each in a suitable basis

Cefradine Oral Solution PoM

(proprietary product: *Velosef Syrup*), cefradine 250 mg/5mL when reconstituted with water

Chlorhexidine Gluconate 1% Gel

(proprietary product: *Corsodyl Dental Gel*), chlorhexidine gluconate 1%

Chlorhexidine Oral Spray

(proprietary product: *Corsodyl Oral Spray*), chlorhexidine gluconate 0.2%

Doxycycline Tablets 20 mg PoM

(proprietary product: *Periostat*), doxycycline (as hyclate) 20 mg

Fluconazole Capsules 50 mg PoM

(proprietary product: *Diflucan*), fluconazole 50 mg

Fluconazole Oral Suspension 50 mg/5 mL PoM

(proprietary product: *Diflucan*), fluconazole 50 mg/5 mL when reconstituted with water

Hydrocortisone and Miconazole Cream PoM

(proprietary product: *Daktacort Cream*), hydrocortisone 1%, miconazole nitrate 2%

Hydrocortisone and Miconazole Ointment PoM

(proprietary product: *Daktacort Ointment*), hydrocortisone 1%, miconazole nitrate 2%

Lidocaine 5% Ointment

lidocaine 5% in a suitable basis

Lidocaine Spray 10%

(proprietary product: *Xylocaine Spray*), lidocaine 10% supplying 10 mg lidocaine/spray

Metronidazole Oral Suspension PoM

(proprietary product: *Flagyl S*), metronidazole (as benzoate) 200 mg/5mL

Mouthwash Solution-tablets

consist of tablets which may contain antimicrobial, colouring and flavouring agents in a suitable soluble effervescent basis to make a mouthwash suitable for dental purposes

Penciclovir Cream PoM

(proprietary product: *Vectavir Cream*), penciclovir 1%

Saliva Stimulating Tablets

(proprietary product: *SST*), citric acid, malic acid and other ingredients in a sorbitol base

Sodium Fluoride Toothpaste 0.619% PoM

(proprietary product: *Duraphat '2800 ppm' Toothpaste*), sodium fluoride 0.619%

Sodium Fluoride Toothpaste 1.1% PoM

(proprietary product: *Duraphat '5000 ppm' Toothpaste*), sodium fluoride 1.1%

Changes to Dental Practitioners' Formulary since September 2007

Additions

Aciclovir Tablets BP, 800 mg

Beclometasone Dipropionate Aerosol Inhalation 50 micrograms/metered dose, DPF

Betamethasone Soluble Tablets, 500 micrograms, DPF

Diclofenac Sodium Tablets, BP

Lidocaine Spray 10%, DPF

Miconazole Cream, BP

Saliva Stimulating Tablets, DPF

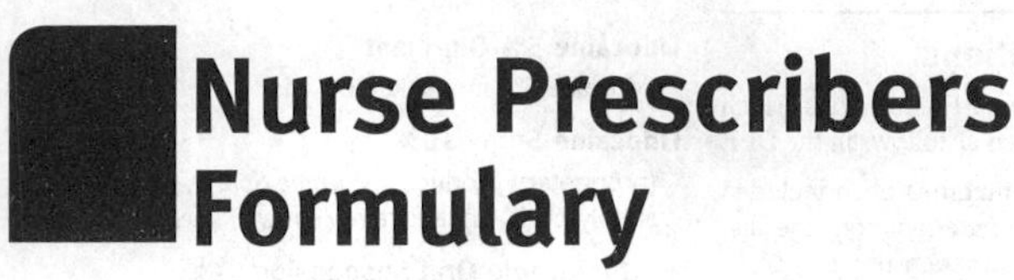

Nurse Prescribers' Formulary

Nurse Prescribers' Formulary for Community Practitioners

Nurse Prescribers' Formulary Appendix (Appendix NPF). List of preparations approved by the Secretary of State which may be prescribed on form FP10P (form HS21(N) in Northern Ireland, form GP10(N) in Scotland, forms FP10(CN) and FP10(PN) in Wales or, when available, WP10CN and WP10PN in Wales) by Nurses for National Health Service patients.

Community practitioners who have completed the necessary training may only prescribe items appearing in the nurse prescribers' list set out below. Community Practitioner Nurse Prescribers are recommended to prescribe generically, except where this would not be clinically appropriate or where there is no approved generic name.

Medicinal Preparations

> Preparations on this list which are not included in the BP or BPC are described on p. 885

Almond Oil Ear Drops, BP
Arachis Oil Enema, NPF
[1]Aspirin Tablets, Dispersible, 300 mg, BP
Bisacodyl Suppositories, BP (includes 5-mg and 10-mg strengths)
Bisacodyl Tablets, BP
Catheter Maintenance Solution, Chlorhexidine, NPF
Catheter Maintenance Solution, Sodium Chloride, NPF
Catheter Maintenance Solution, 'Solution G', NPF
Catheter Maintenance Solution, 'Solution R', NPF
Chlorhexidine Gluconate Alcoholic Solutions containing at least 0.05%
Chlorhexidine Gluconate Aqueous Solutions containing at least 0.05%
Choline Salicylate Dental Gel, BP
Clotrimazole Cream 1%, BP
Co-danthramer Capsules, NPF
Co-danthramer Capsules, Strong, NPF
Co-danthramer Oral Suspension, NPF
Co-danthramer Oral Suspension, Strong, NPF
Co-danthrusate Capsules, BP
Co-danthrusate Oral Suspension, NPF
Crotamiton Cream, BP
Crotamiton Lotion, BP
Dimeticone barrier creams containing at least 10%
Dimeticone Lotion, NPF
Docusate Capsules, BP
Docusate Enema, NPF
Docusate Enema, Compound, BP
Docusate Oral Solution, BP
Docusate Oral Solution, Paediatric, BP
Econazole Cream 1%, BP

1. Max. 96 tablets; max. pack size 32 tablets

Emollients as listed below:
- Aqueous Cream, BP
- Arachis Oil, BP
- Cetraben® Emollient Cream
- Decubal® Clinic
- Dermamist®
- Diprobase® Cream
- Diprobase® Ointment
- Doublebase®
- E45® Cream
- Emulsifying Ointment, BP
- [2]Epaderm®
- Hydromol® Cream
- Hydromol® Ointment
- Hydrous Ointment, BP
- Keri® Therapeutic Lotion
- Linola® Gamma Cream
- Lipobase®
- Liquid and White Soft Paraffin Ointment, NPF
- Neutrogena® Dermatological Cream
- Oilatum® Cream
- Oilatum® Junior Cream
- Paraffin, White Soft, BP
- Paraffin, Yellow Soft, BP
- QV® Cream
- QV® Lotion
- QV® Wash
- Ultrabase®
- Unguentum M®
- Zerobase® Cream

Emollient Bath Additives as listed below:
- Alpha Keri® Bath Oil
- [3]Balneum®
- Cetraben® Emollient Bath Additive
- Dermalo® Bath Emollient
- Diprobath®
- Doublebase® Emollient Shower Gel
- Hydromol® Emollient
- Imuderm® Bath Oil
- Oilatum® Emollient
- Oilatum® Junior Emollient Bath Additive
- Oilatum® Gel
- QV® Bath Oil

Folic Acid 400 micrograms/5 mL Oral Solution, NPF
Folic Acid Tablets 400 micrograms, BP
Glycerol Suppositories, BP
[4]Ibuprofen Oral Suspension, BP
[4]Ibuprofen Tablets, BP
Ispaghula Husk Granules, BP
Ispaghula Husk Granules, Effervescent, BP
Ispaghula Husk Oral Powder, BP
Lactulose Solution, BP
Lidocaine Ointment, BP

2. Included in the Drug Tariff, Scottish Drug Tariff, and Northern Ireland Drug Tariff
3. Except pack sizes that are not to be prescribed under the NHS (see Part XVIIIA of the Drug Tariff, Part XI of the Northern Ireland Drug Tariff)
4. Except for indications and doses that are PoM

Lidocaine and Chlorhexidine Gel, BP
Macrogol Oral Powder, NPF
Macrogol Oral Powder, Compound, NPF
Macrogol Oral Powder, Compound, Half-strength, NPF
Magnesium Hydroxide Mixture, BP
Magnesium Sulphate Paste, BP
Malathion alcoholic lotions containing at least 0.5%
Malathion aqueous lotions containing at least 0.5%
Mebendazole Oral Suspension, NPF
Mebendazole Tablets, NPF
Methylcellulose Tablets, BP
Miconazole Cream 2%, BP
Miconazole Oromucosal Gel, BP
Mouthwash Solution-tablets, NPF
Nicotine Inhalation Cartridge for Oromucosal Use, NPF
Nicotine Lozenge, NPF
Nicotine Medicated Chewing Gum, NPF
Nicotine Nasal Spray, NPF
Nicotine Sublingual Tablets, NPF
Nicotine Transdermal Patches, NPF
Nystatin Oral Suspension, BP
Olive Oil Ear Drops, BP
Paracetamol Oral Suspension, BP (includes 120 mg/5 mL and 250 mg/5 mL strengths—both of which are available as sugar-free formulations)
[1]Paracetamol Tablets, BP
[1]Paracetamol Tablets, Soluble, BP (includes 120-mg and 500-mg tablets)
Permethrin Cream, NPF
Phenothrin Alcoholic Lotion, NPF
Phenothrin Aqueous Lotion, NPF
Phosphate Suppositories, NPF
Phosphates Enema, BP
Piperazine and Senna Powder, NPF
Povidone–Iodine Solution, BP
Senna Granules, Standardised, BP
Senna Oral Solution, NPF
Senna Tablets, BP
Senna and Ispaghula Granules, NPF
Sodium Chloride Solution, Sterile, BP
Sodium Citrate Compound Enema, NPF
Sodium Picosulfate Capsules, NPF
Sodium Picosulfate Elixir, NPF
Spermicidal contraceptives as listed below:
Ortho-Creme® Cream
Sterculia Granules, NPF
Sterculia and Frangula Granules, NPF
Titanium Ointment, BP
Water for Injections, BP
Zinc and Castor Oil Ointment, BP
Zinc Cream, BP
Zinc Ointment, BP
Zinc Oxide and Dimeticone Spray, NPF
Zinc Oxide Impregnated Medicated Bandage, NPF
Zinc Oxide Impregnated Medicated Stocking, NPF
Zinc Paste Bandage, BP 1993
Zinc Paste and Calamine Bandage
Zinc Paste and Ichthammol Bandage, BP 1993

Appliances and Reagents (including Wound Management Products)

Community Practitioner Nurse Prescribers in England, Wales and Northern Ireland can prescribe any appliance or reagent in the relevant Drug Tariff. In the Scottish Drug Tariff, Appliances and Reagents which may **not** be prescribed by Nurses are annotated **Nx**.

1. Max. 96 tablets; max. pack size 32 tablets

Appliances (including Contraceptive Devices[2]) as listed in Part IXA of the Drug Tariff (Part III of the Northern Ireland Drug Tariff, Part 3 (Appliances) and Part 2 (Dressings) of the Scottish Drug Tariff)

Incontinence Appliances as listed in Part IXB of the Drug Tariff (Part III of the Northern Ireland Drug Tariff, Part 5 of the Scottish Drug Tariff)

Stoma Appliances and Associated Products as listed in Part IXC of the Drug Tariff (Part III of the Northern Ireland Drug Tariff, Part 6 of the Scottish Drug Tariff)

Chemical Reagents as listed in Part IXR of the Drug Tariff (Part II of the Northern Ireland Drug Tariff, Part 9 of the Scottish Drug Tariff)

Details of NPF preparations

Preparations on the Nurse Prescribers' Formulary which are not included in the BP or BPC are described as follows in the Nurse Prescribers' Formulary.

Although brand names have sometimes been included for identification purposes, it is recommended that non-proprietary names should be used for prescribing medicinal preparations in the NPF except where a non-proprietary name is not available.

Arachis Oil Enema
(proprietary product: *Fletchers' Arachis Oil Retention Enema*), arachis oil

Catheter Maintenance Solution, Chlorhexidine
(proprietary products: *Uro-Tainer Chlorhexidine*; *Uriflex C*), chlorhexidine 0.02%

Catheter Maintenance Solution, Sodium Chloride
(proprietary products: *OptiFlo S*; *Uro-Tainer Sodium Chloride*; *Uriflex-S*), sodium chloride 0.9%

Catheter Maintenance Solution, 'Solution G'
(proprietary products: *OptiFlo G*; *Uro-Tainer Suby G*; *Uriflex G*), citric acid 3.23%, magnesium oxide 0.38%, sodium bicarbonate 0.7%, disodium edetate 0.01%

Catheter Maintenance Solution, 'Solution R'
(proprietary products: *OptiFlo R*; *Uro-Tainer Solution R*; *Uriflex R*), citric acid 6%, gluconolactone 0.6%, magnesium carbonate 2.8%, disodium edetate 0.01%

Chlorhexidine gluconate alcoholic solutions
(proprietary products: *Hydrex Solution*; *Hydrex spray*), chlorhexidine gluconate in alcoholic solution

Chlorhexidine gluconate aqueous solutions
(proprietary product: *Unisept*) chlorhexidine gluconate in aqueous solution

Co-danthramer Capsules PoM
co-danthramer 25/200 (dantron 25 mg, poloxamer '188' 200 mg)

Co-danthramer Capsules, Strong PoM
co-danthramer 37.5/500 (dantron 37.5 mg, poloxamer '188' 500 mg)

2. Nurse Prescribers in Family Planning Clinics—where it is not appropriate for nurse prescribers in family planning clinics to prescribe contraceptive devices using form FP10(P) (forms FP10(CN) and FP10(PN), or when available WP10CN and WP10PN, in Wales), they may prescribe using the same system as doctors in the clinic

Co-danthramer Oral Suspension PoM
(proprietary product: *Codalax*), co-danthramer 25/200 in 5 mL (dantron 25 mg, poloxamer '188' 200 mg/5 mL)

Co-danthramer Oral Suspension, Strong PoM
(proprietary product: *Codalax Forte*), co-danthramer 75/1000 in 5 mL (dantron 75 mg, poloxamer '188' 1 g/5 mL)

Co-danthrusate Oral Suspension PoM
(proprietary product: *Normax*), co-danthrusate 50/60 (dantron 50 mg, docusate sodium 60 mg/5 mL)

Dimeticone barrier creams
(proprietary products: *Conotrane Cream*, dimeticone '350' 22%; *Siopel Barrier Cream*, dimeticone '1000' 10%; *Vasogen Barrier Cream*, dimeticone 20%), dimeticone 10–22%

Dimeticone Lotion
(proprietary product: *Hedrin*), dimeticone 4%

Docusate Enema
(proprietary product: *Norgalax Micro-enema*) docusate sodium 120 mg in 10 g

Folic Acid Oral Solution 400 micrograms/5 mL
(proprietary product: *Folicare*), folic acid 400 micrograms/5 mL

Liquid and White Soft Paraffin Ointment
liquid paraffin 50%, white soft paraffin 50%

Macrogol Oral Powder
(proprietary product: *Idrolax*), macrogol '4000' (polyethylene glycol '4000') 10 g/sachet

Macrogol Oral Powder, Compound
(proprietary product: *Movicol*; *Movicol Plain*), macrogol '3350' (polyethylene glycol '3350') 13.125 g, sodium bicarbonate 178.5 mg, sodium chloride 350.7 mg, potassium chloride 46.6 mg/sachet

Macrogol Oral Powder, Compound, Half-strength
(proprietary product: *Movicol-Half*), macrogol '3350' (polyethylene glycol '3350') 6.563 g, sodium bicarbonate 89.3 g, sodium chloride 175.4 mg, potassium chloride 23.3 mg/sachet

Malathion alcoholic lotions
(proprietary product: *Prioderm Lotion*), malathion 0.5% in an alcoholic basis

Malathion aqueous lotions
(proprietary products: *Derbac-M Liquid*; *Quellada M Liquid*), malathion 0.5% in an aqueous basis

Mebendazole Oral Suspension PoM
(proprietary product: *Vermox*), mebendazole 100 mg/5 mL

[1]**Mebendazole Tablets** PoM
(proprietary products: *Ovex*, *Vermox*), mebendazole 100 mg

Mouthwash Solution-tablets
consist of tablets which may contain antimicrobial, colouring and flavouring agents in a suitable soluble effervescent basis to make a mouthwash

1. For PoM exemption, see p. 356

[2]**Nicotine Inhalation Cartridge for Oromucosal Use**
(proprietary products: *Nicorette Inhalator*), nicotine 10 mg

Nicotine Lozenge
nicotine (as bitartrate) 1 mg or 2 mg (proprietary product: *Nicotinell Mint Lozenge*) or nicotine (as polacrilex) 2 mg or 4 mg (proprietary product: *NiQuitin CQ Lozenges*)

Nicotine Medicated Chewing Gum
(proprietary products: *Nicorette Gum*, *Nicotinell Gum*, *NiQuitin CQ Gum*), nicotine 2 mg or 4 mg

Nicotine Nasal Spray
(proprietary product: *Nicorette Nasal Spray*), nicotine 500 micrograms/metered spray

[3]**Nicotine Sublingual Tablets**
(proprietary product: *Nicorette Microtab*), nicotine (as a cyclodextrin complex) 2 mg

[4]**Nicotine Transdermal Patches**
releasing in each 16 hours, nicotine approx. 5 mg, 10 mg, or 15 mg (proprietary product: *Nicorette Patch*) or releasing in each 24 hours nicotine approx. 7 mg, 14 mg, or 21 mg (proprietary products: *Nicopatch*, *Nicotinell TTS*, *NiQuitin CQ*)

Permethrin Cream
(proprietary product: *Lyclear Dermal Cream*), permethrin 5%

Phenothrin Alcoholic Lotion
(proprietary product: *Full Marks Lotion*), phenothrin 0.2% in a basis containing isopropyl alcohol

Phenothrin Aqueous Lotion
(proprietary product: *Full Marks Liquid*), phenothrin 0.5% in an aqueous basis

Phosphate Suppositories
(proprietary product: *Carbalax*), sodium acid phosphate (anhydrous) 1.3 g, sodium bicarbonate 1.08 g

Piperazine and Senna Powder
(proprietary product: *Pripsen Oral Powder*), piperazine phosphate 4 g, sennosides 15.3 mg/sachet

Senna Oral Solution
(proprietary product: *Senokot Syrup*), sennosides 7.5 mg/5 mL

Senna and Ispaghula Granules
(proprietary product: *Manevac Granules*), senna fruit 12.4%, ispaghula 54.2%

Sodium Citrate Compound Enema
(proprietary products: *Micolette Micro-enema*; *Micralax Micro-enema*; *Relaxit Micro-enema*), sodium citrate 450 mg with glycerol, sorbitol and an anionic surfactant

Sodium Picosulfate Capsules
(proprietary products: *Dulco-lax Perles*), sodium picosulfate 2.5 mg

2. For use with inhalation mouthpiece; to be prescribed as either a starter pack (6 cartridges with inhalator device and holder) or refill pack (42 cartridges with inhalator device)
3. To be prescribed as either a starter pack (2 x 15-tablet discs with dispenser) or refill pack (7 x 15-tablet discs)
4. Prescriber should specify the brand to be dispensed

Sodium Picosulfate Elixir

(proprietary products: *Dulco-lax Liquid, Laxoberal* [NHS]), sodium picosulfate 5 mg/5 mL

Sterculia Granules

(proprietary product: *Normacol Granules*), sterculia 62%

Sterculia and Frangula Granules

(proprietary product: *Normacol Plus Granules*), sterculia 62%, frangula (standardised) 8%

Zinc Oxide and Dimeticone Spray

(proprietary product: *Sprilon*), dimeticone 1.04%, zinc oxide 12.5% in a pressurised aerosol unit

Zinc Oxide Impregnated Medicated Bandage

(proprietary product: *Steripaste*), sterile cotton bandage impregnated with paste containing zinc oxide 15%

Zinc Oxide Impregnated Medicated Stocking

(proprietary product: *Zipzoc*), sterile rayon stocking impregnated with ointment containing zinc oxide 20%

Nurse Independent Prescribing

Nurse Independent Prescribers (formerly known as Extended Formulary Nurse Prescribers) are able to prescribe any licensed medicine for any medical condition, including some Controlled Drugs (see below).

Nurse Independent Prescribers must work within their own level of professional competence and expertise. They are recommended to prescribe generically, except where this would not be clinically appropriate or where there is no approved non-proprietary name.

Nurse Independent Prescribers are also able to prescribe independently the Controlled Drugs in the table below, *solely for the medical conditions indicated.*

Pharmacist Independent Prescribing

Pharmacist Independent Prescribers can prescribe similarly to Nurse Independent Prescribers, but currently cannot prescribe any Controlled Drug independently.

Up-to-date information and guidance on nurse independent and pharmacist independent prescribing is available on the Department of Health website at www.dh.gov.uk/nonmedicalprescribing

Controlled drugs prescribable by Nurse Independent Prescribers solely for the medical conditions indicated

Drug	Indication	Route of Administration
Buprenorphine	Transdermal use in palliative care	Transdermal
Chlordiazepoxide hydrochloride	Treatment of initial or acute withdrawal symptoms caused by the withdrawal of alcohol from persons habituated to it	Oral
Codeine phosphate	–	Oral
Co-phenotrope	–	Oral
Diamorphine hydrochloride	Use in palliative care, pain relief in respect of suspected myocardial infarction or for relief of acute or severe pain after trauma, including in either case postoperative pain relief	Oral, parenteral
Diazepam	Use in palliative care, treatment of initial or acute withdrawal symptoms caused by the withdrawal of alcohol from persons habituated to it, tonic-clonic seizures	Oral, parenteral, rectal
Dihydrocodeine tartrate	–	Oral
Fentanyl	Transdermal use in palliative care	Transdermal
Lorazepam	Use in palliative care, tonic-clonic seizures	Oral, parenteral
Midazolam	Use in palliative care, tonic-clonic seizures	Parenteral, buccal
Morphine hydrochloride	Use in palliative care, pain relief in respect of suspected myocardial infarction or for relief of acute or severe pain after trauma, including in either case postoperative pain relief	Rectal
Morphine sulphate	Use in palliative care, pain relief in respect of suspected myocardial infarction or for relief of acute or severe pain after trauma, including in either case postoperative pain relief	Oral, parenteral, rectal
Oxycodone hydrochloride	Use in palliative care	Oral, parenteral

Index of manufacturers

3M
3M Health Care Ltd
3M House
Morley St
Loughborough
Leics, LE11 1EP.
tel: (01509) 611611
fax: (01509) 237288

A&H
Allen & Hanburys Ltd
See GSK

A1 Pharmaceuticals
A1 Pharmaceuticals Plc
Units 20+21 Easter Park
Site 8A Beam Reach
Ferrry Lane South, Rainham
Essex, RM13 9BP.
tel: (01708) 528 900
fax: (01708) 528 928
sales@a1plc.co.uk

Abbott
Abbott Laboratories Ltd
Abbott House
Norden Rd, Maidenhead
Berks, SL6 4XE.
tel: (01628) 773 355
fax: (01628) 644 185
ukmedinfo@abbott.com

ABT Healthcare
ABT Healthcare UK Ltd
Springwood Booths Hall
Booths Park
Chelford Rd
Knutsford, WA16 8QZ.
tel: (01565) 757783

Acorus
Acorus Therapeutics Ltd
High Crane Lodge
Hamsterley, Bishop Auckland
Durham, DL13 3QS.
tel: (01388) 710 505
fax: (01388) 710 770
enquiries@acorus-therapeutics.com

Actavis
Actavis UK Ltd
Whiddon Valley
Barnstaple
Devon, EX32 8NS.
tel: (01271) 311 257
fax: (01271) 346 106
medinfo@actavis.co.uk

Actelion
Actelion Pharmaceuticals UK Ltd
BSi Building, 13th Floor
389 Chiswick High Rd, London, W4 4AL.
tel: (020) 8987 3333
fax: (020) 8987 3322

Activa
Activa Healthcare
1 Lancaster Park
Newborough Rd, Needwood
Burton-upon-Trent, Staffs, DE13 9PD.
tel: (0845) 060 6707
fax: (01283) 576 808
advice@activahealthcare.co.uk

Adams Hlth.
Adams Healthcare Ltd
Lotherton Way
Garforth, Leeds, LS25 2JY.
tel: (0113) 232 0066
fax: (0113) 287 1317
enquiries@adams-healthcare.co.uk

ADL
ADL Healthcare Diagnostics
Pitcairn House
Crown Square
1st Avenue, Centrum 100
Burton-on-Trent, Staffs, DE14 2WW.
tel: (01283) 494 300
fax: (01283) 494 304
truetrak@adlhealthcare.co.uk

Advancis
Advancis Medical Ltd
Lowmoor Business Park
Kirkby-in-Ashfield, Nottingham, NG17 7JZ.
tel: (01623) 751 500
fax: (0871) 264 8238
info@advancis.co.uk

Aguettant
Aguettant Ltd
Bishops House
Bishops Rd, Claverham
Somerset, BS49 4NF.
tel: (01934) 835 694
fax: (01934) 876 790
info@aguettant.co.uk

Air Products
Air Products plc
Medical Group
2 Millennium Gate
Westmere Drive, Crewe
Cheshire, CW1 6AP.
tel: (0800) 373 580
fax: (0800) 214 709

Alcon
Alcon Laboratories (UK) Ltd
Pentagon Park
Boundary Way
Hemel Hempstead, Herts, HP2 7UD.
tel: (01442) 341 234
fax: (01442) 341 200

Alembic Products
Alembic Products Ltd
River Lane
Saltney, Chester, Cheshire, CH4 8RQ.
tel: (01244) 680 147
fax: (01244) 680 155

Alexion
Alexion Pharma UK Ltd
3000 Cathedral Hill
Guildford
Surrey, GU2 7YB.
tel: (01483) 246 641
fax: (01483) 245 130
alexion.uk@alxn.com

ALK-Abelló
ALK-Abelló (UK) Ltd
1 Tealgate
Hungerford, Berks, RG17 0YT.
tel: (01488) 686 016
fax: (01488) 685 423
info@uk.alk-abello.com

Allergan
Allergan Ltd
1st Floor Marlow International
The Parkway
Marlow
Bucks, SL7 1YL.
tel: (01628) 494 026
fax: (01628) 494 057

Allergy
Allergy Therapeutics Ltd
Dominion Way
Worthing, West Sussex, BN14 8SA.
tel: (01903) 844 702
fax: (01903) 844 744
infoservices@allergytherapeutics.com

Alliance
Alliance Pharmaceuticals Ltd
Avonbridge House
2 Bath Rd
Chippenham, Wilts, SN15 2BB.
tel: (01249) 466 966
fax: (01249) 466 977
medinfo@alliancepharma.co.uk

Alpharma
See Actavis

Alphashow
Alphashow Ltd
10 South Rd
Amersham
Bucks, HP6 5LX.
tel: (0870) 240 2775
fax: (01672) 515 614
info@alphashow.co.uk

Altana
See Nycomed

Amdipharm
Amdipharm plc
Regency House
Miles Gray Rd
Basildon, Essex, SS14 3AF.
tel: (0870) 777 7675
fax: (0870) 777 7875
medinfo@amdipharm.com

Amgen
Amgen Ltd
240 Cambridge Science Park
Milton Rd, Cambridge, CB4 0WD.
tel: (01223) 420 305
fax: (01223) 426 314
infoline@uk.amgen.com

Anglian
Anglian Pharma Sales & Marketing
Titmore Court
Titmore Green
Little Wymondley, Hitchin
Herts, SG4 7XJ.
tel: (01438) 743 070
fax: (01438) 743 080
mail@anglianpharma.com

Anpharm
See Goldshield

Antigen
See Goldshield

APS
See TEVA UK

Archimedes
Archimedes Pharma UK Ltd
250 South Oak Way
Green Park
Reading
Berks, RG2 6UG.
tel: (0118) 931 5060
fax: (0118) 931 5065
medicalinformation@
archimedespharma.com

Ardana
Ardana Bioscience Ltd
58 Queen St
Edinburgh, EH2 3NS.
tel: (0131) 226 8550
fax: (0131) 226 8551
info@ardana.co.uk

Ardern
Ardern Healthcare Ltd
Pipers Brook Farm
Eastham
Tenbury Wells, Worcs, WR15 8NP.
tel: (01584) 781 777
fax: (01584) 781 788
info@ardernhealthcare.com

Ark Therapeutics
Ark Therapeutics Group Plc
79 New Cavendish St
London, W1W 6XB.
tel: (020) 7388 7722
fax: (020) 7388 7805
info@arktherapeutics.com

Ashbourne
Ashbourne Pharmaceuticals Ltd
The Drummonds
Spring Hill Office Park
Harborough Rd
Pitsford, Northampton, NN6 9AA.
tel: (01604) 883 100
fax: (01604) 881 640

AS Pharma
AS Pharma Ltd
PO Box 181
Polegate, East Sussex, BN26 6WD.
tel: (08700) 664 117
fax: (08700) 664 118
info@aspharma.co.uk

Astellas
Astellas Pharma Ltd
Lovett House, Lovett Rd
Staines, TW18 3AZ.
tel: (01784) 419 615
fax: (01784) 419 401

AstraZeneca
AstraZeneca UK Ltd
Horizon Place
600 Capability Green
Luton, Beds, LU1 3LU.
tel: 0800 7830 033
fax: (01582) 838 003
medical.informationuk@astrazeneca.
com

Auden Mckenzie
Auden Mckenzie (Pharma Division) Ltd
30 Stadium Business Centre
North End Rd
Wembley, Middx, HA9 0AT.
tel: (020) 8900 2122
fax: (020) 8903 9620

Aurum
Aurum Pharmaceuticals Ltd
Hubert Rd
Brentwood
Essex, CM14 4LZ.
tel: (01277) 266600
fax: (01277) 848 976
info@martindalepharma.co.uk

Aventis Pharma
See Sanofi-Aventis

Ayrton Saunders
Ayrton Saunders Ltd
Ayrton House
Commerce Way
Parliament Business Park
Liverpool, Merseyside, L8 7BA.
tel: (0151) 709 2074
fax: (0151) 709 7336
info@ayrtons.com

Bard
Bard Ltd
Forest House
Brighton Rd
Crawley, West Sussex, RH11 9BP.
tel: (01293) 527 888
fax: (01293) 552 428

Bausch & Lomb
Bausch & Lomb UK Ltd
106 London Rd
Kingston-upon-Thames
Surrey, KT2 6TN.
tel: (020) 8781 2900
fax: (020) 8781 2901

Baxter
Baxter Healthcare Ltd
Wallingford Rd
Compton
Newbury
Berks, RG20 7QW.
tel: (01635) 206 345
fax: (01635) 206 071
surecall@baxter.com

Bayer
Bayer plc
Bayer Schering Pharma
Bayer House, Strawberry Hill
Newbury, Berks, RG14 1JA.
tel: (01635) 563 000
fax: (01635) 563 393
medical.science@bayer.co.uk

Bayer Consumer Care
See Bayer

Bayer Diagnostics
See Bayer

BBI Healthcare
BBI Healthcare
Unit A
Kestrel Way
Garngoch Industrial Estate
Gorseinon, Swansea, SA4 9WN.
tel: (01792) 229 333
fax: (01792) 897 311
info@bbihealthcare.com

BCM Specials
BCM Specials Manufacturing
D10 First 114
Nottingham, NG90 2PR.
tel: 0800 952 1010
fax: 0800 085 0673
bcm-specials@bcm-ltd.co.uk

Beacon
Beacon Pharmaceuticals Ltd
85 High St
Tunbridge Wells, TN1 1YG.
tel: (01892) 600 930
fax: (01892) 600 937
info@beaconpharma.co.uk

Becton Dickinson
Becton Dickinson UK Ltd
The Danby Building
Edmund Halley
Oxford Science Park
Oxford, Oxon, OX4 4DQ.
tel: (01865) 781 510
fax: (01865) 731 551

Beiersdorf
Beiersdorf UK Ltd
2010 Solihull Parkway
Birmingham Business Park
Birmingham, B37 7YS.
tel: (0121) 329 8800
fax: (0121) 329 8801

Bell and Croyden
John Bell and Croyden
50-54 Wigmore St
London, W1U 2AU.
tel: (020) 7935 5555
fax: (020) 7935 9605
jbc@johnbellcroyden.co.uk

Berk
See TEVA UK

BHR
BHR Pharmaceuticals Ltd
41 Centenary Business Centre
Hammond Close
Attleborough Fields, Nuneaton
Warwickshire, CV11 6RY.
tel: (024) 7635 3742
fax: (024) 7632 7812
info@bhr.co.uk

Bioaccelerate
Bioaccelerate Ltd
11-12 Charles II St
Savanah House
London, SW1Y 4QU.
tel: (020) 7451 2488
fax: (020) 7451 2459
info@bioaccelerate.com

Bioenvision
Bioenvision Ltd
10 Lockside Place
Edinburgh Park
Edinburgh, EH12 9RG.
tel: (0131) 248 3555
fax: (0131) 2483300
info@bioenvision.com

Biogen
Biogen Idec Ltd
Thames House
Foundation Park
Maidenhead
Berks, SL6 3UD.
tel: (01628) 501 000
fax: (01628) 501 010

Biolitec
Biolitec Pharma Ltd
Unit 2, Broomhill Business Park
Broomhill Rd
Tallaght
Dublin 24, Ireland.
tel: (00353) 14637415
fax: (00353) 14637411
medical.info@biolitec.com

BioMarin
BioMarin Europe Ltd
23-24 Warwick St
London, W1B 5NQ.
tel: (020) 7534 9350
fax: (020) 7534 9351

Biosurgical Research
Biosurgical Research Unit
See ZooBiotic

Blackwell
Blackwell Supplies Ltd
Medcare House
Centurion Close
Gillingham Business Park, Gillingham
Kent, ME8 0SB.
tel: (01634) 877 620
fax: (01634) 877 621

Blake
Thomas Blake & Co
The Byre House
Fearby
Nr. Masham
North Yorks, HG4 4NF.
tel: (01765) 689 042
fax: (01765) 689 042
sales@veilcover.com

BOC
BOC Medical
The Priestley Centre,
10 Priestley Rd
Surrey Research Park
Guildford, Surrey, GU2 7XY.
tel: 0800 111 333
fax: 0800 111 555

Boehringer Ingelheim
Boehringer Ingelheim Ltd
Ellesfield Ave
Bracknell
Berks, RG12 8YS.
tel: (01344) 424 600
fax: (01344) 741 444
medinfo@bra.boehringer-ingelheim.com

Boots
Boots The Chemists
Medical Services
Thane Rd
D90 East S10
Nottingham, NG90 1BS.
tel: (0115) 959 5168
fax: (0115) 959 2565

Borg
Borg Medicare
PO Box 99
Hitchin
Herts, SG5 2GF.
tel: (01462) 442 993
fax: (01462) 441 293

BPC 100
The Bolton Pharmaceutical 100 Ltd
2 Chapel Drive
Ambrosden
Oxfordshire, OX25 2RS.
tel: (0845) 602 3907
fax: (0845) 602 3908
info@bpc100.com

BPL
Bio Products Laboratory
Dagger Lane
Elstree, Herts, WD6 3BX.
tel: (020) 8258 2200
fax: (020) 8258 2601

Braun
B Braun (Medical) Ltd
Brookdale Rd
Thorncliffe Park Estate
Chapeltown, Sheffield, S35 2PW.
tel: (0114) 225 9000
fax: (0114) 225 9111
info.bbmuk@bbraun.com

Braun Biotrol
See Braun

Bray
Bray Health & Leisure
1 Regal Way
Faringdon
Oxon, SN7 7BX.
tel: (01367) 240 736
fax: (01367) 242 625
info@bray.co.uk

Bristol-Myers Squibb
Bristol-Myers Squibb Pharmaceuticals Ltd
Uxbridge Business Park
Sanderson Rd
Uxbridge
Middx, UB8 1DH.
tel: (01895) 523 000
fax: (01895) 523 010
medical.information@bms.com

Britannia
Britannia Pharmaceuticals Ltd
41-51 Brighton Rd
Redhill
Surrey, RH1 6YS.
tel: (01737) 773 741
fax: (01737) 762 672
medicalservices@forumgroup.co.uk

BR Pharma
BR Pharma Ltd
Unit 7, Capital Business Park
Manor Way
Borehamwood
Herts, WD6 1GW.
tel: (020) 8238 6770
fax: (020) 8238 6786
enquiries@brpharmaltd.co.uk

BSIA
See Torbet

BSN Medical
BSN Medical Ltd
PO Box 258
Willerby
Hull, HU10 6WT.
tel: (0845) 1223 600
fax: (0845) 1223 666

Cambridge
Cambridge Laboratories
Deltic House, Kingfisher Way
Silverlink Business Park, Wallsend
Tyne & Wear, NE28 9NX.
tel: (0191) 296 9300
fax: (0191) 296 9368
customer.services@camb-labs.com

Cardinal
Cardinal Health Martindale Products
Hubert Rd
Brentwood
Essex, CM14 4JY.
tel: (01277) 266 600
fax: (01277) 848 976
info@martindalepharma.co.uk

Castlemead
See Sanofi-Aventis

C D Medical
C D Medical Ltd
Aston Grange
Oker, Matlock, DE4 2JJ.
tel: (01629) 733 860
fax: (01629) 733 414

Celgene
Celgene Ltd
Royal Albert House
Sheet St
Windsor
Berks, SL4 1BE.
tel: (08448) 010 045
fax: (08448) 010 046
medinfo.uk.ire@celgene.com

Celltech
See UCB Pharma

Centrapharm
See Derma UK

Cephalon
Cephalon Ltd
1 Albany Place
Hyde Way
Welwyn Garden City
Herts, AL7 3BT.
tel: 0800 783 4869
fax: (01483) 765 008
ukmedinfo@cephalon.com

Ceuta
Ceuta Healthcare Ltd
Hill House
41 Richmond Hill
Bournemouth
Dorset, BH2 6HS.
tel: (01202) 780 558
fax: (01202) 780 559

Chattem UK
Chattem UK Ltd
Guerry House
Ringway Centre
Edison Rd
Basingstoke, RG24 6YH.
tel: (01256) 844 144
fax: (01256) 844 145

Chauvin
See Bausch & Lomb

Chefaro UK
Chefaro UK Ltd
Unit 1, Tower Close
St. Peter's Industrial Park
Huntingdon
Cambs, PE29 7DH.
tel: (01480) 421 800
fax: (01480) 434 861

Chemical Search
Chemical Search International Ltd
29th floor
1 Canada Square
Canary Wharf
London, E14 5DY.
tel: (020) 7712 1758
fax: (020) 7712 1759
info@chemicalsearch.co.uk

Chemidex
Chemidex Pharma Ltd
Chemidex House
Egham Business Village
Crabtree Rd, Egham
Surrey, TW20 8RB.
tel: (01784) 477 167
fax: (01784) 471 776
info@chemidex.co.uk

Chiron
See Novartis

Chiron Vaccines
See Novartis Vaccines

CHS
Cambridge Healthcare Supplies Ltd
14D Wendover Rd
Rackheath Industrial Estate
Rackheath
Norwich, NR13 6LH.
tel: (01603) 735 200
fax: (01603) 735 217
customerservices@typharm.com

Chugai
Chugai Pharma UK Ltd
Mulliner House, Flanders Rd
Turnham Green
London, W4 1NN.
tel: (020) 8987 5680
fax: (020) 8987 5661

Clement Clarke
Clement Clarke International Ltd
Edinburgh Way
Harlow
Essex, CM20 2TT.
tel: (01279) 414 969
fax: (01279) 456 304
resp@clement-clarke.com

CliniMed
CliniMed Ltd
Cavell House, Knaves Beech Way
Loudwater
High Wycombe
Bucks, HP10 9QY.
tel: (01628) 850 100
fax: (01628) 850 331
enquires@clinimed.co.uk

Clinisupplies
Clinisupplies Ltd
9 Crystal Way
Elmgrove Rd
Harrow
Middx, HA1 2HP.
tel: (020) 8863 4168
fax: (020) 8426 0768
info@clinisupplies.co.uk

Clonmel
Clonmel Healthcare Ltd
Waterford Rd
Clonmel
Co. Tipperary
Ireland
tel: (00353) 52 77777
fax: (00353) 52 77799
info@clonmelhealthcare.com

Colgate-Palmolive
Colgate-Palmolive Ltd
Guildford Business Park
Middleton Rd
Guildford
Surrey, GU2 5LZ.
tel: (01483) 302 222
fax: (01483) 303 003

Coloplast
Coloplast Ltd
Peterborough Business Park
Peterborough, PE2 6FX.
tel: (01733) 392 000
fax: (01733) 233 348
gbcareteam@coloplast.com

Community
Community Foods Ltd
Micross, Brent Terrace
London, NW2 1LT.
tel: (020) 8450 9411
fax: (020) 8208 1803
email@communityfoods.co.uk

Complan Foods
Complan Foods Ltd
Imperial House
15–19 Kingsway
London, WC2B 6UN.
tel: (020) 7395 7565
fax: (08704) 434 018

Concord
See Archimedes

ConvaTec
ConvaTec Ltd
Harrington House, Milton Rd
Ickenham
Uxbridge
Middx, UB10 8PU.
tel: (01895) 628 400
fax: (01895) 628 456

Cow & Gate
See Nutricia Clinical

CP
See Wockhardt

Crawford
Crawford Pharmaceuticals
Cheshire House
164 Main Rd
Goostrey
Cheshire, CW4 8NP.
tel: (01477) 537 596
fax: (01477) 534 262

Crookes
See Reckitt Benckiser

CSL Behring
CSL Behring UK Ltd
Hayworth House
Market Place
Haywards Heath
West Sussex, RH16 1DB.
tel: (01444) 447 400
fax: (01444) 447 403
medinfo@cslbehring.com

Daiichi Sankyo
Daiichi Sankyo UK Ltd
Chiltern Place
Chalfont Park
Gerrards Cross, SL9 0BG.
tel: (01753) 893 600
fax: (01753) 893 894
med.info@daiichi-sankyo.co.uk

DDD
DDD Ltd
94 Rickmansworth Rd
Watford
Herts WD18 7JJ.
tel: (01923) 229 251
fax: (01923) 220 728

Denfleet
Denfleet Pharmaceuticals Ltd
260 Centennial Park
Elstree Hill South
Elstree
Herts, WD6 3SR.
tel: (020) 8236 0000
fax: (020) 8236 3501
medical.information@denfleet.com

Dental Health
Dental Health Products Ltd
60 Boughton Lane
Maidstone
Kent, ME15 9QS.
tel: (01622) 749 222
fax: (01622) 744 672

Dentsply
Dentsply Ltd
Hamm Moor Lane
Addlestone
Weybridge
Surrey, KT15 2SE.
tel: (01932) 837 279
fax: (01932) 858 970

Dermal
Dermal Laboratories Ltd
Tatmore Place
Gosmore
Hitchin
Herts, SG4 7QR.
tel: (01462) 458 866
fax (01462) 420 565

Derma UK
Derma UK Ltd
ARC Progress
Mill Lane
Stotfold
Beds, SG5 4NY.
tel (01462) 733 500
fax: (01462) 733 600
info@dermauk.co.uk

De Vilbiss
De Vilbiss Health Care UK Ltd
High Street
Wollaston
West Midlands, DY8 4PS.
tel: (01384) 446 688
fax: (01384) 446 699

De Witt
E C De Witt & Co Ltd
Aegon House
Daresbury Park
Daresbury
Warrington, Cheshire, WA4 4HS.
tel: (01928) 756 800
fax: (01928) 756 818
info@ecdewitt.com

Dexcel
Dexcel-Pharma Ltd
1 Cottesbrooke Park
Heartlands Business Park
Daventry
Northamptonshire, NN11 8YL.
tel: (01327) 312 266
fax: (01327) 312 262
office@dexcelpharma.co.uk

DHP Healthcare
DHP Healthcare Ltd
60 Boughton Lane
Maidstone
Kent, ME15 9QS.
tel: (01622) 749 222
fax: (01622) 743 816
sales@dhphealthcare.co.uk

DiagnoSys
DiagnoSys Medical
Cams Hall
Fareham
Hants, PO16 8AB.
tel: 0800 085 8808
fax: (01329) 227 599

Dimethaid
Dimethaid International
c/o Benoliel Partners
Linden House, Ewelme
Oxfordshire, OX10 6HQ.
tel: (01491) 825 016
fax: (01491) 834 592
medinfo@dimethaid.com

Dr Falk
Dr Falk Pharma UK Ltd
Bourne End Business, Cores End Rd
Bourne End, Bucks, SL8 5AS.
tel: (01628) 536 600

Durbin
Durbin plc
180 Northolt Rd
South Harrow
Middx, HA2 0LT.
tel: (020) 8869 6500
fax: (020) 8869 6565
info@durbin.co.uk

Easigrip
Easigrip Ltd
Unit 13, Scar Bank
Millers Rd
Warwick
Warwickshire, CV34 5DB.
tel: (01926) 497 108
fax: (01926) 497 109
enquiry@easigrip.co.uk

Egis
Egis Pharmaceuticals UK Ltd
127 Shirland Rd
London, W9 2EP.
tel: (020) 7266 2669
fax: (020) 7266 2702
enquiries@medimpexuk.com

Eisai
Eisai Ltd
3 Shortlands
Hammersmith
London, W6 8EE.
tel: (020) 8600 1400
fax: (020) 8600 1401
Lmedinfo@eisai.net

Elida Fabergé
Elida Fabergé Ltd
Coal Rd
Seacroft
Leeds, LS14 2AR.
tel: (0113) 222 5000
fax: (0113) 222 5362

Encysive
Encysive (UK) Ltd
Regus House
Highbridge, Oxford Rd
Uxbridge
Middlesex, UB8 1HR.
tel: (01895) 876 168
fax: (01895) 876 320
enquiries@encysive.co.uk

ENTACO
ENTACO Ltd
Royal Victoria Works,
Birmingham Rd, Studley
Warwickshire, B80 7AP.
tel: (01527) 852 306
fax: (01527) 857 447
sales@entaco.com

Enturia
Enturia Ltd
Reigate Place
43 London Road
Reigate
Surrey, RH2 9PW.
tel: (0800) 043 7546
fax: (01737) 237 950
enquiries@enturia.co.uk

Epiderm
Epiderm Ltd
Wass Lane
Sotby
Market Rasen, LN8 5LR.
tel: (01507) 343 091
fax: (01507) 343 092
djjcovermarkcryo@aol.com

Espire
Espire Healthcare Ltd
The Search Offices
Main Gate Road
The Historic Dockyard
Chatham, ME4 4TE.
tel: (01634) 812 144
fax: (01634) 813 601
info@espirehealth.com

Essential Generics
Essential Generics
7 Egham Business Village
Thorpe Industrial Estate
Egham
Surrey, TW20 8RB.
tel: (01784) 477 167
fax: (01784) 471 776
info@essentialgenerics.co.uk

Ethicon
Ethicon Ltd
P.O. Box 1988
Simpson Parkway
Kirkton Campus
Livingston, EH54 0AB.
tel: (01506) 594 500
fax: (01506) 460 714

Eumedica
Eumedica S.A.
Winston Churchill Avenue 67
1180 Brussels
Belgium
tel: (0208) 444 3377
fax: (0208) 444 6866
enquiries@eumedica.com

EuroGen
EuroGen Pharmaceuticals Ltd
1st Floor, Eagle House
Montpellier Drive
Cheltenham, GL50 1TA.
tel: (01242) 703 646
fax: (01242) 703 648

EUSA Pharma
EUSA Pharma (Europe) Ltd
Building 3, Arlington Business Park
Whittle Way
Stevenage
Herts, SG1 2FP.
tel: (01438) 740 720
fax: (01438) 735 740
medinfo-uk@eusapharma.com

Everfresh
Everfresh Natural Foods
Gatehouse Close
Aylesbury
Bucks, HP19 3DE.
tel: (01296) 425 333
fax: (01296) 422 545

Exelgyn
Exelgyn Laboratories
PO Box 4511
Henley-on-Thames
Oxon, RG9 5ZQ.
tel: (01491) 642 137
fax: (0800) 731 6120

Fabre
Pierre Fabre Ltd
Hyde Abbey House
23 Hyde St
Winchester
Hampshire, SO23 7DR.
tel: (01962) 874 400
fax: (01962) 874 413
contactus@pierre-fabre.co.uk

Fate
Fate Special Foods
Unit E2
Brook Street Business Centre
Brook St, Tipton
West Midlands, DY4 9DD.
tel: (01215) 224 433
fax: (01215) 224 433

Fenton
Fenton Pharmaceuticals Ltd
4J Portman Mansions
Chiltern St
London, W1U 6NS.
tel: (020) 7224 1388
fax: (020) 7486 7258
mail@Fent-Pharm.co.uk

Ferndale
Ferndale Pharmaceuticals Ltd
Unit 605, Thorp Arch Estate
Wetherby
West Yorks, LS23 7BJ.
tel: (01937) 541 122
fax: (01937) 849 682
info@ferndalepharma.co.uk

Ferraris
See nSPIRE

Ferring
Ferring Pharmaceuticals (UK)
The Courtyard
Waterside Drive
Langley
Berks, SL3 6EZ.
tel: (01753) 214 800
fax: (01753) 214 801

Firstplay Dietary
Firstplay Dietary Foods Ltd
338 Turncroft Lane
Offerton
Stockport
Cheshire, SK1 4BP.
tel: (0161) 474 7576
fax: (0161) 474 7576

Flynn
Flynn Pharma Ltd
2nd Floor, The Maltings
Bridge St
Hitchin
Herts, SG5 2DE.
tel: (01462) 458 974
fax: (01462) 450 755

Foodlink
Foodlink (UK) Ltd
2B Plymouth Rd
Plympton
Plymouth, PL7 4JR.
tel: (01752) 344 544
fax: (01752) 342 412
info@foodlinkltd.co.uk

Ford
Ford Medical Associates Ltd
8 Wyndham Way
Orchard Heights
Ashford
Kent, TN25 4PZ.
tel: (01233) 633 224
fax: (01223) 646 595
enquiries@fordmedical.co.uk

Forest
Forest Laboratories UK Ltd
Bourne Rd
Bexley
Kent, DA5 1NX.
tel: (01322) 550 550
fax: (01322) 555 469
medinfo@forest-labs.co.uk

Fournier
See Solvay

Fox
C. H. Fox Ltd
22 Tavistock St
London, WC2E 7PY.
tel: (020) 7240 3111
fax: (020) 7379 3410

FP
Family Planning Sales Ltd
Maerdy Industrial Estate
Rhymney
Gwent, NP22 5PY.
tel: (0870) 4444 620
fax: (0870) 4444 621

Fresenius Kabi
Fresenius Kabi Ltd
Cestrian Court
Eastgate Way
Manor Park, Runcorn
Cheshire, WA7 INT.
tel: (01928) 533 533
fax: (01928) 533 534
med.info-uk@fresenius-kabi.com

Frontier
Frontier Multigate
Newbridge Rd Industrial Estate
Blackwood
South Wales, NP12 2YL.
tel: (01495) 233 050
fax: (01495) 233 055
multigate@frontier-group.co.uk

Galderma
Galderma (UK) Ltd
Meridien House
69-71 Clarendon Rd
Watford
Herts, WD17 1DS.
tel: (01923) 208 950
fax: (01923) 208 998

Galen
Galen Ltd
Seagoe Industrial Estate
Craigavon
Northern Ireland, BT63 5UA.
tel: (028) 3833 4974
fax: (028) 3835 0206

Garnier
Laboratoires Garnier
255 Hammersmith Rd, London, W6 8AZ.
tel: (020) 8762 4000
fax: (020) 8762 4001

GE Healthcare
GE Healthcare
The Grove Centre, White Lion Rd
Amersham, Bucks, HP7 9LL.
tel: (01494) 544 000

Geistlich
Geistlich Pharma
Newton Bank
Long Lane
Chester, CH2 2PF.
tel: (01244) 347 534
fax: (01244) 319 327

General Dietary
General Dietary Ltd
PO Box 38
Kingston upon Thames
Surrey, KT2 7YP.
tel: (020) 8336 2323
fax: (020) 8942 8274

Generics
Generics (UK) Ltd
Albany Gate
Darkes Lane
Potters Bar
Herts, EN6 1AG.
tel: (01707) 853 000
fax: (01707) 643 148

Generpharm
Generpharm Ltd
5 Aberdeen Close
Mount Nod
Coventry
West Midlands, CV5 7NE.
tel: (07963) 625 799

Genus
Genus Pharmaceuticals Ltd
65 London Rd
Newbury
Berks, RG14 1JN.
tel: (01635) 568 400
fax: (01635) 568 401
enquiries@genuspharma.com

Genzyme
Genzyme Therapeutics
4620 Kingsgate
Cascade Way
Oxford Business Park South
Oxford, OX4 2SU.
tel: (01865) 405 200
fax: (01865) 774 172

Gilead
Gilead Sciences
The Flowers Building
Granta Park
Great Abington
Cambs, CB1 6GT.
tel: (01223) 897 300
fax: (01223) 897 291
ukmedinfo@gilead.com

GlaxoSmithKline
See GSK

Glenwood
Glenwood Laboratories Ltd
Jenkins Dale
Chatham
Kent, ME4 5RD.
tel: (01634) 830 535
fax: (01634) 831 345
g.wooduk@virgin.net

Gluten Free Foods Ltd
Gluten Free Foods Ltd
Unit 270 Centennial Park
Centennial Ave
Elstree, Borehamwood
Herts, WD6 3SS.
tel: (020) 8953 4444
fax: (020) 8953 8285
info@glutenfree-foods.co.uk

Goldshield
Goldshield Pharmaceuticals Ltd
NLA Tower
12-16 Addiscombe Rd
Croydon, CR0 0XT.
tel: (020) 8649 8500
fax: (020) 8686 0807

GP Pharma
See Derma UK

Grifols
Grifols UK Ltd
Byron House
Cambridge Business Park
Cowley Road
Cambridge , CB4 0WZ.
tel: (01223) 395 700
fax: (01223) 395 766
reception.uk@grifols.com

Grünenthal
Grünenthal Ltd
2 Beacon Heights Business Park
Ibstone Rd
Stokenchurch
Bucks, HP14 3XR.
tel: (0870) 351 8960
fax: (0870) 351 8961

GSK
GlaxoSmithKline
Stockley Park West
Uxbridge
Middx, UB11 1BT.
tel: 0800 221 441
fax (020) 8990 4328
customercontactuk@gsk.com

GSK Consumer Healthcare
GlaxoSmithKline Consumer Healthcare
GSK House
980 Great West Rd
Brentford
Middx, TW8 9GS.
tel: (0500) 888 878
fax: (020) 8047 6860
customer.relations@gsk.com

Hameln
Hameln Pharmaceuticals Ltd
Nexus
Gloucester Business Park
Gloucester, GL3 4AG.
tel: (01452) 621 661
fax: (01452) 632 732
enquiries@hameln.co.uk

Hartmann
Paul Hartmann Ltd
Unit P2, Parklands
Heywood Distribution Park
Pilsworth Rd, Heywood
Lancs, OL10 2TT.
tel: (01706) 363 200
fax: (01706) 363 201
info@uk.hartmann.info

Healthcare Logistics
See Movianto

Heinz
H. J. Heinz Company Ltd
South Building
Hayes Park
Hayes, UB4 8AL.
tel: (020) 8573 7757
fax: (020) 8848 2325
Farleys_Heinz@Heinz.co.uk

Henleys
Henleys Medical Supplies Ltd
Brownfields
Welwyn Garden City
Herts, AL7 1AN.
tel: (01707) 333 164
fax: (01707) 334 795

Hillcross
AAH Pharmaceuticals Ltd
Sapphire Court
Walsgrave Triangle
Coventry, CV2 2TX.
tel: (024) 7643 2000
fax: (024) 7643 2001

HK Pharma
HK Pharma Ltd
PO Box 105
Hitchin
Herts, SG5 2GG.
tel: (01462) 433 993
fax: (01462) 450 755

Hoechst Marion Roussel
See Sanofi-Aventis

Hospira
Hospira UK Ltd
Queensway
Royal Leamington Spa
Warwickshire, CV31 3RW.
tel: (01926) 820 820
fax: (01926) 821 041

HRA Pharma
Laboratoire HRA Pharma
15 rue Beranger
75003
Paris
France
tel: (0033) 1 40 33 11 30
fax: (0033) 1 40 33 12 31
info@lysodren-europe.com

Hybrand
Hybrand Ltd
Eagle House, The Ring
Bracknell, Berks, RG12 1HB.
tel: (08700) 114 545
fax: (08700) 114 646
customer.services@hybrand.com

Hypoguard
Hypoguard Ltd
Dock Lane
Melton
Woodbridge
Suffolk, IP12 1PE.
tel: (01394) 387 333
fax: (01394) 380 152
enquiries@hypoguard.com

IDIS
IDIS World Medicines
IDIS House
Churchfield Rd
Weybridge
Surrey, KT13 8DB.
tel: (01932) 824 000
fax: (01932) 824 200
idis@idispharma.com

INCA-Pharm
INCA-Pharm UK
PO Box 122
Richmond, DL10 5HX.
tel: (01748) 828 812
fax: (01748) 828 801
info@inca-pharm.com

Infai
Infai UK Ltd
Innovation Centre
University of York Science Park
University Rd
Heslington, York, YO10 5DG.
tel: (01904) 435 228
fax: (01904) 435 229
paul@infai.co.uk

Innovative
Innovative Solutions UK Ltd
Unit 28
Transpennine Industrial Estate
Gorrels Way, Queensway
Rochdale, Lancs, OL11 2QR.
tel: (01706) 746713
enquiries@innovative-solutions.org.uk

Intrapharm
Intrapharm Laboratories Ltd
60 Boughton Lane
Maidstone
Kent, ME15 9QS.
tel: (01622) 749 222
fax: (01622) 744 672
sales@intraphamlabs.com

Ipsen
Ipsen Ltd
190 Bath Rd
Slough
Berks, SL1 3XE.
tel: (01753) 627 777
fax: (01753) 627 778
medical.information@ipsen.com

IVAX
See TEVA UK

J&J
Johnson & Johnson Ltd
Foundation Park
Roxborough Way
Maidenhead
Berks, SL6 3UG.
tel: (01628) 822 222
fax: (01628) 821 222

J&J Medical
Johnson & Johnson Medical
Coronation Rd
Ascot
Berks, SL5 9EY.
tel: (01344) 871 000
fax: (01344) 872 599

J&J MSD
Johnson & Johnson MSD
See McNeil

Janssen-Cilag
Janssen-Cilag Ltd
PO Box 79
Saunderton
High Wycombe
Bucks, HP14 4HJ.
tel: (01494) 567 444
fax: (01494) 567 568

JHC
See Sanofi-Aventis

JLB
B. Braun JLB Ltd
Unit 2A
St Columb Industrial Estate
St Columb Major
Cornwall, TR9 6SF.
tel: (01637) 880 065
fax: (01637) 881 549

Juvela
Juvela (Hero UK) Ltd
19 De-Havilland Drive
Liverpool, L24 8RN.
tel: (0151) 432 5300
fax: (0151) 432 5335
info@juvela.co.uk

K/L
K/L Pharmaceuticals Ltd
21 Macadam Place
South Newmoor
Irvine
Ayrshire, KA11 4HP.
tel: (01294) 215 951
fax: (01294) 221 600

Kappin
Kappin Ltd
Cunard Rd
Park Royal
London, NW10 6PN.
tel: (020) 8961 8511
fax: (020) 8963 7699
hitesh@orbiscpl.com

Kestrel
Kestrel Ltd
Ashfield House
Resolution Rd
Ashby de la Zouch
Leics, LE65 1HW.
tel: (01530) 562 301
fax: (01530) 562 430
kestrel@ventiv.co.uk

Kestrel Ophthalmics
Kestrel Ophthalmics Ltd
Kestrel House
7 Moor Rd
Broadstone
Dorset, BH18 8AZ.
tel: (01202) 658 444
fax: (01202) 659 599

King
King Pharmaceuticals Ltd
2nd Floor, The Maltings
Bridge St
Hitchin
Herts, SG5 2DE.
tel: (01462) 434 366
fax: (01462) 450 755

KoGEN
KoGEN Ltd
Seagoe Industrial Estate
Craigavon, BT63 5UA.
tel: (028) 383 33933
fax: (028) 383 33665
info@kogen.co.uk

KoRa
KoRa Healthcare Ltd
Frans Maas House
Swords Business Park, Swords
Co. Dublin
Ireland
tel: (00353) 1890 0406
fax: (00353) 1890 3016
Kora@ireland.com

Kyowa Hakko
Kyowa Hakko UK Ltd
258 Bath Rd
Slough
Berks, SL1 4DX.
tel: (01753) 566 020
fax: (01753) 566 030

LAB
Laboratories for Applied Biology
91 Amhurst Park
London, N16 5DR.
tel: (020) 8800 2252
fax: (020) 8809 6884
enquiries@cerumol.com

Lederle
See Wyeth

LEO
LEO Pharma
Longwick Rd
Princes Risborough
Bucks, HP27 9RR.
tel: (01844) 347 333
fax: (01844) 342 278
medical-info.uk@leo-pharma.com

LifeScan
LifeScan
50-100 Holmers Farm Way
High Wycombe
Bucks, HP12 4DP.
tel: (01494) 658 750
fax: (01494) 658 751

Lilly
Eli Lilly & Co Ltd
Lilly House
Priestley Rd
Basingstoke
Hampshire, RG24 9NL.
tel: (01256) 315 999
fax: (01256) 775 858

Lincoln Medical
Lincoln Medical Ltd
13 Boathouse Meadow Business Park
Cherry Orchard Lane
Salisbury
Wilts, SP2 7LD.
tel: (01722) 410 443

Linderma
Linderma Ltd
Canon Bridge House
Canon Bridge
Madley
Hereford, HR2 9JF.
tel: (01981) 250 124
fax: (01981) 251 412
linderma@virgin.net

Link
See Archimedes

Lipomed
Lipomed GmbH
Schonaugasse 11
D-79713
Bad Sackingen
tel: (0049) 776 155 9222
fax: (0049) 776 155 9223
lipomed@lipomed.com

LPC
LPC Medical (UK) Ltd
30 Chaul End Lane
Luton, Beds, LU4 8EZ.
tel: (01582) 560 393
fax: (01582) 560 395
info@lpcpharma.com

Lundbeck
Lundbeck Ltd
Lundbeck House
Caldecotte Lake Business Park
Caldecotte, Milton Keynes
Bucks, MK7 8LF.
tel: (01908) 649 966
fax: (01908) 647 888
ukmedicalinformation@lundbeck.com

Maelor
Maelor Pharmaceuticals Ltd
Office Village
Chester Business Park
Chester, CH4 9QZ.
tel: (01244) 625 152
fax: (01244) 625 151
enquiries@maelor.plc.uk

Mandeville
Mandeville Medicines
Stoke Mandeville Hospital
Ayelsbury
Bucks, HP21 8AL.
tel: (01296) 394 142
fax: (01296) 397 223

Manx
Manx Healthcare
Taylor Group House
Wedgnock Lane
Warwick, CV34 5YA.
tel: (01926) 482 511
fax: (01926) 498 711
info@manxhealthcare.com

Marlborough
Marlborough Pharmaceuticals
PO Box 2957
Marlborough
Wilts, SN8 1WS.
tel: (01672) 514 187
fax: (01672) 515 614
info@marlborough-pharma.co.uk

Martindale
See Cardinal

MASTA
MASTA
Moorfield Rd
Yeadon
Leeds, LS19 7BN.
tel: (0113) 238 7500
fax: (0113) 238 7501
medical@masta.org

Mayne
Mayne Pharma plc
Queensway
Royal Leamington Spa
Warwickshire, CV31 3RW.
tel: (01926) 820 820
fax: (01926) 821 041
medinfouk@uk.maynepharma.com

McNeil
McNeil Ltd
Enterprise House, Station Rd
Loadwater, High Wycombe, Bucks,
HP10 9UF.
tel: (01494) 450 778
fax: (01494) 450 487

MDE
MDE Diagnostics Europe Ltd
The Surrey Technology Centre
40 Occam Rd
Surrey Research Park, Guildford
Surrey, GU2 7YG.
tel: (01483) 688 400
info@mdediagnostic.co.uk

Mead Johnson
Mead Johnson Nutritionals
Uxbridge Business Park
Sanderson Rd
Uxbridge
Midcx, UB8 1DH.
tel: (01895) 523 764
fax: (01895) 523 103

Meadow
Meadow Laboratories Ltd
18 Avenue Rd
Chadwell Heath
Romford
Essex, RM6 4JF.
tel: (020) 8597 1203
enquiries@meadowlabs.fsnet.co.uk

Meda
Meda Pharmaceuticals Ltd
Skyway House
Parsonage Rd
Takeley
Bishop's Stortford, CM22 6PU.
tel: (0845) 460 0000
fax: (0845) 460 0002
info@medapharma.co.uk

Medac
Medac (UK)
Scion House, Stirling University
Stirling, FK9 4NF.
tel: (01786) 458 086
fax: (01786) 458 032
info@medac-uk.co.uk

Medical House
The Medical House plc
199 Newhall Rd
Sheffield, S9 2QJ.
tel: (0114) 261 9011
fax: (0114) 243 1597
info@themedicalhouse.com

Medigas
Medigas Ltd
Enterprise Drive
Four Ashes
Wolverhampton, WV10 7DF.
tel: (01902) 791 944
fax: (01902) 791 125

Medihoney
Medihoney (Europe) Ltd
200 Brook Drive
Green Park
Reading, RG2 6UB.
tel: (0800) 071 3912

Medix
See Clement Clarke

Medlock
Medlock Medical Ltd
Tubiton House
Medlock St.
Oldham, OL1 3HS.
tel: (0161) 621 2100
fax: (0161) 627 0932
medical.information@
medlockmedical.com

MedLogic
MedLogic Global Ltd
Western Wood Way
Langage Science Park
Plympton
Plymouth, Devon, PL7 5BG.
tel: (01752) 209 955
fax: (01752) 209 956
enquiries@mlgl.co.uk

Menarini
A. Menarini Pharma UK SRL
Menarini House
Mercury Park
Wycombe Lane, Wooburn Green
Bucks, HP10 0HH.
tel: (01628) 856 400
fax: (01628) 856 402

Menarini Diagnostics
A. Menarini Diagnostics
Wharfedale Rd
Winnersh
Wokingham
Berks, RG41 5RA.
tel: (0118) 944 4100
fax: (0118) 944 4111

Merck
See Merck Serono

Merck Consumer Health
See Seven Seas

Merck Serono
Merck Serono Ltd
Bedfont Cross
Stanwell Rd
Feltham
Middx, TW14 8NX.
tel: (020) 8818 7373
fax: (020) 8818 7274
medinfo.uk@merckserono.net

Merck Sharp & Dohme
See MSD

Merz
Merz Pharma UK Ltd
260 Centennial Park
Elstree Hill South
Herts, WD6 3SR.
tel: (020) 8236 0000
fax: (020) 8236 3501
info@merzpharma.co.uk

Micro Medical
Micro Medical Ltd
Quayside
Chatham Maritime
Chatham
Kent, ME4 4QY.
tel: (01634) 893 500
fax: (01634) 893 600
sales@micromedical.co.uk

Milupa
Milupa Ltd
White Horse Business Park
Trowbridge
Wilts, BA14 0XQ.
tel: (01225) 711 511
fax: (01225) 711 970

Molar
Molar Ltd
The Borough Yard
The Borough
Wedmore
Somerset, BS28 4EB.
tel: (01934) 710 022
fax: (01934) 710 033
info@molarltd.co.uk

Mölnlycke
Mölnlycke Health Care Ltd
The Arenson Centre
Arenson Way
Dunstable
Beds, LU5 5UL.
tel: (0161) 777 2628
fax: (0161) 777 2601
info.uk@molnlycke.net

Morningside
Morningside Healthcare Ltd
115 Narborough Rd
Leicester, LE3 0PA.
tel: (0116) 204 5950
fax: (0116) 247 0756

Movianto
Movianto UK
1 Progress Park
Bedford, MK42 9XE.
tel: (01234) 248 500
fax: (01234) 248 700
movianto.uk@movianto.com

MSD
Merck Sharp & Dohme Ltd
Hertford Rd
Hoddesdon
Herts, EN11 9BU.
tel: (01992) 467 272
fax: (01992) 451 066

Myogen
Myogen GmbH
PO Box 122
Richmond
North Yorks, DL10 5YA.
tel: (01748) 828 812
fax: (01748) 828 801
info@myogen.de

Nagor
Nagor Ltd
PO Box 21, Global House
Isle of Man Business Park
Douglas
Isle of Man, IM99 1AX.
tel: (01624) 625 556
fax: (01624) 661 656
enquiries@nagor.com

Napp
Napp Pharmaceuticals Ltd
Cambridge Science Park
Milton Rd
Cambs, CB4 0GW.
tel: (01223) 424 444
fax: (01223) 424 441

Neolab
Neolab Ltd
57 High St
Odiham, Hampshire, RG29 1LF.
tel: (01256) 704 110
fax: (01256) 701 144
info@neolab.co.uk

Neomedic
Neomedic Ltd
2a Crofters Rd
Northwood
Middx, HA6 3ED.
tel: (01923) 836 379
fax: (01923) 840 160
marketing@neomedic.co.uk

Nestlé
Nestlé Nutrition
St George's House
Park Lane
Croydon
Surrey, CR9 1NR.
tel: (020) 8667 5130
fax: (020) 8667 5616
nutrition@uk.nestle.com

Network
Network Health & Beauty
Network House
41 Invincible Rd
Farnborough
Hants, GU14 7QU.
tel: (01252) 533 333
fax: (01252) 533 344
networkm@globalnet.co.uk

Neutrogena
See J&J

Nordic
Nordic Pharma UK Ltd
Abbey House
1650 Arlington Business Park
Theale
Reading, RG7 4SA.
tel: (0118) 929 8233
fax: (0118) 929 8234
info@nordicpharma.co.uk

Norgine
Norgine Pharmaceuticals Ltd
Chaplin House
Moorhall Rd
Harefield
Middx, UB9 6NS.
tel: (01895) 826 600
fax: (01895) 825 865

Nova
Nova Laboratories Ltd
Martin House
Gloucester Crescent
Wigston
Leicester, LE18 4YL.
tel: (0116) 223 0099
fax: (0116) 223 0120
sales@novalabs.co.uk

Novartis
Novartis Pharmaceuticals UK Ltd
Frimley Business Park
Frimley
Camberley
Surrey, GU16 7SR.
tel: (01276) 692 255
fax: (01276) 692 508

Novartis Consumer Health
Novartis Consumer Health
Wimblehurst Rd
Horsham
West Sussex, RH12 5AB.
tel: (01403) 210 211
fax: (01403) 323 939
medicalaffairs.uk@ch.novartis.com

Novartis Vaccines
Novartis Vaccines Ltd
Gaskill Rd
Speke
Liverpool, L24 9GR.
tel: (08457) 451 500
fax: (0151) 7055 669
serviceuk@chiron.com

Novo Nordisk
Novo Nordisk Ltd
Broadfield Park
Brighton Rd
Crawley
West Sussex, RH11 9RT.
tel: (01293) 613 555
fax: (01293) 613 535
customercareuk@novonordisk.com

nSPIRE Health
nSPIRE Health Ltd
Unit 10, Harforde Court
John Tate Rd
Hertford
Herts, SG13 7NW.
tel: (01992) 526 300
fax: (01992) 526 320
info@nspirehealth.com

Nutricia Clinical
Nutricia Clinical Care
Nutricia Ltd
White Horse Business Park
Trowbridge
Wilts, BA14 0XQ.
tel: (01225) 711 688
fax: (01225) 711 798
cndirect@nutricia.co.uk

Nutricia Dietary
Nutricia Dietary Care
see Nutricia Clinical

Nutrition Point
Nutrition Point Ltd
13 Taurus Park
Westbrook
Warrington
Cheshire, WA5 7ZT.
tel: (07041) 544 044
fax: (07041) 544 055
info@nutritionpoint.co.uk

Nycomed
Nycomed UK Ltd
3 Globeside Business Park
Fieldhouse Lane
Marlow
Bucks, SL7 1HZ.
tel: (01628) 646 400
fax: (01628) 646 401
nycomed@medinformation.co.uk

Octapharma
Octapharma Ltd
6 Elm Court
Copse Drive, Meriden Green
Coventry, CV5 9RG.
tel: (01676) 521 000
fax: (01676) 521 200
octapharma@octapharma.co.uk

Omron
Omron Healthcare (UK) Ltd
Opal Drive
Fox Milne
Milton Keynes, MK15 0DG.
tel: (0870) 750 2771
fax: (0870) 750 2772
info.omronhealthcare.uk@eu.omron.com

OPi
OPi Ltd
2nd Floor, Titan Court
3 Bishop Square
Hatfield
Herts, AL10 9NA.
tel: (01707) 226 094
fax: (01707) 226 194
OPi.UK@orphan-opi.com

Oral B Labs
Oral B Laboratories Ltd
Gillette Corner
Great West Rd
Isleworth
Middx, TW7 5NP.
tel: (020) 8847 7800
fax: (020) 8847 7828

Orbis
Orbis Consumer Products Ltd
See Kappin

Organon
Organon Laboratories Ltd
Cambridge Science Park
Milton Rd
Cambs, CB4 0FL.
tel: (01223) 432 700
fax: (01223) 424 368
medrequest@organon.co.uk

Orion
Orion Pharma (UK) Ltd
Oaklea Court
22 Park Street
Newbury
Berks, RG14 1EA.
tel: (01635) 520 300
fax: (01635) 520 319
medicalinformation@orionpharma.com

Orphan Europe
Orphan Europe (UK) Ltd
Isis House
43 Station Rd
Henley-on-Thames
Oxon, RG9 1AT.
tel: (01491) 414 333
fax: (01491) 414 443
info.uk@orphan-europe.com

Ortho Biotech
Ortho Biotech
PO Box 79
Saunderton
High Wycombe
Bucks, HP14 4HJ.
tel: (0800) 389 2926
fax: (01494) 567 568

Otsuka
Otsuka Pharmaceutical (UK) Ltd
BSi Tower
389 Chiswick High Rd, London, W4 4AJ.
tel: (020) 8742 4300
fax: (020) 8994 8548
medinfo@otsuka.co.uk

Ovation
Ovation Healthcare International Ltd
1 Setanta Place
Dublin 2
Ireland
tel: (00353) 161 39 707
fax: (00353) 161 39 708

Owen Mumford
Owen Mumford Ltd
Brook Hill
Woodstock
Oxford, OX20 1TU.
tel: (01993) 812 021
fax: (01993) 813 466
customerservices@owenmumford.co.uk

Oxford Nutrition
Oxford Nutrition Ltd
Unit 5 Western Units
Pottery Rd
Bovey Tracey, TQ13 9JJ.
tel: (01626) 832 067
fax: (01626) 836 841
info@nutrinox.com

Paines & Byrne
Paines & Byrne Ltd
Lovett House
Lovett Rd
Staines
Middx, TW18 3AZ.
tel: (01784) 419 620
fax: (01784) 419 401

Parema
See Urgo

Pari
PARI Medical Ltd
The Old Sorting Office
Rosemount Ave
West Byfleet
Surrey, KT14 6NE.
tel: (01932) 341 122
fax: (01932) 341 134
parimedical@compuserve.com

Parkside
Parkside Healthcare
12 Parkside Ave
Salford, M7 4HB.
tel: (0161) 795 2792
fax: (0161) 795 4076

Peckforton
Peckforton Pharmaceuticals Ltd
Crewe Hall
Crewe
Cheshire, CW1 6UL.
tel: (01270) 582 255
fax: (01270) 582 299
info@peckforton.com

Penn
Penn Pharmaceuticals Services Ltd
Unit 23 & 24, Tafarnaubach Industrial Estate
Tredegar
Gwent, NP22 3AA.
tel: (01495) 711 222
fax: (01495) 711 225
penn@pennpharm.co.uk

Index of manufacturers

Pfizer
Pfizer Ltd
Walton Oaks
Dorking Rd
Walton-on-the-Hill
Surrey, KT20 7NS.
tel: (01304) 616 161
fax: (01304) 656 221

Pfizer Consumer
See Pfizer

Pharmacia
See Pfizer

Pharma-Global
Pharma-Global Ltd
c/o Iris Healthcare
Nimrod House, Pitfield
Kiln Farm
Milton Keynes, MK11 3LW.
tel: (01908) 423 580
fax: (01908) 423 581
info@irishealthcare.co.uk

Pharma Mar
See IDIS

Pharma Nord
Pharma Nord (UK) Ltd
Telford Court
Morpeth
Northumberland, NE61 2DB.
tel: (01670) 519989
fax: (01670) 534903
info@pharmanord.co.uk

Pharmasol
Pharmasol Ltd
North Way, Walworth Industrial Estate
Andover, Hampshire, SP10 5AZ.
tel: (01264) 363 117
fax: (01264) 332 223
info@pharmasol.co.uk

Pharmasure
Pharmasure Ltd
28 Watford Metro Centre
Dwight Rd
Watford, WD18 9SB.
tel: (01923) 233 466
fax: (01923) 233 113
info@pharmasure.co.uk

Pharmion
Pharmion Ltd
Riverside House
Riverside Walk
Windsor
Berks, SL4 1NA.
tel: (01753) 240 600
fax: (01753) 240 656
info-UK@pharmion.com

Pickles
J. Pickles Healthcare
Beech House
62 High St
Knaresborough
N. Yorks, HG5 0EA.
tel: (01423) 867 314
fax: (01423) 869 177

Pinewood
Pinewood Healthcare
Ballymacabry
Clonmel, Co Tipperary, Eire
tel: (00353) 523 6253
fax: (00353) 523 6311
info@pinewood.ie

PLIVA
PLIVA Pharma Ltd
Vision House
Bedford Rd
Petersfield
Hampshire, GU32 3QB.
tel: (01730) 710900
fax: (01730) 710901
medinfo@pliva-pharma.co.uk

Potters
Potters Ltd
1 Botanic Court
Martland Park
Wigan, WN5 0JZ.
tel: (01924) 219 960
fax: (01924) 219 966
info@pottersherbal.co.uk

Procter & Gamble
Procter & Gamble UK
The Heights
Brooklands
Weybridge
Surrey, KT13 0XP.
tel: (01932) 896 000
fax: (01932) 896 200

Procter & Gamble Pharm.
Procter & Gamble Technical Centres
Medical Dept
Rusham Park
Whitehall Lane
Egham, Surrey, TW20 9NW.
tel: (01784) 474 900
fax: (01784) 474 705

Profile
Profile Pharma Ltd
Chichester Business Park
City Fields Way
Chichester
West Sussex, PO20 2FT.
tel: (0800) 1300 855
fax: (0800) 1300 856
info@profilepharma.com

Profile Respiratory
See Respironics

ProStrakan
ProStrakan Ltd
Galabank Business Park
Galashiels, TD1 1QH.
tel: (01896) 664 000
fax: (01896) 664 001
medinfo@prostrakan.com

Protex
Protex Healthcare (UK) Ltd
Unit 5, Molly Millars Lane
Wokingham
Berks, RG41 2Q2.
tel: (08700) 114 112
orders@protexhealthcare.co.uk

Provalis
See KoGEN

R&C
See Reckitt Benckiser

Ranbaxy
Ranbaxy Ltd
CP House
97-107 Uxbridge Rd
Ealing
London, W5 5TL.
tel: (020) 8280 1600
fax: (020) 8280 1617
medinfoeurope@ranbaxy.com

Ransom
Ransom Consumer Healthcare
Alexander House
40A Wilbury Way
Hitchin
Herts, SG5 1LY.
tel: (01462) 437 615
fax: (01462) 420 528
info@williamransom.com

Reckitt Benckiser
Reckitt Benckiser Healthcare
Dansom Lane
Hull, HU8 7DS.
tel: (01482) 326 151
fax: (01482) 582 526
miu@reckittbenckiser.com

Recordati
Recordati Pharmaceuticals Ltd
Knyvett House
The Causeway
Staines
Middx, TW18 3BA.
tel: (01784) 898 300
fax: (01784) 895 103

Regent Medical
See Mölnlycke

ReSource Medical
ReSource Medical UK Ltd
2 Thorne Rd
Thornton Lodge
Huddersfield, HD1 3JJ.
tel: (01484) 531 489
fax: (01484) 531 584
info@resource-medical.co.uk

Respironics
Respironics (UK) Ltd
Heath Place
Bognor Regis
West Sussex, PO22 9SL.
tel: (0870) 770 3434
fax: (0870) 770 3433
rukmarketing@respironics.com

Rhône-Poulenc Rorer
See Sanofi-Aventis

Richardson
Richardson Healthcare
Richardson House
Crondal Rd
Coventry
Warwickshire, CV7 9NH.
tel: (08700) 111 126
fax: (08700) 111 127

Robinsons
Robinson Healthcare Ltd
Lawn Rd
Carlton-in-Lindrick Industrial Estate
Worksop
Notts, S81 9LB.
tel: (01909) 735 001
fax: (01909) 731 103
enquiries@robinsoncare.com

Roche
Roche Products Ltd
Hexagon Place
6 Falcon Way, Shire Park
Welwyn Garden City
Herts, AL7 1TW.
tel: (0800) 328 1629
fax: (01707) 384 555
medinfo.uk@roche.com

Roche Consumer Health
See Bayer

Roche Diagnostics
Roche Diagnostics Ltd
Charles Avenue
Burgess Hill
West Sussex, RH15 9RY.
tel: (01444) 256 000
fax: (01444) 256 239
burgesshill.accu-chek@roche.com

Rosemont
Rosemont Pharmaceuticals Ltd
Rosemont House
Yorkdale Industrial Park
Braithwaite St
Leeds, LS11 9XE.
tel: (0113) 244 1999
fax: (0113) 246 0738
infodesk@rosemontpharma.com

Rowa
Rowa Pharmaceuticals Ltd
Bantry
Co Cork
Ireland
tel: (00 353 27) 50077
fax: (00 353 27) 50417
rowa@rowa-pharma.ie

S&N Hlth.
Smith & Nephew Healthcare Ltd
Healthcare House
Goulton St
Hull, HU3 4DJ.
tel: (01482) 222 200
fax: (01482) 222 211
advice@smith-nephew.com

Sallis
Sallis Healthcare Ltd
Vernon Works
Waterford St
Basford
Nottingham, NG6 0DH.
tel: (0115) 978 7841
fax: (0115) 942 2272

Sandoz
Sandoz Ltd
Unit 37
Woolmer Way
Bordon
Hants, GU35 9QE.
tel: (01420) 478 301
fax: (01420) 474 427

Sankyo
See Daiichi Sankyo

Sanochemia
Sanochemia Diagnostics UK Ltd
Argentum
510 Bristol Business Park
Coldharbour Lane
Bristol, BS16 1EJ.
tel: (0117) 906 3562
fax: (0117) 906 3709

Sanofi-Aventis
Sanofi-Aventis Ltd
1 Onslow St
Guildford
Surrey, GU1 4YS.
tel: (01483) 505 515
fax: (01483) 535 432
uk-medicalinformation@
sanofi-aventis.com

Sanofi Pasteur
Sanofi Pasteur MSD Ltd
Mallards Reach
Bridge Avenue
Maidenhead
Berks, SL6 1QP.
tel: (01628) 785 291
fax: (01628) 671 722

Sanofi-Synthelabo
See Sanofi-Aventis

Schering Health
See Bayer

Schering-Plough
Schering-Plough Ltd
Shire Park
Welwyn Garden City
Herts, AL7 1TW.
tel: (01707) 363 636
fax: (01707) 363 763
medical.info@spcorp.com

Schuco
Schuco International Ltd
Challenge House
1 Lyndhurst Ave
London, N12 0NE.
tel: (020) 8368 1642
fax: (020) 8361 3761
sales@schuco.co.uk

Schwarz
Schwarz Pharma Ltd
Schwarz House
5 Hercules Way
Leavesden Park
Watford, Herts, WD25 7GS.
tel: (01923) 684 100
fax: (01923) 684 200
medinfo@schwarzpharma.co.uk

Serono
See Merck Serono

Servier
Servier Laboratories Ltd
Gallions
Wexham Springs
Framewood Rd
Wexham, SL3 6RJ.
tel: (01753) 662 744
fax: (01753) 663 456

Seven Seas
Seven Seas Ltd
Hedon Rd
Marfleet
Hull, HU9 5NJ.
tel: (01482) 375 234
fax: (01482) 374 345

Shermond
Shermond
Castle House
Sea View Way
Woodingdean
Brighton, East Sussex, BN2 6NT.
tel: (0870) 242 7701
fax: (01273) 391 028
sales@shermond.com

Shire
Shire Pharmaceuticals Ltd
Hampshire International Business Park
Chineham
Basingstoke
Hants, RG24 8EP.
tel: (01256) 894 000
fax: (01256) 894 708
medinfo@uk.shire.com

SHS
SHS International Ltd
100 Wavertree Boulevard
Wavertree Technology Park
Liverpool, L7 9PT.
tel: (0151) 228 8161
fax: (0151) 230 5365
seve@shsint.co.uk

Sigma
Sigma Pharmaceuticals plc
PO Box 233
Unit 1-7 Colonial Way
Watford
Herts, WD24 4YR.
tel: (01923) 444 999
fax: (01923) 441 998
info@sigpharm.co.uk

Sigma-Tau
Sigma-Tau Pharma Ltd (UK)
Abbey House
1650 Arlington Business Park
Reading
Berks, RG7 4SA.
tel: (0118) 929 8075
fax: (0118) 929 8076
medical.information@sigma-tau.co.uk

Sinclair
Sinclair Pharmaceuticals Ltd
Borough Rd
Godalming
Surrey, GU7 2AB.
tel: (01483) 426 644
fax: (01483) 860 927
info@sinclairpharma.com

SLO Drinks
SLO Drinks Ltd
Unit 1
Torr Top St
New Mills
High Peak, SK22 4BS.
tel: (08452) 22 22 05
fax: (08452) 22 22 06
info@slodrinks.com

SMA Nutrition
See Wyeth

SNBTS
Scottish National Blood Transfusion Service
Protein Fractionation Centre
Ellen's Glen Rd
Edinburgh, EH17 7QT.
tel: (0131) 536 5700
fax: (0131) 536 5781
Contact.pfc@snbts.csa.scot.nhs.uk

Solvay
Solvay Healthcare Ltd
Mansbridge Rd
West End
Southampton, SO18 3JD.
tel: (023) 8046 7000
fax: (023) 8046 5350
medinfo.shl@solvay.com

Sovereign
See Amdipharm

Special Products
Special Products Ltd
Unit 25
Boundary Business Centre
Surrey, GU21 5DH.
tel: (01483) 736 950
fax: (01483) 721 926
graham.march@specprod.co.uk

Specials Laboratory
The Specials Laboratory Ltd
Unit 1, Regents Drive
Lower Prudhoe Industrial Estate
Northumberland, NE42 6PX.
tel: (0800) 028 4925
fax: (0800) 083 4222

Squibb
See Bristol-Myers Squibb

SSL
SSL International plc
Venus, 1 Old Park Lane
Trafford Park
Urmston
Manchester, M41 7HA.
tel: (08701) 222 690
fax: (08701) 222 692
medical.information@ssl-international.com

STD Pharmaceutical
STD Pharmaceutical Products Ltd
Plough Lane
Hereford, HR4 0EL.
tel: (01432) 373 555
fax: (01432) 373 556
enquiries@stdpharm.co.uk

Steraid
Steraid (Gainsborough) Ltd
Unit 42
Corringham Road Industrial Estate
Gainsborough , DN21 1QB.
tel: (01427) 677 659
fax: (01427) 677 654

Sterling Health
See GSK Consumer Healthcare

Sterwin
See Winthrop

Stiefel
Stiefel Laboratories (UK) Ltd
Holtspur Lane
Wooburn Green
High Wycombe
Bucks, HP10 0AU.
tel: (01628) 524 966
fax: (01628) 810 021
general@stiefel.co.uk

Stragen
Stragen UK Ltd
Castle Court
41 London Rd
Reigate
Surrey, RH2 9RJ.
tel: (0870) 351 8744
fax: (0870) 351 8745
info@stragenuk.com

Strakan
See ProStrakan

Sutherland
Sutherland Health Ltd
Unit 1, Rivermead
Pipers Way
Thatcham
Berks, RG19 4EP.
tel: (01635) 874 488
fax: (01635) 877 622

Swedish Orphan
Swedish Orphan International (UK) Ltd
Trinity House
Cambridge Business Park
Cowley Rd
Cambridge, CB4 0WZ.
tel: (01223) 393 512
fax: (01223) 393 501

Synergy Healthcare
Synergy Healthcare (UK) Ltd
Lion Mill
Fitton St
Royton
Oldham, OL2 5JX.
tel: (0161) 624 5641
fax: (0161) 627 0902
patientcare@synergyhealthcare.plc.uk

Syner-Med
Syner-Med (Pharmaceutical Products) Ltd
Beech House
840 Brighton Rd
Purley, CR8 2BH.
tel: (0845) 634 2100
fax: (0845) 634 2101
mail@syner-med.com

Takeda
Takeda UK Ltd
Takeda House, Mercury Park
Wycombe Lane
Wooburn Green
High Wycombe, Bucks, HP10 0HH.
tel: (01628) 537 900
fax: (01628) 526 615

Taro
Taro Pharmaceuticals (UK) Ltd
Lakeside
1 Furzeground Way
Stockley Park East
Uxbridge, Middx, UB11 1BD.
tel: (08707) 369 544
fax: (08707) 369 545
customerservice@taropharma.co.uk

Tarus
See Chemidex

Teofarma
Teofarma S.r.l.
c/o Professional Information Ltd
Olliver
Richmond
North Yorkshire, DL10 5HX.
tel: (01748) 828 857
teofarma@professionalinformation.co.uk

Teva
Teva Pharmaceuticals Ltd
The Gate House
Gatehouse Way
Aylesbury
Bucks, HP19 8DB.
med.info@tevapharma.co.uk

TEVA UK
TEVA UK Ltd
Building V
The London Road Campus
London Rd
Harlow, Essex, CM17 9LP.
tel: (08705) 020 304
fax: (08705) 323 334
medinfo@tevauk.com

Thornton & Ross
Thornton & Ross Ltd
Linthwaite Laboratories
Huddersfield, HD7 5QH.
tel: (01484) 842 217
fax: (01484) 847 301
mail@thorntonross.com

Tillomed
Tillomed Laboratories Ltd
3 Howard Rd
Eaton Socon, St Neots
Cambs, PE19 3ET.
tel: (01480) 402 400
fax: (01480) 402 402
info@tillomed.co.uk

TOL
Tree of Life
Coaldale Rd
Lymedale Business Park
Newcastle Under Lyme
Staff, ST5 9QX.
tel: (01782) 567 100
fax: (01782) 567 199
health@tol-europe.com

TopoTarget
TopoTarget A/S
Symbion Science Park
Fruebjergvej 3
DK-2100
Copenhagen, Denmark
tel: (00 45 39) 178 392
fax: (00 45 39) 179 492

Torbet
Torbet Laboratories Ltd
14D Wendover Rd
Rackheath Industrial Estate
Rackheath
Norwich, NR13 6LH.
tel: (01603) 735 200
fax: (01603) 735 217
torbet@typharm.com

Transdermal
Transdermal Ltd
35 Grimwade Ave
Croydon
Surrey, CR0 5DJ.
tel: (020) 8654 2251
fax: (020) 8654 2252
transdermal@transdermal.co.uk

Trinity
Trinity Pharmaceuticals Ltd
See Trinity-Chiesi

Trinity-Chiesi
Trinity-Chiesi Pharmaceuticals Ltd
Cheadle Royal Business Park
Highfield
Cheadle, SK8 3GY.
tel: (0161) 488 5555
fax: (0161) 488 5565

TSL
Tissue Science Laboratories plc
Victoria House
Victoria Rd
Aldershot
Hants, GU11 1EJ.
tel: (01252) 333 002
fax: (01252) 333 010
enquiries@tissuescience.com

Tyco
Tyco Healthcare
154 Fareham Rd
Gosport
Hants, PO13 0AS.
tel: (01329) 224 000

Typharm
Typharm Ltd
14D Wendover Rd
Rackheath Industrial Estate
Rackheath
Norwich, NR13 6LH.
tel: (01603) 735 200
fax: (01603) 735 217
customerservices@typharm.com

UCB Pharma
UCB Pharma Ltd
208 Bath Rd
Slough, SL1 3WE.
tel: (01753) 534 655
fax: (01753) 536 632
medicalinformationuk@ucb-group.com

Ultrapharm
Ultrapharm Ltd
Centenary Business Park
Henley-on-Thames
Oxon, RG9 1DS.
tel: (01491) 578 016
fax: (01491) 570 001
orders@glutenfree.co.uk

Univar
Univar Ltd
International House
Zenith, Paycocke Rd
Basildon
Essex, SS14 3DW.
tel: (01268) 594 400
fax: (01268) 594 481
trientine@univareurope.com

Unomedical
Unomedical Ltd
Thornhill Rd
Redditch, B98 7NL.
tel: (01527) 587 700
fax: (01527) 592 111

Urgo
Urgo Ltd
Sullington Rd
Shepshed
Loughborough
Leics, LE12 9JJ.
tel: (01509) 502 051
fax: (01509) 650 898
medical@parema.com

Valeant
Valeant Pharmaceuticals Ltd
Cedarwood
Chineham Business Park
Crockford Lane, Basingstoke
Hants, RG24 8WD.
tel: (01256) 707 744
fax: (01256) 707 334
valeantuk@valeant.com

Vegenat
c/o Archaelis Ltd
23 Pembridge Gardens
London, W2 4EB.
tel: (0870) 803 2484
info@vegenat.co.uk

Vernon-Carus
Vernon-Carus Ltd
1 Western Avenue
Matrix Park
Buckshaw Village
Chorley, Lancs, PR7 7NB.
tel: (01772) 299 900
fax: (01772) 299 901
info@vernon-carus.co.uk

Viatris
See Meda

Viridian
Viridian Pharma Ltd
Seales Barn
School Lane
Shuttington, Tamworth
Staffs, B79 0DX.
tel: (01827) 896 996
fax: (0870) 705 8153
info@viridianpharma.co.uk

Vitaflo
Vitaflo Ltd
11 Century Building
Brunswick Business Park
Liverpool, L3 4BL.
tel: (0151) 709 9020
fax: (0151) 709 9727
vitaflo@vitaflo.co.uk

Vitaline
Vitaline Pharmaceuticals UK Ltd
8 Ridge Way
Drakes Drive
Crendon Business Park
Long Crendon, Bucks, HP18 9BF.
tel: (01844) 202 044
fax: (01844) 202 077
vitalineinfo@aol.com

Vitalograph
Vitalograph Ltd
Maids Moreton
Buckingham, MK18 1SW.
tel: (01280) 827 110
fax: (01280) 823 302
sales@vitalograph.co.uk

Wallace Cameron
Wallace Cameron Ltd
26 Netherhall Rd
Netherton Industrial Estate
Wishaw, ML2 0JG.
tel: (01698) 354 600
fax: (01698) 354 700
sales@wallacecameron.com

Wallace Mfg
Wallace Manufacturing Chemists Ltd
Wallace House
New Abbey Court
51-53 Stert St, Abingdon
Oxon, OX14 3JF.
tel: (01235) 538 700
fax: (01235) 538 800
info@alinter.co.uk

Winthrop
Winthrop Pharmaceuticals UK Ltd
PO Box 611
Guildford, Surrey, GU1 4YS.
tel: (01483) 554 101
fax: (01483) 554 810
winthropsales@sanofi-aventis.com

Wockhardt
Wockhardt UK Ltd
Ash Rd North
Wrexham Industrial Estate
Wrexham, LL13 9UF.
tel: (01978) 661 261
fax: (01978) 660 130

Wyeth
Wyeth Pharmaceuticals
Huntercombe Lane South
Taplow
Maidenhead
Berks, SL6 0PH.
tel: (01628) 604 377
fax: (01628) 666 368
ukmedinfo@wyeth.com

Wynlit
Wynlit Laboratories
153 Furzehill Rd
Borehamwood
Herts, WD6 2DR.
tel: (07903) 370 130
fax: (020) 8292 6117

Wyvern
Wyvern Medical Ltd
PO Box 17
Ledbury
Herefordshire, HR8 2ES.
tel: (01531) 631 105
fax: (01531) 634 844

Zeal
G. H. Zeal Ltd
Deer Park Rd
London, SW19 3UU.
tel: (020) 8542 2283
fax: (020) 8543 7840
scientific@zeal.co.uk

Zeneus
See Cephalon

Zeroderma
Zeroderma Ltd
The Manor House
Victor Barns
Northampton Rd, Brixworth
Northampton, NN6 9DQ.
tel: (01604) 889 855
fax: (01604) 883 199
info@ixlpharma.com

ZooBiotic
ZooBiotic Ltd
Biosurgical Research Unit
Surgical Materials Testing Laboratory
Princess of Wales Hospital, Coity Rd
Bridgend, Mid Glamorgan, South Wales, CF31 1RQ.
tel: (0845) 230 1810
fax: (01656) 752 830
maggots@smtl.co.uk

Zurich
See Trinity-Chiesi

Special-order Manufacturers

The following **companies** manufacture 'special-order' products: BCM Specials, Fresenius, Mandeville Medicines, Martindale, Nova Laboratories, Orbis, Phoenix, Rosemont, Special Products, The Specials Laboratory (see Index of Manufacturers for contact details).

Licensed **hospital manufacturing units** also manufacture 'special-order' products as unlicensed medicines, the principal NHS units are listed below. A database (*Profile*) provides information on all medicines manufactured in the NHS.

> The MHRA recommends that an unlicensed medicine should only be used when a patient has special requirements that cannot be met by use of a licensed medicine

England

London

Mr P. Forsey
Production Manager
Guy's and St. Thomas' NHS Foundation Trust
Pharmacy Department
St. Thomas' Hospital
Lambeth Palace Rd
London, SE1 7EH.
tel: (020) 7188 5003
fax: (020) 7188 5013
paul.forsey@gstt.nhs.uk

Mr A. Krol
Director of Commercial Services
Pharmaceutical Manufacturing Unit
Moorfields Eye Hospital NHS Trust
34 Nile St
London, N1 7LX.
tel: (020) 7684 8561
fax: 0800 328 8191
alan.krol@moorfields.nhs.uk

Mr M. Lillywhite
Director of Technical Services
Barts and the London NHS Trust
St. Bartholomew's Hospital
West Smithfield
London, EC1A 7BE.
tel: (020) 7601 7491
fax: (020) 7601 7486
mike.lillywhite@bartsandthelondon.nhs.uk

Dr K. Middleton
Principal Pharmacist, Technical Services
Department of Pharmacy
Northwick Park and St Mark's Hospital
Watford Rd
Harrow
Middx, HA1 3UJ.
tel: (020) 8869 2204/2223
keith.middleton@nwlh.nhs.uk

Ms C. Trehane
Production Manager
Royal Free Hospital
Pond Street
London, NW3 2QG.
tel: (020) 7830 2282 / orders: 2424
christine.trehane@royalfree.nhs.uk

Midlands and Eastern

Mr C. Hanson
Production Manager
Pharmacy Manufacturing Unit
The Ipswich Hospital NHS Trust
Heath Rd
Ipswich, IP4 5PD.
tel: (01473) 703 603
fax: (01473) 703 609
con.hanson@ipswichhospital.nhs.uk

Ms J. Kendall
Assistant Chief Pharmacist
Pharmacy Production Units
Nottingham University Hospitals NHS Trust
Queens Medical Centre Campus
Nottingham, NG7 2UH.
tel: (0115) 875 4521
fax: (0115) 970 9744
jeanette.kendall@nuh.nhs.uk

Mrs R. Newton
Head of Production
Pharmacy Manufacturing Unit
University Hospital of North Staffs
City General Site
Stoke-on-Trent, ST4 6QG.
tel: (01782) 552 290
fax: (01782) 552 916
ruth.newton@uhns.nhs.uk

Dr S. Langford
Principal Pharmacist (Technical Services)
UHB Medicines (SFMU)
32–34 Melchett Rd, Kings Norton Business Centre, Kings Norton
Birmingham, B30 3HS.
tel: (0121) 627 2326
fax: (0121) 627 2168
stephen.langford@uhb.nhs.uk

Dr R. Needle
Chief Pharmacist
Essex Rivers Healthcare NHS Trust
Colchester General Hospital
Turner Rd
Colchester, C04 5JL.
tel: (01206) 742 433
fax: (01206) 742 319
richard.needle@essexrivers.nhs.uk

Mr P.G. Williams
Technical and Support Services Manager
Pharmacy Manufacturing Unit
Queens Hospital
Burton Hospitals NHS Trust
Belvedere Rd
Burton-on-Trent, DE13 0RB.
tel: (01283) 511 511 Extn 5138
fax: (01283) 593 036
paul.williams@burtonh-tr.wmids.nhs.uk

North East

Ms S. Klein
Production Manager
Pharmacy Production Unit
Royal Victoria Infirmary
Queen Victoria Rd
Newcastle-upon-Tyne, NE1 4LP.
tel: (0191) 282 0377
fax: (0191) 282 0376
stephanie.klein@nuth.nhs.uk

North West

Mr M.D. Booth
Principal Pharmacist
Production & Aseptic Services Manager
Stockport Pharmaceuticals
Stepping Hill Hospital
Stockport
Cheshire, SK2 7JE.
tel: (0161) 419 5657
fax: (0161) 419 5664
mike.booth@stockport.nhs.uk

Mr N. Fletcher
Deputy Director of Pharmacy, Technical Services
Preston Pharmaceuticals
Royal Preston Hospital
Fulwood
Preston, PR2 9HT.
tel: (01772) 522 505
fax: (01772) 522 602
neil.fletcher@lthtr.nhs.uk

South East

Mr F. Brown
Head of Production
Pharmacy Department
St Peter's Hospital
Guildford Rd
Chertsey
Surrey, KT16 OPZ.
tel: (01932) 722 886
fax: (01932) 723 209
fraser.brown@asph.nhs.uk

Ms G. Middlehurst
Quality Assurance and Business Manager
Pharmacy Manufacturing Unit
Queen Alexandra Hospital
Southwick Hill Rd
Cosham
Portsmouth
Hants, PO6 3LY.
tel: (02392) 286 335
fax: (02392) 378 288
gillian.middlehurst@porthosp.nhs.uk

Mr M. Sherwood
Principal Pharmacist (Production)
Eastbourne DGH Pharmaceuticals
Eastbourne DGH Hospital
East Sussex Hospitals NHS Trust
Kings Drive, Eastbourne
East Sussex, BN21 2UD.
tel: (01323) 414 906
fax: (01323) 414 931
mike.sherwood@esht.nhs.uk

South West

Mr P. S. Bendell
Pharmacy Manufacturing Services Manager
Torbay PMU
South Devon Healthcare
Kemmings Close, Long Rd
Paignton
Devon, TQ4 7TW.
tel: (01803) 664 707
fax: (01803) 664 354
phil.bendell@nhs.net

Yorkshire

Mr R.W. Brookes
Technical Services Manager
Pharmacy Department
Royal Hallamshire Hospital
Glossop Rd
Sheffield, S10 2JF.
tel: (0114) 271 3104
fax: (0114) 271 2783
roger.brookes@sth.nhs.uk

Dr J. Harwood
Production Manager
Pharmacy Manufacturing Unit
Huddersfield Royal Infirmary
Lindley
Huddersfield
West Yorks, HD3 3EA.
tel: (01484) 342 421
fax: (01484) 342 074
john.harwood@cht.nhs.uk

Northern Ireland

Ms C. McBride
Assistant Director of Pharmaceutical Services
Manufacturing and Royal Group of Hospitals Belfast
77 Boucher Crescent
Belfast, BT12 6HU.
tel: (028) 9063 3310 or (028) 9055 3407
fax: (028) 9055 3498
colette.mcbride@royalhospitals.n-i.nhs.uk

Scotland

Mr G. Conkie
Manager, Pharmacy Production Unit
Western Infirmary
Dumbarton Road
Glasgow, G11 6NT.
tel: (0141) 211 2882
fax: (0141) 211 1967
graham.conkie@northglasgow.scot.nhs.uk

Mr B. W. Millar
General Manager
Tayside Pharmaceuticals
Ninewells Hospital
Dundee, DD1 9SY.
tel: (01382) 632 183
fax: (01382) 632 060
baxter.w.millar@tuht.scot.nhs.uk

Wales

Mr P. Spark
Principal Pharmacist (Production)
Cardiff and Vale NHS Trust
University Hospital of Wales
Heath Park
Cardiff CF14 4XW.
tel: (029) 2074 4828
fax: (029) 2074 3114
paul.spark@cardiffandvale.wales.nhs.uk

Index

Principal page references are printed in **bold** type. Proprietary (trade) names and names of organisms are printed in *italic* type; where the BNF does not include a full entry for a branded product, the non-proprietary name is shown in brackets

A

- Abacavir, 328, **329**
  - lamivudine and zidovudine with, 329
  - lamivudine with, 329
- Abatacept, 552, **553**
  - infusion table, 823
- Abbreviations, *inside back cover*
  - Latin, *inside back cover*
  - of units, 4
  - Symbols, *inside back cover*
- *Abcare*, 366
- Abciximab, **130**
  - infusion table, 823
- Abdominal surgery, antibacterial prophylaxis, 282
- *Abelcet*, 321, 322
- *Abidec*, 528
- *Abilify*, 194
- *Able Spacer*, 157
- Abortion
  - habitual *see* Miscarriage, recurrent, 392
  - haemorrhage, 419
  - induction, 418
- Abrasive agents, acne, 620
- Abscess, dental, 281
- Absence seizures, 245
  - atypical, 245
- Absorbent cotton, bandages, dressings, gauze, 857, 858, 860
- *AC 2000 HI FLO*, 158
- *AC 4000*, 158
- Acamprosate, **269**, 270
- Acanthamoeba keratitis, 566, 581
- Acarbose, 369, **370**
- Acaricides, 634
- ACBS
  - alcoholic beverages, 842
  - foods, 833
  - toilet preparations, 849
- *Accolate*, 165
- *Accu-Chek* preparations, 375
- *Accuhaler*
  - *Flixotide*, 163
  - *Seretide*, 164
  - *Serevent*, 152
  - *Ventolin*, 152
- *Accupro*, 104
- *Accuretic*, 104
- ACE inhibitors, 99
  - heart failure, 99
  - myocardial infarction, 133
  - renal function, 100
- *Acea*, 630
- Acebutolol, **86**
  - *see also* Beta-adrenoceptor blocking drugs
- Aceclofenac, 535, **537**
- Acemetacin, 537
  - postoperative pain, 674
- Acenocoumarol, 127, **128**
- *Acepril* (captopril), 101
- Acetaminophen *see* Paracetamol
- Acetazolamide, **575**
  - diuretic, 78
  - epilepsy, 255
  - eye, 575
  - glaucoma, 572, 575
- Acetic acid, otitis externa, 582
- Acetomenaphthone [ingredient], 528
- Acetylcholine, 579
- Acetylcysteine
  - eye, 577
  - infusion table, 823
  - paracetamol poisoning, 29, **30**, 31
- Acetylsalicylic acid *see* Aspirin
- *Acezide* (co-zidocapt), 101
- Aciclovir, **336**, 337
  - herpes simplex, 336
    - buccal, 593
    - eye, 336, **568**
    - genital, 336, 633
    - labialis, 633
    - skin, 633
  - herpes zoster, 336
  - infusion table, 823
- Acid aspiration, 45
  - surgery, 666
- *Acidex*, 40
- Acidification of urine, 443
- Acidosis
  - metabolic, 505, 508
- Acipimox, **143**
- Acitretin, 612, **615**, 616
- Acknowledgements, iv
- *Aclasta*, 410
- Aclometasone dipropionate, 607
- *Acnamino MR*, 298
- Acne, **618**
- Acne rosacea *see* Rosacea, 618, 630
- *Acnecide*, 619
- *Acnisal*, 621
- *Acnocin* (co-cyprindiol), 621
- *Acomplia*, 217
- Acrolein, 452
- Acromegaly, 401, 410, 488
- ACTH *see* Corticotropin, 398
- *Actiban*, 863
- *Actico*, 863
- *Acticoat* products, 851, 853, 858
- *Actidose-Aqua Advance*, 28
- *Acti-Fast*, 861
- *ActiFormCool*, 853
- *Actilyse*, 134
- *Actinac*, 621
- Actinic keratosis, 625
- Actinomycin D *see* Dactinomycin
- *Actiq*, 232
- *Actisorb Plus*, 859
- *Actisorb Silver*, 859
- *Active*, 374
- *ActivHeal* products, 851, 852, 853, 855, 856
- *Activon Tulle*, 858
- *Acti-Wrap*, 861
- *Actonel* preparations, 409
- *Actos*, 371
- *Actrapid* preparations, 362
- *Acular*, 580
- *Acupan*, 228
- Acute coronary syndrome, 129
- Acute lymphoblastic leukaemia, 468
- *ACWY Vax*, 653
- Acyclovir *see* Aciclovir
- *Adalat* preparations, 115
- Adalimumab, 553
  - Crohn's disease, 52, **57**
  - rheumatic diseases, 551, 552, **553**
- Adapalene, **620**
- *Adartrel*, 261
- *Adcal*, 517
- *Adcal-D$_3$*, 526
- *Adcortyl*
  - in Orabase, 591
  - *Intra-articular/Intradermal*, 545
- Addicts, notification of, 9
- *Add-Ins*, 847
- *Addiphos*, 515
- Addison's disease, 378
- Additives *see* Excipients
- *Additrace*, 515
- Adefovir, **340**
- *Adenocor*, 80
- *Adenoscan* (adenosine), 80
- Adenosine, **80**
- ADH *see* Antidiuretic hormone
- ADHD *see* Attention deficit hyperactivity disorder, 213
- Adhesive
  - dressings, 865
  - films, 856
  - skin tissue, 637
- *Adipine* preparations, 115, 116
- *Adizem* preparations, 113
- Adrenal
  - function test, 398
  - hyperplasia, 379
  - insufficiency, 378
    - dental practice, 21
  - suppression
    - metyrapone, 415
    - systemic corticosteroids, 380
    - topical corticosteroids, 604
- Adrenaline
  - anaphylaxis, 170, **171**
  - cardiopulmonary resuscitation, 122
  - croup, 148
  - eye, 574
  - local anaesthesia, 681, 683
  - parenteral, 172
- Adrenergic neurone blocking drugs, 96
- Adrenoceptor agonists, 149
- *Adriamycin* (doxorubicin), 456
- ADROIT 11
- Adsorbents
  - gastro-intestinal, 51
  - poisoning, 28
- *Adva-Co*, 863
- *Advadraw* products, 860
- *Advagraf*, 477
- Advanced hypereosinophilic syndrome, 468
- *Advantage Plus*, 374
- *Advasil*, 856
- *Advasoft*, 863

Advate (factor VIII fraction), 136
Advazorb Plus, 853
Adverse reactions, reporting, 11
Advisory Committee on Borderline Substances *see* ACBS
Advisory labels *see* Cautionary and advisory labels, 867, 869
AeroBec preparations, 161, 162
AeroChamber, 157
Aerrane, 670
Agalsidase
    alfa, 529, **530**
    beta, 529, **530**
    infusion tables, 823
Agammaglobulinaemia, congenital, 660
Agenerase, 332
Age-related macular degeneration, 580
Aggrastat, 132
Agrippal, 650
AIDS, 327
    vaccines and, 642
Airomir preparations, 152
Airstrip, 865
Aknemin (minocycline), 298
Aknemycin Plus, 620
Alateris, 557
Albendazole, 357
    hydatid disease, 357
    strongyloidiasis, 357
Albumin solution, **509**
Albustix, 375
Albutein preparations (albumin solution), 509
Albuterol *see* salbutamol
Alclometasone dipropionate, 607
Alcohol
    ACBS, 842
    dependence, 269
    hypnotic, 184
    infusion table, 827
    nutrition, 511
    poisoning by, 29
    skin antiseptic, 637
    withdrawal, 269
Alcoholism, 269
    vitamin B, 523
Aldactide preparations (co-flumactone), 78
Aldactone, 77
Aldara, 624
Aldesleukin, 480
Aldioxa, 640
Aldomet, 96
Aldosterone antagonists, 76
Aldurazyme, 531
Alembicol D, 841
Alemtuzumab, **478**
    infusion table, 823
Alendronate sodium *see* Alendronic acid
Alendronic acid, 404, 406, 407
    colecalciferol with, 407
Alfacalcidol, **525**, 526
Alfentanil, 229, 674, **675**
    infusion table, 823
Alfuzosin, **438**
Alginates
    antacids, 38, 40
    dressings, 851, 852
Algisite M products, 851
Algivon, 851
Alglucosidase alfa, **531**
    infusion table, 823
Algosteril products, 851
Alimemazine
    allergic disorders, 166, **167**
    premedication, 167
Alimta, 460
Alione, 855
Aliskiren, **107**
Alkalinisation of urine, 443
Alkeran, 454
Alkylating drugs, 452
Alldress, 856
Allegron, 205
Allergen extract vaccines, 169
Allergy, 379
    anaphylaxis, 170
    angioedema, 171
    conjunctivitis, 570
    food, 57
    rhinitis, 586
Allevyn products, 852, 853
All-Flex diaphragm, 437
Allopurinol, **556**, 557
Almogran, 240
Almond oil, ear, 585
Almotriptan, **239**, 240
Alomide, 571
Alopecia
    cytotoxic drugs, 450
    male-pattern, 627
Aloxi, 223
Alpha Keri Bath Oil, 601
Alpha tocopheryl acetate, 527
Alpha$_2$-adrenoceptor stimulants
    cardiovascular, 95
    eye, 574, 579
    migraine, 243
Alpha-adrenoceptor blocking drugs
    cardiovascular, 97
    urinary tract, 438
Alpha-blockers *see* Alpha-adrenoceptor blocking drugs
Alphaderm, 606
Alphagan, 575
Alphanate (factor VIII fraction), 136
AlphaNine (factor IX fraction), 136
Alphosyl 2 in 1, 626
Alphosyl HC, 614
Alprazolam, 184, **185**
Alprostadil
    ductus arteriosus, 421
    erectile dysfunction, **445**, 446
    infusion table, 823
Altacite preparations (hydrotalcite), 39, 40
Alteplase, 133, **134**
    infusion table, 823
Alternative medicine, 1
Alu-Cap
    antacid, 39
    hyperphosphataemia, 520
Aluminium acetate, ear, 582, **583**
Aluminium chloride, 640
Aluminium hydroxide, 39
    antacid, 39, 40
    hyperphosphataemia, 520
Aluminium oxide, 620
Alupent preparations, 153
Alvedon (paracetamol), 227
Alverine, **42**
Alvesco, 163
Alzheimer's disease, 274
Amantadine
    parkinsonism, **265**
    viral infections, **342**
Amaryl, 368
AmBisome, 321, 323
Ambrix, xiii
Amethocaine *see* Tetracaine
Ametop, 685
Amfebutamone *see* Bupropion, 271
Amfetamine *see* Amphetamines
Amias, 105
Amikacin, 299, **300**
    infusion table, 823
    tuberculosis, 312
Amikin, 300
Amilamont (amiloride), 76
Amil-Co (co-amilozide), 77
Amiloride, **76**
    bumetanide with, 77
    cyclopenthiazide with, 77
    furosemide with, 77
    hydrochlorothiazide with, 77
Aminex, 844
Amino acids
    ACBS, 845, 846, 848
    intravenous nutrition, 511
Aminobenzoic acid, 523, **524**
Aminoglycosides
    ear, 582, 585
    eye, 566
    skin, 628
    systemic, 299
Aminogran, 847
Aminophylline, 154, **155**
    infusion table, 823
    see also Theophylline
Aminoplasmal preparations, 512
Aminosalicylates, 52, 53
Aminoven preparations, 512
Amiodarone, 80, **81**
    cardiopulmonary resuscitation, 122
    infusion table, 823
Amisulpride, 193, **194**
Amitriptyline, **203**, 204
    neuropathic pain, 238
    perphenazine with, 204
    postherpetic neuralgia, 238
Amix (amoxicillin), 288
Amlodipine, **112**
    see also Calcium-channel blockers
    valsartan with, 112
Amlostin (amlodipine), 112
Ammonaps, 532
Ammonia and ipecacuanha mixture, 177
Ammonia, poisoning by, 35
Ammonium chloride, acidification of urine, 443

Amobarbital, 187
  secobarbital with, 187
Amoebiasis, 352
Amoebic
  abscess, 352
  dysentery, 352
Amoebicides, 352
Amoram (amoxicillin), 288
Amorolfine, 630, **631**
Amoxicillin, **287**, 288
  infusion table, 823
  urinary tract infection, 319
Amoxident (amoxicillin), 288
Amoxil preparations, 288
  syrup—discontinued
Amoxycillin *see* Amoxicillin
Amphetamines
  abuse, 8
  poisoning by, 33
Amphocil, 321, 323
Amphotericin, 321, **322**
  bladder infections, 444
  eye, 577
  infusion, 322
    lipid formulation, 321, 322, 323
    liposomal, 323
  infusion table, 823
  leishmaniasis, 353
  mouth, 592, 593
Ampicillin, 287, **288**
  flucloxacillin with [co-fluampicil], 287, **289**
  infusion table, 823
Amprenavir, 328, **332**
Amsacrine, **462**
  infusion table, 824
Amsidine, 462
Amyben (amiodarone), 81
Amylobarbitone *see* Amobarbital
Amyotrophic lateral sclerosis, 267
Anabact, 630
Anabolic steroids, 397
  anaemias, 495
Anaemias, 490
  aplastic, 495
  chronic renal failure, 495
  haemolytic, 495, 499
  hypoplastic, 495
  iron-deficiency, 490
  megaloblastic, 493
  pernicious, 493
  sideroblastic, 495
Anaesthesia
  analgesics, 673
  antimuscarinics, 670
  corticosteroids, 380, 665
  dental practice, 666
  driving, 666
  general
    inhalational, 668
    intravenous, 666
  local, 680
    dental practice, 681
    eye, 577
    mouth, 590
    rectal, 65
    skin, 603
  muscle relaxants, 676
  status epilepticus, 256
Anafranil preparations, 204
Anagrelide, **500**
Anakinra, 552, **553**
Anal fissure, 66
Analeptics, 172
Analgesic-induced headache *see* Medication-overuse headache, 238
Analgesics, 224
  compound, 225
  non-opioid, 224
  NSAIDs, 224, 535
    anaesthesia, 673
    dental pain, 536
    elderly, 20
    orofacial pain, 536
    poisoning by, 29
    rheumatic diseases, 535
    topical, 563
  opioid, 229
    anaesthesia, 674
    cough suppressants, 176
    dependence on, 8
    diabetic neuropathy, 373
    diarrhoea, 51
    equivalent doses, 15
    neuropathic pain, 238
    palliative care, 15, 18
    poisoning by, 31
Analog preparations, 845, 846, 848
Anapen, 171, 172
Anaphylaxis, 170
Anastrozole, 483, **484**, 485
Ancotil, 324
Ancylostomiasis, 357
Androcur, 396
Androgens, 394
  malignant disease, 483
Andropatch, 395
Anectine, 679
Anexate, 680
Angeliq, 387
Angettes 75 (aspirin), 131
Angeze (isosorbide mononitrate), 110, 111
Angilol (propranolol), 86
Angina
  aspirin, 108
  beta-blockers, 85, 107
  calcium-channel blockers, 112
  dental practice, 22, 24
  heparins, 108
  nitrates, 108
  potassium-channel activators, 117
  stable, 107
  statins, 108
  unstable, 108
Angioedema, 171
  hereditary, 171
    danazol, 412
    tranexamic acid, 135
Angiotensin-converting enzyme inhibitors *see* ACE inhibitors
Angiotensin-II receptor antagonists, 105
Angiox, 125
Angitak, 110
Angitil preparations, 113
Angular cheilitis, 593
  bacterial infection, 629
  fungal infection, 630
  inflammation, 604
Anhydrol Forte, 640
Anidulafungin, 322, **323**
  infusion table, 824
Anistreplase, 134
Ankylosing spondylitis, 552
Anogenital warts, 623
Anorectics, 215
Anquil, 190
Antabuse, 270
Antacids
  alginates and, 38
  aluminium, 38
  bismuth, 38
  calcium, 38
  magnesium, 38
  simeticone and, 38
  sodium content, 39
Antazoline, **570**
Antepsin, 47
Anterior uveitis, 571
Anthelmintics, 355
Anthracyclines, 454
Anthralin *see* Dithranol
Anthraquinones, 59
Anthrax, 316
  vaccine, 643, 644
Anti-androgens, 396
Anti-arrhythmic drugs, 78
Antibacterial policies, 278
Antibacterials, 277
  acne, 619, 621
  diarrhoea, 51
  ear, 582
  eczema, 611
  eye, 566
  oral infections, 278
  prophylaxis, 282
  skin, 628
  summary of therapy, 279
  vaginal, 425
Antibiotic policies *see* Antibacterial policies, 278
Antibiotic-associated colitis, **53**
  antibacterial therapy, 279
    clindamycin, in, 303
    metronidazole, in, 315
    vancomycin, in, 305
Antibiotics *see* Antibacterials
Anticholinergic drugs *see* Antimuscarinics
Anticholinergic syndrome, 670
Anticholinesterases, 558
  anaesthesia, 679
Anticoagulant treatment booklets, 128
Anticoagulants
  oral, 127
    dental practice, 25
    reversal, 127
    surgery, 666
  parenteral, 122
Anticonvulsants *see* Antiepileptics
Anti-D (Rh_0) immunoglobulin, 661, 662

Antidepressants, 201
  anxiety, 202
  choice, 203
  obsessive compulsive disorder, 202
  panic disorder, 202
  poisoning by, 31
  post-traumatic stress disorder, 202
  see also Monoamine-oxidase inhibitors
  serotonin re-uptake inhibitors, 208
  social anxiety disorder, 202
  surgery, 666
  tricyclic, 203
    diabetic neuropathy, 373
    enuresis, 443
    MAOIs with, 207
    migraine, 242
    urinary incontinence, 440
  withdrawal, 202
Antidiabetic drugs, 358
  insulin, 359
  oral, 366
Antidiarrhoeal drugs *see* Diarrhoea, 50, 505
Antidiuretic hormone, 402
  antagonist, 404
  inappropriate secretion, 404
Anti-emetics, 217
  cytotoxic therapy and, 449
  migraine, 242
Antiepileptics, 245
  surgery, 665
Antifibrinolytic drugs, 135
Antifungal drugs, 320
  anogenital, 425
  oropharyngeal, 592
  skin, 630
Antigiardial drugs, 353
Antihaemophilic fraction, human, 136
Antihepatitis B immunoglobulin, 661
Antihistamines, 166
  allergic emergencies, 170
  allergy, 166
    eye, 570
    nose, 586
    skin, 604
  cough preparations, 176
  dental, 166
  eczema, 611
  nasal decongestants, 178
  nausea and vertigo, 217, **218**
Antihypertensives, 99
  ACE inhibitors, 99
  adrenergic neurone blockers, 96
  alpha-blockers, 97
  angiotensin-II receptor antagonists, 105
  beta-blockers, 85
  calcium-channel blockers, 112
  centrally-acting, 95
  renin inhibitors, 107
  vasodilator, 93
Anti-inflammatory analgesics *see* Analgesics, NSAIDs
Antileprotic drugs, 314
Antilymphocyte globulin, 495
Antimalarials, 344
  rheumatic diseases, 548
Antimanic drugs, 199
Antimetabolites, 456
Antimigraine drugs, 238
Antimotility drugs, 51
Antimuscarinics
  antipsychotics and, 188
  bronchodilator, 153
  diabetic neuropathy, 373
  eye, 571
  gastro-intestinal, 41
  parkinsonism, 266
  premedication, 670
  quaternary ammonium, 41
  urinary tract, 440
Antineoplastic drugs, 448
  see also Cytotoxic drugs
Anti-oestrogens, 397, 483
Antiperspirants, 640
Antiplatelet drugs, 129
Antiprotozoal drugs, 344
Antipruritics, topical, 604
Antipsychotics, 187
  depot injections, 197
  equivalent doses
    depot, 198
    oral, 189
  high doses, 187
  mania, 199
  withdrawal, 188
Antipyretics, 225
Antirabies immunoglobulin, 661
Antiretrovirals, 327, 328, 335
Antiseptics, 637
  ACBS, 849
  lozenges, 594
  mouthwashes, 594
  sprays, oropharynx, 594
Antiserum, 643, 659
Antispasmodics, 41
Antitetanus immunoglobulin, 661
Antithrombin alfa, 136
Antithrombin III concentrate, **136**
Antithyroid drugs, 377
Antituberculous drugs, 310
Antitussives, 176
Antivaricella-zoster immunoglobulin, 661
Antivenoms, 36
Antiviral drugs, 327
  eye, 568
  mouth, 593
  skin, 633
Anturan, 557
Anugesic-HC, 65
Anusol preparations, 65
Anxiety, 184
  antipsychotics, 187
  chronic, 202
Anxiolytics, 179, **184**
  anaesthesia, 672
  benzodiazepines, 184
  poisoning by, 32
  withdrawal, 179
Anzemet, 221
APD *see* Disodium pamidronate
Aphthous ulcers, 590
Apidra, 362
Aplastic anaemia, 495
APO-go, 260
Apomorphine, **259**, 260
Appetite
  stimulants, 528
  suppressants, 215
Applications, definition, 597
Apraclonidine, 574, **579**
Aprepitant, 218, **223**, 449
Apresoline, 94
Aprinox (bendroflumethiazide), 73
Aproten
  gluten-free, 843
  low-protein, 844
Aprovel, 106
Aptivus, 334
Aquacel products, 855
Aquadrate, 600
Aquafilm, 853
Aquaform, 853
Aquasept, 639
Aqueous cream, 599
Aquilon, 158
Arachis oil
  cradle cap, 626
  enema, 61
  presence of, 170, 2
Aranesp preparations, 496
Arava, 550
Arcoxia, 539
Aredia Dry Powder, 408
Arginine supplement, 848
Argipressin *(Pitressin)*, 403
Aricept, 275
Aricept Evess, 275
Aridil (co-amilofruse), 77
Arilvax, 659
Arimidex, 485
Aripiprazole, 193, **194**
Arixtra, 126
Arlevert, 219
Arnott, 343
Aromasin, 485
Aromatase inhibitors, 484
Arpicolin, 267
Arrhythmias, 78
  beta-blockers, 85
  dental practice, 24
  poisoning and, 27
  supraventricular, 70, 79
  ventricular, 79
Arsenic trioxide, 462, **463**
  infusion table, 824
Artelac (hypromellose), 578
Artelac SDU, 578
Artemether
  lumefantrine with, **349**
Arterial occlusion, 127
Arteritis, giant cell (temporal), 544
Artesunate, 344
Arthritis
  juvenile idiopathic, 546
  psoriatic, 546
  rheumatoid, 534
  septic, 281
Arthrofen (ibuprofen), 540
Arthrotec preparations, 539
Arthroxen (naproxen), 542
Articaine, 681
Artificial saliva, 595
Arythmol, 83
AS Saliva Orthana, 595

5-ASA, 53
Asacol preparations, 54
Asasantin Retard, 131
Ascabiol (benzyl benzoate), 634
Ascaricides, 356
Ascaris, 356
Ascensia products, 366, 374, 375
Ascorbic acid, 524, **525**
    acidification of urine, 443
    iron excretion, 498
Asilone preparations, 40
Askina products, 853, 855, 858, 859
Asmabec preparations, 161, 162
Asmanex, 164
Asmasal preparations, 152
Asparaginase, 464
Aspartame, 516
    presence of, 2
Aspav, 226
Aspergillosis, 321
Aspirin
    analgesia, 225, **226**, 536
    angina, 108
    antiplatelet, 129, **130**, 131
    codeine with, 226
    dipyridamole with, 131
    metoclopramide with, 239
    migraine, 238
    myocardial infarction, 129, 133
    papaveretum with, 226
    rheumatic diseases, 544
Asplenia
    Haemophilus influenzae type b, prophylaxis, 282
    influenza vaccine, 650
    malaria, 346
    pneumococcal infection, 282
    pneumococcal vaccine, 654
    vaccines and, 642
Asthma, 145
    acute severe (table), 147
    $beta_2$ agonists, 149
    chronic (table), 146
    emergency treatment, 148
        dental practice, 22
    exercise-induced, 149
    nocturnal, 149
    pregnancy, 145
    prophylaxis, 164
Astringents
    ear, 582
    skin, 637
AT-10, 526
Atarax, 168
Atazanavir, 328, **332**
Atenix (atenolol) preparations, 87
Atenolol, **86**, 87
    chlortalidone with, 87
    co-amilozide with, 87
    infusion table, 824
    nifedipine with, 87
    see also Beta-adrenoceptor blocking drugs
Athlete's foot, 630
Atimos Modulite, 150
Ativan (lorazepam), 186
Atomoxetine, **213**, 214
Atonic seizures, 245
Atorvastatin, 140, **141**
Atosiban, **423**
    infusion table, 824
Atovaquone, **355**
    malaria, 344, 350, 351
    pneumocystis pneumonia, 354
    proguanil with, 351
Atracurium, 676, **677**
    infusion table, 824
Atrauman products, 858
Atrial fibrillation, 70, **79**, 127
Atrial flutter, 79
Atriance, 460
Atripla, xiii
Atropine sulphate, 41
    anticholinesterases and, 679
    antispasmodic, 41
    beta-blocker poisoning, 32
    bradycardia, 79, 670
    cardiopulmonary resuscitation, 122
    eye, 571
    myocardial infarction, 79
    organophosphorus poisoning, 36
    premedication, 670, 671
Atrovent preparations, 154
ATryn (antithrombin alfa), 136
Attention deficit hyperactivity disorder, 213
Atypical antipsychotics, 193
    prolactin elevation, 193
Augmentin preparations, 289
Auranofin, 546, **547**
Aureocort, 610
Aurothiomalate, **546**
Autolet devices, 366
Autopen, 365
Avance products, 853
Avandamet, 371
Avandia, 371
Avastin, 463
Avaxim, 647
Aveeno preparations, 599, 601
Avelox, 318
Aviva, 374
Avloclor, 349
Avobenzone, 625
Avoca, 623
Avodart, 396
Avomine, 219
Avonex, 480
Axid, 46
Axsain, 564
Azactam, 295
Azamune (azathioprine), 474
Azapropazone, 535, **537**
Azathioprine, 458, **473**, 474
    eczema, 616
    inflammatory bowel disease, 53
    infusion table, 824
    myasthenia gravis, 559
    rheumatic disease, 549
    transplant rejection, 473
Azelaic acid, 619
Azelastine, **570**
    eye, 570
    nose, 586
Azidothymidine, 331
Azilect, 264
Azithromycin, 301, **302**
    trachoma, 566
Azopt, 576
AZT, 331
Aztreonam, **295**
    infusion table, 824

B

Babyhaler, 157
Bacillus Calmette-Guérin
    bladder instillation, 480, 481
    vaccines, 644
Bacitracin
    eye, 568
    skin
        polymyxin with, 629
Back pain, 535
Baclofen, 559, 560
    palliative care, 16
Bacterial vaginosis, 280
Bacteroides fragilis infections
    antipseudomonal penicillins, in, 290
    clindamycin, in, 303
    metronidazole, in, 315
Bactigras, 858
Bactroban, 629
Bactroban Nasal, 590
Baker's Delight, 843
BAL, 34
Balanced Salt Solution, 578
Baldness
    cytotoxic drugs, 450
    male-pattern, 627
Balneum preparations, 600, 601
Balsalazide, 52, 53, **54**
Bambec, 150
Bambuterol, **150**
Bandages, 860, 861, 862, 863, 864
Baraclude, 341
Baratol, 97
Barbiturates, **187**
    anaesthesia, 667
Barkat, 843
Barrier preparations, 602
Basal cell carcinoma, 624, 625
Basiliximab, 474, **475**
    infusion table, 824
Bath additives
    antimicrobial with, 602
    coal tar, 614
    emollient, 601, 602
Baxan, 292
Bazetham MR (tamsulosin), 439
BCG
    bladder instillation, 480
    vaccines, 644
B-D Lancer, 366
BD Micro-Fine products, 366
BD Safe-clip, 366
Becaplermin, **639**, 640
Beclazone (beclometasone) preparations, 161, 162

Beclometasone dipropionate
- asthma, 159, 160, 161, 162
- formoterol with, 162
- nasal allergy, 587
- oral ulceration, 590
- ulcerative colitis, 52, **56**

Beclomethasone dipropionate *see* Beclometasone dipropionate
Becodisks, 161, 162
Beconase preparations, 587
Bedol, 389
Bedranol SR (propranolol), 86
Bedsores, 603
Bee sting allergy preparations, 169
Beeswax, excipient, 598
Begrivac, 651
Belladonna, 41
Bemiparin, 123, **124**
Bendrofluazide *see* Bendroflumethiazide
Bendroflumethiazide, **73**
- hypercalciuria, 518
- potassium with, 78
- timolol with, 91

BeneFIX (factor IX fraction), 136
Benerva (thiamine), 524
Benign fibrocystic breast disease, 412
Benoxinate *see* Oxybuprocaine, **577**
Benperidol, **189**, 190
Benquil, 190
Benzalkonium, 627
- cetrimide with, 602
- chlorhexidine with, 601
- dimeticone with, 602

Benzathine benzylpenicillin, 280, 284
Benzatropine, **266**
Benzbromarone, 556
Benzhexol *see* Trihexyphenidyl
Benzocaine, 685
Benzodiazepines, 179
- anaesthesia, 672
- antagonist, 679
- anxiolytics, 184
- epilepsy, 255
- hypnotics, 180
- mania, 199
- muscle spasm, 559
- poisoning by, 32
- withdrawal, 179

Benzoic acid ointment, compound, 630, 631
Benzoin tincture, compound, 176
Benzoyl peroxide, 618, 619
- clindamycin with, 619
- hydroxyquinoline with, 619

Benzthiazide, 73
- triamterene with, 77

Benztropine *see* Benzatropine, **266**
Benzydamine, 590, **591**
Benzyl alcohol, presence of, 2, 598
Benzyl benzoate, **634**
Benzylpenicillin, 284, **285**
- infusion table, 824
- injection, 285

Beractant, **173**
Besavar XL, 438
Beta$_2$ agonists, 149
Beta-Adalat, 87
Beta-adrenoceptor blocking drugs, 84
- angina, 85, 107
- anxiety, 186
- arrhythmias, 80, 81, 85
- eye, **572**
- heart failure, 85, 99
- hypertension, 85
- migraine, 242
- myocardial infarction, 85, 133
- poisoning by, 32
- thyrotoxicosis, 85, 377
- verapamil and, 117

Beta-adrenoceptor stimulants
- asthma, 149
- premature labour, 423

Beta-blockers *see* Beta-adrenoceptor blocking drugs
Betacap, 607
Beta-Cardone, 90
Betadine
- dry powder spray, 638
- ointment, 639

Betaferon, 480
Betagan, 573
Betahistine, 218, **224**
Betaject Light (interferon beta-1b), 480
Beta-lactamases, 284
Betaloc preparations, 89
Betamethasone, 379, **382**
- mouth, 591
- skin, **607**

Betamethasone dipropionate
- skin, 608
  - calcipotriol with, 613
  - clotrimazole with, 608
  - salicylic acid with, 608

Betamethasone sodium phosphate, 382
- ear, 583
- eye, 569
- infusion table, 824
- nose, 587, 589
- oral ulceration, 382
- rheumatic disease, 545

Betamethasone valerate
- skin, 607, 608
  - clioquinol with, 608
  - fusidic acid with, 608
  - neomycin with, 608

Beta-Prograne, 86
Betaxolol, 572, **573**
Bethanechol
- laxative, 59
- urinary retention, **439**

Betim, 91
Betnelan, 382
Betnesol, 382, 591
- ear, 583
- eye, 569
- injection, 545
- nose, 587

Betnesol-N
- ear, 583
- eye, 569
- nose, 589

Betnovate preparations, 607, 608
Betoptic, 573
Bettamousse, 607
Bevacizumab, **463**
- infusion table, 824

Bexarotene, **463**
Bezafibrate, **139**
Bezalip preparations, 139
Bi-Aglut, 843
Biatain products, 852, 853
Bicalutamide, **487**
Bicarbonate
- intravenous, 508
- oral, 505
- *see also* Sodium bicarbonate

BiCNU, 453
Biguanides, 368
Bilharziasis, 357
Biliary-tract infection, 279
Bimatoprost, 573, **574**
- timolol with, 574

BiNovum, 431
Bioclusive, 856
Biofilm S, 855
Biorphen, 266
Biotène Oralbalance, 595
Biotin, 523, 14
BioXtra, 595
Biphosphonates *see* Bisphosphonates
Bipolar disorder, 200
Birthmarks, ACBS, 849
Bisacodyl, 59
Bismuth chelate, 47
Bismuth subgallate, 64
Bisoprolol, **87**
- *see also* Beta-adrenoceptor blocking drugs

Bisphosphonates, 404, 406
- breast cancer, 484
- hypercalcaemia, 518

Bites
- animal, 281
- human, 281
- snake, 36

Bitters, 528
Bivalirudin, **125**
- infusion table, 824

Bladder
- blood clot dissolution, 444
- irrigations, 443
  - cytotoxic, 444

Blenderm, 865
Bleo-Kyowa (bleomycin), 455
Bleomycin, **455**
- infusion table, 824

Blepharitis, 566
Blepharospasm, **268**
Blisterfilm, 856
Blood incompatibilities, 821
Blood products, 136, 137
Blue line webbing, 863
BM-Accutest, 374
Body-surface, dosage and, 14
Body-weight, dosage and, 14
Boils, 636
Bondronat, 408
Bone metabolism, drugs affecting, 404
Bone tumours, analgesia, 225
Bonefos, 409

Index

Bone-marrow suppression, cytotoxic drugs, 450
Bonjela (choline salicylate), 592
Bonviva preparations, 408
Borderline substances *see* ACBS
Bortezomib, **464**
Bosentan, **93**
Botox, 268
Botulinum
- antitoxin, 645
- hyperhidrosis, 640
- toxin type A, **268**, 269
- toxin type B, **269**

Botulism antitoxin, 645
Bowel
- cleansing solutions, 63
- irrigation, 28
- sterilisation, 299, 308

Bradycardia, 79
- anaesthesia, 670

Bran, 58
Brand names, symbol, 1
Brasivol, 620
Breast
- cancer, **483**
  - bone metastases, 406
  - trastuzumab, 472
- pain, **415**

Breast-feeding, prescribing during, 807
Brevibloc, 88
Brevinor, 431
Brevoxyl, 619
Brexidol (piroxicam), 543
Bricanyl preparations, 153
Brimonidine, **574**, 575
- timolol with, 575

Brinzolamide, **575**, 576
BritLofex, 274
Broflex, 267
Brolene, 568
Bromocriptine, 410, **411**
- acromegaly, 410
- galactorrhoea, 410
- hypogonadism, 411
- lactation suppression, 411
- neuroleptic malignant syndrome, 188
- parkinsonism, 259, **260**
- prolactinoma, 411

Bronchiectasis, 175
Bronchitis, 175, 279
- bronchodilators, 148

Bronchodilators
- adrenoceptor agonist, 149
- antimuscarinic, 153
- surgery, 665
- sympathomimetic, 149
- theophylline, 154

Bronchospasm, 149
Brucellosis, 296, 313
Brufen preparations, 541
Brugia malayi, 357
Bruxism, 225
BSA, 14
Buccastem, 220
Buclizine, 239
Budenofalk, 56
Budesonide, 162
- asthma, 159, **162**
- Crohn's, 52, 56
- croup, **148**
- formoterol with, 163
- inflammatory bowel disease, 52, 56
- nasal
  - allergy, 587
  - polyps, 587

Bumetanide, 74, **75**
- amiloride with, 77
- infusion table, 824

Bupivacaine, **683**
- adrenaline with, 683

Buprenorphine, 230, 231, 273
- intra-operative analgesia, 230
- naloxone with, 273
- opioid dependence, 273
- pain, 229, **230**
- premedication, 230

Bupropion, 271
Burinex, 75
Burinex A, 77
Burns, infected, 628
Buscopan preparations (Hyoscine butylbromide), 42
Buserelin, 414, 487
- endometriosis, 414
- IVF, 414
- prostate cancer, 486, **487**

Busilvex, 453
Buspar, 186
Buspirone, **186**
Busulfan, 452, **453**
- infusion table, 824

Busulphan *see* Busulfan
Butobarbital, 187
Butobarbitone *see* Butobarbital, 187
BuTrans, 230
Butylated hydroxyanisole, excipient, 598
Butylated hydroxytoluene, excipient, 598
Butyrophenones, 189
Byetta, 370

C

C_1 esterase inhibitor, 171
Cabaser, 260
Cabergoline
- hyperprolactinaemia, 410, **411**, 412
- parkinsonism, 259, **260**

Cacit, 407, 517
Cacit D3, 526
Cadesorb, 854
Cadexomer–iodine, 854
Caelyx, 456
Cafergot, 242
Caffeine, 226
Calaband, 864
Calamine, 603
- coal tar with, 614

Calceos, 526
Calcicard CR, 113
Calcichew, 517
Calcichew D3, 526
Calcichew D3 Forte, 526
Calciferol, 525
Calcijex, 526
Calciparine—discontinued
Calcipotriol, 611, **613**
- betamethasone with, 613

Calcitonin, 404
- hypercalcaemia, **405**, 518
- infusion table, 824
- osteoporosis, **405**

Calcitriol, 525, **526**
- osteoporosis, 404
- psoriasis, 611, **613**

Calcium
- colecalciferol with, 525, 526
- ergocalciferol with, 525

Calcium acetate, 520
Calcium alginate dressings, 851
Calcium and vitamin D tablets, 525
Calcium balance, maintenance, 405
Calcium carbonate, 517
- antacid, 38
- disodium etidronate with, 407

Calcium chloride, 517, 518
Calcium folinate, 450, **451**, 494
- infusion table, 824

Calcium gluconate, 517, 518
- infusion table, 824

Calcium lactate tablets, 517
Calcium leucovorin *see* Calcium folinate
Calcium levofolinate, **451**
- infusion table, 824

Calcium phosphate, 526
Calcium polystyrene sulphonate, 504
Calcium Resonium, 504
Calcium salts, 517, 520
Calcium supplements, 517
Calcium-500, 517
Calcium-channel blockers, 111
- angina, 112
- hypertension, 112
- poisoning by, 32

Calcium-Sandoz, 517
Calcort, 383
Calfovit D3, 526
Calluses, 622
Calmurid, 601
Calmurid HC, 606
Calogen, 833
Caloreen, 833
Calpol (paracetamol) preparations, 227
Calprofen (ibuprofen), 541
Calshake, 833
Camcolit preparations, 201
Camouflaging preparations, 626
Campral EC, 270
Campto, 471
Campylobacter enteritis, 279, 301
Cancidas, 323
Candesartan, 105
Candidiasis, 320
- intestinal, 322
- oropharyngeal, 321, 592
- perianal, 64
- skin, 630
- systemic, 321
- vaginal, **425**
- vulval, 425

Index

Candidosis *see* Candidiasis
Canesten
anogenital, 425, 426
ear, 584
HC, 606
Internal Cream (clotrimazole), 426
skin, 631
Cannabis, regulations, 8
Canusal, 126
Capasal, 626
Capastat, 312
Capecitabine, 457, **458**, 459
Caplenal (allopurinol), 556
Capoten, 101
Capozide, 101
Capreomycin, **312**
Caprilon, 841
Caprin (aspirin)
analgesia, 226
antiplatelet, 131
Caps, contraceptive, 437
Capsaicin, 563, 564
diabetic neuropathy, 373, 564
neuropathic pain, 238
osteoarthritis, 534, 563
postherpetic neuralgia, 238, 564
Capsuvac, 60
Capto-co (co-zidocapt), 101
Captopril, **101**
hydrochlorothiazide with, 101
see also ACE inhibitors
Carace preparations, 103
Caramet CR, 263
Carbachol
glaucoma, 576
Carbagen SR, 246
Carbaglu, 532
Carbalax, 63
Carbamazepine
bipolar disorder, 200
diabetes insipidus, 402
diabetic neuropathy, 373
epilepsy, **245**, 246
poisoning, elimination, 28
trigeminal neuralgia, 238
Carbaryl, 634, **635**
Carbetocin, 418, **419**
Carbimazole, **377**
Carbocisteine, **175**
Carbo-Dome, 614
CarboFLEX, 859
Carbomers, 578
Carbomix, 28
Carbon monoxide poisoning, 35
Carbonet, 859
Carbonic anhydrase inhibitors, 78
glaucoma, 575
Carbopad VC, 859
Carboplatin, **466**, 467
infusion table, 824
Carboprost, 419
Carbuncle, 636
Carcinoid tumour, 479, 489
Cardene preparations, 115
Cardiac arrest
see Cardiopulmonary resuscitation, 121
chart, *inside back cover*
Cardiac glycosides, 70
arrhythmias, 80
Cardiac problems, dental practice, 22
Cardiac *see also* Heart
Cardicor, 87
Cardilate MR, 116
Cardioplen XL (felodipine), 114
Cardiopulmonary resuscitation, 121
chart, *inside back cover*
Cardiovascular disease
angina, 107
myocardial infarction, 132
prevention
antiplatelet therapy, 129
diabetes, 92
dyslipidaemia, 140
hypertension, 91
non-drug treatment, 91, 137
obesity, 91
risk assessment, 140
risk prediction charts, *inside back cover*
Cardioxane, 450
Cardura preparations, 97
Carglumic acid, 532
Carisoma, 561
Carisoprodol, **561**
Carmellose
eye, **578**
mouth, 590, **591**
Carmustine, 452, **453**
infusion table, 824
Carnitine, 529
Carnitor, 529
Carobel, Instant, 840
Carpal tunnel syndrome, 545
Carteolol, 572, **573**
Carticaine *see* Articaine, 681
Carvedilol, 84, **87**, 88
see also Beta-adrenoceptor blocking drugs
Carylderm, 635
lotion—discontinued
Cascara, 59
Casilan-90, 841
Casodex, 487
Caspofungin, 321, 322, **323**
infusion table, 824
Castor oil, 59
Catapres, 96
Catarrh, vernal, 570
Catechol-*O*-methyltransferase inhibitors, 264
Catheter maintenance, 444
Catheter patency solutions
chlorhexidine, 444
sodium chloride, 444
solution G, 444
solution R, 444
Cautionary and advisory labels, 867
counselling, 867
list of products, 869
NCL, 867
original packs, 867
Caverject preparations, 446
Cavi-Care, 853
CCNU (lomustine), 454
Ceanel Concentrate, 626
Cedocard Retard, 110
Cefaclor, **291**, 292
Cefadroxil, 291, **292**
Cefalexin, 291, **292**
Cefixime, 291, **292**, 293
Cefotaxime, 291, **293**
infusion table, 824
Cefpodoxime, 291, **293**
Cefradine, 291, **293**
infusion table, 824
Ceftazidime, 291, **294**
eye, 577
infusion table, 824
Ceftriaxone, 291, **294**
infusion table, 825
Cefuroxime, 291, **294**, 295
eye, 577
infusion table, 825
Cefuroxime axetil, 291, 294
Celance, 260
Celebrex, 538
Celecoxib, 536, **537**, 538
Celectol, 88
Celevac, 59
Celiprolol, 84, **88**
see also Beta-adrenoceptor blocking drugs
CellCept, 474
Cellona, 863
Cellulitis, 281
Celluvisc, 578
Celsentri, 335
Central Gard, 857
Central nervous system stimulants, 213
Centyl K, 78
Ceph... *see also* Cef...
Cephalosporins, 291
Ceporex, 292
Ceprotin (protein C concentrate), 137
Cepton, 638
Cerazette, 433
Cerebral oedema, 379
Cerezyme, 530
Cernevit, 515
Cerubidin (daunorubicin), 455
Cerumol, 585
Cervarix, 650
Cetirizine, **166**
Cetostearyl alcohol, excipient, 598
Cetraben, 599, 601
Cetrimide, 602, 636, 637, **638**
benzalkonium with, 602
chlorhexidine with, 638
dimeticone with, 603
Cetrorelix, **412**
Cetrotide, 412
Cetuximab, **464**
CFCs, 149, 159
Chamomile extract, 600
Champix, 272
Charcoal, activated
dressings, 859
poisoning, use in, 28
Charcodote, 28
Cheilitis, angular, 593
bacterial infection, 629
fungal infection, 630
inflammation, 604
Chemydur, 111
Chicken meat, comminuted, 842
Chickenpox, 336
Chilblains, 640

Children
 adverse reactions, 13
 medicine storage, 3
 prescribing for, 13
Child-resistant containers, 3
Chirocaine, 684
Chlamydia
 eye, 566
 genital, 280
 macrolides, in, 301
 quinolones, in, 316
 tetracyclines, in, 296
Chloractil (chlorpromazine), 190
Chloral betaine *see* Cloral betaine, 183
Chloral hydrate, **182**, 183
Chlorambucil, 452, **453**
Chloramphenicol, **304**
 ear, 582, **584**
 eye, 566, **567**
 infusion table, 825
 skin, hydrocortisone with, 621
Chloraprep, 638
Chlordiazepoxide, 184, **185**
Chlorhexidine, 637
 benzalkonium with, 601
 bladder infections, 444
 cetrimide with, 638
 dressing, gauze, 858
 hydrocortisone and nystatin with, 606
 mouth, 590, 593, **594**
 neomycin with, 589, 590
 nose, 589, 590
 skin disinfection, 637, 638
  dressing, 857
  dusting powder, 638
Chlorine poisoning, 35
Chlormethiazole *see* Clomethiazole
Chlorocresol, excipient, 598
Chlorofluorocarbon propellants, 149, 159
Chlorohex, 594
Chloromycetin, 567
Chloroquine, 349
 malaria
  prophylaxis, 346, 347, 348, **349**
  treatment, 345, **349**
 proguanil with, 349
 rheumatic disease, 546, 549
Chloroxylenol, 640
Chlorphenamine, 166, **167**, 168
Chlorpheniramine *see* Chlorphenamine, 166, **167**, 168
Chlorpromazine, 189, **190**
 hiccup, 189
 nausea, **219**
 nausea and vertigo, 217
 psychosis, 189
Chlorpropamide, **367**
 diabetes insipidus, 402
Chlorquinaldol
 hydrocortisone with, 607
Chlortalidone, **73**, **74**
 atenolol with, 87
 diabetes insipidus, 402
 triamterene with, 78
Chlorthalidone *see* Chlortalidone
Cholecalciferol *see* Colecalciferol
Cholera vaccine, 645
 travel, 663
Cholestagel, 138
Cholestyramine *see* Colestyramine
Choline, 523
Choline salicylate
 dental gel, 590, **592**
Cholinergic crises, 558
Cholinesterase inhibitors, 558, 679
Choragon, 398
Choreas, 267
Choriocarcinoma, 456
Choriogonadotropin alfa, **398**
Chorionic gonadotrophin, **398**
Chronic eosinophilic leukaemia, 468
Chronic myeloid leukaemia, 468
Chronic obstructive pulmonary disease, 148, 172
 oxygen, 173, 174
Cialis, 447
Cica-Care, 856
Cicafem, 621
Cicatrin—discontinued
Ciclesonide, **163**
Ciclosporin
 aplastic anaemia, 495
 eczema, 616, **617**
 immunosuppression, 474, **475**, 476
 infusion table, 825
 nephrotic syndrome, 475
 psoriasis, 616, **617**
 rheumatic disease, **549**
 ulcerative colitis, 52
Cidofovir, **338**
 infusion table, 825
Cidomycin, 300
Cigarette smoking, 270
Cilastatin, 295
 imipenem with, 295, **296**
  infusion table, 828
Cilazapril, **101**
 see also ACE inhibitors
Cilest, 432
Cilostazol, **118**, 119
Ciloxan, 567
Cimetidine, **45**, 46
 infusion table, 825
Cinacalcet, 405, **518**, 519
Cinchocaine [ingredient], 65
Cinnarizine, 219
 dimenhydrinate with, 219
 nausea and vertigo, 218
Cipralex, 209
Cipramil, 209
Ciprofibrate, **139**
Ciprofloxacin, 316, **317**, 318
 ear, 585
 eye, 566, **567**
 travellers' diarrhoea, 51
Ciproxin, 318
Cisatracurium, 676, **677**
 infusion table, 825
Cisplatin, 466, **467**
 infusion table, 825
Citalopram, 208, **209**
Citanest, 684
 with Octapressin, 684
CitraFleet, 63
Citramag, 64
Citrugel, 853
Cladribine, 457, **459**
 infusion table, 825
Claforan, 293
Clairette, 621
Clarelux, 608
Clarithromycin, 301, **302**, 303
 infusion table, 825
Clarosip, 302
Classification changes, xii
Clavulanic acid, 287
 amoxicillin with, 287, 288
  infusion table (co-amoxiclav), 825
 ticarcillin with, 290
  infusion table, 831
Cleanlet Fine, 366
Cleansers, skin, 637
Clemastine, **168**
Clenil Modulite, 161, 162
Clexane preparations, 124
Climagest, 387
Climanor, 393
Climaval, 389
Climesse, 387
Clindamycin, **303**, 304
 acne, 619
 benzoyl peroxide with, 619
 infusion table, 825
 malaria treatment, 344, 345
 oral infections, 303
 pneumocystis pneumonia, 354
 vaginal infections, 427
CliniFast, 861
Clinimix preparations, 512
Clinipak syringe, 366
Clinipore, 865
Clinisorb, 859
Clinistix, 375
Clinitar, 614
 shampoo, 627
Clinitek Microalbumin, 375
Clinitest, 375
ClinOleic, 512
Clinorette, 387
Clinoril, 544
Clinutren preparations, 833, 840
Clioquinol
 ear, 582, 583, **584**
 skin
  betamethasone with, 608
  fluocinolone with, 609
  hydrocortisone with, 607
Clipper, 56
CLL *see* Leukaemia, chronic lymphocytic
Clobazam, 184, 245, **255**
 epilepsy, 245, 255
Clobetasol propionate, 608
Clobetasone butyrate
 skin, 608
 tetracycline with, 608
Clodronate sodium *see* Sodium clodronate
Clofarabine, 457, **459**
 infusion table, 825
Clofazimine, **315**
Clomethiazole, **183**
 alcohol withdrawal, 269
Clomid, 397

Index

Clomifene, **397**
Clomiphene *see* Clomifene
Clomipramine, 203, **204**
Clonazepam, 255
epilepsy, 245, **255**
status epilepticus, 255, **256**
infusion table, 825
Clonidine
hypertension, **96**
menopausal flushing, 243, 385
migraine, 242, **243**
Tourette syndrome, 267
Clopamide, 73
pindolol with, 90
Clopidogrel, 129, **131**
Clopixol, 193, 199
Clopixol Acuphase, 193
Clopixol Conc., 199
Cloral betaine, 183
Clostridium botulinum, 645
Clostridium difficile, 53
Clotam, 239
Clotrimazole
anogenital, 425
ear, 584
skin, 630, **631**
betamethasone with, 608
hydrocortisone with, 606
Clozapine, 193, **194**, 195
Clozaril, 195
Cluster headache, 243
CMV, 338
Coal tar, 611, 612, 614
calamine with, 614
dithranol and salicylic acid with, 615
hydrocortisone with, 614
salicylic acid with, 614
scalp, 614, 626, 627
zinc with, 614
Co-amilofruse, 77
Co-amilozide, 77
atenolol with, 87
timolol with, 91
Co-amoxiclav, 287, **288**, 289
infusion table, 825
urinary tract infection, 319
CoAprovel, 106
Cobalin-H (hydroxocobalamin), 494
Coban, 864
Co-beneldopa, **262**, 263
COC *see* Contraception, oral, combined, 427
Cocaine, 215
local anaesthesia, 685
poisoning by, 33
Co-careldopa, **263**
entacapone with, 264
Co-codamol preparations, 227, 228
Co-codaprin preparations, 226
Cocois, 614
Co-cyprindiol, **621**, 622
Cod liver oil
zinc oxide with, 603
Codalax preparations, 60
Co-danthramer preparations, 60
Co-danthrusate preparations, 60
Codeine
aspirin with, 226
buclizine with, 239
cough suppressant, **176**, 177
diabetic neuropathy, 373
diarrhoea, 51
pain, 229, **231**
paracetamol with, 227, 228, 239
Co-Diovan, 107
Codipar, 227
Co-dydramol, 228
Coeliac disease, 516
ACBS, 843
Co-fluampicil, 287, **289**, 290
infusion table, 825
Co-flumactone, 78
Cogentin, 266
Colazide, 54
Colchicine, **555**, 556
Cold sores, 633
Colds, 177, 524
decongestants
nasal, 588
systemic, 178
Colecalciferol, 525, **526**
alendronic acid with, 407
Colesevelam, 137, **138**
Colestid, 138
Colestipol, 137, **138**
Colestyramine, **138**
diarrhoea, 51, **67**
hypercholesterolaemia, 137
hyperlipidaemias, 138
pruritus, 67
Colief, 842
Colifoam, 56
Colistimethate sodium *see* Colistin
Colistin, **308**
eye, 577
infusion table (Colistimethate sodium), 825
Colistin sulphomethate sodium *see* Colistin
Colitis
antibiotic-associated (pseudomembranous), 53
ulcerative, 52
Collodion
definition, 597
flexible, 636
Colloid dressings, 855
Colloidal oatmeal, 599, 601
Colofac preparations (mebeverine), 42
Colomycin, 308
Colpermin, 43
Coma
hyperglycaemic, 372
hyperosmolar nonketotic, 372
hypoglycaemic, 372
hypothyroid, 376
insulin, 372
ketoacidotic, 372
Co-magaldrox, 39
CombiDERM products, 855
Combigan, 575
Combined hormonal contraceptives, 429
see also Contraception
Combivent, 156
aerosol inhalation—discontinued
Combivir, 331
Combur-3 Test, 375
Co-methiamol, 228
Comfeel products, 855
Comfifast products, 861
Comfifoam products, 852, 853
Comfigrip, 861
Compact, 374
Competact, 371
Complan Shake, 833
Complementary medicine, 1
Compliance, 1
Comprilan, 863
Comtess, 265
Concerta XL, 214
Condyline, 624
Condylomata acuminata, 623, 624
Conjugated oestrogens
HRT, 387, 389
vaginal, 425
Conjunctivitis
allergy, 570
infection, 281, 566
Conn's syndrome, 76
Conotrane, 602
Constipation, 57
Contact lenses, 581
Containers, child-resistant, 3
Contents, iii
Contiflo XL (tamsulosin), 439
Contigen, 440
Contraception, 427
devices, 435, 436, 437
contraceptive caps, 437
contraceptive diaphragms, 437
implants, 434
intra-uterine system, 434, 435
oral, **427**
combined, 427
emergency, 437
missed pill, 428, 433
progestogen-only, 432
starting routines, 430, 433
surgery, **429**, 433, 666
travel, 428
parenteral, 433, **434**
perimenopausal, 386
spermicidal, 435
transdermal, 427, 431
detached patch, 428
starting routines, 430
Contreet Foam, 853
Contreet Hydrocolloid, 855
Controlled drugs, 7
see also preparations identified by CD throughout BNF
travel abroad, 9
Conversions, *inside back cover*
Convulex, 254
Convulsions
dental practice, 22
febrile, 258
poisoning and, 28
see also Epilepsy
Coolie, 853
Copaxone, 481
COPD *see* Chronic obstructive pulmonary disease
Copegus, 343
Co-phenotrope, 51

Co-prenozide, 90
Co-proxamol, 226
Coracten preparations, 116
Cordarone X, 81
Cordilox preparations, 117
Corgard, 89
Corlan, 591
Corn flour, 841
Corn starch, 841
Corneal ulcers, 566, 568
Coro-Nitro Pump Spray, 109
Corsodyl preparations, 594
Corticosteroids, 378, 381
  adrenal suppression, 380
  allergic emergencies, 170
  allergy, 379
    nasal, 586
  anaesthesia, 380, 665
  anaphylactic shock, 379
  aphthous ulcers, 590, **591**
  asthma, acute severe, 148
  blood disorders, 495
  breast-feeding, 381
  cancer, 474
  croup, 148
  ear, 582
  equivalent doses, 378
  eye, 566, 568
  gout, 555
  haemorrhoids, 65
  hypercalcaemia, 518
  immunosuppression, 474
  infections, 380
  inflammatory bowel disease, 52
  myasthenia gravis, 557, 559
  nasal
    allergy, 586
    polyps, 586
  neuropathic pain, 238
  osteoarthritis, 535
  pneumocystis pneumonia, 354
  pregnancy, 381
  proctitis, 56
  proctosigmoiditis, 56
  psychiatric reactions, 380
  replacement therapy, 378
  rheumatic disease, 544
  septic shock, 379
  side-effects, 381
  skin
    acne, 620
    eczema, 604, 610
    psoriasis, 605
    suitable quantities, 605
  surgery, 380
  thrombocytopenic purpura, 500
  ulcerative colitis, 56
  withdrawal of, 380
Corticotrophin *see* Corticotropin, 398
Corticotropin, 398
Cortisol, 378
Cortisone acetate, 382
Co-simalcite [ingredient], 40
Cosmegen Lyovac, 455
CosmoFer, 493
Cosmopor E, 858
Cosopt, 576
Cosuric (allopurinol), 556
Co-tenidone, 87
Cotfil, 860
Co-triamterzide, 77
Co-trimoxazole, **308**, 309
  infusion table, 825
  pneumocystis pneumonia, 354
Cotton
  absorbent, 860
  gauze, 860
Cough suppressants, 176
Coumarins, 127
Counter-irritants, 563
Coverflex, 861
Covering creams, 626
Covermark preparations, 626
Coversyl preparations, 103
Cow & Gate Pepti, 842
Cow & Gate Pepti-Junior, 842
Cozaar preparations, 106
Co-zidocapt, 101
Crab lice, 634
Cradle cap, 626
Cramps, nocturnal, 561
Creams
  definition, 597
  suitable quantities, 598
Creatinine clearance, dosage and, 772
Creon preparations, 68, 69
Crestor, 142
Cretinism *see* Hypothyroidism, neonatal, 376
Crinone, 394
Crisantaspase, **464**
Crixivan, 333
Crohn's disease, 52
Cromogen Easi-Breathe—discontinued
Cromoglicate (*or* cromoglycate) *see* Sodium cromoglicate
Crotamiton, 603
  hydrocortisone with, 606
  scabies, 634
Croup, 148
Cryptococcosis, 321
Crystacide, 639
Crystapen, 285
CS gas *see* CS spray, 35
CS spray, 35
Cubicin, 306
Cuplex, 623
Curagel products, 854
Curasorb products, 851
Curatoderm, 613
Curosurf, 173
Cushing's syndrome, 416
  corticosteroid-induced, 381
Cutaneous larva migrans, 357
Cutilin, 858
Cutinova products, 854
Cutisorb Sorbact products, 858
Cutivate, 610
C-View, 856
CX Antiseptic Dusting Powder, 638
Cyanides, poisoning by, 33
Cyanocobalamin, 494
Cyanokit, 33
Cyclimorph, 235
Cyclizine, 218, **219**
Cyclocaps
  beclometasone, 161, 162
  budesonide, 162
  salbutamol, 152
Cyclogest, 394
Cyclohaler
  beclometasone, 161, 162
  budesonide, 162
  salbutamol, 152
Cyclopenthiazide, 73, **74**
  amiloride with, 77
  oxprenolol with, 90
Cyclopentolate, **572**
Cyclophosphamide, 452, **453**
  infusion table, 825
  rheumatic disease, 549
Cycloplegics, 571
Cyclo-Progynova, 387
Cycloserine, **312**
Cyclosporin *see* Ciclosporin
Cyklokapron, 136
Cymbalta, 211
Cymevene, 339
Cyproheptadine, **168**
  migraine, 242
Cyprostat, 487
Cyproterone acetate
  acne, 621
  male hypersexuality, **396**
  malignant disease, **487**
Cystagon, 531
Cysteamine *see* Mercaptamine, **531**
Cystic fibrosis, 68
Cysticide, 357
Cystine Amino Acid Supplement, 846
Cystinosis, nephropathic, 531
Cystinuria, 529
Cystitis, 443
  haemorrhagic, 451
  interstitial, 444
Cystrin, 441
Cytacon (cyanocobalamin), 494
Cytamen (cyanocobalamin), 494
Cytarabine, 457, **459**
  infusion table, 825
Cytokine modulators
  Crohn's disease, 57
  rheumatoid arthritis, 551
  ulcerative colitis, 57
Cytomegalovirus
  infections, 338, 568
Cytotec, 48
Cytotoxic drugs, 448
  alopecia, 450
  bladder instillation, 444
  bone-marrow suppression, 450
  dosage, 449
  extravasation, 449
  handling guidelines, 448
  hyperuricaemia, 449
  nausea and vomiting, 449
  pregnancy, 450
  regimens, 448
  thromboembolism, 450

D

d4T *see* Stavudine, 328, **330**
Dacarbazine, 464, **465**
  infusion table, 825

Index

Daclizumab, 474, **476**
 infusion table, 825
Dactinomycin, **455**
 infusion table, 825
Daktacort, 606
Daktarin
 oral gel, 593
 skin, 632
Dalacin preparations, 304
 acne, 619
 vaginal, 427
Dalfopristin, quinupristin with, **307**, 308
 infusion table, 830
Dalivit, 528
Dalmane, 181
Dalteparin, 123, **124**
Danaparoid, **125**
 infusion table, 825
Danazol, 412, **413**
Dandrazol (ketoconazole), 626
Dandruff, 626
Danlax, 60
Danol, 413
Danthron *see* Dantron, 59, 60
Dantrium, 560
 Intravenous, 680
Dantrolene, **560**
 malignant hyperthermia, **680**
 muscle spasm, 559
 neuroleptic malignant syndrome, 188
Dantron, 59, 60
Daonil, 367
Dapsone, **314**, 315
 dermatitis herpetiformis, 314
 leprosy, 314
 pneumocystis pneumonia, 354
 poisoning, elimination, 28
 pyrimethamine with, 347
Daptomycin, **306**
 infusion table, 825
Daraprim, 351
Darbepoetin, 495, **496**
Darier's disease, 612
Darifenacin, **440**
Darunavir, 328, **332**
Dasatinib, **468**
Daunorubicin, **455**
 infusion table, 825, 826
DaunoXome, 455
DDAVP preparations, 403, 404
DDI *see* Didanosine, **329**
De Vilbiss nebulisers, 158, 159
Deca-Durabolin, 397
Decan, 515
Decapeptyl SR, 415, 488
Decongestants
 nasal, 588
 systemic, 178
Decubal Clinic, 599
Deep-vein thrombosis, 122, 127
DEET *see* Diethyltoluamide, 346
Defective medicines, 13
Defenac (diclofenac), 538, 539
Deferasirox, **498**, 499
Deferiprone, 498, **499**
Deferoxamine *see* Desferrioxamine
Deflazacort, 379, **382**, 383
Delph, 625
Deltacortril Enteric (prednisolone), 384
Deltaprim, 347
Deltastab, 545
Demeclocycline, **297**
 hyponatraemia, 404
Dementia, 274
Demulcent cough preparations, 177
Dendritic ulcer, 568
De-Noltab, 47
Dental Practitioners' Formulary, 882
Dental prescribing
 abscess, 281
 anaesthesia
  general, 666
  local, 681
  vasoconstrictors, 681
 angular cheilitis, 593
 anticoagulation, 25
 anxiety, 180, 672
 caries, prevention, 521
 chronic facial pain, 238
 denture stomatitis, 592
 dry mouth, 595
 endocarditis prophylaxis, 24
 fluoride, 521
 herpes labialis, 336, 633
 herpetic gingivostomatitis, 336
 hypnotic, 180, 672
 infections
  bacterial, 278, 281, 629
  fungal, 592, 630
  viral, 336, 593, 633
 medical emergencies, 21
 medical problems, 23
 nausea and vomiting, 166
 neuropathic pain, 238
 oral hygiene, 594
 oral side-effects, 12
 oral ulceration, 590
 pain, 224, 225, 230, 536
  orofacial, 238, 536
  postoperative, 225
 panic attacks, 180, 672
 postherpetic neuralgia, 238
 premedication, 180, 672
 prophylaxis
  joint prostheses, 283
 sinusitis, 588
 temporomandibular dysfunction, 225
 trigeminal neuralgia, 238
 vitamin deficiency, 522
Dentinox colic drops, 40
Dentomycin, 592
Denture stomatitis, 592
Denzapine, 195
Depakote, 200
Dependence *see* Drug dependence
Depixol preparations, 190, 198
DepoCyte, 459
Depolarising muscle relaxants *see* Muscle relaxants
Depo-Medrone, 384, 545
 with Lidocaine, 545
Deponit, 109
Depo-Provera, 434
 contraception, 433, 434
Depression, 201
 antipsychotics, 187
 manic, 200
Derbac-M, 635
Dermabond ProPen, 637
Dermacare, Vaseline, 600
Dermacolor preparations, 626
Dermalo, 601
Dermamist, 599
Dermatitis
 ACBS, 849
 herpetiformis, 314, 843
 see also Eczema
Dermatix products, 856
Dermatophyte infections, 322
Dermax, 627
Dermol preparations, 601, 602
Dermovate preparations, 608
Deseril, 243
Desferal, 499
Desferrioxamine, **499**
 eye, 577
 infusion table, 826
 iron overload, 498
 poisoning, use in, 32
Desflurane, **669**
Desloratadine, **166**
Desloughing agents, 639
DesmoMelt, 404
Desmopressin, 402, **403**, 404
 fibrinolytic response, 402
 haemophilia, 135
 infusion table, 826
 nocturnal enuresis, **403**, **442**
 von Willebrand's disease, 402
Desmospray, 404
Desmotabs, 404
Desogestrel
 contraception, 431, 432, 433
Destolit, 67
Deteclo—discontinued
Detrunorm preparations, 442
Detrusitol preparations, 442
Dexamethasone, 379, **383**
 croup, 148
 inflammation
  ear, 583
  eye, 569, 577
 infusion table, 826
 nausea and vertigo, 218
 nausea and vomiting, 449
 palliative care, 16, 17
 rheumatic disease, 545
 suppression test, 379
Dexamethasone sodium phosphate, 383
Dexamfetamine, 213, **214**
Dexamphetamine *see* Dexamfetamine, 213, **214**
Dexedrine, 214
Dexfenfluramine, 216
Dexibuprofen, 535, **538**
Dexketoprofen, 535, **538**
Dexomon (diclofenac), 539
Dexrazoxane, **450**
 infusion table, 826
Dexsol (dexamethasone), 383
Dextran
 eye, 578
 intravenous infusions, 509, 510
Dextromethorphan, 176
Dextropropoxyphene, poisoning by, 31

Index

Dextrose monohydrate *see* Glucose
DF-118 Forte, 232
D-Gam, 662
DHC Continus, 232
diabact UBT, 44
Diabetes insipidus, 402
  diagnosis, 402
Diabetes mellitus, 359
  diagnosis, 375
  monitoring, 360
    ketone, 374, 375
    meters, 375
    test strips, 374
Diabetic
  ketoacidosis, **372**, 506, 507
  nephropathy, 373
  neuropathy, 373
    skin ulcers, 639
Diabur Test-5000, 375
DIAGLYK (gliclazide), 367
Dialamine, 841
Dialar (diazepam), 185
Diamicron preparations, 367
Diamorphine, 229, **231**
  infusion table, 826
  morphine equivalence, 15
  pain, 229
    chronic, 229, 16
    myocardial infarction, 133, 231
  pulmonary oedema, 231
Diamox preparations, 575
Dianette, 622
Diaphragms, contraceptive, 437
Diarrhoea, 50, 505
Diastix, 375
Diazemuls (diazepam), 185, 256
Diazepam, **184**, 185
  anaesthesia, **672**
  anxiety, 185
  epilepsy
    status epilepticus, 256
  febrile convulsions, 258
  hypnotic, 181
  infusion table, 826
  muscle spasm, 225, 559, 560
  palliative care, 16
  status epilepticus, **256**
  temporomandibular dysfunction, 225
Diazepam Rectubes, 185, 256
Diazoxide
  hypertension, 93, **94**
  hypoglycaemia, **373**
Dibenyline, 99
Dibucaine *see* Cinchocaine, 65
Diclofenac, **538**, 539
  actinic keratosis, 625
  eye, 579, 580
  gout, 555
  infusion table, 826
  misoprostol with, 539
  postoperative pain, 674
  rheumatic disease, 535, 538
  topical, 563
  ureteric colic, 443, 538
Dicloflex (diclofenac), 538, 539
Diclomax (diclofenac), 539
Diclozip (diclofenac), 538
Dicobalt edetate, 33, **34**
Diconal, 232
Dicyclomine *see* Dicycloverine, **41**
Dicycloverine, **41**
Dicynene, 135
Didanosine, **329**
Didronel preparations, 407
Dietary Specialities, 843
Diethylcarbamazine, 357
Diethylstilbestrol, **482**, 486
Diethyltoluamide, 346
Differin, 620
Difflam, 591
Diffundox XL (tamsulosin), 439
Diflucan preparations, 324
Diflucortolone valerate, 608, 609
Digibind, 72
Digitoxin, **71**
Digoxin, 70, **71**
  heart failure, 99
  infusion table, 826
Digoxin-specific antibody fragments, 71, **72**
  infusion table, 826
Dihydrocodeine, 229, **231**, 232
  paracetamol with, 228
Dihydropyridine calcium-channel blockers, 111
Dihydrotachysterol, 525, **526**
Dihydroxycholecalciferol, 525, 526, 613
Dilcardia SR, 113
Diloxanide furoate, **352**
Diltiazem, **112**, 113, 114
  anal fissure, 66
  poisoning by, 32
  see also Calcium-channel blockers
Dilzem preparations, 113
Dimenhydrinate, cinnarizine with, 219
Dimercaprol, **34**
Dimethicone, activated *see* Simeticone, 38, 40
Dimethyl sulfoxide
  idoxuridine with, 633
  interstitial cystitis, 444
Dimethyl sulphoxide *see* Dimethyl sulfoxide
Dimeticone, 634, **635**
  benzalkonium with, 602
  cetrimide with, 603
  zinc oxide with, 603
  zinc with, 603
Dimeticone, activated *see* Simeticone, 38, 40
Dimetriose, 413
Dinoprostone, 418, 419, 420
  infusion table, 826
Dioctyl, 60
Dioctyl sodium sulphosuccinate *see* Docusate sodium
Dioderm, 606
Dioralyte preparations, 505
Diovan, 107
Dip/Ser, 646
Dipentum, 55
Dipeptiven, 515
Diphenoxylate, 51, 229
  see also Analgesics, opioid
Diphenylbutylpiperidines, 189
Diphosphonates *see* Bisphosphonates
Diphtheria, 284, 645
  antibacterial prophylaxis, 282
  antitoxin, 646
  immunisation
    travel, 645
    vaccines, 645, 646
Dipipanone, 229, **232**
  cyclizine with, 232
Dipivefrine, 574, **575**
Diprivan, 668
Diprobase, 599
Diprobath, 601
Diprosalic, 608
Diprosone, 608
Dipyridamole, 129, **131**
  aspirin with, 131
Discontinued preparations, xii
Disease-modifying antirheumatic drugs *see* DMARDs, 534, 546
Disfiguring skin lesions, ACBS, 849
Disinfectants, 637
  ACBS, 849
Disipal, 266
Diskhaler
  Becodisks, 161
  Flixotide, 163
  Relenza 342
  Serevent, 152
Disodium clodronate *see* Sodium clodronate
Disodium cromoglicate *see* Sodium cromoglicate
Disodium etidronate, 404, 407
  calcium carbonate with, 407
Disodium folinate, **451**
  infusion table, 826
Disodium pamidronate, 407, 408
  infusion table, 826
Disogram SR (diltiazem), 113
Disopyramide, 81, **82**
  infusion table, 826
Disprol (paracetamol) preparations, 227
Distaclor preparations, 292
Distamine, 548
Distigmine
  laxative, 59
  myasthenia gravis, 558
  urinary retention, 439, **440**
Disulfiram, 269, **270**
Dithranol, 611, 612, **615**
  coal tar and salicylic acid with, 615
  salicylic acid and zinc with, 615
Dithrocream, 615
Ditropan, 441
Diumide-K Continus, 78
Diuretics
  carbonic anhydrase inhibitors, 78
  heart failure, 99
  loop, 74
  mercurial, 78
  osmotic, 78
  potassium with, 78, 503
  potassium-sparing, 76
    with other diuretics, 77
  see also Thiazides

Diurexan, 74
Diva, 621
Diverticular disease, 41, **53**
Dixarit, 243
DMARDs (disease-modifying anti-rheumatic drugs), 534, 546
DMPS *see* Unithiol, 34
DMSA *see* Succimer, 34
Dobutamine, 119, **120**
  infusion table, 826
Docetaxel, 470
  infusion table, 826
Docusate sodium
  ear, 585, 586
  laxative, 59, **60**
Docusol, 60
Dolasetron, 218, **221**
  infusion table, 826
Dolmatil, 192
Domette bandage, 861
Domperidone, 220
  diabetic neuropathy, 373
  gastro-intestinal, 43
  migraine, 242
  nausea and vomiting, 217
    cytotoxic drugs, 449
  palliative care, 16
Donepezil, **275**
Dopacard, 120
Dopamine, 119, **120**
  infusion table, 826
Dopamine receptor agonists
  parkinsonism, 259
Dopaminergic drugs
  endocrine, 410
  parkinsonism, 259
Dopexamine, 119, **120**
  infusion table, 826
Dopram, 173
Doralese, 439
Dornase alfa, 176
Dorzolamide, 575, **576**
  with timolol, 576
Dose changes, xi
Doses, 2
  children, 14
  elderly, 20
  liver disease, 762
  renal impairment, 772
Dostinex, 412
Dosulepin, 203, **204**, 205
DOT, 310
Dothiepin *see* Dosulepin, 203, **204**, 205
Doublebase, 599
Dovobet, 613
Dovonex preparations, 613
Doxadura (doxazosin) preparations, 97
Doxapram, 172, **173**
  respiratory depression, 173
Doxazosin
  cardiovascular, **97**
  urinary tract, **438**
Doxepin, 203, **205**
  topical, 603, 604
Doxorubicin, 454, **455**, 456
  bladder, 444
  infusion table, 826
Doxycycline, **297**, 298
  acne, 621
  aphthous ulcers, 590, **591**
  Lyme disease, 287
  malaria
    prophylaxis, 346, 347, 348, **352**
    treatment, 344
  mouth, 591
  oral infections, 297
  periodontitis, 590, 591
  rosacea, 618
Doxylar (doxycycline), 298
Dozic, 191
Drapolene, 602
Dressing packs, 859, 861
Dressings, 850
Dress-it, 859
Driclor, 640
Drisorb, 858
Driver and Vehicle Licensing Agency, *inside back cover*
Driving and drugs, 2
Drogenil, 488
Dromadol preparations, 237
Drospirenone
  contraception, 432
  HRT, 387
Drotrecogin alfa (activated), **136**
Drug
  allergy, 166
  dependence, 7
    management, 269
  interactions, 686
  misusers, notification of, 9
Dry mouth, 595
Duac, 619
Dual block, 678
Ductus arteriosus
  closure, 421
  patency, 421
Dukoral, 645
Dulco-lax (bisacodyl), 60
Dulco-lax (sodium picosulfate), 60, 61
Duloxetine
  depression, **211**
  diabetic neuropathy, **211**, 373
  urinary incontinence, 440, **441**
Duobar, 833
Duocal, 834
DuoDERM products, 855
Duodopa, 263
Duofilm, 623
DuoTrav, 574
Duovent preparations, 156
Duphalac (lactulose), 62
Duphaston preparations, 393
Duraphat preparations, 521, 522
Durogesic DTrans, 232
Durolane, 535
Dusting powders, 598
Dutasteride, **396**
Dyazide, 77
Dydrogesterone, 392, **393**
  HRT, 388, 393
  menstrual disorders, 393
Dynamin (isosorbide mononitrate), 110
Dynastat, 674
Dynepo, 498
Dysentery
  amoebic, 352
  bacillary *see* Shigellosis, 279
Dysmenorrhoea, 225
Dyspepsia, 37, 38
Dysport, 269
Dystonias, drug-induced, 266
Dytac, 76
Dytide, 77

E

E45 preparations, 599, 601
  Itch Relief, 601
  Sun, 625
Ear
  infections, 582
  wax, removal, 585
EarCalm, 582
Easi-Breathe
  Beclazone, 161, 162
  Qvar, 161
  Salamol, 152
Easifast, 862
Easifix products, 861
EasiGRIP, 861
Easiphen, 847
Easyhaler
  beclometasone, 161
  budesonide, 162
  formoterol, 150
  salbutamol, 152
Ebixa, 276
Ebufac (ibuprofen), 540
Ecalta, 323
Eccoxolac (etodolac), 539
Echinocandin antifungal drugs, 322
Echinococcosis, 357
Eclampsia, 519
Eclypse, 857
Econac (diclofenac), 538
Econacort, 606
Econazole
  anogenital, 426
  skin, 630, **631**
    hydrocortisone with, 606
  vaginal, 426
Econoneb, 158
Ecopace (captopril), 101
Ecostatin
  anogenital, 426
  skin, 631
Ecstasy
  controlled drug, 7
  liquid (sodium oxybate), 33
  poisoning by, 33
ECT *see* Electroconvulsive therapy, 202
Ectopic beats, 79
Eculizumab, **499**, 500
  infusion table, 826
Eczema, 610
  ACBS, 849
  ear, 583
Edetic acid, excipient, 598
Ednyt (enalapril), 102

Edronax, 212
Edrophonium
  anaesthesia, **679**
  myasthenia gravis, 558, **559**
Eesiban, 861, 862
Efalizumab, 616, **617**
Efavirenz, 328, **334**
  emtricitabine and tenofovir with, xiii
Efcortelan preparations, 606
Efcortesol, 383
Efexor preparations, 213
Effico, 528
Eflornithine, **627**
Eformoterol *see* Formoterol
Efudix, 626
Elantan preparations, 110, 111
Elaprase, 531
Elastic adhesive
  dressing, 865
  plaster, 865
Elastoplast products, 863, 865
Elastoweb, 863
Eldepryl, 264
Elderly
  diuretics and, 20
  hypertension in, 92
  prescribing for, 19
Eldisine, 462
Electroconvulsive therapy, 202
Electrolade, 505
Electrolyte and water replacement
  intravenous, 506
  oral, 503
Electrolyte concentrations, 503
Elemental-028 preparations, 834
Eletriptan, 239, **240**
Elidel, 617
Elleste Duet preparations, 388
Elleste Solo, 389
Elleste Solo MX, 390
Elocon, 610
Eloxatin, 467
Elset products, 862
Eltroxin (levothyroxine), 376
Eludril preparations, 594
Elyzol, 592
Emadine, 570
Emcor, 87
Emedastine, **570**
Emend, 223
Emergencies, dental practice, 21
Emergency
  contraception, 437
  supply of medicines, 6
Emeside, 247
Emesis, in poisoning, 28
Emflex, 537
Emla, 682
Emollients, 598
  eczema, 610
  psoriasis, 611
Emollin, 600
Emphysema, 148
Emselex, 440
Emsogen, 834
Emtricitabine, 328, **330**
  efavirenz and tenofovir with, xiii
  tenofovir with, 331
Emtriva, 330
Emulsiderm, 602
Emulsifying ointment, 599, 600
Enalapril, **102**
  hydrochlorothiazide with, 102
  see also ACE inhibitors
Enbrel preparations, 554
Enbucrilate, 637
Encephalopathy, hepatic, 62
  drug usage, in, 762
En-De-Kay preparations, 521
Endocarditis, 279, 299
  prophylaxis, 283
    dental practice, 24
Endometrial cancer, 482, 483
Endometriosis, 392, 412
Endophthalmitis, 566
Endoxana, 453
Ener-G
  gluten- and wheat-free, 844
  gluten-free, 843, 844
  low-protein, 844
Energivit, 841
Energy, intravenous nutrition, 511
Enfamil preparations, 840, 842
Enfuvirtide, 328, **335**
Engerix B, 649
Enlive Plus, 834
Enmix Plus Commence, 834
Enoxaparin, 123, **124**
Enoximone, **72**
  infusion table, 826
Enrich preparations, 834
Enshake, 834
Ensure preparations, 834
Entacapone, 264, **265**
Entamoeba histolytica, 352
Entecavir, **340**, 341
Enteral nutrition, 833
Enteric infections, 279
Enterobiasis, 355
Entocort preparations, 56
Entonox, 670
Enuresis, nocturnal, 442
Enzira, 651
Enzyme induction, **686**
Enzymes, fibrinolytic, 133
Epaderm, 600
Epanutin preparations, 251
  Ready Mixed Parenteral, 258
Epaxal, 647, 648
Ephedrine
  anaesthesia, 120, **121**
  bronchospasm, **153**
  diabetic neuropathy, 374
  nasal congestion, 588, **589**
Ephynal (tocopheryl acetate), 527
Epiglottitis, 279, 304
Epiglu, 637
Epilepsy, 245
  dental practice, 22
  driving, 244
  pregnancy, 245
  status epilepticus, 255
    non-convulsive, 256
Epilim preparations, 253
Epimaz (carbamazepine), 246
Epinastine, **570**
Epinephrine *see* Adrenaline
EpiPen, 171, 172
Epirubicin, 455, **456**
  bladder, 444
  infusion table, 827
Episenta preparations, 253
Epistatus (midazolam), 257
Epivir, 330
Eplerenone **76**
Epoetin
  alfa, **496**
  beta, **496**, 497
  delta, **496**, 498
Epoprostenol, 93, **126**
  infusion table, 827
Eposin, 461
Eprex, 497
Eprosartan, **105**
Epsom salts *see* Magnesium sulphate
Eptacog alfa (activated), 136
Eptifibatide 108, 130, **132**
Equanox, 670
Equasym (methylphenidate), 214
Equasym XL, 215
Erbitux, 464
Erdosteine, **175**
Erdotin, 175
Erectile dysfunction, 444
Ergocalciferol, **525**
Ergometrine, 419, **420**
  oxytocin with, 420
Ergot alkaloids, 241
Ergotamine 242
  caffeine with, 242
  cluster headache, 243
  cyclizine and caffeine with, 242
Erlotinib, **468**, 469
Ertapenem, **295**, 296
  infusion table, 827
Erwinase, 464
Erymax, 302
Erysipelas, 281
Erythrocin, 302
Erythromycin, **301**, 302
  acne, 619, 621
    isotretinoin with, 620
    tretinoin with, 620
  infusion table, 827
  rosacea, 618
Erythroped preparations, 302
Erythropoietins, 495
Escitalopram, 208, **209**
Esmeron, 673
Esmolol, 85 **88**
  infusion table, 827
  see also Beta-adrenoceptor blocking drugs
Esomeprazole, **48**, 49
  infusion table, 827
Estracombi, 388
Estracyt, 453
Estraderm MX, 390
Estraderm TTS, 390
Estradiol
  HRT, 387, 388, 389, 390, 391
  implants, 389
  vaginal, 425
Estradiol valerate, 387, 389, 390
Estradot, 390
Estragest TTS, 388

Estramustine, 452, **453**
Estring, 425
Estriol
  HRT, 391
  vaginal, 425
Estrone, 391
Estropipate, 391
Etamsylate, **135**
Etanercept
  psoriasis, 616
  rheumatic diseases, 551, 552, **553**, 554
Ethambutol, 310, 311, **312**
Ethamsylate *see* Etamsylate, **135**
Ethanol, 511
  infusion table, 827
  see also Alcohol
Ethanolamine oleate, **144**
Ethinylestradiol, **391**, 392
  acne *see* Co-cyprindiol, **621**, 622
  contraception, 427, 431, 432
  gestodene with, 431, 432
  HRT, 392
  menstrual disorders, 392
  prostate cancer, 482
Ethinyloestradiol *see* Ethinylestradiol
Ethmozine, 83
Ethosuximide, 245, **247**
Ethyl-2-cyanoacrylate, 637
Ethylene glycol, poisoning by, 34
Ethylenediamine, excipient, 598
Ethynodiol *see* Etynodiol, 433
Etidronate disodium *see* Disodium etidronate
Etodolac, 535, **539**
Etomidate, **667**
Etomidate-Lipuro, 667
Etonogestrel, 434
Etopan XL, 539
Etopophos, 462
Etoposide, **461**, 462
  infusion table, 827
Etoricoxib, 536, **539**
  gout, 555
Etretinate, 612
Etrivex, 608
Etynodiol, 433
Eucardic, 88
Eucerin Intensive, 601
Eudemine
  hypertension, 94
  hypoglycaemia, 373
Euglucon, 367
Eumovate, 608
Eurax, 603
  Hydrocortisone, 606
European viper venom antiserum, 36
Evening primrose oil, 600
Evista, 392
Evohaler
  Flixotide, 163
  Seretide, 164
  Ventolin, 152
Evoltra, 459
Evorel preparations, 388, 390
Evotrox, 376
Evra, 431
Excipients
  details provided, 2
  skin preparations and, 598
  vaccines and, 641
Exelderm, 632
Exelon preparations, 276
Exemestane, 483, 484, **485**
Exenatide, **370**
Exfoliative dermatitis, 379
Exforge, 112
Exjade, 499
Exocin, 568
Exorex, 614
Expectorants, 177
Extemporaneous preparation, 2
Exterol, 585
Extrapyramidal symptoms
  antipsychotics and, 188
  treatment, 266
Extravasation, 562
Exubera—discontinued
Exu-Dry, 857
Eye
  anaesthetics, local, 577
  antibacterials, 566
  antifungals, 568
  antivirals, 568
  contact lenses, 581
  cycloplegics, 571
  drops, 565
  glaucoma, 572
  inflammation, 568, 570
  lotions, 565
  microbial contamination, 566
  miotics, 576
  mydriatics, 571
  ointments, 565
  prostaglandins, 573
Ezetimibe, 138, **139**
  simvastatin with, 143
Ezetrol, 139

F

F16 Wave, 159
Fabrazyme, 530
Fabry's Disease, 529, 530
Factor VIIa (recombinant), 136
Factor VIII fraction, 136
Factor VIII inhibitor bypassing fraction, 136
Factor IX fraction, 136
Factor XIII fraction, 137
Faecal softeners, 61
Fainting, dental practice, 23
Famciclovir, 336, **337**
Familial Mediterranean fever, 556
Famotidine, **46**
Famvir, 337
Fanhdi (factor VIII fraction), 136
Fansidar, 344, 351, 352
Fareston, 486
Farley's Soya Formula, 842
Fasigyn, 316
Faslodex, 485
Fasturtec, 557
Fat emulsions, intravenous, 511, 821
Fate, 844
Faverin, 210
Favism, 500
Febrile convulsions, 258
Fectrim (co-trimoxazole), 309
Feed thickeners, 840
Fefol, 492
FEIBA (factor VIII inhibitor bypassing fraction), 136
Felbinac, 563
Feldene preparations, 543
  gel, 563
  Melt, 543
Felodipine, 112, **114**
  ramipril with, 104
  see also Calcium-channel blockers
Felogen XL (felodipine), 114
Felotens XL (felodipine), 114
Felypressin, 681, 684
Femapak, 388
Femara, 485
Femattrix, 390
FemCap, 437
Femidom, 427
Femodene preparations, 432
Femodette, 431
Femoston preparations, 388
FemSeven preparations, 388, 390
FemTab preparations, 389
Femulen, 433
Fenactol (diclofenac), 538, 539
Fenbid
  Forte Gel, 563
  Spansules, 541
Fenbufen, 535, **540**
Fendrix, 649
Fenfluramine, 216
Fenofibrate, **139**, 140
Fenogal (fenofibrate), 140
Fenoprofen, 535
  pain, **540**
  rheumatic disease, **540**
Fenopron preparations, 540
Fenoterol, 149, **150**
  ipratropium with, 156
Fenpaed (ibuprofen), 541
Fentanyl
  analgesia, 229, **232**
    perioperative, 674, **675**
  infusion table, 827
  injection, 674
  iontophoretic transdermal system, xiii
  lozenge, 232
  patch, 232, 15
Fentazin, 191
Feospan, 491
Feprapax (lofepramine), 205
Fermathron, 535
Ferric salts, 490
Ferriprox, 499
Ferrograd Folic, 492
Ferrograd preparations, 491, 492
Ferrous fumarate, 491
  folic acid with, 492
  vitamins with, 492
Ferrous gluconate, 492
Ferrous salts, 490
Ferrous sulphate, **491**
  ascorbic acid with, 492
  folic acid with, 492

Index

Fersaday, 491
Fersamal, 491
Fertility
 female, 397, 398, 401
 male, 398
 thermometer, 437
Feverfen (ibuprofen), 541
Fexofenadine, **166**
Fibrates, 139
Fibrazate XL (bezafibrate), 139
Fibrelief, 58
Fibrinolytic drugs, 133
Fibrogammin P (factor XIII fraction), 137
Fibrosing alveolitis, 173
Fibro-Vein, 144
Filair (beclometasone), 161
Filair Forte (beclometasone), 162
Filaricides, 357
Filgrastim, **501**, 502
 infusion table, 827
Finacea, 619
Finasteride
 baldness, **627**
 benign prostatic hyperplasia, **396**, 397
Finepoint, 366
Fingertip unit, 605
Fits *see* Epilepsy
Flagyl preparations, 316
Flamatak (diclofenac), 539
Flamazine, 629
Flaminal, 854
Flamrase (diclofenac), 538, 539
Flavour Sachets, 845
FlavourPac, 845
Flavoxate, 440, 441
Flebogamma, 661
Flecainide, 81, **82**
 infusion table, 827
Fleet
 Phospho-soda, 64
 Ready-to-use enema, 63
Fletchers' enemas, 61, 63
Flexi-Ban, 863
Flexible collodion, 636
Flexigran products, 854, 855
FlexiPore, 852
Flexi-T 300, 436
Flexi-T+ 380, 436
Flexoplast, 863, 865
Flexotard MR (diclofenac), 539
Flixonase preparations, 587, 588
Flixotide preparations, 163
Flolan, 126
Flomaxtra XL, 439
Florinef, 378
Flowfusor, 637
Floxapen (flucloxacillin), 286
Flu-Amp (co-fluampicil), 290
Fluanxol, 211
Fluarix, 651
Fluclomix (flucloxacillin), 286
Flucloxacillin, 285, **286**
 ampicillin with [co-fluampicil], 287, **289**
 ear, 582
 infusion table, 827
Fluconazole, 321, 322, **323**, 324
 mouth, 592
Flucytosine, 321, 322, **324**
Fludara, 459
Fludarabine, 457, **459**
 infusion table, 827
Fludrocortisone, **378**
 diabetic neuropathy, 373
Fludroxycortide, **609**
Fluid and electrolyte replacement, 503
Fluid overload, liver disease, 762
Flumazenil, **679**, 680
 benzodiazepine poisoning, 32
 infusion table, 827
Flumetasone, **583**
Flumethasone *see* Flumetasone, **583**
Flunisolide, **587**
Fluocinolone acetonide, 609
 clioquinol with, 609
 neomycin with, 609
Fluocinonide, 609
Fluocortolone, **609**, 610
 [ingredient], 65
Fluor-a-day, 521
Fluorescein, 577, **579**
 lidocaine with, 577
Fluoride, 521
FluoriGard preparations, 521, 522
Fluorometholone, 569
Fluorouracil
 actinic keratosis, 625
 infusion table, 827
 malignant disease, 458, **459**, 460
 skin cancer, 625, **626**
Fluoxetine, 208, **209**, 210
Flupenthixol *see* Flupentixol
Flupentixol, **198**
 depot injections, **198**
 depression, **211**
 psychoses, 189, **190**, 198
Flupentixol decanoate, 198
Fluphenazine, 198
 depot injections, **198**
 tablets—discontinued
Flurandrenolone *see* Fludroxycortide, **609**
Flurazepam, 180, **181**
Flurbiprofen
 diabetic neuropathy, 373
 eye, 579, 580
 pain, **540**
  postoperative, 674
 rheumatic disease, 535, **540**
 sore throat, 590, 591
Flutamide, **487**, 488
Fluticasone propionate
 asthma, 159, **163**
 nasal allergy, 587, 588
 nasal polyps, 588
 salmeterol with, 164
 skin, 610
Fluvastatin, 140, **141**, 142
Fluvoxamine, 208, **210**
FML, 569
Foam dressings, 852
Folate
 deficiency, 493
 rescue, 450
Folic acid, 493, **494**, 495
 iron and, 492
 pregnancy, 492, 494
Folicare (folic acid), 495
Folinic acid
 rescue, 450
 see also Disodium folinate
 see Calcium folinate
Follicle-stimulating hormone, 398
Follitropin, **398**
 alfa, 399
  lutropin alfa with, 399
 beta, 399
Fomepizole, 34
Fondaparinux, **126**
 infusion table, 827
Foodlink Complete, 834
Foods
 enteral, 833
 gluten- and wheat-free, 844
 gluten-free, 843
 intolerance, 842
 low-protein, 844
 metabolic diseases, 845
 special diets, 841
 thickened, 840
Foods for special diets, 516
 ACBS, 833
 vitamin supplements, 528
Foradil, 150
Forceval, 528
Formaldehyde, 622, 623
Formoterol, **149**, **150**
 beclometasone dipropionate with, 162
 budesonide with, 163
Formulary
 Dental, 882
 Nurse, 884
Forsteo, 406
Forticare, 835
Forticreme, 835
Fortifresh, 835
Fortijuce, 835
Fortimel, 835
Fortini preparations, 835
Fortipine LA 40, 116
Fortisip preparations, 835
Fortral (pentazocine), 236
Fortum, 294
Fosamax preparations, 407
Fosamprenavir, 328, **332**
Fosavance, 407
Foscan, 467
Foscarnet, 338, **339**
 infusion table, 827
Foscavir, 339
Fosinopril, **102**
 see also ACE inhibitors
Fosphenytoin, **256**, 257
 infusion table, 827
 status epilepticus, 256
Fosrenol, 520
Fostair, 162
Fostimon, 399
Fragmin, 124
Fragrances, excipient, 598

Framycetin
- ear, 583
- eye, 569

Frangula, 59
Frebini preparations, 835
FreeStyle products, 366, 374, 375
Freeway Freedom, 158
Fresh frozen plasma, 137
Fresubin preparations, 836
Friars' Balsam, 176
Frisium (clobazam), 255
Froben preparations, 540
Froop (furosemide), 75
Frovatriptan, 239, **240**
Fru-Co (co-amilofruse), 77
Fructose, 511, 842
- presence of, 2

Frumil (co-amilofruse), 77
Frusemide *see* Furosemide
Frusene, 78
Frusid (furosemide), 75
Frusol (furosemide), 75
FSH *see* Follicle-stimulating hormone, 398
FTU *see* Fingertip unit, 605
Fucibet, 608
Fucidin, 305
- skin, 629

Fucidin H, 606
Fucithalmic, 567
Full Marks, 636
Fulvestrant, 484, **485**
Fungal infections, 320
- anogenital, 425
- eye, 568
- oral, 321, 592
- skin, 630

Fungilin, 593
Fungizone, 322
Furadantin, 320
Furosemide, 74, **75**
- amiloride with, 77
- infusion table, 827
- potassium with, 78
- spironolactone with, 78
- triamterene with, 78

Fusidic acid, 304, 305
- angular cheilitis, 593
- eye, 566, **567**
- infusion table, 827
- skin, 628, **629**
  - betamethasone with, 608
  - hydrocortisone with, 606

Fuzeon, 335
Fybogel, 58
Fybogel Mebeverine, 42

G

G6PD deficiency, 500
- drugs to be avoided in, 501

Gabapentin, 245, **247**, 248
- diabetic neuropathy, 373
- neuropathic pain, 238
- postherpetic neuralgia, 238
- trigeminal neuralgia, 238

Gabitril, 252
Gadsby's, 843
Galactomin preparations, 842
Galactorrhoea, 411
Galantamine, **275**
Galcodine preparations, 177
Galenamox (amoxicillin), 288
Galenphol, 177
Galfer, 491
Galfer FA, 492
Gallstones, 67
Galpseud, 178
Galsulfase, **531**
- infusion table, 827

Gamgee Tissue, 860
Gammagard S/D, 661
Gamma-hydroxybutyrate (sodium oxybate), 33
Ganciclovir, **338**, 339
- infusion table, 827

Ganfort, 574
Ganirelix, 412, **413**
Gardasil, 650
Gardnerella vaginalis, 315
Gargles, 594
Gas cylinders, 666
Gas-gangrene, 284
- prophylaxis, 282

Gastrectomy
- iron therapy, 490
- vitamin B_{12}, 493

Gastric emptying, poisoning and, 28
Gastrocote, 40
Gastro-enteritis, 51, 279
Gastro-intestinal procedures, antibacterial prophylaxis, 282
Gastro-intestinal stromal tumour, 468
Gastro-intestinal system, electrolytes, 503
Gastro-oesophageal reflux disease, **38**
Gaucher's disease, 530
Gauze
- cotton ribbon, absorbent, 860
- swabs, 860
- viscose ribbon, absorbent cotton and, 860

Gaviscon preparations, 40
G-CSF, 501, 502
Gel FX, 854
Gelatin
- infusion, 509, **510**
- succinylated, 510

Geliperm, 854
Gelofusine, 510
Gels, definition, 597
GelTears, 578
Gemcitabine, 458, **460**
- infusion table, 827

Gemeprost, 418, **420**, 422
Gemfibrozil, 139, **140**
Gemzar, 460
Gencardia (aspirin), 131
Generaid preparations, 841
Generalised anxiety disorder, 202
Generic prescribing, 1
Generpharm products, 843
Genital warts, 623
Genotropin preparations, 400
Gentamicin, 299, **300**
- ear, 584
- eye, 566, **567**, 577
- infusion table, 828

Gentian mixture, alkaline, 528
Genticin
- ear, 584
- eye, 567
- parenteral, 300

Gentisone HC, 584
German measles *see* Rubella
Gestodene, ethinylestradiol with, 431, 432
Gestone, 394
Gestrinone, 412, **413**
GHB (sodium oxybate), 33
Giant cell arteritis, 544
Giardia lamblia, 353
Giardiasis, 353
Gilles de la Tourette syndrome *see* Tourette syndrome, 267
Gingivitis, 594
- acute necrotising ulcerative
  - antibacterial treatment, 281, 315
  - mouthwashes, 594

Givitol, 492
Glamin, 512
Glandosane, 595
Glatiramer, 481
Glaucoma, 572
- steroid, 568

Gliadel, 453
Glibenclamide, 366, **367**
Glibenese, 368
Gliclazide, 366, **367**
Glimepiride, **367**, 368
Glipizide, 368
Glivec 469
Glomerular filtration rate, dosage and, 772
Glossopharyngeal neuralgia, 238
GlucaGen HypoKit, 373
Glucagon, **372**, 373
- beta-blocker poisoning, 32

Glucobay, 370
Glucocorticoids
- equivalent doses, 378
- replacement therapy, 378

GlucoGel, 372
Glucolet, 366
GlucoMen products, 366, 374, 375
Glucophage, 369
Glucosamine, **557**
Glucose, 507
- hypoglycaemia, 372
- infusion, 507
  - potassium and, 508
  - sodium and, 507
- intravenous nutrition, 511
- oral rehydration, 505
- presence of, 2
- special diets, 842
- tests
  - blood, 374
  - tolerance, 375
  - urine, 375

Glucose 6-phosphate dehydrogenase deficiency, 500
- drugs to be avoided in, 501

Glucose syrup, hydrogenated, presence of, 2
Glucotide, 374
Glue ear, 585

Index

Glurenorm—discontinued
Glutafin
 gluten- and wheat-free, 844
 gluten-free, 843, 844
Glutano, 844
Glutaraldehyde, 622, 623
Glutaric aciduria, 845
Glutarol, 623
Gluten, presence of, 2
Gluten-sensitive enteropathies, 843
 wheat-sensitivity and, 844
Glycerin suppositories, 60
Glycerol
 constipation, 59, 60
 glaucoma, 575
Glyceryl trinitrate
 anal fissure, **66**
 angina, 108, **109**, 110
 infusion table, 828
Glycine irrigation solution, **444**
Glycopeptide antibiotics, 305
Glycophos, 516
Glycoprotein IIb/IIIa inhibitors, 130
Glycopyrrolate *see* Glycopyrronium bromide
Glycopyrronium bromide
 hyperhidrosis, 640
 neostigmine with, 679
 palliative care, 18
 premedication, 670, 671
Glycylcycline antibiotic, 298
Glypressin, 404
Glytrin Spray, 109
GnRH *see* Gonadorelin, 401, **402**
Goitre, 376
Gold, 546
Golden Eye Drops (propamidine), 568
Golden Eye Ointment (dibromopropamidine), 568
Golfer's elbow, 545
Gonadorelin, 401, **402**
Gonadorelin analogues, 413
 malignant disease, 486
Gonadotrophin-releasing hormone *see* Gonadorelin, 401, **402**
Gonadotrophins, 398
Gonal-F, 399
Gonapeptyl Depot, 415, 488
Gonorrhoea, 280, 284
 pharyngeal, 280
Gopten, 105
GORD *see* Gastro-oesophageal reflux disease, **38**
Goserelin
 endometriosis, 414
 IVF, 414
 malignant disease, 484, **486**, **488**
Gout, 555
Gramicidin, 567
 ear, 583
 neomycin with, 629
 [ingredient], 584
Gramoxone, poisoning by, 35
Grand mal, 245
Graneodin, 629
Granisetron, 217, **221**, 222
 infusion table, 828
Granocyte, 502
Granuflex products, 855
GranuGel, 854
Granulocyte-colony stimulating factor, 501, 502
Grass pollen allergy preparations, 169
Grazax, 169
Griseofulvin, 321, 322, **324**
 topical, 630, **631**
Grisol AF, 631
Ground-nut oil *see* Arachis oil
Growth factor, platelet derived, 639
Growth hormone, 399
 receptor antagonists, 401
GTN 300-mcg, 109
Guanethidine, **97**
Guillain-Barré syndrome, 660
Gygel, 435
Gyne T, 436
GyneFix, 436
Gyno-Daktarin preparations, 426
Gyno-Pevaryl preparations, 426

H

Haelan preparations, 609
Haem arginate, **532**
 infusion table, 828
Haemaccel, 510
Haemate P (factor VIII fraction), 136
Haemodialysis, 29
Haemolytic anaemia, 495
 G6PD deficiency, 500
Haemolytic disease of newborn, prevention, 661
Haemophilia
 blood products, 136
 desmopressin, in, 402
Haemophilus influenzae type b (Hib), 646
 immunisation, 646
  vaccines, 646, 647
 prophylaxis, 282
Haemorrhage, 135
 abortion, 419
 gastro-intestinal, 45
 postpartum, 419
Haemorrhoids, 64, 65
Haemostatics, 135
HAES-steril, 510
Haldol, 191
 depot injection, 199
Haleraid, 157
Half-Beta-Prograne (propranolol), 86
Half-Inderal LA, 86
Half-Securon SR, 117
Half-Sinemet CR, 263
Halibut-liver oil capsules, 523
Haloperidol, **190**, 191
 hiccup, 189
 movement disorders, **267**
 nausea and vertigo, 217
 palliative care, 16, 18
 psychoses, 189, **190**, **199**
  depot injection, 199
Haloperidol decanoate, 199
Halothane, **669**
Halycitrol, 523
Hansen's disease, 314
Harmogen, 391
Hartmann's solution *see* Sodium lactate, intravenous infusion, compound, 506, 507
Havrix preparations, 648
Hay fever treatment
 systemic, 165
 topical, 586
Hay-Crom preparations (sodium cromoglicate), 571
HBIG *see* Hepatitis B immunoglobulin
HBvaxPRO, 649
HCG *see* Chorionic gonadotrophin, **398**
HCU
 Express, 845
 LV, 845
 gel, 845
Head lice, 634
Headache, 225
 cluster, 243
 migraine, 238
Heaf test, 644
Healthy Start vitamins, 523
Heart failure, 99
 ACE inhibitors, 99
 beta-blockers, 85
 vasodilators, 99
Heart *see also* Cardiac
Hedrin, 635
Height-weight charts, 14
Helicobacter pylori
 eradication, **43**
 tests, 44
Helixate NexGen (factor VIII fraction), 136
Helminth infections, 355
Hemabate, 419
Heminevrin, 183
Hemohes, 510
Heparin, 122, **123**
 flushes, 126
 infusion table, 828
 low molecular weight, 123
 myocardial infarction, 133
Heparinoids
 thrombosis prophylaxis, 125
 topical, 640
Hepatic encephalopathy, 61, 299, 762
Hepatic *see also* Liver
Hepatitis A
 immunisation
  immunoglobulin, normal, 660
  travel, 663
  vaccine, 647, 648, xiii
Hepatitis B
 autoimmune
  corticosteroids, 379
  penicillamine, 529
 chronic, 339
 immunisation
  immunoglobulin, 661
  travel, 663
  vaccine, 648, 649
Hepatitis C, chronic, 340
Hepatolenticular degeneration *see* Wilson's disease, 528
Hepatotoxicity, 762
Hepatyrix, 648
Hepsal, 126
Hepsera, 340
Herbal medicines, 1

Index

Herceptin, 472
Hereditary angioedema *see* Angio-edema, hereditary
Heroin *see* Diamorphine
Herpes infections, 335
- eye, 568
- genital, 336
- immunoglobulin, 661
- mouth, 593
- skin, 633

Herpid, 633
Hetastarch, 509, **510**
Hewletts, 600
Hexamine *see* Methenamine, 319, **320**
Hexetidine, 594, 595
Hexopal, 119
HFAs, 149, 159
HGH *see* Somatropin, 400, 401
Hib, 646
Hibicet Hospital Concentrate—discontinued
Hibiscrub, 638
Hibisol, 638
Hibitane preparations, 638
Hiccup, 189, 267
Hiprex, 320
Hirsutism, 621, 627
Hirudins, 125
Hirudoid, 640
Histamine H_1-antagonists, 165
Histamine H_2-antagonists, 44
Histoacryl, 637
Histoplasmosis, 321
HIV infection, 327
HNIG *see* Immunoglobulins, normal, 659, 660
Hodgkin's disease, 452, 464, 474
Homatropine, 571, 572
Homocystinuria, 845
Hookworm infections, 357
Hormone antagonists
- hypersexuality, 396
- malignant disease, 483

Hormone replacement
- androgens, 394
- oestrogens, 384, **386**
  - vaginal, 424
- progestogens, 384, 392
- surgery, 386

Hormonin, 391
Hosiery, elastic, 866
Hospicrepe products, 862
Hospiform, 861
HPV *see* Human papilloma virus, 649, 650
HRF, 402
HRT, 384, 404
$5HT_1$ agonists, 238, **239**
$5HT_3$ antagonists, 218, 221, 222, 223, 449
HTIG *see* Immunoglobulins, tetanus, **661**
Humalog preparations, 362, 364
Human antihaemophilic fraction, 136
Human chorionic gonadotrophin *see* Chorionic gonadotrophin, **398**
Human factor VIII fraction, 136
Human factor XIII fraction, 137
Human factor IX fraction, 136
Human luteinising hormone *see* Lutropin alfa, 399
Human menopausal gonadotrophins, 399
Human normal immunoglobulin *see* Immunoglobulins, normal, 661
Human papilloma virus, vaccine, 649, 650
HumaPen Ergo, 365
HumaPen Luxura, 365
HumaPen Luxura HD, 365
Humatrope, 401
Humira, 553
Humulin I, 364
Humulin M3, 365
Humulin S, 362
Huntington's chorea, 267
Hyaff, 856
Hyalase, 562
Hyaline membrane disease, 173
Hyalofill products, 856
Hyaluronic acid, 535
- wounds, 856

Hyaluronidase, **562**
Hyate-C (factor VIII inhibitor bypassing fraction), 136
Hycamtin, 471
Hycanthone, 357
Hydatid disease, 357
Hydralazine, 93, **94**
- infusion table, 828

Hydrea, 465
Hydrex, 638
Hydrochlorothiazide, 73
- amiloride with, 77
- captopril with, 101
- enalapril with, 102
- irbesartan with, 106
- lisinopril with, 103
- losartan with, 106
- olmesartan with, 106
- quinapril with, 104
- telmisartan with, 106
- triamterene with, 77
- valsartan with, 107

Hydrocoll, 855
Hydrocolloid dressings, 855, 856
Hydrocortisone, 379, **383**
- colitis, 56
- ear, 584
- eye, 569
- haemorrhoids, 65, 66
- mouth, 590, 591
- oral, 383
- parenteral, 383
  - infusion tables, 828
- pneumocystis pneumonia, 354
- replacement therapy, 378
- rheumatic disease, 545
- skin, 606, 607
  - chloramphenicol with, 621
  - chlorhexidine and nystatin with, 606
  - chlorquinaldol with, 607
  - clioquinol with, 607
  - clotrimazole with, 606
  - coal tar with, 614
  - crotamiton with, 606
  - econazole with, 606
  - fusidic acid with, 606
  - miconazole with, 606
  - nystatin with, 606
  - urea with, 606

Hydrocortistab, 545
Hydrocortone, 383
Hydrofilm, 856
Hydroflumethiazide, 73
- spironolactone with, 78

Hydrofluoroalkane propellants, 149, 159
Hydrogel dressings, 853, 854
Hydrogen peroxide
- cream, 639
- mouthwash, 594, **595**
- solution, **639**

Hydromol preparations, 600, 601
Hydromorphone, **233**, 15
- morphine equivalence, 15

Hydrosorb products, 854
Hydrotalcite, 38, **39**
Hydrous ointment, 599
Hydroxocobalamin, 493, **494**
- cyanide poisoning, 33

Hydroxybenzoates, excipient, 598
Hydroxycarbamide, **465**
- psoriasis, 516
- sickle cell disease, 495

Hydroxychloroquine, 546, **549**
Hydroxycholecalciferol, 525
Hydroxyethyl starch *see* Starch, etherified, 509, 510, 511
Hydroxyethylcellulose, 578
Hydroxyquinoline
- benzoyl peroxide with, 619

Hydroxyurea *see* Hydroxycarbamide
Hydroxyzine, **168**
Hygroton, 74
Hyoscine butylbromide, 41, **42**
Hyoscine hydrobromide, 671
- nausea and vertigo, 218, **224**
- palliative care, 18
- premedication, 670, **671**

Hypafix, 865
Hyperactive children, 213
Hyperaldosteronism, 416
Hyperamine, 512
Hypercalcaemia, 405, 406, 518
Hypercalciuria, 518
Hypercholesterolaemia, 137, 138, 139, 140
Hyperemesis gravidarum, 218
Hyperglycaemia, 359
- coma, 372

HyperHAES, 511
Hyperhidrosis, 640
Hypericum perforatum, 202
Hyperkalaemia, 504
Hyperlipidaemia, 137
Hyperlysinaemia, 846
Hypermethioninaemia, 845
Hyperparathyroidism, 518
Hyperphosphataemia, 520
Hypersensitivity *see* Allergy
Hypersexuality, 396

Hypertension, **91**
    ACE inhibitors, 100
    beta-blockers, 85
    calcium-channel blockers, 112
    crisis, 93
    diabetes, 92
    diuretics, 73
    elderly, 92
    malignant, 93
    poisoning and, 27
    pregnancy, 93
    pulmonary, 93, 126
    renal disease, 93
    systolic, 92
Hyperthermia
    malignant, 680
    poisoning and, 28
Hyperthyroidism *see* Thyrotoxicosis
Hyperuricaemia, 449, 556, 557
Hyperventilation, dental practice, 23
Hypnomidate, 667
Hypnotics, 180
    poisoning by, 32
    withdrawal, 179
Hypnovel, 673
Hypocalcaemia, 517
Hypodermic equipment, insulin, 365
Hypodermoclysis, 506, 562
Hypogammaglobulinaemia, 660
Hypoglycaemia, 360, 372
    acute, 372
    chronic, 373
    dental practice, 23
Hypogonadism, 394
Hypoguard products, 366, 374, 375
Hypokalaemia
    diuretics and, 73
    oral treatment, 503
    parenteral treatment, 507
Hypolar Retard 20, 116
Hypomagnesaemia, 519
Hyponatraemia, 506
Hypoparathyroidism, 525
Hypopituitarism, 378, 394, 398
Hypoproteinaemia, 841
    liver disease, 762
Hyposensitisation, 169
Hypostop Gel, 372
Hypotension
    poisoning and, 27
    sympathomimetics, 120
Hypothalamic hormones, 401
Hypothermia
    antipsychotics and, 188
    poisoning and, 28
Hypothyroidism, 376
    neonatal, 376
Hypovase, 98
Hypovolaemia, 509
Hypoxaemia, 173
Hypromellose, 578
Hypurin Isophane, 363
    biphasic, 365
Hypurin Lente, 363
Hypurin Neutral, 362
Hypurin Protamine Zinc, 364
Hytrin preparations
    cardiovascular, 98
    urinary tract, 439

I

Ibandronic acid, **408**
    infusion table, 828
Ibugel, 563
Ibuprofen
    pain, 535, 536, **540**, 541
        postoperative, 674
    post-immunisation pyrexia, 641
    rheumatic disease, 535, **540**
    topical, 563
Ichthammol, 610, **611**
    zinc with, 611
Ichthopaste, 864
Ichthyosis, 598
Icthaband, 864
Idarubicin, 455, **456**
    infusion table, 828
Idoxuridine, 336
    dimethyl sulfoxide with, **633**
Idrolax, 62
Idursulfase, **531**
    infusion table, 828
Ifosfamide, 452, **453**, 454
    infusion table, 828
Ikorel, 118
Iloprost, 93, **94**
Ilube, 577
Imatinib, 468, **469**
Imdur, 111
Imidapril, **102**
    see also ACE inhibitors
Imidazole antifungal drugs, 321, 322
Imidurea, excipient, 598
Imiglucerase, **530**
    infusion table, 828
Imigran preparations, 241
Imipenem, 295, **296**
    cilastatin with
        infusion table, 828
Imipramine, 203, **205**, 440
Imiquimod, 624
    actinic keratosis, **624**, 625
    genital warts, **624**
    malignant skin disease, **624**, 625
ImmuCyst, 481
Immukin, 663
Immune interferon *see* Interferons, gamma-1b, 663
Immunisation, 641
    international travel, 663
    schedule, 642
Immunity
    active, 641
    passive, 643
Immunodeficiency, 660
    syndrome, acquired, 327
Immunoglobulins, 643, **659**
    anti-D (Rh_0), 661, 662
    aplastic anaemia, 495
    hepatitis B, 661
    myasthenia gravis, 558
    normal, 659, 660
    rabies, 661
    tetanus, **661**
    thrombocytopenic purpura, idiopathic, 500
    varicella-zoster, 661
Immunoprin (azathioprine), 474
Immunostimulants, 477
Immunosuppressants
    malignant disease, 474
    myasthenia gravis, 559
    rheumatic disease, 546, 549
    skin disease, 616
    transplant rejection, 473
Imodium preparations, 52
Impetigo
    systemic treatment, 281
    topical treatment, 628
Implanon, 434
Impotence *see* Erectile dysfunction, 444
Imuderm, 602
Imunovir, 337
Imuran, 474
Imuvac, 651
Inadine, 858
Incontinence, urinary, 440
Increlex, 417
Indapamide, 73, **74**
    perindopril with, 103
Inderal preparations, 86
Indermil, 637
Indian hemp *see* Cannabis, 8
Indinavir, 328, **332**, 333
Indivina preparations, 389
Indocid PDA, 422
Indolar SR (indometacin), 541
Indometacin
    ductus closure, **421**, 422
    gout, 555
    premature labour, 423
    rheumatic disease, 535, **541**
Indomethacin *see* Indometacin
Indoramin
    cardiovascular, **97**
    urinary tract, 438, **439**
Inegy, 143
Infacol, 40
Infanrix-IPV, 646
Infanrix-IPV+Hib, 646
InfaSoy, 842
Infatrini, 836
Infections
    amoebic, 352
    antisera, 643, 659
    bladder, 319
        mycotic, 444
    ear, 582
    eye, 566
    fungal, 320
    helminth, 355
    immunoglobulins, 659
    nail, fungal, 321, 630
    notifiable diseases, 277
    oropharyngeal, 592
        bacterial, 278, 281
    protozoal, 344
    skin, 628
    trichomonal, 353
    vaccines, 641
    vaginal, 425
    viral, 327
    vulval, 425
Infertility
    female, 397, 398, 401
    male, 398

Inflammation, oral, 590
Inflammatory bowel disease, 52
Infliximab
  Crohn's disease, 52, **57**
  infusion table, 828
  psoriasis, 616
  rheumatic diseases, 551, 552, **554**, 555
  ulcerative colitis, 52, **57**
Influenza
  immunisation
    vaccines, 650, 651
  prophylaxis, 341, 342
  treatment, 341
Influvac Sub-unit, 651
Information services
  poisons, 27
Infukoll, 510
Inhalations
  aromatic, 176
  steam, 176, 588
Inhaler devices, 156
Innohep, 125
Innovace, 102
Innovative Solutions, 844
Innozide, 102
Inosine acedoben dimepranol *see* Inosine pranobex
Inosine pranobex, 336, **337**
  anogenital warts, 624
Inositol, 523
Inositol nicotinate, 118, **119**
Inotropic drugs, positive, 70, 119
Inovelon, 251
Insect stings, 166, 36
Insecticides, poisoning by, 35
Insomnia, 180
Inspra, 76
Instillagel, 682
Insulatard preparations, 364
Insulin, 359
  analogues, 361
  aspart, 361, **362**
    biphasic, 363, **364**
  detemir, **363**
  glargine, **363**
  glulisine, 361, **362**
  human, 359
  hypodermic equipment, 365
  infusion table, 828
  injection devices, 365
  isophane, **363**, 364
    biphasic, 363, **364**, 365
  lispro, 361, **362**
    biphasic, 363, **364**
  protamine zinc, 363, **364**
  soluble, **361**, 362
  subcutaneous infusion, 360
  zinc suspension, **363**
    mixed, 363
Insulin-like growth factor, 416
Insuman Basal, 364
Insuman Comb preparations, 365
Insuman Rapid, 362
Insupak, 366
Intal Spincaps, 164
Integrilin, 132
Interactions, 686
Interferons
  alfa, 478, **479**
    chronic hepatitis B, 339
    chronic hepatitis C, 340
    infusion table, 828
  beta, 479, **480**
  gamma, 662
  gamma-1b, 663
  peginterferon alfa, 340, 478, **479**
Interleukin-2 *see* Aldesleukin, 480
Intermittent claudication, 118
International travel, immunisation for, 663
Interpose, 858
Intracranial pressure, raised
  corticosteroids, 379
  palliative care, 16
  thiopental, 667
Intrafusin preparations, 512
Intralipid preparations, 512
Intrasite products, 854
Intra-uterine devices, 435
  copper-bearing, 436, 437
  progestogen-releasing, 434, 435
Intravenous infusions, 506
  addition to, 821
Intravenous nutrition, 511
Intrinsa, 395
IntronA, 479
Invanz, 296
Invega, 196
Invirase, 334
Iocare, 578
Iodine, **377**
  oral solution, 378
  radioactive, 377
  topical, 638, 639
Iodoflex, 854
Iodosorb products, 854
IONSYS, xiii
Iopidine, 579
Ipecacuanha mixture, 28
Ipocol, 54
Ipratropium, **154**
  asthma, 153
  fenoterol with, 156
  rhinorrhoea, 588, **589**
  salbutamol with, 156
  Steri-Neb, 154
IPV, 655, 656
Irbesartan, 105, 106
  hydrochlorothiazide with, 106
Iridocyclitis *see* Anterior uveitis, 571
Irinotecan, **471**
  infusion table, 828
Iron
  deficiency, 490
  folic acid and, 492
  overload, 498
  poisoning by, 32
  therapy
    oral, 490, 491, 492
    parenteral, 492, 493
Iron dextran, **493**
  infusion table, 828
Iron sucrose, 492, **493**
  infusion table, 828
Ironorm, 491
Irriclens, 637
Irripod, 637
Irritable bowel syndrome, 41, **53**
Ischaemic
  attacks, 127
  disease of limbs, 509
ISENTRESS, xiii
Isib 60XL, 111
Island dressings, 865
Ismelin, 97
Ismo preparations, 110, 111
Isocarboxazid, 206, **207**
Isodur preparations, 111
Isoflurane, 669, **670**
Isogel, 59
Isoket preparations, 110
Isoleucine Amino Acid Supplement, 846
Isometheptene, 228
  paracetamol with, 228
Isomil, 842
Isoniazid, 310, 311, **312**, 313
Isophane protamine insulin *see* Insulin, isophane
Isoprenaline, 120
Isopropyl palmitate, excipient, 598
Isopto
  Alkaline, 578
  Plain, 578
Isosorbide dinitrate, 108, **110**
  infusion table, 828
Isosorbide mononitrate, 108, **110**, 111
Isosource preparations, 836
Isotard preparations, 111
Isotretinoin
  acne
    oral, 618, **622**
    topical, 619, 620
  erythromycin with, 620
  rosacea, 618
Isotrex, 620
Isotrexin, 620
Isovaleric acidaemia, 846
Isovorin, 451
Ispagel Orange, 59
Ispaghula
  constipation, **58**, 59
  diarrhoea, 51
  mebeverine with, 42
Isradipine, 112, **114**
  see also Calcium-channel blockers
Istin, 112
Itraconazole, 321, 322, **324**, 325
  infusion table, 828
IUDs *see* Intra-uterine devices
IV3000, 857
Ivabradine, **117**, 118
Ivelip preparations, 512
Ivermectin
  larva migrans, 357
  onchocerciasis, 357
  scabies, 634
  strongyloidiasis, 357
IZS *see* Insulin, zinc suspension

J

Januvia, 372
Japanese encephalitis, 663
Jelonet, 858

Jet nebulisers, 158
Jevity preparations, 836, 837
Joint prostheses
  endocarditis prophylaxis, 283
Juvela
  gluten-free, 844
  low-protein, 844

K

Kabiven preparations, 512
Kala-azar, 353
Kaletra, 333
Kalspare, 78
Kalten, 87
Kaltostat products, 851
Kamillosan, 600
Kaolin, 51
  mixture, 51
  morphine with, 52
  poultices, 564
Kapake, 228
Kaplon (captopril), 101
Karvol preparations, 176
Katya 30/75, 432
Kawasaki syndrome, 660
Kay-Cee-L, 504
K-Band, 861
Kefadim, 294
Keflex, 292
Keftid (cefaclor), 292
Keloc SR (felodipine), 114
Kelo-cote, 856
Keloid dressings, 856
Kemadrin preparations, 267
Kemicetine, 304
Kenalog, 384, 545
Kentera, 441
Kepivance, 451
Keppra, 249
Keral, 538
Keratitis, 566
Keratolytics, warts and calluses, 622
Keratosis follicularis, 612
Keri, 600
Keromask preparations, 626
Kerraboot products, 853
Ketalar, 668
Ketamine, **667**, 668
  infusion table, 828
  neuropathic pain, 238
Ketek, 303
Ketoacidosis, diabetic, 372
KetoCal, 841
Ketocid, 542
Ketoconazole, 321, 322, **325**, 326
  anogenital, 426
  Cushing's syndrome, 416
  scalp, 626
  skin, 630, 631
Ketodiastix, 375
Ketolides, 301
Ketoprofen, **541**
  gout, 555
  pain, 541
    postoperative, 674
  rheumatic disease, 535, 541
  topical, 563
Ketorolac
  eye, 579, 580
  pain, 536
    postoperative, **674**
Ketostix, 375
Ketotifen, 168
  eye, **570**
Ketovail, 542
Ketovite, 528
Ketur Test, 375
K-Four products, 864
Kidney *see* Renal
Kindergen, 837
Kineret, 553
Kivexa, 329
Klaricid preparations, 302, 303
Klean-Prep, 64
Kliofem, 389
Kliovance, 389
K-Lite, 862, 864
Kloref preparations, 504
Knit Fix, 861
Knit-Band, 861
Knit-Firm, 862
Knitted viscose dressing, primary, 858
Ko-Flex, 864
Kogenate Bayer (factor VIII fraction), 136
Kolanticon, 41
Konakion preparations, 527
Kontour, 861
Korsakoff's psychosis, 523
K-Plus, 862, 864
K-Press, 864
K-Soft, 863, 864
K-Tech, 863, 864
K-Two, 864
Kytril, 222

L

Labelling, cautionary and advisory *see* Cautionary and advisory labels, 867, 869
Labetalol, 84, **88**
  infusion table, 829
  see also Beta-adrenoceptor blocking drugs
Labiton, 528
Labour
  analgesia, 230
  induction, 418
  premature, 423
Labyrinthine disorders, 218
Lacidipine, 112, **114**
  see also Calcium-channel blockers
Lacri-Lube, 578
Lactation, suppression
  dopaminergic drugs, 411
  oestrogens, 384
Lactic acid
  hydrocortisone with, 606
  salicylic acid with, 623
Lactugal (lactulose), 62
Lactulose, **62**
Ladropen (flucloxacillin), 286
Laevulose *see* Fructose
Lamictal, 249
Lamisil, 326
  cream, 632
Lamivudine, **330**
  abacavir and zidovudine with, 329
  abacavir with, 329
  chronic hepatitis B, 340
  HIV infection, 328
  zidovudine with, 331
Lamotrigine, 245, **248**, 249
  trigeminal neuralgia, 238
Lancets, 366
Lanolin *see* Wool fat, hydrous, 599
Lanoxin preparations, 71
Lanreotide, 488, **489**
Lansoprazole, **49**
Lanthanum, **520**
Lantus, 363
Lanvis, 461
Larafen CR, 542
Larapam SR, 237
Largactil, 190
Lariam, 350
Laronidase, **530**, 531
  infusion table, 829
LarvE, 639
Laryngojet, 682
Lasikal, 78
Lasilactone, 78
Lasix, 75
Lassar's paste, 615
Latanoprost, 573, **574**
  with timolol, 574
Laxatives, 57
  bulk-forming, 58
  faecal softeners, 61
  osmotic, 61
  stimulant, 59
Laxoberal (sodium picosulfate), 61
Ledclair, 35
Lederfen preparations, 540
Lederfolin (calcium folinate), 451
Ledermycin, 297
Leflunomide, **550**
  rheumatic disease, 549
Left ventricular failure *see* Heart failure
Legionnaires' disease, 301
Leishmaniacides, 353
Leishmaniasis, 353
Lenalidomide, **481**
Lenograstim, 501, **502**
  infusion table, 829
Lepirudin, **125**, 126
  infusion table, 829
Lepra reactions, 314
Leprosy, 314
Leptospirosis, 284, 296
Lercanidipine, 112, **114**, 115
  see also Calcium-channel blockers
Lescol preparations, 142
Letrozole, 483, 484, **485**
Leucine Amino Acid Supplement, 847
Leucovorin *see* Calcium folinate

Index

Leukaemia
acute, 454, 457
lymphoblastic, 456, 464, 474
chronic lymphocytic, 452, 457
chronic myeloid, 452, 465, 479
CNS, prophylaxis, 456
hairy cell, 479
lymphoid, 495
Leukeran, 453
Leukofix, 865
Leukopor, 865
Leukosilk, 865
Leukostrip, 866
Leukotriene receptor antagonists, 165
Leuprorelin
endometriosis, 414
prostate cancer, 486, **488**
uterine fibroids, 413
Leustat, 459
Levamisole, 356
Levemir, 363
Levetiracetam, 245, **249**
infusion table, 829
Levitra, 447
Levobunolol, 572, **573**
Levobupivacaine, **683**, 684
Levocetirizine, 166, **167**
Levodopa, 262
benserazide with, **262**, 263
carbidopa with, 262, **263**
and entacapone with, 264
Levofloxacin, 316, **318**
eye, 566, **567**
Levofolinic acid *see* Calcium levofolinate
Levomenthol, 176
Levomepromazine, **191**
nausea and vertigo, 217
palliative care, 191, 16, 18
psychosis, 191
Levonelle 1500, 438
Levonelle One Step, 437
Levonorgestrel, 434, **437**
contraception, 431, 433
emergency, 437, 438
intra-uterine, 435
HRT, 387, 388, 389
Levothyroxine, 376
Lexpec (folic acid), 495
LH *see* Luteinising hormone, 398
LH-RH *see* Gonadorelin, 401, **402**
Liberty nebuliser, 159
Librium (chlordiazepoxide), 185
Lice, 634
Lidocaine
arrhythmias, **83**, 84
chlorhexidine with, 682
dental, 681
fluorescein with, 577
haemorrhoids, 65, 66
local anaesthesia, **681**, 682, 683
dental, 682
eye, **577**
mouth, 592
postherpetic neuralgia, 238, 682
rectal, 65
urethral, 682
urethral pain, 443
neuropathic pain, 238
phenylephrine with, 683
prilocaine with, 682
Lifestyle preparations, 844
Lignocaine *see* Lidocaine
Lignospan Special , 682
Li-Liquid, 201
Linezolid, **306**, 307
Linola Gamma, 600
Lint, absorbent, 860
Lioresal, 560
Liothyronine, **376**
Lipantil preparations, 140
Lipidem preparations, 512
Lipid-regulating drugs, 137
Lipitor, 141
Lipobase, 600
Lipodystrophy syndrome, 328
Lipofundin preparations, 513
Lipopeptide antibiotic, 306
Liposic, 578
Lipostat, 142
LiquiBand, 637
Liquid and White Soft Paraffin Ointment, 599
Liquid paraffin
constipation, **61**
emulsion, 61
magnesium hydroxide and, 63
eye, lubricant, 578
Liquifilm Tears, 578
Liquigen, 841
Liquivisc, 578
Lisicostad preparations, 103
Lisinopril, **102**, 103
hydrochlorothiazide with, 103
see also ACE inhibitors
Liskonum, 201
Litak, 459
Lithium, 200, 201
cluster headache, 243
mania, 200
poisoning by, 32
recurrent depression, 200
surgery, 666
Lithium carbonate, 200
Lithium citrate, 201
Lithonate (lithium carbonate), 201
Liver disease, prescribing in, 762
Livial, 391
Loa loa, 357
Load 375, 436
Local anaesthetics *see* Anaesthesia, local
Locasol, 842
Loceryl, 631
Locoid preparations, 607
Locorten-Vioform, 583
Lodine, 539
Lodoxamide, 570, **571**
Loestrin-20, 431
Loestrin-30, 432
Lofepramine, 203, **205**
Lofexidine, **273**, 274
Logynon preparations, 431
Lomont (lofepramine), 205
Lomotil, 51
Lomustine, 452, **454**
Loniten, 95
Loop diuretics *see* Diuretics, loop, 74
Lopace (ramipril), 104
Loperamide, 51, 52
palliative care, 16
Lophlex preparations, 847
Lopid, 140
Lopinavir, 328, **333**
ritonavir with, 333
Loprazolam, 180, **181**
Lopresor preparations, 89
Loprofin
low-protein, 845
PKU drink, 847
Loratadine, 166, **167**
Lorazepam
anaesthesia, **672**
anxiety, **184**, **185**, 186
nausea and vomiting, 449
status epilepticus, 255, **257**
Lormetazepam, 180, **181**
Loron, 409
Losartan, 105, **106**
hydrochlorothiazide with, 106
Losec, 50
Lotions
definition, 598
eye, 565
suitable quantities, 598
Lotriderm, 608
Low protein drink, 845
Low sodium content (antacids), 38
Low-protein foods, 844
LSD *see* Lysergide, 8
Luborant, 596
Lubri-Tears, 578
Lucanthone, 357
Lucentis, 581
Lugol's solution, 378
Lumefantrine, 344, **349**
artemether with, 349
Lumigan, 574
Lupus erythematosus
discoid, 546
systemic, 379, 544, 546, 549
Lustral, 211
Luteinising hormone, 398
Lutropin alfa, **399**
follitropin alfa with, 399
Luveris, 399
Lyclear, 636
Lyflex (baclofen), 560
Lyme disease, 287
Lymecycline, **293**
acne, 621
Lymphogranuloma venereum, 296
Lyofoam products, 852, 859
Lyrica, 248
Lyrinel XL, 441
Lysergic acid diethylamide *see* Lysergide, 8
Lysergide, regulations, 8
Lysodren, 466
Lysosomal storage disorder, 529, 530
Lysovir, 342

M

Maalox preparations, 39, 40
MabCampath, 478
Mabron, 237
MabThera, 478
Macrobid, 320
Macrodantin, 320

Index

Macrogol Oral Powder, Compound, NPF, 885, 886
Macrogol Oral Powder, NPF, 885, 886
Macrogols, 62, 64
Macrolides, 301
Macugen, 580
Macular degeneration, age-related, 580
Madopar preparations, 262, 263
Magnapen, 290
Magnesium carbonate, 38, **39**
Magnesium citrate, 63, 64
Magnesium glycerophosphate, 519
Magnesium hydroxide, 38, 40, **63**
  liquid paraffin with, 63
Magnesium sulphate, 63, **519**
  arrhythmias, 519
  asthma, 148
  eclampsia, 519
  infusion table, 829
  injection, 519
  laxative, 63
  myocardial infarction, 519
  paste, 636
Magnesium trisilicate, 38, **39**
Malabsorption syndromes, 53
  electrolytes, 503
  vitamin K, 527
Malaria
  prophylaxis, 346, 347, 348
  treatment, 344, 345
Malarivon, 349
Malarone
  malaria prophylaxis 346, 347, 348, 350, **351**
  malaria treatment, 344, 350, **351**
Malarone Paediatric, 351
Malathion, 634, **635**
Malignant disease, 448
  bladder, 444
  gonadorelin analogues, 486
  hormone antagonists, 483
  pain, 229
    bone, 225
  sex hormones, 482
Malignant effusions, 452
Malignant hyperthermia, 680
  antagonists, 680
Manerix, 208
Manevac, 61
Mania, 187, 199
Manic depression *see* Bipolar disorder, 200
Mannitol, **78**
  glaucoma, 572
  presence of, 2
Mantoux test, 644
Manufacturers, special order, 902
Manusept, 639
MAOIs *see* Monoamine-oxidase inhibitors
Maple syrup urine disease, 846
Mapleflex, 846
Maraviroc, 328, **335**
Marcain preparations, 683
Marevan (warfarin), 128
Marine stings, 36
Marketing authorisation, 1
Marvelon, 432
Mastaflu, 651
Mastalgia, **415**
Matrifen (fentanyl), 232
Maxalt, 240
Maxamaid preparations, 845, 846, 848
Maxamum preparations, 845, 846, 848
Maxepa, 144
Maxidex, 569
Maxijul preparations, 837
Maxisorb, 841
Maxitrol, 569
Maxolon preparations, 221
Maxtrex (methotrexate), 551
MCT Oil, 841
MCT Pepdite, 841
MCT Step 1, 842
MDMA *see* Methylenedioxymethamfetamine
Measles
  immunisation
    immunoglobulin, 660
    vaccines, 651
Measles, mumps and rubella vaccine, 652
Mebendazole, 356
  hookworm infections, 357
  roundworm infections, 356
  threadworm infections, 356
  whipworm infections, 356
Mebeverine, **42**
  ispaghula with, 42
Mecasermin, **416**, 417
Mecillinam, 290
Mecysteine, 175
Medicaid, 602
Medicines information services, *inside front cover*
Medication-overuse headache, 238
Medikinet (methylphenidate), 214
Medikinet XL, 215
Medinol (paracetamol) preparations, 227
Mediplast, 865
Medipore+Pad, 858
Medisafe, 858
MediSense products, 374
Mediterranean fever, familial, 556
Medi-Test products, 375
Medix nebulisers, 158
Medocodene (co-codamol 30/500), 227, 228
Medrone, 383
Medroxyprogesterone
  contraception, 433, **434**
  HRT, 387, 389, 393
  malignant disease, **483**
  menstrual disorders, 392, **393**
Mefenamic acid
  menorrhagia, 542
  pain, 535, **542**
  rheumatic disease, 535, **542**
Mefilm, 857
Mefix, 865
Mefloquine, **350**
  malaria
    prophylaxis, 346, 347, 348
    treatment, 344
Megace, 483
Megestrol, **483**
Melanoma, 464, 479
Melgisorb products, 851
Melolin, 858
Meloxicam, 535, **542**
Melphalan, 452, **454**
  infusion table, 829
Memantine, 275, **276**
Menadiol sodium phosphate, **527**
Mendelson's syndrome, 45, 666
Meniere's disease, 218
Meningeal carcinoma, 456
Meningitec, 653
Meningitis
  cryptococcal, 323
  haemophilus, 280, 304
  immunisation, 652
    Hib with, 647
    vaccine, 653
  initial therapy, 280
  listerial, 280
  meningococcal, 280
    prophylaxis, 282
    travel, 653, 663
  pneumococcal, 280
Meningococcal *see* Meningitis
Menitorix, 647
Menjugate, 653
Menogon—discontinued
Menopausal symptoms, 243, 384
Menopur, 399
Menoring—discontinued
Menorrhagia, 392, 434, 435
  antifibrinolytics, 135
  NSAIDS, 542
Menotrophin, 399
Menthol and eucalyptus inhalation, 176
Mepacrine
  discoid lupus erythematosus, 548
  giardiasis, **353**
Mepiform, 856
Mepilex products, 858
Mepitac, 865
Mepitel, 859
Mepivacaine, 681
Mepore products, 856, 857, 858
Mepradec (omeprazole), 50
Meprobamate, **186**
  muscle spasm, 561
Meptazinol, 229, **233**
Meptid, 233
Merbentyl preparations, 41
Mercaptamine (cysteamine), **531**
Mercaptopurine, 458, **460**
  inflammatory bowel disease, 52
Mercilon, 431
Merional, 399
Meronem, 296
Meropenem, 295, **296**
  infusion table, 829
Mesalazine, 52, 53, **54**, 55
Mesitran products, 854
Mesna, 451, **452**
  infusion fluid, 829
Mesorb, 857
Mesren MR, 54
Mesterolone, **396**
Mestinon, 559
Mestranol, norethisterone with, 432
Metabolic acidosis, 508
Metabolic Mineral Mixture, 842

Index

Metals, poisoning by, 34
Metalyse, 135
Metanium, 602
Metaraminol, **121**
    infusion table, 829
Metastron, 15
Metatone, 528
Meted, 627
Metenix-5, 74
Metformin, **368**, 369
    pioglitazone with, 371
    rosiglitazone with, 371
Methadone, **233**
    cough, 177
    linctus, 177
    opioid dependence, 273, **274**
    oral solution (1 mg/mL), 274
    oral solution, concentrate, 274
    pain, 229, 233
    palliative care, 15
    parenteral, 274
    poisoning by, 31
Methadose, 274
Methaemoglobinaemia, 684
Methanol, poisoning by, 34
Metharose (methadone), 274
Methenamine, 319, **320**
Methicillin-resistant *Staphylococcus aureus see* MRSA
Methionine, 29, **31**
    paracetamol with, 228
Methocarbamol, **561**
Methotrexate
    Crohn's disease, 52, **550**
    infusion table, 829
    malignant disease, 456, 457, **460**
    psoriasis, 616, 617
    rheumatic disease, 546, 549, **550**, 551
Methotrimeprazine *see* Levomepromazine
Methoxy polyethylene glycol-epoetin beta, 495, **498**
Methyl alcohol *see* Methanol, 34
Methyl cysteine *see* Mecysteine, 175
Methyl salicylate, 633, 637
    dithranol and salicylic acid with, 615
Methyl-5-aminolevulinate, 625
Methylated spirit, industrial, 637
Methylcellulose, 216
    constipation, 58, 59
    diarrhoea, 51
    obesity, 59, 216
Methylcysteine *see* Mecysteine, 175
Methyldopa, 95, **96**
Methylene blue *see* Methylthioninium chloride, 684
Methylenedioxymethamfetamine
    controlled drug, 7
    poisoning by, 33
Methylmalonic acidaemia, 846
Methylphenidate, 213, **214**, 215
Methylprednisolone, **383**
    lidocaine with, 545
    rheumatic disease, 545
Methylprednisolone acetate, 384
Methylprednisolone sodium succinate, 384
    infusion table, 829
Methylthioninium chloride, 684
Methysergide, 242, **243**
    cluster headache, 243
Meticillin-resistant *Staphylococcus aureus see* MRSA
Metipranolol, 572, **573**
Metirosine, 98
Metoclopramide
    aspirin with, 239
    diabetic neuropathy, 373
    gastro-intestinal, 43
    infusion table, 829
    migraine, 242
    nausea and vomiting, 217, **220**, 221
        cytotoxic drugs, 449
        postoperative, 218
        pregnancy, 218
    palliative care, 16
    paracetamol with, 239
Metoject, 551
Metolazone, 73, **74**
Metopirone, 416
Metoprolol, **89**
    migraine, 242
    see also Beta-adrenoceptor blocking drugs
Metosyn, 609
Metrogel, 630
Metrolyl, 316
Metronidazole, **315**, 316
    amoebiasis, 352
    Crohn's disease, 53
    giardiasis, 353
    protozoal infections, 353
    skin, 629, 630
    trichomoniasis, 353
    ulcerative gingivitis, 315, 592
    vaginal infections, 427
Metrosa, 630
Metrotop, 630
Metsol (metformin), 369
Metvix, 625
Metyrapone, 415, **416**
Mexiletine, 83, **84**
    infusion table, 829
Mexitil, 84
Mezavant XL, 54
mhi-500, 365
Miacalcic, 405
Mianserin, 203, **206**
Micanol, 615
Micardis preparations, 106
Micolette Micro-enema, 63
Miconazole
    mouth, 592, **593**
    skin, 630, **632**
        hydrocortisone and, 606
    vaginal, 426
Micralax Micro-enema, 63
Micral-Test II, 375
Microalbustik, 375
Microbumintest, 375
Microgynon preparations, 431
Microlance, 366
Micronor, 433
MicroPeak, 156
Micropirin (aspirin), 131
Micropore, 865
Midazolam
    anaesthesia, 672, **673**
    infusion table, 829
    palliative care, 18
    status epilepticus, 256, **257**
Midrid, 228
Mifegyne, 422
Mifepristone, 418, **422**
Migard, 240
Miglustat, **530**
Migraine, 238
    acute attack, 238
    prophylaxis, 242
Migraleve, 239
MigraMax, 239
Migril, 242
Mildison, 606
Milex Arcing Style, 437
Milex Omniflex, 437
Milk, drugs in, 807
Milk-alkali syndrome, 38
Milpar (liquid paraffin emulsion and magnesium hydroxide), 63
Milrinone, **72**
    infusion table, 829
Milupa Low Protein Drink, 845
Milupa PKU preparations, 847
Milward Steri-Let, 366
Mimpara, 519
Minaphlex, 847
Mineralocorticoids, replacement therapy, 378
Mini TT 380 Slimline, 436
Minijet
    Adrenaline, 122, 172
    Aminophylline, 155
    Atropine sulphate, 671
    Calcium Chloride, 518
    Furosemide, 75
    Glucose, 507
    Lignocaine, 84
    Magnesium Sulphate, 519
    Morphine Sulphate, 235
    Naloxone, 31
    Sodium Bicarbonate, 508
Minims
    Amethocaine, 577
    Artificial Tears, 578
    Atropine Sulphate, 571
    Chloramphenicol, 567
    Cyclopentolate, 572
    Dexamethasone, 569
    Fluorescein Sodium, 579
    Gentamicin, 567
    Lignocaine and Fluorescein, 577
    Metipranolol, 573
    Oxybuprocaine, 577
    Phenylephrine, 572
    Pilocarpine Nitrate, 576
    Prednisolone, 570
    Proxymetacaine, 577
    Proxymetacaine and Fluorescein, 577
    Rose Bengal—discontinued
    Saline, 579
    Tropicamide, 572
MiniQuick, 400
Minitran, 109

Miniversol, 637
Mini-Wright, 156
Minocin preparations, 298
Minocycline, 296, **298**
  acne, 621
  preparations, 298
Minodiab, 368
Minoxidil
  hypertension, 93, **94**, 95
  scalp, 627, 628
Mintec, 43
Minulet—discontinued
Miochol-E, 579
Mirapexin, 261
Mircera, 498
Mirena, 434, 435
Mirtazapine, **211**, 212
Miscarriage, recurrent, 392
Misoprostol, 48
  diclofenac with, 539
  naproxen with, 543
  obstetrics, 418
Misuse of drugs
  Act, 7
  Regulations 2001, 7
Mitobronitol, 452
Mitomycin, 455, **456**
  bladder, 444
Mitomycin C Kyowa, 456
Mitotane, **465**, 466
Mitoxana, 454
Mitoxantrone, 455, **456**
  infusion table, 829
Mitozantrone *see* Mitoxantrone
Mivacron, 677
Mivacurium, **677**
  infusion table, 829
Mixtard preparations, 365
Mizolastine, 166, **167**
Mizollen, 167
MMR vaccine, 651, 652
Mobic, 542
Mobiflex, 544
Moclobemide, 207, **208**
Modafinil, 213, **215**
Modalim, 139
Modecate preparations, 198
Modification of Diet in Renal Disease study ('MDRD formula'), 772
Modisal preparations, 111
Moditen—discontinued
Modrasone, 607
Modrenal, 416
Moducren, 91
Modulen IBD, 837
Moduret-25 (co-amilozide), 77
Moduretic (co-amilozide), 77
Moexipril, **103**
  see also ACE inhibitors
Mogadon (nitrazepam), 181
Molcer, 586
Molipaxin, 206
Mometasone
  asthma, 159, **164**
  nasal allergy, 588
  skin, 610
Monigen XL (isosorbide mononitrate), 111
Monoamine-oxidase inhibitors, 206
  reversible, 207
  surgery, 666
  type A, 207
  type B, 264
    parkinsonism, 264
Monoethanolamine oleate *see* Ethanolamine oleate, **144**
Monofluorophosphate, 521
Monogen, 842
Monoject, 366
Monoject Ultra, 366
Monojector, 366
Monolet, 366
Monomax preparations, 111
Monomil XL, 111
Mononine (factor IX fraction), 136
Monoparin preparations, 123
Monosorb XL, 111
Monphytol, 633
Montelukast, **165**
Moracizine, 83
Morhulin, 603
Morphgesic SR, 234
Morphine, 230, **233**, 234, 235
  cough, 177
  cyclizine with, 235
  kaolin with, 52
  pain, 229
  palliative care, 15
Motens, 114
Motifene (diclofenac), 539
Motilium, 220
Motion sickness, 218
Motor neurone disease, amyotrophic lateral sclerosis, 267
Mountain sickness, 78
Mouth ulceration, 590
Mouthwash solution-tablets, 595
Mouthwashes, 594
Movement disorders, 267
Movicol preparations, 62
Moviprep, 64
Moxifloxacin, 316, **318**
Moxisylyte, **119**
Moxonidine, **96**
MPD Ultra Thin, 366
MRSA, 286
  nasal, 589
MST Continus, 234
MSUD preparations, 846
Mucodyne, 175
Mucogel, 39
Mucolytics, 175
  eye, 577
Mucopolysaccharidosis, 530
Mucosa, oral, side-effects on, 12
Mucositis, oral, 449
Multiclix, 366
Multiload IUDs, 436
Multiparin, 123
Multiple myeloma, 464, 479, 495
Multiple sclerosis, 479, 481, 482, 559, 561
Multivitamin preparations, 528
Mumps vaccines, 651, **654**
Mupirocin, **628**
  nose, 589, 590
  skin, 628, 629
Muscle relaxants
  anaesthesia, 676
    depolarising, 678
    non-depolarising, 676
  skeletal, 559
Muscle spasm, 559
  temporomandibular dysfunction, 225
Musculoskeletal disorders, rheumatic, 534
MUSE, 446
Muslin, absorbent, 860
MXL, 234
Myasthenia gravis, 557
  corticosteroids, 559
  diagnosis, 558
  immunosuppressants, 559
Mycobacterium avium complex infections, 310, 313
Mycobutin, 313
Mycophenolate mofetil, 473, 474
  eczema, 616
  infusion table, 829
Mycophenolic acid, 474
Mycoplasma infections, 296
Mycota, 633
Mydriacyl, 572
Mydriatics, 571
Mydrilate, 572
Myeloma, multiple *see* Multiple myeloma, 464, 479, 495
Myfortic, 474
Myleran, 453
Myocardial infarction, 132
  analgesia, 231, 234
  arrhythmias, 79
  beta-blockers, 85
  dental practice, 22, 24
  magnesium sulphate, 519
  secondary prevention, 143
  thrombolytics, 133
Myocet, 456
Myoclonic seizures, 245
Myocrisin 547
Myometrial relaxants, 423
Myotonine, 439
Myozyme 531
Mysoline, 250
Myxoedema, 376

N

N-A Dressing, 858
N-A Ultra, 858
Nabilone, 218, **223**
Nabumetone, 535, **542**
Nadolol, **89**
  cardiovascular, 89
  migraine, 242
  see also Beta-adrenoceptor blocking drugs
  thyrotoxicosis, 377
Nafarelin, 415
Naftidrofuryl, 118, **119**
Naglazyme, 531
Nalcrom, 57

Nalidixic acid, 316, **318**, 319
Nalorex, 274
Naloxone
  anaesthesia, 679, **680**
  buprenorphine with, 273
  infusion table, 829
  poisoning, **31**
Naltrexone, 273, **274**
Name changes, xiv
Nandrolone decanoate, 397
Nappy rash, 602
Napratec, 543
Naprosyn preparations, 543
Naproxen
  gout, 555
  misoprostol with, 543
  pain, 535
  rheumatic disease, 535, **542**, 543
Naramig, 240
Naratriptan, 239, **240**
Narcolepsy, 215
Narcotic analgesics *see* Analgesics, opioid
Narcotic antagonists *see* Opioid antagonists
Nardil, 207
Naropin, 685
Nasacort, 588
Nasal
  allergy, 586
  congestion, 586, 588
  decongestants
    systemic, 165, 178
    topical, 588
  infection, 589
  polyps, 586
Naseptin, 590
Nasobec preparations, 587
Nasofan, 588
Nasonex, 588
Natalizumab, **482**
  infusion table, 829
Nateglinide, 369, **370**
National Institute for Health and Clinical Excellence, 3
Natrilix preparations, 74
Nausea, 218
  cytotoxic drugs, 449
  motion sickness, 218
  palliative care, 17
  postoperative, 218
  pregnancy, 218
Navelbine, 462
Navidrex, 74
Navispare, 77
Navoban, 223
Nebido, 395
Nebilet, 89
Nebivolol, 84, **89**
  see also Beta-adrenoceptor blocking drugs
Nebuchamber, 157
Nebuhaler, 157
Nebulisers, 157
Necatoriasis, 357
Nedocromil
  asthma, 164, 165
  eye, 570, **571**
Needles, insulin, 366
  clipping device, 366
Nefopam, 225, **228**
Negaban, 287
NeisVac-C, 653
Nelarabine, 457, **460**
Nelfinavir, 328, **333**
Neocate preparations, 842, 843
Neoclarityn, 166
Neo-Cortef
  ear, 584
  eye, 569
Neo-Cytamen (hydroxocobalamin), 494
Neofel XL (felodipine), 114
Neo-Mercazole, 377
Neomycin, 299, **300**
  chlorhexidine with, 589, 590
  ear, 582, 583, 584, **585**
    betamethasone with, 583
    prednisolone with, 584
  eye, 566, **567**, 569
    betamethasone with, 569
  nose, 589, 590
    betamethasone with, 589
  skin, 628, **629**
    betamethasone with, 608
    fluocinolone with, 609
    gramicidin with, 629
Neo-NaClex preparations, 73, 78
Neoral, 476
NeoRecormon, 497
Neosporin, 567
Neosport, 862
Neostigmine
  anaesthesia, **679**
  glycopyrronium bromide with, 679
  laxative, 59
  myasthenia gravis, **558**
Neotigason, 616
Neotulle, 858
Nephropathic cystinosis, 531
Nephrotic syndrome, 379
Nepro, 842
Nerisone preparations, 609
Nerve agent, poisoning by, 35
Nestargel, 840
Netillin—discontinued
Neulactil, 191
Neulasta, 502
Neupogen, 502
Neupro, 261
Neural tube defects, prevention, 494
Neuralgia, 203, 238
  glossopharyngeal, 238
NeuroBloc, 269
Neuroleptic malignant syndrome, 188
Neuroleptics *see* Antipsychotics
Neuromuscular blocking drugs, 676
Neuromuscular disorders, 557
Neurontin, 248
Neuropathic pain, 238
Neuropathy, compression, 545
Neutral insulin *see* Insulin, soluble, **361**, 362
Neutrogena Dermatological Cream, 600
Neutropenias, 495, 501
Nevirapine, 328, **334**, 335
New names, xii
New preparations, xii
Nexavar, 469
Nexium, 49
NHS Direct, *inside front cover*
Niaspan, 143
Nicam, 621
Nicardipine, 112, **115**
  see also Calcium-channel blockers
NICE *see* National Institute for Health and Clinical Excellence, 3
Nicef (cefradine), 293
Niclosamide, 356
Nicopass, xiii
Nicopatch, xiii
Nicorandil, 117, **118**
Nicorette preparations, 271
Nicotinamide
  oral, 523, **524**
  topical, 620, 621
Nicotine
  replacement therapy, 270
  smoking cessation products, 271, 272, xiii
Nicotinell preparations, 272
Nicotinic acid, 143
  hyperlipidaemia, **143**
Nicoumalone *see* Acenocoumarol, 127, **128**
Nifedipine, 112, **115**, 116, 118, 423
  atenolol with, 87
  palliative care, 16
  see also Calcium-channel blockers
Nifedipress MR, 116
Niferex preparations, 492
Nifopress Retard, 116
Niko Fix IV, 857
Nimbex, 677
Nimodipine, 112, **116**
  infusion table, 829
Nimotop, 116
Nipent, 466
Niquitin CQ preparations, 272
Niridazole, 357
Nisoldipine, 112, **116**
  see also Calcium-channel blockers
Nitisinone, **532**
Nitrates
  angina, 108
  heart failure, 108
  myocardial infarction, 133
  tolerance to, 108
Nitrazepam, 180, **181**
Nitrocine, 109
Nitro-Dur, 110
Nitrofurantoin, 319, **320**
Nitrolingual Pumpspray, 109
Nitromin, 109
Nitronal, 109
Nitroprusside *see* Sodium nitroprusside
Nitrous oxide, **670**
Nitrous oxide-oxygen, 670
Nivaquine, 349
Nivemycin (neomycin), 300
Nizatidine, **46**
  infusion table, 829
Nizoral, 326
  anogenital, 426
  scalp, 626
  skin, 631
Nocturnal enuresis, 442
Nolvadex preparations, 486
Nonacog alfa, 136

Non-depolarising muscle relaxants *see* Muscle relaxants
Non-nucleoside reverse transcriptase inhibitors, 327, 328
Nonoxinol, 435
Nootropil, 268
Noradrenaline, **121**
  infusion table, 829
Norcuron, 678
Norditropin, 401
Norelgestromin, 431
Norepinephrine *see* Noradrenaline
Norethisterone
  contraception, 431, 432, 433
  HRT, 387
  malignant disease, 483
  menstrual disorders, **393**
Norethisterone acetate
  contraception, 431, 432
  HRT, 388, 389
Norethisterone enantate, 434
  contraception, 434
Norfloxacin, 316, **318**, 319
Norgalax Micro-enema, 60
Norgestimate, 432
Norgeston, 433
Norgestrel
  HRT, 387
  see also Levonorgestrel
Noriday, 433
Norimin, 432
Norimode (loperamide), 52
Norinyl-1, 432
Noristerat, 434
Noritate, 630
Normacol preparations, 59
Normal immunoglobulin *see* Immunoglobulins, normal, 659, 660
Normal saline *see* Sodium chloride
Normasol, 637
Normax, 60
Normosang, 532
Norphyllin SR (aminophylline), 155
Norprolac, 412
Nortriptyline, 203, **205**
  neuropathic pain, 238
Norvir, 333
Norzol (metronidazole), 316
Nose *see* Nasal
Notifiable diseases, 277
Novasource preparations, 837
Nova-T, 436
Novofem, 389
NovoFine, 366
Novogel, 854
Novolizer, 162
NovoMix 30, 364
NovoNorm see Prandin, 371
NovoPen, 365
NovoRapid, 362
NovoSeven (factor VIIa fraction), 136
Noxafil, 326
Nozinan, 191
NPH *see* Insulin, isophane
NSAIDs (non-steroidal anti-inflammatory drugs) *see* Analgesics
NTBC *see* Nitisinone, **532**
NU DERM, 855
Nucleoside analogues *see* Nucleoside reverse transcriptase inhibitors, 327, 328
Nucleoside reverse transcriptase inhibitors, 327, 328
Nuelin SA, 155
Nu-Gel, 854
Nurofen (ibuprofen) preparations, 541
Nurse Prescribers' Extended Formulary, 887
Nurse Prescribers' Formulary, 884
Nurse prescribing, independent, 887
Nu-Seals Aspirin, 131
  analgesia, 226
Nutilis, 840
Nutracel preparations, 513
Nutramigen preparations, 843
Nutraplus, 601
NuTRIflex preparations, 513
Nutrini preparations, 837
Nutriprem preparations, 837
Nutrison preparations, 837, 838
Nutrition, 511
  ACBS, 833
  enteral, 516, 833
  intravenous, 511
  oral, 516
  total parenteral, 511
Nutrizym preparations, 68, 69
NutropinAq, 401
Nuvelle preparations, 389
Nyogel, 573
Nystaform, 632
Nystaform-HC, 606
Nystan, 326
  anogenital, 426
  mouth, 593
  skin, 632
Nystatin, 321, 322, **326**
  anogenital
    perianal, 64
    vaginal, 426
    vulval, 426
  ear, 584
  mouth, 592, 593
  skin, 630, **632**
    chlorhexidine and hydrocortisone with, 606
    hydrocortisone with, 606
    tolnaftate with, 632

O

Obesity, 215
Obidoxime, 35
Obsessive compulsive disorder, 202
Obstetric and gynaecological surgery, antibacterial prophylaxis, 283
Obstructive pulmonary disease *see* Chronic obstructive pulmonary disease
Occlusal, 623
Octagam, 661
Octalbin preparations (albumin solution), 509
Octaplas (fresh frozen plasma), 137
Octim, 404
Octocog alfa, 136
Octreotide, 488, **489**
  palliative care, 18
Octyl 2-cyanoacrylate, 637
Ocufen, 580
Oculotect, 578
Oedema
  cerebral, 78
  pulmonary, 74
Oesophageal varices, 402
Oesophagitis *see* Gastro-oesophageal reflux disease, **38**
Oestradiol *see* Estradiol
Oestriol *see* Estriol
Oestrogel, 390
Oestrogens, 384
  HRT, 384, **386**
    conjugated, 387, 389
  malignant disease, 482
  oral contraceptives, 427
  vaginal, 424
Oestrone *see* Estrone, 391
Ofloxacin, 316, **319**
  ear, 585
  eye, **568**
Oftaquix, 567
Oilatum
  cream, 600
  Emollient, 602
  Fragrance Free, 602
  Plus, 602
  shower emollient, 600
Oily cream, 599
Ointments
  definition, 598
  eye, 565
  suitable quantities, 598
Olanzapine, 193, **195**, **196**
Olbetam, 143
OliClinomel preparations, 513, 514
Olive oil
  cradle cap, 626
  ear, 585
Olmesartan, 105, **106**
  hydrochlorothiazide with, 106
Olmetec preparations, 106
Olopatadine, 570, **571**
Olsalazine, 52, 53, **55**
Omacor, 144
Omalizumab, 169, **170**
Omega-3 fatty acid compounds, 143
Omega-3-acid ethyl esters, **143**, 144
Omega-3-marine triglycerides, **144**
Omegaven preparations, 514
Omeprazole, **49**, 50
  infusion table, 830
Omiderm, 857
Omnic MR (tamsolusin), 439
Omnifix, 865
Omnikan, 366
Omnitrope, 401
Omnopon (papaveretum), 236
Omron nebulisers, 159
Onchocerciasis, 357
OncoTice, 481
Oncovin, 462
Ondansetron, 218, **222**
  infusion table, 830
Ondemet (ondansetron), 222

Index

- *One Touch* products, 366, 374, 375
- *One-Alpha*, 526
- *Onkotrone*, 456
- Onychomycosis *see* Fungal infections
- *Opatanol*, 571
- *Opilon*, 119
- Opioid analgesics *see* Analgesics, opioid
- Opioid antagonists, 679
  - poisoning, 31
- *Opizone*, 274
- *OpSite* products, 857
- *OptiClik*, 365
- *Opticrom* preparations, 571
- *OptiFlo* preparations, 444
- *Optil* (diltiazem), 113
- *Optilast*, 570
- *Optimax*, 212
- *OptiPen Pro*, 365
- *Optium* products, 374, 375
- *Optivate*, 136
- OPV, 656
- *Orabase*, 591
- *Orahesive*, 591
- *Oral balance see Biotène Oralbalance*
- Oral contraceptives *see* Contraception, oral
- Oral hypoglycaemic drugs *see* Antidiabetic drugs, oral, 366
- Oral rehydration, 505
- Oral rehydration salts, 505
  - WHO formula, 505
- Oral syringes, 2
- *Oraldene*, 595
- *Oramorph* preparations, 234
- *Orap*, 192
- *Orbifen* (ibuprofen), 541
- Orciprenaline, 153
- *Orelox*, 293
- *Orencia*, 553
- *Orfadin*, 532
- *Orgalutran*, 413
- Organophosphorus insecticides, poisoning by, 35
- *Orgaran*, 125
- *Orgran*, 844
- *Orlept* (sodium valproate), 253
- Orlistat, **216**
- Oropharynx, 590
  - anti-infective drugs, 592
- Orphenadrine, **266**
- ORS, 505
- ORT, 505
- *Ortho* diaphragm, 437
- *Ortho-Band Plus*, 863
- *Ortho-creme*—discontinued
- *Ortho-Gynest*, 425
- Orthopaedic surgery
  - antibacterial prophylaxis, 283
- *Orthovisc*, 535
- *Orudis*, 541
- *Oruvail* preparations, 541
  - gel, 563
- Oseltamivir, 341, **342**
- *Osmolite* preparations, 838
- *Ostenil*, 535
- Osteoarthritis, 534, 535
- Osteomyelitis, 281, 303, 304
- Osteonecrosis, jaw, 406–9
- Osteoporosis, 404
  - anabolic steroids, 397
  - bisphosphonates, 404, 406
  - calcitonin, 404
  - calcitriol, 404, 525
  - calcium, 404, 517
  - corticosteroid-induced, 405
  - HRT, 404
  - parathyroid hormone, 404
  - postmenopausal, 404
  - raloxifene, 405
  - strontium ranelate, 404
  - teriparatide, 404
- *Otex*, 586
- Otitis externa, 582
  - systemic treatment, 281
  - topical treatment, 582
- Otitis media, 585
  - systemic treatment, 281
  - with effusion, 585
- *Otomize*, 583
- *Otosporin*, 584
- *Otradrops* (xylometazoline), 589
- *Otraspray* (xylometazoline), 589
- *Otrivine* (xylometazoline), 589
- *Otrivine-Antistin*, 570
- *Ovestin*
  - cream, 425
  - tablets, 391
- *Ovitrelle*, 398
- *Ovranette*, 431
- *Ovysmen*, 432
- *Oxactin* (fluoxetine), 210
- Oxaliplatin, 466, **467**
  - infusion table, 830
- Oxamniquine, 357
- Oxazepam, 184, **186**
- Oxazolidinone antibacterials, 306
- Oxcarbazepine, 245, **246**, 247
  - trigeminal neuralgia, 238
- Oxerutins, 119
- Oxidising agents *see* Hydrogen peroxide
- *Oxis*, 150
- Oxpentifylline *see* Pentoxifylline
- Oxprenolol, **89**, 90
  - cyclopenthiazide with, 90
  - *see also* Beta-adrenoceptor blocking drugs
- Oxybenzone, 625
- Oxybuprocaine, **577**
- Oxybutynin, 440, **441**
- Oxycodone, 229, **235**, 15
  - infusion table, 830
  - morphine equivalence, 15
- *OxyContin*, 235
- Oxygen
  - acute asthma, 173
  - anaphylaxis, 170
  - chronic obstructive pulmonary disease, 173, 174
  - cluster headache, 243
  - equipment, 174
  - myocardial infarction, 132
  - nitrous oxide with, 670
  - supply arrangements, 174
- Oxymetazoline, 588
- Oxymetholone, 495
- *Oxymycin* (oxytetracycline), 298
- *OxyNorm*, 235
- Oxytetracycline, **298**
  - acne, 621
  - clobetasone butyrate with, 608
  - oral infections, 297
  - rosacea, 618
- Oxytocin, 419, **420**, **421**
  - ergometrine with, 420
  - infusion table, 830

P

- *Pabal*, 419
- *Fabrinex*, 524
- Pacemakers
  - dental practice, 24
- Paclitaxel, 469, **470**, 471
  - infusion table, 830
- PACT, x
- *Paediasure* preparations, 838
- Paediatric doses, 14
- *Paediatric Seravit*, 842
- Paget's disease, 405
- Pain, 224
  - bone, 225
  - dental, 224, 225, 230, 536
  - dressings, 670
  - musculoskeletal, 225, 563
  - neuropathic, 238
  - obstetric, 670
  - orofacial, 224, 225, 230, 238, 536
    - chronic, 238
  - palliative care, 229, 15, 18
  - perioperative, 230, 673
  - rheumatic, 534
  - sickle-cell disease, 224
  - trigeminal neuralgia, 238
  - urethral, 443
  - visceral, 229
- *Paldesic* (paracetamol) preparations, 227
- Palifermin, **451**
- Paliperidone, 193, **196**
- Palivizumab, 342, **343**
- *Palladone* preparations, 233
- Palliative care
  - prescribing, 15
  - subcutaneous infusion, 17
- Palonosetron, 218, **222**, 223
- *Paludrine*, 351
- *Paludrine/Avloclor*, 349
- *Pamergan-P100*, 237
- Pamidronate disodium *see* Disodium pamidronate
- *Panadeine* (co-codamol 8/500), 227
- *Panadol* (paracetamol) preparations, 227
- *Pancrease HL*, 69
- Pancreatin, **68**, 69
- Pancreatitis, chronic, 68
- *Panerex* preparations, 68
- Pancuronium, **677**, 678
- Panic disorder, 202
- *Panoxyl* preparations, 619
- Panthenol, 523
- Pantoprazole, **50**
  - infusion table, 830

Pantothenic acid, 523
Papaveretum, 236
  anaesthesia, **236**
  aspirin with, 226
  hyoscine with, 236
Papaverine, impotence, 447
Parabens, excipient, 598
Paracetamol, 225, **226**, 227
  buclizine with, 239
  codeine with, 227, 228, 239
  dihydrocodeine with, 228
  febrile convulsions, 258
  infusion table, 830
  isometheptene with, 228
  methionine with, 228
  metoclopramide with, 239
  migraine, 238
  poisoning by, 29
  post-immunisation pyrexia, 641
  postoperative pain, 674
  tramadol with, 237
Paracodol (co-codamol 8/500), 227
Paradote, 228
Paraffin
  eye, 578
  gauze dressing, 858
  liquid and white soft, 599
  oral emulsion, 61
  white soft, 599
  yellow soft, 578, 599
Paragauze, 858
Paraldehyde, 257
  status epilepticus, 256, **257**
Paramax, 239
Paramol (co-dydramol), 228
Paranet, 858
Paraplatin, 467
Paraproteinaemias, 495
Paraquat, poisoning by, 35
Parasiticidal preparations, 634
  suitable quantities, 633
Parasympathomimetics
  anaesthesia, 679
  eye, 576
  laxatives, 59
  myasthenia gravis, 558
  urinary retention, 439
Paratex, 858
Parathyroid hormone, 404, 405, **406**
Paratulle, 858
Pardelprin (indometacin), 541
Parecoxib, 536, **674**
Parenteral nutrition, 511
  preparations, 515, 516
PARI
  nebulisers, 158
  Vortex Spacer, 157
Paricalcitol, 525, **526**, 527
Pariet, 50
Parkinsonism, 258
  drug-induced, 188, 266
  idiopathic, 258
Parlodel, 411
Parmid XL (felodipine), 114
Paromomycin, 353
Paroven, 119
Paroxetine, 208, **210**
Paroxysmal nocturnal haemoglobinuria, 499
Partial seizures, 245
Partobulin SDF, 662
Parvolex, 31
Pastes, definition, 598
Patents, 3
Patient group direction, 3
Patient packs, x
Pavacol-D (pholcodine), **177**
Peak flow meters, 156
Peanut oil *see* Arachis oil
PEC high compression bandage, 862
Pediacel, 646
Pediculosis, 634
Peditrace, 516
Pegaptanib, **580**
Pegasys, 479
Pegfilgrastim, 501, **502**
Peginterferon alfa, 340, **479**
PegIntron, 479
Pegvisomant, **401**
Pegzerepoetin alfa *see* Methoxy polyethylene glycol-epoetin beta, 495, **498**
Peha Crepp E, 861
Pelvic inflammatory disease, 280
Pemetrexed, 458, **460**
  infusion table, 830
Pemphigus, 379
Penbritin, 288
Penciclovir, 336, **633**
Penfine, 366
Penicillamine, 548
  autoimmune hepatitis, **529**
  cystinuria, **529**
  poisoning, **34**
  rheumatic disease, 546, **547**
  Wilson's disease, 528, **529**
Penicillin G *see* Benzylpenicillin
Penicillin V *see* Phenoxymethylpenicillin, 284, **285**
Penicillin VK *see* Phenoxymethylpenicillin, 284, **285**
Penicillinases, 285
Penicillins, 284
  antipseudomonal, 290
  broad spectrum, 287
  penicillinase-resistant, 285
  penicillinase-sensitive, 284
Penlet II, 366
Pennsaid, 563
Pentacarinat, 355
Pentamidine isetionate, **355**
  infusion table, 830
  leishmaniasis, 353
  pneumocystis pneumonia, 354
Pentasa, 54
Pentastarch, 509, **510**
Pentazocine, 229, **236**
Pentostam, 354
Pentostatin, **466**
  infusion table, 830
Pentoxifylline, **119**, 862
Pentrax, 627
Pepcid (famotidine) preparations, 46
Pepdite, 843
Peppermint oil, 42, **43**
Peptac, 40
Peptamen preparations, 838
Peptimax (cimetidine), 45
Peptisorb, 838
Perative, 838
Percutol, 110
Perdix, 103
Perfalgan, 227
Perfan, 72
Pergolide, 259, **260**
Pergoveris, 399
Periactin, 168
Pericoronitis, 281
Pericyazine, **191**
Perinal, 65
Perindopril, **103**
  indapamide with, 103
  see also ACE inhibitors
Periodontitis, 590
  antibacterial treatment, 281
Periostat, 590, 591
Peripheral vascular disease, 118
Peritonitis, 279
PermaFoam products, 852, 853
Permethrin, 634, **635**, 636
Permitabs, 639
Peroxyl, 595
Perphenazine, 189, **191**
  amitriptyline with, 204
  nausea, **219**
  nausea and vertigo, 217
  psychoses, 191
Persantin preparations, 131
Pertussis
  immunisation
    vaccines, 646, **654**
  prophylaxis, 282
Pethidine, 230
  anaesthesia, 236
  analgesia, 230, **236**
  preparations, 236
  promethazine with, 237
Petit mal, 245
Petroleum jelly, 599
Petroleum products, poisoning by, 28
Pevaryl, 531
Peyronie's disease, 524
PGD *see* Patient group direction, 3
Phaeochromocytoma, 85, **98**
Pharmacist prescribing, independent, 887
Pharma-Ject Morphine Sulphate, 230
Pharmagen, 169
Pharmapore-PU products, 857
Pharmorubicin preparations, 456
Pharyngitis *see* Throat infections
Pharynx *see* Oropharynx
Phenelzine, 206, **207**
Phenergan preparations, 168
Phenindione, 127, **128**
Phenobarbital, 250
  epilepsy, **250**
    status epilepticus, **257**
  poisoning, elimination, 28
Phenobarbital sodium, 258
Phenobarbitone *see* Phenobarbital
Phenol, 66
  haemorrhoids, 66
  injection, oily, 66

Index

Phenothiazines, 189
  classification, 189
  nausea and vertigo, 217, 218
  poisoning by, 33
  psychoses, 189
Phenothrin, **636**
Phenoxybenzamine, **98**, 99
  infusion table, 830
Phenoxymethylpenicillin, 284, **285**
Phentermine, 216
Phentolamine, 98, **99**
  impotence, **447**
  papaverine with, 447
  preparations, 99
Phenylephrine, 572
  eye, **572**
  hypotension, 121
  infusion table, 830
  injection, 121
  lidocaine with, 683
Phenylketonuria, 516, 847
Phenytoin
  diabetic neuropathy, 373
  epilepsy, **250**, 251
    status epilepticus, 256, **258**
  infusion table, 830
  trigeminal neuralgia, 238
Phlexy-10, 847
Phlexy-Vits preparations, 847
Phobia, 206
Pholcodine, 176, **177**
Phosex, 520
Phosgene, poisoning by, 35
Phosphate supplements, 519
Phosphate-binding agents, 520
Phosphates, 63, 520
  enemas, 62
  intravenous, 520
  rectal, 63, 64
Phosphate-Sandoz, 520
Phosphodiesterase inhibitors
  erectile dysfunction, 446
  heart failure, 72
  pulmonary hypertension, 95
Phosphorus, 519
Photodamage, skin, 625
Photodermatoses, 624
  ACBS, 849
Photodynamic therapy, 467
Photofrin, 467
Phototherapy, psoriasis, 612
Phyllocontin Continus, 155
Physeptone (methadone), 233, 274
Physiological saline *see* Sodium chloride
Physiotens, 96
Physiotulle products, 859
Phytex, 632
Phytomenadione, 527
  infusion table, 830
Phytosterolaemia, 138
Picolax, 64
Piggy-back technique, 822
Piko-1, 156
Pilocarpine
  dry eyes, 595, **596**
  dry mouth, 595, **596**
  eye, **576**
Pilogel, 576
Pimecrolimus, 616, **617**
Pimozide, 189, **192**
  Tourette syndrome, 267
Pindolol, **90**
  clopamide with, 90
  see also Beta-adrenoceptor blocking drugs
Pinetarsol, 614
Pinworm infections, 355
Pioglitazone, 369, **370**, 371
  with metformin, 371
Piperacillin, **290**
  tazobactam with, 290
    infusion table, 830
Piperazine, **356**
  roundworm infections, 356
  threadworm infections, 356
Piperazine oestrone sulphate *see* Estropipate, 391
Piportil Depot, 199
Pipothiazine *see* Pipotiazine, **199**
Pipotiazine, **199**
Piracetam, 255, **267**, 268
Pirenzepine, 47
Piriton, 168
Piroxicam, **543**
  rheumatic disease, 535, 543
  topical, 563
Pitressin, 403
Pituitary
  function test, 415
  hormones
    anterior, 398
    posterior, 402
Pityriasis versicolor, 321, 630
Pivmecillinam, 290, **291**
Pizotifen, **242**, 243
PK Aid 4, 847
PK Foods preparations, 847
PKU preparations, 847, 848
Plaque, 594
Plaquenil, 549
Plasma concentrations, electrolytes, 503
Plasma substitutes, 508
Plasma, fresh frozen, 137
Plasma-Lyte preparations, 514
Plasmapheresis, myasthenia gravis, 558
Plasters, 865
Plastic wound dressing
  impermeable, 865
  permeable, 865
Plastipak, 366
Plavix, 131
Plendil, 114
Pleniday, 844
Pletal, 119
Pneumococcal infection
  antibacterial prophylaxis, 282
  immunisation
    vaccines, 654, 655
Pneumocystis pneumonia, 354
Pneumonia, 173, 279, 280
  pneumococcal, 654
Pneumovax II, 655
Pocket Chamber, 157
Pocketpeak, 156
PocketScan products, 374, 375
Podagra, 555
Podophyllin, 622, **624**
Podophyllotoxin, 623, 624
Podophyllum resin, 622
  see also Podophyllin
  see also Podophyllotoxin
Poisoning, 27
  active elimination, 28
  adsorbents, 28
  hospital admission, 27
Polial, 844
Polihexanide, 581
Poliomyelitis, 655
  immunisation
    travel, 655, 663
    vaccines, 646, 655, 656
Pollinex, 169
Polyacrylic acid *see* Carbomers, 578
Polyarteritis nodosa, 379, 544
Polycal, 838
  glucose tolerance test, 376
Polycose, 839
Polycystic ovary syndrome, 368
Polyene antifungal drugs, 321
Polyethoxylated castor oil *see* Polyoxyl castor oil, 2
Polyethylene glycols, 62
  [ingredient], 64
Polyfax, 629
  eye, 568
Polyfield Nitrile Patient Pack, 859
Polyfield Soft Vinyl Patient Pack, 859
Polygeline, 510
Polyhexamethylene biguanide *see* Polihexanide, 581
Polyhexanide *see* Polihexanide, 581
PolyMem products, 852, 853
Polymethylmethacrylate, 637
Polymyalgia rheumatica, 544
Polymyositis, 544, 549
Polymyxins, 308
  ear, 584, 585
  eye, 566, 567, 568, 569
  skin, 628, 629
Polyoxyl castor oil, presence of, 2
Polyps, nasal, 586
Polysaccharide–iron complex, 492
Polyserositis, 556
Polyskin products, 857
Polysorbates, excipient, 598
Polystyrene sulphonate resins, 504
Polytar
  AF, 627
  Emollient, 614
  Liquid, 627
  Plus, 627
Polyurethane foam dressing, 852, 853
Polyvinyl alcohol, 578
Pompe disease, 531
Ponstan preparations, 542
POP *see* Progestogens, contraceptives, oral, 427, 432, **433**
Poractant alfa, 173
Porfimer sodium, 467
Pork Actrapid, 362
Pork Insulatard, 364
Pork Mixtard-30—discontinued
Porphyrias, acute, 532
  drugs to be avoided in, 532, 533

Portal hypertension, 86
Porta-Neb, 158
Posaconazole, 322, **326**
Posalfilin, 623
Postherpetic neuralgia, 238, 336
Post-traumatic stress disorder, 202
Potaba, 524
Potable water, 2
Potassium aminobenzoate, 524
Potassium bicarbonate, 505, **506**
  tablets, effervescent, 506
Potassium chloride, 504, 507, 508
  concentrate, sterile, 508
  infusion
    glucose and, 508
    sodium chloride and, 508
    sodium chloride, glucose and, 508
    table, 830
  oral preparations, 504
Potassium citrate, 443
Potassium permanganate, 611, 637, **639**
Potassium supplements, 503
  diuretic with, 78
Potassium tablets, effervescent, 506
Potassium-channel activators, 117
  angina, 107
Povidone, eye, 578
Povidone-iodine
  skin, 637, **638**, 639
    dressing, 857, 858
Powergel, 563
Prader-Willi syndrome, 399, 400
Pralidoxime chloride, 35, **36**
Pramipexole, 259, **260**, 261
Pramocaine [ingredient], 65
Pramoxine *see* Pramocaine, 65
Prandin, 371
Pravastatin, 140, **142**
Praxilene, 119
Praziquantel, 357
Prazosin, **97**
  cardiovascular, 97
  preparations, 98
  urinary tract, 438, **439**
Precocious puberty, 413
Pred Forte, 569
Predenema, 56
Predfoam, 56
Prednisolone, 379, **384**
  asthma, acute severe, 148
  Crohn's disease, 56
  ear, 584
    neomycin with, 584
  eye, 569, 570
  haemorrhoids, 65
  injection, 545
  lepra reactions, 314
  malignant disease, 474
  myasthenia gravis, 559
  palliative care, 17
  pneumocystis pneumonia, 354
  rectal, 56, 57
  rheumatic disease, 544, 545
  ulcerative colitis, 56
  withdrawal of, 380
Predsol
  ear, 584
  eye, 569
  rectal, 57
Predsol-N
  ear, 584
  eye, 570
Pre-eclampsia, 93, 519
Preface, iii
Pregabalin, 245, **248**
  epilepsy, 247
  generalised anxiety disorder, 248
  neuropathic pain, 238
Pregaday, 492
Pregestimil, 843
Pregnancy
  anticoagulants, 128
  asthma, 145
  epilepsy and, 245
  folate supplements, 492, 494
  hypertension in, 93
  iron, 490
    folic acid and, 492
  nausea and vomiting, 218
  prescribing in, 787
  termination, 418
Pregnyl, 398
Prejomin, 843
Premarin
  oral, 389
  vaginal, 425
PremCare, 839
Premedication, 670
  children, 672
  dental procedures, 180, 672
Premenstrual syndrome, 392, 523
PremierPore VP, 857
Premique preparations, 387
Prempak-C, 387
Preotact, 406
Prepadine (dosulepin), 205
Prescal, 114
Prescribing, x
  ACBS, 833
  addicts, 9
  analyses and cost, x
  breast-feeding, 807
  children, 13
  computer-generated, 5
  controlled drugs, 8
  dental practice, 4
  drug misusers, 9
  elderly, 19
  generic, 1
  instalments, 8
  liver disease, 762
  non-proprietary, 1
  palliative care, 15
  patient packs, x
  pregnancy, 787
  renal impairment, 772
Prescription forms, 8
  controlled drugs, 7
  dental, 4
  nurses, 884
  security, 3
Prescription only medicines *see* preparations identified by PoM throughout BNF
Prescription writing, 4
Preservex, 537
Presinex (desmopressin), 403
Pressure sores, 603
Prestige Smart System, 374, 375
Prestim, 91
Prevenar, 655
Prexige—discontinued
Prezista, 332
Priadel, 201
Prialt, 225
Priapism, 445
Prices, x
Prilocaine, **684**
  felypressin with, 681, 684
  lidocaine with, 682
Primacine (erythromycin), 302
Primacor, 72
Primapore, 858
Primaquine, 345, **350**
  pneumocystis pneumonia, 354
Primaxin, 296
  infusion table, 828
Primene, 514
Primidone, **250**
Primolut N, 393
Prioderm, 635
Priorix, 652
Pripsen, 356
Pro-Banthine, 42
Probenecid, **556**, 557
Procainamide, 81, **82**, 83
  infusion table, 830
Procaine, **684**
Pro-Cal preparations, 839
Procarbazine, **467**
Prochlorperazine
  nausea and vertigo, 217, 218, **220**
  psychoses, **192**
Procoralan, 118
Proctofoam HC, 65
Proctosedyl, 65
Procyclidine, **266**, 267
Prodose, 94
Product licence, 1
Pro-Epanutin, 257
Proflavine cream, 636
Profore products, 858, 862, 863, 864
Progesterone, 392, **393**, 394
Progestogen-only pill *see* Progestogens, contraceptives, oral, 427, 432, **433**
Progestogens, 392, 484
  contraceptives
    intra-uterine, 434, **435**
    oral, 427, 432, **433**
    parenteral, 433, **434**
  HRT and, 392
  malignant disease, 483
Prograf, 477
Proguanil, 346, 347, 348, 349, **350**, 351
  atovaquone with, 344, 351
ProGuide products, 859, 863, 864
Progynova, 390
Progynova TS, 390
Proleukin, 480
Promazine, 189, **192**
Promethazine
  allergic disorders, 166, **168**
  hypnotic, **183**
  nausea and vertigo, 218, **219**
  premedication, 168
Promethazine teoclate, 219

Promin, 845
Promixin, 308
Promogran products, **854**
Pronestyl, 83
Prontosan, 854
Propafenone, 81, **83**
Propamidine isetionate, 566, **568**
Propantheline, 42
  gastro-intestinal, 41, 42
  urinary tract, 440, 442
Propax SDP, 859
Propecia, 627
Propess, 420
Prophylaxis, antibacterial, 282
Propine, 575
Propionibacterium acnes, 619
Propionic acidaemia, 846
Propiverine, 440, 442
Propofol, 667, **668**
  infusion table, 830
Propofol-Lipuro, 668
Propoven, 668
Propranolol, **85**, 86
  cardiovascular, 85
  migraine, 242
  see also Beta-adrenoceptor blocking drugs
  thyrotoxicosis, 377
  tremor, 267
Proprietary names, symbol, 1
Propylene glycol, presence of, 2, 598
Propylthiouracil, 377, **378**
Proscar, 397
Prosobee, 843
Prostacyclin *see* Epoprostenol
Prostaglandins
  anticoagulant, 126
  ductus arteriosus, 421
  eye, 572, 573
  gastro-intestinal, 48
  obstetrics, 418, 419, 420, 421
Prostap SR, 488
Prostap-3, 488
Prostate cancer, 452, **486**, 488
Prostatic hyperplasia, benign 396, 438
Prostatitis, 280, 319
Prostin E2 preparations, 420
Prostin VR, 421
Prosulf, 129
ProSure, 839
Protamine sulphate, 123, 128, **129**
Protease inhibitors, 327, 328
Protease modulating matrix, 854
Proteasome inhibitors, 464
ProtectFilm, 857
Protein C concentrate, 137
Protein kinase inhibitors, 468
Protein, intravenous nutrition, 511
Protelos, 410
Prothiaden, 205
Prothionamide *see* Protionamide, 312
Prothrombin complex concentrate, 127
Protifar, 841
Protionamide, 312
Protirelin, **402**
Protium, 50
Proton pump inhibitors, 48
Protopam, 36
Protopic, 618
Protozoal infections, 344
Provera
  gynaecology, 393
  malignant disease, 483
Provide, 839
Provigil, 215
Pro-Viron, 396
Proxymetacaine, **577**
Prozac, 210
Prozep (fluoxetine), 210
Pruritus, 166, 603
  ACBS, 849
Pruritus ani, 65
Pseudoephedrine, **178**
Pseudomembranous colitis, 53
  antibacterial therapy, 279
    metronidazole, in, 315
    vancomycin, in, 305
  clindamycin, in, 303
Pseudomonas aeruginosa infections, 295, 299, 308
  antipseudomonal penicillins, in, 290
  cephalosporins, in, 291
  eye, 566
Psittacosis, 296
Psoriasis, 611
  corticosteroids, 605
Psoriatic arthropathy, 549
Psoriderm preparations, 614
  scalp, 627
Psorin preparations, 615
Psychoses, 187
Puberty
  delayed, 394, 398
  precocious, 413, 415
Pubic lice, 634
Pulmicort preparations, 162
Pulmonary
  embolism, 122, 133, 173
  hypertension, 93, 126, 174
  oedema, 74
  surfactants, 173
Pulmozyme, 176
Pulvinal Beclometasone Dipropionate, 161, 162
Pulvinal Salbutamol, 152
Puregon, 399
Purilon, 854
Puri-Nethol, 460
Purpura, thrombocytopenic, 500
Pyelonephritis, 280, 319
Pylobactell, 44
Pyralvex, 592
Pyrazinamide, 310, 311, **313**
Pyrexia, 225
  post immunisation, 641
Pyridostigmine, 558, **559**
  laxative, 59
Pyridoxine, 523, **524**
  anaemias, 495
  status epilepticus, 255
Pyrimethamine, **351**
  malaria, 351
  sulfadoxine with, 351, 352
  toxoplasmosis, 354
Pyrithione zinc shampoos, 626

Q

Q-fever, 296
Quaternary ammonium compounds, 41
Quaternium 15, excipient, 598
Quellada M, 635
Questran preparations, 138
Quetiapine, 193, **196**
QuickCal, 839
Quinagolide, 410, **412**
Quinapril, **103**, 104
  hydrochlorothiazide with, 104
  see also ACE inhibitors
Quinil (quinapril), 104
Quinine, **352**
  infusion table, 830
  malaria, 344, 352
  nocturnal cramps, 561
  poisoning
    elimination, 23
Quinoderm, 619
Quinolones, 316
  eye, 566
Quinupristin, dalfopristin with, **307**, 308
  infusion table, 830
QV preparations, 600, 602
Qvar preparations, 161

R

Rabeprazole, **50**
Rabies
  immunisation, 656
    travel, 663
  immunoglobulin, **661**
  vaccine, 656
Rabipur, 656
Raloxifene, **392**, 405
Raltegravir, xiii
Raltitrexed, 458, 461
  infusion table, 830
Ramipril, **104**
  felodipine with, 104
  see also ACE inhibitors
Ranibizumab, **580**, 581
Ranitic (ranitidine), 47
Ranitidine, **46**, 47
  infusion table, 831
Rantec (ranitidine), 47
Rapamune, 476
Rapifen, 675
Rapilysin, 134
Rapitil, 571
Rapolyte, 505
Raptiva, 617
Rasagiline, **264**
Rasburicase, 449, **557**
  infusion table, 831
Rashes, urticarial, 166
Rasilez, 107
Raynaud's syndrome, 98, 115, 118
Rebetol, 343
Rebif, 480
Reboxetine, 211, **212**
Recombinant activated protein C, **136**
Rectogesic, 66
Red eye, 566, 568

Index

Red line webbing, 863
Redoxon (ascorbic acid), 525
Reductil, 217
ReFacto (factor VIII fraction), 136
Reflexions, 437
Refludan, 126
Reflux oesophagitis *see* Gastro-oesophageal reflux disease, **38**
Refolinon (calcium folinate), 451
Regaine, 628
Regal, 860
Regranex, 640
Regulan, 59
Regulose (lactulose), 62
Regurin, 442
Rehydration
 oral, 505
 parenteral, 506
Relaxit, 63
Release, 858
Relenza, 342
Relestat, 570
Relifex, 542
Relpax, 240
Remedeine, 228
Remicade, 555
Remifentanil, 229, 674, **675**, 676
 infusion table, 831
Reminyl preparations, 275
Remnos (nitrazepam), 181
Renagel, 520
Renal colic *see* Ureteric colic, 443
Renal excretion, interactions affecting, 686
Renal impairment, prescribing in, 772
Renamil, 842
Renapro, 841
Renilon 7.5, 839
Renin inhibitors, 107
Rennie Duo, 40
ReoPro, 130
Repaglinide, 369, **371**
Repevax, 646
Replagal, 530
Replenate (factor VIII fraction), 136
Replenine-VF (factor IX fraction), 136
Replens, 425
Replicare Ultra, 855
Requip, 261
RescueFlow, 510
Resonium A, 504
Resource preparations, 839, 840
Respiratory depression
 poisoning, 27
 postoperative, 679
Respiratory distress syndrome, 173
Respiratory failure, 172
Respiratory stimulants, 172
Respiratory syncytial virus infections, 342
Respontin, 154
Resprin, 226
Restandol, 394
Restless legs syndrome
 pramipexole, 260
 ropinirole, 261
Resuscitation
 cardiopulmonary, 121
 dental practice, 666
Reteplase, 133, **134**
Retin-A, 620
Retinoids
 acne
  oral, 622
  topical, 619
 leukaemia, 472
 psoriasis, 612, **615**
Retinol *see* Vitamin A
Retrovir, 331
Revatio, 95, 447
Revaxis, 646
Revlimid, 481
Rexocaine, 682
Reyataz, 332
Reye's syndrome, aspirin and, 226
Rhesus incompatibility, 661
Rheumatac Retard (diclofenac), 539
Rheumatic diseases, 534, 544
 corticosteroid injections, 545
 rubefacients, 563
Rheumatic fever
 prophylaxis, 282
Rheumatism, palindromic, 546
Rheumatoid arthritis, 379, 534
Rheumox, 537
Rhinitis
 allergic, 165, 586
 medicamentosa, 588
 vasomotor, 165, 588
Rhinocort Aqua, 587
Rhinolast preparations, 586
Rhophylac, 662
Rhumalgan (diclofenac), 539
Riamet, 344, 349
Ribavirin, **343**
 chronic hepatitis C, 340, 342
 respiratory syncytial virus, 342
Riboflavin, 523
Rickets, hypophosphataemic, 519
Rickettsia, 296
Ridaura, 547
Rifabutin, 311, **313**
Rifadin, 313
Rifampicin, **313**, 314
 compound preparations, 314
 infusion table, 831
 leprosy, 314
 tuberculosis, 310, 311
Rifamycins, 310, 311, 313
Rifater, 310, 314
Rifinah, 310, 314
Rilutek, 268
Riluzole, 267, **268**
RIMA, 207
Rimacid (indometacin), 541
Rimacillin (ampicillin), 288
Rimactane, 314
Rimactazid 300—discontinued
Rimafen (ibuprofen), 540
Rimapam (diazepam), 185
Rimapurinol (allopurinol), 556
Rimexolone, **570**
Rimonabant, **216**, 217
Rimoxallin (amoxicillin), 288
Rimso-50, 444
Rinatec, 589
Ringer's solution, 507
Ringer-Lactate solution, 507
Ringworm infection *see* Dermatophyte infection, 322
Risedronate sodium, 404, **408**, 409
Risperdal preparations, 197, 199
Risperidone, 193, **196**, 197
 depot injection, 199
Ritalin, 214
Rite-Diet
 gluten-free, 844
 low protein, 845
Ritodrine, 423, 424
 infusion table, 831
Ritonavir, 328, **333**
 lopinavir with, 333
 see also Kaletra
Rituximab, 478
 infusion table, 831
 malignant diseases, 477, **478**
 rheumatic diseases, 552, 555
Rivastigmine, 275, **276**
Rivotril, 255, 256
Rizatriptan, 239, **240**
Roaccutane, 622
Robaxin, 561
Robinson Primary, 858
Robinul, 640, 671
Robinul-Neostigmine, 679
Rocaltrol, 526
Rocephin, 294
Rocuronium, 677, **678**
 infusion table, 831
Roferon-A, 479
Rogitine, 99
Ropinirole, 259, **261**
Ropivacaine, **684**, 685
Rosacea, 618, 630
Rosidal K, 863
Rosiglitazone, 369, **371**
 metformin with, 371
Rosuvastatin, 140, **142**
Rotarix, 657
Rotavirus vaccine, 657
Rotigotine, 259, **261**
Roundworm infections, 356
Rowachol, 67
Rowatinex, 443
Rozex, 630
rt-PA *see* Alteplase
Rubefacients, 563
Rubella, 657
 immunisation
  immunoglobulin, 660
  vaccines, 657
Rufinamide, **251**
Rusyde (furosemide), 75
Rutosides, 119
Rynacrom, 588
Rythmodan preparations, 82

S

Sabril, 254
Saizen, 401
Salactol, 623
Salagen, 596
Salamol (salbutamol) preparations, 151, 152
Salapin (salbutamol), 151
Salatac, 623

Salazopyrin, 55, 555
    retention enema—discontinued
Salbutamol, **151**, 152
    asthma, 149
    infusion table, 831
    ipratropium with, 156
    premature labour, 424
Salcatonin *see* Calcitonin
Salicylates
    aphthous ulcers, 592
    rheumatic disease
        topical, 563
Salicylic acid, 615
    acne, 620, 621
    betamethasone with, 608
    coal tar and dithranol with, 615
    fungal infections, 632
        undecenoates with, 633
    hyperkeratoses, 622
    podophyllum with, 623
    psoriasis, 612
        coal tar with, 614, 626
        dithranol and zinc with, 615
        sulphur with, 627
        zinc with, 615
    scalp, 626
    warts and calluses, 623
Saline *see* Sodium chloride
Salinum, 596
Saliva, artificial, 595
Saliveze, 596
Salivix, 596
Salmeterol, 149, **152**
    fluticasone with, 164
Salmonellosis, 279
Salofalk preparations, 55
Salpingitis, 296
Salt substitutes, 503
Sandimmun, 476
Sandocal preparations, 517
Sandoglobulin preparations, 661
Sando-K, 504
Sandostatin, 489
Sandostatin LAR, 489
Sandrena, 391
Sanomigran, 243
Saquinavir, 328, **334**
Savene, 450
Savlon Dry powder, 639
Scabies, 634
Scandishake, 839
Scandonest, 681
Scanpor, 865
Schar, 844
Scheriproct, 65
Schistosoma, 357
Schistosomicides, 357
Schizophrenia, 188
Scleroderma, 524
Sclerosants, 144
Scopoderm preparations, 224
Scopolamine *see* Hyoscine, 41, **42**
Scottish Medicines Consortium, 3
Scottish Prescribing Analysis, x
Scurvy, 524
SeaSorb products, 851
Sebco, 614
Sebivo, 341
Sebomin, 298
Seborrhoeic dermatitis, 611
Seborrhoeic eczema, 611
Secobarbital, 187
    amobarbital with, 187
Seconal Sodium, 187
Sectral, 86
Securon, 117
    tablets—discontinued
Sedation, anaesthesia, 671
Sedatives, 179
    see also Anxiolytics
Select-A-Jet Dopamine, 120
Selegiline, **264**
Selenase, 522
Selenium, **522**
Selenium sulphide, 626, 627, 630
Selexid, 291
Selsun, 627
Semi-Daonil—discontinued
Semi-permeable adhesive film, 856
Semisodium valproate, 200
Senna, **60**, 61
Senokot, 61
Septanest, 681
Septic arthritis, 281
Septicaemia
    catheter-related, 281
    community-acquired, 280
    hospital-acquired, 280
    meningococcal, 281
Septrin, 309
Seractil, 538
Seravit, Paediatric, 842
Serc, 224
Serdolect, 197
Serenace, 191
Seretide, 164
Serevent, 152
Seroquel, 196
Serotonin re-uptake inhibitor antidepressants *see* Antidepressants
Seroxat, 210
Sertindole, 193, 197
Sertraline, 208, **210**, 211
Sesame oil, presence of, 2
Setocrepe, 862
Setoplast, 865
Setopress, 862
Setoprime, 858
Sevelamer, **520**
Sevoflurane, 669, **670**
Sevredol, 234
Sex hormones
    androgens, 394
        antagonists, 396
    malignant disease, 482
    oestrogens, 384
        antagonists, 397
    progestogens, 392
Sexual deviation, 189, 396
Shampoos, 626
Shared care, 4
Sharpsbin, 366
Shigellosis, 279
Shingles, 336
Shock, 120
    anaphylactic, 170
        dental practice, 21
    cardiogenic, 120
    metabolic acidosis, 508
    plasma substitutes, 509
    septic, 120, 379
SHS Modjul Flavour, 845
Sibutramine, 216, **217**
Sicca syndrome, 595
Sickle-cell disease, pain, 224
Sidestream Durable, 158
Sigma ETB, 861
Significant changes, xi
Sildenafil, 447
    erectile dysfunction, 446, **447**
    pulmonary hypertension, 93, **95**
Silgel, 856
Silicone gel, 856
    sheets, 856
Silicone spray, 856
Silkis, 613
Silkolan, 863
Silver nitrate, 622, **623**
Silver sulfadiazine, 628, **629**
Silver sulphadiazine *see* Silver sulfadiazine, 628, **629**
Silvercel, 856
Simeticone, 38, 40
Simple eye ointment, 578
Simple linctus, 177
    paediatric, 178
SimpleXx, 401
Simulect, 475
Simvador (simvastatin), 143
Simvastatin, 143, 140, **142**, 143
    ezetimibe with, 143
Sinemet preparations, 263
Sinepin, 205
Singulair, 165
Sinthrome, 128
Sinusitis, 588
    antibacterial treatment, 281
    inhalation, 176
Siopel, 603
Sirolimus, 474, **476**
Sitagliptin, 369, **371**, 372
Sitaxentan, 93, **95**
Sitosterolaemia, 138
Skelid, **409**
Skin preparations
    anaesthetic, 603
    antibacterials, 628
    antipruritic, 604
    antiviral, 633
    barrier, 602
    cleansing, 637
    corticosteroids, 604
    emollient, 598
    excipients, 598
    tissue adhesive, 637
    ulcers, 639
Skinoren, 619
Skintact, 858
Slinky, 861
SLO Drinks, 841
Slocinx XL (doxazosin), 97
Slofenac (diclofenac), 539
Slo-Indo (indometacin), 541
Slo-Phyllin, 155
Slo-Pro (propranolol), 86
Slow-K, 504
Slow-Sodium, 504
Slow-Trasicor, 90
Slozem, 113
SMA preparations, 840, 841, 843

Index

Smallpox vaccine, 657
SMC *see* Scottish Medicines Consortium, 3
SMOFlipid preparations, 514
Smoking cessation, 270
Snake bites, 36
  antivenom, 36
Sno Tears, 578
Sno-Pro, 845
Social anxiety disorder, 202
Social phobia *see* social anxiety disorder
Sodiofolin, 451
Sodium acid phosphate, 520
Sodium alendronate *see* Alendronic acid
Sodium Amytal, 187
Sodium aurothiomalate, **546**, 547
Sodium benzoate, 14
Sodium bicarbonate
  antacid, 38
  ear, 585
  ear, 585
  intravenous, 508
  oral, 505, 506
  urine alkalinisation, 443
Sodium calcium edetate, **34**, 35
  infusion table, 831
Sodium calciumedetate *see* Sodium calcium edetate
Sodium carboxymethylcellulose *see* Carmellose
Sodium chloride
  bladder irrigation, 444, 637
  eye irrigation, 565, **578**, 579
  infusion, 506, 507
    glucose and, 506, 507
    hypercalcaemia, 518
    potassium chloride and, 508
    potassium chloride, glucose and, 508
  mouthwash, compound, 594, **595**
  nasal solution, 588
  nebuliser solution, 159
  oral, 504
  skin cleansing, **637**
Sodium citrate
  acid aspiration prophylaxis, 666
  bladder irrigation, **444**
  rectal, 63
  urine alkalinisation, 443
Sodium clodronate, 409
  infusion table, 831
Sodium content, antacids, 39
Sodium cromoglicate
  asthma, **164**
  eye, 570, **571**
  food allergy, 57
  nose, 586, **588**
Sodium cromoglycate *see* Sodium cromoglicate
Sodium docusate *see* Docusate sodium
Sodium feredetate, 492
Sodium fluoride, **521**, 522
Sodium fusidate, **304**
  angular cheilitis, 593
  skin, 629
Sodium hyaluronate
  intra-articular, 535
  intra-ocular, 579
Sodium ironedetate *see* Sodium feredetate, 492
Sodium lactate, 508
  intravenous infusion, 508
    compound, 506, 507
Sodium metabisulphite, excipient, 598
Sodium nitrite, 33, **34**
Sodium nitroprusside, 93, **95**
  infusion table, 831
Sodium oxybate, **184**, 33
Sodium phenylbutyrate, 532
Sodium picosulfate, **61**, 63, 64
Sodium picosulphate *see* Sodium picosulfate, **61**, 63, 64
Sodium pidolate, 600
Sodium polystyrene sulphonate, 504
Sodium risedronate *see* Risedronate sodium, 404, **408**, 409
Sodium stibocaptate, 357
Sodium stibogluconate, **353**, 354
Sodium tetradecyl sulphate, **144**
Sodium thiosulphate, 33, **34**
Sodium valproate *see* Valproate
Soffcrepe, 862
Sofradex
  ear, 583
  eye, 569
Soft tissue disorders, 534
Soft Touch, 366
Softclix products, 366
Softexe, 863
Softpore, 858
Solaraze, 625
Solian, 194
Solifenacin, 440, **442**
Soliris, 500
Solivito N, 516
Solpadol, 228
Soltamox (tamoxifen), 486
Solu-Cortef, 383
Solu-Medrone, 384
Solvaline N, 858
Solvazinc, 522
Solvents, ear wax removal, 585
Somatomedins, 416
Somatostatin analogues, 488
Somatotrophin *see* Somatropin, 400, 401
Somatropin, 400, 401
Somatuline Autogel, 489
Somatuline LA, 489
Somavert, 401
Somnite (nitrazepam), 181
Sonata, 182
Soneryl, 187
Sorafenib, 468, **469**
Sorbalgon products, 851
Sorbic acid, excipient, 598
Sorbitol, 511
  presence of, 2
Sorbsan products, 851, 859
Sotacor, 90
Sotalol, **90**
  cardiovascular, 85
  infusion table, 831
  see also Beta-adrenoceptor blocking drugs
Soya oil, 601
SPA, x
Spacer devices, 157
Spasmonal preparations, 42
Spasticity, 559
SpectraBan, 625
Spermicides, 435
SPF, 625
Spinhaler, 157, 164
Spiramycin 301, 354
Spirit
  industrial methylated, 637
  surgical, 637
Spiriva preparations, 154
Spironolactone, **76**, 77
  furosemide with, 78
  heart failure, 99
  hydroflumethiazide with, 78
Splenectomy *see* Asplenia
Sporanox, 325
Sporanox-Pulse, 325
Sports card, 26
Sprilon, 603
Sprycel, 468
SQ-PEN, 365
SSRIs *see* Antidepressants, serotonin re-uptake inhibitor, 208
SST, 596
St John's Wort, 202
Stalevo, 264
Stamaril, 659
Stannous fluoride, 522
Starch, etherified, 509, 510, 511
Staril, 102
Starlix, 370
Statins, 140
  angina, 108
Status epilepticus, 255
  non-convulsive, 256
Stavudine, 328, **330**
Stayform, 861
STD injection see *Fibro-Vein*
Steam inhalations, 588
Stelazine 193
Stemetil, 220
Sterculia, 59
  constipation, 58, 59
  diarrhoea, 51
Stericlens, 637
Sterifix, 858
Sterile larvae, 639
Steri-Neb
  ipratropium, 154
  Salamol, 152
  sodium chloride, 159
Steripaste, 864
Steripod (sodium chloride), 637
Steripoule (sodium chloride), 159
Steri-strip, 866
Steroid cards, 381
Ster-Zac Bath Concentrate, 639
Stesolid (diazepam), 185, 256
Stibocaptate *see* Sodium stibocaptate, 357
Stiemycin, 619
Stilboestrol *see* Diethylstilbestrol, **482**, 486
Still's disease *see* Arthritis, juvenile idiopathic, 546
Stilnoct, 182
Stimulants
  central nervous system, 213
  respiratory, 172

Index

Stings, 36
Stockinettes, 861, 862
Stoma, drugs and, 66
Stomatitis
  denture, 592
  herpetic, 593
Strappal, 865
Strattera, 214
Strefen, 591
Streptase, 135
Streptococcal infection
  antibacterial prophylaxis, 282
Streptogramin antibiotics, 307
Streptokinase, 133, **134**, 135
  infusion table, 831
Streptomycin, 310, 311, **314**
Striant SR, 395
Stronazon MR (tamsulosin), 439
Strongyloidiasis, 357
Strontium ranelate, 404, **410**
StructoKabiven preparations, 514
Structolipid, 514
Stugeron, 219
Subcuvia, 660
Subgam, 660
Sublimaze, 675
Suboxone, 273
Subutex, 273
Succimer, 34
Sucralfate, **47**
Sucrose, presence of, 2
Sudafed, 178
Sudocrem, 603
Sugar, 2
Sugar-free liquid medicines *see* preparations identified by 'sugar-free' throughout BNF
Sugar-free, definition, 2
Sulazine EC (sulfasalazine), 55, 555
Sulconazole, 630, **632**
Sulfa... *see also* Sulpha...
Sulfadiazine, **309**
  infusion table, 831
  toxoplasmosis, 354
Sulfadiazine, silver, 629
Sulfadoxine
  malaria, 351
  pyrimethamine with, 352
  pyrimethamine with, *see Fansidar*
Sulfamethoxazole, trimethoprim with, *see* Co-trimoxazole
Sulfasalazine, 52
  Crohn's disease, 55
  inflammatory bowel disease, 53, **55**
  rheumatic disease, 546, 555
  ulcerative colitis, 53, **55**
Sulfinpyrazone, 556, **557**
Sulindac, 536, **543**, 544
  gout, 555
  preparations, 544
Sulpha... *see also* Sulfa...
Sulphadiazine *see* Sulfadiazine
Sulphasalazine *see* Sulfasalazine
Sulphinpyrazone *see* Sulfinpyrazone, 556, **557**
Sulphonamides, 308
Sulphonylureas, 366
Sulphur, 612, 620
  salicylic acid with, 627
Sulphur dioxide, poisoning, 35
Sulpiride, 189, **192**
  Tourette syndrome, 267
Sulpor, 192
Sumar products, 860
Sumatriptan, 239, **241**
  cluster headache, 243
  migraine, 239
Sun protection factor, 625
Sunitinib, 468, **469**
Sunnyvale, 844
Sunscreens, 624
  ACBS, 849
Sunsense Ultra, 625
Sunya 20/75, 431
Superinfection, 279
Suplasyn, 535
Suplena, 842
Supplementary preparations, 515
Supralip, 140
Suprane, 669
Suprasorb products, 852, 854, 856, 857
Suprax, 293
Suprecur, 414
Suprefact, 487
Suramin, 357
SurePress, 863
Surgam preparations, 544
Surgery
  antibacterial prophylaxis, 282, 283
  diabetes and, 361
  long-term medication and, 665
  tetanus vaccine, 657
Surgical adhesive tapes, 865
Surgical spirit, 637
Surgipad, 859
Surmontil, 206
Survanta, 173
Survimed OPD, 840
Suscard, 109
Sustac—discontinued
Sustanon preparations, 395
Sustiva, 334
Sutent, 469
Suxamethonium, **678**, 679
  infusion table, 831
Swabs, 860
Sylk, 425
Symbicort, 163
Symbols, *inside back cover*
Symmetrel, 265
Sympathomimetics
  asthma, 149
  decongestants, 588
  eye, 572, 574
  inotropic, 119
  premature labour, 423
  vasoconstrictor, 120
Synacthen, 398
Synacthen Depot, 398
Synagis, 343
Synalar preparations, 609
Synarel, 415
Synastone (methadone), 233, 274
Syncope, dental practice, 23
Synercid, 308
Syner-KINASE, 135
Synflex, 543
Syncrom, 535
Synphase, 432
Syntaris, 587
Synthamin preparations, 515
Syntocinon, 418, 421
Syntometrine, 419, 420
Synvisc, 535
Syphilis, 280
Syprol (propranolol), 86
Syringe drivers, palliative care, 17
Syringes
  insulin, 366
    blind patients, 366
  oral, 2
Syscor MR, 116
System 4 products, 864
System 22 nebulisers, 159
Sytron, 492

T

Tabphyn MR (tamsulosin), 439
Tacalcitol, 611 **613**
Tachycardias *see* Arrhythmias
Tacrolimus
  eczema, 616, **618**
  infusion table, 831
  transplant rejection, 474, **476**, 477
Tadalafil, 446, **447**
Taenicides, 356
Tagamet preparations, 46
Tambocor, 82
Tamiflu, 342
Tamoxifen, 483, 484, **485**, 486
  breast pain, 415
  infertility, 397
Tamsulosin, 438, **439**
Tanatril, 102
Tapes, surgical adhesive, 865
Tapeworm infections, 356
Tar, 614
  see also Coal tar
Tarceva, 469
Tardive dyskinesia, 188
Targocid, 306
Targretin, 463
Tarivid, 319
Tarka, 105
Tartrazine, presence of, 2
Tasmar, 265
Tavanic, 318
Tavegil, 168
Taxanes, 469
Taxol, 471
Taxotere, 470
Tazarotene, 612, 613
Tazobactam, 290
  piperacillin with, 290
    infusion table, 830
Tazocin, 290
  infusion table, 830
3TC *see* Lamivudine
Tear deficiency, 577
Tear gas, 35
Tears Naturale, 578

Tears, artificial, 577
Tegaderm products, 852, 853, 855, 856, 857, 859
Tegafur, 458, 461
- uracil with, 461

Tegagen, 852
Tegapore, 859
Tegasorb, 856
Tegretol preparations, 246
Teicoplanin, **305**, 306
- infusion table, 831

Telangiectasia, hereditary haemorrhagic, 391
Telbivudine, 340, **341**
Telfa products, 857, 858
Telfast, 166
Telithromycin, 301, **303**
Telmisartan, 105, **106**
- hydrochlorothiazide with, 106

Telzir, 332
Temazepam, 180, **181**
- anaesthesia, 672, **673**

Temgesic, 230
Temocillin, 285, **287**
- infusion table, 831

Temodal, 465
Temoporfin, **467**
Temozolomide, 464, **465**
Temporomandibular dysfunction, 225
Tendinitis, 545
Tenecteplase, 133, **135**
Tenif, 87
Tennis elbow, 545
Tenofovir, 328, **330**, 331
- efavirenz and emtricitabine with, xiii
- emtricitibine with, 331

Tenoret-50, 87
Tenoretic, 87
Tenormin, 87
Tenoxicam, 536, **544**
TENS, 16
Tensipine MR, 116
Tensium (diazepam), 185
Tensogrip, 861
Tensopress, 863
Tensopril (captopril), 101
Tentrini preparations, 840
Teoptic, 573
Teratogenesis, 787
Terazosin
- cardiovascular, 97, **98**
- urinary tract, 438, **439**

Terbinafine, 321, 322, **326**
- topical, 630, **632**

Terbutaline
- asthma, 149, **152**
- infusion table, 831
- premature labour, 424
- preparations, 153

Teriparatide, 404, 405, **406**
Terlipressin, 404
Terminal care *see* Palliative care
Terpenes, gall bladder, 67
Tertroxin—discontinued
Testim, 395
Testogel, 395
Testosterone
- buccal tablets, 395
- enantate, 394, 395
- esters, 394
- gel, 395
- implants, 395
- injection, 395
- malignant disease, 483
- oral, 394
- patches, 395
- propionate, 394, 395
- undecanoate, 394, 395

Tetanus, 284
- immunisation
  - immunoglobulin, **661**
  - vaccines, 646, **657**
- muscle spasm, 560
- travel, 663

Tetany, hypocalcaemic, 517
Tetrabenazine, 267, **268**
Tetracaine, 65, 685
- eye, **577**
- local anaesthetic, **685**

Tetracosactide, **398**
Tetracosactrin *see* Tetracosactide, **398**
Tetracycline, 296, **297**
- acne, 621
- diabetic neuropathy, 373
- oral infections, 297
- rosacea, 618

Tetracyclines *see* Tetracycline
Tetralysal-300, 298
Tetrastarch, 509, **511**
Teveten, 105
Textube, 861
T-Gel, 627
Thalassaemia, 498
Thalidomide, 481
- lepra reactions, 314

Thelin, 95
Theophylline, 154, **155**
- poisoning, 33
  - elimination, 28
- *see also* Aminophylline

Thermometer, fertility, 437
Thiamine, 523, 524
- status epilepticus, 255

Thiazides, 73
- diabetes insipidus, 402
- *see also* Diuretics

Thiazolidinediones, 369
Thick and Easy, 841
Thioguanine *see* Tioguanine, 458, **461**
Thiopental, **667**
Thiopentone *see* Thiopental, **667**
Thiopurine methyltransferase, 473
Thiotepa, 444, 452, **454**
Thioxanthenes, 189
Thixo-D, 841
Threadworm infections, 355
Throat infections, 281
- gonorrhoea, 280

Thrombocythaemia, 500
Thrombocytopenia, 495
Thrombocytopenic purpura, 500
- immunoglobulin, 660

Thromboembolism, 127
- pulmonary, 122, 133, 173

Thrombolytics, 133
Thrombosis
- antiplatelet drugs, 129
- deep-vein, 122, 127
- prophylaxis, 122
- venous, 133

Thrush *see* Candidiasis
Thymol, 595
Thymoxamine *see* Moxisylyte, **119**
Thyrogen, 401
Thyroid
- antagonists, 377
- carcinoma, 376
- function test, 402
- hormones, 376
- stimulating hormone, 401
- storm, 377

Thyroidectomy, 377
Thyrotoxic crisis, 377
Thyrotoxicosis, 377
- beta-blockers, 85, 377

Thyrotrophin, 401
Thyrotrophin-releasing hormone *see* Protirelin, **402**
Thyrotropin alfa, **401**
Thyroxine *see* Levothyroxine, 376
Tiagabine, 245, **251**, 252
Tiaprofenic acid, 535, **544**
Tibolone, 384, **391**
Ticarcillin, **290**
- clavulanic acid with, 290
  - infusion table, 831

Tick-borne encephalitis, 663
- immunisation, vaccine, 658

TicoVac, 658
Tics, 267
Tielle products, 852, 853
Tigecycline, **298**, 299
- infusion table, 831

Tilade CFC-free Inhaler, 165
Tildiem preparations, 113
Tilofyl (fentanyl), 232
Tiloket CR, 542
Tiloryth (erythromycin), 301
Tiludronic acid, 409
Timentin, 290
- infusion table, 831

Timodine, 606
Timolol, 90, 91
- bendroflumethiazide with, 91
- cardiovascular, 90
- co-amilozide with, 91
- eye, 572, **573**
  - bimatoprost with, 574
  - brimonidine with, 575
  - dorzolamide with, 576
  - latanoprost with, 574
  - travoprost with, 574
- migraine, 242
- *see also* Beta-adrenoceptor blocking drugs

Timoptol, 573
Timoptol LA, 573
Tinaderm-M, 632
Tinea infections, 321, 630
Tinidazole, 315, **316**
- amoebiasis, 352
- giardiasis, 353
- protozoal infections, 353
- trichomoniasis, 353

Tinzaparin, 123, **125**

Index

Tioconazole, 630, **632**
Tioguanine, 458, **461**
Tiotropium, 153, **154**
Tipranavir, 328, **334**
Tirofiban, 108, 130, **132**
  infusion table, 831
Tisept, 638
Tissue adhesive, 637
Titanium dioxide, 602
Tixycolds preparations, 589
Tizanidine, 559, **561**
Tobi, 301
Tobradex, 569
Tobramycin, 299, **300**, 301
  eye, 569
  infusion table, 831
Tocopherols, 527
Tocopheryl, 527
Toilet preparations, ACBS, 849
Tolbutamide, 366, **368**
Tolcapone, 264, **265**
Tolfenamic acid, **239**, 536
Tolnaftate, 630, 632
Tolterodine, 440, **442**
Tomudex, 461
Tonic seizures, 245
Tonic-clonic seizures, 245
Tonics, 528
Tonsillitis *see* Throat infections
Topal, 41
Topamax, 252
Topiramate, 242, 245, **252**
Topotecan, **471**
  infusion table, 831
Toradol, 674
Torasemide, 74, **75**
Torem, 75
Toremifene, 484, **486**
Torsade de pointes, **79**, 519
  magnesium sulphate, 519
Torsion dystonias, 268
Tostran, 395
Total parenteral nutrition, 511
Totaretic (co-tenidone), 87
Tourer, 159
Tourette syndrome, 267
TOXBASE, 27
Toxoplasma choroidoretinitis, 354
Toxoplasmosis, 354
TPA *see* Alteplase
TPN, 511
Trabectedin, **471**, 472
Trachoma, 296, 566
Tracleer, 93
Tracrium, 677
Tractocile, 423
Trade marks, symbol, 1
Tradorec XL, 237
Tramacet, 237
Tramadol, 230, **237**
  infusion table, 832
  paracetamol with, 237
Tramake preparations, 237
Trandate, 88
Trandolapril, **104**, 105
  see also ACE inhibitors
  verapamil with, 105
Tranexamic acid, **135**, 136
  infusion table, 832
Trangina XL (isosorbide mononitrate), 111
Tranquillisers, 179
Transcutaneous electrical nerve stimulation, 16
Transfusion reactions, 495
Transiderm-Nitro, 110
Transorbent, 852
Transplant rejection, 473, 474
Transtec, 231
Tranylcypromine, 206, **207**
Trasicor, 90
Trasidrex, 90
Trastuzumab, **472**
  infusion table, 832
Trasylol—discontinued
Travasept-100, 638
Travatan, 574
Travel, vaccination for, 663
Travellers' diarrhoea, 663
Travoprost, 573, **574**
  with timolol, 574
Traxam preparations, 563
Trazodone, 203, **206**
Treatment cards, anticoagulant, 128
Tree pollen allergy preparations, 169
Tremors, 267
Trental, 119
Treosulfan, 452, **454**
  infusion table, 832
Tretinoin
  acne, 619, 620
    erythromycin with, 620
  leukaemia, 472
TRH *see* Protirelin, **402**
Tri-Adcortyl, 610
Tri-Adcortyl Otic, 584
Triadene, 432
Triamcinolone
  ear, 584
  injection
    allergic conditions, **384**
    rheumatic diseases, 545
  mouth, 591
  nasal allergy, 588
  skin, 610
Triam-Co (co-triamterzide), 77
Triamterene, **76**
  benzthiazide with, 77
  chlortalidone with, 78
  furosemide with, 78
  hydrochlorothiazide with, 77
Triapin preparations, 104
Triazole antifungal drugs, 321, 322
Tribavirin *see* Ribavirin
Trichomonacides, 353
Trichomonal infections, 353
Triclofos, 182, **183**
Triclosan, 637, 639
Tricotex, 858
Tricyclic antidepressants *see* Antidepressants, tricyclic
Tridestra, 389
Trientine, **529**
Trifluoperazine
  nausea and vertigo, 217, **220**
  psychoses, 189, **192**, 193
Trigeminal neuralgia, 238
Trihexyphenidyl, 266, **267**
  movement disorders, 267
Tri-iodothyronine, 377
Trileptal, 247
Trilostane, **416**
  malignant disease, 484
Trimeprazine *see* Alimemazine
Trimethoprim, 308, **309**, 319
  acne, 621
  pneumocystis pneumonia, 354
  sulfamethoxazole with, *see* Co-trimoxazole
Tri-Minulet—discontinued
Trimipramine, 203, **205**, 206
Trimopan (trimethoprim), 309
Trimovate, 608
Trinordiol, 431
TriNovum, 432
Trintek, 110
Tripotassium dicitratobismuthate, **47**
Triptafen preparations, 204
Triptans *see* $5HT_1$ agonists, 238, **239**
Triptorelin
  endometriosis, 415
  prostate cancer, 486, **488**
  uterine fibroids, 413, 415
Trisenox, 463
Trisequens preparations, 389
Tritace 104
Tritamyl, 844
Trizivir 329
Tropical diseases, advice, 344
Tropicamide, 571, **572**
Tropisetron, 218, **223**
  infusion table, 832
Tropium (chlordiazepoxide), 185
Trospium, 440, **442**
Trosyl, 632
TrueTrack products, 374, 375
Trufoam products, 852, 853
Trusopt 576
Truvada, 331
Trypanocides, 354
Trypanosomiasis, 354
Tryptophan, 211 **212**
T-Safe CU 380 A, 436
TT 380 Slimline, 437
Tubegauz, 862
Tuberculin, 644, 645
Tuberculosis, 310
  diagnosis, 644
  immunisation
    travel, 663
    vaccines, 644
  prophylaxis, 282
Tubifast, 862
Tubigrip, 861
Tubipad, 861
Tuinal, 187
Tulle dressings, 858
Tumour lysis syndrome, 449
Turbohaler
  Bricanyl, 153
  Oxis 150
  Pulmicort, 162
  Symbicort, 163
Turboneb 159
Turner's syndrome, 399, 400
Twinrix preparations, 648
TwoCal HN, 840
Tygacil, 299

Index

Tylex, 228
Typherix, 658
Typhim Vi, 658
Typhoid
  antibacterial treatment, 279
  immunisation
    travel, 663
    vaccines, 658
TYR cooler, 848
TYR express, 848
TYR gel, 848
Tyrosinaemia, 848
Tyrosine kinase inhibitors, 468
Tyrosine supplement, 848
Tysabri, 482

U

Ubretid, 440
Ucerax, 168
Uftoral, 461
Ulcerative colitis, 52
Ulcerative gingivitis
  antibacterial treatment, 281, 315
  mouthwashes, 594
Ulcer-healing drugs, 43
Ulcers
  aphthous, 590
  corneal, 566, 568
  duodenal, 43, 44
  gastric, 43, 44
  Hunner's, 444
  mouth, 590
  NSAID-associated, 44
  skin, 639
Ultec Pro, 856
Ultima, 159
Ultiva, 676
Ultra bandages, 863, 864
Ultra foods
  gluten-free, 844
  low-protein, 845
Ultra Neb-2000, 159
Ultrabase, 600
Ultralanum Plain, 610
Ultraproct, 65
Ultrasonic nebulisers, 159
Ultraviolet radiation, 624
Undecenoates, **632**, 633
Unguentum M, 600
Unifine products, 366
Unilet products, 366
Uniphyllin Continus, 155
Uniroid-HC, 65
Unisept, 638
Unistik products, 366
Unithiol, 34
Unitulle, 858
Univer, 117
Universal, 366
Unresectable dermatofibrosarcoma protuberans, 468
Uracil, tegafur with, 461
Urdox, 67
Urea, 599, 600, 601
  hydrocortisone with, 606
Urea cycle disorders, 532
  arginine supplement, 848
Ureteric colic, 443
Urethritis, non-gonococcal, 280, 296
Urgosorb products, 852
Urgotul products, 859
Uriben, 318
Uricosuric drugs, 556
Uriflex preparations, 444
Urinary
  frequency, 440
  incontinence, 440
  infections, 280, 319
  pH adjustment, 443
  retention, 438
Urine tests, 375
Urispas-200, 441
Uristix, 375
Urofoliitropin, 399
Urofollitrophin *see* Urofollitropin, 398
Urofollitropin, 398
Urokinase, 133, **135**
  infusion table, 832
Urological procedures
  antibacterial prophylaxis, 283
Uromitexan, 452
Uro-Tainer preparations, 444
Urothelial toxicity, 451
Ursodeoxycholic acid, **67**
Ursofalk, 67
Ursogal, 67
Urticaria, 166
UT 380 Short, 437
UT 380 Standard, 437
Uterine
  bleeding, 419
  relaxants, 423
  stimulants, 418
Utinor, 319
Utovlan, 393
Utrogestan, 394
UVB, psoriasis, 612
Uvistat preparations, 625

V

Vaccination
  HIV-positive subjects, 642
  schedule, 642
  travel, 663
Vaccines
  active immunity, 641
  allergen extract, 169
  contra-indications, 641
  post-immunisation pyrexia, 641
  pregnancy, 641
  side-effects, 641
  storage and use, 643
Vacunet, 854
Vacuskin, 857
Vacutex, 860
Vagifem, 425
Vaginitis
  candidal, 425
  herpes simplex, 427
  menopausal, 384, 424
  non-specific *see* Vaginosis, bacterial, 280
  trichomonal, 426
Vaginosis, bacterial, 280
Vaginyl (metronidazole), 316
Valaciclovir, 336, **337**, 338
Valclair (diazepam), 185
Valcyte, 339
Valganciclovir, 338, 339
Valine Amino Acid Supplement, 846
Vallergan, 167
Valoid, 219
Valpiform, 844
Valproate
  bipolar disorder, **200**
  epilepsy, 245, **252**, 253, 254
  infusion table, 831
  migraine, 242
Valproic acid *see* Valproate
Valsartan, 105, **107**
  amlodipine with, 112
  hydrochlorothiazide with, 107
Valtrex, 338
Vamin preparations, 515
Vaminolact, 515
Vancocin, 305
Vancomycin, **305**
  eye, 577
  infusion table, 832
Vancomycin-resistant enterococci, 298, 306
Vaniqa, 627
Vapour-permeable adhesive film, 856
Vaqta, 648
Vardenafil, 446, **447**
Varenicline, 270, **272**
Variceal bleeding, 402, 488
Varicella-zoster, 336
  immunisation
    vaccine, 658, 659, 661
  immunoglobulin, **661**
Varicose veins, 144, 640
Varilrix, 659
Varivax, 659
Vascace, 101
Vascalpha (felodipine), 114
Vascular surgery
  antibacterial prophylaxis, 283
Vaseline Dermacare, 600
Vasoconstrictors
  local anaesthesia, 681
    dental practice, 681
  sympathomimetic, 120
Vasodilators
  antihypertensive, 93
  peripheral, 118
Vasogen, 603
Vasopressin, **402**
  infusion table, 832
VEC high compression bandage, 863
Vectavir, 633
Vecuronium, 677, **678**
  infusion table, 832
Vegenat-med, 840
Veil preparations, 626
Velband, 863
Velbe, 462
Velcade, 464
Velosef, 293
Venlafaxine, 211, **212**, 213
Venofer, 493
Venofundin, 511
Venta-Neb, 94
Ventavis, 94
Ventilatory failure, 172

Ventmax SR (salbutamol), 151
Ventolin preparations, 151, 152
Ventstream, 158
Vepesid, 462
Veracur, 623
Verapamil, **116**, 117
  angina, 111
  arrhythmias, 80
  beta-blockers and, 117
  cluster headache, 243
  hypertension, 111
  poisoning by, 32
  see also Calcium-channel blockers
  trandolapril with, 105
Verapress MR, 117
Vermox, 356
Vernaid, 859
Verrucas, 622
Verrugon, 623
Versatis, 682
Versiva, 856
Vertab SR 240, 117
Verteporfin, 580, **581**
  infusion table, 832
Vesanoid, 472
Vesicare, 442
Vestibular disorders, 218
Vexol, 570
Vfend, 327
Viagra, 447
ViATIM, 648
Viazem XL, 113
Vibramycin preparations, 298
Videne, 639
Videx preparations, 329
Vigabatrin, **254**
Vigam preparations, 661
Vigranon B, 524
Vinblastine, 461, **462**
  infusion table, 832
Vinca alkaloids, 461
Vincent's infection
  antibacterial treatment, 281, 315
  mouthwashes, 594
Vincristine, 461, **462**
  infusion table, 832
Vindesine, 461, **462**
  infusion table, 832
Vinorelbine, 461, **462**
  infusion table, 832
Vioform-Hydrocortisone, 607
Viracept, 333
Viraferon, 479
ViraferonPeg, 479
Viramune, 335
Virazole, 343
Viread, 331
Viridal Duo, 446
Viroflu, 651
Virormone injection, 395
Virovir (aciclovir), 337
Virus infections, 327
Visclair, 175
Viscopaste PB7, 864
Viscotears, 578
Viskaldix, 90
Visken, 90
Vistabel, 269
Vista-Methasone
  ear, 583
  eye, 569
  nose, 587
Vista-Methasone N
  ear, 583
  eye, 569
  nose, 589
Vistide, 338
Visudyne, 581
Vita Bite, 845
Vitajoule, 840
Vitalograph peak flow meters, 156
Vitamin
  multivitamin preparations, 528
Vitamin A, **523**
  vitamin D and, 523
Vitamin B group, 523, 524
  B and C injection, 524
    infusion table, 832
Vitamin B_{12}, 493, 494
Vitamin C *see* Ascorbic acid
Vitamin D, 525
  psoriasis, 611
Vitamin deficiency, 522
Vitamin E, 527
Vitamin K, 527
Vitamins, 522
  children's drops, 523
  multivitamin preparations, 528
    infusion table, 832
  parenteral nutrition, 515
Vitapro, 841
Vitaquick, 841
Vitasavoury, 840
Vitiligo, 626
  ACBS, 849
Vitlipid N, 516
Vitrex products, 366
Vivacor (bisoprolol), 87
Vivaglobin, 660
Vividrin (sodium cromoglicate)
  eye, 571
  nose, 588
Vivotif, 658
Volmax, 151
Volplex, 510
Volsaid (diclofenac), 539
Voltarol preparations, 538, 539
  Emulgel, 563
  eye, 580
  Gel patch, 563
  Ophtha, 580
  Rapid, 539
Volumatic, 157
Volume expansion, 509
Voluven, 511
Vomiting, 217
  cytotoxic drugs, 449
  palliative care, 17
  postoperative, 218
  pregnancy, 218
von Willebrand's disease, 403
Voriconazole, 321, 322, **327**
  infusion table, 832
Vulvitis, candidal, 425
VZIG *see* Immunoglobulins, varicella-zoster, 661

W

Waldenstrom's macroglobulinaemia, 452
Warfarin, 127, **128**
Warticon preparations, 624
Warts, 622
Wasp sting allergy preparations, 169
Water
  for injections, 508
  potable, 2
Waxsol, 586
Webbing, blue line, 863
Webbing, red line, 863
Welldorm, 183
Wellvone, 355
Wernicke's encephalopathy, 523
West's syndrome, 254
Wheat sensitivity, gluten-sensitive enteropathy with, 844
Whooping cough *see* Pertussis
Wilson's disease, 528
Wilzin 529
WinRho SDF, 662
Withdrawal
  alcohol, 269
  anxiolytics, 179
  corticosteroids, 380
  hypnotics, 179
  nicotine, 270
  opioids, 273
Wolff-Parkinson-White syndrome, 80
Wool fat, excipient, 598
Wool fat, hydrous, 599
World Traveller HI FLO, 159
Worm infestation, 355
Wound dressings, 850
  pads, 857
Wuchereria bancrofti, 357
Wysoy, 843

X

Xagrid, 500
Xalacom, 574
Xalatan, 574
Xanax (alprazolam), 185
Xanthine bronchodilators *see* Theophylline
Xanthine-oxidase inhibitor, 556
Xatral preparations, 438
Xeloda, 459
Xenazine, 268
Xenical, 216
Xepin, 604
Xerostomia, 595
Xigris (drotrecogin alfa (activated)), 136
Xipamide, 73, **74**
Xismox XL (isosorbide mononitrate), 111
XLEU
  Analog, 846
  Faladon, 846
  Mazamaid, 846

Index

XLYS
Analog, 846
Maxamaid, 846
XLYS Low TRY
Analog, 845
Maxamaid, 845
XMET
Analog, 845
Homidon, 845
Maxamaid, 845
Maxamum, 845
XMTVI
Analog, 846
Asadon, 846
Maxamaid, 846
Maxamum, 846
Xolair, 170
XP
Analog, 848
Maxamaid, 848
Maxamaid, Concentrate, 848
Maxamum, 848
XP LCP Analog, 848
XPHEN TYR
Analog, 848
Maxamaid, 848
Tyrosidon, 848
XPTM
Analog, 848
Tyrosidon, 848
Xupad, 858
Xylitol, presence of, 2
Xylocaine, 592, 682, 683
Xylometazoline
eye, 570
nose, 588, **589**
Xyloproct, 66
Xyrem, 184
Xyzal, 167

Y

8Y (factor VIII fraction), 136
Yasmin, 432
Yeasts, 321
Yellow fever
immunisation
travel, 663
vaccine, 659
Yentreve, 441
Yondelis, 472
Yutopar, 424

Z

Zacin, 563
Zaditen, 168, 570
Zafirlukast, **165**
Zaleplon, 181, **182**
Zamadol preparations, 237
Zanaflex, 561
Zanamivir, 341, **342**
Zanidip, 115
Zantac, 47
Zapain (co-codamol 30/500), 227
Zaponex, 195
Zarontin, 247
Zavedos, 456
Zavesca, 530
ZeaSORB, 640
Zeffix, 330
Zelapar, 264
Zemon preparations, 111
Zemplar, 527
Zemtard preparations, 114
Zenalb preparations (albumin solution), 509
Zenapax, 476
Zerit, 330
Zerobase, 600
Zestoretic preparations, 103
Zestril, 103
Zetuvit E, 857
Ziagen, 329
Zibor, 124
Ziconotide, 225
Zidoval, 427
Zidovudine, **331**
abacavir and lamivudine with, 329
infusion table, 832
lamivudine with, 331
Zimbacol XL (bezafibrate), 139
Zimovane, 182
Zinacef, 295
Zinc
bandages, 864
calamine and, 864
ichthammol and, 610, 611, 864
stocking, 864
deficiency, **522**
eye, 577, 579
skin
benzyl benzoate with, 603
castor oil and, 602
coal tar with, 614
cod liver oil with, 603
cream, 602
dimeticone with, 603
ichthammol with, 611
ointment, 602
salicylic acid with, 615
tape, adhesive, 865
Wilson's disease (zinc acetate), **529**
Zincaband, 864
Zindaclin, 619
Zineryt, 619
Zinnat, 295
Zipzoc, 864
Zispin preparations, 212
Zithromax, 302
Zocor, 143
Zocor Heart-Pro (simvastatin), 143
Zofran, 222
Zoladex preparations, 488
endometriosis, 414
IVF, 414
Zoledronic acid, **409**, **410**
infusion table, 832
Zoleptil, 197
Zollinger–Ellison syndrome, 44
Zolmitriptan, 239, **241**
Zolpidem, 181, **182**
Zolvera (verapamil), **117**
Zomacton, 401
Zometa, 410
Zomig preparations, 241
Zomorph, 235
Zonegran, 255
Zonisamide, 245, **254**, 255
Zopiclone, 181, **182**
Zorac, 613
Zoster *see* Herpes infections
Zotepine, 193, **197**
Zoton, 49
suspension—discontinued
Zovirax preparations
cream, 633
eye ointment, 568
injection, 337
tablets, 337
Zuclopenthixol, 189, 199
depot injections, 198, 199
injection, 193
tablets, 193
Zuclopenthixol acetate, **193**
Zuclopenthixol decanoate, **199**
Zuclopenthixol dihydrochloride, **193**
Zumenon, 391
Zuvogen, 633
Zyban, 271
Zydol preparations, 237
Zyloric, 556
Zyomet, 630
Zyprexa, 196
Zyvox, 307

Yellowcard

COMMISSION ON HUMAN MEDICINES

In Confidence

MHRA

SUSPECTED ADVERSE DRUG REACTIONS

If you suspect that an adverse reaction may be related to a drug, or a combination of drugs, you should complete this Yellow Card or complete a report on the website at www.yellowcard.gov.uk. For *intensively monitored medicines* (identified by ▼) report **all** suspected reactions (including any considered not to be serious). For *established drugs* and *herbal remedies* report **all serious** adverse reactions in adults; report **all serious and minor** adverse reactions in **children** (under 18 years). You do not have to be certain about causality: if in doubt, please report. Do not be put off reporting just because some details are not known. See BNF (page 11) or the MHRA website (www.yellowcard.gov.uk) for additional advice.

PATIENT DETAILS Patient Initials: ____________ Sex: M / F Weight if known (kg): ____________

Age (at time of reaction): ____________ Identification (Your Practice / Hospital Ref.)*: ____________

SUSPECTED DRUG(S)

Give brand name of drug and batch number if known	Route	Dosage	Date started	Date stopped	Prescribed for

SUSPECTED REACTION(S)

Please describe the reaction(s) and any treatment given:

Outcome

Recovered ☐
Recovering ☐
Continuing ☐
Other ☐

Date reaction(s) started: ____________ Date reaction(s) stopped: ____________

Do you consider the reaction to be serious? Yes / No

If *yes*, please indicate why the reaction is considered to be serious (please tick all that apply):

Patient died due to reaction ☐ Involved or prolonged inpatient hospitalisation ☐
Life threatening ☐ Involved persistent or significant disability or incapacity ☐
Congenital abnormality ☐ Medically significant; please give details:

* This is to enable you to identify the patient in any future correspondence concerning this report

Please attach additional pages if necessary

Please list other drugs taken in the last 3 months prior to the reaction (including self-medication & herbal remedies)

Was the patient on any other medication? Yes / No If *yes*, please give the following information if known:

Drug (Brand, if known)	Route	Dosage	Date started	Date stopped	Prescribed for

Additional relevant information e.g. medical history, test results, known allergies, rechallenge (if performed), suspected drug interactions. For congenital abnormalities please state all other drugs taken during pregnancy and the date of the last menstrual period.

REPORTER DETAILS

Name and Professional Address: ______________________

Post code: ______________ Tel No: ______________

Speciality: ______________________

Signature: Date:

CLINICIAN (if not the reporter)

Name and Professional Address: ______________________

Post code: ______________

Tel No: ______________ Speciality: ______________

If you would like information about other adverse reactions associated with the suspected drug, please tick this box ☐

If you report from an area served by a Yellow Card Centre (YCC), MHRA may ask the Centre to communicate with you, on its behalf, about your report. See BNF (page 11) for further details on YCCs. If you want only MHRA to contact you, please tick this box. ☐

Send to **Medicines and Healthcare products Regulatory Agency, CHM FREEPOST, LONDON SW8 5BR**

Yellowcard

COMMISSION ON HUMAN MEDICINES

In Confidence

MHRA

SUSPECTED ADVERSE DRUG REACTIONS

If you suspect that an adverse reaction may be related to a drug, or a combination of drugs, you should complete this Yellow Card or complete a report on the website at www.yellowcard.gov.uk. For *intensively monitored medicines* (identified by ▼) report **all** suspected reactions (including any considered not to be serious). For *established drugs* and *herbal remedies* report **all serious** adverse reactions in adults; report **all serious and minor** adverse reactions in **children** (under 18 years). You do not have to be certain about causality: if in doubt, please report. Do not be put off reporting just because some details are not known. See BNF (page 11) or the MHRA website (www.yellowcard.gov.uk) for additional advice.

PATIENT DETAILS Patient Initials: ________ Sex: M / F Weight if known (kg): ________

Age (at time of reaction): ________ Identification (Your Practice / Hospital Ref.)*: ________

SUSPECTED DRUG(S)

Give brand name of drug and batch number if known	Route	Dosage	Date started	Date stopped	Prescribed for

SUSPECTED REACTION(S)

Please describe the reaction(s) and any treatment given:

Outcome

Recovered ☐
Recovering ☐
Continuing ☐
Other ☐

Date reaction(s) started: ________ Date reaction(s) stopped: ________

Do you consider the reaction to be serious? Yes / No

If *yes*, please indicate why the reaction is considered to be serious (please tick all that apply):

Patient died due to reaction ☐
Life threatening ☐
Congenital abnormality ☐
Involved or prolonged inpatient hospitalisation ☐
Involved persistent or significant disability or incapacity ☐
Medically significant; please give details:

* This is to enable you to identify the patient in any future correspondence concerning this report

Please attach additional pages if necessary

Please list other drugs taken in the last 3 months prior to the reaction (including self-medication & herbal remedies)

Was the patient on any other medication? Yes / No If *yes*, please give the following information if known:

Drug (Brand, if known)	Route	Dosage	Date started	Date stopped	Prescribed for

Additional relevant information e.g. medical history, test results, known allergies, rechallenge (if performed), suspected drug interactions. For congenital abnormalities please state all other drugs taken during pregnancy and the date of the last menstrual period.

REPORTER DETAILS

Name and Professional Address: __________

Post code: __________ Tel No: __________

Speciality: __________

Signature: Date:

CLINICIAN (if not the reporter)

Name and Professional Address: __________

Post code: __________

Tel No: __________ Speciality: __________

If you would like information about other adverse reactions associated with the suspected drug, please tick this box ☐

If you report from an area served by a Yellow Card Centre (YCC), MHRA may ask the Centre to communicate with you, on its behalf, about your report. See BNF (page 11) for further details on YCCs. If you want only MHRA to contact you, please tick this box. ☐

Send to **Medicines and Healthcare products Regulatory Agency, CHM FREEPOST, LONDON SW8 5BR**

Yellowcard

COMMISSION ON HUMAN MEDICINES

In Confidence

MHRA

SUSPECTED ADVERSE DRUG REACTIONS

If you suspect that an adverse reaction may be related to a drug, or a combination of drugs, you should complete this Yellow Card or complete a report on the website at www.yellowcard.gov.uk. For *intensively monitored medicines* (identified by ▼) report **all** suspected reactions (including any considered not to be serious). For *established drugs* and *herbal remedies* report **all serious** adverse reactions in adults; report **all serious and minor** adverse reactions in **children** (under 18 years). You do not have to be certain about causality: if in doubt, please report. Do not be put off reporting just because some details are not known. See BNF (page 11) or the MHRA website (www.yellowcard.gov.uk) for additional advice.

PATIENT DETAILS Patient Initials: ______ Sex: M / F Weight if known (kg): ______

Age (at time of reaction): ______ Identification (Your Practice / Hospital Ref.)*: ______

SUSPECTED DRUG(S)

Give brand name of drug and batch number if known	Route	Dosage	Date started	Date stopped	Prescribed for

SUSPECTED REACTION(S)

Please describe the reaction(s) and any treatment given:

Outcome

Recovered ☐
Recovering ☐
Continuing ☐
Other ☐

Date reaction(s) started: ______ Date reaction(s) stopped: ______

Do you consider the reaction to be serious? Yes / No

If *yes*, please indicate why the reaction is considered to be serious (please tick all that apply):

Patient died due to reaction ☐ Involved or prolonged inpatient hospitalisation ☐
Life threatening ☐ Involved persistent or significant disability or incapacity ☐
Congenital abnormality ☐ Medically significant; please give details:

* This is to enable you to identify the patient in any future correspondence concerning this report

Please attach additional pages if necessary

Please list other drugs taken in the last 3 months prior to the reaction (including self-medication & herbal remedies)

Was the patient on any other medication? Yes / No If *yes*, please give the following information if known:

Drug (Brand, if known)	Route	Dosage	Date started	Date stopped	Prescribed for

Additional relevant information e.g. medical history, test results, known allergies, rechallenge (if performed), suspected drug interactions. For congenital abnormalities please state all other drugs taken during pregnancy and the date of the last menstrual period.

REPORTER DETAILS

Name and Professional Address: ______

______

______

Post code: ______ Tel No: ______

Speciality: ______

Signature: Date:

CLINICIAN (if not the reporter)

Name and Professional Address: ______

______

______ Post code: ______

Tel No: ______ Speciality: ______

If you would like information about other adverse reactions associated with the suspected drug, please tick this box ☐

u report from an area served by a Yellow Card Centre (YCC), MHRA may ask the Centre to communicate with you, on its behalf, about your t. See BNF (page 11) for further details on YCCs. If you want only MHRA to contact you, please tick this box. ☐

Send to **Medicines and Healthcare products Regulatory Agency, CHM FREEPOST, LONDON SW8 5BR**

Cardiovascular Risk Prediction Charts

Heart 2005; **91**(Suppl V): v1–v52

How to use the Cardiovascular Risk Prediction Charts for Primary Prevention

These charts are for estimating cardiovascular disease (CVD) risk (non-fatal myocardial infarction and stroke, coronary and stroke death and new angina pectoris) for individuals who have **not** already developed coronary heart disease (CHD) or other major atherosclerotic disease. They are an aid to making clinical decisions about how intensively to intervene on lifestyle and whether to use antihypertensive, lipid lowering and anti-platelet medication, but should **not replace clinical judgment**.

- The use of these charts is **not appropriate** for patients who have existing diseases which already put them at high risk such as:
  - coronary heart disease or other major atherosclerotic disease;
  - familial hypercholesterolaemia or other inherited dyslipidaemias;
  - renal dysfunction including diabetic nephropathy;
  - type 1 and 2 diabetes mellitus.
- The charts should **not** be used to decide whether to introduce antihypertensive medication when blood pressure is persistently at or above 160/100 mmHg or when target organ damage due to hypertension is present. In both cases antihypertensive medication is recommended regardless of CVD risk. Similarly the charts should **not** be used to decide whether to introduce lipid-lowering medication when the ratio of serum total to HDL cholesterol exceeds 6. Such medication is generally then indicated regardless of estimated CVD risk.
- To estimate an individual's absolute 10-year risk of developing CVD choose the chart for his or her sex, lifetime smoking status and age. Within this square identify the level of risk according to the point where the coordinates for systolic blood pressure and the ratio of total cholesterol to high density lipoprotein (HDL) cholesterol meet. If no HDL cholesterol result is available, then assume this is 1.0 mmol/litre and the lipid scale can be used for total cholesterol alone.
- Higher risk individuals (red areas) are defined as those whose 10-year CVD risk exceeds 20%, which is approximately equivalent to the coronary heart disease risk of > 15% over the same period.
- The chart also assists in identifying individuals whose 10-year CVD risk is moderately increased in the range 10–20% (orange areas) and those in whom risk is lower than 10% over 10 years (green areas).
- Smoking status should reflect lifetime exposure to tobacco and not simply tobacco use at the time of assessment. For example, those who have given up smoking within 5 years should be regarded as current smokers for the purposes of the charts.
- The initial blood pressure and the first random (non-fasting) total cholesterol and HDL cholesterol can be used to estimate an individual's risk. However, the decision on using drug therapy should generally be based on repeat risk factor measurements over a period of time.

(Continued over)

- Men and women do not reach the level of risk predicted by the charts for the three age bands until they reach the ages 49, 59, and 69 years respectively. The charts will overestimate current risk most in the under 40s. Clinical judgement must be exercised in deciding on treatment in younger patients. However, it should be recognised that blood pressure and cholesterol tend to rise most and HDL cholesterol to decline most in younger people already with adverse levels. Left untreated, their risk at the age 49 years is likely to be higher than the projected risk shown on the age-under-50-years chart. From age 70 years the CVD risk, especially for men, is usually ≥ 20% over 10 years and the charts will underestimate true total CVD risk.

- These charts (and all other currently available methods of CVD risk prediction) are based on groups of people with **untreated** levels of blood pressure, total cholesterol and HDL cholesterol. In patients already receiving antihypertensive therapy in whom the decision is to be made about whether to introduce lipid-lowering medication, or vice versa, the charts can only act as a guide. Unless recent pre-treatment risk factor values are available it is generally safest to assume that CVD risk is higher than that predicted by current levels of blood pressure or lipids on treatment.

- CVD risk is also higher than indicated in the charts for:
  - those with a family history of premature CVD or stroke (male first-degree relatives aged < 55 years and female first-degree relatives aged < 65 years) which increases the risk by a factor of approximately 1.3;
  - those with raised triglyceride levels (> 1.7 mmol/litre);
  - women with premature menopause;
  - those who are not yet diabetic, but have impaired fasting glycaemia (6.1–6.9 mmol/litre) or impaired glucose tolerance (2 hour glucose ≥ 7.8 mmol/litre but < 11.1 mmol/litre in an oral glucose tolerance test).

- The charts have not been validated in ethnic minorities and in some may underestimate CVD risk. For example, in people originating from the Indian subcontinent it is safest to assume that the CVD risk is higher than predicted from the charts (1.4 times).

- An individual can be shown on the chart the direction in which his or her risk of CVD can be reduced by changing smoking status, blood pressure, or cholesterol, but it should be borne in mind that the estimate of risk is for a group of people with similar risk factors and that within that group there will be considerable variation in risk. It should also be pointed out in younger people that the estimated risk will generally not be reached before the age of 50, if their current blood pressure and lipid levels remain unchanged. The charts are primarily to assist in directing intervention to those who typically stand to benefit most.

(Continued over)

NONDIABETIC MEN

Non-smoker | Smoker

Age under 50 years

SBP 180 160 140 120 100

3 4 5 6 7 8 9 10
TC : HDL

SBP 180 160 140 120 100

3 4 5 6 7 8 9 10
TC : HDL

Age 50–59 years

SBP 180 160 140 120 100

3 4 5 6 7 8 9 10
TC : HDL

SBP 180 160 140 120 100

3 4 5 6 7 8 9 10
TC : HDL

Age 60 years and over

SBP 180 160 140 120 100

3 4 5 6 7 8 9 10
TC : HDL

SBP 180 160 140 120 100

3 4 5 6 7 8 9 10
TC HDL

CVD risk <10% over next 10 years

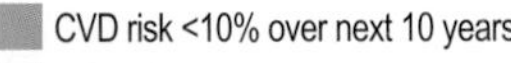

CVD risk 10-20% over next 10 years

CVD risk >20% over next 10 years

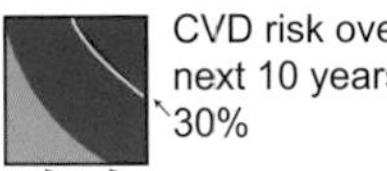

SBP = systolic blood pressure mmHg
TC : HDL = serum total cholesterol to HDL cholesterol ratio

(Continued over)

NONDIABETIC WOMEN

Non-smoker | Smoker

Age under 50 years

SBP 180 160 140 120 100

3 4 5 6 7 8 9 10
TC : HDL

SBP 180 160 140 120 100

3 4 5 6 7 8 9 10
TC : HDL

Age 50–59 years

SBP 180 160 140 120 100

3 4 5 6 7 8 9 10
TC : HDL

SBP 180 160 140 120 100

3 4 5 6 7 8 9 10
TC : HDL

Age 60 years and over

SBP 180 160 140 120 100

3 4 5 6 7 8 9 10
TC : HDL

SBP 180 160 140 120 100

3 4 5 6 7 8 9 10
TC : HDL

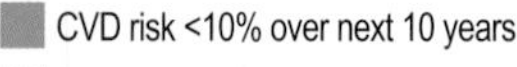

CVD risk <10% over next 10 years

CVD risk 10-20% over next 10 years

CVD risk >20% over next 10 years

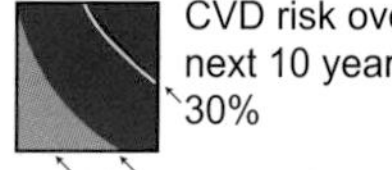

CVD risk over next 10 years

SBP = systolic blood pressure mmHg
TC : HDL = serum total cholesterol to HDL cholesterol ratio

ADULT ADVANCED LIFE SUPPORT ALGORITHM

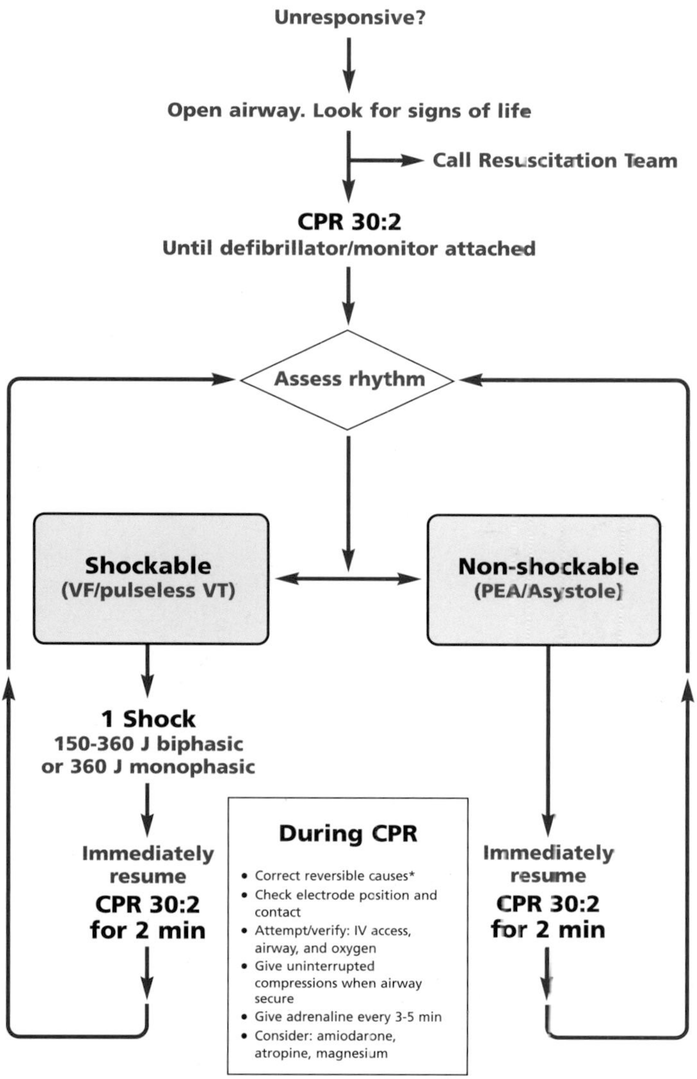

Unresponsive?

↓

Open airway. Look for signs of life

→ Call Resuscitation Team

↓

CPR 30:2
Until defibrillator/monitor attached

↓

Assess rhythm

Shockable
(VF/pulseless VT)

Non-shockable
(PEA/Asystole)

Shockable:

1 Shock
150-360 J biphasic
or 360 J monophasic

↓

Immediately resume
CPR 30:2
for 2 min

↑ (return to Assess rhythm)

Non-shockable:

↓

Immediately resume
CPR 30:2
for 2 min

↑ (return to Assess rhythm)

During CPR

- Correct reversible causes*
- Check electrode position and contact
- Attempt/verify: IV access, airway, and oxygen
- Give uninterrupted compressions when airway secure
- Give adrenaline every 3-5 min
- Consider: amiodarone, atropine, magnesium

***Reversible causes**

Hypoxia	Tension pneumothorax
Hypovolaemia	Tamponade, cardiac
Hypo/hyperkalaemia/metabolic	Toxins
Hypothermia	Thrombosis (coronary or pulmonary)

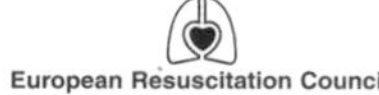

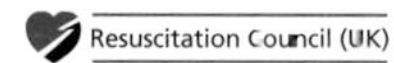

Medical emergencies in the community

Drug treatment outlined below is intended for use by community healthcare professionals. Only drugs that are used for immediate relief are shown; advice on supporting care is not given. Where the patient's condition requires investigation and further treatment, the patient should be transferred to hospital promptly.

Anaphylaxis

(section 3.4.3)

Adrenaline injection 1 mg/mL (1 in 1000)

- By intramuscular injection
  CHILD UNDER 6 YEARS 150 micrograms (0.15 mL), repeated every 5 minutes if necessary
  CHILD 6–12 YEARS 300 micrograms (0.3 mL), repeated every 5 minutes if necessary
  CHILD 12–18 YEARS 500 micrograms (0.5 mL), repeated every 5 minutes if necessary
  ADULT 500 micrograms (0.5 mL), repeated every 5 minutes if necessary

Chlorphenamine injection 10 mg/mL

- By intravenous injection over 1 minute
  CHILD 1 MONTH–1 YEAR 250 micrograms/kg (max. 2.5 mg) up to 4 times in 24 hours
  CHILD 1–6 YEARS 2.5–5 mg up to 4 times in 24 hours
  CHILD 6–12 YEARS 5–10 mg up to 4 times in 24 hours
  CHILD 12–18 YEARS 10–20 mg up to 4 times in 24 hours (max. 40 mg in 24 hours)
  ADULT 10–20 mg up to 4 times in 24 hours (max. 40 mg in 24 hours)

High-flow **oxygen** should be given if required.

Hydrocortisone by intravenous injection (section 6.3.2) has delayed action but should be given to severely affected patients to prevent further deterioration.

Angina: unstable

(section 2.6)

Aspirin dispersible tablets 75 mg, 300 mg

- By mouth (dispersed in water or chewed)
  ADULT 300 mg

Plus

either **Glyceryl trinitrate** aerosol spray 400 micrograms/metered dose

- Sublingually
  ADULT 1–2 sprays, repeated as required

or **Glyceryl trinitrate** tablets 300 micrograms, 500 micrograms, 600 micrograms

- Sublingually
  ADULT 0.3–1 mg, repeated as required

Asthma: acute

(section 3.1)

Regard each emergency consultation as being for **acute severe asthma** until shown otherwise; failure to respond adequately **at any time** requires immediate referral to hospital

Either **salbutamol** aerosol inhaler 100 micrograms/metered inhalation

- By aerosol inhalation via large-volume spacer (and face mask in young children)
  CHILD UNDER 18 YEARS 1 puff every 15–30 seconds, up to max. 10 puffs; repeat after 20–30 minutes if necessary
  ADULT 4–6 puffs each inhaled separately, dose repeated every 10–20 minutes if necessary

or **salbutamol** nebuliser solution 1 mg/mL, 2 mg/mL

- By inhalation of nebulised solution (via oxygen-driven nebuliser)
  CHILD UNDER 18 MONTHS 2.5 mg every 20–30 minutes if necessary
  CHILD 18 MONTHS–18 YEARS 2.5–5 mg every 20–30 minutes if necessary
  ADULT 2.5–5 mg every 15–30 minutes if necessary

or **terbutaline** nebuliser solution 2.5 mg/mL

- By inhalation of nebulised solution (via oxygen-driven nebuliser)
  CHILD UNDER 3 YEARS 2 mg every 20–30 minutes if necessary
  CHILD 3–6 YEARS 3 mg every 20–30 minutes if necessary
  CHILD 6–8 YEARS 4 mg every 20–30 minutes if necessary
  CHILD 8–18 YEARS 5–10 mg every 20–30 minutes if necessary
  ADULT 5–10 mg every 15–30 minutes if necessary

Plus (in all cases)

either **prednisolone** soluble tablets 5 mg

- By mouth
  CHILD UNDER 18 YEARS 1–2 mg/kg (max. 40 mg) once daily for 3 days; if child already taking oral corticosteroids, give prednisolone 2 mg/kg (max. 60 mg) once daily
  ADULT 40–50 mg once daily for 5 days

or **hydrocortisone**

- By intravenous injection
  CHILD UNDER 1 YEAR 25 mg
  CHILD 1–6 YEARS 50 mg
  CHILD 6–18 YEARS 100 mg
  ADULT 100 mg

High-flow **oxygen** if available (via face mask in children)

Monitor response 15 to 30 minutes after nebulisation; if any signs of acute asthma persist, arrange hospital admission. While awaiting ambulance, repeat nebulised beta$_2$ agonist (as above) and give with

ipratropium nebuliser solution 250 micrograms/mL

- By inhalation of nebulised solution (via oxygen-driven nebuliser)
  CHILD UNDER 2 YEARS 125–250 micrograms every 20–30 minutes if necessary
  CHILD 2–12 YEARS 250 micrograms every 20–30 minutes if necessary
  CHILD 12–18 YEARS 500 micrograms repeated as necessary
  ADULT 500 micrograms, repeated as necessary

Or if nebuliser not available, **salbutamol** aerosol inhaler 100 micrograms/metered inhalation

- By aerosol inhalation via large-volume spacer (and face mask in young children)
  CHILD UNDER 18 YEARS 1 puff every 15–30 seconds, up to max. 10 puffs; repeat after 20–30 minutes if necessary
  ADULT 1 puff, repeat 10–20 times

Croup

(section 3.1)

Dexamethasone oral solution 2 mg/5 mL

- By mouth
  CHILD 150 micrograms/kg as a single dose

Convulsions

(section 4.8.2)

Either **diazepam** rectal solution 2 mg/mL, 4 mg/mL

- By rectum
  CHILD BODY-WEIGHT OVER 10 KG 500 micrograms/kg up to max. 30 mg, repeated after 15 minutes if necessary
  ADULT 500 micrograms/kg, up to max. 30 mg (ELDERLY 250 micrograms/kg up to max. 15 mg), repeated after 15 minutes if necessary

or **midazolam** buccal liquid 10 mg/mL or injection solution given by buccal route

- By buccal administration
  NEONATE 300 micrograms/kg (max. 2.5 mg), repeated once if necessary
  CHILD 1–6 MONTHS 300 micrograms/kg (max. 2.5 mg), repeated once if necessary
  CHILD 6 MONTHS–1 YEAR 2.5 mg, repeated once if necessary
  CHILD 1–5 YEARS 5 mg, repeated once if necessary
  CHILD 5–10 YEARS 7.5 mg, repeated once if necessary
  CHILD 10–18 YEARS 10 mg, repeated once if necessary
  ADULT 10 mg, repeated once if necessary

Diabetic hypoglycaemia

(section 6.1.4)

Glucose or **sucrose**

- By mouth
  CHILD 2–18 YEARS approx. 10–20 g (2–4 teaspoonfuls of sugar *or* 3–6 sugar lumps *or*
  55–110 mL *Lucozade® Energy Original or*
  90–180 mL *Coca-Cola®*—both non-diet versions *or*
  GlucoGel® one or two 25-g tubes (containing glucose 10 g/25-g tube)) repeated after 10–15 minutes if necessary
  ADULT approx. 10–20 g (2–4 teaspoonfuls of sugar *or* 3–6 sugar lumps *or*
  55–110 mL *Lucozade® Energy Original or*
  90–180 mL *Coca-Cola®*—both non-diet versions *or*
  GlucoGel® one or two 25-g tubes (containing glucose 10 g/25-g tube)) repeated after 10–15 minutes if necessary

or if hypoglycaemia unresponsive *or* if oral route cannot be used

Glucagon injection 1 mg/mL

- By subcutaneous, intramuscular, or intravenous injection
  CHILD BODY-WEIGHT UNDER 25 KG 500 micrograms (0.5 mL)
  CHILD BODY-WEIGHT OVER 25 KG 1 mg (1 mL)
  ADULT 1 mg (1 mL)

or if hypoglycaemia prolonged *or* unresponsive to glucagon after 10 minutes

Glucose intravenous infusion 10%

- By intravenous injection into large vein
  CHILD 1 MONTH–18 YEARS 2–5 mL/kg (glucose 200–500 mg/kg)

Glucose intravenous infusion 20%

- By intravenous injection into large vein
  ADULT 50 mL

Febrile convulsions lasting longer than 15 minutes

(section 4.8.3)

Diazepam rectal solution 2 mg/mL, 4 mg/mL

- By rectum
  CHILD BODY-WEIGHT OVER 10 KG 500 micrograms/kg up to max. 30 mg, repeated after 15 minutes if necessary

Meningococcal disease

(Table 1, section 5.1)

Benzylpenicillin injection 600 mg, 1.2 g

- By intravenous injection (or by intramuscular injection if venous access not available)
  NEONATE 300 mg
  CHILD 1 MONTH–1 YEAR 300 mg
  CHILD 1–10 YEARS 600 mg
  CHILD 10–18 YEARS 1.2 g
  ADULT 1.2 g
  Note Give single dose and transfer urgently to hospital

or if history of delayed allergy to penicillin

Cefotaxime injection 1 g

- By intravenous injection (or by intramuscular injection if venous access not available)
  NEONATE 50 mg/kg
  CHILD 1 MONTH–12 YEARS 50 mg/kg (max. 1 g)
  CHILD 12–18 YEARS 1 g
  ADULT 1 g
  Note Give single dose and transfer urgently to hospital

or if history of immediate allergy (including anaphylaxis, angioedema, or urticarial reaction) to penicillin or cephalosporins

Chloramphenicol injection 1 g

- By intravenous injection
  CHILD 1 MONTH–18 YEARS 12.5–25 mg/kg
  ADULT 12.5–25 mg/kg
  Note Give single dose and transfer urgently to hospital

Myocardial infarction

(section 2.10.1)

Aspirin dispersible tablets 75 mg, 300 mg

- By mouth (dispersed in water or chewed)
  ADULT 300 mg

Glyceryl trinitrate aerosol spray 400 micrograms/metered dose

- Sublingually
  ADULT 1–2 sprays, repeated as required

or **Glyceryl trinitrate** tablets 300 micrograms, 500 micrograms, 600 micrograms

- Sublingually
  ADULT 0.3–1 mg, repeated as required

Metoclopramide injection 5 mg/mL

- By intravenous injection
  ADULT (UNDER 60 KG) 18–19 YEARS 5 mg
  ADULT (OVER 60 KG) 18–19 YEARS 10 mg
  ADULT OVER 19 YEARS 10 mg

Diamorphine injection (5 mg powder for reconstitution)

- By slow intravenous injection (1 mg/minute)
  ADULT 5 mg followed by a further 2.5–5 mg if necessary; ELDERLY or FRAIL patients, reduce dose by half

Oxygen, if appropriate

Pneumonia: uncomplicated

(Table 1, section 5.1)

Amoxicillin oral suspension 125 mg/5 mL, 250 mg/5 mL; capsules 250 mg

- By mouth
  CHILD 6 MONTHS–1 YEAR 125 mg 3 times daily
  CHILD 1–5 YEARS 250 mg 3 times daily
  CHILD 5–18 YEARS 500 mg 3 times daily
  ADULT 0.5–1 g 3 times daily

or if allergic to penicillin or atypical organism suspected

Erythromycin oral suspension 125 mg/5 mL, 250 mg/5 mL; tablets 250 mg

- By mouth
  CHILD 6 MONTHS–2 YEARS 125 mg 4 times daily
  CHILD 2–8 YEARS 250 mg 4 times daily
  CHILD 8–18 YEARS 250–500 mg 4 times daily
  ADULT 500 mg 4 times daily

Approximate conversions and units

lb	kg	stones	kg	mL	fl oz
1	0.45	1	6.35	50	1.8
2	0.91	2	12.70	100	3.5
3	1.36	3	19.05	150	5.3
4	1.81	4	25.40	200	7.0
5	2.27	5	31.75	500	17.6
6	2.72	6	38.10	1000	35.2
7	3.18	7	44.45		
8	3.63	8	50.80		
9	4.08	9	57.15		
10	4.54	10	63.50		
11	4.99	11	69.85		
12	5.44	12	76.20		
13	5.90	13	82.55		
14	6.35	14	88.90		
		15	95.25		

Length

1 metre (m)		= 1000 millimetres (mm)
1 centimetre (cm)		= 10 mm
1 inch (in)		= 25.4 mm
1 foot (ft)	=12 inches	= 304.8 mm

Mass

1 kilogram (kg)	= 1000 grams (g)
1 gram (g)	= 1000 milligrams (mg)
1 milligram (mg)	= 1000 micrograms
1 microgram	= 1000 nanograms
1 nanogram	= 1000 picograms

Volume

1 litre	= 1000 millilitres (mL)
1 millilitre (1 mL)	= 1000 microlitres
1 pint	≈ 568 mL

Other units

1 kilocalorie (kcal)	= 4186.8 joules (J)
1000 kilocalories (kcal)	= 4.1868 megajoules (MJ)
1 megajoule (MJ)	= 238.8 kilocalories (kcal)
1 millimetre of mercury (mmHg)	= 133.3 pascals (Pa)
1 kilopascal (kPa)	= 7.5 mmHg (pressure)

Plasma-drug concentrations in the BNF are expressed in mass units per litre (e.g. mg/litre). The approximate equivalent in terms of amount of substance units (e.g. micromol/litre) is given in brackets.

Prescribing for children

Weight, height and body surface area

The table below shows the **mean values** for weight, height and body surface area by age; these values may be used to calculate doses in the absence of actual measurements. However, an individual's actual weight and height might vary considerably from the values in the table and it is important to ensure that the value chosen is appropriate. In most cases the actual measurement should be obtained as soon as possible and the dose re-calculated.

Age	Weight kg	Height cm	Body surface m²
Full-term neonate	3.5	50	0.24
1 month	4.2	55	0.27
2 months	4.5	57	0.28
3 months	5.6	59	0.33
4 months	6.5	62	0.36
6 months	7.7	67	0.41
1 year	10	76	0.49
3 years	15	94	0.65
5 years	18	108	0.74
7 years	23	120	0.87
10 years	30	132	1.10
12 years	39	148	1.30
14 years	50	163	1.50
Adult male	68	173	1.80
Adult female	56	163	1.60

Recommended wording of cautionary and advisory labels

For details see Appendix 9

1 Warning. May cause drowsiness
2 Warning. May cause drowsiness. If affected do not drive or operate machinery. Avoid alcoholic drink
3 Warning. May cause drowsiness. If affected do not drive or operate machinery
4 Warning. Avoid alcoholic drink
5 Do not take indigestion remedies at the same time of day as this medicine
6 Do not take indigestion remedies or medicines containing iron or zinc at the same time of day as this medicine
7 Do not take milk, indigestion remedies, or medicines containing iron or zinc at the same time of day as this medicine
8 Do not stop taking this medicine except on your doctor's advice
9 Take at regular intervals. Complete the prescribed course unless otherwise directed
10 Warning. Follow the printed instructions you have been given with this medicine
11 Avoid exposure of skin to direct sunlight or sun lamps
12 Do not take anything containing aspirin while taking this medicine
13 Dissolve or mix with water before taking
14 This medicine may colour the urine
15 Caution flammable: keep away from fire or flames
16 Allow to dissolve under the tongue. Do not transfer from this container. Keep tightly closed. Discard 8 weeks after opening
17 Do not take more than ... in 24 hours
18 Do not take more than ... in 24 hours or ... in any one week
19 Warning. Causes drowsiness which may continue the next day. If affected do not drive or operate machinery. Avoid alcoholic drink
21 ... with or after food
22 ... half to one hour before food
23 ... an hour before food or on an empty stomach
24 ... sucked or chewed
25 ... swallowed whole, not chewed
26 ... dissolved under the tongue
27 ... with plenty of water
28 To be spread thinly ...
29 Do not take more than 2 at any one time. Do not take more than 8 in 24 hours
30 Do not take with any other paracetamol products
31 Contains aspirin and paracetamol. Do not take with any other paracetamol products
32 Contains aspirin
33 Contains an aspirin-like medicine